Willard & Spackman's

Occupational Therapy

ELEVENTH EDITION

WILLARD & SPACKMAN'S
Occupational Therapy

Elizabeth Blesedell Crepeau, PhD, OTR, FAOTA
England Professor of Occupational Therapy
Occupational Therapy Department
College of Health and Human Services
University of New Hampshire
Durham, New Hampshire

Ellen S. Cohn, ScD, OTR, FAOTA
Clinical Associate Professor
Occupational Therapy Department
Sargent College of Health and Rehabilitation Sciences
Boston University
Boston, Massachusetts

Barbara A. Boyt Schell, PhD, OTR, FAOTA
Professor & Graduate Coordinator
Occupational Therapy Department
Brenau University
Gainsville, Georgia

Wolters Kluwer | Lippincott Williams & Wilkins
Health
Philadelphia • Baltimore • New York • London
Buenos Aires • Hong Kong • Sydney • Tokyo

Acquisitions Editor: Emily Lupash
Managing Editor: Matt Hauber / Laura Horowitz
Marketing Manager: Allison Noplock
Production Editor: Gina Aiello
Designer: Holly McLaughlin
Compositor: Circle Graphics

11th Edition

351 West Camden Street   530 Walnut Street
Baltimore, MD 21201   Philadelphia, PA 19106

Printed in the United States.

9 8 7 6 5 4 3 2

Library of Congress Cataloging-in-Publication Data

Willard & Spackman's occupational therapy. — 11th ed. / [edited by] Elizabeth Blesedell Crepeau, Ellen S. Cohn, Barbara A. Boyt Schell.
        p. ; cm.
    Includes bibliographical references and index.
    ISBN-13: 978-0-7817-6004-1
    ISBN-10: 0-7817-6004-6
1. Occupational therapy. I. Willard, Helen S. II. Crepeau, Elizabeth Blesedell. III. Cohn, Ellen S., OTR. IV. Schell, Barbara A. Boyt. V. Title: Occupational therapy. VI. Title: Willard and Spackman's occupational therapy.
    [DNLM: 1. Occupational Therapy. 2. Rehabilitation, Vocational. WB 555 W692 2008]
    RM735.W5 2008
    615.8'515—dc22

                                    2007049604

DISCLAIMER

Care has been taken to confirm the accuracy of the information present and to describe generally accepted practices. However, the authors, editors, and publisher are not responsible for errors or omissions or for any consequences from application of the information in this book and make no warranty, expressed or implied, with respect to the currency, completeness, or accuracy of the contents of the publication. Application of this information in a particular situation remains the professional responsibility of the practitioner; the clinical treatments described and recommended may not be considered absolute and universal recommendations.

The authors, editors, and publisher have exerted every effort to ensure that drug selection and dosage set forth in this text are in accordance with the current recommendations and practice at the time of publication. However, in view of ongoing research, changes in government regulations, and the constant flow of information relating to drug therapy and drug reactions, the reader is urged to check the package insert for each drug for any change in indications and dosage and for added warnings and precautions. This is particularly important when the recommended agent is a new or infrequently employed drug.

Some drugs and medical devices presented in this publication have Food and Drug Administration (FDA) clearance for limited use in restricted research settings. It is the responsibility of the health care provider to ascertain the FDA status of each drug or device planned for use in their clinical practice.

When citing chapters from this book, please use the appropriate form. The APA format is as follows:

[Chapter author last name, I.] (2009). Chapter title. In E. B. Crepeau, E. S. Cohn, & B. A. B. Schell (Eds.), *Willard and Spackman's occupational therapy* (11th ed., pp. x – x). Philadelphia: Lippincott Williams & Wilkins.

Dickie, V. (2009). What is occupation? In E. B. Crepeau, E. S. Cohn, & B. A. B. Schell (Eds.). *Willard and Spackman's occupational therapy* (11th ed., pp. 15 – 21). Philadelphia: Lippincott Williams & Wilkins.

Colonel Brandon to Miss Dashwood:
"What can it do?
Give me an occupation or I shall run Mad!"

JANE AUSTEN, *Sense and Sensibility*

Dedication

**Helen Hopkins, Ed.D, OTR, FAOTA and
Helen D. Smith, MS, OTR, FAOTA**

Co-Editors, Willard and Spackman's Occupational
Therapy 5th through 8th editions

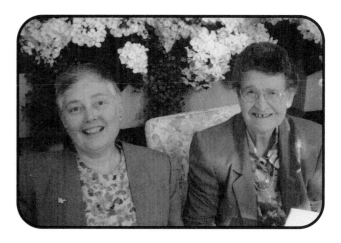

Helen Hopkins and Helen D. Smith edited the 5th through the 8th editions of *Willard and Spackman's Occupational Therapy.* Helen Hopkins was a founding member of the Occupational Therapy Department at Temple University. She chaired this program for many years prior to her retirement in 1986. Helen Smith was a long time faculty member at Tufts University—Boston School of Occupational Therapy retiring in 1998. The two "Helen's" were both dedicated and caring teachers who were deeply committed to the learning of their students. They were equally dedicated to occupational therapy. For many years we could count on seeing them together at the AOTA Annual Conference. Whether talking to and sharing stories with former students, *Willard and Spackman* contributors, or to their many colleagues, they always were encouraging and thought provoking. Even after passing the editorship of *Willard and Spackman* to their successors, they remained interested in the evolution of the book and supportive of our work as editors. We are grateful for their many years of service and dedicate this edition to them to honor their contribution to the profession.

Preface

Willard & Spackman's Occupational Therapy has a long tradition that extends back to the 1st edition published in 1947. Helen Willard and Clare Spackman, colleagues who taught together at the Occupational Therapy Program at the University of Pennsylvania, co-edited the 1st through the 4th editions. They turned the editorial responsibilities over to Helen Hopkins and Helen Smith, faculty members at Temple University and Tufts University, respectively. They edited the 5th through the 8th editions. Maureen Neistadt and Elizabeth Crepeau, faculty colleagues at the University of New Hampshire, edited the 9th edition and began work on the 10th edition. After Maureen's death, Ellen Cohn at Boston University and Barbara Schell at Brenau University joined Betty in editing the 10th and this edition.

We revised and updated the 11th edition to highlight the advances in knowledge in occupational therapy and occupational science in the past five years. This edition includes significant changes in both the scope and nature of content from the 9th and 10th editions. These changes are derived from the evolution of the field, results of surveys of faculty and students using the book, and three focus groups of occupational therapy students, occupational therapy faculty, and occupational therapy visionaries held during the 2004 AOTA Annual Conference in Minneapolis, Minnesota. Information from these sources indicated that people use the book to gain a broad understanding of the field and for its encyclopedic content. We were encouraged to include more information about occupational science and the occupational nature of human beings and to provide a more international perspective of the field. In addition to providing a broad overview of the profession, we were urged to include a critical perspective, examining the profession relative to whose interests were being served (and whose overlooked) by the field's current practices. We also discovered that the pediatric and adult units of the 10th edition were less important to readers, most likely due to the emergence of many more specialized texts in occupational therapy. Readers also appeared to be using different resources for theories other than occupation-based theories. Our revision incorporates these observations and

recommendations. In this edition, we have attempted to balance the tradition of the encyclopedic function of *Willard & Spackman* as the "place to start" while providing sufficient depth in coverage of topics critical for an introductory text.

This new edition of *Willard & Spackman's Occupational Therapy* is structured to make navigation through the text easier. This has been accomplished by

1. The new sequence of units;
2. The elimination of multi-section chapters;
3. The integration of theory, evaluation, and intervention into single units; and
4. The addition of specific resources for common conditions and practice settings.

Additionally, this edition reflects trends in the field regarding the centrality of occupation as the basis for practice. Finally, there is more explicit attention to the influence of the broader social and political environment on participation in the day-to-day lives of people.

Units I–II introduce readers to the concepts of occupation, the personal narratives of people with disabilities, and the relationship of society to occupation. This organization of chapters places important core concepts of occupation early in the book as the foundation for understanding occupational therapy practice. Feedback from the 10th edition indicated that Mary Feldhaus-Weber's chapter (*The Book of Sorrows, Book of Dreams*) was very effective. Mary's first person account vividly describes her personal experience with acquired brain injury, making her story accessible to readers who may have little understanding of what it may be like to live with a disability. Building on this success, Unit II includes six new chapters beginning with a brief overview of narrative theory. Subsequent chapters provide first person accounts from three different individuals. The first chapter is Mary's account of living with acquired brain injury; the second chapter describes growing up with cerebral palsy from the perspective of the child (now a young adult) and his parents; and the third chapter is the narrative of a person living with chronic mental illness. The caregiver perspective is represented in a fourth chapter. The unit closes with two chapters from international authors reflecting community-based occupational therapy practice that involves the development of client narratives as a way of promoting understanding and change.

Unit III: Occupation and Health in Society addresses important social and health policy issues, health promotion, community integration, and occupational justice. These chapters provide background information promoting the broad societal responsibilities of the occupational therapy profession. These chapters support the ideal that every individual has a right to be able to meet basic needs and to have equal opportunities and life chances to reach toward her or his potential through engagement in diverse and meaningful occupation

Unit IV: Profile of the Occupational Therapy Profession begins with a review of the history of the profession and then provides the reader with an overview of contemporary occupational therapy practice. The remainder of this unit consists of new chapters: one provides an overview of occupational therapy practice in the world, a second chapter addresses the organization of the profession within the USA, and a third chapter describes concepts of professional competence and competency. A substantially revised chapter on fieldwork is placed in this unit as well. The final chapter in this unit provides a critical perspective of occupational therapy practice today.

Units V through IX introduce readers to the building blocks of practice from content related to the values and beliefs of the profession itself, to the core reasoning and analytic processes inherent in practice. In addition to substantially updated chapters about occupational analysis, interviewing, and teamwork, new chapters address therapeutic relationships and communication with clients as well as professional communications and presentations. Unit VIII: Conceptual Basis for Practice includes expanded chapters on the major occupation-based theories, emphasizing the centrality of occupation as the core of practice.

Units X through XII introduce readers to occupational therapy evaluation and intervention in relation to occupations, personal factors, and the environment. Each chapter reviews relevant theoretical perspectives and integrates these perspectives with evaluation and intervention processes, demonstrating the integrated nature of practice. These chapters provide examples of evaluation and intervention of clients which cross the life course as well as the continuum of occupational therapy practice. Authors provide a summary of important evidence guiding practice as well as a critical analysis of gaps in the available evidence. A new chapter addressing personal factors provides a list of body functions and structures useful in prompting consideration of the many factors affecting performance.

Unit XIII: Therapists in Action: Examples of Expert Practice is entirely new, taking a narrative perspective of occupational therapy practice from the point of view of expert practitioners discussing their work. This unit provides insights into the professional reasoning of expert practitioners and helps readers understand the challenges and complexities of occupational therapy practice in different practice settings, including school-based practice, shelters for people who are homeless, long term care, and outpatient medical settings.

Unit XIV: Managing Practice addresses basic management principles in occupational therapy practice. All new chapters in this section address basic management functions, including supervision with specific attention to occupational therapists, occupational therapy assistants, and aides. An overview of payment for services describes the many options for payment and provides the context for understanding reimbursement structures in the USA. The final chapter on consultation brings the insights of current practitioners to readers who may consider this form of practice.

Unit XV: Common Conditions: Related Resources and Evidence includes brief summaries of many common conditions seen in occupational therapy practice with basic information about signs and symptoms, diagnostic criteria, medical/social interventions, occupational therapy evaluation and intervention, review of the evidence supporting practice, and caregiver considerations. Additional resources are listed for further reading. Information about additional conditions are posted on the *Willard and Spackman* website.

Unit XVI: Occupational Therapy Resource Summaries: Practice Settings provides a basic overview of the various settings in which occupational therapy practitioners provide services. This overview is in an accessible table format, including descriptions of settings, clients, length of stay, reimbursement mechanisms, etc. Units XV and XVI provide readers with a "place to start"—a characteristic of the book we felt was important to retain.

Unit XVII: Table of Assessments returns and includes all assessment instruments mentioned in the chapters in the book in alphabetical order by title. This resource contains information about the assessment, including author, purpose, age range, areas assessed, and publisher information.

The **Glossary** includes definitions of key words from chapters and important terminology from the August 2007 draft of the 2nd edition of the Occupational Therapy Practice Framework.

This edition includes the terminology of the International Classification of Function and the draft versions of the 2nd edition of the Occupational Therapy Practice Framework. At the time this book went to press the Framework was still under review, consequently some of our terminology may not reflect the final version.

Because we are aware of the power of language to influence the way we think, we have attempted to be as inclusive as possible in the descriptors of individuals. To the extent possible, we used the term occupational therapy practitioners to represent the certified occupational therapist and certified occupational therapy assistant.

We have tried to avoid language that exhibits bias and labels people with disabilities. We have used nonmedical language to the extent that this was appropriate.

Throughout the book are special features that expand and extend the text of the chapter. In addition to case studies and Practice Dilemmas, readers will find Commentaries on the Evidence, Ethical Dilemmas, and Provocative Questions to foster greater processing of the material in the book. The companion website to this book has additional supports for learning, including PowerPoint presentations, class-based and out of-class learning activities, case studies, and figures from the book suitable for use by instructors for class activities.

We are grateful to our many colleagues who have given us feedback about the 10th edition. Our efforts have been to create a book that represents the best aspects of our field—and that reflects positively on the important heritage of this book. The former editors and the current and former contributors have provided a strong foundation for us to build upon. It is our hope that this edition honors the past and provides a pathway for future generations of occupational therapy practitioners.

Elizabeth Blesedell Crepeau
Ellen S. Cohn
Barbara A. Boyt Schell

Contributors

Alyssa Wells Arnold, MS, OTR
University of New Hampshire
Durham, NH

Sara Baker, MS, OTR/L
Occupational Therapist
Radius Specialty Hospital
Roxbury, MA

Kim Bennet
Brenau University
Athens, GA

Sue Berger, MS, OTR/L
Clinical Assistant Professor
Boston University
Sargent College of Health and Rehabilitation Sciences
Occupational Therapy Department
Boston, MA

Christy Billock, PhD, OTR/L
Assistant Professor
Occupational Therapy Department
School of Allied Health Professions
Loma Linda University
Loma Linda, CA

Cheryl Lynne Trautmann Boop, MS, OTR/L
Occupational Therapist
Athens Regional Medical Center
Athens, GA

Brent Braveman, PhD, OTR/L, FAOTA
Clinical Professor
University of Illinois at Chicago
Chicago, IL

Sara Jane Brayman, PhD,OTR, FAOTA
Professor and Chair
Brenau University
Gainesville, GA

Catana Brown, PhD, OTR, FAOTA
Associate Professor
Touro University—Nevada
Henderson, NV

Mary Ellen Buning, PhD, OTR, ATP
Assistant Professor
University of Colorado, Denver
School of Medicine, Department of Physical Medicine
    & Rehabilitation
Assistive Technology Partners
Denver, CO

Jim Charlton
Lecturer, Disabilities Studies
University of Chicago
Chicago, IL
Founder, Access Living
Chicago, IL

Florence Clark, PhD, OTR/L, FAOTA
Associate Dean and Professor
University of Southern California
Los Angeles, CA

Ellen S. Cohn, ScD, OTR/L, FAOTA
Clinical Associate Professor
Boston University
Sargent College of Health and Rehabilitation Sciences
Occupational Therapy Department
Boston, MA

Elizabeth Blesedell Crepeau, PhD, OTR, FAOTA
England Professor of Occupational Therapy
Occupational Therapy Department
College of Health and Human Services
University of New Hampshire
Durham, NH

Terry Crowe, PhD, OTR/L, FAOTA
Director and Professor
The University of New Mexico School of Medicine
Albuquerque, NM

Debora Davidson, PhD, OTR/L
Associate Professor and Administrator
    of Professional Programs
Department of Occupational Science
    and Occupational Therapy
College of Health Sciences
Saint Louis University
Saint Louis, MO

Gloria Dickerson
Recovery Specialist
Institute for Homelessness and Trauma
Newton, MA

Virginia Dickie, PhD, OTR/L, FAOTA
Associate Professor and Director
Division of Occupational Science
The University of North Carolina at Chapel Hill
Chapel Hill, NC

Regina Ferraro Doherty, OTD, OTR/L
Lecturer
Occupational Therapy Department
Graduate School of Arts and Science
Tufts University
Medford, MA

Laura J. Dossett, MS, OTR/L
Occupational Therapist
Evergreen Healthcare
Tacoma, WA

Brian J. Dudgeon, PhD, OTR, FAOTA
Associate Professor
University of Washington
Seattle, WA

Winnie Dunn, PhD, OTR, FAOTA
Professor and Chair
Department of Occupational Therapy Education
University of Kansas Medical Center
Kansas City, KS

Mary Evenson, MPH, OTR/L
Academic Fieldwork Coordinator
Tufts University
Medford, MA

Mary Feldhaus-Weber
Writer, Painter, Head Injury Survivor
Jamaica Plain, MA

Rachel W. Fleming
The Schenck School
Atlanta, GA

Kimberly Fletcher, OTR/L
Occupational Therapist
Eastern Suffolk BOCES
Suffolk County, NY

Kirsty Forsyth, PhD, OTR
Senior Lecturer
Occupational Therapy
Queen Margaret University
Edinburgh, Scotland

Karen R Garren, MS, OTR/L, CHT
Certified Hand Therapist
New Milford, CT

Clare Giuffrida, PhD, OTR/L, FAOTA
Chair and Associate Professor
Department of Occupational Therapy
Rush University
Rush University Medical Center
Chicago, IL

Coralie "Corky" Glantz, OT/L, BCG, FAOTA
Co-Owner
Glantz/Richman Rehabilitation Associates
Riverwoods, IL

Kathleen Golisz, OTR, MA
Associate Professor
Mercy College
Dobbs Ferry, NY

Don Gordon, PhD, OTR/L
Assistant Professor
University of Southern California
Los Angeles, CA

Yael Goverover, PhD, OT
Assistant Professor
New York University
New York, NY

Stephanie Grant, MS,OTR/L
Project Development
United Osteoporosis Centers
Gainesville, GA

Meredith Grinnell, MS, OTR/L
Centre for Neuro Skills,
Bakersfield, CA

Lou Ann Griswold, PhD, OTR, FAOTA
Associate Professor
University of New Hampshire
Durham, NH

Stacey Halpern, MS, OTR/L
Senior Occupational Therapist
New York City Department of Education
New York, NY

Joy Hammel, PhD, OTR/L, FAOTA
Associate Professor
University of Illinois at Chicago
Chicago, IL

Alexis D. Henry, ScD, OTR/L, FAOTA
Research Assistant Professor
Center for Health Policy and Research
University of Massachusetts Medical School
Shrewsbury, MA

Clare Hocking, PhD, MHSc(OT)
Associate Professor
AUT University
Auckland, New Zealand

Margo B. Holm, PhD, OTR/L, FAOTA, ABDA
Professor and Director of Post-Professional Education
Occupational Therapy Department
School of Health and Rehabilitation Sciences
University of Pittsburgh
Pittsburgh, PA

Justina Hsu, MS, OTR/L
Occupational Therapist
Rapid City Regional Hospital
Rapid City, SD

Pai-Chuan Huang, MS, OT
Doctoral Candidate
Boston University
Boston, MA

Ruth Humphry, PhD, OTR/L, FAOTA
Professor
Division of Occupational Science
University of North Carolina
Chapel Hill, NC

Karen Jacobs, EdD, OTR/L, CPE, FAOTA
Clinical Professor
Boston University
Sargent College of Health and Rehabilitation Sciences
Occupational Therapy Department
Boston, MA

S. Essie Jacobs, PhD, OTR/L
Seattle, WA

Anne Birge James, PhD, OTR/L
Professor
Bay Path College
Longmeadow, MA

Robin A Jones, MPA, COTA/L, ROH
Project Director and Instructor
DBTAC–Great Lakes ADA Center
Department of Disability and Human Development
University of Illinois at Chicago
Chicago, IL

Alisa Jordan, MSOT, OTR/L
Occupational Therapist
London Children's Practice
London, England

Bridget Kane, MS, OTR/L
West Springfield, MA

Jennifer Keller, MS, OTR/L
Boston University
Boston, MA

Gary Kielhofner, PhD, OTR, FAOTA
Professor and Wade-Meyer Chair
University of Illinois at Chicago
Chicago, IL

Phyllis King, PhD, OT, FAOTA
Professor
University of Wisconsin, Milwaukee
Milwaukee, WI

Kristin Knesek, MS, OTR/L
Rehabilitation Director
Forum at Memorial Woods
Five Star Rehabilitation & Wellness
Houston, TX

Jessica M. Kramer, MS, OTR/L
PhD Candidate, Disability Studies
Head Research Assistant
MOHO Clearinghouse University of Illinois at Chicago
Chicago, IL

Hsin-yu Kuo
Doctoral Candidate
Boston University
Boston, MA

Amy Jo Lamb, OTD, BS, OTR/L
AJ Lamb Consulting
Blair, NE

Mary C. Lawlor, ScD, OTR, FAOTA
Professor
Division of Occupational Science
    and Occupational Therapy
University of Southern California
Los Angeles, CA

Lori Letts, PhD, OT Reg. (Ont.)
Associate Professor
School of Rehabilitation Science
McMaster University
Hamilton, Ontario, Canada

Ling-Yi Lin, MS, OT
Doctoral Candidate
Boston University
Boston, MA

Helene Lohman, OTD, OTR/L
Associate Professor
Creighton University
Omaha, NE

Theresa Lorenzo, BSc (OT), PhD
Senior Lecturer
Occupational Therapy Department
University of Cape Town
Cape Town, South Africa

Cathy Lysack, PhD, OT(C)
Associate Professor
Wayne State University
Detroit, MI

Karen Marticello, MS OTR/L
Dallas Children's Medical Center
Dallas, TX

Cheryl Mattingly, PhD
Professor
University of Southern California
Los Angeles, CA

Juli McGruder, PhD, OTR
Distinguished Professor
University of Puget Sound
Tacoma, WA

Alexander McIntosh
Undergraduate
University of New Hampshire
Durham, NH

Laurie S. McIntosh, MS, OTR/L
Occupational Therapist
Supervisory Union 16
Exeter, NH

Lou McIntosh
Parent Consultant
Merrywing Corporation
Eliot, ME

Jane Melton, MSc, DipCOT
Consultant Occupational Therapist in Mental Health
Gloucestershire Partnership NHS Trust
Gloucester, United Kingdom

Penelope A. Moyers, EdD, OTR/L, BCMH, FAOTA
Professor and Chair
Department of Occupational Therapy
University of Alabama at Birmingham
Birmingham, AL

Mary Muhlenhaupt, OTR/L, FAOTA
Clinical Research Coordinator,
    Child and Family Studies Research Programs
Adjunct Instructor, Occupational Therapy Program
Thomas Jefferson University
Philadelphia, PA

Donald Murray
Professor Emeritus
English Department
University of New Hampshire
Durham, NH

Jan Nisbet, PhD
Director, Institute on Disability
University of New Hampshire
Durham, NH

Darcie L. Olson, MHS, OTR, CHT
Madison Area Technical College
Madison, Wisconsin

Jan Miller Polgar, PhD, OT Reg (Ont.), FCAOT
Associate Professor and Graduate Chair
The University of Western Ontario
London, ON

Nick Pollard, BA, DipCOT, PGCE, MA, MSc
Senior Lecturer in Occupational Therapy
Faculty of Health and Wellbeing
Sheffield Hallam University
United Kingdom

Janet Poole, PhD, OTR/L, FAOTA
Professor
Occupational Therapy Graduate Program
University of New Mexico
Alburquerque, NM

Pollie Price, PhD, OTR/L
Assitant Professor
University of Utah, Division of Occupational Therapy
Salt Lake City, UT

Loree A. Primeau, PhD, OTR, FAOTA
Occupational Therapist
Treehouse Pediatric Center
San Antonio, TX
Formerly
Associate Professor
Department of Occupational Therapy
School of Allied Health Sciences
University of Texas Medical Branch
Galveston, TX

Kirsten M. Protos
Brenau University
Gainesville, GA

Martin S. Rice, Ph.D., OTR/L
Associate Professor
The University of Toledo
Toledo, OH

Patty Rigby
Associate Professor and Graduate Coordinator
Department of Occupational Science
    and Occupational Therapy
University of Toronto
Toronto, Ontario, Canada

Laurie Ringaert
Senior Researcher,
Canadian Centre on Disability Studies
Winnipeg, Manitoba, Canada

**Pamela S. Roberts, PhD, OTR/L,
SCFES, CPHQ, FAOTA**
Manager, Rehabilitation, Neurology,
    and Neuropsychology
Cedars-Sinai Medical Center
Los Angeles, CA

Joan C. Rogers, PhD, OTR/L, FAOTA
Professor and Chair
University of Pittsburgh
Pittsburgh, PA

Susan Ayres Rosa, PhD, OTR
Clinical Instructor
Occupational Therapy Program,
    Department of Kinesiology
University of Wisconsin, Madison
Madison, WI

Graham D. Rowles, Ph.D.
Professor and Director
Graduate Center for Gerontology
University of Kentucky
Lexington, KY

Karen M. Sames, MBA, OTR/L
Associate Professor
The College of St. Catherine
St. Paul, MN

Barbara A. Boyt Schell, PhD, FAOTA, OTR
Professor and Graduate Coordinator
Occupational Therapy Department
Brenau University
Gainesville, GA

Sally A. Schreiber-Cohn, MTS
Editor and friend
Minister, Sufi Order International Boston Area
Marblehead, MA

Sally Schultz, PhD, OTR, LPC
Professor and Director
School of Occupational Therapy
Texas Woman's University
Denton/Dallas/Houston, TX

**Winifred Schultz-Krohn, PhD, OTR/L, BCP,
FAOTA**
Professor of Occupational Therapy
San Jose State University
San Jose, CA

Sharan L. Schwartzberg, EdD, OTR/L, FAOTA
Professor Occupational Therapy
Graduate School of Arts and Sciences
Adjunct Professor Psychiatry
School of Medicine
Tufts University
Medford, MA

Janie B. Scott, MA, OT/L, FAOTA
Occupational Therapy and Aging-in-Place Consultant
Columbia, MD

Susanne Smith Roley, MS, OTR/L, FAOTA
Project Director, USC USC/WPS Comprehensive
    Program in Sensory Integration
Los Angeles, CA
Coordinator of Education and Research,
    Pediatric Therapy Network
Torrance, CA

Susan Stark, PhD, OTR/L, FAOTA
Assistant Professor of Occupational Therapy
    and Neurology
Washington University School of Medicine
St. Louis, MO

Perri Stern, EdD, OTR/L, FAOTA
Consultant
Pittsburgh, PA

Kate-Lyn Stone
Occupational Therapy Master's Student
University of New Hampshire
Durham, NH

Yvonne Swinth
Professor
University of Puget Sound
Tacoma, WA

Kayoko Takahashi, MS, OT
Doctoral Candidate
Boston University
Boston, MA

Linda Tickle-Degnen, PhD, OTR/L, FAOTA
Professor and Chair
Tufts University
Medford, MA

Joan Toglia, PhD, OTR
Associate Professor
Mercy College
Dobbs Ferry, NY

Elizabeth Townsend, PhD, OT (C), Reg. NS, FCAOT
Professor and Director
School of Occupational Therapy
Dalhousie University
Nova Scotia, Canada

Grace M. Trudeau, MS, OTR/L
Thom Child and Family Services
Boston-Metro Early Intervention
Boston, MA

Barbara Prudhomme White, PhD, OTR/L
Associate Professor
University of New Hampshire
Durham, NH

John A. White, Jr., PhD, OTR/L
Program Director and Associate Professor
Pacific University School of Occupational Therapy
Forest Grove, OR

Ann A. Wilcock, PhD, FCOT
Honorary Professor
Occupational Science and Therapy
Deakin University, Geelong
Victoria, Australia

Tom Wilson, MA
Personal Assistant and Health Care Team Leader
Access Living
Chicago, IL

Mary Jane Youngstrom, MS, OTR/L, FAOTA
Occupational Therapist and Health Care
    Management Consultant
Overland Park, KS

Acknowledgments

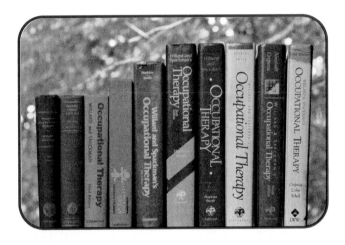

T his edition of *Willard & Spackman* was accomplished through the collective efforts of the contributors, focus group members, editorial review board, photographers, students, colleagues, friends, and family. Well over 120 people have directly contributed to the development of this book. We are grateful for their many contributions to this effort and know that their generosity has improved the quality of the work presented here. We are pleased that Anne James agreed to take on the role of editor for web-based instructional materials and are thankful for her work in expanding the horizons of this text into the virtual context of cyberspace.

Our work as a team has also been essential to the development of the book. We have engaged in many conversations about the structure of the text, the content, how to approach issues which lack agreement in the field, and how to represent the breadth, scope and depth of the evolving knowledge base of the field. This work did not go on in a vacuum, but was enmeshed in our day-to-day lives of our families, our work, and our community involvements. The past 5 years have brought new grandchildren: to Betty (Naomi, Owen, and Theo) and Barb (Samarra and Akhasa). Ellen's girls have become vibrant and mature young women, participated in national and international synchronized skating competitions. Adrienne

has gone off to college and Maggie started driving. We have experienced the challenges of receiving health care and the benefits of competent rehabilitation services when Betty had both knees replaced, Barb received a new hip and Ellen worked to restore an injured knee. Our husbands have tolerated our time spent on this book far more patiently than we could ever expect. In the midst of already full professional and personal lives, we have practiced what Elizabeth Larson refers to as occupational orchestration as we worked on this book. Sometimes this orchestration has required us to withdraw from some valued occupations to which we plan to return—Betty to her garden, knitting, and sewing, Ellen to the courts, trails, roads and beaches, and Barb to her golf, artwork, and walks with the family dogs. None-the-less, editing this book has been a privilege. We have worked with contributors equally devoted to sharing their knowledge of the field with the next generation of occupational therapy practitioners. Our relationships with the contributors have brought us into contact with some of the leading scholars in the field which has enriched our understanding of the changes in the field and the challenges we face in the future. We thank all who have supported us and who have contributed to this endeavor and hope that our efforts to represent these contributions live up to the fine tradition the *Willard & Spackman* has in the field.

While working on this book has been a serious undertaking, the infusion of humor has lightened the load. Like many cohesive teams, we have developed slogans and catch phrases that are a way for us to mark special issues and moments. Some of these include

- *Putting the hay down where the goats can get it*—This phrase was a reminder to remember our primary audience, occupational therapy students, and challenged us to make complex topics relevant and accessible to them.
- *The horses are smelling the barn*—This phrase refers to the fact that as horses approach home, they speed up because they know that food and water will be available in the barn. We chanted the phrase when we reached important milestones in the book such as completion of the initial book proposal, critical chapters or units, etc.

◆ *PIGASI (Paint it gray and ship it)*—This nonsensical phrase we adopted from Linda Duncombe of Boston University. It reminded us that while we wanted everything in the book to be perfect—sometimes we just had to PIGASI.

We thank those listed below for their generous assistance in helping us conceptualize this book and bring it to fruition.

Photographs and Historical Documents

John Adams, Gary Samson, Ron Bergeron, Doug Prince, Lisa Nugent, University of New Hampshire Photographic Services Department, Durham, NH.
Linda Anderson, Wisconsion Occupational Therapy Association
Lori Andersen & Barbara Kornblau
Ellen Cohn
Laura Collins and Bob Sacheli, American Occupational Therapy Association
Roderick Crepeau
Mindy Hecker, American Occupational Therapy Foundation
Barbara and John Schell

Secretaries and Administrative Support

Janice Mutschler and Renate Jurden, Occupational Therapy Department, University of New Hampshire
Elaine Chu and David Richie, Occupational Therapy Department, Boston University, Sargent College
Vivian Gammell and Alicia Kinsey of Brenau University
Donna Rinaldi and Meg Trafton, Dover Secretarial Services, Dover, NH

Professional Colleagues and Students

With gratitude and appreciation, we acknowledge our colleagues at Boston University, Brenau University, and the University of New Hampshire for their assistance, support, insightful feedback, and willingness to listen to endless conversations about *Willard & Spackman*

Boston University

◆ Sue Berger, Sharon Cermak, Wendy Coster, Linda Duncombe, Karen Jacobs, Nancy Lowenstein, Deane McCraith, Naomi Moran, Gael Orsmond and Elsie Vergara
◆ Patricia Nemec for recommending Gloria Dickerson as an author
◆ Occupational therapy students: Pamela Errico, Christine Hegarty, Brooke Howard, and Kate Runge
◆ Rebecca Hanson for outstanding attention to detail, proofing, and conceptual clarity
◆ HP 870: Theory and Research in the Health and Rehabilitation Sciences graduate seminar students, Spring 2005

Brenau University

◆ Faculty colleagues M. Irma Alvarado, Lori Andersen, Sara Brayman, Mary Shotwell and Robin Underwood,
◆ Classes of 2007 and 2008

University of New Hampshire

◆ Kasey Dutra, Kristy Golt, Meredith Grinnell, Christine Leonard, Hilary Maynes, Amanda Neill, Kate-Lyn Stone,
◆ Classes of 2007 and 2008
◆ Sajay Arthanat, Lou Ann Griswold, Susan Merrill, Shelley Mulligan, Douglas Simmons, Elizabeth Stewart, Barbara Prudhomme White, Kerryellen Vroman, and Therese Willkomm

Lippincott Williams & Wilkins

◆ Current and former Lippincott Williams and Wilkins personnel contributed to the development of this book
◆ Pamela Lappies, Susan Katz, Nancy Peterson, Emily Lupash, and Matt Hauber
◆ Laura Horowitz of Hearthside Publishing Services provided overall guidance of the development of the manuscript through the production of the book. Her steady guidance, expertise, patience, and good humor provided significant support to our efforts.
◆ Gina Aiello and Eve Malakoff-Klein, production editors, who collaborated with us in the final steps of transforming the manuscript to finished text.
◆ Barbara Willette, copy editor, whose careful work caught our confusing language, misplaced commas, and errors in APA format.
◆ Gelya Frank at the University of Southern California inspired our epigraph.

Editorial Review Board

Brief Contents

Contents

Features

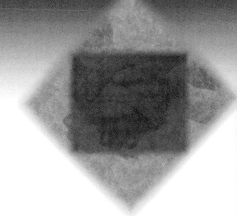

Provocative Questions

I

OCCUPATIONAL SCIENCE AND THE OCCUPATIONAL NATURE OF HUMANS

> " I believe that the ordinary rhythm of daily living is the deep primordial nourishment of our existence. It is the "truth"—the primary reality for each one of us. After all, everyday occupation is present in our lives at *all* times and in *all* places. "
>
> *Betty Risteen Hasselkus*

The Making and Mattering of Occupational Science

FLORENCE CLARK AND MARY C. LAWLOR

Learning Objectives

After reading this chapter, you will be able to:

1. Describe the recent history in the development of occupational science.
2. Demonstrate an understanding of the domains of concern of the discipline of occupational science.
3. Discuss the linkages between occupational science and occupational therapy.
4. Identify ways in which knowledge generated through research in occupational science informs occupational therapy practice.

Occupational science has been described as both an emergent discipline (Molke, Laliberte-Rudman, & Polatajko, 2004; Wilcock, 2001; Yerxa, 1993; Yerxa et al., 1989) and an evolving discipline (Zemke & Clark, 1996a). Even though the discipline of occupational science is still in its infancy, compared to other more established disciplines, a number of exciting developments both illustrate the shape the field is taking and foreshadow future possibilities. In this chapter, we discuss the nature of this discipline, describe its evolution, analyze the interrelationships of occupational science and occupational therapy, and provide evidence of the contributions of the discipline to occupational therapy. We also discuss how an understanding of occupational science, including the recent history of the field, informs and influences innovative occupational therapy practice.

The name of the discipline itself warrants further unpacking, as both the terms *occupational* and *science* have been the focus of much consideration and, at times, debate. Words matter. Although these words might seem self-explanatory, the interpretations of the meanings continue to influence understandings. In the following passages, we will frame the definitional issues and the implications for future development. Occupational science was grounded in the interdisciplinary social sciences and continues to sustain interrelationships with a number of these disciplines, including sociology, anthropology, philosophy, and psychology. As the discipline has evolved, new and productive conceptual and practical linkages have been formed with disciplines in other academic traditions, including neuroscience, biology, preventive medicine, rehabilitation science, gerontology, biomedical engineering, public health, and physiology. Occupational science is also recognized for its unique relationship with occupational therapy and, in a more general way, the remarkable success of this young discipline in navigating the intersection of academic disciplines and practice professions. This achievement marks occupational science as a new form of discipline, a discipline that is poised to facilitate the application or translation of new knowledge and theory into efficacious solutions to real-world problems.

DOMAINS OF CONCERN OF OCCUPATIONAL SCIENCE

Definitions are designed to clarify what something, in this case occupational science, is or means. Although definitions can be helpful, they tend to oversimplify the nature of a discipline, its domains of concern, and perhaps more important, what a discipline does, the utility of a science, the ways in which a science addresses the needs of society. As we describe later in this chapter, occupational science now has a global presence and at local and national levels there is considerable diversity in the defining or foregrounding of characteristics as scholars and practitioners adapt theoretical assumptions to the needs of local societies.

Definitions can provide a snapshot of the domains of concern of a discipline. Taken collectively, definitions also offer insights into a range of perspectives that relate to the identification of the most salient dimensions of the field. Occupational science has been defined as "a basic science devoted to the study of the human as an occupational being" (Yerxa, 1993, p. 5) and, similarly, as "the rigorous study of humans as occupational beings" (Wilcock, 1998, p. 257). The phrase *occupational science* is most often approached by defining the terms *occupation* or *occupations.* One of the earliest and most cited definitions is as follows: "chunks of culturally and personally meaningful activity in which humans engage that are named in the lexicon of the culture" (Clark et al., 1991, p. 4). Occupation has also been described as "a synthesis of doing, being, and becoming" (Wilcock, 1999, p. 3).

Yerxa (1993) placed issues of skill development, holism, and experience in the foreground in describing the founding principles of occupational science. Occupational science addresses the centrality of engagement in occupations and in human life, particularly as they relate to health and well-being, and social participation. Concep-

tualized broadly as the activities that constitute everyday experience, occupations include the kinds of purposive activity that make up people's lives, such as activities of daily living, interpersonal activities, physical activities, restorative activities, and social and cultural practices. Because occupations are so far ranging, they are conceived as crossing the spectrum of human needs and desires from survival and reproduction to economic subsistence, participation in social life, and artistic and spiritual expression (e.g., Wilcock, 2005; Yerxa et al., 1989; Zemke & Clark, 1996a, 1996b). But the focus of occupational science is not only on the activity per se, but also on the social actors who are engaged in occupations within the social, cultural, and historical particulars of their lived world—in essence, how people live and learn in everyday life; the relationships among activity, participation, and health; and how social engagements and social structures afford and constrain health, participation, quality of life, and human experience (e.g., Dickie, Cutchin, & Humphry, 2006; Farnworth, 1998; Hocking, 2000; Lawlor, 2003; Molineux & Whiteford, 1999). In accord with this perspective, occupational science might be thought of as addressing the variety of ways in which people are occupied as human beings and the impact that such engagement has on bodies, selves (Abbott, 2004),[1] communities, and the world.

METHODOLOGICAL APPROACHES

Modes of inquiry and methodological approaches in occupational science have developed in ways that reflect the evolving nature of the discipline and the strengthening of the interrelationships between occupational science and occupational therapy. When occupational science was established, efforts were devoted to differentiating this science from traditional, positivistic approaches that relied on experimental paradigms to generate knowledge and test theory (Zemke & Clark, 1996b). There appeared to be a natural affinity between research questions in occupational science and qualitative, phenomenological, and narrative modes of inquiry (Gray, 1997; Hocking, 2000; Lentin, 2002; Mattingly & Lawlor, 2000; Wicks & Whiteford, 2003). Although these approaches have produced new

---

[1]This statement draws on a quote from Dr. Andrew Abbott's paper "Creating an Academic Discipline That Supports Practice," which was presented at the 16th annual Occupational Science Symposium at USC on January 16, 2004. In his thoughtful and provocative paper, Dr. Abbott argued that the discipline should develop by moving : "towards organizing occupational science around a general theory of the immediate daily activities with which we occupy our bodies and ourselves" (p. 12). We are deeply indebted to Dr. Abbott for his scholarship, including his other published work, and we continue to be influenced, intrigued, and challenged by his insights.

3

knowledge and enhanced theory development, they only partially represent the range of methodological approaches that are inherent in occupational science research.

In their efforts to generate new theoretical understandings of the occupational, social, cultural, political, and historical dimensions of participation in everyday life, occupational scientists have expanded methodological approaches to studying occupation and its relationship to health and social participation. Occupational science is designed to systematize knowledge about occupation, especially in relation to health and well-being. In addition, occupational scientists are collaborating with scholars in other disciplines to provide methodological and theoretical support in interdisciplinary research programs where issues related to understanding engagement, activity, participation, experience, and health provide unique challenges. The study of occupations requires complex analytic frames to capture the multifaceted aspects of occupations, particularly in naturalistic settings. As Glass and McAtee (2006) have argued, understanding relationships between behaviors and health requires a contextual orientation that is multidimensional, examining individual and distal social features, biological features on multiple levels, human action, and other characteristics across time. The *science of occupational science* is grounded in multiple methods and reflects a recent trend to avoid differentiation of research into the overly simplistic categories of basic and applied (e.g., Flyvberg, 2001).

One of the most significant developments in occupational science is the development of new methods that are scientifically rigorous, span the continuum of paradigms from ethnography to randomized controlled trials, and facilitate translation into practice. In addition, occupational scientists have designed research programs that evaluate and utilize mixed method approaches in innovative ways. These developments combine both conceptual approaches to inquiry and the application of new technologies in research endeavors. Later in this chapter, we provide exemplars of this work, drawing on the University of Southern California (USC) Well Elderly Study and USC/Rancho Los Amigos National Rehabilitation Center Pressure Ulcer Prevention Study (PUPS).

THE GROWTH OF OCCUPATIONAL SCIENCE

Although occupational science is a mere 18 years old, there is no doubt that it is flourishing. In this short period of time, more than 45 scholars have received their PhD degrees in occupational science at USC alone, and most of them are now in academic leadership positions in the United States and worldwide. Furthermore, 20 occupational therapy academic programs have been renamed to include occupational science in their titles. Consistent with this trend, several programs now offer degrees at various levels in occupational science. For example, Towson State University now awards a ScD in Occupational Science, the University of North Carolina (UNC) and USC grant the PhD in the discipline and a joint MSc/PhD in Occupational Science can be earned at the University of Western Ontario. Other colleges and universities have chosen to offer occupational science undergraduate major and minor programs that aimed at providing a strong foundation for entry into occupational therapy professional programs. In total, 20 programs throughout the world are identified as occupational science university programs (www.jos.edu.au). Finally, founded at the University of South Australia in 1993, first as the *Journal of Occupational Science: Australia* (JOS:A), the *Journal of Occupational Science* (JOS) is now in its 15th year of publication. Unlike journals that have the words *occupational therapy* in their title, JOS is dedicated to publishing articles about humans as occupational beings and has a policy that bars publishing manuscripts that are strictly focused on therapy (Wilcock, 2003).

Arguably, one of the most impressive aspects of occupational science is the magnitude with which it has taken root internationally (Clark, 2006; Hocking, 2000; Mounter & Ilott, 1997, 2000; Wilcock, 2005; Yerxa, 2000). In 1999, just 10 years after the founding of the discipline, the International Society of Occupational Scientists (ISOS) was established by 32 occupational scientists who wished to further the discipline by building international bridges. The aims of ISOS are designated on its Website (http://isos.nfshost.com/aims.php) as follows:

◆ To promote study and research of humans as occupational beings within the context of their communities and the organization of occupation in society
◆ To disseminate information to increase a general understanding of people's occupational needs and the contribution of occupation to the health and well-being of communities
◆ To advocate for occupational justice internationally
◆ To encourage a range of disciplines to consider and frame their own research from an occupational perspective so they may expand their influence on sociocultural, political, medical, environmental, and occupational processes

Soon after ISOS was established, national or regional societies began to be formed that were modeled to a considerable extent on ISOS but also were tailored to address the priorities of each one's particular stakeholders. Table 1.1 lists the Website addresses and founding dates of the 10 organizations and societies worldwide that have as one of their chief aims furthering occupational science. As the table reveals, these organizations are relatively new, all having been established between the years 2000 and 2006. The various Websites provide a broad-based sense of the commonalities shared by these organizations and the differences in their focuses. While all of the organizations

TABLE 1.1   INTERNATIONAL OCCUPATIONAL SCIENCE ORGANIZATIONS

Name	Year Founded	Website
International Society of Occupational Scientists (ISOS)	1999	http://isos.nfshost.com/
Australasian Society of Occupational Scientists (ASOS)	2000	http://asos.nfshost.com/
Continuing Education and Research: Occupational Science Project Group ENOTHE (European Network of Occupational Therapy in Higher Education)	2000	http://www.enothe.hva.nl/cer/index.html
Occupation UK: The British Institute for Occupation and Health	2000–2001	http://www.occupationuk.org/
Canadian Society of Occupational Scientists (CSOS)	2001	http://occupationalsciencecanada.dal.ca/home.html
The Society for the Study of Occupation: USA (SSO:USA)	2002	http://www.sso-usa.org/
Australasian Occupational Science Center (AOSC)	2004	http://shoalhaven.uow.edu.au/aosc/whatis.html
European Cooperative in Occupational Therapy Research and Occupational Science (ECOTROS)	2006	http://www.enothe.hva.nl/cer/research.htm
Japanese Society for the Study of Occupation	2006	http://www.amrf.or.jp/jsso./.indexe.htm
WFOT International Advisory Group: Occupational Science	2006	http://www.wfot.org.au/

have as primary aims promoting research on occupation, particularly as it relates to health, they differ in the degree of emphasis they place on other aims such as multidisciplinarity, promoting social justice, or linking occupational science to occupational therapy. A promising new development is that in 2006 and 2007, two international Think Tanks were held, the first in Australia (Wicks, 2006) and the second in the United States, with representatives from as many as 14 countries and five continents, most of whom were from the organizations listed in Table 1.1, to explore the ways in which the various organizations might relate with one another and support ISOS. The key result of the Think Tanks was the unanimous decision to move forward in seeking affiliative relationships among the organizations and in supporting ISOS as a potential umbrella organization.

Another indicator that occupational science is flourishing is the number and quality of scientific symposia that are being held. For 19 consecutive years, an annual occupational science symposium has been held at USC featuring over 100 presentations on interdisciplinary occupational science–related themes and relevant research. These symposia have typically included presentations from world-renowned scientists, philosophers, and scholars. Among the most eminent presenters have been primatologist Jane Goodall, neuroscientist Antonio Damasio, sociologist Andrew Abbott, rehabilitation scientist Margaret Stineman, neuroscientist Candace Pert, philosopher John

Searle, psychologist Mihaly Csikszentmihalyi, psychologist Jerome Bruner, anthropologist and linguist Mary Catherine Bateson, and physicist Stephen Hawking.

As scientific societies have been established throughout the world devoted to furthering occupational science, they too have held annual symposia. Between 2000 and 2007, 18 such symposia were convened. Collectively, these symposia (including those held at USC in this time period) have included over 300 presentations, with speakers from over a dozen countries. It is interesting to note the most frequently addressed topics included occupation and health, occupation and the environment, cultural influences on occupations, occupational justice, time use, work, arts and creativity, parenting, and the importance of everyday activities. The populations that were most frequently addressed were women; individuals with chronic illnesses or disabilities; and infants, children, and adolescents. People who are homeless, inmates and ex-inmates, college students, individuals identifying as gay, lesbian, bisexual, or transgender, and refugees and immigrants were also participants in occupational science research presented at these symposia.

Finally, perhaps the key indicators of the vitality of occupational science are the number and the quality of papers that its scholars produce annually in peer-reviewed journals. These benchmarks, of course, are difficult to track thoroughly for several reasons. First, papers that occupational scientists produce are often not identified in databases as occupational science. Second, it is difficult to develop criteria for inclusion of articles as occupational science. Third, certain publications in occupational science are authored by non–occupational scientists and/or are published in journals that are not affiliated with occupational therapy. Additionally, occupational scientists might publish their work in interdisciplinary journals without indicating in the manuscript that their study or piece of scholarship is occupational science.

Nevertheless, two studies have recently been undertaken that identify publication trends in occupational science. Molke, Laliberte-Rudman, and Polatajko (2004) focused on the years 1990 and 2000 to detect changes in publication patterns between these two points in time. To be included in the study, the publications had to meet the following criteria: (1) the phrase *occupational science* or *science of occupation* was in the title, identified as a key word in the abstract, or in a collective title, and (2) the publication was not a book review, letter to the editor, or workshop summary. The authors found that only 10 publications qualified in 1990 (one year after occupational science had been founded) but that in 2000, 44 papers were identified, a fourfold increase. Moreover, in the second time period, there was a pronounced expansion in the number of authors from countries other than the United States compared to the author pool in 1990. Also, in 2000, the publications had appeared in a wider range of journals and showed a growth trend in the numbers employing qualitative methods in contrast to quantitative or mixed methods. Despite this, the percentage of publications that was data-based as distinguished from discussion-focused remained at 30% in the two time periods. Finally, the most common themes emerging from the review that were perceived to be shaping the direction of the emergent field were identified: (1) providing a broad and general understanding of occupation, (2) nurturing occupational therapy by providing it with a science-based foundation, (3) seeing occupational science as a vehicle for defending occupational therapy's commitment to certain values or ideals, and (4) describing the discipline as one that achieves social reform by championing occupation's place in social justice, a theme that was seen largely in the latter set of publications and in those written by Canadian and Australian authors.

The second study, which has just been completed by Glover (2007), builds on the preceding one by examining many more years to gain a finer-grained picture of publication trends. To be included in the study, the publication had to have appeared in a journal in any of the years between 1996 and 2006. As in the first study, the publication had to use the term *occupational science* or *science of occupation* in its title, key words, or abstract. However, in this study, only articles that appeared in peer-reviewed journals were included because these are considered by the scientific community to be the most legitimate vehicle for disseminating new findings. The selection process resulted in the identification of 244 articles. When publications from the earlier years were compared to those in later years, Glover found that although publication numbers fluctuated from year to year, in general, more articles were published in more recent years. Furthermore, over time the proportion of data-based articles increased, most being qualitative in nature. Also, the majority of publications addressed adults 18 to 64 years of age and without disability, although a hefty 26.8% did concern people with disabling conditions, a larger representation than would typically be found in traditional social sciences (such as anthropology or geography). Authors tended to be from the United States, Canada, and Australia, although other countries were also represented. Finally, in later years, a greater proportion of articles indicated that the work reported had been supported by extramural funding. This trend is particularly important because the prestige and growth of an academic discipline are largely contingent on receiving grants from federal and other agencies. In summary, although these two studies represent only a first cut in assessing how occupational science publications are developing, they nevertheless suggest that the discipline has grown impressively as it enters its third decade.

LINKAGES BETWEEN OCCUPATIONAL SCIENCE AND OCCUPATIONAL THERAPY

In 2017, the profession of occupational therapy will be 100 years old. In anticipation of this landmark occasion, the American Occupational Therapy Association (AOTA) has adopted the following Centennial Vision:

> By the year 2017, we envision that occupational therapy is a powerful, widely recognized, science-driven, and evidence-based profession with a globally connected and diverse workforce meeting society's occupational needs. (AOTA, 2007, paragraph 1)

How does occupational science relate to this vision? Or, to back up a bit, what is the relationship between occupational science and occupational therapy? We will make the case that the relationship between occupational science and occupational therapy is symbiotic, that each contributes to the survival of the other (Clark, 2006), and that occupational science is the vehicle through which the profession is becoming more science-driven and evidence-based.

The founders of occupational science, as we have explained, originally conceived of the discipline as basic in nature but as existing, in part, to nurture occupational therapy (Clark et al., 1991; Wilcock, 1991; Yerxa, 1993; Yerxa et al., 1989). Designating the science as basic at the time made sense for two reasons: First, the founders saw the advantage of building theory on occupation (basic science), in the general sense, without concern for its specific application in therapy (applied science). At that time, no discipline had occupation as its core subject matter, and it was clear that a science devoted to the study of occupation could have benefits that went well beyond occupational therapy practice. For example, this discipline could contribute new knowledge on occupation and synthesize existing interdisciplinary knowledge for use by those who are interested in preventing chronic illness and disability, promoting global health, or simply expanding our understanding of this central feature of human existence. The second reason was more practical. Universities in the decade of the 1980s privileged basic science over applied science. The climate was such that the chances of being able to establish a new basic science rather than an applied one were better. However, it should be reiterated that in the founders' original conceptualization, occupational science was always intended to furnish knowledge that could be used to theoretically inform, and thereby refine and develop, occupational therapy interventions.

Although a debate initially took place on whether or not occupational science should be independent of occupational therapy (Carlson & Dunlea, 1995; Clark, 1993; Clark et al., 1993; Lunt, 1997; Mosey, 1992, 1993), the two have subsequently become closely interlinked. Much attention has been placed on the relationship between occupational therapy and occupational science in the beginning, a kind of creation story, in which occupational science is purported to have grown out of occupational therapy. Lunt (1997) somewhat provocatively proposed that occupational science might have been created as a vehicle for elevating status of the study of occupation and distancing the field from the "dirty work" of a practicing field such as occupational therapy, a perspective that we and others would dispute.

In fact, the ties between occupational science and occupational therapy were reinforced in 1997 (nine years after the founding of the discipline) when Zemke and Clark (1996a, 1996b) moved away from defining occupational science as a basic science, recommending that its focus be not only on the nature of occupation, but also on how it is used in occupational therapy contexts. The fruitful ways in which occupational science has contributed to the profession of occupational therapy and to the addressing of societal needs have increased the excitement surrounding the discipline and the sense of its worthiness (Carlson & Dunlea, 1995; Clark, 1993; Jackson, Carlson, Mandel, Zemke, & Clark, 1998). Generation of knowledge for occupational therapy is frequently described as the primary aim or purpose for the discipline, and the need for more theory about occupation within occupational therapy curricula has also been noted (Whiteford & Wilcock, 2001; Yerxa, 1993). Interest in the study of occupation as related to the practice of occupational therapy has surged in recent years, and many people in the field consider it to be part of a kind of course correction to return current practice to its philosophical roots, overcoming the reductionism that

marked the tight coupling of the field with biomedicine, particularly around the 1970s (e.g., Wilcock, 2001).

Basic research on the nature of occupation, including its observable and phenomenological aspects, can be catalytic for improving existing therapeutic approaches and creating new ones, moving the profession away from reliance on "adhoc, recipe-based knowledge" (Abbott, 2004, p. 4). Similarly, studies on the impact of occupation on the health of individuals, communities, and the global arena can result in an expansion in occupational therapy's scope of practice. In addressing a wide variety of topics that are relevant to the general population, occupational science can broaden occupational therapy's professional jurisdiction while appropriating the profession greater stature and credibility. For example, as scientific evidence is produced that demonstrates the ways in which health-promoting activity lessens the risk for developing chronic diseases or disability, occupational therapy will become better positioned to stake a claim in the prevention arena. Just as much of dental practice (since the discovery of fluoride) is dedicated to prevention, so too could a significant amount of occupational therapy practice be aimed at preventing the very diseases and disabilities that its practitioners have traditionally remediated. In this way, the profession will be able to stake out new territory for its therapeutic work (Abbott, 2004). Finally, the applied arm of occupational science can produce the much-needed outcome studies on intervention effectiveness. This broader conceptualization of occupational science, that is, as a comprehensive translational science, is the way in which the discipline is now taking shape in the United States, a development that provides a goodness-of-fit with what is required for realization of AOTA's Centennial Vision.

Figure 1.1 depicts graphically the ways in which occupational science is related to other disciplines as well as to occupational therapy, its primary practice arm. In this model, occupational science is seen as contributing its subject matter and research findings to the universe of knowledge. In doing so, it enriches other academic disciplines and professions, simultaneously creating widespread understanding of its focus. Reciprocally, these fields supply intellectual content and research findings that are of relevance to occupation back to occupational science. Occupational science is also shown as being highly intermeshed with occupational therapy. The various kinds of knowledge that are generated by the field, overall, are seen as bolstering the scientific credibility of the profession and could lead to increased growth in third-party payment for occupational therapy services and the enactment of public policies that render occupational therapy services more widely available. Syntheses of interdisciplinary knowledge and basic science on occupation can be translated into innovative treatment advances or used to refine existing protocols. They can also provide justification for expanding professional jurisdictional claims (Abbott, 2004).

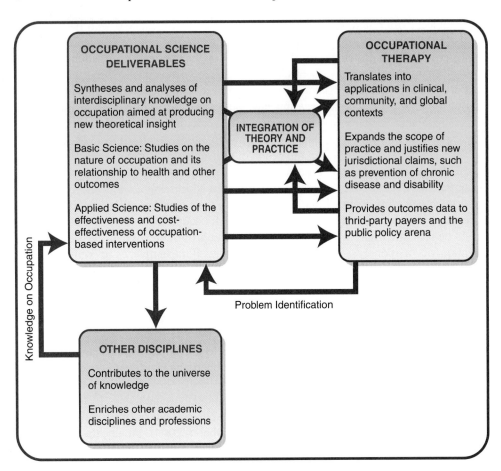

FIGURE 1.1 Interlinks between occupational science, occupational therapy, and other academic disciplines and fields: a mechanism for furthering the Centennial Vision.

As can be seen in Figure 1.2, we believe that the confluence of these activities will lead to greater public awareness and valuing of the occupational therapy profession, ultimately generating benefits to society. However, for occupational science and occupational therapy to be intermeshed in this way and to further key aspects of the Centennial Vision, a carefully thought-out division of labor is required. In Figure 1.3, a diverse occupational therapy/ occupational science workforce (including scientists, educators, and practitioners) is depicted. Practitioners (occupational therapy assistants and occupational therapists) are depicted as working across diverse settings, where they will implement traditional and new models of practice for individuals, groups, and communities. They may also be invited to share their up-to-date clinical expertise in educational programs or become interventionists on clinical trial research teams. Occupational scientists with PhD or ScD degrees are seen as constituting the core tenure-track faculty and the main cadre of researchers developing the body of occupational science knowledge, doing large-scale outcome studies, and infusing findings in curricula. Practitioners and faculty who have Doctor of Occupational Therapy (OTD) degrees are pictured as being in the lead position for drawing from occupational science to develop intervention models and study their effectiveness, as well as for joining faculty who have PhDs in updating curricula in accord

with new scientific breakthroughs. We conceive of this new breed of OTDs as pioneer experts in clinical practice and as leaders in facilitating education, policy, or administrative changes to create alignments with the Centennial Vision.

AN ILLUSTRATION OF THE RESEARCH PROCESS: THE USC WELL ELDERLY STUDY

To explicate one way in which occupational science has nurtured occupational therapy, we will now describe a template for conducting translational research that is used by the USC Well Elderly Study group (Clark et al., 1997; Clark, Azen et al., 2001; Hay et al., 2002; Jackson et al., 1998; Mandel, Jackson, Zemke, Nelson, & Clark, 1999). A research team that has been funded through federal grant support. The trajectory of research activities as designed by this team is depicted in Figure 1.4. The research program begins by identifying a problem worthy of investigation (Step 1). For example, in the USC Well Elderly Study, the problem was framed as whether or not an activity (occupation) based intervention could slow down the declines that are normally associated with aging or improve health in the elderly (Clark et al., 1997; Mandel et al., 1999). The group used qualitative research meth-

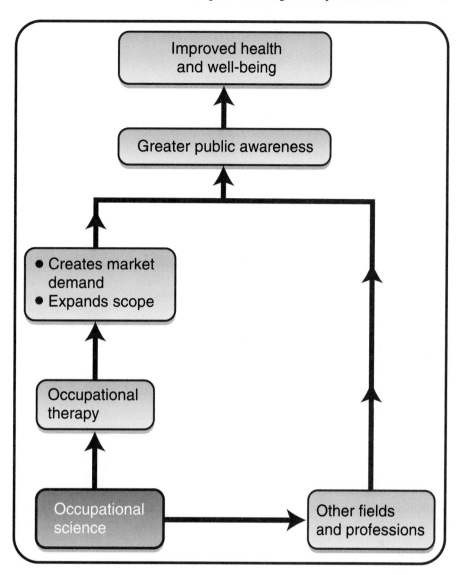

FIGURE 1.2   Overview of linkages that can support public awareness of occupational therapy.

ods to obtain a detailed and complex understanding of the contextual factors that needed to be taken into consideration (Step 2) (Mandel et al., 1999). Following this qualitative work, which can be thought of as more basic than applied science, the findings were then used to enhance aspects of occupational therapy practice, by refining existing approaches or creating new interventions (Step 3) (Mandel et al., 1999).

The research group sought federal funding to conduct a large-scale clinical trial (Step 4) that employs quantitative methods to demonstrate the cost-effectiveness (Step 5) of the new or refined therapeutic approach (applied science). If the results of the trial demonstrate effectiveness, the next step is to obtain funding to conduct subsequent studies on the mechanisms that account for the positive outcomes (Step 6). This work, in turn, can lead to further theory development and practice improvements (Step 7). The process, which initially might have seemed disconnected from practice, culminates in therapeutic innovation and the delivery of outcomes data that can have a

positive effect on reimbursement for services and public policy decisions. Ultimately, the Well Elderly Study demonstrated the cost-effectiveness of a preventive occupational therapy program, entitled Lifestyle Redesign®, in improving health outcomes in the elderly (Clark et al., 1997; Clark, Azen, et al., 2001; Hay et al., 2002).

REFRAMING OCCUPATIONAL SCIENCE AND BIOMEDICAL CONDITIONS THROUGH THE USC/RANCHO LOS AMIGOS NATIONAL REHABILITATION CENTER PRESSURE ULCER PREVENTION STUDY

One commonly held misconception is that occupational science is too "soft" a discipline to create substantive innovation in the treatment of biomedical conditions. This line

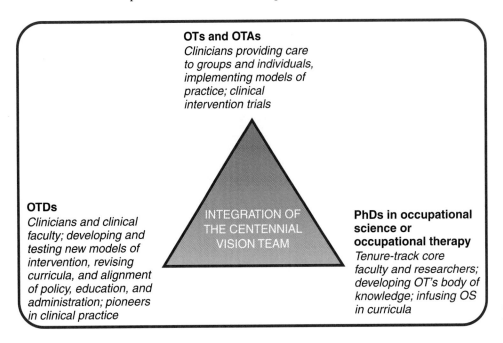

OTs and OTAs
Clinicians providing care to groups and individuals, implementing models of practice; clinical intervention trials

INTEGRATION OF THE CENTENNIAL VISION TEAM

OTDs
Clinicians and clinical faculty; developing and testing new models of intervention, revising curricula, and alignment of policy, education, and administration; pioneers in clinical practice

PhDs in occupational science or occupational therapy
Tenure-track core faculty and researchers; developing OT's body of knowledge; infusing OS in curricula

FIGURE 1.3 Primary contributions to Centennial Vision.

of thinking assumes that contextual factors and other complex life circumstances are not particularly relevant to the care of patients who have, or are at risk for, discrete biologically based impairments, diseases, or disabilities. It also is grounded in the preconception that a discipline that is focused on explaining occupation and its impact on health is too removed in its emphases from traditional biomedical procedures and practices to have genuine payoffs in the provision of care. We will try to illustrate that such circumscribed reasoning is limiting and problematic. To accomplish this, we will describe the methods that are used as well as the findings and resources that have been generated through the USC/Rancho Los Amigos National Rehabilitation Center Pressure Ulcer Prevention Study (PUPS) study (Clark et al., 2006). Not only has this research program resulted in innovations in occupational therapy treatment in the area of pressure ulcer prevention, but it has also generated resource materials (USC/RLRPUPP, 2006a, 2006b, 2006c) that are intended to improve best practices for the wider community of rehabilitation professionals.

The PUPS study team selected the problem of pressure ulcer prevention in people with spinal cord injury to work on for three reasons (Step 1 in Figure 1.4). First, the general area of pressure ulcer prevention had been identified as a significant national health concern. For example, both Healthy People 2010 and the Joint Commission on Accreditation of Health Care Organizations identified it as a key priority (Martucci, 2006). Second, existing best practices have failed to address the problem adequately with the costs of wound management soaring. Once pressure ulcers are at advanced stages, the cost of care is astronomical with surgical costs reaching as much as $70,000 per wound (Clark et al., 2006). Having the expertise to do

cost-effectiveness studies, the PUPS research team was attracted to this research area in part because of the potential through scientific discovery to reduce the burden of these health care costs. However, finally, and perhaps most importantly, a literature review had revealed that recurrent pressure ulcers were serious threats to the quality of life of people with spinal cord injuries, compromising their potential to express themselves as occupational beings (Clark et al., 2006; Clark, Sanders, Carlson, Jackson, & Imperatore-Blanche, in press; Consortium for Spinal Cord Medicine, 2000; Cutajar & Roberts, 2005). Typically, the occurrence of an advanced pressure ulcer requires months of confinement to bed, creates a decrease in functional ability because of muscle loss due to surgery, and can cause depression and an overwhelming sense of helplessness. The PUPS team therefore decided to use a fullfledged occupational science–based strategy incorporating the steps in the translational research template shown in Figure 1.4 for investigating this seemingly intractable problem, which manifests itself proximally as skin breakdown, a discrete biomedical condition, but then has radiating distal effects on both private lives and the public reimbursement sector.

In executing the second step of the translational research template (see Figure 1.4), the PUPS team secured a Field Initiated Research Grant (#H133G000062) from the National Institute of Disability and Rehabilitation Research to conduct a qualitative study to obtain new and detailed understandings of the complex interplay of life circumstances and other contextual factors that contribute to the development of pressure ulcers in people with spinal cord injury. The methodology entailed conducting in-depth interviews and participant observation of events that led to pressure ulcer development in the lives of 19 people with

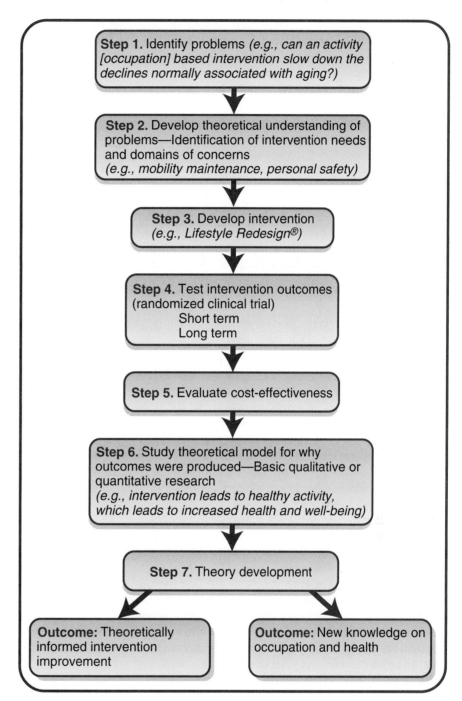

FIGURE 1.4 Blueprint for a translational science research program.

spinal cord injury and one person with spinal myelitis, all of whom had had a history of recurrent pressure ulcer development. The findings underscored the significant degree to which a complex cluster of factors led to the emergence of pressure ulcers (Clark et al., 2006). Results revealed several principles that addressed the complexity of contextual concerns that tended to explain pressure ulcer development in people with spinal cord injury (USC/RLRPUPP, 2006c). They also led to the creation of a set of models that described the daily lifestyle factors that influenced the likelihood of incurring a pressure ulcer (Clark et al., 2006). From the findings, it was clear that focusing on convention-

ally linked factors such as equipment breakdowns or failure to comply with the pressure relief procedures was insufficient in explaining how the participants developed pressure ulcers. Factors related to occupation, such as moment-to-moment decision making on whether or not to engage in a high-risk activity, negotiating tradeoffs between pursuing a passion and resting when an ulcer was in an early stage, or problem solving in unanticipated and unusual circumstances such as being trapped in an airport for 16 hours, were often pivotal in contributing to pressure ulcer development. To date, this research program has demonstrated that prevention efforts need to take into account the unique constellations of circumstances in a person's everyday life (Clark et al., 2006), that traditional assessments of pressure ulcer risk need to be broadened to include factors related to life situations (Seip, Carlson, Jackson, & Clark, 2007), and that more attention needs to be given to the decisions people make about their daily activity engagement when a pressure ulcer is in an early stage, to minimize the likelihood that it will advance to a stage for which surgery is required (Dunn, Carlson, Jackson, & Clark, 2007).

While the thrust of the PUPS study described above leans on the side of being basic in nature, in that the primary goal of the initial study was descriptive, the research team has translated the findings into applications that might turn out not only to expand occupational therapy's stake in the area of wound prevention and care, but also to yield practical benefits for other rehabilitation professionals, and real-life, real-world benefits to people who are prone to pressure ulcer development. First, the PUPS team used the findings to develop an innovative Lifestyle Redesign® Pressure Ulcer Prevention Program (USC/RLRPUPP, 2006a) that was intended for use by occupational therapists. Second, it produced a Rehabilitation Professionals Manual and a Companion Manual, which exist in hard copy and CD-ROM formats, that were intended as a resource for all rehabilitation professionals working in this area (USC/RLRPUPP, 2006c). These manuals contain narratives of the life circumstances that led to the development of pressure ulcers in the 20 study participants. The format is interactive, containing elements such as decision trees, questions addressing various dilemmas related to pressure ulcer risk with a choice of several possible solutions of varying degrees of correctness, and highlighted words embedded in the stories that represent factors that place particular participants at risk for pressure ulcer development. Clicking on the highlighted text in the Rehabilitation Professionals Manual takes the reader to a corresponding article in the Companion Manual that summarizes recent research on the topic of interest. Finally, the PUPS team drew from the findings to create a manual for consumer use, which can be easily accessed at http://www.pressureulcerprevention.com and contains articles on 46 factors that were found to contribute to the development of pressure ulcers in the actual lives of the study participants.

At this point, with a manual of interventions in hand that incorporates traditional occupational therapy approaches to pressure ulcer prevention with new strategies derived from the PUPS study, the research team is now attempting to secure federal funding to conduct a large-scale randomized clinical trial with hopes of demonstrating the intervention's cost-effectiveness. Members of the team also intend to develop an assessment based on the findings that will be capable of predicting risk with more exactitude than is typical of currently used pressure ulcer risk assessments. Assuming that they are successful, the PUPS study will be able to demonstrate the way in which occupational science supports the development of state-of-the-art rehabilitation interventions, contributes to a complex understanding of pressure ulcer risk, translates into concrete occupational therapy approaches, and provides consumer access to new information on the factors that lead to the development of pressure ulcers.

CONCLUSION

The PUPS study has the potential to illustrate how a detailed understanding of daily lives and occupations, acquired through science, can lead to strong, multifaceted theoretically informed intervention approaches that go well beyond traditional biomedical protocols. In this way, occupational science can fortify occupational therapy. In turn, occupational therapy, strengthened by occupational science, will be better positioned for securing new reimbursement streams and expanding its scope. As occupational therapy becomes recognized as a scientifically driven and evidence-based practice, its clinicians will go on to identify the next problem areas that need to be tackled by occupational scientists.

PROVOCATIVE QUESTIONS

1. How is the described relationship between occupational science and occupational therapy mutually beneficial?
2. What do you think are the most pressing problems to address through the proposed translational science research program?
3. In your mind, jump ahead 10 years. Envision yourself to be writing a section describing recent developments in occupational science over the past decade. What might you be able to say or hope to be able to say?

ON THE WEB

◆ See http://www.pressureulcerprevention.com for more information about the Pressure Ulcer Prevention Project.

ACKNOWLEDGMENTS

(For PUPS) This study was funded by a grant (#H133G000062) from the National Institute on Disability and Rehabilitation Research. We thank all the members of the USC/Rancho Los Amigos National Rehabilitation Center Pressure Ulcer Prevention Study group for their contributions to the PUPS study, some of the content of which is covered in this chapter. Specifically, we thank Jeanne Jackson, PhD, OTR, who served as co-PI on the project, and Michael Scott, MD, Mike Carlson, PhD, Michal Atkins, MA, OTR/L, Debra Uhles-Tanaka, MA, Salah Rubayi, MD, Erna Blanche, PhD, OTR/L, Rod Adkins, PhD, Kathleen Gross, MA, OTR/L, Clarissa Saunders-Newton, MA, OTR/L, Stephanie Mielke, OTD,

OTR/L, Mary Kay Wolfe, OTD, OTR/L, Paul Bailey, MSc, Elizabeth Crall, MA, OTR/L, Aaron Eakman, PhD, OTR/L, and Faryl Saliman Reingold, MA, OTR/L.

(For Well Elderly) This study was funded by a grant (#1R01 AG021108-01A3) from the National Institutes of Health. We thank all the members of the USC Well Elderly Study group for their contributions to the Well Elderly study, some of the content of which is covered in this chapter. Specifically, we thank Jeanne Jackson, PhD, OTR, who served as co-PI on the project, and Stan Azen, PhD, Ruth Zemke, PhD, OTR, Mike Carlson, PhD, Deborah Mandel, MS, OTR, Joel Hay, PhD, Karen Josephson, MD, Barbara Cherry, PhD, Colin Hessel, MS, Joycelynne Palmer, MS, Loren Lipson, MD, Geyla Frank, PhD, Laurie Nelson, MA, OTR, Laurie LaBree, MS, Brian Young, MA, OTR, Shan-Pin Fanchiang, PhD, OTR, Karen Patterson, MA, OTR/L, Bridget Larson Ennevor, MA, OTR, LuAn Hobson, MA, OTR/L, Jennifer Crandall, MA, OTR/L, Allyn Rankin-Martinez, MA, OTR, Roger Luo, PhD, Jeanine Blanchard, MA, OTR, Karen McNulty, MA, OTR/L, Gitu Bhatvani, MA, OTR/L, Joan Vartanian, BS, OTR, Patricia Gonzalez, MA, OTR, and Aisha Mohammed, MA, OTR.

REFERENCES

Abbott, A. (2004, January). Creating an academic discipline that supports practice. Keynote lecture delivered at the 16th Annual USC Occupational Science Symposium, Los Angeles, CA.

American Occupational Therapy Association. (2007). *AOTA's Centennial Vision.* Retrieved July 1, 2007, from http://www.aota.org/News/Centennial/Background/36562.aspx

Carlson, M., & Dunlea, A. (1995). Further thoughts on the pitfalls of partition: A response to Mosey. *The American Journal of Occupational Therapy, 49*(1), 73–81.

Clark, F. (1993). Occupation embedded in real life: Interweaving occupational science and occupational therapy. 1993 Eleanor Clarke Slagle Lecture. *The American Journal of Occupational Therapy, 47*(12), 1067–1078.

Clark, F. (2006). One person's thoughts on the future of occupational science. *Journal of Occupational Science, 13*(3), 167–179.

Clark, F., Azen, S. P., Carlson, M., Mandel, D., LaBree, L., Hay, J., et al. (2001). Embedding health-promoting changes into the daily lives of independent-living older adults: Long-term follow-up of occupational therapy intervention. *Journal of Gerontology: Psychological Sciences and Social Sciences, 56B,* 60–63.

Clark, F., Azen, S. P., Zemke, R., Jackson, J., Carlson, M., Hay, J., et al. (1997). Occupational therapy for independent-living older adults: A randomized controlled trial. *Journal of the American Medical Association, 278*(16), 1321–1326.

Clark, F., Jackson, J., Scott, M., Atkins, M., Uhles-Tanaka, M., & Rubayi, S. (2006). Data-based models of how pressure ulcers develop in daily-living contexts of adults with spinal cord injury. *Archives of Physical Medicine and Rehabilitation, 87,* 1516–1525.

Clark, F. A., Parham, D., Carlson, M. E., Frank, G., Jackson, J., Pierce, D., et al. (1991). Occupational science: Academic innovation in the service of occupational therapy's future. *The American Journal of Occupational Therapy, 45*(4), 300–310.

Clark, F., Sanders, K., Carlson, M., Jackson, J., & Imperatore-Blanche, E. (in press). Synthesis of habit theory. *Occupational Therapy Journal of Research.*

Clark, F., Zemke, R., Frank, G., Parham, D., Neville-Jan, A., Hendricks, C., et al. (1993). Dangers inherent in the partition of occupational therapy and occupational science. *The American Journal of Occupational Therapy, 47*(2), 184–186.

Consortium for Spinal Cord Medicine. (2000). *Pressure ulcer prevention and treatment following spinal cord injury: A clinical practice guideline for health-care professionals.* Waldorf, MD: Paralyzed Veterans of America.

Cutajar, R., & Roberts, A. (2005). Occupations and pressure sore development in Saudi men with paraplegia. *British Journal of Occupational Therapy, 68,* 307–314.

Dickie, V., Cutchin, M. P., & Humphry, R. (2006). Occupation as transactional experience: A critique of individualism in occupational science. *Journal of Occupational Science, 13*(1), 83–93.

Dunn, C. A., Carlson, M., Jackson, J. M., & Clark, F. A. (2007). *Response factors surrounding progression of low-grade pressure ulcers in community-residing adults with spinal cord injury.* Unpublished manuscript, University of Southern California, Los Angeles.

Farnworth, L. (1998). Doing, being, and boredom. *Journal of Occupational Science, 5*(3), 140–146.

Flyvberg, B. (2001). *Making social sciences matter: Why social science fails and how it can succeed again.* Cambridge, UK: Cambridge University Press.

Glass, T. A., & McAtee, M. J. (2006). Behavioral science at the crossroads in public health: Extending horizons, envisioning the future. *Social Science & Medicine, 62,* 1650–1671.

Glover, J. (2007). The literature of occupational science: Peer-reviewed publications from 1996–2006. Unpublished manuscript, University of Southern California, Los Angeles.

Gray, J. M. (1997). Application of the phenomenological method to the concept of occupation. *Journal of Occupational Science: Australia, 4*(3), 5–17.

Hasselkus, B. R. (2006). 2006 Eleanor Clarke Slagle Lecture— The world of everyday occupation: Real people, real lives. *American Journal of Occupational Therapy, 60,* 627–640. Quote from p. 638. *(unit opening quote)*

Hay, J., LaBree, L, Luo, R., Clark, F., Carlson, M., Mandel, D., et al. (2002). Cost-effectiveness of preventive occupational therapy for independent-living older adults. *Journal of the American Geriatrics Society, 50*(8), 1381–1388.

Hocking, C. (2000). Occupational science: A stock take of accumulated insights. *Journal of Occupational Science, 7*(2), 58–67.

Jackson, J., Carlson, M., Mandel, D., Zemke, R., & Clark, F. (1998). Occupation in lifestyle redesign: The well elderly study occupational therapy program. *The American Journal of Occupational Therapy, 52*(5), 326–336.

Lawlor, M. C. (2003). The significance of being occupied: The social construction of childhood occupations. *American Journal of Occupational Therapy, 57*(4), 424–434.

Lentin, P. (2002). The human spirit and occupation: Surviving and creating a life. *Journal of Occupational Science, 9*(3), 143–152.

Lunt A. (1997). Occupational science and occupational therapy: Negotiating the boundary between a discipline and a profession. *Journal of Occupational Science: Australia, 4*(2), 56–61.

Mandel, D. R., Jackson, J. M., Zemke, R., Nelson, L., & Clark, F. A. (1999). *Lifestyle redesign: Implementing the well-elderly program.* Bethesda, MD: American Occupational Therapy Association.

Mattingly, C., & Lawlor, M. (2000). Learning from stories: Narrative interviewing in cross cultural research. *Scandinavian Journal of Occupational Therapy, 7*(1), 4–14.

Martucci, N. (2006). An ounce of prevention: Arresting the occurrence of pressure ulcerations in individuals with disabilities. *Rehab Magazine, 19*(10), 36–39.

Molineux, M. L., & Whiteford, G. E. (1999). Prisons: from occupational deprivation to occupational enrichment. *Journal of Occupational Science, 6*(3), 124–130.

Molke, D. K., Laliberte-Rudman, D., & Polatajko, H. (2004). The promise of occupational science: A developmental assessment of an emerging academic discipline. *Canadian Journal of Occupational Therapy, 71*(5), 269–281.

Mosey, A. C. (1992). Partition of occupational science and occupational therapy. *American Journal of Occupational Therapy, 47*, 851–853.

Mosey, A. C. (1993). Partition of occupational science and occupational therapy: Sorting out some issues. *The American Journal of Occupational Therapy, 47*(8), 751–754.

Mounter, C., & Ilott, I. (1997). Occupational science: A journey of discovery in the United Kingdom. *Journal of Occupational Science: Australia, 4*(2), 50–55.

Mounter, C. R., & Ilott, I. (2000). Occupational science: Updating the United Kingdom journey of discovery. *Occupational Therapy International, 7*(2), 111–120.

Seip, J. G., Carlson, M., Jackson, J., & Clark, F. A. (2007). *Pressure ulcer risk assessment in adults with spinal cord injury: The need to incorporate daily lifestyle concerns.* Unpublished manuscript, University of Southern California, Los Angeles.

USC/Rancho Lifestyle Redesign® Pressure Ulcer Prevention Project. (2006a). *Lifestyle Redesign® for Pressure Ulcer Prevention.* Unpublished manuscript, USC/Rancho Lifestyle Redesign® Pressure Ulcer Prevention Project, Los Angeles.

USC/Rancho Lifestyle Redesign® Pressure Ulcer Prevention Project. (2006b). *Pressure ulcer prevention project consumer manual online.* Retrieved June 6, 2007, from http://www.usc.edu/pups

USC/Rancho Lifestyle Redesign® Pressure Ulcer Prevention Project. (2006c). *PUPS study rehabilitation manual.* Unpublished manuscript, USC/Rancho Los Amigos, Los Angeles.

Whiteford, G. E., & Wilcock, A. A. (2001). Centralizing occupation in occupational therapy curricula: Imperative of a new millennium. *Occupational Therapy International, 8*(2), 81–85.

Wicks, A. (2006). *Occupational science: Generating an international perspective.* Report on the Inaugural International Science Think Tank. Shoalhaven Campus, University of Wollongong, July 19–21, 2006.

Wicks, A., & Whiteford, G. (2003). Value of life stories in occupation-based research. *Australian Occupational Therapy Journal, 50*, 86–91.

Wilcock, A. A. (1991). Occupational science. *British Journal of Occupational Therapy, 54*(8), 297–300.

Wilcock, A. A. (1998). *An occupational perspective on health.* Thorofare, NJ: Slack.

Wilcock, A. A. (1999). Reflections on doing, being, and becoming. *Australian Journal of Occupational Therapy, 46*, 1–11.

Wilcock, A. A. (2001). Occupational science: The key to broadening horizons. *British Journal of Occupational Therapy, 64*(8), 412–417.

Wilcock, A. A. (2003). Occupational science: The study of humans as occupational beings. In P. Kramer, J. Hinojosa, & C. B. Royeen (Eds.), *Perspectives in human occupation: Participation in life* (pp. 156–180). Baltimore: Lippincott Williams & Wilkins.

Wilcock, A. A. (2005). Occupational science: Bridging occupation and health. 2004 CAOT Conference Keynote Address. *Canadian Journal of Occupational Therapy, 72*(1), 5–11.

Yerxa, E. J. (1993). Occupational science: A new source of power for participants in occupational therapy. *Occupational Science, 1*(1), 3–9.

Yerxa, E. J. (2000). Occupational science: A renaissance of service to humankind through knowledge. *Occupational Therapy International, 7*(2), 87–98.

Yerxa, E. J., Clark, F., Frank, G., Jackson, J., Parham, D., Pierce, D., Stein, C., & Zemke, R. (1989). An introduction to occupational science, A foundation for occupational therapy in the 21st century. In J. Johnson & E. Yerxa (Eds.), *Occupational science: The foundation for new models of practice* (pp. 1–17). New York: Haworth Press.

Zemke, R., & Clark, F. (Eds.). (1996a). *Occupational science: The evolving discipline.* Philadelphia: F. A. Davis.

Zemke, R., & Clark, F. (Eds.). (1996b). Preface. In *Occupational science: The evolving discipline* (pp. vii–xviii). Philadelphia: F. A. Davis.

What Is Occupation?

VIRGINIA DICKIE

2

> **Mr. Jourdain.** You mean to say that when I say "Nicole, fetch me my slippers" or "Give me my nightcap" that's prose? **Philosopher.** Certainly, sir. **Mr. Jourdain.** Well, my goodness! Here I've been talking prose for forty years and never known it . . .
>
> —MOLIERE (1670)

Learning Objectives

After reading this chapter, you will be able to:

1. Identify and evaluate ways of knowing occupation.
2. Articulate different ways of defining and classifying occupation.
3. Describe the relationship between occupation and context.

KNOWING AND LEARNING ABOUT OCCUPATION

Reading the paper, washing hands, throwing a Frisbee, walking through a colorful market in a foreign country, telling a story (in poetry or prose)—all are occupations people do without ever thinking about them as being occupations. Many occupations are ordinary and become part of the context of daily living. Such occupations are generally taken for granted and most often are habitual (Aarts & Dijksterhuis, 2000; Bargh & Chartrand, 1999; Wood, Quinn, & Kashy, 2002). In the myriad of activities people do every day, they do *occupation* all their lives, perhaps without ever knowing it.

Occupations are ordinary, but they can also be special when they represent a new achievement such as driving a car or when they are part of celebrations and rites of passage. Preparing and hosting Thanksgiving dinner for the first time and baking the pies for the annual family holiday for the twentieth time are examples of special occupations. Occupations tend to be special when they happen infrequently and carry symbolic meanings such as representing achievement of adulthood or one's love for family. Occupations are also special when they form part of a treasured routine such as reading a bedtime story to one's child, singing "Twinkle, Twinkle, Little Star," and tucking the covers around the small, sleepy body. But even special occupations, while heavy with tradition, may change over time. Hocking, Wright-St. Clair, and Bunrayong (2002) illustrated the complexity of traditional occupations in their study of holiday food preparation by older women in Thailand and New Zealand. The study identified many similarities between the groups (such as the activities the authors named "recipe work"), but the Thai women valued maintenance of an invariant tradition in what they prepared and how they did it, while the New Zealand women changed the foods they prepared over time and expected such changes to continue. Nevertheless, the doing of food-centered occupations around holidays was a tradition for both groups.

To be human is to be occupational. Occupation is a biological imperative, evident in the evolutionary history of humankind, the current behaviors of our primate relatives, and the survival needs that must be met through occupation (Clark, 1997; Krishnagiri, 2000; Wilcock, 1998; Wood, 1998). Fromm (as cited by Reilly, 1962), asserted that people had a "physiologically conditioned need" to work as an act of self-preservation (p. 4). Humans also have occupational needs beyond survival. Addressing one type of occupation, Dissanayake (1992, 1995) argued that making art, or, as she describes it, "making special," is a biological necessity of human existence. According to Molineux (2004), occupational therapists now understand humans, their function, and their therapeutic needs in an occupational manner in which *occupation is life itself* [emphasis added]. Townsend (1997) described occupation as the "active process of living: from the beginning to the end of life, our occupations are all the active processes of looking after ourselves and others, enjoying life, and being socially and economically productive over the lifespan and in various contexts" (p. 19).

THE NEED TO UNDERSTAND OCCUPATION

Occupational therapy practitioners need to base their work on a thorough understanding of occupation and its role in health. Understanding occupation is more than having an easy definition (which is a daunting challenge in its own right). To know what occupation is, it is necessary to examine what humans do with their time, how such activities are organized, what purposes they serve, and what they mean for individuals and society.

Personal experience of doing occupation, whether consciously attended to or not, provides a fundamental understanding of occupation—what it is, how it happens, what it means, what is good about it, and what is not. This way of knowing is both basic and extraordinarily rich.

Looking Inward to Know Occupation

If you had asked me about gardening when I was young, I would have described the hard work of weeding the family garden on hot summer days, emphasizing that gar-

dening was a *chore*. In my parents' garden I learned a great deal about how to garden, such as varieties of flowers and vegetables, sunshine and rain requirements, weed identification, and how to grasp a weed to pull it out with all its roots. This is *knowledge* of rules and techniques, of how to *do* gardening. Now, many years later, I know gardening in a very different way. Weeding is one of my great pleasures. I understand the challenges of learning to garden in new places, the patience required to discover what will grow where, and the right time of year to plant. Between my youth and the present, gardening has taken on a different *form* (no longer a chore assigned by my parents but now creating and maintaining a low-tillage series of small gardens with herbs, shrubs, flowers, and selected vegetables on my own initiative or with my husband), *function* (then I gardened to avoid displeasing my parents, and now I garden to meet my own needs for aesthetic pleasures and satisfying "doing"), and *meaning* (from being a neutral to disagreeable series of chores to being a source of relaxation, reflection, shared time, and gratifying hard work). These elements—the form, function, and meaning of occupation—are the basic areas of focus for the science of occupation (Larson, Wood, & Clark, 2003).

To be useful to occupational therapy practitioners, knowledge of occupation based on personal experience demands examination and reflection. What do we do, how do we do it, when and where does it take place, and what does it mean? Who else is involved directly and indirectly? What capacities does it require in us? What does it cost? Is it challenging or easy? How has this occupation changed over time? What would it be like if we no longer had this occupation? My gardening example illustrates how occupation is a *transaction* with the *environment* or *context* of other people, plants, earth, and weather. It includes the *temporal* nature of occupation—seasonal variations but also change over time and perhaps some notion of occupation filling time. That I call myself a gardener exemplifies how occupation has become part of my *identity* and suggests that it might be difficult for me to give up gardening.

Basic as it is, however, understanding derived from personal experience is insufficient as the basis for practice. Reliance solely on this source of knowledge has the risk of expecting everyone to experience occupation in the same manner as the therapist. So while occupational therapy practitioners will profit in being attuned to their own occupations, they must also turn their view to the occupation around them and to understanding occupation through study and research.

Looking Outward to Know Occupation

Observation of the world through an occupational lens is another rich source of occupational knowledge. Connoisseurs of occupation can train themselves to new ways of seeing a world rich with occupations: the way a restaurant hostess manages a crowd when the wait for seating is long, the economy of movement of a construction worker

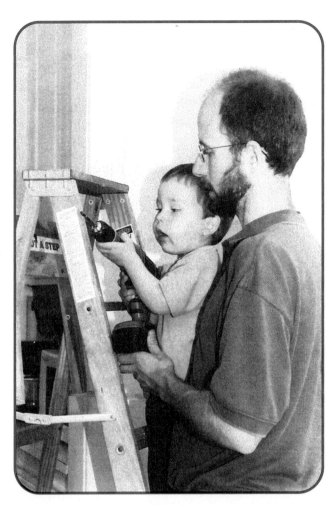

FIGURE 2.1 What occupations are represented in this picture?

doing a repetitive task, the activities of musicians in the orchestra pit when they are not playing. People like to talk about what they do, and the student of occupation can learn a great deal by asking for information about people's work and play. By being observant and asking questions, people increase their repertoires of occupational knowledge far beyond the boundaries of personal interests, practices, and capabilities (Figure 2.1).

Observation of others' occupations enriches the occupational therapy practitioner's knowledge of the range of occupational possibilities and of human responses to occupational opportunities. But while this sort of knowledge goes far beyond the limits of personal experience, it is still bounded by the world any one person is able to access, and it lacks the depth of knowledge that is developed through research and scholarship.

Turning to Research and Scholarship to Understand Occupation

Knowledge of occupation that comes from personal experience and observation must be augmented with understand-ing of occupation drawn from research in occupational therapy and occupational science as well as other disciplines. Hocking (2000) developed a framework of needed knowledge for research in occupation, organized into the categories of the "essential elements of occupation . . . occupational processes . . . [and the] relationship of occupation to other phenomena" (p.59). This research is being done within occupational therapy and occupational science, but there is also a wealth of information to be found in the work of other disciplines. For example, in anthropology, Orr studied the work of copy machine repairmen (1996), and Downey (1998) studied computer engineers and what they did. Consumer researchers have studied Christmas shopping (Sherry & McGrath, 1989), motorcycle riding (Schouten & McAlexander, 1995), and many other occupations of consumption. Psychologists have studied habits (Aarts & Dijksterhuis, 2000; Bargh & Chartrand, 1999; Wood, Quinn, & Kashy, 2002) and a wealth of other topics that relate to how people engage in occupation. Understanding of occupation will benefit from more research within occupational therapy and occupational science and from accessing relevant works of scholars in other fields.

DEFINING OCCUPATION

For many years, the word *occupation* was not part of the daily language of occupational therapists; nor was it prominent in the profession's literature (Hinojosa, Kramer, Royeen, & Luebben, 2003). According to Kielhofner and Burke (1977), the founding paradigm of occupational therapy was occupation, and the occupational perspective focused on people and their health "in the context of the culture of daily living and its activities" (p. 688). But beginning in the 1930s, occupational therapy strove to become more like the medical profession, entering into a paradigm of **reductionism** that lasted into the 1970s with occupation, both as a concept and as a means and/or outcome of intervention, essentially absent. With time, a few professional leaders began to call for occupational therapy to return to its roots in occupation (Schwartz, 2003), and since the 1970s, acceptance of occupation as the foundation of occupational therapy has grown (Kielhofner, 1997). With that growth, professional debates about the definition and nature of occupation emerged, and they continue to this day.

Defining occupation in occupational therapy is challenging because the word is part of common language with meanings that the profession cannot control. The term *occupation* and related concepts such as *activity, task, employment,* and *work* are used in many ways within occupational therapy. It seems quite logical to think of a job, or cleaning house, or bike riding as an occupation, but the concept is fuzzier when we think about the smaller components of these larger categories. Is dusting an occupation, or is it part of the occupation of house cleaning? Is riding a bike a skill that is part of some larger occupation, such as physical conditioning or getting from home to school, or is it an occupation in its own right? Does this change over time?

The founders of occupational therapy used the word *occupation* to describe a way of "properly" using time that included work and worklike activities and recreational activities (Meyer, 1922/1977). Breines (1995) pointed out that the founders chose a term that was both ambiguous and comprehensive to name the profession, and she argued that this choice was not accidental. The term was open to holistic interpretations that supported the diverse areas of practice of the time, encompassing the elements of occupation defined by Breines (1995) as "mind, body, time, space, and others" (p. 459). The term *occupation* spawned ongoing examination, controversy, and redefinition as the profession has matured.

Nelson (1988, 1997) introduced the terms *occupational form*, "the preexisting structure that elicits, guides, or structures subsequent human performance," and *occupational performance*, "the human actions taken in response to an occupational form" (1988, p. 633). This distinction separates individuals and their actual doing of occupations from the general notion of an occupation and what it requires of anyone who does it.

Yerxa et al. (1989) defined occupation as "specific 'chunks' of activity within the ongoing stream of human behavior which are named in the lexicon of the culture. . . . These daily pursuits are self-initiated, goal-directed (purposeful), and socially sanctioned" (p. 5). Yerxa (1993) further elaborated this definition to incorporate an environmental perspective and a greater breadth of characteristics. "Occupations are units of activity which are classified and named by the culture according to the purposes they serve in enabling people to meet environmental challenges successfully. . . . Some essential characteristics of occupation are that it is self-initiated, goal directed (even if the goal is fun or pleasure), experiential as well as behavioral, socially valued or recognized, constituted of adaptive skills or repertoires, organized, essential to the quality of life experienced, and possesses the capacity to influence health" (p. 5).

According to the Canadian Association of Occupational Therapists (as cited in Law, Steinwender, & Leclair, 1998), occupation is "groups of activities and tasks of everyday life, named, organized and given value and meaning by individuals and a culture. Occupation is everything people do to occupy themselves, including looking after themselves (self-care), enjoying life (leisure), and contributing to the social and economic fabric of their communities (productivity)" (p. 83). More recently, occupational scientists Larson, Wood, and Clark (2003) provided a simple definition of occupation as "the activities that comprise our life experience and can be named in the culture" (p. 16).

The previous definitions of occupation from occupational therapy literature help in explaining why occupation is the profession's focus (particularly in the context of therapy), yet they are open enough to allow continuing research on the nature of occupation. Despite, and perhaps because of, the ubiquity of occupation in human life, there is still much to learn about the nature of occupation through systematic research using an array of methodologies (Hocking, 2000; Molke, Laliberte-Rudman, & Polatajko, 2004). Such research should include examination of the premises that are built into the accepted definitions of occupation.

CONTEXT AND OCCUPATION

The photograph of the two young boys playing in the garden sprinkler evokes a sense of a hot summer day and the experience of icy cold water coming out of the sprinkler, striking and stinging the boys' faces and tongues (Figure 2.2). Playing in the sprinkler has a context with temporal elements (summer, the play of children, and the viewer's memories of doing it in the past), a physical environment (grass, hot weather, hose, sprinkler, cold water), and a social environment (a pair of children and the likelihood of an indulgent parent). Playing in the sprinkler cannot be described or understood—or even happen—without its context. It is difficult to imagine that either boy would enjoy the activity as much doing it alone; the social context is part of the experience. A sprinkler might be set up for play on an asphalt driveway but not in a living room. Parents would be unlikely to allow their children to get soaking wet in cold weather. The contexts of the people viewing the picture are important too; many will relate the picture to their own past experiences, but someone who lives in a place where lawn sprinklers are never used might find the picture meaningless and/or confusing. This example illustrates how occupation and context are enmeshed with one another.

It is generally accepted that the specific *meaning* of an occupation is fully known only to the individual engaged

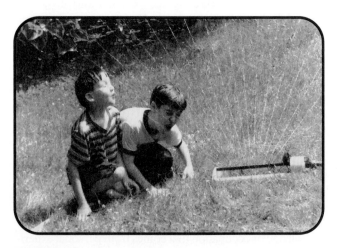

FIGURE 2.2 Two boys on a hot summer day.

in the occupation (Larson, Wood, & Clark, 2003; Pierce, 2001; Weinblatt, Ziv, & Avrech-Bar, 2000). But it is also well accepted that occupations take place in *context* (sometimes referred to as the environment) (e.g., Baum & Christiansen, 2005; Kielhofner, 2002; Law, Cooper et al., 1996; Schkade & Schultz, 2003; Yerxa et al., 1989) and thus have dimensions that consider other humans (in both social and cultural ways), temporality, the physical environment, and even virtual environments (American Occupational Therapy Association, 2002).

Description of occupation as taking place *in* or *with* the environment or context implies a separation of person and context that is problematic. In reality, person, occupation, and context are inseparable. Context is changeable but always present. Cutchin (2004) offered a critique of occupational therapy theories of adaptation-to-environment that separate person from environment, and proposed that John Dewey's view of human experience as "always situated and contextualized" (p. 305) was a more useful perspective. According to Cutchin, "situations are always inclusive of us, and us of them" (p. 305). Occupation occurs at the level of the situation and thus is inclusive of the individual and context (Dickie, Cutchin, & Humphry, 2006). Occupational therapy interventions cannot be context free. Even when an occupational therapy practitioner is working with individuals, the contexts of other people, the culture of therapist and client, the physical space, and past experiences are present.

IS OCCUPATION ALWAYS GOOD?

In occupational therapy, occupation is associated with health and well-being, both as a means and as an end. But occupation can also be unhealthy, dangerous, maladaptive, or destructive to self or others and can contribute to societal problems and environmental degradation. For example, the seemingly benign act of using a car to get to work, run errands, and pursue other occupations can limit one's physical activity and risk injury to self and others. Furthermore, Americans' reliance on the automobile contributes to urban sprawl, the decline of neighborhoods, air pollution, and over use of nonrenewable natural resources.

Personal and societal occupational choices have consequences, good and bad. In coming to understand occupation, we need to acknowledge the breadth of occupational choices and their effects on individuals and the world itself.

ORGANIZING OCCUPATION

Categorization of occupations (for example, into areas of activities of daily living, work, and leisure) is often problematic. Attempts to define work and leisure demonstrate that distinctions between the two are not always

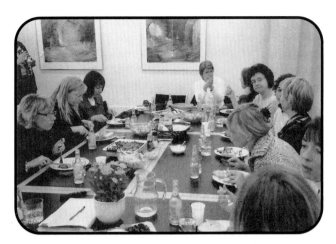

FIGURE 2.3   A complex social occupation.

clear (Csikszentmihalyi & LeFevre, 1989; Primeau, 1996). Work may be defined as something people *have* to do, an unpleasant necessity of life, but many people enjoy their work and describe it as "fun." Indeed, Hochschild (1997) discovered that employees in the work setting she studied often preferred the homelike qualities of work to being in their actual homes and consequently spent more time at work than was necessary. The concept of leisure is problematic as well. Leisure might involve activities that are experienced as hard work, such as helping a friend to build a deck on a weekend.

Similar problems can be described with any categorization scheme. The photograph of the women around a table illustrates the difficulty in applying categories to a real situation (Figure 2.3). Some individuals are eating, so perhaps they are engaged in an activity of daily living. Others are talking or listening, so their occupation might be social participation. The tables pushed together and the folder and pen suggest that the meal might be a meeting of some sort, so perhaps this eating is work. Notice the hand positions of the women eating; the European style of eating with fork in left hand and knife in right used by some (but not all) could be a clue that this meal involves international travel. Does this make it a leisure occupation? No simple designation of what is happening in the picture will suffice.

Another problem with categories is that an individual may experience an occupation as something entirely different from what it appears to be to others. Weinblatt, Ziv, & Avrech-Bar (2000) described how an elderly woman used the supermarket for purposes quite different from provisioning (which would likely be called an instrumental activity of daily living). Instead, this woman used her time in the store as a source of new knowledge and interesting information about modern life. What should we call her occupation in this instance?

The construct of occupation might very well defy efforts to reduce it to a single definition or a set of categories.

Just as the photograph of the women eating illustrates the pitfalls of trying to fit occupations into a single category, examples of occupations can be found that challenge other theoretical approaches and definitions. Nevertheless, the richness and complexity of occupation will continue to challenge occupational therapists to know and value it through personal experience, observations, and scholarly work. The practice of occupational therapy depends on this knowledge.

PROVOCATIVE QUESTIONS

1. Why should a national health care system (however that system is organized) be concerned about occupation and support occupational therapy services? Construct an argument that focuses on occupation.

2. Is it of major importance for the profession of occupational therapy to use a single definition of occupation? Defend your answer.

REFERENCES

Aarts, J., & Dijksterhuis, A. (2000). Habits as knowledge structures: Automaticity in goal-directed behavior. *Journal of Personality and Social Psychology, 78,* 53–63.

American Occupational Therapy Association. (2002). Occupational therapy practice framework: Domain and process. *American Journal of Occupational Therapy, 56,* 609–639.

Bargh, J., & Chartrand, T. (1999). The unbearable automaticity of being. *American Psychologist, 54,* 462–479.

Baum, C., & Christiansen, C. (2005). Person-environment-occupation-performance: An occupation-based framework for practice. In C. Christiansen & C. Baum (Eds.), *Occupational therapy: Performance, participation, and well-being* (pp. 243–266). Thorofare, NJ: SLACK.

Breines, E. (1995). Understanding "occupation" as the founders did. *British Journal of Occupational Therapy, 59,* 458–460.

Clark, F. (1997). Reflections on the human as an occupational being: Biological need, tempo and temporality. *Journal of Occupational Science: Australia, 4,* 86–92.

Csikszentmihalyi, M., & LeFevre, J. (1989). Optimal experience in work and leisure. *Journal of Personality and Social Psychology, 56,* 815–822.

Cutchin, M. (2004). Using Deweyan philosophy to rename and reframe adaptation-to-environment. *American Journal of Occupational Therapy, 58,* 303–312.

Dickie, V., Cutchin, M., & Humphry, R. (2006). Occupation as transactional experience: A critique of individualism in occupational science. *Journal of Occupational Science, 13,* 83–93.

Dissanayake, E. (1992). *Homo aestheticus: Where does art come from and why.* Seattle: University of Washington Press.

Dissanayake, E. (1995). The pleasure and meaning of making. *American Craft, 55* (April/May), 40–45.

Downey, G. (1988). *The machine in me.* New York: Routledge.

Hinojosa, J., Kramer, P., Royeen, C., & Luebben, A. (2003). Core concept of occupation. In P. Kramer, J. Hinojosa, & C. Royeen (Eds.), *Perspectives in human occupation: Participation in life* (pp. 1–17). Philadelphia: Lippincott Williams & Wilkins.

Hochschild, A. (1997) *The time bind: When work becomes home and home becomes work.* New York: Metropolitan Books.

Hocking, C. (2000). Occupational science: A stock take of accumulated insights. *Journal of Occupational Science, 7,* 58–67.

Hocking, C., Wright-St. Clair, V., & Bunrayong, W. (2002). The meaning of cooking and recipe work for older Thai and New Zealand women. *Journal of Occupational Science, 9,* 117–127.

Kielhofner, G. (1997). *Conceptual foundations of occupational therapy.* Philadelphia: F. A. Davis.

Kielhofner, G. (2002). *Model of human occupation: Theory and application* (3rd ed.). Philadelphia: Lippincott Williams & Wilkins.

Kielhofner, G., & Burke, J. (1977). Occupational therapy after 60 years: An account of changing identity and knowledge. *American Journal of Occupational Therapy, 31,* 675–689.

Krishnagiri, S. (2000). Occupations and their dimensions. In J. Hinojosa & M. Blount (Eds.), *The texture of life: Purposeful activities in occupational therapy* (pp. 35–50). Bethesda, MD: American Occupational Therapy Association.

Larson, E., Wood, W., & Clark, F. (2003). Occupational science: Building the science and practice of occupation through an academic discipline. In E. B. Crepeau, E. S. Cohn, & B. A. B. Schell (Eds.), *Willard & Spackman's occupational therapy* (10th ed., pp. 15–26). Philadelphia: Lippincott Williams & Wilkins.

Law, M., Cooper, B., Strong, S., Stewart, D., Rigby, P., & Letts, L. (1996). The person-environment-occupation model: A transactive approach to occupational performance. *Canadian Journal of Occupational Therapy, 63,* 9–23.

Law, M., Steinwender, S., & Leclair, L (1998). Occupation, health and well-being. *Canadian Journal of Occupational Therapy, 65,* 81–91.

Meyer, A. (1922/1977). The philosophy of occupational therapy. *American Journal of Occupational Therapy, 31,* 639–642.

Molineux, M. (2004). Occupation in occupational therapy: A labour in vain? In M. Molineux (Ed.), *Occupation for occupational therapists* (pp. 1–14). Oxford, UK: Blackwell.

Molke, D., Laliberte-Rudman, D., & Polatajko, H. (2004). The promise of occupational science: A developmental assessment of an emerging academic discipline. *Canadian Journal of Occupational Therapy, 71,* 269–281.

Nelson, D. (1988). Occupation: Form and performance. *American Journal of Occupational Therapy, 42,* 633–641.

Nelson, D. (1997). Why the profession of occupational therapy will flourish in the 21st century. The 1996 Eleanor Clarke Slagle Lecture. *American Journal of Occupational Therapy, 51,* 11–24.

Orr, J. (1996). *Talking about machines.* Ithaca, NY: Cornell University Press.

Pierce, D. (2001). Untangling occupation and activity. *American Journal of Occupational Therapy, 55,* 138–146.

Primeau, L. (1996). Work and leisure: Transcending the dichotomy. *American Journal of Occupational Therapy, 50,* 569–577.

Reilly, M. (1962). Occupational therapy can be one of the great ideas of 20th century medicine. *American Journal of Occupational Therapy, 16,* 1–9.

Schkade, J., & Schultz, S. (2003). Occupational adaptation. In P. Kramer, J. Hinojosa, & C. Royeen (Eds.), *Perspectives in human occupation: Participation in life* (pp. 181–221). Philadelphia: Lippincott Williams & Wilkins.

Schouten, J., & McAlexander, J. (1995). Subcultures of consumption: An ethnography of the new bikers. *Journal of Consumer Research, 22,* 43–61.

Schwartz, K. (2003). History of occupation. In P. Kramer, J. Hinojosa, & C. Royeen (Eds.), *Perspectives in human occupation: Participation in life* (pp. 18–31). Philadelphia: Lippincott Williams & Wilkins.

Sherry, J., & McGrath, M. (1989). Unpacking the holiday presence: A comparative ethnography of two gift stores. In E. Hirschmann (Ed.), *Interpretative consumer research.* Provo, UT: Association for Consumer Research.

Townsend, E. (1997). Occupation: Potential for personal and social transformation. *Journal of Occupational Science: Australia, 4,* 18–26.

Weinblatt, N., Ziv, N., & Avrech-Bar, M. (2000). The old lady from the supermarket—Categorization of occupation according to performance areas: Is it relevant for the elderly. *Journal of Occupational Science, 7,* 73–79.

Wilcock, A. (1998). *An occupational perspective of health.* Thorofare, NJ: SLACK.

Wood, W. (1998). Biological requirements for occupation in primates: An exploratory study and theoretical synthesis. *Journal of Occupational Science, 5,* 68–81.

Wood, W., Quinn, J., & Kashy, D. (2002). Habits in everyday life: Thought, emotion, and action. *Journal of Personality and Social Psychology, 83,* 1281–1297.

Yerxa, E. (1993). Occupational science: A new source of power for participants in occupational therapy. *Journal of Occupational Science: Australia, 1,* 3–9.

Yerxa, E., Clark, F., Frank, G., Jackson, J., Parham, D., Pierce, D., Stein, C., & Zemke, R. (1989). An introduction to occupational science, a foundation for occupational therapy in the 21st century. In J. Johnson & E. Yerxa (Eds.), *Occupational science: The foundation for new models of practice* (pp. 1–17). New York: Haworth Press.

Occupation and Development: A Contextual Perspective

3

RUTH HUMPHRY

Learning Objectives

After reading this chapter, you will be able to:

1. Reflectively explore the origins and nature of your own knowledge about children, development, and what children of certain ages like to do.
2. Explain the societal nature of everyday activities of children and culture made for children.
3. Engage in analysis of children's interpersonal interactions during a shared occupation and describe the forces that influence the acquisition of and transformation in occupations.
4. Describe how children's experiences of meaning and purpose shape occupational engagement and serve as change mechanisms.
5. Recognize the complex transactions of children with their environments as functional systems.

INTRODUCTION AND DEFINITIONS

As you have learned, the construct of *occupation* has defied definition and categorization (see Chapter 2). This applies as well to children's occupations. The general idea that occupations are the everyday activities and special events named by the culture captures an adult-centered definition (Spitzer, 2003). What about the idiosyncratic activities that children find to be interesting ways to spend their time, such as walking on a seesaw (Figure 3.1) or jumping on a bed (Figure 3.2). These "invented occupations" might be accepted in special situations, such as at grandmother's home, but are not typically encouraged. Here, *occupations* are defined as coherent patterns of action that emerge through transactions between the child and environment and are things the child wants to do or is expected to do (Humphry, 2002; Spitzer, 2003). The environment is composed of people, materials, time, and

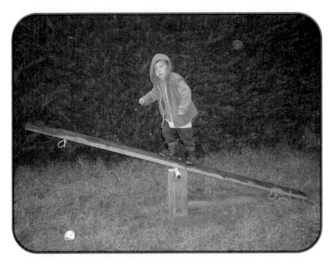

FIGURE 3.1 Walking on the seesaw is a child's "invented occupation" that is not typically encouraged.

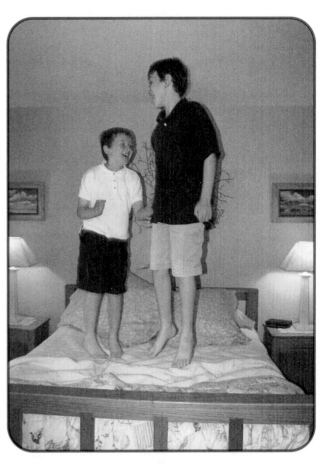

FIGURE 3.2 Jumping on the bed is another "invented occupation" that might be tolerated by a relative and not permitted by the parents.

space that have meaning relative to children's potential occupations. Thus, children's occupational performance emerges from both their capacities to act and their interpretations of these meanings. Reasons for engaging in occupations can be the child's interest as well as to achieve an outcome. Or children may engage in occupations because other people create situations that make engagement meaningful. The definition of *occupation* is broad to include children's exploration and play behaviors that have no other names. However, these child- and situation-specific occupations do not reflect broader **cultural practices**, a community's routine way of doing things and common appreciation of an occupation's importance (Gallimore & Lopez, 2001; Miller & Goodnow, 1995; Rogoff, 2003). Cultural practices are seen in more conventional occupations, such as playing tea party (Figure 3.3). This chapter focuses on the development of conventional occupations, those expected of children by their communities, but I encourage you to consider the role unconventional occupations have in children's well-being.

WHAT IS DEVELOPING AND WHAT IS DEVELOPMENT?

By engaging in occupations, children meet their current interests and needs while also learning from their environments, mastering skills and ways of behaving they will need when they are older. When children are at risk for not doing the valued and expected occupations or do not perform to their own or others' satisfaction, occupational therapy practitioners work with families, teachers, and other team members to advance the children's performance in conventional occupations. Critical to successful practice with children is the way in which occupational therapy practitioners conceptualize development and the change

process. These ideas are organized into different models of practice that lead to alternative forms of service. This chapter explores different ways of thinking about development, contrasting assumptions about what determines the things children do, and the forces that transform their occupations. I suggest that a way of framing the issues is

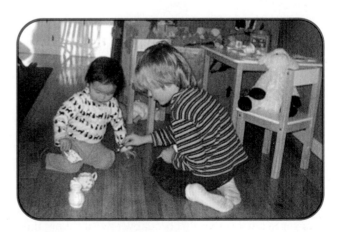

FIGURE 3.3 Playing tea party is a conventional occupation for children.

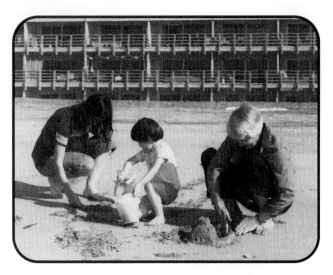

FIGURE 3.4   Building sandcastles is an intergenerational occupation for this grandmother, her daughter, and her granddaughter.

to shift the focus from development of an individual's performance capacities to development of occupations in a social context.

Before discussing the change process, it is important to think about what it means to develop an occupation. To explore what this entails, consider Figure 3.4, in which a grandmother, her adult daughter, and her preschool-age granddaughter are making sandcastles. The grandmother learned the practice of making sandcastles as a way of being at the beach from her parents, and she shared it with her children. Thus, though it is new for this preschooler, the occupation of making sandcastles on the beach has roots that cross generations. Development of an occupation builds on a framework of other people's experiences.

Though the picture captures a moment in time, the reader can imagine that making a sandcastle with a child unfolds as a communal project with an uncertain outcome. However, the grandmother and the adult daughter share an unspoken appreciation of the essential characteristics that define a sandcastle, procedural knowledge, and a sense of why it is meaningful to build one. To varying degrees, these ideas are shared by other people who have made sandcastles. Cultural practices then organize and coordinate the adults' actions, their tool use, and how they guide the preschooler's participation in making sandcastles. The preschooler, without explicit teaching by her mother or grandmother, comes to share their ideas about sandcastles, the options for actions offered by toy shovels and buckets, and what is significant about making sandcastles at the beach. Development of an occupation then is part of an unfolding social situation and mastery of cultural practices.

Finally, development captures both continuity and changes in occupations that occur over two different time spans. In the context of working beside two other sandcastle makers, the girl modifies her performance to enact

her evolving understanding of the occupation. Within the time frame of a day at the beach, the preschooler's knowledge and performance undergo transformations that can be described as learning. Over months and years, she will make sandcastles with other people and on her own, and these cumulative experiences will further inform her understanding of making sandcastles and her experiences of what is significant about building them, and she will eventually create intricately designed and innovative structures. Development of occupation reflects changes in knowledge, meaning, and performance over these longer periods of time during which the girl comes to identify herself as an experienced sandcastle maker with a particular style of her own. Though different in the time frames, learning is connected to developmental change with many of the same origins, so learning can be thought of as microdevelopment (Granott & Parziale, 2002; Siegler, 2000).

The developmental mechanisms that need to be understood are those forces that initially lead to doing an occupation and how microdevelopment transforms how it is done and experienced. For centuries, generations of children have learned to do the valued occupations of their communities. The reader might wonder whether this knowledge is not already available; after all, parents, teachers, older siblings, and coaches help children learn to do their occupations all the time. But not all children have parents or teachers who can help them to master occupations. There may also be special circumstances that prevent children from developing the occupations needed for participation. So what should an occupational therapy practitioner know?

Our knowledge about children and what they do at certain ages arises from different sources. First, there are "commonsense" ideas that are generated by adults who care for and work with children. People make observations and talk among themselves about children's age-related behaviors and their changing occupations. In essence, people construct a set of ideas about childhood occupations. Because everyone in that community sees children and their occupations in a similar manner, commonsense knowledge is accepted as fact. Another source of knowledge about children and their occupations is anecdotal testimony of experienced people viewed as having authoritative knowledge. Individuals who have years of experience with many children may be viewed as having dependable knowledge. In occupational therapy, master clinicians frequently offer anecdotal information to new clinicians as they serve as clinical supervisors or give workshops based on their practice experiences. But can these forms of knowledge be applied more broadly than the situations in which they are formed?

Commonsense knowledge and anecdotal information are socially constructed, shaped by how a society views children at that time in history. This means that ideas about children and what they do change over time (Davis, Polatajko, & Ruud, 2002). These belief systems vary between communities, so children may engage in very different occupations (Larson & Verma, 1999; LeVine et al., 1994). For example, some societies believe that play has little importance for children's future, and 6-year olds are considered responsible enough to tend to livestock or care for a younger sibling (Rogoff, 2003). In the United States, 6-year-olds are seen as immature, and parents encourage their play as a way to learn skills. Diverse ideas such as these are so readily accepted locally that they are not held up to scientific critique. In an era in which professionals are expected to offer services based on evidence, occupational therapy guided only by common sense or anecdotal information is inadequate.

In an effort to have informed practice, occupational therapy has turned to the literature about children generated by researchers in other disciplines. Developmental theories of psychologists are seen as useful to occupational therapy, and students are encouraged to learn them (Edwards & Christiansen, 2005; Law, Missiuna, Pollock, & Stewart, 2005). The profession needs to consider several issues, however. First, much of the work has been carried out in North America and Europe, which limits generalization to other cultures. Second, scientists who study children come with questions based on the interests of their disciplines. Developmental psychology tends to emphasize the individual, and the theories are devised to explain changing psychological functions. Third, these classic theoretical models are dated and not considered by psychologists to be cutting-edge science (Lerner, 2002).

TWO PERSPECTIVES IMPORTED FROM DEVELOPMENTAL PSYCHOLOGY

Service providers, parents, and scientists start with different philosophical worldviews about how things work, which in turn shape the body of knowledge they use to explain what changes children's behaviors (Lerner, 2002; Meacham, 2004; Super & Harkness, 2003). Sometimes, change is explained as a product of forces in the environment. Other authors take a biological view of the child, explaining development as the result of a genetically driven program to become more mature. Both perspectives on how development works appear in psychology and occupational therapy literature.

Originally expressed in an almost mechanical, cause-and-effect perspective, learning theory focused on the power of positive or negative rewards in shaping the behaviors of animals and children (Lerner, 2002; Skinner, 1971). Bandura (1978) expanded on the social nature of learning and how self-directed behavior occurs as children strive to achieve observed outcomes. Royeen and Duncan (1999) noted that a behavioral perspective is not often identified in the occupational therapy literature but is frequently implied. In writing about a skill acquisition approach, these authors suggest that practitioners create environmental

supports and positive feedback to help children learn skills or subskills of targeted occupations. A developmental approach adds an understanding of the hierarchy from immature to more mature skills and uses positive encouragement so that the child practices the youngest skill level or occupational performance the child is not able to do (Hinojosa & Kramer, 1999). The form and frequency of feedback about performance are not stressed; rather, the body of knowledge emphasizes the sequence of changing behaviors. Lists of typical age-related milestones in play and self-care domains and the associated fine motor, gross motor, cognitive, and social skills are available (e.g., Case-Smith, 2005). Basing services on typical development, however, overlooks the reality that children with special needs may have their own unique ways of doing things. In addition, conceptualizing development as following a continuum and practicing the most immature form that the child cannot do might be developmentally appropriate, but it might not be age appropriate, leaving the child open to stigmatization.

In contrast, other developmental theorists have described the forces for systematic change as the result of an innate drive or a self-regulating program within the child. What generates this intrinsic drive to achieve an individual's potential has been a source of speculation among psychologists. Classic theorists in developmental psychology have alluded to an intrinsic need for psychosocial adjustment, knowledge, or mastery (Erikson, 1982; Piaget, 1952; White, 1959). In occupational therapy, a child's drive to engage in occupation is seen as the medium through which the child brings about development of his or her own abilities to do occupations (Primeau & Ferguson, 1999). When children have occupational performance difficulties, practitioners are encouraged to work for an optimal match between person, task, and environment. This may include remediation of underlying performance components using neurodevelopmental approaches. Instead of occupation, the focus then became one of using therapeutic activities to change the organization of the nervous system and develop ability (Law et al., 2005). However, therapeutic activities that are created for sensory or motor experiences lack contextual meaning that arises from the child's natural environment; thus, they are contrived rather than being children's true occupations (Fisher, 1998).

Without evidence that either a developmental skills approach or neurodevelopmental interventions are effective (Mahoney, Robinson & Fewell, 2001), occupational therapy practitioners have adopted eclectic practices. For example, Case-Smith (2000) describes preparatory therapeutic activities drawing on a sensory integration approach and then graded motor practice to build fine motor skills using playful interactions to reinforce the child's efforts in challenging occupations Other authors suggest that young children's development may be explained by experiences that somehow trigger biological growth of their capacities but that development of school-age children is explained

TABLE 3.1   PROPOSED MECHANISMS BRINGING ABOUT CHANGE IN OCCUPATIONS

Broad Categories	Proposed Change Mechanisms in Development of an Occupation
Societal investment in children's occupations	Communities invest in childhood occupations and express normative expectations that children at particular ages participate in these occupations. People in the community hold socially designated roles with responsibility for orchestrating children's time and supporting valued occupations.
Interpersonal influences on occupational engagement	Vicarious learning from familiar people engaged in their occupations informs children about occupation. As active onlookers, children learn about possible outcomes and what is significant in occupations. During shared occupation performance demands are distributed between participants and children learn new information about the outcomes and meanings of the occupation. Explicit teaching and scaffolding of the occupation brings the child's performance to a higher level. The more experienced partner introduces more culturally influenced ideas about outcome and meaning.
The dynamics of doing an occupation	Challenges to familiar ways of doing things lead children to try to new combinations of their capacities, contributing to discovery of new performance strategies. Gradually, children learn to select performance strategies to fit particular situations. Altered experiences of outcome and significance of the occupation leads the child to find new performance strategies. Performance and capacities are interrelated with reciprocal influences from multiple levels of change. In this way, experiences in occupation furthers development at multiple levels, which is then available so that the child's performance in the occupation reflects the practices of the community.

by forces in their environments (Cronin, 2005). If this were the case, then neurodevelopmental approaches would be appropriate for infants and preschoolers but not for school-age children. In summary, the strategy of adopting developmental psychology's theories about children has not generated a coherent body of knowledge that focuses on development of occupations.

A THIRD PERSPECTIVE ON THE DEVELOPMENTAL PROCESS

Recall the example at the beginning of the chapter, in which a preschooler learns from her mother and grandmother to make sandcastles. This and other conventional occupations are socially constructed, determined by children's cultures. Thus, the body of knowledge that informs occupational therapy cannot be just about development of capacities of individual children. Our understanding needs to be contextual, seeing the person-situation as a functional whole system (Dickie, Cutchin, & Humphry, 2006). From this perspective, occupation is the way in which a person engages with the environment. Research on people's occupations and theories of development that grew out of the ideas of Russian psychologists such as Vygotsky and Luria and the writing of the pragmatist philosopher Dewey

(e.g., Engestrom, Miettinen, & Punamaki, 1999; Gallimore & Lopez, 2002, Goncu, 1999; Rogoff, 2003) contributed to the ideas presented below.

I asked what constitutes an appropriate model to guide occupation-centered practice with children and engaged in a series of two observational studies of children in child-care situations to find out how children learn to do the things that they do. A different way of thinking is outlined below, with examples drawn from my observations (using pseudonyms). First, I studied typically developing infants in a child-care classroom. Then I observed preschoolers with special needs and their classmates who showed typical development. I watched while children in both groups learned cultural practices such as "Ring Around the Rosie" and do songs with associated gestures or movements. These occupations became classroom routines and a way in which children connected with each other (McNamara & Humphry, in press).

Developmental mechanisms identified in this chapter are forces that act synergistically to bring about engagement in an occupation and transform how it is done and experienced (Humphry, 2005). These changes occur on a micro-developmental time scale, and gradually, over months and years, the occupations develop. For the reader's ease in tracking major concepts, the mechanisms are listed in Table 3.1, organized into three broad categories.

Societal Resources Bringing About Development of Childhood Occupations

By moving the focus away from development of the individual to development of occupation, it is easier to see sociocultural features in everyday occupations and how these are part of the developmental process. Ann Wilcock (1998) argues for the concurrent evolution of *Homo sapiens'* occupational and cultural nature so that as groups of people worked collaboratively, their shared goals, values and standards created cultural practices. Singing to or sharing music with children reflects a cultural practice that takes many forms around the world and occurs regularly in the United States (Custodero, Britto, & Brooks-Gunn, 2003). The societal investment in children's occupations is reflected by creation of things for children to do and manufactured objects for their occupations (Mouritsen, 2002). In the infants' class, there were toy radios adapted to the developmental abilities of young children. The preschool had child-sized musical instruments. Songs written for children, such as "The Wheels on the Bus," were a regular part of the preschoolers' circle time.

Another societal investment in children's occupations is the commitment of human resources. Every community has people who hold socially designated roles to oversee children's engagement in occupations that are valued and expected of children. Rogoff, Paradise, Arauz, Correa-Chavez, and Angelillo (2003) observed that when children are not routinely brought into the adult occupations of their communities, special child-focused occupations are created for them. In the United States, parents manage the space at home, offer child-focused occupations, and serve as play partners (Pierce & Marshall, 2004; Rogoff et al., 2003). In the classrooms, the lead teachers in each classroom had degrees in early childhood education and took charge of organizing classroom routines on the basis of their educational objectives. For the preschoolers, doing songs was designated as part of "circle time," while music was less formal for the infants; their teacher sat with a couple of children and engaged them in songs.

In occupational therapy, understanding the societal influences on development of occupation is informative. Part of the commonsense information that is shared in a community is what children like to do at different ages. These occupations carry **normative expectations**, through which a community shares the understanding that by a certain age, children will behave in a particular way. So parents and educators may refer children for services if children are not participating in expected occupations. Also, children are rarely part of just one community, so the cultural practices and normative expectations of their families and those of the child-care centers and educational programs can be different. The occupational therapy practitioner will want to hear about the occupations that are expected in different situations.

Interpersonal Influences on Occupational Engagement

Before moving into the interpersonal processes, I first consider children's experiences of occupation. Children's behaviors in doing different occupations are organized into intentional efforts in order to experience effects that are significant to them or to achieve the outcomes that they have in mind (Humphry, 2002; Spitzer, 2003). Infants who were a year old had ideas about specific occupations and asked adults to do something in particular. For example, Helen approached a visitor, carrying a book on the ABCs. She handed the book to the visitor and sat beside the woman, who obliged by reading the first pages. However, Helen stood, took back the book, and gave it to her teacher, who sang the ABCs. Helen seemed satisfied and sat through the song, looking at the pictures. In essence, the book was Helen's way of naming what she wanted to do. When her communicative act failed to elicit the expected routine from the visitor, Helen sought out a more informed companion for her occupation. The example illustrates young children's awareness of occupations as distinct, with unique significance and expected outcomes. This section addresses how children build this understanding in the context of their everyday lives.

As was seen in the earlier example of learning to build a sandcastle, interpersonal connections in a social situation with familiar people are critical to the development of occupations. Occupational therapy practitioners seek indicators of learning about occupations and capitalize on these processes in working with children who are at risk for delays (Humphry & Wakeford, 2006). The social milieu created by people who are engaged in a variety of occupations forms a powerful interpersonal change mechanism. The act of watching supports vicarious participation in occupations before young children actually do things. Children, anticipating that they will one day do particular occupations, watch other people do things with a higher degree of intensity (Rogoff et al., 2003). In this context, children acquire information about how to do the occupation and what constitutes satisfactory performance. They also develop ideas about the outcomes and gain a sense about the occupation's significance. Children, in onlooker roles, are active participants, learning about an occupation well before they engage in it.

There is controversy over children's abilities to interpret what other people do as intentional (Reddy & Morris, 2004). One group of developmental psychologists suggests that before children interpret other people's actions as intentional, they need to have the mental appreciation that another person's actions are guided by that person's mind ("theory of mind"). An alternative, more contextual argument is that young children are not separated from familiar people who are engaged in their occupations. Children do not need abstract concepts such as how other people's actions are guided by thoughts before understanding another's acts as purposeful; rather, children are sensitive to the organized, focused flow of people through their emotional engagement (Reddy & Morris, 2004). There may be a physiological basis for this assertion. Recent work on so-called mirror neurons supports the possibility of vicarious participation, even among other primates. Rizzolatti, Fogassi, and Gallese (2006) explained that they found, in nonhuman primates and human volunteers, a subset of neurons that respond, by becoming active, to observations of a researcher moving to pick up food. The pattern of activation was the same as it would have been if the nonhuman primate or person was himself or herself reaching for food. In other words, the observers were mentally sharing the experience of moving in a functional manner. These scientists argue that through the activation of mirror neurons, a person has firsthand experiences of another person's act, intention, and emotions. Though further research is needed, it could explain how children are able to learn about how to do occupations by watching.

For example, one of the preschoolers, Joshua, was physically and intellectually challenged and was unable to stand unaided because of his fluctuating muscle tone. He frequently participated in circle time while positioned in a stander, so he was unable to move his legs. He could and did join his classmates by raising his arms in the part of the "The Ants Go Marching" song about the ants climbing out of the ground and watched as they marched to other parts of the song. Joshua demonstrated that he had not been a passive onlooker when one of the classroom aides helped him to join the group by holding him under his arms in supported standing. He grinned and stepped at the time in the song when the ants were marching. Both the aide and the teacher commented on his glee at doing what he had seen other children do.

In Table 3.1, in the category of interpersonal influences, the second and third proposed change mechanisms have many common features. Children can move back and forth between learning through vicarious engagement and joining in a shared occupation with either a peer or a more experienced partner. There are two ways in which sharing an occupation promotes its development. First, when children do something together, they organize their performance around their shared situation, in essence, cocreating the occupation. In coordinating their actions to sustain their engagement, the performance demands are distributed among participants. Thus, one child may model, point to, or offer hints to support a peer who is having performance problems (Johnson-Pynn & Nisbet, 2002). In this way, performance challenges are shared among participants, contributing to their acquisition of new performance skills. While supporting one another in their occupation, children also introduce variability, challenging each other to invent new ways of doing things.

The second aspect in the interpersonal change mechanism is the progression of a child's sense of the significance and expected outcome in the occupation. A child's ideas about the occupation are part of how the child interprets what is happening, part of his or her "situation definition" (Wertsch, 1999, p. 69). As peers coordinate their actions, individual situation definitions are shared through facial expressions, words, and actions, so as the occupation unfolds, they exchange feelings about meaning and purpose. In this way, participants in an occupation achieve a mutual understanding that is different from their original situation definition. These altered or new experiences of significance and expected outcomes change performance and become part of the child's situation definition the next time the opportunity for that occupation is perceived.

Lawlor (2003) pointed out that at times, the significance of an occupation rests primarily in the sense of being socially engaged. Even when the child might hesitate to do something, the fact that it includes another person might be sufficient to get the child to take up the occupation. This phenomenon, finding meaning in being part of a group, is described as "togetherness" and is thought to be linked to a feeling of belonging (van Oers & Hannikainen, 2001). What is important is that as part of the child's situation definition, even if the child is engaged in the occupation alone the next time, he or she retains a sense of belonging to a larger group defined by the occupation.

For example, in the infant classroom, Anya sat with a toy radio on a mattress. She turned the radio on by pushing a lever, and it played "She'll Be Coming 'Round the Mountain." A younger classmate walked over and sat beside Anya. In sitting, Anya swung her arms and twisted her shoulder to the music. She looked at the classmate, who rocked back and forth at the waist while the music played. They smiled as they looked at each other dancing. Observations of Anya dancing were repeated throughout the study, and I concluded that her situation definition when she used musical toys included belonging to a group of dancers.

One of the commonsense ideas that occupational therapy practitioners may hear is that children have to demonstrate readiness skills before they engage in an occupation. For example, one might argue that before a young child or person with intellectual challenges can understand the meaning and outcomes of a shared occupation, he or she needs communication skills. An alternative is to recognize that in the context of experiencing dancing together, the infants' communicative acts (gestures, rhythmic movements, child-to-child regard, smiling) defined their togetherness as a significant element of dancing to music. Their coordinated interactions are transactional; one child gestured or looked, and the other child interpreted the expression and smiled communicating her experiences to the first child (Budwig, 2003; Reddy & Morris, 2004). Rather than defining abilities as prerequisite to occupation, the occupational therapy practitioner realizes that by shar-

BOX 3.1

How an Experienced Person Can Support a Child's Engagement in a Challenging Occupation

1. Playfully encourage the child to do an activity that otherwise has little meaning.
2. Fill in performance gaps, doing difficult parts of the activity.
3. Suggest different ways to do the activity.
4. Introduce and model the use of new objects in the activity.
5. Add relevant information about the activity.
6. Introduce alternative outcomes.
7. Bring in more culturally shaped meanings regarding why the activity is significant.

ing an occupation, the child enters a situation in which the needed abilities are elicited and practiced.

The power of a shared occupation takes on additional weight as a change mechanism when the other person holds a socially identified role with expectations for explicitly teaching, scaffolding, or guiding children's participation in occupations (Rogoff, 2003; Valsiner, 1997). As adults and children coconstruct an occupation, the adult initially adjusts to the situation definition of the child (Wertsch, 1999). Once the connection of doing the occupation together is established, the adult introduces new definitions of significance and expected outcomes reflecting the cultural practices of the community. Box 3.1 lists ways in which the experienced person contributes to development of occupation.

In my observations, the presence of other people was a central element to the development of occupations, and the teacher sometimes took advantage of group situations. For example, when engaging the toddlers in "Ring Around the Rosie," the teacher called the attention of younger children to the behavior of the older classmate who had learned to squat when the song came to "we all fall down." Peer learning did not always occur, though, when the teacher thought an occupation belonged to an individual. When Joshua was set up with a switch that activated a musical toy, he showed limited interest and did not persist in reaching for the button. When the teacher left, Joshua lost all interest until a classmate used the switch and toy. This refocused Joshua's attention on the music. He watched his classmate push the switch and play music until the teacher returned and told the classmate, "Don't touch this toy, it's for Joshua." Sending his classmate away so that Joshua could practice reaching for the switch interrupted

his learning about the expected outcome of using the switch and the social significance of music.

The Dynamics of Doing

The societal and interpersonal change mechanisms discussed above are integrated with an understanding of the dynamic and contextual nature of occupational performance (Case-Smith, 2005, Humphry, 2002, Kielhofner, 2002). The coherent patterns of action in occupation reflect **emergent performance,** the unique integration of abilities in actions. Different combinations are brought together at that time and in a particular situation. Thus, how something is done is not predetermined, and the combined use of the child's sensorimotor, psychosocial, and cognitive abilities in acting are interdependent, influencing each other. Furthermore, a child's ideas about the occupation and affordances in the environment determine occupational performance (American Occupational Therapy Association, 2002; Law et al., 1996). This stands in contrast to thinking of occupational performance as being determined just by the maturation of particular abilities intrinsic to the child. At one time, the appearance of a new skill, such as picking up a Cheerio between the index finger and thumb or skipping, was thought to reflect the maturation of motor section of the nervous system. However, it is now recognized that performance is influenced simultaneously by a variety of body structures and functions and by various features of the situation (Thelen, 1995). Kevin, for example, knew the lyrics of a song about the ABCs. He sang it while jumping on a trampoline in the preschool classroom. However, his occupational performance, singing, was changed by the context. When the same song was sung as part of circle time, Kevin participated as an onlooker, finding the social situation too demanding for singing. This phenomenon— that occupational performance emerges from the child-environment as a functional system—is the basis for the change mechanisms described below. These changes primarily reflect microdevelopment, subtle shifts in performance strategies that accumulate over time to transform performance, reflecting development of occupation.

Three interlinked change mechanisms occur as a child engages in doing an occupation (see Table 3.1). First, in response to performance challenges, a child recruits and rearranges his or her abilities, using existing abilities in new ways to continue engagement. Challenges arise from new environments, novel objects used in the occupation, or changes in how another person collaborates in doing it (as was suggested above). When a familiar way of doing the occupation fails, the child tries different combinations of capacities. In a trial-and-error process, the child functions sometimes at higher end of his or her performance range (Siegler, 2000). The child learns which new combinations of capacities work and in what conditions, employing more often the strategies that achieve the expected outcome and selecting more accurately what strategy fits a particular situation. In this way, engagement in the occupation leads to more refined performance and builds towards generalization across contexts.

For example, during circle time, the teacher sang the song "Where Is Thumbkin?" and encouraged the children to hold their fists up and extend their thumbs. Ari held up both hands, pointing with his index fingers at the ceiling (a familiar hand movement). The teacher modeled again and said "thumbs up." Ari held up an open hand and watched as he closed his fingers. (He used visual feedback to get his thumbs extended.) The next week, when his teacher announced that the next song was "Thumbkin," Ari seemed to remember what he needed to do. That time, though, he started with his left fist and pried his thumb up with his right hand. However, he could not maintain the left hand fisted when he shifted his effort and tried the same prying procedure with his right hand. That day, he did the song with one hand. With repeated practice of different strategies, Ari eventually used sensory feedback from muscles and joints to maintain his hands in the correct position so that he could do "Thumbkin."

Changes in a child's understanding of the outcome or ideas about significance in doing an occupation also alter performance (Humphry, 2002). As was discussed above, watching other people do things and coconstructing an occupation with others alters the child's situation definition about an occupation. Children can also discover their own new ideas about the outcomes or experience some aspect of the occupation as more interesting than before. Even when an occupation seems to be routine, a new meaning changes how it is done. For example, part of the circle routine was to sing a good morning song, and each verse greeted one of the preschoolers by name. The children sat and clapped their knees as the teacher sang a verse. In time, Molly realized that one verse specifically named her. From then on, instead of clapping her knees when it was her turn to be named, she smiled and shook her head for that verse.

Finally, though maturation of capacities does not completely explain changes in occupational performance, capacities do change with use. In a broad biological sense, development of a child occurs simultaneously at several levels, including genetic activity, body structure, the functions of body systems, capacities, and performance (Gottlieb, 2000). Furthermore, there are reciprocal influences across levels. This means that as children use their capacities, repeated experiences changes these levels and directly or indirectly bring their capacities and performance to higher states of maturity. Subsequently, more mature capacities become available and occupational performance changes. However, the situated and emergent nature of performance in context needs to be remembered. When occupational performance was thought to be a product of the maturity of certain parts of the nervous system, any therapeutic activity that challenged the functional capacity that was thought to be "immature" was believed to lead to further maturation of that part of the brain. This assumption that performance comes from within the child and is uninfluenced by the child's the situation and occupational opportunities led to the developmental skills approach that emphasized components of performance.

For example, Lyle, who was born with Down syndrome, watched his preschool classmates doing songs by clapping, raising their arms or marching. He participated only when adults took his hands in theirs and helped him to clap or do hand gestures. His interest in the occupation but inability to plan and sequence movements efficiently is consistent with his genetic disorder (Fidler, Hepburn, Mankin & Rogers, 2005). Using a developmental skills approach, intervention might include therapeutic activities with repetitive, sequenced acts such as stacking blocks and drawing circles on a chalkboard to remediate Lyle's problems with planning. In light of what we now understand about the emergent and situated nature of performance, the most effective way to draw on developmental mechanisms described here is to help Lyle participate in songs. This could be done by using hand over hand, direct teaching, or slower songs or by giving him time to move and approximate others while doing songs.

CONCLUSION

Occupational therapy is indicated when a child is unable to do conventional occupations such as spending time at the art table, engaging with a parent in bedtime routines, or eating lunch with classmates in the cafeteria. How occupational therapy practitioners conceptualize the change process determines how they practice. This chapter outlines a way of thinking about development that takes a contextual perspective in which occupations are a way of connecting the person with their environments (Dickie et al., 2006). Understanding the developmental process requires knowledge of the circumstances surrounding childhood occupations. Conditions to consider include the origins of the occupation and an appreciation of the child's present situations. For example, children are members of a variety of communities that create different occupational opportunities. Thus, distinctive occupations can be coconstructed and shared with a range of people in different contexts. These ideas are important, since development of occupation occurs because children and their environments form a functional system, something that is understood in its entirety. The forces of change include the societal, interpersonal, and dynamical processes and work synergistically. Application of these ideas has been made to practice with children (Humphry & Wakeford, 2006). Microdevelopment and development occur over the entire life course, and implications of this developmental model for work with people of other ages await further exploration.

PROVOCATIVE QUESTIONS

1. Children in other countries perform differently from children in the United States on standardized assessments that are thought to measure internal capacities such as manual dexterity, balance, and perceptual-motor skills. On the basis of the developmental mechanisms described in this chapter, what explains this finding? What are the implications for children who have special needs?

2. Select one of your childhood occupations (e.g., drawing pictures, soccer, eating dinner with the family). What were societal and interpersonal influences that contributed to development of your occupation?

3. In this chapter, you were encouraged to think about the importance of idiosyncratic occupations that children find to be interesting ways to spend their time. How do these occupations contribute to their well-being? Given the nature of the developmental mechanisms discussed above, would you expect these unconventional occupations to change over time?

REFERENCES

American Occupational Therapy Association. (2002). Occupational therapy practice framework: Domain and process. *American Journal of Occupational Therapy, 56,* 609–639.

Bandura, A. (1978, April). The self system in reciprocal determinism. *American Psychologist, 33,* 344–358.

Budwig, N. (2003). Context and the dynamic construal of meaning in early childhood. In C. Raeff & J. B. Benson (Eds.), *Social and cognitive development in the context of individual, social and cultural processes* (pp. 101–130), New York: Routledge.

Case-Smith, J. (2000). Effects of occupational therapy services on fine motor and functional performance in preschool children. *American Journal of Occupational Therapy, 54,* 372–380.

Case-Smith, J. (2005). Development of childhood occupations. In J. Case-Smith (Ed.), *Occupational therapy for children* (5th ed., pp. 88–116). St. Louis: Elsevier Mosby.

Cronin, A. (2005). Middle childhood and school. In A. Cronin & M. B. Mandich (Eds.), *Human development and performance throughout the lifespan* (pp. 199–216). Clifton Park, NY: Thomson Delmar Learning.

Custodero, L. A., Britto, P. R., & Brooks-Gunn, J. (2003). Musical lives: A collective portrait of American parents and their young children. *Applied Developmental Psychology, 24,* 553–572.

Davis, J. A., Polatajko, H. J., & Ruud, C. A. (2002). Children's occupations in context: The influence of history. *Journal of Occupational Science, 9,* 54–64.

Dickie, V., Cutchin, M. P., & Humphry, R. (2006). Occupation as transactional experience: A critique of individualism in occupational science. *Journal of Occupational Science, 13,* 83–93.

Edwards, D., & Christiansen, C. H. (2005). Occupational development. In C. H. Christiansen, C. M. Baum, & J. Bass-Haugen (Eds.), *Occupational therapy: Performance, participation, and well-being* (3rd ed., pp. 43–63). Thorofare, NJ: Slack.

Engestrom, Y. Miettinen, R., & Punamaki, R. L. (Eds.). (1999). *Perspectives on activity theory.* New York: Cambridge University Press.

Erikson, E. H. (1982). *The life cycle repeated: A review.* New York: Norton.

Fidler, D. J., Hepburn, S. L., Mankin, G., & Rogers, S. J. (2005). Praxis skills in young children with Down syndrome, other developmental disabilities, and typically developing children. *American Journal of Occupational Therapy, 59,* 129–138.

Fisher, A. (1998). The 1998 Eleanor Clarke Slagle lecture: Uniting practice and theory in an occupational framework. *American Journal of Occupational Therapy, 52,* 509–521.

Gallimore, R., & Lopez, E. M. (2002). Everyday routines, human agency, and ecocultural context: Construction and maintenance of individual habits. *Occupational Therapy Journal of Research, 22*(Supplement), 70S–77S.

Goncu, A. (Ed.). (1999). *Children's engagement in the world: Sociocultural perspectives.* Cambridge, UK: Cambridge University Press.

Gottlieb, G. (2000). Understanding genetic activity within a holistic framework. In L. R. Bergman, R. B. Cairns, L. Nilsson, & L. Nystedt (Eds.), *Developmental science and the holistic approach* (pp. 179–201). Mahwah, NJ: Lawrence Erlbaum Associates.

Granott, N., & Parziale, J. (2002). Microdevelopment: A process-oriented perspective for studying development and learning. In N. Granott & J. Parziale (Eds.), *Microdevelopment: Transition processes in development and learning.* New York: Cambridge University Press.

Hinojosa, J., & Kramer, P. (1999). Developmental perspective: Fundamentals of Developmental theory. Acquisition frame of reference. In P. Kramer & J. Hinojosa (Eds.), *Frames of reference for pediatric occupational therapy* (2nd ed., pp. 3–8). Philadelphia: Lippincott Williams & Wilkins.

Humphry, R. (2002). Young children's occupational behaviors: Explicating developmental processes. *American Journal of Occupational Therapy, 56,* 171–179.

Humphry, R. (2005). Model of processes transforming occupations: Exploring societal and social influences. *Journal of Occupational Science, 12,* 36–41.

Humphry, R., & Wakeford, L. (2006). An occupation-centered discussion of development and implications for practice. *American Journal of Occupational Therapy, 60,* 258–268.

Johnson-Pynn, J. S., & Nisbet, V. S. (2002). Preschoolers effectively tutor novice classmates in a block construction task. *Child Study Journal, 32,* 241–255.

Kielhofner, G. (2002). *Model of human occupation: Theory and application* (3rd ed.). Philadelphia: Lippincott Williams & Wilkins.

Larson, R. W., & Verma, S. (1999). How children and adolescents spend time across the world: Work, play, and developmental opportunities. *Psychological Bulletin, 125,* 701–736.

Law, M., Cooper, B., Strong, S., Stewart, D., Rigby, P., & Letts, L. (1996). The person-environment-occupation model: A transactive approach to occupational performance. *Canadian Journal of Occupational Therapy, 63,* 9–23.

Law, M., Missiuna, C., Pollock, N., & Stewart, D. (2005). Foundations for occupational therapy practice with children.

In J. Case-Smith (Ed.), *Occupational therapy for children* (5th ed., pp. 53–87). St. Louis: Elsevier Mosby.

Lawlor, M. (2003). The significance of being occupied: The social construction of childhood occupations. *American Journal of Occupational Therapy, 57,* 424–434.

Lerner, R. M. (2002). *Concepts and theories of human development* (3rd ed.). Mahwah, NJ: Lawrence Erlbaum Associates.

LeVine, R. A., Dixon, S., LeVine, S., Richman, A., Leiderman, P. H., Keefer, C. H., et al. (1994). *Child care and culture: Lessons from Africa.* New York: Cambridge Press.

Mahoney, G., Robinson, D., & Fewell, R. (2001). The effects of early motor intervention on children with Down syndrome or cerebral palsy: A field-base study. *Journal of Developmental and Behavioral Pediatrics, 22,* 153–162.

McNamara, P., & Humphry, R. (in press). Now this is what you do: Developing structured routines. *OTJR Occupation, Participation and Health.* (Supp. 3).

Meacham, J. A. (2004). Action, voice, and identity in children's lives. In P. B. Pufall & R. P. Unsworth (Eds.), *Rethinking childhood* (pp. 69–84). New Brunswick, NJ: Rutgers University Press.

Miller, P. J., & Goodnow, J. J. (1995). Cultural practices: Toward an integration of culture and development. In J. J. Goodnow, P. J. Miller, & F. Kessel (Eds.), *Cultural practices as the contexts for development* (pp. 5–16). San Francisco: Jossey Bass.

Mouritsen, F. (2002). Child culture-play culture. In F. Mouritsen & J. Quortrup (Eds.), *Childhood and children's cultures* (pp. 14–39). Odense: University Press of Southern Denmark.

Piaget, J. (1952). *The origins of intelligence in children.* New York: International Universities Press.

Pierce, D., & Marshall, A. (2004) Maternal management of home space and time to facilitate infant/toddler play and development. In S. A. Esdaile, & J. A. Olson (Eds.), *Mothering occupations: Challenge, agency and participation* (pp. 73–94). Philadelphia: F. A. Davis.

Primeau, L. A., & Ferguson, J. M. (1999). Occupational frame of reference. In P. Kramer & J Hinojosa (Eds.), *Frames of reference for pediatric occupational therapy* (2nd ed., pp. 469–516). Philadelphia: Lippincott Williams & Wilkins.

Reddy, V., & Morris, P. (2004). Participants don't need theories. *Theory and Psychology, 14,* 647–665.

Rizzolatti, G., Fogassi, L., & Gallese, V. (2006, November). Mirrors in the mind. *Scientific American, 295,* 54–61.

Rogoff, B. (2003). *The cultural nature of human development.* New York: Oxford University Press.

Rogoff, B., Paradise, R., Arauz, R. M., Correa-Chavez, M., & Angelillo, C. (2003). Firsthand learning through intent participation. *Annual Review of Psychology, 54,* 175–203.

Royeen, C. B., & Duncan, M. (1999). Acquisition frame of reference. In P. Kramer & J. Hinojosa (Eds.), *Frames of reference for pediatric occupational therapy* (2nd ed., pp. 377–400). Philadelphia: Lippincott Williams & Wilkins.

Siegler, R. S. (2000). The rebirth of children's learning. *Child Development, 71,* 26–35.

Skinner, B. F. (1971). *Beyond freedom and dignity.* New York: Knopf.

Spitzer, S. L. (2003). With and without words: Exploring occupation in relation to young children with autism. *Journal of Occupational Science, 10,* 67–79.

Super C. M., & Harkness S. (2003). The metaphors of development. *Human Development, 46,* 3–23.

Thelen, E. (1995). Motor development: A new synthesis, *American Psychologist, 50*(2), 79–95.

Valsiner, J. (1997). *Culture and the development of children's actions: A theory of human development* (2nd ed.). New York: John Wiley & Sons.

van Oers, B., & Hannikainen, M. (2001). Some thoughts about togetherness: An introduction. *International Journal of Early Years Education, 9,* 101–108.

Wertsch, J. V. (1998). *Mind as action.* New York: Oxford University Press.

Wertsch, J. V. (1999). The zone of proximal development: Some conceptual issues. In P. Lloyd & C. Fernyhough (Eds.), *Lev Vygotsky: Critical assessments* (Vol. III, pp. 67–78). London: Routledge.

White, R. W. (1959). Motivation reconsidered: The concept of competence. *Psychological Review, 66,* 297–333.

Wilcock, A. A. (1998). *An occupational perspective of health.* Thorofare, NJ: Slack.

Understanding Family Perspectives on Illness and Disability Experiences

MARY C. LAWLOR AND CHERYL MATTINGLY

Learning Objectives

After reading and reflecting on this chapter, you will be able to:

1. Discuss ways in which family members experience illness and disability and how these experiences are situated in family life.
2. Recognize the expertise that family members have and bring to health care encounters, including occupational therapy sessions.
3. Understand the health care encounter as a complex social arena in which perceptions and decisions about care are created, contested, and negotiated by multiple social actors.
4. Describe knowledge, skills, and behaviors that facilitate effective "partnering up" and collaboration.

So, what I did is, I became very personal with my therapist. She just wasn't a lady I saw once a week; she was adopted into my family. And I brought my family to therapy with me. I brought children. I brought my grandma (laughs), so that she could be in on what it is that we would be trying to achieve. What it was that we need my daughter to accomplish. I brought children, aunties, uncles, close neighbors—everybody that was a part of my close daily surroundings, went to therapy. And that's just the way it was. So that the therapy was not just once a week, it was seven days a week. It was from the minute we woke up to the minute we went to bed.

The above quote is an excerpt from a transcribed interview with a mother who was telling a story about her daughter's occupational therapy program. It is drawn from an ethnographic research study conducted by the authors and an interdisciplinary research team that will be described in more detail below.[1] This brief passage illustrates the ways in which health care encounters, including occupational therapy, are collaborative efforts that are centrally situated in family life. Health care encounters are not only specific events, but also episodes in the histories of client and family life and, conceivably, also episodes that are embedded in practitioners' lives and institutional cultures. Encounters such as occupational therapy sessions, particularly ones in which significant experiences happen, are events in longer illness and developmental trajectories. Significant moments in therapy sessions may resonate across time to other moments in one's life and across place to the extent that the impact is felt in other contexts, such as life at home, school, or work. In a similar way, salient moments in home and family life may influence health care encounters and the happenings that occur in occupational therapy sessions.

This chapter addresses the need to attend to family perspectives in providing services to people with chronic illnesses or disabilities and the experiences of family members that are related to their participation in occupational therapy services. The **family-centered care** movement, cost containment initiatives, and technological advancements in care delivery have fundamentally altered the expectations of families and practitioners, the nature of health care and caregiving practices, and outcomes of interventions. Health care encounters, once characterized by dyadic communication between a patient and doctor, are now complex social arenas in which multiple social actors, including family members, convene. Health care encounters involving family members are sites of intense **boundary crossing** where families and practitioners create, negotiate, contest, and/or modify perceptions, perspectives, and caregiving and treatment practices. Multiple perspectives on health care events are both anticipated and managed within often relatively brief moments of interaction. Some of the interesting dilemmas and opportunities that emerge when practitioners involve families actively in the therapeutic process are highlighted in this chapter.

We begin by arguing for the need to bring families into the picture in a central way and by discussing the recent movement (largely in pediatrics) toward family-centered care, raising some questions about what this term might mean in practice. We look at why families have been so peripheral in the way in which most health care professions have defined their practice and discuss how involvement of family members in health care fundamentally changes the nature of the encounter. The heart of the chapter moves from these more general considerations to the intricacies, dilemmas, surprises, and riches of therapeutic work that takes seriously the illness and disability experiences of families. Processes related to "partnering up" between practitioners and family members are also examined.

WHY ARE FAMILIES IMPORTANT IN HEALTH CARE?

Common sense tells us that most people who come to occupational therapy live in social worlds that include families of some kind. Even when people live apart from their families, it is very likely that some family members will be instrumental in caregiving in some way. Even in those instances in which no family member is actively involved in care, it is likely that someone from the client's family will be concerned with this care, including the services of the occupational therapy practitioner. Furthermore, the way in which clients experience disability and how it affects their functioning in the world often depend heavily on the clients' relationships with family members and other significant people in their social worlds. This is most obvious in pediatric care when the client is a very young child and in geriatric care when spouses and adult children become involved in care. Families, in various forms and partnership arrangements, tend to matter for most people who experience illness or disability, no matter what the age, ethnicity, socioeconomic status, or geographical location. Not only do families matter, but families shift in response to the issues raised by having a family member with an illness or disability. Roles change. Power relations change. Activities change. The way in which meals are eaten, vacations are taken, disputes are negotiated, beds are made, money is earned, and houses are organized, as well as other aspects of family life, are likely to be affected.

The implementation of federal initiatives related to providing services for children with special health care needs and their families was documented as early as 1912, with the establishment of the Children's Bureau in Maternal and Child Health (Hanft, 1991) and expanded with the implementation of Title V legislation in 1935 (Colman, 1988). The implementation of P.L. 94-142, Part B, an amendment to the Education for the Handicapped Act (EHA) in 1975, and P.L. 99-457, Part H, an amendment to the EHA in 1986, prompted dramatic changes in the nature of service delivery to children in educational and

---

[1]The data that are used in this chapter are drawn from a longitudinal study funded through three sources: *Crossing Cultural Boundaries: An Ethnographic Study* (MCJ Grant # MCJ 060745); *Boundary Crossing: A Longitudinal and Ethnographic Study* (NICHD, NIH, #1 R01 38878); and *Boundary Crossings: Re-Situating Cultural Competence* (NICHD, NIH, #2 R01 38878). Pseudonyms are used to provide greater confidentiality.

early childhood settings (Hanft, 1991; Lawlor, 1991). In 1990, EHA was renamed the Individuals with Disabilities Act (IDEA, P.L. 101-476). Implementation of these services placed new demands on practitioners to reframe traditional medical models of practice to accommodate to the needs of families as well as the child who was referred for services (American Occupational Therapy Association, 1999). In 2004, IDEA was reauthorized, and although much of the language around family participation has changed, many of the earlier principles have been retained. For example, the new statute still incorporates an Individual Family Service Plan as one of the minimum requirements for a statewide system's provision of services for each infant or toddler with a disability and the family of that child (108th Congress, 2004).

Family-Centered Care

Although the development of services that center on the needs and values of families began in early childhood programs through family-centered care initiatives (Hanft, 1991; Lawlor & Mattingly, 1998), many of the principles apply to services for people of all ages (Humphry, Gonzales, & Taylor, 1993). As human service systems moved into the community and family members began providing home care, practitioners developed a deeper appreciation of the centrality of families in healing, recovery, and adaptation. Practitioners also recognized that family members often had different perspectives from those of the professionals about the needs, priorities, and strengths. This recognition led to a shift from perceiving family members as people who will carry out the doctors' and practitioners' orders to perceiving family members as people who are most knowledgeable about the client and who are partners in decision making. Family members' perspectives about how the client is doing, what the client needs, what the family needs, and what is most important and meaningful in everyday life have become part of the clinical dialogue.

Family-centered care involves much more than thinking of adding family members into the therapy session; occupational therapy practice is fundamentally altered when family members are brought into the therapeutic process in a central way (Lawlor & Mattingly, 1998). Family members, including parents, often have powerful roles in the creation of significant experiences in therapy (Mattingly & Lawlor, 2001). The challenge for the occupational therapy practitioner is to collaborate with clients, their families, and other team members in designing a program that builds on strengths and addresses needs. When done successfully, intervention services are individualized to each family and reflect their unique cultural world. Drawing on the work of Dunst, Trivette, and Deal (1988), we have defined family-centered care as *an experience that happens when practitioners effectively and compassionately listen to the concerns, address the needs, and support the hopes of people and their families* (Lawlor & Cada, 1993; Lawlor & Mattingly,

1998). Sometimes practitioners can best involve clients and families in the decision-making process by offering multiple options for interventions (Rosen & Granger, 1992). This type of engagement is often described as a means of enabling and empowering families (e.g., Deal, Dunst, & Trivette, 1989).

Family-centered care is enacted through the collaborative efforts of family members and practitioners (Edelman, Greenland, & Mills, 1993; Lawlor & Mattingly, 1998) and typically is provided through multidisciplinary and interdisciplinary team structures. Partnerships are created on the basis of the establishment of trust and rapport as well as respect for family values, beliefs, and routines (Hanft, 1989). Additional elements of successful collaboration include clarity and honesty in communication, mutual agreement on goals, effective information sharing, accessibility, and absence of blame (McGonigel, Kaufmann, & Johnson, 1991). Successful collaboration occurs when practitioners and family members form relationships that foster a shared understanding of the needs, hopes, expectations, and contributions of all partners (Lawlor & Cada, 1993).

The Processes of "Partnering Up" and Collaboration

Collaboration is much more than being "nice" (Lawlor & Mattingly, 1998; Mattingly, 1998). It involves complex interpretative acts in which the practitioner must understand the meanings of interventions, the meanings of illness or disability in a person and family's life, and the feelings that accompany these experiences. Collaboration is also dependent on the development of a quality of interrelatedness that is evident in many therapy sessions that is not merely a question of establishing good rapport, eliciting cooperation, or prompting a client or patient to buy into a particular agenda in order for him or her to perform required tasks (Lawlor, 2003). The central question for practitioners, clients and their families is "How can we come to know enough about each other to effectively partner up?" (Lawlor & Mattingly, 2001). For therapists, the nature of the work in collaboration "is not merely technical in the sense that a procedure is done or a therapy or other intervention is provided, nor does the work just entail drawing upon clinical expertise. Rather, 'partnering-up' requires skilled relational work and involves the drawing upon a range of social skills including, intersubjectivity, communication, engagement, and understanding" (Lawlor, 2004, p. 306). Assumptions about race, culture, ethnicity, social status, economic level, and education (and frequently the contesting of these assumptions) often powerfully influence the process of "partnering up" between families and professionals. Family members and practitioners live and operate in a multiplicity of cultural domains that are shaped by their profession, economic class, ethnicity, and community affiliations. When practitioners and family members interact, their values, assumptions, and perceptions about the interaction are shaped by their membership in these cultures.

"Partnering up" also involves bridging differences, establishing points of common interests and mutuality, and capitalizing on complementarities. This aspect of collaboration is particularly important when family members and practitioners perceive that they come from seemingly differently lived worlds. Mattingly (2006), drawing on reconceptualizations of culture that are prevalent in current anthropology, argues that health care encounters are like border zones, where there is often heightened engagement related to marking differences, finding commonalities, and creating understanding. Families in many ways are the consummate travelers in border zones with the daunting task of coming to understand biomedical, institutional, and practitioner cultural worlds and practices and participating in these practices in such a way that their nonbiomedical conceptualizations of their children, their families, and illness and disability can shape health care encounters.

Developing Understandings of Illness and Disability Experiences

Although increasing attention is being paid to family members, families are systematically underconsidered when it comes to health care. Professional training, institutional structures, reimbursement procedures, and reward systems all tend to contribute to the marginalization of families. When occupational therapy practitioners do try to consider the needs of their clients and of family caregivers, they can find themselves addressing a range of issues and facing a number of dilemmas for which they might not feel prepared.

The easiest way to understand why families have not traditionally been better included in decisions about health care is to remember that health care professionals, including occupational therapy practitioners, are members of professional cultures and work in settings that have institutional cultures. All health care professions have been powerfully influenced by what anthropologists sometimes call the "culture of Western biomedicine" (B. Good, 1994; Hahn & Gaines, 1985; Jackson, 2000; Locke & Gordon, 1988; Rhodes, 1991). It is a bit deceptive to speak of one monolithic culture of biomedicine, as though this were some single homogeneous entity. Occupational therapy practitioners, for example, might find that they live only partly in the same professional culture as, say, neurosurgeons. And practitioners working within one setting might find that this institutional culture is quite different from another setting in which they have practiced. This can hold true even if both organizations appear outwardly similar— two different rehabilitation hospitals, for instance. But even if all these differences and nuances are kept in mind, there are a number of powerful assumptions that are shared at some level by many health professionals working across a wide variety of settings.

Not only do professionals such as occupational therapy practitioners learn professional skills when they enter the field, they also assimilate a set of values and beliefs that make them members of a professional culture or community of practice (M. J. Good, 1995; Wenger, 1998). The culture of biomedicine has developed over the past 250 years.[2] Biomedicine has provided a powerful view of what it means to be ill and what is expected of the client, the health care professional, and the client's family or key caregivers (B. Good, 1994). There are some deeply held beliefs about what constitutes an appropriate relationship among professional, client, and family caregivers. These assumptions about the professional-client-caregiver relationship are influenced, in turn, by other basic assumptions about the nature of illness and how it is best treated. Some of these assumptions are especially problematic for rehabilitation professionals such as occupational therapy practitioners who treat clients with chronic illnesses and disabling conditions.

Attempts to understand illness and disability experiences have been facilitated by the "narrative turn" in medicine (Garro & Mattingly, 2000a; Hurwitz, Greenhalgh, & Skultans, 2004). As Garro and Mattingly (2000b) note, "An important thread in the literature which has emerged from or is directed toward the clinical community and aspires to reorient medical practice in society, is the need to distinguish disease, as phenomena seen from the practitioner's perspective (from the outside), from illness, as phenomena seen from the perspective of the sufferer" (p. 9). Literature in anthropology, particularly medical anthropology, occupational science and occupational therapy, medicine, and other health-related fields are increasingly drawing on narrative approaches to (1) enhance understanding of illness and disability from the perspectives of the individuals and their families who are living with illnesses or disabilities (e.g., Bluebond-Langer, 1978; A. Frank, 1995; G. Frank, 2000; Kleinman, 1988, 2006; Monks & Frankenberg, 1995; Murphy, 1990); (2) analyze how narrative modes of reasoning or narrative-based ethics influence health and therapeutic practices (e.g., Becker, 1997; Cain, 1991; Charon & Montello, 2002; Fleming & Mattingly, 1994; Hurwitz et al., 2004); and (3) recognize narrative as a structure for creating significant experiences in therapeutic practices (Clark, 1993; Mattingly, 1998).

Occupational therapists have also found it helpful to read and reflect on first-person accounts of illness and disability experiences (e.g., Bauby, 1997; Greenfeld, 1978, 1986; Hockenberry, 1995; Park, 1982, 2001; Williams, 1992). At times, popular media, including films and television shows, can generate insights that support practitioners' reflections on their clinical practices. Even films or television shows that present portrayals of illnesses or disabilities or health and therapeutic practices that may be

---

[2]For a detailed reading of this history as a cultural phenomena, see, for example, Foucault, (1973, 1979).

disturbing, demeaning, or inaccurate can provide important experiences for clarifying beliefs and philosophies that are critical to the provision of efficacious, collaborative, and compassionate family-centered care.

TROUBLESOME ASSUMPTIONS ABOUT DISABILITY, ILLNESS EXPERIENCES, AND FAMILIES

Several key assumptions that are particularly potent and particularly tenacious (Gordon, 1988) in the culture of biomedicine and in occupational therapy have significantly influenced the way in which families are drawn into the therapeutic process. Although over the past twenty years there has been increasing attention toward understanding the ways in which family members participate in health care practices (e.g., Hinojosa, Sproat, Mankhetwit, & Anderson, 2002; Lawlor & Mattingly, 1998), much additional knowledge and reflection are needed (e.g., Cohn, 2001; Ochieng, 2003). Many practitioners who work in multicultural settings recognize the complexity of organizing health care and therapy practices in such a way as to understand and address the specific needs of family members who have diverse backgrounds. The following sections illustrate how problematic or flawed assumptions about the illness and disability experiences of family members can affect care.

The Disability Belongs to the Individual

One of the most pervasive assumptions in biomedicine is that the professional's task is to treat the individual who has the illness. Sometimes, this is narrowly interpreted among health professionals as "treating the pathology," but occupational therapy practitioners usually try to remember that they are also treating a person who has a disabling condition. The hand therapist is treating not only a hand injury, for example, but also an out-of-work auto mechanic who has a wife and three children. The therapist recognizes that this client whose hand was injured on the job is fearful about his ability to regain his role as family breadwinner.

Put differently, practitioners try to treat what anthropologists speak of as *the illness experience* rather than simply the disease (B. Good, 1994; B. Good & M. J. Good, 1994; Kleinman, 1988; Luhrmann, 2000). In the context of occupational therapy, a more accurate term is probably *the disability experience*, for it is certainly possible to have a disability, even one that requires therapy, without being ill. Practitioners try to attend both to the disability as a physiological condition and to the meaning this particular condition carries for the person who has the disability (Mattingly, 1998, 2000; Mattingly & Fleming, 1994). If a practitioner knows that a client wants to relearn how to drive, dress independently, eat out at restaurants, or continue to work as an auto mechanic, the practitioner may be able to organize therapeutic tasks that aid the client in carrying out these activities.

However, some goals are far less tangible. This is especially true for goals that concern the client's social world and the connection between functional skills and social relationships. It is artificial to treat only narrowly defined functional skills as though they were unrelated to a client's social world, for a key aspect of the meaning of a condition is how it affects an individual's personal relationships, which is one of the trickier aspects of therapeutic work. By contrast, with such goals as learning how to dress oneself and learning wheelchair mobility, goals and concerns that are connected to family relations are much more difficult to define, and they are certainly likely to be hard to measure. Helping a client to reclaim his identity as a good father to his 5-year-old daughter even though he has a spinal cord injury, for example, is harder to translate into discrete, skill-based goals than is learning how to increase upper body strength or learning how to eat independently. However, learning what family members hope for—what they would like to see happen—is critical to the development of collaborative therapy practices with families. As Cohn, Miller, and Tickle-Degnan (2000) found in their qualitative study of parents of children with sensory modulation disorders, skillful listening to parents' perspectives can generate insights that promote therapy that is meaningful in terms of family goals and values.

Family-oriented goals are likely to be tied to outcomes that are diffuse, complex, subtle, and difficult to measure, even when they are deeply significant to the client and family. When a client's goals and concerns are tied to shifting family relationships, these might seem out of professional bounds for the occupational therapy practitioner. Despite the many difficulties in trying to understand a disabling condition as it pertains to a client's role in the family, ignoring this aspect often means being blind to the most significant aspects of the illness (or disability) experience. Ignoring family-oriented goals or the meaning of a disability as it ties to family concerns and family relationships can mean ignoring the person altogether.

There Is Only One Perspective per Family

Although much of the literature on family-centered care presumes that practitioners come to know all members of the family, we have found that often one member of the family, typically a mother or spouse, serves as the primary contact for the practitioner. It is this individual's perspective that practitioners come to know. However, this might be only one of several perspectives held by family members. Practitioners sometimes get to know other family members, but in many settings, the primary contact is the family member who brings the child to therapy or accompanies an adult or parent to therapy. Often, the family member who comes to the therapy session has a complicated culture-brokering role in which the person needs to both represent home, family, and community life in the clinic world and represent the clinic and institutional world back in home and family life. Such questions as, "So, what happened?" are indicative of the information requests that spouses, significant others, grandparents, and other family members might ask.

Family members may also have quite divergent perspectives on the nature of the problem, priorities for intervention, and meanings of illness and disability in daily life. These within-family differences often generate within-family negotiations and a kind of "partnering up" within family life that will influence family-practitioner partnerships. The dynamics of these multiple perspectives and within-family negotiations will likely change over time and be influenced by changes in illness trajectories, developmental agendas, household configurations, and constellation of household resources and needs. In addition, illness and disability might be only one subplot or drama in family life, competing with other pressing concerns and needs.

Illness and Disability Generate Only Negative Experiences

There has been, and continues to be, an assumption that all the effects of illness and disability on a family are negative. This belief leads to the erroneous conclusion that family reactions to illness and disability are both predictable and shared. In other words, the practitioner might presume to know about the effect of an illness or disability on the family without fully understanding a particular family. These notions get dismissed once one listens to families talk about their experiences. We have been struck by the incredible richness of their stories and the difficulty people have in reducing their complex reactions to a few discrete categories such as stress, grief, or acceptance. Some theorists have also attempted to develop theories based on stages of reactions, but the fixedness of these stages has been criticized (Moses, 1983).

Much of the research that has been conducted that relates to the response of family members to illness or disability has been conducted with parents of children who have special health care needs. Recently, parents and other family members have offered critiques of this body of research (e.g., Lipsky, 1985), citing the failure of researchers to recognize positive outcomes from these experiences. Researchers have tended to measure such predetermined variables as maternal depression and stress. Critics note that personal reports of other effects, including positive changes in family life, have been discounted. Advocates of the family-centered care movement note the failure of many researchers and practitioners to understand the unique features of family adaptation and coping and assert the need for further research that is grounded in the perspectives of family members. Although it is beyond the scope of this chapter to summarize this body of literature, the assumption that the effects of disability are unilateral and negative must be challenged as both simplistic and inadequate.

Practitioners need to seek understanding of the effects of illness and disability on the families of the people who come to them for assistance. These effects will likely change over time, and the perceptions of the relative stress of families will be shaped by other events in the family and the availability of resources. The presumption that the entirety of a family's experience can be summarized as stressful often leads to misunderstandings and lost opportunities to promote any positive aspects and celebrate successes (Lawlor & Cada, 1993; Lawlor & Mattingly, 1998; Mattingly & Lawlor, 2000).

The Professional Is the Expert

Traditionally, Western biomedicine has been concerned with curing people. The notion of the professional as healer is important here. The healer is an expert who can both ascertain what is wrong (assess and diagnose) and identify the correct intervention to cure the ailment (treat) (Biesele & Davis-Floyd, 1996; Davis-Floyd & Sargent, 1997; M. J. Good, 1995). The patient's role has been viewed as a submissive one, offering information as requested, submitting to physical examination, and following the expert's directives for treatment. In this view, health care professionals make people healthy by curing disease. The concern of the professional is largely with the disease rather than with the person who has the disease (the oncologist fighting the cancer cells with radiation, for instance). The patient's personal history, family situation, and work history might be only of peripheral importance in the healer's task of diagnosing and treating the pathologic condition that is causing the illness. Whereas the hope of medicine has been curing or healing, which implies the ability of the health professional to bring a person from a state of illness to some state of "normalcy" or premorbidity, occupational therapy practitioners are rarely in a position to cure anyone. The people they treat may have rich, full lives, but they are usually living these lives with an impairment or chronic condition that cannot be totally eradicated or fixed.

Practices steeped in Western biomedical traditions frequently adopt professional-client relationships that are based on hierarchical models or expert-driven models. The expert model remains prevalent in early childhood practices, despite increasing recognition that elements of this model create barriers to developing collaborative partnerships and understanding family life. The expert model tends to promote dependence within recipients of services, to limit opportunities for families to contribute insights and have their specific concerns and needs addressed, to burden the professional with the unrealistic expectation of always having the expertise to respond to all issues (Cunningham & Davis, 1985), and to organize services in ways that are self-serving to the expert (Howard & Strauss, 1975).

Practitioners know that therapy will be successful only if their clients (and often the key family caregivers as well) become motivated to work hard at it. But even as active participants, the clients and family members are often assigned a role as recipients of the instructions offered by occupational therapy practitioners and other rehabilitation experts. While these "active recipients" are sometimes offered a range of choices of goals or preferred activities and practitioners often try to accommodate therapeutic goals into the life of the client or family, practitioners still tend to equate good patients and good families with compliant ones. Thus, a quite typical scenario is for the practitioner to assign homework for the client to do between therapy sessions. When family members are involved in therapy, they are assigned roles as facilitators of the home therapy program. Even though there is nothing necessarily wrong with this kind of collaborative relationship between practitioner and family, it carries some dangers, especially when practitioners are unaware of their power to shift family dynamics and family relationships by pressing family caregivers to become responsible for therapeutic gains. One critical danger is that both practitioners and family members might unconsciously begin to presume that the family's primary role is as a kind of adjunct practitioner.

It is not surprising that reliance on expert models fosters relationships between practitioners and family members that incorporate compliance and coercion strategies. This leads to considerable confusion about whether the "story" is one of collaboration, coercion, or compliance (Lawlor & Mattingly, 1998). The issue is not merely a semantics problem. Each approach to working relationships creates distinctly different experiences for all parties. Practitioner judgments that a person is noncompliant or, in the terms used by family members, "bad parent," "bad daughter," and the like, divert energies away from more reflective analysis or direct attempts to understand alternative perspectives (Trostle, 1988). Comments such as "they are just in denial" often indicate a breach in understanding, a dismissal of family or personal perspectives. Families typically have tremendous expertise and knowledge related to their family members, family life, the illness or disability of their family member, and the ways in which treatment recommendations can most likely be implemented in the home. As Bedell, Cohn, and Dumas (2005) note, parents are well situated to promote and support their child's development in home and community life and able to modify or develop effective strategies.

FAMILY EXPERIENCES AND OCCUPATIONAL THERAPY PRACTICE

We have spent many hours watching occupational therapy practices, primarily with children. In addition, we have interviewed many parents and other family members and practitioners. These data have been gathered as part of a longitudinal, urban, ethnographic research project currently entitled *Boundary Crossings: Re-Situating Cultural Competence.* We have been following a cohort of African American children with illnesses and/or disabilities, their primary caregivers, family members, and the practitioners who serve them for approximately 10 years. This is a multifaceted study that includes analysis of meanings of illness and disability in family and clinical worlds; cross-cultural communication in health care encounters; health care practices including occupational therapy; health disparities; processes of "partnering up" and how illness and disability, family life, health care, and development are interrelated (Lawlor, 2003; Lawlor, 2004; Mattingly, 2006). The conceptual framework for the study draws heavily on narrative, interpretive, and phenomenological approaches to understanding human experience.

One of our most striking discoveries is the way in which seemingly casual conversation, brief moments of social engagement, attention to connectedness, and shared moments in the course of therapy sessions can deeply affect the experiences of family members and practitioners and, perhaps most important, the outcomes of therapy. These moments can be quite subtle and appear to be a kind of backdrop to the real work in therapy time or in health care encounters. Their seemingly mundane nature can belie their impact. As is illustrated below, there are also times of heightened engagement in which there is intensity around the learning or insights to understanding that are unfolding. There are, of course, other kinds of moments in family-centered care that are also consequential and appear to be marked by conflict, tension, drama, or highly charged emotion. As Laderman and Roseman (1996) remind us, "Medical encounters, no matter how mundane are dramatic events" (p.1).

In the following passages, we provide examples of family experiences related to illness and disability and their interactions with practitioners, including occupational therapists. Occupational therapists have shared many stories that relate to how they or their practice has been influenced by their experiences with families. We will begin by returning to the quote that was used to introduce this chapter. In that quote, this mother shared her strategy for ensuring that her family, including extended members, was knowledgeable about her child's therapy program and the clinical world in which therapy takes place. The following passages, excerpted from interviews with the occupational therapist, provide insights into her experiences related to meeting this family and her deep appreciation for lessons learned through this partnership. The occupational therapist credits this mother, whom we will call Leslie, with helping her to learn how to engage with Leslie's daughter, a toddler, who initially would not let the therapist come near her to work with her. As the following quote reveals, this successful partnership began with a rather precarious start:

> And it, it was just such a nice relationship, building of a relationship and then to come back and have her do her therapy with me was a really nice thing. But the

first, um, four months of therapy I couldn't touch her. And that was interesting. I think that almost was successful, because I had to work through Leslie. Leslie did all the therapy and I sort of sat . . . It was really funny [laughter]. I wish we could have some videotape, this was so funny. In the room I would sit in the corner. I had . . . I even couldn't approach her (the child) or she would start to cry. And I would sit a certain distance, which got closer and closer each session and I would direct Leslie what to do. And I think that that taught her so much about what she needed to do and gave her that physical, um, experience that just doing something with her daughter and knowing what it was, what the goals were, rather than sitting back and watching it. That might have been . . . I don't know. 'Cause I just see her as so successful with that and I wonder sometimes if that wasn't part of it. . . . 'Cause she had to, to do her daughter's therapy [laughter]. I, I couldn't. I couldn't get . . . you know. Then finally, and it was Leslie's idea and my idea, too, to bring her other children in because we couldn't get her to move. She wouldn't . . . she was terrified . . . climb up in things or any normal things that would . . . a normal child would explore. She was terrified. So when you see her today, it's like not the same. It was really, really interesting.

At another time, the therapist elaborated on what she had learned from this mother:

And so she taught me a lot about that. And she also— what happens when you work with a mother like that, they, they teach you about the power of negotiation and respecting an individual's rights. Because sometimes as a therapist, when the therapist doesn't have children, I can take more of the teacherly role and put my foot down and push through. And, and I can do that. And as a mother, I don't think that works so much in a household. You just get confrontation. You don't have that kind of power over your kids like a teacher. And she has the most incredible way of negotiating with the personality and she actually taught me how to do that with her daughter. So if I, there were situations where I would kinda be more teacherly and put my foot down and this is the rules and here we go. And Leslie would sort of pull me into a more productive understanding of how she raises her kids and that was really helpful.

The therapist, whom we will call Megan, further clarifies how knowledge about family life facilitates the therapeutic process. Leslie's strategy to bring family members into the therapy world not only enabled the family members to understand more about therapy, but also provided Megan with information that helped her to picture possibilities of family life. Megan also skillfully incorporated sto-

ries into therapy conversations that further illuminated life outside the clinic world. In one interview, she commented:

but it's not like in Leslie's case where you just get this just fabulous, you know, understanding of what's going on here. And this sort of communication and commitment and feedback about what's happening there in this other world. Like I have such a knowledge of what's happening in Leslie's world. I mean, I feel like I almost have pictures of their family life and I imagine, you know, she'll tell me a story about the Christmas tree and how Kylie's (the child), you know, she's making her put ornaments in this one section high up because then she has to use her arm in that way. And I can just see the family and I, I. . . .

As part of our research, we are trying to understand more about how practitioners and families do come to know and understand enough about each other to effectively partner up and what attributes influence partnerships. Leslie shares her perspective as follows:

It has nothing whatsoever to do with how much schooling you've had. It's just all from your life experience. And that makes a difference. Because I think my experience that I had with Megan as far as us having to communicate with one another. . . . I don't know a lot—I don't know and I didn't know an awful lot about her personal life. Okay, but I knew enough to know that whatever has happened to her in her life has either made her stronger, or, I don't know if that's what I'm looking for—it gave her a sense of caring about people. Whether it was something that really bad, that she said, Okay I'm not gonna be like that, or something that was really good because she was brought up in a nurturing environment, it just made her personality care. And, and that made a big difference. 'Cause that's what she brought to the table. You know? And, my strong sense of family, and 'course, that's my baby we're talking about, you know. And you have those two, us two bringing back to the table . . . when we sit down to discuss what is best for a child. I think that made a big difference. If—if Megan would have been more of just all business, keep it very technical . . . you know, I think the outcome would have been different. And I probably would have told somebody, I don't want her to be my therapist for my baby. You know, I mean 'cause I wouldn't have felt that, that nurturing that's within her. That's needed as far as I'm concerned, to deal with every child, not just mine. But, oh it's, oh, that is so great!

We now want to just briefly describe a portion of an occupational session that illustrates the often subtle but highly effective participation of family members in therapy sessions. The moment that we describe in the Case Study occurred partway through a session in which an occupational therapist was working with a young boy with a brachial plexus injury. The activity that she planned provided an opportunity to evaluate his sensation, fine motor abilities, and bilateral coordination. This vignette shows the narrative structuring of therapy sessions and the ways in which family members can contribute through both co-narration and their participation as social actors in the therapy scene (Lawlor, 2003; Mattingly, 1998). Even though we are describing only several minutes within a therapy session here, we are excerpting key aspects. Therapy time, particularly sessions with heightened engagement and family participation, is too rich and too complex to provide all the detail and description.

It is always a bit difficult in written text to convey social action among engaged social actors. In the brief passages in the Case Study, we have attempted to evoke the kinds of animation, attunement, engagement, enjoyment, and joint

---

CASE STUDY: *The Magic Box*

The therapist, whom we will call Georgia, announces a guessing game and presents a rather elaborately decorated box, approximately 9 inches square and 12 inches tall. Micah, who is approximately four years old, his brother Damian, who is several years older, and his mother, Sheana, are all present, along with one of the authors, who is videotaping. Sheana, who is sitting off to the side, says, "Oooh," with dramatic intonation. Georgia further proclaims that it is a "magic box." The two brothers join her in a fairly tight circle on the floor mat. Georgia instructs Micah that he must reach into the box without peeking and find things (these things are small objects that are buried among beans). By touching his left arm, she cues him that this is the arm she wants him to use. (Micah's brachial plexus injury is on his left side.) "See if you can find anything. Move your arm in there. I'll tell you when you have something. No. [whispers] It's a secret box. No, you cannot peek. It's a secret. Find anything in there?" Micah has tried to look under the lid of the box as an adaptive strategy, as he is apparently having trouble feeling the objects buried in the beans. Micah whines a bit in frustration and slips his right hand into the box and quickly retrieves an object. Georgia says, "No, no this hand may not . . . ," and his mother says, "Only lefty can, Micah," thus supporting the therapist's agenda that he use his left arm. Georgia takes the retrieved object and places it in Micah's left hand. She then asks him to show and give the object to his brother, thus smoothly incorporating Micah's older brother into this therapy activity that clearly has potential for further intrigue.

The activity unfolds with continued skillful co-narration and participation of Sheana and Damian. The brothers are highly engaged, and Damian at times seems to scaffold for his brother, thus heightening Micah's potential for success. For example, as Micah reaches into the box, Damian comments, "They might be all the way down," thus facilitating Micah's attempts to move deeper into the box. Sheana, at times, skillfully co-manages the session, seemingly vigilant that Damian does not take over or become too involved, thus disrupting Micah's session, or become disengaged in a way that limits his ability to support the therapeutic activity. For example, she calls out Damian's name when she wants him to pull back a bit or, conversely, to pay more attention.

The action that all four of these actors produce is almost seamless, almost choreographed in its fluidity, but also obviously spontaneous and organized in the flow of therapy. The work that the mother, brother, and therapist do to help make this session so effective is not merely related to promoting the desired behavior, though this is important. Both mother and brother skillfully use changes in tone of voice to support Micah's efforts. The transcript of the session is peppered with comments such as "You did it!" and "Oooh," a kind of quieter admiration. They also seem to be heightening the engagement in the doing, making the "guessing game" more appealing, more dramatic. For example, Damian becomes a kind of announcer about the characters that are retrieved from the box. What seemed initially to be a box of farm animals becomes a box with oddities such that Mickey Mouse, lions, and gorillas appear with considerable puzzlement and humor. As Damian comments when Mickey is found, "What's he doing here?"

At other times in this session, Damian was given many of the same tasks as his brother, such as swinging on the trapeze or picking up the beans that had been strewn on the floor while Micah was digging in the "magic box." Damian's inclusion not only helped to make the session more fun, but also provided many opportunities for reciprocity, turn taking, and sharing between these two brothers. Sheana's careful attention to the session and her sons' behaviors, as well as her skillful co-narration, further added to the perception that this was a family event.

Near the end of the activity, Sheana comments, "It's a very cute thing." Georgia responds with both a smile and the comment "It's something you really could enjoy at home." This is a replay of a conversation that occurred partway through the game when Damian had said, "Let's take it home" in the midst of his enjoyment, after his mother's comment "That's a cute little idea—I like that." A brief exchange follows about whether beans or rice would be better. Interspersed throughout this activity had been comments from Georgia related to the ways in which this was a therapeutic activity for Micah.

coordination that marked these moments. These family members and this therapist created a therapeutic experience that addressed Micah's challenging clinical needs while affording an opportunity for engaging moments. These moments were engaging enough that this family was actively designing ways to replicate the experience at home, to recreate this event in the clinic as a family experience at home.

CONCLUSION

In this chapter, we highlighted many of the challenges that are involved in attempting to respond to the needs of clients and their families. Challenges are coupled with opportunities. As practitioners discover ways of getting to know families and understanding their perspectives, opportunities emerge for practitioners to construct richer, more meaningful experiences. The more meaningful the experience is, the more likely it is that treatment will be efficacious.

We have found that discussions of opportunities must be tempered with specific cautions. Approaches to getting to know families must be noninvasive, sensitive, nonjudgmental, and respectful of the parameters for privacy and disclosure that individuals indicate. Understanding a perspective does not presume that as an occupational therapy practitioner, you are responsible for intervening in every dimension of that perspective. Family-centered care is implemented most effectively in situations in which interdisciplinary efforts are well coordinated and effectively communicated. In situations in which practitioners are working in relative isolation, caution must be exercised to ensure that they are practicing within the bounds of their expertise and appropriately facilitating access to other resources as needed.

One of the greatest challenges for practitioners is to understand how their own lived experience shapes their interactions with family members in the course of providing services. Conceptual models of practice and theory regarding family systems and human development, ethics, and public and institutional policies all contribute to our framework for family-centered interventions. However, practitioners, as the instruments for intervention, bring their own selves and their cultural views of families into clinical interactions.

We intuitively recognize that such things as our ethnicity, nationality, geographical home, and perhaps even religion provide us with powerful cultural worlds. These aspects of our background help to make us who we are, culturally speaking. We are often not fully aware that our profession and our family also offer cultural worlds that shape some of our deepest assumptions, beliefs, and values. This chapter concerns a kind of cultural intersection between the practitioner (acting as a member of a professional culture) and a client (acting as a member of a family culture). Practitioners, of course, have families, and clients often have professions. However, when practitioners and clients meet during occupational therapy intervention, the practitioner's professional and institutional cultures are particularly significant in shaping how the practitioner defines good intervention and a good professional-client relationship.

Occupational therapy practitioners come to their profession with life experiences of being a member of a family. This lived experience of growing up in a family significantly shapes who we are as practitioners, particularly in situations in which practitioners are getting to know a family and seeking to understand their needs, priorities, values, hopes, and resources. These assumptions about family life tend to be quite tacit, and we are often not aware of their influence unless we actively reflect on our actions. Guided reflection through mentorship and supervision, as well as discussions with other team members concerning beliefs about specific families, are essential components of intervention planning and implementation with clients and their families.

ACKNOWLEDGMENTS

This chapter was supported by work related to four research projects. One study was supported by grant MCJ-060745 from the Maternal and Child Health Program (Title V, Social Security Act), Health and Services Administration, Department of Health and Human Services. Appreciation is expressed to the American Occupational Therapy Foundation for their support of pilot work related to that study. Research was also supported by *Boundary Crossing: A Longitudinal and Ethnographic Study* (# R01 HD 38878) and *Boundary Crossings: Re-Situating Cultural Competence* (# 2R01 HD 38878) funded through the National Institute of Child Health and Human Development (NICHD), National Institutes of Health (NIH). The contents of this chapter are solely the responsibility of the authors and do not necessarily represent the official views of any of these agencies. We also would like to express our appreciation to the many children, families, therapists, and practitioners who have participated in these research efforts and who have willingly shared their experiences. We would also like to specifically thank Melissa Park, Beth Crall, Cristine Carrier, Kim Wilkinson, Jesus Diaz, Lisa Hickey, Cynthia Strathmann, Emily Areinoff, and Claudia Dunn for their contributions and assistance in preparing this chapter.

PROVOCATIVE QUESTIONS

1. Reflect on the quotations from Leslie and Megan and comment on what surprised you most.
2. What do you think helped to make this relationship work?

3. How do you think your own life and family life experiences might affect how you "partner up" with families?
4. Can you identify any additional problematic assumptions that might influence your collaboration with families?

REFERENCES

108th Congress. (2004). Pub. L. No. 108-446: An act to reauthorize the individuals with disabilities education act, and for other purposes.

American Occupational Therapy Association. (1999). *Occupational therapy services for children and youth under the Individuals with Disabilities Education Act* (2nd ed.). Bethesda, MD: Author.

Bauby, J. D. (1997). *The diving bell and the butterfly.* New York: Random House.

Becker, G. (1997). *Disrupted lives: How people create meaning in a chaotic world.* Berkeley: University of California Press.

Bedell, G. M., Cohn, E. S., & Dumas, H. M. (2005). Exploring parents' use of strategies to promote social participation of school-age children with acquired brain injuries. *American Journal of Occupational Therapy, 59*(3), 273–284.

Biesele, M., & Davis-Floyd, R. (1996). Dying as a medical performance: The oncologist as Charon. In C. Laderman & M. Roseman (Eds.), *The performance of healing* (pp. 291–321). New York: Routledge.

Bluebond-Langer, M. (1978). *The private worlds of dying children.* Princeton, NJ: Princeton University Press.

Cain, C. (1991). Personal stories: Identity acquisition and self-understanding in Alcoholics Anonymous. *Ethos, 19,* 210–253.

Charon, R., & Montello, M. (2002). *Stories matter: The role of narrative in medical ethics.* New York: Routledge.

Clark, F. (1993). Occupation embedded in real life: Interweaving occupational science and occupational therapy: 1993 Eleanor Clarke Slagle Lecture. *American Journal of Occupational Therapy, 47*(12), 1067–1078.

Cohn, E. S. (2001). From waiting to relating: Parents' experiences in the waiting room of an occupational therapy clinic. *American Journal of Occupational Therapy, 55,* 167–174.

Cohn E. S., Miller, L. J., & Tickle-Degnan, L. (2000). Parental hopes for therapy outcomes: Children with sensory modulation disorders. *American Journal of Occupational Therapy, 54*(1), 36–43.

Colman, W. (1988). The evolution of occupational therapy in the public schools: The laws mandating practice. *American Journal of Occupational Therapy, 42,* 701–705.

Cunningham, C., & Davis, H. (1985). *Working with parents: Frameworks for collaboration.* Philadelphia: Open University Press.

Davis-Floyd, R., & Sargent, C. (1997). *Childbirth and authoritative knowledge: Cross-cultural perspectives.* Berkeley: University of California Press.

Deal, A., Dunst, C., & Trivette, C. (1989). A flexible and functional approach to developing individualized family support plans. *Infants and Young Children, 1*(4), 32–43.

Dunst, C., Trivette, C., & Deal, A. (1988). *Enabling and empowering families: Principles and guidelines for practice.* Cambridge, MA: Brookline.

Edelman, L., Greenland, B., & Mills, B. (1993). *Building parent professional collaboration: Facilitator's guide.* St. Paul, MN: Pathfinder Resources.

Fleming, M., & Mattingly, C. (1994). *Clinical reasoning: Forms of inquiry in therapeutic practice.* Philadelphia: F. A. Davis.

Foucault, M. (1973). *The birth of the clinic: An archaeology of medical perception.* New York: Vintage.

Foucault, M. (1979). *Discipline and punish: The birth of the prison.* New York: Vintage.

Frank, A. (1995). *The wounded storyteller: Body, illness, and ethics.* Chicago: University of Chicago Press.

Frank, G. (2000). *Venus on wheels: Two decades of dialogue on disability, biography, and being female in America.* Berkeley: University of California Press.

Garro, L., & Mattingly, C. (2000a). Narrative turns. In C. Mattingly & L. C. Garro (Eds.), *Narrative and the cultural construction of illness and healing* (pp. 259–269). Berkeley: University of California Press.

Garro, L., & Mattingly, C. (2000b). Narrative as construct and construction. In C. Mattingly & L. C. Garro (Eds.), *Narrative and the cultural construction of illness and healing* (pp. 1–49). Berkeley: University of California Press.

Good, B. (1994). *Medicine, rationality, and experience.* Cambridge, UK: Cambridge University Press.

Good, B., & Good, M. J. (1994). In the subjunctive mode: Epilepsy narratives in Turkey. *Social Science in Medicine, 38,* 835–842.

Good, M. J. (1995). *American medicine: The quest for competence.* Berkeley: University of California Press.

Gordon, D. (1988). Clinical science and clinical experience: Changing boundaries between art and science in medicine. In M. Locke & D. Gordon (Eds.), *Biomedicine examined* (pp. 257–295). Dordrecht: Kluwer Academic.

Greenfeld, J. (1978). *A place for Noah.* New York: Henry Holt.

Greenfeld, J. (1986). *A client called Noah: A family journey continued.* New York: Henry Holt.

Hahn, R. A., & Gaines, A. D. (Eds.). (1985). *Physicians of Western medicine.* Norwell, MA: Reidel.

Hanft, B. (1989). *Family-centered care: An early intervention resource manual.* Rockville, MD: American Occupational Therapy Association.

Hanft, B. E. (1991). Impact of public policy on pediatric health and education programs. In W. Dunn (Ed.), *Pediatric occupational therapy: Facilitating effective service provision* (pp. 273–284). Thorofare, NJ: Slack.

Hinojosa, J., Sproat, C. T., Mankhetwit, S., & Anderson, J. (2002). Shifts in parent-therapist partnerships: Twelve years of change. *American Journal of Occupational Therapy, 56*(5), 556–563.

Hockenberry, J. (1995). *Moving violations: War zones, wheelchairs, and declarations of independence.* New York: Hyperion.

Howard, J., & Strauss, A. (1975). *Humanizing health care.* New York: Wiley.

Humphry, R., Gonzales, S., & Taylor, E. (1993). Family involvement in practice: Issues and attitudes. *American Journal of Occupational Therapy, 47*(7), 587–593.

Hurwitz, B., Greenhalgh, T., & Skultans, V. (2004). Introduction. In B. Hurwitz, T. Greenhalgh, & V. Skultans (Eds.), *Narrative research in health and illness* (pp. 1–20). Malden, MA: Blackwell.

Jackson, J. (2000). *Camp pain: Talking with chronic pain patients.* Berkeley: University of California Press.

Kleinman, A. (1988). *The illness narratives: Suffering, healing, and the human condition.* New York: Basic Books.

Kleinman, A. (2006). *What really matters: Living a moral life amidst uncertainty and danger.* New York: Oxford University Press.

Laderman, C., & Roseman, M. (1996). Introduction. In C. Laderman & M. Roseman (Eds.), *The performance of healing* (pp. 1–16). New York: Routledge.

Lawlor M. C. (1991). Historical and societal influences on school system practice. In A. Bundy (Ed.), *Making a difference: OTs and PTs in public schools* (pp. 1–15). Chicago: University of Illinois.

Lawlor, M. C. (2003). The significance of being occupied: The social construction of childhood occupations. *American Journal of Occupational Therapy, 57*(4), 424–434.

Lawlor, M. C. (2004). Mothering work: Negotiating health care, illness and disability, and development. In S. Esdaille & J. Olson (Eds.), *Mothering occupations: Challenge, agency, and participation* (pp. 306–322). Philadelphia: F. A. Davis.

Lawlor, M. C., & Cada, E. (1993). Partnerships between therapists, parents, and children. *OSERS News in Print, 5*(4), 27–30.

Lawlor, M. C., & Mattingly, C. (1998). The complexities in family-centered care. *American Journal of Occupational Therapy, 52,* 259–267.

Lawlor, M. C., & Mattingly, C. F. (2001). Beyond the unobtrusive observer. *American Journal of Occupational Therapy, 55*(2), 147–154.

Lipsky, D. K. (1985). A parental perspective in stress and coping. *American Journal of Orthopsychiatry, 55,* 614–617.

Locke, M., & Gordon, D. (Eds.). (1988). *Biomedicine examined.* Dordrecht: Kluwer Academic.

Luhrmann, T. M. (2000). *Of two minds: The growing disorder of American psychiatry.* New York: Knopf.

Mattingly, C. (1998). *Healing dramas and clinical plots: The narrative structure of experience.* Cambridge, UK: Cambridge University Press.

Mattingly, C. (2000). Emergent narratives. In C. Mattingly & L. C. Garro (Eds.), *Narrative and the cultural construction of healing* (pp. 181–211). Berkeley: University of California Press.

Mattingly, C. (2006). Pocahontas goes to the clinic: Popular culture as lingua franca in a cultural borderland. *American Anthropologist, 106*(3), 494–501.

Mattingly, C., & Fleming, M. (1994). *Clinical reasoning: Forms of inquiry in a therapeutic practice.* Philadelphia: F. A. Davis.

Mattingly, C., & Lawlor, M. (2000). Learning from stories: Narrative interviewing in cross-cultural research. *The Scandinavian Journal of Occupational Therapy, 7,* 4–14.

Mattingly, C., & Lawlor, M. (2001). The fragility of healing. *Ethos, 29*(1), 30–57.

McGonigel, M. J., Kaufmann, R. K., & Johnson, B. H. (Eds.). (1991). *Guidelines and recommended practices for the individualized family service plan.* Bethesda, MD: Association for the Care of Children's Health.

Monks, J., & Frankenberg, R. (1995). Being ill and being me: Self, body, and time in multiple sclerosis narratives. In B. Ingstad & S. R. Whyte (Eds.), *Disability and culture* (pp. 107–134). Berkeley: University of California Press.

Moses, K. L. (1983). The impact of initial diagnosis: Mobilizing family resources. In J. Mulick & S. Pueschel (Eds.), *Parent-professional partnerships in developmental disability services* (pp. 11–34). Cambridge, MA: Academic Guild.

Murphy, R. F. (1990). *The body silent.* New York: W. W. Norton.

Ochieng, B. M. N. (2003). Minority ethnic families and family-centered care. *Journal of Child Health Care, 7*(2), 123–132.

Park, C. C. (1982). *The siege: The first eight years of an autistic child.* Boston: Little, Brown.

Park, C. C. (2001). *Exiting Nirvana: A daughter's life with autism.* Boston: Little, Brown and Company.

Rhodes, L. (1991). *Emptying beds: The work of an emergency psychiatric unit.* Berkeley: University of California Press.

Rosen, S., & Granger, M. (1992). Early intervention and school programs. In A. Crocker, H. Cohen, & T. Kastner (Eds.), *HIV infection and developmental disabilities: A resource for service providers* (pp. 75–84). Baltimore: Brookes.

Trostle, J. A. (1988). Medical compliance as an ideology. *Social Sciences in Medicine, 27,* 1299–1308.

Wenger, E. (1998). *Communities of practice.* Cambridge, UK: Cambridge University Press.

Williams, D. (1992). *Nobody nowhere: The extraordinary autobiography of an autistic.* New York: Avon Books.

Contribution of Occupation to Health and Well-Being

CLARE HOCKING

Learning Objectives

After reading this chapter, you will be able to:

1. Explain how health is both a resource supporting participation in occupation and an outcome of participation.
2. Define what is meant by health and how health differs from well-being.
3. Explain health in terms of biological needs, skills, and capacities.
4. Identify physical, mental, and social aspects of well-being and how these might be influenced by a person's physical, social, and attitudinal environment.
5. Discuss the ways in which people's occupations and how those occupations are organized might support or undermine health and well-being.
6. Explain how having an impairment might affect well-being, taking into account present-day occupational experiences, expectations for the future, and the influence of environmental barriers.

Jane: I always make fruit-mince pies at Christmas. I make quite a big deal out of it I guess, because I make my own fruit-mince and put lots of brandy in it. It really is delicious, even if I do say so myself. I'll cook up quite a number when I get going, four or five dozen I suppose. I have a bit of a production line going. When I go and visit my friends, I make up a little package of two or four of them depending on the number of people. It doesn't constitute a present. We're not into Christmas presents, you can spend so much on them it's ridiculous. It's just a little something.

Brenda: It works very well.

Dawn: I like your idea of it not being a present as such. It's not costly and it doesn't give the receiver a feeling that "Oh, I've got to get you something."

Jane: It does work well. That's what people like to have and they like my mince pies. They're eaten on the day, and I have enough left over for Boxing Day.

(Wright-St. Clair & Hocking, unpublished data, 2000)

Jane, Brenda, and Dawn agree that Christmas fruit-mince pies are the perfect gift. Jane has the pleasure of savoring the smell of the minced fruit as it matures over several weeks and enjoys the process of efficiently baking all the pies. She knows that her friends appreciate the time and effort she puts into her gift but do not feel obligated to buy something to give her in return. Best of all, because they are fresh and delicious, Jane knows that her pies are eaten straight away. In this ordinary yet thoughtful **occupation**, Jane exercises her skills as a cook, employs her knowledge of the meaning of Christmas, and reinforces relationships that make her world a warm and welcoming place. In return, she receives feedback that her effort, expertise, and friendship are appreciated.

The feelings of competence and social relatedness that Jane experiences through baking and gifting food contribute to her overall sense of **well-being**. Despite her advancing years, Jane continues this annual tradition along with many other occupations she considers important. Although her daily routines and occupational choices are different from those of other times in her life, she is generally satisfied with her life and circumstances. Moreover, when she is fully engaged in and enjoying what she is doing, such as when she is parceling up her fruit-mince pies, Jane experiences a welcome sense of vitality and involvement with friends, family, and her community.

OCCUPATION AND HEALTH

Jane's experience aligns with popular understandings of **health** and well-being. Unlike biomedical views of health, which tend to emphasize the absence of disease (Glanze, 1990), people in Western societies commonly perceive themselves to be physically and mentally healthy when they are able to do the things that are important to them. In fact, people often claim to be in good health despite having quite severe health conditions, restricted life circumstances, and clearly apparent limitations in **functioning** (World Health Organization [WHO], 2001). For example, one woman who declared that she was "very healthy apart from this arthritis" was described by a researcher as a "crippled and housebound woman of 61" (Blaxter, 1990, p. 22). People generally equate their health with appearance, physical fitness, energy levels, psychosocial well-being, social relationships, and being able to carry out their normal round of occupations (Blaxter, 1990). It is this occupational view of health that is the focus of this discussion.

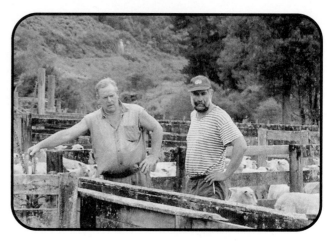

FIGURE 5.1   Bruce and John at work drafting sheep.

The first point to note is that being in good health clearly supports the ability to do normal, day-to-day occupations. That is, it helps if people are sufficiently fit, strong, and flexible; able to focus their thoughts and attention; and not too fatigued to do what needs to be done. For example, Bruce and John (Figure 5.1) rely on being healthy to complete tasks around the farm. It also helps if their efforts are not unduly hampered by pain, deformity, breathlessness, malnutrition, confusion, despair, or the apathy that comes of boredom or hopelessness. In this sense, health is a resource, albeit one that many people take for granted. One illustration of treating health as a resource for occupation is the response to illness. For many people, being sick is a legitimate reason not to do the things they usually do. Illness often means being released from responsibilities and that others will do things on the sick person's behalf. Thus, mothers cook chicken soup or the cultural equivalent for their sick family members, and workmates take on extra tasks to ensure that essential aspects of the ill person's job are completed on time.

Needs, Skills, and Capacities

While health facilitates **participation**, the opposite is also true: Participation in occupation contributes to good health. At the level of individual and species survival, as Wilcock (1993) has cogently argued, occupation is essential because the basic **biological needs** for sustenance, self-care, shelter, and safety are met through the things people do. In meeting these needs and through other occupations of daily life, people develop "skills, social structures and technology aimed at superiority over predators and the environment" (Wilcock, 1993, p. 20). These skills include, for example, growing and cooking nutritious food and constructing warm clothing and dry houses. Also important, though not always achieved, is the skill of living peacefully with neighbors. Depending on the circumstances, many other skills are also relevant to health. Reading and writing, for example, are important means of conveying information relevant to sustaining health and seeking health care in Western societies but may be less relevant in other places. It is also important to note that not everyone needs all the skills that are relevant to survival. Rather, health depends on being part of a family or community of people who together have the skills necessary to survive, and perhaps to flourish, as well as access to the resources to put their skills to use.

Meeting survival needs and becoming skilled are not sufficient to ensure good health; of equal importance is the contribution that occupation makes to developing and exercising personal **capacities** (Wilcock, 1993, 1995). These capacities spring from the biological characteristics shared by all humans: walking upright, opposing thumb and fingers to grasp objects, learning to speak, and so on. People have the capacity to, among other things, carry loads, design new tools and find novel uses for old ones, understand the workings of the universe, accumulate and pass on knowledge, predict what might happen and prepare for the future, form relationships, and express themselves artistically and spiritually. People also have the capacity to play, as Jamie shows us, caught in the moment of throwing a petanque ball (Figure 5.2).

Each person's capacities reflect this human potential, via his or her genetic inheritance, brought into being through the developmental process and a unique life history of occupational opportunities, preferences, and choices. On the basis of their history of doing things and expectations of what they might do in the future, people are generally aware of the capacities they have: whether they are better at sport, art, or music; whether they find schoolwork or practical tasks more congenial; and whether they prefer solitary occupations or mixing socially.

The capacities that are most often cited in relation to being healthy are those relating to physical performance. For example the estimated 20 million to 30 million Americans who regularly run say that they do so to enhance their physical fitness, that is, their capacity for intense physical activity, as well as for the benefits it bestows on weight control and feeling good (Primeau, 1996). Not everyone likes to run, however, and many people do not regularly engage in other physically demanding occupations such as gardening, swimming, riding a bicycle, playing a sport, or cleaning. In short, people who do not exercise are not maintaining the capacity to exert themselves physically. The consequences are potentially serious. As well as not being able to sustain physical exertion, should they need to, people who do not engage in sufficient physical exercise have increased risk of cardiovascular disease and cancer (Wallis, Miranda, & Park, 2005). Lack of exercise is also associated with the looming crisis of childhood obesity (see the case study). For those who do not exercise in other ways, walking reasonably quickly for at least 30 minutes a day, five days a week, is considered the minimum requirement to maintain health (Wallis, Miranda, & Park, 2005). Estimates of the number of people who achieve this level of activity vary. Only 6% of Norwegians over 65 years of age

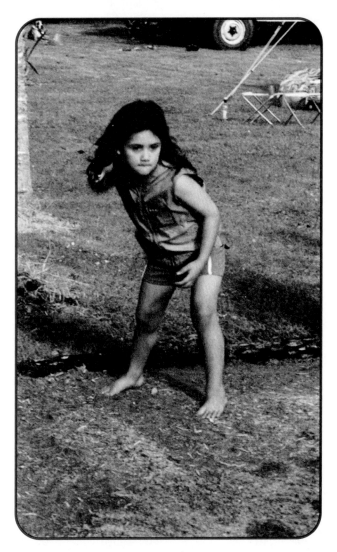

FIGURE 5.2   Jamie intent on playing petanque.

meet this exercise guideline (Loland, 2004). In the United States, 22.4% of adults engage in vigorous physical activity five times a week; the percent by age range decreases from 31.7% for people age 18–24 to 6.2% for people 75 years and older (Centers for Disease Control and Prevention [CDC], 2005a). These statistics indicate that many people's lifestyle does not support optimal health.

Although less emphasized in the literature, exercising mental and social capacities in order to maintain cognitive functioning, psychological health, and positive social networks is also important. Indeed, participating in occupations can generate benefits that cross physical, mental, and social aspects of health. For instance, a large-scale study of older Americans showed that social and productive occupations decreased their risk of mortality as much as physical activities did (Glass, de Leon, Marottoli, & Berkman, 1999). Likewise, older people in residential care in Britain live longer and are less likely to be depressed if they are aware of opportunities to be occupied and enjoy the things they do (Mozley, 2001). Similarly, the more older Americans garden, dance, play golf or bowl, swim, cycle or jog, or walk for exercise, the better their cognitive functioning is likely to be. Participating in these occupations seems to reduce the likelihood of depression and to strengthen social networks (Vance, Wadley, Ball, Roenker, & Rizzo, 2005).

Developing Skills and Exercising Capacities

What stimulates people to engage in occupations that enhance their chances of survival, develop skills, and exercise capacities is much debated. One suggestion, first advanced by Wilcock in 1993, is that humans experience biological needs that stimulate occupation, which in turn promotes health. These needs relate, first, to correcting threats to our physiological state, such as being excessively hot or cold or feeling hungry or thirsty. The discomfort of these sensations stimulates us to action: to find some shade, put on more clothing, or seek out food or drink. (See Figure 5.3.)

The second set of needs is protective and preventive, such as the need to develop skills and exercise capacities. These are experienced as a surge of energy that propels us to acquire and practice the skills required to solve problems and plan, interact with others, do whatever generates our livelihood, and so on. In so doing, at least before technology removed many of the physical demands of earlier lifestyles, people exercised their capacity for physical, mental, and social functioning. The third and final set of needs prompts and rewards engagement in occupation. Meeting these needs gives a sense of purpose, satisfaction, and fulfillment. More typically associated with higher levels of health and well-being, these concepts are addressed later in the discussion.

HEALTH AND WELL-BEING

While no definitive description of well-being exists, it is generally understood to be a person's subjective perception of his or her health. In Western societies, in which individualistic values prevail, well-being is commonly associated with concepts such as self-esteem, happiness, a sense of

belonging, and personal growth and encompasses people's feelings about their physical, mental, and social health (Wilcock, 1998). The cultures of indigenous populations frequently also include notions of spiritual well-being, community spirit, and connection to the land (Aguis, 1993; Durie, 1994). Taking an ecological perspective, Wilcock (1998) has suggested that people's well-being is inextricably bound to the health of local and global ecosystems.

Acknowledging that health and well-being are affected by factors outside an individual suggests that something can be learned about individuals' health and well-being by examining relevant measures of population health. Accordingly, when considered in relation to mortality statistics, well-being seems to relate to employment, prosperity, and ethnicity, since people who are employed, those with higher incomes, and members of the dominant ethnic group in a society have lower incidences of most chronic diseases and better health care outcomes (CDC, 2005b; Ministry of Health Manatū Hauora, 2005). Moreover, their children are more likely to survive (Whitehead, 1988).

This is not to say that well-being is incompatible with disease and injury. Indeed, even people with a terminal illness can put that fact aside, at least for a while, and thoroughly enjoy themselves (Hasselkus, 2002). It does acknowledge, however, the additional burden of having a health condition, particularly if the person's physical, social, or attitudinal context is less than supportive of participation in the normal range of occupations others enjoy (WHO, 2001). Examples of such circumstances include inaccessible buildings, poverty and high levels of unemployment, and the stigma attached to conditions such as AIDS, leprosy, and mental illness. Facing these barriers, particularly when they persist, might well challenge perceptions of well-being.

OCCUPATION AND WELL-BEING

In the previous section, well-being was defined as the subjective experience of health or people's feelings about their health. From an occupational perspective, feelings of well-being arise from the things people do that provide a sense of vitality, purpose, satisfaction, or fulfillment. Occu-

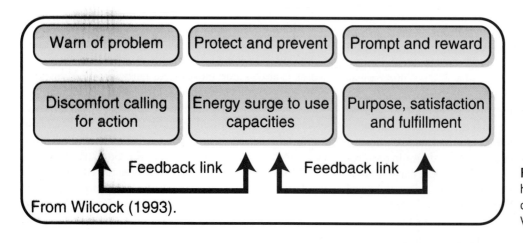

FIGURE 5.3 Biological hierarchy of need for occupation. (From Wilcock, 1993.)

pational well-being also relates to the things people envision doing in the future. Well-being is expressed in terms of feeling on top of the world; feeling nourished, contented, transformed, at peace, strong, interested, and fully alive; or experiencing intense concentration (Wilcock, 1998). Such views are largely in keeping with the Ottawa Charter, which asserts that to attain complete well-being, "an individual or group must be able to identify and to realize aspirations, satisfy needs, and cope with the environment" (WHO, 1986, p. 1). As was discussed earlier, the mechanism by which people achieve these things is through occupation.

Not surprisingly, however, attempts to equate well-being with frequency or extent of participation in valued occupations have been largely unsuccessful (see for example, Christiansen, 1996; Stanley, 1995). This finding supports the notion that well-being relates more to the quality or intensity of the experience itself (Csikszentmihalyi, 1993; Persson, Eklund, & Isacsson, 1999). Examples of people experiencing a sense of well-being through occupation abound. Within the occupational science literature, they include the claims that dance is a transformative occupation that can awaken people to their spiritual essence (Graham, 2002) and that cake decorating both reduces stress and gives rise to immense satisfaction. Moreover, recipients interpret the time put into decorating their cake as a gift of love, which implies a positive impact on their sense of well-being (Scheerer, Cahill, Kirby, & Lane, 2004). Similarly, quilting unlocks creativity, even as women work within the structure of traditional quilting patterns, and for some becomes an all-consuming pursuit. In addition, it fosters learning and sharing and feeds curiosity (Dickie, 2003, 2004). Equally, women who attend book clubs in Australia relish the opportunity to "let their hair down" (Howie, 2003, p. 135) and freely express ideas and feelings.

As is suggested by the recipients of decorated cakes, occupations also afford opportunities to influence others' well-being. One example is the older women in Northern Thailand who cook kha nom jok, a sweet or savory snack, for the New Year celebration (Figure 5.4). The literal meaning of the name of this dish is "togetherness" or "wrapped together." By willingly undertaking the task of preparing this dish and ensuring that it is of the very best quality, these women hope to confer this epitome of social well-being on their family (Hocking, Wright-St. Clair, & Bunrayong, 2002). In addition, by sharing the food they have cooked with friends and neighbors, older Thai women enact traditional values of making a good and generous society (Wright-St. Clair, Bunrayong, Vittayakorn, Rattakorn, & Hocking, 2004).

Half a world away, in a suburb in North London, housewives strive to achieve more individually targeted improvements in well-being. This means purchasing healthier foods than their children might select for themselves, choosing better-quality clothing than their children prefer, and occasionally buying treats for themselves and other family members (Miller, 1998). Of course, a single occupation can influence well-being in multiple ways. For

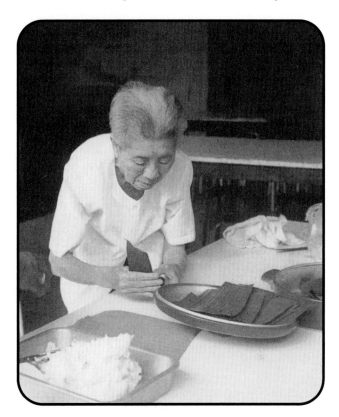

FIGURE 5.4 Wrapping kha nom jok ingredients together symbolizes bringing people together.

instance, while cooking dinner for the family can be a pleasant experience in itself, consuming it together around the table might provide sustenance and create a sense of connection with others. Depending on the menu, it might also serve as a reward, a family celebration, and a potent symbol of affection (De Vault, 1991). Although most of these examples relate to women's occupations, there is no reason to think that men do not experience similar benefits from masculine pursuits. Trevor, for example, willingly climbed a ladder to lend a hand, fixing the guttering on the shower block at the campground where he was holidaying (Figure 5.5).

TIME USE AND WELL-BEING

As well as the contribution specific occupations make to well-being, the impact of overall patterns of occupations is important. One trend that has been widely noted is the increasing tempo of modern lifestyles. This phenomenon, in which people rush from one occupation to the next, is associated with high workloads, limited access to leisure time pursuits, and increasing levels of stress and stress-related illness (Zuzanek, 1998). Perhaps more significant, because they do not have time to reflect on and experience meaning in living, people are channeled toward culturally constructed occupations such as shopping at the mall rather than pastimes they might find more absorbing and rewarding (Clark, 1997). Such lifestyles appear incompatible with

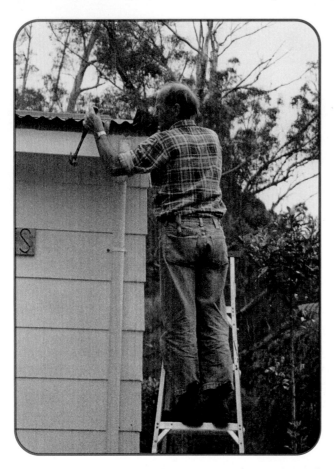

FIGURE 5.5   Trevor fixing the guttering at the campground.

high-level well-being. In response to such concerns, Cusick (1990) suggested categorizing the routine occupations that are undertaken in a typical week as enjoyable, boring, disliked, or performed automatically, in hopes that people might understand the relationship between the things they do and their lack of well-being.

Three further insights in relation to occupation and the ways in which people use time are also pertinent here. The first is the link Erlandsson (2003) established between time use and well-being. Her study traced 100 Swedish women's daily occupations, focusing particularly on transitions from one activity to another. It showed that highly complex patterns of occupation characterized by frequent interruptions and changes of task correlate with lower levels of reported well-being than are found in women with less complex occupational patterns. The second relates to the temporal demands of shift work and the reasons female nurses who work the night shift sacrifice sleep to fulfill their responsibilities as mothers, caregivers, and home-makers (Gallew & Mu, 2004). The long-term impact of disrupted occupational routines and sleep deprivation once again appear incompatible with well-being. The third consideration in relation to time use is the boredom that results from lack of occupation. Drawing from her study of young offenders, Farnworth (1998) proposed that boredom

is perhaps "endemic in Western industrialized nations" (p. 145). The short- and long-term impact of boredom on health and well-being is unknown, in part because boredom itself is poorly understood. Nonetheless, workplace boredom has been associated with low morale, depression, and engagement in destructive and unauthorized activities (Long, 2004).

Over a longer time span, occupational scientists and others have suggested, people become what they do. Two studies in particular lend support to a relationship between what people do over their lifetime and well-being. They first proposed the concept of occupational persona, which is described as an aspect of self that "is shaped, and to some extent reinvented" through engagement in occupation (Whiteford & Wicks, 2000, p. 48). Of note in the context of this discussion are several themes used to depict these personas, variously described as having a passion, seizing opportunities, creating fun, feeling proud and satisfied, and creating a better world, which echo definitions of well-being.

The second study addressed the occupational potential that each person realizes, in the context of personal, historical, sociocultural, and political influences (Wicks, 2001, 2005). Looking back over a lifetime, the person might or might not derive a sense of well-being depending on the person's evaluation of his or her choices and accomplishments and the person's restrictions and regrets. As this discussion implies, it is the evaluation of their choices and accomplishments that influences the extent to which people experience well-being. As Casey (1995) observed, some "experiences restrict opportunities for personal control, skill-use and intimacy" (p. 81). If, in addition, opportunities for personal development are few and use of "initiative, thought and independent judgment . . . [is not welcomed, then] what people do in their work directly affects their cognitive functioning, their values, their conceptions of self, and their orientations to the world around them" (p. 82). Although Casey's focus was on people's employment experiences, it is conceivable that other people experience similar restrictions in other realms of life.

OCCUPATION, IMPAIRMENT, AND WELL-BEING

It is well known that occupation can harm people. Indeed, to shock the nation into legislative reform, nineteenth century social reformers graphically exposed the ways in which working in Britain's coal mines stunted, maimed, and sickened workers (Wilcock, 2001). Although safety standards, working hours, and the grueling physical demands of previous decades have substantially improved (Guber, 1995), the risks that workplace occupations pose to health and well-being remain a focus for unions and governments alike. Less attention has been paid to the risks that nonwork occupations may pose and people's experience of participation in day-to-day occupations when they have an **impairment**.

The term *impairment*, in everyday language, suggests an injury, flaw, or imperfection or that some harm has occurred. In this context, a more precise meaning is implied, consistent with the World Health Organization's *International Classification of Functioning, Disability and Health* (2001). That is, an impairment is any problem with normal psychological or physiological function or with a body structure such as a joint or organ. In this sense, health conditions may cause impairments, for example, loss of power in an arm after a stroke. In addition, impairments may put people at risk of a health condition, such as a person who becomes depressed when denied access to work because of a cognitive impairment.

Although few studies have explored the relationship between occupation, impairment, and well-being, a small body of occupationally focused studies suggests that the presence of impairment may or may not undermine well-being. One determining factor seems to be the effect impairment has on participation in occupation. For instance, older people who were admitted to the hospital after an acute health episode discovered by trying to do things how their impairments had changed their capacity for occupation. This knowledge underscored the seriousness of their condition. However, as their health stabilized and they mastered new ways of completing tasks, they grew more hopeful and sought opportunities to test and strengthen their returning function (Gooder, 2001). Theirs was an experience of return to well-being. Similarly, while men with dyspraxia struggle to complete once familiar tasks such as putting on socks and shoes or making a hot drink, their small successes and signs of improvement elicited expressions of triumph and renewed hopefulness for the future (Blijlevens, 2005).

In contrast, adults with a rapidly advancing neurological disease experienced their impairments as losses, evidencing not only diminishing occupational capacity but also loss of valued aspects of identity, inability to access occupational settings that gave variety to life, and an inevitable decline toward dependency and death (Brott, 2004; Hocking, Brott, & Paddy, 2006). Expressions of courage, humor, gratitude for remaining abilities, and appreciation for the support received from family and health care workers were overshadowed by fatigue, frustration, distress over loss of the future they had envisaged, and fear of becoming a burden. Each of these has an occupational component:

◆ Fatigue from basic self-care tasks
◆ Frustration over declining occupational capacity, barriers to valued occupations, and long hours that were no longer filled with productive activity
◆ Regret for occupations they had looked forward to and would now not achieve, such as holding a grandchild

As their health declined, their sense of well-being was under constant threat.

Considered together, these studies suggest that whether impairments detract from well-being is influenced as much by a person's expectations for the future as by his or her present-day experiences.

Despite enjoying what they do and being hopeful for the future, however, people who have an impairment can face external barriers that undermine well-being. Roulstone (1998) found that 90% of people with a disability who used enabling technologies at work identified ways in which technology directly benefited them. Nonetheless, they reported continued barriers to employment, including problems with "limited workplace access, inadequate training, under use and misuse of new technology, and the continued presence of disabling attitudes" (p. 125). They reported being made to feel like an inferior worker, instances of physical impairment being equated with low intellect, and a general expectation that they "should feel lucky that their employers have the heart to employ them" (p. 115). In addition, they faced begrudging attitudes and resentment toward the provision of technology when they were given technology that was not available to able-bodied workers.

In addition to these workplace issues, people with an impairment that affects occupational performance find that societal factors make participation in work more difficult. The women in Jakobsen's (2004) study, for instance, battled with the lack of recognition of the additional physical and psychological rigors of self-care and domestic tasks for those who are not able-bodied. They also reported difficulty managing appointments with health care workers, home help, wheelchair maintenance personnel, and care assistants, who were available only during work hours. Despite being highly motivated to work and deriving all the benefits of employment that others report, all three women found participation in work too strenuous and resigned their positions. In sum, Roulstone's and Jakobsen's studies suggest that the benefits most people derive from employment might not be sufficient to support well-being in the face of unavoidable barriers in the physical, social, and attitudinal environment.

STRUCTURING OCCUPATION TO ENHANCE WELL-BEING

Even if workplace experiences do not always support well-being, people are surprisingly resourceful in structuring their occupations to support and enhance well-being. For instance, immigrant women, recently arrived in New Zealand from India, adopted three key strategies to help them settle in and feel at home. They consciously preserved some occupations from their home country, stuck to familiar routes and venues for repeat occupations such as grocery shopping, and asked for advice about how things are done in their adopted country (Nayar, 2005).

Similarly, as people recovered from mental illness, they reported progressing from a disintegrated experience

CASE STUDY: *Do or Die*

Dennis is 11 years old and lives in a low-socioeconomic-level suburb of a large city in Sweden. He likes to watch television and, as he has grown older, has started to play computer games and to surf the Internet. On average, he spends around 3 hours a day on the computer (Magnusson, Hulthén, & Kjellgren, 2005). If he lived in Israel, that figure might have been as high as 4½ or 5 hours per day (Nemet et al., 2005). While he watches, plays games, or surfs, Dennis likes to have a glass of fruit juice or lemonade. Like the other 30% of children in his suburb who are overweight or obese, he also tends to skip breakfast. Despite the health risks adults associate with low levels of physical activity, high calorie intake, and starting the day without food, Dennis does not believe that his lifestyle has any effect on his health (Magnusson, Hulthén, & Kjellgren, 2005).

Is Obesity So Bad?

Were he located in New Zealand, the health risks Dennis faces would be well recognized. If he were one of the 26% of boys of Pacific Island heritage aged 7–14 years who are obese, he would face well-documented risks of joining those already presenting with type II diabetes (Ministry of Health, 2003). In a few years, he might well contribute to the skyrocketing figures for life-threatening cardiovascular disease and, rather than following the trend of increasing longevity recorded over recent decades, have a substantially reduced life expectancy.

What If Dennis Were American?

If he were American, we might suspect that Dennis's obesity was associated with some well-known features of the urban landscape. As reported in *Time* magazine, most American cities were designed for automobiles (Wallis, Miranda, & Park, 2005). That means that most suburbs lack sidewalks and bike paths. No wonder that between 1991 and 1995, walking anywhere became 40% less likely and the chances of walking to school were reduced by 60%. Indeed by 2001, the statistics report, walking and riding a bicycle accounted for only 13% of trips to school. All this suggests that even if Dennis lived less than a mile from school, he would not have walked.

In fact, locating Dennis in the United States rather than in Sweden might have meant a lifestyle with very little physical effort, especially given that many schools with tight budgets have trimmed physical education classes from the curriculum. Furthermore, his parents might be among the 65% of Americans who would like to exercise more but do not have enough time, find exercise boring (28%), or do not have access to a convenient place to exercise (24%). One advantage of being in the United States, however, is that Dennis would be in the midst of a growing awareness that lack of physical exercise might be an even greater threat to health than obesity (Wallis, Miranda, & Park, 2005).

Can Anything Be Done?

Perhaps if he lived in Israel, Dennis might have been one of the 54 obese children recruited to a research group (Nemet et al., 2005). With a little luck and the right attitude, he might have found his way into the active treatment group and been one of 20 participants to complete a three-month exercise program and one-year follow-up. In that case, Dennis would have had the privilege of joining in games led by former members of the national track and field team for two hours each week. To supplement that program, Dennis and his parents would have participated in counseling sessions focusing on food choice and behavior change. That advice would have included cutting his food intake by about 30%. He would also have been encouraged to walk or engage in some other physical exercise for another 30 to 45 minutes a week.

At follow-up, it is likely that Dennis would have gained less than a kilo in weight, compared to the average 5.2 kilos put on by children in the control group. He would have significantly less body fat and more important, significantly increased activity levels and physical endurance. In addition, he would have cut his TV and video game time by more than an hour a day (Nemet et al., 2005).

Questions and Exercises

- Research results cited in this case study identify calorie intake, physical inactivity, and urban design as factors contributing to childhood obesity and its associated health problems. What other parental, environmental, societal, or legislative factors can you identify as contributing to the problem?
- The program implemented in Israel might or might not be feasible in your context. If you were working with children between 6 and 16 years old, what features of the Israeli program would you hope to replicate and which would you modify?

of doing and being they described as nondoing, through different levels of occupational engagement characterized variously as half-doing, engaged doing, and absorbed doing. This progression enabled their participation in the human and nonhuman world at an intensity they could sustain and that contributed to their reconnection with the environment, structuring of time and space, reintegration of a sense of self, and the opening up of future possibilities in the everyday world (Sutton, 2006).

At a community level rather than an individual level, an elder of the Windjingare tribe in Australia described how he drew on traditional ideas about socially useful work to help his people break the cycle of welfare dependency, alcoholism, and violence. The venture focused on vocational opportunities in the bush, where young people learned traditional skills and values and built culturally appropriate housing, using their own labor and incorporating bush materials. A key element, in line with long-established practices, was the intention to move between different locations and occupations for the wet and dry seasons (Shaw & Dann, 1999).

CONCLUSION

The things we do meet our biological needs for sustenance and shelter. Occupation keeps us alive. In the longer term, occupation can provide the physical activity, mental stimulation, and social interaction we need to keep our bodies, minds, and communities healthy. In addition, through participation in occupation, we express ourselves, develop skills, experience pleasure and involvement, and achieve the things we believe to be important. In short, we have opportunities for enhanced levels of well-being. Being healthy supports engagement in occupation, and it is often in the process of doing things that we realize how healthy we are and enjoy a heightened sense of well-being.

Equally, occupation can threaten or destroy health. Doing too much, doing too little, and doing things that expose us to risk can all have deleterious effects. It is also important to recognize that it is often through having trouble doing things that we become aware of health issues and the full impact of impairments. Furthermore, physical, social, or attitudinal barriers in the environment can exacerbate the impact of a health condition or impairment, sometimes to the point at which participation in occupation is unsustainable. However, if we carefully structure the things we do, review lifestyle choices, and address barriers to participation, engagement in occupation can improve people's health and well-being.

PROVOCATIVE QUESTIONS

1. Wilcock proposed that people have needs that serve as warnings, protect us, and reward participation in occupation. Why, then, do most people in postindustrial societies fail to get sufficient exercise?
2. If immigrant women, people recovering from mental illness, and community leaders can structure occupations to enhance their own and others' health and well-being without help from an occupational therapist, are occupational therapists necessary?
3. Which of your occupations support your health and well-being? Which threaten them? How could you change your lifestyle or environment to maximize well-being?
4. If you could change one thing in the physical, social, and attitudinal environment of your country to enhance the nation's health and well-being, what would you change? How would the change you propose affect people's occupations?

REFERENCES

Aguis, T. (1993). Aboriginal health in aboriginal hands. In J. Fuller, J. Barclay, & J. Zollo (Eds.), *Multicultural health-care in South Australia* (pp. 127–135). Adelaide: University of South Australia.

Blaxter, M. (1990). *Health and lifestyles.* London: Travistock/Routledge.

Blijlevens, H. (2005). *The experience of dyspraxia in everyday life.* Unpublished master's thesis, Auckland University of Technology, Auckland, New Zealand.

Brott, T. (2004). *Living with motor neurone disease: An interpretive study.* Unpublished master's thesis, Auckland University of Technology, Auckland, New Zealand.

Casey, C. (1995). *Work, self and society: After industrialism.* London: Routledge.

Centers for Disease Control and Prevention. (2005a). *Heath behaviors of adults: United States, 1999–2000* (Series 10, N. 219, 2003). Washington, DC: U.S. Department of Health and Human Services. Retrieved August 2, 2005, from www.cdc.gov/nchs/dataseries/sr_10/gr10_219.pdf

Centers for Disease Control and Prevention. (2005b). *Summary health statistics for the U.S. population: National health interview survey* (Series 10, N. 224, 2003). Washington, DC: U.S. Department of Health and Human Services. Retrieved August 2, 2005, from www.cdc.gov/nchs/date/series/gr_10224.pdf

Christiansen, C. (1996). Three perspectives on balance in occupation. In R. Zemke & F. Clark (Eds.), *Occupational science: The evolving discipline* (pp. 417–435). Philadelphia: F. A. Davis.

Clark, F. (1997). Reflections on the human as an occupational being: Biological need, tempo and temporality. *Journal of Occupational Science: Australia, 4*(3), 86–92.

Csikszentmihalyi, M. (1993). Activity and happiness: Toward a science of occupation. *Journal of Occupational Science: Australia, 1*(1), 38–42.

Cusick, A. (1990). *Choices: What am I doing with my life?* Sydney, Australia: Simon & Schuster.

De Vault, M. L. (1991). *Feeding the family: The social organization of caring as gendered work.* Chicago: University of Chicago Press.

Dickie, V. A. (2003). The role of learning in quilt making. *Journal of Occupational Science, 10*(3), 120–129.

Dickie, V. A. (2004). From drunkard's path to Kansas cyclones: Discovering creativity inside the blocks. *Journal of Occupational Science, 11*(2), 51–57.

Durie, M. (1994). Māori perspectives on health and illness. In J. Spicer, A. Trlin, & J. A. Walton (Eds.), *Social dimensions of health and disease: New Zealand perspectives* (pp. 194–203). Palmerston North, New Zealand: Dunmore Press.

Erlandsson, L.-K. (2003). *101 women's patterns of daily occupations.* Lund, Sweden: Lund University.

Farnworth, L. (1998). Doing, being, and boredom. *Journal of Occupational Science, 5*(3), 141–146.

Gallew, H. A., & Mu, K. (2004). An occupational look at temporal adaptation: Night shift nurses. *Journal of Occupational Science, 11*(1), 23–30.

Glanze, W. D. (Ed.). (1990). *Mosby's medical, nursing, and allied health dictionary* (3rd ed.). St. Louis: Mosby.

Glass, T. A., de Leon C. M., Marottoli, R. A., & Berkman, L. F. (1999). Population based study of social and productive activities as predictors of survival among elderly Americans. *British Medical Journal, 310,* 478–483.

Gooder, J. (2001). *Becoming human again: Older adults' experience of rehabilitation in hospital.* Unpublished master's thesis. Auckland University of Technology, Auckland, New Zealand.

Graham, S. F. (2002). Dance: A transformative occupation. *Journal of Occupational Science, 9*(3), 128–134.

Guber, H. E. (1995). Visionary realism, lifespan discretionary time, and the evolving role of work. In L. M. W. Martin, K. Nelson, & E. Tobach (Eds.), *Sociocultural psychology: Theory and practice of doing and knowing* (pp. 383–404). New York: Cambridge University Press.

Hasselkus, B. R. (2002). *The meaning of everyday occupation.* Thorofare, NJ: Slack.

Hocking, C., Brott, T., & Paddy, A. (2006). Caring for people with motor neurone disease. *International Journal of Therapy and Rehabilitation, 13*(8), 351–355.

Hocking, C., Wright-St. Clair, V., & Bunrayong, W. (2002). The meaning of cooking and recipe work for older Thai and New Zealand women. *Journal of Occupational Science, 9*(3), 117–127.

Howie, L. (2003). Ritualising in book clubs: Implications for evolving occupational identities. *Journal of Occupational Science, 10*(3), 130–139.

Jakobsen, K. (2004). If work doesn't work: How to enable occupational justice. *Journal of Occupational Science, 11*(3), 125–134.

Loland, N. W. (2004). Exercise, health, and aging. *Journal of Aging and Physical Activity, 11,* 170–184.

Long, C. (2004). On watching paint dry: An exploration of boredom. In M. Molineux (Ed.), *Occupation for occupational therapists* (pp. 78–89). Oxford, UK: Blackwell.

Magnusson, M. B., Hulthén, L., & Kjellgren, K. I. (2005). Obesity, dietary pattern and physical activity among children in a suburb with a high proportion of immigrants. *Journal of Human Nutrition & Dietetics, 18*(3), 187–194.

Miller, D. (1998). *A theory of shopping.* Cambridge, UK: Polity Press.

Ministry of Health. (2003). NZ food, NZ children: Findings of the 2002 national children's nutrition survey. Wellington, New Zealand: Author. Retrieved July 21, 2005, from http://www.moh.govt.nz/moh.nsf/49ba80c00757b8804c256673001d47d0/064234a7283a0478cc256dd60000ab4c/$FILE/NZ_Food,_NZ_Children_sectionE.pdf

Ministry of Health Manatū Hauora. (2005). Decades of disparity II: Socio-economic mortality trends in New Zealand, 1981–1999. Wellington, New Zealand: Author.

Mozley, C. G. (2001). Exploring the connections between occupation and mental health in care homes for older people. *Journal of Occupational Science, 8*(3), 14–19.

Nayar, S. (2005). *Two becoming one: Immigrant Indian women sustaining self and well-being through doing: A grounded theory study.* Unpublished master's thesis, Auckland University of Technology, Auckland, New Zealand.

Nemet, D., Barkan, S., Epstein, Y., Friedland, O., Kowen, G., & Eliakim, A. (2005). Short- and long-term beneficial effects of a combined dietary-behavioral-physical activity intervention for the treatment of childhood obesity. *Pediatrics, 115,* 43–449.

Persson, D., Eklund, M., & Isacsson, A. (1999). The experience of everyday occupations and its relation to sense of coherence: A methodological study. *Journal of Occupational Science, 6*(1), 13–26.

Primeau, L. (1996). Running as an occupation: Multiple meanings and purposes. In R. Zemke & F. Clark (Eds.), *Occupational science: The evolving discipline* (pp. 275–286). Philadelphia: F. A. Davis.

Roulstone, A. (1998). *Enabling technology: Disabled people, work and new technology.* Philadelphia: Open University Press.

Scheerer, C. R., Cahill, L. G., Kirby, K., & Lane, J. (2004). Cake decorating as occupation: Meaning and motivation. *Journal of Occupational Science, 11*(2), 68–74.

Shaw, K., & Dann, J. (1999). Work is sacred: The journey out of welfare. *Journal of Occupational Science, 6*(2), 80–87.

Stanley, M. (1995). An investigation into the relationship between engagement in valued occupations and life satisfaction for elderly South Australians. *Journal of Occupational Science: Australia, 3*(3), 100–114.

Sutton, D. (2006, July). *The lived experience of occupational performance during recovery from mental illness.* World Federation of Occupational Therapists Congress, Sydney, Australia.

Vance, D. E., Wadley, V. G., Ball, K. K., Roenker, D. L., & Rizzo, M. (2005). The effects of physical activity and sedentary behavior on cognitive health in older adults. *Journal of Aging and Physical Activity, 13,* 294–313.

Wallis, C., Miranda, C. A., & Park, A. (2005). Get moving! *Time, 165*(23), 46–51.

Whiteford, G., & Wicks, A. (2000). Occupation: Person, environment, engagement and outcomes. An analytic review of the *Journal of Occupational Science* profiles. Part 2. *Journal of Occupational Science, 7*(2), 48–57.

Whitehead, M. (1988). *The health divide.* New York: Penguin.

Wicks, A. (2001). Occupational potential: A topic worthy of exploration. *Journal of Occupational Science, 8*(3), 32–35.

Wicks, A. (2005). Understanding occupational potential. *Journal of Occupational Science, 12*(3), 130–139.

Wilcock, A. (1993). A theory of the human need for occupation. *Journal of Occupational Science: Australia, 1*(1), 17–24.

Wilcock, A. (1995). The occupational brain: A theory of human nature. *Journal of Occupational Science: Australia, 2*(1), 68–73.

Wilcock, A. A. (1998). *An occupational perspective of health.* Thorofare, NJ: Slack.

Wilcock, A. A. (2001). *Occupation for health, Volume 1: A journey from self health to prescription.* London: British Association and College of Occupational Therapy.

World Health Organization. (2001). *International classification of functioning, disability and health.* Geneva: Author.

World Health Organization, Health and Welfare Canada, Canadian Public Health Association. (1986). *Ottawa charter for health promotion.* Ottawa: WHO.

Wright-St. Clair, V., Bunrayong, W., Vittayakorn, S., Rattakorn, P., & Hocking, C. (2004). Offerings: Food traditions of older Thai women at Songkran. *Journal of Occupational Science, 11*(3), 115–124.

Zuzanek, J. (1998). Time use, time pressure, personal stress, mental health, and life satisfaction from a life cycle perspective. *Journal of Occupational Science, 5*(1), 26–39.

Culture, Race, Ethnicity, and Other Forms of Human Diversity in Occupational Therapy

6

JULI McGRUDER

" What sets worlds in motion is the interplay of differences, their attractions and repulsions. Life is plurality, death is uniformity. By suppressing differences and peculiarities, by eliminating different civilizations and cultures, progress weakens life and favors death. The ideal of a single civilization for everyone, implicit in the cult of progress and technique, impoverishes and mutilates us. Every view of the world that becomes extinct, every culture that disappears, diminishes a possibility of life. "

—OCTAVIO PAZ (1967)

Learning Objectives

After reading this chapter, you will be able to:

1. Discuss culture in terms of a list of six agreed-on attributes.
2. List and discuss five reasons for occupational therapists to strive for an accurate understanding of culture and other forms of diversity.

3. Distinguish between cultural awareness and cultural sensitivity and examine one's own levels of each.

CULTURE AND OTHER FORMS OF HUMAN DIVERSITY IN OCCUPATIONAL THERAPY

My friend Lizzi grew up in rural Oregon, surrounded by plants and animals. Now an adult, living in the suburbs, Lizzi plants dozens of flower bulbs and "puts up" scores of quarts of fruits and vegetables every year. She even cans foods that she does not eat, such as fish. She has a rambunctious young Labrador retriever, an elderly cat, and a noisy parrot. Lizzi also has tetraplegia, from a C5–6 spinal cord injury, and very compromised hand function. She admits that snapping beans and peeling peaches are laborious and difficult activities for her and that managing the hot water bath for her canned goods has led to so many burns that she now delegates this part of the canning activity to her goddaughter. Still, she would never choose to give up her canning. While she notes that Bijou, the Labrador, could easily tip her wheelchair, she persists in her routine of coming home from a long day of advocacy work to patiently train the young dog.

When I visit Lizzi, I stand in awe of the power of culture to influence occupational choice. If I had Lizzi's physical limitations, I would give up the bit of gardening I do. I would not take on the care routines of three pets or the laborious tasks of canning. Yet Lizzi chooses to reenact with her sisters, nieces, and goddaughters the productive social activity of gathering in the kitchen several times each year to preserve foods, just as her mother and aunts did. She chooses to pass on the cultural tradition of canning the best pickled green beans. This is culture at work. The high value attached to home-processed foodstuffs, the knowledge of recipe contents and processes, the form of the gendered social gathering, and even the idea that vegetable matter steeped in vinegar and salt is delicious have all been culturally transmitted. Because culture underlies occupational choice, it is of central interest to occupational therapy practitioners.

Culture is a notoriously difficult concept to define. A recent dialogue in *American Journal of Occupational Therapy* reviewed definitions of culture, the history of their use by anthropologists, and their current utility for occupational therapy practitioners (Bonder, Martin, & Miracle, 2004; Dickie, 2004). In occupational therapy, *culture* has been defined as learned, shared experience that provides "the individual and the group with effective mechanisms for interacting both with others and with the surrounding environment" (Krefting & Krefting, 1991, p. 102) and as evident in both group patterns and individual variations in occupational behavior (Bonder, Martin, & Miracle, 2004). The American Occupational Therapy Association (AOTA) defines culture as "customs, beliefs,

activity patterns, behavior standards and expectations accepted by the society of which the individual is a member" (2002, p. 623). Frank and colleagues prefer a definition that recognizes the contested status of cultures "as composed of competing discourses and practices within social fields characterized by the unequal distribution of power" (2001, p. 503). Occupational therapy practitioners aim to discover and support clients' agency in making meaning in everyday actions and activities, which necessitates interaction with the cultural worlds into which their clients have been socialized (Mattingly & Beer, 1993).

Culture is just one distinguishing human characteristic, however, and cannot be relied on to explain all kinds of difference. Dyck (1992) cautioned occupational therapy practitioners not to confuse culture and other sources of difference when she wrote:

> A reliance on culture as distinct beliefs, values, and customary practices to explain nonadherence and difficulties in the therapeutic process is misguided. The everyday social and work conditions that shape health experiences and behaviors must also be recognized. These, in turn, are forged within a socioeconomic and political environment. (p. 696)

Dyck (1993) and Fitzgerald (2004) have raised this specific caution in the use of the culture concept in occupational therapy. Their concern is informed by three more general criticisms of conceptualizations of culture: that the concept, misused, has a tendency to essentialize, reify, and mystify human difference. To *essentialize* is to take complex multifaceted phenomena, such as the lifeways, ideas, and all that a group of humans has acquired by learning, and reduce them to a few basic and inherent "essences" that purport to explain this group in totality. Descriptions that essentialize are often ahistorical, and in that way, they distort. To *reify* is to "thing-ify," to take an abstract and to treat it as a fixed and concrete thing with definable boundaries. Treating culture as a thing can promote stereotyping. Reifying culture ignores the interactive nature of humans as creators of culture situated in environments that change. Reifying fails to notice that many humans have incorporated ideas from more than one culture. To *mystify* is to obscure important causes, contributing factors, or results of a phenomenon. For example, when Senator Daniel Patrick Moynihan (1965) referred to the African-American family as a "tangle of pathology," he obscured the economic and political factors that underlay cultural phenomena he was criticizing. Dyck, quoted above, was specifically concerned that differences in seeking and following health care advice noted among Chinese immigrant women in Canada not be misunderstood as cultural when in fact the source of difference was related to economics and work situations. She documented a similar concern related to health promotion research with Indo-Canadian Sikh mothers (Dyck,

1993). Attempts to define or discuss culture should try not to reproduce common errors and fallacies. With that precaution in mind, let's examine a list of agreed-on defining attributes of culture.

WHAT CULTURE IS: AN AGREED-ON LIST

Culture Is Real

While not concrete or tangible, culture is real. When someone falls ill because of a curse, the illness is real. When someone feels peace or joy because appropriate rituals have appeased supernatural beings, the emotional state is significant and real. When people stand in ritual costumes in front of a representative of the Almighty or the State, recite traditional word strings, and exchange specifically ordained pieces of jewelry, they achieve a different social status that affects their kin relations and their economic and social status with the government: They are married! That is the power of culture, and each culture shapes, among other things, the forms and meanings of changes in social status in the group. We cannot see or touch culture, but its effects surround us, rendering culture a very real force.

Culture Is Not Inherited, It Is Learned

Beliefs and values are taught to us both explicitly and tacitly in our families and communities and by mass media. Most readers will not have learned much about spirits, curses, or propitiation rituals but will have been taught in thousands of ways that they are each unique individuals with inalienable rights. The idea that we are individuals with a free will and a "natural" right to our own opinions seems a given to Americans, but it is a cultural idea, quite foreign to others. Observers from other cultures have commented on the ways in which we entrain this idea of individual self-determination in children. I once counted how many decisions a middle-class European-American preschooler was offered in her first waking hour of the day. The decisions—about what to wear, where to dress, what to eat—numbered around 20. The child was actively being taught about her individuality and her right to choose. Later that evening, as adults were discussing where to go for dinner, this child announced, "Those are your ideas, and I have ideas of my own." At age 3, she had already internalized the dominant cultural ideal of individual intellectual independence.

Culture Is Not Idiosyncratic But Is Shared in Human Society

Although it may be carried in the minds of individuals, as some have argued, culture's manifestations are social.

How do you greet your grandfather? With a verbal greeting only, with a hug, or with a kiss on the cheek or his hand? How many such kisses? Do you bend down to touch his feet? Do you shake his hand, then kiss your own and place it over your heart, as a respectful child in coastal East Africa would? Do you seek or avoid eye contact with him? Or do you ignore him? Scholars of culture may dispute whether it is the greeting behavior itself or the shared understanding that underlies it that is the locus of culture, but all agree that culture is shared socially. As such, it is most easily perceived in interactions between and among people. Dickie (2004) reminded occupational therapists that while our focus may be the effects of cultural socialization on individual agency and action, we must not ignore the collective and social nature of culture.

Culture Changes, Usually Slowly

Culture has incredible staying power, is conservative, and does not easily change (Dickie, 2004). But culture is not static, fixed, or immutable. Values, attitudes, aesthetics, lifeways, arts, morals, customs, laws, and the many other things that are included in culture can change in response to the forces of history, politics, and economics. Culture is malleable and dynamic.

Even a cursory glance at the advertising media of the United States in the twenty-first century would reveal that we are encouraged to think that light brown or beige skin, narrow muscular buttocks, large chests, and full lips are aesthetically pleasing in either gender. But it was not always so. For example, before the Industrial Revolution, when European peasants labored outdoors, suntanned skin was not considered aesthetically pleasing; it was considered a mark of low class. The North American and European leisured classes of the preindustrial era took pains to protect the whiteness of their skins even while enjoying outdoor activities. It was not until workers went indoors to sunless factories that suntanning became a mark of expendable income and leisure time and thus became culturally valued. A review of racialized mass media, as done by Marlon Riggs (1986) in the film "Ethnic Notions," shows that full lips were a feature of African origin that was once hyperbolized and demeaned. Now film actresses and models get collagen injections to make their lips fuller. Aesthetics are cultural, and cultures change as human groups encounter each other. When groups of humans come into contact, they influence each other's cultures by imitation, innovation, and even coercion. When the political and economic environment changes, cultures adapt to that change. Dickie (2004) includes a wonderful example of both the changing and changeless aspects of an American cultural ritual, the family reunion. Among the unchanging aspects is the preference for summer outdoor venues, with the elders sitting in the shade reminiscing and the children playing. What has changed for many families is the more inclusive definition of family, with people invited who would have been excluded just decades ago: same-sex couples, unmarried couples living together, divorced spouses, and step-grandparents.

Culture Drives Values

Culture shapes human values. We rely on our enculturation in one or more cultural worlds to determine what is right and wrong, good and bad, beautiful and ugly, included and excluded, appropriate and inappropriate, safe and dangerous. The cultural values that we have internalized guide our occupational choices and our daily routines for getting things done. Breaking cultural norms that were learned early can provoke a visceral reaction. When traveling in a Muslim country, if I hand someone something with my left hand, I immediately feel wrong and embarrassed because I have been taught to use my right hand for exchanges in Muslim cultures. When I return to the United States, I experience this same feeling of "wrongness" until I readjust to American expectations, usually after a couple of fumbling exchanges with perplexed-looking clerks.

As occupational therapy practitioners, we are often in contact with people who, because of misfortune or a time of crisis, are trying hard to decide what is right and good. We respect their cultures by giving them a psychologically supportive space in which to make meaningful what has happened to them and to apply the values they have lived by.

Culture Is Invisible

Culture is invisible, especially to those who participate in it. It is taken for granted. A common analogy used is "as the water is to the fish." We are often blind to our own cultures, but when we encounter cultural ways that are different from our own, we perceive the otherness, the strangeness of the other group's ways. Still, it takes repeated experiences with entering other cultural spaces, coupled with introspection, just to make our own cultural assumptions visible to us.

Whiteford and Wilcock (2000) point out that the person who is most likely to be blind to his or her own cultural assumptions is white, heterosexual, and middle class. Often, members of minority groups have been socialized into both their own groups' ways and the ways of the dominant majority group, giving them an early experience with crossing cultural boundaries. Majority group therapists might mistakenly think that only minority group "others" have a culture that must be taken into account in therapy. Dickie (2004) suggests that the focus on culture as a problem issue in our clinical interactions could productively shift from the culture of the clients to that of the therapist. That is, rather than seeing that culture must be addressed because some clients come from backgrounds unlike that of therapists, we might shift focus and see that the limited cultural excursions of the majority of therapists hinder their ability to understand and help all of their clients.

One manifestation of our profession's occasional culture blindness that is repeatedly remarked on in our literature is the emphasis on independence as if it were a naturally valued status. Several authors remind us that interdependence with, or dependence on, particular family members in particular activities may be valued, and hence valid, options for clients (Fitzgerald, 2004; Whiteford & Wilcock, 2000). This often-noted potential clash between therapists' cultural and professional values and those of client families is but one of many areas in which difficulties in cross-cultural collaboration can arise.

Even the "nature" of human nature is a culturally constructed entity, invisible to us because we are immersed in it. In Western culture, we accept without question the unity of consciousness and continuity of personhood as obvious and natural. Many cultures include ideas about consciousness and personhood that would strike us as unusual. Most of us do not believe, for example, that we physically travel in our dreams to other places, that spirits of deceased ancestors inhabit the landscape around us, or that our bodies can be literally taken over—possessed—by other active entities. Still, our popular culture in recent years includes stories of angels helping humans, and we seem to be increasingly fascinated by such possibilities. Ideas about spirits, malign or beneficent, and the perhaps permeable limits of the person are part of spiritual practices or cosmologies, and as the Occupational Therapy Practice Framework directs, understanding these ideas as they pertain to clients is within the realm of our practice.

HUMAN DIFFERENCES THAT MAY INFLUENCE CULTURE BUT ARE NOT PRECISELY CULTURAL

Ethnic and Racial Diversity

Culture is not the same as **ethnicity** or race. *Culture* is not a polite synonym for the word *race*, although people who are uncomfortable with discussing race and ethnicity sometimes use it that way. Many occupational therapy authors caution against making this mistake (Bonder, Martin, & Miracle, 2004; Evans, 1992; Fitzgerald 2004). Ethnic groups, according to Weber's (1922/1968) classic definition, are groups that "entertain a subjective belief in their common descent because of similarities of physical type or of customs or of both, or because of memories of colonization and migration" (p. 389). Ethnic identity can be self-selected and built from within a group, imposed from outside it, or both. It is dynamic and fluid, changing in response to social change (Cornell & Hartmann, 1998).

Race and ethnicity are socially constructed categories, concepts agreed on in public and private discourse that can be understood only in the context of the history of their employment in a particular place.

When ethnic labels are assigned from outside the group, the group's phenotype or appearance is the basis for group assignment. **Phenotype**, the actual physical appearance of an individual, is different from **genotype**, which is the exact genetic makeup of an individual. Even identical twins, whose genotypes are exact copies of one another, have subtle phenotypic differences, including their fingerprints.

In the sad history of human atrocities, a particular phenotype or appearance is often featured in propaganda aimed at isolating or destroying an ethnic group. Thus, Hitler's propaganda included descriptions of the "Jewish type." Hutus in Rwanda massacred those they perceived as Tutsis, people who were said to be taller, with narrower, longer noses. For centuries before, under Belgian and German colonialism, Tutsis—or those perceived as Tutsis—had been favored with land and employment and helped to oppress those perceived as Hutus. Individuals who do not fit the propagandized phenotype in situations of ethnic conflict or genocide are more likely to escape.

Race—although an operative concept in American social life, politics, economics, and entertainment marketing—is not a biological entity. Biologists have shown that there is more variation within than between the so-called races of humans, thus invalidating the categorization on a statistical basis. Moreover, with race as with ethnicity, there is often a difference between phenotype and genotype. To say that race is a bogus concept biologically or that it is socially constructed, however, does not mean that race is not psychologically or socially real. Dealing with race relations is a very real part of life. Humans are killed on the basis of race. Humans are denied or given rights and privileges on the basis of race. Although race and ethnicity are not the same as culture, the historical experience of oppression—or, for that matter, of privilege—based on racial, ethnic, religious, or other group membership can shape culture. Therefore, although race, ethnicity, or religion and culture are distinct concepts, they may overlap, interact, and intersect with each other.

Large groups, such as those based on race, language, religion, or national origin, are often more heterogeneous than homogeneous and might not share much overlap in cultural beliefs, attitudes, and practices. For example, though African Americans are grouped in a racial category, cultural practices vary within the group (Llorens, 1971). American citizens of African descent who have recently and voluntarily migrated from Africa or who have come from the Caribbean have cultural beliefs, practices, and lifeways that are different from those of African Americans whose families have been in the United States since being forced there by enslavement; nevertheless, these groups share a racial designation in our social sys-tem of labeling race. Teasing apart race, ethnicity, and culture becomes more tricky when we realize that social forces or practices that are used to isolate a racial or ethnic group will affect that group's culture. Racial bias or discriminatory treatment is something that most Americans of African descent have experienced. Some commonly held cultural beliefs and practices have been organized in response to this experience and have functioned to protect family members in a hostile environment.

Race, ethnicity, class, religion, language group, sexual orientation, and gender diversity all interact and affect the cultural adaptation of groups of people. Cultural traditions often carry with them an emphasis on a shared language, just as language is shaped by culture. Consider all speakers of Spanish as a first language. It would not be accurate to say that they share a "Spanish" culture. Still, many of their cultural values, health practices, and occupational traditions employ terms unique to Spanish that do not have a simple, precise translation in other languages.

Our nation includes increasing numbers of families and individuals who are multiracial and multicultural. The 2000 Census allowed multiracial Americans for the first time to check all of the categories that apply in describing their race. In the past, such citizens were forced to pick one race. Approximately 2.4% of Americans, nearly 7 million, identify themselves as of more than one race.

Language Group Diversity

Because occupational therapy practitioners rely on interviews for gathering data relevant to treatment planning, perhaps the diversity that most complicates the treatment process is language diversity. According to the 2000 census, nearly 47 million Americans speak a language other than English at home. Some practitioners are naive about issues surrounding cross-cultural communication (Wardin, 1996). Wardin surveyed occupational therapists to identify both difficulties in cross-lingual communication and examples of successful interaction during the evaluation process. She found that when family members or professional translators were not available, gestural communication was considered reliable. Yet, gestures are not universal, and without an understanding of what gestures mean in different cultural contexts, therapy practitioners risk insulting their clients. In North America, when we gesture for someone to come close, we flex the index finger, and the more pleading and apologetic we are, the more likely we are to minimize the range and the size of this beckoning gesture. In East Africa, a polite "come here" signal must be made with the whole hand and forearm, and using a digit or minimizing the size of the gesture is a serious insult. Signaling "okay" with thumb and index finger or with a thumbs-up seems positive and benign to many of us, but in some cultures these gestures are obscene. Even a smile can be misinterpreted. Smiles may be seen as sly indications of the smiler's superiority

TIPS TO FOLLOW WHEN USING AN INTERPRETER

◆ A trained medical interpreter is held to the same standards of confidentiality that any other health professional must follow. If using a family member or bilingual staff member instead of a trained interpreter, remind the interpreter in front of the client that everything that you and your client say is confidential information, not to be repeated.

◆ Address the client directly. Do not converse with the interpreter about the client.

◆ Do not ask for a summary or expect the interpreter to filter important from nonessential details. It is the interpreter's job to preserve and convey the client's speech and emotional tone in as much detail as possible. A professional medical interpreter conveys not only what is said, but also how it is said. This takes time, so allow extra time.

◆ Pause frequently and ask whether the client has questions. It is both your role and the interpreter's role in a health care situation to minimize the client's discomfort and to ensure mutual understanding.

or that the one smiled at is appearing foolish. One foreign student in the United States noted that he felt that he should return to his room to make certain his trouser fly was closed, because he could think of no other reason for his fellow students to persist in grinning at him so. Clearly, nonverbal communication is an inadequate basis on which to form a therapeutic relationship across cultures.

Many respondents to Wardin's (1996) research worked in systems in which they relied on family members for translation. Problems occur, however, when family members serve as interpreters, frequently because they give help or suggest responses on evaluations. Furthermore, junior family members may experience role strain when required to ask personal questions of, or assertively give directions to, senior family members. Federal legislation mandates provision of translation services in primary health care facilities that accept federal funds (National Center for Cultural Competence, 2000). In some areas, medical interpreter services are available by telephone. See Box 6.1 for tips on using interpreters effectively.

Compared to citizens of other nations, those of the United States are more often monolingual and less aware of cross-cultural communication issues. Wardin's (1996) study showed that practitioners who were functionally bilingual reported more effective practice strategies, even with clients whose languages they did not speak. Thus, there is evidence that language study sensitizes practitioners to issues surrounding limited English proficiency.

Communication is not a simple or straightforward process. When analyzed closely, it can be seen as fraught with so many complications that one is amazed that we understand each other at all. Practitioners acknowledge the need for skillful use of interpreters and for active listening to check that the meaning received is the one intended and to attend to both verbal and nonverbal aspects of communication.

Diversity of Sexual Orientation

Sexual orientation is the physical and emotional attraction toward intimacy with others, seen in spontaneous feelings and erotic desires (Hall, 2001). Sexual orientation, whether heterosexual, homosexual, bisexual, or asexual, is not a choice or a preference (McNaught, 1993a). To say, for example, that a man has a homosexual orientation is not to say that he finds all other men sexually attractive, that he cannot control his sexual impulses toward them, or that he finds women repugnant. It simply means that the individuals to whom he finds himself amorously attracted are male. Homosexual people do not have a particular "lifestyle" or culture; neither do heterosexual people. Both groups comprise people who have many different lifestyles, cultures, races, ethnicities, social classes, and occupations. The experience of group persecution, however, is a strong stimulus to developing shared cultural understandings and values and to the formation of communities, shared rituals such as the annual Gay Pride parades, and unique vocabularies.

The 2000 Census reported that 594,391 households in the United States were made up of same-sex couples who defined themselves as partners; this was 1% of all coupled households. We do not know what makes the majority of the population heterosexual. Similarly, we do not know causes of other sexual orientations, and it is useful to realize that the range of sexual orientations may be an expression of simple natural variations in humans (Hall, 2001). There is nothing that parents, families, friends, or lovers do to "make" people have one orientation or another, and it is difficult if not impossible to change a person's sexual orientation (Hall, 2001). Many myths and stereotypes surround sexual orientation. Dominant cultural disapproval (including harassment and murder of gay individuals) makes it difficult for those who realize that they are not attracted to people of the opposite sex to apply a sexual orientation label to themselves. Self-acceptance is challenged, and the process of reaching psychosexual maturity is complicated for many young people with something other than a heterosexual orientation because our mainstream culture is steeped in images that depict some varieties of sexual expression and sexual orientation as evil or wrong (McNaught, 1993b). This is not to say that gay or lesbian young people are less psychologically healthy but rather that they may find reaching sexual maturity to be fraught with more challenges (Crepeau, 1998; Walsh & Crepeau. 1998). There are many good video, print, and Internet resources for those who want more information on sexual orientation; I recommend books and videos by Brian McNaught (a complete list can be found at http://www.brian-mcnaught.com/resources. html) and the interactive website Sex 101 (http://www. yforum.com/sex101.html), which allows readers to post questions and responses.

Occupational therapy scholars have observed that understanding sexual orientation is important as a theme of meaning and identity in clients' lives and that, as such, it is often expressed in choices of occupations (Jackson, 1995; Wood, 1992). Because their lives are about more than just their sexualities, many people prefer terms such as *gay* and *lesbian* to the term *homosexual*. As we strive to understand the fullness of our clients' lives and occupations, we cannot ignore the sexual dimensions of their personhood. That does not mean that we need to know the specifics of the sexual activities in which they engage— except at times when we might become involved in helping people with disabilities to solve kinesiological problems involved in sexual expression. For all clients, skilled practitioners create an environment in which acceptance of sexuality, as with acceptance of culture, is clear and invites true collaboration. In establishing accurate empathy with our diverse clientele, skilled occupational therapy practitioners avoid **homophobia**, just as they avoid racism and ethnocentricity. Creating a climate of tolerance and acceptance in the workplace also means that gay, lesbian, and bisexual coworkers can focus their efforts on patient care and not on having to keep their identities secret (McNaught, 1993a)

MYTHS, STEREOTYPES, XENOPHOBIA, AND GENERALIZATIONS

With regard to multicultural awareness, a **myth** is an unfounded or poorly founded belief that is given uncritical acceptance by members of a group. Myths operate in support of existing or traditional practices and institutions. **Stereotypes** are mental pictures based on myths that lead people to associate a characteristic or set of characteristics with particular groups of people. **Xenophobia** is an unreasonable fear or hatred of those different from ourselves. Is xenophobia just part of human nature, as some have argued, or is it taught and learned, handed down from adults to children as part and parcel of a social group's culture? The fact that xenophobia can be unlearned and that some humans are consistently attracted to those who are different from themselves argues against a view of humans as naturally suspicious of other humans not of their own group.

The tendencies to generalize, however, and to cluster perceptions in memory do appear to be inherent parts of the human mental apparatus. Piaget (1969) described the development of children's thinking in terms of forming and refining schemata for grouping objects and creatures in the natural world around them. Thinking about such cognitive clustering can provide some insights into how myths and stereotypes about groups of others are formed. It is a way to begin to undo some of the myths and stereotypes we might have incorporated into our own thinking about human diversity.

Let's say that at some point in your youth, you heard the phrase *woman driver*. The circumstances under which you heard this term employed allowed you to understand quickly that it was a phrase meant to disparage the abilities of women to operate motor vehicles safely and efficiently. Having heard the phrase used once or twice, you internalized this concept, even if just on a trial basis. With the concept embedded in your mental apparatus, you were readily able to incorporate and file away in this conceptual category any and all instances you noted personally or heard about in which a female did indeed operate a motor vehicle in an unskilled or unsafe manner. Conversely, there was no handy cognitive schema in which you might mentally record, in a ready-made category, all incidents or reports of males driving badly. Challenged to recall instances of or anecdotes about bad driving by females and by males, you would much more readily retrieve from memory all those precoded instances of bad driving by females. A concept is introduced, and as with a self-fulfilling prophecy, evidence begins to be amassed through experience— experience filtered through previously learned cognitive categories. You might well conclude that women are worse drivers than men. Then you would be confronted with a different reality. Insurance actuarial tables show that, in fact, women are better drivers than men, and insurance companies, large and small, honor that truth in the way they structure differential rates for coverage by gender in certain age groups and where allowed under state law.

Humans apparently cannot turn off the grouping, generalizing, and schemata-building aspects of their minds. However, we can rigorously examine the generalizations we make about other humans and the conclusions we draw. To practice competently and ethically with a diversity of individuals and groups, health care professionals accept the responsibility of examining their generalizations, because adhering to myths and stereotypes leads to poor health care outcomes for stigmatized groups. For example, people of color have less access to health care, receive inferior health care services, and experience worse outcomes of care, including increased rates of mortality and morbidity in many disease categories (Williams, Lavizzo-Mourey, & Warren, 1994).

Generalizations about cultural or racial groups are not all negative or destructive. Health care professionals have sometimes found it useful to generalize from published lists of characterizations of particular ethnic, cultural, or language groups. Recent discussions in occupational therapy literature have joined this text in stating that such lists ought to be used with caution but that learning specifics about cultural groups is a place to start in attaining multicultural competence (Bonder, Martin, & Miracle, 2004; Dickie, 2004; Wells & Black, 2000, Whiteford & Wilcock, 2000) As an example, here is a list that contrasts beliefs, values, and practices of Native Americans with those of Anglo-European Americans, so all the statements are considered relative comparisons. In contrast to European Americans, Native Americans are characterized as (Joe & Malch, 1992):

- More group oriented than individual oriented
- Having respect for elders and experts
- Viewing time and place as permanent and settled
- Being introverted and avoiding ridicule or criticism of others
- Being pragmatic and accepting of what is
- Emphasizing responsibility for family and self more than authority over or responsibility for larger social groups
- Attending to how others behave more than to what they say they think or feel, and seeking harmony

This may be useful information to have as a starting point for observations of and conversations with a particular Native American client or family, but it is important to remain open to the possibility that the individual or various family members may espouse and enact all, some, or none of these beliefs and values. If, for example, the hypothetical client were an urban American Indian Movement activist leader, it is unlikely that she would concern herself only with self and family or pragmatically accept the status quo. The more information that you have about the social history and context of an individual or family group, the better able you will be to discern whether published descriptions of these cultural others apply.

Attempts to generalize from knowledge of another's religion present particular difficulties. While North Americans and Europeans tend to give a religious tradition complete allegiance, excluding the possibility of participating in religious practices springing from other traditions, this is not the rule worldwide. Muslims in North, West, and East Africa, for example, do not experience rituals aimed at recognizing or propitiating capricious and problematic spirits as contradictory to or disrespectful of their Islamic faith. Similarly, spirit possession and animal sacrifice practices by Brazilians practicing candomblé or Cubans practicing santeria, both of which blend elements of Christianity with worship of West African deities, do not see these as interfering with their practice of Roman Catholicism. Conservative orthodox leaders of Sunni Islam or of Roman Catholicism may frown on such practices, but their disapproval is somewhat moot from the perspective of the practitioner–client relationship and attempts at cross-cultural understanding. Medical anthropologists have long observed that, faced with adversity, humans generally try any remedies they perceive as useful, even if those remedies do not fit into one systematic worldview or set of beliefs in the supernatural.

It is also wise to consider the forces of assimilation in applying generalizations. As was noted above, mass media and interactions with other social group members provide a powerful impetus for cultural or racial minorities to adopt dominant group values, beliefs, and practices. This is seen most readily in generations born to immigrant citizens. A client's personal ethos (worldview and approach to life) might well be a creative blend of cultural elements from the previous society or older generation's culture and the new society and culture the client has entered (see Case Study 7.A on the Willard & Spackman Website).

Finally, it is important to realize that the process of generalizing about culturally different others is multi-directional. As you interact with those who are different from you and test hypotheses based on your learned generalizations, others will be doing the same in regard to you. Myths and stereotypes about all cultural and racial groups, including European Americans, abound. Books such as Henry Louis Gates's *Colored People* (1994), Anne Fadiman's *The Spirit Catches You and You Fall Down* (1997), and Anna Deavere Smith's *Twilight, Los Angeles, 1992* (1994) and *Fires in the Mirror* (1993) provide priceless insights into cultural and racial myth making and stereotyping in America. *Distant Mirrors* (DeVita & James, 2002) includes many essays that detail immigrants' and visitors' impressions of American culture. Some of them will probably surprise you.

CULTURE AND OTHER FORMS OF DIVERSITY IN OCCUPATIONAL THERAPY THEORY AND PRACTICE

Mattingly and Beer (1993) offered two reasons for occupational therapy practitioners to strive for an accurate understanding of their clients' cultural backgrounds: to allow for collaboration in goal setting and treatment planning and to individualize therapy. I would add three others: to ensure accurate assessment, to refine occupational therapy theory in ways that take all humans into account, and to increase the likelihood of equitable treatment. Underlying all of these goals of culturally sensitive treatment is the imperative that we establish accurate empathy for our clients.

African Americans, Hispanic and Latino Americans, and Native Americans are underrepresented in our profession. More than 90% of occupational therapy practitioners are white, whereas 76% of the U.S. population is white. Although race and ethnicity are not the same as culture, they are attributes that, like culture, are marked as differences in North American society. As such, they can create challenges to interpersonal understanding between individuals who come from different groups, just as class and culture do. Moreover, occupational therapy practitioners come from a narrower range of class backgrounds than do their clients, and all practitioners share the socializing influence of higher education. If we do not pay attention to differences in a respectful way and do not reflect on our own potential for bias, we will fail at establishing accurate empathy for our clients and good working relationships with them. Occupational therapists of different races responding to a survey agreed on a list of beliefs and values but ascribed different sets of values to ethnic groups other than their own (Pineda, 1996).

We attend to cultural differences during the process of assessment and attempt to choose evaluation instruments and strategies that are not culturally biased and to interpret results correctly. By their very nature, standardized norm-referenced assessment tools make assumptions about normalcy that may be culture bound. Most testing instruments assume characteristics of modal individuals, often based on middle-class European-American lifeways and experiences. For example, Law (1993) found that assessments of activities of daily living (ADL) and instrumental activities of daily living reflected North American dominant cultural values regarding independence and individual rights. Occupational therapy researchers have studied locus of control—a measure of feeling self-determined and empowered—in a variety of populations and found that people of color often score lower (or more externally controlled) than anticipated, perhaps because of the demoralizing influences of racism (Elliot & McGruder, 1995; Janelle, 1992; Spadone, 1992). Occupational therapy practitioners have found that pediatric assessment tools normed in the United States may be biased, inapplicable, or simply not useful in evaluating poor children, ethnic minorities, disadvantaged orphans overseas, or recent immigrants (Bowman & Wallace, 1990; Colonius, 1995; Fudge, 1992; Miller, 1992; Myers, 1992). Even scales of infant behavior might not apply where child-rearing practices differ with culture (Packir, 1994).

A concern with removing cultural bias, insofar as possible, from assessments of ADL in adults inspired the design of the Assessment of Motor and Process Skills, an occupational therapy assessment tool that allows clients choice in what activities to perform and how to perform them. Work is ongoing to determine whether this approach does indeed eliminate bias and lead to cross-cultural validity; results to date are promising (Goto, Fisher, & Mayberry, 1996; Stauffer, Fisher, & Duran, 2000).

Humphry (1995) described how chronic poverty, an experience that is unequally shared across cultural and racial groups in the United States, depersonalizes and erodes the sense of self, alters children's developmental progression, and causes potential conflicts between practitioners and clients or their caregivers around the five universal problems of time orientation, activity, human relationships, human nature, and control of natural forces. These values conflicts have implications, not only for testing that purports to measure locus of control, human motivation, or ADL performance, but also for how we represent humans and human occupation in occupational therapy theory.

Occupational therapy theoreticians continually build and refine models for practice. The profession values this scholarly activity. Refinement takes place as scholars open their work for criticism and debate among their peers. Rigorously examining the culture-based assumptions of a practice model is one way to test it.

The model of human occupation, one of the more encompassing theories in occupational therapy, incorporates multiple levels of data gathering about humans' skills, habits and roles, interests, and motivations embedded in a social and cultural environment. The model emphasizes humans' relationships to time and includes locus of control and belief in personal effectiveness as elements in the volitional regulation of playful and productive output (Kielhofner, 2002). Yet making statements about what is normal, universal, functional, or adaptive in these realms is almost impossible, for these areas are largely defined by culture. Some theoreticians working on the model of human occupation have moved away from standardized, quantification oriented-assessments of volition in favor of a more qualitative approach of eliciting narratives (Helfrich & Kielhofner, 1994; Helfrich, Kielhofner, & Mattingly, 1994). Others have questioned the adequacy of attention to the cultural and social environment, much mentioned but little analyzed in earlier descriptions of the model, and have called into question the assumed hierarchy among subsystems with volition driving habituation and skill performance (Haglund & Kjelberg, 1999).

From its inception, occupational science has embraced narrative, or story making, as the best means to understand clients' experiences of their illness or disability (Clark, 1993). The emphasis in occupational science on emic (insiders') perspectives gives it the potential to cross cultural barriers. Concern with the client's own account of his or her life is part of the occupational therapy tradition (Frank, 1996). In the application of narrative methods of assessment across cultures, however, it is important to recognize that what is a satisfying narrative to Western minds has a particular linear structure. That structure has been discussed (and prescribed) in Western culture since Aristotle's time. Proponents of narrative methods of evaluation admit that the "story" arrived at by the client (and family) and practitioner is the result of a negotiation between the client's telling and the practitioner's reconstruction of the story (Frank, 1996). When occupational therapy practitioners interview clients to discover their activity goals or the meanings that activities hold for them, they sometimes elicit stories that make no sense to the practitioners. The task for ethical practitioners is to push themselves outside the comfortable but invisible confines of their own culture and class to attempt an accurate understanding of their clients' worldviews and life situations. Doing so is a necessary step in collaborative goal setting, accurate assessment, individualized treatment planning, and equitable treatment provision.

See Case Study 7.B on the Willard & Spackman website for one example of the process of cross-cultural negotiation across several kinds of diversity.

ACHIEVING MULTICULTURAL COMPETENCE AS AN OCCUPATIONAL THERAPY PRACTITIONER

There are almost as many definitions of cultural competence as there are of culture. Fortunately for the length of this chapter, there is a great deal of agreement on what is involved in becoming a culturally competent practitioner. Most models of multicultural competence encompass the idea that knowledge of self and realization of one's own cultural values and orientations constitute a necessary first step. This aspect is often referred to as *cultural awareness* (Dillard, Andonian, Flores, MacRae, & Shakir, 1992). In tandem with cultural awareness is the need for *cultural sensitivity*, defined as an openness to the cultural values of others (Dillard et al., 1992).

Programs aimed at increasing awareness of one's own culture often begin with examination of dominant North American cultural values, to make those values less invisible to those who have assimilated them and to diminish ethnocentrism or the tendency to see one's own culture as the norm and expectation against which others are compared. The list below includes some observations about dominant North American cultural values (DeVita & James, 2002; Humphry, 1995; Pineda, 1996; Sanchez, 1964). In some cases, the values orientation of the dominant culture and that of the occupational therapy profession coincide, creating a strong bias that we must be aware of—and be willing to give up—when working with those whose values may be different.

In comparison with other cultural groups, dominant group members in the United States of America have been said to:

◆ Value the future over the present and value long-range planning and delaying gratification

◆ Value individuality and place the good of one individual over that of the rest of the social group

◆ Value independence over interdependence and group members doing for themselves over being served by others

◆ Be more secretive and private about their money and property than about their sexual behavior

◆ Resist sharing space or food without prior notice and planning and dislike "drop-in" visitors

◆ See the locus of identity as the individual and define the social unit primarily as the nuclear family

◆ Desire and value a sense of being in control and not to readily acquiesce to situations others may see as fate

◆ See science and technology as a source of control over the natural world, including humans

◆ Value physicality and doing over introspection and being

◆ Believe that humans are nearly perfectible and value discipline and learning as a means toward that end

For European-American practitioners, increasing cultural awareness and learning to establish accurate empathy begin with acknowledgment of the privileges and advantages inherent in membership in the dominant group (Evans, 1992; Matala, 1993). This is not an easy step, but it is a necessary one. Dominant cultural group members might have been raised with the myths that humans may pull themselves up by their bootstraps and that hard work always pays off. Moreover, they might have worked very hard for their achievements. Thus, they come to see their status as a just reward and wonder why others have not achieved similarly. The privileges, small and large, that accompany dominant group membership status might be invisible to them. Box 6.2 shows a sampling of such privileges, taken from a longer list by McIntosh (1997).

Cultural sensitivity follows when learners are aware of their own value orientations and are ready to explore those of others nonjudgmentally. Contact with empowered individuals whose culture, race, ethnicity, class, gender, or sexual orientation is different from their own is the most highly valued sort of activity for increasing cultural sensitivity.

While some discussions of cultural competence emphasize this dyad of awareness and sensitivity, others include a third dimension: skill (Wells & Black, 2000). The inclusion of the dimension of skill reminds us that multicultural competence is more than a set of attitudes or a general understanding; rather, it encompasses a learned set of actions that can be practiced and refined. Bonder and colleagues (2004) recommend three general actions therapists can practice for increasing multicultural competence: (1) carefully attending to the "interactional moment," taking into account as many verbal and nonverbal aspects of the communication as possible; (2) being curious about the meaning of all that one notices in so doing; and (3) engaging in reflective assessment of one's own com-

BOX 6.2 ACKNOWLEDGING PRIVILEGE INHERENT IN DOMINANT GROUP MEMBERSHIP

- If I wish, I can arrange to be in the company of people of my race most of the time.
- I can avoid spending time with people whom I was trained to mistrust and who have learned to mistrust my kind or me.
- If I should need to move, I can be pretty sure of renting or purchasing housing in an area that I can afford and in which I would want to live.
- I can be pretty sure that my neighbors in such a location will be neutral or pleasant to me.
- I can go shopping alone most of the time, pretty well assured that I will not be followed or harassed. Whether I use checks, credit cards, or cash, I can count on my skin color not to work against the appearance of financial reliability.
- I can turn on the television or open to the front page of the paper and see people of my race widely represented.
- When I am told about our national heritage or about "civilization," I am shown that people of my color made

it what it is. . . . I can be sure that my children will be given curricular materials that testify to the existence of their race.
- I can arrange to protect my children most of the time from people who might not like them.
- I do not have to educate my children to be aware of systemic racism for their own daily physical protection.
- I can be pretty sure that my children's teachers and employers will tolerate them if they fit school and workplace norms; my chief worries about them do not concern others' attitudes toward their race.
- I am never asked to speak for all the people of my racial group.
- I can remain oblivious of the language and customs of persons of color who constitute the world's majority without feeling in my culture any penalty for such oblivion

Adapted from McIntosh, P. (1997). White privilege and male privilege: A personal account of coming to see correspondences through work in women's studies. In R. Delgado & J. Stefancic (Eds.), Critical white studies: Looking behind the mirror (pp. 291–299). Philadelphia: Temple University Press.

---

munication in interactions. While face-to-face contact and immersion in culturally distinct environments is extremely useful, much can also be learned from reading autobiographies and novels written by those different from oneself.

CONCLUSION

Developing multicultural competence is a challenge, but the learning that occurs along the way can be a joy. Nothing is more interesting than the varieties of ways humans use to solve the problems of daily living and the variety of occupations that they choose. An appreciation of culture allows the skilled practitioner insight into how something as mundane as home canning can take on great importance to individuals as they write through occupation the stories of their lives.

Looking for culture through careful observation of and interaction with others, coupled with introspection of self, enables the establishment of accurate empathy between practitioner and client. Cultural difference then becomes a basis for understanding and working together and not a barrier to therapeutic gains. One of the encouraging developments in our profession has been the con-

scious use of cultural understanding in developing health promotion programs for healthy and at-risk populations. For example, see DeMars's (1992) description of community consulting in a Native Canadian village; Frank and colleagues' (2001) description of an occupation-based multidisciplinary program focused on helping black and Latino youngsters become the producers of culture, not just the passive consumers of mass cultural products; and Barnard and colleagues' (2004) description of a project aimed at enhancing wellness in a predominantly black rural farming community in North Carolina.

There are many excellent resources to help you on your personal journey toward multicultural competence. Websites abound. Book-length works on health care and culture by occupational therapists include Wells and Black's (2000) *Cultural Competency for Health Professionals* and Bonder, Martin, and Miracle's (2001) *Culture in Clinical Care.*

ON THE WEB

- Case Study 6.A: Negotiating Across Multiple Layers of Diversity
- Case Study 6.B: Examining Generalizations and Assumptions

ACKNOWLEDGEMENTS

The author wishes to thank her own multiracial and multicultural family for increasing her awareness of the matters discussed above. I thank in particular Mrs. Mary Frances Evans and the late Rev. Banks Evans, Sr. and Banks Evans, Jr., to whose memories this chapter is dedicated.

REFERENCES

American Occupational Therapy Association. (2002). Occupational therapy practice framework: Domain and process. *American Journal of Occupational Therapy, 56,* 609–639.

Barnard, S., Dunn, S., Reddic, E., Rhodes, K., Russell, J., Tuitt, S., Velde, B. P., Walden, J., Wittman, P. P., & White, K. (2004). Wellness in Tillery: A community-built program. *Family and Community Health, 27,* 151–157.

Bonder, B., Martin L., & Miracle, A. W. (2001). *Culture in Clinical Care.* Thorofare, NJ: Slack.

Bonder, B., Martin, L, & Miracle, A. W. (2004). Culture emergent in occupation. *American Journal of Occupational Therapy, 58,* 159–168.

Bowman, O. J., & Wallace, B. A. (1990). The effects of socioeconomic status on hand size and strength, vestibular function, visuomotor integration and praxis in preschool children. *American Journal of Occupational Therapy, 44,* 610–622.

Clark, F. (1993). Occupation embedded in a real life: Interweaving occupational science and occupational therapy. *American Journal of Occupational Therapy, 47,* 1067–1078.

Colonius, G. (1995). *Measurement accuracy of the FirstSTEP: A comparison between Alaska native children and the First-STEP norms.* Unpublished master's thesis, University of Puget Sound, Tacoma, WA.

Cornell, S., & Hartmann, D. (1998). *Ethnicity and race: Making identities in a changing world.* Thousand Oaks, CA: Pine Forge.

Crepeau, E. B. (1998). Clinical interpretation of "My Secret Life": The emergence of one gay man's authentic identity. *American Journal of Occupational Therapy, 52,* 570–572.

DeMars, P. A. (1992). An occupational therapy lifeskills curriculum model for a Native American tribe: A health promotion program based on ethnographic research. *American Journal of Occupational Therapy, 46,* 727–736.

DeVita, P. R., & James, J. D. (Eds.). (2002). *Distant mirrors: America as a foreign culture* (3rd ed.). Belmont, CA: Wadsworth.

Dickie, V. A. (2004). Culture is tricky: A commentary on culture emergent in occupation. *American Journal of Occupational Therapy, 58,* 169–173.

Dillard, M., Andonian, L., Flores, O., MacRae, A., & Shakir, M. (1992). Culturally competent occupational therapy in a diversely populated mental health setting. *American Journal of Occupational Therapy, 46,* 721–726.

Dyck, I. (1992). Managing chronic illness: An immigrant woman's acquisition and use of health care knowledge. *American Journal of Occupational Therapy, 46,* 696–705.

Dyck, I. (1993). Health promotion, occupational therapy and multiculturalism: Lessons from research. *Canadian Journal of Occupational Therapy, 60,* 120–129.

Elliot, S., & McGruder, J. (1995). Locus of control in African-Americans and European Americans. In *Conference Abstracts and resources, 1995, American Occupational Therapy Association Conference.* Lewiston, ID: Lewiston Rehabilitation and Care Center.

Evans, J. (1992). Nationally speaking: What occupational therapists can do to eliminate racial barriers to health care access. *American Journal of Occupational Therapy 46,* 679–683.

Fadiman, A. (1997). *The spirit catches you and you fall down: A Hmong child, her American doctors and the collision of two cultures.* New York: Farrar, Straus & Giroux.

Fitzgerald, M. H. (2004). A dialogue of occupational therapy, culture and families. *American Journal of Occupational Therapy, 58,* 489–498.

Frank, G. (1996). Life histories in occupational therapy clinical practice. *American Journal of Occupational Therapy, 50,* 251–264.

Frank, G., Fishman, M., Crowley, C., Blair, B., Murphy, S. T., Montoya, J. A., Hickey, M. P., Brancaccio, M. V., & Bensimon, E. M. (2001). The New Stories/New Cultures afterschool enrichment program: A direct cultural intervention. *American Journal of Occupational Therapy, 55,* 501–508.

Fudge, S. (1992). A perspective on consulting in Guatemala. *Occupational Therapy in Health Care, 8,* 15–37.

Gates, H. L. (1994). *Colored people: A memoir.* New York: Knopf.

Goto, S., Fisher, A. G., Mayberry, W. L. (1996). The assessment of motor and process skills applied cross-culturally to the Japanese. *American Journal of Occupational Therapy, 50,* 798–806.

Haglund, L., & Kjelberg, A. (1999). A critical analysis of the Model of Human Occupation. *Canadian Journal of Occupational Therapy, 66,* 102–108.

Hall, L. A. (2001). Sexual orientation. In E. C. Blakemore & S. Jennett (Eds.), *The Oxford Companion to the Body.* Oxford, UK: Oxford University Press, 2001. *Oxford Reference Online.* Oxford University Press. Retrieved June 9, 2006, from http://www.oxfordreference.com/views/ENTRY.html?subview=Main&entry=t128.e850

Helfrich, C., & Kielhofner, G. (1994). Volitional narratives and the meaning of therapy. *American Journal of Occupational Therapy, 48,* 319–326.

Helfrich, C, Kielhofner, G., & Mattingly C. (1994). Volition as narrative: Understanding motivation in chronic illness. *American Journal of Occupational Therapy, 48,* 311–317.

Humphry, R. (1995). Families who live in chronic poverty: Meeting the challenge of family-centered services. *American Journal of Occupational Therapy, 49,* 687–693.

Jackson, J. M. (1995). Sexual orientation: Its relevance to occupational science and the practice of occupational therapy. *American Journal of Occupational Therapy, 49,* 669–680.

Janelle, S. (1992). Locus of control in nondisabled versus congenitally physically disabled adolescents. *American Journal of Occupational Therapy, 46,* 334–342.

Joe, J. R., & Malach, R. S. (1992). Families with Native American roots. In E. W. Lynch & M. J. Hanson (Eds.), *Developing cross-cultural competence: A guide for working with young children and their families* (pp. 127–164). Baltimore, MD: Brookes.

Kielhofner, G. (2002). *A model of human occupation: Theory and application* (3rd ed.). Philadelphia: Lippincott, Williams and Wilkins.

Krefting, L., & Krefting, D. (1991). Cultural influences on performance. In C. Christiansen and C. Baum (Eds.), *Occupational therapy: Overcoming human performance deficits* (pp. 101–124). Thorofare, NJ: Slack.

Law, M. (1993). Evaluating activities of daily living: Directions for the future. *American Journal of Occupational Therapy, 47,* 233–237.

Llorens, L. (1971). Black culture and child development. *American Journal of Occupational Therapy, 25,* 144–148.

Matala, M. R. (1993). Race relations at work: A challenge to occupational therapy. *British Journal of Occupational Therapy, 56,* 434–436.

Mattingly, C., & Beer, D. (1993). Interpreting culture in a therapeutic context. In H. Hopkins & H. D. Smith (Eds.), *Willard and Spackman's occupational therapy* (8th ed., pp. 154–161). Philadelphia: Lippincott.

McIntosh, P. (1997). White privilege and male privilege: A personal account of coming to see correspondences through work in women's studies. In R. Delgado & J. Stefancic (Eds.), *Critical white studies: Looking behind the mirror* (pp. 291–299). Philadelphia: Temple.

McNaught, B. (1993a). *Homophobia in the workplace* [videorecording]. Provincetown, MA: TRB Productions.

McNaught, B. (1993b). *Growing up Gay and Lesbian* [videorecording]. Provincetown, MA: TRB Productions.

Miller, L. (1992). Evaluating the developmental skills of Cambodian orphans. *Occupational Therapy in Health Care, 8,* 73–87.

Moynihan, D. P. (1965, March). *The Negro Family: The case for national action* [The Moynihan Report]. Washington, DC: U.S. Department of Labor, Office of Planning and Research.

Myers, C. (1992). Hmong children and their families: Consideration of cultural influences in assessment. *American Journal of Occupational Therapy, 46,* 737–744.

National Center for Cultural Competence. (2000). Policy Brief 2. Developed by T. Goode, S. Sockalingam, M. Brown, & W. Jones. Linguistic Competence in Primary Health Care Delivery Systems: Implications for Policy Makers. Retrieved July 1, 2005, from http://gucchd.georgetown.edu/nccc/ncccpolicy2.html.

Packir, R. (1994). *Comparison of Sri Lankan and American mother-child dyads on the NCAST.* Unpublished master's thesis, University of Puget Sound, Tacoma, WA.

Paz, O. (1967). *The labyrinth of solitude.* London: Penguin Press.

Piaget, J. (1969). *Science of education and the psychology of the child* (D. Coltman, Trans.). New York: Viking.

Pineda, L. (1996). *Occupational therapists' multicultural competence and attitudes toward ethnically and culturally different clients.* Unpublished master's thesis, University of Puget Sound, Tacoma, WA.

Riggs, M. T. (1986) *Ethnic Notions* [videorecording]. San Francisco: California Newsreel. (Note: Riggs is writer, director, and producer.)

Sanchez, V. (1964). Relevance of cultural values for occupational therapy programs. *American Journal of Occupational Therapy, 18,* 1–5.

Smith, A. D. (1993). *Fires in the mirror: Crown Heights, Brooklyn and other identities.* New York: Dramatists Play Service, Inc.

Smith, A. D. (1994). *Twilight Los Angeles, 1992: On the road: A search for American character.* New York: Doubleday.

Spadone, R. (1992). Internal-external control and temporal orientation among Southeast Asians and White Americans. *American Journal of Occupational Therapy, 46,* 713–719.

Stauffer, L. M., Fisher, A. G., & Duran, L. (2000). ADL performance of black Americans and white Americans on the assessment of motor and process skills. *American Journal of Occupational Therapy, 54,* 607–613.

Walsh, A. L., & Crepeau, E. B. (1998) "My Secret Life": The emergence of one gay man's authentic identity. *American Journal of Occupational Therapy, 52,* 563–569.

Wardin, K. (1996). A comparison of verbal assessment of clients with limited English proficiency and English speaking clients in physical rehabilitation settings. *American Journal of Occupational Therapy, 50,* 816–825.

Weber, M. (1968). *Economy and society: An interpretive sociology* (E. Fischoff, Trans.; G. Roth & C. Wittich, Eds.). New York: Bedminster. (Original work published 1922)

Wells, S. A., & Black, R. M. (2000). *Cultural competency for health professionals.* Bethesda, MD: American Occupational Therapy Association.

Whiteford, G. E., & Wilcock, A. A. (2000). Cultural relativism: Occupation and independence reconsidered. *Canadian Journal of Occupational Therapy, 67,* 324–336.

Williams, D. R., Lavizzo-Mourey, R., & Warren, R. C. (1994). The concept of race and health status in America. *Public Health Reports, 109,* 26–41.

Wood, W. (1992). Temporal adaptation and self-identification as lesbian or gay. Paper presented at the Annual Conference of the American Occupational Therapy Association, Houston, TX, March 1992.

Socioeconomic Factors and Their Influence on Occupational Performance

7

CATHY LYSACK

Learning Objectives

After reading this chapter, you will be able to:

1. Distinguish between socioeconomic status, socioeconomic position, and class.
2. Understand that health is related to the person's position in the social hierarchy.
3. Identify client groups that are at greater risk for occupational performance difficulties related to socioeconomic disadvantage.
4. Name the mechanism by which social inequalities adversely affect health.
5. Describe five major social determinants of health that influence the occupational performance of clients.
6. Describe three actions that occupational therapy practitioners can take to reduce the impact of social inequalities and health disparities in clients' lives.

INTRODUCTION

The focus of this chapter is the social causes of health and disability and how socioeconomic factors influence people seeking and receiving occupational therapy services. As the case study illustrates, the environment in which Annie and Desmond lived influenced their chances for health. Desmond might have contracted his illness in an unhealthy workplace. Like Annie and Desmond, their children attended inner-city public schools that might

Annie is 72 years old and spent 11 days in the hospital. She "took a spell" and tumbled down her basement steps, fracturing her left hip and two ribs on her right side. She is using a wheelchair now but hopes that it is temporary. Annie is worried about managing at home. To make matters worse, she is still coping with the consequences of a mild stroke two years ago. Annie lives in inner-city Detroit. Her house has two small bedrooms and a bathroom on the second floor, with laundry facilities in the basement. She is a widow, and her only surviving child, a son, lives in Chicago. Throughout her life, Annie stayed home to raise three children while her husband Desmond worked at an automotive supply company. Unfortunately, after 31 years of work, Desmond was laid off at age 52. Shortly afterward, he became ill with lung cancer and died. Desmond was a nonsmoker, and workers in his plant wondered whether their jobs had made them sick. This was never determined. Making things worse, the company's financial problems brought changes in pension benefits transferred to surviving spouses. Shortly after Des passed away, Annie learned that she would have to get by on her monthly Social Security check and Medicare. She would receive nothing from her husband's pension.

Just before being discharged from the hospital, Annie was assessed by an occupational therapist and was given recommendations about how to bathe and dress and how to cook and clean safely and independently once she returned home. She was also given information about Dial-a-Ride, a transportation service for older adults and people with disabilities, and the name of a senior center where she could take exercise classes and participate in social activities on a drop-in basis. Annie was disappointed that she would not receive an in-home evaluation as several other women she met in the hospital had had. According to Annie, these women were getting "nice solid bathseats and grab bars." It was also rumored that some might get "adjustments to their kitchen cupboards" and even "a fancy ramp." Annie's insurance covered none of this, not even the raised toilet seat her therapist told her would help to avoid another fall. In addition, her doctor said that her mobility problems were "too mild" to qualify for further rehabilitation.

After three weeks at home, Annie is more worried than ever about the slowness of her recovery and her mounting out-of-pocket expenses for medications. Friends at Annie's church are bringing meals and helping with groceries, but Annie is anxious to be more self-sufficient. Still, she doesn't trust her legs "not to buckle out from under me." In a phone call to her son, she even expressed fear about going out in her neighborhood, saying that she felt like "a sitting duck" for anyone who "took it into their heads to get up to no good." Annie wonders whether the women she met weeks ago in hospital are faring better than she is and how different it would be if she could get even a little more help. She is praying that the good Lord will "see her through."

not have provided an optimal education. In addition, since medical benefits are linked to employment, the family might not have had an equal chance to achieve good health. How good has Annie's family's health care been through the years? How does this compare to the families of the women Annie met during her hospital stay? It is also worth asking how fair it is that Annie does not qualify for home support services and why there is no accessible public transportation or Meals-on-Wheels programs in her neighborhood.

Annie is struggling to regain mobility and independence after her fall, but it is not her bodily impairments that dictate her future now. Rather, it is her socioeconomic resources, shaped by a range of physical and social conditions over a lifetime and her place in the social hierarchy, which is dictated by the differences and inequalities among the groups Annie belongs to. These differences systematically advantage some and burden others. In this chapter, we will focus on those people who are systematically disadvantaged—those rendered most vulnerable by underlying social structures and political, economic, and legal institutions. Groups that are known to experience disadvantage in this sense include women, but even more so, visible minorities, the poor, and people with disabilities. As others have pointed out, occupational therapy practitioners as a group are overwhelmingly white and middle-class (Wells & Black, 2000). In general, we live more privileged lives than nearly all our clients do. One of the responsibilities of a competent and ethical practitioner is to recognize that such differences have deep historical roots that shape the health choices and behaviors of clients of well as the responses as health professionals. The reality of social and economic influences on health calls for a vigorous examination and discussion of the array of factors that influence health and disability in society and how these influence our practice.

DEFINING THE SOCIAL CAUSES OF HEALTH AND ILLNESS

What Do We Mean by Socioeconomic Position, Class, and Social Mobility?

Several terms are used to signal the influence of social and economic factors on health, and each term has a slightly different meaning. One of the most familiar terms is **socioeconomic status** (SES). This term refers to occupational, educational, and income achievements of individuals and groups. SES may overemphasize social prestige and underemphasize the role of material resources in shaping one's life chances, particularly related to health. Thus, as Krieger (2001) suggests, it might be time to replace the term *SES* with the term **socioeconomic position**.

The term **class** is also used to indicate social differences, as in *lower class*, *working class*, *middle class*, and *upper class*. Class is not easily defined. To some, class denotes culture and taste or particular attitudes and assumptions, lifestyle, or source of identity. To others, it just means having money. Classes are groups of people with similar economic means, especially those with similar levels of ownership of property and capital. To varying degrees, all societies are stratified by class. Since the United States is an industrialized free-market economy, the degree to which we move up or down the social ladder, something sociologists call **social mobility**, is in large part dictated by our class, that is, by our income and wealth.

What Are Social Inequalities, the Social Gradient, and Health Disparities?

The terms *social inequalities, the social gradient,* and *health disparities* come to us from the public health literature and are closely related to class. **Social inequality** refers to the pattern of unequal rewards and opportunities that accrue to different individuals and groups in society, particularly those rewards and opportunities that are judged to be unfair, unjust, avoidable, and unnecessary (Krieger, 2001). While some differences between people in society are fixed and cannot be changed, others are morally wrong and can be improved. For example, discrimination against people on the basis of gender or sexual orientation is morally wrong. Social inequalities are a regrettable reality in the United States, and much work needs to be done to address the underlying factors that create these inequalities.

One reason that social inequalities are of great concern to health professionals is that social inequalities put people at risk for poorer health. Life expectancy is shorter and most diseases are more common farther down the social ladder. The reality that health diminishes with each step down in the social hierarchy has been called the **social gradient**. Decades of research has shown this is true in both rich and poor societies (Marmot & Wilkinson, 1999). Making matters worse is the fact that "upward mobility," that is, doing better and having more than our parents, is happening less than we thought. Americans are more likely, not less likely, than they were 30 years ago to remain in the same class into which they were born (Bradbury & Katz, 2002). While equality and reward are embodied in the ideal of the American dream, the dream is accessible only to some.

Health disparities refer to differences of treatment and health care services that are unfair and may be the direct result of either underlying social inequalities or improper actions by professionals within the health system. The *Healthy People 2010* report (U.S. Department of Health and Human Services, 2000a) defines disparities as differences that occur by gender, race or **ethnicity**, education or income, disability, geographic location, or sexual orientation. The factors that contribute to health disparities are a major preoccupation in the United States because there is mounting evidence that members of minorities receive substandard levels of health care and have much poorer health. Studies have found that even after symptoms and insurance coverage are controlled for, doctors are more likely to offer whites life-preserving treatments, including angioplasty and bypass surgery for cardiac disease, and are more likely to offer minorities various less desirable procedures such as amputations for diabetes (Institute of Medicine, 2002). This research indicates that clinical encounters between members of minorities and health care professionals may be the source of additional poor treatment. Stereotyping and institutional racism are widely recognized as unjust forces in the health care environment that must be changed. The longer-term consequences of a lifetime of perceived racism are also coming to be understood as adversely influencing health (Clark, 2004). Differences in age, gender, and ethnicity will always exist; it is wrong, however, when these differences lead to unequal care. To what extent do occupational therapy practitioners discriminate against minorities, the poor, and the elderly? Do their attitudes restrict access to high-quality occupational therapy services for these individuals?

The Intersections of Gender, Ethnicity, Age, and Disability

The notion of class differences and social inequalities is not an appealing one. Americans typically avoid talking about this problem (Fussell, 1983; hooks, 2000). The notion that we all have equal chances and opportunities is an idea that we want to believe is true. For example, we want to believe that we can all go to the schools of our choice, enter any occupation we desire, and be free to participate in any leisure activity that appeals to us. On the other hand, we know from experience that we often have to change our plans or reconsider our goals because we lack the necessary means to achieve them. The ability to achieve what we want out of life depends on our resources—quite often, financial resources, but not entirely. A positive outlook on life or a strong family support system, for example, may get us through a difficult period more successfully than having a large amount of money. Other factors that influence health outcomes are inextricably linked to the social categories we belong to, including whether we are male or female; what our age, ethnicity, and sexual orientation is; and whether we are disabled or not. These factors dictate our future too, and they are not so easily changed.

Gender Inequalities

For many women, the gendered experience of being a woman continues to be one of inequality. For example, women have found it difficult to enter some professions because of gender bias. Others have felt trapped in roles that are perceived to be "women's work" (Apter, 1993; Hesse-Biber & Carter, 2000). *The Economist* (2005) reports that women account for fewer than 8% of all CEOs in the United States even though women constitute 46% of the national workforce. This is only very marginally better than the situation a decade ago. Research also confirms a wage gap between men and women. Analysis of U.S. Census data shows that, on average, women's pay is still only 77 cents for every $1 a man earns (Economic Policy Institute, 2005). While this can be partly explained by the kinds of jobs women have and the lower salaries associated with these jobs, this does not explain the entire difference.

Gender also exerts a strong influence on health. Currently, women enjoy a longer average life expectancy than men do. However, once the patterns of illness and disability are examined by gender, the picture is more ambiguous. Although men die earlier than women overall, women experience higher rates of chronic illness at each age. For example, women age 15 years and older account for 60% of all people diagnosed with arthritis (National Center for Health Statistics, 2004). Similarly, depression is nearly twice as common in women as in men. Some of these gender differences are accounted for by biological differences between the sexes; others are related to differences in gender roles. For example, since women live longer than men and have fewer financial resources in retirement (owing to a lifetime of lower wages and less time in the paid labor force as a result of child rearing), women have less money to take care of their health (Collins, Estes, & Bradsher, 2001).

Ethnic Inequalities

Ethnicity significantly affects the life chances of individuals. We use the term *ethnicity* here, rather than *race*, to signal cultural rather than biological explanations for differences in social and economic opportunity. First, and most basically, ethnicity affects educational opportunities. The extent and quality of education are critical factors in life because employment opportunities and thus income are tied to early educational attainment (Miringoff & Miringoff, 1999; Shonkoff & Phillips, 2000). But neither educational opportunities nor the quality of educational experiences is equitably distributed. The U.S. government recognized this fact as early as the 1950s, when it established the Head Start program, a national network of comprehensive child development programs that targeted low-income families and their communities. It should not be that hard to understand that poor minority children are at an educational disadvantage compared with children of wealthier parents from predominantly white fam-

ilies (Young, 1997). Poor children grow up in poor neighborhoods, which have poorer-quality schools, staffed by teachers with fewer resources to enrich the learning environment. Individuals with diminished chances in the early years seldom catch up. This has a particularly dramatic impact on visible minorities, who are more likely to be poor.

Poverty affects health even more than ethnicity does, though the two factors are often found together. Nowhere are the inequalities more clear than in studies of infant mortality. The Population Reference Bureau (2005) publishes data on the infant mortality rates in many countries. These data show that Sweden's infant mortality rate is 3.1 per 1,000 live births, while the U.S. average is 6.6. For black Americans in the United States, however, the figure is a startling 14.4 deaths per 1,000 live births (National Center for Health Statistics, 2004). There are disparities in mortality rates and disease-specific risks too. Census data show, for example, that the prevalence of hypertension is about 40% higher in black Americans than in white Americans, while the prevalence of diabetes is nearly 60% higher in black Americans (National Center for Health Statistics, 2004).

Age Inequalities

Age is another factor that shapes societal opportunity and, in turn, individual health. All societies have some sort of shared cultural expectations of its members based on age. For example, it is commonly accepted that the Japanese treat their elders with more respect and honor than we do in North America. **Ageism** is the term used to describe discrimination based on age (Estes, 2001). Aging is not perceived particularly positively in the United States. Despite substantial research to the contrary, people in the age category we might call "young-old" are often seen as "over the hill." Although it is against the law to discriminate in hiring people, the 60-year-old who wants or needs to find a new job does not find many open doors, regardless of his or her experience. That said, we might see a decrease in ageism as the full impact of the aging Baby Boom generation is felt. Baby Boomers are healthier, wealthier, better educated, and more politically savvy than previous generations were (Soto, 2005). They will likely exert a considerable influence on age-appropriate social roles, including what it means to be "old."

Health and aging are tightly intertwined. Not surprisingly, "age is the single most important predictor of mortality and morbidity" (Weitz, 2004, p. 52). Mortality rates drop dramatically after birth and rise again only at about age 40. Not until age 65 do chronic illnesses overcome acute illnesses as the major cause of death. However, because age and illness are so closely tied, when the average age of the population increases, so does the prevalence of health problems. The proportion of Americans age 65 or older is projected to reach 18% by 2020

(U.S. Administration on Aging, 2005). The health problems associated with aging populations and the financial means to address them are anticipated to be among the biggest health challenges many nations have ever encountered.

Inequalities Due to Disability

Disability is associated with disadvantage, regardless of individual skills or financial resources. In the 2000 Census, disability was defined as a chronic health condition that makes it difficult to perform one or more activities generally considered appropriate for individuals of a given age: play or school for children, work for adults, and basic activities of daily living for the elderly. In 2003, the Census counted 49.7 million people with disability. This represented 19.3% of the population, or 257.2 million people age 5 years and older living in the community (U.S. Census, 2003). The same census revealed employment inequities for people with disability: 79% of working-age men without a disability were employed in 2000, but only 60% of those with a disability were employed. The percentage drops sharply for people with more severe disabilities. Of those with mental disabilities, 41% are employed. For wheelchair users, the figure is 22% (Stoddard, Jans, Ripple, & Kraus, 1998). Medical and technological advances have enabled people to live longer and be more independent, but full social integration and inclusion cannot be achieved without access to schools, jobs, and leisure. The actions at the basis of the Americans with Disabilities Act and earlier legislation reflect the long-standing efforts of the disability rights movement and its allies (including occupational therapy practitioners) to improve life conditions for people with disabilities. Some of the main goals of the disability rights movement are to change attitudes, public policies, and the law (Colker, 2005; Trattner, 1994).

Finally, people with disabilities have poorer health than their able-bodied counterparts. Higher rates of diabetes, depression, elevated blood pressure and blood cholesterol, obesity, and vision and hearing impairments have all been reported (U.S. Department of Health and Human Services, 2000b). Lower rates of recommended health behaviors such as cardiovascular fitness have been found too, as have low rates of patient education and treatment for mental illness.

Because of the intersections of age, ethnicity, and poverty, it is possible to identify specific subgroups of disabled people who are at particular risk. One such group is elderly women living in the inner city, many of whom are minorities. Remember Annie, who lives alone in her home in the inner city after her fall? Lysack and colleagues (2003) found that older urban African-American women who live alone are at increased risk for physical problems, including falls, and cognitive decline, both of which can precede a complete loss of independence and institutionalization. Older adults have also been shown to have less access to specialized rehabilitation services than younger working adults with similar rehabilitation needs (Neufeld & Lysack, 2006). Are occupational therapy practitioners aware of and sufficiently responsive to these particularly disadvantaged groups?

In summary, regardless of our professed beliefs in equal opportunity and despite legislation intended to prevent discrimination, life choices and chances are not equal; they are mediated by an array of powerful social and economic variables that can dramatically dictate the fate of individuals and their health. The foregoing discussion reminds us that these variables are not easily changed or overcome through individual desire and effort. Much larger forces in society, including the health system, play an integral role.

THE POLITICAL ECONOMY OF THE HEALTH CARE SYSTEM

To fully appreciate the influence of socioeconomic factors in individual lives, these factors must be set against the backdrop of the health care system, which has been described as a highly dynamic and fragmented system of competition, regulation, and reimbursement (Shi & Singh, 1998). It is also the most expensive health care system in the world. Health expenditures in the United States in 2004 totaled $1.7 trillion, or 14.6% of gross domestic product, and averaged $5,274 per capita per year (Anderson, Hussey, Frogner, & Waters, 2005).

International Comparisons

Despite the huge amount spent on medical care, the United States ranks low on many health indicators (World Health Organization, 2005), and there is mounting evidence that the system is plagued with serious problems at all levels (Moss, 2000; Rylko-Bauer & Farmer, 2002). Life expectancy in the United States stands at 77.2 years, below the average of 77.8 years for the 30 developed countries that belong to the Organization for Economic Cooperation and Development (OECD, 2005). This lags behind countries such as Poland, Korea, and Mexico. Infant mortality rates, too, though they have fallen greatly over the past few decades, have not fallen as much as the rates in most other OECD countries. Infant mortality stood at 7 deaths per 1,000 live births in 2002, above the OECD average of 6.1 and well behind countries such as Japan, Iceland, Finland, and Sweden. As citizens of one of the richest countries in the world, Americans have a right to expect better health (Whiteis, 2000).

The Role of Health Insurance

Health insurance (or, more accurately, medical insurance) is important because access to health care in the mostly private U.S. system requires either a job with health benefits or the financial means to pay out of pocket. A substantial number of Americans lack both. Nearly 45 million Americans are estimated to have no health insurance, and another 52 million are thought to have insufficient coverage (Brouwer, 1998; Cutler, 2004). Minorities make up a disproportionate part of the uninsured: Blacks are twice as likely as whites and Hispanics are three times as likely as whites to be uninsured because of type of employment and lower income (Centers for Disease Control and Prevention, 2003). Insurance matters because the uninsured and underinsured have reduced access and less appropriate care, are in poorer health, and are more likely to die prematurely (DeNavas-Walt, Proctor, & Lee, 2005; Institute of Medicine, 2002; Krieger, 1999).

The health disadvantage associated with lack of health insurance is not only a poor person's problem. The Kaiser Family Foundation (2003) found that over half of all uninsured workers in the United States in 2002 worked full-time that year. The problem is increasing because fewer middle-class jobs are coming with employer-sponsored health benefits (Lee, Soffel, & Luft, 1994; Shi & Singh, 1998). A recent *New York Times* series showed just how hard the middle class is being squeezed by factory closures, layoffs, and large-scale economic downturns (Scott, 2005). This is linked to health. For example, in 2003, more than 27 million working adults had medical debt, yet only 62% of those had health insurance (Doty, Edwards, & Holmgren, 2005).

In programs in which people have health insurance paid for by the government, such as Medicare and Medicaid, the impact of out-of-pocket expenses can still be significant. Researchers at the American Association of Retired Persons (Caplan & Brangan, 2004) found that Medicare beneficiaries (age 65+) spent an average of $3,455, or 22% of their income, on unreimbursed health care. The largest cost was prescription drugs. The situation is even worse for uninsured workers with chronic conditions. Nearly half of the total of 6.6 million uninsured chronically ill Americans report medical bill problems, making them much more likely to forgo or delay needed medical care (Ha, 2004). This is leading to major hardships for many. A study found that 28.3% of all personal bankruptcies in the United States today are substantially caused by illness or injury; the comparable rate in Canada is lower than 7% (Himmelstein, Warren, Thorne, & Woolhandler, 2005).

There is no question that Americans need to care about the uninsured and rising costs of health care, whether on the basis of social justice or simply as a matter of dollars and cents. Kawachi and Berkman (2003) warn that the least fortunate in society must be cared for, or spillover effects will adversely affect everyone. Wide income disparities lead to stress, family disruption, and mass frustration, which in turn lead to violence and crime. According to Lynch and colleagues (1998), if this trend

is left unchecked, the economic prosperity of the nation could be permanently compromised.

MECHANISMS OF DISADVANTAGE ACROSS THE LIFE COURSE

There is an untested assumption that disparities in health arise from disparities in health care. Of course, there is a gap in this logic: The fact that there are defects in a medical system does not mean that the system caused the problems. So why are there differences in health status across different groups in society? Part of the problem is poverty and income inequality.

Money Matters: Economic Deprivation and Health

Poverty is bad for health. The term *poverty* refers to the lack of material resources that are necessary for subsistence. Poverty increases exposure to factors that make people sick, and it decreases the chances of having high-quality medical insurance (and thus care) when the person needs it. Children, older adults, new immigrants, disabled people, and members of ethnic minorities are at greatest risk of poverty (U.S. Census, 2003). Perhaps most alarming is the fact that the official poverty rate in the United States increased in each of the last four consecutive years that were measured, from a 26-year low of 11.3% in 2000 to 12.7% in 2004. As of 2004, 37 million Americans lived below the official poverty threshold (U.S. Census, 2005).

Economics and health policy experts are asking whether pronounced levels of income inequality take a lasting toll on other aspects of people's lives, not just health. A report published in the *New York Times* in 2003 (Browning, 2003) pointed out that the richest 1% of Americans in 2000 had more money to spend after taxes than the bottom 40% put together. That's roughly three million people outearning 110 million—a rather staggering figure. Perhaps this has fueled the entry of two new terms into the popular lexicon: *the working poor* and *the new poor*. The **working poor** are people who work full-time but whose wages do not raise them above the poverty line. Nearly 6% of U.S. workers currently earn the federal minimum wage of $5.15 an hour (U.S. Department of Labor, 2005). Based on a 40-hour week, this provides an annual income of $10,700. Many critics have asked how the working poor even get by (Ehrenreich, 2001; Shipler, 2005; Wilson, 1997). The **new poor** are those people who have fallen into poverty because of sudden and unexpected circumstances such as serious illness, divorce, or sudden job layoffs. Sidel (1996) describes the situation of one woman who, after 23 years of marriage, was divorced by her husband. When he left the state and refused to pay child support, the family's annual income fell from

$70,000 to $7,000. Her part-time job was not enough to keep her out of poverty.

The working poor and the new poor stand in sharp contrast to the wealthiest individuals in the United States. Did you know that the average CEO's pay in the United States is $11.8 million? Since the average American worker earns only $27,460 per year, this is an astounding 431-to-1 ratio (Institute for Policy Studies and United for a Fair Economy, 2005). Recall Annie's struggle to regain her mobility after her hip fracture and how she must rely on limited financial and medical resources (see Figure 7.1). Will Annie join the ranks of the new poor? What affordable suggestions would you give Annie if you were her occupational therapist? What kinds of barriers should you anticipate as Annie tries to implement your recommendations?

The case study about Annie that opened this chapter reminds us that money matters in efforts to achieve good health. But money is not the only thing. A variety of other factors matter too. In a set of famous studies commonly referred to as the Whitehall studies, Marmot, Shipley, and Rose (1984) studied British civil servants over three decades to ascertain more precisely how one's place in the occupational hierarchy influences health. Because occupation is shaped by both economic circumstances and other factors in the social environment, this turned out to be highly influential research. Results of the Whitehall studies showed that men in the lowest levels of the civil service, office support workers, had a mortality rate four times greater than that of men in the highest administrative jobs. The findings were consistent across the spectrum of job categories. Being on the top rung was clearly best for your health, but every step closer to the top mattered too (i.e., the social gradient). This work and studies that followed laid the groundwork for an entire new branch of epidemiology called the **social determinants of health**. Today, it is widely accepted that whatever the importance of biological and genetic factors and even personal lifestyle factors and access to health care, the social and physical environment is of tremendous significance too.

Proponents of a social determinants perspective argue that the mechanism by which health is adversely affected is through physiological stress. The lower people are in the social hierarchy, the more common and pronounced are their stress-related problems. The disadvantages concentrate among the same people, and the effects of these disadvantages on health are cumulative (Lynch et al., 1998). Simply put, the longer people live in stressful social and economic circumstances, the greater is their physiological wear and tear and the less likely they are to enjoy a healthy old age. The implications of this are tremendous. Most basically, it means that "fixing" the health care system by addressing disparities in treatment is only part of the solution. If we really wish to improve the health of those who are most disadvantaged in society, we must work to reduce various forms of social inequalities and social

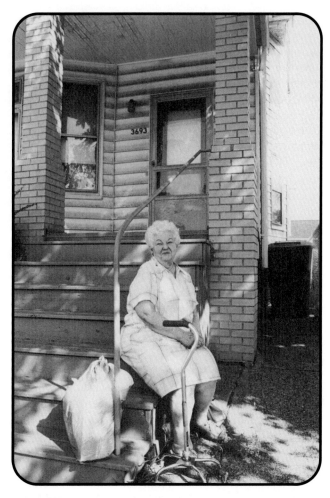

FIGURE 7.1   Many older women living in the inner city lack financial resources to modify their homes to improve safety and independence. What can feasibly be done at low cost to facilitate community mobility and participation in this group? (Source: Lee Ann Johnson, photographer, Wayne State University, Detroit, used with permission.)

deprivation that exist in society. This would need to begin in early childhood and continue throughout life.

Deprivation Across the Life Course

A plethora of observational research and intervention studies show that the foundations of adult health are laid in early childhood, even before birth (Brown et al., 2004; Young, 1997). This combination of a poor start and slow growth "become embedded in biology during the processes of development, and form the basis of the individual's biological and human capital, which affects health throughout life" (Wilkinson & Marmot, 2003, p. 14). Studies have demonstrated that as cognitive, emotional, and sensory inputs program the brain's responses, insecure emotional attachment and poor stimulation can lead to low educational attainment, problem behavior, and the risk of social marginalization in adulthood (Barker, 1998). Slow physical growth in infancy is also associated with reduced cardiovascular, respiratory, pancreatic, and kidney function, which increases the risk of serious illness in adulthood (Shonkoff & Phillips, 2000).

Children also learn and develop through play. Not only does play help them to learn about themselves as individuals, it also helps them to acquire their fundamental socialization skills and many motor and cognitive skills. Kozol (1991, 1995) describes neighborhoods overrun by poverty, crime, and economic neglect. In such neighborhoods, parents are afraid to let their children play outdoors because of high rates of violence and heightened exposure to environmental toxins, injuries, and disease (Kozol, 1991, 1995). The cumulative damage is such that some argue that no amount of therapy and treatment can undo the consequences (Brown et al., 2004).

Social inequalities over the life course also contribute to deprivation in adults. This occurs primarily in the realm of work. While work is in many ways a marker of good health, work can also be the source of poor health. Anxiety, substance abuse, and depression rates are all higher in populations in which unemployment is high (Lawrence, Chau, & Lennon, 2004). For those who are employed, there are other stress-related problems; research has shown that lack of personal autonomy and control in one's work is significantly related to cardiovascular disease (Bosma, Peter, Siegrist, & Marmot, 1998). The mechanism for this appears to be related to excessive production of cortisol or "stress hormones." Beyond the workplace, the news for workers is hardly better: leisure time is decreasing. A recent international travel survey by Expedia.com (2005) found that Americans work the most hours of any affluent country. Americans earn an average of 12 vacation days annually, lagging behind Canada with 21 days and Germany and France with 27 and 39 vacation days, respectively. Even so, 31% of Americans do not take all of their accrued annual vacation time, with 10% saying they are "too busy at work" to get away.

OCCUPATIONAL THERAPY SERVICES: ARE WE EQUITABLE? ARE WE RESPONSIVE?

Townsend and Wilcock (2003) asserted that it is an occupational injustice to ignore the social and economic determinants of health. Others have called on occupational therapists to address the segregation of groups of people based on lack of meaningful participation in daily life occupations, something that Kronenberg and Pollard (2005) have provocatively called **occupational apartheid**. There is little doubt that socioeconomic factors are real and exert a powerful influence on health, but what is the average occupational therapist to do in the face of what appear to be intractable problems on a very large scale? Even if we develop greater awareness of the influence of social in-

equalities on health and the extent of health disparities in the clients we serve, what are the next practical steps?

First, we can apply the small but growing body of evidence we have from occupational therapy research that focused interventions can bring meaningful benefits. For example, occupational therapy with children can effectively address sensory motor performance deficits (Case-Smith, 2002), peer play relationships (Tanta, Dietz, White, & Billingsley, 2005), and family interactions (Bedell, Cohn, & Dumas, 2005), which all may be more prevalent in socioeconomically disadvantaged families. Occupational therapists can also support parents to better understand their children's emotional and cognitive needs and modify school and home environments to facilitate occupational performance (Letts, Rigby, & Stewart, 2003). Occupational therapists working in gerontology can help to design supportive environments for older adults that facilitate aging in place.

Occupational therapists are experts at person-environment fit and recognize the centrality of meaningful occupations to facilitate good health. Yet there are serious gaps in our knowledge. For example, we know very little about meaningful occupational engagement for chronically unemployed people and what kinds of interventions might be effective for them. We know even less about occupational deprivation due to immigration, geographical isolation, and incarceration (Whiteford, 2000). Much more research is needed if we expect to extend beneficial therapeutic interventions to these groups of people, who might be the most occupationally disadvantaged of all.

A second concrete and immediate step we can take is to move past an all-too-pervasive "occupational hazard" in occupational therapy, which is to think of our clients in depersonalized categories and our practice as politically neutral. With respect to the first issue, we tend to treat "a really interesting traumatic brain injury" or complain about "an old stroke that has plateaued." These phrases are shorthand abstractions of what we really intend to offer in the occupational therapy process. We like to say that one of the unique strengths of the profession is our holistic approach. That phrase does not simply mean that we address the physical and psychosocial domains in our therapeutic goals with our clients. It means that we have to learn about our clients just like Annie, in the terms of her world, her perceptions, her experiences, and her realities. This is easy to say and much more difficult to do. Purtilo and Haddad (2002) describe many difficulties that arise between practitioners and clients because of socioeconomic and cultural differences. These differences influence how we feel about our clients, including the degree to which we empathize with them and even understand their daily routines.

Occupational therapy practice is not value-neutral. Socioeconomic and cultural differences affect practice in very real ways on a daily basis. Fitzgerald, Williamson, Russell, and Manor (2005) describe the dilemmas therapists encounter as they try to balance their professional concern and protection of clients with the wishes clients express for themselves. In reviewing these dilemmas, the investigators reported that while every occupational therapist "wants to wear a cloak of competence" and "wants others to see it as fine and good" (p. 344), there is no denying the force of moral judgments in their work. Therapists cannot help but be shaped by the prevailing cultural attitudes of their times and they would be remiss not to recognize how these attitudes and values, at times, operate to further disadvantage their clients. At minimum, this research reminds occupational therapists of the fundamental importance of critical reflective practice.

Third, to be able to act on issues of occupational deprivation and occupational injustice requires that therapists become much more educated about socioeconomic barriers to treatment and optimal health outcomes. More than a decade ago, Dunn, Brown, and McGuigan (1994) referred to the need to consider the effect of context and questioned whether "standardized functional assessments are valid for capturing what is actually known about the person's performance in the natural context" (p. 605). The context to which these authors referred was the home and community context. But context can be extended further to include the adequacy of neighborhoods and communities to provide a safe and secure living environment, the accessibility of transportation and housing, and even the availability of work for individuals with disabilities. Do we routinely use or even have appropriate assessments of neighborhood safety and community mobility? What about measures of the adequacy of public housing and transit for patients who are discharged home? Are occupational therapists prepared to expand their scope of practice into the social and economic environment, even if reimbursement issues can be overcome?

Another issue is the financial ability of our clients to implement actions aimed at enhancing their independence and participation in daily life. In a study focused on home modification recommendations, Lysack and Neufeld (2003) found that patients who relied solely on Medicaid and Medicare received fewer recommendations from their occupational therapists than did privately insured patients, even when their health conditions were similar. Mathieson, Kronenfeld, and Keith (2002) found that having supplemental health insurance acted as an enabling factor with respect to using equipment and implementing home modification recommendations. Taken together, studies like these suggest that clients who lack the ability to pay or even are perceived to lack the ability to pay may lose out. Their functional independence and even their participation in society may be compromised as a result. More research is needed to determine how prevalent these practices are and how important a factor income really is in determining rehabilitation outcomes over time. This work is urgently needed if we wish to understand the socioeconomic dis-

advantage that some of our clients confront every day and to identify effective pathways of redress.

In addition to being evidence-based practitioners who identify and use new assessments that tap into the socioeconomic realities of clients more deeply, occupational therapists can leverage their position within the health care system to help reduce the impact of socioeconomic disadvantage. For example, therapists can enlighten insurance payers about the needs of their low-income clients by listing occupational therapy services recommended as the ideal for their clients alongside the documentation required for services currently eligible for reimbursement. This kind of documentation practice keeps the gaps between the ideal and the real in the forefront of the minds of decision makers who have the power to affect wider change.

Lohman and Brown (1997) addressed the issue of therapists' ethical obligations and moral stance in the context of managed care and urged clinicians to vigorously represent and advocate for patients—not only in direct service situations, but also at policy levels. Many occupational therapists working in inner-city environments already pursue alternative modes of funding to implement home safety recommendations (Pynoos, Tabbarah, Angelelli, & Demiere, 1998). Another strategy is to employ the specific rules and language of insurance companies much more strategically so that occupational therapy interventions have the best chance of being accepted by payers (Uili & Wood, 1995). Efforts like this take commitment and persistence, but these efforts can be effective—and not only for a single client around a single issue. A successful change in policy can benefit thousands if not tens of thousands of clients, making these efforts more than worthwhile.

CONCLUSION

The majority of health care professionals would say that they learned their most important lessons from their clients. These stories are usually about how the professional lacked an understanding of the situation and how the client set the professional straight about how things really were. This means that we have to listen, and we have to ask the right questions and give the time and space for the answers (Law, 1998; Lawlor, 2003; Wood, 1996). But while listening to and learning from individual clients are paramount to effective occupational therapy interventions, we must remember that this approach individualizes the underlying problems of health disparities and inequalities that are fundamentally social in nature. Occupational therapists who work with socioeconomically disadvantaged clients are well acquainted with this tension. And while some experts have argued that the path forward lies in large-scale professional coalitions aimed at major transformations of the health care system (Cutler, 2004), this takes time to achieve, if it can be achieved at all. In the meantime, occupational therapists must work in a system that is imperfect, knowing full well that it does not meet many of their clients' pressing needs.

Recall once more Annie's struggle to recover from a lifetime of social and economic disadvantage. There are many Annies in occupational therapy practice, and you will likely meet more than one. To accomplish the true promise of occupational therapy undoubtedly requires better knowledge of the communities from which our clients come and the socioeconomic and historical and political forces that have shaped their lives and their health. The onus is on us to identify inequalities and disparities where they exist and work to ameliorate them. This is the only way to advance health for all.

REFERENCES

Anderson, G. F., Hussey, P. S., Frogner, B. K., & Waters, H. R. (2005). Health spending in the United States and the rest of the industrialized world. *Health Affairs, 24*(4), 903–914.

Apter, T. (1993). *Working women don't have wives: Professional success in the 1990s.* New York: St. Martin's Press.

Barker, D. (1998). *Mothers, babies and disease in later life* (2nd ed.). Edinburgh: Churchill Livingstone.

Bedell, G. M., Cohn, E. S., & Dumas, H. M. (2005). Exploring parents' use of strategies to promote social participation of school-age children with acquired brain injuries. *American Journal of Occupational Therapy, 59,* 273–284.

Bosma, H., Peter, R., Siegrist, J., & Marmot, M. (1998). Two alternative job stress models and risk of coronary heart disease. *American Journal of Public Health, 88,* 68–74.

Bradbury, K., & Katz, J. (2002). Women's labor market involvement and family income mobility when marriage ends. *New England Economic Review, Q4,* 41–74.

Brouwer, S. (1998). *Sharing the pie: A citizen's guide to wealth and power in America.* New York: Holt.

Brown, B., Bzostek, S., Aufseeser, D., Berry, D., Weitzman, M., Kavanaugh, M., Bagley, S., & Auinger, P. (Eds.). (2004). *Early child development in social context: A chartbook.* New York: The Commonwealth Fund. Retrieved April 7, 2006, from http://www.cmwf.org/publications/publications_show.htm?doc_id=237483

Browning, L. (2003, September 28). Divide between rich, poor widens. *The New York Times, Special Section,* p.1.

Caplan, C., & Brangan, N. (2004). *Out-of-pocket spending on health care by Medicare beneficiaries age 65 and older in 2003.* Washington, DC: AARP Public Policy Institute.

Case-Smith, J. (2002). Effectiveness of school-based occupational therapy intervention on handwriting. *American Journal of Occupational Therapy, 56,* 17–25.

Centers for Disease Control and Prevention. (2003). *Fact sheet: Racial and Ethnic disparities in health status.* Atlanta: Author. Retrieved April 7, 2006, from http://www.cdc.gov/od/oc/media/pressrel/fs020514b.htm

Clark, R. (2004). Significance of perceived racism: Toward understanding the ethnic group disparities in health, the later years. In N. Anderson, R. Bulato, and B. Cohen (Eds.), *Critical perspectives on racial and ethnic differences in health in late life* (pp. 540–566). Washington, DC: National Academies Press.

Colker, R. (2005). *The disability pendulum: The first decade of the Americans with Disabilities Act.* New York: New York University Press.

Collins, C. A., Estes, C. L., & Bradsher, J. E. (2001). Inequality and aging: The creation of dependency. In Estes, C. L., & Associates (Eds.), *Social policy & aging: A critical perspective* (pp. 137–163). Thousand Oaks, CA: Sage.

Cutler, D. (2004). *Your money or your life: Strong medicine for American healthcare system.* New York: Oxford University Press.

DeNavas-Walt, C., Proctor, C., & Lee, C. H. (2005). *U.S. Census Bureau, current population reports, P60-229, Income, poverty, and health insurance coverage in the United States: 2004,* Washington, DC: U.S. Government Printing Office. Retrieved April 8, 2006, from http://www.census.gov/prod/2005pubs/p60-229.pdf

Doty, M., Edwards, J., & Holmgren, A. (2005). *Seeing red: Americans driven into debt by medical bills.* New York: The Commonwealth Fund. Retrieved April 8, 2006, from http://www.cmwf.org/publications/publications_show.htm?doc_id=290074

Dunn, W., Brown, C., & McGuigan, A. (1994). The ecology of human performance: A framework for considering the effect of context. *American Journal of Occupational Therapy, 48,* 595–607.

Economic Policy Institute. (2005). *State of working in America 2004/2005. Fact & figures: Wages.* Retrieved April 8, 2006, from http://www.epinet.org/books/swa2004/news/swafacts_wages.pdf

Ehrenreich, B. (2001). *Nickel and dimed: On (not) getting by in America.* New York: Henry Holt.

Estes, C. (2001). *Social policy & aging: A critical perspective.* Thousand Oaks, CA: Sage.

Expedia.com. (2005). Vacation deprivation survey. Released online May 17, 2005, at http://press.expedia.com/index.php?s=press_releases&item=220

Fitzgerald, M., Williamson, P., Russell, C., & Manor, D. (2005). Doubling the cloak of (in)competence in client/therapist interactions. *Medical Anthropology Quarterly, 19,* 331–347.

Fussell, P. (1983). *Class: A guide through the American status system.* New York: Touchstone.

Ha, T. (2004). *Rising health costs, medical debt and chronic conditions* (Issue Brief No. 88). Washington, DC: Center for Studying Health System Change. Retrieved December 8, 2005, from http://hschange.org/CONTENT/706/

Hesse-Biber, S., & Carter, G. (2000). *Working women in America: Split dreams.* New York: Oxford University Press.

Himmelstein, D., Warren, E., Thorne, D., & Woolhandler, S. (2005, February 2). Illness and injury as contributors to bankruptcy. *Health Affairs.* Retrieved April 8, 2006, from http://content.healthaffairs.org/cgi/content/full/hlthaff.w5.63/DC1

hooks, b. (2000). *Where we stand: Class matters.* New York: Routledge.

Institute for Policy Studies and United for a Fair Economy. (2005, August 5). *Executive excess 2005: Defense contractors get more bucks for the bang* (12th annual CEO compensation survey). Washington, DC: Author.

Institute of Medicine. (2002). *Unequal treatment: Confronting racial and ethnic disparities in health care.* Washington, DC: National Academies Press.

Kaiser Family Foundation. (2003). *Health Insurance Coverage in America: 2002 Data Update.* Retrieved March 22, 2006, from http://www.kff.org/uninsured/4154.cfm

Kawachi, I., & Berkman, L. (2003). *Neighborhoods and health.* New York: Oxford University Press.

Kozol, J. (1991). *Savage inequalities: Children in America's schools.* New York: HarperCollins.

Kozol, J. (1995). *Amazing grace.* New York: Crown.

Krieger, N. (1999). Embodying inequality: A review of concepts, measures, and methods for studying health consequences of discrimination. *International Journal of Health Services, 29,* 295–352.

Krieger, N. (2001). A glossary for social epidemiology. *Journal of Epidemiology and Community Health, 55,* 693–700.

Kronenberg, F., & Pollard, N. (2005). Overcoming occupational apartheid: A preliminary exploration of the political nature of occupational therapy. In F. Kronenberg, S. Algado, and N. Pollard (Eds.), *Occupational therapy without borders: Learning from the spirit of survivors* (pp. 58–86). New York: Elsevier.

Law, M. (1998). *Client-centred occupational therapy.* Thorofare, NJ: Slack.

Lawlor, M. (2003). Gazing anew: The shift from a clinical gaze to an ethnographic lens. *American Journal of Occupational Therapy, 57,* 29–39.

Lawrence, S., Chau, M., & Lennon, M. C. (2004, June). *Depression, substance abuse, and domestic violence: Little is known about co-occurrence and combined effects on low-income families.* New York: National Center for Children in Poverty. Retrieved September 19, 2005, from http://www.researchforum.org/media/RFdsd04.pdf

Lee, P., Soffel, D., & Luft, H. (1994). Costs and coverage: Pressures toward health care reform. In P. Lee and C. Estes (Eds.), *The nation's health* (4th ed., pp. 204–213). Boston: Jones & Bartlett.

Letts, L., Rigby, P., & Stewart, D. (2003). *Using environments to enable occupational performance.* Thorofare, NJ: Slack.

Lohman, H., & Brown, K. (1997). Ethical issues related to managed care: An in-depth discussion of an occupational therapy case study. *Occupational Therapy in Health Care, 10*(4), 1–12.

Lynch, J. W., Kaplan, G. A., Pamuk, E. R., Cohen, R. D., Heck, K. E., Balfour, J. L., & Yen, I. H. (1998). Income inequality and mortality in metropolitan areas of the United States. *American Journal of Public Health, 88*(7), 1074–1080.

Lysack, C., & Neufeld, S. (2003). Occupational therapist home evaluations: Inequalities, but doing the best we can? *American Journal of Occupational Therapy, 57,* 369–379.

Lysack, C., Neufeld, S., Mast, B. MacNeill, S., & Lichtenberg, P. (2003). After rehabilitation: An 18-month follow-up of elderly inner-city women. *American Journal of Occupational Therapy, 57,* 298–306.

Marmot, M., Shipley, M., & Rose, G. (1984). Inequalities in death: Specific explanations of a general pattern. *Lancet, i*(May 5), 1003–1006.

Marmot, M., & Wilkinson, R. (Eds.). (1999). *Social determinants of health.* London: Oxford Press.

Mathieson, K. M., Kronenfeld, J. J., & Keith, V. M. (2002). Maintaining functional independence in elderly adults: The roles of health status and financial resources in predicting home modifications and use of mobility equipment. *The Gerontologist, 42*(1), 24–31.

Miringoff, M., & Miringoff, M. (1999). *The social health of the nation: How America is really doing.* New York: Oxford University Press.

Moss, N. (2000). Socioeconomic disparities in health in the US: An agenda for action. *Social Science and Medicine, 51,* 1627–1638.

National Center for Health Statistics. (2004). *Health, United States, 2004, with chartbook on trends in the health of Americans.* Hyattsville, MD: Author.

Neufeld, C., & Lysack, C. (2006). Investigating differences among older adults' access to specialized rehabilitation services, *Journal of Aging and Health, 18*(4), 584–623.

Organisation for Economic Co-operation and Development. (2005). *Health Data 2005: Statistics and indicators for 30 countries. How does the United States compare.* Paris: Author. Retrieved March 22, 2006, from http://www.oecd.org/dataoecd/15/23/34970246.pdf

Population Reference Bureau. (2005). *The 2005 world population data sheet.* Washington, DC: Author. Retrieved February 23, 2005, from http://www.prb.org/pdf05/05WorldDataSheet_Eng.pdf

Purtilo, R., & Haddad, A. (2002). *Health professional and patient interaction.* Philadelphia: Saunders.

Pynoos, J., Tabbarah, M., Angelelli, J., & Demiere, M. (1998). Improving the delivery of home modifications. *Technology and Disability, 8,* 3–14.

Rylko-Bauer, B., & Farmer, P. (2002). Managed care or managed inequality?: A call for critiques of market-based medicine. *Medical Anthropology Quarterly, 16*(4), 476–502.

Scott, J. (2005, May 16). Class matters: Life at the top in America isn't just better, it's longer. *The New York Times, Special Section,* p.1.

Shi, L., & Singh, D. (1998). *Delivering health care in America: A systems approach.* Gaithersburg, MD: Aspen.

Shipler, D. (2005). *The working poor: Invisible in America.* New York: Knopf.

Shonkoff, J., & Phillips, D. (2000). *From neurons to neighbourhoods: The science of early childhood development.* Washington, DC: National Academies Press.

Sidel, R. (1996). *Keeping women and children last: America's war on the poor.* New York: Penguin.

Soto, M. (2005, March). *Will baby boomers drown in debt?: Just the facts on retirement issues* (Issue 15). Boston: Center for Retirement Research at Boston College.

Stoddard, S., Jans, L., Ripple, J., & Kraus, L. (1998). *Chartbook on work and disability in the United States, 1998: An inhouse report.* Washington, DC: U.S. National Institute on Disability and Rehabilitation Research. Retrieved February 22, 2005, from http://www.infouse.com/disabilitydata/workdisability/2_1.php

Tanta, K., Deitz, J., White, O., & Billingsley, F. (2005). The effects of peer-play level on initiations and responses of preschool children with delayed play skills. *American Journal of Occupational Therapy, 59,* 437–445.

The Economist. (2005, July 21). Women in business: The conundrum of the glass ceiling. *The Economist* (from print edition). Retrieved April 8, 2006, from http://www.economist.com/business/displaystory.cfm?story_id=4197626

Townsend, E., & Wilcock, A. (2003). Occupational justice. In C. Christiansen & E. Townsend (Eds.), *Introduction to occupation* (pp. 243–273). Saddle River, NJ: Prentice Hall.

Trattner, W. (1994). *From poor law to welfare state: A history of social welfare in America* (5th ed.). New York: Free Press.

Uili, R. M., & Wood, R. (1995). The effect of third-party payers on the clinical decision making of physical therapists. *Social Science and Medicine, 40*(7), 873–879.

U.S. Administration on Aging. (2005). *A profile of older Americans: 2004.* Retrieved April 8, 2006, from http://www.aoa.gov/prof/Statistics/profile/2004/profiles2004.asp

U.S. Census. (2003). *Disability Status: 2000: A Census 2000 Brief.* Issue March 2003. Retrieved April 8, 2006, from http://www.census.gov/prod/2003pubs/c2kbr-17.pdf

U.S. Census. (2005). *Disability and American Families: 2000.* Census 2000 Special Reports. Retrieved April 8, 2006 from http://www.census.gov/prod/2005pubs/censr-23.pdf

U.S. Department of Health and Human Services. (2000a). *Healthy people 2010: Understanding and improving health* (2nd ed.). Washington, DC: U.S. Government Printing Office. Retrieved April 8, 2006, from http://www.healthypeople.gov/Document/pdf/uih/2010uih.pdf

U.S. Department of Health and Human Services. (2000b). Disability and secondary conditions. In *Healthy people 2010.* Retrieved June 1, 2005, from http://www.healthypeople.gov/Document/HTML/Volume1/06Disability.htm

U.S. Department of Labor. (2005). *Employment standards administration wage and hour division.* Retrieved May 30, 2005, from http://www.dol.gov/esa/minwage/america.htm

Weitz, R. (2004). *The sociology of health, illness, and health care.* Belmont, CA: Wadsworth.

Wells, S., & Black, R. (2000). *Cultural competency for health professionals.* Bethesda, MD: American Occupational Therapy Association.

Whiteford, G. (2003). Occupational deprivation: Global challenge in the new millennium. *British Journal of Occupational Therapy, 63*(5), 200–204.

Whiteis, D. (2000). Poverty, policy, and pathogenesis: Economic justice and public health in the U.S. *Critical Public Health, 10*(2), 257–271.

Wilkinson, R., & Marmot, M. (2003) *Social determinants of health: The solid facts* (2nd ed.). Copenhagen: World Health Organization, Regional Office for Europe.

Wilson, W. (1997). *When work disappears: The world of the new urban poor.* New York: Alfred A. Knopf.

Wood, W. (1996). Delivering occupational therapy's fullest promise: Clinical interpretations of "Life domains and adaptive strategies of a group of low-income, well older adults." *American Journal of Occupational Therapy, 50,* 109–112.

World Health Organization. (2005). *The world health report 2005.* Geneva: Author.

Young, M. E. (1997). *Early childhood development.* Washington, DC: The World Bank Development.

The Meaning of Place

GRAHAM D. ROWLES

8

Learning Objectives

After reading this chapter, you will be able to:

1. Identify, define, and explain the dimensions of a person's relationship with environment and the phenomenon of being in place.
2. Describe and explain life course–related changes in the manner in which people experience their environment as they progress from infancy to old age.
3. Explain the role of the physical environment and personal artifacts in defining and sustaining the self.
4. Describe the primary effects of environmental change and relocation and explain the mechanisms that individuals use to accommodate to environmental change and reestablish themselves in new environments.
5. Understand and explain the critical significance of an understanding of environment and place for effective occupational therapy practice.

THE PERSON-ENVIRONMENT RELATIONSHIP IN OCCUPATIONAL THERAPY

Place in Human Experience

Increased recognition of the role of the environment in conditioning human experience began to permeate occupational therapy during the 1980s (Barris, 1986; Barris, Kielhofner, Levine, & Neville, 1985; Kiernat, 1982, 1987). It is now widely acknowledged that full understanding of a person cannot be achieved independently of an appreciation of environmental context—the place where the person dwells. Occupational therapists have proposed several theories of the person-environment relationship that emphasize this interdependence (Christiansen & Baum, 1997; Dunn, Brown, & McGuigan, 1994; Kielhofner, 1995; Law et al., 1996; Schkade & Schultz, 1992). These transactional theories, as well as more recent ascendant perspectives that focus on the phenomenology of "being in place" (Rowles, 1991, 2000), "physical comminglings" (Seamon, 2002), and holistic Deweyan perspectives on "place integration" (Cutchin, 2004; Dickie, Cutchin, & Humphry, 2006), represent a shift from simple sequential stimulus-response conceptualizations of the individual as influenced by the environment or the environment as modified by human action. We are now moving toward directly acknowledging the degree to which the relationship involves blending person and place in human experience. Indeed, it is now widely accepted that the self evolves through activity that is in and of rather than being separate from the environment and that lives are intimately and inextricably defined by and immersed in place.

There is also increasing recognition that each person's relationship with environment cannot be considered independent of its historical context and the accumulation of experiences of place over time (Settersten, 1999, 2003; Wheeler, 1995). Each person is born in a particular location, into a particular family configuration, into a particular culture, and into a specific birth cohort. Over the course of life, each individual is molded by experience—a melding of physiological capability, individual agency, and circumstance—in a manner that profoundly influences the person he or she becomes (Jonsson, Josephson, & Kielhofner, 2000).

Phenomenological Perspective

Effective occupational therapy practice requires more than cursory inspection of a physical setting and compilation of a brief personal history. Probing deeper, it is important to understand each person from the perspective of an experienced context—the life world within which he or she defines the self, conducts daily activities, and receives occupational therapy intervention. From such a phenomenological perspective, how does the person experience his or her world? To what extent has the person created the physical setting of home, with its familiar furniture, memorabilia, and photographs, as an expression of self, perhaps over the course of decades (Rowles & Chaudhury, 2005)? To what extent is the person continuing to manipulate the setting to accommodate changing needs and abilities in ways that facilitate maintaining a sense of self, agency, and a meaningful life? Alternatively, in what ways is the person a prisoner of space, constrained by the configuration and accoutrements of the setting and trapped in a place that is increasingly confining and restrictive? In essence, what is the meaning of dwelling in a particular place and what are the implications of this meaning for the practice of occupational therapy? To answer such questions, it is important to understand complex dimensions of meaning that characterize the phenomenon of dwelling and that nurture a therapeutically desirable sense of being in place (Rowles, 1991, 2000).

 BOX 8.1

DIMENSIONS OF BEING IN PLACE

Use of Space

◆ Immediate physical activity: Range of motion and functional capability-related movement in the proximal environment.

◆ Everyday activity: Routine and often repeated daily trips along familiar pathways involved in the conduct of daily life.

◆ Occasional trips: Vacations and long-distance trips, generally involving overnight stays.

Orientation in Space

◆ Personal schema: A physiologically based axial orientation that enables the individual to maintain balance and distinguish left from right, front from back, and up from down.

◆ Specific schemata: Cognitive linear maps of regularly traveled pathways including an awareness of environmental cues that facilitate successfully traversing these pathways.

◆ General schema: An implicit cognitive map of the world as known, which can be evoked and mentally constituted at diverse scales and in diverse manifestations that vary according to the circumstances in which it is invoked.

Emotional Affiliations with Place

◆ Personal: Emotions evoked by personal experiences within particular locations that imbue settings with meaning and significance for the individual (may be positive or negative).

◆ Shared: Mutually developed emotions for place developed and refined through interaction over time among residents of a shared environment or through shared experience of an environment.

Vicarious Participation in Spatially and/or Temporally Displaced Environments

◆ Reflective: Involvement in places of one's past (either the current environment as it was in the past or previously experienced places located elsewhere).

◆ Projective: Vicarious projection into contemporary places that are geographically separated from the individual's current location.

Relevance to Occupational Therapy

Developing a sense of environmental, life course, and phenomenological context and blending this sense within a holistic understanding of each person's situation is of paramount importance to practitioners because occupational therapy interventions are invariably framed within a unique set of social and environmental circumstances (Gitlin, Corcoran, & Leinmiller-Eckhardt, 1995) and against the backdrop of a person's integration of these circumstances within a unique sense of self and of being in place. Interventions that take an individual out of place—for example, those that involve radical reconfiguration of the residence (e.g., significant rearrangement of furniture) or those that occur in a hospital, clinic, or rehabilitation environment—are invariably compromised because the person's agenda is necessarily expanded to cope with accommodation to a new and unfamiliar setting. In some cases, treatment in a hospital or clinical setting is inevitable because of the availability of specialized equipment and personnel. This does not obviate the need for understanding the dimensions of a person's being in place. Rather, it makes such understanding even more important in order to design treatment settings that create a level of environmental comfort that is conducive to effective occupational therapy practice.

DIMENSIONS OF BEING IN PLACE

A person's sense of being in place is a complex and dynamic phenomenon (Rowles, 1978, 1991, 2000; Rubinstein & Parmalee, 1992; Tuan, 1977). Several underlying themes or dimensions can be identified, as described in Box 8.1.

Using Space

At its most fundamental and easily observable level, being in place involves patterns of activity in using space. Space is utilized on multiple levels. First is the domain of immediate physical activity or range of motion. This involves activities of daily living, such as the functional ability to reach for a high shelf or to crouch without difficulty to don socks or tie shoelaces. Use of space on this level becomes a primary focus of occupational therapy when activity becomes limited through illness or accident and basic movement is impaired.

On a larger scale, we traverse the physical environment and trace regular pathways of everyday activity that over time become habitual (Rowles, 1978, 2000; Seamon, 1980). Each weekday morning, we walk to the corner of our street to catch the bus to work. On Sundays we drive a familiar route to church. Over time, we tend to develop a regular time-space rhythm and routine in use of the physical environment that becomes taken for granted and subconscious as our body adapts to the setting (Figure 8.1). Occupational therapy research suggests that deeper understanding of habits and habituation might hold the key to important therapeutic interventions (American Occupational Therapy Foundation, 2000, 2002).

The regular routine of everyday behaviors is enriched or disrupted by occasional trips that take us beyond our daily round. We vacation in a distant state or make an annual visit to stay with a relative. After an automobile accident, we might spend a period recuperating in a rehabilitation hospital some distance from our home.

Over the life course, patterns of using space gradually evolve in concert with changing capabilities and resources.

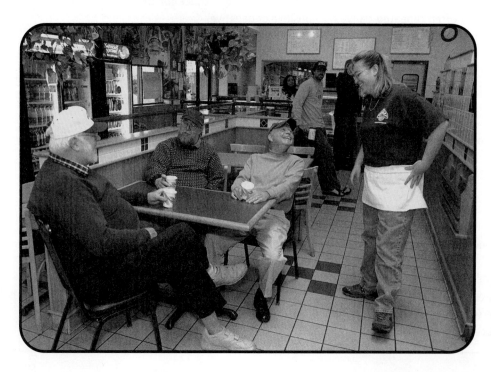

FIGURE 8.1   The everyday habit of breakfast at a local eatery forms important relationships. (Courtesy of D. Prince, University of New Hampshire Photographic Services, Durham, NH.)

The infant is restricted to a crib or playpen. The child, under a parent or sibling's watchful eye, might be permitted to play in the yard or in the neighborhood. Access to a first automobile significantly increases spatial range and in adulthood might lead to increased propensity to roam far and wide. With advancing years, the space within which we physically reside and travel might become limited once again as we become environmentally vulnerable.

Patterns of using space are closely intertwined with the manner in which we cognitively orient ourselves in the environment. This involves a physiological orientation within the axial system of the human body that provides the ability to discriminate up from down, left from right, and front from back. This personal schema is taken for granted. Its critical role might be fully recognized only when we become disoriented through a health condition such as Meniere's disease, excessive consumption of alcohol, or the secondary effects of medication.

Physiologic orientation is a necessary but not sufficient condition for moving around in the environment. We must also develop mental images, that is, cognitive maps of the configuration of the environment that guide us as we traverse space (Downs & Stea, 1973). Over time, we develop detailed cognitive awareness of paths we trace each day. This awareness may involve an array of environmental cues, comprising specific schemata that mark each route we take: The more familiar the journey, the more implicit are the schemata. The first time we walk an unfamiliar route, we are acutely aware of directions and environmental cues that mark the places to turn or to cross the street. As we repeatedly pass along this way, the need to use these cues recedes into the subconscious.

Cognitive awareness of regular pathways is embedded within a general schema. This implicit cognitive map of the world as we know it is characteristically centered on our residence. It involves detailed awareness of zones of immediately adjacent space, for example, the surveillance zone—the area within the visual field in which we may develop strong visual or mutually supportive relationships with neighbors characterized by a high level of everyday reciprocity (Rowles, 1981) (Fig. 8.2). We may also be familiar with space beyond the visual field, which becomes identified as our neighborhood. As we move farther away from home, cognitive awareness of space becomes progressively more fragmented and sketchier. There may be limited cognitive knowledge of the configuration of spaces beyond our own community, city, or town. The exception is a limited number of "beyond spaces." These are places we have visited on occasional trips, settings where we lived in the past, or familiar places where relatives reside. We might retain detailed images of the configuration of such noncontiguous places despite lack of everyday exposure.

Life course transitions in the use of space are paralleled by evolution in the manner in which we orient ourselves within space. In childhood, the imaged environment might be limited to our home and surroundings in the immediate vicinity. As experience increases and we become geographically liberated, our cognitive world becomes more extensive. A cosmopolitan mobile pattern of life in adulthood may lead to familiarity with environments throughout the world and an acute sense of their configuration and spatial relationship to one another. If we lead a life that is focused on a single urban neighborhood or rural community, our orientation might be equally rich and detailed but more locally focused. Finally, as we grow older, the tricks of memory and the sheer volume of accumulated place experiences can result in complex overlapping cogni-

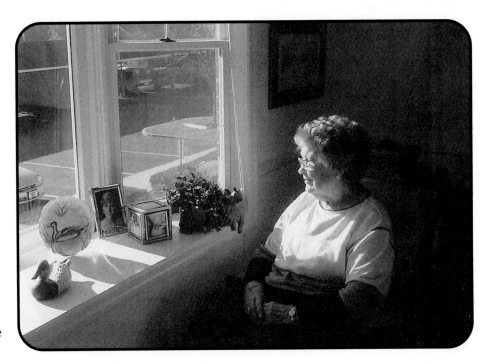

FIGURE 8.2 The surveillance zone. (Courtesy of G. Rowles.)

tive images within which specific locations may be known simultaneously as they were during a series of different times in their existence. Our awareness of a less frequently visited location might be a residual memory of its past rather than an accurate image of its current configuration.

Meaning in Place

Patterns of use and cognitive orientation to place parallel the development and reinforcement of distinctive place-related emotions (Altman & Low, 1992; Seamon, 1984). Some of these are individual and highly personal meanings. They may express a sense of affinity with places where key life events transpired—where we first met our future spouse, made love for the first time, or experienced a traumatic event. Mere presence in such places can evoke memories, the resurrection in consciousness of key incidents in our lives, and strong visceral emotions. As life experiences accumulate, frequently inhabited places where multiple events occurred over an extended period of time become suffused with an array of emotions that reflect a place biography of self and setting (Cattell, 2005).

Other place-related emotions reflect shared meanings. They arise from common habitation of a space—for example, an inner-city neighborhood or residential suburb—by a cohort of residents who, through their interaction and shared experiences, gradually come to imbue the place with its own personality, identity, and meanings as a social space (Després & Lord, 2005; Peace, Holland, & Kellaher, 2005; Rowles, 1978; Suttles, 1969). Long-time residents of changing neighborhoods may share complex emotional identification with a collage of the many different places it has been over the course of their lives, ranging from vibrant new development to rundown and largely abandoned slum.

Recognition of the critical role of time in human experience allows us to understand being in place as far more than the physical occupation of a space, the use of orientation skills, and the development of emotional affiliation with particular locales. Through the uniquely human capacity to remember, to imagine, and to project ourselves mentally into spaces beyond our immediate visual field, we can vicariously participate in spaces that have been displaced in space and time. We can return in our minds to the places of our childhood through a process of reflective vicarious reimmersion (Chaudhury, 1999). We can also engage in projective vicarious participation within the contemporary environments of family members and imagine what they might be doing half a continent away as we watch a televised national weather forecast that informs us that it is raining where they live (Rowles, 1978).

The ability to traverse space and time in our mind and inhabit an experiential world that is much larger than the immediate and contemporary physical setting is nurtured and reinforced by the artifacts with which we surround ourselves. Particular items of furniture, treasured per-

sonal possessions, scrapbooks, and photographs all serve as cues to the resurrection or stimulation of place experience in consciousness (Belk, 1992; Boschetti, 1995; Sherman & Dacher, 2005). Such items convey a sense of identity, capture essential elements of our autobiography, and, in so doing, help us to define and maintain a sense of self. We become the places of our lives—where we live and what we own.

To summarize, the spaces of our life become transformed into the places of our life through a variety of physical, cognitive, emotional, and imaginative processes of habitation that imbue existence with meaning and personal significance. Contemporary physical presence is only a small part of being in place. It is merely the overtly observable and most readily apparent aspect of a complex self that has gradually evolved over the life course, with the accumulation and integration of a plethora of life-shaping and person-forming experiences in the different places we have occupied from birth until the present.

Meaning of Home

The most intense expression of being in place characteristically involves our relationship with home—usually, although not invariably, the dwelling where we reside. In this location, we find the most sophisticated expressions of human relationship with the environment with respect to all levels of being in place: use, cognitive orientation, emotional affiliation, and vicarious involvement (Marcus, 1995; Rowles & Chaudhury, 2005; Rubinstein, 1989; Sixsmith, 1986; Zingmark, Norberg, & Sandman, 1995). Indeed, being in place entails being "at home."

Home is territory—a place of possession and ownership that may be fiercely defended. Home is a place of privacy, safety, and security. Often, home is the spatial fulcrum of our life, a place of comfort and centering that may become the core of our being and a location from which we venture forth into a potentially hostile world outside and beyond and to which we return for shelter. Home is a place of freedom, a location where we can let go and be ourselves. Home is a repository of the items we have accumulated that catalogue our history and define who we are. Beyond the personal significances with which such items can be imbued, home often also becomes a locus of expression as we present ourselves to visitors, neighbors, and those who pass by, through the way in which we maintain and decorate the property and care for our yard.

Because of the complex interweaving of these themes over an extended period of residence, home may come to be viewed as a sacred place and the seat of a person's very being and identity (Eliade, 1959; Rowles, 2006). For many people, to abandon one's home is not only to become homeless and placeless (Hasselkus, 2002; Relph, 1976; Watkins & Hosier, 2005), but also, in a quite literal sense, to experience a severance from self.

MAKING SPACES INTO PLACES OVER THE LIFE COURSE

Being in place and its relationship to self is a dynamic phenomenon. Throughout the life course, as we move from location to location, we are constantly creating and recreating place as a component of personal identity. With every move, we slough off elements of our past. With every move, we carry selected elements of this past with us and meld them with new experiences and the influence of new environments in creating a contemporary lifestyle and sense of being in place in the present. This selective process of transference allows us to maintain a continuity of self and identity that is reinforced by an evolving relationship with the places of our life (Rowles & Watkins, 2003; Twigger-Ross & Uzzell, 1996).

Transitions and Disruptions of Being in Place

A variety of circumstances result in changes in an individual's relationship with place that have important consequences for sense of self and well-being. Among the most profound are changes in personal capability. During the first portion of life, such changes are generally liberating. As we progress from infancy through childhood and into adolescence, the geographical world tends to expand as physical and mental capabilities develop and access is gained to an ever-wider array of resources (education, income, transportation). Competence tends to increase within an increasingly diverse array of environments. At the other end of the life course, as we grow old, physical and sensory decrements may become restrictive and confining, at least with respect to our physical use of space. It might become more difficult to venture abroad, to maintain our home, even to climb the stairs to an upstairs bedroom.

Lives are also lived within the context of constantly changing environments. New roadways slice disruptively through neighborhoods, the physical landscape changes with the addition of new buildings or the deterioration and demolition of old ones, new populations migrate into formerly stable residential enclaves, and both natural and human-made disasters transform the landscapes of our life. In youth, such change might be a source of stimulation and new opportunity; but as we grow older, we might become less resilient in accommodating to external environmental changes. Regardless of its source, change in people's relationship with the environment, whether in situ change or relocation, has become a predominant motif of life in contemporary Western societies.

Creating and Recreating Place

A fundamental human tension exists between the need for familiarity, security, and a sense of continuity and an urge to explore and to venture forth into the unknown (Balint, 1955; Buttimer, 1980). This tension is expressed in sequential habitation of the environments of our life through processes whereby we constantly create and recreate place as an expression of an evolving self (Rowles & Watkins, 2003). Most people exhibit residential inertia and reluctance to move. The intensity of this inertia may vary over the life course and among different generations; many young people exhibit greater enthusiasm for relocation, and many elders express a desire to age in place (Callahan, 1992; Tilson, 1990). When relocation does occur, there are certain constancies in the manner in which people accommodate to change.

People who have a history of frequent relocation often become experienced place-makers. With every relocation, they become more adept at sustaining links with places of their past even as they accommodate to opportunities provided by new settings. The process involves several overlapping elements, and each serves to preserve a continuity of self. First, there is a tendency for "holding on," which is manifest in routine ways of accommodating to the stress of separation from environments of our past. Contact with previous settings may be maintained through periodic return visits, telephone calls to former neighbors, or maintaining ongoing correspondence. Maintaining links with the places and the self of the past may also involve transferring treasured artifacts, including photographs and memorabilia, that serve as cues to key events and locations in personal history (Boschetti, 1995; Paton & Cram, 1992).

A second element of creating and recreating place is a recurring process of "moving on"—personal growth through active investment in each new setting (Leith, 2006). Often, this involves lifestyle change as a result of accommodation to illness, disability, or other changed circumstances. The process may involve the use of learned strategies for making new friends and becoming involved in the local social milieu such as making conscious efforts to visit new neighbors or coresidents (Reed & Payton, 1996). It may entail efforts, sometimes subconscious, to recreate elements of the familiar in each new setting. For example, some people facilitate maintaining a comfortable routine in the use of space by arranging their furniture in a configuration similar to that which existed in their previous residence (Hartwigsen, 1987; Toyama, 1988). Re-creation of place may also involve the selective transfer of artifacts and possessions and their arrangement within a new space in ways that serve to define and reinforce an evolving sense of self (Belk, 1992; Boschetti, 1995). Finally, moving on may involve a determined, conscious and adaptive phenomenological reformulation of the meaning of home through an ongoing process of merging lifelong expectations and experiences of previous places of residence with the potentialities and limitations of each new environment "thereby creating an essence of home that is at once old and new" (Leith, 2006, p.331).

Creating and recreating place is a lifelong process. During the first part of life, processes of accumulation tend to be dominant. Thus, a student apartment gives way to the condominium of the young professional, the first single-family home, and a series of progressively larger dwellings in parallel with changing needs as we find a partner and establish a family. We tend to accumulate more and more possessions—possessions that can come to define our persona. As we grow older, in many cases, we are obliged to move from spacious dwellings to residences with progressively less space. This process may gradually give way to processes of household disbandment and divestiture that involve a carefully reasoned but often emotionally taxing reduction of inventory (Eckerdt, Sergeant, Dingel, & Bowen, 2004; Morris, 1992). A priority may be placed on retaining items of particular personal and self-defining significance while selectively giving other items to children and others in the process of establishing a legacy that will allow aspects of the self to endure after death (Hunter, 2005). For elders, a continuing sense of being in place may be closely related to the ability to accomplish these processes in a manner that facilitates the retention of ongoing identity.

THE PLACE OF PLACE IN OCCUPATIONAL THERAPY

This chapter suggests that understanding a person's sense of self and well-being is intimately linked to a phenomenological life course–based understanding of an evolving person-environment transaction. Within this rubric, the definition of *person* has been expanded to emphasize the role of autobiography in defining the self. The concept of environment is elaborated and recast as the experiential notion of place. This reconfiguration is more than semantic novelty. Rather, it provides the basis for deeper understanding of human "being in the environment as a whole" aspects of the experienced world of the client that have important implications for practice (Dickie, Cutchin, & Humphry, 2006).

At the most fundamental level, there is a need for occupational therapy practitioners to become more intimately attuned and sensitive to the complexity of each client's being in place. It is not enough solely to observe a person's contemporary architectural setting and identify the physical barriers that interfere with performance of daily occupational tasks. Admittedly, it is important for practitioners to become advocates for client-centered environmental design that enhances occupational performance through design modification and the use of assistive devices. While this might be necessary as a first step in seeking interventions to improve functional performance, it is not sufficient if the goal is to enable the client to realize his or her full potential for attaining the highest possible quality of life. To accomplish this more sophisticated objective, it is necessary to embrace a broader understanding of place as a component of therapy—to develop place therapy (Scheidt & Norris-Baker, 1999).

What would an occupational place therapy look like? More than a rigid set of prescribed procedures, such a therapy would focus primarily on attitude and the practitioner's manner of relating to each client. It would focus on identifying customary patterns in the use of space, the role of habit and routine in these behaviors, and ways in which interventions can minimize disruption of habits and routines or create new ones that are consonant with a client's personal history. It would focus on identifying the manner in which each client cognitively orients daily behaviors in relation to the places of his or her life and normatively uses such constructions in accommodating to personal or environmental change. It would focus on developing client-sensitive appreciation of the disruptions of being in place at home that occurs as, with the increasing prevalence of home care, residences become physically and socially transformed into places of care provided by intruders from outside (Dyck, Kontos, Angus, & McKeever, 2005).

Such information would enable the practitioner to provide appropriate support and reorientation in response to changed circumstances. It would explicitly focus on the implications of disrupting long-standing emotional attachments to specific environments and to the artifacts that these environments contain and would seek ways of compensating for such disruptions, such as facilitating the transfer of key personal possessions when relocation is necessary (Wapner, Demick, & Redondo, 1990). And it would focus on framing interventions within the constraints and opportunities provided by the myriad environments that clients vicariously inhabit in their mind—environments that have been displaced in space and or time—that often are key elements in their definition of self. In this domain, key occupational therapy intervention might include reminiscence therapy or other types of activity that serve to maintain clients' connection with the places of their life that constitute their experiential world (Burnside & Haight, 1994; Chaudhury, 1999).

The question becomes how to translate such lofty aspirations into practical terms in the context of home and relocation. Possibilities for facilitating adjustment to either reduced physical capability in situ or a needed relocation include preparation strategies ranging from anticipatory modeling of change (Hunt & Pastalan, 1987) through processes of "constructing familiarity" (Reed & Payton, 1996) to psychotherapy based on "ecoanalysis of the home" (Peled & Schwartz, 1999). Such strategies are designed to prepare clients to deal with the consequences of separation from familiar place and routine and to facilitate the re-creation of place in a manner consistent with changed circumstances.

It is important to add words of caution at this point. First, for some people, expressions of self and of being in the world derive from dimensions of life other than place and home. It can be argued that such "placeless" people might be alienated from their environment and perhaps, by extension, from self. Nonetheless, it is important to avoid the dangers of romanticism and to avoid a stereotypical view of the role of place in people's lives. Second, occupational place therapy might be more appropriate for some clients than for others. For example, people with lengthy histories and multiple experiences of accommodating to change both within their indigenous environment and through experience in place-making gained from frequent relocations might be very adept at accommodating to lifestyle and behavioral changes necessitated by a needed occupational therapy intervention. But what about those who have been more residentially stable and are accustomed to lifelong routines of using a single space and relating to only a few places? Such individuals might experience great difficulty in abandoning familiar routines, adjusting the nature of their being in place in a familiar residence or, should relocation be necessary, transforming a new space into a place. For these individuals, change might be particularly traumatic.

CONCLUSION

There is a tendency in contemporary society to assume that successful rehabilitation is achieved merely by returning individuals to former levels of physical functioning and behavioral competence. Such a view is myopic and demeaning with respect to the richness of human experience. When a practitioner advocates removal of a potentially hazardous throw rug from a client's hallway, offers assistance in rearranging the client's space to accommodate a disability, or provides training in the use of the latest occupational therapy gadget, the practitioner might be enhancing the safety of the home and the physical competence of the client while also diminishing the client's sense of control and autonomy. These interventions might mean discarding a rug that was inherited from a favorite grandmother and transported from home to home over a lifetime—an artifact that is an enduring symbol of family history and continuity. Rearranging the space might move important family photographs beyond the visual field of a favorite chair that, itself, was formerly by the window but has been moved to a safer location that no longer affords a view of activities in the surveillance zone outside. The gadget that the therapist finds so innovative and helpful might achieve its overt purpose but reinforce a sense of inadequacy and incompetence in an individual who might be even better served by accommodating to his or her disability through a less overtly intrusive strategy.

With the hindsight of history, the past few decades might come to be known as an era in which our technology exceeded our humanity as humankind lapsed into hedonistic obsession with material and technological ingenuity. By reinvesting in meaning through place, occupational therapy might be able to help us rediscover our humanity. By seeking new ways to enable individuals to maintain an enduring sense of being in place as a component of the self, the practice of occupational therapy can become elevated to a higher plane.

PROVOCATIVE QUESTIONS

1. How does your relationship to place differ from that of your parents? Your grandparents? Your children?
2. In what ways are the dimensions of being in place outlined in Box 8.1 modified under circumstances in which multiple individuals inhabit a shared residence?
3. In an increasingly mobile society, how will the greater frequency of relocation during the life course affect individual's ability to establish and maintain a sense of being in place? Will the outcome be alienation from place? What are the implications of this for occupational therapy?
4. How can occupational therapy intervention ease the process of relocation?

REFERENCES

Altman, I., & Low, S. M. (Eds.). (1992). *Place attachment.* New York: Plenum Press.

American Occupational Therapy Foundation. (2000). *The Occupational Therapy Journal of Research 20*(Suppl. 1), 2S–143S.

American Occupational Therapy Foundation. (2002). *The Occupational Therapy Journal of Research 22*(Suppl. 1), 3S–112S.

Balint, M. (1955). Friendly expanses—horrid empty spaces. *International Journal of Psychoanalysis, 36*(4/5), 225–241.

Barris, R. (1986). Activity: The interface between person and environment. *Physical and Occupational Therapy in Geriatrics, 5,* 39–49.

Barris, R., Kielhofner, G., Levine, R. E., & Neville, A. M. (1985). Occupation as interaction with environment. In G. Kielhofner (Ed.), *A model of human occupation: Theory and application* (pp. 42–62). Baltimore: Williams & Wilkins.

Belk, R. W. (1992). Attachment to possessions. In I. Altman & S. M. Low (Eds.), *Place attachment* (pp. 37–62). New York: Plenum Press.

Boschetti, M. A. (1995). Attachment to personal possessions: An interpretive study of the older person's experiences. *Journal of Interior Design, 21*(1), 1–12.

Burnside, I., & Haight, B. (1994). Reminiscence and life review: Therapeutic interventions for older people. *Nurse Practitioner, 19*(4), 55–61.

Buttimer, A. (1980). Home, reach and the sense of place. In A. Buttimer & D. Seamon (Eds.), *The human experience of space and place* (pp. 166–187). New York: St. Martin's Press.

Callahan, J. J. (1992). Aging in place. *Generations, 16,* 5–6.

Cattell, M. G. (2005). African reinventions: Home, place and kinship among Abaluyia of Kenya. In G. D. Rowles & H. Chaudhury (Eds.), *Home and identity in late life: International perspectives* (pp. 317–340). New York: Springer.

Chaudhury, H. (1999). Self and reminiscence of place: A conceptual study. *Journal of Aging and Identity, 4*(4), 231–253.

Christiansen C., & Baum, C. (1997). Person-environment-occupational performance: A conceptual model for practice. In C. Christiansen & C. Baum (Eds.), *Occupational therapy: Enabling function and well-being* (pp. 46–70). Thorofare, NJ: Slack.

Cutchin, M. P. (2004). Using Deweyan philosophy to rename and reframe adaptation-to-environment. *American Journal of Occupational Therapy, 58*(3), 303–312.

Després, C., & Lord, S. (2005). Growing older in postwar suburbs: The meanings and experiences of home. In G. D. Rowles & H. Chaudhury (Eds.), *Home and identity in late life: International perspectives* (pp. 317–340). New York: Springer.

Dickie, V., Cutchin, M. P., & Humphry, R. (2006). Occupation as transactional experience: A critique of individualism in occupational science. *Journal of Occupational Science, 13*(1), 83–93.

Downs, R. M., & Stea, D. (Eds.). (1973). *Image and environment: Cognitive mapping and spatial behavior.* Chicago: Aldine.

Dunn, W., Brown, C., & McGuigan, A. (1994). The ecology of human performance: A framework for considering the effect of context. *American Journal of Occupational Therapy, 48*(7), 595–607.

Dyck, I., Kontos, P., Angus, J., & McKeever, P. (2005). The home as a site for long-term care: Meanings and management of bodies and spaces. *Health and Place, 11,* 173–185.

Eckerdt, D. J., Sergeant, J. F., Dingel, M., & Bowen, M. E. (2004). Household disbandment in later life. *Journals of Gerontology: Social Sciences, 59S*(5), S265–S273.

Eliade, M. (1959). *The sacred and the profane.* New York: Harcourt, Brace & World.

Gitlin, L. N., Corcoran, M., & Leinmiller-Eckhardt, S. (1995). Understanding the family perspective: An ethnographic framework for providing occupational therapy in the home. *American Journal of Occupational Therapy, 49,* 802–809.

Hasselkus, B. R. (2002). *The meaning of everyday occupation.* Thorofare, NJ: Slack.

Hartwigsen, G. (1987). Older widows and the transference of home. *International Journal of Aging and Human Development, 25*(3), 195–207.

Hunt, M. E., & Pastalan, L. A. (1987). Easing relocation: An environmental learning process. In V. Regnier & J. Pynoos (Eds.), *Housing the aged: Design directives and policy considerations* (pp. 421–440). New York: Elsevier.

Hunter, E. G., & Rowles, G. D. (2005). Leaving a legacy: Toward a typology. *Journal of Aging Studies, 19,* 327–347.

Jonsson, H., Josephson, S., & Kielhofner, G. (2000). Evolving narratives in the course of retirement: A longitudinal study. *American Journal of Occupational Therapy 54,* 463–470.

Kielhofner, G. (1995). *A model of human occupation: Theory and application* (2nd ed.) Baltimore: Williams & Wilkins.

Kiernat, J. M. (1982). Environment: The hidden modality. *Physical and Occupational Therapy in Geriatrics 2,* 3–12.

Kiernat, J. M. (1987). Promoting independence and autonomy through environmental approaches. *Topics in Geriatric Rehabilitation 3,* 1–6.

Law, M., Cooper, B., Strong, S., Steward, D., Rigby, P., & Letts, L. (1996). The person-environment occupation model: A transactive approach to occupational performance. *Canadian Journal of Occupational Therapy, 63,* 9–23.

Leith, K. H. (2006). "Home is where the heart is . . . or is it?": A phenomenological exploration of the meaning of home for older women in congregate housing. *Journal of Aging Studies, 20,* 317–333.

Marcus, C. C. (1995). *House as a mirror of self: Exploring the deeper meaning of home.* Berkeley, CA: Conari Press.

Morris, B. R. (1992). Reducing inventory: Divestiture of personal possessions. *Journal of Women and Aging, 4*(2), 79–92.

Paton, H., & Cram, F. (1992). Personal possessions and environmental control: The experiences of elderly women in three residential settings. *Journal of Women and Aging, 4*(2), 61–78.

Peace, S. M., Holland, C., & Kellaher, L. (2005). The influence of neighborhood and community on well-being and identity in later life: An English perspective. In G. D. Rowles & H. Chaudhury (Eds.), *Home and identity in late life: International perspectives* (pp. 297–315). New York: Springer.

Peled, A., & Schwartz, H. (1999). Exploring the ideal home in psychotherapy: Two case studies. *Journal of Environmental Psychology, 19,* 87–94.

Reed, J., & Payton, V. R. (1996). Constructing familiarity and managing the self: Ways of adapting to life in nursing and residential homes for older people. *Ageing and Society, 16,* 543–560.

Relph, E. (1976). *Place and placelessness.* London: Pion Limited.

Rowles, G. D. (1978). *Prisoners of space? Exploring the geographical experience of older people.* Boulder, CO: Westview Press.

Rowles, G. D. (1981). The surveillance zone as meaningful space for the aged. *The Gerontologist, 21*(3), 304–311.

Rowles, G. D. (1991). Beyond performance: Being in place as a component of occupational therapy. *American Journal of Occupational Therapy, 45*(3), 265–271.

Rowles, G. D. (2000). Habituation and being in place. *Occupational Therapy Journal of Research, 20*(Suppl. 1), 52S–67S.

Rowles, G. D. (2006). A house is not a home: But can it become one? In H.-W. Wahl, H. Brenner, H. Mollenkopf, D. Rothenbacher, & C. Rott (Eds.), *The many faces of health, competence and well-being in old age* (pp. 25–32). Dordrecht, The Netherlands: Springer.

Rowles, G. D., & Chaudhury, H. (Eds.). (2005). *Home and identity in late life: International perspectives.* New York: Springer.

Rowles, G. D., & Watkins, J. F. (2003). History, habit, heart and hearth: On making spaces into places. In K. W. Schaie, H.-W. Wahl, H. Mollenkopf, & F. Oswald (Eds.), *Aging in the community: Living environments and mobility* (pp. 77–96). New York: Springer.

Rubinstein, R. (1989). The home environments of older people: A description of the psychosocial processes linking person to place. *Journal of Gerontology, 44,* S45–S53.

Rubinstein, R., & Parmalee, P. A. (1992). Attachment to place and the representation of the life course by the elderly.

In I. Altman & S. M. Low (Eds.), *Place attachment* (pp. 139–163). New York: Plenum Press.

Scheidt, R. J., & Norris-Baker, C. (1999). Place therapies for older adults: Conceptual and interventive approaches. *International Journal of Aging and Human Development, 48*(1), 1–15.

Schkade, J. K., & Schultz, S. (1992). Occupational adaptation: Toward a holistic approach for contemporary practice: Part 1. *American Journal of Occupational Therapy, 46,* 829–837.

Seamon, D. (1980). Body subject, time-space routines, and place ballets. In A. Buttimer & D. Seamon (Eds.), *The human experience of space and place* (pp. 148–165). London: Croom Helm.

Seamon, D. (1984). Emotional experience of the environment. *American Behavioral Scientist, 27*(6), 757–770.

Seamon, D. (2002). Physical comminglings: Body, habit and space transformed into place. *Occupational Therapy Journal of Research, 22,* 42S–51S.

Settersten, R. A. (1999). *Lives in time and place: The problems and promises of developmental science.* Amityville, NY: Baywood.

Settersten, R. A. (Ed). (2003). *Invitation to the life course: Toward new understandings of later life.* Amityville, NY: Baywood.

Sherman, E., & Dacher, J. (2005). Cherished objects and the home: Their meaning and roles in later life. In G. D. Rowles & H. Chaudhury (Eds.), *Home and identity in late life: International perspectives* (pp. 63–79). New York: Springer.

Sixsmith, J. (1986). The meaning of home: An exploratory study of environmental experience. *Journal of Environmental Psychology, 6,* 281–298.

Suttles, G. D. (1969). *The social order of the slum.* Chicago: University of Chicago Press.

Tilson, D. (Ed.). (1990). *Aging in place: Supporting the frail elderly in residential environments.* Glenview, IL: Scott, Foresman.

Toyama, T. (1988). *Identity and milieu: A study of relocation focusing on reciprocal changes in elderly people and their environment.* Stockholm, Sweden: Department for Building Function Analysis, the Royal Institute of Technology.

Tuan, Y. F. (1977). *Space and place: The perspective of experience.* Minneapolis: University of Minnesota Press.

Twigger-Ross, C., & Uzzell, D. L. (1996). Place and identity processes. *Journal of Environmental Psychology, 16,* 205–220.

Wapner, S., Demick, J., & Redondo, J. P. (1990). Cherished possessions and adaptation of older people to nursing homes. *International Journal of Aging and Human Development, 31*(3), 219–235.

Watkins, J. F., & Hosier, A. F. (2005). Conceptualizing home and homelessness: A life course perspective. In G. D. Rowles & H. Chaudhury (Eds.), *Home and identity in late life: International perspectives* (pp. 197–216). New York: Springer.

Wheeler, W. M. (1995). *Elderly residential experience: The evolution of places as residence.* New York: Garland.

Zingmark, A., Norberg, K., & Sandman, P.-O. (1995). The experience of being at home throughout the lifespan: Investigation of persons 2 to 102. *International Journal of Aging and Human Development, 41*(1), 47–62.

Spirituality, Occupation, and Occupational Therapy

CHRISTY BILLOCK

> "In a way all sacred experience and all journeys of soul lead us to the smallest moment of the most ordinary day"
>
> —SUE MONK KIDD (1996)

Learning Objectives

After reading this chapter, you will be able to:

1. Develop an understanding of the meaning of spirituality as related to occupational therapy practice, including definition, related themes, and distinction from religion.
2. Recognize the relationship between spirituality, occupation, health, and well-being.
3. Identify the relationship of spirituality to occupational therapy's history.
4. Understand the relevance of individual experiences of spirituality. through occupation by examining important factors such as context, reflection and intention, and occupational engagement.
5. Describe strategies to integrate spirituality into occupational therapy practice.
6. Explore how spirituality and occupation might intersect in your own life experiences.

INTRODUCTION

As occupational therapy continues to evolve as a profession rooted in the rich and complex notion of occupation, spirituality emerges as an interconnected relevant theme that deserves further exploration. No strangers to confronting complexity, occupational therapists and occupational scientists grasp the necessity of creating a deeper theoretical and practical base for understanding spirituality as it relates to occupational engagement, intervention, and professional practice. This chapter serves as an introductory resource for understanding spirituality in occupational therapy practice. I begin by asking the fundamental question: What is spirituality and how does it relate to occupational therapy? Second, I will discuss the multiple ways in which spirituality is experienced through occupation. Third, I will integrate spirituality into occupational therapy practice. Last, I will pose reflective questions that will allow readers to explore their own views of spirituality.

FRAMING SPIRITUALITY FROM AN OCCUPATIONAL THERAPY PERSPECTIVE

The multidimensional and complex nature of spirituality defies simple definition. According to Hasselkus (2002):

> Spirituality cannot be directly observed in the physical sense. We are not even at all sure what behaviors we might identify that represent this phenomenon. We have trouble finding the words to describe what we think we mean when we use the word *spirituality*. Yet we probably all acknowledge the existence of some sort of spiritual nature in ourselves and in the lives of all human beings. (p. 102)

Definitions typically emphasize spirituality as a metaphysical and individually experienced internal phenomenon involving an essential spirit, soul, or essence of a person (Egan & DeLaat, 1994; Hasselkus, 2002; Moore, 1992). Individuals might experience spirituality as a sense of connectedness that relates them to a transcendent being, a belief, themselves, others, or the physical world. Recurring themes related to spirituality within occupational therapy and other health professions' literature are hope, faith, coping, and self-transcendence (Haase, Britt, Coward, Leidy, & Penn, 1992; Kelly, 2004; Spencer, Davidson, & White, 1997).

Spirituality can be defined as a deep experience of meaning (Urbanowski & Vargo, 1994) brought about by engaging in occupations that involve the enacting of personal ideologies, reflection, and intention within a supportive contextual environment. Occupational therapy places meaning as a central tenet of the profession, and meaning-making, in its essence, is a spiritual process that seeks expression through occupation (Peloquin, 1997). People often experience spirituality through engagement in everyday activities (Moore, 1992); consequently, occupation creates meaning and helps to answer larger existential questions of the meaning of life (Christiansen, 1997; Frankl,

1959). Recently, the American Occupational Therapy Association (AOTA) included spirituality in the practice framework as a context for occupation, which is "the fundamental orientation of a person's life, that which inspires and motivates that individual" (AOTA, 2002, p. 633). The notion of a "fundamental orientation" evokes an understanding of spirituality as the deepest and most central kind of meaning a person experiences.

Religion is often linked with spirituality and can inform a person's understanding and experience of meaning. Religion is defined as an integrated system of beliefs with their attendant practices (Engquist, Short-DeGraff, Gliner, & Oltjenbruns, 1997). As a set of individual and communal practices, religion permeates many people's experiences of spirituality on a daily basis through occupations such as prayer, meditation, reading theological books, and attending religious services. Not only do religions provide followers with practices that directly relate to theological beliefs, but religious beliefs often ascribe spiritual meaning to daily occupations such as food preparation, work, and intimacy, especially if they are "understood as commanded by God" (Frank et al., 1997, p. 201). Although many people use religion as a tool for framing spirituality in their lives, individual spiritual experience is not dependent on religious affiliation or practice.

Spiritual and religious practices are linked to well-being and health (Low, 1997; Miller & Thoresen, 2003). Spiritual health takes on many definitions but generally connotes being able to experience meaning, fulfillment, and connection with self, others, and a higher power or larger reality (Hawks, Hull, Thalman, & Richins, 1995). These viewpoints also recognize that illness and disease affect the whole person, including the body, mind, and spirit, and all need to be addressed to restore health (do Rozario, 1997). Experiences of occupational alienation (Townsend & Wilcock, 2004), that is, an inability to create meaning and express one's spirit through occupation, demonstrates a lack of spiritual health or well-being for a person (Simo Algado et al., 2002).

It is important to address the right of marginalized populations such as people with disabilities, mental illness, and the aged to experience spirituality and practice religion (Eisland & Saliers, 1998; Koenig, George, & Peterson, 1998; Richards, 1990). These issues of access to occupations as a fundamental human right connect the principles of occupational justice and spirituality (Wilcock, 2001).

Exploring the historical roots of occupational therapy reveals traces of spirituality from the profession's founding. Moral treatment influenced the founders of occupational therapy in the early twentieth century (Bockhoven, 1971). Advocates of moral treatment valued ideals such as holism, humanism, and a recognition that engagement of the mind, body, and spirit through occupation promoted health and brought meaning to life (Meyer, 1922/1977). In the 1920s and 1930s, the medical establishment criticized occupational therapy for its lack of theory grounded in scientific principles (Gritzer & Arluke, 1989). In an attempt to legitimize the profession, occupational therapists adopted reductionistic models through the 1950s, thereby minimizing the emphasis on recognition of the human spirit as expressed in occupation (Yerxa, 1992). In 1962, Reilly expressed concern that the reductionistic view of occupational therapy could not capture the role that occupation could play in facilitating health. Reilly's words proved to be a catalyst for the reemergence of a holistic perspective valuing spirituality as a central concept of occupational therapy (Atler, Fisher, Moret, & White, 2000).

In the late twentieth century, the Canadian Association of Occupational Therapy (CAOT) explicitly integrated spirituality into theories about client-centered practice and occupational performance, placing spirituality at the center of theoretical constructs of occupation that guide occupational therapy practice (CAOT, 1991, 1997). In the United States, the AOTA in 1997 devoted an entire issue of the *American Journal of Occupational Therapy* to the topic of spirituality. Spirituality gained inclusion in the Occupational Therapy Practice Framework (AOTA, 2002) as a context for occupation ushering in the official recognition of the importance of spirituality to occupational therapy in the United States.

EXPERIENCING SPIRITUALITY THROUGH OCCUPATION

A person's ability to create and experience a deep sense of meaning through engagement in occupation makes spirituality compelling. Although spirituality can be experienced outside of occupation, engaging in occupation is the most common and effective mechanism for these experiences because it is through occupational engagement that spirituality becomes more tangible. Peloquin (1997) refers to occupation as an act of making that represents an extension and animation of the human spirit:

> To see such radical making in the acts that we commonly name *doing* purposeful activities, *performing* life roles and tasks, *adapting* to the environment, *adjusting* to disability, and *achieving* skills or mastery, is to discern the spiritual depth of occupation. (p. 167)

Linking occupation and spirituality together with the notion of "making" implies a fluid and active approach to the phenomenon. In making, a person expresses tangibly the intangible yet vital realities of life. This expression, though invariably interconnected with the social world, is ultimately created and interpreted internally by each individual. These internal representations about the meaning of reality and the world drive people to orchestrate occupations to express those meanings (Kroeker, 1997).

Trends within Western society signify a moving away from practices directed by organized religion and toward personal construction of practices for the foundation of spiritual life (Wuthnow, 1998). McColl (2002) contends that given the erosion of meaning in work from industrialization and the prevalence of secular pluralism in modern society, occupation "may be the most effective medium available through which individuals can affirm their connection with the self, with others, with the cosmos, and with the divine" (p. 352). Orchestration of and engagement in everyday occupation holds the potential of helping people to meet the fundamental need for spiritual expression. For example, the busy executive's attending a yoga class, receiving a massage, or taking a hike might serve the vitally important role of facilitating his or her experiences of spirituality.

Contextual Factors

Spiritual experiences through occupation are dependent on and vulnerable to several contextual factors, including the physical and social world. Symbolism is a potent nexus of meaning-making embedded within these contextual factors (Fine, 1999). Places, objects, and communities hold symbolic meanings to individuals that are informed by past history, both individual and communal (Holland, Lachicotte, Skinner, & Cain, 1998).

The physical world can serve to potentially facilitate or block spiritual experiences (Jackson, 1996). Many people communicate experiences of spirituality through occupations in nature such as hiking in the mountains, fly-fishing in a stream, or walking along the beach. Built spaces such as churches, houses, and other structures serve to refine and make more vivid human feeling, perception, and comprehension of reality (Tuan, 1977). Out of experiencing those spaces and the objects within them, a person draws a sense of place that is "an organized world of meaning" (Tuan, 1977, p. 179). For example, a home filled with memories of family gatherings and decorated with special pieces of art and pictures of loved ones can provide support for experiencing spirituality through the occupations that are engaged in within the space. Gathering around a table appointed with grandmother's linens and pottery made by friends, then lighting candles when friends come to share a meal, marks the event as one with special meaning and spiritual import. Whereas home can support one person's experiences of spirituality, for another person, the home might be a place of strained memories and relationships. For a woman who is physically abused by her husband in the privacy of their home, experiences of occupation within her home may show little potential for spiritual experience.

The social world can significantly influence spiritual experience because meaning is both personally and socially constructed (Hasselkus, 2002). Therefore, attempts to understand spiritual experience involve looking at the doer of the occupation in reference to the social and cultural worlds of engagement. Engaging in occupations with others, or co-occupation (Zemke & Clark, 1996), can potentiate the likelihood of a spiritual experience. Religions recognize the importance of believers practicing their faith with others as a means of mutual support and affirmation of belief (Howard & Howard, 1997). Communal occupations such as attending sporting events, concerts, or political protests as well as family celebrations such as weddings or graduations can be rich environments for spiritual experience.

The Centrality of Reflection and Intention

Spiritual experience also relies on personal reflection and intention. Reflection refers to the exploration of one's inner world and necessarily involves recognition of feelings, emotions, and motivations to act. Reflection also becomes a tool of interpretation that can lead to a setting apart of spiritual experiences as different from everyday life, something special or transcendent (Bell, 1997). Intention involves a conscious imbuing of meaning or directing occupational experience toward something such as a value, belief, or ideology. Reflection or intention in an occupational experience does not necessarily need to be labeled "spiritual"; rather, it may be sensed as deeply satisfying or meaningful.

Occupations engaging a person's creativity offer the opportunity for deep levels of reflection, intention, and ultimately spiritual experience. Kidd (1996), speaking of creativity and spirituality, says, "my creative life is my greatest prayer" (p. 123). Cameron (1992) shares a similar view of the intertwining of spirituality and creativity,

> Creativity is an experience—to my eye, a spiritual experience. It does not matter which way you think of it: creativity leading to spirituality or spirituality leading to creativity. In fact, I do not make a distinction between the two. (p. 2)

Infusing occupation with creativity allows for expression of internal states innately spiritual in nature (Simo Algado et al., 2002). Whereas artistic occupations such as painting, making pottery, or writing poetry show high potential for spiritual experience, numerous other everyday occupations can be filled with creativity as well (Hasselkus, 2002). Occupations such as cooking, conversing with others, or planning a party, along with countless others, can be occupations in which creativity is expressed.

Occupational Engagement

Not all occupations are experienced as spiritual, but all occupations hold the potential to be spiritual. Although people often name occupations stemming from religious traditions as spiritual, the lived experience of such occupations might not be spiritual. Everyday occupations such as work, walking the dog, or gardening might be experienced as spiritual but likely would not be named as religious (Howard & Howard, 1997; Unruh, 1997). Occupations that are deeply meaningful to the person, imbued with personal reflection and intention, and carried out within a supportive contextual environment offer the highest potential for spiritual experience. Kidd (1996) describes the fleeting nature of spirituality in the midst of the details of a normal morning:

> I rose to make the coffee. I walked to the door and paused. When I looked back, I saw my life shining within every ordinary thing. And I was seized by the same feeling I get whenever I see the ocean—the feeling that it is all too much to behold, too beautiful, too much to bear—and I was filled with an aching love for it. In the next instant the moment was gone, and I was climbing down the stairs, walking into the kitchen, into a day of small, humble, distracting things, and somehow nothing seemed more holy to me than just being there, naturally myself, in the midst of it. Such moments are not as common for me as I might wish. But when they come, they leave me with a willingness to relate to my ordinary space—my work and family and friends and all the mundane duties—more authentically. (p. 222)

The demands of routine activities that must be done often blocks the ability to reflect, be intentional, and find deep meaning in the moment (Norris, 1998).

People frequently experience rituals as spiritual, and throughout history, many ordinary activities such as serving food have been used in ritual (Bell, 1997). Common to understandings of ritual are the notions of repetition, fixedness, and predictability that are usually embedded in the doing of religion (Hasselkus, 2002). Outside of religion, any occupation can take on ritualistic characteristics of formalism, tradition, invariance, sacral symbolization, and performance. It is these characteristics that differentiate sacred experience from the more mundane aspects of life (Bell, 1997). Depending on an individual's engagement, an occupation such as taking a bath could be experienced as spiritual owing to ritualized characteristics. Bell recognizes the importance of rituallike performances because they "communicate on multiple sensory levels, usually involving highly visual imagery, dramatic sounds, and sometimes even tactile, olfactory, and gustatory stimulation" (p. 160). For example, engagement in the occupations of a holiday celebration with its attendant ritual practices involving food and particular actions offers the possibility of spiritual experience in bringing together personal, familial, social, religious, and cultural aspects of life (Luboshitzky & Gaber, 2001).

INTEGRATING SPIRITUALITY INTO OCCUPATIONAL THERAPY PRACTICE

As a profession rooted in holistic and humanistic values, occupational therapy holds a unique opportunity to help clients restore meaning to their lives, a vitally important and essentially spiritual task. Although most occupational therapists recognize spirituality as an important aspect of life, integrating a spiritual perspective into occupational therapy practice proves problematic because of its ambiguity and the large diversity of therapists' understanding of the notion (Enquist et al., 1997). Also, in light of the drive toward evidence-based practice, inclusion of spirituality in the core of occupational performance has become increasingly controversial (Unruh, Versnel, & Kerr, 2002). These challenges lead to role ambiguity and a lack of confidence in addressing spirituality in practice in spite of a recognized need for its inclusion (Belcham, 2004). As Howard and Howard (1997) indicate, "occupational therapists need not look beyond the tools, theories, and values of the profession to provide a context for acknowledging the spiritual in the clinic" (p. 185). If spirituality is a deep experience of meaning effectively experienced through occupational engagement, then occupational therapy intervention strategies that uphold holism through occupation-based and client-centered techniques will likely promote clients' spiritual health and well-being.

Recognizing the difficulty of integrating spirituality into practice, Egan and Swedersky (2003) identified four strategies used by occupational therapists who successfully achieve this integration:

♦ Addressing clients' religious concerns
♦ Assisting clients' in dealing with suffering
♦ Helping clients to recognize their own worth and efficacy
♦ Recognizing their own transformations brought about by working with clients

Integrating spirituality into practice starts with the occupational therapy practitioner (Townsend et al., 1999). Practitioners must consider their own understanding of spirituality and how their spirituality plays out in their occupations and experiences. Additionally, this self-reflective process may lead to the recognition of personal biases or beliefs that could interfere with the crucially needed openness to clients' diverse beliefs and experiences. Self-reflection also aids in the ethically important need for therapeutic interventions to be consistent with the client's spiritual life, not the therapist's (Rosenfeld, 2001). Those who practice therapeutic use of self through active listening, empathy, tolerance, unconditional acceptance, and flexibility toward the client's desires and needs demonstrate a spiritual approach to therapeutic interaction.

Many consumers of occupational therapy have experienced disruptions to and loss of the occupations through which they experience spirituality and meaning. By honoring the subjective experiences of clients in the evaluation, goal-setting, and intervention-planning processes, the practitioner moves toward integrating spirituality into practice and will likely increase the client's motivation (Townsend et al., 1999). Tools such as the Canadian Occupational Performance Measure allow for a client-centered and occupation-based approach that can address spiritual needs through actively integrating the client into the phases of evaluation and intervention (Law, et al., 1994).

A client-centered occupational therapy approach that draws spirituality into practice requires close attention to the client's culture (Simo Algado et al., 2002) as well as the form, function, and meaning of the occupations used in intervention (Larson, Wood, & Clark, 2003). Practitioners sometimes feel uncomfortable integrating clients' religious occupations into intervention. If these occupations are important aspects of a client's daily life, religious occupations such as prayer or reading sacred texts can be integrated into intervention sessions as deeply meaningful occupations. Addressing culture might call for learning more about rituals and religious traditions different from the practitioner's own religious experience or exposure. Clergy from the client's religion as well as family members can serve as resources for the practitioner to increase cultural and religious competence (Rosenfeld, 2001). For clients who are dealing with emotional trauma, occupations that encourage reflection and expression of internal states, such as artistic pursuits and storytelling, can provide opportunity for spiritual insight and coping (Simo Algado et al., 2002).

CONCLUSION

The rich concept of spirituality provides occupational therapists with a valuable tool for understanding the deep meaning of engaging in occupation. Important to clients' health and well-being, integrating spirituality into occupational therapy practice proves relevant to the profession's goal of providing holistic occupation-based and client-centered care.

PROVOCATIVE QUESTIONS

1. How do you personally define spirituality? What life experiences or occupations would you call spiritual?
2. Think of your favorite occupation. How do you feel when you are doing it? How would you feel if you could no longer do it?
3. Think about your favorite places. How do you feel when you are there? What makes them special to you?
4. Bring one of your most special objects to class to share. Why is it special to you? How do you feel when you look at it?
5. What occupations do you engage in that address your spiritual needs?

6. What values led you to choose occupational therapy as your profession?
7. Tell your life story from a spiritual perspective.

ON THE WEB

Spirituality in Occupational Therapy Practice: Justine and Hazel.

REFERENCES

American Occupational Therapy Association. (2002). Occupational therapy practice framework: Domain and process. *American Journal of Occupational Therapy, 56,* 609–639.

Atler, K., Fisher, C., Moret, S., & White, J. (2000, March). *Combining spirituality and storytelling: Changing lives and enhancing practice.* Institute presented at the annual meeting of the American Occupational Therapy Association, Seattle, WA.

Belcham, C. (2004). Spirituality in occupational therapy: Theory in practice? *British Journal of Occupational Therapy, 67,* 39–46.

Bell, C. (1997). *Ritual: Perspectives and dimensions.* Oxford, UK: Oxford University Press.

Bockhoven, J. S. (1971). Legacy of moral treatment: 1800's to 1910. *American Journal of Occupational Therapy, 25,* 223–226.

Cameron, J. (1992). *The artist's way: A spiritual path to higher creativity.* New York: Penguin Putnam.

Canadian Association of Occupational Therapy. (1991). *Occupational therapy guidelines for client-centered practice.* Toronto: Author.

Canadian Association of Occupational Therapy. (1997). *Enabling occupation: An occupational perspective.* Toronto: Author.

Christiansen, C. (1997). Nationally speaking: Acknowledging a spiritual dimension in occupational therapy practice. *American Journal of Occupational Therapy, 51,* 169–172.

do Rozario, L. A. (1997). Spirituality in the lives of people with disability and chronic illness: A creative paradigm of wholeness and reconstitution. *Disability and Rehabilitation, 19*(10), 427–434.

Egan, M., & DeLaat, M. D. (1994). Considering spirituality in occupational therapy practice. *Canadian Journal of Occupational Therapy, 61*(2), 95–101.

Egan, M., & Swedersky, J. (2003). Spirituality as experienced by occupational therapists in practice. *American Journal of Occupational Therapy, 57,* 525–533.

Eisland, N. L., & Saliers, D. E. (Eds.). (1998). *Human disability and the service of God: Reassessing religious practice.* Nashville, TN: Abingdon.

Enquist, D. E., Short-DeGraff, M., Gliner, J., & Oltjenbruns, K. (1997). Occupational theorists' beliefs and practices with regard to spirituality and therapy. *American Journal of Occupational Therapy, 51,* 173–180.

Fine, S. B., (1999). Symbolization: Making meaning for self and society. In G. Fidler & B. Velde (Eds.), *Activities: Reality and symbol* (pp. 11–25). Thorofare, NJ: Slack.

Frank, G., Bernardo, C. S., Tropper, S., Noguchi, F., Lipman, C., Maulhardt, B., & Weitze, L. (1997). Jewish spirituality through actions in time: Daily occupations of young orthodox Jewish couples in Los Angeles. *American Journal of Occupational Therapy, 51,* 199–206.

Frankl, V. (1959). *Man's search for meaning.* New York: Washington Square Press.

Gritzer, G., & Arluke, A. (1989). *The making of rehabilitation: A political economy of medical specialization: 1890–1980.* Los Angeles: University of California Press.

Haase, J., Britt, T., Coward, D., Leidy, N., & Penn, P. (1992). Simultaneous concept analysis of spiritual perspective, hope, acceptance, and self-transcendence. *IMAGE: Journal of Nursing Scholarship, 24*(2), 141–147.

Hasselkus, B. R. (2002). *The meaning of everyday occupation.* Thorofare, NJ: Slack.

Hawks, S. R., Hull, M. L., Thalman, R. L., & Richins, P. M. (1995). Review of spiritual health: Definition, role and intervention strategies in health promotion. *American Journal of Health Promotion, 9,* 371–378.

Holland, D., Lachicotte, W., Skinner, D., & Cain, C. (1998). *Identity and agency in cultural worlds.* Cambridge, MA: Harvard University Press.

Howard, B. S., & Howard, J. R. (1997). Occupation as spiritual activity. *American Journal of Occupational Therapy, 51,* 181–185.

Jackson, J. M. (1996). Living a meaningful existence in old age. In R. Zemke & F. Clark (Eds.), *Occupational science: The evolving discipline* (pp. 339–361). Philadelphia: F. A. Davis.

Kelly, J. (2004). Spirituality as a coping mechanism. *Dimensions of Critical Care Nursing, 23*(4), 162–168.

Kidd, S. M. (1996). *Dance of the dissident daughter: A woman's journey from Christian tradition to the sacred feminine.* San Francisco: HarperCollins.

Koenig, H. G., George, L. K., & Peterson, B. L. (1998). Religiosity and remission of depression in medically ill older patients. *American Journal of Psychiatry, 155*(4), 536–542.

Kroeker, T. (1997). Spirituality and occupational therapy in a secular culture. *Canadian Journal of Occupational Therapy, 64,* 122–126.

Larson, B., Wood, W., & Clark, F. (2003). Occupational science: Building the science and practice of occupation through an academic discipline. In E. B. Crepeau, E. S. Cohn, & B. A. B. Schell (Eds.), *Willard & Spackman's occupational therapy* (10th ed., pp. 15–26). Philadelphia: Lippincott Williams & Wilkins.

Law, M., Baptiste, S., Carswell, A., McColl, M. A., Polatajko, H., & Pollock, N. (1994). *Canadian Occupational Performance Measure.* Toronto, Canada: CAOT Publications.

Low, J. (1997). Religious orientation and pain management. *American Journal of Occupational Therapy, 51,* 215–219.

Luboshitzky, D., & Gaber, L. B. (2001). Holidays and celebrations as a spiritual occupation. *Australian Occupational Therapy Journal, 48,* 66–74.

McColl, M. A. (2002). Occupation in stressful times. *American Journal of Occupational Therapy, 56,* 350–353.

Meyer, A. (1977). The philosophy of occupation therapy. *American Journal of Occupational Therapy, 31,* 639–642. (Original work published 1922)

Miller, W. R., & Thoresen, C. E. (2003). Spirituality, religion, and health: An emerging research field. *American Psychologist, 58,* 23–35.

Moore, T. (1992). *Care of the soul.* New York: Harper Perennial.

Norris, K. (1998). *The quotidian mysteries: Laundry, liturgy, and "women's work."* New York: Paulist Press.

Peloquin, S. M. (1997). Nationally speaking: The spiritual depth of occupation: Making worlds and making lives. *American Journal of Occupational Therapy, 51,* 167–168.

Reilly, M. (1962). Eleanor Clarke Slagle Lecture: Occupational therapy can be one of the great ideas of 20th century medicine. *American Journal of Occupational Therapy, 16,* 1–9.

Richards, M. (1990). Meeting the spiritual needs of the cognitively impaired. *Generations, 14*(4), 63–64.

Rosenfeld, M. S. (2001). Exploring a spiritual context for care. *OT Practice, 6*(11), 18–26.

Simo Algado, S., Mehta, N., Kronenberg, F., Cockburn, L., & Kirsh, B. (2002). Occupational therapy intervention with children survivors of war. *Canadian Journal of Occupational Therapy, 69*(4), 205–215.

Spencer, J., Davidson, H., & White, V. (1997). Helping clients develop hopes for the future. *American Journal of Occupational Therapy, 51,* 191–198.

Townsend, E., DeLaat, D., Egan, M., Thibeault, R., & Wright, W. A. (1999). *Spirituality in enabling occupation: A learner-centered workbook.* Ottawa, Canada: CAOT Publications.

Townsend, E., & Wilcock, A. (2004). Occupational justice and client-centered practice: A dialogue in practice. *Canadian Journal of Occupational Therapy, 71*(2), 75–85.

Tuan, Y. (1977). *Space and place: The perspective of experience.* Minneapolis, MN: University of Minnesota Press.

Unruh, A. M. (1997). Spirituality and occupation: Garden musings and the Himalayan blue poppy. *Canadian Journal of Occupational Therapy, 64*(3), 156–160.

Unruh, A. M., Versnel, J., & Kerr, N. (2002). Spirituality unplugged: A review of commonalities and contentions, and a resolution. *Canadian Journal of Occupational Therapy, 69*(1), 5–19.

Urbanowski, R., & Vargo, J. (1994). Spirituality, daily practice and the occupational therapy performance model. *Canadian Journal of Occupational Therapy, 61*(2), 88–94.

Wilcock, A. (2001). Occupational utopias: Back to the future. *Journal of Occupational Science, 1,* 5–12.

Wuthnow, R. (1998). *After heaven: Spirituality in America since the 1950's.* Los Angeles: University of California Press.

Yerxa, E. J. (1992). Some implications of occupational therapy's history for its epistemology, values, and relation to medicine. *American Journal of Occupational Therapy, 46,* 79–83.

Zemke, R., & Clark, F. (1996). Section V: Co-occupations of mothers and children: Introduction. In R. Zemke & F. Clark (Eds.), *Occupational science: The evolving discipline* (pp. 213–215). Philadelphia: F. A. Davis.

II

NARRATIVE PERSPECTIVES ON OCCUPATION AND DISABILITY

" A story presumes both a teller and a community of listeners, such that the act of telling the story and responding to it is a reciprocal exercise designed in part to strengthen community bonds. "

Howard Brody

Narrative as a Key to Understanding

10

ELIZABETH BLESEDELL CREPEAU AND ELLEN S. COHN

Learning Objectives

After reading this chapter, you will be able to:

1. Explain why listening to clients' stories is an essential component of occupational therapy practice.
2. Explain the relationship between experience, narrative, and the interpretive process.
3. Discuss narrative types.
4. Describe the role of narratives in occupational therapy practice.

Think back over the past few days. How many times have you told a story about an experience you had? How many times have you listened to a story told to you by a friend or family member? We tell stories all the time about the things that we did or that happened to us and to others as a way to share and interpret our experience. In fact, we could be called *Homo narratus* rather than *Homo sapiens* because of the centrality of storytelling to human experience (Fisher, 1984). Some people are better storytellers than others. Good storytellers can infuse their narratives with tension, drama, and suspense, but regardless of how well the story is told, it is human nature to share stories with others. Consequently, it is not surprising that occupational therapy clients and their family members have stories to tell about their experiences with injury, disease, or disability. This unit is devoted to these stories, written by the people themselves, their family members, or occupational therapists who incorporate a narrative perspective into their work with clients. That we devote an entire unit to these narratives indicates the importance of the narrative perspectives of the people who seek occupational therapy and how essential narrative is to the entire occupational therapy process.

In the 1980s, social scientists were rediscovering the significance of narrative as a way to understand human experience, and there was a tremendous growth of interest in patients' stories in the health care fields (J. A. Clark & Mishler, 1992; Kleinman, 1980; Mishler, 1984; Polkinghorne, 1988). The interest in patients' stories of their experiences living with illness emerged from a "dehumanized" and highly technological approach to health care that lacked sufficient attention to the human aspects of experience. This "narrative turn" in occupational therapy occurred in the mid-1980s when an anthropologist, Cheryl Mattingly, directed the AOTA/AOTF Clinical Reasoning Study, an ethnographic study of occupational therapists in a large teaching hospital (Mattingly, 1994, Mattingly & Fleming, 1994). Mattingly and the research team used observation, interviews with therapists and clients, and videotaped occupational therapy sessions to analyze and uncover the stories that emerged during occupational therapy intervention. In her observations of therapists throughout their work day, Mattingly noted that therapists utilized different forms of talk to discuss their work with clients. Therapists used what Mattingly referred to as "chart talk," a formal reporting register that typically occurred during team meetings and other structured situations to describe the technical and reimbursable aspects of practice. In contrast, therapists told stories during lunch and other times to describe the rich, more interpretive aspects of their meaningful interactions with clients. These stories had all the elements that we have come to expect from a story: a plot, drama, suspense, action, and a moral or lesson. Mattingly's work legitimized the telling of stories as an interpretive process that helped therapists to make sense of their experience. Mattingly's influential work focused attention on the value of therapists listening to clients' stories and explicated how clients and occupational therapy practitioners collaboratively create new or different "meaningful" life narratives in the context of living with disease or disability. She introduced the idea that occupational therapy intervention itself involved a "narrative" process in which the therapy was a dramatic plot to transform the moment toward a path of recovery, healing, or new potential while living with a health condition.

Since then, a significant amount of research in occupational therapy has examined narrative from the perspective of clients (Braveman & Helfrich, 2001; Jonsson, Kielhofner, & Borell, 1997; Knutas & Borell, 1995; Price-Lackey & Cashman, 1996), their families (Cohn, 2001; Kautzmann, 1993), and therapists (Labovitz, 2003; Mattingly, 1991). The narrative turn has even influenced research on meetings (Boje, 1991; Schwartzman, 1998) and team meetings in health care (Atkinson, 1995, 1997; Griffiths & Hughes, 1994; Opie, 1997) and how storytelling influences the clinical reasoning of team members (Crepeau, 1994, 2000).

NARRATIVE AND STORY

There are numerous ways to define *narrative* and *story*. In some traditions, particularly literary theory, *narrative* and *story* refer to distinct phenomena. However, in this chapter, we will use *narrative* and *story* equivalently (as do Hamilton, 2008, Mattingly & Garro, 2000; and Polk-inghorne, 1988). In everyday speech, stories are quite common, perhaps so "natural" that they do not need explaining. Although common, stories are incredibly complex and quite difficult to describe. In a very fundamental way, stories concern action and offer a way to make sense of experiences. By linking narrative, act, and consequence, stories offer us windows on social life and human character. Some literary theorists claim that through a chaining of events, stories offer causal explanations of events. In this chapter, we will draw on Mattingly's definition: "stories are about someone trying to do something, and what happens to her and others as a result" (Mattingly, 1998, p. 7). Consider an excerpt from Alex McIntosh's chapter (see Chapter 12). Alex's story has numerous features that make stories especially appealing for understanding his experiences in living with cerebral palsy. Alex's story is event centered, concerns human action and interaction, and includes the social aspects of human behavior. As the narrator of this story, Alex knows the ending and carefully selects the relevant details to direct our attention to his plot. He narrates the story in a particular way to convey his message and ultimately communicates to the reader that he has an amazing imagination and that walking with crutches is secondary to who he is as a person. His story even has a deeper moral message: Alex's story teaches us that peoples' ideas about disability are not rationally determined but socially constructed. Alex shows us that a disability is determined by social expectations rather than by diagnostic conditions.

In this story, Alex tells what happened to him and how he and his mother shared an unspoken secret about a naïve woman's social construction and understanding of who Alex really is.

> When I was about seven years old, I was firmly convinced that I was a werewolf. I had never actually undergone any physical transformation at the full of the moon, but seven-year-olds are not bothered by such trifles. The crowning touch was that my crutches acted as a second pair of legs, and although when wearing them I could never really manage a wolf-like lope, I made do instead with a sort of galloping skip. Nevertheless, it was fast enough (to me) to reinforce fantasies of running swiftly through the forest on silent paws, seeking unsuspecting prey.
>
> The technical term for the condition of being a werewolf is *lycanthropy*, after the mythical Greek king Lycaon, whom the god Zeus transformed into a wolf as punishment for his tyranny. I knew the word at the age of seven, having read every book on werewolves that I could both find and understand. I was proud to declare myself a lycanthrope to everyone I met.
>
> One day that year, my mother, my younger brother, and I attended a fund-raising boat race, the object of which was to allow wealthy yacht owners to raise money for the disabled. I was skipping around

the lobby of the yacht club where the event was being held, giving long, mournful, ear-splitting howls, as a proper werewolf should. Mom was over in a corner with my brother, trying to pretend that I was someone else's child.

One of the yacht owners saw me, and she said, "Look at you, doing so well. What's your disability, honey?"

"I have lycanthropy!" I said, beaming.

A few minutes later, she was chatting with my mother and said, "I just met your son. What a nice boy. It's so sad that he has lycanthropy."

Mom smirked. "Um, I think there's something you should know . . ."

That is what happens to people who are lacking in disability awareness.

Alex, now a twenty-year-old, starts his story by orienting us to the characters and setting, placing himself at a younger age. This particular story serves a referential function. In telling about the things that happened to them and others, people connect their experience to the world beyond themselves and provide a retrospective glance at past events. Alex, a seven-year-old boy, who, using his words "could never really manage" a particular gait, transforms himself into a wolf, "running swiftly through the forest, sneaking up on unsuspecting prey" (the yacht owner) to describe to the reader who he is and what he does in this world. Alex has imaginatively transformed himself from a young boy walking with crutches to a werewolf "skipping" and "howling" around the lobby. He communicates his experience, one in which he is not a child with a disability but a competent and clever young boy playing a trick and perhaps educating an adult who does not understand "disability." Alex draws us into his werewolf fantasy as a means to communicate his experience. Yet the narrative moment in this story is not even in the story and has no words. We can only imagine the ironic pleasure that Alex and his mother shared in their unspoken words, "If she only knew." Alex's ending creates an experience for us, the audience, and allow us to infer something about what it feels like to be in his world. Alex's story is worth telling because it conveys to the reader a particular outcome that he feels is important for us to understand. We can share in the joy, imagining what it might be like to have some fun while teaching others that Alex is a clever and imaginative child who happens to use crutches.

We have learned a lot about Alex in his story. We know that he has a vivid imagination, that he has loved to read since he was quite young, and that he is an effective storyteller who can incorporate drama, comedy, and irony into his storytelling. By listening to our clients' stories, we can understand their interpretation of their experience and begin to discern who they are as individuals, their illness or disability experience, and how this experience has shaped their daily occupations. The interpretive process of storytelling helps to differentiate our clients from each other, even those with very similar medical and social histories. While we may work with many clients with the same diagnosis, their lived experience and the stories they tell about their lives will be as important as their particular occupational problems in shaping the way in which we work with them to plan and implement their occupational therapy intervention.

NARRATIVE AS AN INTERPRETIVE PROCESS

Creating stories or narratives is an interpretive process that involves selecting aspects of past experience and representing that experience to others in the present (Bruner, 1986, 1990, 1991). Because storytelling is interpretive, the way in which an individual interprets the past may be strongly influenced by present circumstances. This does not mean that storytelling is a fabrication; rather, stories are constructed to present a coherent interpretation of the past in light of the present.

Drawing on Reissman's (1993) delineation of the multiple levels of representation of experience in narrative analysis, we propose that the chapters in this unit have several levels of representation. These levels are (1) the author's attention to the experience in the moment, (2) the telling of this experience in the writing of the chapter, (3) the editorial process, and (4) the interpretation derived from reading the chapter. First of all, just as Alex was selective, others cannot observe everything in the environment; rather, they select what is important or meaningful to them at that moment, which is then available for a future story. Second, we asked our chapter authors to tell their story to make it accessible to you. In doing so, they have ordered and interpreted events to create a coherent account that you, as the reader, can understand. Because they were asked to write about their experience for occupational therapy students, their stories are told from that standpoint. Their chapters might have a different focus if they were writing for a different audience. In this sense, the chapters are "constructed" for a certain purpose, to convey their experience to readers who will someday be working with people who might have had similar experiences with illness or disability. Thus, the chapters are positioned to reflect experience from a particular interpretive lens: "let me tell you my story so that you will understand the experience of your future clients." In fact, some authors end their chapters by addressing you directly as future occupational therapists to be sure that you understand the importance of their message. The third level of the process involves editing the chapter, which may further shape the story. As editors of these chapters, we tried to sustain the perspective of the authors while helping them to bring clarity and order to their writing. This is a delicate process because in editing, we ran the risk of changing the representation of their experience by our shaping of it. Finally, you will bring your own interpretive process to your reading of these chapters based on your own life experience.

Telling stories is important. We knew this when we decided to have personal narratives in this edition of *Willard and Spackman.* But working with the authors of these chapters brought the importance of narratives home to us as the authors reminded us of the value to the authors themselves of writing their narratives. Laurie McIntosh said that the chapter she wrote with her son and husband (Chapter 12) helped them to realize the distinctiveness of their perspectives—being a child with a disability, the child's mother, or the child's father. Writing the chapter provided an opportunity to reflect on their individual experience of raising Alex from the perspective of his departure for college, an important developmental milestone. Should they revise this chapter for the next edition of *Willard and Spackman,* they might interpret Alex's childhood differently because of the events in the intervening years. You will see some of this reinterpretation in Mary Feldhaus-Weber's chapter (Chapter 11) in the sections in which she writes about her brain injury at various times from the accident to the present. The basic elements of Mary's story remain the same, but the passage of time and experience have shifted Mary's interpretation. In working on the chapter for this edition, she said that she felt that she could reveal some of the "darker" aspects of her experience because she no longer felt that it was essential to project a strong image. Don Murray wrote his chapter a year after the death of his wife (see Chapter 14). Although he was a professional writer who wrote frequently about Minnie Mae in his *Boston Globe* column, this chapter provided him with a broader vehicle for integrating and synthesizing the experience of her illness, his care giving, and her death. He thanked us for this opportunity and said that it helped him to mourn during the year after her death. Gloria Dickerson's chapter (see Chapter 13) illustrates her exquisite ability to make sense of incredibly painful life experiences and actions that she did not understand as a child. She places her experiences within the context of grand narratives of racism and sexism within our culture and ultimately shows the readers how she shapes her future actions by reflecting on her experience to rewrite and live out a new life story. How you react to these powerful and inspirational stories will teach you much about how your interpretive lenses influence your worldview.

Frank (1995, 2002) argues that in listening to patients' stories, health care practitioners bear witness to suffering as well as to personal strengths and triumphs. The chapters in this unit provide you with a way to begin to think about your clients' stories and what these stories tell you about the clients' character and the meaning they ascribe to their experience. On the basis of listening to stories of others and reading personal accounts of illness and disability, Frank identified three types of illness narratives: the restitution, chaos, and quest narratives (see Table 10.1

for definitions of these narrative types). Frank asserts that these narrative types might not be the only types of illness narratives but that they presented themselves in many of the stories he listened to and read. Individuals may use one or more of the types in one story or may shift narrative types depending on the particular standpoint from which they are telling the story. Frank's purpose in delineating various types of narrative is to sensitize others and to assist them in listening to patients' narratives more effectively. Keeping in mind the three narrative types as you listen to client stories can help you to achieve a better sense of their experience.

Clients telling a restitution story are showing how medicine has resolved their problems to return them to health (Frank, 1995). Clients often tell restitution stories retrospectively, but they might also use this story form to project themselves into the future. A plotline might involve a major surgical intervention, such as a joint replacement, followed by rehabilitation and ultimate return to former occupational pursuits. These stories are easy to listen to because they represent the triumph of Western medicine. In contrast, Frank (1995) asserts that chaos narratives are the most difficult to hear because, unlike the restitution narrative, they are not sequenced by a plotline that we are socialized to follow. Rather, the person who tells a chaos narrative is so embedded in the experience that little order or interpretation is possible. Chaos narratives represent a life that is out of control with no solutions in sight. They are characterized by events that are connected by phrases such as "and then . . . and then . . . and then. . . ." This lack of causal ordering or plot renders the telling hard to understand because the person is still enmeshed in the experience. Quest narratives, in contrast, show the personal transformation that can occur when clients confront serious illness and disability and, as a result, make fundamental changes in their lives. Most of the published illness narratives are quest narratives. For example, Phillip Simmons's book *Learning to Fall: Reflections on an Imperfect Life* (2000) provides a vehicle for him to use his diagnosis of amyotrophic lateral sclerosis as a tool, to understand the way in which he lived in the past and how he pursued a meaningful life despite increasing disability, which would eventually lead to death. By providing clients with the opportunity to tell their stories, no matter how chaotic, health care providers can open an opportunity for reflection or interpretation. This may be as important as medical intervention.

THE ROLE OF NARRATIVE IN OCCUPATIONAL THERAPY PRACTICE

Storytelling

Occupational therapy practice provides many opportunities to listen to and elicit stories from clients and to tell

TABLE 10.1 TYPES OF ILLNESS NARRATIVES

Type	Definition	Characteristic	Basic Storyline
Restitution narrative	A restitution narrative is a common illness narrative that delineates the course of illness from early symptoms and diagnosis through treatment and recovery. These stories may be told by patients or their families and friends. Hospitals and other health care institutions may also use restitution narratives to demonstrate the power of medicine to heal.	A typical plot demonstrates the power of medicine to heal. The focus is on the role of medicine to heal, demonstrating the transitory nature of illness. While the individual tells the story, the primary focus is on the restorative power of medicine.	"Yesterday I was healthy, today I'm sick, but tomorrow, I'll be healthy again" (Frank, 1995, p. 77).
Chaos narrative	A chaos narrative, as its title suggests, represents the lack of control and vulnerability an individual who is ill experiences. These narratives display few elements of typical stories, such as a logical sequence or plot. People telling these stories are so embedded in the illness that they have limited ability to order or interpret their experience. Because these stories tend to be painful and lack the typical conventions expected of stories, they are difficult to hear. Consequently, listening carefully rather than interrupting or changing the topic is especially important.	There is no story line or plot. While the story is about the individual, the person is not an active character in the story. Illness predominates, with a corresponding lack of control by the storyteller or health care personnel.	"Just as the chaos narrative is an anti-narrative, so it is a non-self story. Where life can be given narrative order, chaos is already at bay" (Frank, 1995, p. 105).
Quest narrative	Quest narratives, as their title suggests, represent the transformative journey of a person experiencing serious illness or disability. Like restitution narratives, these narratives capture the diagnosis and course of illness; however, the outcome of the story is focused not on a return to health but on the transformation of the storyteller. Quest narratives focus on how illness has fundamentally changed the person's character, values, and outlook on life.	The voice of quest narratives is the person's, and the quest involves the person's transformation. Illness experience is part of the story; however, the focus is on how this illness transformed the person's life in fundamental ways.	"Whatever has happened to me or will happen . . . the purpose remains mine to determine" (Frank, 1995, p. 131).

Source: Frank, A. W. (1995). *The wounded storyteller: Body, illness and ethics*. Chicago: University of Chicago Press.

clients stories as a form of motivation or to help them see themselves in particular kinds of therapeutic plots (Mattingly, 1998). Occupational therapists also tell stories to each other while socializing and during team meetings and other interdisciplinary forms of communication (Crepeau, 1994, 2000). They might tell puzzling stories to each other to make sense of what happened or determine how they should proceed with a particular client. They may also use stories to persuade others of a particular point of view or insight about a client. For example, an occupational therapist used a very persuasive account of a patient in a geropsychiatric unit to reformulate the patient's problem from one of refusal to participate in the milieu to one of an inability to participate. The occupational therapist's interpretation of the client's story proved to be a turning point for the team in planning care for this client (Crepeau, 2000). Consequently, the therapist's interpretation of the patient's behavior reconstructed the team's view and plans for her care.

Storymaking

While this chapter has focused on storytelling as a way to interpret and share experience, stories do not simply look back and interpret past events in light of the present, Mattingly proposed that narratives can shape action and that occupational therapy intervention involves a prospective "therapeutic emplotment" in which clients and therapists create new narratives; that is, new "stories are created in clinical time" (Mattingly, 2000, p. 183). She argued that therapists and clients create a collaborative intervention process to understand and enable clients to move from where or who they are to where or who they want to be (Mattingly, 1991, 1998). Elaborating on Mattingly's argument, Clark introduced the term *occupational storymaking* to describe how occupational therapists engage people in desired occupations to rewrite, revise, or re-create their life story and image new possibilities. As clients engage in desired occupations and experience their potential to participate in desired activities, a new story is enacted in the intervention process (F. Clark & Ennevor, 1996). Clark (1993) described her intervention with Penny Richardson, a colleague who experienced a cerebral aneurysm at the age of 47. Because Clark listened to Penny and understood her life story, Clark and Penny were able to identify Penny's challenges to engagement in desired occupations and rewrite potential solutions to occupational problems. In one example of the process, Clark and Penny identified the walker as a constant reminder of Penny's continued balance problems and symbol of disability. Before the aneurysm, Penny enjoyed outdoor activities, was an avid hiker, and pushed herself to be physically competent. Recycling her familiar story lines and attending to her motives to remove stigmatizing barriers, Penny began what she called "cane hiking" to transition herself from walking with a walker to using a cane. To rewrite the narrative, Clark and Penny engaged in occupations that allowed Penny to connect her former self to her new self.

Many of the chapters in this unit provide vivid illustrations of occupational "storytelling" and "storymaking." Nick Pollard (Chapter 15) shows how storytelling in a supported setting enabled people with intellectual difficulties to write, publish, and share their stories with others. These stories provide a window on the lived experience of the participants in the *Voices Talk, Hands Write* project. Theresa Lorenzo (Chapter 16) tells of the therapeutic power of storymaking, which enabled poor South African women with disabilities to recognize their strengths and build more autonomous lives through occupational engagement.

CONCLUSION

Our purpose in writing this chapter is to give you a very brief overview of the importance of narrative to occupational therapy practice. Our hope is that you will read the chapters in this unit and will approach working with others with a respect for the importance of narrative to understand how people interpret their experience and how storytelling and storymaking can be used as part of the therapeutic process. As you read the following chapters, consider the questions listed below.

PROVOCATIVE QUESTIONS

1. What is the plot of the chapter and what is the moral of the story?
2. What are major themes represented in the story?
3. What insights have you gained from the stories in these chapters?
4. If you were an occupational therapist for these individuals, how would their narratives shape your work with them?

REFERENCES

Atkinson, P. (1995). *Medical talk and medical work.* London: Sage.

Atkinson, P. (1997). Narrative turn or blind alley? *Qualitative Health Research, 17*(3), 325–344.

Boje, D. M. (1991). The storytelling organization: A study of performance in an office supply firm. *Administrative Science Quarterly, 36,* 106–126.

Braveman, B., & Helfrich, C. A. (2001). Occupational identity: Exploring the narratives of three men living with AIDS. *Journal of Occupational Science, 8*(2), 25–31.

Brody, H. (1987). *Stories of sickness.* New Haven, CT: Yale University Press, p. 15. *(unit opening quote)*

Bruner, J. (1986). *Actual minds, possible worlds.* Cambridge, MA: Harvard University Press.

Bruner, J. (1990). *Acts of meaning.* Cambridge, MA: Harvard University Press.

Bruner, J. (1991). The narrative construction of reality. *Critical Inquiry, 18,* 1–21.

Clark, F. (1993). Occupation embedded in a real life: Interweaving occupational science and occupational therapy. *American Journal of Occupational Therapy, 47,* 1069–1078.

Clark, F., & Ennevor, B. L. (1996). A grounded theory of techniques for occupational storytelling and occupational storymaking. In R. Zemke & F. Clark (Eds.), *Occupational science: The evolving discipline* (pp. 373–392). Philadelphia: F. A. Davis.

Clark, J. A., & Mishler, E. G. (1992). Attending to patients' stories: Reframing the clinical task. *Sociology of Health & Illness, 14,* 344–372.

Cohn, E. S. (2001). From waiting to relating: Parents' experiences in the waiting room of an occupational therapy clinic. *American Journal of Occupational Therapy, 55,* 168–175.

Crepeau, E. B. (1994). Three images of interdisciplinary team meetings. *The American Journal of Occupational Therapy, 48,* 717–722.

Crepeau, E. B. (2000). Reconstructing Gloria: A narrative analysis of team meetings. *Qualitative Health Research, 10*(6), 766–787.

Fisher, W. R. (1984). Narration as a human communication paradigm: The case of public moral argument. *Communication Monographs, 51,* 1–22.

Frank, A. W. (1995). *The wounded storyteller: Body, illness and ethics.* Chicago: University of Chicago Press.

Frank, A. W. (2002). "How can they act like that?": Clinicians and patients as characters in each other's stories. *Hastings Center Report, 32,* 14–22.

Griffiths, L., & Hughes, D. (1994). "Innocent parties" and "disheartening" experiences: Natural rhetorics in neuronrehabilitation admission conferences. *Qualitative Health Research, 49*(4), 385–410.

Hamilton, T. B. (2008). Narrative reasoning. In B. A. Schell & J. W. Schell (Eds.), *Clinical and professional reasoning in occupational therapy* (pp. 125–126). Baltimore: Lippincott Williams & Wilkins.

Jonsson, H., Kielhofner, G., & Borell, L., (1997). Anticipating retirement: The formation of narratives concerning an occupational transition. *American Journal of Occupational Therapy, 51,* 49–56.

Kautzmann, L. N. (1993). Linking patient and family stories to caregivers' use of clinical reasoning. *American Journal of Occupational Therapy, 47,* 169–173.

Kleinman, A. (1980) *Patients and healers in the context of culture: An exploration of the borderland between anthropology, medicine, and psychiatry.* Berkeley: University of California Press.

Knutas, A., & Borell, L. (1995). The meaning of stroke in everyday life: A comparative case study of two persons. *Scandinavian Journal of Occupational Therapy, 2,* 56–62.

Labovitz, D. R. (Ed.). (2003). *Ordinary miracles: True stories about overcoming obstacles and surviving catastrophes.* Thorofare, NJ: Slack.

Mattingly, C. (1991). The narrative nature of clinical reasoning. *American Journal of Occupational Therapy, 45*(11), 998–1005.

Mattingly, C. (1994). The narrative nature of clinical reasoning. In C. Mattingly & M. H. Fleming (Eds.), *Clinical reasoning: Forms on inquiry in a therapeutic practice* (pp. 239–269). Philadelphia: F. A. Davis.

Mattingly, C. (1998). *Healing dramas and clinical plots: The narrative structure of experience.* New York: Cambridge University Press.

Mattingly, C. (2000). Emergent narratives. In C. Mattingly & L. C. Garro (Eds.), *Narrative and the cultural construction of illness and healing* (pp. 181–211). Berkeley: University of California Press

Mattingly, C., & Fleming, M. H. (1994). *Clinical reasoning: Forms of inquiry in a therapeutic practice.* Philadelphia: F. A. Davis.

Mattingly, C., & Garro, L. C. (2000). *Narrative and the cultural construction of illness and healing.* Berkeley: University of California Press.

Mishler, E. G. (1984). *The discourse of medicine: Dialectics of medical interviews.* Norwood, NJ: Ablex.

Opie, A. (1997). Teams as author: Narrative knowledge creation in case discussions in multidisciplinary health teams. *Sociological Research Online, 2*(3), 1–18.

Polkinghorne, D. E. (1988). *Narrative knowing and the human sciences.* Albany, NY: State University of New York Press.

Price-Lackey, P., & Cashman, J. (1996). Jenny's story: Reinventing oneself through occupation and narrative configuration. *American Journal of Occupational Therapy, 50,* 306–314.

Reissman, C. K. (1993). *Narrative analysis: Qualitative research methods* (Vol. 30). Newbury Park, CA: Sage.

Schwartzman, H. B. (1989) *The meeting: Gatherings in organizations and communities.* New York: Plenum.

Simmons, P. (2000). *Learning to fall: The blessings of an imperfect life.* New York: Bantam Books.

An Excerpt from *The Book of Sorrows, Book of Dreams:* A First-Person Narrative

11

MARY FELDHAUS-WEBER

Sally Schreiber-Cohn, CHAPTER EDITOR

UNIT EDITOR'S PROLOGUE

Mary Feldhaus-Weber was in her thirties; lived in Boston; and was a successful playwright, filmmaker, and television producer. She had produced documentaries for the Public Broadcasting System (PBS). Her plays had been produced off-off-Broadway. She had just finished making *Joan Robinson: One Woman's Story,* an award-winning documentary film about her friend's three-year struggle with and death from ovarian cancer. In December 1979, three weeks before this film was to be telecast on PBS, Mary was the passenger in a car that was struck by a drunk driver. Mary was taken from the demolished car and was rushed to a hospital emergency room. Although her head had smashed the car window during the accident, she was released from the hospital that very night. Just three days later, Mary began to have seizures. Months later, she was diagnosed as having epilepsy, a seizure disorder, caused by traumatic brain injury. Her brain had been injured when she hit her head during the car accident. She was never hospitalized for this traumatic injury. Her seizures initially were not well controlled with medication. New medication recently has brought them largely under control; however, she has never been able to return to work.

What follows is Mary Feldhaus-Weber's story of her struggle to live with the effects of her brain injury and seizure disorder—in her own words.

These excerpts were taken from her book in progress, *The Book of Sorrows, Book of Dreams*. The first part of the story covers the years 1979 to 1981. Mary dictated this part of her story to friends and occupational therapy students who were working with her. Mary was able to write the final three parts of her story by herself. Noted throughout the chapter are references to color plates of Mary's painting.

1979 TO 1981

The Accident

Now let me tell you about this. My friend Sally was driving me home at 3:00 A.M. after working on the Joan Robinson film, getting it ready for its national air date. A large American car, going at a high rate of speed, hit the small foreign car we were in, on the passenger side.

I was the passenger. The car we were in was hit with such intensity that both cars were demolished, totaled (see Color Plate 1, "Intersection"). My head went through the passenger window sideways. The side of my head above the temple totally shattered the glass, hit with such impact that every piece of glass had been knocked out (see Color Plate 2, "The Shattering"). People in the emergency room were astonished that I had no facial cuts. I told them my hard Scandinavian head was harder than glass—like stone or a diamond.

I can remember the car lights coming at us. I can remember the sense that we could not get out of the way. I can remember shouting to my friend, "watch out," and then the impact of the car. But strangely, when the car hit, I had the sense that it had not really hit me or the car I was in, that there had been a buffer that was made of time and space. Eternal. Would not break. A shield.

I was also sure that the driver of my car, my friend Sally Schreiber-Cohn, had reached out at the moment of impact and shielded me with her own body. I was absolutely sure this happened. When we got to the hospital, I asked her. She said, "Oh no, I kept both hands on the wheel, of course." If the other car had hit a few inches further back, I probably would have been decapitated. But it hit where it hit. Sally was bruised and badly shaken up. All the damage has been inside my brain.

One doctor described it as if someone were to have taken Jell-O, the consistency of the brain, and thrown it at a wall as hard as one could. That's how hard the brain hit one side of the skull and then ricocheted back and hit the other side of the skull, leaving me with right- and left-side brain injuries. Even though only one side of my head hit the window, both sides of my brain are damaged (see Color Plate 3, "Damaged Brain").

Six Months After the Accident

Six months after the accident, when I started to have more and more seizures, it became clear that I could no longer live alone, so I had to ask my mother to come from South Dakota to stay with me. I did this with great reluctance because she was 78 and my father wanted her there, taking care of him. When she got here, the thing I remember her saying was that she hadn't realized it had been so bad. Why hadn't I called her sooner? This was the time before the seizures were under any kind of control at all, which is to say, I was very sick.

I sat in the corner day after day, noticing that it was light or dark, noticing that my mother was busy, or sleeping, or crying, noticing that sometimes the phone rang or that it was the day to see the doctor, noticing that sometimes I had pain in my head. My mother said, "I wonder if a cold wet towel on your head would help?" I think we both remembered that if a horse sprains its leg, you wrap its leg in towels. And so Mother would get wet towels from the bathroom and wrap them around my head, my brain becoming like a sprained leg, a muscle that wasn't working. Cramped and tense. Convulsing. Filled with fear.

And then because things change and time moves on, the pain would stop, and I would become briefly aware that the couch cover was blue, or that the dog had been rolling in the dust, or that Mother wanted to fix soup for lunch. And we discovered that after I had a seizure, or as one doctor called them "spells," I didn't have the coordination, or was too confused, to drink soup or hold a spoon. Because Mother liked soup so much, we seemed to try this many times, larger spoons, smaller spoons, bigger cups, smaller cups. It was decided that tomato soup was the easiest. Why, I'm not sure. Finally, I told Mother I did not like soup and had not for years. Therefore, could we try something else?

At this time, I was having constant seizures. There was no time that I was not either having one, getting ready to have one, feeling "spacey," with a strong metallic taste in my mouth, or feeling confused and disoriented after having had one. I felt like the seizures were a powerful force outside of me that suddenly grabbed my brain, me, the essence of me, and with the kind of fury of winds, blizzards, and driving rain, held me under ice (see Color Plate 4, "Blue Seizure"). While the *me* that was present could breathe the water under the ice, I knew I was caught, forced to be there. I knew if I struggled even slightly, the pain, the terror, became worse. And for the time the active seizure was roaring on inside me, I had to concentrate on total stillness until the fury dissipated and I was released.

All the drive and the tenacity, the ambition, the creativity, all of the things that had made me who I was did not help in this place. I was terrified, and I was alone. I no longer knew the words to ask or tell anyone what I was living through. I could just sense what hurt, and it hurt less to be absolutely still until the force chose to release me. I had no control of when it seized me or when it chose to release me.

My friend Sally tells me now that looking at me was like watching a candle about to go out. It seemed to her that only 3 percent of me was left.

I felt that I was being annihilated. The *me* that I had become, lived with, was ceasing to be, over and over and over again. It occurred to me that this was what it felt like to die and, for whatever reason, I was dying again and again.

One Year After the Accident

My mother had to return to South Dakota, so I was living alone. One day at the neurologist's office a year after the accident, still confused and in a deep fog, I noticed the doctor's tie. It was a bright, clear yellow Marimekko tie. I stared at the color yellow. It was the first thing to make sense to me since the accident. I understood what I was seeing. The color yellow. The fog lifted for a minute. I understood something, and I had not had to struggle to understand it. I can remember thinking: I am going to be all right.

When I got home that day, someone got me a set of poster paints, and I painted a small, bright, vivid, yellow daisy (see Color Plate 5, "Daisy"). And I started painting. When I began painting, I was surprised to find that it didn't turn out so badly, even though I had never painted before. Painting was one thing I could do all by myself, whether anyone was there or not. It didn't matter if I was spacey or sick. I could just lay down the piece of paper I was working on and continue again after the seizure had come and gone.

Some days, I did as many as ten paintings. Looking back, I realize that I was desperate to understand my situation. I could hear people talk, but nothing made sense. I looked at their faces. I watched their mouths move, but I could not concentrate on what they were telling me. I can remember thinking: I have to try to explain all this to myself—what is happening to me—because I can't understand anyone else. So I painted. The only time I felt like the person I used to be was when I was painting.

I started finger painting with acrylic paint, wet tissue paper, and poster paints. I was drawn to the colors and shapes of things. I started to paint brains. I tried to paint the experience of seizures, which I did over and over again (see Color Plate 6, "Hemisphere"). In a strange kind of way, it was like having an artist's model for myself—not a model I could see, but a model which was myself, an internal experience that I then tried to translate into color. The painting gave me something to talk about other than myself. Something to talk about when people came to the house. It was a relief to have something to show someone, to have them look at pieces of paper, not to look at me. It also gave me a way to try to talk about what I was living through. Part of me hoped that the paintings weren't pitiful, because of all the things I did not want to be, to be pitied seemed the very worst.

I was also aware that I had to start from scratch with painting. I had been at the top of my career in film, and now I had to struggle to squeeze the paint tubes. I had to learn to be patient with myself. I was at the very beginning and grateful to be there.

Two Years After the Accident

I still had no real picture of what happened to my brain, to I spent a great deal of time thinking about it. Trying to think about it (see Color Plate 7, "Dendrites"). I had listened to explanations from doctors, nurses, and social workers, and none of them had made sense. All I knew was that I was unable to do the simplest thing—make a bed, tell time, count. Add or subtract. Recognize faces. Tell right from left. Read. Understand what people said to me. Remember things. And perhaps worst of all, I did not feel like myself, like *me*. I felt like someone, but not like any one I knew. I was a stranger to myself. I was lost (see Color Plate 8, "Self-Portrait").

On days that I had constant seizures, I had to ask my friend Sally to come and stay with me. It was at these times that we were aware that I was not getting better; in fact, I was barely hanging on.

The everyday litany was long and grim: I fell all the time; I was covered with black and blue marks everywhere. I would come to from a seizure to find that I had bitten the inside of my mouth and was bleeding and had a shard of my broken front tooth sticking out of my bottom lip. Sometimes, I would put my finger in my eyes during a seizure, and the eye would be red and swollen for days. I hit my head. I broke my elbow. It did not seem safe for me to live alone.

I had lost my income when my film company closed after the accident, and I had lost my health insurance with it. Because of these factors, my only option would have been to go on welfare and go into a nursing home. My neurologist felt that if I did that, I would likely never come out. I think he had seen too many people become institutionalized. In other words, they had become helpless and had given up. I still had some small fight left in me; I had been a functional, successful adult. The 3 percent of me that was left was 3 percent of a fighter. We were all counting on the fact that I would keep fighting and I would get better. That somehow I would manage. I also knew I desperately needed someone to help me help myself.

Finally, more than two years after the accident, we found someone to help me. Sally had called a therapist friend who said that she did know someone who was a gifted occupational therapist and liked dogs. And who was kind. When Sally called the occupational therapist—Anna Deane Scott—she said that she knew very little about head injury. She was a professor at Boston University and the coauthor of a famous occupational therapy textbook, and, yes, she did like dogs. She agreed to come to my house to meet me.

When she first met me, Anna Deane told me later, I was sitting in the dark on a couch, crying. We talked; she admired my dogs and told me about her own dog. After she left, I called her to ask what she thought of the meeting. I was afraid that she might have felt I was beyond help. I asked her how she felt about meeting me. Anna

Deane said, "I felt sad." She told me the truth. I knew I could trust her.

Every time Anna Deane came over, we talked about things in the house that were a problem for me. I was afraid of falling in the shower when I was getting spacey from a seizure, so we got a shower chair and a metal bar on the wall and rubber rugs inside the tub and outside the tub. Each one of these areas we worked on took months to identify the problem and with trial and error find the solutions. But in the case of the shower, finally I was able to take a shower, and I was no longer afraid. I was also afraid of burning myself on the flames of my gas stove if I was feeling confused, so we got a large electric hot plate, and I could heat something up without being afraid of lighting myself or my clothes on fire.

I had lost the ability to do things; I knew there were steps to take to do any task, but I had no idea which step came first. I later learned that I had lost the ability to sequence, a loss that sometimes occurs when you have had an injury to the frontal lobe of the brain.

Anna Deane and I set out to discover how to teach me to do things again. She said that there was always another way to do something. First we had to find out how I was still able to learn. You will notice when I speak of Anna Deane and myself, I always say WE did this, WE decided that. Unlike many other health professionals, Anna Deane felt her role was not to tell me what to do, but to work with me, to empower me. She asked me constantly what was important to me. What did I think of something? What did I want to do? And she LISTENED to me. Extraordinary!

One problem in my life was how to unlock my front door. My house has two doors, an outside door and an inner door, and therefore I have two different keys. If someone would bring me home from the doctor's office, one of the few places that I went, I would often try to get the key in the lock and not be able to. I would try to unlock the door for what felt like hours, over and over again, desperately trying to get into my own house. I asked whoever dropped me off to see that I got into the house before they drove off. Often they would have to open the door for me. I felt stupid, unable to do the simplest thing.

Anna Deane watched me try to get into the house and said she understood what the problem was. She said when I couldn't get in the outside door with one key, that I should try the other key. It had not occurred to me to try the other key. I would stand endlessly with the wrong key doing it over and over again, but when I had this new strategy, it freed me to get into my own house, and each time I opened the door myself, it was such a victory. And I began to feel hope for myself.

Anna Deane and I discovered that it was impossible for me to just follow or understand verbal directions, but if I could also watch someone do a task, listen to the directions, even place my hands on the things at the same time, I could, after a number of tries, do it again myself.

Anna Deane said that we could not be sure which parts of my brain were still working, but we had the best chance for success if we used as many senses as possible, hoping that we could tap into the areas in my brain that still functioned. When Anna Deane first said this, it sounded like the most primitive kind of investigation into unknown territories, all of which were inside me. We were searching for the *me* that was still there. But she was right. With Anna Deane's help, I have learned to do everything (day-to-day self-maintenance activities) over again—absolutely everything. It is not too strong to say that she gave me my life back.

Another thing that Anna Deane and I worked on was a chart that monitored my daily activities. One of the problems was that I had lost any sense of time. With epilepsy, it is important that you take a certain amount of pills at a certain time every day. It's very simple—if you don't, the seizures come back. You also have to eat and rest regularly in relationship to taking the pills, and before I met Anna Deane, I could not remember whether I had taken a pill, had lunch, let the dogs out; I couldn't tell if it was afternoon or morning or what day it was.

Gradually, over a period of months and many failures, we worked out a chart on a magnetic blackboard that we divided into morning, afternoon, and evening. We used different colored magnets for different parts of the day, as we discovered that I could understand colors better than words. For every victory, such as the discovery that I still remembered colors, there were dozens of defeats. Anna Deane said over and over that there was always another way to do something. We just had to find the other way. And every time we failed, she learned that much more about my brain, what still worked and how it was working. She said there was no such thing as a "failure." She learned something each time we tried something new.

I, on the other hand, felt the failures very keenly. Because I had been quick and life had come easily to me, I was not used to trying and failing at something simple again and again and again. The things we were trying to do, such as a system to get me to remember to take my pills, were both very simple and very important. I was impatient with myself and judged myself by who I had been. For each failure, I shed many tears.

I tried not to cry in front of Anna Deane. My dogs, Desmond and Todd, listened to my crying. I would go to pet them, and their fur would be wet. I would be puzzled at first and then remembered I had been crying. And they had been sitting beside me on the couch, wet with my tears.

Anna Deane said that I was doing what I needed to do, grieving over my losses. I had lost a great deal. And that if one didn't grieve and let the past go, it was harder to do new things. That grief could stand in the way of progress (see Color Plate 9, "The Color of My Grief"). But on the other hand, I also needed to look at the balance of things. I needed to find things that still made me happy, gave me pleasure. It became my job each day to do one thing that gave me pleasure (see Color Plate 10, "Goblin"). This sometimes was as hard to do as the task of grieving. It became obvious to me that the two were connected.

So we refined the magnetic board system further: colored magnets for each time of day, further divided into take pill, have lunch, feed dogs, and so on. When the activity had been completed, I moved the magnet from the not-done category to the done category. The chart is large and colorful, and I can look at it from across the room and tell what I have done and what I haven't done yet and how I'm doing. And so, eventually, time and memory seemed somewhat under my control again (see Color Plate 11, "Healing Brain").

Anna Deane came to my house every week for an hour, and we talked on the phone a number of times between the visits. In the year that I worked with her, I could see small changes in my life; and as I got greater control over the details of my life again, the person who I had been started to reemerge. I wasn't making films, but I could change the sheets on my bed. I wasn't writing poetry, but I could dress myself. These may seem like small things, but with each skill I regained, I could feel life flowing back into me again.

Another triumph that stands out was the ability to get into and out of buildings. There are many buildings in Boston where you have to buzz the company or office that you are going to, and then they buzz you back and the door opens. I was no more able to decipher this than the Rosetta Stone. It was impossibly complex for me and therefore overwhelming, and therefore tear-producing, and therefore one more thing that I couldn't do.

Anna Deane and I talked about every possible kind of solution and came up with one that worked. The solution was to stand and watch until someone else came along and pushed a button and got in the door, watch how they did it, and either go in with them or do the same thing they did. And it worked.

In large buildings, it's still a problem finding the correct office if I haven't been there before, because in the elevator, I am not able to understand whether 5 is the same as 7 is the same as 9 when the elevator opens. So I have been lost in the best hospitals in Boston. The people who had taken me went to park their car and against their better judgment let me out, me telling them not to worry about it, that I would meet them at the office. And then, 45 minutes later when I did not show up at the office, and it became clear that there was a problem, various people would be sent to find me. For my part, I would be asking people if this was the fourth floor, etc., etc.

Among the least helpful people to give this kind of simple direction are doctors, nurses, or anyone else from "the allied health professions." Among the most helpful, of course, are the other patients and all the cleaning and maintenance people. However, Anna Deane and I have not figured a way around this problem, a way to make me independent, to do it all on my own. It is still, sadly, something that makes me cry.

With Anna Deane's help, I listened to talking books for reading and used a calculator to add and subtract, told time with a digital clock, asked people to take me places and not just give me directions, and used the brightly colored arrows that told me which way to turn the thermostat to heat my house and to turn on the water faucets in the shower. In other words, many victories. And more to come.

Sometimes people ask me what kind of fee Anna Deane charged me for this amount of work and of devotion. The answer is—not one cent. She told me that she did not know enough about brain injury to charge for her services; it was a learning experience for her too. And she did not say it, but I knew she knew that I did not have a cent to my name.

MAY 1996: SEVENTEEN YEARS AFTER THE ACCIDENT

How am I now? I was told that if a function did not come back after a year, it would not come back. They were wrong about this in some cases. I have continued to regain things over a period of 16 years. I can discriminate between right and left again, I am much better at recognizing faces—not perfect, but better. I can understand poetry and most abstractions again. I regained my sense of smell. I can read a bit if the print is big. I can write again.

I still can't count. I still can't do multiplication tables or months of the year. I still see double out of one eye. I still have to sit and think a long time about what steps go into a task such as putting the laundry in the washing machine and what order those steps should take. I still have balance problems. I still have a lot of seizures— several a day most of the time. I have learned to live with these things—the things that are lost to me and the things that have come back but are different.

I had a battery of neuropsychological tests done on me recently, and I still do badly on a number of them. You are reading the writing of someone who now has an IQ still considerably under 100.

I was surprised how many strong feelings I had when I started to answer the simple sounding question—"How are you?" First of all, it is not until I started to get better that I realized how much I had lost. Before that, I was too sick or too overwhelmed to notice, to understand the breadth of the loss. In broad strokes, I lost 10 years of my life where I almost ceased to exist. And I still grieve over that loss; some days it feels like a very big loss, other days it doesn't (see Color Plate 12, "Broken Dreams").

So how am I now? I am doing better without having gotten better. In other words, I learned to do a lot of things in new ways just as Anna Deane Scott, the occupational therapist who worked with me, said I would—tell time with a digital clock, read with talking books, write with a large-screen, large-print computer. I feel like myself again. I am happy most of the time—in fact I seem to be one of the more happy and contented people I know. I have become grateful for things large and small. I am more appreciative of other people. In fact, I think we should all gets stars and bluebirds for getting up in the morning. The head injury has forced me to look at myself. Look at all the sad, angry parts of me that I did not consider when I was a hotshot television producer. I was too busy working 18-hour days. Being very busy in a high-visibility job can be seductive. What you are doing seems so important that you can easily push everything else into a corner. But when you are sitting home, day after day, when the phone isn't ringing off the hook, it is less possible to ignore things.

Being brain injured has given me time to look at who I was, how I got there, and to ask myself what I want to do about my life. Counseling also helped me to survive many assaults on the spirit that can occur when you are forced to endlessly deal with health care providers. Being a patient can be a grueling life. I know that this will seem strange; it seems strange to me even as I write it down. There is a belief that if you have one sense such as sight taken away, your hearing becomes more acute to compensate. To understand my own suffering, I have come to better understand the suffering of others.

I also laugh more, am made happy more easily. I am much more at ease with myself. I feel quite literally that I walked and walked and walked through the valley of the shadow of death, stumbling, crying, falling, breaking bones, and finally came out on the other side. When asked about the brain injury, I tell people I would not wish it on my worst enemy. Yet strangely, I am also grateful for the journey.

JULY 2001: TWENTY-TWO YEARS AFTER THE ACCIDENT

I continue to live with the physical problems that came from the original injury. And there are still the problems I have because I am who I am. I was on the phone recently with a spit-and-polish person that I don't particularly like. At a point in the conversation, I was not able to understand what she was saying. And then I started perseverating—saying the same word over and over again, which she didn't notice. These signals told me that I was probably about to have a seizure.

I felt frustrated and ashamed. I could do nothing to stop the seizure. Worse still, I thought I might start crying, but I forced myself to be polite. I finally hung up when I began losing the ability to speak. And I felt terrible about myself. I could hear Anne Deane Scott's voice when I used to tell her about this kind of social situation: "Just hang up the phone. And if they don't like it, too bad

for them!" A life lesson I have yet to learn. Even after these 22 years, I still need to please others at my own expense.

I have had the best help in the world, so why don't I learn these lessons? I suppose that is because I am a human being and I still carry the same baggage I had before the accident.

And now I think it is time to tell you about good things.

About five years ago. a new antiseizure medicine came on the market that has made a large, positive difference in the quality of my life. At long last, I have fewer seizures and am more clear-headed. I am *me* more of the time. It's wonderful. I have a computer and like it for all the same reasons that everyone else does. Even though I am mostly house-bound, I have the world in front of me.

I have always loved animals, and now I am active with animal rescue and finding homes for abused, homeless animals (see Color Plate 13, "I Stand by While Good Dogs Die"). Since a large part of this can be done on the phone or the Internet, I can do this when I am feeling okay. I have become part of a network of people who care about animals as much as I do. They have no idea that I used to be a filmmaker or even that I was in a terrible accident, although I do tell them about the brain injury if there is a reason to. I never have to fear that anyone will feel sorry for me. I am just one more person who is dedicated to helping animals.

I love this part of my life.

In the 22 years since the accident, I have gone from not being able to read and write at all or to even turn the pages in a book to be able to write what you are reading right now. I write easily now.

Finally, there is something unexpected that I seldom hear discussed by brain-injured survivors or the people who work with them.

The car accident was a crushing, wrenching assault on me. For the first few years after the accident, the question that I asked over and over was this: How could God do this to me?

Before the accident, I had been a spiritual person. I believed in a compassionate, wise God who cared about each sparrow that fell and each lily of the field.

After, it seemed like God cared about everything but me. I was shocked and heart-broken that God let this happen. I thought about it constantly and talked to anyone who would listen. I felt twisted and damaged inside and out (see Color Plate 14, "When I Think of Dying")—and angry. Angry. Angry. You can see this in my paintings (see Color Plate 15, "Pain#2").

The years went by, and I never came to any understanding. After a time, my sorrow blew away like smoke (see Color Plate 16, "White Brain"),

I understand now that the greatest damage I experienced was the damage no one can see. It left me feeling afraid of things, not trusting in life, not being able to believe in a kind, loving God. I felt alone.

I have had the best occupational therapy and counseling and profited from them. I have learned to do many of the skills of daily living again. I have changed and grown.

And there is more.

My spirit has been the last to heal.

I am still healing.

JULY 2007: TWENTY-EIGHT YEARS AFTER THE ACCIDENT

When I first heard the term *occupational therapy,* it made me think of a black-and-white photograph from the turn of the century with dozens of sturdy young women working at looms. It was the word *occupational,* of course. As it turns out, occupational therapy deals with all the things that make us feel human—the delicate interchange between mind and body. I've heard brain-injured people say, "I don't feel like myself." And I've said the same. I had experienced a shocking, terrible interior change that took away my ability to be and do. Occupational therapy helps us to realign ourselves, cell by cell.

When Anna Deane Scott started working with me, she first had me tested. The doctors in 1982 were perplexed because I had been unconscious only for a few seconds. Usually, there is more lack of consciousness to have so much damage. Of the many problems that the tests pinpointed, my ability to *sequence* proved to be the most damaged. In other words, I knew there were steps to do things but had no idea what order they came in. Therefore, I literally couldn't count, couldn't say the months of the year, the days of the week. I couldn't tell time. I couldn't read. Unfortunately, the world is made of sequences.

Another problem was an inability at times to find a name for an object or even recognize it. To work with this, Anna Deane said that we should try all of my senses—touch, sound, and so on. One time she put a number of things—lipstick, comb, pencil, spoon—into a sack. I was not able to recognize them with my eyes. When I used my sense of touch, I was able to recognize them, to understand them, and to give them their names with my fingers. I told Anna Dean I felt like Helen Keller when she signed the word WATER for the first time. It was victory for me. It was hope. It was making the undamaged cells take up another function. And they did, even though it has taken years.

Experts in the field of brain injury in 1982 told me that young adult males were most likely to have head injury. And being young, they were quicker to heal. Women my age, on the other hand, statistically did not often suffer brain injury and, being older, did not heal as quickly. These young people hadn't lived very long and therefore did not have life experience and, because of this, did not have as many life skills as an adult does. I, on the other hand, an older woman—me—had developed a set of work skills. I knew how to do a lot of things. I had been a television producer and filmmaker. To be a successful television producer and filmmaker, you have to have tremendous drive, know how to make things happen, and be a hard worker. The accident had not crushed those parts of me. That and the creative part of me were still there, although at the time, I didn't know this. I was just trying to fill my days, which were also filled with seizures and confusion.

If you look at my paintings, you can see how simply they started. I used finger paint, water, and torn tissue paper. I painted at least 10 paintings a day. Make a painting, lie down, and rest. Make a painting, pet the dogs. Make a painting, cry. Make a painting, stare at the ceiling. And gradually, and with the grace of God, I began healing. There was another plus to my painting. When an artist friend and other friends came over, we often talked about paintings. I had something other than pain and suffering to talk about. Above all, I didn't want people to feel sorry for me.

I have thought so many times that I was lucky to have been born at this time and this place. I was lucky to have lived at a time when people were starting to understand head injury. Head injury—people call it brain injury now. One hundred years ago, if I had this kind of brain injury, I might not have lived through it. Or if I had lived, I would have been tied to a chair in some dreary institution.

On the other side, there were many dark times when I often thought it would have been easier to die. Because life had become an unendurable burden. I didn't feel like myself. I had lost myself. I felt that I would always be caught in this terrible web. It seemed that there was no way out of it. And how could God have done this to me? What did I do to deserve this? I thought of suicide constantly. I didn't talk about this. Not to my parents. Not to Sally. Early on, a man who was educated and sophisticated about the ins and outs of the head injury world visited me. He was kind and reassuring. He also had a brain injury and epilepsy. He told me not to tell anyone you feel suicidal—you would be pink-slipped "for your own good." Meaning you would be put in the insane asylum. Particularly do not tell any of the doctors, he said; and I believed him. You can bet I believed him. That was all I needed, to be in an asylum.

For a time I was in a discussion group of people with seizures and brain injury. I listened to far too much horrifying "for your own good" that had been done to people. But that is another book.

I am speaking in my own voice right now—not the voice of the overwhelmed, defeated person. In fact, at the time, I was still unable to do the simplest things. And Anna Deane Scott, bless her heart, sent out some of her occupational therapy students to my house to work with me for academic credit. They were wonderful. We all gained. They learned firsthand about brain injury and I learned to do things that I was not able to do on my own. I wanted to write a story about my Jack Russell terrier, Todd. The students wrote down the Todd stories that I was not able to read or write myself. I said the words one by one, and the students wrote them down one by one.

The story was named "Todd and the Stars." I was painting and the students went to the store to get yellow paint for me. And they helped me. They were like sunshine coming into a dark room. Anna Deane was so smart. I kept painting. I could see that my pictures were getting better. And though I didn't know it at the time, I was getting better.

I was healing. I lived and went on to tell this story. And I am glad to be alive.

It has been 28 years since the car accident. I had learned to live with my brain injury. For the most part I'm fine at home, with my friends, in familiar places. But I forget that I am not okay in the eyes of the world. I do not do well with new situations. Several years ago, I needed a knee replacement and went to a highly thought-of hospital and rehabilitation facility. After the surgery, I was brought back to my room, groggy, crying, confused, and in pain. The nurse on duty told me that there was a way of controlling my pain—I only had to push a button by my hand and I would receive the right amount of pain meds. She demonstrated it and left. The pain went on and on. My friend Sally could see that I did not understand the sequential steps to make the pain machine work. She called the nurse and told her that I couldn't understand how to use the pain button because I had a brain injury. Sally asked—could she push the pain button for me? The nurse said Sally most certainly could NOT touch the machine and that I had to do it for myself.

A frustrated Sally repeated about my inability to deal with sequences and because of that, I wasn't able to use the pain machine. The nurse told us that everyone is capable of using the pain device—even people 80 years old can do this and "so can you." The nurse left. The pain continued. Sally called for the nurse and again explained about my brain injury. This sequence went on a number of times. I am not sure how it resolved itself, but finally another nurse came in and started to give me shots for the pain. This was the first of many other such episodes. The staff seemed to think that if I was able to talk, I should be able to understand what they wanted me to do.

Next was getting out of bed. There are steps to learn to get out of a bed after knee replacement surgery. A nurse and a nurse's aide told me what to do over and over. I asked over and over and tried to understand what they were telling me. And, worse still, when I struggled to explain something my speech became garbled and confused. The nurse's aide turned to the nurse and asked what was wrong with me. The nurse looked right at me, put her finger making a circle around her ear—the sign that children use to mean "crazy."

This, even though Sally had told all the nursing staff about my brain injury, had put a sign over the bed to that effect, and had made sure the information was added to my medical file along with my own doctor's evaluation of my situation. Most of the nursing and medical staff were not interested in anything we had to say about my brain injury. They completely dismissed what Sally and I said. Further, alas, they were quick to criticize and say that I wasn't trying hard enough. They talked about me in front of me and others. They talked to me like I was a badly behaved child.

Some of the more frightening situations came up when the rehabilitation people were trying to teach me to do things on my own: go up stairs, get in and out of the bathtub, or walk with the walker. I was frightened because they didn't listen to a word I said. I know how dangerous this situation can be for me. At home, I have fallen and broken bones, broken teeth, bitten the inside of my mouth, and put my fingers in my eyes. These people didn't listen to me about my brain injury. I asked to speak to the supervisor and described the situation I was in. I talked to her about the rehabilitation staff not listening to me. The supervisor said that they must have been tired that day. I talked to my doctor about the same thing. He said to write to the president of the hospital and that no one listened to him either.

Finally, thank God, I got out of that place. It had been a nightmare. All too often this must be how some people—the old, the retarded, the insane, the poor, people who don't speak English—are treated. What they have to endure. And so did I.

Time passed, and I needed to go to a hospital for pneumonia. This new hospital was a far different experience. It is known for its innovative work with brain trauma. The staff took detailed information about my brain injury. They were as interested in it as the other place was not. I sighed with relief. I didn't have to struggle to communicate. When I said I had temporal lobe brain damage, they understood. It was like coming to a different country. And I no longer had to be in a defensive posture. Better than that—they believed me when I described the characteristics, albeit very strange even to me, of my brain injury.

And now on television, I see our men and woman soldiers, damaged, crushed, brought back to many armed services hospitals and rehabilitation facilities where there might be very little or no concept of brain injury or how to deal with it. I would guess that these people coming back from the war and their families are going to run into problems similar to the ones I had and that my friend Sally encountered on my behalf. A recent article in *DISCOVER* Magazine entitled "Dead Men Walking: What Sort of Future Do Brain-Injured Iraq Veterans Face?" by Michael Mason (2007) describes the situation faced by these veterans. When I read this article, it broke my heart because I know brain injury can be a lifelong tragedy.

In a flash, the blast incinerates air, sprays metal, burns flesh. Milliseconds after an improvised explosive device (IED) detonates, a blink after a mortar shell blows, an overpressurization wave engulfs the human body, and just as quickly, an underpressure wave follows and vanishes. Eardrums burst, bubbles appear in the blood-

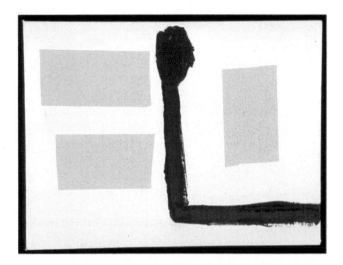

PLATE 1. Intersection: For a long time after the accident my mind played and replayed the car crash. I finally painted it to get the memory outside of myself. Here was the inter-section, and here was the car I was in. Then the collision, the smashing of the car and of me. (Color plate courtesy of Mary Feldhaus-Weber)

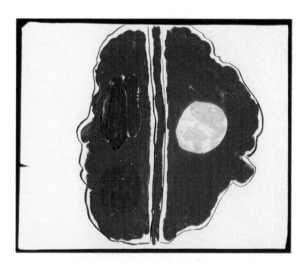

PLATE 3. Damaged Brain: 1981—When I started paint-ing, I painted what I thought my own brain must look like. In this painting I painted a brain that was terribly hurt on both sides—like mine, I thought. Much later, when the doctor ran my CAT scans, indeed my brain was damaged on both sides. (Color plate courtesy of Mary Feldhaus-Weber)

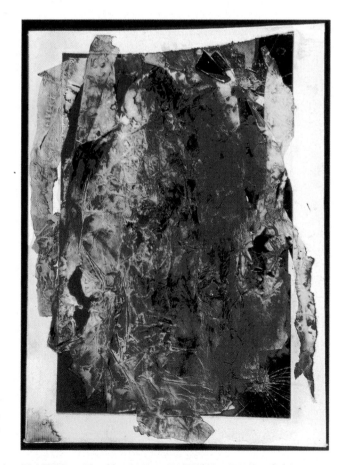

PLATE 2. The Shattering: 11/20/83—I painted this on the fifth anniversary of the accident. I still felt like I was bleeding to death. (Color plate courtesy of Mary Feldhaus-Weber)

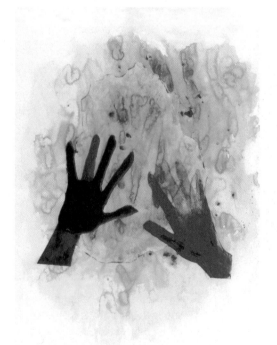

PLATE 4. Blue Seizure: Before we discovered an epilepsy medication that worked I was having constant seizures. This is a picture of what it felt like: a force outside myself (the hands) held my brain under ice. It held me there, terrified, desperate, helpless. Until it chose to release me. One of the fingers was red because I sometimes felt pain during the seizures. This picture broke through to a lot of people. My friend Sally said she had witnessed many of my seizures, but never understood how I felt. This painting, she said, was the only thing that helped her "get it." (Color plate courtesy of Mary Feldhaus-Weber)

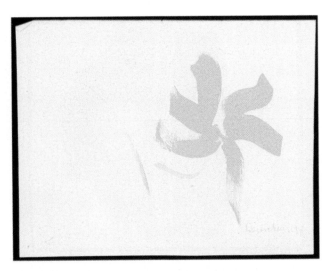

PLATE 5.   **Daisy:** December, 1980—The first picture I painted. One year after the accident I painted this modest yellow daisy. I came to this with great desperation. I had never studied painting, but I knew I had to fight to survive or I would be lost. The color of the daisy was the color of my neurologist's tie. (Color plate courtesy of Mary Feldhaus-Weber)

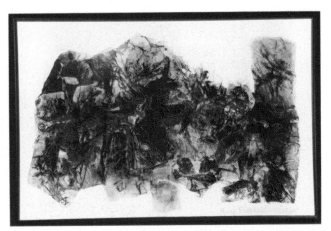

PLATE 7.   **Dendrites:** Painted when I was starting to get better. I began to pick up the jargon of the neurology team I was working with. They explained how parts of the brain communicate. I came home and painted what I thought dendrites might look like. Beautiful and strange. This is one of my favorite paintings. (Color plate courtesy of Susan Mc Ginley)

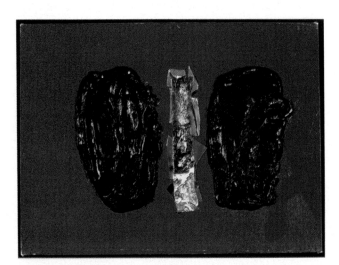

PLATE 6.   **Hemisphere:** Someone told me that for the brain to heal, the two hemispheres of the injured brain had to learn to communicate with each other again—find new pathways that worked. The right side had to take up what the left side used to do. In this picture, I put broken mirrors between the two hemispheres. The idea of my brain ever getting better seemed impossible, painful, exhausting. (Color plate courtesy of Mary Feldhaus-Weber)

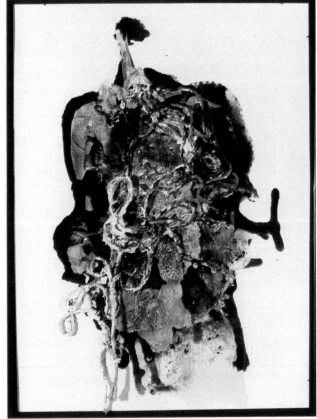

PLATE 8.   **Self Portrait:** The tiny knob was my head. I felt I had ceased to have intelligence. I was just a confused, tattered body. No part of me worked. (Color plate courtesy of Mary Feldhaus-Weber)

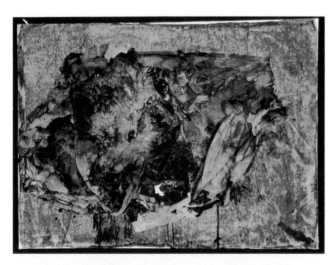

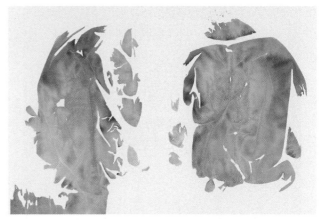

PLATE 11. **Healing Brain:** Early 1983—This picture shows what I imagined the damaged brain and the healed brain would look like, side by side. (Color plate courtesy of Mary Feldhaus-Weber)

PLATE 9. **The Color of My Grief:** I connected with a woman in the field of education rehabilitation. With her help I was able to understand the concept of counting again. After several months I was able to count to four. I was thrilled. For some reason I never understood, the agency she was with fired her out of the blue. It was a huge loss to me. Grief upon grief. When you find someone who can help you, they are like gold. I was furious at the people who fired her, and sad beyond words. (Color plate courtesy of Mary Feldhaus-Weber)

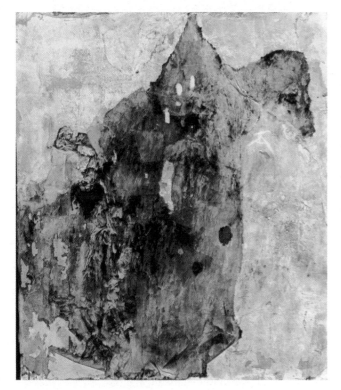

PLATE 10. **Goblin:** Done for fun. (Color plate courtesy of Mary Feldhaus-Weber)

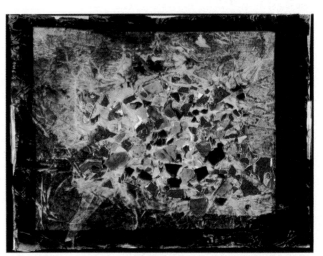

PLATE 12. **Broken Dreams:** I painted this when I saw a friend's film on TV and I realized that the people I worked with in TV production were moving ahead. I, on the other hand, was sitting at home, having seizures and only able to dial the telephone after many tries. (Color plate courtesy of Mary Feldhaus-Weber)

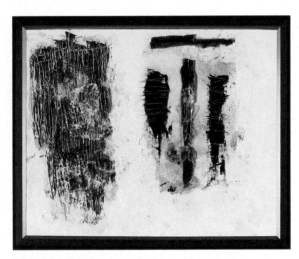

PLATE 13. I Stand By While Good Dogs Die: June, 2001—I have always liked dogs more than anything. I now work as a volunteer with an animal rescue group. I work from home on the telephone when I am able to. Many of the dogs we try to rescue cannot be saved, in spite of our best efforts. There are simply not enough homes to go around. In this picture, I am the figure on the left covered with mica (shiny sheets of mineral), which represents my good intentions. The dogs on the right represent the dogs we cannot save. Their spirits are moving upward toward the shining mica, which represents life beyond life. This is my most recent painting. (Color plate courtesy of Mary Feldhaus-Weber)

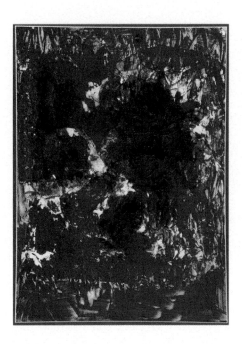

PLATE 15. Pain #2: 1987—More pain, more feeling trapped and desperate. I felt this way a long, long time. My painting was often the only way I had to express it. (Color plate courtesy of Mary Feldhaus-Weber)

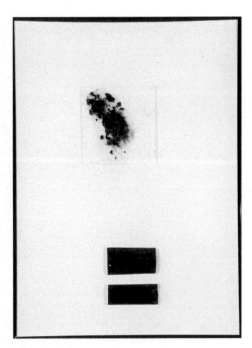

PLATE 14. When I Think of Dying: 10/15/83—As I started to get better, I realized how much I had lost. It was at this time that I thought about suicide. This picture was what I imagined the soul might look like upon leaving the dying body. (Color plate courtesy of Mary Feldhaus-Weber)

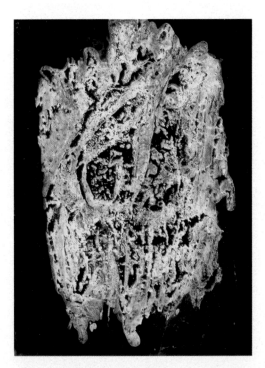

PLATE 16. White Brain: At a certain point I began to make my brain pictures more "decorative," artistic. I was no longer so obsessed with understanding the damage. I was beginning to integrate my feelings about the head injury. (Color plate courtesy of Mary Feldhaus-Weber)

stream, the heart slows. A soldier or a civilian can survive the blast without a single penetrating wound and still receive the worst diagnosis: traumatic brain injury, or TBI, the signature injury of the Iraq War.

But in the same instant that the blast unleashes chaos, it also activates the most organized and sophisticated trauma care in history. Within a matter of hours, a soldier can be medevaced to a state-of-the-art field hospital, placed on a flying intensive care unit, and receive continuous critical care a sea away. (During Vietnam, it took an average of 15 days to receive that level of treatment. Today the military can deliver it in 13 hours.) Heroic measures may be yielding unprecedented survival rates, but they also carry a grim consequence: No other war has created so many seriously disabled veterans. Soldiers are surviving some brain injuries with only their brain stems unimpaired. (Mason, 2007, paragraphs 1–2).

Later in the article, Mason goes on to write about the rehabilitation possibilities for brain-injured soldiers. When I read this part, I thought about all the things occupational therapists could bring to their suffering. In an interview, Marilyn Price Spivack asserted that

Men and women in the military will receive excellent care for a time, but eventually, they are going back to their communities. "The military is doing an extraordinary job in saving young soldiers and treating them through the acute rehabilitation phase," says Spivack, who works with the brain-injured population at Spaulding Rehabilitation Hospital in Boston. In the early 1980s she founded the Brain Injury Association, today the foremost advocacy organization for TBI survivors. "Now the government must make a commitment to help them in their recovery, but where are the resources going to come from? As brain-injury professionals, we know that TBI services aren't available in many places across the country, and we are aware of huge holes in the system," she says. "Frankly, I'm frustrated and angry about the government's refusal to give the TBI population the support it desperately needs."

Spivack is not being glib; the giant holes are glaringly apparent. Many states do not have a single brain-injury rehabilitation center, and of the states that do offer some level of TBI treatment, few actually provide enough assistance to acquire even the most basic level of specialized care. At rates that can exceed a thousand dollars a day for postacute TBI rehabilitation, there aren't many American families that can afford a month's worth of treatment, much less the recommended minimum of 90 days.

As recently as mid-July 2006, the VA Office of the Inspector General admitted that patients and families were dealing with major inadequacies. The reality is that a fundamental level of care is simply absent in most states. (Mason, 2007, paragraphs 29–31)

I encourage you to read Mason's powerful article (see on the ON THE WEB, p. 115). I fear that these veterans will come up against the worst kind of ignorance—people who don't know that they don't know. This is an enormous situation that has no easy answers.

HOW AM I NOW?

I often wonder how things would have been if there hadn't been a car accident. As it is, I have lost many years of my life. Some of those years were complete dropouts, because there are not words for what I went through. I felt that I had fallen into a deep, deep pit. I was alive but not alive. Gradually I have gotten better in many ways.

I have four or five hours in a day—good hours when I can do things. If I go past that, my speech becomes garbled, my coordination is bad, and I have to worry if I will fall. I have to be SO careful about hanging onto things so I won't fall. I have handles and grab bars all over the house that help me walk. But if I am too exhausted, I have to stay in bed. If I do a small thing that's just too much, my brain becomes frozen, rigid, or like an old car, or a cranky baby. I never know when it will choose to give out. When this happens, I have to be quiet and let it rest.

There are things I wish I could do. I would like to go horseback riding. I'd love to go to movies. I'd like to go to Sweden and see the midnight sun again. I'd like to go to a symphony orchestra again. I'd like to see the cherry blossoms in Washington. And the redwood trees. And Animals in Africa. And sit through five days of a film festival. And go dancing with a good-looking man—a rascal.

The one movie that I tried to go to, I had to leave and sit in the accessible ladies room because of overload from the pictures and sound. I had to say to the people I was with that I had to go home. It was the *Pirates of the Caribbean,* and I enjoyed the 30 minutes tremendously.

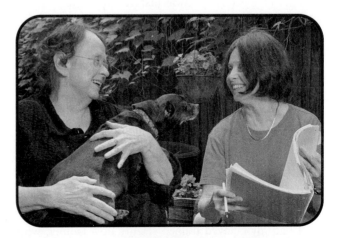

FIGURE 11.1   Mary, Sally, and LaBeam chatting in the garden. (Photo courtesy of L. Nugent, Photographic Services, University of New Hampshire, Durham, NH.)

But all that said, I can watch television at home because I can put the sound down if necessary.

And if this fails, I listen to my Talking Books, which have all kinds of subjects. I can listen to poetry or essays or history with the lights off with my four dogs on the bed, and I am very, very happy.

I'm going to a meeting tomorrow in my wheelchair, and if I have to go to the bathroom, I have to have help, because most restrooms are not accessible for people who have disabilities. I don't talk about the ins and outs of this, but trust me, its true. People want to think that all of this has changed and the bathrooms are accessible and all of the sidewalks have curb cuts so you don't have to deal with a curb. NOT.

And I don't do as many things as I am able to do because of the complexity of managing the comings and goings.

I live alone and have people who help me. I have my groceries delivered. I have people help me with the housework. I have people who take me to the doctor, if I can make this happen—both coordinating and paying people to take me to the doctor. Many times I can't get someone to take me to the doctor for love or money.

So getting back to more interesting things. Many of my friends and I rescue animals, and we find good homes for them. When we see a dog that has been starved and beaten become a healthy, happy dog, it is a great experience. And I do gardening on my front porch. And like everyone else, I have a computer, and like everyone else, it is my link to the world.

I have most recently started working with people in the inner city. They have been giving Christmas parties for children for years. Last Christmas we got toys, books, tasty things to eat for 800 children. I was told that these presents might be the only ones the children would receive. This event was wonderful. I sat at a special Christmas gift table with books about animals and toys for the children's pets. I felt I was just exactly where I should be—with children who liked animals as much as I do. One little boy asked if I had any books about snakes, and luckily I did. He was delighted when he opened the present and said, "**SNAKES**!!!" There we were. The child. The snake book. And me. This was one of the happiest moments of my life.

I started to paint again, I laugh with my friends, I am lucky to have come this far.

I had the luck to meet Anna Deane Scott, who had the belief that there was always another way to do something. And indeed that was the case.

I met Maureen Neistadt, who asked me to speak to her OT students and show them my paintings.

I had my beloved trained seizure dog Timmy, who helped me to walk, stopped me from falling, made me feel safe. He was an incredible gift for me when I was frightened and lonely.

In the early years right after the accident, Dr. Thomas Glick, a neurologist, was important to me. He encouraged me, was kind to me, was generous with his time, and listened to my many, many tears. Dr. Glick was a remarkable man.

My Mother and Father in South Dakota kept me afloat financially and emotionally. They called me every day after day. I can't imagine what would have happened to me without their help, when I had next to nothing. They had been so proud of me—of my plays, my films—that had drawn honor and acclaim and added meaning to their lives. I knew what had happened to me had broken their hearts. I could hear it in their voices when they talked to me on the phone.

If I had lived 100 years ago or had been born in the third world, I would never have survived.

Instead here I am having the honor of talking to you.

And who am I now? I'm a human being. Just like everyone else.

POSTSCRIPT: THOUGHTS FOR OCCUPATIONAL THERAPY PRACTITIONERS

I have one final thought that I want to share with you. I have spent a lot of time thinking about what "helps" in the kind of situation I have been in with my brain injury. Why could some people get through to me and not others? Why did some people comfort and heal me and other seemingly well-meaning people shame or humiliate me? In other words: What works? What heals? What helps?

I discovered that power is at the heart of living with an injury, and power is at the heart of getting better. Many of us, particularly women, don't think of ourselves as having power. It is just a word, not something we own or think much about. Yet power is the ability to make things happen.

When I was at my most diminished, it felt as though everyone was more powerful than I was—from the secretary in the doctor's office who had to take the time to push the right elevator button for me to the cab driver I had to trust to give back the correct change because I could not count. The people who had to show me to the restroom when I was not capable of finding it. The doctors who filled out the insurance forms so that I would get disability payments to buy food and pay the rent. It was a very long list, and I was at the bottom. I had to depend on everyone.

Because of the power issues (who has it, who wants it, who needs it, who can share it), I think it is important to check why you are going into the healing professions. Ask yourself tough questions and keep asking them. Questions like "What do I get out of this work?" "How does this situation make me feel about myself?" "Do I need to have things in black and white or can I bear the uncertainty of all the shades of gray that illness and sorrow present us with?" "Can I trust people, however damaged, to know what is best for themselves?"

So the question I am asking you is this: Can you give over power to another person? Can you honor their own wishes, dreams, abilities? Can you be as interested in their abilities as you are in their disabilities? Can you give them the tools to get their own lives back on track?

And do you listen to people? Do you *hear* what they are telling you? I believe that we are far wiser than we give ourselves or each other credit for. So I am telling you that the two most important things you can do as occupational therapy practitioners are to listen and to empower. The people who helped me the most did both of those things. I continue to bless them and to use what they have taught me every day.

Since I first started occupational therapy with Anna Deane in 1982, books have been written about brain injury, and classes have been given. There are whole hospitals for people with brain injury. Because of the war in Iraq, this is a new time for brain injury, and this is the time when you as occupational therapy practitioners are going to have to think new and think large—because there is such a desperate situation. I think it is a disgrace that every injured soldier might not receive occupational therapy. When I read that returning soldiers were not even evaluated for brain injury—it's like the Dark Ages. And so much suffering has been needless.

So then, dear friends who are reading this, I think your calling could be taking care of the soldiers who are coming back from the war. These are times to stand beside the soldiers and to advocate for them.

You have chosen a profession that helps, restores, teaches, and gives comfort. Some of the finest human beings I have ever met are occupational therapy practitioners. You speak for us, the people you serve. You are in our corner. You are needed. Each and every one of you is desperately needed. I am glad that you have chosen this profession. I am proud of you. Bless you. Bless you all.

ACKNOWLEDGMENT

Let me tell you about my friend Sally. Sally Schreiber-Cohn has helped me to make this chapter happen, from taking some of the original dictation when I was too sick to do it myself to bringing me art supplies for my painting. Sally and I were friends before the accident, and she has stayed my friend through these 28 years. Sally, an artist herself, stuck with me on a day-by-day basis, patient, kind, and worked to see that the artist in me did not die. She has always been in my corner.

Sally is a large part of why I came through all this.

ON THE WEB

For an additional perspective on rehabilitation for veterans with brain injury, see the report on the Palo Alto Veterans' Administration at http://www.pbs.org/newshour/bb/health/july-dec06/brain_09-14.html

REFERENCE

Mason, M. (2007, February 23). Dead men walking: What sort of future do brain-injured Iraq veterans face? *Discover Magazine*. Retrieved June 4, 2007, from http://discovermagazine.com/2007/mar/dead-men-walking

He's Not Broken—He's Alex: Three Perspectives

**ALEXANDER McINTOSH,
LAURIE McINTOSH, AND
LOU McINTOSH**

In every lifetime, there are directions to take and choices to make. Each one of us carries a vision of our future. When something unexpected happens that takes us down an unfamiliar path, we have to adjust our vision and change our expectations while maintaining our self-identity. When parents discover that their child has a disability, they must adapt to this change and create a new vision for themselves and their child. This is the story of Alex, a person with cerebral palsy, told from three perspectives. Laurie, Alex's mother, begins the chapter. Then comes Lou, Alex's father. Alex has the last word, because it is his story that we want you to remember.

LAURIE

Before Alex was born, it had been easy to slip into fantasies of his future. I could picture him toddling around the deck of our sailboat. (I would have to remember to look into safety netting.) I would have to be careful to watch him around our home, which was also a boatyard. When he got old enough, we would get him his first toolbox and hand tools. He would bang his little toy hammer side by side with his dad while he worked on boats.

Alex was born twelve weeks before his due date. He weighed two pounds and needed all the medical support of the neonatal intensive care unit (NICU) to stay alive. Ten days after his birth, my husband Lou and I were ushered into the conference room near the nurses' station. I remember that the room was darkened. The shades had been drawn against the bright sunlight outside, and no one had turned on the lights. I was surprised to see that the social worker and the neonatologist were joining us—all the players. The neurologist was friendly but somber as he showed us pictures of Alex's latest brain ultrasound. As he used words like *periventricular leucomalacia,* I tried to swim to the surface by putting on my professional hat and being the occupational therapist that I was trained to be. Yes, I knew all about spastic diplegia. He would have trouble moving his arms and legs. Of course, I could help explain this to my husband. Cognition would probably be undamaged. Well, that's something good. Of course, there is always the chance. . . . the brain does amazing things. I was in a fog as I left the room, trying to make sense of the news.

Lou and I walked back to Alex's isolette. We peered in at the uncomfortable little being who was still pulling at his feeding tube and now making a faint mewing sound. I put my hands through the portholes in the side of the box and stroked his arms down away from the tube. I couldn't get myself to talk to him. I stared at him but could not make sense of what I was seeing. Who was this new person? . . . "Spastic diplegia." Would he even walk? I couldn't picture anything. I left the hospital that day with an empty feeling. It was almost as if Alex had died.

However, Alex didn't die. He grew and changed. He developed a unique personality before he even left the NICU. When he finally came home, near the time of his due date, he seemed like a typical baby. I loved showing him off to people and telling them what a miracle baby he was. There were days when I completely forgot about the brain scan and pictured Alex as I had in my dreams before he was born. On other days I would panic over his inability to roll over or sit up. I would imagine him having to use a wheelchair or being unable to get a job. The part of Alex that was his future was completely cloudy to me. All I could do was focus on the Alex that was present.

Throughout Alex's youth, we repeatedly cycled through the stages of grieving. Once, when I was furious with a neurologist, I remembered reading about anger being one of the typical stages, along with denial, bargaining, guilt, and others. In my practice, I frequently heard health professionals scoffing about this parent being in denial or that parent "just going through the anger phase." They sounded so superior, as if they would never handle a situation like this in such an unhealthy manner. Had I been in denial about Alex? Sometimes. Was that a bad thing? Did that make me weak or neurotic? Absolutely not. Professionals who criticize parents for going through the stages of grieving should have a chance to try it themselves. Telling someone that she should not be in denial or not be angry is like trying to tell her to self-actualize. It is just not something that you can do on command.

Our best health professionals were those who listened carefully, recognized where we were coming from on any particular day, and accepted that that was the reality of the day. Some days I was optimistic, and on other days I didn't see how we could possibly manage. Some days I would be full of energy and ask for more exercises or suggestions for activities, and on other days I hid my head in shame because I had not done Alex's stretches faithfully. I was grateful to the professionals who could adapt to my changes and who were patient and knew when to push and when to rest.

As Alex developed into a little person, we began to be able to visualize his future. Our circle of friends began to include other families of children with disabilities. We attended support groups and special activities that were offered through our local agency. Lou began working on some national disabilities issues that brought him into contact with adults with disabilities who were making important changes in legislation. Lou and I were able to get advice from other parents and ask successful adults with disabilities what we should be doing to help Alex. It was this exposure to others in the disability community that allowed us to begin to picture Alex as a successful adult. My training and experience as an occupational therapist helped me to focus on creating a home environment with typical expectations. In my occupational therapy courses, I had learned how a person's habits, routines, attitudes, and values are rooted in the experiences of childhood. I wanted to make sure that Alex grew up with the habits, attitudes, and values that would make him a successful adult.

As Alex became a preschooler, I wanted to give him experiences that were as typical as possible. At this point, he was an incredibly verbal and imaginative child who used a tiny wheelchair. His left hand was nearly typical, but his right hand did not have skilled movements. He needed exercises to strengthen and stretch his legs and to improve his hand use. I found it much easier to embed therapeutic activities into our daily routines than to set aside special times to do "exercises." When I cooked meals, I would give Alex packages to open, mixtures to stir, and food to place in bowls. For example, I would chop green beans and put handfuls of chopped pieces on his tray so that he could place them in the pan. He helped me to fold and sort laundry. His specialty was matching socks. I gave him a radio-frequency remote control switch so that he could control electrical appliances such as the vacuum cleaner, the blender, the radio, or the Christmas tree lights. I supported him in standing at the kitchen sink so that he could "help" with the dishes. He loved washing the car with the hose. This kind of "work" was "play" for Alex. He often pretended to be an adult such as a chef, machine operator, or "car wash guy" as he performed these tasks.

I found out later, while doing research for my master's thesis, that preschoolers have a strong drive to imitate their caregivers. Not only are household chores motivating for young children, but they also help children to feel like part of the family. It is one of the first opportunities that children have to contribute and to feel gratified by helping others. By this point, Alex was in grade school, busy with homework and after-school activities and not as interested in helping me around the house. I wanted him to feel a sense of responsibility and to realize that he could be a person on whom other people depended.

Because of his physical limitations, it was difficult to find a task that he could do completely independently. I gave him the job of cleaning the bathroom sink. We soon discovered that he needed to wear an apron for this task to keep the cleanser from getting all over his shirt. He became "Myrtle the Maid." It took several weeks to train him to do all the aspects of cleaning the sink. He had to learn to regulate the amount of cleaning powder that he poured out. He learned to hold the sponge at the correct angle to wipe the sink clean. He learned to work in an organized pattern so that he did not mess up an area that he had just cleaned. When he finished cleaning the sink, he would call me in for the "white glove" test to see whether I approved of his work. Alex was proud of his work, but that pride did not motivate him to clean the sink on his own. When I chose this task for him, I had to commit to never cleaning the sink myself. I needed him to understand that our family depended on him to do it. This was a challenge for me when we had company and I realized that the sink was not clean. I learned to warn Alex when company was coming so that he could clean it before they arrived. Lou and I put Post-it notes addressed to "Myrtle the Maid" on the mirror, asking her to please clean the sink. Alex took his responsibility seriously and, despite complaining, did his job well. After mastering sink cleaning, he moved on to toilet cleaning, dusting, and vacuuming.

Alex always managed to make household chores into something fun, but he did not like his daily living tasks, such as dressing himself. Alex started to realize that I was not really sure how much he could do on his own. He learned that if he had lots of difficulty with a task, I would probably finish it for him. Like any child, he would rather play than work, and putting on his clothes was work. I would watch him struggle with some part of dressing, trying over and over and getting more frustrated by the minute. We were always in a hurry, since everything took a long time for Alex. Inevitably, I would give up and rescue him. The next day, he would not have to struggle as hard to get me to help him because he was unconsciously training me to respond to his frustration and anger. All he had to do was get angry and frustrated sooner. Finally, I caught on to the pattern and decided to pick my battles carefully. On the weekends, when there was plenty of time, I would have him practice some aspect of dressing so that I knew that he could do it. Then, during the week, I would do all the parts of dressing that he had mastered and let him spend the time on the one skill that most needed practice. Some days, I would have him do only the parts of dressing that I knew he could do quickly. Only when there was plenty of time did I ask him to dress himself completely. Eventually, he put it all together and was able to dress himself, although it still took a long time and required lots of patience.

Lou and I knew the power of learned dependence, and we worked hard to create an environment in which Alex felt responsible for himself even when he needed help with some things. We tried to make sure that he felt the consequences of his choices. Behavior plans became part of our lives. For instance, in the mornings, Alex assumed that we would pack up all of his things, make his bed, put a coat on him, and send him out to the bus. At first, we had to help him with these things because they were physically difficult and time-consuming, but gradually, we tried to fade our assistance. Once we knew that he was capable of doing things on his own, we had to enforce that independence and make it part of his routine. For many years, he had to complete all the tasks on a checklist and get out to the bus on time in order to earn a reward. The reward for Alex was usually a book to read on the bus. Lou and I found that well-thought-out behavior plans worked for us as well as for Alex. We needed constant reminders to let him do things on his own and not jump in to help when things got a little tough.

As parents, we had a fairly good idea of what Alex's capabilities were at any particular time. It was much easier for Alex to take advantage of the well-meaning staff at school. People wanted to help him all the time, especially people in the cafeteria or the bus line. Every year, we had to meet with teachers and staff to explain to them how important it was for Alex to learn to think on his own. One late fall day when Alex was in middle school, I brought him back to school after a dentist appointment. After we checked in at the office, I told Alex to go to class and I would carry his backpack for him. I realized that Alex had no idea how to find his classroom. He had always had an aide or student carry his backpack, and he simply followed them. The next day, he came to school with a backpack on wheels so that he could pull it himself. However, he still had someone with him because there was a policy that a disabled student could not ride the elevator alone. It took a few phone calls to change the policy, and Alex was soon getting around the school completely independently.

Occupational therapy and physical therapy were available to Alex at school, but it was always difficult to balance therapies with academics. Alex was an extremely good student, and he wanted to be in the classroom as much as possible. In elementary school, he was seen outside the classroom for physical therapy, but occupational therapy was done on a consultation basis. Eventually, Alex's physical therapy was changed to a consultation model, which meant that he had to take more responsibility for his own stretching and exercises at home. By the time Alex was in high school, he was switched from an Individual Education Plan to a 504 plan because he did not require special education, merely modifications to regular education. Alex learned to advocate for himself by meeting with his teachers to adjust program requirements as needed. Assistive technology became a necessity in high school. Alex's handwriting and typing were slow, so he used a voice recognition program on the computer that converted his voice to text for taking notes and writing essays. He also found that a digital voice recorder was helpful for taking notes, recording assignments, and remembering tasks that needed to be done.

Recreation activities were another area that required thoughtful planning. My first instinct was to have Alex be involved only in "typical" recreation activities for "typical" children. I did not want him to grow up feeling separate and different from other children. Alex took karate lessons and attended a karate day camp in the summer. He swam at the town pool and attended a theater/puppetry class. He even became a Cub Scout. All these activities were great for him, although they came at a cost. Even though the adults who were in charge of these activities had good intentions, they had difficulty planning the activities with Alex's skills in mind. I became his aide during many activities in order for him to be fully included. Field trips and special activities required special planning to make sure that accessibility was considered and that Alex would be able to stay with the group. We had a few disasters with trips to places that we thought would be accessible but were not or leaders who planned activities that were too physically demanding for him.

It was a great relief to relax my standards and allow Alex to try specialized recreation activities. He participated in adapted horseback riding, hand-cycling, wheelchair court sports, and adapted skiing (Figure 12.1). At these specialized programs, I did not have to worry about making modifications because everything was set up for children with disabilities. Volunteers and program leaders were trained to deal with everything from transfers to helping a child in the bathroom. At many of these programs, parents were able to drop their children off and pick them up two hours later. That was a new experience for me! When I did choose to stay, I loved being able to sit back and watch my child having a good time while I stayed on the sidelines and chatted with other parents. It felt so "normal." Alex enjoyed the camaraderie of being with other children who had similar challenges, and many of the friendships that began at these activities have lasted for years.

Preparing for Alex to go to college took a lot of planning and creativity. Alex decided that he wanted to be within a three-hour drive of home, so we looked at colleges throughout the Northeast. Several of them were willing to accommodate students with disabilities but did not have much experience with this, and the campuses were not fully wheelchair accessible. Alex decided to attend a university near our home. This school had an access office, which coordinated accommodations for students with disabilities. He wanted to live on campus and have a typical college experience, including living on his own in a dorm. In the summer before he moved on campus, we checked out his dorm room, which had been carefully chosen to meet his needs. He spent several afternoons driving his new three-wheeled scooter around the campus and learning how to get through doors and operate elevators. Alex decided not to hire a personal care attendant even though it was still taking him over an hour to shower and dress in the morning. We carefully set up his room with a special stand for his reacher, sock-aide, and dressing stick. We bought a carpet for the room so that he could push his feet into his braces and shoes without having them slide. The dorm already had a fully equipped accessible shower. We purchased special shelves for the closet so that Alex could reach his supplies. We put up several plastic hooks to make it easier for him to hang his bathrobe and coat. A small folding shopping cart doubled as a hamper and a means of getting the laundry down to the laundry room. We practiced washing and folding laundry at a local laundromat during the summer.

The first few weeks of college were difficult for Lou and me as we waited at home to hear how things were going. Like many college students, Alex was enjoying being on his own and did not feel like calling home. When we finally heard from him, he was doing just fine. There had been a few problems with automatic doors not working, but Alex had contacted the right people to get things fixed. Crossing busy streets in his scooter had been a challenge at first, but he learned to use the crosswalks that were equipped with pedestrian signals. Lou and I were pleased to admit that we had passed the test. Alex was ready to be on his own. We had learned a lot as parents and made many mistakes along the way, but we knew that we had done some things right: Alex grew up feeling like a typical person who happened to have a physical disability. He knew that there were obstacles to overcome, but there were also people to help him when he asked for it. He knew that nothing is impossible and that there is always a way to modify and adapt things for success. He knew that he could help others and contribute to the world. Most of all, he learned that he was in charge of his own life.

LOU

When Alex was born, I suppose I was a typical new father in most respects. I didn't have a clear idea what fatherhood would be like. As far as I knew, dads were supposed to do

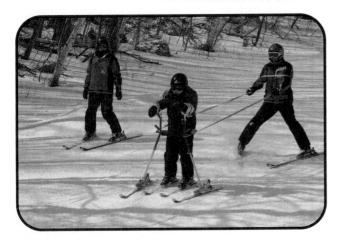

FIGURE 12.1   Alex skiing with the slider. (Photo courtesy of Maine Handicapped Skiing.)

what they were told by moms, who somehow "just knew" all about babies and young children. I was sure I would be informed of my role when it was time for me to know. My pictures certainly didn't include the possibility that my own child might be born with special needs. I thought I would be playing catch with my six-year-old in a few years and arguing about access to the car in another few years. I hoped I would be an adequate dad and not let my child down.

So the news that Alex had an abnormal ultrasound scan and probable brain damage was completely outside my experience. I had no idea what to do. I had expected to be less important than Mom, but now I was irrelevant. Mom was an occupational therapist and had professional knowledge about disability. I didn't. There wasn't much that I could contribute to the family except for diaper changes and a paycheck.

I remember feeling utterly marginalized almost from the beginning. Doctors and nurses would talk to Mom, not to me. Mom got the pamphlets and lectures about how to care for Alex. When I went to an appointment with Alex, I was always asked gently whether Mom was planning to arrive later, or . . . ? After all, it was Mom's job to take care of this child, to know about disability, to learn about social services, to make appointments, and to make the decisions about Alex's care. So I began to act the part: I spent less time with my family, had a few too many beers in the evening, and began to hear everything that was said to me as a reproof or insult.

In the years since that time, I have learned that my experience was typical. New dads of children with special needs discover immediately that the world of children's services is focused on the moms. That's unfortunate, because for our own mental health, let alone our ability to support our families emotionally and financially, dads need recognition that their role extends beyond "making sure Mom is listened to" and "pinch hitting." We need recognition that a "dad" is not merely an inferior form of a "mom." (Of course, since so many of the physicians are male, so many of those males are patronizing and condescending, and so many of them seem to know almost nothing about the experience of disability except for the medical part, moms get marginalized in their children's care too and have their own horror stories to share. But I'm telling the dads' story.)

On the other hand, this marginalization can also be very important in allowing dads to think independently about their children's disabilities. One of my memories is about Alex's first pediatrician, who loved babies. When Alex first came home from the hospital, the doctor proudly carried him out and paraded him around the waiting room, exclaiming how perfect he was. But as Alex grew older and his legs and arms didn't work quite the same way as other children's, the doctor seemed to become more and more reluctant to deal with him. He assured Mom and me that our child was "going to be fine! He'll be just fine, you'll see!" When Alex was a year old and unable to roll over, let alone crawl, the doctor warned us that we needed to make sure every part of the house was childproofed. When Alex was three, still unable to stand up without assistance and able to walk only a few steps on crutches, the doctor lectured us about making sure to hold his hand so that he wouldn't dash out into traffic. The doctor even counseled me, "as one dad to another," that I must "not give up hope" about my son.

At last, during an office visit when Alex was four years old, I suddenly realized what was going on. This doctor loved *perfect* babies, but he regarded my "imperfect" son as a failure—a baby he hadn't managed to rescue completely from the results of prematurity, a child he needed to *fix*. I lost my temper and told the doctor that *despite* an inability to run out in traffic, my child was *already* fine, *and* he had cerebral palsy; and that I did not need *hope*, I needed *routine medical advice*. Since Alex wasn't *broken* and didn't need to be *fixed*, I felt that it was time the doctor stopped giving me warnings about dire possibilities that weren't possibilities at all for Alex.

After that experience, I began to notice that the medical and therapeutic worlds have a "broken/fixed" paradigm: "This limb *doesn't work* and we must *restore it to health*." That's fine for rehabilitation situations, but it doesn't fit the facts when we're talking about a child or adult who is *already just fine* and whose legs or arms don't work. As a Dad, I certainly want advice and support on how to make my child's movements more functional, but please don't waste my spirit or his self-esteem by trying to tell me he's *broken*! I know better: He is *absolutely fine*, just the way he is.

Families of children with disabilities often claim that our stress levels and divorce rates are higher than those of typical families. The data I have seen tend to suggest, surprisingly, that we're wrong about the divorce rates, but there's no doubt that we're right about the stress levels. The early years of parenting children with disabilities are a very lonely and challenging time for both parents, and dads have very few role models and not much support. It is especially difficult for dads to admit their own weakness. We don't always know how to seek support appropriately, and sometimes our ways of asking are not very clear. Sometimes they're abrupt, and sometimes they're scary. The result is that we antagonize the people from whom we need the most understanding and support. Like many other dads, I slipped into marginalization and irrelevance during Alex's first years of life, and I was very lucky to escape from the trap. The experiences that rescued me were the opportunities I had to contribute in a special way to Alex's life. Those experiences are the most important things I have to share with you, because they transformed my life.

One day when Alex was about three years old, his mom and I had our usual fight in which she accused me (correctly) of avoiding the family and spending hour after hour "playing" in the workshop instead of "doing a fair share." At the end, she said something like this:

I know you're going to just run away again and hide out in that shop; so while you're there, if you actually want to be useful, you could prove it by building something for Alex to sit on. It needs to be some kind of a chair, with a foot rest ten inches below the seat, and a seat depth of eleven inches, and a seat back with a couple of corner pieces to pull his scapulas forward and break up the hyperextension pattern. Oh, yes, and it needs a pommel so he can't arch out of it—and it needs a seat belt—and it would be *really nice* if you could make it light enough so that I could pick it up and move it—you always overbuild everything.

These were fightin' words, but Mom had grown up in a woodshop and was entitled to her opinion even if I didn't agree with it.

So I went out to the workshop, in a very sour mood, and sawed and fitted and fastened for a couple of hours and built a little portable seat with all the dimensions she had given me. It not only was portable, but also could actually be taken apart, and all the loose pieces could be stowed away underneath the chair. I was quite proud of my invention, although of course I was absolutely sure it wouldn't be appreciated.

I brought this creation into the house, and Mom carefully put Alex in the chair and positioned him at the kitchen table with some paper and a couple of crayons. To my utter astonishment, Alex picked up one of the crayons and began to color and draw on his paper independently—skills I had never seen him use before. There must be something good about this "proper positioning" I had been hearing about! Suddenly, I realized that I had actually done something that was directly, obviously related to making Alex successful in overcoming some of the effects of his disability. Perhaps I wasn't as utterly useless as I had thought (Figure 12.2).

Of course, there is a limit to how many chairs a dad can build before he runs out of baby butts to park in them, so if that was to be my only dad skill, I was still quite a useless fellow. But it was a good start, and I was lucky enough to be able to keep going. Within the next few years, I became an advocate not only for my own family, but also for others in the early intervention world. I developed an electronic network for families of special-needs children; I became part of a national committee to oversee early-intervention services for young children across the country; and eventually, I became a professional special education advocate. I know I would not have had any of these experiences if it weren't for that little chair and for the opportunity I was given, as a dad, to contribute to my child's life.

Today, as an advocate, I see moms and dads playing the same stereotyped roles that Alex's mom and I played when he was small. Mom keeps the records, Mom deals with the school folks and the doctors, and Mom goes to the meetings. There is often a feeling that if Dad goes to a meeting, there must be something wrong. Even today, most of

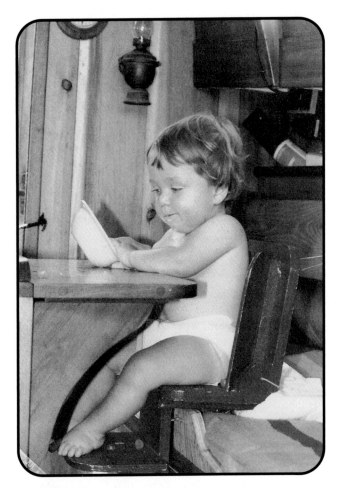

FIGURE 12.2   Alex sitting in his chair on the sailboat. (Photo courtesy of Laurie McIntosh.)

the people at educational team meetings are women, and Dad is not likely to feel welcome; in fact, he's often seen as a very scary person who doesn't understand how hard everyone is trying and who doesn't "know how to be reasonable." He is marginalized and excluded, sometimes kindly and sometimes out of fear and hostility, and Mom is left to deal with the child's disability without his assistance.

That is particularly unfortunate because we know from research that it is bad for the children. Longitudinal studies of children with disabilities have shown that family cohesion is one of the best predictors of good outcomes for children with disabilities (Hauser-Cram et al., 1999; Shonkoff & Philips, 2000). Any time we exclude dads from their children's lives or do anything to diminish dads' importance, we have a direct negative impact on those children's prospects for success in life.[1] If you care about the children, that is unacceptable.

---

[1] An excellent resource on father involvement is the Head Start Bureau's June 2004 Bulletin, *Father Involvement: Building Strong Programs for Strong Families,* available for download at http://www.headstartinfo.org/pdf/father_involvement.pdf.

At the same time, I have also learned to remember that Dad's job is to be a parent and Mom's job is also to be a parent. Neither Mom nor Dad needs to be a doctor, therapist, or teacher in order to have credibility. What we bring to the table as "mere parents" is sufficient, because we are the keepers of the dreams and visions for our children, and we will be their advocates and companions long after all their childhood caregivers and teachers have retired. Mom and Dad may *also* be professionals with titles and credentials and lots of education, but the most important hat we will ever wear is the Parent Hat.

ALEX

When I was about seven years old, I was firmly convinced that I was a werewolf. I had never actually undergone any physical transformation at the full of the moon, but seven-year-olds are not bothered by such trifles. The crowning touch was that my crutches acted as a second pair of legs, and although when wearing them I could never really manage a wolf-like lope, I made do instead with a sort of galloping skip. Nevertheless, it was fast enough (to me) to reinforce fantasies of running swiftly through the forest on silent paws, seeking unsuspecting prey.

The technical term for the condition of being a werewolf is *lycanthropy,* after the mythical Greek king Lycaon, whom the god Zeus transformed into a wolf as punishment for his tyranny. I knew the word at the age of seven, having read every book on werewolves that I could both find and understand. I was proud to declare myself a lycanthrope to everyone I met.

One day that year, my mother, my younger brother, and I attended a fund-raising boat race, the object of which was to allow wealthy yacht owners to raise money for the disabled. I was skipping around the lobby of the yacht club where the event was being held, giving long, mournful, ear-splitting howls, as a proper werewolf should. Mom was over in a corner with my brother, trying to pretend that I was someone else's child.

One of the yacht owners saw me, and she said, "Look at you, doing so well. What's your disability, honey?"

"I have lycanthropy!" I said, beaming.

A few minutes later, she was chatting with my mother and said, "I just met your son. What a nice boy. It's so sad that he has lycanthropy."

Mom smirked. "Um, I think there's something you should know . . ."

That is what happens to people who are lacking in disability awareness.

When I was about fifteen, I decided to try my hand at metalwork. My father has a workshop next to the house, and he found me the gloves, jacket, goggles, and apron necessary for working with heated metal. My primary objective during my first experiment was to make a three-inch-long model sword out of nails.

I learned how to manage a coal fire those first few days and, later, a propane blowtorch. I learned not to leave a nail in the fire for more than a minute or two for fear of burning the metal and that heat dissipates very quickly from a nail after it has been taken out of the fire. I also learned (the hard way) that just because a nail isn't glowing red anymore doesn't mean that it's not hot enough to burn flesh through a glove.

Because I had to strike the nail quickly while the heat was retained, there was a great deal of tension in my hands when I was hammering. My cerebral palsy kept the muscles in my hands rather tight to begin with. Try as I might, I couldn't strike the metal at the right angles to make an even, straight blade or hilt. The nails kept twisting into a corkscrew shape. What I ended up having to do was hammer out the rough shapes as best I could, quench them (dunk them in a bucket of water to cool them), take them out of the vice grips I held them in and clamp them in a vice, then use the vice grips to straighten the twisted parts (Figure 12.3).

Sometimes the twists were so subtle that I could barely see them. In these instances, I had to make very small, precise movements with my hands, which are difficult enough even for those who don't have cerebral palsy. I often didn't affect the metal at all, and I even more often overshot the mark and twisted it more than it had been originally. I am still learning this skill; I have a long way to go before I can correct subtle flaws in metal.

My father says that the minds of people who have learned to use tools and build things work in a fundamentally different way from other people's minds. Builders' minds have a better combination of practicality and creativity, and they are better able to analyze a problem and come up with a solution. As I become more involved in metalwork, I hope I begin to think this way as well (Figure 12.4).

I have been involved in the Maine Handicapped Skiing Program since I was six years old. During most of my

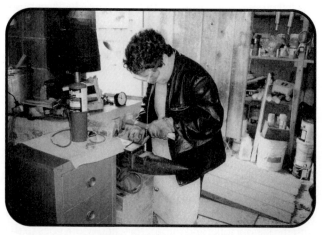

FIGURE 12.3 Alex engaged in metal working. (Photo courtesy of Laurie McIntosh.)

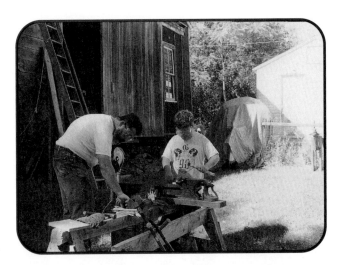

FIGURE 12.4 Alex and his dad doing metal work in the boatyard. (Photo courtesy of Laurie McIntosh.)

time there (twice-monthly lessons from January through March each year), I used normal skis combined with outriggers, devices that resemble crutches with skis attached. I used the same ground for each lesson: the end of a trail right outside the Maine Handicapped Skiing lodge.

I learned very quickly that there is nothing so apt to make one acutely aware of one's own body as the fear of crashing into something. I have learned to use this awareness to judge turns and to move my legs, skis, and outriggers in just the right way to make myself stop. However, in eleven of my twelve years of skiing, my ability to turn came and went.

When I used the outriggers, I had to put a great deal of weight on my arms to hold myself upright on the snow. This did not leave me free to put as much weight on my skis as I needed to turn at will and in the direction I chose. Therefore, my ability to turn on any given day depended largely on how willing I was to take the weight off my arms and, to my mind, increase the risk of falling.

This past year, I tried a new method, using skis and a device called a slider, patterned on the walkers used by the elderly. The slider acts as a support system for my upper body, leaving me free to shift the weight on my legs as needed. I am also tethered to one of my ski instructors, who helps me slow down on especially steep slopes.

With the help of the slider-and-tether system, I am able to travel farther on ski trails than I did in all my eleven previous years of skiing. I can maneuver through rough terrain. In consequence, I believe I am even more in control of my body.

In elementary school and high school, gym class was seldom a productive time for me. This fact hinged on my not being able to run. I used crutches rather than a wheelchair at school. Although the instructor sensibly assigned me the position of flag keeper in games of capture-the-flag, the members of the opposing team who ran past me were always just a little too far away for me to reach out and tag them, which was extremely frustrating. I must admit that sometimes my inability to tag people had more to do with my attention span than my disability.

There were instances in which my teachers came up with creative modifications to such activities, but these were so few and far between that I cannot now clearly recall them. Most of the time, my participation in such games consisted chiefly of my hopping around on my crutches while everyone else ran and making the motions of what the other students were doing. I probably looked ridiculous.

The exception was baseball. I never learned the rules of the game quite as well as my peers, but I could bat as well as anyone in my class. When it came time to run the bases, either I had someone else represent me or my opponent was required to hop on one foot to even the odds.

On the whole, I am glad I no longer have to take physical education courses.

I have recently enrolled at a state university, which is ten minutes away from my hometown. The process of moving in began with evaluating the accessibility of my dorm: the ease or difficulty of entering and moving around the rooms in an electric scooter and on foot and the accessibility of the bathrooms, laundry room, and lounge areas. Even though we went to the dorm in the summer to see how everything would work, it still took me a while to get used to the new routines once school actually started. I had to remember to grab my little bucket of bathroom supplies before heading down the hall to the bathroom. My schedule now had to include time to get to the dining hall for meals and time to do laundry on the weekends. In short, I had to plan ahead for almost everything.

One of the biggest challenges for me was learning to find my way around the campus. I think that my lack of mobility as a child kept me from learning some fundamental lessons about directions. When I was a young child, I was pushed long distances in a wheelchair, and the distances I walked were very short. I was never left on my own to find my way around because of safety issues. As a teenager, I would go for walks in my neighborhood, but it was a familiar area, and I usually just walked around the block.

The summer before I went to high school, my mother took me to the empty building to practice my routes at least three times before I felt secure. When I arrived on the university campus, I realized that I had a very poor aptitude for map reading. I had no idea how to get from one place to another by looking at a map. Even when I asked people for directions, I would often have to ask several other people along the way before I found my destination. Since I got my new three-wheeled electric scooter right before school started, I had not had much opportunity to practice driving it. I was not a car driver and had never had a power vehicle. Most of the time, I managed to get places without ruining too much sheetrock or crushing too many toes. Small elevators were a challenge, as was maneuvering in the crowded dining hall without knocking over piles of dishes and spilling drinks. The automatic doors for the buildings on campus usually worked, but there were always a few that were out of commission. Sometimes I would be lucky enough to find someone to hold the door for me, but I soon learned to hold the door open with one hand while driving the scooter through with the other. Since my door-holding hand is weak, I fear that I may have left some scratches on a few doors. The most difficult problem was parking on the shuttle buses. They were accessible and had lovely ramps, but once inside, I found myself required to parallel park in a specific and confined spot in order for my scooter to be properly tied down. I wished I had had scooter-driving lessons in high school.

My dorm is set up with automatic doors that have remote controls. Students with mobility problems are given small remote control units to attach to our key rings. It gives me such a great sense of power to approach the dorm door at full speed, push the little button and cruise right in without even stopping. Of course, I do this only when there is no one around to run over. Other students stand at the door and fumble for their identification cards in order to run them through the door-opening machine. Most of the other students don't know that I have this remote control device, so I can "magically" open the doors for attractive girls when I'm twenty feet away.

Given that I am late for class more often than I would like (because my morning routine always takes longer than I plan for), I often have to drive my scooter very quickly across the campus. This sometimes proves to be unsafe. At one point, I was racing toward the building in which my class was taking place, and my overfull backpack, hanging on the back of my scooter, caused the scooter to tip sideways. I crashed onto the concrete path, swearing inaudibly but profusely. Fortunately, the noise attracted the attention of two kindhearted passersby, who helped me to my feet and also laboriously got the scooter right side up again. Since that time, I have been more careful to carry less weight in my backpack and take the corners more slowly (Figure 12.5).

The university has been good about making sure that my classes are all held in wheelchair-accessible rooms. There is an access office that coordinates all the services and modifications for students with disabilities. They move classes to accessible rooms for specific students. The access office also coordinates student note takers so that students with disabilities can have other students take notes for them. The note takers never know which student in their class is receiving their notes. The note takers deliver the notes to the access office, and the notes are distributed to the students who need them. At this university, the accommodations that are listed on the student's high school Individual Education Plans or 504 plans are respected. For instance, in high school, I was allowed to have extra time to take tests, and I have the same accommodation at the university.

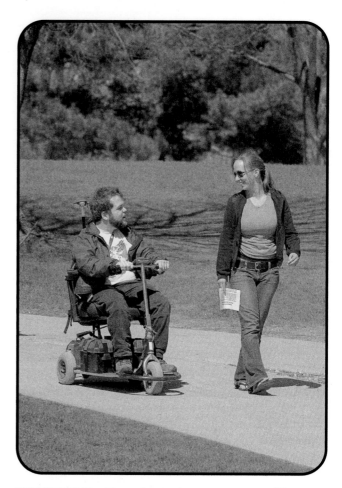

FIGURE 12.5   Alex going to classes on campus. (Photo courtesy of Lisa Nugent, Photographic Services, University of New Hampshire.)

As buildings on campus are renovated, they are made accessible. Unfortunately, the English Department building has not been renovated yet, and since I am majoring in English, this has presented some problems. The department offices, including my advisor's office, are up a flight of stairs. If I need to pick up forms or drop things off, I call on my cell phone, and someone comes downstairs. If I want to see my advisor I have to e-mail her to set up a specific appointment because I can't just show up during her office hours or drop by to see whether she's in. So far this system seems to work, although it is just one more way in which my life requires more planning.

The teachers and students on campus treat me just like any other student. It is obvious that this school is used to students with disabilities because the community is very accepting. I don't feel patronized or disrespected at all. My teachers expect the same work from me that they would get from someone else except that they are nice enough to give me more time to do it. There are a number of students with various disabilities on the campus, and we all just seem to fit in like anyone else.

CONCLUSION

Many people, including many new parents of children with disabilities, assume that a disability is like a shadow that hangs over a child's life, forever reminding him or her of things that cannot be done or achieved. As my behavior during the Lycanthropy Incident proved, I couldn't have cared less, as a child, about my disability in terms of what it prevented me from doing. I was just having fun and living my own life. I was able to do this freely because of what my parents learned, and taught to me, when I was growing up: *I am not broken; I don't need to be fixed.* Knowing this, I was, and am, able to choose who and what to be: werewolf, blacksmith, skier, college student, writer. The list is still being added to.

QUESTIONS FROM ALEX

1. What did you expect to find in this chapter? How did it meet, or differ from, your expectations?
2. Can you recall any instance in which the actions of someone with a disability contradicted your assumptions about how that person was going to behave?
3. List some common stereotypes about people with disabilities, and identify information in this chapter that negates those stereotypes.
4. Imagine for a moment that you have been in a horrible accident and your legs have had to be amputated. Brainstorm some modifications to your favorite (physical) recreational activity that will enable you to keep doing it.
5. Research currently available examples of what you came up with in Question 4. What are the similarities and differences between these and your own ideas? Have you come up with something that you think is innovative? If so, why are you still doing this exercise instead of promoting your idea?

QUESTIONS FROM LOU

1. To have a successful and fulfilling role in the life of a child with a disability, each family member needs to have the opportunity to contribute to that child's quality of life. Assigning "homework" is not the same thing and can be very damaging to the family. What is the difference? How can the occupational therapist's intervention support the creation of opportunities instead of the mere assignment of tasks?
2. What can an occupational therapist do to support family cohesion, and why is it important to the child?

3. In this chapter, Alex's father says that "Alex wasn't *broken* and didn't need to be *fixed*." How would you reconcile this perspective with the rehabilitation model of service? Can you reconcile it with the model of human occupation or another occupational therapy model? Why or why not?
4. Parents and siblings of a child with a disability often have no knowledge of occupational therapy and no understanding of why therapeutic interventions are necessary. Yet these "mere parents" bring a vital perspective to the planning process. What is that perspective, and how should the occupational therapist integrate that perspective into the child's treatment plan?

QUESTIONS FROM LAURIE

1. Learned dependence can be a more serious disability than cerebral palsy. People who never learn to be responsible for themselves might need assistance for the rest of their lives. How can occupational therapists prevent situations that lead to learned dependence?
2. We used household chores to give Alex a sense of responsibility and an important role in the family. What can occupational therapists do to help parents find useful roles for their children with disabilities?
3. We made sure that all the necessary modifications were in place for Alex to live in a dorm and attend classes at the university. Should some of this have been the responsibility of the high school occupational therapist as part of Alex's transition plan? Why or why not?
4. What was the difference in how Alex felt about himself in physical education classes versus handicapped skiing? How could his physical education classes been set up differently so that he felt better about himself?

QUESTIONS FROM THE EDITOR

1. This chapter presents three perspectives of Alex's life. How do these perspectives differ, and why is it important to have an appreciation of each perspective?

REFERENCES

Hauser-Cram, P., Warfield, M. E., Shonkoff, J. P., Krauss, M. W., Upshur, C. C., & Sayer, A. (1999). Family influences on adaptive development in young children with Down syndrome. *Child Development, 70,* 979–989.

Shonkoff, J. P., & Philips, D. A. (Eds.). (2000). *From neurons to neighborhoods: The science of early childhood development.* Washington, DC: National Academies Press.

While Focusing on Recovery I Forgot to Get a Life

13

GLORIA DICKERSON

Hello! My name is Gloria. I am a fifty-four year old Black woman living in Boston. Most of my life, I have meandered along within the bubble of mental health treatment under a variety of designated attributes of being ill. To date, my sole primary and trusted relationships have been with providers of health services. At age 15, I was introduced to the mental health system as a patient. Now I look back and revisit my journey through a life of treatment in the light of today. From this vantage point, my life seems to have been an initiation into the land of never good enough, never quite arrived, filled with cyclical pain-filled struggles and some rays of sun. My birth seems to have hurled me into a predesignated life sentence of less than and a never-ending journey of repetitive bouts of trying to rise.

I have endured a life of injustice and mistreatment that was made bearable by my religious upbringing and years of therapy. My religious upbringing was both extremely painful and exquisitely inspiring. The deep, profound hope that is imbedded in the words and concepts of the Black Church and Bible gave me a foundation of hope that serves as a compass and, although sorely tested, has never been destroyed. The idea that we are all connected, obligated, and encompassed in a mission greater than each of us gives my life purpose and meaning. I have tried to turn away from my faith and connectedness many times, but life always brought me back to center.

In addition to religion, therapy is a primary source for hope in the goodness of people, for staying alive, and for trying to find a way to live well. The expert help of my therapist has helped to reduce the effects of parental mistreatment, torture, and sexual and physical abuse. Effective therapy is only as good as the quality of the relationship between the therapist and the consumer, paired with a "goodness of fit" between the need of the consumer and the specific therapeutic tools utilized. My therapy was effective or "good" only when there was collaboration between my therapist and myself. My most effective therapist knew the difference between her intention to help and my perception of being helped. She understood that my perception of being helped is a subjective state of feeling helped that can be discerned only by me.

126

My therapist is extremely respectful. She knows that any attempts to help me must be based on my stated wishes, desires, and needs. She allows me to choose, to take risks, and sometimes even to fail. The intention to "help," "being helpful," or "giving help" is only one part of the helping process. The "end" of the helping process is achieved when the person being helped feels "helped." The ability to make choices has been critical to my relearning skills of self-reliance and safety when engaging with others. Engagement and building trust have always been elusive concepts. For me, trusting a therapist begins for me with warm greetings, kindness, and acknowledgment of my rights as an adult. I can endure conflicts, misgivings, errors, hurts, and slights if I feel connected and valued as an adult.

There are some basic and essential qualities of all effective therapists regardless of theoretical orientation. Therapists must like people, access the ability to personally censor, be curious, respect difference, create a repertoire of skills, and have the ability to maintain commitment over time. Therapists must learn to acknowledge personal biases, avoid harm, and use their personal self knowledge to educate for change. Skilled therapists use all of their knowledge, skills, and personal gifts and deficits gleaned from their own life journey and operate from the position of being a change agent and healer. It is not enough to be correct theoretically. Therapists must be skilled human beings who care about and like others. The therapists I love have all these qualities. My therapy, though freeing, was very concentrated and focused. Unfortunately for me, all of us forgot one little thing: a therapeutic relationship is an assist to learning to establish other relationships that become a source of primary sustenance. Therapeutic relationships should never become a substitute for intimate, loving family and friends.

Life is bigger than the therapy relationship. Stabilization and maintenance are great goals to awaken hurt souls. However, once an individual grasps and mourns the losses and pain that brought her or him into therapy, then what? We need to remember that the primary pain associated with having severe mental illness and trauma often comes out of failed and abusive relationships. My primary "disconnect" emerged over time. Like a stealth bomber, silent at first, it soared in the night and then swooped down, blowing my insides into shards, simply changing the course of my life forever

My first years in the South as a young girl were riddled with incidents of trauma. I consider myself to be a Southerner because, up to the age of 5, my ancestral roots, my psyche and consciousness spring from events that occurred within a small town in Alabama. The family relationships and life in this small town caused essential disconnections within myself, with others, and with the world. My experiences include parental abuse resulting in the birth of my daughter, long inpatient stays in mental hospitals, graduation from college, more hospital-

izations, suicide attempts, five different postcollege graduate programs, work throughout the human services field, and 39 years of therapy. These are only a few of the most influential and important experiences that dot the course of my life.

In this writing, I am going to tell you about who I am and where I have been. I will attempt to explain how I learned who I was and how this has affected every aspect of my being, from my excess weight to my choices of occupations and even to my dress. My present gifts and my abilities, my pain and my hope, as well as my deficits and despair, can be traced back to events during the first few years of my life. As with everyone on the planet, every event and experience, good or bad, has shaped me and culminated in making me the person that I am. After learning the facts of my life, people who have come to know me are surprised and astonished that I have survived with my intellect and hope intact. After hearing what I have lived through, most people react with jaw-dropping awareness and awe and silence. As people get to know me, they recognize that my life has been filled with extreme horror and that my endurance and survival are amazing.

I begin with accounts of memories about my family of origin and my early years. For years, I was the only girl child of my parents. My daddy (James) was born in 1925. My ma (Stella) was born in 1927. My brother Andrew is one year older and was born in 1949. I was the oldest girl and was born in 1951. My brother Roger was born 11 months later, in 1952. We often joked that this close proximity in our birth made us almost twins. We have always felt closest to each other. My brother Junior was born in July 1953, and he was the baby for many years. My brother Donnie was born in 1955. He died tragically and suddenly, and his existence has been erased from all family accounts. My sister Daisy was born in 1958. Her birth was my dream come true. I always thought she was a personal gift from God. Her choice to become and to remain estranged from me has been one of the greatest losses of my life. My brother George was born in 1962. Amazingly, he still fails to be recognized as a valued and independent person by my family system. My brother David was born in 1967. Although he is nearly 40, his life continues to affirm his status as my mom's "baby." As a Black man with untreated dyslexia, he makes do and escapes all aspects of being an adult, except procreation, and he lives without income on his relationships with others.

As for most of our neighbors, Black and White, life in the South meant Sundays in church, life as a sharecropper, and extremes of joy, violence, calmness, and pain. The residues of lives touched by violent, chaotic nights and the hard-fought-for appearance of calm, peaceful days set the stage for a culture of fear. The minister was pivotal in helping individuals caught in the maze of violence find meaning and maintain hope necessary for endurance. There are at least two types of ministers. Some ministers believe in, are motivated by, and love

"God" and all the things that a good "God" stands for. A minister operating from powerful needs to nurture "a loving and hopeful life-affirming world" will make mistakes, but her or his intention is to promote relationships between people that rest on ideals of love and hope. The conscious actions of a good minister start from deep-seated basic beliefs such as "Love your neighbor as you would yourself" and "Do no intentional harm." Other ministers beam out their fears of confronting feelings and thoughts that they deem evil and project negative intentions and motivations onto others. My grandfather was the second type: a fire-and-brimstone type minister. He could not have designed a better-suited context (the ministry) in which he could hide and insinuate his personal brand of fear and pain. Under the cover of the prevailing myths of goodness, high praise, and quality attributes of a "Minister," he operated unquestioned. He could do no wrong. His motives were never questioned. His actions were revered. His destruction is immeasurable.

My mother's and my father's children can be understood by looking at my parents' life context. Knowing how we learned to be the people we are is not an excuse for our failures and our deficits. It teaches us how to make meaning and find understanding. The meanings we make tell us how to understand our "self," others, and our relationships in the world. This is the foundation from which we begin to act or not act, choose or not choose, know or not know. We learn what it is to be a human being early. We learn about relationships from those around us. We learn what is important, what our value is, and what is right and what is wrong from our early relationships. They form the lens through which we see and know everything. What follows are some of the experiences that make up my lens. This is my beginning.

My mother was 23 years old and my father 25 years old when I was born. My mother tells a story about my birth and early days of life that has been critical to forming my vision of myself, my character, and my strength that has at different times both supported and diminished my assessment of my worth in my own eyes. I have heard this story since . . . well . . . the beginning. She said,

> When you were born, you weighed 4 pounds and 10 ounces. Your father came to see you. He said you were so small that he was scared to hold you. When he first saw you he looked at you and said, "God, she's so hairy and looks just like a little rat." And while you were in the hospital you lost down to three pounds. Everyone thought you were going to die. You stayed in the hospital for one month in a makeshift incubator. Dr. Everage was so good. He made an incubator from odds and ends and pumped oxygen into it to keep you alive. But you were not gaining weight so they sent you home. I think they thought you were going to die. I was so scared and I put you in a dresser drawer with a hot water bottle. I had to stay up all night with you and

> I kept pinching you to make you cry because I was so afraid you were going to die. I had to struggle and work so hard to keep you alive. You put me through so much.

My mother has reminded me of this story periodically and with precision throughout my life, reiterating the fact that my father thought I looked like a rat and keeping the wounds of this image alive and potent. Her pronouncements of her great sacrifice and the extreme imposition and burden of my birth have weighed heavily and occasionally tipped the scales in favor of trying to secure my early demise through serious suicide attempts. Often, to make a point during times I "got too big for my britches" or became "too full of myself" by thinking that I was smart or worthy of high praise or love, she would remind me of my botched entrance into the world, reducing me to the reality of her perception that I was "filthy and less than dirt." Her spiel often concluded with pronouncements that the debt I owed her could never be repaid and I was lucky to be alive. The picture my mother painted about how she and my father greeted me and her feelings about me combine with the full weight of subsequent events leave me with profound feelings of guilt and terror and periods of dissociated pain and thoughts that plunged me into depths of despair and my own personal brand of hell all my life.

My mother's family worked as sharecroppers on a farm in Alabama in 1954. My grandfathers on both sides of the family were ministers. As a minister's family, we had some social status among other poor Black families in the area. Yet my grandmother's predicament seemed to be no different from that of other Black women in the area. Most of the women of the South lived as silent subjects in the land of domineering husbands. But Black women that I grew up with had the additional burden of being alternately longed for, sexually desired, while at the same time their essence as beings was despised, sometimes by their husbands and most of the time by all men and women within this slice of society. I learned at a very early age that a woman's safety depended on the repertoire of defensive maneuvers of women and on the emotional state, whims, and actions of men. Unfortunately for my mom, she grew up with men who became enraged and physically abusive to any woman who dared think and act as if she was as intelligent and entitled to rights as any other human being, particularly a man. My mom tells stories that show her radical insistence on saying what she wanted, when she wanted, relentlessly voicing her opinions and naming what was unacceptable. To my great despair, her tales of bravery often concluded with epic depictions of her getting "beat down to the ground." Yet to my amazement, she took great delight in the struggle—in the standing up. The defeat seemed to be incidental. The pride she beamed out every time she tossed her head back and recounted her defiance, blow after blow, left its mark on my heart and mind. I resonate with her physical strength and resilience but mostly with her pride of being defiant. This defying of "the beat down" reminds me that I come from a long line of survivors. The need to fight injustice has often thrilled me, motivated me. Overall, my mother's life taught her that she was inferior. She learned that her pain and terror were caused because she was Black and a female. Depending on the context, her Blackness or her womanhood or both got her mercilessly victimized. She had to endure, cajole her way out of, and fight against rape and verbal and physical assault from early childhood by her father, brother, and other male relatives. Later, as a woman, she entered the world of having to fight off White men in the households where she worked. These are the things that infiltrated my mother's heart, made my mother who she was, and caused her to hate that which came from her: her first-born girl.

It is as if every time my mother looked at me, she saw a girl with all the qualities and characteristics that she imagined that every person saw that led them to hurt and hate her. My face was a mirror. She looked into my face at one week, at one year, and for the rest of my life, and she could only see the vile, filthy little girl that got her beat and brutalized and kept her from the life she wanted. I have always felt hated by my mother. I could see that when she looked at me, she felt tremendous hatred and rage. There was no escaping the consequence of my meaning for her. I was everything that she thought others saw that made them hurt her. And I was gonna pay!

The life context in which my family lived overwhelmed their human potential and capacity for being hopeful. In this context, their actions can be understood, though it can never be a justification. The context shows how I learned to make meanings that sustain my life throughout recovery from devastating and unimaginably hurtful events in my life.

The phrase *keeping time in chaos* adequately describes my life during and for years after the emergence of my mental illness. My first five years of daily life in the South contained moments of exquisite pleasure, of running through the fields, pulling up peanuts when I wanted, and finding buried treasure by digging deep in the ground and pulling up unsuspecting sweet potatoes or carrots. Sitting by the water at one of the only swimming and fishing areas near our house, I often watched ants. My eyes went back and forth as I followed them as they went scurrying. I remembered wondering what could they possibly be thinking about.

I have always settled for the basic tenets of life, making lemonade out of lemons. Knowing that I missed out on love from a family and from friends, I lacked a viable self that is based on knowing that one is safe and loved. I am left knowing that I substituted therapy for a life and therapeutic relationships for love. My having a mental illness, PTSD and depression, could not have been avoided. Life circumstances and early relationships made this inevitable. I was lucky and unlucky—lucky because I got mental health treatment. I was unlucky because my disorders are PTSD and dissociative identity disorder (DID). The emergence of DID was a lifesaving technique. I learned that I could live through overwhelming experiences by "turning around inside myself," and soon I had a host of friends and loved ones of my own creations. Having DID allowed me to compartmentalize my life—the tasks, developmental stages, reactions, feelings, thoughts, and reality. I learned to put away what I could not deal with so that I could get through the day and keep functioning with a modicum of sanity. DID, my prize possession, was a great skill. I could, in my mind, change myself to fit any situation, provide for other people's needs, avoid threats, and as for the chameleon, change was a great tool for functioning.

This survival technique, like all maneuvers to change reality, became a doubled-edged sword. The downside of dissociation, like all actions to change internal states by various techniques of avoidance, was that it took on a life of its own. My "functioning" was based on "magical thinking" and the appearance of functioning well. Changing my state by magical thinking replaces my adult consciousness with a child's-eye view, a child's reactions and a child's feelings, which are out of place. Yesterday's solution is a barrier now. Along with magical shifts in my consciousness come the pain and horror images, thoughts and feelings, and my deep immersion in "memory hell." Being in memory hell is like being locked in a closet full of feelings and thought patterns from the most torturous times in my life. Themes of abandonment, terrors, humiliations, pain-filled body states, and loss fill my vision and cloud my judgment. I walk through life in a 54-year-old body pretending— pretending so well that even I am not aware of the incongruence between being 54 and acting like I am 5 years old.

As a young adult, I had only a few vague recollections about my past. I never knew when or how my dissociation began. Even a month ago, I did not understand the implication of my trauma reaction and how it affected my perceptions, thoughts, feelings, and daily life. I have great shame and humiliation about being in a 54-year-old body with no ability to monitor elapses in time and no way to place things in chronological order. When asked to remember when an event occurred, confusion and embarrassment erupt, and I usually respond by saying, "Well, I believe it was a couple of weeks ago." Often, I wake up to find that I have been able to justify using an abusive tone and questioning of my allies' commitment, integrity, and moral stance because I was triggered.

The ability to divide my consciousness and convince myself that the shift is real began early in my life. I remember witnessing my brother getting shot by my mother. Later, I saw the rape and brutal murder of my best friend. I experienced sexual abuse and torture at the hands of my mother and father. I witnessed the lynching of my uncle. This all occurred before I turned 6 years old. After my baby brother was killed, before my friend died, and before my uncle was killed, my family left our home in Birmingham.

We went to live in my grandfather's home in Alabama. I believe my family was running away from questions about the death of my baby brother.

Life had started over. My brothers, my parents, and I never mentioned the name or existence of my brother again. I became best friends with a little white girl, named Paula. We both knew that we could never be seen together. One day, we were playing in the barn, and Paula, my best friend in the world, was killed. Her slaying was brutal, and today my mother's words still haunt me: "See what happens to your friends." I have come to believe that her death occurred because she was White and a needed target for sexual abuse. After Paula was killed, one night while sleeping, I was awakened by yelling and loud bangs on the door. My family was hauled out into the dark and beaten. I was raped before my family. My uncle was tortured and lynched and eviscerated. My heart was broken as a child. As an adult, I get to relive every gut-wrenching episode, try to metabolize that pain, and free myself from the memory by knowing what it was like through the repetition compulsion and then the frantic attempts to undo that come with hypervigilance.

I believe that the level of trauma my parents experienced and their demoralization are directly responsible for the abuse they heaped on my siblings, on me, and on others in their world. My father and mother gave words to high spiritual values and had a core work ethic that informed them. My father worked in construction, and my mother worked as a presser in a laundry and, in her later life, as a home health aide. My mother demonstrated that maintaining your life is the prime task of life. I am a survivor, and I come from a long line of survivors. We survived physically—some of us with hope and love intact but most often not. Like other victims of racism and genocide, I believed that traumatic and abusive relationships were the only model of how to live. Racism and postslavery oppression created a caustic environment, showing my parents that hope for a better future and rights of Americans to full citizenship seemed bound to remain a theoretical illusion simply because of the color of their skin. The illusion of freedom and acceptance of all within society made the reality all the harder to bear. Like a knife twisting and distorting their soul, words of freedom, equality, and acceptance remained great high-sounding values that never seemed to make their way into their lives.

I came to Boston when I was approaching my sixth birthday, leaving behind my maternal stepgrandmother. On arriving in Boston, I became more immersed in living in my head, because I believed that my stepgrandmother was all that stood between my death and me. When I entered school, I lost all hope of being safe in the world. School was terrifying because I was never allowed to be around White people in the South, especially after the murder of my best friend on the farm where my grandfather was a sharecropper. Terror interfered with my functioning as I entered school and I saw my teachers and met the principal. They were all White people, and all the kids were Black.

I was basically nonverbal but had a great imagination. Living in my head created an oasis from chaos, terror, and pain created by adults who were sexually abusive and often enraged for reasons that I could not understand. During September of that year, I heard my birth name, "Gloria," for the first time when my mother took me to kindergarten. On entering kindergarten, I already knew how to write my name. My older brother taught me how to make letters and write my name. He was teaching me that the letters meant something. He would say, "Now Fay," because they all called me "Fay," "make a straight line down, like a pole. Now, make a line on the top of the pole like a hat. That is how you make a 'T.'" I learned to hate messing up because my brother was good at everything. My mother loved everything he did. My father liked what he did. My grandparents thought he was so smart. He was everything to all of them. After all, he was lucky. He was a boy. The difference between how my mother looked at him and how she looked at me made me work harder to overcome my primordial defect of being a girl. So I learned I would have to work extra hard to be liked, to become, to finally deserve to be alive. My prized secrets were that I really was better than my brother and that I could do anything as well as my older brother and any boy or man. This notion that I was deemed inferior by all those I loved was critical to my development. I have lived a life of striving and overcoming. I was going to show everyone that I was as good as a boy. Anyone who stated or indicated in any way that I was inferior to a boy because of my gender could count on my angry protestation. Any authority figure making such accusations could count on my secret retribution for what I felt was a most heinous assault against my very being. I tried to do everything that a boy could do. I rebelled against my lot in life because of the unalterable fact that I happened to be a girl.

As the teacher discovered my skills, she made a decision, and I was placed in first grade. Then the tide turned. The teacher's enthrallment with my gifts was short-lived, and I was demoted and returned to kindergarten. This event precipitated seeds of doubt about my intelligence that has followed me all my life. It is not every child who can say she or he was demoted in first grade. My teacher's explanation was that I was extremely "immature." My persistent hysterical crying, flailing about, and screams for my mother led them to conclude that I was very babyish. This first entry into school began to show that my sorrow and pain were deeply entrenched.

When I was 15, my mother and father fought over money, accusations of extramarital affairs, infidelity, and alcohol-related distress. They also fought over my father's excessive attention and sexual abuse of me. I had been an A student, and up until age 15, I had found school to be a sanctuary. At 15, I became terrified of school. I slept little. During the night, I would literally run out of my house to

Boston City Hospital. I would sit in the lounge area with sick people who were waiting to see a doctor. I only went to the hospital because I was aware that as a young girl on the streets of Boston, I was still unprotected prey. Every night for months, I ran away after becoming frightened while trying to sleep. Each night, I envisioned that as soon as I fell asleep, a man would come and stand over me. He would wait until my sleep was deep, and when terror peaked and fear of surprise imminent, I knew he would spring upon me. I knew as sure as I can see the words on this page that he would end my life in torturous ways. It became safer to stay up all night in the emergency room. I slept during the day. I missed a lot of school. I was able to forge notes from my mom and escaped consequences of unexcused absences for almost a year. My physical and emotional state became unmanageable and my distress apparent. I cried for days. I felt so alone, trapped, and abandoned. There was no one I could tell without getting into trouble. I went to school one day and collapsed on the gym floor. I had a miscarriage. My friend Wanda recently told me that I was curled up in a ball on the floor. I was whispering to her, "Wanda, please don't let them come and get me . . . please . . . please!" She cites this as my introduction to the mental health system. All I know is that in 1966, at age 15, I had my first visit with a psychiatrist.

The psychiatrist was a woman who came from another country. She had a heavy accent. I was too shy to tell her that often I did not understand a word she was saying. I wanted to trust her. I immediately acted as if she loved and cared about me even though I did not really know. I was starved for affection and love. I was so lonely I could die. I wanted someone to trust and love so much that any semblance of trustworthiness and any inquiry into what I wanted passed for love and caring. Simple courtesy and proximity with another human being who asked me questions were soothing. These simple acts of kindness and professionalism were the salve and balm that soothed my wounds emanating from torture, abandonment, and neglect. I learned to glean hope and security from her gestures, pseudo-trust, and questions that I thought were enough for me to prove that she loved me. The professionals became surrogate family with all the attending loyalties and conflicts, and later therapeutic relationships were enough.

At age 16, I entered a public psychiatric institution and started on my path of receiving professional services in lieu of mutual loving nurturing relationships, with the goal of reducing pain and fear. I was terrified on entering Boston State Hospital, but from the first moment that adults asked me what I thought, what had hurt me, and what I needed, I was hooked on treatment. The focus was on me, and people said they wanted to help me feel better. I have stayed in mental health treatment for 39 years because I settled for the promise of caring. Professional caring was, and still is, the only caring that has felt safe enough for me to allow in my life. This is the only caring that I felt I could get.

My treatment for symptoms of mental illness has been successful in that it allowed me to go to Tufts University and learn from five graduate programs, even though I have not completed a master's degree. I have been able to work and live on the periphery of life, settling for the love of my therapist and an apartment, and substituting work and getting well for getting a life. If appearance was the test of having fully recovered, I often passed with flying colors. As for most of us with a mental illness, recovery is full of relapses and recurrences of illness. The journey of recovery is full of moratoriums and plateaus in between mountains and valleys. The journey becomes less tumultuous for most, but eruptions of symptoms can never be ruled out. Life with mental illness is precarious and a terrible predicament in which to find oneself.

Think of what I have told you about my early life: the accounts of witnessing the death of my brother before age 6, the murder and rape of my best friend, the sexual abuse and torture I experienced, and the lynching of my uncle. Some doctors find my statements unbelievable and preposterous. One doctor even chided me saying, "Now Gloria, think about what you are saying. Don't you believe that the police would have intervened?" I would laugh except I know that his thinking is caused by the fact that most people have forgotten what life was like for Black people in 1955. This lack of historical knowledge, paired with a pervasive need to "not know" the pain of racism and family dysfunction, is extremely prevalent in our society. It always feels like a personal affront when helpers replace my real-life experiences with their theories of what "really" went on. This not being believed simply because what happened to me is out of the experience of my professional friends continually causes me the most pain in my life. The questioning of the truth of my experience occurs because my professional friends believe in the severity of the impact of my trauma and because their training requires them to dissect every statement I make in an attempt to find the errors in my thinking and judgment. This sophisticated way of "nulling and voiding" my experience and replacing it with theoretical guessing is really based only on the fantasy in their heads. These interactions always leave me feeling isolated, discriminated against, and demoralized, leaving me hopeless to ever gain credibility when my life experience is diminished because it is so radically different from that of most people.

I realize that once I entered into the contract of therapy and treatment, like a binding contract with the devil—it is perpetual, and its course is certain. It is rare that anyone who enters mental health treatment will ever escape or ever lose the devastating moniker and attributes associated with the status of being a "mental patient." After years of faithful immersion in and commitment to therapeutic treatment, I find myself left feeling tricked, deceived, and abandoned. I believe these feelings are primarily the result of my feelings of being hurt by powerful administrators within the mental health system and worsened when my brother Junior, at age 46, died unnecessarily because of the negligence of staff within a vendor agency of the mental health system.

My interface with medical health providers has added an additional burden to my recovery. I am older and require medical care from doctors who stigmatize and humiliate me because I have been diagnosed as "mentally ill," then react with anger, hostility, and retribution to my complaints about their hurtful behavior. My other professional helpers have not responded to my pleas to help me access basic rights to humane and decent treatment in medical settings. All these factors culminate in leaving me with profound feelings of despair. I missed out on structuring a life that supports and sustains me after the nine-to-five professional friends go home. My previous therapists all said that my past traumas were too devastating for me ever to marry. Therapy and the psychiatric hospitals have created a cocoon that kept me in isolation, with a fear of living. The stigma of being an older mental patient now fills me with sadness.

My lot in America meant that my life was going to be difficult. The additional burden of abuse, 39 years of mental health treatment, and an active, curious, and generally very fine mind left me disillusioned. With the awareness of what could have been, my losses test my resilience, hope, and faith. I now exist without my many disguises, my alternate selves, and without the benefit of a loving support system. This life of having to make lemonade out of lemons created habitual responses of resilience that now keep me on the planet, however unhappy and striving for better. My personal existential crisis is how do I endure, do no harm, and wait—after all I have been through? I still have hope in the goodness of people.

At Boston University Center for Psychiatric Rehabilitation Center, I met people who happened to be professionals. They were outrageously radical professionals. Their theories of how to help were not based on seeking out what is wrong with me. They did not think that it was impossible that I was their equal. They did not label me defective or tell me how was sick I was. They spoke of my having options and a valued role in life. They told me that my inability to succeed was caused by barriers. They had requirements and expectations. They made plans based on my needs, wants, and preferences, requiring me to make choices. They believed that I would achieve and grow. They inspired me and sided with my resilience, leaving me feeling energized, ready to act in my own behalf, and hopeful for a better outcome. Dr. Spaniol mentored me and gave me a valued role facilitating recovery groups and cofacilitating statewide workshops. He provided knowledge and

skills to increase my competence, and pairing this with doable expectations, he increased my overall life functioning and satisfaction exponentially. I now have a newly found identity of educator. This was a dream of mine when as a little girl, I played school with my childhood friends. These experiences allowed me a glimpse into the land of being accepted and well respected. And now, I am forever changed, and giving up is simply harder because of them. Their use of the universal concept that difficulties are caused by barriers took me out of the land of a defective human being failing to function and placed me squarely back in the land of human beings striving to overcome environmental obstacles without judgments about my intellect, character, or motivation. I was on an equal playing field with all others. I was a person who needed help, knowledge, skills, and support. I am not an inferior being treated by superiors. Many of the conflicts and power struggles embedded in traditional therapy are no longer an issue. This subtle and exquisite shift in perspective allows practitioners to have a better chance of greeting a real live person rather than a collection of symptoms.

I am an equal partner with responsibilities to participate to ensure a good outcome. As a partner with the practitioner, I do not sit passively by, awaiting my rescue. The knowledge that my counselors at Boston University cared created a feeling in me that their theories about me, their interventions, and the specific treatment outcomes were never as healing as their personhood, their stated desire and intention. Without their genuine curiosity that allowed them to listen, their respect that kept them from judging, and the high regard for my individualism that allowed them to tolerate me being me, I could not have withstood facing my woundedness and despair. The words "I don't always know how to help but I really want to help you" feel like balm on an open sore and soothe me in ways that I can only approximate by saying, "It healed my soul." This is one of the many supreme gifts of human connection that I have found only in my relationship with my therapist and my counselors at Boston University.

I have had a lot of experiences that showed me how to "make meaning" and transform injury and devastation into hopeful scenarios. Routinely affirming hopefulness and habitually responding to devastation with resilience are skills that helped me to transform evil and rise from the ashes. "The phoenix rising" is my life metaphor. As life plunges me into the depths of despair, I look inside and find a light of hope to try and live well. I have repeatedly risen from the ashes, and with my faith intact, I can envision no other response.

The Privilege of Giving Care

14

DONALD M. MURRAY

"**I** don't know who he is, but every morning and afternoon, a man comes to see me and he is awfully nice." The woman who said those words was Minnie Mae, my wife of 54 years, and I have lived by those words in the months ever since she broke through her dementia on a Friday afternoon and told the hospice nurse, "No more water. No food. No pills."

Fourteen years earlier, when she was 72, she was given her annual physical. There seemed to be none of the surprises during this exam that had tested Minnie Mae's courage, sense of humor, and ability to survive pain in the past. The doctor's calm and professional "hum's, uh-huh's, mmm's" during the exam reassured us. The doctor studied the lab reports—another comforting "mmm"—and, smiling, our doctor went to the examining room door, turned and told my wife, "You have Parkinson's," stepped out into the corridor, and shut the door behind him.

This not a story of "the elderly" and the global difficulties and pleasures of old age. I have no theories. No statistics. I have not read books, studies, or journal articles on aging. This is simply an account of the final intimacy and love of one couple facing the challenge of Parkinson's, a long-lasting fatal disease for which there is no cure. Like so many of us in our eighties, Minnie Mae was an experienced patient. Before this last illness, she had suffered life-threatening toxemia with our first child, an appendix attack with three separate infections, an emergency hysterectomy, nine—I believe—eye operations, and skin and breast cancer.

We didn't really know what Parkinson's was, but we knew that it wasn't good. There seem to be two types of elderly patients: those who worry and predict and research about what might happen and those like us who simply face each "surprise" with as much acceptance, courage, and toughness as we can summon. We take life a step at a time. Now we had a new challenge: Parkinson's.

We drove immediately to my cardiologist, who referred us to a neurologist. That didn't help as much as we hoped. We wanted to learn how to treat Parkinson's, how it might evolve, how it would affect our daily lives and our future. Instead of answers, we ran into the sort of professional terminology debate that interests doctors but not us.

Our neurologist carried on a debate with himself in front of us. Minnie Mae might have "Parkinsonism," or she might have Parkinson's itself. It was never clear what the difference was and how it might affect Minnie Mae's life. Would Parkinson's or Parkinsonism move toward death at a different speed? We were never able to understand the difference, except we were told that a blood pressure drug Minnie Mae had previously used was associated with "Parkinsonism" or "Parkinson's" in about 25% of the patient's who were prescribed that medication. Minnie Mae (a direct person who like direct answers) asked, "What caused my Parkinsonism or Parkinson's, or whatever it is?" The doctor answered, "I'll know when I slice your brain."

Looking back, we seemed remarkably innocent and calm. The unspoken medical message was that aging is tough, but so were we (Figure 14.1).

Wet your pants?

"I have many older patients who have that problem."

Tremor getting worse?

"As you age, you'll have doctors' penmanship."

Stagger?

"That happens. My father was a minister, but when he grew old, he walked like he had two too many."

Bent neck?

"Arthritis. It comes with age."

The neurologist prescribed Sinemet. Minnie Mae took it at lunch and felt better within the hour. The specialist may have been a cold fish, but there was a pill for whatever she had. Our personalities, our genes, and our personal experience with death and illness had taught us not to seek problems. Trouble would come in its time, and we would face it head on. I think this pragmatic stoicism is typical of our Depression and World War II generation, but I also believe that many of my generation develop a passive fatalism together with the belief that the more challenges they face and survive, the stronger they become. There may be something to this. We were stoics, steeling ourselves to confront medical problems and do what was necessary to deal with them. We were not happy with our neurologist's personality, but the pills worked. He must know something even if he didn't know how to relate to his patients. Then he planned, since Minnie Mae was doing so well, to prescribe a new, more powerful drug.

At that moment, we experienced a fortunate coincidence. I was invited to speak at Beth Israel Hospital in

Boston because of my *Boston Globe* column on aging. After I spoke, a reader talked to me about the column and mentioned that she was a neurologist. I asked what doctor she would recommend to a member of her family with Parkinson's, and she referred us to a kind doctor who has been called the best neurologist in Boston. He was a listener and an explainer who told us they had tested the new drug our neurologist planned to give Minnie Mae and that it would have irrevocably damaged her brain. We remained his patient until Minnie Mae could no longer make the trip from New Hampshire to Beth Israel.

When we asked him about the future—we prided ourselves on being realists—he explained that each case was so different that there was no way to predict the future. Furthermore, he told us that there was only "treatment." We did not shy away from his diagnosis, ask God why me, search the Internet for miracles, or join one of the therapy groups that help so many. We just did what had to be done hour by hour. I learned new skills, knowing that new demands would be made on those skills in the years ahead.

We learned that the most efficient way to help Minnie Mae up after a fall was to have me plant my size 15 feet on hers to keep her feet from skidding away, then, taking her hands in mine, lift trying to keep the pressure on each equal. Sometimes it took many attempts to get Minnie Mae on her feet. She used her favorite curse, "Shit fire and save matches," and many times we sat on the floor laughing at our clumsy failures. And when we couldn't get her up, we called for help from a young neighbor.

We survived by our own black humor. "You used to struggle getting my bra off, now you have trouble getting it on." We continued to go out to eat as long as it was possible. We liked The Olive Garden with its sliding chairs. One day, driving to the restaurant, Minnie Mae said, "We should bring a bottle of wine." As she traveled further and further into the confusion of dementia, she kept her humor and I kept mine. She was never a "patient" but the woman I loved.

As the disease inevitably grew worse, we realized that our geography had changed. We avoided stairs without railings, sloping sidewalks, uneven surfaces of grass and sand, and wind that could push Minnie Mae sideways. I still tell people I am with to watch the curb.

The days passed, as a poet said, like a giant water wheel that tumbled slowly, one bucket after another. I never questioned my obligation, and it did not feel like duty. It was another stage in our lives. The most difficult tasks—bladder and bowel accidents, tumbles, falls, getting Minnie Mae to take her pills—became further intimacies in our long life together.

I tried to keep Minnie Mae's life as normal as possible. A friend of mine with good intentions took over all the cooking, shopping, and cleaning. He was caring—too caring. Minnie Mae lost all purpose in her life. She was unneeded, and her mental health suffered.

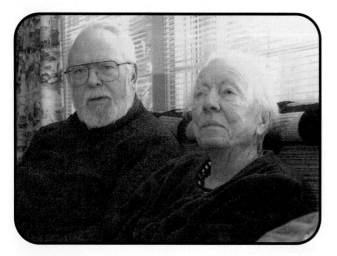

FIGURE 14.1 Don and Minnie Mae Murray in their home. (Courtesy of Donald M. Murray.)

I helped Minnie Mae with the shopping, but she was in charge. For years, she scooted between the supermarket aisles at full speed with the help of a grocery cart. She had been a great cook, but her meals became ordinary or worse. She knew it, but it was important that she was still in charge of the kitchen. Eating out allowed her to see different people and the beautiful New Hampshire countryside. For a long time, Minnie Mae could still shop for groceries and attend UNH hockey games, loudly coaching from the stands far longer than I thought possible. And she would stagger across the lawn with a cane, trying to work in her beloved garden (Figure 14.2).

All the time, I continued to write my column, books, and poetry. I needed to lose myself in the exercise of my craft and its deep concentration. Novelist Bernard Malamud explained, "If it is winter in the book, spring surprises me, when I look up."

It was tragic to see Minnie Mae's world grow small, but neither of us focused on the past. We focused on what could we do now—this morning, this afternoon, this evening. My daughters and I tried to treat Minnie Mae as the acerbic woman with the biting dry humor she had always been.

Many elderly people refuse to allow help to come into their home when they need it. That is a mistake. We were fortunate in having Dot Benson, who came in two or three times a week. She continued to be our cleaning woman, but as the Parkinson's increased, so did Dot's contributions to the quality of our life. She became more friend than employee. She took over the tasks that Minnie Mae could no longer do and I did not have the time to do if I was to continue to be a publishing writer. She also was a therapist, bringing the world to Minnie Mae, whose horizon grew closer and closer. She gave each of us the physical and emotional support we needed. When a couple she was caring for passed away, my psychiatric social worker daughter said, "Grab her. Right now. Get those hours." I resisted, I now recognize, because I didn't want to admit that Minnie Mae was in the early stages of dying. We needed Dot, and I am grateful for my daughter's command.

As Minnie Mae needed more and more care, a daughter, with the best of intentions, hired a team of additional caretakers. That didn't work. They didn't arrive on time or arrived ahead of time, they brought food we didn't need or like, they asked for advances on their pay that they didn't return, and worst of all, they talked to Minnie Mae in baby talk. Dot Benson was just the opposite in every way, and we increased her hours when they became available and then placed her on salary. I was 80 years old when Minnie Mae died. Dot stayed on to help me by taking over my bookkeeping and by providing computer assistance. She makes an offering of good humor each time she shows up. No cheeriness, no baby talk, just a down-to-earth model in how to live a life with acceptance while making the most of each day. I can't imagine my life before and after Minnie Mae's death without her help.

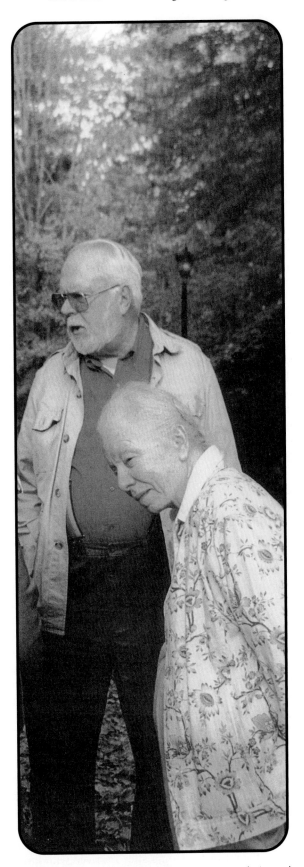

FIGURE 14.2 Don and Minnie Mae Murray in their garden. (Courtesy of Donald M. Murray.)

The years of care became normal and accelerated at the same time. I was uncomfortable with the term *demands*. There were no demands, just the increasing need for closeness and sharing. In my case, the time I had in combat as a paratrooper helped. At the front, you do what needs to be done, no question, no evasion, no excuses. The compliments of friends and neighbors who said how wonderful I was embarrassed and puzzled me. I was not wonderful. I loved Minnie Mae, simple as that. We had enjoyed better, and with the death of our daughter in 1977, we had survived worse. Who else should take care of her but the man who met her when she was a substitute blind date 54 years before?

I was fortunate to be retired from the University and had the time to care for her as I continued to write at home. Caring for someone with Parkinson's and so many other chronic diseases is a matter of small tasks—delivering pills on time, changing clothes, getting to the doctor—that accumulate so slowly that you hardly notice their increase. We had to develop our own tricks for this unplanned new trade of caregiver: how we could brace our feet against each other's so I could lift her efficiently and painlessly after inevitable falls, how a gentle hand under the armpit (developed from a not so gentle hold I learned as a military policeman) could tell Minnie Mae I was there, ready to help if she needed it, how I could wake in the night and watch her blanket so I could tell if she was still breathing.

We were, of course, both patients. She had to learn to protect her feisty, aggressive approach of life. I had to tune my Type A personality to a C while caring for someone who was living in slow motion. I had to learn not to invade her territory and, for example, take over the cooking early on. It became gradually more difficult for her, but cooking was her pride. I could not take it away from her. We had to discover how to calm or sustain each other at moments of terror or despair. When humor or yet another "Law & Order" rerun didn't work, a trip to get a dish of ice cream did. Ginger ice cream was the most therapeutic. Minnie Mae refused to worry about how her more obvious handicaps might disturb people, and we ate out a lot. I should add that everyone, wait staff and fellow customers alike, offered her respect, kindness, good humor, and help when necessary.

I suffered more stress than I felt or admitted. I did what needed to be done, but when my daughters, close friends, and doctors urged me to take care of myself, I shrugged off their counsel. I had had a cardiac bypass years before, and when I felt some heart symptoms, I went to my cardiologist, who examined me and said he would see me in three months. The symptoms continued, so a few days later I arranged for Dot to be with Minnie Mae and called 911 at three in the morning. Hours after I arrived with flashing lights at the hospital, I had a new cardiologist, and the next day I had six stents placed in the arteries near my heart. There must have been more stress than I realized.

I am surprised to find I miss the caregiving, now it is over, while enjoying the freedom to browse in a bookstore or play my music at top volume. In some way I cannot yet understand, the erotic intimacy of our first years seemed to flow into the intimacy of helping Minnie Mae dress and undress. There was nothing we did not know about each other and no moment when we were not available to the other. My job was to keep Minnie Mae from feeling shame or embarrassment as her body betrayed her. It is what she would have done for me.

The grand landscape of Parkinson's was fearful. But the day-to-day tasks that became essential as we traveled this landscape became intimate and appropriate. These were not years of hope. There are pills that can slow Parkinson's, but there is no cure. We had to accept the reality, but that did not make them dark years. When Minnie Mae started to call her cane a ladder, we laughed. No bother. I didn't correct her but simply brought the cane. Now I realize that dementia had arrived a long time before we admitted it. This was not denial but simply that we kept adapting to the language as we had adjusted to our daughters' first efforts to speak, which only we could understand. I would have expected an incapacitating horror to see the brain of such a smart, quick, opinionated woman change. Of course, it was what we had both feared the most, but it wasn't like that at all.

There are many marriages within a long marriage: no children, three children, moves to new cities and states, promotions and firing, manuscript acceptance and rejection, the children leaving, retirement, and now Parkinson's. Eventually, Minnie Mae's neurologist suggested that she be examined at a psychiatric and geriatric facility at a nearby hospital. As soon as we arrived and I saw Minnie Mae with the nine other patients, I knew we had entered a new territory some time before. Minutes after the chief psychiatrist began what would be a long examination, he turned to me and said I must activate my power of attorney. It was a chilling moment. After days of tests, it was clear that she would not come home. The fear we all have of ending our days filed away in a nursing home had come true for her. They sent her to a nursing home connected with the hospital that was as bad as any I have seen. I was beside Minnie Mae the first day when she was strapped in a chair while two nurses had a fistfight in front of us. She said, "Get me out of here." I answered, "We certainly will."

Dot and I raced from one facility to another in a day and half. Obviously, we should have visited more of them early on, but our "one step at a time" policy kept us from looking too far ahead. Perhaps we were right. Parkinson's varies radically between patients, and neither the doctors nor we could predict the care she would need. Luckily, we found a small assisted living facility—32 patients maximum—seven miles from our home. Minnie Mae had said she would kill herself before she would go to a nursing home, but she moved in without complaint. She seemed, despite the dementia, to know she needed this level of care.

When Minnie Mae was admitted to Kirkwood Corners, an outstanding assisted living facility, a nurse told me that my wife's dementia produced fascinating fantasies. She said Minnie Mae had told the nurse that she had been one of the first people to work in the Pentagon, that she had relayed messages from Secretary of War George Marshall to General Walter Bedell Smith in London, who then told General Dwight D. Eisenhower what to do. My wife added that she was a professional mezzo-soprano who had soloed in Washington, D.C., and Boston. She said she had Q Clearance, the highest possible security status. She added that she might lose that status, since she was, according to the Associated Press, the first person in the country to get people on the sidewalk to sign a petition calling for President Richard Nixon's impeachment.

I told the nurse it was all true, not the product of dementia. The staff got to know her as a woman of accomplishment and not just another patient. "I don't know why these people treat me so well," said my wife, who had promised to kill herself if she had to go to a nursing home. The staff at Kirkwood Corners treated all their patients with respect, but Minnie Mae felt she got special attention.

Understandably, many dedicated doctors, nurses, therapists, aides, and the blessed people from hospice focus on the patient. The care is intense and continual. They are patients, men and woman, who have chronic and terminal illnesses that demand care and love. The Kirkwood Corners staff realized that the patients see themselves not so much as they are but what they were: cabinetmakers, soldiers, parents and grandparents, lawyers, bakers, secretaries, corporate executives, gardeners, researchers, gamblers, teachers, salespeople.

If those who treat the elderly get to know the worlds in which they have been productive, then respect is easy, and all the treatments are given in the context of their entire lives. During my bypass surgery, I was seen as a combat paratrooper who was familiar with pain. It helped me to return, with the staff, to another life.

Minnie Mae's father had been a baker, and when she opened an imaginary bakery in the basement of Kirkwood Corners, the cook discussed recipes as if the business really existed. Staff members took care of Minnie Mae's imaginary pack of strawberry dogs. Office staff helped with flight schedules when she had to fly to London on a secret mission for the CIA. They treated her as if she has Q Clearance. Minnie Mae was obviously happier than at home. She had better care than we could provide, and she was not isolated, as she had become at home. She would watch the daily parade of staff, residents, and visitors with some understanding and a great deal of amusement.

And how did I feel visiting her twice a day? I put aside the larger picture, as I had in combat, and focused entirely on the woman I loved. She recognized me less and less, but when I held her hand, she would give a sudden, tight squeeze, and I knew that somewhere in her clotted brain was an "I love you."

What did I learn from the years of increasing caregiving? There is as much intimacy, caring, and love at the end of a lifetime together as when we first discovered each other and grew our lives together, perhaps more. An elderly couple facing a long struggle without a terminal illness needs a calm, detailed explanation of illness. They do not need evasions. They have lived a long life together and are usually tougher than they—or you—think. Truth is better, no matter how hard it is, than the imagination of the patient and gossip about the disease related by friends. What else did I learn?

◆ Don't yank. Minnie Mae was tugged and painfully hauled up from her falls by many caring passers-by. I learned to allow her to do all she could and then be nearby to help if she needed it: hand barely touching her armpit tells her that help is at hand—if SHE needs it.
◆ Share some of yourself. Minnie Mae was delighted to hear stories about children, grandchildren, and dogs.
◆ Do not correct someone with dementia, saying, "That didn't happen in Atlanta but Utica." They can't understand, and what difference does it make anyway?

Those of us who find ourselves as caregivers will discover that we have strengths and skills of which we were not aware. What I did and every other caregiver does is done not out of duty, responsibility, and obligation but, above all, love.

Suddenly one Friday afternoon, Minnie Mae's dementia lifted, and she gave the staff clear orders: "No pills. No food. No water." It is what she had wanted, documented in writing, and my daughters and I felt she had the right to die her way, in command to the end. Hospice and the Kirkwood Corner staff were experienced, loving, and professional. Minnie Mae's daughters and I were with her most of the 11 days it took her to sleep away her life. She was treated with dignity, and she suffered no pain. I was holding her hand when she gave one last quick puff of air and was gone.

AFTERWORD

On January 2, 2007 shortly after completing this chapter, Donald M. Murray died while visiting friends. He was an Emeritus Professor of English at the University of New Hampshire. He won the Pulitzer Prize for editorial writing in 1954, and wrote the weekly column "Now and Then" for the *Boston Globe*, which explored his reactions to the process of aging. He also published memoirs, novels, short stories, poetry, and textbooks on the writing process. I asked him to write this chapter because he was a well-known faculty member at the University of New Hampshire. I was acquainted with his work because I had attended several of his writing workshops and knew a

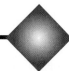

NOW AND THEN

Friends Caring and Sharing Show the Way

Donald M. Murray

For those of us who are introspective, life is a continuous exploration into the self, where we hope to find the person we are and the person we may become. Of course, the apple does not fall far from the tree, and we discover we have become a mixed breed of our parents, grandparents, uncles, and aunts. I found this discouraging. I had thought I had made my escape.

Now I accept my genes but imagine I have a tuning dial so that I can adjust their instincts and standards to the life, far different than theirs, I have constructed. This new life has been created by friends who have seen me as I have not yet been able to see myself. With Yankee respect they have mostly kept their distance, but when they have spoken, or touched a shoulder, or given a smile of encouragement, it has been important to me.

When we lost our daughter Lee at 20, it was the subtle but sturdy support of friends that got us through those first years. They saw us as strong when we felt weak. They said we had done more than enough, when we felt we had done far too little. They gave us a future when we thought there was none.

And then came the years of Minnie Mae's Parkinson's. We attended to the hour-by-hour physical demands of living, and then the dementia arrived, and again it was friends who supported and guided me. I often felt like a huge ship being nudged into port by friendly tugs.

These friends and neighbors, too many to name, were there when I began a new life alone. First they eliminated much of the alone with invitations and visits. They approved future relationships before I had imagined them. They suggested small steps of independence and supported me when I took them.

And what have I learned? To pass friendship on. To speak out, to touch, to be there when others need me.

Donald M. Murray, "Now and Then: Friends Caring and Sharing Show the Way." The Boston Globe, December 29, 2006, reprinted with permission.

number of his former students who revered his contribution to their education and careers. Over the years, I purchased several of his books on writing and his memoirs. Every Tuesday morning I looked for his column, "Now and Then," in the *Boston Globe*.

It was only after his death that I realized how many people he influenced through his teaching, mentorship, and writing. Many of the letters to the editor detailed the personal connection people felt to Don and Minnie Mae from his columns. Many of his former students are newspaper editors, writers, and teachers. He submitted his last column to the *Boston Globe* on December 29th, just a few days before his death. We have reprinted it here as it represents much of his grace and character.

—Elizabeth Crepeau

Voices Talk, Hands Write

15

NICK POLLARD WITH THE VOICES TALK, HANDS WRITE WRITING GROUP

BRIAN HAUGHIE

I was born in Dumfries 42 years ago. When I was a little boy I went to Carnforth School and I was happy there. My favourite lesson was maths, 'cos I learned to add things up. I made loads and loads of friends, I had lots.

I live in a flat by myself now. I like reading the *Telegraph* every night at home to find out the news and like reading adverts. I write letters about problems like how it is difficult for disabled people to use the buses and sometimes they are printed. I sit in my favourite chair to watch television and find out what's going on.

Where I live the neighbours are sometimes nice to me and some of them are not very nice to me, they call me names. They tell me to do things when I can't do them. When I've got some shopping in my hands they tell me to use the stairs when I can't. I say, I have to use the lift for my safety, to stop me from falling.

I like going to the pub to have a drink of Coke on my own and going to the cinema to see films. I like going shopping for food in Asda and Kwik Save and going to town to look at the shops (Figure 15.1). I like going ten pin bowling at Cleethorpes Bowling Alley. I win sometimes.

Life of Wearing My Suit *by* Brian Haughie*

The first time I wore a suit I was one of two Best Men at my brother Scott's wedding and the other Best Man was my twin brother Alan.

The *Telegraph* came to my brother's wedding and took pictures. My brother Scott's wedding took place on 22nd December 1990 and the picture appeared in the Telegraph on 27th December, the last day me and my brother Alan were 26 years old. I wore a tie with the suit.

The second time I wore the suit was for my Grandma's funeral on 13th June 1994 in Bolton which wasn't a nice day for my cousin Jacqueline because it was her birthday then, but I was pleased when my cousin Jacqueline put her hand on my shoulder when she saw me crying my eyes out when I came out of the church. I wore a tie with the suit.

The third time I wore the suit was when I went to one of my annual Christmas parties. The Christmas party I wore the suit for was the Christmas party I have been going to for years since I was a little boy and that

*From Haughie, Brian. (2005). *Stories*. Grimsby, UK: Voices Talk and Hands Write.

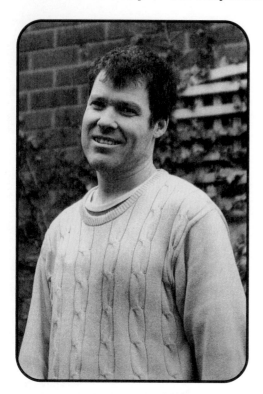

FIGURE 15.1 Brian Haughie. (Courtesy of N. Pollard.)

christmas party is the Spastics' Society christmas party. The christmas party was held on 10th December 1994 at Heneage Road Youth Service Centre. It was my Mum's idea for me to wear the suit for the christmas party in 1994 and because my brother Alan came to visit and Alan put the tie on me before I went to the party.

The fourth time I wore the suit was over eight years ago for my Mum's funeral. My Mum's funeral took place at Grimsby Crematorium on April 23rd 1996 which was on a Tuesday. I was once again crying at my Mum's funeral. I started crying when I saw the hoist with my Mum's coffin on it. My Mum liked the *Sound of Music*. At the funeral they played "My Favourite Things" at the beginning of the funeral and "So Long, Farewell" at the end of the funeral.

I have been to Steels Corner House Restaurant wearing the suit. I wore a tie with the suit. And finally I wore the suit again this year on 16th July when I was told to write this story about me wearing my suit. The *Telegraph* came to take a picture and the picture appeared in the paper on 29th July which is one of my Auntie's birthday. I was very surprised to find myself in the paper on one of my Auntie's birthdays.

And that's the story of me wearing the suit.

ERICKA TURNER

I live with three men, all three come to this centre at Queen's Road. We are tenants in our own home.

I like watching *Black Beauty* on the video and *Mary Poppins*. I watch *Dirty Dancing* as well. I watch these videos at weekends. I like my breakfasts on a Saturday mornings, my favourite food is shepherd's pie, potatoes and carrots.

I like watching "Neighbours," "EastEnders," "Emmerdale Farm," and "Coronation Street" on telly. My favourite programme is "Coronation Street," all my favourite stars are there.

I type on a computer at home. I like doing gardening, I like to go out at night time. I go to the pub with Keith and Paul, I drink coke and I play pool. My favourite place to go is the youth club.

Walking Talking Doll *by* Ericka Turner*

My Mam and Dad bought me a doll with long black hair. They brought it to me when I was in bed. I wasn't very well. The doll walked and talked. It said, "tell them to find me when I run off." When I went upstairs to the toilet, it ran out!

I called it Susan. I bought some clothes for her, some dresses and some trousers. I played with her on my own. When I put her back in my bedroom and went to lie down she was downstairs, my Mam said, "she's down here."

If she had batteries in she would do it, but if you didn't put batteries in she wouldn't work. She walked downstairs and out of the house.

I went and found her in the back garden on her own, pulling flowers up. I thought "what are you doing in our back garden?" She said, "I'm picking flowers." I tried to take her with me when I went out, but she wanted to stay with my Mam. "I want to stay with your Mam and your Dad, I don't want to go out," she said. I went to the shop to buy her some shoes.

I wanted to tie them on but she wouldn't let me tie them on her. I said, "if you don't want to have them on then I'll have them off you." She said, "if you want them you can have them."

My brother broke her. He pulled all her hair off because he didn't like the colour. It was nice, it wasn't dirty because I had washed it. Then my Mam told him off about it. I had to carry on playing with her with no hair. "All my hair's gone, so I'll have to buy a wig," she said. So I bought her one.

IRIS GARRITY

I am 66, 67 next birthday, and live in Cleethorpes (Figure 15.2). There is lots of shops down our street. Our house is a big one, it is a council place. Mine has three rooms, one big and two small. I live with my friend Jayne, the two of us, but we do have a little help.

*From *Voices Talk Hands Write*. (2004). Stoke on Trent, UK: The Federation of Worker Writers and Community Publishers.

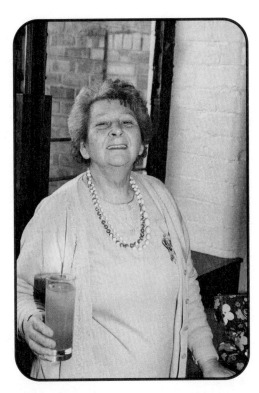

FIGURE 15.2 Iris Garrity. (Courtesy of N. Pollard.)

I like sewing and cooking. Tuesday afternoons, we go to Fort School. I do table cloths and tapestries and do my computers and games. I go shopping to Sainsbury's and go to the market to buy some fruit. I like oranges, peaches and strawberries and cream. I like doing cooking, scones to eat but I can't eat them because I am a diabetic. I eat baked potatoes with cheese and meat pie with vegetables. I like housework, doing cleaning especially my bedroom.

What I'd Do, What I'd Really, Really Do *by* Iris Garrity*

I'd like to be Tony Blair for a week, to go and meet people and helping people as he says, and to the Houses of Parliament to talk about meetings and other things, about the war and when people get hurt and go to hospitals to get better, and to see how they are getting on. Talking about the news how they've been getting on.

Lots of people are talking about that car bomb last night and that debris, there's a good few people what died last night.

Then there's Michael Jackson, the story about him and his baby.

I would change other things, like change staffing in the hospital so there's more staff, and it's more safer.

*From Voices Talk Hands Write. (2004). Stoke on Trent, UK: The Federation of Worker Writers and Community Publishers.

The doctors there I would change. I would take the old ones out because they're not very good and put more younger male doctors and nurses in. I'd change the beds to be better and the floors better than what they are.

More cleaners and better hoovers and better dinners than what they are now.

Better receptionist at the hospitals, and the Houses of Parliament because they're not much good when you see them on the telly.

And Tony, he goes round talking to people and shaking hands to other people. I would change that because he's always showing off.

He's always showing off to other people.

He does, yes.

And better cars to what they are now.

I would take the old ones out and put the new ones in to make more cars safer than what they are now.

I would change the police and put more and better ones in because they're not much good they're never around when you want them.

And about them lollipop ladies as well, I'd change everything around. I'd make it safer because it's not very good, as they get knocked down, two of them did.

I would change the hairdressers. I'd put new ones in and old ones out because, they're alright, but not as good as they used to be and different hair styles and different kinds of hair dryers would be good.

I would change the Farnhurst staff upstairs. I'd put new ones in and olds ones out, but not Mandy Ives. I'd get rid of all the old ones from upstairs and new ones in, because they're not much good them upstairs, because I can't go up there. I can't always get up the stairs and this makes me feel that I'm not welcome.

DISCUSSION

It is often assumed that people with learning difficulties cannot really express themselves. This chapter demonstrates how occupational therapists can provide a client-centered program that enables people with learning difficulties this opportunity. Voice Talk, Hands Write was negotiated as a community arts and education initiative with social services—in other words, outside a health context. The project involved complex input from the Federation of Worker Writers and Community Publishers (or Fed) and some of its member groups: Pecket Well College (a cooperative adult and basic education facility), the Grimsby Writers group, and local support workers. It secured funding for a twelve-session writing group with a day center and other local clients with learning difficulties who chose to come. The project focused on the development of creative, expressive, and social abilities. Its principal aims were:

- ◆ To form a writing group for people with learning difficulties

♦ To produce community publications of the participants writing

♦ To publish the project in professional media with the participants' agreement.

What Are Community Publishing Practices?

Creative writing is often used in occupational therapy (Pollard, 2004a), but writing and community publishing involve a complex range of other occupations. The purpose and meaning of the writing activity described here are a vehicle for addressing multiple occupational goals, which are contained in the Fed's own purpose of "making writing and publishing accessible to all" (FWWCP, 2005). This international association of people who write about life in their communities includes many writers with experiences of disabling conditions. This project came about because the Fed wanted to enable more people to experience the benefits of community publishing.

A key aim of the project was to enable the group and its supporters to develop skills for sustainability. Community publishing originated in the politically radical counterculture of the 1970s, through alliances with marginalized sections of the population on the basis of inequalities of gender, race, class, or low literacy (Courtman, 2000; Mace, 1995). Because marginalized people have often not known how to approach arts funders, activities have depended on volunteer commitment and the ability to publish cheaply by learning to do it yourself. Until it decides to publish, a writing group needs only pens and paper, which people generally provide themselves. The greatest cost is the meeting space and the input of support workers. This is important in working among people with disabilities, who often have contact only with paid workers and therefore are excluded from building "real relationships within their own communities" (Mason, 2002, p. 56), an essential element to being an active community publisher.

Grimsby offered potential for these essential connections. The Fed's then chairperson worked in the Grimsby Social Services Department and proposed working with a local day center for people with learning difficulties. She convened the large and strong local writers' workshop, with people who were interested in developing new activities around writing (Figure 15.3). The Fed's magazine editor is an occupational therapist who was then working as a part-time research development worker in the mental health trust that served Grimsby.

As a consequence of its origins, community publishing is a very open activity. Two principles are that writing can include oral composition that is not necessarily transmitted to paper and that community publication includes any means of reaching an audience, including performance. Cassette tapes and, increasingly, CD-ROM formats (with both sound and text) can be cost-effective and more accessible than print (Pollard, 2003, 2004b, 2004c). This range of media combined with the participative and

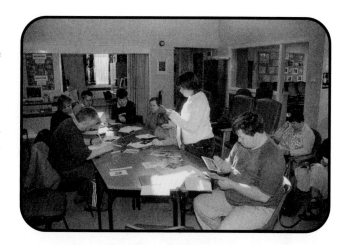

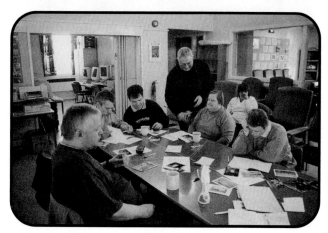

FIGURE 15.3   The group works on their writing during the meetings, but many members also write at home. (Courtesy of N. Pollard.)

diverse nature of making community publishing accessible offers many extensions of the writing process and links to new occupational roles (Pollard, 2004a; Pollard, Smart & Voices Talk and Hands Write, 2005).

Not Therapy but Empowerment: Why Take Writing Seriously?

Writing is a private activity that makes truths clear only to the writer, but publishing makes these truths available to others. In mental health contexts, therapeutic writing projects have been used to assist in the promotion of community and trust (Philips, Linington & Penman, 1999), even after war, particularly among children (Simo Algado & Burgman, 2005). Some (e.g., Foster, 1988) have included a subsequent community publication (Cox & Duffin, 1988), while the mental health survivors movement (see web addresses at end of the chapter) have encouraged publications that aim at a broad audience. Those produced with and for people with learning difficulties have mostly been intended for their own local groups rather than wider communities, partly through apprehension about exposing these individuals to public prurience. Often, these publications are difficult to obtain; consequently, they remain hidden. There are exceptions: *Our Lives, Our Group* (The Thursday Club, 2002), produced by adult women with learning difficulties, was an inspiration for this project.

For community publishers, writing is a socially inclusive political act that promotes the artistic expression and exploration of feelings for the appreciation of others through writing and dissemination. The word is treated "as if it counted in the world" (Willinsky, 1990, p. 187), the writer with learning difficulties is taken at face value as a *writer* (Sampson & Hunt, 1998). The connection of community publication with therapeutic activities can be controversial and problematic. The responsibilities associated with this stance should be carefully negotiated:

- Collaboration on publication projects raises professional and ethical concerns about publishing "the unsifted contents of a troubled mind" (Bolton, 1999, p. 225).
- Publication may create an intense local prominence, which individuals are sometimes ill-equipped to deal with (Pollard 2004c). This may lead to libel action and even physical retaliation if community members feel that they have been maligned.
- The cathartic and therapeutic aspects of writing activities have been used to dismiss the value and content of "worker writing" (Morley & Worpole, 1982), especially when the writer has disabilities or is an adult learner.
- Publication of their work means publicly acknowledging a stigmatizing illness or that they are literacy learners; consequently, some people have not participated in the celebration of their publications (Fitzpatrick, 1995).

Us in Our Town *by* VTHW Group

We like to live in our community
With our friends we have real unity
We choose to live in Grimsby, Cleethorpes and about
We live in houses. From high rise flats we have to shout
We don't let vandals get us down
We can move to other parts of town
In community gardens there are flowers and trees
We can be as quiet as we please
This is why we live in our town.

Voices Talk, Hands Write are a group who directly raise local awareness of the real needs and lives of people with learning difficulties through the publication and performance of writing (Figure 15.4). Once established and with local volunteers to support them, the group then decided to continue meeting, although funding has been difficult to obtain. The group could not have been sustained without committed volunteer input. Writing is usually produced in group sessions in response to a topic that is chosen and negotiated between the members. The finished pieces are immediately read back to other members, but some members also write at home about subjects of their own choice. All the members have taken part in public performances at venues ranging from the town hall to the local pub and even local radio. In December 2005, one of the group members, Brian Haughie, was awarded a laptop computer and printer by a local charity in recognition of his achievements, while a second anthology was about to go to print. This continuity is a significant indication of the group's sustained interest, commitment, and sense of achievement.

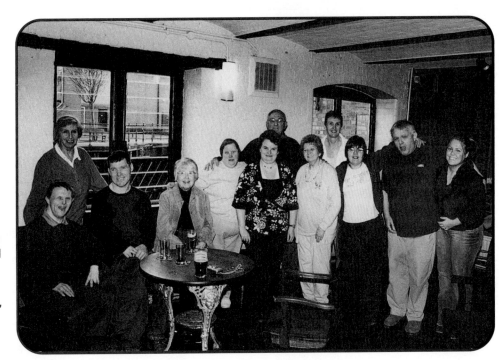

FIGURE 15.4 Voices Talk, Hands Write Group in their local pub, the Tap and Spile, Grimsby. Writing groups are also about socializing, and Voices Talk, Hands Write often go out together, just for a change. (Courtesy of N. Pollard.)

CASE STUDY: *Mark Wainwright: A Writer with Learning Difficulties*

Mark Wainwright is a 35-year-old man with learning difficulties who lives with his parents. He has a part-time job at the local market, where he works in a greengrocer's stall. Sometimes he goes to the pub after work with the other people from the market.

Two days a week, Mark attends a day center for people with learning difficulties, where he meets his girlfriend and attends a writing group that is led by an occupational therapist. The group has given performances at the center and at residential units and has now published a collection of poems. Mark and his fellow workshop members have been told that their collection will be ready to coincide with the town's literature festival. They are so excited about having their work in print and organize a launch party. The occupational therapist is very proud of the group's achievements and can't wait to begin distributing the poetry collection, which her managers are very pleased with.

The following day the occupational therapist receives a phone call from Mark's mother. She objects to his poem about getting drunk with his mates from the market. She says that she should have had advance warning that his work would be published. Had she known, she would have stopped him participating. She asks for an apology.

1. Does the right of people with learning difficulties to write and publish compromise their carers' or relatives' right to confidentiality? How does an occupational therapist determine whether community publication is an appropriate occupational activity?

The occupational therapist takes the group and some support workers to a reading event at the library. The group members are in their best clothes and have carefully rehearsed their performances. The receptive audience give enthusiastic applause, even though some readings are difficult to understand. However, Mark becomes upset when he overhears the remark "I came to hear some literature, not a bunch of clowns from a therapy group."

2. What are the barriers for people with learning difficulties who want to participate in artistic and creative activities in the wider community and how would an occupational therapist empower individuals and groups to overcome these barriers?

Several months later, the group reviews its achievements. They recall the things they have written about and the events in which they have participated. Many of the anthologies are still unsold. They decide to have a "press conference" with the social services press officer to celebrate one year since the group started and to promote the remaining anthologies through a day center magazine. Their interview is also reported in the local paper, but they find that the articles have concentrated on the occupational therapist rather than the group. Many of the responses articulated by group members have been ignored. "They've made us look stupid," Mark says.

3. If they are community based, arts projects that involve people with disabilities can have unpredictable outcomes. How can an occupational therapist structure the experience to enable everyone to get the most benefit from participation?

ACKNOWLEDGMENTS

The authors are indebted to Jim White for his valuable comments and suggestions and the participation of June Baxendale, Matthew Blastard, Mandy Carpenter, Claire Clayton, Jayne Fletcher, Sally Fox, Gary Gant, Iris Garrity, Trevor George, Michael Hardaker, Brian Haughie, Ellen Jebsen, Maggie Macdonald, Kenny Money, Andy Murdoch, Fiona Murdoch, Trevor Parkinson, Kim Stowe, and Ericka Turner, as well as Jo Barnes, Tim Diggles, and Pat Smart.

REFERENCES

Bolton, G. (1999). *The therapeutic potential of creative writing: Writing myself.* London: Jessica Kingsley Publishers.

Courtman, S. (2000). Frierian liberation, cultural transaction and writing from 'the working class and the spades.' *The Society for Caribbean Studies Annual Conference Papers.* Retrieved March 27, 2006, from http://www.scsonline.freeserve.co.uk/olv1p6.pdf

Cox, A., & Duffin, P. (1988) *Day in, day out: Memories of North Manchester from women in Monsall Hospital.* Manchester, UK: Gatehouse Project.

Fitzpatrick, S. (1995). Sailing out from safe harbours: Writing for publication in adult basic education. In J. Mace (Ed.), *Literacy, language and community publishing: Essays in adult education* (pp. 1–22). Clevedon, UK: Multilingual Matters Ltd.

Foster, L. (1988). Writers workshops, the word processor and the psychiatric patient, *British Journal of Occupational Therapy, 51*(6), 191–192.

FWWCP. (2005). *The FWWCP constitution.* Retrieved March 28, 2006, from http://www.thefwwcp.org.uk/pages/constitution.php

Mace, J. (1995). Introduction. In J. Mace (Ed.), *Literacy, language and community publishing: Essays in adult education* (pp. ix–xx). Clevedon, UK: Multilingual Matters Ltd.

Mason, M. (2002). *Incurably human.* London: Working Press.

Morley, D., & Worpole, K. (Eds.). (1982). *The republic of letters: Working class writing and local publishing.* London: Comedia/MPG.

Philips, D., Linington, L., & Penman, D. (1999). *Writing well: Creative writing and mental health.* London: Jessica Kingsley Publishers.

Pollard, N. (2003). DIY publishing: Part 1, *Federation, 26:* 27–30. Retrieved March 27, 20006, from http://www.thefwwcp.org.uk/magazines/26mag.pdf

Pollard, N. (2004a). Notes towards a therapeutic use for creative writing in occupational therapy. In F. Sampson (Ed.), *Creative writing in health and social care* (pp. 189–206). London: Jessica Kingsley Publishers.

Pollard, N. (2004b). DIY Publishing: Part 2, *Federation, 27,* 28–29. Retrieved March 27, 2006, from http://www.thefwwcp.org.uk/magazines/27mag.pdf

Pollard, N. (2004c). DIY Publishing: Part 3, *Federation, 28,* 27–30. Retrieved March 27, 2006, from http://www.thefwwcp.org.uk/magazines/28mag.pdf

Pollard, N., Smart, P., & Voices Talk and Hands Write. (2005). Voices talk and hands write. In F. Kronenberg, S. Simo Algado, & N. Pollard (Eds.), *Occupational therapy without borders: Learning from the spirit of survivors* (pp. 295–310). Oxford, UK: Elsevier.

Sampson, F., & Hunt, C. (1998). Towards a writing therapy?: Implications of existing practice and theory. In C. Hunt & F. Sampson (Eds.), *The self on the page: Theory and practice of creative writing in personal development* (pp. 198–210). London: Jessica Kingsley Publishers.

Simo Algado, S., & Burgman, I. (2005). Occupational therapy intervention with children survivors of war. In F. Kronenberg, S. Simo Algado, & N. Pollard (Eds.), *Occupational therapy without borders: Learning from the spirit of survivors* (pp. 152–165). Oxford, UK: Elsevier.

The Thursday Club. (2002). *Our lives our group.* Sheffield, UK: Author.

Willinsky, J. (1990). *The new literacy: Redefining reading and writing in the schools.* New York: Routledge

SUGGESTIONS FOR FURTHER READING

Pecket Well College http://www.pecketwell-college.co.uk/

Sampson, F. (1998). 'Men wearing pyjamas': Using creative writing with people with learning disabilities. In C. Hunt & F. Sampson (Eds.), *The self on the page: Theory and practice of creative writing in personal development* (pp. 63–77). London: Jessica Kingsley Publishers.

Survivors' Poetry (U.K. group for survivors of mental distress) http://www.survivorspoetry.com/pages/home.php

Mobilizing the Collective Action of Disabled Women in Developing Contexts to Tackle Poverty and Development

THERESA LORENZO

Learning Objectives

After reading this chapter, you will be able to:

1. Share narratives of South African women with disabilities who participated in a series of narrative action reflection workshops
2. Describe a human rights approach to equalizing opportunities for disabled women, with particular focus on women who live in developing contexts
3. Illustrate the shift from individual focus in rehabilitation to a population approach in addressing disability issues

This chapter shares the human development narratives of disabled women who live in wooden shacks in the periurban areas of Khayelitsha and Greater Nyanga, in Cape Town in the Western Cape Province of South Africa. Human development is

> a process of change that enables people to take charge of their own destinies and realise their full potential. It requires building up in the people the confidence, skills, assets and freedoms necessary to achieve this goal. (Taylor, 2000, p. 49)

An important aspect of this definition of human development is the access citizens of a country have to an environment in which they are able to obtain opportunities and resources and makes choices to live decent lives. Taylor (2000) adds that human development recognizes that people need economic, social, cultural, political, and human rights in order to develop to their fullest potential and to live meaningful lives. She identified access to water, knowledge, health care, employment, and other productive resources as basic ingredients for human development. In South Africa, human development has been impaired because these rights have been denied to the majority of the people. South Africa's rate of poverty is 45%, which means that more than 18 million citizens (or 3,126,000 households) live below the poverty line, which is pegged at an income of R353 [approximately US$59] per adult per month (Taylor, 2000). In rural areas, the poverty rate rises above 50%. Besides experiencing simultaneous oppression related to race, gender, and disability, poverty creates a fourth form of oppression.

Over a period of two and a half years, many disabled women participated in narrative action reflection (NAR) workshops led by the author (an occupational therapist herself), another occupational therapist, and a disabled woman. We planned these workshops to combine action learning (Taylor, Marais & Kaplan, 1997) and storytelling (Slim and Thompson, 1993) with narrative inquiry to enable participants to describe the meaning of human actions and link them to larger social concerns (Clandinin and Connelly, 2000). We facilitated the workshops in a way that enabled the women to tell their stories and to analyze the stories to raise their awareness of the root causes of their oppression. This cycle of action and reflection occurs within a single workshop, as well as between and across workshops (Hope and Timmel, 1995). In this way, the process aims to enable each woman to feel heard in a way that mobilizes her to take action toward social change (Figure 16.1).

The women who participated in these workshops are mostly single mothers who look after more than just their own children. They are also responsible for members of their extended families. Many have migrated from the rural areas of the Eastern Cape in the hope of finding better medical care and economic opportunities to alleviate their poverty.

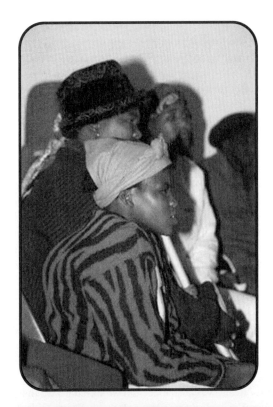

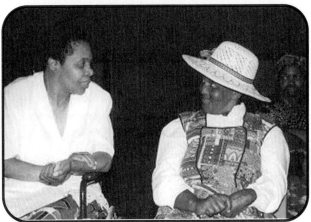

FIGURE 16.1 Women in workshops learn to listen to each other's stories with Marjorie as facilitator.

BULELWA: I SEE MYSELF AS A LIGHT FOR OTHER DISABLED PEOPLE

Bulelwa is a vibrant entrepreneur, very hard-working while being very concerned for the well-being and growth of the other women in the workshops. She shares her story:

> After the first workshop where I told my story, I felt much stronger. I realized these workshops could really help other women in the same situation as me. Our rehabilitation did not help us return and settle back with

our families or communities. Here I made a clay sculpture of a plate and two women to share how I changed from gaining knowledge of disability rights and advocacy skills. The workshops helped us to find knowledge and information for each other. We felt happier. We recognized the gains we've made in changing our living conditions. These skills have led to a better life together. I made myself using clay. I want to show you that before I became disabled, my body was thin. I was small before and you can now see how big I am. So I want to share the good news so that others can be big like me. I must be the light, even in the community and preach about disability and how they can treat disabled people. I talk about disability. I became more confident and gained skills in being able to change things. I was used to speaking in church and sharing my testimony. Now I speak about disability. I also loved to sing and dance.

I see myself as a light for other disabled people and I'm not afraid. I know I'm able to talk. I'm usually shy, but since I've been here I am free. I used to worry a lot at home, but since I've been here I'm much better. When I see my neighbours quarrelling, I say to them "Call your family and sort this out." Later they say to me "Really we called them and we solved it." So that is why I'm saying I'm a lamp. I see that even with the women, there is change. I'm able to see how they were before and how they are now. Ever since they have been meeting in the groups, the load was taken away and everything has been lighter.

So I was not the only one who wanted to shine a light to change attitudes to disability ourselves, amongst our families and our neighbours. The workshops also helped us see how we could heal each other. The workshops gave us courage to be visible in our families and community again. I told a story from the Bible: "I identify myself with the person who was next to the dam and people were coming and going not helping him. So Jesus asked him, 'do you want to be well?' 'I want to, but I don't have a person who will help me and put me in this dam.' Jesus said 'take your mat and go and by those words you are healed.' " So now I'm well, but it's sad when you see others having problems.

THANDISWA: NOW I FEEL I CAN DO ANYTHING

After her discharge from a general hospital where she received physical rehabilitation following a stroke, Thandiswa stayed at home and felt quite isolated from her community. She told the group how much her participation in the workshops had helped her at personal, family, and community levels:

I experienced deep changes about how I feel. I used to cry a lot, but since I met other women, I got new ideas.

I joined the Nobantu group.[1] When Bulelwa introduced me to the group, I was happy and I became one of them. I understand more about this impairment now. When I became disabled, I always undermined myself when I was with my friends. I always sat in one place. But when I met with the other women I became stronger and that thing of always feeling sorry for myself is gone. My in-laws did not love me but today my house is always full. I'm strong. Today I'm not crying. Now no one can believe that I used crutches before. No one can say I'm disabled now. I identify myself with the sun because before it was dark and I didn't want to accept my disability. I couldn't even sit in the sun. Now I can do things with my hands and I got a certificate in business skills. After that I could do things for myself. Now I'm like a mother in the house even when the children are not there. I never used to be like that. I used to wait for them to come back from school. Now I feel that I can do anything.

GLORIA: THEY SEE A MOTHER WHO IS A ROLE MODEL

Gloria had been disabled by polio as a child. She told how her children had found support from the workshops as well as they also felt the pressure to change the stigma of disability. Gloria said:

I'm receiving a lot of support from my family. My two children always show interest in what I'm doing. At school they used to be laughed at by other children because of my disability. But they told them that with their mother, they can't see any disability, but they see a mother who is a role model and who can afford everything unlike nondisabled mothers who can't afford the basics. You see nondisabled mothers who can't even afford buying their children shoes. As mothers we learnt to teach our children respect and good social skills. Your child has a right to ask for things from you, but you need to teach them to talk nicely when they are asking for something. They mustn't go and ask for something from other people because they think you can't do things since you are disabled.

NONTSIDISO: A PILLAR OF STRENGTH

Nontsidiso had a tubercular spinal deformity as a child, leaving her with a hunchback. However, it was not her impairment that made her feel different from other children, but rather the poverty and the loneliness she expe-

---

[1]A small business group that was initiated in Khayelitsha in 1996 that started with some of the disabled men with the support of the community rehabilitation workers.

rienced after the death of her parents as a young child. Nontsidiso was unable to complete her schooling because of poverty. As an adult and single parent, she also faced the absence of spousal support. Her abbreviated story follows.

I am Nontsidiso. I am *intsika,* a pillar of strength, because now there is nothing that I cannot do. I cried a lot when I told my story in the beginning, as I had never shared my story with other women before. I didn't feel I was different from other children when I grew up with a hunchback. We lived in the Transkei.[2] I came to Cape Town with my mother because she was sick. My mother died leaving me alone with her youngest child. Now I felt lonely and powerless because I had no mother, no father, not even an older brother who could help me. I don't have a sister. I had no money and used to ask for food from the neighbours. Now I saw that I was not like other children. Other children were not hungry; I was hungry. I dropped out of school because of money problems. Then I had two children of my own, but their father didn't help me. He is a drunkard and drug addict and he beats me. I called the police one day and they beat him. I have also reported my problem of being beaten in the community, but no one does anything. I was suffering and my children were suffering. Sometimes, friends and neighbours help me with food. I couldn't get a disability grant. Then I heard from the social worker about the women's group. I came because I wanted advice to help my children.

I was also in the group that went to the catering workshops as part of skills development in business (Figure 16.2). I didn't know that so much would come up with so little popcorn. I got a certificate now so that I can get a job in catering and do something with my hands. I didn't know that I could be taught and become educated. I see how I was able to change inside from believing that I could not manage to work. Now I am able to make mats that I learnt about at Philani Nutrition Centre.[3] I work on my own. Another man has promised to take me to a place to get material. Even with the beads, I don't ask anyone. I make them on my own.

My confidence increased, so did my hope and belief that the feelings and beliefs of my family and neighbours towards me would change. I wanted to change being called names. Even if I'm walking, people say "shame, that cripple." I wanted to change the way they say when I'm talking "Don't listen to her, she's handicapped." I wanted to be seen on TV or to take a flight and then my family would say, "oh her, we were looking down on her." The opportunity came for me to go with Marjorie to the national Disabled People South Africa (DPSA)

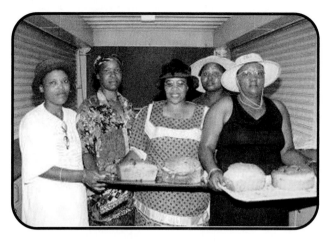

FIGURE 16.2 Women participate in catering workshops to develop skills in entrepreneurship.

Women Achiever Award ceremony. The group was excited with me, clapping and rejoicing. Now it was my first time to go to Johannesburg. I was really excited about taking a flight. Now I'm not scared of disability. I'll be someone one day. My family began to see me participating in national DPSA conferences. Before I could not go to occasions in the community because I was shy. Now I'm used to sharing with people from different areas. I forgot totally that I don't have parents. I really appreciate what I get from other people. So if people are laughing at me now, I don't cry, so up with Marjorie.

As disabled women, we didn't know what to do after being disabled. The job of women in the community is to make the traditional African beer that is drunk by the men at special ceremonies. We were very excited when one of the women made a clay sculpture of the pot from which the men drink different African brews. The pot reminded other women of what they could do. When we sat down and thought about our future, we realized we could make *mqombothi* [African beer] and sell it. We realized that in this group we would succeed. We could make *marewu* [sour milk] in this calabash whilst we're still alive so that we can succeed. So this pot (group) gave us life and a name in our community.'

SELF-DEVELOPMENT, CREATIVITY, AND ADVOCACY

The women found that the workshops were a good space where they felt nurtured. One woman made a clay sculpture of a tree to symbolize the potential among them. The tree's roots represented the women growing as different people from different areas. They made friends as they have been together in the workshops. The passion and energy for advocacy and spreading the message revealed an evangelical zeal. The women grew in confidence to speak about disability to other disabled and nondisabled women as well

---

[2]A rural area in the Eastern Cape.
[3]An NGO in Khayelitsha that provide nutrition programs for children and skills development in income generation for mothers and women.

as the wider community organizations (Figure 16.3). It inspired their self-development. They mobilized each other to rethink their images of disability and challenge public stereotypes. They acted collectively to raise awareness and advocate for change in attitudes towards disability.

These stories portray some of the tensions of personal and social change, which disabled women have to negotiate in pursuit of freedom, inclusion, and equal participation. Disability and innate potential, realism and anticipation, fact and faith, permanence and transience are juxtaposed throughout a poem, "Waiting to Succeed," which was composed from the women's responses to a question, "What are you waiting for?" that was posed by the facilitators. The poem is an edited extract from a published correction of their stories about living with a disability in Khayelitsha (Lorenzo et al., 2002).

Waiting to Succeed

> *I am waiting for success in my life,*
> *whereby God will give me power to succeed in my struggles*
> *so that one day I can help other people who are struggling*
> *and teach them that they must take what they have,*
> *even if it's small,*
> *and know that success lies within themselves.*
> *I am waiting for success in my heart;*
> *As a disabled person, even if I'm sitting,*
> *I have hope inside.*
> *I am waiting for success in my problems;*
> *Since I became disabled, things are slow,*
> *now I must first think*
> *about how I'm going to get something,*
> *then wait until I get it . . .*
> *I am waiting for God*
> *to give me freedom*
> *to get a job, to get money*
> *so that I can buy small things to sell . . .*
> *so that I can have a perm*
> *and be beautiful more than this.*
> *I am waiting for happiness,*
> *for hope that God will add more years to my life . . .*
> *I am waiting to be helped with my disability,*
> *for a walking stick to help me walk,*
> *because my legs are too lame to walk on my own . . .*
> *Some hardships in this world come and go.*
> *I am waiting for Jesus to come and free me*
> *from my ties and problems.*
> *The devil is waiting for big things from me*
> *but he will never get them*
> *because I don't belong to him.*
> *I pray and worship the One above who helps me.*
> *I am waiting to succeed*
> *in all that I wish and hope and pray for.*
> *And I will see the results of all these things*
> *in my disability and in my children.*[4]

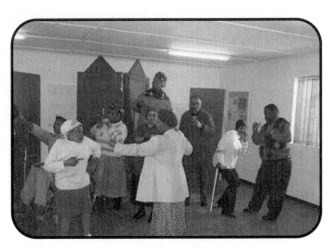

FIGURE 16.3   Disabled women and men are trained in drama for disability awareness and advocacy by the Community Arts Project.

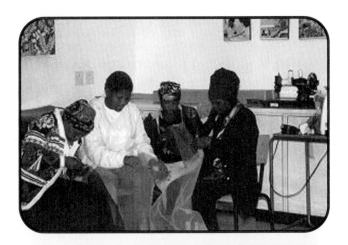

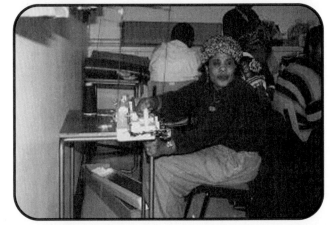

FIGURE 16.4   Disabled women participate in a skills development workshop to demonstrate sewing and machine knitting skills as a means for small business development.

---

[4]"Waiting to Succeed," from a creative activity with women in a NAR workshop. The poem is an edited extract from a published collection of their stories about living with a disability in Khayelitsha (Lorenzo et al., 2002).

REFLECTIVE SUMMARY

The workshops created a space for the women to make their voices heard. Their stories reveal that disability is a human rights issue in the struggle of disabled people for opportunities to participate as equal citizens of their community and country. The complexity and multidimensional nature of poverty require a collective approach of individuals, families, communities, organizations, and institutions to sustain change initiatives. The stories in this chapter show that it is feasible for occupational therapists, as professionals and academics, to engage with disabled people in partnerships for research and development that leads to social action and change.

Fifteen women who had participated regularly in the monthly NAR workshops published their stories about the changes that happened in a book titled *On the Road of Hope: Stories of Disabled Women in Khayelitsha* (Lorenzo, Saunders, January, & Mdlokolo, 2002).[5] The women were excited and proud when they received copies of the book, which raised their morale and self-esteem. Profits from the book go back into the Disabled Women's Development Project of DPSA for other development initiatives.

This chapter suggests that there is not much about these stories that would distinguish these women from other nondisabled women. Such evidence supports the fact that their impairments do not make the women unable to learn and achieve. The potential for responding to rebuilding the social fabric of our communities would be applicable to any other disadvantaged groups as well. The power of the collective to foster change through engage-ment in occupations at individual and societal levels was evident, as it facilitates an inward journey that leads to outward actions. The spirituality of the women reinforced their resilience to address the obstacles they encountered. Occupational therapists should move from the comfortable zone of individual rehabilitation to embrace the sociopolitical and economic challenges that face many of the people with whom we work. Such shifts to a population approach will foster optimal human development and engagement in occupations that will contribute to the promotion of healthy lifestyles and an inclusive, just society.

REFERENCES

Clandinin, D. J., & Connelly, F. M. (2000). *Narrative inquiry: Experience and story in qualitative research* San Francisco: Jossey-Bass Publishers.

Hope, A., & Timmel, S. (1995). *Training for transformation: A handbook for community workers* (rev. ed.). Zimbabwe: Mambo Press.

Lorenzo, T., Saunders, C., January, M., & Mdlokolo, P. (Eds.). (2002) *On the road of hope: Stories told by disabled women in Khayelitsha.* Cape Town: Division of Occupational Therapy, University of Cape Town.

Slim, H., & Thompson, P. (1993). *Listening for a change: Oral testimony and development* London: Panos Publications Ltd.

Taylor, J., Marais, D., and Kaplan, A (1997). *Action learning for development: Use your experience to improve your effectiveness.* Cape Town: Juta and CDRA.

Taylor, V. (2000). *South Africa: Transformation for human development 2000.* Pretoria: United Nations Development Programme.

---

[5]The book was sponsored by the Centre for the Book and formed part of Adult Literacy Week in September 2002.

III

OCCUPATION AND HEALTH IN SOCIETY

"Occupational therapy is a profession concerned with promoting health and well being through occupation. The primary goal of occupational therapy is to enable people to participate in the activities of everyday life. Occupational therapists achieve this outcome by enabling people to do things that will enhance their ability to participate or by modifying the environment to better support participation."

World Federation of Occupational Therapy

Social and Health Policies in the United States

17

JAN NISBET

Learning Objectives

After reading this chapter, you will be able to:

1. Understand social and health policies and the major U.S. agencies responsible for people with health conditions and/or disabilities and their families.
2. Understand the role of advocacy in the development of public policies and associated regulatory processes.
3. Distinguish between general health care and long-term care.
4. Understand public entitlement programs and how they affect the lives of people with health conditions and/or disabilities and their families.
5. Articulate legislative initiatives that created programs and services for people with health conditions and/or disabilities and their families.

PUBLIC POLICY

Put simply, "public policy is anything a government chooses to do or not to do" (Dye, 1972, p. 2.) The public or social policy decisions take form in laws, regulations, funding decisions, and other actions that serve to communicate to the citizens or constituents. Public policymaking requires choices about the role of government in the lives of people and the responsibility engendered by citizens, states, and/or the federal government. The policies reflect attitudes, opinions, interests, and ideologies (Howlett & Ramesh, 2003). Theories suggest that policymakers as well as citizens are guided by self-interest and make choices according to "best advantage." For example, the Americans with Disabilities Act (1990) was passed after people with disabilities organized to gained access to public and private facilities and services. Many businesses opposed the ADA because they feared that ensuring access and providing accommodations was too costly. Policymakers made a decision to support the law with caveats such as "to the maximum extent possible," thereby appeasing businesses and individuals with disabilities and assuring constituent satisfaction. Clearly, private and public organizations and groups influence public policies, but they do not enact laws. Elected officials in the legislature have that responsibility. However, understanding how to influence public policy is critical. Equally important is understanding the nature of influence and the role that organized groups with organized resources can have.

Silverstein (2000) identified five categories of laws affecting people with disabilities:

- Civil rights statutes (e.g., ADA, Fair Housing Act of 1968)
- Entitlement programs (e.g., Medicaid, vocational rehabilitation)
- Discretionary grant programs (e.g., Individuals with Disabilities Education Act, Centers for Independent Living)
- Regulatory statutes (e.g., Voter Registration Act of 1973, Family Leave Act)
- Miscellaneous provisions (e.g., Targeted Jobs Credit, Disabled Access Tax Credit).

He also summarized the core underlying principles that provide the framework for disability policy in the United States. These include (1) equality of opportunity; (2) full participation, empowering individuals and families; (3) independent living; and (4) economic self-sufficiency. These core principles have been articulated by advocates and legislators in many legislative actions and efforts, and they continue to be reframed and reemphasized in emerging policy initiatives.

ADVOCATING FOR CHANGE

Numerous advocates of community organizing to influence public policy (Alinsky, 1989; Biklen, 1982) make clear the role of powerful corporations and interests in the development of policies and practices that are not congruent with community welfare. Our inability, as a nation, to move toward universal health care can be blamed in part on powerful private markets, including health insurance, private medicine, and pharmaceutical companies (Johnson & Broder, 1996). Advocacy groups, such as ADAPT, represent individuals with disabilities who want affordable and accessible transportation and the removal of the **institutional bias** in the Medicaid program. Institutional bias refers to the fact that dollars can be expended on institutional care, nursing home care, or other segregated settings but cannot be expended in community-based settings. Advocacy groups have used effective strategies that require organized efforts to confront powerful interest groups. Each year, members of ADAPT protest at the annual meeting of the American Hospital Association, another group that has opposed removing the institutional bias in the Medicaid program. Federal legislation designed to support and more fully fund community-based services has been opposed by the powerful nursing home industry and, as a result, has not been passed and implemented. ADAPT is an example of one kind of advocacy group. Others exist to represent the interests of organizations such as community health care clinics, and service providers (e.g., American Occupational Therapy Association) as well as specific populations, such as children, retirees, people with Alzheimer's, and people with amyotrophic lateral sclerosis, multiple sclerosis, Down syndrome, autism, and others.

Organized protests are one form of advocacy. Christopher Kush (2004) in his book *The One-Hour Activist* recommends 20 strategies that anyone can use to influence policies:

1. Learn how grassroots advocacy works.
2. Pick your issues and your angle.
3. Identify and meet with your senators and representatives.
4. Join an interest group.
5. Create a legislative agenda.
6. Analyze a bill.
7. Conduct opposition research.
8. Write an effective letter.
9. Send a powerful e-mail.
10. Make a compelling phone call.
11. Persuade others to act.
12. Get out the vote.
13. Contribute money to candidates who support your cause.
14. Start a press clippings file.
15. Write a letter to the editor.
16. Have a face-to-face meeting with your representative.
17. Testify at a public hearing.
18. Participate in a protest.
19. Volunteer for a political campaign.
20. Pitch a news story or give an interview (p. viii).

Each of these strategies, alone or combined, can move a public policy agenda forward. Although individuals can make a difference acting alone, organized groups have proved more effective in influencing the outcomes of elections and public policy reforms.

PUBLIC HEALTH: THE FEDERAL ROLE

The World Health Organization (1946) defines health as a state of complete physical, mental, and social well-being, not merely the absence of disease or infirmity. Public health emphasizes population-based interventions and measures as well as prevention of both primary and secondary conditions and disabilities. Public health can be viewed broadly and interpreted to encompass prevention, both acute and long-term care, and overall community infrastructure and is focused on the health of the population rather than on that of any specific individual. According to the Institute of

Medicine (1988, 2002), the mission of public health is defined as "fulfilling society's interest in assuring conditions in which people can be healthy." Gordon (1997) defines *pubic health* as the art and science of preventing disease and injury and promoting health and efficiency through organized community effort. In contrast, *health care* involves the diagnosis, treatment, or rehabilitation of a patient who is under care, accomplished on a one-to-one basis (as cited in Patel & Rushefsky, 2005, p. xii) Only 2–3% of all health care expenditures in the United States are directed at public health (McFarlane, 2005). The vast majority of dollars are spent on curative health rather than preventive health (Patel & Rushefsky, 2005). Despite this disparity in funding, Americans' life expectancy has increased by 30 years in the last century. Twenty-five of these years are attributable to public health campaigns to increase seatbelt use and to reduce coronary artery disease, more family planning, improved oral health, fluoridation of drinking water, decline in smoking, better sanitation, improved safety in the workplace, vaccines, and improved pregnancy practices (Patel & Rushefsky, 2005).

Medicaid, for example, is a federal and state program that many people consider to be a public health program and that is targeted to people who have lower incomes and those with disabilities. Yet one could argue that it focuses primarily on health care but funds many things that are considered to be in the realm of public health, such as screening and vaccinations. It supports parents, children, seniors, and people with disabilities. Administered by the **Centers for Medicaid and Medicare Services (CMS)** in the U.S. Department of Health and Human Services, Medicaid provides a useful lens through which to understand public health and health care policies involving people who are poor, are elderly, and/or have disabilities. Medicare, the federally funded insurance program for individuals over the age of 65 years and for younger individuals with specific disabilities, is also considered a public health program by some yet funds primarily treatment-related activities. Because there are so many definitions of public health, it is sometimes difficult to describe exactly what it is and why it needs to be supported (Patel & Rushefsky, 2005).

The **Centers for Disease Control (CDC)** "is the principal agency in the United States government for protecting the health and safety of all Americans and for providing essential human services, especially for those people who are least able to help themselves" (CDC, 2006). Founded in 1948 to help the United States combat the threat of malaria, the CDC today has far-reaching goals (see Box 17.1). The CDC addresses these goals through public awareness, dissemination of evidence-based practices, research, and working with other public and private entities to advance prevention and wellness (Lang, Moore, Harris, & Anderson, 2005). It makes the public aware of "threats" to their health such as tobacco use, overconsumption of alcohol, risky sexual behavior, poor

---

BOX 17.1	CDC GOALS

1. Healthy people at every stage of life
2. Healthy people in healthy places
3. People prepared for emerging health threats
4. Healthy people in a healthy world

---

nutrition, inactivity, obesity, and environmental toxins. The CDC also serves as an important source to inform and alert policymakers about impending public health threats. For example, the CDC has focused on improving the health infrastructure necessary to respond to the avian flu virus, bioterrorism, and natural disasters such as hurricanes.

The **Health Resources and Services Administration (HRSA)** in the U.S. Department of Health and Human Services is the primary federal agency for improving access to health care services for people who are uninsured, isolated or medically vulnerable (HRSA, 2007). It has seven goals (see Box 17.2). It accomplishes these goals by funding numerous programs such as community health centers, the national health service corps, training for diversity and disparities in health care, public health workforce development, nursing programs, the maternal and child health block grant, programs for people with traumatic brain injuries, Healthy Start, universal newborn hearing screening, genetic services, and emergency services for children's rural health programs. The HRSA works closely with other agencies such as the CDC, the Food and Drug Administration, the Environmental Protection Agency, the Indian Health Service, the Occupational Safety and Health Administration, and the National Institutes of Health to advance its goals.

BOX 17.2	HRSA GOALS

1. Improve access to health care.
2. Improve health outcomes.
3. Improve the quality of health care.
4. Eliminate health disparities.
5. Improve the public health and health care systems.
6. Enhance the ability of the health care system to respond to public health emergencies.
7. Achieve excellence in management practices.

PUBLIC HEALTH INITIATIVES

There are numerous public health initiatives and programs, many of them underfunded. For example, in 1988, the Institute on Medicine (IOM), which has as a mission "to serve as an unbiased and objective advisor to the nation to improve health," undertook a study of our nation's public health system. Many members believed that the U.S. system was in disarray and that the United States was ignoring such issues as HIV-AIDS, exposure to toxic chemicals, the aging of America, chronic illness, and disability. The IOM reported that millions of Americans (over 25%) do not have a regular source of health care or have difficulty obtaining it. The Kaiser Commission on Medicaid and the Uninsured (2006) reported that 17% of people with moderate incomes, 36% of the poor, and 30% of the near-poor were uninsured in 2003, an increase of 1.4 million from 2002. This amounts to a total of 44.7 million non-elderly (under age 65 years) who are uninsured in the United States. The uninsured have poorer health outcomes, more unnecessary hospitalizations, and higher rates of emergency room utilization; get diagnosed later with significant illnesses; and have higher mortality rates than those with insurance. (Bodenheimer & Grumbach, 2002).

The IOM followed up on the earlier study conducted in 1988 and made a number of recommendations regarding the public health system that address the multiple factors that affect the population. Each of these recommendations has implications for public policy refinement and development (Institute of Medicine, 2002, p. 4):

1. Adopting a population health approach that considers the multiple determinants of health
2. Strengthening the governmental public health infrastructure, which forms the backbone of the public health system
3. Building a new generation of intersectoral partnerships that also draw on the perspectives and resources of diverse communities and actively engage them in health action
4. Developing systems of accountability to ensure the quality and availability of public health services
5. Making evidence the foundation of decision making and the measure of success
6. Enhancing and facilitating communication within the public health system (e.g., among all levels of the governmental public health infrastructure and between public health professionals and community members)

THE HEALTH CARE WORKFORCE

Clearly, one of the factors necessary to improve public health is the workforce. Unlike clinical health workers, public health professionals are educated specifically to

have a population versus a patient or individualized focus. Gebbie, Rosenstock, and Herandez (2003) report that these professionals are taught by using an ecological model of health that emphasizes the interaction among multiple determinants of health and emphasizes the core disciplines of biostatistics, epidemiology, environmental health, health services administration, and social and behavioral science. New disciplines are emerging and are increasingly part of public health curricula. Areas such as informatics, genomics, communication, cultural competence, community-based participatory research, policy and law, global health, and ethics are considered essential tools to track population trends, identify population and regionally specific health issues, and understand the impact of new technologies on health outcomes. Schools and programs in public health are and will have to continue to adapt to the global forces and emergent threats and issues such as avian flu, drug resistant tuberculosis, AIDS, and environmentally induced illnesses. Public policymakers, primarily through the HRSA, have targeted public dollars for the purposes of training health professionals. These policy responses, however, have not met the need expressed by both the IOM and the American Public Health Association.

PUBLIC HEALTH PRIORITIES

The **Office of the Surgeon General** (2006) has identified seven public health priorities (see Box 17.3). Each of these priorities will require policies, regulations, and funding by the U.S. government, state governments, and, increasingly, private foundations such as the Robert Wood Johnson Foundation, the Kaiser Family Foundation, and the numerous health conversion foundations that resulted from the sale of not-for-profit entities such as Blue Cross/Blue Shield and/or hospitals to for-profit entities.

INVOLVEMENT OF THE PRIVATE SECTOR

Access to employment-based health insurance has decreased over the past 10 years. The U.S. economy has transitioned to a lower-wage, increasingly part-time, and nonunionized workforce. As a result, there are increasing numbers of Americans without health insurance. Yet the United States relies heavily on the private sector to fund and support health care. Our pluralistic health care system is the result of numerous policy decisions without a comprehensive restructuring of the system composed of public health, private providers including physicians and hospitals, and the public and private insurance markets. Rosenbaum (2003) argues that our public health is threatened by the overreliance on the private insurance market. Medicare Part D, the prescription drug benefit program

BOX 17.3 · PRIORITIES OF THE OFFICE OF THE SURGEON GENERAL

1. Disease prevention (HIV-AIDS, tobacco use, birth defects, preventing injury, obesity, and increasing physical activity)
2. Eliminating health disparities (eliminating the greater burden of death and disease from breast cancer, prostate cancer, cervical cancer, cardiovascular disease, diabetes, and other illnesses in minority communities)
3. Public health preparedness (terrorism, emerging infections, natural disasters, mental health, and resilience)
4. Improving health literacy (the ability of an individual to access, understand, and use health-related information and services to make appropriate health decisions)
5. Organ donation
6. Encouraging children and adolescents to make healthy choices
7. Bone health and osteoporosis (10 million Americans over the age of 50 years have osteoporosis, the most common bone disease, while another 34 million are at risk for developing osteoporosis, and each year, roughly 1.5 million people suffer a bone fracture related to osteoporosis)

for individuals over the age of 65 years, is an example of a public policy that relies on private markets—in this case, the pharmaceutical industry to provide health care. Health maintenance organizations (HMOs) have attempted to reduce health care costs by focusing on prevention and managing care. Bodenheimer and Grumbach (2002) argue that HMOs currently see themselves as responsible for individual enrollees but should also have the responsibility for offering comprehensive preventive health care to the entire enrolled population.

CASE STUDY: *Living with Amyotrophic Lateral Sclerosis*

This case study is designed to illustrate the variety of public health issues and public policies that a person and his or her family can confront during an illness or the onset of a disability.

Toby is a 57-year-old man who was recently diagnosed with amyotrophic lateral sclerosis (ALS). Before his diagnosis, he was working as a restaurant manager without health care benefits. He is able to work but fatigues easily. His physicians say that the course of his illness is unpredictable and that he might need to be in a wheelchair by the end of the year. He did not have medical insurance through his job and was unable to pay the premiums for an individual plan. His two adolescent children qualified for the State Children's Health Insurance Plan and receive routine medical care. His wife, who also works full-time, has a limited health insurance plan through her employer. When Toby first noticed his symptoms, growing weakness and clumsiness, he went to the emergency room, where a number of tests were administered. He was sent home with no diagnosis. He returned several times, each time complaining that he was getting worse. After his third visit, he was diagnosed with ALS, a neurodegenerative disease that usually attacks both upper and lower motor neurons and causes degeneration throughout the brain and spinal cord. A common first symptom is a painless weakness in a hand, foot, arm, or leg, which occurs in more than half of all cases. Other early symptoms include difficulty in speech, swallowing, or walking. Most commonly, the disease strikes people between the ages of 40 and 70, and as many as 30,000 Americans have the disease at any given time. ALS is progressive and generally fatal (Amyotrophic Lateral Sclerosis Association, 2004). The emergency room physician recommended that Toby apply for Social Security Disability Insurance (SSDI) and Medicaid. Toby did not know about these programs and went to the Social Security Office to ask for an application. This is what he learned about SSDI, Medicaid, and Medicare.

Entitlement Programs: Social Security Disability Insurance, Supplemental Security Income, Medicaid, and Medicare

Social Security Disability Insurance (SSDI) is a public program for people who meet the medical definition of "disability" and who have worked at least 10 years and paid FICA taxes for 5 of the past 10 years of employment. To be considered disabled, a person must prove that he or she is unable to engage in substantial gainful activity for a period that has lasted 12 months or is expected to last 12 months. Once an authorized physician has made the determination that the person is disabled, a benefit based on wages earned over time is calculated. The amount is approximately 85% of the highest wages earned during the past several years. This program is different from Supplemental

CASE STUDY: *Living with Amyotrophic Lateral Sclerosis* *Continued*

Security Income (SSI). Supplemental Security Income is available to people who meet the statutory definition of disability, are also unable to engage in substantial gainful activity, and are "indigent." This means that they have less than $2,000 in assets and do not have a history of earning substantial wages. The State Children's Health Insurance Program (P.L. 105-33), Title XXI of the Social Security Act, allows states to expand Medicaid eligibility to uninsured low-income children. As a result of the act, states have expanded eligibility to larger numbers of children. For the adult with a disability, the income cap is around $690 per month, depending on the source of income (unearned or earned). Above that cap, the person can be eligible for Medicaid but is responsible for a certain amount of costs per month (called a *spend down*). For example, an adult who receives $1,800 from SSDI would have to spend down about $1,300 each month to qualify for Medicaid. Each of his children would be allocated an exemption, and states have options to exempt various types of incomes and medically necessary expenses.

If the person is eligible for a waiver, the income caps are higher to qualify for Medicaid, but the person must pay a monthly fee (called *cost of care*). Medicaid waivers are authorized under Section 1915(c) of the Social Security Act and allow the Secretary of the U.S. Department of Health and Human Services to waive certain Medicaid statutory requirements. As a result, states can pay for home and community-based services (HCBS) for specific populations. Under the Deficit Reduction Act of 2006, services that once required a waiver may be offered as an optional benefit. However, if states choose to implement this provision, they may also cap the number of people receiving services, which many believe undermines the Medicaid entitlement to services. In many families, as a result, children have health insurance while their parents do not. For example, in New Hampshire, the children can receive "Healthy Kids" Medicaid if the family's income is under 300% of the federal poverty level (based on number of people in the household). For a family of two parents with two children, this is approximately $28,000 per year of income. The adults will not receive Medicaid unless the family is low-income and the adults have a disability.

Individuals are eligible for Medicare if they or their spouses worked at least 10 years and paid payroll taxes and are 65 years of age or in a special disability category. People who have ALS also qualify for Medicare even though they are not 65 years of age. There is a special provision for this population. In these situations, they are eligible for both Medicaid and Medicare. Medicare is a federal public health insurance program provided to every American over the age of 65 and to some other groups, including those who have received SSDI for two years, those with renal failure, and those with

ALS prior to that age. There are other specific groups, as described in regulation, that also qualify. Medicare pays for hospitalizations and medical expenses and, most recently through Part D, prescription drug coverage. It is funded through employee and employer payroll taxes and monthly premiums deducted from Social Security checks. It does not pay for many expenses associated with long-term care.

Toby qualifies for SSDI, according to his physician and the Social Security Office. He is told that the disability determination process will likely take 60 to 90 days, and from that date he will have a six-month waiting period from the time he is deemed eligible to receive his first SSDI check. In the meantime, Toby needs ongoing medical care, including adaptive equipment to help him with daily tasks. He will need a walker and eventually a wheelchair, and he will need physical and occupational therapy in the future. There are also several drugs that were recommended that are very expensive. Toby will have to rely on his wife's wages and their savings until he begins to receive the monthly SSDI check. Toby is eligible for Medicare because he has ALS. He might be able to qualify for Medicaid because he meets the definition of disability. But he must also qualify on the basis of his income (income under $13,330 for a family of three). To qualify, he might have to spend down some of his income, and he must have $2,500 or less in liquidatable assets.

Medicaid

Medicaid, or Title XIX of the Social Security Act, is a state-administered program for people who meet certain eligibility categories and have limited incomes. These categories include children, pregnant women, and individuals with disabilities and/or over the age of 65 years. The federal government matches the state allocation, using a complicated formula based on the state's demographic characteristics. The Medicaid program was not designed for people who are simply poor. They must also be in one of the eligible categories. The Kaiser Commission (2006) reported that in 2005, Medicaid provided insurance coverage to 52 million individuals. Its budget has grown by one third since 2001. The growth is related to an increase in the number of people in poverty and those without private health insurance. The following are categorically needy groups (Centers for Medicaid and Medicare Services, 2006):

- Individuals who meet the Aid to Families with Dependent Children (AFDC) program that were in effect in their state on July 16, 1996
- Children under age 6 years whose family income is at or below 133% of the federal poverty level (FPL)
- Pregnant women whose family income is below 133% of the FPL (Services to these women are limited to
Continued

CASE STUDY: *Living with Amyotrophic Lateral Sclerosis*   *Continued*

those related to pregnancy, complications of pregnancy, delivery, and postpartum care.)

♦ Supplemental Security Income (SSI) recipients in most states (Some states use more restrictive Medicaid eligibility requirements that predate SSI.)

♦ Recipients of adoption or foster care assistance under Title IV of the Social Security Act

♦ Special protected groups (typically individuals who lose their cash assistance due to earnings from work or from increased Social Security benefits but who may keep Medicaid for a period of time)

♦ All children born after September 30, 1983, who are under age 19 years and are in families with incomes at or below the FPL

♦ Certain Medicare beneficiaries

There are also optional groups (CMS, 2006) to which states can elect to provide Medicaid coverage. They include the following:

♦ Infants up to age 1 and pregnant women not covered under the mandatory rules whose family income is no more than 185% of the FPL (the percentage amount is set by each state)

♦ Children under age 21 who meet criteria more liberal than the AFDC income and resources requirements that were in effect in their state on July 16, 1996

♦ Institutionalized individuals eligible under a "special income level" (the amount is set by each state—up to 300% of the SSI federal benefit rate)

♦ Individuals who would be eligible if institutionalized but who are receiving care under HCBS waivers

♦ Certain aged, blind, or disabled adults who have incomes above those requiring mandatory coverage but below the FPL

♦ Recipients of state supplementary income payments

♦ Certain working and disabled individuals with family income less than 250% of the FPL who would qualify for SSI if they did not work

♦ TB-infected individuals who would be financially eligible for Medicaid at the SSI income level if they were within a Medicaid-covered category (However, coverage is limited to TB-related ambulatory services and TB drugs.)

♦ Certain uninsured or low-income women who are screened for breast or cervical cancer through a program administered by the CDC. The Breast and Cervical Cancer Prevention and Treatment Act of 2000 (P.L. 106-354) provides these women with medical assistance and follow-up diagnostic services through Medicaid

♦ "Optional targeted low-income children" included within the State Children's Health Insurance Program established by the Balanced Budget Act of 1997 (P.L. 105-33)

♦ "Medically needy" individuals

Because each state designs and administers it own programs, eligibility and benefits vary. A person could be eligible in one state and found to be ineligible in another. In addition, a person could receive one set of services in one state and a different set in another. Medicaid pays for medical services, both acute and long-term care. This includes the following:

♦ Inpatient hospital services

♦ Outpatient hospital services

♦ Prenatal care

♦ Vaccines for children

♦ Physician services

♦ Nursing facility services for persons aged 21 years or older

♦ Family-planning services and supplies

♦ Rural health clinic services

♦ Home health care for individuals who are eligible for skilled nursing services

♦ Laboratory and X-ray services

♦ Pediatric and family nurse-practitioner services

♦ Nurse-midwife services.

♦ Federally qualified health center services

♦ Early and periodic screening, diagnostic, and treatment services for children under age 21 years

States may also choose to receive federal Medicaid matching dollars for optional services. These include diagnostic services, clinic services, intermediate care facilities for the mentally retarded, prescribed drugs and prosthetic devices, optometrist services and eyeglasses, nursing facility services for children under age 21, transportation services, occupational and physical therapy services, home and community-based care to certain individuals with chronic impairments, and others (CMS, 2006). The level of reimbursement for these services varies. In some cases, private physicians will refuse to see Medicaid recipients because the reimbursement for their care is less that 25% of the cost of providing the services. This is a huge barrier to accessing good-quality health care, including dental care.

Currently, Toby is not able to qualify for Medicaid services based on the state plan. He has too many assets and has been saving for his children's education. His wife's income is also deemed to be available to him. To receive Medicaid services, he will have to spend down his savings. His house and vehicle do not count against his assets. His anticipated monthly SSDI check will not be more than approximately $1,800 per month. He will quickly become indigent as his nonreimbursable medical costs increase with his illness. At that point, he will qualify financially for Medicaid. Toby's doctors told him that he could end up in a nursing home. He does not want this. He wants to remain at home with his family and receive care there. A state Medicaid program designed through an option called the Elderly and Chronically Ill (ECI) Waiver pays for

CASE STUDY: *Living with Amyotrophic Lateral Sclerosis*   *Continued*

long-term care expenses and could help him. Toby calls the Medicaid Office to inquire about getting waiver services. He has been told that in his state, the limit for home and community-based care under the ECI Waiver is that the cost of services has to be less than 50% of what it costs for a nursing home. This means that if his services exceed the 50% limit, he will have to go to a nursing home to receive the necessary care, even if it can be provided at home. Some critics refer to this as the institutional bias in the Medicaid program. Because Toby has a disability, he can receive Medicaid but will have to spend down his assets over time to remain qualified.

Community-Based Care

The fields of disabilities, chronic illness, and aging have seen numerous changes over the past decade. This ideological and legislative trend away from institutionalization toward home and community-based services has been only partially supported by fiscal policies with major incentives in Title XIX (Grants to States for Medical Assistance) and Title XVIII (Health Insurance for the Aged and Disabled) of the Social Security Act programs and fiscal structures that support institutional care. Resource allocation has varied extensively with groups and across states not necessarily favoring community supports. The imbalance has produced an institutionalized population of people with developmental disabilities as well as numerous elders in nursing homes. It has also established a divided set of interests within the professionals and direct care staff employed in this arena. There is a powerful nursing home lobby in this country that has rejected removing the institutional bias in the Medicaid program. People in need of long-term services and supports desperately need some alternative in order to overcome the current institutional funding biases. Under the Deficit Reduction Act (2005), states can provide home and community-based services as part of their state plan without seeking a specific waiver to do so. This has the potential to improve the availability of home and community-based care and remove the institutional bias in Medicaid services. However, there are ongoing efforts to restrict the entitlement to Medicaid because of its rapid growth.

Toby realizes that he and his family face significant challenges. He has sought assistance from an ALS support group, which meets monthly. He feels as though he is learning more about the disease and his disability. One of the group members suggested that he contact the Independent Living Center to help with benefits counseling and personal assistance services. These services consist of formal and informal help provided to people with disabilities to assist them in activities of daily living. The Independent Living Center provides personal assistance services. The group also suggested that Toby contact the Assistive Technology Center to learn about devices

that might help him. He contacts both and is provided with numerous ideas and supports for the present and the future.

Contemporary Disability Policy: Independent Living, Inclusion, and Choice

The core values of contemporary disability policy are based on independent living, equal opportunity, self-determination, community inclusion, and participation. Statutes at the federal and state levels widely embody principles of nondiscrimination; least restrictive environment; access to education, employment, and housing; and consumer direction and control. The Americans with Disabilities Act (1990) promotes access to public and private facilities and programs while prohibiting discrimination against people with disabilities. Many states have already included statutory language in legislation affecting people with disabilities and those who are aging that ensure consumer choice, control, and planning. In 1999, the U.S. Supreme Court ruled in *Olmstead v. L. C. & E. W.* (1999). Writing for the majority, Justice Ruth Bader Ginsburg said that under Title II of the federal Americans with Disabilities Act, "states are required to place persons with mental disabilities in community settings rather than in institutions when the State's treatment professionals have determined that community placement is appropriate, the transfer from institutional care to a less restrictive setting is not opposed by the affected individual, and the placement can be reasonably accommodated, taking into account the resources available to the State and the needs of others with mental disabilities."

This court ruling as well as other state legal cases provided the needed impetus to motivate states to develop "Olmstead Plans" that identified barriers to living independently in the community. These barriers, attitudinal, fiscal, and policy-related, are being addressed in a systematic fashion in many states. More and more people are rejecting nursing home care and other forms of institutionalized care in favor of home and community-based options. Furthermore, they seek more control over the services and supports that they do receive. New solutions such as personal assistance services, cash and counseling, and self-directed services and supports are being developed throughout the United States. Cash and Counseling, for example, is a program that provides dollars in the form of vouchers to individuals who want to purchase their own services outside of the service system that exists.

Other laws and policies support the principles of inclusion and self-determination. The Individuals with Disabilities Education Improvement Act (2006) promotes access to general education curricula for students with disabilities. The Rehabilitation Act of 1973 prohibits discrimination by entities that receive federal assistance from discriminating on the basis of disability. Title VII of the Act authorized the creation

Continued

of Independent Living Centers: nonresidential, community-based not-for-profit agencies run by and for people with disabilities that provide peer support, advocacy, independent living skill training, and information and referral. The development of these centers empowered members of the disability community to identify and help to develop policy solutions to existing policy barriers and gaps in services. Many centers provide assistive technology, equipment repair, personal assistance services, and housing assistance, including home modification. This ability was enhanced by the Technology-Related Assistance for Individuals with Disabilities Act of 1988, which "provides financial assistance to States to undertake activities that assist each State in maintaining and strengthening a permanent comprehensive statewide program of technology-related assistance, for individuals with disabilities of all ages, that is designed to increase the availability of, funding for, access to, and provision of, assistive technology devices and assistive technology services." Access to assistive technology enables many individuals to participate more fully in education, employment, and the community. Yet it does not necessarily address issues related to universal design. Mace, Hardie, and Place (1991) defined *universal design* as the design of products and environments to be usable by all people, to the greatest extent possible without the need for adaptation or specialized design. One area in which universal design has been applied is housing. Houses are being designed so that people who use wheelchairs or need mobility support can get in the front doors and use the bathrooms and kitchens. The visitability movement acknowledges that our houses should be able to accommodate our aging relatives and friends who have disabilities. (See Chapters 19 and 61 for more on visitability.)

It is three years since Toby was diagnosed with ALS. He is now using a wheelchair and needs assistance in dressing and eating. His disease seems to have slowed in the last three months. Because of excessive medical expenses, over a year ago Toby qualified for Medicaid and was able to qualify for the HCBS waiver under the ECI Waiver offered by the state. He continues to receive Medicare, which does not adequately cover all of his medical expense, and even with the new Medicaid prescription drug option (Part D), he must pay out of pocket for many of the prescriptions and generic drugs he needs. Under the waiver, he is receiving nursing and home health services in his home. However, under the waiver, he can receive only a maximum of $16,000 per year for all of his services. The home health agency bills the state for services at $30.00 per hour. This means that Toby can receive only 533 hours of services per year, or 44 hours of service each month. Toby's wife and children are helping out as well, but the amount of service is insufficient for his needs. His wife has to keep her full-time paid employment to pay expenses.

Additionally, there have been many times when a nurse has not been available. There are frequent changes in personnel, and on several occasions, Toby's wife has had to be late or miss work to care for Toby. His extended family provides some help, but they are unable to fill in all of the gaps. Toby and his wife, with support from the Independent Living Center, are directing their own services and have decided that the nursing level of care is not necessary. They are arranging to have a personal care assistant under the Consumer Directed Care Option provide the support at half the cost of home health services. This means that Toby and his family will receive approximately twice as much service, or 88 hours each month. They wonder how long they can get by with only 22 hours of service each week.

Transportation is also a problem. Although the family has a van, it is the only vehicle. When Toby has a medical appointment, his wife must take a day off from work, or Toby must use specialized transportation services. Going out simply to get out of the house when his wife is working is almost impossible because of lack or either fixed route or para-transit accessible transportation. Toby is essentially homebound.

Self-Direction and Consumer Directed Care

Control over one's life has been positively correlated with good health and self-esteem. Wagner, Nadash, Friedman, Litvak, and Eckels (1996) articulated principles of consumer-directed home and community-based services for elders and people with disabilities. Wehmeyer and Schwartz (1997) found in a follow-up study that young adults with mental retardation who exhibited more self-determined behaviors were more effective problem solvers; were more assertive and self-aware; and held significantly more adaptive perceptions of control, self-efficacy, outcome expectancy, and self-esteem. These findings have been supported by others studying empowerment and general health status. Therefore, the design of any public health system should reduce people's dependency on formal medical structures and integrate principles of consumer control and self-determination. Cash and Counseling is a nationally recognized approach that provides Medicaid participants the ability to directly pay for their own supports and services through a voucher-like system with support from service coordinators or case managers. In an evaluation of three state Cash and Counseling demonstration projects (Dale, Brown, & Shapiro, 2005), participants cited the following reasons for participation: more control over the hiring of caregivers, hiring family and friends, receiving care at more convenient times, and more and better-quality care. Cash and Counseling has been implemented in three states and is now being replicated with support from the Robert Wood Johnson Foundation in an additional 12 states. The approach to service delivery is supported by the CMS through the Independence Plus Waiver. This waiver was specifically informed

CASE STUDY: *Living with Amyotrophic Lateral Sclerosis* *Continued*

by the Cash and Counseling Demonstrations as well as the Self-Determination demonstrations that were implemented in 12 states. CMS reports that: "these programs afforded service recipients or their families the option to direct the design and delivery of services and supports, avoid unnecessary institutionalization, experience higher levels of satisfaction, and maximize the efficient use of community services and supports" (CMS, 2006). For states to receive an Independence Plus Waiver, they must include the following components in their Medicaid Plan:

♦ **Person-centered planning:** A process, directed by the participant, intended to identify the strengths, capacities, preferences, needs, and desired outcomes of the participant.

♦ **Individual budgeting:** The total dollar value of the services and supports, as specified in the plan of care, under the control and direction of the program participant.

♦ **Self-directed services and supports:** A system of activities that help the participant to develop, implement, and manage the support services identified in his or her individual budget.

♦ **Quality assurance and quality improvement (QA/QI):** The QA/QI model will build on the existing foundation, formally introduced under the CMS Quality Framework, of discovery, remediation, and continuous improvement (CMS, 2006).

Toby is requiring more and more care. He has made clear that he does not want to go to a nursing home. He is having difficulty swallowing, and he is using some alternative feeding methods. He has for several years used nighttime breathing support. His doctors believe that he will not survive for more than three more months. His children, now in college, visit frequently. His wife continues to work. Medicare is paying for his in-home medical care. Medicaid is paying for personal assistance services. Toby remains in control of his life and the decisions about his care.

Conclusion

Toby and his family have had to traverse the complicated health care and social service systems. The lack of coordination of care by human service agencies and the lack of access within the community have challenged the family's intellectual, physical, and financial resources. However, new models that emphasize self-direction, community engagement, and coordinated care can provide new opportunities for professionals and people with disabilities to work together to achieve better public policies that result in better health outcomes for all people. These models are part of a larger public health system that remains fragmented, difficult to traverse, and focused on treatment rather than prevention. Changes to these systems will be made only through organized advocacy efforts on behalf of and with people who lack health insurance and need community-based personal assistance services and income support programs. There are powerful interests that must be organized before there is any fundamental shift in our nation's health care system.

REFERENCES

Alinsky, S. (1989). *Rules for radicals.* New York: Vintage Press.

American Hospital Association. (2005). *Taking the pulse: The state of America's hospitals.* Retrieved July 6, 2006, from http://www.aha.org/resource-center

Americans with Disabilities Act of 1990, P.L. 101-336, 2(a), 42 U.S.C. §12101.

Amyotrophic Lateral Sclerosis Association. (2004). *About ALS.* Retrieved April 6, 2007, from http://www.alsa.org

Balanced Budget Act of 1997. P.L. 105-33.

Biklen, D. (1982). *Community organizing: Theory and practice.* New York: Prentice Hall

Bodenheimer, T. S., & Grumbach, K. (2002). *Understanding health policy: A clinical approach.* New York: Lange Medical Books/McGraw-Hill.

Breast and Cervical Cancer Prevention and Treatment Act of 2000. P.L. 106-354, 42 U.S.C. §1305.

Centers for Disease Control and Prevention. (2006). *About CDC.* Retrieved July 6, 2006, from http://www.cdc.gov/about/default.htm

Centers for Medicaid and Medicare Services. (2006). *CMS programs and information.* Retrieved July 6, 2006, from http://www.cms.hhs.gov

Dale, S., Brown, R., & Shapiro, R. (2005). *Assessing the appeal of the cash and counseling demonstration in Arkansas, New Jersey, and Florida.* Princeton, NJ: Mathematica Policy Research.

Deficit Reduction Act of 2005. P.L. 109-171, 120 Stat. 4.

Dye, T. (1972). *Understanding public policy.* Englewood Cliffs, NJ: Prentice-Hall.

Gebbie, K., Rosenstock, L., & Herandez, L. (Eds.). (2003). *Who will keep the public healthy?: Educating public health professionals for the 21st century.* Washington, DC: National Academies Press.

Gordon, L. J. (1997). Environmental health and protection. In F. D. Scutchfield and C. W. Keck (Eds.), *Principles of public health practice* (p. 301). Albany, NY: Delmar Publishers

Health Resources and Services Administration. (2007). *About HRSA.* Retrieved April 9, 2007, from http://www.hrsa.gov

Howlett, M. & Ramesh, M. (2003). *Studying public policy.* Don Mills, Ontario, Canada: Oxford University Press.

Johnson, H. & Broder, D. (1996). *The system.* Boston: Little Brown & Co.

Individuals with Disabilities Education Improvement Act of 2006, HR 1350, 20 U.S.C., 1400 *et seq.*

Institute of Medicine, Committee for the Study of the Future of Public Health, Division of Health Care Services. (1988).

The future of public health. Washington, DC: National Academies Press.

Institute of Medicine. (2002). *The future of the public's health in the 21st century: Shaping the future for health.* Washington, DC: National Academies Press.

Kaiser Commission on Medicaid and the Uninsured. (2006). *Deficit Reduction Act of 2005: Implications for Medicaid.* Washington, DC: Author.

Kush, C. (2004). *The one hour activist.* San Francisco, CA: Jossey-Bass.

Lang, J. E., Moore, M. J., Harris, A. C., & Anderson, L. A. (2005). Healthy aging: Priorities and programs of the Centers for Disease Control and Prevention. *Generations, 29*(2), 17–20.

Mace, R. L., Hardie, G. J., & Place, J. P. (1991). *Accessible environments: Toward universal design.* Raleigh, NC: Center for Universal Design, North Carolina State University.

McFarlane, D. R. (2005). Foreword. In Patel, K., & Rushefsky, M. E., *The politics of public health in the United States* (p. xii). Armonk, NY: M. E. Sharpe.

Office of the Surgeon General. (2006). Retrieved May 5, 2006, from http://www.surgeongeneral.gov/publichealth priorities.html

Olmstead v. L. C. & E. W. (98-536) 527 U.S. 581 (1999). 138 F.3d 893.

Patel, K., & Rushefsky, M. (2005). *The politics of public health in the United States.* Armonk, NY: M. E. Sharpe.

Rehabilitation Act of 1973, 29 U.S.C. § 720.

Rosenbaum, S. (2003). New directions for health insurance design: Implications for public health policy and practice. *Journal of Law, Medicine & Ethics.* Special supplement to Volume 31, Number 4: The public health and law in the 21st century.

Silverstein, R. (2000). Emerging disability framework: A guidepost for analyzing public policy. *Iowa Law Review, 85*(5), 1691–1797.

Technology-Related Assistance for Individuals with Disabilities Act of 1988 (P.L. 100-407), 29 U.S.C. 3001 *et seq.*

Wagner, D., Nadash, P., Friedman, A., Litvak, S., & Eckels, K. (1996). *Principles of consumer-directed home and community-based services.* Washington, DC: National Council on Aging.

Wehmeyer, M. L., & Schwartz, M. (1997). Self-determination and positive adult outcomes: A follow-up study of youth with mental retardation and learning disabilities. *Exceptional Children, 63,* 245–255.

World Health Organization (1946). *Constitution,* United Nations, Treaty Series, vol. 14, p. 185.

Health Promotion

LORI LETTS

Learning Objectives

After reading this chapter, you will be able to:

1. Understand definitions and approaches to health.
2. Become familiar with common terminology used in relation to health and health promotion.
3. Understand the principles and process of health promotion.
4. Understand how occupational therapists can be involved in promoting health.

INTRODUCTION

Health promotion seems like something that occupational therapists should be able to do quite easily. The goal of the profession is to promote health through engagement in meaningful occupations. This goal applies equally to people who are experiencing challenges in occupational performance, people with disabilities, and those who are healthy and independent. Because occupational therapy is premised on the importance of health through occupation, it seems natural for occupational therapists to be involved in health promotion; to promote health through meaningful engagement in occupation for all. However, health promotion is understood in many different ways, as is health itself. The purpose of this chapter is to provide definitions of health, health promotion, and related terms and to share ideas on how occupational therapists can apply the principles of health promotion in practice.

DEFINITIONS OF HEALTH

Health can be defined in many ways, although the definition from the World Health Organization (WHO) is probably the most frequently cited: "health is a state of complete physical, mental and social well-being and not merely the absence of disease or infirmity" (WHO, 1948).

Although frequently cited by many involved in health care and health promotion, the WHO definition of health has also been criticized. Seedhouse (2001) notes numerous problems with this definition. It implies that people cannot be healthy if they have a disease or infirmity; the definitions of physical, mental, and social well-being are unclear; and the definition of health is so ideal that it is impossible to achieve. Callahan (as cited in

Raeburn & Rootman, 1998) has suggested that the WHO definition of health has threatened the direction and costs of health services by suggesting that anything can be related to health. Nursing and academic definitions of health tend to be multidimensional, with emphasis on biopsychosocial components (Raeburn & Rootman, 1996). Evans and Stoddart (1990) suggest that definitions of health can be placed on a continuum with the WHO definition at one end and the traditional absence of disease definition at the other.

APPROACHES TO HEALTH

Depending on how health is understood, and even if the WHO definition is accepted, there are varying ways to approach health. Labonte (1993) provides a framework to describe how different understandings of health lead to different actions or approaches to address health problems. These include medical, behavioral, and socioenvironmental approaches to health. Labonte notes that the distinctions between these approaches are not always clear; nor do health professionals subscribe to one approach only. Rather, they represent global approaches that shed light on the various ways in which health problems are understood and addressed. These are summarized in Table 18.1.

The Medical Approach to Health

In the medical approach, health problems are understood primarily in relation to disease states, including common health problems such as cancer, cardiovascular disease, diabetes, mental illnesses, hypertension, and AIDS, as well as injuries that need to be treated in emergency departments. The medical approach to health promotion identifies risk factors for these disease states and works to prevent the diseases by decreasing the risk factors. This is done through interventions such as medications, illness care in hospitals, physician-supervised smoking reduction or diet regimens, and screening for other risk factors such as cholesterol or blood pressure levels. In terms of **prevention**, the focus of the medical approach is on preventing a person from becoming more ill or dying, which is sometimes referred to as *tertiary prevention*. The medical approach focuses on outcomes such as morbidity rates, mortality rates, and decreased prevalence of risk factors for disease (Labonte, 1993).

Occupational therapists working with people with posttraumatic hand injury or rehabilitation centers for people who have had strokes often adopt a medical approach to health. In many situations, this is very appropriate, since clients come to therapists with an acute or recent injury that is amenable to intervention; to assist them to return to their preinjury state. Splints, work conditioning, and constraint-induced movement therapy may all be interventions that are adopted by occupational therapists working from a medical approach to health.

The Behavioral Approach to Health

A behavioral approach to health focuses on individual lifestyle choices, health often being closely linked to wellness. Health problems are primarily related to behavioral risk factors, and this approach addresses behaviors such as smoking, poor fitness, drug and alcohol abuse, or limited abilities to cope with stress. The behavioral approach

TABLE 18.1   APPROACHES TO HEALTH

Approach	Medical	Behavioral	Socioenvironmental
Health definition	Biomedical; absence of disease or disability	Individualized; physical functional ability, physical well-being	Positive state; ability to do things that are important and have meaning
Targets for health initiatives and health problems	Individuals with health problems or at high risk for health problems such as cancer, diabetes, obesity	Individuals at high risk for health problems and children, to deal with health problems such as smoking, lack of fitness, limited life skills	High-risk conditions or environment with health problems such as poverty, unemployment, pollution, hazardous working conditions.
Strategies to improve health	Treating health problems through: surgery, drugs, illness care, medically managed behavior changes	Improving lifestyles or creating healthy lifestyles through health education, social marketing, advocacy for public policies supporting lifestyle choices	Creating healthy environments and creating healthy lifestyles through: personal empowerment, community organization, small group development, political action, coalition advocacy

involves health education, stress management or coping skills training, social marketing to help people make healthier lifestyle choices that will in turn improve their health, and encouraging children to adopt healthy lifestyles from early stages of life. Strategies are often implemented at the level of communities, although most frequently, health concerns are identified and strategies are developed by professionals. If the focus of the intervention is on preventing disease or injury by changing unhealthy behaviors, this is referred to as *secondary prevention*. If the focus is on developing and maintaining healthy behaviors, this is *primary prevention*. Success is benchmarked on the basis of behavioral changes and reducing behavioral risk factors (Labonte, 1993).

The American Occupational Therapy Association (AOTA) (2001) provides numerous examples that illustrate strategies to address health through a behavioral approach, including (to name only a few) educating and training to prevent secondary disabilities through such strategies as regular blood sugar checks and foot inspections for people with diabetes, educating caregivers about proper body mechanics for lifting a family member with a disability, teaching self-management to people with chronic conditions, and leading falls prevention sessions with older adults.

The Socioenvironmental Approach to Health

The socioenvironmental approach to health focuses on health as a positive state that has as a major priority social connections to family, friends, and communities. Health problems are understood as being tied to environmental risk conditions and psychosocial risk factors. Examples of risk conditions include poverty, limited education, unemployment, and hazardous living or working conditions. Psychosocial risk factors include such things as isolation, stress, and limited social networks. Labonte (1993) discusses five strategies to address health problems from the socioenvironmental perspective: personal care, small group development, community organization, coalition building and advocacy, and political action. These will be discussed later in this chapter specifically related to health promotion. The socioenvironmental approach is focused on primary prevention (creating healthy lifestyles) and health promotion (creating healthy living conditions). Success from a socioenvironmental perspective is based on indicators such as environmentally sustainable practices at personal and public levels, improved social networks, and more equitable social distribution of power and resources (Labonte, 1993).

Many occupational therapists who work with community organizations have adopted a socioenvironmental approach to health. For example, the Canadian Association of Occupational Therapists (CAOT) Seniors' Health Promotion Project (Letts, Fraser, Finlayson, & Walls, 1993) included initiatives such as an oral history program in which senior volunteers, trained by the occupational therapist, visited and collected oral histories from homebound seniors in Newfoundland. The aims of the oral history program were to address social isolation for homebound seniors and to foster skill development for the senior volunteers. In Manitoba, the occupational therapist provided an educational workshop to staff in a community recreation center to enable the inclusion of older adults with disabilities into the regular recreation programming at the center.

The three approaches to health described here are complementary. They can be applied in various ways to meet health goals. Problems are more likely to arise when too many resources are devoted to one approach to the detriment of the others. The following parable illustrates this point and demonstrates the value of each of the three approaches.

THINKING UPSTREAM: A POWERFUL METAPHOR

A number of health promotion documents cite a metaphor to explain how health promotion can be conceived as being different from traditional medical approaches to health. The metaphor, although varied depending on its source, can also be used to illustrate the different approaches to health described by Labonte (1993) and how each has its own place in efforts to optimize health for individuals and communities.

> One day a group of villagers was working in the fields by the river. Suddenly, someone noticed a man coming downstream, flailing in the water. A group of people rushed out and rescued the man and brought him to shore. One woman who helped rescue him brought him home to care for him.
>
> The next day, there were two people, a man and a woman flailing in the water, and the people who rescued them took them home to care for them. On the third day, there were three people. Before long, there was a steady stream of people needing rescue downstream. Soon the whole village was involved in the business of pulling flailing people out of the stream and ensuring that they were rehabilitated.
>
> One day someone decided to go upstream to find out how or why the people were ending up in the river. A huge controversy erupted. One group argued that every possible hand was needed to save the people in the river, since they were barely keeping up with the current flow. Others argued that if they found out how people were ending up in the water, they could stop them and would not need to rescue people anymore—or at least not with the same frequency. (Saskatoon District Health Community Development Team and Dr. Ron Labonte, 1999, p. 1. Adapted with permission from Prairie Regional Health Promotion Research Centre.)

This parable can be used to illustrate the different approaches to health that were previously described. A medical approach would result in action that the people downstream first implemented; that is, providing treatment and rehabilitation to people who were rescued from the river. Using a behavioral approach, there might be attempts to provide secondary prevention to people after their recovery. For example, people could be taught to swim after their rescue so that they do not have to flail in the water; they could be instructed to behave in safer ways so that they do not fall in; or the rocks in the water could be removed or padded so people will not be hurt when they fall in. At a primary prevention level using a behavioral approach, the focus would be on helping young children to live healthy lifestyles, including swimming and overall fitness so that they could better cope if they fell in, and teaching them safe water practices early in their lives. From a socioenvironmental approach, the focus at the primary prevention level would be on promoting healthy lifestyles in young children. It would also include a focus on the circumstances that result in people falling in the river. For example, are the docks poorly designed? Are people forced to work close to the water's edge for their very survival? What can be changed in their setting to make their survival possible without putting them at risk of falling in the water?

The parable also illustrates the need to consider the "upstream" issues related to health problems, regardless of the approach that is taken to address health. All three approaches consider risk factors for health problems, although they take different perspectives on how risk is defined and understood. Regardless, there is acceptance of the need to consider the sources of health problems. In recent years, the **determinants of health** have received significant attention in the literature and in the fields of **public health** and health promotion. Exploring the determinants of health is a way to look upstream, to better understand the source of health problems.

DETERMINANTS OF HEALTH

Considering the need for upstream thinking and the various approaches to health, it is important to understand the factors that determine what makes people healthy. If these factors can be identified, multiple sectors and approaches can be mobilized to improve the health of individuals and communities.

Health is determined by many factors. In a U.S. national report entitled *Healthy People 2010*, determinants of health are described within six broad categories: biology, behaviors, social environment, physical environments, policies and interventions, and access to high-quality health care (U.S. Department of Health and Human Services, 2000). A number of goals and objectives relate to the overall health of the nation and are relevant to occupational therapy. For example, objectives focus on reducing the proportion of adults with chronic joint symptoms who experience a limitation in activity due to arthri-

tis and increasing the proportion of adults with disabilities who participate in social activities. In *Healthy People 2010*, health disparities are acknowledged, although they are not labeled as determinants of health. Significant health differences or disparities are noted among groups of people based on their gender, race and ethnicity, income and education, disability, geographic location, and sexual orientation. While these are not described as determinants of health in this report, there are clear differences between groups of people based on these factors. Other documents have described many of these factors as key determinants of health (Hamilton & Bhatti, 1996; WHO Regional Office for Europe, 2002). Lists of the determinants of health frequently include the following factors:

◆ Income and social status
◆ Social supports
◆ Gender
◆ Education
◆ Working conditions
◆ Physical environments
◆ Air quality
◆ Food safety
◆ Water
◆ Biology and genetics
◆ Personal health practices and coping skills
◆ Nutrition
◆ Physical activity
◆ Healthy child development
◆ Health services

Research and information related to the determinants of health are often found in literature related to **population health**. Population health data can help policymakers to identify the major factors within a community that are contributing to health challenges and may lead to policies and initiatives to promote health.

HEALTH PROMOTION

The determinants of health can be used as a foundation to consider how health can then be promoted. *Health promotion* is a term that has received significant attention from the World Health Organization and nations around the world. Health promotion has commonly been defined as the "process of enabling people to increase control over and improve their health" (WHO, 1986, p. 2). Although the definition of health promotion does not directly acknowledge determinants of health, the Ottawa Charter identifies prerequisites for health which include "peace, shelter, education, food, income, a stable eco-system, sustainable resources, social justice and equity" (WHO, 1986, p. 2). Clearly, some of the environmental and social determinants of health are considered so vital to health that they are in fact prerequisites, factors that are foundational to any improvements in health.

The Ottawa Charter includes three strategies that can be implemented in health promotion initiatives: advocacy for conditions that are favorable for health, enablement of people to achieve their health potential, and mediation between differing interests in society. The Ottawa Charter also describes five areas of health promotion action: build healthy public policy, create supportive environments, strengthen community action, develop personal skills, and reorient health services.

Principles

Underlying the definition, strategies, and actions of health promotion as described in the Ottawa Charter (WHO, 1986) are a number of principles related to health promotion that are not explicitly stated in the charter. These principles have been articulated by others, including de Leeuw (1989) and Thibeault and Hebert (1997).

The first principle relates to *community participation.* Health promotion needs to involve community members throughout all phases, from identifying the health issue of concern to determining how best to address it and then to evaluating whether or not it has been addressed. At heart, health promotion is participatory. All phases of health promotion processes involve community participation as an integral component.

The second principle of health promotion relates to *empowerment,* which is linked closely with the first principle of community participation. Empowerment implies that people and communities that are involved in health promotion processes will gain knowledge and skills and, through that, a sense of self-efficacy and empowerment. While Labonte (1994) notes that health promotion can sometimes become bureaucratic and disempowering, the underlying purpose of health promotion initiatives should be community participation and ownership so that empowerment occurs.

Underlying the principles of community participation and empowerment is a principle of *respect for diversity.* Groups and communities that are interested in participating in health promotion processes are very diverse and may represent groups that face marginalization for a number of reasons, such as age, race or ethnicity, or sexual orientation. Health promotion involves respect for all stakeholders in addressing a health issue and respect for diversity that occurs within and between communities.

Social justice is another underlying principle of health promotion. Many of the social determinants of health, such as poverty, education, and discrimination based on race or gender, can best be addressed through social justice initiatives. In occupational therapy, Townsend and Wilcock (2004) describe *occupational justice* and suggest that it is related to, but distinct from, social justice. They describe social justice as "a concept that recognizes humans as social beings who engage in social relations" and suggest that advocacy in social justice "favors equitable (same)

access to opportunities and resources in order to reduce group differences" (Townsend & Wilcock, 2004, p. 262). Occupational justice is "a concept to guide humans as occupational beings who need and want to participate in occupations in order to develop and thrive" with the advocacy related to "enablement of different access to opportunities and resources in order to acknowledge individual differences" (Townsend & Wilcock, 2004, p. 262). Occupational therapists who are involved in health promotion aim for social justice in trying to ensure access to opportunities that are equitable across and between groups (social justice) and those that meet the unique needs of individuals (occupational justice). (See Chapter 20 for an in-depth discussion of occupational justice).

The determinants of health go well beyond the health sector alone. Health care services can contribute to improved health, but other sectors are also key stakeholders and need to be involved in initiatives to improve health. For example, the availability and accessibility of transportation systems in large urban centers can influence people's abilities to access education, recreation, and employment. The media can have significant involvement in health promotion initiatives through public service announcements. Schools can also play significant roles in influencing health and addressing health issues. Because health is influenced by many sectors, health promotion initiatives are best implemented if they are *intersectoral.* For example, addressing the social isolation of older adults might involve transportation systems, cultural and religious organizations, social services, welfare, and housing.

Health promotion is also an *integrative* process, one that includes many strategies to address the health concern, including education, legislation, and **community development.** For example, workplace health promotion involves legislation through laws that ensure basic workplace safety, organizational policies (e.g., through employee assistance programs), educational initiatives (e.g., safe lifting in-service workshops), as well as organizational initiatives to create a collaborative workplace based on principles of respect and empowerment.

Finally, health promotion is *continuous.* Ideally, successful health promotion initiatives will result in strengthened communities and healthy public policy that can lead to further initiatives to promote health either by addressing new health issues or by building on one initiative to create another to further address the original issue. Practitioners who are committed to health promotion need to be committed to change (Letts et al., 1993). While occupational therapy practitioners do not necessarily have to be involved in all health promotion initiatives after one interaction with a group or community, they need to understand that health promotion is seldom constrained to one activity or initiative.

Process

Health promotion should be considered a process rather than a specific one-time standardized intervention. The stages of the process are not always clearly defined, but common elements or phases of health promotion can be described. Letts and colleagues (1993) described the initial phases of the health promotion process as including the following:

- Networking (within communities to identify stakeholders and communities or sectors)
- Consulting (to identify health issues)
- Collaborating (to select a specific health issue to address) and
- Planning (to specifically plan actions and develop objectives).

Actions are then implemented in partnership and can be evaluated by the group. Raeburn and Rootman (1998) describe a thirteen-step process of engaging in people-centered health promotion, from beginning initial consultations, conducting needs assessment, setting goals, planning resources and actions, and evaluating progress. The overall process of health promotion generally includes a process of consulting a community or group to identify the health issue (epidemiological or community statistics can also provide information about health issues), conducting needs assessments, identifying priorities, and planning actions in partnership with communities to address the identified health issue.

Approaches to Health Promotion

How can the ideas of the Ottawa Charter (WHO, 1986) and the principles of health promotion be implemented with individuals, groups, and communities? What does it look like, and how should occupational therapists be involved? The notions of enablement, mediation, and advocacy as described in the Ottawa Charter provide a place to begin. Within a health promotion framework, occupational therapists can use their skills and knowledge in numerous ways.

Wilcock (1998) suggests five models that represent different but not mutually exclusive approaches to health promotion. These include wellness, preventive medicine, community development, social justice, and ecological sustainability. These approaches range from individually focused initiatives to help people make healthier choices (wellness) through community-based consultations that promote communitywide responsibility for health (community development), to initiatives at the global level to promote healthy relationships between humans and all other organisms to sustain life on the planet (ecological sustainability).

McComas and Carswell (1994) developed a model to describe the process for health promotion action based on an initiative with women with disabilities. Their model was based on Labonte's (1994) framework for health professionals to think about how to apply health promotion concepts in practice, ranging from strategies of individual empowerment, through small group development, community organization, coalition advocacy, and political action. The Labonte model has similarities with the Wilcock (1998) model in that there is a range from individual focus to broader focus, although Labonte does not address the health of the planet.

Labonte's (1994) model described the empowerment strategies as following a continuum from working with individuals who face health challenges to political advocacy to address health inequities. He described the model as a holosphere, with each strategy as a sphere overlapping with the others. In working with individuals, for example, Labonte notes that personal care for individuals based on health promotion principles would be supportive and noncontrolling, with health professionals providing information and resources to individuals. Group development involves helping groups of individuals to organize around their health issues. Health professionals need to be aware of groups that might be appropriate to refer individual clients but also be willing to act as a facilitator or guest. Community organization involves groups of people coming together as communities to address health issues. Although health professionals may be involved in such initiatives, Labonte cautions them to ensure that this does not become bureaucratic. Coalition advocacy occurs when links between organizations are formed to address health issues through advocacy, by linking communities around a common interest to change structures or policy. Political action is often the next step after coalition advocacy and frequently involves conflict and a need for someone to take a role as facilitator in organizing collaboratively.

Building on Labonte's ideas, McComas and Carswell (1994) suggest that the actions can be thought of as a series of circles that become increasingly large as the initiatives expand and build on one another. Further, the notions of participation, supportive environments, personal and group control, and personal competence suggest underlying principles or foundations that need to be in place for the process of health promotion action to be successful (Figure 18.1).

The process for health promotion action as described by McComas and Carswell (1994) provides a way for occupational therapists to consider how their knowledge and skills can be applied at many different levels through health promotion. It also demonstrates how the different approaches or levels of action are related to one another. Further examples of initiatives by occupational therapists will be described later in the chapter.

CONCEPTS RELATED TO HEALTH PROMOTION

This section provides a summary of terms that are commonly used in conjunction with health promotion, their most common use, and key points about their links to health promotion. A helpful resource on health promotion termi-

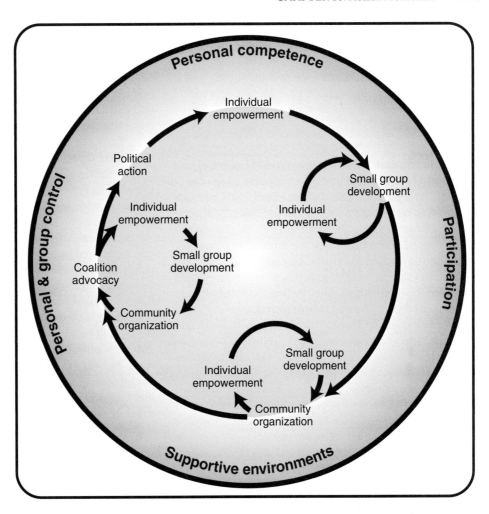

FIGURE 18.1   Process for health promotion action.

nology is the *Health Promotion Glossary,* which was written by Nutbeam (1998) for the World Health Organization.

Population Health

Most recently, population health has been strongly associated with research on the determinants of health, in particular the work of Evans, Barer, and Marmor (1994) and Evans and Stoddart (1990). Population health has been defined as "the health outcomes of a group of individuals, including the distribution of such outcomes within the group" (Kindig & Stoddart, 2003, p. 381). The focus of population health research tends to be on health indicators or outcomes at the level of populations and is frequently conducted by epidemiologists.

Critiques of population health have noted that it attempts to be nonpolitical while providing justification for reduced funding to the health care sector without necessarily calling for reallocation of those funds to address social determinants of health (Robertson, 1998); it does not adequately attempt to understand the underlying social conditions that result in the differences between groups of people in health and it does not provide a vision for how

changes can be made at the level of individuals or communities (Coburn et al., 2003).

Hamilton and Bhatti (1996) describe the complementary nature of population health and health promotion, highlighting the importance of considering the determinants of health to understand health issues that might be addressed through health promotion initiatives. Their three-dimensional model describes the link between determinants of health, levels of activity, and the five strategies articulated in the Ottawa Charter for Health Promotion (WHO, 1986). However, what are missing from Hamilton and Bhatti's discussion are some of the underlying principles of health promotion that were discussed previously in this chapter, including community participation, empowerment, and social justice. Although they are related and probably complementary concepts, population health and health promotion are distinct from one another.

Public Health

Health promotion has its roots in public health. Nutbeam (1998, p. 3) has defined public health as "a social and political concept aimed at improving health, prolonging life and improving the quality of life among whole populations through health promotion, disease prevention and other forms of health intervention." Public health incorporates health promotion but also health protection, through such things as restaurant inspections and disease prevention through childhood immunization programs.

Primary Health Care

Primary health care, defined by the World Health Organization in 1978, is "essential health care made accessible at a cost a country and community can afford, with methods that are practical, scientifically sound and socially acceptable" (Nutbeam, 1998, p. 3). More recently, primary health care reform has been underway in a number of countries, including the United Kingdom, Canada, Australia, and Sweden. In Canada, a 2004 conference on primary health care noted that there are problems when the terms *primary care* and *primary health care* are used interchangeably, since primary care is limited to health care service delivery and primary health care is a more expansive term that addresses health but also social issues (Lewis, 2004). Many definitions of primary health care appear to overlap significantly with health promotion. A difference may be in emphasis more than in approach or understandings of health or its determinants, although this has yet to be determined or debated in the health promotion literature.

Disability Postponement

Disability postponement has been described as "those intervention activities that focus on delaying physical or mental decline, service use or long-term care utilization among people who have an existing chronic illness" (Finlayson & Edwards, 1997, p. 457). Occupational therapists who work with people with preexisting conditions and disabilities might find the idea of disability postponement useful when considering opportunities to apply health promotion principles in practice.

Disease and Injury Prevention

Prevention is a concept that is closely linked to health promotion, especially when a behavioral approach to health is adopted. While most descriptions of prevention focus on disease prevention, occupational therapists might find it helpful also to consider injury prevention as a potential role (Finlayson & Edwards, 1997). Although there is sometimes significant overlap between health promotion and disease and injury prevention, prevention initiatives tend to be initiated in the health sector and focus on risk factors and behaviors that result in health problems.

Community Development and Capacity Building

Wilcock (1998, p. 238) describes community development as "community consultation, deliberation, and action

to promote individual, family, and community-wide responsibility for self-sustaining development, health and well-being. It is a holistic, participatory model, aimed at facilitating a community's social and economic development, based on community analysis, use of local resources, and self-sustaining programs." Although some community development issues relate to health, community development is not limited to health; rather, it may result in initiatives that promote the economic development of a community. Community development initiatives are intended to expand the capacity of a community in terms of the knowledge and skills that are required for the community to survive and thrive.

In the case of community development, communities may be defined by the geographic location, but they are also defined by members with a common shared interest. For example, older adults in an amalgamating city might not live in the same neighborhood but come together as a community based on a common concern about how their voices will be heard in a new metropolitan area (Letts, 2003a). Communities can define themselves in a variety of ways. Bulmer (1987) notes that *community* is a normative as well as an analytic and descriptive concept and that communities are diverse and changing in how they are understood, making it important to describe the community that is the focus of any community development initiative.

Community development is at the basis of community-based rehabilitation (CBR), which emerged at about the same time as primary health care and is described as a community development strategy for rehabilitation (Kronenberg, Fransen, & Pollard, 2005). Through a recent position statement on CBR (World Federation of Occupational Therapists (WFOT), 2004) and other activities to gather information about occupational therapists' roles in CBR, WFOT has taken a lead role in demonstrating how community development can be used to promote community participation with people with disabilities around the world.

Not all health promotion initiatives fall within a community development framework. For example, individually focused initiatives that use a behavioral approach to health would not necessarily involve a participatory consultation process with community members to implement. However, many health promotion initiatives that occupational therapists describe do fall within a community development framework (Banks & Head, 2004; Letts et al., 1993; Wilcock, 1998).

HEALTH PROMOTION AND OCCUPATIONAL THERAPY

So how should occupational therapists take the broad body of knowledge and models of health promotion and apply them in their own practice? de Leeuw (1989) suggested that "health professionals should realize that their personal involvement in health promotion should not mean they give up their disciplinary training and work area but rather that they should acquire some kind of framework of reference in which they could put their own efforts in the integrated, intersectoral health promotion context" (p. 103). In applying this quote to occupational therapy, Letts and colleagues (1993) suggested that rather than thinking about "doing" health promotion, occupational therapists should think about "doing" occupational therapy but within a health promotion framework.

Occupational therapists have applied health promotion frameworks, demonstrating a role for occupational therapists in varying contexts. Reitz (1992) documented ideas related to preventive health and wellness in the earliest foundations of occupational therapy. Wilcock (2001) documented the idea of the Regimen Sanitatis, which was influential from the twelfth to the nineteenth centuries. The Regimen includes a set of six rules for health that include such things as eating and drinking and getting adequate sleep. She demonstrates the link between these historical rules and the principles and strategies expressed in the Ottawa Charter (WHO, 1986) as well as occupational therapy's underlying premise of occupation for health, that is, that engagement in occupation is a prerequisite for health and also may have restorative benefits for people with health concerns.

Occupational therapy was founded on ideas related to promoting health and well-being through occupation, and a resurgence of discussions on the contributions that occupational therapists could make to prevention and health promotion began in the late 1960s (Reitz, 1992). In the next section, examples of occupational therapists using a health promotion framework are put into a conceptual context, and the challenges and opportunities of health promotion are considered.

Conceptual Links

The roots and underlying philosophy of client-centered occupation-based occupational therapy practice align well with the principles and models of health promotion. Thibeault and Hebert (1997) compared health promotion and occupational therapy principles, highlighting many areas of consistency in the approaches (see Table 18.2). For example, the participatory processes that are described as a principle of health promotion are very similar to the client-centered processes that occupational therapists have adopted for use with clients in a variety of settings. The links between social justice as a principle of health promotion and occupational justice and social justice that are valued by occupational therapists are also highlighted. Townsend (2003) has similarly focused attention on ideas of justice in client-centered occupational therapy practice. Both health promotion and occupational therapy practice have underlying principles related to respect for diversity in working with individuals and communities.

Community is one of the major foci of health promotion. Health promotion is implemented in partnership with a variety of communities and most frequently occurs within community contexts rather than within medical institutions. Initiatives that emphasize individual wellness often are undertaken in community contexts in order to reach the people who are the targets of the initiatives. Occupational therapy has a natural fit within community settings as well (Baum & Law, 1998; Scaffa, 2001). Thibeault and Hebert (1997) note that one difference between health promotion

TABLE 18.2   COMPARISON OF THE MAIN TENETS OF HEALTH PROMOTION AND OCCUPATIONAL THERAPY

Health Promotion	Occupational Therapy
Community participation	Worth of the individual with his or her unique nature, needs, potential, and growth, active within his or her own environment and community; occupation as the pivot of human life
Empowerment	Empowerment and enablement; occupational therapists, clients, and community members as equals
Social justice	Social justice
Greater autonomy for the community	Greater autonomy for the individual and the community
Importance of active and meaningful lifestyles	Importance of active and meaningful lifestyles; therapeutic dimension of occupation
Respect for cultural diversity	Respect for cultural diversity and marginalized groups

Source: Reproduced with permission from Thibeault, R., & Hebert, M. (1997). A congruent model for health promotion in occupational therapy. *Occupational Therapy International, 4,* 271–293. © John Wiley & Sons Limited.

and occupational therapy is that health promotion is frequently focused on working with communities, while occupational therapy models tend to focus on individuals. They note that many models in occupational therapy are applicable with communities and groups but are seldom explicitly applied in that way. Occupational therapy practice in community settings is not necessarily grounded in health promotion principles or models. However, occupational therapists in community settings are well placed to challenge existing models of service delivery and work to share skills and knowledge using a health promotion framework.

Wilcock (1998, 2001) has provided a rich overview of the conceptual links between the underlying importance of occupation as a determinant of health and as a means to improve it, described as "occupation for health." Thibeault and Hebert (1997, p. 277) reinforce this by observing that occupation is viewed as the "pivot of human life" and note that occupational therapy considers the therapeutic dimension of occupation.

Occupational therapy's emphasis on client-centered occupation-based practice with increasing numbers of therapists in community settings means that occupational therapists are poised to apply their skills and knowledge within a health promotion framework. The sections that follow provide examples of occupational therapists who are involved in health promotion initiatives in different community contexts.

Practice Examples: Healthy Aging

Excellent examples that demonstrate the role of occupational therapists in promoting health when working with older adults are described in the literature. The Well Elderly Study in California demonstrated through a randomized clinical trial design that a preventive occupational therapy intervention (Lifestyle Redesign) resulted in benefits in health, function and quality of life (Clark et al., 1997), and these results were sustained after a six-month follow up (Clark et al., 2001). The nine-month occupational therapy intervention in the Well Elderly study focused on helping older adults to build positive changes into their lifestyles, covering areas such as transportation, safety, finances, and social relationships (Carlson, Clark, & Young, 1998). The processes that were used in the intervention included presentations of information to individuals and groups, peer exchange, and personal exploration. This same approach to intervention has been applied (with some modifications) in other settings, including a medical-model adult day program (Horowitz & Chang, 2004), and with middle- and upper-class older adults living in seniors' apartments (Matuska, Giles-Heinz, Flinn, Neighbor, & Bass-Haugen, 2003). The reports of applications to other populations have tended to be pilot studies, with small groups of older adults and no comparison or control groups. Despite the lack of rigor in the research designs, the studies do provide evidence that the Lifestyle Redesign

Program can be adapted and applied in a variety of contexts to promote health with older adults.

In the CAOT Seniors' Health Promotion Project (Letts et al., 1993), occupational therapists worked in seniors' organizations in two Canadian provinces (Manitoba and Newfoundland) to explore how occupational therapy skills and knowledge could be used in a health promotion framework. A diverse range of initiatives were undertaken, including a large initiative in Newfoundland to improve health through improved transportation for older adults in the city of St. John's and education sessions in Manitoba provided through cable television, print media, and presentations to seniors' organizations on senior-generated topics such as maintaining physical activity, home safety, and managing arthritis. Barnard and colleagues (2004) describe an initiative that was developed by occupational therapy faculty and students in partnership with older adults in a small North Carolina town. They developed a five-week wellness program focused on physical activity, using spirituality as a means of expression, increasing awareness of nutrition and cooking, and increasing cognitive functions. Miller and colleagues (2001) describe the Microwave Project, in which occupational therapy students worked with an interdisciplinary team and older adults who received Meals on Wheels to address a challenge that some recipients were having in reheating their meals adequately and safely. Older adults who were at risk of health problems because of difficulty with food preparation were involved in a luncheon program (if they were able to leave their homes to attend) or the homebound program so that they could gain skills in food preparation and reheating using a microwave oven (Figure 18.2). Community outreach was undertaken to give older adults with low incomes access to microwave ovens.

Additionally, numerous occupational therapists participate in falls prevention initiatives with older adults in the community (e.g., Clemson, et al., 2004; Tolley & Atwal, 2003). Overall, the occupational therapy literature suggests that there is a strong role for occupational therapy in adopting a health promotion framework with older adults. The initiatives range from those that take a behavioral and preventive approach (e.g., Lifestyle Redesign, falls prevention) to those that are more aligned with a socio-environmental approach to health (e.g., the CAOT Seniors' Health Promotion Project and the Microwave Project).

Practice Examples: Workplace Health Promotion

In 1986, a number of articles described the contribution of occupational therapy to workplace programs, including employee assistance programs (Maynard, 1986), health education programming to employees (Hollander Kaplan & Burch-Minakan, 1986), and workstation or office re-design (Allen, 1986). More recently, Moyers and Coleman (2004) identified strategies that occupational therapists

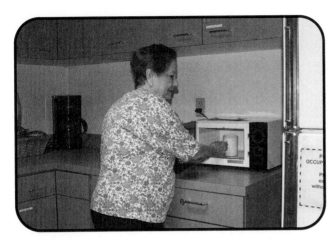

FIGURE 18.2   Older adult practices reheating coffee in microwave.

can implement in partnership with workers and employers to promote the health of aging workers, including job redesign, organizational restructuring, and health promotion initiatives that include wellness and physical activity programs as well as ergonomics, maintenance of abilities, and promoting ongoing interest in work. Kirsh, Cockburn, and Gewurtz (2004) describe roles for occupational therapists in promoting health in the workplace, including analyzing job demands and employer skills and designing workplace accommodations. Initiatives such as these are believed to promote healthy work and workers.

Although occupational therapists are among many professionals who are involved in workplace health promotion, the role of occupational therapy is not well established internationally. In one review of the effectiveness of workplace health promotion, occupational therapy was not an explicit component of any of the 35 multicomponent workplace health promotion programs that were reviewed (Heaney & Goetzel, 1997). Moreover, there seems to be limited rigorous evidence that demonstrates the effectiveness of occupational therapists using their skills and knowledge in this way. Occupational therapists need to demonstrate with rigorous data the effectiveness of contributions using a health promotion framework.

Challenges and Opportunities for Occupational Therapy in Health Promotion

Healthy aging and workplace health promotion are not the only health promotion initiatives in which occupational therapists are involved. Examples that are cited in the literature include partnerships with organizations that serve the needs of people with physical disabilities (Neufeld & Kniepmann, 2001) and a campaign to promote safe backpack selection and use for children (Jacobs, 2003) (Figure 18.3).

Another area of occupational therapy practice is mental health promotion (Creek, 2002). Although mental health promotion might not be a common area of occupational therapy practice in the United States, examples from other countries illustrate the contributions occupational therapists can make. For example, Russell and Lloyd (2004) describe an initiative in Australia that focused on physical and mental health promotion among people with mental illness. Each session included a physical activity component and didactic presentations on self-esteem and self-image, life skills, nutrition, relaxation, and stress management. Babiski, Sidle, and McColl (1996) described a health promotion role for occupational therapists and community support workers who provided support services to boarding home operators and tenants. The goal was to improve the tenants' quality of life by addressing individual, group, and environmental barriers to mental health. Olson, Heaney, and Soppas-Hoffman (1989) describe the role of an occupational therapist in a parent-child activity group, which was designed in collaboration between a teaching hospital and a local child care center to meet the needs of at-risk families. An occupational therapist and a counseling therapist developed and facilitated the activity group to help children to elicit positive attention from parents and to help parents respond effectively to the needs of the child. The group included discussion of parent-child activity interactions and facilitated play between the mothers and children.

Despite the potential and hope that such examples offer, occupational therapists who are interested in working from a health promotion framework face challenges. Occupational therapists frequently find themselves working in medical contexts, in which a socioenvironmental approach to health is not easily adopted. Further, many policies that are related to health promotion fall within behavioral and institutionally driven models of service delivery. Even community-based practices are often focused on short-term interventions with individual clients to address specific occupational performance concerns. Scriven and Atwal (2004) state that occupational therapy roles in health promotion most commonly involve tertiary health promotion (downstream work), facilitating individuals to develop personal skills to cope with disability or chronic illness. For occupational therapists who are interested in more community development approaches, it can be difficult to find support within existing models of service delivery (Spalding, 1996).

Funding for occupational therapy services from a health promotion framework is equally a challenge. When occupational therapy services are most frequently offered and billed on the basis of service provision to individual clients, it is challenging to link funding to working with communities on health issues in a participatory, empowering, intersectoral manner (Spalding, 1996). Related to funding is the availability of occupational therapy resources and how these are distributed to meet the health needs of

COMMENTARY ON THE EVIDENCE

Evaluating the Effectiveness of Occupational Therapy and Health Promotion

Establishing evidence to support the effectiveness of health promotion implemented by occupational therapists or anyone can be challenging in light of traditional approaches to research and evaluation and the underlying principles of health promotion.

Randomized controlled trials are frequently described as the most rigorous way to evaluate the effectiveness of interventions. However, they are best designed when the population receiving an intervention (and a control group) is well defined, the intervention is standardized, and the timelines for outcomes are reasonably short. In contrast, health promotion initiatives are often grounded in communities that have fluctuating memberships (making it very difficult to define intervention and control groups) and interventions that fluctuate depending on the responses of the community (making standardization of the intervention difficult) and may require significant lengths of time to result in change in community or individual health.

Furthermore, considering the principles underlying health promotion, there is a potential lack of fit between health promotion and traditional methods of evaluation. Lincoln (1992, p. S10) notes that "it does no good to improve the health of an individual if we simultaneously undermine her or his self-esteem and sense of agency" through research or evaluation. Traditional methods of evaluation may reinforce power imbalances that health promotion seeks to redress (Coombe, 1997).

Despite these challenges, it is important to demonstrate the effectiveness of health promotion. In health promotion evaluation, a randomized control trial might not always be the best approach to adopt. Gillies (1998, p. 114) notes that this design "simply cannot capture the richness of the process . . . they simply are not sufficiently sophisticated to deal with the complexity and diversity of the process and outcome of health promotion at community level [sic]."

As a result of the concerns about traditional evaluation methods, a number of sources have called for the adoption of participatory or empowerment evaluation (Green et al., 1995; Papineau & Kiely, 1996; Thibeault & Hebert, 1997; WHO European Working Group on Health Promotion Evaluation, 1998). In occupational therapy, participatory research has also been receiving increasing attention (Cockburn & Trentham, 2002; Letts, 2003b; Taylor, Braveman, & Hammel, 2004). Participatory evaluation involves participants in the evaluation throughout all stages, relies on the knowledge and expertise of all participants, and implements changes to the health promotion initiative resulting from the evaluation. These characteristics align well with principles of health promotion.

In all evaluations, the approach that is chosen needs to reflect the process that is being undertaken. Depending on the approach to health that is used in developing a health promotion initiative, a randomized controlled trial might be appropriate. For example, a randomized controlled trial can be useful in circumstances in which a well-defined intervention is offered to a distinct group of people, with a control group available. The Well Elderly Study (Clark et al, 1997, 2001) and falls prevention initiatives (e.g., Clemson et al, 2004) are examples of interventions that have been evaluated through randomized controlled trials. In other situations, a participatory, community, or capacity-building health promotion initiative might be better evaluated by using a participatory approach (Letts, 2003b; Taylor et al., 2004). Regardless of the type of evaluation, there is a need for occupational therapists who are involved in health promotion to plan evaluations of these initiatives to build a body of evidence to support the role of occupational therapy in health promotion.

communities. If more occupational therapy services are to be offered upstream, focused on primary health promotion with communities that are well and independent, would there be adequate therapy provision to meet the needs of people with disabilities (Scriven & Atwal, 2004)? There will almost undoubtedly always be a need for occupational therapists to provide services based on all three approaches to health: medical, behavioral and socioenvironmental. The challenge is to find the balance of resources that optimizes health and utilization of occupational therapy services.

Finally, if health promotion is to be valued as a role for occupational therapists, there needs to be more evidence

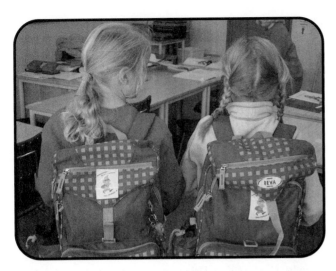

FIGURE 18.3   Students in Iceland model safe backpacks.

to support its adoption. The work of Clark and colleagues (1997) provides one example of an initiative to rigorously evaluate the effectiveness of occupational therapy in a prevention role with healthy older adults. Similar evidence is needed in other areas of occupational therapy practice. There are debates in the health promotion literature as to the best strategies to evaluate community-based health promotion initiatives (see Commentary on the Evidence). Regardless, systematic data gathering and analyses are needed to generate a body of evidence that supports the role of occupational therapy in health promotion.

Challenges can also be viewed as opportunities, and from those, strategies can be formulated to address them. If occupational therapists face challenges in using a health promotion framework, forming alliances with other groups is a useful strategy to consider. Other groups of health professionals may be allies in developing new roles in health promotion. For example, social workers, public health nurses, and community developers may be partners with occupational therapists. Working at the level of the multidisciplinary team is familiar to occupational therapists, and they have skills in optimizing health through partnerships (Spalding, 1996). Furthermore, community groups can be important allies in creating demand for occupational therapists to use their skills and knowledge in a health promotion framework (Fraser, Letts, & Carswell, 1993). Partnerships and alliances can be created at various levels. For example, individual occupational therapists can volunteer to work with a group of older adults at a community recreation center. At a broader level, professional organizations such as the American Occupational Therapy Association can partner with consumer groups, such as the American Association of Retired Persons to advocate for more occupational therapists working with well older adults to maintain and improve their health.

When applying occupational therapy skills and knowledge in a health promotion framework, occupational ther-

apists might also need to assess whether they have all of the necessary knowledge. For example, in consulting with communities and groups about their health issues, occupational therapists need to describe themselves in terms that focus on health rather than illness and disability (Letts et al., 1993). Further, occupational therapists need to understand the public policy process if they are involved in community organizing, coalition advocacy, or political action. For example, the AOTA developed a comprehensive advocacy initiative to remove Medicare caps on outpatient rehabilitation. The strategy involved the association as well as its members to advocate with the federal government and legislators to remove the caps. Any advocacy requires an understanding of what message needs to be conveyed, to whom, and how can it be delivered effectively. Finally, skills in program evaluation are needed to ensure that health promotion initiatives are evaluated.

CONCLUSIONS

Health promotion has evolved in recent decades, and this chapter has demonstrated congruence between health promotion and occupational therapy. Occupational therapists can apply their skills and knowledge using a health promotion framework, but they face a number of challenges to do so. It is important to begin by understanding approaches to health, health promotion, and related concepts such as population health, public health, community development, and primary health care. To develop partnerships in health promotion, occupational therapists need to be able to describe occupational therapy in a way that focuses on health rather than disability. Occupational therapists need to work with individuals, groups, and communities to identify the health issues that need to be addressed. Funding for occupational therapists to work from a health promotion framework continues to be a challenge and may require creativity and searching for funding outside of traditional sources. For example, foundations that are interested in community organizing might fund an occupational therapist in a coordinating function. Finally, as work in the area of health promotion increases, rigorous evaluations need to demonstrate the effectiveness of occupational therapy in health promotion.

PROVOCATIVE QUESTIONS

1. "Unless professionals think simultaneously in both personal and structural ways, they risk losing sight of the simultaneous reality of both. If they focus only on the individual, and only on crisis management or service delivery, they risk privatizing by rendering personal the social and economic underpinnings to poverty and powerlessness. If they only focus on the structural issues, they risk ignoring the immediate pains and personal woundings of the powerless and

people in crisis" (Labonte, 1994, p. 259). What does this quote say to you about the role of occupational therapy in health promotion? Consider examples in which occupational therapists might be overemphasizing individual or structural issues and how a balance between the two can be maintained.

2. Examples of health promotion in occupational therapy often seem to be grounded in a behavioral approach to health. Critics of the behavioral approach note that this approach, more than either a medical or a socioenvironmental approach, is at risk of blaming the victim. For example, suppose a person becomes injured because he or she used an improper lifting technique even after receiving education on proper lifting techniques from an occupational therapist. Furthermore, despite receiving information about the importance of abdominal exercise and general fitness to prevent back injuries, suppose the person chose a more sedentary lifestyle with limited physical fitness activities. When the person is injured at work, it might result in a conclusion that the injured worker is to blame for the injury and a belief that the person deserves less compensation or rehabilitation because he or she should have known better. Do you agree that the injured worker is to blame? How does this affect your perception of the person in general and as an occupational therapist?

REFERENCES

Allen, V. R. (1986). Health promotion in the office. *American Journal of Occupational Therapy, 40,* 764–770.

American Occupational Therapy Association. (2001). Occupational therapy in the promotion of health and the prevention of disease and disability statement. *American Journal of Occupational Therapy, 55,* 656–660.

Babiski, L., Sidle, N., & McColl, M. (1996). Challenges in achieving health for all in the boarding home sector. *Canadian Journal of Occupational Therapy, 63,* 33–41.

Banks, S., & Head, B. (2004). Partnering occupational therapy and community development. *Canadian Journal of Occupational Therapy, 71,* 5–7, 10.

Barnard, S., Dunn, S., Reddic, E., Rhodes, K., Russell, J., Tuitt, T. S., et al. (2004). Wellness in Tillery: A community-built program. *Family and Community Health, 27,* 151–157.

Baum, C., & Law, M. (1998). Community health: A responsibility, an opportunity, and a fit for occupational therapy. *American Journal of Occupational Therapy, 52,* 7–10.

Bulmer, M. (1987). *The social basis of community care.* London, UK: Allen & Unwin.

Carlson, M., Clark, F., & Young, B. (1998). Practical contributions of occupational science to the art of successful ageing: How to sculpt a meaningful life in older adulthood. *Journal of Occupational Science, 5,* 107–118.

Clark, F., Azen, S. P., Carlson, M., Mandel, D., LaBree, L. Hay, J., et al. (2001). Embedding health-promoting changes into the daily lives of independent-living older adults: Long-term follow-up of occupational therapy intervention. *Journal of Gerontology: Psychological Sciences, 56B,* P60–P63.

Clark, F., Azen, S. P., Zemke, R., Jackson, J., Carlson, M., Mandel, D., et al. (1997). Occupational therapy for independent-living older adults: A randomized controlled trial. *Journal of the American Medical Association, 278,* 1321–1326.

Clemson, L., Cumming, R. G., Kendig, H., Swann, M, Heard, R., & Taylor, K. (2004). The effectiveness of a community-based program for reducing the incidence of falls in the elderly: A randomized trial. *Journal of the American Geriatrics Society, 52,* 1487–1494.

Coburn, D., Kenny, K., Mykhalovskly, E., McDonough, P., Robertson, A., & Love, R. (2003). Population health in Canada: A brief critique. *American Journal of Public Health, 93,* 392–396.

Cockburn, L., & Trentham, B. (2002). Participatory action research: Integrating community occupational therapy practice and research. *Canadian Journal of Occupational Therapy, 69,* 20–30.

Coombe, C. M. (1997). Using empowerment evaluation in community organizing and community-based health initiatives. In M. Minkler (Ed.), *Community organizing and community building for health* (pp. 291–307). New Brunswick, NJ: Rutgers University Press.

Creek, J. (2002). A mental health promotion role for occupational therapy. *British Journal of Occupational Therapy, 65,* 157.

de Leeuw, E. (1989). *The sane revolution—health promotion: Backgrounds, scope, prospects.* Assen, The Netherlands: van Gorcum.

Evans, R. G., Barer, M. L., & Marmor, T. R. (1994). *Why are some people healthy and others not?: The determinants of health of populations.* New York: Aldine de Gruyter.

Evans, R. G., & Stoddart, G. L. (1990). Producing health, consuming health care. *Social Science and Medicine, 31,* 1347–1363.

Finlayson, M., & Edwards, J. (1997). Evolving health environments and occupational therapy: Definitions, descriptions and opportunities. *British Journal of Occupational Therapy, 60,* 456–460.

Fraser, B., Letts, L., & Carswell, A. (1993). Health promotion issue paper—Effective change: The education, demand, opportunity equation. *The National (Canadian Association of Occupational Therapists' Newsletter), 10*(2), insert.

Gillies, P. (1998). Effectiveness of alliances and partnerships for health promotion. *Health Promotion International, 13*(2), 99–120.

Green, L. W., George, M. A., Daniel, M., Frankish, C. J., Herbert, C. J., Bowie, W., R., et al. (1995). *Study of participatory research in health promotion: Review and recommendations for the development of participatory research in health promotion in Canada.* Vancouver, BC: Royal Society of Canada.

Hamilton, N., & Bhatti, T. (1996). *Population health promotion: An integrated model of population health and health promotion.* Ottawa, ON: Health Promotion Development Division, Health Canada.

Heaney, C. A., & Goetzel, R. Z. (1997). A review of health-related outcomes of multi-component worksite health promotion programs. *American Journal of Public Health, 11,* 290–308.

Hollander Kaplan, L., & Burch-Minakan, L. (1986). Reach out for health: A corporation's approach to health promotion. *American Journal of Occupational Therapy, 40,* 777–780.

Horowitz, B. P., & Chang, P. F. J. (2004). Promoting well-being and engagement in life through occupational therapy lifestyle redesign: A pilot study within adult day programs. *Topics in Geriatric Rehabilitation, 20*(1), 46–58.

Jacobs, K. (2003). Occupational therapy national awareness campaign to promote health in student backpack users. *Orthopedic Physical Therapy Practice,* 40–42.

Kindig, D., & Stoddart, G. (2003). What is population health? *American Journal of Public Health, 93,* 380–383.

Kirsh, B., Cockburn, L., & Gewurtz, R. (2004). Doing work well: Preserving and promoting mental health in the workplace. *Occupational Therapy Now, 6*(5), 25–27.

Kronenberg, F., Fransen, H., & Pollard, N. (2005). The WFOT position paper on community-based rehabilitation: A call upon the profession to engage with people affected by occupational apartheid. *WFOT Bulletin, 51*(May), 5–13.

Labonte, R. (1993). *Health promotion and empowerment: Practice frameworks.* Toronto, ON: Centre for Health Promotion, University of Toronto.

Labonte, R. (1994). Health promotion and empowerment: Reflections on professional practice. *Health Education Quarterly, 21,* 253–268.

Letts, L. (2003a). Enabling citizen participation of older adults through social and political environments. In L. Letts, P. Rigby, & D. Stewart (Eds.), *Using environments to enable occupational performance* (pp. 71–80). Thorofare, NJ: Slack.

Letts, L. (2003b). Occupational therapy and participatory research: A partnership worth pursuing. *American Journal of Occupational Therapy, 57,* 77–87.

Letts, L., Fraser, B., Finlayson, M., & Walls, J. (1993). *For the health of it!: Occupational therapy within a health promotion framework.* Ottawa, ON: CAOT Publications ACE.

Lewis, S. (2004). *A thousand points of light? Moving forward on primary health care: A synthesis of the key themes and ideas from the National Primary Health Care Conference, Winnipeg, Manitoba, May 16–19, 2004.* Retrieved July 22, 2005, from http://www.phcconference.ca/synthesis.pdf

Lincoln, Y. (1992). Fourth generation evaluation: The paradigm revolution and health promotion. *Canadian Journal of Public Health, 18*(Suppl.), S6–S10.

Matuska, K., Giles-Heinz, A., Flinn, N., Neighbor, M., & Bass-Haugen, J. (2003). Outcomes of a pilot occupational therapy wellness program for older adults. *American Journal of Occupational Therapy, 57,* 220–224.

Maynard, M. (1986). Health promotion through employee assistance programs: A role for occupational therapists. *American Journal of Occupational Therapy, 40,* 771–776.

McComas, J., & Carswell, A. (1994). A model for action in health promotion: A community experience. *Canadian Journal of Rehabilitation, 7,* 257–265.

Miller, P. A., Hedden, J. L., Argento, L., Vaccaro, M., Murad, V., & Dionne, W. (2001). A team approach to health promotion of community elders: The microwave project. *Occupational Therapy in Health Care, 14*(3/4), 17–34.

Moyers, P. A., & Coleman, S. D. (2004). Adaptation of the older worker to occupational challenges. *Work, 22,* 71–78.

Neufeld, P., & Kniepmann, K. (2001). Gateway to wellness: An occupational therapy collaboration with the National Multiple Sclerosis Society. *Occupational Therapy in Health Care, 13*(3/4), 67–84.

Nutbeam, D. (1998). *Health promotion glossary.* Geneva: World Health Organization. Retrieved July 22, 2005, from http://whqlibdoc.who.int/hq/1998/WHO_HPR_HEP_98.1.pdf

Olson, L., Heaney, C., & Soppas-Hoffman, B. (1989). Parent-child activity group treatment in preventive psychiatry. *Occupational Therapy in Health Care, 6*(1), 29–43.

Papineau, D., & Kiely, M. C. (1996). Participatory evaluation in a community organization: Fostering stakeholder empowerment and utilization. *Evaluation and Program Planning, 19*(1), 79–93.

Raeburn, J., & Rootman, I. (1996). Quality of life and health promotion. In R. Renwick, I. Brown, & M. Nagler (Eds.), *Quality of life in health promotion and rehabilitation: Conceptual approaches, issues and applications* (pp. 14–25). Thousand Oaks, CA: Sage.

Raeburn, J., & Rootman, I. (1998). *People-centred health promotion.* New York: John Wiley & Sons.

Reitz, S. M. (1992). A historical review of occupational therapy's role in preventive health and wellness. *American Journal of Occupational Therapy, 46,* 50–55.

Robertson, A. (1998). Shifting discourses on health in Canada: From health promotion to population health. *Health Promotion International, 13,* 155–166.

Russell, A., & Lloyd, C. (2004). Partnerships in mental health: Addressing barriers to social inclusion. *International Journal of Therapy and Rehabilitation, 11,* 267–274.

Saskatoon District Health Community Development Team and Dr. Ron Labonte. (1999). *Working upstream: Discovering effective practice strategies for community development in health.* Saskatoon, SK: Prairie Region Health Promotion Research Centre, University of Saskatoon.

Scaffa, M. (2001). *Occupational therapy in community-based practice settings.* Philadelphia: F. A. Davis.

Scriven, A., & Atwal, A. (2004). Occupational therapists as primary health promoters: Opportunities and barriers. *British Journal of Occupational Therapy, 67,* 424–429.

Seedhouse, D. (2001). *Health: The foundations for achievement* (2nd ed.). New York: Wiley.

Spalding, N. (1996). Health promotion and the role of occupational therapy. *British Journal of Therapy and Rehabilitation, 3,* 143–147.

Taylor, R. R., Braveman, B., & Hammel, J. (2004). Developing and evaluating community-based services through participatory action research: Two case examples. *American Journal of Occupational Therapy, 58,* 73–82.

Thibeault, R., & Hebert, M. (1997). A congruent model for health promotion in occupational therapy. *Occupational Therapy International, 4,* 271–293.

Tolley, L., & Atwal, A. (2003). Determining the effectiveness of a falls prevention programme to enhance quality of life: An occupational therapy perspective. *British Journal of Occupational Therapy, 66,* 269–276.

Townsend, E. (2003). Reflections on power and justice in enabling occupation. *Canadian Journal of Occupational Therapy, 70,* 74–87.

Townsend, E., & Wilcock, A. (2004). Occupational justice. In C. H. Christiansen & E. A. Townsend (Eds.), *Introduction to occupation: The art and science of living* (pp. 243–273). Upper Saddle River, NJ: Prentice Hall.

U.S. Department of Health and Human Services. (2000). *Healthy people 2010: Understanding and improving health* (2nd ed.). Washington, DC: U.S. Government Printing Office.

Wilcock, A. A. (1998). *An occupational perspective of health.* Thorofare, NJ: Slack Incorporated.

Wilcock, A. A. (2001). Occupation for health: Re-activating the regimen sanitatis. *Journal of Occupational Science, 8*(3), 20–24.

World Federation of Occupational Therapists. (2004). *Position Paper on Community Based Rehabilitation (CBR).* Retrieved July 23, 2005, from http://www.wfot.org/officefiles/CBR position%20Final.pdf

World Health Organization. (1948). Preamble to the Constitution of the World Health Organization as adopted by the International Health Conference, New York, 19–22 June, 1946; signed on 22 July 1946 by the representatives of 61 States (Official Records of the World Health Organization, no. 2, p. 100) and entered into force on 7 April 1948.

World Health Organization. (1986). *Ottawa charter for health promotion.* Geneva: Author.

World Health Organization European Working Group on Health Promotion Evaluation. (1998). *Health promotion evaluation: Recommendations to policymakers.* Geneva: World Health Organization.

World Health Organization Regional Office for Europe. (2002). *The European Health Report 2002.* Copenhagen, Denmark: WHO Regional Publications, European Series, No. 97. Retrieved July 5, 2005, from http://www.euro.who.int/document/e76907.pdf

Community Integration

BRIAN J. DUDGEON

Learning Objectives

After reading this chapter, you will be able to:

1. Define disability and identify challenges to participation that those with disability are likely to experience as part of community living.
2. Contrast client-centered and community-centered approaches to practice.
3. Distinguish between clinical service and advocacy roles regarding community integration.
4. Discuss approaches to community-centered assessment and identify coalitions that may be formed as part of advocacy for access and acceptance.

INTRODUCTION

To design goals and interventions that promote participation in communities, it is important to consider concerns for specific individuals as well as needs of the entire community. In promoting participation, both client- and community-centered approaches are used. These approaches have common issues and goals but have distinct intervention strategies. This chapter presents the continuum of client-centered and community-centered interventions to facilitate participation for people with disability.

On an individual basis, intervention may focus on community integration of a child with disability or reintegration of an adult with onset of disability. This client-centered approach emphasizes developing, restoring, or adapting the individual's skills as well as organizing and using assistance available in natural supports from family and friends (Law & Mills, 1998). It also includes the creation of accessible environments that promote the individual's membership, belonging, and sense of having a constructive role.

On a population or community basis, intervention emphasizes accessibility and acceptance within physical, social, and cultural environments. **Community-centered** approaches generally involve advocacy, creating universal or accessible design throughout the community, and the promotion of understanding and inclusion of those with differing characteristics or abilities.

PARTICIPATION IN COMMUNITY: DEFINITIONS

Difficulty in carrying out activities is regarded as **disability**, and various impairments of body systems can contribute to one's inability to carry out activities in an expected or accepted manner. While many activities are private, disability is also associated with problems in **participation**, or an individual's involvement in life situations in communities. Activity limitation as well as environmental barriers may contribute to restrictions in participation. Environmental factors include the physical, social, and attitudinal settings in which people live and conduct their lives (World Health Organization, 2001).

Community reintegration has been formally defined as the process of becoming part of the mainstream of family and community life, participating in normal roles and responsibilities, and being an active and contributing member of one's social groups and society as a whole (Dijkers, 1998). Moves toward focusing on participation rather than integration are now acknowledged (Brown et al., 2004). The community integration construct has been called into question through examination of clinical and research measures (Minnes et al., 2004), and similar dilemmas are seen with multidimensional aspects of participation as part of community living (Dumont, Bertrand, Fougeyrollas, & Gervais, 2003). Whereas integration denotes membership, participation implies sharing as an active and dynamic process, and this description might better characterize views of individuals with disability.

Contexts termed *community* have been debated as well. Definitions of **community** include a people's sharing of an area (e.g., locality, district, government) as well as interests and interactions and perhaps a sense of shared identity (Oxford English Dictionary, 2001). Community is also defined by the designation of rural, suburban, and urban communities, which is based on metropolitan statistical area or measurements of population density. These designations are sometimes used to contrast communities in terms of resource availability as well as lifestyles and diversity (Fazio, 2001).

Traditional views of community are helpful in conceptualizing both the needs of individuals as well as groups within the community. Toennies (translated in 1957) used the German term *gemeinschaft* to characterize the relationships between individuals that are private and based on shared interests with kin or family, neighborhoods and groups of friends. Such personalized community elements were contrasted with *gesellschaft*, the term used to characterize system resources and actions that are a public expression or response to a duty or to an organization within society. While both *gemeinschaft* and *gesellschaft* are present in contemporary societies, urban settings are often viewed as having fewer personalized supports in place and rural settings as having fewer system resources

(Christenson, 1979). The rural versus urban, personal versus system contrasts might be overly simplistic, particularly in modern times as intentional or virtual communities form based on shared interests and identity, with connections that are electronic and not dependent on shared geography (Fellowship for Intentional Community, 1996; Rheingold, 1998). For some, participation through the Internet can make disability invisible, along with other aspects of identity (Bowker & Tuffin, 2002).

Nevertheless, these definitions of community remind practitioners to draw on natural helpers and supports in the environment while also informing clients about their rights, responsibilities, and entitlements to participate within community programs and systems. Uses of natural helpers and supports are hallmarks of community integration and can play a key role in assessment and intervention planning (Hagner, Rogan, & Murphy, 1992; Israel, 1985).

Another useful characterization of community is found in Bronfenbrenner's model (1977), which recognizes the interdependencies that exist between people and their social settings. According to Bronfenbrenner, the individual lives in a microsystem, the immediate settings involving factors of place, time, physical features, activity, participants, and roles. Interrelations between microsystems such as home, school, and workplaces are designated a mesosystem and include personal groupings such as family and friends, schoolmates, and coworkers. Formal and informal social systems at the local level are termed exosystems and include influences of neighborhood, mass media, agencies of government, business, communication and transportation systems, and other social networks. At the societal level is the macrosystem, the overarching patterns of the culture or subculture that often guide or organize the economy as well as educational, social, legal, and political systems.

The complex interdependence between individuals and their environmental surroundings is important for understanding issues and developing interventions that include all levels of community. Client-centered approaches focus on microsystems (e.g., the home), and community-based approaches include mesosystems as well (e.g., local stores, school, work settings). Community-centered approaches are focused on exosystems (e.g., public health programs) and macrosystems (e.g., public policy, rules and regulations) that may optimize accessibility and acceptance within communities. An individual's success with transition toward community participation will likely involve change at both the individual and community levels and points to a necessary blending of client-centered and community-centered approaches.

The term *community (re)integration* suggests that a poor fit exists between the individual and the community in which he or she seeks a connection. The individual might feel different, excluded, and perhaps not welcome. Therapeutic and social efforts seek to afford individuals a right to become a participating member within a community and give guidance in understanding responsibilities and duties

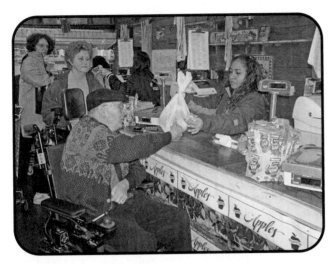

FIGURE 19.1 A customer shops with his wife and pays for groceries at a local market for vegetable growers. Both accessibility and acceptance are a part of community participation. Photo by Jackie Hall, M.S., OTR, VA Puget Sound Health Care System.

to the community. When these efforts are successful, full participation allows unrestricted and equal association, access, and acceptance into a community (Figure 19.1). Inclusion may be used to describe one's presence in a group or an opportunity to fully participate. With a strong understanding of person-environment interactions, occupational therapy practitioners are well prepared to promote community integration (Collins, 1996).

For occupational therapists and other practitioners, tension exists between scope of practice and context of practice. We have seen moves from institutional care to center-based care to community-based care. Institutional care, now generally frowned on, began as a thoughtful strategy to congregate and protect people who were perceived as being vulnerable. However, protection resulted more in segregation, alienation, and stigmatization (Priestly, 1999). Moves toward deinstitutionalization lead to center-based care, in which buildings were created for purposes of congregating services, with an effort made to have centers considered a part of the regional or local community. Dissatisfaction still exists with centers, due to perceived disconnection with natural contexts. So now a **community-based** orientation is promoted with a focus on actual environments of function and participation (e.g., homes, schools, businesses, parks, and transportation) (Law & Mills, 1998; McColl, 1998). Advocacy for community-based rehabilitation is also part of the World Health Organization's mission in promoting inclusion and opportunities for people with disability worldwide (WHO, 2004).

Client-centered and family-centered approaches can be community-based (Scaffa, 2001) but are distinct from community-centered approaches, in which community systems, places, or attitudes are addressed. These approaches have specific focuses of concern and different evaluation and intervention practices.

Client-Centered Approaches

Concern for the individual's community participation typically involves analysis of personal environments such as home accessibility, safety, supervision needs, and personal as well as social engagements. Reorganization of such environments, additions of durable medical equipment, and architectural modifications are sometimes necessary, as are family training and counseling regarding provision of assistance. **Client-centered** or family-centered approaches may include accessing, advising, and/or training to support performance in local community settings such as the grocery store, movie theater, park, and community bus or rail system. Sometimes attention is focused specifically on performance and participation in educational programs, volunteer or paid work settings, or involvement with organized city or county recreational facilities and programs. Citizenship activities such as access to voting also may be addressed.

The individual's and family's means of making changes in the home, communication systems, means of transportation, and returning or new participation in community activity is planned with and around the client and his or her resources. Values that are supported in that effort are client-specific and culturally sensitive. For some people, independence and a reduced burden of care and/or economic burden on one's personal network (e.g., family) are priorities. Sometimes the choices and ultimate decisions made by clients and families might differ from the practitioner's recommendations, but in client-centered care, the client's authority and preferences are supported by the practitioner's teaching and guidance rather than the practitioner's directing or commanding (Scaffa, 2001). The practitioner uses a nondirective style and a phenomenological approach in having individuals describe their experiences and their reality (Law & Mills, 1998). Respect for client and families and making sure that enough time is devoted to active listening are essential components of a client-centered approach. Self-efficacy is also at the core of client-centered practice (Baum, 1998), but clients and families will differ in how much they want to participate in a partnership. Regardless, being treated with respect and receiving information that will help in decision making is likely to increase client and family satisfaction.

Community-Centered Approaches

Concern about integration of all community members with disability calls for different orientations and intervention strategies. Community-focused strategies are discussed, but for understanding needs and setting priorities, it is helpful to review the community participation challenges that people with disability experience. A recent survey reports that nearly 49 million people (19% of the U.S. population) have a disability or limitation in one or more activities of daily living (ADL) or instrumental activities of daily living (IADL) (Kraus, Stoddard, & Gilmartin, 1996). Over 12% of the U.S. population has what is regarded as a severe disability, and almost 4% need personal assistance during their daily lives. IADL problems are more common than are ADL difficulties for people with disability, and adults with IADL problems are most often challenged by problems of mobility, cognition, manipulation, and activities involving vision, hearing, and communication. Another common characteristic of people in the community with disability is unemployment. For many groups with disability, the community wide rate of unemployment is well over 60%, and the poverty rate for people ages 25 to 64 years with severe disability is nearly 28%, compared to 8% for those without disability. Although older age and residence in a rural setting are indicative of greater rates and severity of disability, the prevalence of disability and needs for addressing health challenges appear to be on the increase in all age groups (Lollar, 2002; Rimmer & Braddock, 2002).

A move from a client-centered to a community-centered focus on health and well-being brings attention to the reality that while health is a personal issue, one's health status and functional well-being involve a dynamic interaction between personal factors and community factors. The latter can be explored through addressing the **independent living movement (ILM)** practices of public health and other efforts to create safe, healthy, and accessible communities that enable full participation.

Independent Living Movement

During the latter half of the twentieth century, as larger numbers of individuals with disability sought opportunities within communities, the ILM was created and gave rise to a number of public changes in views about disability (DeJong, 1979). For example, the Americans with Disabilities Act of 1990 brought a sense of civil rights to all communities, an extension of the rights that had previously been associated only with government programs (e.g., Rehabilitation Act of 1973, Education for All legislation [PL 94-142] of 1975). The ILM is a social movement that was conceived and aimed toward a better quality of life for people with disability. The ILM is heavily indebted to other contemporary social movements such as civil rights, consumerism, self-help, demedicalization of self-care, and deinstitutionalization. The self-empowerment of people with disability is credited with a shifting of traditional policy values to integrated living values. Examples include shifts from concepts of care to participation, from segregation to integration, from normalization to self-determination, from charity to civil

rights, and from caseload to citizenship (Priestly, 1999). The ILM recognizes the following:

> Each person has the right to independence through maximum control over his or her life, based on an ability and opportunity to make choices in performing everyday activities. These activities include: managing one's personal life; participating in community life; fulfilling social roles, such as marriage, parenthood, employment, and citizenship; sustaining self-determination; and minimizing physical or psychological dependence on others. Community integration incorporates ideas of both place and participation, so that a person is physically located in a community setting, and participates in community activities. Issues of consumer direction and control also are integral to concepts of community integration. (National Center for the Dissemination of Rehabilitation Research, 2006)

The ILM continues to be a social force that acknowledges changing community systems. For example, during the rise in health care costs nationwide, people with disability are put at particular risk. Medical expenditure per capita for people reporting two or more disabling chronic conditions can be five times the amount incurred by those with no limiting conditions and almost two times the amount incurred by those with one limiting condition (Rice & LaPlante, 1992). Those with disabilities caused by chronic conditions have higher-than-average health care costs and are considered a high-risk population that calls for rehabilitation specialists to partner with consumers to effectively advocate for services (Batavia, 1999). Moves toward managed care have put a squeeze on individuals and groups of people with disability, which results in Medicaid (i.e., publicly funded health insurance) being the single largest provider of health care financing for people with disability (DeJong, Palsbo, Beatty, Jones, Kroll, & Neri, 2002).

Public Health Perspective

Financial dilemmas associated with health care costs and particular challenges associated with disability draw attention to another important community orientation. A **public health** perspective recognizes the value of medical care as only one level of intervention, bringing attention to prevention of community-wide health challenges. In public health, the **target condition** is the health or disease outcome that the preventive care intervention avoids (primary prevention), identifies early (secondary prevention), or treats effectively (tertiary prevention). **Risk factors** are the attributes associated with the target condition and may include demographic variables, behavioral risk factors, and environmental factors. The most promising role for prevention in current practice may lie in changing the personal health behaviors of individuals prior to disease or injury onset. For example, about half of all disability and deaths may be attributed to tobacco, alcohol, and illicit drug use; diet and activity patterns; motor vehicles; and sexual behavior. Prevention practice can involve all health and education professionals (U.S. Preventive Services Task Force, 1996).

Although public health practices are found in various agencies outside of hospitals or other health care settings, important roles for all practitioners are acknowledged. Physicians, for example, are encouraged to provide brief advice during routine visits and to refer clients to allied health professionals with special counseling skills in their areas of expertise (e.g., occupational therapy for automobile driver safety). For all practitioners, principles of prevention follow along with ideas of patient activation (Hibbard, 2003) and include those in Box 19.1.

Every opportunity should be taken to deliver preventive services, especially to people who have limited access to care. Delivering preventive services at every visit is recommended. For some health problems, community-level interventions might be more effective than clinical preventive services. An important role for clinicians is their participation in community systems that address various types of health problems.

Public health practices are often described by using the analogy of a continuous flowing river (Orleans, Gruman, Ulmer, Emont, & Hollendonner, 1999). Downstream tactics or programs seek to make a change in individual behaviors of people in targeted groups that are at risk and sometimes all groups within communities. Midstream strategies are designed to influence those who might have an influence on individuals. Physicians and other health practitioners as well as educators may be recruited to deliver prevention practice information. Upstream concerns confront public policy and regulatory mechanisms that have a population focus. Examples include pollution and other environmental issues as well as roadway safety and manufacturing of devices for public use.

Healthy People 2010

Within the United States, public health strategies are a part of the development of national health priorities. Sponsored by the U.S. Surgeon General and building from previous national health priorities, Healthy People 2010 identifies 10 public health priorities for the country (Office of Disease Prevention and Health Promotion, 2001). Health People 2010 seeks to augment the health of each individual, the health of communities, and the health of the nation. The report serves as a basis for developing community plans to address two paramount goals for individuals of all ages: (1) Increase quality and years of healthy life, and (2) eliminate health disparities that exist within the population. Stark differences in health exist on the basis of gender, race or ethnicity, education or income, disability, geographic location, and sexual orientation. Ten health indicators are designated to serve as targets for individual and community action, and focus areas call for specific attention to key activities to reduce or eliminate illness, disability, and premature death among individuals within communities (Box 19.2).

Health promotion and disease prevention activities have long been advocated within occupational therapy, and Healthy People 2010 calls for community-centered application of those ideals (Hildenbrand & Froehlich, 2002). Areas of focus can become widespread and include efforts to promote uses of assistive technology, accessible design, and access to health-promoting occupations for all people. While different from traditional client-centered services,

---

BOX 19.1 ACTIVATION PRINCIPLES

- Assisting individuals to assume greater responsibility for their own health and personal health practices.
- Seeing individuals as the principal agents in primary prevention and empowering and counseling individuals to change health-related behaviors.
- Understanding that when people have the confidence to affect their health, they are more likely to do so than are those without such confidence (Schwarzer, 1992).
- Shared decision making and respect for values about possible outcomes.
- Education and consideration of choices, preferences, and uncertainty as part of decision making rather than a uniform policy for all people.

BOX 19.2 PUBLIC HEALTH CHALLENGE TARGETS

- Promote regular physical activity.
- Promote healthier weight and good nutrition.
- Prevent and reduce tobacco use.
- Prevent and reduce substance abuse.
- Promote responsible sexual behavior.
- Promote mental health and well-being.
- Promote safety and reduce violence.
- Promote healthy environments.
- Prevent infectious disease through immunization.
- Increase access to high-quality health care.

many efforts that address community-centered concerns can be approached though cost-effective collaborations (Merryman, 2002).

National organizations, such as the American Occupational Therapy Association, are called on to develop programs that empower individuals to make informed health care decisions and promote community-wide safety, education, and access to health care (e.g., backpack safety for school-aged children) (American Occupational Therapy Association, 2005). Primary prevention is a priority for community action. To address Healthy People 2010 objectives, arenas for programmatic interventions include places where people congregate and interact. These may include school settings, worksite settings, health care settings, and the community at large through public facilities, local government agencies, and social services as well as faith-based and civic organizations to reach people where they live, work, and play.

EVALUATION AND INTERVENTION TO ENABLE COMMUNITY PARTICIPATION

Evaluation and intervention services can be provided on a continuum using both client-centered and community-centered perspectives. Intervention initially may focus on the individual and a shift from institution or clinical context of care to the client's own community. This shift moves intervention to natural environments in which clients conduct their lives and encounter and adapt to realities of physical, social, and political contexts. At the other end of the continuum, intervention may focus primarily on the community, where one takes action to change community systems to enable full participation by all individuals, including those with disability (Figure 19.2).

Client-Centered Evaluation and Intervention

Evaluation of the individual includes a traditional approach of addressing the client's skills and needs but also includes people who are in the client's personal network (e.g., family, friends, and neighbors). An individual's place of residence and local settings in the community and transportation systems are also assessed.

Assessment of participation can focus on a single care recipient or on a sampling of individuals with specific diagnostic conditions or classifications of disability. While the International Classification of Functioning, Disability and Health (ICF) model directs that greater attention be given to participation as an outcome, the effective measurement of participation is viewed as problematic and in need of new assessment approaches (Granlund, Eriksson, & Ylven, 2004; Jette & Haley, 2005; Okochi, Utsunomiya & Takahashi, 2005; Salter, Jutai, Teasell, Foley, Bitensky, & Bayley, 2005). Although a variety of measures have been

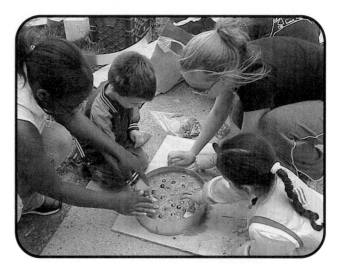

FIGURE 19.2 Children, including those who have social isolation challenges due to autism or emotional disorders, participate in making mosaic steppingstones to honor family members in a neighborhood revitalization project. Photo by Roger Ideishi, Ph.D., OTR, University of the Sciences in Philadelphia.

proposed to evaluate community integration and participation, critiques of those measures reveals that it is often difficult to measure activity and participation levels separately (Perenboom & Chorus, 2003). Approaches to community participation assessment do indicate that the phenomenon is best addressed as a self-reported outcome. How the individual views his or her level of success and the individual's identification of barriers with participation are important features of assessment.

Shifting from a center-based to community-based approach requires shifting practice environments as well as shifting one's philosophy. Practitioners must be expert in consultation and program development and focus on issues that are broader than typical direct service (Dudgeon & Greenberg, 1998). Working through teachers in schools, supervisors in jobs, and other natural supports in the community might be necessary to be effective. In transitioning to community-based practice, Fazio (2001) suggests that natural settings might be the most effective arena for service delivery. Community-based approaches, such as evaluating people's needs in their homes, are encouraged (Freeman, 1997; Sabari, Meisler, & Silver, 2000) and are sometimes found to be effective for stroke rehabilitation and for individuals with brain injury (Anderson et al., 2000; Willer, Button, & Rempel, 1999).

Community-Centered Evaluation and Involvement

Community assessment may involve exploration of incidence and prevalence of occupational dysfunction needs within populations. However, assessing dysfunction could backfire and not support a community because it focuses on deficiency rather than potential. Kretzmann and McKnight (1993) suggest that we need to move away from focusing on community deficiencies (e.g., unemployment, crime, illiteracy, gangs, and dropouts). Instead, moves can be made toward recognizing and utilizing relationships between community assets such as those that exist in individuals (e.g., the elderly, youth, artists), citizen organizations (e.g., cultural groups, churches), and local institutions (e.g., schools, businesses, parks, hospitals). A "needs survey" becomes a deficiency inventory, whereas a "capacity inventory" moves toward empowerment of communities (Kretzmann & McNight, 1993). McKnight (1994) argues that health care organizations can behave as community members (e.g., through advocacy, financing, volunteerism, and space availability) and address community needs by focusing not on an epidemiological or diagnostic ideology but on an individual, family, or community's capacities and assets.

Kretzmann (2000) contends that health is a product of four determinants: (1) the behavior of the individual, (2) the strength of individual social relationships, (3) the healthfulness of the physical environment, and (4) the economic status of the individual. He proposes "asset-based community assessment and development." Skills of local residents, power of voluntary citizens' associations, and resources of public, private and nonprofit institutions should be harnessed to promote health within a community. For example, to address the influence of local associations, practitioners might explore partnerships with schools, youth organizations, local businesses, and associations that promote participation by those with disability. Such partnerships might include collaborations with Coalitions of Citizens with Disability, the National Alliance for the Mentally Ill, ARC (the national organization of and for people with mental retardation and related developmental disabilities and their families), the Arthritis Foundation, or other support and advocacy organizations.

Occupational therapy practitioners have much to contribute to community accessibility and acceptance of people with disabilities. Contributions may involve developing community partnerships with a "new cadre of colleagues including people with disabilities, engineers, architects, personal assistants, independent living counselors, recreation and exercise personnel, city planners, law enforcement, and transportation specialists" (Baum & Law, 1997, p. 280). Community change can be approached through county and city councils, business and visitor bureaus, and local media and advocacy organizations.

Advocacy About Accessibility

Advocacy, a key element of community-centered care, brings attention to issues and educates potential members of a community, ultimately drawing them into problem-solving actions that may resolve or lessen barriers to participation. At the community level, advocacy may focus on accessibility and acceptance. Community accessibility involves the application of accessible design rules that have been established over the years at the federal, state, and local levels through building codes. In both new construction and remodeling, accessibility guidelines help to create access for those who are challenged in the areas of mobility, cognition, manipulation, hearing, vision, and/or communication. Access applies to the building environment as well as to products and other community systems such as transportation, communication, and information systems. For example, for people with any combination of sensory, motor, or cognitive difficulties, access to the Internet is challenged by Web designs that restrict accessibility options and may restrict individuals' access to information and participation in virtual communities (World Wide Web Consortium, 2001).

Although accessibility guidelines have been in place for several decades, some dissatisfaction continues to exist with design because codes dictate a minimal approach to access rather than a universal application of design that may apply to a more inclusive community. **Universal design** concepts and principles suggest that environments and products be designed to be usable by all people, to the greatest extent possible, without the need for special arrangements, adaptations, or greater cost (Center for Universal Design, 1997; Iwarsson & Stahl, 2003).

Accessible and universal design needs to have advocates in the community. While many people with disability do advocate on behalf of themselves and others, greater community awareness and improved timing of attention to accessibility need to occur. Both design and manufacturing of buildings and other systems are expensive ventures, and a lack of attention to access or universal design becomes cost prohibitive if applied too late. As an advocate, one needs to practice what one preaches. Such an attitude may include doing business with those who provide access and boycotting those who fail to address accessibility. One can also apply accessibility and universal design to one's own environment. In recent years, the concept of **visitability** has been suggested and sometimes mandated (Smith, 2003). Visitability applies simple design elements to residential settings. The concept and practice creates at least one level entrance to a dwelling and access (e.g., 32 inches wide) to one bathroom on that level. Other suggestions for universal design in homes are the creation of floor space for toilet and tub transfers as well as structural supports in walls for the mounting of grab bars that might become necessary for safety and independence. A shortage of accessible living settings in neighborhoods is a recognized problem, and creation of visitability might help to overcome such shortages.

Advocacy About Acceptance

Addressing community acceptance of people with disability can be a harder advocacy role to assume. The "differentness" that disability entails often creates mystery and uneasiness. Comfort within a community is sometimes based on similarity rather than on differentness (Whyte & Ingstad, 1995). A more accessible environment could provide people with disability a greater feeling of acceptance, but disability also can evoke feelings of blame, shame, pity, and avoidance. Physical, cognitive, sensory, and behavioral differences might need to be addressed by educating for understanding and the practice of inclusion in residential, educational, employment, and recreational settings. One of the hallmarks of community-based rehabilitation is the recognition that barriers to full participation exist in the community and that one can increase community awareness of the needs of members with disability, providing changes that create occupational opportunities (Baker &

Brownson, 1999). Access to opportunities for citizenship, housing, employment, transportation, education, and other social structures give people with disabilities opportunities to be successful. Occupational therapy practitioners can support the initiatives of people with disabilities or advocacy groups that promote social development and lead toward institutional, political, and social frameworks that support full participation. For example, practitioners could hold forums to educate employers in the local community about the workplace accommodations that are most useful to people with psychiatric disabilities. Unlike a physical accommodation such as a wheelchair ramp, accommodations for people with psychiatric disabilities are often social in nature and need ongoing attention and retraining.

CASE STUDY: *Jason's Story: Living with a Spinal Cord Injury*

Jason is a young man who experienced C-6 complete spinal cord injury one and a half years ago in a motor vehicle crash. As a 23-year-old, Jason had completed high school and had worked in various entry-level service jobs before his injury. With nearly complete loss of sensation and movement from C-7 down, his medical rehabilitation involved development of wheelchair mobility skills and adapted performance of activities of daily living, including self-catheterization and a bowel program. Jason was also instructed to do regular skin inspection, follow diet and weight control measures, and engage in fitness activities.

To address independent living and community integration as part of discharge planning, the Craig Handicap Assessment and Reporting Tool (CHART) (Whiteneck, Charlifue, Gerhart, Overholser, & Richardson, 1992) was used as part of assessment and intervention planning. Jason scored well on all mobility items but had lower than expected scores related to occupation, economic, and social outcomes. As part of care planning, therapists were involved in doing a home assessment, staging of independent living trials within the hospital, and going out with Jason and others on various community outings to explore transportation and community functioning.

Jason would be discharged to apartment living in a building his family owned, which his sister-in-law lived in and managed. He would have reduced rent, and both his sister-in-law and his brother would be nearby to provide assistance as needed.

Within the hospital setting, a trial apartment-style unit was available for Jason to stay in and practice routine living activities toward the conclusion of his stay, with nursing and therapy services readily available as necessary. Community outings were coordinated through recreational therapy and occupational therapy. These included shopping at a grocery store as part of a meal preparation and cooking activity,

viewing a movie at a local theater, and shopping for clothes in a department store. Orientation to city bus services was provided, and Jason was encouraged to use the bus, with the plan that he would later be referred for driver's training. Jason also works with vocational rehabilitation and is planning to enroll in college to enhance his potential for employment that would require fewer physical demands.

Jason's experiences were reflected best by his later return for outpatient therapy and interview by his therapist, who asked about community functioning.

Regarding his transition, Jason said, "I mean it's such night and day between when I got discharged from the hospital and now as to how fast I can do things. It just frees up so much time. I mean, it's amazing how much more free time I have, and time to concentrate on living life rather than getting through life. I mean, taking care of myself used to be all of my day right there. And now I can be at home and maybe get something to eat and get a second wind again, and go out with friends or something, but it's definitely a large stamina issue." Jason went on to say, "I really enjoy the company of my friends, but I can't hang out with them for more than a couple of days at a time because they'll run me dry. I mean . . . I'll start getting haggard and tired and falling asleep sitting in my wheelchair."

Reflecting on his inpatient rehabilitation, Jason was positive about "the support group that was there, the therapy, the people coming in the middle of the day to try and get you up and get you about. I mean those early stages are pretty important. Without that, it's easy to just stay down and not really have a desire to get better and strive for more." Jason said, "It definitely, sort of feels like I've been taken under wing by a community. I definitely could not have done what I have . . . without that support."

Jason described rehabilitation as "just learning all over again . . . something that you unconsciously learn when you are a toddler." Jason mentioned the importance of exposure to various pieces of equipment and learning how to use adaptive devices. He remarked, "It definitely can be huge in someone's life, and so I think it's good and important to have those things shown to you."

About his discharge, he said, "It feels like you're getting tossed out somewhere. I mean, I definitely knew they weren't just saying bye; I knew I was still going to be signing up for out patient therapy. Yet at the same time, you do kind of feel like you're definitely tossed out on your own."

Source: Adapted from Davidson, Dudgeon, & Carpenter (submitted).

Jason reported that he "definitely has more of a feeling of . . . unconditional love" and that the compassion he had been shown had made him "see a more loving side to the world." He also reported feeling "more at peace" with himself, but he continued to be challenged with being different. About being in the community, Jason said, "It's the last place I want to be, like, I'm this kid in a wheelchair in a sports athletic store, and it's just so frustrating. I just want to hide from everybody. It's just working on trying to be comfortable with myself again."

SUMMARY

Community well-being is both behavioral and social in nature and includes individual lifestyle behaviors, the environment, socioeconomic factors, and local, state, and federal regulations and policies. Promoting participation in community life includes client and community approaches. One way to conceive of community care is to apply a public health model, with practitioners providing midstream and upstream interventions. Primary prevention measures are those that prevent the onset of a targeted condition (e.g., antismoking, promotion of activity and fitness). Such practices may be advocated and taught in community centers, senior programs, schools, and workplaces. Secondary prevention measures identify and treat asymptomatic people who have developed risk factors or preclinical disease before the condition is clinically evident. Examples include backpack safety for school children, ergonomics for at-risk workers, fall prevention among the elderly, and violence prevention in various settings. Tertiary prevention measures focus on intervention with people with clinical illnesses, health conditions, and disaster relief needs. Traditionally, occupational therapy practitioners focused on development, recovery, or adaptation as well as prevention of secondary complications, and maintenance of skills in community living. More recently, practitioners are shifting their focus to include community-centered intervention approaches to promote participation for all people, regardless of their ability status.

PROVOCATIVE QUESTIONS

The International Classification of Function and Disability places an emphasis on participation as an important characteristic in measurement of health. *Participation* is defined as "involvement in a life situation," and *participation restrictions* are defined as "problems an individual may have with involvement in life situations." Some problems can be due to environmental factors, which include all aspects of the physical, social, and attitudinal world.

Although defined, the measurement of participation is more challenging and is the subject of some controversy. Brown and colleagues (2004) have suggested that *community integration*, a construct that first emerged as part of deinstitutionalization of people with developmental and mental health disabilities, be replaced by or amended with the term *community participation*. *Community integration* may be viewed as a term that outsiders use in describing successful or unsuccessful fitting in to community living. In contrast, *community participation* can suggest a more dynamic status as part of community living.

1. Have you, a family member, or a friend experienced a difference or disability that caused a problem with participation? What was the nature of that problem, and in what ways could have participation been enhanced?

2. Ask that same question using the term *integration*. Have you, a family member, or a friend experienced a difference or disability that caused a problem with integration? What was the nature of that problem, and in what ways might integration have been enhanced?

3. The terminology above in some ways reflects a tension between the medical model and the social model of disability. In the medical model, disability reflects a deficit in the person who is unable to lead life in traditional or accepted ways. In the social model, fault for dysfunction is shifted to society, wherein systems and environments are viewed as enabling or disabling, such as creating barriers to performance and effective participation. Occupational therapists may appraise environments as being enabling or disabling, yet there is continuing tension between devoting resources to "fixing the person" and devoting them to "fixing the environment." For example, accessible and universal design are promoted as a means to create more enabling environments for everyone, yet the

expenses of retrofitting the existing built environment and designing with universal design ideas from the start are often viewed as excessively costly and unachievable. After its passage, the ADA was soon regarded as one of the U.S. government's largest *unfunded mandates*. What are your thoughts (and conflicts) relative to fixing the community to enable better participation, versus fixing the person or enabling the person to deal better with participation challenges in unaltered communities?

ON THE WEB

◆ Educational activities

REFERENCES

American Occupational Therapy Association. (2005). *National School Backpack Awareness Day was a huge success.* Retrieved October 25, 2005, from http://www.promoteot.org/AI_BackpackAwareness.html

Anderson, C., Rubenbach, S., Mhurchu, C. N., Clark, M., Spencer, C., & Winsor, A. (2000). Home or hospital for stroke rehabilitation? Results of a randomized controlled trial. 1: Health outcomes at 6 months [Electronic version]. *Stroke, 31,* 1024–1031.

Baker, E. A., & Brownson, R. C. (1999) Defining characteristics of community-based health promotion programs. In R. C., Brownson, E. A. Baker, & L. F. Novick (Eds.), *Community-based prevention: Programs that work* (pp. 7–19). Gaithersburg, MD: Aspen.

Batavia, A. I. (1999). Independent living centers, medical rehabilitation centers, and managed care for people with disabilities. *Archives of Physical Medicine and Rehabilitation, 80,* 1357–1360.

Baum, C. (1998). Client-centered practice in a changing health care system. In M. Law (Ed.), *Client-centered occupational therapy* (pp. 29–45). Thorofare, NJ: Slack.

Baum, C., & Law, M. (1997). Occupational therapy practice: Focusing on occupational performance. *American Journal of Occupational Therapy, 51,* 277–288.

Bowker, N., & Tuffin, K. (2002). Disability discourses for online identities. *Disability & Society, 17,* 327–344.

Bronfenbrenner, U. (1977). Toward an experimental ecology of human development. *American Psychologist, 32,* 513–531.

Brown, M., Dijkers, M. P., Gordon, W. A., Ashman, T., Charatz, H., & Cheng, Z. (2004). Participation objective, participation subjective: A measure of participation combining outsider and insider perspectives. *Journal of Head Trauma Rehabilitation, 19,* 459–481.

Center for Universal Design. (1997, April 1). *What is universal design?* Raleigh: North Carolina State University, Center for Universal Design. Retrieved May 7 2007, from http://www.ncsu.edu/www/ncsu/design/sod5/cud/about_ud/udprinciples.htm

Christenson, J. A. (1979). Gemeinschaft and Gesellschaft: Testing the spatial and communal hypothesis. *Social Forces, 63,* 160–168.

Collins, L. F. (1996). Easing client transition from facility to community. *OT Practice, 1,* 36–39.

Davidson, C. A., Dudgeon, B. J., & Carpenter, C. M. (submitted). Surviving to living: The transition from rehabilitation to community participation after spinal cord injury. *OTJR: Occupation, Participation and Health.*

DeJong, G. (1979). Independent living: From social movement to analytic paradigm. *Archives of Physical Medicine and Rehabilitation, 60,* 435–446.

DeJong, G., Palsbo, S. E., Beatty, P. W., Jones, G. C., Kroll, T., & Neri, M. T. (2002). The organization and financing of health services for individuals with disabilities. *Milbank Quarterly 80,* 261–301.

Dijkers, M. (1998). Community integration: Conceptual issues and measurement approaches in rehabilitation research. *Topics in Spinal Cord Injury Rehabilitation, 4,* 1–15.

Dudgeon, B. J., & Greenberg, S. L. (1998). Preparing students for consultation roles and systems. *American Journal of Occupational Therapy, 52,* 801–809.

Dumont, C., Bertrand, R., Fougeyrollas, P., & Gervais, M. (2003). Rasch modeling and the measurement of social participation. *Journal Applied Measurement, 4,* 309–325.

Fazio, L. S. (2001). *Developing occupation-centered programs for the community: A workbook for students and professionals,* Upper Saddle River, NJ: Prentice Hall.

Fellowship for Intentional Communities. (1996, October). *What's true about intentional communities: Dispelling the myths.* Retrieved October 25, 2005, from http://www.ic.org/pnp/myths.html

Freeman, E. A. (1997). Community-based rehabilitation of the person with a severe brain injury. *Brain Injury, 11,* 143–153.

Granlund, J., Eriksson, L., & Ylvén, R. (2004). Utility of international classification of functioning, disability and health's participation dimension in assigning ICF codes to items from extant rating instruments. *Journal Rehabilitation Medicine, 36,* 130–137.

Hagner, D., Rogan, P., & Murphy, S. (1992). Facilitating natural supports in the workplace: Strategies for support consultants. *Journal of Rehabilitation, 58,* 29–34.

Hibbard, J. H. (2003). Engaging health care consumers to improve the quality of care. *Medical Care, 41*(1, Suppl.), 161–170.

Hildenbrand, W. C., & Froehlich, K. (2002). Promoting health: Historical roots, renewed vision. *OT Practice, 7,* 5, 10–15.

Israel, B. A. (1985). Social networks and social support: Implications for natural helpers and community level interventions. *Health Education Quarterly, 12,* 1, 65–80.

Iwarsson, S., & Stahl, A. (2003). Accessibility, usability and universal design-positioning and definition of concepts describing person-environment relationships. *Disability and Rehabilitation, 25,* 57–66.

Jette, A. M., & Haley, S. M. (2005). Contemporary measurement techniques for rehabilitation outcomes assessment. *Journal Rehabilitation Medicine, 37,* 339–345.

Kraus, L., Stoddard, S., & Gilmartin, D. (1996). *Chartbook on disability in the United States, 1996.* An InfoUse Report. Washington, DC: U.S. National Institute on Disability and Rehabilitation Research. Retrieved October 25, 2005, from http://www.infouse.com/disabilitydata/disability/1_1.php

Kretzmann, J. P. (2000). Co-producing health: Professionals and communities build on assets. *Health Forum Journal, 43,* 42.

Kretzmann, J. P., & McKnight, J. L. (1993). *Building communities from the inside out: A path toward finding and mobilizing a community's assets.* Evanston, IL: Northwestern University.

Law, M., & Mills, J. (1998). Client-centered occupational therapy. In M. Law (Ed.), *Client-centered occupational therapy* (pp. 1–18). Thorofare, NJ: Slack.

Lollar, D. J. (2002). Public health and disability: Emerging opportunities. *Public Health Report, 117,* 131–136.

McColl, M. A. (1998). What do we need to know to practice in the community? *American Journal of Occupational Therapy, 52,* 11–18.

McKnight, J. L. (1994). Hospitals and the health of their communities. *Hospitals and Health Networks, 68,* 40–41.

Merryman, M. B. (2002). Networking as an entrée to paid community practice. *OT Practice, 7*(9), 10–13.

Minnes, P. M., Buell, M. K., Nolte, M. L., McColl, M. A., Carlson, P., & Johnston, J. (2001). Defining community integration of persons with brain injury as acculturation: A Canadian perspective. *NeuroRehabilitation, 16,* 3–10.

National Center for the Dissemination of Rehabilitation Research. (2006). National Institute on Disability and Rehabilitation Research (NIDRR): Long-Range Plan for Fiscal Years 2005–2009. Retrieved May 6, 2007, from http://www.ncddr.org/new/announcements/lrp/fy2005–2009/index.html#ccl

Office of Disease Prevention and Health Promotion, Department of Health and Human Services. (2001, April). *Healthy people 2010: Understanding and improving health* (Stock no. 017-001-00550-9). Retrieved October 25, 2005, from http://www.healthypeople.gov/Document/pdf/uih/uih.pdf

Okochi, J., Utsunomiya, S., & Takahashi, T. (2005). Health measurement using the ICF: Test-retest reliability study of ICF codes and qualifiers in geriatric care. *Health and Quality of Life Outcomes, 3,* 46.

Orleans, C. T., Gruman, J., Ulmer, C., Emont, S. L., & Hollendonner, J. K. (1999). Rating our progress in population health promotion: Report card on six behaviors. *American Journal of Health Promotion, 14,* 75–82.

Oxford English Dictionary. (2001). [Electronic version]. Cary, NC: Oxford University Press.

Perenboom, R., & Chorus, A. (2003). Measuring participation according to the International Classification of Functioning, Disability and Health (ICF). *Disability and Rehabilitation, 25,* 577–587.

Priestly, M. (1999). *Disability politics and community care.* Philadelphia: Jessica Kingsley Publisher.

Rheingold, H. (1998). *The virtual community: Homesteading on the electronic frontier.* Retrieved October 25, 2005, from http://www.rheingold.com/vc/book

Rice, D. P., & LaPlante, M. P. (1992). Medical expenditures for disability and disabling comorbidity. *American Journal Public Health, 82,* 739–741.

Rimmer, J. H., & Braddock, D. (2002). Health promotion for people with physical, cognitive and sensory disabilities: an emerging national priority. *American Journal Health Promotion, 16,* 220–224.

Sabari, J. S., Meisler, J., & Silver, E. (2000). Reflections upon rehabilitation by members of a community based stroke club. *Disability Rehabilitation, 22,* 330–336.

Scaffa, M. (2001). *Occupational therapy in community-based practice settings.* Philadelphia: F. A. Davis.

Schwarzer, R. (1992). Self-efficacy in the adoption and maintenance of health behaviors: Theoretical approaches and a new model. In R. Schwarzer (Ed.), *Self-efficacy: Thought control of action* (pp. 217–243). Washington, DC: Hemisphere.

Salter, K., Jutai, J. W., Teasell, R., Foley, N. C., Bitensky, J., & Bayley, M. (2005). Issues for selection of outcome measures in stroke rehabilitation: ICF participation. *Disability and Rehabilitation, 27,* 507–528.

Smith, E. (2003, November). *Visitability defined 2003.* Retrieved October 25, 2005, from http://www.concretechange.org/Definition_of_Visitability.htm

Toennies, F. (1957). *Community & society (gemeinschaft and gesellschaft)* (C. P. Loomis, Trans.). New Brunswick, NJ: Transaction Publishers.

U.S. Preventive Services Task Force. (1996). *Guide to clinical preventive services* (2nd ed.). Washington, DC: U.S. Department of Health and Human Services. Retrieved July 19, 2001, from http://odphp.osophs.dhhs.gov/pubs/guidecps

Whiteneck, G. G., Charlifue, S. W., Gerhart, K. A., Overholser, J. D., & Richardson, G. N. (1992). Quantifying handicap: A new measure of long-term rehabilitation outcomes. *Archives of Physical Medicine and Rehabilitation, 73,* 519–526.

Whyte, S. R., & Ingstad, B. (1995). Disability and culture: An overview. In B. Ingstad, & S. R. Whyte (Eds.), *Disability and culture* (pp. 3–32). Berkeley: University of California Press.

Willer, B., Button, J., & Rempel, R. (1999). Residential and home-based postacute rehabilitation of individuals with traumatic brain injury: A case control study. *Archives of Physical Medicine and Rehabilitation, 80,* 399–406.

World Health Organization (WHO). (2004). *Community based rehabilitation (CBR).* Retrieved October 25, 2005, from, http://www.who.int/disabilities/publications/cbr/en/

World Wide Web Consortium. (2001, September 14). *Web accessibility initiative.* Retrieved October 25, 2005, from http://www.w3.org/WAI/

Occupational Justice

20

ANN A. WILCOCK AND ELIZABETH A. TOWNSEND

Learning Objectives

After reading this chapter, you will be able to:

1. Describe occupational justice.
2. Describe the integration of occupational justice within occupational therapy.
3. Identify occupational injustices with regard to clients.
4. Discuss approaches to advocate and mediate for change to enable clients to participate in occupations according to their needs.

Occupational justice is an integral but only recently acknowledged aspect of occupational therapy. From the profession's beginnings, therapists based their interventions on the idea that occupations contribute to health and that people have both a need and a right to participate in meaningful occupations (Dunton, 1915; LeVesconte, 1935; Meyer, 1922; Wilcock, 1998). To illustrate the power and potential of occupational justice, three intervention scenarios using an occupational justice perspective are presented.

The concept of occupational justice gives voice to occupational therapists' implicit historical and ethical stance to address potential or real injustices (Wood, Hooper, & Womack, 2005). In the mid-1990s, the concept of occupational justice arose from two directions of study in two different parts of the globe. One direction, concerned with understanding the relationship between occupation and health, discovered that beneficial or negative health outcomes related to occupations are dependent on sociopolitical and cultural determinants that can be framed in justice terms (Wilcock, 1993, 1995, 1998). The other direction, concerned with critical social analyses of client-centered practice, discovered that the work of enabling client empowerment through occupation is congruent with social justice work (Townsend, 1993, 1996, 1998). Both research directions generated reflections on occupation and social justice and whether or not social justice sufficiently addresses the rights of persons, individually and collectively, to participate in meaningful occupations. Occupational therapists around the world are currently discussing whether occupational justice is but one important aspect of social justice or a concept on its own. Some argue that both concepts envisage ideal societies governed by a set of ethical, moral, and civic principles about the rights and responsibilities between people; the ways in which they treat and relate to each other; societal liberties and freedoms; and the distribution of human and financial resources. Others argue that because social justice does not sufficiently address the difference between individual occupational natures and needs, occupational justice and social justice should be thought of as separate entities so that important aspects of occupational justice are not overlooked. Both perspectives acknowledge that all people are occupational beings with differing natures and needs and that meeting those needs is a matter of health, which makes it a matter of justice.

HOW TO DESCRIBE OCCUPATIONAL JUSTICE

There are no simple translations for the English terms *occupation* and *justice* to transcend cultural, linguistic, and social differences. Instead, consideration of four related terms is called for: *occupation, justice, social justice,* and, finally, *occupational justice.*

Occupation

Occupational therapists tend to hold different views about what the word *occupation* embraces. Here, *occupation* is used to mean all the things that people want, need, or have to do, whether of a physical, mental, social, sexual, political, spiritual, or any other nature, including sleep and rest activities. Occupation enables populations and communities to participate actively in shaping their own destinies (Thibeault, 2002) and can be health-enhancing or health-threatening. The duality of health or harm in occupation is a central tension that underlies occupational therapy.

Occupation is shaped by time, place, and social conditions and is a unit of economy. It is the practical, everyday medium of self-expression or of making or experiencing meaning because it is the activist element of human existence whether contemplative, reflective, and meditative or action-based performance. Occupation can provide the means to suppress the self, identity, being, belief, spirit, and autonomy as well as the means to express it. As a fundamental means of achieving implicit or explicit goals, power relations are central to possibilities and limitations. The power to participate in occupations may be controlled through physical force or invisibly through regulation and cultural expectations.

Justice

Justice has been defined in many ways throughout history. It has been equated with words such as *rights, equity,* and *fairness,* and Benjamin Disraeli (1851) described it as "truth in action." The term *justice* is most often applied to legal systems, but it is also used in arguing for equal dis-

tribution of resources and positive discrimination in terms of marginalized persons (Norton, 1994).

Social Justice

Social justice is a concept about rights, equity, and fairness. An accepted part of postmodern societies, this concept of justice centers on just social relations and conditions regardless of difference in race, class, gender, income, or disability. Social justice is applied to the ethical distribution and sharing of resources, rights, and responsibilities between people recognizing their equal worth as citizens, "their equal right to be able to meet basic needs, the need to spread opportunities and life chances as widely as possible, and finally the requirement that we reduce and where possible eliminate unjustified inequalities" (Commission on Social Justice, 1994, p. 1).

Occupational Justice

Occupational justice is also equated with words such as *rights, equity,* and *fairness.* It, too, is applied to the right of every individual to be able to meet basic needs and to have equal opportunities and life chances to reach toward her or his potential but specific to the individual's engagement in diverse and meaningful occupation. Occupational justice is a justice of difference because people have different natures, needs, and capacities that are expressed through what they do. Therefore, occupational justice requires ethical distribution and sharing of resources, rights, and responsibilities with regard to what individuals want, need, or are obliged to do within the social and ethical standards of a community. Occupation is what brings us to the reality of daily life, where we can talk about the everyday individual, group, and population experiences of occupation that occur within broad social conditions and structures that shape options for and against justice.

Social and occupational justice provide different perspectives for raising questions around a shared interest in justice (Figure 20.1). An exploratory theory of occupational justice proposed by Townsend and Wilcock (2004) suggests how these four ideas—occupation, justice, social justice, and occupational justice—relate to each other.

The theory presented in Figure 20.2 assumes that people are occupational beings, that they participate in occupations as autonomous beings, that participation is interdependent and contextual, and that it is a determinant of health and quality of life. The theory proposes the principles of empowerment through occupations; an inclusive classification of all occupations; individual and collective enablement of occupational potential; and diversity, inclusion, and shared advantage in occupational participation.

The primary purpose for developing the theory of occupational justice was to draw attention to the fact that

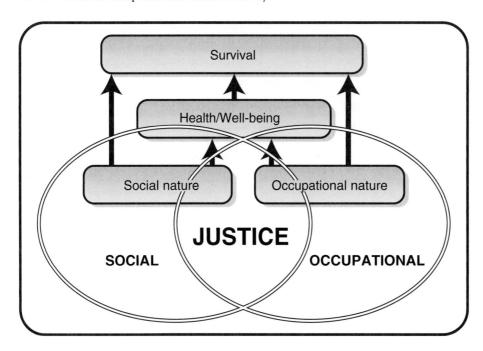

FIGURE 20.1 Occupational justice and social justice enabling the meeting of biological needs.

throughout the world, people are constrained, deprived, and alienated from engaging in occupations that provide personal, family, and/or community satisfaction, meaning, and balance through what they do. In many cases, people are unable to provide the necessities of life that are prerequisites to health:

The fundamental conditions and resources for health are peace, shelter, education, food, income, a stable eco-system, sustainable resources, social justice and equity. (World Health Organization [WHO], Health and Welfare Canada, Canadian Public Health Association, 1986, p. 2)

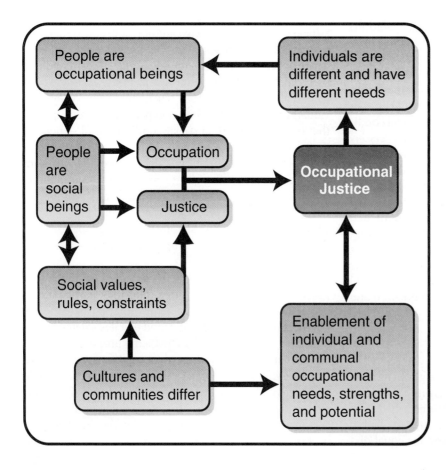

FIGURE 20.2 An exploratory theory of occupational justice: intersecting ideas. (Reproduced with permission from Prentice Hall.)

The World Health Organization (WHO) recommends action to promote health for all in many of its directives, such as the Ottawa Charter for Health Promotion (WHO et al., 1986), which calls not only for the satisfaction of needs and coping with the environment, but also for the realization of aspirations of physical, mental, and social well-being. *Health for All in the Twenty-first Century* (WHO, 1998) validates "the uniqueness of each person and the need to respond to each individual's spiritual quest for meaning, purpose and belonging" as part of health and as a matter of justice.

During the 1990s, the development of "active societies" and "enabling states" was addressed within international organizations (Gilbert, 1995; Kalisch, 1991, pp. 3–9; Organization for Economic Cooperation and Development [OECD], 1989). The Clinton Administration, for example, encouraged a Progressive Policy Institute "blueprint for a new America" in which

> the enabling state be organized around the goals of work and individual empowerment. . . . Above all, it should help poor Americans develop the capacities they need to liberate themselves from poverty and dependence. . . . An enabling strategy should see the poor as the prime agents of their own development, rather than as passive clients of the welfare system. (Marshall & Schram, 1993)

The Universal Declaration of Human Rights (United Nations [UN], 1998) advocates for all people to have a standard of living that is adequate for health and well-being. Advocacy is for people to have equal rights to work; to free choice of employment; to rest, leisure and holidays; to participate in the cultural life of a community; to engage in the arts and scientific advancement; to take part in national governments; and to fully develop the human personality. This declaration of fundamental rights for all provides topics for debate centering on notions of empowerment, choice, and opportunity; the tension between individual and community rights; and the tension between justice for individuals and the common good. The need for such rights to be considered part of intervention in health care is worthy of debate at all levels. Occupational therapists can enter this debate by addressing the need for participation in occupations that meet people's individual natures, capacities, and choice and how these relate to health and well-being.

RECOGNIZING THE PLACE OF OCCUPATIONAL JUSTICE WITHIN OCCUPATIONAL THERAPY

In addition to occupational therapy publications that focus on justice, such as *Spirit of Survivors: Occupational Therapy Without Borders* (Kronenberg, Algado, & Pollard, 2005), occupational justice ideas are influencing the governance, planning, and professional policies of occu-

pational therapy's professional organizations. The British College of Occupational Therapists (COT, 2002) put forward a strategic plan founded on contemporary ideas of health and social justice. In 2005, COT argued that equality and social justice are central to the professions' conceptual framework in that "occupational therapists have long worked with the most excluded and disadvantaged people to enable them to achieve fulfilling lives as members of communities." COT goes on to state:

> The profession uses the term 'occupational justice' to refer to the concept that acts as a complementary extension to social justice. Occupational justice provides a framework for asking questions about inequities of opportunity for occupational development, or inequities related to lack of appropriate enablement for those living with a disability (p. 2–3).

The European Network of Occupational Therapists in Higher Education embraced occupational justice as the theme of its 2003 annual conference. At that meeting, Townsend (2003) asked, "Why would occupational therapists be concerned with occupational justice?" Responses centered on the injustices that occur when humans are barred, trapped, confined, segregated, restricted, prohibited, unable to develop, disrupted, alienated, imbalanced, deprived, or marginalized in ways that exclude them from participating optimally in the occupations they need and want to do to sustain health throughout the life course.

The World Federation of Occupational Therapists (WFOT) also recognizes an increasing need for occupational justice to counter the sociopolitical and economic factors that underlie and are a consequence of disability. The WFOT affirms that "many people with disabilities are restricted in or denied access to dignified and meaningful occupation in their daily life and their well-being is sometimes compromised through occupational apartheid and/or occupational deprivation" (WFOT, 2004–2005, p. 2). In addition the international professional body has drawn up a Human Rights Position Statement that addresses issues of occupational justice (WFOT, 2006).

Today's practice of occupational therapy may actually rest on the profession's success in putting occupational injustice explicitly on the public agenda and showing what an occupation-focused, justice-driven profession can accomplish. Imagine, for instance, the power of reducing occupational disruptions for workers who have lost their jobs because of work-related injuries, of minimizing the occupational alienation and imbalances of people who live with severe and persistent mental illnesses, of fostering the occupational development of children with disabilities. Further, imagine the potential impacts of advocating for and participating in a restructuring of global economics and practices on the collective crises of war, refugees, dislocation of cultural groups, or natural disasters in which occupational deprivation, marginalization, or apartheid is the implicit and often taken-for-granted result.

WHAT TO DISCUSS WITH OTHERS ABOUT THE NATURE OF OCCUPATIONAL JUSTICE OR INJUSTICE

Occupational justice draws together two powerful biological needs: the need to do and the need to be part of a social group. Both are innate survival mechanisms, as archaeological and anthropological research demonstrates (Wilcock, 1998, 2006). The association of well-being with supportive relationships is strongly supported by research (Argyle, 1987; Blaxter, 1990; Cohen et al., 1982; Isaksson, 1990; Warr, 1990). The association of well-being with occupation is less well recognized but was supported in a survey in which participants were asked to define their concept of well-being (Wilcock et al., 1998, 2006). The most common responses to a question about the situation or environment they associated with feelings of well-being related to occupation, although the word *occupation* was not used. Instead, participants spoke of leisure, achievement, work, rest, selfless activity, self-care, and religious practices. The next most common response was related to relationships, suggesting that what people do and having others to do it with are central to well-being.

The term *occupational justice* can be used to attract media attention to issues that might otherwise be ignored by those concentrating on technical aspects of recovery or concerned with cost containment and efficiency in intervention. After the first Canadian Symposium on Occupational Science, the Canadian Broadcasting Corporation interviewed Patricia Manuel (2003) about the potential occupational deprivation that is experienced when natural areas used for informal play by children living in the city are usurped by housing developments. Manuel's references to occupational justice reframed the implications of urban planning.

MAKING OCCUPATIONAL JUSTICE EXPLICIT IN OCCUPATIONAL THERAPY PRACTICE

Three scenarios illustrate occupational therapy practice with clients whose justice concerns are related to aging, social problems, and immigration.

Occupational Injustice and Old Age

Older adults can be trapped in a narrow life with limited opportunity, little chance of fulfillment, poor health, reduced well-being, reduced quality of life, and feelings of disempowerment to determine their own destiny. As a matter of justice, all older adults require options for health-enhancing occupations. To deny them options for such participation is more than a matter of medical care. Not all older people are infirm, demented, or unable to strive

toward personal goals, as some managers of services to the aging population might imply. Many older adults remain interested in the future and the part they will play in it. They remain interested in doing whatever has meaning to them unless, as too commonly happens, they are confined in or shackled to restricting, disempowering situations in the care of patronizing, "for your own safety," overzealous caregivers. Provision of opportunity to meet unique occupational wants and needs is a matter of justice as part of an active aging process. There is little emphasis in health, social welfare, or popular literature on encouraging older people to engage actively in the aging process. There are exceptions perhaps with regard to those who do exceptional things at a very advanced age and are deemed extraordinary. The increasingly litigious nature of Western societies is, in itself, counter to occupational justice for older people. Fear of legal action should accidents occur if older people engage in more than self-care occupations has resulted in many excellent programs being axed owing to risk management concerns. From an occupational perspective, program limitations or an overemphasis on risk for seniors is discriminatory and unjust (Wilcock, 2005).

These everyday struggles are situated in a social context. Thus, occupational therapists would analyze more than physical or mental impairments and might raise critical questions to make explicit matters of occupational justice, as illustrated with reference to seniors in Box 20.1.

BOX 20.1 OCCUPATIONAL INJUSTICE AND SENIORS: A CHECKLIST

1. Sitting alone in nursing homes or other confined settings with nothing to do except to watch others in the same situation or a television that shows program after program that they did not choose
2. Taken for outings they have no interest in
3. Not attended to when they talk about what they have done in their lives
4. Not asked for advice or listened to when they give it
5. Given no chance to help others
6. Prevented from doing what they want in the name of risk management
7. Told they can't do something they would enjoy "for their own good"
8. Not allocated resources, helpers, services, or support to find satisfying occupations
9. Social contact only with paid service providers who bring food and change their bedding
10. Restricted, deprived, or alienated by the policies of people in authority or by legislation

Occupational Injustice and Social Problems

Economic rationalism and bureaucratic legislation have led to many people being unable to obtain regular paid employment that meets their interests and skills or to be self-employed. Condemned to living on social support or to engage in unsatisfying, often part-time employment, they experience long-term, negative health effects. For example, some people lose the self-esteem required to take personal responsibility for promoting their own health. Other negative effects may include the loss of income to eat healthy food, or disconnectedness from coworkers with whom occupations were previously shared. People might prefer to accept social security instead of paid employment because there are no financial or social incentives to work part-time. Families might be caught in employment policies that expect them to do too much or lose their jobs. Unemployment may actually be welcomed by those with alternative, subsistence occupational skills, such as growing vegetables, chopping wood, and repairing goods for reuse and recycling. People without such skills or the opportunities to engage in subsistence occupations may live unhealthy, occupationally deprived, unbalanced, or alienating lifestyles.

An occupational perspective can bring new insights to social problems. Thus, occupational therapists would attend to occupational injustices by raising questions about daily life, as illustrated in the case study that follows.

Occupational Injustice, Environmental Degradation, Refugeeism, and Immigration

In agricultural economies, many people are in dire need of help to obtain the prerequisites of health because of environmental degradation caused, at least in part, by the greed of multinational organizations and citizen disempowerment. Many people are occupationally deprived owing to war, political upheavals, and rigid dictatorships or because of natural disasters. The effects of occupational injustice in the immediacy of people driven from their homes by war or environmental disasters may take time to manifest and, because of this, are unrecognized or unheeded. Large numbers of displaced people are warehoused in refugee camps where they have very little to do or where life consists of subsistence occupations and occupations of persistent self-protection from violence and abuse. Some people recognize the impossibility of remaining in restrictive or alienating conditions and seek a better future in another land. There, they may be disadvantaged by refugee protocols, even to the extent of being segregated in detention centers while seeking right of entry. During formal immigration processes, most people will have access to a very restricted range of occupations. They continue to experience occupations that are far from health giving and that are unjust in terms of either human rights or health needs. Quality of life, empowerment, and social inclusion in occupations

---

CASE STUDY: *Petra: Occupational Injustices and Social Problems*

Eight-year-old Petra is a small, thin, shy, pleasant girl with poor school performance. She attends an after-school day care program run by municipal community services in part because of her need for extra school support and in part because no one is available at home for her after school. Her mother Juliana, age 35, works at two jobs just to keep her daughter rather than accepting the social worker's advice and putting Petra in a foster home. Petra's 12-year-old sister, Aggie, is becoming a wild teenager whose school performance is satisfactory, although her attendance is dropping rapidly. Aggie gets Petra ready for school because Juliana's first job starts at 5:00 A.M. Weekend time for Juliana is virtually nonexistent, because of the extra sewing that she does to make ends meet. A women's career development center has referred Juliana to a Job Skills for Women Program operated by the municipal community services. The municipal welfare office has employed an occupational therapist consultant to work with the five after-school and ten job skill development programs they operate. The professional team includes resource and special education teachers as well as social workers.

An occupational perspective can bring new insights to social problems. Thus, occupational therapists would attend

to occupational injustices by raising questions about daily life, as illustrated in the case study of Petra.

Sample Questions to Analyze Occupational Injustices and Social Problems

1. Who would the occupational therapist name as clients: Petra or Aggie, Juliana as a single mother, after-school programs, job skills programs, the municipality?

2. What documentation will demonstrate accountability for occupational therapy practice: Assessment of spirituality and the physical, mental, and cognitive occupational performance of individuals; program consultation descriptions; population data on children and single parents; program costs and outcomes?

3. What are the occupational concerns for children and adolescents who are not thriving in poor social conditions? For single women or men?

4. Who are the occupational therapists' allies in working for occupational justice?

CASE STUDY: *The El Khalil Family: Occupational Injustices and Immigration*

The El Khalil family were overjoyed when they arrived as refugees and new immigrants in Canada. Both parents are physicians, and the four children, aged 13, 12, 9, and 5, had been successful in school in their North African homeland. After two years of immigration challenges to their refugee status, the parents are both employed as school crossing guards. With little income, they live in a rundown one-bedroom apartment in a tough neighborhood, where the 13-year-old son has just been charged with assault as a young offender. He has been sent for observation to a youth detention center, where an occupational therapist is employed on a mental health team.

Sample Questions to Analyze Occupational Injustices and Immigration

1. What changes in occupational routines, locations, and supports have likely occurred for the family since immigration?
2. What occupational concerns are the family juggling?
3. From an occupational perspective, what will the boy gain and lose by admission to a detention center?
4. What public education would highlight the occupational issues associated with immigration and youth detention and the need to address occupational injustices?

---

are matters of justice and of health, as the case study above illustrates.

HOW TO ADVOCATE OR MEDIATE TO ENABLE CLIENTS TO PARTICIPATE IN MEANINGFUL OCCUPATION

Delivering occupationally just programs may entail keeping awareness of the occupational nature of clients in the forefront during any interaction; engaging people in dialogue about their perceived occupational needs; assessing according to those needs; and implementing programs that ensure that needs are met. Delivering occupationally just programs also entails advocating for occupational justice and mediating between competing intervention and resource priorities. The use of powerful arguments and the media to increase awareness may be called for. This entails being cognizant of and using occupational language, being available for public dialogue about enabling and inclusive social structures and occupation policies, knowing when and how to talk about occupational justice issues, and being ready to advance public understanding.

Both the UN and WHO are useful sources of accepted "health speak" and "justice speak." The WHO's (2002, p. 2) theme of Active Ageing, for example, provides a Policy Framework for discussion and action to promote healthy aging. The framework examines the need to prevent discriminatory action that can be counterproductive to well-being and to enabling those who are able to continue to contribute to society in important ways, posing questions that might be useful advocacy tools (WHO, 2002). Raising awareness among the general public is just as important as writing for occupational therapists or other health professionals. On any and every occasion, it is important to introduce the notion of occupational justice

and the view of people as occupational beings. All people need to be able or enabled to engage in the occupations of their need and choice; to grow through what they do; and to experience independence or interdependence, equality, participation, security, health, and well-being.

REFERENCES

Argyle, M. (1987). *The psychology of happiness.* New York: Methuen.

Blaxter, M. (1990). *Health and lifestyles.* London: Tavistock/ Routledge.

Cohen, P., Struening, E. L., Genevie, L. E., Kaplan, S. R., Muhlin, G. L., & Peck, H. B. (1982). Community stressors, mediating conditions and wellbeing in urban neighborhoods. *Journal of Community Psychology, 10,* 377–390.

College of Occupational Therapists. (2002). *From interface to integration: A strategy for modernising occupational therapy services in local health and social care communities.* London: College of Occupational Therapists. Retrieved January 2003 from http://www.cot.org.uk

College of Occupational Therapists. (2005). *Making the connections: Delivering better services for Wales* (Clause 3.1.4.). London: College of Occupational Therapists. Retrieved February 2006 from http://www.cot.org.uk

Commission on Social Justice. (1994). *Social justice: Strategies for national renewal. The report of the Commission on Social Justice.* London: Vintage.

Disraeli, B. (1851). Speech in the House of Commons, 11 February, 1851. London.

Dunton, W. R., Jr. (1915). *Occupational therapy: A manual for nurses.* Philadelphia: W. B. Saunders.

Gilbert, N. (1995). *Welfare justice: Restoring social equity.* New Haven, CT: Yale University Press.

Isaksson, K. (1990). A longitudinal study of the relationship between frequent job change and psychological well-being. *Journal of Occupational Psychology, 63,* 297–308.

Kalisch, D. (1991). The active society. *Social Security Journal,* August, 3–9.

Kronenberg, F., Algado, S. S., & Pollard, N. (Eds.). (2005). *Spirit of survivors: Occupational therapy without borders.* Edinburgh: Elsevier/Churchill Livingstone.

LeVesconte, H. (1935). Expanding fields of occupational therapy. *Canadian Journal of Occupational Therapy, 3,* 4–12.

Manuel, P. (2003). Occupied with ponds: Exploring the meaning, bewaring the loss for kids and communities of nature's small spaces. *Journal of Occupational Science, 10*(1), 31–39.

Marshall, W., & Schram, M. (Eds.). (1993). *Mandate for change.* New York: Berkley, p. 228.

Meyer, A. (1922). The philosophy of occupational therapy. *Archives of Occupational Therapy, 1,* 1–10.

Norton, A. L. (Ed.). (1994). Justice. In *The Hutchinson Dictionary of Ideas.* Oxford, UK: Helicon Publishing.

Organization for Economic Cooperation and Development. (1989). The path to full employment: Structural adjustment for an active society (Editorial). *Employment Outlook, July.*

Thibeault, R. (2002). Occupation and the rebuilding of civic society: Notes from the war zone. *Journal of Occupational Science, 9*(1), 38–47.

Townsend, E. A. (1993). Muriel Driver Memorial Lecture: Occupational therapy's social vision. *Canadian Journal of Occupational Therapy, 60,* 174–184.

Townsend, E. A. (1996). Enabling empowerment: Using simulations versus real occupations. *Canadian Journal of Occupational Therapy, 63,* 113–128.

Townsend, E. A. (1998). *Good intentions overruled: A critique of empowerment in the routine organization of mental health services.* Toronto, ON: University of Toronto Press.

Townsend, E. A. (2003). *Occupational justice: Ethical, moral and civic principles for an inclusive world.* Paper presented at Annual Meeting of the European Network of Occupational Therapy in Higher Education, Prague, Czech Republic. Retrieved October 2003 from www.enothe.hva.nl/meet/ac03/acc03-text03.doc

Townsend, E. A., & Wilcock, A. A. (2004). Occupational justice. In C. H. Christiansen & E. A. Townsend (Eds.), *Introduction to occupation: The art and science of living.* Upper Saddle River, NJ: Prentice Hall.

United Nations. (1998). *Universal declaration of Human Rights.* Geneva: General Assembly of the United Nations.

Warr, P. (1990). The measurement of well-being and other aspects of mental health. *Journal of Occupational Psychology, 63*(4), 193–210.

Wilcock, A. (1993). A theory of the human need for occupation. *Journal of Occupational Science: Australia, 1*(1), 17–24.

Wilcock, A. (1995). The occupational brain: A theory of human nature. *Journal of Occupational Science: Australia, 2*(1), 68–73.

Wilcock, A. A. (1998). *An occupational perspective of health.* Thorofare, NJ: Slack.

Wilcock, A. A. (2005). Older people and occupational justice. In A. McIntyre, & A. Atwal (Eds.), *Occupational Therapy and Older People.* Oxford, UK: Blackwell Publishing.

Wilcock, A. A. (2006). *An occupational perspective of health.* Second edition. Thorofare, NJ: Slack.

Wilcock, A. A., van der Aren, H., Darling, K., Scholz, J., Siddall, R., Snigg, C., et al. (1998). An exploratory study of people's perception and experiences of well-being. *British Journal of Occupational Therapy, 61*(2), 75–82.

Wood, W., Hooper, B., & Womack, J. (2005). Reflections on occupational justice as a subtext of occupation-centred education. In F. Kronenberg, S. S. Algado, & N. Pollard, N. (Eds.), *Spirit of survivors: Occupational therapy without borders.* Edinburgh: Elsevier/Churchill Livingstone, pp. 378–389.

World Federation of Occupational Therapists. (2004–2005). *The World Federation of Occupational Therapists approved project plan: Data collection about occupational therapists involved in community based rehabilitation* (December 2004, revised 3/21/05). Retrieved August 2005 from http://www.wfot.org.au/officefiles/CBR%20data%20collection%20project%20plan1.pdf

World Federation of Occupational Therapists (2006). Human rights position paper. Retrieved 7 October 2006 from www.netf.no/onternasjonalt/Human_Rights_Position_Statement Final.pdf

World Health Organization. (1997). Jakarta Declaration on Leading Health Promotion into the 21st Century. 4th International Conference on Health Promotion, Jakarta, Indonesia, 21–25th July.

World Health Organization. (1998). *Health for all in the twenty-first century.* (Document A51/5). Geneva: World Health Organization.

World Health Organization. (2002). *Active ageing: A policy framework.* Second United Nations World Assembly on Ageing. Madrid, Spain.

World Health Organization, Health and Welfare Canada, Canadian Public Health Association. (1986). *Ottawa charter for health promotion.* Ottawa, Canada.

IV

PROFILE OF THE OCCUPATIONAL THERAPY PROFESSION

"The integrity of the profession is in your hands."

Eleanor Clarke Slagle

The History of Occupational Therapy

21

DON M. GORDON

Learning Objectives

After reading this chapter, you will be able to:

1. Articulate the relationship of moral treatment to the founding of occupational therapy.
2. Understand how new ideas concerning the relationship between the mind, body, and health created an environment that was ripe for the emergence of occupational therapy.
3. Understand how the world wars influenced the growth and development of occupational therapy.
4. Understand how ongoing projects in the occupational therapy community relate to historical concerns.

INTRODUCTION

The history of occupational therapy is integrally linked to the time of its origination and development. Although occupational therapy is a relatively recent idea, generated in the early years of the twentieth century, the recognition of the healing effects of occupation goes back thousands of years. The history of occupational therapy itself is also a story of the development of a scientific understanding of occupation. This look at the history of occupational therapy will begin with a look at the origins of the understanding that occupation influenced health. Then we will track the development of the profession of occupational therapy. This will include understanding the growth of science and professionalism in the larger culture and how these factors affected the development of occupational therapy. Uncovering these issues is fundamental to understanding how the expanding influence of science and medicine led to the origin of occupational therapy.

THE PREHISTORY OF OCCUPATIONAL THERAPY

Early observations of the healing effects of occupation are virtually as old at the written word itself; the first references to the use of occupation in healing go back to the Egyptians (American Occupational Therapy Association, 1967; Pinel, 1806/1962). The oldest observations of the healing effects of occupation and their use as part of a therapeutic program began in the treatment of "madness" or "insanity"—what is today known as mental illness. For example, Thomas Willis (1621–1675), who coined the word *neurology* and is immortalized in the term *circle of Willis* recognized the value of occupation in the treatment of insanity. He advocated directing patients toward occupations that promoted "cheerfulness and joy," such as music, dancing, singing, hunting, fishing, and even chemical and mathematical studies (Hunter and Macalpine, 1963). However, this understanding was less than widespread, and medical treatment of the insane consisted primarily of bloodlettings and "nausea treatment," the use of purgatives and emetics to weaken and help control patients. Daily whippings or beatings were also utilized, given that physical abuse was the most expedient means of controlling behavior (Kraepelin, 1917/1962). It was not until the beginning of the nineteenth century that a greater understanding of the healing potential of occupation was utilized in a more widespread manner. Then, with the birth of the asylum, a fundamental advance in the treatment of the insane came about: moral treatment.

THE BIRTH OF THE ASYLUM AND MORAL TREATMENT

With the birth of the asylum in the beginning of the nineteenth century, the treatment of the insane underwent a fundamental shift toward a more humanitarian approach. The word *asylum* is derived from the Greek and Latin root signifying a place of refuge and protection (*Oxford English Dictionary*, 1971). The asylum was viewed as a reformative institution that represented an optimistic and hopeful possibility for the humane treatment of insanity (Porter, 1997). The birth of the asylum also brought medicine formally into the treatment of the insane. In 1808, Riel coined the term *psychiaterie* for the new discipline directed toward the cure of mental disorders (Shorter, 1997). Its most fundamental practice was moral treatment, intended to replace brutality with kindness and idleness with occupation. Moral treatment described a general approach to care of the insane summarized nicely by William Browne in 1837: "moral treatment . . . may be summed up in two words, kindness and occupation" (as cited in Shorter, 1997, p. 43).

The history of occupational therapy has long been associated with moral treatment (for some examples, see Bing, 1981; Bockoven, 1963, 1971; Hopkins, 1978, 1988; Kielhofner and Burke, 1977; Peloquin, 1989, 1994). Moral treatment was a social reform movement concerning the care of the insane that was a blend of Enlightenment optimism (Bockoven, 1963; Peloquin, 1989, 1994; Szasz, 1974) and folk wisdom (Porter, 1997). A fundamental belief that the insane remained creatures of reason meant that their treatment demanded compassion rather than cruelty. This reform was part of a larger social reform movement that included the penal system, working conditions, and the rights of children (Rosen, 1968). There were also very practical reasons for the changes in the treatment of the insane patient. Many superintendents of "madhouses" recognized that the daily whippings and beatings accompanied by the widespread use of emetics, purgatives, and bloodlettings that were common in the treatment of the insane led to the demise of those in their care more frequently than cure. It was observed by some that a focus on the management of behavior while minimizing the use of medical treatments restored a greater number of those in their care (Hunter and Macalpine, 1963). Out of these observations and the spirit of reform generated by the times, moral treatment was born. Moral treatment has been considered one of the three most significant advances in medicine in the nineteenth century, along with antisepsis and anesthesia (Hunter and Macalpine, 1963).

Occupations were an essential element of the moral treatment of the insane. Some doctors initially favored the use of agriculture (Rush, 1812/1964), but as the nineteenth century progressed, the occupations that were used in the application of moral treatment expanded. Various forms of manual labor, including agriculture, tailoring, working in the shoe shop, and sewing, were among the various occupations utilized. Many occupations were also related to the maintenance of the institution and even as contracted labor in the community, a practice that was certainly utilitarian though at times controversial (Bockoven, 1963; Dain, 1971; Grob, 1966). Religious worship was also a common component, as many asylum superintendents in the United States were men of strong religious underpinnings (Dain, 1971; Grob, 1966).

Although moral treatment was truly a remarkable advance in the treatment of the insane, it had faded from the limelight by the end of the nineteenth century. The concept that the insane deserved humane treatment was not lost but remained as one of the basic practices and principles in the practice of psychiatry (Hunter and Macalpine, 1963). The term *moral treatment* fell into disuse for several reasons. One fundamental reason for this decline in the use of this term was that moral treatment was not specifically a medical treatment. Clergymen, philosophers, and jurists all claimed authority over the practice of moral treatment (Vandermeersch, 1994). In addition, the authority of the moral treatment superintendent emanated from the moral and social order, not from scientific knowledge

(Grob, 1994). In the latter half of the nineteenth century, medicine continued to garner power, and its practices became increasingly linked to scientific knowledge (Kimball, 1992; Starr, 1982). This exposed another fundamental problem with the foundation of moral treatment, for it was not scientifically based. By the close of the nineteenth century, science was becoming one of the most powerful elements of American culture (Bledstein, 1976; Burnham, 1987; Daniels, 1971; Ellenberger, 1970; Kimball, 1992; Reingold and Reingold, 1981, Rosenberg, 1997). As medicine took over the practice of treating the mentally ill, the unscientific jargon of moral treatment fell by the wayside and was replaced by a new treatment approach: psychotherapy. While many have argued that moral treatment was discredited and discarded (Bockoven, 1963, 1971; Peloquin, 1989, 1994), this appears not to be entirely the case. The growth of science and the birth of psychotherapy set the stage for the emergence of a new profession: occupational therapy.

THE BIRTH OF OCCUPATIONAL THERAPY

The genesis of occupational therapy occurred during a remarkably dynamic time of cultural change in American history as well as the history of medicine, marked by dramatic changes in lifestyles and habits (Allen, 1952). Science and modernization held the promise of improvement. "Science, efficiency, speed, and movement—these were the ideals" (Jones, 1971, p. 150). Darwin's theory of evolution illustrated the potential for science to address issues that had previously been considered outside of its reach (Hollinger, 1995). Science came to play a much larger role in social policies, prompting W. J. Mcgee to claim in 1898 that "America has become a nation of science" (as cited in Daniels, 1971, p. 295). Though the relationship of science to social thought is often overlooked (Rosenberg, 1997), science was possibly the most powerful cultural force in the twentieth century (Daniels, 1971; Fuller, 1991; Shumway and Messer-Davidow, 1991).

Until the latter part of the nineteenth century, consideration of the psyche or mental processes in the role of health had essentially been ignored by medicine. Mental illness was viewed as the product of somatic disease or dysfunction. The prevalent belief in a Lockean concept of consciousness, the "tabula rasa," meant that all mental processes were believed to be under conscious control, precluding unconscious psychic processes (Hunter and Macalpine, 1963). At the end of the nineteenth century, new ideas about "nervous energy" and the role of the psyche in mental illness and health were revolutionary. Views of consciousness and the unconscious changed dramatically. Then a confluence of events occurred that propelled the psyche into the forefront of medical practice: (1) the success of the rest-cure, (2) the successes of the

Christian Science movement, and (3) the psychodynamic revolution and the birth of psychotherapy. With the birth of psychotherapy, the stage was set for the introduction of a new profession: occupational therapy (Gordon, 2002).

After the discovery of the electrical nature of the nervous system in 1852, many theories were developed to explain the regulation of one's nervous energy (Rosenberg, 1997). One of the more influential practices was generated by Silas Weir Mitchell's "rest-cure." The rest-cure was envisioned as a somatic treatment, with rest and a milk diet theorized as being integral to the restoration of one's "nervous battery." This treatment was devised to cure the physical exhaustion that led to nervous illness and was immediately successful and much copied. However, physicians soon recognized that the most powerful element of the cure was the suggestive power of the physician, intensified by the isolation that was part of the treatment (Shorter, 1997). This somatically based treatment thus was one factor that demonstrated the psychological element of healing, helping to stimulate the recognition of the role of the mind in healing and the mind-body connection.

To appreciate this emerging recognition of mind-body unity, one must also consider the cultural events that supported these concepts. Faith healing, "mind-cures," and New Thought movements represented a variety of alternative schemas of healing that were designed to replace or supplement traditional medical beliefs (Haller, 1981). The most significant of these mind-cures was the Christian Science movement, or Eddyism, named after its founder, Mary Baker Eddy (1821–1910). This movement sought to scientifically master the teachings of Christ in order to reestablish his mission to heal the sick. A tenet of Christian Science was that disease was an abnormal condition that could be remedied through proper exercises of the mind. Christian Science became very popular, reporting countless cures.

However, these claims of cure were considered an outrage to the medical community of the time, which was now fervently engaged in the pursuit of developing the science of medicine. Though these claims to healing were rejected, they could not be ignored. To address this issue, Henry Goddard of Clark University conducted a study in 1898, which found that there was nothing incompatible in the simultaneous use of both drug therapies and mental therapeutics; in fact, the two were found to be mutually reinforcing (Haller, 1981). Goddard's findings helped to open the door to stake a claim to mental therapeutics in the science of medicine. The successes of faith healers were viewed not as displacing medicine but as highlighting the medical community's disregard concerning the role of the mind in healing, with medicine emphasizing drug therapies up until this time. The success of Christian Science set the stage for medicine to take a more holistic stance regarding human health that incorporated both the mind and body (Haller, 1981).

The late nineteenth and early twentieth century were also marked by the emergence of dynamic psychiatry. At this time in history, the treatment of mental disease was in the midst of radical change. The ideas of Emile Kraepelin, Pierre Janet, Sigmund Freud, and William James were changing the way in which nervous illness and the path to cure were conceptualized. Theories of nervous energy and how the psychic forces influenced physical and mental health were generated to further understand the mechanisms behind health and illness. The word *psychotherapy* was coined in 1891 to describe a new and groundbreaking form of medical treatment (Ellenberger, 1970). The new profession of occupational therapy, which was initially considered by some as a form of psychotherapy (see Barker, 1908; Carroll, 1910; Schwab, 1907), emerged from the world of dynamic psychiatry.

OCCUPATIONAL THERAPY: A NEW TREATMENT APPROACH

The early founders of occupational therapy endeavored to create a new role for occupation in the process of healing both the mind and the body. Although early writers certainly acknowledged the age-old tradition of the use of occupation as a curative measure, including moral treatment (for early examples, see Dunton, 1919b; Slagle, 1914), the systematic use of occupation was seen not as a continuation of past practices but as a truly new endeavor in therapeutics (Dunton, 1919b; Hall, 1910a). The critical difference between prior practices and occupational therapy was the systematic nature of how occupation was utilized and the integration of scientific knowledge formations in understanding the therapeutic effect of occupation (Gordon, 2002).

From the time that physicians began to utilize occupation as a therapeutic measure in the early twentieth century, they endeavored to understand the healing effect of occupation in scientific terms. Scientific knowledge is not only the foundation of professional legitimacy (Bledstein, 1976; Kimball, 1992), but possibly the most powerful cultural force in the twentieth century (Daniels, 1971; Fuller, 1991; Shumway and Messer-Davidow, 1991). What was considered science in the early twentieth century was quite different from our current conceptualization of science. An older view of science persisted into the early twentieth century that perceived knowledge gained of the natural world as "science." This meant that virtually any technique or process that produced positive results was viewed as "science." In the United States, those who were involved in occupations related to scientific disciplines and applied professions such as medicine or engineering were considered scientists, and their work was considered to be science (Reingold and Reingold, 1981). The attempt to understand the therapeutic effect of occupational therapy

in scientific terms was certainly integral to the profession from its early implementation.

At the dawn of the twentieth century, the rest-cure remained the preeminent treatment for nervous illness. However, this treatment supported by a somatic rationale came under fire from a physician who had a staunch belief in the power of occupation: Herbert Hall. Hall was a physician who treated nervous illness and one of the early leaders of occupational therapy. For him, the rationale for the rest-cure failed to recognize the fundamental role of the psyche and one's day-to-day behavior in the etiology of nervous illness. Hall (1905a) constructed the "work-cure" as "a practical protest against the almost universal application of rest in the treatment of neurasthenia and allied conditions." (p. 29). For Hall (1905b), poor lifestyle adjustment and worry meant that "the patient's whole personality is at war with the environment" (p. 48). The resulting nervous depletion was not the same as the rest-cure postulated by Mitchell, but Hall considered nervous illness as having psychic causes in addition to somatic etiologies. In these early writings, we see the combination of somatic and psychic concepts of illness and healing, producing a conceptual unification of mind and body.

In the early twentieth century, scientific rationales for treatment ranged from the purely physical to the exclusively psychic, though a blend of the two factors is generally seen in the early literature. For example, by exercising, the body occupation restored physical health, which in turn restored mental health (Cohn, 1908; Moher, 1907; Neff, 1910). Occupation helped to boost the nutrition of nerve cells and rid them of toxins en route to addressing nervous illness (Hall, 1905b; Moher, 1907; Willson, 1908). Neff (1910) argued that occupation improved happiness, which in turn fortified the blood, stimulated the metabolism, and improved sleep, digestion, and the functioning of every organ in the body.

Psychic explanations viewed the therapeutic use of occupation as taking a "synthetic" approach (Hall, 1910b; Thayer, 1908). This terminology distinguished this synthetic school of thought from the analytic approach commonly associated with Freudian psychotherapy. Rather than searching for "first causes" of psychopathology in an attempt to ultimately restore unity to one's psychic functioning, the synthetic approach addressed the behavior problems manifest in an unbalanced lifestyle, aiming to achieve synthesis through the unity of thought and action (Hall, 1910b). This addressed a concern of many of the physicians of the time with the analytic method, for morbid introspection was a common malady in those with nervous illness. Given that unhealthy attention to "self-consciousness and self-concern" (Hall, 1910b) only worsened the disease process, a therapeutic technique that was based on intense self-analysis appeared dangerous in the hands of all but the most highly trained physicians (Atwood, 1907; Hall, 1910b, 1923; Schwab, 1908; Thayer, 1908). Therapeutic occupation produced its therapeutic effect by redirecting one's thought down healthier channels, avoiding "useless self-analysis" (Hall, 1910b). While this collection of scientific rationales for the effectiveness of treatment might seem rather insubstantial by today's standards, scientific investigation had a very different meaning at the beginning of the twentieth century from that of today.

THE FORMATION OF OCCUPATIONAL THERAPY'S PROFESSIONAL ORGANIZATION AND BIRTH OF THE PROFESSION

In March 1917, a small group of individuals, including medical doctors, nurses, architects, social workers, secretaries, and teachers of arts and crafts, were brought together by the idea that occupation could play an important role in healing and health (Figure 21.1). (Dunton, 1918a, 1918b).

The practices that made up the future profession of occupational therapy were scattered throughout the medical community, but with this meeting in 1917, the National Society for the Promotion of Occupational Therapy (NSPOT), later renamed the American Occupational Therapy Association (AOTA), brought these practices together. This meeting marked the origins of the profession of occupational therapy. To understand just what this means, it is important first to define *profession*. Kimball (1992) defines a profession as "a dignified occupation espousing an ethic of service, organized into an association, and practicing functional science" (p. 16). The fledg-

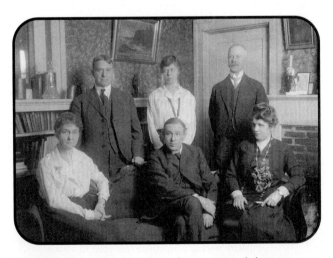

FIGURE 21.1 The founders of occupational therapy at Consolation House, Clifton Springs, New York, March 1917. Front row (left to right): Susan Cox Johnson, George Edward Barton, and Eleanor Clarke Slagle. Back row (left to right): William Rush Dunton, Isabelle Newton, and Thomas Bessell Kidner. (Photo courtesy of the archives of AOTA, Bethesda, MD.)

ling profession of occupational therapy endeavored to fashion itself in this image. George Barton, the first president of NSPOT, was in fact pivotal in the naming of the profession, having the foresight to insist on the term *therapy* in the organizations name (Barton, 1917, personal communication to William Rush Dunton). Therapy is defined as "the medical treatment of disease" (*Oxford English Dictionary*, 1971, p. 3284). Barton's insistence on the use of the term *occupational therapy* reinforced the future profession's inclusion within the realm of medical science. He also promoted the use of medical language to promote the legitimacy of the professional base of occupational therapy. Occupational therapy closely allied itself with the medical profession, envisioning prescription and medical supervision as necessities (Dunton, 1928; Hall, 1923; Kelleher, 1925; Richardson, 1926). The new profession of occupational therapy rooted itself in medical science to establish legitimacy, for "Any form of therapy that does not rest upon science in the true sense of the word becomes a cult or worse, quackery" (Robinson, 1925, p. 2).

However, the founders were somewhat ambivalent toward the name of this new profession. William Rush Dunton, one of the founders of NSPOT and visionary figure in the first decades of the profession struggled with "the cumbersomeness of the term occupational therapy" (1919a, p. 36), as it lacked the "exactness of meaning which is possessed by scientific terms" (p. 36). Other titles such as "work-cure," "ergotherapy" (*ergo* being the Greek root for "work"), and "creative occupations" were discussed as substitutes, but ultimately, none possessed the broad meaning that the practice of occupational therapy demanded in order to capture the many forms of treatment that existed from the beginning (Gordon, 2002). Though practitioners continue to struggle with the abstract nature of the term *occupational therapy* to this day, the name of the profession appears to have been well chosen.

In the early years of occupational therapy, the predominant therapeutic activities that were used comprised a great variety of handcrafted goods and activities (Figure 21.2). At times, the salability of these goods was critical to the economic viability of the institution (see Hall, 1905a, 1905b, 1910a, 1910b). However, this was a point of contention even among early leaders, who were fearful that this would diminish the therapeutic mission of the new profession (Barton, 1917, personal communication to William Rush Dunton; Kidner, 1932). Other forms of therapeutic interventions were encouraged from the beginning of the profession, including the use of recreation, music, and art. Although crafts were initially the principal form of occupational therapy used with children (Clark, 1925; Conrick, 1930), the fundamental value of play as the most fundamental occupation for children was quickly recognized (Clark, 1925; Mackay, 1933; Obrock, 1932).

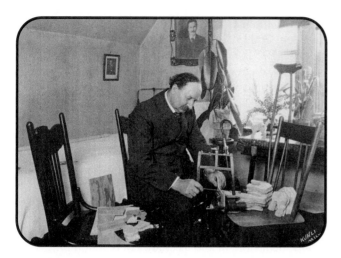

FIGURE 21.2   Crafts were commonly used as a form of therapy in the early years of the profession. (Photo courtesy of the Wisconsin Occupational Therapy Association Archives.)

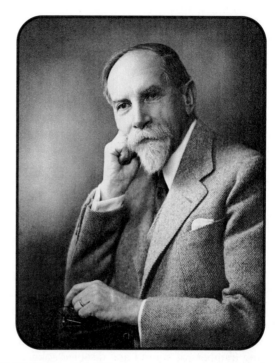

FIGURE 21.3   Adolf Meyer, renowned psychobiologist and author of The Philosophy of Occupation Therapy (1922). (Photo courtesy of the archives of AOTA, Bethesda, MD.)

THE PHILOSOPHY OF OCCUPATIONAL THERAPY

From the time that physicians began to articulate a concept of the therapeutic application of occupation, a scientific philosophy of work and occupation began to be developed. New ideas such as Darwin's theory of evolution were changing conceptions of human nature in unforeseen ways (Hollinger, 1995). Physicians endeavored to understand the role of occupation within the span of human evolution. The human capacity for work was seen as being a defining factor, "Work is truly life, and any treatment which ignores every means which will make possible such life in greater abundance, cannot be comprehensive." (Carroll, 1910, p. 2033). Human beings had evolved through work and action, making these elements of life a fundamental human need (Gordon, 2002).

But it was Adolph Meyer who most clearly articulated the philosophy of occupational therapy in his landmark article of the same title published in 1922 (Figure 21.3). Embodying the "Pollyanna spirit" that was widespread among health reformers of the time (Burnham, 1987), Meyer (1922) espoused the potential for scientific thought and progress to improve the human condition. The fundamental change in psychiatry had come about in viewing "mental problems as problems of living" (p. 4). He notes how the previous 30 years had yielded great gains in scientific understanding, particularly in physics with the rise of energetics and understanding the "applications of work" (p. 5). His seminal paper introduced occupational therapy's concern for coming to a fuller understanding of the role of time in one's life, or temporal adaptation. Meyer (1922) noted that just as our heart beats in a rhythm, so do we respond to the greater rhythms of day and night, sleeping and waking, and hunger and

satiation, all centered on the fundamental activities of human life: "work and play and rest and sleep" (p. 8). These ideas remain as touchstones of occupational therapy thought and practice to this day.

KEY EVENTS IN THE HISTORY OF THE PROFESSION

A variety of key events and relevant cultural forces were elemental to the growth and development of the profession of occupational therapy. In the early twentieth century, the newfound world of the psyche and medical treatment via psychotherapy opened up a new world of possibilities for treatment of the mentally ill and improving the quality of life of the general population. While Americans embraced science and technology, the rapid cultural changes and increasing pace to life were seen as a factor in the genesis of nervous illness. William James (1899/1918) believed that American "overtension and jerkiness and breathlessness" (p.59) was a "bad habit" that had slowly been acquired over the years. The challenge was to find a way to replace these traits with an appreciation of "harmony, dignity, and ease" (James, 1899/1918, p. 65). Herbert Hall (1910b) believed that the proper use of occupation could address these societal concerns, asserting that "many people are suffering in mind and body because of the attempt to accomplish too much, or from idleness which is not necessary, that a therapeutic readjustment would mean preventive and curative medicine on a large and important scale." (p. 297). These remain challenging issues.

The early twentieth century was a time in which the rising incidence of disability related to industrial accidents, tuberculosis, World War I, and mental illness brought about an increasing social awareness of the issues involved. This created a growing concern about the need to increase societal efficiency, giving birth to the efficiency movement (Daniels, 1971). George Barton was a vocal proponent of efficiency techniques, including the "motion study method" (Barton, 1916, p. 82) of Kenneth and Lillian Gilbreth, efficiency experts during the early twentieth century. This attention to analyzing and understanding the ways in which to streamline activity marked the beginning of energy conservation practices in occupational therapy.

The entry of the United States into World War I was also a crucial event in the history of the profession. Up until this time, occupational therapy had been concerned primarily with the treatment of people with mental illness. However, U.S. involvement in the Great War and the escalating numbers of injured and disabled soldiers presented a daunting challenge to those in command. The military enlisted the assistance of NSPOT to recruit and train over 1,200 "reconstruction aides" to help with the rehabilitation of those wounded in the war. Given that "shell shock" was a common cause of disability during the First World War, these forerunners of occupational therapy provided treatment that was significant for its holistic approach, healing not only the body of the patient but the mind as well (Figure 21.4). This provided the boost in attention and interest that would help to eventually propel occupational therapy into the status of a profession (Gordon, 2002; Quiroga, 1995).

The 1920s and 1930s were a time of establishing standards of education and laying the foundation of the profession and its organization. Eleanor Clarke Slagle proposed a 12-month course of training in 1922, and these standards were adopted in 1923 (Hopkins, 1978). Educational standards were expanded to a total training time of 18 months in 1930 to place the requirements for professional entry on par with those of other professions (Kidner, 1930). During this time, the psychodynamic paradigm continued to grow in influence, becoming the dominant schema for the scientific understanding of the therapeutic effect of occupation regarding one's mental health. Behaviorism and its studies of reaction time were seen as groundbreaking means for understanding human behavior and were influential in these early years as well (for examples, see Amar, 1922; Meyer, 1922). Various psychological schemas were incorporated and blended, concepts being taken from Adolph Meyer, Sigmund Freud, Carl Jung, Alfred Adler, and other influential thinkers in the world of psychology and psychiatry in this era. Incorporation of the most influential ideas concerning human psychology served to reinforce occupational therapy's claims to professional legitimacy and its alliance with medicine (Gordon, 2002). While the Great Depression of the 1930s presented a challenging time for the new profession, occupational therapy remained viable, continuing to raise educational standards. Then with the advent of World War II, the demand for occupational therapists again exploded, prompting new education programs and expanding membership in the field from a

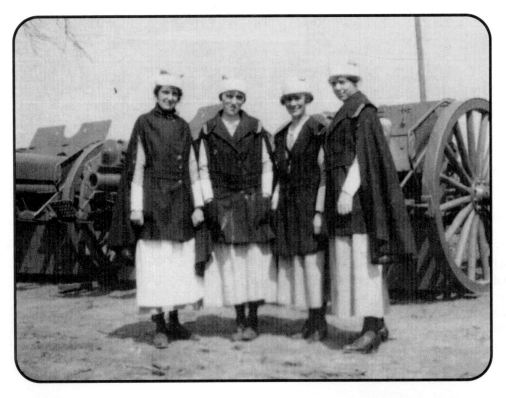

FIGURE 21.4 Reconstruction aides in official uniform capes of grey with maroon lining. (Photo courtesy of the American Occupational Therapy Association, Inc. Photograph G4.119A.97.)

mere 1,144 registered therapists in 1941 to 2,265 in 1946 (Hopkins, 1978).

WORLD WAR II AND THE GROWTH OF REHABILITATION

With entry into World War II and the ensuing skyrocketing demand for therapists to treat those injured in the war, the field of occupational therapy underwent dramatic growth and change (Figure 21.5). Occupational therapists needed to be skilled not only in the use of constructive activities such as crafts, but also increasingly in the use of activities of daily living (Hopkins, 1978). The changing science that surrounded the practices of rehabilitation of physical disabilities required accredited schools to undergo intense reorganization of their educational curricula. This prompted the publication of the first textbook in the United States written principally for occupational therapists to be published in 1947, edited by Helen S. Willard and Clare S. Spackman (Spackman, 1968) (Figure 21.6). Occupational therapy also began to expand its educa-

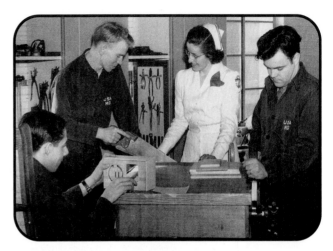

FIGURE 21.5 Wilma L. West, head of orthopedics occupational therapy, Walter Reed General Hospital, Washington, DC, 1943–1944. West was a founder of the American Occupational Therapy Foundation and its president from 1972 to 1982. She was also president of AOTA from 1961 to 1964 and Eleanor Clarke Slagle lecturer in 1967. (Photo courtesy of the archives of AOTA, Bethesda, MD.)

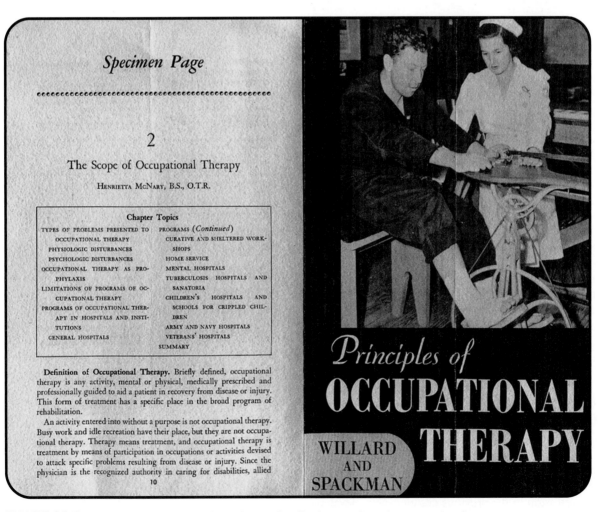

FIGURE 21.6 Advertisement for the first edition of *Willard & Spackman's Occupational Therapy*. (Photo courtesy Dr. Lori Anderson & Dr. Barbara Kornblau.)

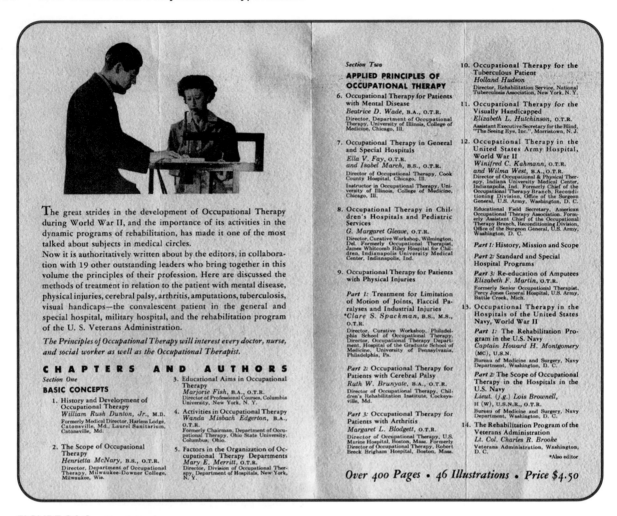

FIGURE 21.6 *Continued*

tion into the graduate level, the first master's degree in occupational therapy being offered at the University of Southern California in 1947.

The profession continued to grow and redefine itself in the 1950s. Educational programs and the number of individuals entering the profession continued to increase, from 13 accredited schools in 1938 to 24 schools in 1960 (Hopkins, 1978). The profession also began to assess the potential for the use of trained assistants in the attempt to address the ongoing shortage of qualified therapists, and educational standards for occupational therapy assistants were implemented in 1960 (Hopkins, 1978).

CHANGES IN THE 1960S THROUGH THE 1980S

The 1960s and 1970s were a time of ongoing change and growth for the profession as it struggled to incorporated new knowledge and cope with the recent and rapid growth of the profession in the previous decades. New developments in the areas of neurobehavioral research led to new conceptualizations and new treatment approaches, possibly the most groundbreaking being the sensory integrative approach developed by A. Jean Ayres (Ayres, 1972, 1979). Ayres was influenced early on by the work of Margaret Rood and Carl and Berta Bobath in the treatment of neuromuscular dysfunction and Piaget, who examined the developmental process through a sensorimotor lens (Baloueff, 2003). Ayres incorporated an evolutionary perspective in her attempt to articulate how sensory experiences are understood, incorporated, and utilized by human beings to allow for adaptation in one's behavior. Her pioneering work in this area was remarkable in many ways, integrating new ideas about neuronal plasticity and the importance of sensory input into the normal and healthy development of the brain and nervous system. She continued to refine her ideas until her death in 1988. Her ideas continue to be further developed and increasingly incorporated in the understanding of child behavior and occupational therapy interventions to this day.

There had been profound growth in the profession in many ways since the Second World War, with growing ranks among occupational therapists, the introduction of occupational therapy assistants, and the accompanying increase in educational programs. However, all this growth and change came at a cost, and some within the profession of occupational therapy felt that the profession had lost its moorings and had drifted from its originally charted course. Mary Reilly (1962) was one such voice (Figure 21.7).

Reilly believed that the profession had lost its focus on occupation and challenged the profession to work more diligently toward understanding occupation from an interdisciplinary perspective, including recent findings in sociology, psychology, philosophy, economics, and biology. She called for a return to the founding belief of occupational therapy "that man through the use of his hands as they are energized by mind and will, can influence the state of his own health" (Reilly, 1962, p. 2). Citing recent research on sensory deprivation, Reilly (1962) postulated that the human nervous system requires a wide variety of stimuli to maintain healthy sensory processing and that occupation is the vehicle through which we may experience this basic need.

The 1960s and 1970s appear to have been a time of introspection for many leaders in the field. In addition to Reilly's influential questions for the profession, others followed in her footsteps. Fidler (1966/2005) challenged the profession to recognize the professional commitment to learning, critical thinking, and creativity. She cautioned that the educational process must teach more than technical skills; instead, it should focus on basic principles and concepts that can be applied differentially in varied settings. Wilma West (1968/2005) exhorted the profession to look ahead and seek innovative avenues for treatment in response to the changing needs of society. West argued that the profession needed to move into the new role of "health agent," as prevention needed to become a more integral element of the health care system.

Elizabeth June Yerxa further extended this call to address our professional goals and status (Figure 21.8). Yerxa (1967/2005) noted that "the scientific attitude is not incompatible with concern for the client as a human being but may be one of the best foundations for acting upon that concern." (p. 128). However, she warned that occupational therapy had often not met the challenge of the profession, simply being content to apply knowledge at the level of technical skills and interventions. Yerxa believed that the profession must focus on its unique assets, such as allowing the client to exercise choice in the engagement of "self-initiated, purposeful activity" (1967/2005, p. 134). Ultimately, the goal of practice is to provide "authentic occupational therapy" (1967/2005, p. 138).

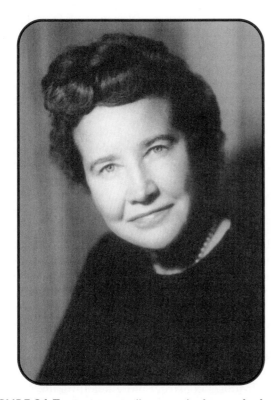

FIGURE 21.7 Dr. Mary Reilly created a frame of reference known as occupational behavior. She was the Eleanor Clarke Slagle Lecturer in 1961 and a charter member of the Academy of Research of the American Occupational Therapy Foundation. (Photo courtesy of the archives of AOTA, Bethesda, MD.)

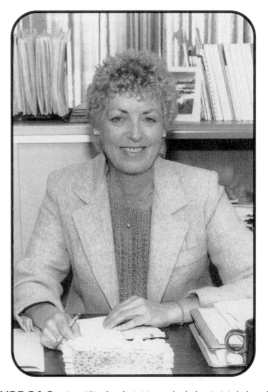

FIGURE 21.8 Dr. Elizabeth J. Yerxa led the initial development of the academic discipline of occupational science. Dr. Yerxa received many awards for her work, including the AOTA Award of Merit for her leadership of the profession. (Photo courtesy of the archives of AOTA, Bethesda, MD.)

In achieving this goal, we may be truly committed to the client's goals, with a sincere involvement in their healing experience while establishing a mutual and meaningful relationship with our clients during their recovery process. This certainly remains a gold standard of practice to this day.

Jerry Johnson (1973) continued along these lines, which harkened back to the ideas of the founders, proclaiming that the knowledge base of occupational therapy was well suited to address both individual and societal needs. Johnson emphasized the need for occupational therapy to reexamine the profession's relationships with other professions to better adapt to a changing world. This included a concern over the closeness of the relationship of occupational therapy to medicine, stating that occupational therapy should look to market services outside of the hospital, including community health care centers, school systems, and day care centers. Advances in the behavioral sciences were seen as having tremendous potential for the enrichment of the profession and its practices, helping to address the feeling among some in the profession that it had become lost in the medical model during the rapid growth of the post–World War II era (Dasio, 1971). Josephine Moore (1976/2005) echoed this theme of integrating new knowledge from the behavioral sciences to better understand ourselves and our clients. In a similar vein, Lorna Jean King (1978/2005) expressed the belief that the knowledge regarding behavior should be integrated into a theory base specific to the understanding of adaptation and adaptive processes to meet the needs of the profession. The leaders of this time had a profound influence on the next generation of occupational therapy leaders and practitioners.

In 1977, Kielhofner and Burke's historical analysis characterized this rift with the conceptual model of medicine in terms of competing paradigms of professional thought. Theirs was probably the most comprehensive history of the profession written up to that time, looking at the first 60 years of the profession. The roots of occupational therapy were characterized as being largely humanistic but gravitating toward an increasingly reductionistic or mechanistic practice, focusing more on body parts and isolated functions than on larger sets of occupations and the meaning associated with engagement. This rift was characterized as creating a growing crisis in professional thought. Kielhofner and Burke (1977) discussed the need for the profession to continue to develop a paradigm of occupation that takes into account the active nature of the human adaptive process with attention to ongoing research concerning developmental and social theory. This need continues to be a focus of Gary Kielhofner's (2002) work in the form of the model of human occupation. Since publication of the first edition of his book in 1985, Kielhofner and his colleagues have been working to further the scientific understanding of the human need for occupation and its application to the practice of occupational therapy.

The model of human occupation has kept an eye on the past, striving for a holistic perspective in the endeavor to understand human occupation, while incorporating contemporary theories and concepts. The model of human occupation respects the past while incorporating current knowledge formations.

ONGOING GROWTH AND DEVELOPMENT OF THE PROFESSION AND ITS RELATIONSHIP TO HISTORY

The profession of occupational therapy has continued to develop in new directions, one influential innovation being the development of occupational science. Occupational science traces its roots back to the ideas of the founders, who believed that occupation and knowledge of its capacity to promote health and well-being may be used throughout the broader population to improve quality of life. Spearheaded by Elizabeth June Yerxa in 1989, the first occupational science program was developed at the University of Southern California with the intent to further understand the complexity of human occupation. Occupational science was developed with the intention of informing and providing inspiration for occupational therapy practice while attempting to look at occupation in new ways, infusing new concepts and ideas into the understanding of occupation (Clark, Wood, and Larson, 1998). This includes utilizing varied research approaches, including case studies that allow for more naturalistic inquiry and experience sampling methods, in addition to more standard research approaches such as randomized clinical trials.

Occupational science's unique focus on the broader issues of human occupation, rather than an exclusive focus on occupational therapy practice, has been designed to meet the goal of producing more powerful therapeutic interventions which can be utilized by occupational therapists in both traditional and innovative treatment settings (Clark et al., 2005). A prime example of this occupation-based intervention is the well-elderly study (Clark et al., 1997). This research project broke new ground in the world of occupational therapy, demonstrating that preventive occupational therapy could help to prevent the declines normally associated with aging. Out of this study came the concept of "lifestyle redesign." This new intervention relies on fundamental occupational therapy ideas and ongoing occupational science research and theory development that provide individualized intervention to help individuals construct more healthful life routines and foster more meaningful engagement, the end result being improved quality of life. For example, research is now being directed toward understanding how occupations influence the risk of pressure sores among those with spinal cord injury. Another application of lifestyle redesign principles is in the area of weight loss. Using an occupational science perspective on the issues of weight gain and modulation of one's activity, the lifestyle redesign program to help individuals lose and control weight shows potential for being one way to address the growing public health concern about obesity in the United States. Just as those associated with the founding of occupational therapy hoped that knowledge of occupation would help to address the growing public health concerns about mental health at the dawn of the twentieth century, so do practitioners of occupational science hope to help occupational therapy address the growing public health concerns of the twenty-first century (Clark et al., 2005).

Evidenced-based practice is another recent and powerful development in society and in the profession of occupational therapy as the profession strives to hone its skills and understanding of the therapeutic value of our interventions (Holm, 2000). Although evidence-based practice might appear to be a new issue in many ways, it is truly an ideal that resonates with the founding of the profession. From the beginning of the profession, many physicians were able to see the beneficial effects of occupation on the recovery of their patients. Using the science of the time, they struggled to understand the mechanism of healing in those they served. Evidenced-based practice is closely related, being the vehicle of our own time to understand what are the most effective means of helping those whom we serve and understanding the means and pathways that our interventions help to produce gains in health and quality of life.

CONCLUSION

When one considers the history of the profession of occupational therapy, a number of consistent themes emerge. First, the profession has always had an altruistic mission, sought a scientific foundation for practice, and utilized the strength of its professional organization to establish itself as a true profession. Occupational therapy began during a unique time in which a dynamic integration of mind and body was at the forefront of the medical profession, and our profession continues to incorporate a therapeutic perspective in which mind and body are integrated in the concept of health and wellness. Occupational therapy was seen as having the potential to be an important contributor to society from its inception, and it continues to have a potentially powerful role in enhancing the lives of individuals throughout the life course.

PROVOCATIVE QUESTIONS

1. The social challenges of changing lifestyles and growing concerns over the general health of the population were important factors in the early conceptual development of occupational therapy. Has occupational therapy met the challenge of helping the general public to lead healthier lifestyles? How can we improve on our performance in this area?

2. At the dawn of the twentieth century, Americans were concerned that life was too fast paced, that people suffered from a lack of energy, and that lifestyle changes were necessary to address this growing concern. How would you compare the social issues and concerns of 100 years ago with those in our current cultural discussion?

3. The incorporation of scientific theory and ideas is a critical element of professional status for any profession. How is current knowledge development supporting our scientific understanding of occupational therapy? Do you feel that you have a strong scientific understanding of your own therapy practices?

REFERENCES

Allen, F. C. (1952). *The big change.* New York: Harper and Brothers.

Amar, J. (1922). The psychograph as an instrument to measure working capacity. *Archives of Occupational Therapy, 1,* 265–267.

American Occupational Therapy Association. (1967). *Occupational therapy: Then—and now.* New York: American Occupational Therapy Association.

Atwood, C. E. (1907). The favorable influence of occupation in certain nervous disorders. *New York Medical Journal, 86,* 1101–1103.

Ayres, A. J. (1972). Sensory integration and learning disorders. Los Angeles: Western Psychological Services.

Ayres, A. J. (1979). Sensory integration and the child. Los Angeles: Western Psychological Services.

Baloueff, O. (2003). Sensory integration. In E. B. Crepeau, E. S. Cohn, & B. A. Boyt Schell (Eds.), *Willard and Spackman's occupational therapy* (10th ed., p. 247–252). Philadelphia: Lippincott, Williams & Wilkins.

Barker, L. F. (1908). Psychotherapeutics. In proceedings of societies. *New York Medical Journal, 87,* 1219.

Barton, G. E. (1916). *Occupational Therapy.* New York: Lakeside.

Bing, R. K. (1981). Occupational therapy revisited: A paraphrastic journey. *American Journal of Occupational Therapy, 35,* 499–518.

Bledstein, B. (1976). *The culture of professionalism: The middle class and the development of higher education in America.* New York: W. W. Norton.

Bockoven, J. S. (1963). *Moral treatment in American psychiatry.* New York: Springer.

Bockoven, J. S. (1971). Legacy of moral treatment: 1800's to 1910. *American Journal of Occupational Therapy, 25,* 223–225.

Burnham, J. C. (1987). *How superstition won and science lost: Popularizing science and health in the United States.* New Brunswick, NJ: Rutgers University Press.

Carroll, R. S. (1910). The therapy of work. *Journal of the American Medical Association, 54,* 2032–2035.

Clark, F., Azen, S. P., Zemke, R., Jackson, J., Carlson, M, Mandel, D., Hay, J., Josephson, K., Charry, B., Helles, C., Palmer, J., & Lipson, L. (1997). Occupational therapy for independent living older adults: A randomized controlled trial. *Journal of the American Medical Association, 278*(16), 1321–1326.

Clark, F., Jackson, J., Wolfe, M. K., & Salles-Jordan, K. (2005). *Lifestyle redesign research and practice with the elderly, pressure sore prevention, and weight loss.* Paper presented at American Occupational Therapy Annual Conference and Expo, 2005.

Clark, F., Wood, W., & Larson, E. A. (1998). Occupational science: Occupational therapy's legacy for the 21st century. In M. Neistadt, & E. Crepeau. (Eds.), *Willard and Spackman's occupational therapy* (9th ed., pp. 13–21). Philadelphia: Lippincott.

Clark, M. (1925). Occupational therapy for children. *Archives of Occupational Therapy, 4,* 61–67.

Cohn, E. (1908). The systematic occupation and entertainment of the insane in public institutions. *Journal of the American Medical Association, 50,* 1249–1251.

Conrick, W. (1930). Occupational therapy at James Whitcomb Riley hospital for children. *Occupational Therapy and Rehabilitation, 9,* 93–102.

Dain, N. (1971). *Disordered minds.* Williamsburg, VA: Colonial Williamsburg Foundation.

Daniels, G. (1971). *Science in American society: A social history.* New York: Alfred A. Knopf.

Dasio, K. (1971). The modern era: 1960 to 1970. *American Journal of Occupational Therapy, 25,* 237–242.

Dunton, W. R., Jr. (1918a). National Society for the Promotion of Occupational Therapy. *Maryland Psychiatric Quarterly, 7,* 55–56.

Dunton, W. R., Jr. (1918b). N.S.P.O.T. *Maryland Psychiatric Quarterly, 8,* 68–74.

Dunton, W. R., Jr. (1919a). Wanted. A name. *Maryland Psychiatric Quarterly, 9,* 35–36.

Dunton, W. R., Jr. (1919b). Problems in occupational therapy. *Maryland Psychiatric Quarterly, 9,* 37–45.

Dunton, W. R., Jr. (1928). *Prescribing occupational therapy.* Baltimore: Charles C. Thomas.

Ellenberger, H. (1970). *The discovery of the unconscious: The history and evolution of dynamic psychiatry.* London: Allan Lane.

Fidler, G. (1966/2005). Learning as a growth process: A conceptual framework for professional education. In R. Padilla (Ed.), *A professional legacy: The Eleanor Clarke Slagle lectures in occupational therapy, 1955–2004* (2nd ed., pp. 115–126). Bethesda, MD: AOTA Press.

Fuller, S. (1991). Disciplinary boundaries and the rhetoric of the social sciences. *Poetics Today, 12,* 301–325.

Gordon, D. (2002). *Therapeutics and science in the history of occupational therapy.* Doctoral dissertation, University of Southern California. (UMI Microform 3094328)

Grob, G. (1966). *The state and the mentally ill.* Chapel Hill: University of North Carolina Press.

Grob, G (1994). The history of the asylum revisited: Personal reflections. In M. S. Micale & R. Porter (Eds.), *Discovering the history of psychiatry* (pp. 260–281). New York: Oxford University Press.

Hall, H. J. (1905a). The systematic use of work as a remedy in neurasthenia and allied conditions. *Boston Medical and Surgical Journal, 152,* 29–31.

Hall, H. J. (1905b). Neurasthenia: A study of etiology. Treatment by occupation. *Boston Medical and Surgical Journal, 153,* 47–49.

Hall, H. J. (1910a). Work-cure. *Journal of the American Medical Association. 54,* 12–14.

Hall, H. J. (1910b). Manual work in the treatment of the functional nervous diseases. *Journal of the American Medical Association, 55,* 295–297.

Hall, H. J. (1923). *O.T.: A new profession.* Concord, NH: Rumford Press.

Haller, J. S. (1981). *American medicine in transition: 1840–1910.* Chicago: University of Illinois Press.

Hollinger, D. A. (1995). Scientism and cognitivism. In R. W. Fox and J. T. Kloppenberg (Eds.), *A companion to American thought* (pp. 616–618). Cambridge, MA: Blackwell.

Holm, M. B. (2000). Our mandate for the new millennium: Evidence-based practice. *American Journal of Occupational Therapy, 54,* 575–585.

Hopkins, H. L. (1978). An historical perspective on occupational therapy. In H. L. Hopkins & H. D. Smith (Eds.), *Willard and Spackman's occupational therapy* (5th ed., pp. 3–23). Philadelphia: J. B. Lippincott.

Hopkins, H. L. (1988). An historical perspective on occupational therapy. In H. L. Hopkins & H. D. Smith (Eds.), *Willard and Spackman's occupational therapy* (7th ed., pp. 16–37). Philadelphia: J. B. Lippincott Company.

Hunter, R., & Macalpine, I. (1963). *Three hundred years of psychiatry.* New York: Oxford University Press.

James, W. (1899/1918). *On vital reserves. The energies of men: The gospel of relaxation.* New York: Henry Holt.

Johnson, J. (1973). Occupational therapy: A model for the future. *American Journal of Occupational Therapy, 27,* 1–7.

Jones, H. M. (1971). *The age of energy. Varieties of American experience: 1865–1915.* New York: Viking Press.

Kelleher, J. P. (1925). Motivation of social interest. *Archives of Occupational Therapy, 4,* 365–371.

Kidner, T. B. (1930). The progress of occupational therapy. *Occupational Therapy and Rehabilitation, 9,* 221–224.

Kidner, T. B. (1932). Occupational therapy: Its aims and developments. *Occupational Therapy and Rehabilitation, 11,* 233–239.

Kielhofner, G. (2002). *Model of human occupation* (3rd ed.). Baltimore: Lippincott, Williams & Wilkins.

Kielhofner, G., & Burke, J. (1977). Occupational therapy after 60 years: An account of changing identity and knowledge. *American Journal of Occupational Therapy, 31*(10), 675–689.

Kimball, B. A. (1992). *The "true professional ideal" in America: A history.* Cambridge, MA: Blackwell.

King, L. J. (1976/2005). Toward a science of adaptive responses. *A professional legacy: The Eleanor Clarke Slagle lectures in occupational therapy, 1955–2004* (pp. 253–266). Bethesda: AOTA Press.

Kraepelin, E. (1917/1962). *One hundred years of psychiatry.* New York: Citadel Press.

Mackay, R. (1933). Therapy for children. *Occupational Therapy and Rehabilitation, 12,* 299–304.

Meyer, A. (1922). The philosophy of occupational therapy. *Archives of Occupational Therapy, 1,* 1–10.

Moher, T. J. (1907). Occupation in the treatment of the insane. *Journal of the American Medical Association, 48,* 1664–1666.

Moore, J. (1976/2005). Behavior, bias, and the limbic system. *A professional legacy: The Eleanor Clarke Slagle lectures in occupational therapy, 1955–2004* (pp. 226–239). Bethesda, MD: AOTA Press.

Neff, M. L. (1910). Occupation as a therapeutic agent in insanity. *Medical Record, 78,* 996–1000.

Obrock, I. (1932). Occupational therapy for crippled children. *Occupational Therapy and Rehabilitation, 11,* 203–211.

Oxford English Dictionary. (1971). New York: Oxford University Press.

Peloquin, S. (1989). Moral treatment: Contexts considered. *American Journal of Occupational Therapy, 42*(8), 537–544.

Peloquin, S. (1994). Moral treatment: How a caring practice lost its rationale. *American Journal of Occupational Therapy, 48,* 167–173.

Pinel, P. (1806/1962). *A treatise on insanity.* New York: Hafner.

Porter, R. (1997). *The greatest benefit to mankind.* New York: Oxford University Press.

Quiroga, V. (1995). *Occupational therapy: The first 30 years, 1900–1930.* Bethesda, MD: American Occupational Therapy Association.

Reilly, M. (1962). Occupational therapy can be one of the great ideas of 20th-century medicine. *American Journal of Occupational Therapy, 16,* 1–9.

Reingold, N., & Reingold, I. H. (1981). *Science in America: A documentary history, 1900–1939.* Chicago: University of Chicago Press.

Richardson, H. K. (1926). Occupation and psychopathy. *Occupational Therapy and Rehabilitation, 5,* 95–109.

Robinson, G. C. (1925). The relation of occupational therapy and medicine. *Archives of Occupational Therapy, 4,* 1–5.

Rosen, G. (1968). *Madness in society.* London: Routledge and Kegan Paul.

Rosenberg, C. E. (1997). *No other gods: On science and American social thought.* Baltimore: Johns Hopkins University Press.

Rush, B. (1812/1964). *Medical inquiries and observations upon the diseases of the mind.* New York: Hafner.

Schwab, S. I. (1907). The use of social intercourse as a therapeutic agent in the psychoneuroses, a contribution to the art of psychotherapy. *Journal of Nervous and Mental Diseases, 34,* 497–503.

Shorter, E. (1997). *A history of psychiatry: From the era of the asylum to the age of Prozac.* New York: John Wiley and Sons.

Shumway, D., & Messer-Davidow, E. (1991). Disciplinarity: An introduction. *Poetics Today, 12,* 201–225.

Slagle, E. C. (1914). History of the development of occupation for the insane. *Maryland Psychiatric Quarterly, 4,* 14–19.

Slagle, E. C. (1922). Training aides for mental patients. *Archives of Occupational Therapy, 1,* 11–17.

Spackman, C. S. (1968). A history of the practice of occupational therapy for restoration of physical function: 1917–1967. *American Journal of Occupational Therapy, 22,* 67–71.

Starr, P. (1982). *The social transformation of American medicine.* New York: Basic Books.

Szasz, T. (1974). *The myth of mental illness.* New York: Harper & Row.

Thayer, A. S. (1908). Work cure. *Journal of the American Medical Association, 55,* 1485–1487.

Vandermeersch, P. (1994). "Les mythes d'origine" in the history of psychiatry. In M. S. Micale and R. Porter (Eds.), *Discovering the history of psychiatry* (pp. 219–231). New York: Oxford University Press.

West, W. (1968/2005). Professional responsibility in times of change. *A professional legacy: The Eleanor Clarke Slagle lectures in occupational therapy, 1955–2004* (pp. 141–151). Bethesda, MD: AOTA Press.

Willson, R. N. (1908). The pathogenesis and treatment of neurasthenia in the young. *American Journal of Medical Science, 135,* 178–187.

Yerxa, E. J. (1967/2005). Authentic occupational therapy. In R. Padilla (Ed.), *A professional legacy: The Eleanor Clarke Slagle lectures in occupational therapy, 1955–2004* (pp. 127–140). Bethesda: AOTA Press.

Contemporary Occupational Therapy Practice in the United States

22

ELIZABETH BLESEDELL CREPEAU,
BARBARA A. BOYT SCHELL, AND
ELLEN S. COHN

" People are most true to their humanity when engaged in occupation. "

—YERXA ET AL. (1989)

Learning Objectives

After reading this chapter, you will be able to:

1. Define occupational therapy.
2. Describe examples of the range of services provided in the
   United States.
3. Identify common core aspects of practice.
4. Consider possible futures for the profession.

♦ Linda is a 35-year-old carpenter who accidentally cut the tendons across
the back of her right, dominant, hand at work. She lives with her partner, Susan, in a house surrounded by a garden to which they devote
considerable time and energy. Robin, an occupational therapist, custom-
made a hand splint for Linda that positions and protects her hand while
it is healing. Robin also showed her how to manage her wound care as
part of her daily self-care routine. Together they discussed what activities Linda could realistically and safely do, both at home and at work.
Robin encouraged Linda to use the two fingers on her injured hand that

216

were not involved as much as possible and suggested that she might want to use the coming weeks to do the computer work needed to get her year-end taxes ready, since Linda owns her own business.

- Lauro is a 14-year-old junior high student with developmental disabilities. He has been successfully included in the public school setting, but he, his family, and his educational team must begin planning for his transition from school to life after graduation. At a recent educational-planning meeting Lauro stated that he would like to take the local bus with his peers to his weekly after-school sports program rather than driving with his mother each week. Lauro has never used public transportation and has little understanding of how to manage money. He is not sure what he would like to do when he grows up but knows he wants to live in his own apartment someday.
- Jack, Pete, and Harry like to attend the Bridges program at the local recreation center. Bridges is a member-directed program for people who are living with mental illness. This morning, the newspaper group discussed ideas for articles for the next monthly issue. Members selected topics and went to the recreation center's computer room to search the Web for ideas. When they arrived at the computer room, Sally, a certified occupational therapy assistant, helped each member set up a computer with the appropriate adaptations.
- Maplewood Industries is a furniture company whose employees have experienced many work-related repetitive trauma injuries. John, an occupational therapist, has a contract with Maplewood to conduct a work-site assessment to identify how the various workstations could be changed to avoid repetitive trauma injuries. He also has been working with the company health nurse to develop and implement an employee-training program to prevent the onset of these injuries.
- Mrs. Oak is a retired schoolteacher whose husband of 52 years died the past spring. She has just moved into a small apartment in a life-care community. Her daughter, who lives in another state, is concerned that her mother seems depressed and is not adjusting to her new setting, even though there are many activities there for her to enjoy. Pam, the occupational therapist, interviewed Mrs. Oak about her lifelong interests and activities and is helping Mrs. Oak adapt her routines to this setting.
- Mary works with the Mayor and City Council to help shape policies and funding priorities designed to make the town safer and easier for everyone to access public services and engage in healthy behaviors. As a result of her advocacy, there are now safe and well-lit walking paths with frequent resting places that senior citizens and families with young children are enjoying. Additionally sidewalks and bicycle paths within a one-mile radius of schools are monitored by school guards and volunteers to encourage children to walk or bike to school, thus the children are getting more exercise and

parents are saving time in transportation. Currently Mary is working on a grant with the recreation department director to obtain playground equipment designed to make it easier for children with mobility impairments to use the public playgrounds.

These six scenarios represent the diversity of occupational therapy intervention for occupational therapy clients, be they individuals, groups, organizations or populations. Linda wants to be able to return to work and her garden. Like most adolescents, Lauro wants to be more autonomous from his parents, use public transportation, live in his own apartment someday, and learn job skills to prepare him for life after high school. The members of the Bridges program want to be able to contribute to their group and the broader community and to enjoy time with their friends. The manager at Maplewood Industries wants to be sure that his employees do not develop repetitive trauma injuries because of his concern for them as human beings and for the company's productivity. Mrs. Oaks wants to find a way to live meaningfully in her new life, and her daughter wants her to be as comfortable as possible. Mary and the leaders of her community want a healthy population that is able to participate fully in public areas. As these scenarios demonstrate, occupational therapy practitioners provide services to a variety of clients in many settings, from hospitals and schools to community programs and businesses. These services include direct intervention with individuals to programming for groups to consultation within organizations and public advocacy. In all cases, the overarching goal of occupational therapy is to engage people in meaningful and important occupations to support health and to participate as fully as possible in society.

DEFINITION OF OCCUPATIONAL THERAPY

Occupational therapy is the art and science of helping people do the day-to-day activities that are important and meaningful to their health and well-being through engagement in valued occupations. The *occupation* in occupational therapy comes from an older use of the word, meaning how people use or "occupy" their time. Hasselkus (2006) in her Slagle lecture spoke about everyday occupation as something that is so ordinary and embedded in the everyday that we may fail to appreciate its complexity and how our occupations constitute an interwoven network of all we do on a daily basis. Occupational therapy, drawing on the centrality of occupation to daily life, refers to all of the activities that occupy people's time, construct identity through doing, and provide meaning (Christiansen, 1999, Zemke, 2004). Occupation includes the complex network of day-to-day activities that enable people to sustain their health, to meet their needs, to contribute to the life of their family, and to participate in the broader society (American Occupational Therapy Association [AOTA], in press).

Finally, occupational engagement is important because it has the capacity to contribute to health and well-being (Clark et al., 1997; Glass, Mendes de Leon, Marottoli, & Berkman, 1999; Law, Seinwender, & Leclair, 1998). As the scenarios that opened this chapter illustrate, occupational therapy practitioners provide individual or group intervention as well as consultative services that foster community participation, prevention, and wellness of groups in a wide range of settings. The desired outcome of occupational therapy intervention is that people will live their lives engaged in occupations that sustain themselves, support their health, and foster involvement with others in their social world.

Contemporary occupational therapy practice draws on the historical roots of the profession, filtered through current occupational therapy, health, and human service research and practice. Meyer (1977/1922), for example, in his oft-quoted address to the National Society for the Promotion of Occupational Therapy asserted, "Our role consists in giving opportunities rather than prescriptions. There must be opportunities to work, opportunities to do, to plan and create, and to use material" (p. 641). Englehardt (1977), and more recently Pörn (1993), asserted that health is measured by an individual's adaptive capacity and engagement in daily activities. In her Eleanor Clarke Slagle Lecture, Yerxa (1967) explained that authentic occupational therapy focuses on clients' humanity and their ability to choose and initiate activities that provide the basis for the discovery of meaning. She further argued that authentic occupational therapy requires that the practitioner "in every professional act defines the profession" and, in doing so, enters into a reciprocal relationship characterized by mutual care and that "to care means to be affected just as surely as it means to affect" (p. 8). Later in her address, Yerxa called for practitioner engagement in research to promote the development of the knowledge base of the profession. These themes translate into three principles to guide contemporary occupational therapy:

1. Client-centered practice
2. Occupation-centered practice
3. Evidence-based practice

CLIENT-CENTERED PRACTICE

At the core of occupational therapy is the commitment to focus on the client as an active agent seeking to accomplish important day-to-day activities. Occupational therapy practitioners often work with people who are disempowered (Kronenberg & Pollard, 2005; Townsend, 1996). Clients seek care and professional help to "gain mastery over their affairs" (Rappaport, 1987, p. 122). To be client centered, practitioners must be willing to enter the client's world to create a relationship that encourages the other to enhance his or her life in ways that are most meaningful to that person. Practitioners strive to understand the client as a person embedded in a particular context consisting of family and friends, socioeconomic status, culture, etc.

In a client-centered model, practitioner and client collaboratively engage in the therapeutic process (Law, 1998). Mattingly (1991) asserted that this process is narrative in nature, which means the practitioner and client create an understanding of the client's past, present, and future story. Mattingly further asserted that the future story is co-constructed and constantly revised in the midst of therapy. Practitioners strive to understand human feelings and intentions as well as the deeper meaning of people's lives through what Clark (1993) called occupational storytelling. In contrast, occupational storymaking occurs in the midst of therapy. It is that imaginative process through which clients create and then enact new occupational identities (Clark, 1993).

OCCUPATION-CENTERED PRACTICE

Contemporary occupational therapy emphasizes occupational engagement. Clients seek occupational therapy because they need help engaging in their valued occupations. The emphasis on occupational engagement stems from the profession's beliefs, substantiated by emerging research, that people's occupations are central to their identity and that they can reconstruct themselves through their occupations (Jackson, 1998). Occupations are not isolated activities but are connected in a web of daily activities that help people fulfill their basic needs and contribute to their family, friends, and broader community (Hasselkus, 2006). Occupation-centered practice focuses on meaningful occupations selected by clients and performed in their typical settings (Fisher, 1998; Pierce, 1998). Systematic assessment of clients' occupations and priorities are vital to occupation-centered practice. This information—when coupled with careful analyses of the person's capacities, the task's demands, and the performance context—provides the basis for intervention. Intervention goals are directly connected to the person's occupational concerns, and intervention methods capitalize on the person's occupational interests. In this way, both the means (methods) and the ends (goals) of therapy involve intervention grounded in the occupations of the client (Fisher, 1998; Gray, 1998; Trombly, 1995).

Consistent with client-centered and occupation-based practice, Ann Wilcock and Elizabeth Townsend, leaders in occupational therapy from two different part of the world, introduced the concept of occupational justice to acknowledge that all people are occupational beings and that meeting all peoples' need for engagement in meaningful occupation is a matter of justice (see Chapter 20). Wilcock and Townsend equate occupational justice with rights, equity, and fairness and argue that every individual has the right to have equal opportunities and access. To address injustices, occupational therapy practitioners have begun to develop interventions and advocate for people who are disempowered by legislation, war, political upheavals, dictatorships or natural disasters. While many of the occupational therapy initiatives to address instances of occupational injustice have been developed in other parts of the world, practitioners in the United States have begun to embrace the ideals of an "occupationally just" world and develop interventions with these goals in mind.

EVIDENCE-BASED PRACTICE

One of the important trends in health care is the growing requirement to base intervention decisions on "the conscientious, explicit, and judicious use of current best evidence" (Sackett, Rosenberg, Muir Grany, Haynes, & Richardson, 1996, p. 71). This process, called evidence-based practice, entails being able to integrate research evidence into the clinical-reasoning process to explain the rationale behind interventions and predict probable outcomes—or, as Gray asserted, "doing the right things right" (cited in Holm, 2000, p. 576). Beyond "doing the right things right," evidence-based practice involves being able to explain occupational therapy recommendations to clients in a language clients will understand (Tickle-Degnen, 2000). Furthermore, intervention grounded in the customs of the field no longer meets the ethical requirement to "fully inform the service recipients of the nature, risks, and potential outcomes of any interventions" (American Occupational Therapy Association [AOTA], 2000, p. 614).

The challenge for occupational therapy practitioners is threefold.

◆ First, to practice occupational therapy based on research evidence, practitioners must know how to access, evaluate, and interpret relevant research.

◆ Second, practitioners must have the capacity to collect data to support their intervention recommendations.

◆ Third, once practitioners understand the possible interventions and related outcomes, they need to communicate the probable outcomes to clients and/or their care providers, so clients can decide whether to participate in occupational therapy intervention.

Not only must practitioners be willing to examine intervention practices to see if they are effective but also they must be open to changes in their intervention patterns when the evidence suggests more effective approaches than the ones they typically use.

OCCUPATIONAL THERAPY PRACTITIONERS

Clients are, of course, an essential component of occupational therapy intervention, but occupational therapy practitioners are the other part of the equation. Practitioners use their professional reasoning abilities to actualize their knowledge and skills in practice. Just as clients have an occupational history, so do practitioners. They are also embedded in personal, social, and cultural contexts that shape their worldview. These include their preferred theories and intervention techniques, the practical realities of the setting in which they practice, and the team members with whom they work (Schell, 2007).

Like clients, practitioners come with particular strengths and limitations that influence their interactions with others. These strengths and limitations influence how practitioners frame client problems and use the intervention context to benefit clients.

VISION FOR THE FUTURE

In 2017 the American Occupational Therapy Association will celebrate its 100th Anniversary. In recognition of this milestone, the AOTA spent several years in an extensive visioning process, designed to guide the profession toward maximizing its potential to be of service to society. The Centennial Vision was approved by the AOTA Representative Assembly at the 2006 annual conference. The vision statement states:

> We envision that occupational therapy is a powerful, widely recognized, science-driven and evidence-based profession with a globally connected and diverse workforce meeting society's occupational needs. (AOTA, 2006)

The Centennial Vision lists key points to achieve this vision by 2017. These elements address the preparation and diversity of the occupational therapy workforce so that it is more visible, powerful and able to collaborate with others to improve the health and well-being of individuals and the broader society. In addition, our leaders envision greater innovation based on science to guide practice and to provide the evidence to support occupational therapy intervention. Finally, membership in AOTA will be seen as a professional responsibility because it is through a strong member involvement that the potential of occupational therapy to meet society's occupational needs will become a reality (AOTA, 2006). In her Farewell Presidential Address Carolyn Baum, AOTA president from 2004–2007, said:

> Those who founded our profession had a vision: that occupational therapy would study and use occupation as it influences health, and would educate people about its value. Many, many advances are making our founders' vision a reality. As we get closer to the actual Centennial celebration, it is a time for occupational therapists and occupational therapy assistants to seize the opportunities of those changes in the health care system that place value on health and par-

ticipation. We must use our knowledge and skills to be very visible with our contributions, which improve the quality of the lives of those we serve. (Baum, 2007)

CONCLUSION

Occupational therapy is a complex process that involves collaborative interaction between the practitioner and the client embedded in the intervention context. Occupational therapy intervention must be grounded in research and focused on the client as an occupational being. The therapeutic process evolves as the practitioner and client work together to analyze carefully the client's occupations and performance limitations. Because occupational therapy is a "doing with" and not a "doing to" profession, there is an improvisational aspect of intervention that requires the practitioner and client to coordinate their actions to achieve the client's goal. The rest of this book delineates the various aspects of occupational therapy. It emphasizes consistently that best practice involves (1) understanding and respecting clients, (2) collaborating with clients to achieve their occupational goals, and (3) using interventions that are supported by research.

As you start your career, our challenge to you is to strive to achieve the ideals of the profession. First, be aware of the influence of your beliefs and your personal and professional contexts and how these influence your actions. Second, consistently challenge yourself to listen to your clients so that you can facilitate their autonomy and engagement in desired occupations. Third, use the most effective assessment instruments and interventions to support the progress of your clients. Fourth, advocate for your clients so they can obtain the services they need and learn to advocate for themselves. Finally, systematically evaluate your practice to ensure that your interventions enable your clients to engage in those occupations they value most. The people whose scenarios opened this chapter remind us that we have the responsibility to live up to the ideals of the profession. Peloquin, one of our philosophers, concluded her 2005 Eleanor Clarke Slagle with the following statement:

> The ethos of occupational therapy restores our clear-sightedness so that we see what is essential: We are pathfinders. We enable occupations that heal. We cocreate daily lives. We reach for hearts as well as hands. We are artists and scientists at once. If we discern this in ourselves, if we act on this understanding everyday, we will advance into the future embracing our ethos of engagement. And we will have reclaimed our magnificent heart. (2005, p. 623)

We welcome you to the path of occupational therapy.

REFERENCES

American Occupational Therapy Association [AOTA]. (2000). Occupational therapy code of ethics. *American Journal of Occupational Therapy, 54,* 614–615.

American Occupational Therapy Association. (2006). *AOTA adopts centennial vision.* Retrieved July 31, 2007, from www.aota.org/News/Media/PR/2006/38538.aspx

American Occupational Therapy Association. (in press). Occupational therapy practice framework: Domain and process (2nd ed.). *American Journal of Occupational Therapy.*

Baum, C. M. (2007, April 28). *Farewell presidential address.* American Occupational Therapy Association Annual Conference, St. Louis, MO.

Christiansen, C. H. (1999). Defining lives: Occupation as identity: An essay on competence, coherence, and the creation of meaning. *American Journal of Occupational Therapy, 54,* 547–558.

Clark, F. (1993). The 1993 Eleanor Clarke Slagle Lecture—Occupation embedded in a real life: Interweaving occupational science and occupational therapy. *American Journal of Occupational Therapy, 47,* 1067–1078.

Clark, F., Azen, S. P., Zemke, R., Jackson, J., Carlson, M., Mandel, D., Hay, J., Josephson, K., Cherry, B., Hessel, C., Palmer, J., & Lipson L. (1997). Occupational therapy for independent-living older adults: A randomized controlled trial. *Journal of the American Medical Association, 278,* 1321–1326.

Engelhardt, H. T. (1977). Defining occupational therapy: The meaning of therapy and the virtues of occupation. *American Journal of Occupational Therapy, 31,* 666–672.

Fisher, A. G. (1998). The 1998 Eleanor Clarke Slagle Lecture—Uniting practice and theory in an occupational framework. *American Journal of Occupational Therapy, 52,* 509–521.

Glass, T. A., Mendes de Leon, C., Marottoli, R. A., & Berkman, L. F. (1999). Population based study of social and productive activities as predictors of survival among elderly Americans. *British Medical Journal, 319,* 478–483.

Gray, J. M. (1998). Putting occupation into practice: Occupation as ends, occupation as means. *American Journal of Occupational Therapy, 52,* 354–364.

Hasselkus, B. R. (2006). The 2006 Eleanor Clarke Slagle Lecture—The world of everyday occupation: Real people, real lives. *American Journal of Occupational Therapy, 60,* 627–640.

Holm, H. B. (2000). The 2000 Eleanor Clarke Slagle Lecture—Our mandate for a new millennium: Evidence-based practice. *American Journal of Occupational Therapy, 54,* 575–585.

Jackson, J. (1998). The value of occupation as the core of treatment: Sandy's experience. *American Journal of Occupational Therapy, 52,* 466–473.

Kronenberg, F., & Pollard, N. (2005). Introduction: A beginning. In F. Kronenberg, S. Simo Algado, & N. Pollard (Eds.), *Occupational therapy without borders: Learning from the spirit of survivors* (pp. 1–13). Edinburgh: Elsevier Churchill Livingstone.

Law, M. (1998). *Client-centered occupational therapy*. Thorofare, NJ: Slack.

Law, M., Seinwender, S., & Leclair, L. (1998). Occupation, health, and well-being. *Canadian Journal of Occupational Therapy, 65,* 81–91.

Mattingly, C. (1991). The narrative nature of clinical reasoning. *American Journal of Occupational Therapy, 45,* 979–986.

Meyer, A. (1977/1922). The philosophy of occupational therapy. *American Journal of Occupational Therapy, 31,* 639–642.

Peloquin, S. M. (2005). The 2005 Eleanor Clarke Slagle Lecture—Embracing our ethos, reclaiming our heart. *American Journal of Occupational Therapy, 59,* 611–625.

Pierce, D. (1998). What is the source of occupation's treatment power? *American Journal of Occupational Therapy, 52,* 490–491.

Pörn, I. (1993). Health and adaptedness. *Theoretical Medicine, 14,* 295–303.

Rappaport, J. (1987). Terms of empowerment/exemplars of prevention: Toward a theory for community psychology. *American Journal of Community Psychology, 15*(2), 121–145.

Sackett, D. L., Rosenberg, W. M. C., Muir Granny, J. A., Haynes, R. B., & Richardson, W. S. (1996). Evidence-based medicine. What it is and what it isn't. *British Medical Journal, 312,* 71–72.

Schell, B. A. B. (2008). Pragmatic reasoning. In B. A. B. Schell & J. W. Schell (Eds.), *Clinical and professional reasoning in occupational therapy*. Baltimore: Lippincott Williams and Wilkins.

Tickle-Degnen, L. (2000). Communicating with clients, family members, and colleagues about research evidence. *American Journal of Occupational Therapy, 54,* 341–343.

Townsend, E. (1996). Institutional ethnography: A method for showing how the context shapes practice. *Occupational Therapy Journal of Research, 16,* 179–199.

Trombly, C. A. (1995). The 1995 Eleanor Clarke Slagle Lecture—Purposefulness and meaningfulness as therapeutic mechanisms. *American Journal of Occupational Therapy, 49,* 960–972.

Yerxa, E. J. (1967). The 1967 Eleanor Clarke Slagle Lecture—Authentic occupational therapy. *American Journal of Occupational Therapy, 21,* 1–9.

Yerxa, E. J., Clark, F., Frank, G., Jackson, J., Parham, D., Pierce, D., Stein, C., & Zemke, R. (1989). An introduction to occupational science: The foundation for occupational therapy in the 21st century. *Occupational Therapy in Health Care, 6*(4), 1–17.

Zemke, R. (2004). The 2004 Eleanor Clarke Slagle Lecture—Time, space, and the kaleidoscopes of occupation. *American Journal of Occupational Therapy, 58,* 608–620.

Contemporary Occupational Therapy Practice Worldwide

23

TERRY K. CROWE

Learning Objectives

After reading this chapter, you will be able to:

1. Review the historical development of the World Federation of Occupational Therapists (WFOT)
2. Recognize the functions and structure of WFOT
3. View the diversity of professional practice and entry-level occupational therapy education through a world lens
4. Understand requirements and opportunities for international work
5. Reflect about the future trends of occupational therapy internationally

As the world becomes "smaller" through communication connections and globalization influences, we can learn from the occupational therapy perspectives and activities at a world level. This chapter focuses on the growth and future trends of occupational therapy internationally.

HISTORICAL OVERVIEW

In 1952, the World Federation of Occupational Therapists (WFOT) was created (Spackman, 1967). WFOT is the key international representative for occupational therapy and the official international organization for the promotion of occupational therapy (World Federation of Occupational Therapists, 2006a). The founding members of WFOT were Australia, Canada, Denmark, Great Britain (England and Scotland), India, Israel, New Zealand, South Africa, Sweden, and the United States (Spackman, 1967). Helen Willard and Clare Spackman were part of the original WFOT leaders (Mendez, 1986). Spackman became the first WFOT delegate from the American Occupational Therapy Association (AOTA) and went on to become the WFOT president from 1959 to 1961.

WFOT Congresses

Only two years after WFOT was founded, the first WFOT Congress was held in Edinburgh, Scotland. It was attended by almost 400 participants from 21 countries (Paterson, 1994). The conference themes reflected the major areas of occupational therapy at that time: tuberculosis, poliomyelitis, psychiatry, cerebral palsy, and rehabilitation and resettlement. The international issues facing the profession were summarized as an inadequate number of educational programs; a shortage of occupational therapists; lack of governmental, medical, and civil support; and the lack of unification of educational standards and terms of service. The WFOT Congresses continue to be held every four years, bringing together occupational therapists from around the world. At the 14th Congress in Australia, in 2006, over 2,000 occupational therapists from 80 nations learned from each other (Crowe, 2006a). The next Congress will be held in Santiago, Chile, in 2010.

WFOT Organization

WFOT comprises 66 organizational members, 10 associate members, and over 6,000 individual members, 2,038 of whom are from the United States (Table 23.1) (Evert & Cronin, 2007; World Federation of Occupational Ther-

apists, 2006b). WFOT is structured in five main program areas: education and research, promotion and development, standards and quality, international cooperation, and the executive program (World Federation of Occupational Therapists, 2006c). Specific projects within these programs are undertaken by occupational therapists from around the world. The federation is managed by volunteer leadership using a virtual office. AOTA elects three individuals to represent the United States in the World Federation (American Occupational Therapy Association, 2005). The delegate is the voting member at the WFOT Council meetings. The first alternate delegate sits in the Representative Assembly to represent AOTA members who practice in foreign countries. The second alternate delegate acts as a liaison helping therapists who would like to work temporarily or permanently in other countries. All three delegates plan and implement the International Day at the AOTA Annual Conference.

GLOBAL GROWTH IN OCCUPATIONAL THERAPY

Occupational therapy continues to expand worldwide. For example, professionals in Georgia, a former Soviet Republic that has a population of 4.7 million people (World Factbook, 2006), recognized the need to develop occupational therapy in 2001 (World Federation of Occupational Therapists, 2005a). With help from the European Network of Occupational Therapy, eight Georgian students were

TABLE 23.1   WFOT MEMBERSHIP CATEGORIES

Category	Requirements
Full Country Membership	◆ Have an occupational therapy association with an approved constitution ◆ Have at least one WFOT approved entry-level educational program ◆ Can vote on WFOT agenda items ◆ 66 WFOT Member nations
Associate Country Membership	◆ An occupational therapy association with an approved constitution ◆ Cannot vote on WFOT agenda items ◆ 10 WFOT Associate Member Countries
Individual Membership	◆ Open to Occupational Therapy and Occupational Therapy assistants who are members of their country professional Occupational Therapy association (i.e. AOTA) ◆ Dues paid to WFOT through national association ◆ Receive WFOT Bulletin ◆ Access to member only aspects of WFOT webpage ◆ Eligible for WFOT Research Awards ◆ Can participate in WFOT Project Teams ◆ 6,749 individual members ◆ Of this, 2,038 are from the United States + 490 student members

[From World Federation of Occupational Therapists (2006d).]

locally educated and graduated in 2004, and the Georgian Occupational Therapy Association was formed. Practice areas in Georgia and other former Soviet Republic countries include integrating children and adults into the community and upgrading the intervention that is provided to people who reside in institutions. In 2006, Georgia became a member of WFOT. Similarly, assisted by WFOT, Egypt, which has 78.9 million residents (World Factbook, 2006), plans to develop occupational therapy education programs in three Egyptian universities (World Federation of Occupational Therapists, 2005e).

EDUCATION OF OCCUPATIONAL THERAPISTS WORLDWIDE

Education of occupational therapists at the international level is critical to the advancement and global expansion of occupational therapy worldwide (Figure 23.1). Many of these educational programs are guided by the educational standards set by WFOT. The first WFOT Educational Minimal Standards were published in 1958 (Hockings & Ness, 2002). The 2002 Revised WFOT Minimum Standards are visionary and address the challenge of making higher education relevant to each country's cultural uniqueness, social and economic structure, and prevailing health needs and priorities (Hockings & Ness, 2004a). These standards highlight the centrality of occupation, the realization of cultural differences in occupation and health care practice, and the power of occupation in building healthy communities. They emphasize that educational programs need to disseminate local as well as international knowledge related to the profession. The local context refers to the geographical area of the country, the characteristics of health and welfare needs and systems, and the diversity of cultural backgrounds. The AOTA Educational Standards meet or exceed the WFOT Educational Minimal Standards (American Occupational Therapy Association, 1998).

Currently, WFOT recognizes 566 occupational therapy educational programs (World Federation of Occupational Therapists, 2006e). Internationally, there are numerous other occupational therapy educational programs that teach occupational therapy but that have not been reviewed or approved by WFOT. Educational programs for occupational therapy vary widely in their intensity and level of content. The minimum requirement recommended by WFOT for occupational therapy education is 90 weeks (Hocking & Ness, 2004b). Educational programs may be housed in universities, colleges, private institutions, or medical facilities. Students may graduate at a certificate, diploma, undergraduate, or graduate degree levels. The United States and Canada have the highest educational degree requirement: Entry-level occupational therapists must have a master's degree (American Occupational Therapy Association, 1998; Canadian Association of Occupational Therapists, 2005). Only the United States, the United Kingdom, and South Africa have recognized educational programs for occupational therapy assistants (American Occupational Therapy Association, 1998; British Association/College of Occupational Therapist, 2006; Van der Reyden, 2005).

WORKING INTERNATIONALLY

Occupational therapists can work in other countries if they meet the requirements of the specific country. Many countries will employ occupational therapists only if they have graduated from a WFOT-approved school (World Federation of Occupational Therapists, 2007). A great way to connect with international occupational therapy work and volunteer opportunities is through the Occupational Therapy International Outreach Network (OTION), a forum for information exchange (Newton & Fuller, 2005). OTION's goal is to form partnerships between occupational therapists in resource-rich countries and organizations serving people with disabilities in resource-poor countries. There are many pathways to working internationally, including volunteering with the Peace Corps (Crowe, 2005a, 2007), working with an international nongovernmental organization, volunteering short or long term (Crowe, 2005b, 2005c, 2006b), or working in a facility that provides occupational therapy.

COUNTRY PROFILES

Although occupational therapy is now a worldwide profession, the nature of practice is shaped to meet the different cultures and resources within each country. Table 23.2 provides brief profiles of the practice of occupational therapy

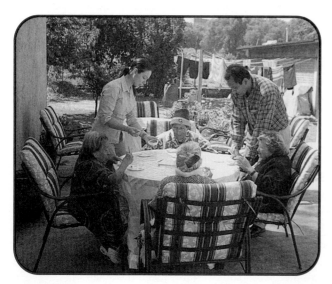

FIGURE 23.1 Occupational therapy students in Mexico City facilitate participation in a home for elderly people.

TABLE 23.2   OCCUPATIONAL THERAPY FACTS FOR AUSTRALIA, CHILE, INDIA, UGANDA, & THE UNITED KINGDOM

	Australia (www.ausot.com.au)	Chile (www.terapia-ocupacional.cl)	India (www.aiota.org)	Uganda (ott@infocom.co.ug)	United Kingdom (www.cot.co.uk)
Population	20.3 million	16.1 million	1.1 billion	28.2 million	60.6 million
Number of Occupational Therapists	11,500	900	5,000	70	26,031
Year of WFOT membership	1952	2005	1952	1998	1952
Professional Journal	Australian Occupational Therapy Journal, 4 issues/year	Revista Chilena de Terapia Ocupacional, one issue/year	Indian Journal of Occupational Therapy, 3 issues/year	none, newsletter produced one time a year	British Journal of Occupational Therapy (BJOT), 12 issues/year
Number of WFOT approved education programs	17	1	20	1	56 in 34 different Universities
Organization strategic priorities	◆ Strengthen, enhance and unify the partnership between OT AUSTRALIA National and all member associations to develop and deliver quality member outcomes	◆ Strengthen the labor, ethical, social, and political commitment in order to address the public health issues of the country ◆ Make sure that OT services will be available in the new health	◆ Increase awareness of Occupational Therapy in medical, governmental and public sectors ◆ Increase employment opportunities in	◆ Developing OT interventions that are relevant to rural residents ◆ Raising awareness of occupational therapy with the government	◆ Develop the workforce to meet new service delivery challenges ◆ Integrate and reform Occupational Therapy services to provide more effective and

Continued

TABLE 23. 2   OCCUPATIONAL THERAPY FACTS FOR AUSTRALIA, CHILE, INDIA, UGANDA, & THE UNITED KINGDOM   *Continued*

Australia (www.ausot.com.au)	Chile (www.terapia-ocupacional.cl)	India (www.aiota.org)	Uganda (ott@infocom.co.ug)	United Kingdom (www.cot.co.uk)
◆ Actively promote and facilitate the development of excellence in the profession in all areas of practice ◆ Be an efficient, effective and financially viable organization through excellence in practice ◆ Maximize the relevance, effectiveness and profile of OT AUSTRALIA through quality professional representation and marketing activities/ initiatives (M. Pattison, personal communication, Oct. 13, 2006)	systems and assure greater OT participation ◆ Continue working in cooperation with different organizations, groups and other professional associations to develop greater civic participation ◆ Advance the professional certification to a national level to assure high quality Occupational Therapy interventions ◆ Enhance the continuous specialization and training of occupational therapists (E. Henny and O. Castro, personal communication, Dec. 16, 2006)	governmental and non-governmental organizations ◆ Increase occupational therapy research ◆ Assure that the Indian Council of Occupational Therapy govern the profession in respect to occupational therapy education and practice ◆ Increase community-based and evidence-based occupational therapy (A. Srivastava, personal communication, Nov. 21, 2006)	(S. Shann, personal communication, Nov. 9, 2006)	efficient service delivery ◆ Increase the role for Occupational Therapy in vocational rehabilitation and employment ◆ Assure that occupation is central to service delivery ◆ Create more roles for occupational therapists related to health promotion and public health (B. Steeden, personal communication, Oct. 13, 2006)

on each of the five world continents. One country is high-lighted on each continent. Notice that very different health issues face each country. The WFOT Website provides similar information on many countries in the world.

FUTURE OF OCCUPATIONAL THERAPY WORLDWIDE

Since only 76 of the world's 271 nations and other recog-nized territories have established practices in occupational therapy as acknowledged by WFOT, a significant amount of growth is needed for occupational therapy to reach the world's estimated 6 billion, 538 million people (U.S. and World Population Clocks, 2007). For example, in Bangladesh, a country of 147 million people (World Fact-book, 2006), in 2005, there were only 25 locally trained occupational therapists and two occupational therapists who had been trained in other countries (Newton & Fuller, 2005). Other countries, such as Cambodia, Vietnam, and Bermuda, do not have any locally trained occupational therapists (Crowe, 2005c; M. Patterson, personal commu-nication, August 26, 2005), although there may be some foreign occupational therapists working on special projects or local therapists who have been educated outside of their country (Figure 23.2). Many countries around the world provide opportunities to develop occupational therapy that is culturally relevant. Occupational therapy needs to be contextualized and acknowledge traditional and cultural beliefs around health, illness, and disability. This offers occupational therapists a chance to develop innovative practice and educational models to assist people around the world to have occupationally rich lives.

An inspiring development in occupational therapy on the world stage is the involvement in community-based rehabilitation, an approach that is used primarily in coun-tries with limited resources (Fransen, 2005; Sinclair, Sakellariou, Kronenberg, Fransen & Pollard, 2006). Pro-fessionals including occupational therapists implement rehabilitation at a community level, attempting to equalize opportunities and promote social integration of people with disabilities (Figure 23.3). Human rights are an issue even in countries with established occupational therapy ser-vices where many marginalized people are not able to access services. Examples are people without health insurance, refugees, survivors of violence, indigenous people, or peo-ple who are homeless (Algado & Burgman, 2005; Algado & Cardona, 2005; Davis & Kutter, 1998; Kronenberg, 2005; Petrenchik, 2006; Simmond, 2005). Challenges include tremendous personal, occupational, and environ-mental adversity. Occupational therapy needs to expand service delivery models to meet these challenges and to embrace more people internationally. Peloquin (2005) ele-

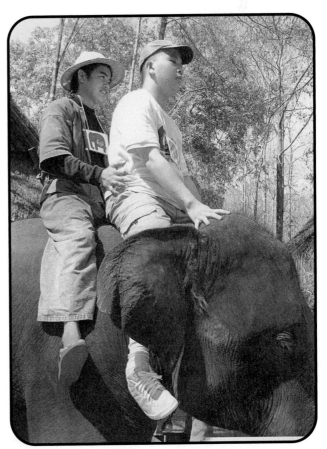

FIGURE 23.3 A child with an autism spectrum disorder participates in an elephant camp implemented by occupa-tional therapists in Thailand. Through carefully monitored interactions with the elephants, the outcomes include higher levels of adaptive responses and social/communication abilities in the children.

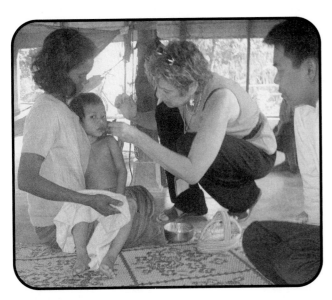

FIGURE 23.2 The author works with a child and her mother while consulting with a visiting nurse in a Cambodian village.

PRACTICE DILEMMA

PROVIDING SERVICES IN ANOTHER COUNTRY

You have volunteered to work in an educational program for children with disabilities in Oaxaca City, Oaxaca, Mexico. Oaxaca has only a handful of occupational therapists, mostly working in a nearby government rehabilitation hospital. You speak intermediate-level Spanish. You have graduated from an educational program approved by the American Association of Occupational Therapy (AOTA).

1. Can you practice in Mexico without any additional qualifications? How do you know?
2. Since you are not fluent in Spanish, how will you understand a family's occupational needs and views of health, illness, and disability? How will you develop occupational priorities for children that are specifically relevant to the children and their families within their cultural context?

gantly states: "Through the use of empowering occupations, our therapy programs transform settings. In a world grown small because of easier travel and widespread media coverage, those who are poor, disenfranchised, socially isolated and marginally cared for beckon to us (as occupational therapists) as they have never done before" (p. 101). It is the responsibility of all of us to promote the participation of people with disabilities in all countries.

SUMMARY

Occupational therapy has expanded widely throughout the world since its beginning in 1917. With the currently increasing global professional networking and international collaboration, occupational therapists will be spearheading international cooperative efforts to improve responses to natural and human-made disasters, improve the health and well-bring of all worldwide citizens, and provide meaningful occupations to all. In the next decade, we will see many countries joining WFOT. In addition, occupational therapy will strengthen its role and continue to expand service delivery approaches to meet the needs of more people on an international level. Yerxa (2003) stated that "occupational therapy is committed to improving the life opportunities, health and capability of all people, including those with chronic impairments by employing occupation as therapy, contributing new knowledge of occupation to society, and

by influencing public policy for people" (p. 976). This needs to take place internationally so that people with occupational challenges can lead more meaningful lives.

REFERENCES

Algado, S. S., & Burgman, I. (2005). Occupational therapy intervention with children survivors of war. In F. Kronenberg, S. S. Algado, & N. Pollard (Eds.), *Occupational therapy without borders: Learning from the spirit of survivors* (pp. 245–260). Edinburgh: Elsevier Churchill Livingstone.

Algado, S. S., & Cardona, C. E. (2005). The return of the corn men: An intervention project with a Mayan community of Guatemalan retornos. In F. Kronenberg, S. S. Algado, & N. Pollard (Eds.), *Occupational therapy without borders: Learning from the spirit of survivors* (pp. 336–350). Edinburgh: Elsevier Churchill Livingstone.

American Occupational Therapy Association. (1998). *Standards for an accredited educational program for the occupational therapist and occupational therapist assistant.* Retrieved December 20, 2006, from http://www.aota.org/nonmembers/area613/links/link13.asp

American Occupational Therapy Association. (2005). *Bylaws.* Retrieved December 15,2006, from http://www.aota.org/members/area6/docs/bylaws101304.pdf, 20–21

British Association/College of Occupational Therapists. (2006). *Careers handbook introduction: Part 1.* Retrieved September 14, 2006, from http://www.cot.org.uk

Canadian Association of Occupational Therapy. (2005). *CAOT academic accreditation standards and self-study guide.* Retrieved December 18, 2006, from http://www.caot.ca/pdfs/GuideComplete.pdf

Crowe, T. K. (2005a). How about joining the Peace Corps?: International Perspective Column. *Advance, 21,* 14.

Crowe, T. K. (2005b). Volunteering internationally: International Perspective Column. *Advance, 21,* 13.

Crowe, T. K. (2005c). Rehabilitation in Vietnam: International Perspective Column. *Advance, 21,* 10.

Crowe, T. K. (2006a). Professional growth down under: International Perspective Column. *Advance, 22,* 7.

Crowe, T. K. (2006b). Preparing for international consultation: International Perspective Column. *Advance, 22,* 11.

Crowe, T. K. (2007). The adventure of a lifetime: International Perspective Column. *Advance, 23,*

Davis, J., & Kutter, C. J. (1998). Independent living skills and posttraumatic stress disorder in women who are homeless: Implications for future practice. *American Journal of Occupational Therapy, 52,* 39–44.

Evert, M. M. & Cronin, A. (2007). Report of the World Federation of Occupational Therapists to the Representative Assembly. Retrieved April 12, 2007, http://www.aota.org.

Fransen, H. (2005). Challenges for occupational therapy in community-based rehabilitation: Occupation in a community approach to handicap in development. In F. Kronenberg, S. S. Algado, & N. Pollard (Eds.), *Occupational therapy without borders: Learning from the spirit of survivors* (pp. 166–182). Edinburgh: Elsevier Churchill Livingstone.

Hocking, C., & Ness, H. E. (2002). Introduction to the revised minimum standards for the education of occupational therapists: 2002. *WFOT Bulletin, 46,* 30–33.

Hocking, C., & Ness, H. E. (2004a). WFOT minimum standards for the education of occupational therapist: Shaping the profession. *WFOT Bulletin, 50,* 9–17.

Hocking, C., & Ness, H. E. (2004b). *Advise for the establishment of a new programme or the education of occupational therapists.* Retrieved December 18, 2006, from http://www.wfot.org

Kronenberg, F. (2005). Occupational therapy with street children. In F. Kronenberg, S. S. Algado, & N. Pollard (Eds.), *Occupational therapy without borders: Learning from the spirit of survivors* (pp. 261–276). Edinburgh: Elsevier Churchill Livingstone.

Mendez, M. A. (1986) *A chronicle of the World Federation of Occupational Therapists: The first 30 years: 1952—982: Part I.* Retrieved September 19, 2005, from http://www.wfot.org.

Newton, E., & Fuller, B. (2005). The Occupational Therapy International Outreach Network: Supporting occupational therapists working without borders. In F. Kronenberg, S. S. Algado, & N. Pollard (Eds.) *Occupational therapy without borders: Learning from the spirit of survivors* (pp. 361–373). Edinburgh: Elsevier Churchill Livingstone.

Paterson, C. F. (1994). The first international congress of the World Federation of Occupational Therapist—Edinburgh, 1954. *The British Journal of Occupational Therapy, 57,* 115–120.

Peloquin, S. M. (2005). The art of occupational therapy: Engaging hearts in practice. In F. Kronenberg, S. S. Algado, & N. Pollard (Eds.), *Occupational therapy without borders: Learning from the spirit of survivors* (pp. 99–109). Edinburgh: Elsevier Churchill Livingstone.

Petrenchik, T. (2006). Homelessness: Perspectives, misconceptions, and considerations for occupational therapy. *Occupational Therapy in Health Care, 20,* 9–30.

Simmond, M. (2005). Practicing to learn: Occupational therapy with the children of Viet Nam. In F. Kronenberg, S. S. Algado, & N. Pollard (Eds.), *Occupational therapy without borders: Learning from the spirit of survivors* (pp. 277–286). Edinburgh: Elsevier Churchill Livingstone.

Sinclair, K., Sakellariou, D., Kronenberg, F., Fransen, H., & Pollard, N. (2006). Reporting on the WFOT-CBR master project plan: The data collection subproject. *WFOT Bulletin, 54,* 37–45.

Spackman, C. S. (1967). The World Federation of Occupational Therapists: 1952–1967, *American Journal of Occupational Therapy, 21,* 301–309.

Van der Reyden, D. (2005). Auxiliary staff in the field of psychiatry: Requirement, functions and supervision. In R. Crouch & V. Alers (Eds.), *Occupational therapy in psychiatry and mental health* (4th ed.) London: Whurr Publishers Ltd.

U.S. and World Population Clocks. (2007). Retrieved January 8, 2007, from http://www.census.gob/main/www/popclock.html

World Factbook. (2006). Retrieved December 15, 2006, from http://www/cia.gov/cia/publications/factbook/fields/2119.html

World Federation of Occupational Therapists. (2005a). *Development of occupational therapy in Georgia.* Retrieved August 29, 2005, from http://www.wfot.org

World Federation of Occupational Therapists. (2005b). *CDOT newsletter #2.* Retrieved October 2, 2005, from http://www.wfot.org

World Federation of Occupational Therapists. (2006d). *Membership.* Retrieved September 15, 2006, from http://www.wfot.org

World Federation of Occupational Therapists. *Recognized programs and schools.* (2006e). Retrieved December 15, 2006, from http://www.wfot.org/schoolLinks.asp

World Federation of Occupational Therapists. (2006c). *Annual Report 2004/2006.* Retrieved December 15, 2006, from http://www.wfot.org

World Federation of Occupational Therapists. (2006a). *Welcome.* Retrieved October 11, 2006, from http://www.wfot.org

World Federation of Occupational Therapists. (2006e). *WFOT council meeting.* Retrieved December 15, 2006, from http://www.wfot.org

World Federation of Occupational Therapists. (2007). *Country profiles.* Retrieved January 8, 2007, from http://www.wfot.org

Yerxa, E. J. (2003). Dreams, decisions and directions for occupational therapy in the millennium of occupation. In E. B. Crepeau, E. S. Cohn, & B. A. Boyt Schell (Eds.), *Willard & Spackman's occupational therapy.* (pp 976–980). Philadelphia: Lippincott Williams & Wilkins

Occupational Therapy Professional Organizations

24

SARA BRAYMAN

Learning Objectives

After reading this chapter, you will be able to:

1. Describe the roles of AOTA, NBCOT, and state regulatory boards in the credentialing of occupational therapy practitioners in the United States.
2. Appreciate the roles that both volunteer and paid staff members in professional organizations play in developing and supporting all aspects of the profession and its members.
3. Understand how professional and regulatory organizations serve the consumers of occupational therapy through standard setting and education.

O ccupational therapy students, occupational therapy assistants, and occupational therapists are, by virtue of their education, license, and/or certification, eligible to be members of the occupational therapy profession. The formation of professional identity is a developmental process that begins at the point at which an individual chooses occupational therapy. It builds while he or she is in school, beginning to learn the theories, techniques, and procedures of practice. This developmental process does not cease when the individual graduates and enters practice but continues to develop throughout his or her professional life. Being a professional requires that an individual recognize and adhere to that profession's code of ethics, practice within its defined scope, and contribute to the evolving development of knowledge and skills that are necessary to continually refine that profession. The entire process is supported by professional organizations that set standards and provide support to individuals and the profession as a whole. The following Case Study provides an example that illustrates the various organizations that support the entry into the profession of occupational therapy. As you read this chapter, refer back to this case.

Kanesha is a senior in high school. She has just discovered that she would like to be an occupational therapist who works with children with special needs. She learned about occupational therapy (OT) from a video and a presentation by OT students during a career fair at her school. The students invited her to come to the university, sit in on a class, and meet some of the professors. They also suggested that she visit the Website of the American Occupational Therapy Association (AOTA) to learn more about OT. Perusing the Website only served to heighten Kanesha's interest in OT, so she made arrangements to visit the university and to speak with one of the OT faculty members. She completed the application process and was accepted into the freshman class as a pre-occupational therapy student. She worked hard to maintain a good grade point average and was careful to take all of the courses needed to enter the OT program.

Kanesha was very excited when she was accepted to the program. Her first courses were very challenging, and she was pleased to learn more about her chosen profession. She joined AOTA as a student member and became increasingly interested in all of the different areas in which occupational therapists practice. She took advantage of one of the benefits of belonging to AOTA as a student member. She found that the *American Journal of Occupational Therapy, OT Practice,* and the Special Interest Section Quarterlies contained interesting articles that were relevant to her coursework. Additionally, she used the OT Search through the AOTA's Website to quickly find OT resources for research papers.

While completing her coursework, Kanesha and her clinical fieldwork coordinator worked together to find a Level II fieldwork site in Florida so that she could complete the last of her fieldwork while living with her grandparents. Using the AOTA e-mail list, her coordinator found other fieldwork coordinators in Florida and was able to locate an appropriate fieldwork placement. During her final Level II fieldwork placement, Kanesha contacted the National Board for Certification of Occupational Therapists (NBCOT®) and applied to take her certification examination after completing her fieldwork. She could take the examination at a site that was close to her home. During this time, she studied by reviewing information from her textbooks and from the portfolio of all of her course work. She was glad that she had studied because the examination was rigorous.

Kanesha began to answer advertisements for occupational therapists. She interviewed at several places and finally narrowed her choices down to a position in South Carolina and another closer to home in Texas. Because she was not sure which of the positions she would accept, she contacted the state regulatory boards in both states to apply for licensure. She asked NBCOT to send her examination results to both of them. She anxiously awaited word from NBCOT and, after a couple of weeks, was thrilled to learn that she had passed the examination and was now a registered occupational therapist. She accepted the offer from a private practice group in Texas and began her new job working with children with autism. There was so much to learn! When her student membership expired, she renewed her AOTA membership and joined both the Developmental Disabilities and the School System Special Interest Sections so that she could communicate with other occupational therapists who worked with this population. Kanesha welcomed the information and resources provided by these therapists and by her supervisor and coworkers. She joined the Texas Occupational Therapy Association so that she would get to know other OTs in her state and become an active part of her profession.

This chapter introduces the reader to the major professional occupational therapy organizations in the United States. Because many of the profession's major standards and policies are developed by the American Occupational Therapy Association, much of this chapter focuses on the various components of that organization. State and international organizations and legal entities that affect occupational therapy are also briefly discussed, including how the AOTA relates to the World Federation of Occupational Therapy, which was discussed in Chapter 23.

AMERICAN OCCUPATIONAL THERAPY ASSOCIATION

American Occupational Therapy Association (AOTA) is the member organization in the United States that is responsible for guiding and developing occupational therapy's standards and code of ethics and for defining the profession's scope of practice. It was incorporated in New York in 1917 as the Society for the Promotion of Occupational Therapy. Its name was changed in 1927 to the American Occupational Therapy Association. Its membership comprises individual occupational therapists, occupational therapy assistants (OTAs), and students from all areas of practice. The members develop and refine AOTA's mission, education and practice standards, and code of ethics, all of which shape the profession. This is accomplished by individual members working together as volunteers serving on association committees.

The volunteer leaders as well as the members of the association are supported by staff employed by AOTA. The staff is supervised by the AOTA Executive Director, who in turn is supervised by the AOTA Board of Directors. Because most of the profession's policies, resources and standards are developed by volunteers, it is helpful to understand the many leaders and groups within the association. Table 24.1 provides a summary of the key volunteer offices and groups within AOTA. Table 24.2 summarizes some of the common acronyms that are used to refer to related groups.

AOTA Officers and Directors

AOTA has four officers: the president, vice president, secretary, and treasurer. The president presides over the Board of Directors (BOD) and the annual business meeting and is the primary spokesperson of the profession. The vice president's primary responsibility is to guide the development and direction of the strategic and long-range plans of the association. For example, in recent years, the AOTA president and vice president led the association in defining a vision of where the profession should be by the year 2017. The secretary is responsible for keeping the official minutes and documents of the association, and the treasurer has the responsibility for guiding the budgetary processes.

TABLE 24.1   LEADERSHIP ROLES AND FUNCTIONS IN AOTA

Leadership Role	Function	How Elected or Appointed
AOTA officers ◆ President ◆ Vice president ◆ Secretary ◆ Treasurer	Lead the association	Elected by all AOTA members.
Board of Directors ◆ AOTA officers ◆ Speaker of the Representative Assembly ◆ Directors (OT/OTA) ◆ Public advisor ◆ Consumer advisor	Provide oversight to organization; legally responsible for association actions and finances	Elected by all AOTA members except the consumer member, who is appointed by the president.
Representative Assembly ◆ Representatives from states/election areas ◆ Chairs of Commissions ◆ Chair of Special Interest Section Standing Committee ◆ Delegate from Affiliated State Association Presidents ◆ Delegate from the Assembly of Student Delegates ◆ OTA delegate ◆ Delegate for therapists residing in foreign countries	Make and approve policies guiding the organization and profession	Representatives elected by state/election area AOTA members. Students elect student delegates.
Commissions ◆ Commission on Practice ◆ Commission on Standards and Ethics ◆ Commission on Education ◆ Commission on Continuing Competence and Professional Development	Develop guidelines and respond to issues related to practice Address issues related to ethics and professional standards Develop guidelines and respond to issues related to education Develop guidelines and respond to issues related to advanced competency	Chair elected by all AOTA members. Commission members appointed or designated per AOTA policy.
Affiliated State Association Presidents	Coordinate activities of state occupational therapy organizations	Chair elected by state association presidents.

TABLE 24.2 COMMON ACRONYMS FOR AOTA-RELATED GROUPS

ACOTE	Accreditation Council for Occupational Therapy Education
AOTF	American Occupational Therapy Foundation
ASAP	Affiliated State Association Presidents
ASD	Assembly of Student Delegates
AOTA	The American Occupational Therapy Association, Inc.
BOD	The Board of Directors
CCCPD	Commission on Continuing Competence and Professional Development
COE	Commission on Education
COP	Commission on Practice
NBCOT	National Board for Certification in Occupational Therapy
OT	Occupational Therapist
OTA	Occupational Therapy Assistant
RA	Representative Assembly
SCB	Specialty Certification Board
SEC	Commission on Standards and Ethics
SIS	Special Interest Section
WFOT	World Federation of Occupational Therapists.

Adapted from American Occupational Therapy Association. (2004). *The reference manual of the official documents* (10th ed.). Bethesda: Author.

The BOD has the financial responsibility for the association and is legally responsible for the actions of AOTA. In between meetings, business is conducted online or via telephone conference call. The president often invites others to serve as resources to the BOD so that many points of view are considered. Those individuals cannot vote but may enter into the discussions.

Representative Assembly

The largest body of AOTA, the Representative Assembly (RA), makes the policies that govern the association. The RA meets face to face each spring at the AOTA Annual Conference and Exposition and also conducts business in an online meeting each fall. Every faction of the membership is represented in this legislative body. Each representative is elected either nationally or by the AOTA members who reside in the particular state or jurisdiction. Before these meetings, the representatives seek input from their members about important policy decisions facing the profession. Issues such the move from a bachelor's degree to a graduate degree requirement for professional entry had to be approved by the assembly. Practice standards in general, as well as statements about the role of occupational therapy in various specialty areas, such as driving and neonatal intensive care, are ultimately approved by this group. (See Box 24.1 for a look behind the scenes about the controversy that sometimes occurs in the process of setting policy.) Each representative serves for a term of three years, and terms are staggered on a rotational basis to ensure continuity. Representatives elect leaders within the group to guide the business of the assembly.

Commissions

There are four commissions in AOTA: Practice, Education, Standards and Ethics, and Continuing Competency and Professional Development. The chair of each is a member of the RA. Each commission serves a major role in shaping the profession's identity. The chair of each commission appoints individuals to serve on the commission, selecting AOTA members who represent various areas of expertise and geographic diversity. The number of individuals on each commission varies. Each commissioner is a voting member of the RA.

Commission on Practice (COP)

This commission is charged with developing standards and other documents such as position papers, roles and functions papers, practice guidelines, and white papers that are related to and define the practice of occupational therapy. For example, the Standards of Practice for Occupational Therapy serves to define the profession by describing how occupational therapists respond to referrals, screen and evaluate their clients, plan and execute intervention, transition the client to other needed services, and discontinue services when appropriate. Also included is the practice related to education and certification credentials needed (AOTA 2005).

Commission on Education (COE)

This commission generates education-related policy recommendations to the RA for deliberation. For example, this commission has defined the role competencies for faculty teaching in occupational therapy programs, such as the one Kanesha attended (see the preceding Case Study). COE identifies, analyzes, and anticipates issues related to education in conjunction with the Education Special Interest Section.

Commission on Standards and Ethics (SEC)

This commission develops the association's code of ethics and recommends standards and ethics for the profession.

BOX 24.1 BEHIND THE SCENES

When you read a chapter such as this, it might seem that all these organizations and the policies that they promote "just happen." Nothing could be farther from the truth. Not only is there a great deal of work by volunteers and staff alike, there is also a lot of discussion, negotiation, and sometimes professional tension that occur in the making of policies and standards. One of the best ways to see this is to watch the discussions of the RA in action. Hotly contested topics over the years have included the following:

◆ Whether AOTA should support state licensure of occupational therapists: Many therapists thought that it would be better to maintain a national certification so that therapists would not be hampered when moving from state to state. However, over time, the argument for becoming licensed won, as therapists wanted legal standing in their states. Until therapists were licensed in their states, anyone could say that her or she was an occupational therapist, whether the person had the professional credentials or not.

◆ Whether the educational level for occupational therapists should move from bachelor's to master's level: This discussion went on for over 20 years, until the move was made to postgraduate entry for occupational therapists. Those who were against the move were concerned that it would reduce the number of therapists, thus making access to services even more of a problem during times of shortage. Those who supported the move thought that many programs were requiring so many credit hours that it was like getting a postgraduate education without the degree. Although occupational therapists now must enter at the master's level, the dialogue about the appropriate standards and role of the occupational therapy doctorate is front and center while this book is being written.

◆ The scope of occupational therapy: A perennial concern is related to guidelines for what sorts of evaluations and interventions are "really occupational therapy" and what ones go beyond the scope of practice. For example, one question was whether it is appropriate for occupational therapists to utilize physical agent modalities or complementary and alternative interventions in their practice.

◆ The role of the Certified Occupational Therapy Assistant (COTA): Although AOTA policies are pretty clear that the COTA functions under the supervision of a registered occupational therapist (OTR), the exact nature of that supervision is frequently reexamined as practice evolves and new arenas emerge.

It serves as an oversight body related to complaints about unethical practice of members.

Commission on Continued Competency and Professional Development (CCCPD)

This commission's role is to develop the criteria and certification examinations for advanced areas of practice. It recommends standards for continuing competence and develops strategies for communicating information to stakeholders about issues of continuing competence and competency affecting occupational therapy. The CCCPD also develops tools to assist members in the development and implementation of continuing competence plans.

Special Interest Sections

In addition to the four commissions, there is a network of AOTA members representing eleven special interest sections. The special interest sections (SIS) are designed to respond to practice needs by focusing on a specific component of practice, at the same time recognizing that all occupational therapy personnel must practice within the general scope of the profession. The special interest sections are defined by the individual client served, the age of persons served, a particular area of skill or expertise, practice role, and location of practice. Table 24.3 lists the special interest sections that were in existence at the time of this writing. More than likely, no one special interest section will address all of a therapist's practice needs because practice is an integration of knowledge from many areas (AOTA, 2007a). For instance, in the case study, Kanesha chose to belong to two groups to help keep up with practice issues related to children with autism.

Each SIS provides its members with the opportunity for dialogue through its newsletters and through e-mail lists that are available to its members. These are invaluable tools for therapists who want to communicate with other therapists who have similar practice interests. Members of

TABLE 24.3 AOTA SPECIAL INTEREST SECTIONS BY FOCUS	
Focus	**Special Interest Section**
Client health condition	Developmental Disabilities (DDSIS) Mental Health (MHSIS) Physical Disabilities (PDSIS) Sensory Integration (SISIS)
Client age	Gerontology (GSIS)
Therapy skills	Technology (TSIS) Work Programs (WPSIS)
Practice roles	Administration and Supervision (AMSIS) Education (EDSIS)

the special interest sections often work collaboratively with the various commissions on projects such as defining roles and functions of occupational therapists in a particular practice arena, guiding the development of advanced competencies and specialized skills, or developing standards for education of occupational therapy personnel. Each chair belongs to the Special Interest Section Steering Committee (SISSC), which works to coordinate the efforts and collaborate on issues of mutual importance. The chair of SISSC sits on the RA with voice and vote.

Affiliation of State Association Presidents

There is an occupational therapy association in each state. These organizations are independent from AOTA but work with AOTA to advance the profession in that particular state and to advocate for the people and populations who are served by occupational therapy. The president of each state association belongs to the Affiliation of State Association Presidents. This group provides a venue for the presidents to communicate with and support each other.

Assembly of Student Delegates

Students are valued members of AOTA and belong to the Assembly of Student Delegates (ASD). Each educational program may select a student as its delegate to the ASD meeting that takes place during the AOTA Annual Conference and Exposition. ASD provides a platform for students to share their perspectives on issues that affect the profession. A representative of ASD serves in the RA and on each of the commissions.

AOTA Staff

All of the efforts of this large volunteer network of members would not be possible without a highly competent and dedicated staff at the national headquarters housed in Bethesda, Maryland (Figure 24.1). The staff includes occupational therapists, attorneys, accountants, policy specialists, and administrative, clerical, and technical personnel. The national headquarters staff is led by an executive director who is responsible for all of the personnel and operations of the national headquarters. This person reports directly to the AOTA president and attends all board meetings and meetings of the RA and has voice but cannot vote. The purpose of the national headquarters is to support the efforts of the association by providing the personnel and expertise required to accomplish the association's mission and the policies and positions enacted by the RA. Some of its key operations include supporting the work of the member volunteer groups, designing and delivering continuing education, compiling evidence-based practice information, monitoring and influencing public policy, and advocating for the profession and the persons it serves and maintaining sound business operations.

Staff members who are occupational therapists serve as a liaisons to the RA, to each of the commissions, and to the special interest section steering committee. Other staff members serve as liaisons to the various committees,

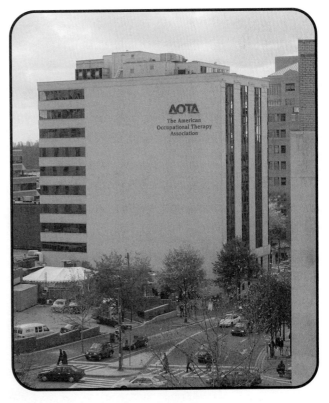

FIGURE 24.1 AOTA's national office building in Bethesda, Maryland.

commissions, and volunteer groups in the association. The liaisons provide knowledgeable and consistent support to the committee chairs, which enables each volunteer group to address its tasks with the assurance that the necessary administrative and clerical support is available to accomplish the tasks. Staff also responds to countless requests for information from members about specific issues related to the profession.

Continuing Education and Professional Development

Another whole group of staff members develop and coordinate continuing education offerings, including live and online workshops, seminars, online courses, and self-paced clinical courses. Many of these are offered throughout the country and in varied formats designed to best meet the needs of the participants. The most evident and widely publicized event is the AOTA Annual Conference and Exposition (Figure 24.2). This major undertaking involves solicitation and selection of continuing education presentations that address the needs of the membership, recruitment of vendors for the conference marketplace, and coordination of housing and meeting rooms to accommodate the thousands of participants. AOTA members may attend at a reduced cost. This Conference and Exposition is planned and implemented by staff from the national headquarters, although volunteer members review and rank presentations that are submitted for inclusion at conference and help provide needed human resources during the actual conference.

Evidence for Practice

Another major initiative of the AOTA staff is researching the literature to locate and gather the data that provide evidence for the practice of occupational therapy. As this data are collected, they are compiled into Evidence Based Briefs that therapists and others can use to support occupational therapy intervention. In addition to the Evidence Based Briefs, AOTA maintains a Practice Directory that provides links to various publications and Internet sources containing additional information that supports practice. This directory is a valuable resource that is available to AOTA members.

Public Policy and Advocacy

An important staff role is to represent and advocate for the interests of occupational therapists and their clients in the areas of public policy. This work involves lobbying with legislators regarding initiatives that are important to the profession and to the people who are served by occupational therapy. At the federal level, this may also involve working with the policymakers from the Office of Special Education, the Rehabilitation Services Administration, and other governmental agencies regarding eligibility for service as well as guidelines for reimbursement. AOTA staff is often called on to provide information and testimony before congressional committees who make recommendations regarding the interpretation and implementation of legislation.

This group also supports the activities of state and local occupational therapy associations and licensure boards to

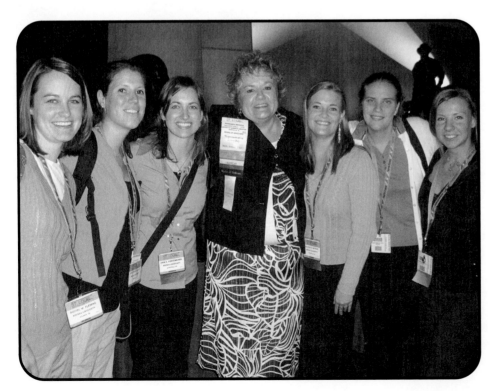

FIGURE 24.2 Students from Brenau University meet Dr. Penelope Moyers, president of AOTA, during the 2007 AOTA Conference and Exposition.

ensure that language supportive of occupational therapy is included in state legislation and that occupational therapy is supported and not inappropriately restricted by encroachment by other professions. AOTA staff members also provide educational materials and individual support to members and state associations to prepare them to effectively lobby, testify, and advocate for the profession and those who are served in their area by occupational therapy.

Business Operations

A number of AOTA staff members manage the business operations of the association. Income comes primarily from member dues, publications, conference registrations, and vendor fees. AOTA owns an eight-story office building in Bethesda, Maryland, that houses the national headquarters. Space in the building that is not used by the association is rented, and rental fees are a major source of the association's income. The largest category of AOTA expenses is travel and per diem support for the many members who volunteer to serve on the committees, boards, and commissions that support the work of the association. Other major expenses fund the initiatives passed by the RA and pay for staff salaries and benefits (AOTA, 2007b).

Accreditation Council for Occupational Therapy Education

Working under the umbrella of AOTA is the Accreditation Council for Occupational Therapy Education (ACOTE®). Members of the council are occupational therapists and occupational therapy assistants who are AOTA members who represent both clinical and academic interests. There is also a representative from the public. The role of ACOTE is to develop and implement the standards for all occupational therapy and occupational therapy assistant educational programs. ACOTE standards are related to all aspects of the program, including the curriculum, the credentials of faculty and staff, the content of courses, the physical facilities and resources, and the administrative policies of the school that relate to the occupational therapy program. To become accredited and to maintain accreditation, every OT and OTA program is evaluated on a regular basis by ACOTE. Completion of an occupational therapy program that is accredited by ACOTE is an eligibility requirement for students taking the certification examination (AOTA, 2007c). In the Case Study, Kanesha graduated from an ACOTE-accredited program as part of becoming an occupational therapist.

Publications

The official publication of the Association is the *American Journal of Occupational Therapy* (AJOT®). This peer-reviewed journal is available to all association members,

as it is included in their professional dues. The BOD selects the AJOT editor, who in turn selects an editorial board composed of occupational therapy scholars and practitioners, who solicit and review each submission.

The association also publishes *OT Practice,* a bimonthly magazine that includes informative articles about the profession. In addition to this magazine and the AJOT, AOTA publishes Special Interest Section Quarterlies, Newsletters on State Policy, monthly updates on legislative issues, and biweekly updates on current events that are of interest to members of the profession (AOTA, 2007d). Many of these publications are distributed electronically.

In addition to its regular ongoing publications, AOTA Press publishes books, manuals, monographs, and consumer guides that address topics of concern to occupational therapists and their consumers. AOTA also maintains a marketplace or clearinghouse for these publications, videos, and other documents as well as items that are appropriate for marketing occupational therapy. The cost of most of these items is reduced for AOTA members.

Summary

As should be obvious from this review, AOTA is an important partner for every member of the profession, providing services that range from educational standards to resources that support professional development to the advocacy needed to ensure that occupational therapists and the clients they serve are well represented in national policy decisions. Although this section has focused on AOTA, there are many parallel organizations in the countries where occupational therapy is a well accepted profession.

STATE REGULATORY BOARDS

Each state or jurisdiction regulates occupational therapy in some way. Most do this through a licensure board or regulatory agency. The definitions and guidelines are enacted by the legislature in that particular state. AOTA is a valued resource for these regulatory agencies, providing information about the profession. When students complete their Level II fieldwork and successfully pass the certification examination of the National Board for Certification of Occupational Therapists, they are eligible to apply for licenses to practice.

OTHER IMPORTANT ORGANIZATIONS

In addition to AOTA, there are other occupational therapy organizations with missions that support the profession of occupational therapy. There are two such organizations in the United States; one is a charitable foundation, and the other is the profession's credentialing body. There is also the World Federation of Occupational Therapy, which was discussed in Chapter 23.

American Occupational Therapy Foundation

The American Occupational Therapy Foundation (AOTF) is a charitable organization that was established in 1965 to advance the science of occupational therapy and to increase public understanding of its value. The foundation comprises occupational therapists and its corporate partners that support the profession. It is financially supported by contributions and corporations that value occupational therapy. Each year, the foundation holds special events at the AOTA annual conference and exposition to raise money to support its work.

As part of its mission to advance the science of occupational therapy, AOTF publishes a scholarly journal, *Occupational Therapy Journal of Research: Occupation, Participation and Health* (OTJR). The foundation also maintains the Wilma West Library, a national clearinghouse for occupational therapy information. In addition to the excellent library, the foundation maintains OT SEARCH, a comprehensive electronic search engine for literature related to occupational therapy. OT SEARCH and the other library services are housed in the same building as AOTA headquarters in Bethesda and are available to all members of AOTA.

AOTF supports scholarship and research through scholarships and financial assistance to students whose research advances the field. Small grants are available to students for funding their research. Larger amounts are granted to scholars to fund innovative studies that may affect the profession and build understanding of occupational science. Finally, the foundation partners with higher education to fund centers of scholarship and research (AOTF, 2007).

National Board for Certification of Occupational Therapists

The profession is also supported through the work of the National Board for Certification of Occupational Therapists (NBCOT®). This board is the credentialing body for therapists and assistants practicing in the United States. Registered occupational therapists, certified occupational therapy assistants, and consumers serve on this board. NBCOT develops and administers the initial certification examinations that occupational therapists and occupational therapy assistants take following their Level II fieldwork. The examinations are comprehensive and are designed to measure the knowledge and skills required for an OT or OTA to enter practice. The items in the certification examinations are based on an extensive practice analysis of novice occupational therapists from throughout the country. The certification examination includes items that reflect occupational therapy evaluation and intervention with diverse popula-

tions in a variety of practice environments. Examination results are shared with individual state licensure boards. Achievement of a passing score on the certification examination is required in almost every state in order to be eligible to obtain a license to practice. OTs and OTAs from other countries who wish to practice in the United States must successfully complete the certification examination (NBCOT, 2007).

World Federation of Occupational Therapy

Occupational therapy is a global profession. As was discussed in the previous chapter, the World Federation of Occupational Therapy (WFOT) was created as the "official international organization for the promotion of occupational therapy." The United States is one of 57 member countries belonging to the WFOT (WFOT, 2007).

AOTA, NBCOT, and WFOT are the principal organizations in the United States concerned with occupational therapy. AOTA also actively seeks and participates in partnerships with many other groups to address areas of common concern. These organizations collaborate with AOTA to work on meeting common goals. For example, the American Society of Speech and Hearing Association (ASHA) and the American Physical Therapy Association (APTA) and AOTA have formed the TriAlliance of Health and Rehabilitation Professions, which collaborates to advocate for issues that may affect all the members of those three professions.

In addition to the TriAlliance, AOTA collaborates with other associations, nonprofit groups and coalitions to address issues of mutual concern. The primary concern of some of these groups. such as the American Arthritis Foundation, the American Foundation for the Blind, and the Alzheimer's Association, might be people who have a particular disease or condition, while other groups might collaborate with AOTA on specific issues. For example the American Association of Retired Persons (AARP), the American Automobile Association (AAA), and AOTA are working together to address the issues related to community mobility and the needs of older drivers. AOTA also collaborates with AARP and the National Association of Home Builders around home modifications and aging in place for older adults. Similarly, AOTA frequently works with coalitions of advocacy and professional groups such as the Consortium for Citizens with Disabilities (CCD) and the Mental Health Liaison Group on critical public policy issues (F. Sommers, personal communication, February 28, 2007).

CONCLUSION

It is clear that the profession of occupational therapy involves many different areas of practice and opportunity. As occupational therapists, occupational therapy assistants, and occupational therapy students, we are supported by AOTA and the other organizations that provide the resources and information that we need in order to practice. As professionals, we also have the opportunity and responsibility to support and participate in our professional organizations so that we can work toward continually developing, shaping, and promoting our chosen profession.

REFERENCES

American Occupational Therapy Association. (2005). Standards of practice for occupational therapy. *American Journal of Occupational Therapy, 59,* 663–665.

American Occupational Therapy Association. (2007a). *Special interest sections.* Retrieved January 21, 2007, from www.aota.org/members/area3/index.asp

American Occupational Therapy Association. (2007b). Retrieved July 25, 2007 http://www.aota.org/Govern/RefDocs.aspx

American Occupational Therapy Association. (2007c). *Accreditation.* Retrieved from http://www.aota.org/nonmembers/area13/links/LINK13.asp

American Occupational Therapy Association. (2007d). *Publications.* Retrieved January 21, 2007, from www.aota.org/non-members/area7/index.asp

American Occupational Therapy Foundation. (2007). *Scholarships.* Retrieved February 15, 2007, from http://www.aotf.org/#

National Board for Certification of Occupational Therapy. (2007). *About us.* Retrieved February 12, 2007, from http://www.nbcot.org/webarticles/anmviewer.asp?a=45&z=12

World Federation of Occupational Therapy. (2007). *History.* Retrieved February 28, 2007, from http://www.wfot.org.au/linkresource/asp

ADDITIONAL RESOURCES

To learn more about the profession of occupational therapy and the organizations that support it, check out the following Websites:

American Occupational Therapy Association: www.aota.org
American Occupational Therapy Foundation: www.aotf.org
National Board for Certification of Occupational Therapy: www.nbcot.org
World Federation of Occupational Therapy: www.wfot.org (Note: There are links or contact information to professional organizations in countries throughout the world at this site.)

Each of these Websites contains numerous links that will aid in your exploration of the profession.

Occupational Therapy Practitioners: Competence and Professional Development

PENELOPE MOYERS

Learning Objectives

After reading this chapter, you will be able to:

1. Understand the entry-level competencies for both occupational therapists and occupational therapy assistants.
2. Appreciate the multiple variables influencing the complexity of continuing competence and competency.
3. Differentiate among the terms continuing competence and competency, being competent, and professional development.
4. Understand and apply the Triangular Model of Continuing Competency and Competence.
5. Determine the importance of licensure and credentialing as an aspect of competence while accepting one's own responsibility for this process.
6. Be able to develop a learning plan and select the best learning activities for plan implementation.
7. Become aware of the evidence supporting continuing competency and competence.
8. Consider whether advanced and specialty certifications would be important for your practice.

Society expects practitioners to render services that reflect the standards of their profession. Changing practice settings, changes in health care technology, and new evidence all demand that practitioners must frequently develop new knowledge and skills. Practitioners are expected to take responsibility for their ongoing professional development and to carefully assess the degree to which their knowledge and skills are adequate to meet the demands of their current or anticipated practice environments. This chapter discusses aspects of that professional responsibility, primarily from the perspective of practice in the United States. The general concepts are likely to be of use internationally and include discussions of entry-level competency and the difference between competence and continuing competency. Subsequent sections of the chapter discuss the various factors associated with developing and maintaining both continuing competence and competency, ending with a discussion of advanced certification and specialty certification.

ENTRY-LEVEL COMPETENCIES

The occupational therapist and the occupational therapy assistant have different entering-level **competencies** when each begins practice. The occupational therapist receives a post-baccalaureate degree, which may either be a master's or entry-level doctorate degree; and the occupational therapy assistant receives an associate's degree. While there are differences in the depth of learning, both practitioners receive education in the liberal arts; take prerequisites in the biological, physical, social and behavioral sciences; and learn about the basic tenets of occupational therapy (Accreditation Council for Occupational Therapy Education [ACOTE®], 2007). The occupational therapist comprehends and knows how to apply the various theoretical perspectives of occupational therapy and understands the evaluation process, which emphasizes the interpretation of assessments in terms of the underlying factors contributing to problems of occupational performance as well as how the environment provides barriers to and supports for participation in daily life. The occupational therapy assistant helps with the screening and assessment process through data collection.

The occupational therapist uses the interpretation of the assessment data to formulate an intervention plan—in collaboration with the client and the occupational therapy assistant—designed to improve occupational performance and daily life participation. Both practitioners may implement the intervention plan, but the occupational therapist is ultimately responsible for the entire occupational therapy process. The occupational therapist is trained in service management within various types of service delivery models. The occupational therapy assistant supports the occupational therapist in service management and understands the influence of these service delivery

models, such as educational, medical, or community. Both practitioners read the professional literature, but the occupational therapist is able to determine how to use and apply research within practice. There is an emphasis in the education of both practitioners on advocacy, lifelong learning, professional ethics, values, and responsibilities. (See Table 25.1 for the comparison and contrast of the roles between the occupational therapist and occupational therapy assistant.)

LEARNING AND IMPROVED PRACTICE PERFORMANCE

Occupational therapy practice changes rapidly in response to up-to-date information, new knowledge, and modern technologies. Consequently, consumers and clients, employers, accreditation agencies, licensure boards, and other stakeholders expect occupational therapists and occupational therapy assistants to work actively to maintain their **continuing competency** and **competence** within specific areas of practice and within specific service delivery contexts. However, occupational therapy practitioners are challenged to assure their continuing competency and competence for many reasons:

◆ The skills and abilities of all practitioners fade with lack of practice, feedback, or administrative/system support
◆ The explosion of knowledge makes it difficult to maintain and focus learning
◆ Significant sophistication is required to translate these knowledge discoveries into practice, particularly given that knowledge must attend to the need for client-centered care within a confluence of cultures.
◆ Added to this is the pressure from complex health care and social systems that prevent change in practice (Moyers, 2005).

Additionally, there is not a linear relationship between learning and improved practice performance. Instead, there may be periods of time when there is either no improvement or even a slight decrease in performance. The dynamic interaction among the client, the practitioner, the nature of the occupation-based therapeutic intervention, and the context in which therapy is occurring influences the way in which new knowledge and skills may be applied to the practice situation. Each client situation is different; thus practitioner performance is highly context dependent. The practitioner may have better outcomes in one situation compared to another similar situation (Handfield-Jones, et al., 2002). Applying new learning to practice typically requires cognitive reorganization involving abandonment of previously held ideas and principles or incorporating this learning to restructure previously held ways of thinking. Consequently, there are periods of little change followed by sudden jumps in practice performance rather than learning demonstrated as continuous and gradual change

TABLE 25.1   DIFFERENCES IN OCCUPATIONAL THERAPISTS AND OCCUPATIONAL THERAPY ASSISTANT STANDARDS OF PRACTICE

Standards of Practice for Occupational Therapy (AOTA, 2005c)

Occupational Therapy Process	Occupational Therapist	Occupational Therapy Assistant
Screening, Evaluation, and Re-evaluation		
1. Accepts and responds to referrals in compliance with state laws or other regulatory requirements.	X	
2. In collaboration with the client, evaluates the client's ability to participate in daily life activities by considering the client's capacities, the activities, and the environments in which these activities occur.	X	
3. Initiates and directs the screening, evaluation, and re-evaluation process and analyzes and interprets the data in accordance with law, regulatory requirements, and AOTA documents.	X	Contributes
4. Follows defined protocols when standardized assessments are used.	X	X
5. Completes and documents occupational therapy evaluation results.	X	Contributes
6. Communicates screening, evaluation, and re-evaluation results within the boundaries of client confidentiality to the appropriate person, group, or organization.	X	X
7. Recommends additional consultations or refers clients to appropriate resources when the needs of the client can best be served by the expertise of other professionals or services.	X	
8. Educates current and potential referral sources about the scope of occupational therapy services and the process of initiating occupational therapy services.	X	X
Intervention		
1. Has overall responsibility for the development, documentation, and implementation of the occupational therapy intervention based on the evaluation, client goals, current best evidence, and clinical reasoning.	X	
2. Ensures that the intervention plan is documented within the time frames, formats, and standards established by the practice settings, agencies, external accreditation programs, and payers.	X	
3. Selects, implements, and makes modifications to therapeutic activities and interventions that are consistent with the occupational therapy assistant's demonstrated competency and delegated responsibilities, the intervention plan, and requirements of the practice setting.	X	X
4. Reviews the intervention plan with the client and appropriate others regarding the rationale, safety issues, and relative benefits and risks of the planned interventions.	X	X
5. Modifies the intervention plan throughout the intervention process and documents the changes in the client's needs, goals, and performance.	X	Contributes
6. Documents the occupational therapy services provided within the time frames, formats, and standards established by the practice settings, agencies, external accreditation programs, payers, and AOTA documents.	X	X

TABLE 25.1   DIFFERENCES IN OCCUPATIONAL THERAPISTS AND OCCUPATIONAL THERAPY ASSISTANT STANDARDS OF PRACTICE   *Continued*

Standards of Practice for Occupational Therapy (AOTA, 2005c)

Occupational Therapy Process	Occupational Therapist	Occupational Therapy Assistant
Outcomes		
1. Responsible for selecting, measuring, documenting, and interpreting expected or achieved outcomes that are related to the client's ability to engage in occupations.	X	
2. Responsible for documenting changes in the client's performance and capacities and for discontinuing services when the client has achieved identified goals, reached maximum benefit, or does not desire to continue services.	X	Contributes
3. Prepares and implements a discontinuation plan or transition plan based on the client's needs, goals, performance, and appropriate follow-up resources.	X	Contributes
4. Facilitates that transition process in collaboration with the client, family members, significant others, team, and community resources and individuals, when appropriate.	X	X
5. Responsible for evaluating the safety and effectiveness of the occupational therapy processes and interventions within the practice setting.	X	Contributes

(Handfield-Jones, et al., 2002). There seem to be periods where practice performance improves in some areas, while simultaneously deteriorating in others.

To facilitate understanding of the complex issues of remaining updated, this chapter examines the Triangular Model of Competency and Continuing Competence (Figure 25.1). The goal is to become familiar with AOTA *Standards for Continuing Competence* (2005) and the way in which they serve as indicators of achieving the competencies associated with one's professional responsibilities. The *AOTA Professional Development Tool* (PDT) (AOTA, May, 2003) is described as a guideline for constructing a reflective portfolio useful in documenting one's efforts toward continuing competence. The National Board for Certification in Occupational Therapy (NBCOT) processes for initial certification and certification renewal are briefly explained along with AOTA's board and specialty certification programs, which use self-assessment and self-appraisal approaches. The importance of state licensure is highlighted.

WHAT DOES IT MEAN TO BE COMPETENT?

There is an important difference between the terms *continuing competence* and *continuing competency;* however, the word *continuing,* in front of each term, indicates the significant focus on lifelong learning. **Continuing com-** **petence** "refers to an individual's capacity to perform job [professional] responsibilities" (McConnell, 2001, p. 14). For instance, Maria, who is an occupational therapist, is working with persons with schizophrenia within an inpatient setting, and she plans to develop a club house model program for her clients who return to the community. She needs to focus her learning on the theoretical aspects of the club house model, evidence of the approach's effectiveness, and the business models for its implementation. This building capacity involving the preparation for significant change in practice is continuing competence.

"**Continuing competency** focuses on an individual's actual performance in a particular situation" (McConnell, 2001, p. 14). *Competency* implies a determination of whether one is competent to perform a behavior or task as measured against a specific criterion (Hinojosa, et al., 2000a). Tiffany, an occupational therapy assistant, has just taken a position at the local hospital. Before she can begin seeing clients with occupational performance problems related to the upper extremity, she must demonstrate her skills or competency to the supervising occupational therapist in using standardized hand therapy assessments, splinting, and implementing interventions according to evidence-based and occupation-based protocols developed for each type of diagnosis or surgical intervention.

Being **competent** involves the ability to select the best assessment tools, intervention approaches, and outcome measures according to the evidence indicating effectiveness and efficacy as well as to skillfully provide the appro-

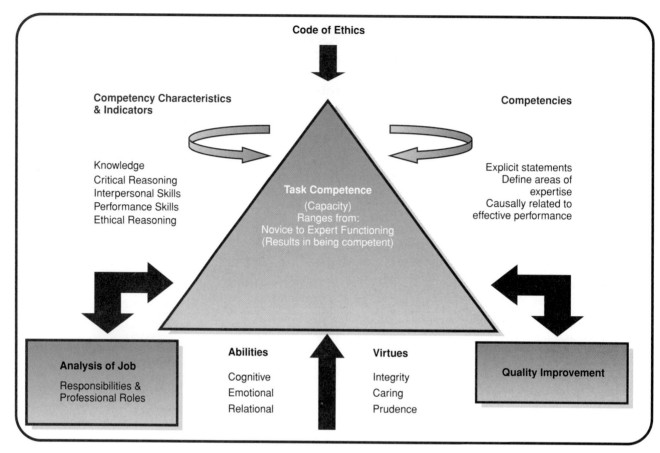

FIGURE 25.1 Triangular Model of Continuing Competency & Competence.

priate services to meet the needs of the client (Moyers, 1999). Competent occupational therapy practitioners have the prerequisite knowledge, skills, and attitudes that authorize them to perform restricted, skilled activities resulting in defined client outcomes. Only someone licensed or regulated in a given profession or technical trade may perform a restricted activity, or those processes and procedures ascribed to particular professions or job classifications where specific education and training is required (Moyers & Hinojosa, 2003).

The next important distinction in terms is contrasting *professional development* with *continuing competence* and *continuing competency*. **Professional development** is a career development process and focuses on what the occupational therapy practitioner wants to learn in order to achieve future career aspirations, such as becoming an expert clinician, administrator, educator, researcher, consultant, or private practitioner. The focus of professional development is on determining the future roles you would like to develop and the kinds of tasks and knowledge that are included in these roles. With an understanding of the possible tasks within these future roles, you can begin to determine the skills and reasoning needing further development as well as the criteria used for measuring successful performance.

FACTORS AFFECTING CONTINUING COMPETENCY AND COMPETENCE

Ultimately, the interest in competence is because there are risks associated with poor intervention. When interventions are provided incompetently, they may harm the client, the results of which may in turn raise a further risk of a legal liability for malpractice. Providers, payers, business and industry, social service agencies, and service recipients expect effective intervention leading to desired outcomes. Although there are many factors contributing to unsatisfactory outcomes, practitioners who have not consistently updated their knowledge and skills could be a source of practice errors. The triangular model of continuing competency and competence explains the elements contributing to one's success in remaining proficient (Moyers, 2005). (see Figure 25.1)

The Case Study about José helps in understanding why job task competence is situated at the center of the Triangular Model for Continuing Competency and Competence (Figure 25.1). Occupational therapy practitioners may perform a variety of duties including those of a practitioner, fieldwork supervisor, manager or administrator, consultant, entrepreneur, advocate, educator, researcher,

CASE STUDY: *José: A Therapist Improving Competence and Competencies*

José is an occupational therapist with three years of experience working with clients with brain injury providing both inpatient rehabilitation and outpatient community re-entry programs. His past performance evaluations from his supervisor indicate José enjoys learning, relates well with others, and exudes a calming and rational influence on staff and clients alike. These are all important abilities underlying continuing competence and competency. He displays the necessary virtues in that he genuinely cares for his clients, has the integrity to focus learning on areas of weakness, and the prudence to select learning methods that will help him apply learning to practice. According to the analysis of his responsibilities, the competencies primarily related to his job involve evidence-based evaluation, intervention planning and implementation, discharge planning, community re-entry program implementation, and outcome measurement, all with a focus on occupational performance in daily life participation.

Although no longer being a novice in performing these competencies, his client outcomes indicate that there is a group of clients with high no-show rates in the community re-entry program. When surveying this group of clients, they indicate feelings of depression and unresolved problems with vision. The caregivers of these clients describe their behavior as being difficult to manage because the clients are often argumentative and angry, and often refuse to perform many daily living tasks in which they had previously engaged prior to their head injuries. José schedules a meeting with his supervisor to develop some learning goals related to training caregivers in behavior management, and evaluation and intervention for depression and visual problems. His supervisor agrees that this learning plan will improve his competency, but also wants to bring to the attention of José that the hospital will be putting in place a new documentation and outcome measurement system, with a phase-in process over the next two years. José agrees to add this continuing competence issue into his learning plan.

In order to more fully develop his learning plan, José realizes that he needs to decide how to break-down his learning goals so that he will select the best learning methods that will help him apply the learning to his practice so that

his client no-show rate in the community re-entry program will decline. He decides that he knows a lot about behavior management (competency characteristic), but needs to learn the best way to teach this knowledge (performance skill) to the caregivers so that they will be able to implement these strategies to better support their clients' daily performance. He is worried about how to give feedback in a way that is constructive and does not ruin rapport (interpersonal skill) when working with the caregivers in their practice of these new behavior management skills. Thus, he has identified some potential mismatches between his current competency and knowledge and those needed in the future. He also realizes that he received only basic information (competency characteristic) in his entry-level program about the vision issues of persons with head injuries and that he needs to begin improving his knowledge and critical reasoning through some continuing education courses, reading the research literature, and studying some case studies. As his knowledge and critical reasoning improves, he decides to contact a local occupational therapist with expertise in the vision issues of persons with head injuries to mentor him in his critical and ethical reasoning, and to perhaps provide some observational opportunities and supervised practice experiences (performance skills).

His supervisor provided some of the resources for learning in terms of paying for one continuing education course in low vision and providing the training in the new documentation and outcome measurement systems; however, José knew it was his ethical responsibility to search out and implement other learning opportunities beyond what his employer was willing to provide. His employer, however, was prepared to purchase the recommended supplies or equipment to support application of his learning to practice as she knew José had carefully researched which equipment would most likely be economical as well as effective in evaluating and providing intervention for persons with vision problems affecting their occupational performance. José worked out with his supervisor a plan for program changes in the community re-entry program as well as how to incorporate the new documentation and measurement system.

scientist, or scholar. Regardless of the variety of professional roles held, the occupational therapist and occupational therapy assistant must successfully manage the multiple responsibilities inherent in the job. Job task competence ranges from being a novice to being an expert not only depending upon experience with the task, but depending on the various contextual factors dynamically interacting with the job task. New work tasks or projects or working within new contexts, even though the occupational therapy practitioner might have a lengthy tenure in

a particular job, result in the employee being considered a novice. Even though normally being an expert in a particular job task, a client from a culture different from any clients one has previously provided intervention, may create a task situation in which the expert is performing more at the novice end of the continuum because of the cultural complexities added to the situation.

According to Principle 4 of the *Occupational Therapy Code of Ethics* (AOTA, 2005b), it is the duty of the occupational therapy practitioner to achieve and continually maintain high standards of competence. Therefore, when encountering work tasks, projects, or contexts in which one is a novice, the occupational therapy practitioner must engage in a self-initiated approach to develop and implement an individualized plan for learning (Hinojosa, et al., 2000b). A learning plan is based on an analysis of the job and quality improvement data to determine the explicit statements or competencies that are causally related to effective job performance or client outcomes.

Competencies typically address those that are generic across all jobs in an organization (e.g., a customer service orientation), those that are related to management or supervision roles (e.g., budgeting or personnel management), those that are threshold or that are the minimum requirements of a job (e.g., being able to evaluate a client), and those that are specific to a job (e.g., being able to conduct a feeding and swallowing evaluation) (Decker & Strader, 1997).

Once competencies and outcomes are determined, the next step is to delineate the indicators fundamental to these competencies (Decker & Strader, 1997). The triangular model of competency and continuing competence uses the *Standards for Continuing Competence* (AOTA, 2005a) as indicators. These include knowledge, critical and ethical reasoning, and performance and interpersonal skills. For example, the competency of client evaluation requires selecting the most appropriate assessment instruments given the client's condition, selecting goals and preferences for specific outcomes, and requiring the adept administration of the tools to yield accurate and reliable data. This competency requires knowledge of a variety of assessment instruments, the critical and ethical reasoning skills to determine which would be the best test given the nature of the instrument and the client circumstances, and the interpersonal and performance skills to conduct the assessment properly while developing empathy with the client. Competency characteristics are intrinsic to the occupational practitioner and include such aspects as expert knowledge and skills, motivation to change performance, positive self-concept that one can become proficient, and attitudes conducive for and a value of learning. If there is a mismatch between the competency statement and the competency characteristics, such as being unaware of available assessment instruments, the occupational therapist in this instance must devise a plan to improve the knowledge needed for achievement of the competency.

Remaining competent and pursuing competence depends upon the occupational therapy practitioner's cognitive, emotional and relational abilities. In order to learn, the occupational therapy practitioner must use the requisite cognitive and intellectual abilities to understand and synthesize complex information. The occupational therapy practitioner must demonstrate a well-adjusted personality, which involves the emotional abilities of open-mindedness, flexibility, and self-monitoring or self-regulation. In addition, the occupational therapy practitioner must have the relational abilities to successfully establish rapport with and advocate for clients and their families or relevant others.

There are also specific virtues related to competence where the occupational therapy practitioner is called upon to aspire toward ideals and to develop virtues of character enabling achievement of those ideals. Integrity involves honesty and sincerity, caring involves the understanding of the altruistic responsibility associated with client service provision, and prudence involves the ability to govern and discipline oneself through the use of reason (AOTA, 1993). These virtues help motivate the occupational therapy practitioner to learn because of the desire to perform better on behalf of the client (caring). Prudence facilitates the disciplined implementation of the learning plan developed in an honest way in terms of making a sincere attempt to achieve job competence as opposed to implementing a plan that focuses on what is easiest or most convenient to learn.

WHO DETERMINES WHETHER SOMEONE IS COMPETENT?

Credentialing, such as state licensure, is an indicator to the public that the health care practitioner has some level of competence to provide skilled services within a specified scope of practice; however, the public is increasingly aware that licensure reflects the minimal standards of competence necessary to protect the public (Grossman, 1997). State licensure boards are primarily responsible for entry into practice by requiring occupational therapy practitioners to pass the examination administered by the National Board for Certification in Occupational Therapy (NBCOT) after completing an accredited educational program in occupational therapy and the required fieldwork. Background checks and fingerprinting may be required as well.

Renewal of the license to practice in a jurisdiction occurs when the practitioner pays a fee. Renewal of the license may also be dependent upon evidence of continuing education, adherence to ethical standards, and evidence of knowledge about the laws and regulations governing occupational therapy practice (jurisprudence tests). The occupational therapy practitioner also has to attest prior to renewal that he or she has never been sued or had an award for malpractice or negligence made against him or her, and never had the license or practice privileges revoked or suspended. If answers to these questions are positive, the licensure board launches an investigation to determine whether the license to practice should be renewed.

While state licensure focuses upon restricting entry to practice in a given jurisdiction to those who are appropriately qualified and who regularly maintain their license, NBCOT, a private credentialing body, awards the ability of occupational therapists to use the initials OTR® and the occupational therapy assistant to use the initials COTA®. Ability to use the credentials depends upon the initial successful completion of the entry examination and then upon regularly renewing the certification. This certification renewal program is voluntary, is not required by most state regulatory boards, and is not required to receive Medicare or Medicaid reimbursement for the delivery of occupational therapy services. Some employers may require renewal with NBCOT. Renewal of the NBCOT certification involves the collection and documentation of professional development units (PDUs), (some of which must have direct bearing on occupational therapy), through engagement in a variety of learning activities (NBCOT, 2006).

Licensure boards and certification granting organizations tend to use the most common approach in determining competence, which is through testing, credentialing and requiring the appropriate continuing education. However, quality of care is an example of a construct that cannot be directly observed nor measured in all aspects. Certification tests used by many certification programs cannot evaluate how well the applicant actually performs in a given practice situation.

Therefore, understanding the emerging concept of context specificity creates debate regarding the way competence is currently defined and measured. Context specificity indicates that "an individual's performance on a particular problem or in a particular situation is only weakly predictive of the same individual's performance on a different problem or in a different situation" (Eva, 2003, p. 587). According to this definition, competence is best determined by observing the occupational therapy practitioner complete the key competencies important to successful job performance and client outcomes. Due to the expense and impracticality of performance-based testing, the methodology and resources are not feasible at this time for use by licensure boards and other credentialing bodies. Instead, employers may be in the best position to actually determine competency, which has been a recent focus of such organizational accreditation programs as the Joint Commission on the Accreditation of Healthcare Organi-

zations (JCAHO). According to these standards, health care organizations have to prove, track, and improve the competence of employees (Herringer, 2002). The renewal programs of licensure boards and other credentialing bodies are really focusing on pursuit of continuing competence and capacity to perform in the certification area.

WHO IS RESPONSIBLE FOR ENSURING WHETHER SOMEONE IS COMPETENT?

Regardless of legal requirements associated with licensure for maintaining competence and the importance of competence to employers, it is the professional duty of the practitioner, according to the AOTA Code of Ethics (2005b), to assess, maintain, and document his or her own competence. Given that competence is the primary responsibility of the professional, Hinojosa et al. (2000b) outlined AOTA's Continuing Competence Plan for Professional Development as involving nine components, each of which is described in Box 25.1.

Development and implementation of the continuing competence plan can be guided through the use of AOTA's Professional Development Tool (AOTA, May, 2003) which is a framework for building a portfolio that can be used with licensure boards, employers, NBCOT, and AOTA advanced and specialty certifications.

As AOTA's plan for continuing competence suggests, the professional should judge his or her competence according to the current job responsibilities. Does the practitioner have the required knowledge, critical and ethical reasoning ability, and interpersonal and performance skills necessary to perform successfully and to facilitate client achievement of specified outcomes? There is need to maintain skills required for implementing the core of occupational therapy, to develop a specialized knowledge

---

BOX 25.1 — COMPONENTS OF CONTINUING COMPETENCE PLAN

1. Recognition of triggers that signal the need to examine competence
2. Examination of one's practice responsibilities
3. Self-assessment of one's competence status for a given responsibility
4. Identification of competence-related educational needs in light of the *Standards for Continuing Competence* (AOTA, 2005a)
5. Development of a competence improvement plan
6. Implementation of the competence plan
7. Documentation of professional development and change in competence
8. Implementation of changes in practice based on new competence, and
9. Demonstration of continuing competence

Adapted from Hinojosa et al (2000b, p. CE-1). Used courtesy of AOTA.

and skill base, and to obtain advanced abilities. For instance, although the core of occupational therapy does not change, the technology related to promoting a client's adaptation or to analyzing an occupation and its associated activities may change.

HOW DO YOU KNOW HOW TO SELECT THE MOST EFFECTIVE LEARNING ACTIVITIES?

In order to develop an effective learning plan, you need to be aware of the best methods for learning performance and interpersonal skills, gaining knowledge, and developing critical and ethical reasoning related to your job competencies. For example, reading may lead to increased knowledge, but role-playing and simulation strategies may be more effective in enhancing interpersonal abilities. The critical issue in selecting learning methods is to use cognitive processes similar to the creative thinking typical of the intricacy of today's practice environment (Fraser, & Greenhalgh, 2001). Therefore, learning approaches should help the practitioner "appraise the situation as a whole, prioritize issues, and then integrate and make sense of many different sources of data to arrive at a solution" (p. 801). These creative learning approaches often involve story telling, case histories, reflection, and problem-based learning strategies. There is an emphasis on self-directed learning where content in the subject matter varies depending on the needs of the learner and there is a use of a variety of learning approaches including experiential learning, networking, list serves for professional interest groups, opportunities to teach others, and time for feedback on the application of the learning (Fraser & Greenhalgh, 2001, p. 802).

COMMENTARY ON THE EVIDENCE

Do Continuing Education and Audits Improve Professional Practice?

O'Brien, et al. (2001) completed a systematic evidence review of randomized trials and quasi-experimental studies to examine the effect of continuing education meetings (including lectures, workshops, and courses) on the clinical practice of health professionals or health care outcomes. Included were thirty-two studies involving from 13 to 411 health professionals (total N = 2995). Within these studies, there was substantial variation in the targeted behaviors, methods for measuring baseline performance, the characteristics of the learning interventions, and the results. The types of planned educational activities studied included meetings, conferences, lectures, workshops, seminars, symposia, and courses that occurred off-site from the practice setting. These educational activities were classified into the general learning methods of interactive workshops, combined workshops and didactic presentations, and those with only didactic presentations. The authors concluded from their analysis that interactive workshops resulted in moderately large changes in professional practice, while didactic sessions alone were unlikely to change professional practice.

Jamtvedt, Young, Kristoffersen, O'Brien, and Oxman (2006) conducted another systematic review of randomized trials to assess the effects of audit and feedback on the practice of health care professionals and patient outcomes.

Audit and feedback was defined as any summary of clinical performance over a specified period of time that reported objectively measured professional practice outcomes. They investigated the variation in the effectiveness of interventions across: the type of intervention (audit and feedback alone, audit and feedback with educational meetings, or multifaceted interventions that included audit and feedback), the intensity of the audit and feedback, the complexity of the targeted behavior, the seriousness of the outcome, baseline compliance and study quality. Based upon the 118 studies reviewed, the authors concluded that providing health care professionals with data about their performance (audit and feedback) may help improve their practice; however, the effects were variable and, when effective, produced a small to moderate impact on client outcomes.

These two systematic reviews are important in that it is clear that the learning methods chosen may have differential ability to positively impact client outcomes. Learners must therefore be clear whether they are trying to gain knowledge, improvements in critical and ethical reasoning, or enhanced performance and interpersonal skills. Didactic or lecture style presentations may augment knowledge, but may not lead to application of this knowledge to practice in comparison to more active learning methods and use of feedback on performance.

WHAT DOES ADVANCED AND SPECIALTY CERTIFICATION MEAN?

Specialization refers to becoming proficient in a particular practice area, diagnostic category, or intervention approach. However, specialization is often confused with advanced practice. The public typically views the advanced practitioner as an independent practitioner who possesses a high degree of skill because of more complicated responsibilities. Madill and Hollis (2003) described the key competency characteristics of the advanced health care practitioner as possessing a breadth and depth of knowledge with concerted efforts to continuously add new knowledge, an appreciation of the wider environmental context, the ability to use critical thinking and analysis, extensive contribution to one or more areas of practice, commitment to quality, motivation to continually develop new skills, and advanced qualifications (p. 32). One may be at the entry-level of a specialized area or may be at the advanced level of a specialized area. Whether specialized or advanced, competence includes the practitioner's abilities to implement the core of occupational therapy practice, as well as abilities to work within specialized practice areas, ranging from the entry to the advanced levels, depending on the requirements of the job (Youngstrom, 1998, p. 719).

The AOTA board (mental health, pediatrics, gerontology, and physical rehabilitation) and specialty certifications (low vision; feeding, eating, and swallowing; environmental modification; and driving and community mobility) are examples of ways to stimulate an occupational therapy practitioner's continuing competence, which involves the development of capacity and competency characteristics needed for the future. There are specialty certifications offered through other organizations, such as the Certified Hand Therapist credential from the Hand Therapy Certification Commission (www.htcc.org). See Table 25.2 for examples of advanced and specialty certifications.

TABLE 25.2   ENTRY LEVEL AND POST-ENTRY LEVEL CERTIFICATIONS IN THE UNITED STATES

Credentials		Granting Organization
Entry-Level Credentialing & Certification Renewal		
ACOTE Accredited	Refers to the status of an occupational therapy education program that is fully accredited	ACOTE
OTR	Occupational therapist, registered (professional level)	NBCOT
COTA	Certified occupational therapy assistant (technical level)	NBCOT
Advanced Practice Certifications		
BCG	Board Certification in Gerontology	AOTA-BASC
BCMH	Board Certification in Mental Health	AOTA-BASC
BCP	Board Certification in Pediatrics	AOTA-BASC
BCPR	Board Certification in Physical Rehabilitation	AOTA-BASC
Specialty Certifications		
ATP	Assistive Technology Practitioner	RESNA
CCM	Certified Case Managers	CCMC
CDRS	Certified Driving Rehabilitation Practitioner	ADED
CHT	Certified Hand Therapist	HTCC
CLVT	Certification in Low Vision Therapy	ACVREP
CPE	Certified Professional Ergonomist	BCPE
CVE	Certified Vocational Evaluation Specialist	CCWAVES
SCDCM	Specialty Certification in Driving & Community Mobility	AOTA-BASC
SCEM	Specialty Certification in Environmental Modification	AOTA-BASC
SCFES	Specialty Certification in Feeding, Eating, & Swallowing	AOTA-BASC
SCLV	Specialty Certification in Low Vision	AOTA-BASC

ACOTE, Accreditation Council for Occupational Therapy Education; AOTA-BASCP, American Occupational Therapy Association: Board and Specialty Certification programs; ACVREP, Academy for Certification of Vision Rehabilitation and Education Professionals; ADED, Association for Driving Rehabilitation Specialists; BCPE, Board of Certification in Professional Ergonomics; CCMC, Commission for Case Management Certification; CCWAVES, Commission on Certification of Work Adjustment and Vocational Evaluation Specialists; HTCC, Hand Therapy Certification Commission; RESNA, Rehabilitation Engineering & Assistive Technology Society of North America

These AOTA certifications require the applicant to develop a reflective **portfolio**. These are growing in popularity as "[professional development] tools that aggregate assessment information across time" (Melnick, 2004, p. s44). A reflective portfolio archives for each competency carefully appraised learning activities, the appropriate evidence of this learning, reflections on this learning, and for board only, a **self-assessment** or identification of needs for and a plan for new learning. **Self-appraisal** of learning activities answers the question: What evidence would best indicate I have acquired the competencies needed for specialized or advanced practice? In other words, the portfolio is not a collection or scrapbook of everything one has done, but requires careful selection of learning activities thought most likely to contribute to one's capacity for achieving the competency in a given context.

Self-appraisal thus begins with examining the competency statement and the client outcomes in order to make decisions about how best to learn. A wide variety of learning activities may be used to achieve each competency. Multiple methods of learning are encouraged and rewarded as the learner determines how best to enable the following results (Miller, 1990):

◆ *Knowing and knowing why:* Learning methods that increase the knowledge needed to have a significant impact on improved client outcomes.

◆ *Knowing how, when, and with whom:* Learning methods that are focused on the learner developing and using critical and ethical reasoning, in other words, knowing not only the steps, but when and with whom to use the procedures.

◆ *Showing how:* Learning methods that facilitate skill development so that one can actually perform the steps and procedures in various contexts.

◆ *Doing:* Learning methods that facilitate application of knowledge, critical and ethical reasoning and interpersonal and performance skills to practice in a consistent manner. This application results in a change in client outcomes.

CONCLUSION

Continuing competence and competency and professional development are the responsibility of the practitioner, educator, administrator, and researcher. The public, our clients, our colleagues, and our employers expect that competent occupational therapists and occupational therapy assistants are providing high quality services. Learning must be managed systematically through careful self-assessment of one's client outcomes, job responsibilities, and future trends in service delivery. Self-assessment helps the practitioner devise a learning plan complete with learning activities most likely to lead to a change in practice. The plan must be properly implemented with the help from administration to apply and evaluate the consequence of the new learning in practice.

PROVOCATIVE QUESTIONS

1. How does one avoid engaging only in learning activities one finds interesting rather than what one needs to know to practice more effectively?
2. What are some ways to ensure new learning is applied to practice?
3. How will you know if your new learning application to practice is effective?

REFERENCES

Accreditation Council for Occupational Therapy Education [ACOTE®], (2007), Accreditation Council for Occupational Therapy Education (ACOTE®) Standards and Interpretative Guidelines. Retrieved June 2, 2007, from http://www.aota.org/nonmembers/area13/docs/acotestandards107.pdf

American Occupational Therapy Association. (2003, May). Professional development tool. Bethesda, MD: Author. Retrieved August 1, 2007, from http://www.aota.org/pdt

AOTA. (1993). Core values and attitudes of occupational therapy practice. *American Journal of Occupational Therapy, 54,* 614–616.

AOTA. (2005a). Standards for continuing competence. *American Journal of Occupational Therapy, 59,* 661–662.

AOTA (2005b). Occupational therapy code of ethics (2005) (revised Ethics document). *American Journal of Occupational Therapy, 59,* 639–642.

AOTA. (2005c). Standards of practice for occupational therapy (revised). *American Journal of Occupational Therapy, 59,* 663–665.

Decker, P. J., & Strader, M. K. (1997). Beyond JCAHO: Using competency models to improve healthcare organizations, Part 1. *Hospital Topics, 75,* 1–23.

Eva, K. W. (2003). On the generality of specificity. *Medical Education, 37,* 587–588.

Fraser, S. W., & Greenhalgh, T. (2001). Complexity science. Coping with complexity: Education for capability. *British Medical Journal, 323*(6), 799–803.

Grossman, J. (1997). *A study of the professions.* White Plains, NY: MAGI Educational Services.

Handfield-Jones, R. S., Mann, K. V., Challis, M. E., Hobma, S. O., Klass, D. F., McManus, I. C., Paget, N. S., Parboosingh, I. F., Wade, W. B., & Wikinson, T. F. (2002). Linking assessment to learning: A new route to quality assurance in medical practice. *Medical Education, 36,* 949–958.

Herringer, J. M. (2002). Once isn't enough when measuring staff competence. *Nursing Management, 33*(2), 22.

Hinojosa, J., Bowen, R., Case-Smith, J., Epstein, C. F., Moyers, P., & Schwope, C. (2000a). Standards for continuing competence for occupational therapy practitioners. *OT Practice, 5*(20), CE-1–CE-8.

Hinojosa, J., Bowen, R., Case-Smith, J., Epstein, C. F., Moyers, Pl, & Schwope, C. (2000b). Self-initiated continuing competence. *OT Practice, 5*(24): CE1–CE8.

Jamtvedt, G., Young, J. M., Kristoffersen, D. T., O'Brien, M. A., & Oxman, A. D. (2006). Audit and feedback: Effects on professional practice and health care outcomes. *Cochrane Database of Systematic Reviews* 2006, Issue 2. Art. No.: CD000259. DOI: 10.1002/14651858.CD000259.pub2.

Madill, H. M., & Hollis, V. (2003). Developing competencies for advanced practice: How do I get there from here? In G. Brown, S. A. Esdaile, & S. E. Ryan (Eds.). *Becoming an advanced healthcare practitioner,* New York: Butterworth Heinemann.

McConnell, E. A. (2001). Competence vs. competency. *Nursing Management, 32*(5), 14.

Melnick, D. E. (2004). Effect of physician performance and assessment on continuing medical education and continuing professional development. *Journal of Continuing Education of Health Professionals, 24*(suppl 1), s38–s49.

Miller, G. E. (1990). The assessment of clinical skills/competence/performance. *Academy of Medicine, 65*(9), s63–s67.

Moyers, P. A. (2005). The ethics of competence. In R. B. Purtilo, G. M. Jensen, & C. B. Royeen (Eds.), *Educating for moral action: A sourcebook in health and rehabilitation ethics.* Philadelphia, PA: F. A. Davis Company, 21–30.

Moyers, P. A., & Hinojosa, J. (2003). Continuing competency. In G. L. McCormack, E. G. Jaffe, & M. Goodman-Lavey (Eds.), *The occupational therapy manager (4th ed.).* Bethesda, MD: AOTA Press, 463–489.

NBCOT. (2006). Certification renewal handbook for the occupational therapist registered OTR® and the certified occupational therapy assistant COTA®. Gaithersburg, MD: NBCOT.

O'Brien, M. A., Freemantle, N., Oxman, A. D., Wolf, F., Davis, D. A., & Herrin, J. Continuing education meetings and workshops: effects on professional practice and health care outcomes. *Cochrane Database of Systematic Reviews* 2001, Issue 1. Art. No.: CD003030. DOI: 10.1002/14651858.CD003030.

Youngstrom, M. J. (1998). Evolving competence in the practitioner role. *American Journal of Occupational Therapy, 52,* 716–720.

Fieldwork: The Transition from Student to Professional

26

MARY E. EVENSON

Learning Objectives

After reading this chapter, you will be able to:

1. Comprehend how fieldwork is integral to the educational curriculum and one's own professional development.
2. Realize the requirements and levels of fieldwork education in U.S. and international academic occupational therapy programs.
3. Become familiar with traditional and innovative types of fieldwork settings and supervision models.
4. Grasp the dynamic nature of the personal and professional transitions that are inherent in the role shifts from that of being a student to assuming the role of a professional.
5. Appreciate the roles and responsibilities of those stakeholders who are involved in the fieldwork education process.
6. Gain an understanding of the process and types of competencies that are used to evaluate student fieldwork performance.

Fieldwork can be defined as "Work done or firsthand observations made in the field as opposed to that done or observed in a controlled environment" (Pickett, 2000). For occupational therapy education, fieldwork is most often referred to as work done outside of the classroom. The consensus within the occupational therapy profession is that the fieldwork experience plays an integral role in professional development. In 1923, the first standards requiring fieldwork experiences were approved by the American Occupational Therapy Association (AOTA) (Pressler, 1983). Fieldwork continues to function as the critical link between the academic world of theory and the world of practice, demonstrating the value the profession places on experience-based curricula (Cohn & Crist, 1995; Lewis, 2005).

Fieldwork experiences are intended to provide students with opportunities to carry out professional responsibilities under supervision of professionals who also act as role models (Accreditation Council for Occupational

Therapy Education, 2007). Working in the context of real-life practice, students develop a multitude of skills that enable them to establish the foundations of their future practice career. The two main categories of skill development that are inherent in participating in fieldwork are (1) the core skills and techniques that are relevant to occupational therapy service delivery for a given setting and (2) the personal skills that evolve and transform one's level of professional behavior (Missiuna, Polatajko & Ernest-Conibear, 1992). Fieldwork provides a venue for enculturation into the field as the interplay between the student as a person, the profession, and the environment support the development of a professional identity along with a set of basic professional competencies (Alsop & Donald, 1996). This component of education functions as the gateway into the profession because it enables students to establish the fundamental skills of the profession that will support them in transitioning from the practice context of fieldwork into employment. Furthermore, students in Canada and the United States, for example, must complete fieldwork requirements to become eligible to take the respective national certification examinations.

The process and content of fieldwork experiences have been debated over the years. Yet the value of having an opportunity to integrate academic knowledge with application skills at progressively higher levels of performance and responsibility has always been acknowledged (AOTA, 2003; Pressler, 1983). Christie, Joyce, and Moeller (1985) highlighted that value by documenting the fieldwork experience as having the greatest influence on the development of a therapist's preference for a specific area of clinical practice. Of the 131 therapists who were surveyed, 55% indicated that clinical practice preferences were either formed or changed during the fieldwork experience, and another 24% noted that fieldwork experience expanded their interests to other areas of practice. Similarly, Crowe and Mackenzie (2002) examined the influence of fieldwork on preferred future practice areas of occupational therapy students. This study also demonstrated that "students use the fieldwork experience to guide their decision to enter an area of practice" (Crowe & Mackenzie, 2002, p. 25). Thus, the fieldwork experience can be rich and rewarding, and as such, it is likely to have a tremendous bearing on a student's career choices.

PURPOSE AND LEVELS OF FIELDWORK: UNITED STATES

The purpose of fieldwork education is to provide students with opportunities to apply the knowledge, skills, and attitudes that they learn in the classroom into their practice in the fieldwork setting (Costa, 2004). The Accreditation Council for Occupational Therapy Education (ACOTE) Standards and Interpretative Guidelines (ACOTE, 2007)

outline the general fieldwork requirements for students. The requirements are divided into two classifications: Level I and Level II fieldwork. Level I fieldwork offers students practical experiences that are integrated throughout the academic program. The ACOTE standards describe **Level I fieldwork** as "experiences designed to enrich didactic course work through directed observation and participation in selected aspects of the occupational therapy process" (ACOTE, 2007). For both occupational therapy and occupational therapy assistant students, the goal of Level I fieldwork is to introduce students to the experience, "to apply knowledge to practice, and to develop understanding of the needs of clients" (ACOTE, 2007).

Level I Fieldwork Experience

Through Level I fieldwork experiences, students are exposed to the values and traditions of occupational therapy practice and have the opportunity to examine their reactions to clients, systems of service delivery, related personnel, and potential role(s) within the profession. Because the academic Level I performance expectations and specific purposes of the Level I fieldwork experience vary in each occupational therapy curriculum, the timing, length, requirements, and specific focus of the experience are determined by each academic program on an individual basis (AOTA, 1999a). For example, schedule options may include full or half days throughout an academic term, a one-week placement, or otherwise prearranged visits to fieldwork sites.

A study of contexts and perceptions of Level I fieldwork in current practice revealed that the number of placements in emerging practice is growing and that students generally rated their Level I fieldwork experiences as positive (Johnson, Koenig, Piersol, Santalucia, & Wachter-Schutz, 2006). In examining the types of learning opportunities that are afforded to Level I students, observation and communication skills were the most commonly practiced skills across all types of settings (Johnson et al., 2006). Practice of additional clinical skills during Level I fieldwork most frequently included fine and gross motor activities (94%) in pediatrics, range of motion (82%) in physical disabilities, interviewing (77%) in emerging practice settings, and behavioral management (73%) in mental health settings (Johnson et al., 1006, p. 281). Overall, students felt that their learning experience was maximized when they had an opportunity to practice skills and to experience occupation-based practice.

One model of fieldwork that can support students in practicing skills on Level I fieldwork and carrying them over into their Level II placements is the **Same Site Model of Fieldwork** (Evenson, Barnes, & Cohn, 2002). This unique approach provides continuity in structuring learning whereby a student completes a Level I and Level II fieldwork experience at the same training site. Exploratory investigation has shown that students and fieldwork educators identified the perceived benefits of this model to include becoming familiar with the setting, increasing comfort by lessening anxiety, and gaining preparation for Level II fieldwork.

Level II Fieldwork Experience

The goal of **Level II fieldwork** for the occupational therapy and occupational therapy assistant student is "to develop competent, entry-level generalist" practitioners (ACOTE, 2007). ACOTE (2007) Accreditation Standards state that "Level II fieldwork must be integral to the program's curriculum design and must include an in-depth experience in delivering occupational therapy services to clients, focusing on the application of purposeful and meaningful occupation." The goal of students participating in administration and management of occupational therapy services and research is differentiated for occupational therapy Level II fieldwork when applicable. Additional learning outcomes for occupational therapy Level II fieldwork are to "promote clinical reasoning and reflective practice; to transmit the values, beliefs, that enable ethical practice; and to develop professionalism and competence as career responsibilities" (ACOTE, 2007). For occupational therapy assistant students, the purpose of Level II fieldwork is to "promote clinical reasoning, appropriate to the occupational therapy assistant role" as well as to achieve professionalism and competence (ACOTE, 2007).

Initially working under direct supervision, students test firsthand the theories and facts that they learned in academic study and have a chance to refine skills through interaction with clients across the life course, with clients' families, and with team members while working in various service delivery settings and systems. As the students' abilities grow, supervision may become less direct as appropriate for the setting and the severity of the client's condition. A **developmental model of supervision** can be applied as an approach for planning, intervening, and evaluating the students' readiness for learning and participation throughout the trajectory of a fieldwork placement. Within a developmental framework, the learner and supervisor relationship progresses through four different phases: directive, coaching, supportive, and delegation (Barnes & Evenson, 2000). In all, supervision of students must meet existing local, state/provincial, and/or federal/national safety and health requirements for relevant policies, laws, and regulations for occupational therapy practice.

For students, the overall purpose of the fieldwork experience is to gain mastery of occupational therapy clinical reasoning and techniques to develop entry-level competence. Effective oral and written communication of ideas and objectives that are relevant to the roles and duties of an occupational therapist or occupational therapy assistant, including professional interaction with clients and staff, is expected of all students. Students are responsible for demonstrating a sensitivity to and respect for client con-

fidentiality, establishing and sustaining therapeutic relationships, and working collaboratively with others. Another expectation-more internal to the students' development of positive professional self-images-includes taking responsibility for maintaining, assessing, and improving self-competence. Students are responsible for articulating their understanding of theoretical information and identifying their abilities to implement evaluation or intervention techniques. Moreover, the ability to benefit from supervision as a resource for self-directed learning is *crucial* to professional development.

The requirements established by ACOTE (2007) include a minimum of the equivalent of 24 weeks full-time of Level II fieldwork for occupational therapy students in a minimum of one setting if it is reflective of more than one practice area, or in a maximum of four different settings and a minimum of the equivalent of 16 weeks full-time for occupational therapy assistant students in a minimum of one setting if it is reflective of more than one practice area or in a maximum of three settings. Level II fieldwork may be completed on a part-time basis "as defined by the fieldwork placement in accordance with usual and customary personnel policies as long as it is at least 50% of a full-time equivalent at that site" (ACOTE, 2007). Alternatives to full-time fieldwork, such as part-time models or 12-month experiences, are becoming more common (Adelstein, Cohn, Baker, & Barnes, 1990; Phillips & Legaspi, 1995).

FIELDWORK: INTERNATIONAL PERSPECTIVES

Internationally, the World Federation of Occupational Therapy (WFOT) Minimum Standards for the Education of Occupational Therapists (Hocking & Ness, 2002) require that students complete a minimum of 1,000 hours of approved clinical fieldwork that is spread throughout all years of an academic program. The WFOT requires that fieldwork placements be in locations that offer different levels of health care, such as acute care, rehabilitation, disability, community, and wellness settings. Within these types of settings, fieldwork must provide students with the opportunity to work with people of different ages who have acute and chronic health needs, delivering interventions that focus on the person, the occupation, and the environment (Hocking & Ness, 2002). At least some fieldwork placements must be of up to eight weeks' duration to enable a comprehensive learning experience. Targeted learning outcomes for graduates of WFOT-approved educational programs are to demonstrate knowledge, skills, and attitudes in the following competencies: the person-occupation-environment and its relationship to health, therapeutic and professional relationships, occupational therapy processes, professional reasoning and behavior, and the context of professional practice (Hocking & Ness, 2002).

FIELDWORK SETTINGS AND MODELS

Traditionally, fieldwork has taken place in the context of a hospital or primary health care setting, in which students spend six weeks to three months at one facility with a single supervisor. However, a number of factors, such as increasing demand for occupational therapy services, personnel shortages, and increasing needs for student placements, are influencing the profession to develop and expand innovative fieldwork opportunities (AOTA, 2000; Thomas, Penman, & Williamson, 2005). Academic programs are developing fieldwork in contexts of emerging practice such as community-based day treatment programs, senior centers, assisted living facilities, sheltered workshops, homeless shelters, after-school programs, home health care, rural settings, and international placements (AOTA, 1999b; Johnson et al., 2006). In particular, **project-focused fieldwork** provides a viable approach to developing new programs or resources or, in evaluating existing programs, for prevention or health promotion settings (Fortune, Farnworth, & McKinstry, 2006).

Additionally, various innovative models of supervision have been proposed as approaches to promote self-direction among students and to better equip them to become lifelong learners as alternatives to the model of one-to-one supervision, which can reinforce dependency (Thomas et al., 2005). The development of three models of supervision has been identified: role-emerging, collaborative, and interagency. The impetus for these alternative approaches to supervision is to foster the profession's goal of new graduates being innovative and effective reflective practitioners and critical thinkers (Bonello, 2001). **Role-emerging supervision**, which occurs in a placement in which there is no occupational therapist on site, provides opportunities for students to be more autonomous and independent, promoting increased professional growth. The WFOT Standards (Hocking & Ness, 2002) and the ACOTE (2007) Standards both note that fieldwork can occur in sites where occupational therapy is emerging. ACOTE requires that students in this type of placement receive a minimum of eight hours of supervision each week from a practitioner who has a minimum of three years of experience. Under these circumstances, a member of the facility's staff assumes the responsibilities of day-to-day supervision.

Collaborative supervision is another model used in fieldwork that may entail one or more supervisors working with multiple students "with all participants viewed as more equal partners in the learning process" (Thomas et al., 2005, p. 80). This model encourages students to assume greater responsibility for their learning through peer teaching and mutual problem solving (Ladyshewsky, 1995). In the case of more than one supervisor, it is useful to identify who will serve as the primary supervisor in order to be responsible for managing the overall fieldwork experience, including the evaluation process.

Another approach to supervision is to merge the traditional one-to-one model in an area of emerging practice; this has been described as the **Interagency Model of Fieldwork** (Fisher & Savin-Badin, 2002). In this approach, occupational therapists who have a vision for the development of a new position for occupational therapy work in partnership with community agencies or industry to establish a fieldwork placement. This model is deserving of further study to determine how to offer high-quality learning experiences, including funding the necessary education and training of both fieldwork supervisors and students in order for this model to be successful. Such experiences hold the promise of building skills that will enable individual practitioners as well as the profession to manage opportunities and transitions that lie ahead in the future.

TRANSITION FROM STUDENT TO PROFESSIONAL

The shift from the academic setting to the fieldwork setting is an obvious, yet often underestimated, life change. Occupational therapy students are making the environmental transition from the classroom to the fieldwork setting while simultaneously emerging from the role of student into the role of occupational therapy practitioner. As with any transition, occupational therapy students leaving academia face a process of change from one structure, role, or sense of self to another. The struggle to assimilate into a new environment and to develop a new role can jolt students into disequilibrium, and some students have trouble adjusting to the new role. As is true of all life changes, this disequilibrium can be an opportunity for growth, especially in the context of a supportive supervisory relationship.

This time of transition for students results in changes in assumptions about themselves and the world and requires a corresponding change in behaviors, relationships, learning styles, and self-perceptions. As they move into fieldwork settings, students may begin to reassess their suppositions about occupational therapy, the theories they learned in school, and their views of themselves as practitioners, learners, and individuals. Because individuals differ in their ability to adapt to change and because each student is placed in a different fieldwork setting, the transition has a different effect on each student.

The nature of the fieldwork environment is fundamentally different from that of the academic environment. Knowing and acknowledging some of the distinctions between the two settings can ease the transition and provide students with support to accept the challenges of fieldwork experiences (see Table 26.1). Within the fieldwork environment, the learning focus shifts to the application or implementation of therapy techniques in an applied interpersonal context. Techniques that were introduced in a simulated context now must be mastered and applied with attention to the client's emotional needs.

TABLE 26.1 DISTINCTIONS BETWEEN ACADEMIC AND FIELDWORK SETTINGS

Characteristic	Academic Setting	Fieldwork Setting
Purpose	Dissemination of knowledge, development of creative thought, student growth	Provide high-quality client care
Faculty/supervisor accountability	To student, to university/college	To client and significant others, to fieldwork center and team, to student
Student accountability	To self	To clients and significant others, to supervisor and team, to fieldwork center
Pace	Depends on curriculum, adaptable to student and faculty needs	Depends on clients' needs, less adaptable, shaped by facility procedures
Student: educator ratio	Many students to one faculty member	One student to one supervisor, small group of students to one supervisor, one or two student(s) to two supervisors
Source of feedback	Summative at midterm or end of term, provided by faculty	Provided by clients and significant others, supervisor, and other staff; formative
Degree of faculty/supervisor control of educational experience	Able to plan, controlled	Limited control, various diagnoses and length of client stay, pace of setting and size of caseload varies from setting to setting
Primary learning tool	Books, journal articles, lectures, audiovisual aids, case studies, simulations, technology, Internet	Situation of practice; clients, families, significant others, and staff; may be face to face or electronic (e.g., webcams, e-mail)
Conceptual learning	Abstract, theoretical	Pragmatic, applied in interpersonal context
Learning process	Teacher-directed	Client, self, peer, supervisor-directed
Tolerance for ambiguity	High	Low
Lifestyle	Flexible, able to plan time around class schedule	Structured, flexible time limited to evenings and weekends
Contexts	University or college classroom, online learning	Hospitals, schools, nursing homes, day care centers, day treatment programs, community-based agencies, clients' homes

Abstract questions that are appropriate in the academic environment shift to pragmatic questions to reduce the possibility of error in one's thinking. For example, rather than thinking about a client's function in the kitchen from an abstract perspective, the student has to think about the client's function in the context of a specific kitchen in a certain small apartment and attend to the client's concerns about his or her roles, activities, family, and home environment. Because the student recognizes that his or her actions have an influence on the client's life, tolerance for ambiguity or uncertainty declines during fieldwork.

In the academic setting, students are accountable primarily to themselves, and performance is evaluated on a summative basis through tests, assignments, and grades. Students choose whether to disclose their grades to family or peers, and their performance does not affect others. In the fieldwork center, a student's performance is evaluated on a formative basis and may be observed by the entire health care team, especially at team meetings. Performance is no longer the private matter that it was at school but is publicly observed because it has direct and critical consequences for clients. Colleagues, clients, and their families may offer meaningful feedback. Although all these opportunities may create disequilibrium or tension, they also constitute new ways in which students learn about themselves and their profession. The broad and diverse experience within the fieldwork setting challenges students to redefine their sense of self.

Fieldwork takes place in a situation over which fieldwork educators have little control. The organizational factors of the health care setting, combined with client care factors, such as the nature and complexity of the client's problem, the length of stay, and fluctuation in the client load, make planning difficult, especially in acute care settings. In settings that provide extended care for clients, however, the fieldwork educators are able to plan ahead, because the client population is more constant and the fieldwork educator knows which clients will be available during student placements.

Fieldwork educators' primary responsibility is client care; they have an ethical imperative to ensure the welfare of clients. This appropriate professional ethic may constrain activities that are desirable from the standpoint of education. However, the supervisory relationship allows fieldwork educators to adapt to the constraints of the setting. This unique relationship is a positive aspect of the fieldwork environment because fieldwork educators can adapt the fieldwork experiences to meet the learner's needs.

Examination of supervisors' perceptions of successful fieldwork students showed important themes of active experimentation as part of the learning process, including adaptability and doing, as well as being flexible and engaging in teamwork (Herzberg, 1994). A literature review on fieldwork success identifies a number of positive attributes to promote student participation (Sladyk, 2002, p. 8), as summarized in Box 26.1. Awareness of these attributes

and characteristics, in addition to positive coping strategies, can aid students in preparing for and participating in their fieldwork placements.

Exploration of students' coping strategies and their perceptions of fieldwork has shown that a majority of students view the experience as important, while more than half found the experience to be stressful (Mitchell & Kampfe, 1993). Level II fieldwork students invested significantly more effort in the positive coping strategies of being problem-focused, making a plan of action and following it, and seeking social support to obtain information, advice, or emotional support. These results verify healthy approaches and "coping skills for dealing with fieldwork transition and stress" (Mitchell & Kampfe, 1993, p. 537). Students less frequently used negatively regarded strategies such as blaming, wishful thinking, or avoidance, implying that students have healthy coping skills available to them to support their participation in the transitions associated with fieldwork.

An **occupational adaptation model of professional development** as applied to Level II fieldwork outlines three classes of adaptive response behaviors: primitive, transitional, and mature, which are typically demonstrated among all students (Garrett and Schkade, 1995). When faced with situations that they perceive as too difficult or too unfamiliar, students tend to revert to lower-level behaviors. This model can be a useful resource both for fieldwork students, to self-assess their own behavior, and for their supervisors, to help understand the implications and timing for increasing workload assignments and providing new learning challenges during fieldwork.

ROLES AND RESPONSIBILITIES OF STUDENTS AND EDUCATORS

After completion of the prerequisite academic coursework, occupational therapy and occupational therapy assistant students are eligible to begin their fieldwork experiences.

BOX 26.1   POSITIVE ATTRIBUTES OF SUCCESSFUL FIELDWORK STUDENTS

- Showing interest in the area of practice and the profession
- Demonstrating concern for the client's needs and issues
- Regarding safety as a priority
- Taking responsibility for one's attitude and behaviors
- Managing time
- Adhering to timelines and due dates
- Seeking additional information

- Practicing skills
- Listening
- Using supervision time effectively
- Exchanging feedback with one's supervisor
- Accepting criticism
- Avoiding excuses
- Exploring new approaches or projects
- Engaging in creative problem solving

Sladyk (2002).

Generally, academic fieldwork coordinators are responsible for administrative arrangements to support students' participation in fieldwork experiences, commensurate with the goals of the curriculum as well as with the policies of affiliated practice settings and health care systems. Clearly defined objectives and guidelines help students to organize their efforts toward achieving professional competence. Working toward mastery of the entry-level skills required for high-quality client care is a mutual undertaking between the fieldwork educators and the students. Both assume primary responsibility for the process of evaluating students' progress and modifying the learning experience within the environment, in consultation with the academic fieldwork coordinator, as appropriate. See Table 26.2 to gain insight into how each person contributes to and participates in the overall fieldwork process.

Fieldwork Educator Guidelines

The role for the people who are responsible for supervising students is formally titled *fieldwork educator,* although the terms *clinical educator, fieldwork supervisor,* and *student supervisor* are also commonly used (AOTA, 2000). The people who are responsible for the fieldwork education program and direct supervision of occupational therapy students must be occupational therapists who meet state practice acts and regulations and have a minimum of one year of practice experience, subsequent to the requisite initial certification (ACOTE, 2007; CAOT, 2005). For occupational therapy assistant students, supervision can be provided by a registered occupational therapist or a certified occupational therapy assistant, also with a minimum of one year of experience. Although the minimum require-

ment is one year of experience, fieldwork educators should be competent practitioners who can serve as good role models or mentors for future practitioners. Ultimately, the fieldwork educator strives to develop and provide the best opportunity for the implementation of theoretical concepts offered as part of the academic educational program while creating an environment that facilitates learning, inquiry, self-direction, and reflection on one's practice.

Fieldwork Evaluation

Frequently, students receive informal feedback during supervision meetings; however, formal mechanisms for providing feedback and evaluation of a student's performance, judgments, and attitudes are built into the fieldwork experience. Fieldwork evaluation has two distinct purposes. One is the formative, ongoing process of directing student learning throughout the fieldwork experience; the other is summative, documenting the level of skills attained at the completion of the fieldwork experience. Although these two processes are different, they are not mutually exclusive. The formative process occurs throughout the fieldwork experience so that students and fieldwork educators can compare perceptions, assess which student activities are important and which are less so, review objectives, plan new learning opportunities, and make necessary modifications in behaviors. The second process, which is cumulative, requires documentation of a student's performance at the midpoint of the placement and after completion of the fieldwork experience.

In the United States, the Fieldwork Performance Evaluation for the Occupational Therapy Student (FWPE/OTS) (AOTA, 2002b) and the Fieldwork Performance

TABLE 26.2   ROLES AND RESPONSIBILITIES IN FIELDWORK

Roles	Responsibilities
Academic Fieldwork Coordinator (AFWC)	◆ Serve as a liaison and collaborator with faculty and fieldwork educators to ensure integration of curricular goals with fieldwork (ACOTE, 2007) ◆ Select training sites and assigns students ◆ Oversee administrative requirements, such as contracts and student health records ◆ Available for consultation to fieldwork educators and students
Fieldwork Educator	◆ Meet requisite eligibility for supervisory role, as applicable (ACOTE, 2007; Canadian Association of Occupational Therapy, 2005) ◆ Engage in administrative collaboration with AFWC to determine and schedule assignments ◆ Provide day-to-day student supervision ◆ Complete evaluation of student performance, as designated ◆ Structure learning and create a positive learning environment
Student	◆ Fulfill all duties identified by the fieldwork educators and academic fieldwork coordinators within the designated timelines ◆ Comply with the professional standards identified by the fieldwork facility, the education program, and the Occupational Therapy Code of Ethics (AOTA, 2005)

Evaluation for the Occupational Therapy Assistant Student (FWPE/OTAS) (AOTA, 2002a) are companion instruments, adopted by AOTA's Commission on Education in 2002 (Atler, 2003). Apart from a numeric rating system, the forms provide space for supervisors to add or qualify their scoring with written descriptions and comments (Atler, 2003). The intent of the fieldwork evaluation is not to differentiate between students, but to measure their achievement of specific entry-level competencies. A profession usually defines its boundaries by setting up criteria for entry. In occupational therapy, the fieldwork experience is an essential component of the entry criteria. Successful completion of Level II fieldwork is a requirement for certification as a registered occupational therapist (OTR) or certified occupational therapy assistant (COTA) (National Board for Certification in Occupational Therapy, 2007). Fieldwork provides students with situations in which to practice interpersonal skills with clients and staff and to develop characteristics that are essential to productive working relationships (AOTA, 2000). Future employers want assurance that students satisfy the entry-level requirements. The FWPE data may be synthesized to provide the foundation for employment references.

Internationally, there is a trend toward the use of standardized approaches for the evaluation of student fieldwork performance. The Competency Based Fieldwork Evaluation for Occupational Therapists (CBFE-OT) (Bossers, Miller, Polatajko & Hartley, 2001), widely used across Canada and the United Kingdom, is designed for use in any level of fieldwork and within any placement area. This instrument is used in conjunction with a learning contract associated with each competency. In Australia, eight out of ten academic programs have adopted the use of the Student Placement Evaluation Form (SPEF) (Allison & Turpin, 2004; University of Queensland, 1998). A unique aspect of this tool is banks of items, grouped according to types of practice settings, from which supervisors can select the most relevant learning objectives and items for evaluating student performance. It is noteworthy that each of these fieldwork evaluation tools is intended to be used across and within all practice settings. Furthermore, similar content and competency areas are evident among these tools, as noted in Table 26.3.

Student Evaluation of the Fieldwork Experience

Students also have the opportunity to provide the fieldwork educators and the fieldwork facility with feedback. AOTA (2006) recommends the Student Evaluation of Fieldwork Experiences (SEFWE) form. This form allows students to provide feedback about orientation, caseload, occupational therapy process; theory, frames of reference, and models of practice; fieldwork assignments; supervisor interactions; aspects of the environment, such as team relationships; and how the entire learning expe-rience related to the academic curriculum and their own professional development. The fieldwork sites use this information to improve fieldwork programs, and the academic programs share the information with future students who are interested in training at those sites. In Canada, a similar form is used for students to provide feedback to fieldwork sites. Overall, documentation of students' feedback regarding their fieldwork experiences is information that is valuable to both the training site and the academic program.

CONCLUSION

Fieldwork is the beginning of a lifelong process of connecting theory with practice. The depth of the experience depends greatly on the degree to which students and fieldwork educators share the responsibility for teaching and learning. Today's rapidly changing health and human service delivery systems are providing new opportunities for occupational therapy practice and fieldwork education. Globally, the profession is giving attention to innovative approaches to improving the quality of fieldwork while taking into consideration each country's health, economic, educational, and social status (Bonello, 2001). To be successful in these dynamic and complex situations, practitioners must be able to make judgments based on thoughtful inquiry, analysis, and reflection on practice in order to support their clients in improving their participation in daily and social activities and overall quality of life.

ACKNOWLEDGMENT

A sincere thanks to Ellen S. Cohn for her long-time mentorship and for providing the foundational concepts as the basis of this chapter from the tenth edition of *Willard & Spackman's Occupational Therapy.*

PROVOCATIVE QUESTIONS

1. How can the profession reconcile the tension between the evolution of fieldwork in emerging practice, where there might not be an occupational therapy supervisor on site, and the trend for increased regulations requiring direct supervision, such as Medicare in the United States?
2. You are a student who is interested in a Level II fieldwork placement opportunity working in a health and wellness setting. However, your academic program has established fieldwork arrangements with only hospitals, schools, and private health care facilities. How might you proceed to communicate your learning goals and develop a plan of action to explore the feasibility of developing a new type of Level II fieldwork experience?

TABLE 26.3 FIELDWORK EVALUATION IN THE UNITED STATES, AUSTRALIA, CANADA, AND THE UNITED KINGDOM

Fieldwork Evaluations and Authors	FWPE/OT (U.S.) (AOTA, 2002b)	FWPE/OTA (U.S.) (AOTA, 2002a)	SPEF (Australia) (University of Queensland, 1998)	CBFE-OT (Canada, U.K.) (Bossers et al., 2001)
Purpose	To measure entry-level competence of the occupational therapy student	To measure entry-level competence of the occupational therapy assistant student	To assess student fieldwork performance	To evaluate a student's performance and learning
Content: Areas of Competency	◆ Fundamentals of practice ◆ Basic tenets ◆ Evaluation/ screening ◆ Intervention ◆ Management of OT services ◆ Communication ◆ Professional behavior	◆ Fundamentals of practice ◆ Basic tenets ◆ Evaluation/ screening ◆ Intervention ◆ Communication ◆ Professional behavior	◆ Professional practice ◆ Self-management skills ◆ Communication skills ◆ Documentation ◆ Assessment/ information gathering ◆ Intervention ◆ Evaluation ◆ Group skills (optional)	◆ Practice knowledge ◆ Clinical reasoning ◆ Facilitating change with a practice process ◆ Professional interactions ◆ Communication ◆ Professional development ◆ Performance management
Number of Items	42	25	Variable; item bank, selected by supervisor; items vary for: ◆ direct client contact ◆ case management ◆ project management/ consultancy	Variable; learning objectives are written by each fieldwork site as relevant to the setting
Rating scale	4 points	4 points	5 points	3 points
Evaluation	Midterm, final	Midterm, final	Midterm (halfway), final	Midterm, final

REFERENCES

Accreditation Council for Occupational Therapy Education. (2007). *Standards and interpretative guide for an entry-level educational program for the occupational therapist and the occupational therapy assistant.* Bethesda, MD: American Occupational Therapy Association. Available at: http://www.aota.org/nonmembers/area13/links/link13.asp

Adelstein, L. A., Cohn, E. S., Baker, R. C., & Barnes, M. A. (1990). A part-time level II fieldwork program. *American Journal of Occupational Therapy, 44,* 60–65.

Allison, H. & Turpin, M. (2004). Development of the student placement evaluation form: A tool for assessing student fieldwork performance. *Australian Occupational Therapy Journal, 51,* 125–132.

Alsop, A., & Donald, M. (1996). Taking stock and taking chances: Creating new opportunities for fieldwork education. *British Journal of Occupational Therapy, 59*(11), 498–502.

American Occupational Therapy Association, Commission on Education. (1999a). *Guidelines for an occupational therapy fieldwork experience: Level I.* Bethesda, MD: Author.

American Occupational Therapy Association, Education Department. (1999b). *Innovative fieldwork annotated bibliography.* Bethesda, MD: Author. Available at: http://www.aota.org/Educate/EdRes/Fieldwork/38240.aspx

American Occupational Therapy Association, Commission on Education and Fieldwork Issues Committee. (2000). *Guidelines for an occupational therapy fieldwork experience: Level II.* Bethesda, MD.

American Occupational Therapy Association. (2002a). *Fieldwork performance evaluation for the occupational therapy assistant student.* Bethesda, MD: Author.

American Occupational Therapy Association. (2002b). *Fieldwork performance evaluation for the occupational therapy student.* Bethesda, MD: Author.

American Occupational Therapy Association. (2003). Purpose and value of occupational therapy fieldwork education. *American Journal of Occupational Therapy, 57,* 644.

American Occupational Therapy Association. (2005). Occupational therapy code of ethics. *American Journal of Occupational Therapy, 59,* 639–642.

American Occupational Therapy Association, Student Evaluation of Fieldwork Experience Task Force. (2006). *Student evaluation of fieldwork experience.* Bethesda, MD: Author.

Atler, K. (2003). *Using the fieldwork performance evaluation forms: The complete guide.* Bethesda, MD: American Occupational Therapy Association.

Barnes, M. A. & Evenson, M. E. (2000). Supervision and mentoring. In S. C. Merrill & P. A. Crist (Eds.), *Meeting the fieldwork challenge: A self-paced clinical course, Lesson 5* (pp. 9–12). Bethesda, MD: American Occupational Therapy Association.

Bonello, M. (2001). Fieldwork within the context of higher education: A literature review. *British Journal of Occupational Therapy, 64,* 93–99.

Bossers, A., Miller, L. T., Polatajko, H. J., & Hartley, M. (2001). *Competency based fieldwork evaluation for occupational therapists CFE-OT.* Albany, NY: Delmar Thomson Learning.

Canadian Association of Occupational Therapy. (2005). *Academic accreditation standards and self-study guide.* Ottawa, ON: Author. Available at: http://www.caot.ca/pdfs/Guide Complete.pdf

Christie, B. A., Joyce, P. C., & Moeller, P. L. (1985). Fieldwork experience 1: Impact on practice preference. *American Journal of Occupational Therapy, 39,* 671–674.

Cohn, E. S., & Crist, P. (1995). Back to the future: New approaches to fieldwork education. *American Journal of Occupational Therapy, 49,* 103–106.

Costa, D. (Ed.). (2004). *The essential guide to occupational therapy fieldwork education: Resources for today's educators and practitioners.* Bethesda, MD: American Occupational Therapy Association.

Crowe, M. J., & Mackenzie, L. (2002). The influence of fieldwork on the preferred future practice areas of final year occupational therapy students. *Australian Occupational Therapy Journal, 49,* 25–36.

Evenson, M. Barnes, M. A., & Cohn, E. S. (2002). Brief report: Perceptions of level I and level II fieldwork in the same site. *American Journal of Occupational Therapy, 56,* 103–106.

Fisher, A. & Savin Badin, M. (2002). Modernizing fieldwork, part 2: Realizing the new agenda. *British Journal of Occupational Therapy, 65,* 275–282.

Fortune, T., Farnworth, L., & McKinstry, C. (2006). Project-focused fieldwork: Core business or fieldwork fillers? *Australian Occupational Therapy Journal, 53,* 233–236.

Garrett, S. A., & Schkade, J. K. (1995). Occupational adaptation model of professional development as applied to Level II fieldwork. *American Journal of Occupational Therapy, 49,* 119–126.

Herzberg, G. L. (1994). The successful fieldwork student: Supervisor perceptions. *American Journal of Occupational Therapy, 48,* 817–823.

Hocking, C. & Ness, N. E. (2002). *Minimum standards for the education of occupational therapists.* Forrestfield, Australia: World Federation of Occupational Therapists.

Johnson, C. R., Koenig, K. P., Piersol, C. V., Santalucia, S. E., & Wachter-Schutz, W. (2006). Level I fieldwork today: A study of contexts and perceptions. *American Journal of Occupational Therapy, 60,* 275–287.

Ladyshewsky, R. K. (1995). Enhancing service productivity in acute care inpatient settings using a collaborative clinical education model. *Physical Therapy, 75,* 53–58.

Lewis, L. M. (2005, September). Fieldwork requirements of the past, present, and future. *Education Special Interest Section Quarterly, 15,* 1–4.

Missiuna, C. A., Polatajko, H. I., & Ernest-Conibear, M. (1992). Skill acquisition during fieldwork placements in occupational therapy. *Canadian Journal of Occupational Therapy, 59*(1), 28–39.

Mitchell, M. M. & Kampfe, C. M. (1993). Student coping strategies and perceptions of fieldwork. *American Journal of Occupational Therapy, 47,* 535–540.

National Board for Certification in Occupational Therapy. (2007). *Certification examination handbook and application.* Gaithersburg, MD: Author.

Phillips, E. C., & Legaspi, W. S. (1995). A 12-month internship model of level II fieldwork. *American Journal of Occupational Therapy, 49,* 146–149.

Pickett, J. (Ed.). (2000). *The American Heritage® dictionary of the English language* (4th ed.). Boston: Houghton Mifflin.

Pressler, S. (1983). Fieldwork education: The proving ground of the profession. *American Journal of Occupational Therapy, 3,* 163–165.

Sladyk, K. (Ed.). (2002). *The successful occupational therapy fieldwork student.* Thorofare, NJ: Slack.

Thomas, Y., Penman, M., & Williamson, P. (2005). Australian and New Zealand fieldwork: Charting the territory for future practice. *Australian Occupational Therapy Journal, 52,* 78–81.

University of Queensland, Division of Occupational Therapy. (1998). *Student placement evaluation and handbook.* Brisbane: Author.

Questions for Occupational Therapy Practice

JOHN WHITE

Learning Objectives

After reading this chapter, you will be able to:

1. Describe examples of current practice from individual to population-based occupational therapy.
2. Reflect on and discuss key questions that help to inform decisions about current and future occupational therapy practice.
3. Develop questions that support critiques of current occupational therapy practice.
4. Identify possible directions for the development of future occupational therapy practice.
5. Describe threats and opportunities to the future development of occupational therapy.
6. Identify and describe who is optimally served by existing occupational therapy resources and how those services will best be delivered and distributed.

> *I dwell in Possibility–*
> *A fairer house than Prose–*
> *More numerous of Window–*
> *Superior–for Doors–*
>
> *Of Chambers as the Cedars–*
> *Impregnable of Eye–*
> *And for an Everlasting Roof–*
> *The Gambrels of the Sky–*
>
> *Of Visitors–the fairest–*
> *For Occupation–This–*
> *The spreading wide my narrow Hands–*
> *To gather Paradise–*
>
> —EMILY DICKINSON

27

"**D**welling in possibilities" is as natural to practitioners of occupational therapy as is the belief in the link between occupation and health (Meyer, 1977; Rebeiro, 2001; Wilcock, 1993, 1998a, 1998b; Yerxa, 1998). Occupational therapy confronts limitations that environments, circumstances, impairments, policies, and sociocultural situations place on people and imagines possibilities for creating full and satisfying lives. In this chapter, we will explore visions of possible futures for occupational therapy from individual and organizational perspectives.

OPENING QUESTIONS

How are we doing as a profession at creating possibilities for the clients who most need our services? Are we doing our best? If not, what is holding us back? Who is being served through our activities: clients, health care systems, third-party reimbursers, ourselves? Where are we going in the future? This chapter addresses these and related queries in order to prompt therapists to reflect on the relevance of our current practice and how well it corresponds to the most appropriate needs of those we serve. In addressing these questions, occupational therapy practice in the United States will be the primary reference point, but examples of practice in other countries will also be used. I will first address examples of change in the field and then identify some significant threats to our viability. Throughout the chapter, I will pose questions for reflection as we move forward into a rapidly changing future.

RAPID CHANGE

Society is changing at a dramatic and unpredictable pace and increasing in complexity in areas such as technology, knowledge, politics, and culture. Occupational therapy is part of this "hyperchange"—change that is rapid, unpredictable, chaotic, and turbulent (Hinojosa, 2007; Weiner & Brown, 2006). In the 30 years that I have been in practice, especially in the last 15 years, there has been an explosion of changes in occupational therapy. These changes have occurred in occupational therapy education and practice as well as in health care, policy, and technology. We will consider examples of changes in theory, research, and technology.

Some of the change in occupational therapy education and practice has been driven by changes in occupational therapy–related theories. For example, many of the theoretical changes and some of the changes in practice have been fueled by the advent of **occupational science** (e.g., the theories that are featured in Unit I), as well as new approaches to assessment, intervention, education, and research. Occupational science is only one of many influences on changing theory and practice. Practice and theory in Canada, for example, were prompted to change

by the Canadian health ministry's charge to the national occupational therapy association to develop more client-centered practice guidelines (Law et al., 2005). One outcome was the Canadian Model of Occupational Performance (Law, 1998; Law, Baptiste, & Mills, 1995), which brought the concept of spirituality into occupational therapy's domain of concern (Christiansen, 1997; Collins, 1998; Crepeau, 1991; Egan & De Laat, 1994; Townsend, De Laat, Egan, Thibeault, & Wright, 1999; Urbanowski & Vargo, 1994) and ensured a process for person-centered assessment and intervention.

The approach to conducting and using research in occupational therapy changed dramatically with the advent of evidence-based practice (EBP) as a modified form of evidence-based medicine (EBM). Though EBM was first introduced in the 1970s (Cochrane, 1972), it did not have a significant influence in occupational therapy until the late 1990s. EBP began at that time in the United Kingdom (Culshaw, 1995; Eakin, 1997) and spread rapidly to the United States and Canada (Hayes & McGrath, 1998; Law, 1998; Ottenbacher & Maas, 1999). EBP is now becoming a driving force in occupational therapy education and practice (Baum, 2006; Corcoran, 2006) and in other fields. I explore questions concerning EBP later in this chapter.

In the realm of changing technology, home or office-based computers still seemed like science fiction in 1976, yet less than 10 years later, I was using simple cognitive retraining programs on an Apple® computer and learned about a voice-recognition system that cost $25,000 (similar software now retails for about $100). Assistive technology today is evolving faster than many therapists can keep up with, and technological innovation is making participation in a range of occupations possible for people with disabilities that were only dreamed about 20 years ago (Cate & Perez, 2004; Gentry, 2005; Lange & Brians, 1995). How do we best incorporate technology in our field, which has long celebrated the human-to-human connection?

Changes in technology, the role of EBP, and theories are only a few of the many examples that have potentially profound effects on the profession and the status of practice. When we consider the combined force of all the possible global and local changes that affect practice, we begin to see the influence of hyperchange. Change is often said to be good for us, but it is usually challenging, and it can be threatening if we feel that our security or established routines and roles are at risk. If some change is good, is hyperchange better—or just more threatening? Our response is largely determined by how prepared we are to cope with, and adapt to, the changes. "Futurethink" or anticipatory thinking and problem solving, is an approach that Weiner and Brown (2006) recommend as the most effective way to avoid the stresses and negative outcomes in the midst of the turbulent events surrounding hyperchange. Following are some steps in futurethink:

1. Conduct a thorough analysis of the situation by asking good questions, and don't just look for the answers

that you hope to see, but look for the ones that are there in reality.

2. Look for the big picture in its most holistic context by linking events and trends for the broadest patterns and key connections.

3. Link information to action. Once you understand the big picture in its full context and have an idea of how to proceed, take action to implement the solution in order to avoid blocks that lead to inaction (Weiner & Brown, 2006).

THREATS TO PRACTICE

Considering the extent of current change, it might be that change itself is a threat to the profession. We will now analyze some external and internal threats to occupational therapy.

External Threats

External threats to the success of the global profession are most easily identified. These threats warrant action if we are to fulfill our "potential to create a significant impact on tomorrow's world" (Yerxa, 2003, p. 979) by promoting a "new concept of health" that promotes agency and participation for those we serve (Yerxa, 2003, p. 978). One of the biggest external challenges to sustained growth and success in occupational therapy is the source of payment for occupational therapy services, whether in free-market or government-sponsored health systems, along with the ever-growing pressure and related ethical challenges to increase therapist productivity (Howard, 1991; Slater, 2006). For example, in the United States, reimbursement for rehabilitation services in skilled nursing facilities was severely curtailed in 1999. In that case, government policy was primarily responsible for significantly decreased payment for services (Daus, 1999). This change in payment for services followed close behind changes in health care systems, such as the advent of managed care practices (Christiansen, 1996). These professional crises (Baptiste & Martin, 1994; Fine, 1998; Wood, 1998) were preceded by a constantly changing approach to reimbursement by federal, state, and private insurers that have dictated what work occupational therapists would and would not be paid for (Walker, 2001). Tighter budgets for therapy services drive the need for greater productivity in terms of "treatment units" (the unit of intervention time that is charged to the client's account) ever higher. A different sort of resource crisis occurs in some developing nations when occupational therapists leave their native countries to pursue practice in nations where salaries are much higher, sometimes after being recruited by companies in developed countries (Sinclair, 2005). Considering our commitment to ethical, high-quality service, what is our response to a trend that is essentially taking from the poor to give to

the rich? How do we balance the individual freedom to practice where one chooses with the need to provide services where they are most needed?

Professional "turf" competition, often played out at the professional licensure level, is an increasing threat as other professional groups claim practice areas that have traditionally been held sacred by occupational therapy (see the "practice alerts" section on www.aota.org for various turf issues). These are certainly challenges that must be addressed by the members of the profession through individual and organizational activity and advocacy. When challenged in this way by groups that feel that they can do work that occupational therapists have traditionally claimed, it is critical for us to ask ourselves, "What are we doing that is unique to occupational therapy and not redundant to related professions?" For example, what can make hand therapy a unique and obviously a special part of occupational therapy? There are examples of occupation-based hand therapy in the literature that begin with client-centered assessment (Amini, 2004; Earley & Shannon, 2006). Will they prove to be uniquely occupational therapy and simultaneously more effective than more pathology-focused approaches? What differentiates occupational therapy service in a long-term care facility from activity therapy or physical therapy (Atwal, 2003) or makes it distinct from social work in a community mental health program (Rebeiro, Day, Semeniu, O'Brien, & Wilson, 2001)?

Considering innovative and emerging practice models from international examples, how are our resources best applied to relatively new populations? New models of practice are seen with occupational therapy for children who survived war in Kosovo (Algado & Burgman, 2005), and advocating and promoting participation through play for children with HIV/AIDS in South Africa (Ramugondo, 2005). Yet one more example is through power-sharing, using approaches such as community-based rehabilitation (CBR), which applies traditional rehabilitation approaches in community settings to address **occupational apartheid** and **occupational deprivation** (Kronenberg & Pollard, 2005).

If we can successfully address the questions in this section, we should be able to avoid the risk that Mary Reilly identified when she described a potential dilemma for the profession in that the need for occupationally relevant services will always exist, but it is up to occupational therapy to make the most of its unique contribution to society to ensure the profession's survival. Reilly asserted that even if occupational therapy were to fail as a profession, another similarly situated group would emerge to "serve society's need for action" (Reilly, 1962, p. 2).

However, as significant as these examples of external threats are, if we allow internal professional threats to prevent us from developing our fullest potential to serve those who most need our services, there will be little force or structure that we can use to find ways to meet the external challenges.

Internal Threats

What internal forces threaten to diminish our effectiveness in a world of need for our services? A few examples to be explored here are the question of unification versus diversification, the tension between general practice and specialization, and the role of professional associations. A search for agreement about our common purpose, core values, and unifying theory is perhaps one of the most significant challenges with which occupational therapists have wrestled for at least the past 30 years (Engelhardt, 1977; Hocking, Whiteford, Henare, & Hansen, 1995; Kimura, 1987; Nelson, 1997; Polatajko, 2006; Whiteford, Townsend, & Hocking, 2000). Do we gain more strength, credibility, and value as a profession through the diversity of many approaches to practice, or will we benefit more from a universal approach?

Occupational science has contributed to the search for a common unifying core that began with a spirited debate about whether the new discipline should be partitioned off from occupational therapy (Clark et al., 1993; Mosey, 1992, 1993). Time has shown that increasingly, the evolution of the science and therapy are intricately intertwined, leading to new theories, applications, and research endeavors. There is a growing global presence in that there are now at least eight societies promoting various aspects of occupational science that are influencing occupational therapy practice worldwide (see http://isos.nfshost.com/links.php).

How ultimately successful the interaction between occupational science and occupational therapy will be has yet to be determined, but several examples demonstrate early influences. One is the landmark USC Well-Elderly Study (Clark et al., 1997; Mandel, Jackson, Zemke, Nelson, & Clark, 1999), which demonstrated the value of occupational therapy interventions enhanced by occupational science research to improve health and life satisfaction in community-dwelling elders. Another example of the influence of occupational science on practice is evident in the change in focus of national conference presentations in North America, the United Kingdom, and the World Federation of Occupational Therapy (WFOT). Before the development of doctoral and other occupational science programs since 1989 (Clark et al., 1991; Yerxa et al., 1989), the use of the term *occupation* in national occupational therapy conference papers was rare. *Occupation* is now featured prominently in program titles, yet the challenge to develop a universally agreed-upon definition of *occupation* and its distinction from *activity* persists (American Occupational Therapy Association, 1995; Baum & Edwards, 1995; Evans, 1987; Pierce, 2001; Wilcock & Townsend, 2000; Wu & Lin, 1999). Entry-level educational programs are incorporating occupational science into curricula in hopes of preparing students to better understand and apply occupation in practice (Behr, Bass-Haugen, Gordon, Bennett, & Henderson, 2003; Hender-

son, 2004; Hilton & Randolph, 2003; Wilcock, 2003; Wood et al., 2000). Finally, professional associations in several countries have adopted practice guidelines that reflect the influence of occupational science research and theory development (College of Occupational Therapists, 2004; Youngstrom et al., 2002). The summary question arising from this discussion is: Will occupational science be a force that is capable of uniting the occupational therapy profession through its international focus on understanding occupation and promoting new and more effective approaches to applying that understanding in practice?

Specialization is another phenomenon that could be a strength or could present a potential threat to the profession. While helping individual practitioners to develop the expertise they need to address highly complex specific problems, specialization can also dilute a common professional identity and potentially lead to a scramble for resources. The debate is not unique to the United States and is linked to the power of the national occupational therapy organizations to control the issue of specialization (Chacksfield, 2006; Crawford-White, 1996; Cromwell, 1979; Knutsson, 1980). Former American Occupational Therapy Association (AOTA) president Mary Foto presented a comprehensive review of arguments for and against specialization that have been extant in the United States since at least 1952. She proposed a compromise position in which the profession could embrace "specialists, generalists, and assistants." However, much work is still needed to clearly define the different roles and develop clear competencies for each (Foto, 1996). Foto proposed that such work would most appropriately be done by AOTA.

AOTA has apparently responded to Foto's recommendation through the development of board certifications in various practice areas such as mental health, pediatrics, and physical rehabilitation, as well as certification in specialty practices related to driving, low vision, and dysphagia (AOTA, 2007). Other organizations also offer specialty certifications with widely varying criteria for earning the certificate. For example, the American Society of Hand Therapists (ASHT) supports certification in hand therapy through a rigorous and lengthy process (American Society of Hand Therapists, 2007; Hand Therapy Certification Commission, 2007). Some for-profit companies offer certification in specialized testing techniques such as the Sensory Integration and Praxis Test (Western Psychological Services, 2007) or treatment procedures such as lymphedema management (Coast to Coast School of Lymphedema Management, 2007). What are the implications for such specialization, and who is being optimally served through these certifications? At what point does a person become a hand therapist or lymphedema specialist and lose his or her identity as an occupational therapist? If the specialist is helping the client, does it matter what professional name is used to identify the therapist? Would the client be served better if the specialty were delivered through the context of authentic occupational therapy (Wilcock,

1998a; Yerxa, 1967)? We must also ask ourselves about the legal and ethical issues that arise when a person who is certified as an occupational therapist is providing services that have little resemblance to occupational therapy, but are being charged in the name of occupational therapy. I believe that the name under which one practices and the kinds of practice one performs do matter and that specialization should add value to a service that is delivered in keeping with the guiding principles of occupational therapy, not supplant or replace it so that the professional identity as an occupational therapist is lost.

Threats can be the paradoxical side of strength. Such is the case with professional associations that are generally seen as a strength in advancing the field but can also be seen as holding back progress through entrenched traditions and bureaucracies. What are the most appropriate roles of our professional organization in helping us face a rapidly changing world? Hinojosa (Hinojosa, 2007) suggested that if we are to flourish in an age of hyperchange, we will need to consider challenging questions related to the structure of our professional organizations, more critically and rapidly scrutinize our practices, and create innovative paradigms to cope with rapid social and scientific change. One way in which AOTA is charting a course for the future of occupational therapy in the United States is through development and promotion of a Centennial Vision for 2017 that states, "we envision that occupational therapy is a powerful, widely recognized, science-driven, and evidence-based profession with a globally connected and diverse workforce meeting society's occupational needs" (AOTA, 2006) with suggested actions to accomplish these goals. Does this vision capture the unique nature and contribution of occupational therapy? If so, will such a vision be adequate to meet the challenges of hyperchange? Is the profession prepared to step up to do the work that is needed to be ready to embody the vision? In taking action, will the profession practice good "future-think" (Weiner & Brown, 2006)? For example, will our professional associations push us to unquestioningly embrace evidence-based practice as a key to professional validation?

Evidence-Based Practice

One factor that has been imposed from outside the field but is being supported by professional organizations and adopted in practice is that of evidence-based practice (Holm, 2000, 2003). What began as an epidemiologist's proposal to use appraisals of relevant medical research to guide systematic decision making (Cochrane, 1972), eventually called evidence-based medicine (EBM), has grown into a worldwide phenomenon that most health care professions have adopted as the singular most important hallmark of best practice. The EBM agenda promotes effectiveness, efficiency, and equality in the delivery of health services and grew out of a social ethic of care and

equitable distribution of services (Cochrane, 1972). Other fields, including occupational therapy, adopted an approach related to EBM called evidence-based practice (EBP). EBP clearly has the potential to improve clinical decision making and foster the growth and acceptance of the field of occupational therapy. However, there is a risk inherent in the rush to embrace EBP that threatens our ability to demonstrate the effectiveness of our outcomes. That risk occurs when we uncritically adopt the hierarchy of levels of evidence, and it is compounded when the client's perspective is ignored (Coster, 2005; Sudsawad, 2006).

Fortunately, there are leaders in the EBM/EBP fields who are promoting a more integrated approach to EBP. This approach helps practitioners and researchers to value the client's collaboration in the clinical decision-making process and rely on their own practice expertise while appraising the best scientific evidence available. David Sackett, a leader in the practice and teaching of EBM, and his colleagues have updated the definition thus: "Evidence-based medicine (EBM) is the integration of best research evidence with clinical expertise and patient values." (Sackett, Straus, Richardson, Rosenberg, & Haynes, 2000, p. 1). They emphasize that practitioners must incorporate the patient's unique expectations, preferences, and concerns if practice decisions are to truly serve the individual.

Qualitative methodologies can be one form of research evidence that informs practitioners of client values and experiences (Sackett et al., 2000; Sudsawad, 2006; Tickle-Degnen & Bedell, 2003; Whiteford, 2005, 2007). However, qualitative studies are still considered to be at the lowest level in the hierarchy of levels of evidence (Mykhalovskiy, & Wier, 2004; Tickle-Degnen & Bedell, 2003; Whiteford, 2007). Evidence-based medicine is appropriately reliant on strict quantitative scientific method to study questions of pathophysiology. However, those reductionistic methods are likely to fall short in studying the complex phenomena associated with human behavior, meaning, and occupation. In a strict EBP approach, qualitative research methods that are more descriptive, narrative, or interpretive in nature are more easily discounted, and the credibility of much of the core of occupational therapy service (i.e., restoration of a meaningful life of action (Yerxa, 1991, 1998)) is thus diminished.

Occupational therapy needs an approach to EBP that supports **integrated practitioners** who use "integrated science." An integrated practitioner is one who considers the best scientific evidence while simultaneously attending to the humanistic aspects of the client's narrative and lived experience (Yerxa, 2005). Whether or not occupational therapists develop such an EBP approach and earn the respect of others in its use will likely depend on our skill in using currently defined best practice, demonstrating the value of our practices with multiple research methods, and collaboratively guiding the change to a more inclusive model of the types of evidence that are needed in a holistic and integrated field of practice such as occupational therapy.

Across professions, there are calls for new approaches to incorporate multiple methods and factors into the research appraisal process (Clarke, 1999; Kuzel & Engel, 2001; McGuire, 2005; Mykhalovskiy & Wier, 2004; Upshur, VanDenKerkhof, & Goel, 2001). Tickle-Degnen and Bedell (2003) offer an alternative appraisal model in their **heterarchical** approach, which suggests that therapists consider a network of factors for clinical decision making instead of a hierarchy of levels. Humphris (2000) suggests that the levels of evidence be viewed along a continuum in which the significance of the level is determined by the nature of the question or clinical situation being considered. In this approach, the congruity between the research or clinical question and the research methodology takes precedence in appraising the evidence (Ottenbacher, 1992).

Even if more inclusive and integrated models are created, they will be useful only if therapists adopt them as standard practice. McCluskey (2006) describes the barriers to implementing EBP in occupational therapy and the process of managing change in a fast-changing world. How will therapists find enough time and develop adequate skills (the most oft-cited barriers) to integrate EBP into their practices? These challenges cannot be addressed by individual practitioners alone but must be taken on by professional organizations, employers, and educational institutions to attain systematic change in the use of EBP. Occupational therapy theory development also needs to incorporate these concepts to support best evidence-based practice.

Theories and Models of Practice

Our theories themselves, if not constantly questioned, tested from new perspectives, and validated through research and practice, can be limits to our success. Kuhn (1970) argued that fields that tenaciously hold onto inadequate paradigms to support their theories and practices are likely to miss opportunities to envision new and more suitable paradigms, thus risking becoming ineffective. How well do our theories explain our most important phenomena of concern, such as occupation, life balance, adaptation, independence, and performance? How universally can theories that are developed in one country be applied elsewhere? How open are we to consider alternative explanatory theories?

Michael Iwama, an occupational therapist of Japanese ancestry who was raised in Canada, was confronted by just such a paradigm dilemma while on an extended teaching assignment in Japan. The result was the development, with his students, of the Kawa (River) model (Iwama, 2003, 2006). This model was developed because of the difficulty his students in Japan had in understanding and applying some Western concepts and models of occupational therapy and occupational science to their own lives. The Kawa model was built on assumptions about Japanese culture, which is more collectivist, naturalistic, interdependent, and hierarchically structured than is typical in Western cultures, and demonstrates the value of **cultural relativism**. If we envision occupational therapy becoming universally relevant, we must understand the cultural implications of our understandings of occupation and intervention (Iwama, 2005) and be open to reinterpreting or revising them. Iwama's own questions prompt important challenges for consideration:

> With whose cultural norms do we view our clients—especially those clients who fall outside of our conceptions of the normal? Do our current epistemologies, ideologies, theories and practice in occupational therapy truly abide within the lived realities of those we serve? To what extent do occupational therapists situated outside of the mainstream social spheres of experience participate in our knowledge production and discourse? (Iwama, 2005, p. 252)

Many other commonly used occupational therapy concepts need such critical scrutiny. Balance is one such idea that needs elaboration through research and theory development as well as a means of clearly applying it in practice, should it prove useful. Early work is being done to examine what life balance is (Blessing, 2004; Matuska & Christiansen, 2003), how to measure it (Erickson & Matuska, 2006; Matuska & Christiansen, 2003), and how to use it in practice (Davis, 2004). Occupational therapy has repeatedly emphasized the importance of independence as a goal of practice, yet the concept has not been fully explicated or researched. Alternatives to independent functioning such as the notion of interdependence (Gage, 1997; Higgs & Titchen, 2001) are emerging, especially as occupational therapists consider more inclusive cultural views (Iwama, 2006). Occupational justice is a relatively new idea that demands greater cultural competence and is providing a means of considering population-based occupational therapy.

OCCUPATIONAL JUSTICE

If we have difficulty in understanding the cultural differences of our clients, how well will we be able to serve them? So far in this chapter, the question of who is being served has focused more on the individual, the traditional unit of interest in occupational therapy. However, with the advent of the concept of occupational justice (Townsend & Wilcock, 2004; Wilcock, 1998b), occupational therapists are increasingly considering larger groups and entire populations in terms of opportunities for occupation and the social, cultural, political, economic, and geographic factors that control or affect access to participation. Significant numbers of the world's population experience occupational deprivation, the lack of opportunity to participate in needed or desired occupations; for example, over half the people of the world are malnourished and lack basic health care (World Health Organization, 2002). When such basic needs are not met, it is difficult to pursue higher-level needs (Maslow, 1943), ones that are usually associated with occupational fulfillment. People who are experiencing disability are often deprived of occupational opportunities either related directly to the impairment underlying the disability or, in many cases, due to the social construct of disability (Beer, 1998; Higgins, 1992; Liachowitz, 1988) in which political, attitudinal, physical, or social barriers limit occupational opportunities.

Often when I am teaching about occupational justice, students or therapists seem to be inspired by the concept of improving justice in the world through occupational therapy. However, a common question arises: "With so much need for occupational therapy in traditional settings, why should we be looking to do this kind of work?" My response is that once a practitioner has embraced the basic philosophy of the profession, (i.e., that occupational engagement and meaningful occupation are essential for health and well-being (Wilcock, 1998a, 1998b) and the environment either supports or constrains occupational performance), it is difficult to think about how occupational therapy would *not* be used to promote occupational justice. In other words, occupational justice is fundamental to our practice. Furthermore, whenever the occupational therapy process is used to help a person achieve occupational goals, it is assumed that occupational deprivation is remediated or prevented and thus occupational justice is advanced for that person.

What is our responsibility for addressing the problems of the world's people who are "constrained, deprived, and alienated from engaging in occupations that provide personal, family, and/or community satisfaction, meaning and balance through what they do" (Wilcock & Townsend, 2000, p. 85)? Do we accept the charge from the World Health Organization to "respond to each individual's spiritual quest for meaning, purpose, and belonging" along with the individual's rights to employment, rest, and leisure (World Health Organization, 1998, p. 2) by promoting participation and supporting pursuit of meaningful activities, that is, by applying an occupational therapy process to help correct injustices in these areas? If we, as an international profession do embrace occupational justice, there are many challenges to its admittedly utopian vision. However, if we are not in pursuit of an ideal world, we risk settling for less than the best of what occupational therapy has to offer.

There is, however, a growing awareness of occupational justice through publications and projects on health disparities (Braveman, 2006; Ford, Waring, & Boggis, 2006). International attention to the occupational justice–related projects featured in *Occupational Therapy Without*

Borders: Learning from the Spirit of Survivors (Kronenberg, Algado, & Pollard, 2005), as well as WFOT's adoption of CBR (Kronenberg, 2003), are useful examples. Currently, occupational justice is best known in circles of educators and those who are actively involved in international professional activities. Therefore, a key question to consider is whether or not concepts related to occupational justice will eventually be adopted by mainstream therapists and incorporated into what Kronenberg has called **political activities of daily living** (Kronenberg & Pollard, 2005). "The availability of occupational justice is determined by political factors in the occupational environment" (Kronenberg & Pollard, 2005, p. 67), and Kronenberg believes that those with political freedoms must take political action at whatever level is available to them to help resolve occupational injustices. The practice of political activities of daily living extends beyond writing letters to lawmakers, raising funds for a political cause, or voting regularly, as important as those activities are. Understanding the political nature of human relations and societies and then embodying that understanding so that political awareness and action for justice become activities of daily life is a key to achieving occupational justice.

When considering occupational justice in occupational therapy, one envisions practice as applied to large populations, although the concept does apply to individuals as well. However, to achieve the ambitious goals of an occupational justice vision, by thinking and working at the population level, occupational therapy can have a much greater impact than its usual focus on the individual. Yet what will it take to create a critical mass of therapists who view practice in this way to be able to realize significant gains for a more occupationally just world? How significantly will the educational process need to change for occupational therapists? Can it be integrated into an already crowded curriculum in a way that still allows graduates to competently enter more typical practice areas? Does occupational justice present a threat to the profession through taking the focus off our traditional unit of interest (the individual), or does it offer a potential boon by reaching greater numbers of individuals through population work, thus demonstrating greater value to society? Would an occupational therapist working strictly at the policy level in a national government still be doing occupational therapy? If he or she is promoting occupational justice through the policy work, does it matter? These are among the questions for pondering and reflection.

SUMMARY

This chapter provided an overview of occupational therapy practice with examples that present a small sample of the incredibly wide range of ways in which occupational therapy is practiced and pose many questions (and a few answers), designed to assist us in appraising the status of the field currently and into the future. The chapter began with an eye toward the many possibilities that exist for the profession, then examined some of the factors that threaten our realization of those possibilities. Throughout, we periodically considered the question of who is being served by our actions, which is perhaps the most crucial question we should continuously be asking ourselves.

The overview that was presented here is designed to help in creating a big picture of occupational therapy practice. A big picture, yes, but within the confines of this brief chapter, it is a necessarily incomplete one. Keeping an accurate vision of the big picture is one of the three steps that are recommended for successfully coping with the hyperchange (Weiner & Brown, 2006) in which we are all immersed. In keeping with that recommendation, I encourage you, the reader, to seek to complete this big picture of practice through your reading of this text and the many other sources of information about practice and international occupational therapy. Join your state and national association, as well as the World Federation of Occupational Therapists. Attend conferences to meet others in your field and hear firsthand your fellow occupational therapists' stories of research, practice, theory, and dreams. In doing so, you will likely learn, as I have, that the big picture of occupational therapy is ever changing, ever growing. Understanding the big picture of occupational therapy is like the view from an airplane leaving the earth: You see more and more of the world, but the more you take in, the more there is to see, and you realize that you will never get the whole picture—but how much fascination there is in seeking it!

I hope that you are prompted to reflect on these questions and press yourself and your fellow students and colleagues for answers and to use those answers to help chart the future of the profession. So I will leave you with two final questions:

1. What possibilities will occupational therapy realize?
2. What constraints and threats will we allow to hold us back or face creatively and adaptively to realize the promise of our unique field?

PROVOCATIVE QUESTIONS

1. Where does the greatest potential lie for occupational therapy to realize its greatest good for society? How should the profession pursue that potential?
2. Assuming that the current models of EBP do not optimally serve occupational therapy practice, what form of EBP will best serve the development of occupational therapy?

REFERENCES

Algado, S. S., & Burgman, I. (2005). Occupational therapy intervention with children survivors of war. In F. Kronenberg, S. S. Algado, & N. Pollard (Eds.), *Occupational therapy without borders: Learning from the spirit of survivors* (pp. 245–260). London: Elsevier.

American Occupational Therapy Association. (1995). Position paper: Occupation. *American Journal of Occupational Therapy, 49*(12), 1015–1018.

American Occupational Therapy Association. (2006). *AOTA's centennial vision.* Bethesda, MD: American Occupational Therapy Association.

American Occupational Therapy Association. (2007). *AOTA board certification & specialty certification.* Retrieved June 10, 2007, from http://www.aota.org/nonmembers/area15/links/link12.asp

American Society of Hand Therapists. (2007). *American Society of Hand Therapists home page.* Retrieved June 11, 2007, from http://www.asht.org/

Amini, D. (2004). Renaissance occupational therapy and occupation-based hand therapy. *OT Practice, 9*(3), 11–15.

Atwal, A. J. (2003). Struggling for occupational satisfaction: Older people in care homes. *British Journal of Occupational Therapy, 66*(3), 118–124.

Baptiste, S., & Martin, A. (1994). Maintaining a balance in service and education in a climate of fiscal crisis. *Canadian Journal of Occupational Therapy, 61*(1), 44–46.

Baum, C. (2006). Centennial challenges, millennium opportunities. *American Journal of Occupational Therapy, 60*(6), 609–616.

Baum, C., & Edwards, D. (1995). Occupational performance: Occupational therapy's definition of function; A position paper. *American Journal of Occupational Therapy, 49*(12), 1019–1020.

Beer, D. W. (1998). The illness and disability experience from an individual perspective. In M. E. Neistadt & E. B. Crepeau (Eds.), *Willard & Spackman's occupational therapy* (9th ed., pp. 32–53). Philadelphia: Lippincott.

Behr, S., Bass-Haugen, J., Gordon, C., Bennett, O., & Henderson, M. L. (2003, October). *Bachelor of science in occupational science: The evolution of a new degree.* Paper presented at the 2nd Annual Research Conference of the Society for Study of Occupation: USA, Park City, UT.

Blessing, L. (2003, October). *The impact of caregiving on lifestyle balance on elderly women.* Paper presented at the 2nd Annual Research Conference of the Society for Study of Occupation: USA, Park City, UT.

Braveman, B. (2006). AOTA's statement on health disparities. *American Journal of Occupational Therapy, 60*(6), 679.

Cate, Y. I., & Perez, M. R. (2004). Assistive technology for persons with low vision. *Technology Special Interest Section Quarterly, 14*(4), 1–4.

Chacksfield, J. (2006). COT should keep its hands off the specialist groups ... "Groups win clout through OT link." *Therapy Weekly, 33*(16), 4.

Christiansen, C. (1996). Nationally speaking. Managed care: Opportunities and challenges for occupational therapy in the emerging systems of the 21st century. *American Journal of Occupational Therapy, 50*(6), 409–412.

Christiansen, C. H. (1997). Acknowledging a spiritual dimension in occupational therapy practice. *American Journal of Occupational Therapy, 51*, 169–172.

Clark, F., Azen, S. P., Zemke, R., Jackson, J., Carlson, M., Mandel, D., et al. (1997). Occupational therapy for independent-living older adults. *Journal of the American Medical Association, 278*, 1321–1326.

Clark, F., Parham, D., Carlson, M., Frank, G., Jackson, J., Pierce, D., et al. (1991). Occupational science: Academic innovation in the service of occupational therapy's future. *American Journal of Occupational Therapy, 45*(4), 300–310.

Clark, F., Zemke, R., Frank, G., Parham, D., Neville-Jan, A., Hedricks, C., et al. (1993). Dangers inherent in the partition of occupational therapy and occupational science. *American Journal of Occupational Therapy, 47*(2), 184–186.

Clarke, J. (1999). Evidence based practice: A retrograde step? The importance of pluralism in evidence generation for the practice of healthcare. *Journal of Clinical Nursing, 8,* 89–94.

Coast to Coast School of Lymphedema Management. 2007. *Certification.* Retrieved May 25, 2007, from www.lymph edemamanagement.com/certification.asp

Cochrane, A. L. (1972). *Effectiveness and efficiency: Random reflections on health services.* London: Nuffield Provincial Hospitals Trust.

College of Occupational Therapists. (2004). *College of Occupational Therapists Practice Guidelines Development Manual.* London: College of Occupational Therapists.

Collins, M. (1998). Occupational therapy and spirituality: Reflecting on quality of experience in therapeutic interventions. *British Journal of Occupational Therapy, 61*(8), 280–284.

Corcoran, M. (2006). Dissemination or knowledge translation? *American Journal of Occupational Therapy, 60*(5), 487–488.

Coster, W. (2005). The foundation. International Conference on Evidence-Based Practice: A collaborative effort of the American Occupational Therapy Association, the American Occupational Therapy Foundation, and the Agency for Healthcare Research and Quality. *American Journal of Occupational Therapy, 59*(3), 356–358.

Crawford-White, J. (1996). Are primary health-care occupational therapists specialists or generalists? *British Journal of Therapy & Rehabilitation, 3*(7), 373–374, 376–379.

Crepeau, E. B. (1991). Achieving intersubjective understanding: Examples from an occupational therapy treatment session. *American Journal of Occupational Therapy, 45*(11), 1016–1025.

Cromwell, F. S. (1979, May). Should occupational therapists be generalists or specialists? *WFOT Bulletin,* 11–13.

Culshaw, H. M. S. (1995). Evidence-based practice for sale? *British Journal of Occupational Therapy, 58*(6), 233.

Daus, C. (1999). Fighting the good fight . . . to challenge Medicare outpatient cap on physical therapy, occupational therapy, and speech therapy. *Rehab Management: The Interdisciplinary Journal of Rehabilitation, 12*(2), 50, 52–53.

Davis, J. A. (2004). An occupational perspective on work-life balance. *Occupational Therapy Now, 6*(3), 3–5.

Eakin, P. (1997). Shifting the balance: Evidence-based practice. The Casson Memorial Lecture 1997. *British Journal of Occupational Therapy, 60*(7), 290–294.

Earley, D., & Shannon, M. (2006). The use of occupation-based treatment with a person who has shoulder adhesive capsulitis: A case report. *American Journal of Occupational Therapy, 60*(4), 397–403.

Egan, M., & De Laat, M. D. (1994). Considering spirituality in occupational therapy. *Canadian Journal of Occupational Therapy, 61,* 95–101.

Engelhardt, H. T. (1977). Defining occupational therapy: The meaning of therapy and the virtues of occupation. *American Journal of Occupational Therapy, 31*(10), 666–672.

Erickson, B., & Matuska, K. (2006, October, 2006). *How Do Adults With Multiple Sclerosis Experience Life Balance?* Paper presented at the Annual Research Conference of the Society for the Study of Occupation: USA, St. Louis, MO.

Evans, K. A. (1987). Definition of occupation as the core concept of occupational therapy: Hierarchy, developmental sequence, biopsychosocial unity, and adaptive capacities. *American Journal of Occupational Therapy, 41*(10), 627–628.

Fine, S. B. (1998). Surviving the health care revolution: Rediscovering the meaning of "good work." *Occupational Therapy in Mental Health, 14*(1/2), 7–18.

Ford, K., Waring, L., & Boggis, T. (2006). Living on the edge: The hidden voices of health disparities. *OT Practice, 12*(6), 17–22.

Foto, M. (1996). Nationally speaking. Generalist versus specialist occupational therapies. *American Journal of Occupational Therapy, 50*(10), 771–774.

Gage, M. (1997). From independence to interdependence: Creating synergistic health care teams. Muriel Driver Lectureship. *Canadian Journal of Occupational Therapy, 64*(4), 174–183.

Gentry, T. (2005). A brain in the palm of your hand: Assistive technology for cognition. *OT Practice, 10*(19), 10–12.

Hand Therapy Certification Commission. (2007). *Welcome to the Hand Therapy Certification Commission-HTCC.* Retrieved July 21, 2007, from http://www.htcc.org/

Hayes, R. L., & McGrath, J. J. (1998). Evidence-based practice: The Cochrane Collaboration, and occupational therapy. *Canadian Journal of Occupational Therapy, 65*(3), 144–151.

Henderson, M. L. (2004, October 29–31, 2004). *Program assessment of an undergraduate occupational science major.* Paper presented at the Society for the Study of Occupation: USA 3rd Annual Research Conference, Warm Springs, OR.

Higgs, J., & Titchen, A. (2001). Rethinking the practice-knowledge interface in an uncertain world: A model for practice development. *British Journal of Occupational Therapy, 64*(11), 526–533.

Higgins, P. C. (1992). *Making disability: Exploring the social transformation of human variation.* Springfield, IL: Charles C. Thomas.

Hilton, C. L., & Ranolph, D. S. (2003, October). *Context: An occupational science baccalaureate course.* Paper presented at the Society for the Study of Occupation: USA 2nd Annual Research Conference, Park City, UT.

Hinojosa, J. (2007). *Becoming innovators in an era of hyperchange: Eleanor Clarke Slagle Lecture.* Paper presented at the American Occupational Therapy Association's 87th Conference and Expo. St. Louis, MO. April 22, 2007.

Hocking, C., Whiteford, G., Henare, D., & Hansen, R. (1995). What constitutes core values in occupational therapy practice?: Core values and attitudes of occupational therapy practice. *American Journal of Occupational Therapy, 49*(2), 175–176.

Holm, M. B. (2000). Our mandate for the new millennium: Evidence-based practice. The 2000 Eleanor Clarke Slagle Lecture. *American Journal of Occupational Therapy, 54*(6), 575–585.

Holm, M. B. (2003). Evidence-based practice: Top 10 reasons for becoming an evidence-based practitioner. *OT Practice, 8*(3), 9–11.

Howard, B. S. (1991). How high do we jump?: The effect of reimbursement on occupational therapy. *American Journal of Occupational Therapy, 45*(10), 875–881.

Humphris, D. (2000). Types of evidence. In S. Hamer & G. Collinson (Eds.), *Evidence based practice: A handbook for practitioners.* (pp. 79–91) Edinburgh: Bailliere Tindall.

Iwama, M. (2003). The issue is: Toward culturally relevant epistemologies in occupational therapy. *American Journal of Occupational Therapy, 57,* 582–588.

Iwama, M. (2005). Occupation as a cross-cultural construct. In G. Whiteford & V. Wright-St. Clair (Eds.), *Occupation and practice in context* (pp. 242–253). London: Elsevier Churchill Livingstone.

Iwama, M. (2006). *The Kawa model: Culturally relevant occupational therapy.* New York: Churchill Livingstone.

Kimura, N. (1987). Establishing the core of occupational therapy. *WFOT Bulletin, 16,* 18–21.

Knutsson, H. (1980). Specialization versus generalization in occupational therapy treatment in Iceland. *WFOT Bulletin*(May), 22–25.

Kronenberg, F. (2003). *WFOT Draft position paper on community based rehabilitation.* Perth, Australia: World Federation of Occupational Therapists.

Kronenberg, F., Algado, S. S., & Pollard, N. (2005). *Occupational therapy without borders: Learning from the spirit of survivors.* London: Elsevier Churchill Livingstone.

Kronenberg, F., & Pollard, N. (2005). Overcoming occupational apartheid: A preliminary exploration of the political nature of occupational therapy. In F. Kronenberg, S. Simi-Algado, & N. Pollard (Eds.), *Occupational therapy without borders: Learning from the spirit of survivors* (pp. 58–86). London: Elsevier Churchill Livingstone.

Kuhn, T. S. (1970). *The structure of scientific revolutions* (2nd ed.). Chicago: University of Chicago Press.

Kuzel, A., & Engel, J. (2001). Some pragmatic thoughts about evaluating qualitative health research In J. Morse, J. Swanson & A. Kuzel (Eds.), *The nature of qualitative evidence* (pp. 114–138). Thousand Oaks, CA: Sage.

Lange, M. L., & Brians, D. (1995, April 8–12, 1995). *Environmental control systems: Conference abstracts and resources.* Paper presented at the American Occupational Therapy Association's 1995 annual conference and exposition, Denver, CO.

Law, M. (Ed.). (1998). *Client-centered occupational therapy.* Thorofare, NJ: Slack.

Law, M., Baptiste, S., Carswell, A., McColl, M., Polatajko, H. J., & Pollock, N. (2005). *The Canadian Occupational Performance Measure* (4th ed.). Toronto, Ontario: CAOT.

Law, M., Baptiste, S., & Mills, J. (1995). Client-centred practice: What does it mean and does it make a difference? *Canadian Journal of Occupational Therapy, 62*(5), 250–257.

Liachowitz, C. H. (1988). *Disability as a social construct: Legislative roots.* Philadelphia: University of Pennsylvania Press.

Mandel, D., Jackson, J. M., Zemke, R., Nelson, L., & Clark, F. (1999). *Lifestyle redesign: Implementing the well elderly program.* Bethesda, MD: AOTA.

Maslow, A. (1943). A theory of human motivation. *Psychological Review, 50,* 370–396.

Matuska, K., & Christiansen, C. (2003, October). *A model of occupational balance.* Paper presented at the 2nd Annual Research Conference of the Society for Study of Occupation: USA, Park City, UT.

McCluskey, A. (2006). Managing change and barriers to evidence-based practice. In G. Kielfhofner (Ed.), *Research in occupational therapy: Methods of inquiry for enhancing practice* (pp. 685–596). Philadelphia: F. A. Davis.

McGuire, W. L. (2005). Beyond EBM: New directions for evidence-based public health. *Perspectives in Biology and Medicine, 48*(4), 557–569.

Meyer, A. (1977). The philosophy of occupational therapy. *American Journal of Occupational Therapy, 31*(10), 639–642.

Mosey, A. C. (1992). Partition of occupational science and occupational therapy. *American Journal of Occupational Therapy, 46*(9), 851–853.

Mosey, A. C. (1993). Partition of occupational science and occupational therapy: Sorting out some issues. *American Journal of Occupational Therapy, 47*(8), 751–754.

Mykhalovskiy, E., & Wier, L. (2004). The problem of evidence-based medicine: Directions for social science. *Social Science and Medicine, 59,* 1050–1069

Nelson, D. (1997). Why the profession of occupational therapy will flourish in the 21st century. 1996 Eleanor Clarke Slagle Lecture. *American Journal of Occupational Therapy, 51*(1), 11–24.

Ottenbacher, K. J. (1992). Confusion in occupational therapy research: Does the end justify the method? *American Journal of Occupational Therapy, 46*(10), 871–874.

Ottenbacher, K. J., & Maas, F. (1999). Qualitative research series. How to detect effects: Statistical power and evidence-based practice in occupational therapy research. *American Journal of Occupational Therapy, 53*(2), 181–188.

Pierce, D. (2001). Untangling occupation in activity. *American Journal of Occupational Therapy, 55*(2), 138–146.

Polatajko, H. J. (2006). Our core business: Occupational therapy research our core focus: occupation . . . limiting or not? *OTJR: Occupation, Participation and Health, 26*(3), 86–87.

Ramugondo, E. L. (2005). Unlocking spirituality: Play as a health-promoting occupation in the context of HIV/AIDS. In F. Kronenberg, S. S. Algado, & N. Pollard (Eds.), *Occupational therapy without borders: Learning from the spirit of survivors* (pp. 313–325). London: Elsevier.

Rebeiro, K. L. (2001). Enabling occupation: The importance of an affirming environment. *Canadian Journal of Occupational Therapy, 68*(2), 80–89.

Rebeiro, K. L., Day, D. G., Semeniu, B., O'Brien, M. C., & Wilson, B. (2001). Northern Initiative for Social Action: An occupation-based mental health program. *American Journal of Occupational Therapy, 55*(5), 493–500.

Reilly, M. (1962). Occupational therapy can be one of the great ideas of 20th century medicine. Eleanor Clarke Slagle Lecture. *American Journal of Occupational Therapy, 16,* 1–9.

Sackett, D. L., Straus, S. E., Richardson, W. S., Rosenberg, W., & Haynes, R. B. (2000). *Evidence based medicine: How to practice and teach EBM* (2nd ed.). Edinburgh: Churchill Livingstone.

Sinclair, K. (2005). World connected: The international context of professional practice. In G. Whiteford & V. Wright-St. Clair (Eds.), *Occupation and practice in context* (pp. 104–126). London: Elsevier Churchill Livingstone.

Slater, D. Y. (2006). The ethics of productivity: Occupational therapy practitioners have a legal and ethical responsibility to their clients, regardless of facility policies. *OT Practice, 11*(19), 17–20.

Sudsawad, P. (2006). Definition, evolution, and implementation of evidence-based practice in occupational therapy. In G. Kielfhofner (Ed.), *Research in occupational therapy: Methods of inquiry for enhancing practice* (pp. 656–662). Philadelphia: F. A. Davis.

Tickle-Degnen, L., & Bedell, G. (2003). Heterarchy and hierarchy: A critical appraisal of the "levels of evidence" as a tool for clinical decision making. *American Journal of Occupational Therapy, 57*(2), 234–237.

Townsend, E., De Laat, D., Egan, M., Thibeault, R., & Wright, W. A. (1999). *Spirituality in enabling occupation: A learner-centered workbook.* Ottawa, Ontario: CAOT.

Townsend, E., & Wilcock, A. A. (2004). Occupational justice. In C. H. Christiansen & E. Townsend (Eds.), *Introduction to occupation: The art and science of living* (pp. 206–225). Upper Saddle River, NJ: Prentice-Hall.

Upshur, R. E., VanDenKerkhof, E. G., & Goel, V. (2001). Meaning and measurement: A new model of evidence in health care. *Journal of Evaluation in Clinical Practice, 7*(2), 91–96.

Urbanowski, R., & Vargo, J. (1994). Spirituality, daily practice, and the occupational performance model. *Canadian Journal of Occupational Therapy, 61*(2), 88–94.

Walker, K. F. (2001). Adjustments to managed health care: Pushing against it, going with it, and making the best of it. *American Journal of Occupational Therapy, 55*(2), 129–137.

Weiner, E., & Brown, A. (2006). *FutureThink: How to Think Clearly in a Time of Change.* Upper Saddle River, NJ: Pearson Education/Prentice Hall.

Whiteford, G. (2005). Knowledge, power, evidence: A critical analysis of key issues in evidence based practice. In G. E. Whiteford & V. Wright-St. Clair (Eds.), *Occupation & context in practice* (pp. 34–50). London: Elsevier.

Whiteford, G. (2007). Autonomy, accountability, and professional practice: contemporary issues and challenges. *New Zealand Journal of Occupational Therapy, 54*(1), 11–14.

Whiteford, G., Townsend, E., & Hocking, C. (2000). Reflections on a renaissance of occupation. *Canadian Journal of Occupational Therapy, 67,* 61–69.

Wilcock, A. (1993). A theory of the human need for occupation. *Occupational Science: Australia, 1*(1), 17–24.

Wilcock, A. (1998a). Occupation for health. *British Journal of Occupational Therapy, 61*(8), 340–345.

Wilcock, A. (1998b). *An occupational perspective of health.* Thorofare, NJ: Slack.

Wilcock, A. (2003). Occupational science and therapy: A new course at Deakin University, Geelong, Australia. *WFOT Bulletin, 47,* 28–31.

Wilcock, A. A., & Townsend, E. (2000). Occupational terminology interactive dialogue: Occupational justice. *Journal of Occupational Science, 7*(2), 84–86.

Wood, W. (1998). It is jump time for occupational therapy. *American Journal of Occupational Therapy, 52*(6), 403–411.

Wood, W., Nielson, C., Humphry, R., Coppola, S., Baranek, G., & Rourk, J. (2000). A curricular renaissance: Graduate education centered on occupation. *American Journal of Occupational Therapy, 54*(6), 586–597.

World Health Organization. (1998). *Health for all in the 21st century.* Geneva: World Health Organization.

World Health Organization. (2002). *Reducing risks, promoting healthy life.* Geneva: World Health Organization.

Western Psychological Services. 2007. Sensory Integration and Praxis Test (SIPT). Retrieved June 9, 2007, from http://portal.wpspublish.com

Wu, C.-Y., & Lin, K.-C. (1999). Defining occupation: A comparative analysis. *Journal of Occupational Science, 6*(1), 5–12.

Yerxa, E. J. (1967). The Eleanor Clark Lectureship-1966: Authentic occupational therapy. *American Journal of Occupational Therapy, 21*(1), 1–9.

Yerxa, E. J. (1991). Nationally speaking: Seeking a relevant, ethical, and realistic way of knowing for occupational therapy. *American Journal of Occupational Therapy, 45*(3), 199–205.

Yerxa, E. (1998). Health and the human spirit for occupation. *American Journal of Occupational Therapy, 52*(6), 412–418.

Yerxa, E. (2003). Dreams, decisions, and directions for occupational therapy in the millennium of occupation. In E. B. Crepeau, E. S. Cohn, & B. B. Schell (Eds.), *Willard & Spackman's occupational therapy* (10th ed., pp. 975–980). Philadelphia: Lippincott Williams & Wilkins.

Yerxa, E. (2005). *The infinite distance between the "I" and the "it."* Unpublished manuscript.

Yerxa, E., Clark, F., Frank, G., Jackson, J., Parham, D., Pierce, D., et al. (1989). An introduction to occupational science, a foundation for occupational therapy in the 21st century. *Occupational Therapy and Health Care, 6,* 1–15.

Youngstrom, M. J., Brayman, S. J., Anthony, P., Brinson, M., Brownrigg, S., Clark, G. F., et al. (2002). Occupational therapy practice framework: Domain and process. *American Journal of Occupational Therapy, 56*(6), 609–639.

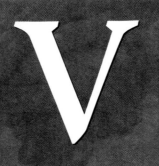

OT VALUES AND BELIEFS IN ACTION

❝ We are smart, talented people who have a passion to improve the lives of those we serve. We can provide leadership to our institutions, our communities, and to society. The work we do is so important. ❞

M. Carolyn Baum

Ethical Decision Making in Occupational Therapy Practice

28

REGINA F. DOHERTY

"The tools of ethical decision making include developing 'habits of thought' for reflection on complex, changing situations that are part of everyday practice."

—JENSEN (2005)

Learning Objectives

After reading this chapter, you will be able to:

1. Recognize the ethical issues that occupational therapy practitioners encounter in clinical practice.
2. Understand basic ethical theories and approaches to ethics.
3. Understand and apply an ethical decision-making guide for case analysis.
4. Understand and apply ethical reasoning as a construct within the clinical decision-making process.
5. Identify and know how to access ethics resources.
6. Understand effective communication strategies for difficult conversations.

WHY ETHICS?

Ask yourself the following questions:

- What would I do if a client told me that he had stopped taking his medication but he didn't want me to tell his doctor because the client had been giving the prescription to his girlfriend who "needs the drug more" but cannot afford it?

274

- How would I feel if the family of an infant with Down syndrome told me that they wanted to discontinue the infant's feeding tube because they did not think she would have a good quality of life?
- What would I say to a colleague who asked me to change my documentation to indicate that a client is worse than he really is so that the client can qualify for additional services?

Ethical questions like these often arise for occupational therapy practitioners in their day-to-day clinical practice. These questions must be attended to so that normal care delivery is not disrupted and best practice is achieved. This requires practitioners to recognize ethical situations and to have both the capacity and the willingness to address these situations systematically. This chapter discusses ethical issues that arise in occupational therapy practice. It serves as a foundation to aide the reader in understanding, recognizing, and reasoning through ethical issues. Occupational therapy practitioners in all professional roles will encounter ethical problems. Ethics is about reflecting, thinking, critically reasoning, justifying, acting on, and evaluating decisions. Ethical problems are often dynamic and complex, requiring additional knowledge and consultation with various resources. Consequently, knowledge and understanding of ethical reasoning and decision making are essential for competent occupational therapy practice.

ETHICS, MORALITY, AND MORAL REASONING

The terms *ethical* and *moral* are often used interchangeably in clinical practice, and though related, they have slightly different meanings. The term *ethics* stems from the Greek word *ethos,* meaning "character." Ethics is a branch of philosophy that involves systemic study and reflection providing language, methods, and guidelines to study and reflect on morality (Purtilo, 2005). In contrast, the term *morality* refers to social conventions about right and wrong human conduct and sets the stage for ethical behavior. Values, duty, and moral character guide reasoning and inform ethical decisions (Beauchamp & Childress, 2001). Values are the beliefs or objects a person holds dear (e.g., life). Duties describe an action that is required (e.g., provide food and shelter to care for ones family). Moral character describes traits or dispositions that facilitate trust and human flourishing (e.g., compassion, honesty) (Purtilo, 2005). There are three types of morality: personal, group or professional, and societal (Glaser, 2005). Personal morality includes individual beliefs and values. Group morality is the morality of the profession or group to which an individual belongs. A professional organization, such as the American Occupational Therapy Association (AOTA), maintains collective values that guide group decisions. For occupational therapists, this might be the emphasis on occupational performance. Societal morality is the morality of society as a whole. Societal values may change over time, and different communities may fight for the protection of different values and rights. It is important to reflect on how these different types of morality interrelate, because in a pluralistic society, no single vision of morality prevails, making ethical decision making ever challenging.

We use moral reasoning to reflect on ethical issues. Moral reasoning is about norms and values, ideas of right and wrong, and how practitioners make decisions in professional work (Barnitt, 1993). Ethics provides the mechanisms for this reflective process (Purtilo, 2005), which ultimately results in a course of action that practitioners feel is the most ethical to pursue. Ethical practice requires a commitment to personal conduct and an appreciation of its effect on others (Jennings, 2003).

Occupational therapy practice involves collaborating with clients to help them to optimize their independence and quality of life. This work consists of personal encounters that may bring with them difficult situations that challenge the value system of practitioners and society. Consequently, effective moral reasoning and ethical decision making are closely linked to effective practice (Bebeau, 2002; Hartwell, 1995; Sisola, 2000).

ETHICAL IMPLICATIONS OF TRENDS IN HEALTH CARE AND OCCUPATIONAL THERAPY PRACTICE

Health care systems are increasingly complex. New technologies, including those utilized in intensive care, life-sustaining treatment, reproductive medicine, genetics, and organ transplantation, have created ethical dilemmas for health care professionals relative to patient autonomy and the allocation of resources. Improved lifestyle choices, managed care, and changes in health care legislation also complicate occupational therapy practice, increasing the likelihood of encountering ethical dilemmas. Practitioners may face dual obligations regarding clients and the institutions that the practitioners serve centering on limited resources related to health care access and coverage. Tensions between what is good for society as a whole and what is best for the individual also arise in care delivery (Smith, Hiatt, & Berwick, 1999; World Health Organization, 1994). Common ethical issues that occupational therapy practitioners encounter include the following:

1. Confidentiality and disclosure
2. Quality of life
3. Clients' decision-making capacity
4. Personal and professional boundaries
5. Use of power
6. Resource allocation and priorities in treatment
7. Cultural, religious, and family considerations
8. Balancing benefits and harm in the care of patients (Barnitt, 1998; Fletcher, Miller, & Spencer, 1997; Foye, Kirschner, Wagner, Stocking, & Siegler, 2002; Purtilo, 2005).

The most frequently cited ethical issues that rehabilitation practitioners encounter are related to health care reimbursement, conflicts around goal setting, and patients' and/or caregivers' refusal to follow the team's recommendations (Foye et al., 2002). Occupational therapy practitioners often face competing demands between access to care and reimbursement for services. Balancing obligations to both patients and non-patient-related groups (e.g., payers, administrators) is a common struggle, and ethical issues arise when obligations to both cannot be met (Foye et al., 2002; Triezenberg, 2005).

VIRTUES OF HEALTH CARE PROFESSIONALS

Health care professionals hold a unique societal role because the public expects them to uphold particular virtues. These include the virtues of benevolence, competence, objectivity, caring, and compassion (Devettere, 2000; Fletcher et al., 1997; Pellegrino, 1995, 2002; Purtilo, 2005). First, the occupational therapy practitioner must be benevolent and focus on the good of the client. This often requires subordination of self-interest to that of the client. Second, the practitioner must be competent. All practitioners are responsible for achieving and maintaining competence in their area of clinical practice. Third, practitioners must be objective and use evidence to guide practice decisions. Fourth, practitioners must be caring because care enhances comfort and recovery (Fry & Veatch, 2000). While most practitioners recognize that caring is inherent in the health care professional's role, there are times when professionals must deal with difficult clients or families. There may be lack of reciprocity and mutuality caused by the condition itself, such as combativeness resulting from a head injury, which can erode the caring relationship. Erosions in care relationships can also occur when acuity rises and staffing diminishes (Maupin, 1995). Finally, practitioners must be compassionate. Compassion is the ability to enter into the experience of illness with the client (Pellegrino, 1982). Compassion is being kind, understanding, genuine, empathetic, caring, considerate, and professional in carrying out a task or duty. From time to time, all health care providers will experience complex situations and conflicting demands. It is during these times that practitioners must call on both character and conduct to provide compassionate care.

DISTINGUISHING AMONG CLINICAL, LEGAL, AND ETHICAL PROBLEMS IN PRACTICE

Practitioners must learn to distinguish ethical questions from other questions that they encounter in the care of clients. Many times, what might appear to be an ethical issue is in fact something else, such as a miscommunication or a clinical or a legal issue. For example, a clinical question would be "Can clients with severe dysphasia due to end-stage amyotrophic lateral sclerosis (ALS) eat?" This is a clinical question because there is a diagnostic answer to the question. Clients who pass a modified barium swallow (MBS) test are clinically able to eat. If they fail this test but want to continue eating orally, an ethical question could arise. The ethical question would be "Should clients with end-stage ALS who fail a MBS test eat?" This is an ethical question, as it raises questions relative to quality of life and the risks and benefits of eating with diminished swallowing capacity.

Legal questions may also arise in decision making in patient care. Law and ethics are related fields; however, they have different goals and sanctions. Both rely on analytical processes and ground rules for good decision making; however, laws are legislated and are legally enforceable (Horner, 2003). Laws prescribe what we cannot do. What may be permitted legally might not be justified ethically and vice versa. In the case of clients with ALS, a legal question would be "Do competent clients have the right to refuse medical advice and continue eating orally despite the recommendation of the team?" This example highlights the importance of distinguishing the type of question to more critically reason through the problem.

Reflection and Ethical Practice

Recognizing the morally significant features of a situation is the first step in ethical reflection. Reflection is a form of self-assessment that can be used to improve practice. Developing reflective capacity is a critical element in professional development and competence (Jensen & Richert, 2005). When reflecting on ethical aspects of practice, practitioners must consider their own values and how those values might influence their work. A value is a belief or an ideal to which an individual is committed (Kanny, 1993). Values clarification is commonly used to aid providers in reflection. Clarifying values and opinions allows practitioners to see elements of a situation that they did not see before, allowing for better appreciation of the complexity of decisions. For a values clarification exercise see Exercise 28.A on the Willard & Spackman Website.

Another form of reflection is mindfulness. Mindful practice entails metaprocessing—thinking about thinking or feeling about feelings. Mindful practice enables practitioners to listen more attentively to clients' distresses, recognize their own errors, refine their technical skills, make evidence-based decisions, and recognize the values necessary to act with compassion, competence, presence, and insight (Epstein, 1999).

Use of narratives, both written and oral, is another form of reflection. Telling stories allows therapists to reason through the moral features of a situation and develop a judgment about what ought to be done (Mattingly, 1998).

Guided narrative review with a mentor is an effective way to infuse ethical reasoning into clinical practice.

Identifying Different Types of Ethical Problems

When reflecting on an ethical issue, it is important to distinguish among the different types of ethical problems that occur in clinical practice. An ethical problem is a situation that is believed to have negative implications regarding cherished moral values and duties *and* that will pose an extremely difficult choice to an individual or group of individuals (Purtilo, 2005). It may be manifested by an emotional reaction such as discomfort, anxiety, or anger. An ethical issue is often captured when the clinician says, "This just doesn't feel right." This "not right" feeling is an emotional response that serves as a trigger to initiate ethical reflection. These feelings are often moral challenges and must be worked out beyond gut feelings to reasoned alternatives and actions.

Ethical distress is a type of problem that occurs when clinicians know the right thing to do but cannot achieve it because of external barriers or uncertainty about the outcome (Purtilo, 2005). Often, multiple stakeholders are involved in the care of the client (e.g., the primary care physician, consulting specialists, rehabilitation practitioners, the organizational administrator, the private insurer, and the family). Ethical distress occurs when stakeholders hold different opinions regarding the goals of care, leaving practitioners with no clear course of action. While conflict may arise in the care of patients, the paramount goal should always be patient's welfare. Ethical distress must be worked through so that this goal can be achieved.

An ethical dilemma is slightly different from an ethical distress. A dilemma is a situation that is marked by conflict between ethical beliefs and involves choice between alternatives that appear to be equally morally unacceptable (Purtilo, 2005). An ethical dilemma exists when the individual has obligations to do both X and Y but cannot do both (Horner, 2003). In a true dilemma, there is a strong persuasive argument both for and against a course of action, posing a moral conflict for the individual.

ETHICAL THEORIES AND PRINCIPLES THAT APPLY TO CLINICAL PRACTICE

Theories provide support for clinical decision making. Ethical theories and principles provide us with language for diagnosing, communicating, and problem solving ethical questions in clinical practice. Ethical theories are well-developed, systematic frameworks of rules and principles (R. J. Nash, 2002). They provide reasons and ideals for ethical standards. Many ethical approaches and theories serve as a reference point for guiding clinical decision making. The most commonly used ethical approaches in health care ethics are principle-based approaches, virtue- and character-based ethics, utilitarianism, and deontology.

Principle-Based Approach

A principle-based approach to ethics relies on ordinary shared moral beliefs as theoretical content. Principles are duties, rights, or other moral guidelines that provide a logical approach to analyzing ethical issues for a given situation. In case analysis, principles are identified, applied, and compared to weigh one principle against another in deciding a course of action. The following principles are commonly used in clinical ethics:

◆ Autonomy. Autonomy is the ability to act independently on one's own decisions (Beauchamp & Childress, 2001). Because autonomy is so highly valued in Western society and medicine, it is often regarded as the most important element in health care decision making (Pellegrino, Siegler, & Singer, 1991).
◆ Beneficence. Beneficence refers to actions done on or for the benefit of others.
◆ Nonmaleficence. Nonmaleficence is the duty not to harm others.
◆ Fidelity. Fidelity means being faithful to both implicit and explicit promises or commitments.
◆ Justice. Justice refers to equal treatment. It deals with the proper distribution of benefits, burdens, and resources. Procedural justice is often used to reflect impartial decision-making procedures. Distributive justice refers to the equitable allocation of societal resources such as health care (Horner, 2003).
◆ Veracity. Veracity refers to telling the truth.
◆ Paternalism or parentalism. Paternalism or parentalism occurs when an individual assumes to know best and makes decisions for the client (rather than with a client). Paternalism can limit clients' access to information and violates their autonomy.

Virtue- and Character-Based Ethics

Virtues are dispositions of character and conduct that motivate and enable clinicians to provide good care (Fletcher, Miller, & Spencer, 1997). Virtue ethics, derived from Aristotle and Thomas Aquinas, focuses on moral agents and their good character. Using this approach, moral goodness is achieved when behaviors are chosen for the sake of virtue (caring and kindness) rather than obligation.

Utilitarianism

Utilitarianism derived from the work of Jeremy Bentham and John Stuart Mill is concerned with actions that maximize good consequences and minimize bad consequences. From this perspective, morally right acts produce the best overall results; that is, the ends justify the means. Utilitarianism is often used in public policy development. A common criticism of utilitarianism is that it deemphasizes relationships to maximize outcomes for as many people as possible.

Deontology

Deontology is a duty-based moral theory that is based primarily on the work of Immanuel Kant. In this theory, moral rules are universal and never to be broken; consequently, doing one's duty is considered primary, regardless of the consequences. For example, truthfulness is an unconditional Kantian duty. A practitioner would never protect a client from the truth even if the truth would harm the client in some way. From a Kantian perspective, respect for people is a moral imperative; therefore, withholding the truth disrespects clients' right to know. A common criticism of deontology is that it overlooks the potential for conflicting obligations, overemphasizes rules, and underemphasizes the consequences of action.

ETHICAL RESOURCES AND JURISDICTION

Resources

Practitioners who face ethical issues must be knowledgeable about the resources that exist to support them in this dimension of their clinical reasoning. Resources are crucial for sharing the uncertainties related to ethical issues that practitioners encounter at all levels of practice.

Ethics Committees

Ethics committees support practitioners who need assistance in reasoning about ethical dimensions of care. The three primary roles of ethics committees are consultation, education, and policy review and development. The courts, the President's Commission for the Study of Ethical Problems in Medicine and Biomedical and Behavioral Research, and accrediting agencies such as the Joint Commission on the Accreditation of Hospital Organizations recommend consultation with ethics committees (Aulisio, Arnold, & Younger, 2000). Ethics committees provide an environment for safe and open discussion of basic moral questions, ease the feelings of staff, provide knowledgeable resources, and empower clinicians to make morally justified decisions.

Effective ethics committees are interdisciplinary and have strong institutional support. They analyze cases from many different perspectives to ensure the best outcome for clients. Occupational therapy practitioners who are either interested novices or experts in ethics should serve as members of ethics committees because they can bring broad perspectives to ethics discussions, are resources for topics related to values clarification and quality of life, and are skilled in group facilitation. Practitioners in settings without ethics committees should use their mentors, managers, administrative supports, and professional organizations

for assistance with ethical issues. Other organizational resources, such as the office of patient care advocacy (also known as the ombudsman), office of social work, chaplaincy service, and office of legal counsel, can also provide guidance with ethical issues.

Institutional Review Boards

Increased impetus for research and attention to evidence-based practice have resulted in an increase in the number of occupational therapy practitioners involved in clinical research. All clinicians who are involved in research activity have a moral obligation to familiarize themselves with the rules, regulations, and ethical obligations of conducting responsible research. There are many ethical considerations in research (e.g., data integrity, conflict of interest, authorship), but the most compelling pertains to human subjects as research participants.

To ensure an objective review of ethical issues related to human subject research, any institution that receives federal funding is required to have an Institutional Review Board (IRB). An IRB is a panel of diverse individuals, including organization staff and at least one community member, who are responsible for reviewing all research proposals and grants to ensure that adequate protections for research participants are in place. These protections include informed consent, research design and methodology, recruitment, the balance of risks and benefits, and confidentiality. The three fundamental principles that guide the ethical conduct of research involving human participants are respect for persons (autonomy), beneficence, and justice (National Commission for the Protection of Human Subjects of Biomedical and Behavioral Research, 1979). Occupational therapy practitioners should refer to their organization's specific policies and regulations regarding oversight and training in ethical conduct in research.

Codes of Ethics

Codes of ethics embody professional ethics (Banks, 2004). They are written documents produced by professional associations, organizations or regulatory bodies that state the commitment to a service ideal or core purpose. Ethical codes ensure public trust and safeguard the reputation of a profession. Codes of ethics are often aspirational, educational, and regulatory in nature (Banks, 2004). The values articulated in the ethical code serve to guide professional practice.

The AOTA's Occupational Therapy Code of Ethics (AOTA, 2005) serves as a guide to professional conduct. It is supported by the Guidelines to the Occupational Therapy Code of Ethics (AOTA, 2006) and the Core Values and Attitudes of Occupational Therapy Practice (AOTA, 1993). Together, these three documents, known as the Ethics Standards, serve as resources to all occupational therapy practitioners encouraging them to attain the highest level of professional behavior. These documents reflect the values and beliefs of the profession and provide clarification and support when an ethical issue arises. Additional information about the code and related documents and the AOTA Ethics Commission can be found at www.aota.org.

Regulatory Agencies

Three types of organizations provide oversight for occupational therapy practice: the AOTA, the National Board of Certification in Occupational Therapy, and state regulatory boards. Each has distinct concerns, sanctions, and jurisdiction, but one commonality is their concern for ethical practice.

The American Occupational Therapy Association

The AOTA, the professional association for occupational therapy, is the primary vehicle for influencing, promoting, and developing the profession's services to society (Doherty, Peterson, and Braveman 2006). The AOTA develops standards of practice for all occupational therapy practitioners. These standards are an essential resource for clinicians, students, educators, and researchers. As health care professionals, occupational therapy practitioners have an obligation to understand, respect, and demonstrate the values and ethics of the profession (Slater, 2006).

Within AOTA, the Ethics Commission reviews the AOTA Occupational Therapy Code of Ethics every five years. Its primary responsibility is to recommend the ethics standards for the profession. It also educates members and consumers regarding ethics standards. Ethics Commission members and staff of the AOTA Ethics Program are resources for students, clinicians, educators, and consumers. They provide assistance with the interpretation of relevant ethical principles via advisory opinions, consultation, articles, and presentations. Finally, the Ethics Commission is responsible for the process of developing and implementing the enforcement procedures for the code. Disciplinary actions apply to members of AOTA and include reprimand, censure, probation, suspension of membership, and permanent revocation of membership.

National Board for Certification of Occupational Therapy

The National Board for Certification in Occupational Therapy (NBCOT) is a credentialing agency that provides certification for the occupational therapy profession (NCBOT, 2006). Its mission is to serve the public interest by assuring the competency of all certified occupational therapy practitioners. NBCOT establishes minimum standards for certification to enter practice and ongoing recertification standards, including continuing competency through professional development. The NBCOT Certifi-

cant Code of Conduct outlines professional responsibilities for certified occupational therapy practitioners. As in many organizational codes of conduct, the NBCOT Certificant Code of Conduct includes ethics-related principles such as fairness, honesty, truthfulness, and technical competence. Violation of this code of conduct is grounds for sanction, which may entail reprimand, probation, or suspension or revocation of certification. Suspension or revocation of certification prohibits sanctioned individuals from practicing occupational therapy.

The NBCOT Qualifications and Compliance Review Committee oversees certification violation issues such as breaches of ethics and unprofessional practice. NBCOT notifies state regulatory boards and the public of any complaints it receives and the disciplinary action it takes in response to these complaints. Additional information about NBCOT and the NBCOT Certificant Code of Conduct can be found at www.nbcot.org.

State Regulatory Boards

State regulatory or licensing boards (SRBs) safeguard and promote the public welfare by ensuring that qualifications and standards for professional practice are properly evaluated, applied, and enforced (Doherty, Peterson, & Braveman, 2006). Occupational therapy is regulated in all 50 states and in three U.S. territories. The level of regulation varies; therefore, all occupational therapy practitioners must be aware of the specific provisions and statutes for the state in which they work. Most states use professional licensure to regulate practice, but several have certification, registration, or simply trademark requirements. Licensure is a means of defining a lawful scope of practice. It ensures patient protections and legally articulates the domain of practice for the profession. Licensure also prevents nonqualified individuals from practicing occupational therapy or using the title "occupational therapist" or "occupational therapy assistant." Many states include codes of ethics or codes of ethical conduct) statements in their licensure law or regulations. SRBs have the authority by state law to discipline occupational therapy clinicians who violate regulations, including the state's code of ethics. Practitioners have the responsibility to understand the regulations under which they work and the procedure for processing a complaint.

THE ETHICAL DECISION-MAKING PROCESS

The ethical decision-making process, like the clinical reasoning process, aids in reasoning through a problem in a structured and systematic way. This process provides a way for practitioners to give due consideration to issues, reflect on them, formulate possible alternatives, and make thoughtful choices. Common aspects of ethical decision-making models are the need for the clinician to do the following:

1. Identify the ethical question
2. Gather the relevant data
3. Formulate a moral diagnosis
4. Problem-solve practical alternatives and decide on an alternative for action
5. Act on the choice and evaluate the results (Bailey & Schwartzberg, 2003; Gervais, 2005; Hansen & Kyler-Hutchison, 1989; Miller, Fletcher, & Fins, 1995; Purtilo, 2005; Scanlon & Glover, 1995).

CASE STUDY: *Dual Obligations and Difficult Conversations: Ethical Issues in Confidentiality and Refusal of Services*

Maura is an occupational therapist working for an early intervention (EI) program. She received a referral on a 2 ½ year old girl named Jen Stone who was recently discharged from the hospital. Jen is the youngest of five children, and the reason for her referral to EI was a recent hospital admission following a home accident. Jen was injured when the Stones were moving. During the move, they removed a door from its hinges to move several large pieces of furniture. The door fell on Jen, resulting in head trauma. Maura's initial evaluation noted that Jen was profoundly delayed in all developmental milestones. Her vocabulary was limited to about 10 words, and she demonstrated a mild left hand weakness and significant delays in fine motor skills. Jen rarely smiled and demonstrated significant stranger anxiety during the evaluation. Ms. Stone reported that all her children were "slow talkers." Ms. Stone thinks that Jen needs medication because of the way she hit her head. In subsequent conversation with Ms. Stone, Maura realized that Ms. Stone was talking about phenobarbital, an anticonvulsant medication that is prescribed to prevent seizures and not designed to foster development. Maura explained the purpose of the medicine and that Jen needs extensive therapy to assist with her neurological recovery. Ms. Stone told Maura that everyone in the hospital wanted Jen to go to a rehabilitation facility but that she really wanted to take Jen home. Maura concluded that Ms. Stone had a poor understanding of typical child development and how this head injury would affect Jen.

Maura left the Stones troubled by the case and with serious questions about Jen and her family. In her monthly meeting with the EI team, Maura brought up her concerns. Shoshona, the caseworker assigned to Jen's case, reported that "this is a high-risk family" and that other siblings had been admitted to the hospital in the past only to be taken home against medical advice. After that meeting, Maura and some of her coworkers went for a quick cup of coffee. As Maura waited in the line at the coffee shop, Shoshona said, "Stick with that Stone case. Make sure you do whatever you need to stay involved. Remember this is a high-risk family." Maura was shocked at this breach of confidentiality and said, "Remember, we are not at the office anymore."

The following week when Maura went to see Jen, Ms. Stone would not let her in, saying that her husband had overheard some people talking about them in a coffee shop. Mr. Stone had told his wife, "If you let *them* in the house again, *you* will regret it." Maura quickly apologized and left, embarrassed, upset, and concerned about Jen and her family.

This case highlights how in clinical ethics, a client's story often begins in one setting and continues to unfold in another. It also highlights the imperative nature of facts in complex ethical decision making. To ensure a professional and caring response to this situation Maura must carefully analyze the ethical issues. The ethical decision-making process serves to help guide her thinking and actions. The following sections describe that process.

Identify the Ethical Question

The first step in addressing an ethical issue is to determine that the problem has an ethical dimension separate from other dimensions (clinical, legal, and political). The occupational therapy practitioner must identify and reflect on the ethical questions that have emerged in the case. This often begins with the question "What should I do?" In the case of Jen and Maura, some of the ethical questions are as follows:

- Should Maura persist in seeking to follow up with Ms. Stone and Jen? If she does, will she be doing more harm than good?
- Should the Stones have the right to refuse services for their daughter?
- Should the facility discuss the breach in confidentiality with the Stones? With their overseeing agencies? Could the facility regain the trust of the family despite this breach?
- Should Maura advocate for the organization or for Jen and the Stones? How can she balance her dual obligations to the Stone family and the organization?

In clinical practice, ethical questions often occur alongside clinical and legal questions. Our emphasis here is on the ethical analysis of this case. However, practitioners must also be aware of the legal and clinical dimensions to effectively analyze complex cases. One of the ethical questions identified above is "*Should* the Stones have the right to refuse services for their daughter?" This is different from the legal question "*Do* the Stones have the right (legally) to refuse services for their daughter?" One of the clinical questions in this case is "What would be the impact of denied therapeutic intervention on Jen's development?" Another is "What is the evidence to support timing of intervention following head injury?" The practitioner must consider these various dimensions and reflect on the contribution of each to the overall critical reasoning process, the goal being to achieve the best outcome for the client.

Gather the Relevant Data

The next step in ethical analysis is to gather the relevant data identifying the known facts and beliefs about the case. It is important to distinguish between the two. Facts are needed to make judicious decisions. Facts regarding medical information and factors such as family context, client preferences, social and cultural issues, institutional factors, and provider considerations should be confirmed for accuracy. Additional information should be sought if needed.

Some of the facts regarding the current problem are as follows:

◆ Jen presents with developmental skills that are well below the norm for her chronological age.
◆ The Stones took Jen home against the advice of hospital staff members, who recommended transferring Jen to an inpatient rehabilitation facility.
◆ Ms. Stone has a low education level.
◆ Maura has been denied access to the home.
◆ The caseworker broke confidentiality and violated client privilege when talking about the case at the coffee shop.

Some of the beliefs are as follows:

◆ There might be neglect or abuse in the home.
◆ Jen's parents are not acting in her best interests by refusing inpatient rehabilitation and early intervention.
◆ Jen's baseline status was one of significant developmental delay.
◆ Jen would have made more progress in a rehabilitation facility than at home.
◆ The Stones believe that the caseworker's breach of confidence was intentional. (In most cases, breaches in confidentiality are not malicious in nature but rather are either unintentional disclosures with the goal of bringing about a good result or the result of carelessness.)

Formulate a Moral Diagnosis

Once the information has been gathered, a moral diagnosis must be formulated by identifying the type of ethical problem and the principles that apply to the case. If there is more than one problem, they should be ranked in order of importance.

Having considered the ethical questions in the case of Jen, Maura must decide whether the ethical problem is distress or dilemma. As is common in clinical practice, many cases pose distress; however, Jen's case is a true dilemma because Maura is faced with two courses of action, both of which appear to be unacceptable. If she returns, Jen and Ms. Stone might be harmed by Mr. Stone. If she does not return, Jen's development is at risk. Maura is having difficulty deciding what to do that will both honor the principles of beneficence (doing good for Jen) and nonmaleficence (not causing harm to Jen and Ms. Stone). Maura knows that Shoshona's breach of confidentiality violated the family's trust (fidelity) and that she must take steps at her facility to ensure that the confidentiality of others is not violated in this way again (justice). Maura is also in a position in which she might need to balance organizational and professional responsibilities.

There are many stakeholders in this case, and there are multiple issues of power between and among Mr. and Ms. Stone, Maura, Shoshona, and the EI agency.

Problem-Solve Practical Alternatives and Decide on a Course of Action

Now that Maura has delineated the facts and beliefs about the problem, she must begin to identify practical alternatives and decide what do. Maura must ask herself, "What is the good or right thing to do?" She would be wise to seek out ethics resources in her facility and to ask her mentors for guidance in this ethical analysis. She might consult with various stakeholders, such as the social work office, the EI service director, Jen's pediatrician, and the team, to identify strategies to engage the family and regain their trust. She could also meet with the agency's ethics committee or read resources such as the AOTA Occupational Therapy Code of Ethics. These resources will help to guide Maura's reflection and subsequent actions. Generating a list of alternatives enables evaluation of the positive and negative consequences. Once the alternatives have been identified, ethical theory should be applied to support and justify the proposed action.

Maura brainstormed a list of possible alternatives:

◆ Approach Ms. Stone one last time to clarify the facts and ensure that she is making an informed refusal of services
◆ Apologize for the breach in confidentiality in an attempt to move forward
◆ Tell the family about the steps the agency has taken to ensure that this breach in confidentiality does not happen again

Continued

◆ Offer an alternative practitioner to work with Jen
◆ Offer an alternative agency or setting to provide services

Maura will need to reason through the alternatives, apply ethical theory to support her actions, and come to a judgment on the best approach. Maura and her employer might also need to consult with agency's legal counsel, since the confidentiality breach represents a HIPAA (Health Insurance Portability and Accountability Act) violation. Having virtue, sensitivity to ethical issues, and a process for analyzing ethical questions are important elements in ethical decision making. Maura weighs all of the alternatives and, after conversations with multiple resources, decides to reapproach Ms. Stone ensure that she is making an informed refusal and, if so, to offer her alternative agencies to service Jen and social service resources, should she wish to pursue them.

Act on That Choice and Evaluate the Results

Now that Maura has decided on the course of action, she must act on the decision, bridging the gap between knowing what she ought to do and actually doing it. This is where the Aristotelian notion of practical wisdom and moral argument join together with clinical judgment for action. Often, this is the most difficult step because it requires calling on moral courage to take positions that are unpopular or contrary to the interest of others (Aulisio et al., 2000). Moral courage is a skill. It involves facing and overcoming fear to uphold an ultimate good.

Maura will need courage to talk with Ms. Stone. She must uphold the virtue of humility and acknowledge the error in the EI system. Maura must also have the fortitude and skill to engage the family in regaining trust so that Jen will have access to therapy. She will need to be attentive to the interests and emotions of the family and remember the ultimate goal, which is to get Jen the therapy she needs. Maura must justify her action with moral reasons. If the social worker and Maura gather evidence of abuse or neglect in the home, they will need to familiarize them-

selves with EI agency and state policies on mandated reporting. Maura will need to be creative in coming up with alternatives to this complex situation so that the ultimate goal of caring for Jen is achieved. She might also have to make sacrifices for Jen's benefit. This could include withdrawing from the case and turning it over to a different EI agency so that Jen will receive intervention.

Finally, Maura must evaluate the results of her action. Evaluation includes both current and retrospective analysis. Seeking the input of knowledgeable colleagues and even ethics committee members can be helpful in evaluating the outcome of the actions taken. This analysis can guide future action by either avoiding or preventing a similar situation or knowing how to act should a similar situation arise in the future. Questions Maura might ask are as follows:

◆ What have I learned from this case to help improve future patient care?
◆ What have I learned that will contribute to my own moral life and to my virtues as a practitioner?
◆ How has this case affected me as a care provider?
◆ What additional knowledge do I need to be more effective in handling future ethical dilemmas?

Evaluation of the decision-making process in cases such as this one has the potential to change clinical practice, policies, education, or service delivery systems. Evaluation provides the opportunity for personal and professional reflection that can lead to further professional development and greater confidence to respond to future ethical dilemmas. Maura could also work with her colleagues and agency to make changes in policies (such as confidentiality and disclosure) and staff education so that a similar breach of confidentiality does not occur in the future. Maura should also consider how those she consulted with contributed to the case and should critique her own decision-making process to improve her future practice.

DIFFICULT CONVERSATIONS

The case of Maura and Jen highlights how practitioners must engage in difficult conversations. Some of these are with clients, some with families, and some with colleagues. While these conversations may be uncomfortable and awkward, through development of effective listening and communication strategies, practitioners can become more skillful and confident in meeting this challenge.

Occupational therapy practitioners who are empathetic are better prepared for difficult conversations. The discus-

sion of empathy is relevant in ethical decision making as it can help practitioners appreciate the experience of those who seek their care. However difficult these discussions might be, clients also have difficult choices. Developing the ability to evaluate a client or family's behavior requires practitioners to appreciate and accept a different perspective and different choices (Cohen, 2004). This is the first step in demonstrating moral sensitivity.

Open communication and empathy are key components to the delivery of compassionate care. The following are suggestions for effective communication:

1. **Be present.** Always respect others. Try to minimize interruptions and ensure that the environment is as free of distractions as possible. Choose an appropriate communication style for the situation. Establish rapport by making good eye contact, sitting close to the person, and/or touching the person as appropriate to communicate support.

2. **Use open-ended communication and listen quietly.** We often say too much, which does not allow time for the other person to speak. Phrases such as "go on" can encourage the person to examine issues at a deeper level (Cameron, 2004).

3. **Remain focused on the person and the goals of intervention.** Are the goals appropriate and achievable? Do they maximize benefit and minimize burden? If the conversation begins to stray off the topic, bring it back by stating, "While I appreciate you sharing that interesting information, it diverts us from our focus today, which is on. . . ."

4. **Be contrite and humble.** If you do not know the answer to a question, say so and assure the person that you will find the answer. Then find the answer and follow up with the person. Share your uncertainty about the case or prognosis.

5. **Legitimize the losses that the person is experiencing.** It is important to acknowledge the person's experience. Many clients are not prepared to cope with their newly diagnosed condition. They did not expect ever to be in a compromised state, and their family might not be able to cope with the personal or financial implications of this change. Denial, depression, and anger are common responses to disease and disability. Practitioners need to acknowledge these emotions openly by stating, "What I am hearing you say is that you are angry that you can no longer cook" or "Let me see if I can summarize what your daughter is trying to say. . . . . Is that correct?"

6. **If you are having difficulty with an issue, think how the problem might be experienced from the client's perspective** (L. Nash, 1981). By listening more openly to the other side of the argument, one can appreciate it for what it is (Cohen, 2004).

7. **Acknowledge 'the elephant in the room'** (Quill, 2000). Questions surrounding quality-of-life and end-of-life issues can be especially complex. Occupational therapy practitioners who have established relationships with their clients are obligated to fully inform clients of the likelihood of the success or failure of therapeutic interventions. It is important to engage clients in shared decision making. Practitioners should keep questions straightforward, listen carefully to answers, and follow the person's lead by asking focused follow-up questions using the person's own words. Asking questions such as "What are your most important hopes?" and "What are your biggest fears?" can assist both practitioner and client in setting appropriate goals for care (Quill, 2000).

8. **Pay attention to the words you use and how you use them.** Be aware of your tone, facial expressions, and body language. Use calm and composed language (Weeks, 2001). If the content of your message is clear, the listener can better process the information.

CONCLUSION

Ethical issues are ever present in professional practice and will continue to challenge occupational therapy practitioners as the fields of medicine, technology, and health care delivery evolve. Occupational therapists must recognize, critically reason, act, and reflect on ethical issues that arise in their professional roles. Occupational therapy practitioners who are reflective and knowledgeable in ethical decision-making processes are best prepared to successfully address ethical aspects of practice. Ethical behavior is the responsibility of all occupational therapy professionals.

> You have chosen a career path that will require complex (and at times perplexing) judgments about morality regarding patient care, health policy and other aspects of professional life. Many such judgments will have significance in terms of your own moral life, that of your profession, and that of society. But the path is not one you must forge anew every step of the way. (Purtilo, 2000)

ON THE WEB

See the Willard & Spackman Website for additional case studies and exercises.

- Case Study 28.A: Academic Honesty in a Community Placement
- Case Study 28.B: Ethical Issues Surrounding Decision-Making Capacity and Home Safety
- Case Study 28.C: Balancing Burden and Benefit: Should Judy Be Allowed to Refuse Care?
- Exercise 28.A: Values Clarification Exercise

REFERENCES

American Occupational Therapy Association. (1993). Core values and attitudes of occupational therapy practice. *American Journal of Occupational Therapy, 47,* 1085–1086.

American Occupational Therapy Association. (2005). Occupational therapy code of ethics. *American Journal of Occupational Therapy, 59,* 639–642.

American Occupational Therapy Association. (2006). *Guidelines to the OT code of ethics.* In D. Y. Slater (Ed.), *Reference guide to the occupational therapy code of ethics* (pp. 15–21). Bethesda, MD: Author.

Aulisio, M. P., Arnold, R. M., & Younger, S. J. (2000). Health care ethics consultation: Nature, goals, and competencies: A position paper from the Society for Health and Human

Values–Society for Bioethics Consultation Task Force on Standards for Bioethics Consultation. *Annals of Internal Medicine 133,* 59–69.

Bailey, D. M., & Schwartzberg, S. L. (Eds.). (2003). Ethical and legal dilemmas in occupational therapy (2nd ed). Philadelphia: F. A. Davis.

Banks, S. (2004). *Ethics, accountability, and the social professions.* NY: Palgrave Macmillan.

Barnitt, R. E. (1993). Deeply troubling questions: The teaching of ethics in undergraduate courses. *British Journal of Occupational Therapy, 56,* 404–406.

Barnitt, R. (1998). Ethical dilemmas in occupational therapy and physical therapy: A survey of practitioners in the UK National Health Service. *Journal of Medical Ethics, 24,* 193–199.

Baum, M. C. (2006). Presidential Address 2006: Centennial challenges, millennium opportunities. *American Journal of Occupational Therapy, 60,* 609–616.

Beauchamp, T. L., & Childress, J. F. (2001). *Principles of biomedical ethics* (5th ed.). New York: Oxford University Press.

Bebeau, M. J. (2002). The Defining Issues Test and the four component model: Contributions to professional education. *Journal of Moral Education, 3,* 271–293.

Cameron, M. (2004). Ethical listening as therapy. *Journal of Professional Nursing, 20,* 141–142.

Cohen, S. (2004). *The nature of moral reasoning: The framework and activities of ethical deliberation, argument and decision making.* New York: Oxford University Press.

Devettere, R. J. (2000). *Practical decision making in health care ethics: Cases and concepts* (2nd ed.). Washington, DC: Georgetown University Press.

Doherty, R., Peterson, E. W., & Braveman, B. (2006). Responsible participation in a profession, In Braveman, B. (Ed.), *Leading and managing occupational therapy services:* An evidence-based approach. Philadelphia: F. A. Davis.

Epstein, R. M. (1999). Mindful practice. *Journal of the American Medical Association, 282,* 833–839.

Fletcher, J. C., Miller, F. G., & Spencer, E. M. (1997). Clinical ethics: History, content and resources. In J. C. Fletcher, P. A. Lombardo, M. F. Marshall, & F. G. Miller (Eds.), *Introduction to clinical ethics,* (2nd ed., pp. 3–20). Hagerstown, MD: University Publishing Group.

Foye, S. J., Kirschner, K. L., Wagner, L. C. B., Stocking, C., & Siegler, M. (2002). Ethics in practice: Ethical issues in rehabilitation: A qualitative analysis of dilemmas identified by occupational therapists. *Topics in Stroke Rehabilitation, 9,* 89–101.

Fry, S. T., & Veatch, R. M. (2000). *Case studies in nursing ethics.* Sudbury, MA: Jones & Bartlett.

Gervais, K. G. (2005). A model for ethical decision making to inform the ethics education of future professionals. In R. Purtilo, G. M. Jensen, & C. B. Royeen (Eds.), *Educating for moral action: A sourcebook in health and rehabilitation ethics* (pp. 185–190). Philadelphia: F. A. Davis.

Glaser, J. W. (2005). Three realms of ethics: An integrating map of ethics for the future. In R. Purtilo, G. M. Jensen, & C. B. Royeen (Eds.), *Educating for moral action: A sourcebook in health and rehabilitation ethics* (pp. 169–184). Philadelphia: F. A. Davis.

Hansen, R., & Kyler-Hutchison, P. (1989, April). *Light at the end of the tunnel.* Workshop presented at the annual conference of the American Occupational Therapy Association, Baltimore, MD.

Hartwell, S. (1995). Promoting moral development through experiential teaching. *Clinical Law Review, 1,* 505–539.

Horner, J. (2003). Morality, ethics and law: Introductory concepts. *Seminars in Speech and Language, 24,* 263–274.

Jennings, B. (2003). A strategy for discussing ethical issues in public health. In B. Jennings, J. Kahn, A. Mastroianni, & L. S. Parker (Eds.), *Ethics and public health: model curriculum.* Retrieved January 20, 2006, from www.asph.org

Jensen, G. M. (2005). Mindfulness: Applications for teaching and learning in ethics education. In R. Purtilo, G. M. Jensen, & C. B. Royeen (Eds.), *Educating for moral action: A sourcebook in health and rehabilitation ethics* (pp. 191–202). Philadelphia: F. A. Davis.

Jensen, G. M., & Richert, A. E. (2005). Reflection on the teaching of ethics in physical therapist education: Integrating cases, theory, and learning. *Journal of Physical Therapy Education, 19,* 78–85.

Kanny, E. (1993). Core values and attitudes of occupational therapy practice. *American Journal of Occupational Therapy, 47,* 1085–1086.

Mattingly, C. (1998). In search of the good: Narrative reasoning in clinical practice. *Medical Anthropology Quarterly, 12,* 273–297.

Maupin, C. R. (1995). The potential for noncaring when dealing with difficult patients: Strategies for making moral decisions. *Journal of Cardiovascular Nursing, 9,* 11–22.

Miller, F. G., Fletcher, J. C., & Fins, J. J. (1995). Clinical pragmatism: A case method of moral problem solving. In J. C. Fletcher, P. A. Lombardo, M. F. Marshall, & F. G. Miller (Eds.), *Introduction to clinical ethics* (2nd ed., pp. 21–38). Hagerstown, MD: University Publishing Group.

Nash, L. (1981). Ethics without the sermon. *Harvard Business Review, 59*(6), 79–90.

Nash, R. J. (2002). *Real world ethics: Frameworks for educators and human service professionals* (2nd ed.). New York: Teachers College Press.

National Board for Certification of Occupational Therapy. (2006). *About us.* Retrieved December 12, 2006, from, www.NBCOT.org

National Commission for the Protection of Human Subjects of Biomedical and Behavioral Research. (1979). *The Belmont report.* Retrieved April 1, 2006, from, http://www.hhs.gov/ohrp/humansubjects/guidance/belmont.htm

Pellegrino, E. D. (1982). Being ill and being healed: Some reflections on the grounding of medical morality. In V. Kestenbaum (Ed.), *The humanity of the ill: Phenomenological perspectives* (pp. 157–166). Knoxville: University of Tennessee Press.

Pellegrino, E. D. (1995). Toward a virtue-based normative ethics for the health professions. *Kennedy Institute of Ethics Journal 5,* 253–277.

Pellegrino, E. D. (2002). Professionalism, profession and the virtues of the good physician. *The Mount Sinai Journal of Medicine, 69,* 378–384.

Pellegrino, E. D., Siegler, M., & Singer, P. A. (1991). Future directions in clinical ethics. *The Journal of Clinical Ethics, 2,* 5–9.

Purtilo, R. B. (2000). Thirty-first Mary McMillan lecture. A time to harvest, a time to sow: Ethics for a shifting landscape. *Physical Therapy, 80,* 1112–1119.

Purtilo, R. (2005). *Ethical dimensions in the health professions* (4th ed.). Philadelphia: Elsevier Saunders.

Quill, T. E. (2000). Initiating end of life discussions with seriously ill patients: Addressing the "elephant in the room." *Journal of the American Medical Association, 284,* 2502–2507.

Scanlon, C., & Glover, J. (1995). Ethical issues: A professional code of ethics: Providing a moral compass for turbulent times. *Oncology Nursing Forum, 10,* 1515–1521.

Sisola, S. W. (2000). Moral reasoning as a predictor of clinical practice: The development of physical therapy students across the professional curriculum. *Journal of Physical Therapy Education, 14*(3), 26–34.

Slater, D. Y. (2006). *Reference guide to the occupational therapy code of ethics.* Bethesda, MD: American Occupational Therapy Association.

Smith, R., Hiatt, H., & Berwick, D. (1999). Shared ethical principles for everybody in health care: A working draft from the Tavistock group. *British Medical Journal, 318,* 248–251.

Triezenberg, H. L. (2005). Examining the moral role of physical therapists. In R. B. Purtilo, G. M. Jenson, & C. B. Royeen (Eds.), *Educating for moral action: A sourcebook in health and rehabilitation ethics* (pp. 85–98). Philadelphia: F. A. Davis.

Weeks, H. (2001). Taking the stress out of stressful conversations. *Harvard Business Review, 79*(7), 112–119.

World Health Organization (1994, October). *The teaching of medical ethics: Fourth consultation with leading medical practitioners.* Geneva: World Health Organization.

Client-Centered Collaboration

29

SUSAN AYRES ROSA

Learning Objectives

After reading this chapter, you will be able to:

1. Discuss the terms *collaboration, client-centered care*, and *autonomous moral agency* in the context of health care.
2. Describe the benefits to clients and practitioners of client-centered collaboration.
3. Identify environmental and personal factors that can pose challenges to using client-centered principles in occupational therapy practice.
4. Discuss the importance of client advocacy, communication skills, and negotiating differences with clients over therapy goals and expectations to client-centered practice.

INTRODUCTION

Prominent among the values reflected in the official documents of the American Occupational Therapy Association (AOTA) is an appreciation of and respect for the uniqueness of individual clients and each client's right to exercise choice and self-direction (AOTA, 1998, 2002, 2005). The AOTA Code of Ethics (AOTA, 2005) specifically mandates that practitioners respect their clients' rights to influence decisions that affect them. One way in which practitioners act in accordance with these ideals and ethical mandates is by encouraging clients to participate in all phases of the therapeutic process, including problem identification, goal setting, intervention planning, and evaluating outcomes. Working together with clients in this way is at the heart of collaborative models of care and client-centered practice in occupational therapy (Corcoran, 1993; Law, 1998).

In this chapter, we examine the terms *collaboration* and *client-centered* and review the research evidence on the outcomes of client-centered practices. We also explore some of the challenges facing practitioners that may help to explain why being client-centered remains elusive for occupational therapists.

COLLABORATION IN HEALTH CARE

To collaborate with clients in health care means working with them to find common ground regarding health-related problems and what to do about them. Collaboration involves a dynamic process of information sharing and negotiation in which both clients and practitioners are active partners. Clients must be able and willing to express their concerns. Practitioners must strive to understand those concerns while also sharing their expertise and technical knowledge.

Collaborative models of care, such as client-centered practice, are grounded in the conviction that clients are capable of acting as autonomous moral agents on their own behalf (Bartholome, 1992). This is the notion that clients not only have the right and the capacity to contribute to the decisions that affect them, but also are the experts on their own illness-related experiences. Because of the personal knowledge that clients have of their own situation, they are likely to know better than health care professionals can what will work for them. As our profession struggles to glean knowledge from relatively scant research evidence to guide decisions about best practices, practitioners must strive to seek out and honor the personal knowledge that clients bring to the therapy encounter; it may be the best and most relevant evidence available to them.

BEING CLIENT-CENTERED

In occupational therapy, the ideal of collaboration is incorporated in the concept of client-centered practice (Law, Baptiste, & Mills, 1995). The term *client-centered practice* dates back to the late 1930s and the writings of the psychologist Carl Rogers, who championed an approach to counseling that focused on the concerns that clients themselves identified (Law & Mills, 1998). The foundation of Rogers's approach is a respect for the unique cultural values of clients and a belief that clients both desire and have the capacity to take an active role in directing their own care. Rogers ardently believed that clients know best their own needs and experiences.

The following seven concepts are common to all occupational therapy models of client-centered practice:

1. Respect for clients and their families and the choices they make
2. Recognition that clients and families have the ultimate responsibility for decisions about daily occupational and occupational therapy services
3. Provision of information, physical comfort, and emotional support with an emphasis on person-centered communication
4. Facilitation of client participation in all aspects of occupational therapy service
5. Delivery of flexible, individualized occupational therapy services
6. Facilitation of the capacity of clients to solve their occupational performance issues
7. Recognition of and focus on the person-environment-occupation relationship (Law & Mills, 1998)

This list clearly reflects a respect for clients as autonomous moral agents and the principles that Rogers espoused.

RESEARCH EVIDENCE

While research evidence is scant that addresses the effectiveness of a specifically client-centered approach in occupational therapy, an emerging body of research findings suggests multiple benefits to be derived from incorporating client-centered principles. Moreover, this evidence suggests that both clients and practitioners benefit.

The benefits that have been reported for occupational therapy clients from using a client-centered approach include improved functional performance in areas of interest to them, resumption of life roles, decreased pain, improved safety and physical health, and increased levels of satisfaction with therapy and the outcomes of intervention (Case-Smith, 2003; Horowitz, 2002; Van Leit & Crowe, 2002). A greater awareness on the part of clients of their therapy goals and increased adherence to intervention recommendations have also been associated with treatment approaches that incorporate client-centered principles (Case-Smith, 2003; Law, Baptiste, & Mills, 1995; Wressle, Eeg-Olofsson, Marcusson, & Henriksson, 2002).

A number of studies have examined client perspectives on occupational therapy generally (McKinnon, 2000; Palmadottir, 2003) and client-centered practices specifically (Corring & Cook, 1999; Darragh, Sample, & Krieger, 2001; Sumsion, 2005). These, like the personal testimonial of Mary Feldhaus-Weber printed in Chapter 11, teach us how important it is to clients and how empowering it can be for them when practitioners are willing to listen carefully to clients' concerns, honor their abilities, and trust their knowledge about what is best for themselves.

Research has also shown that working in a client-centered way can have important consequences for practitioners. Occupational practitioners who feel that they have helped clients in ways that are meaningful to the clients report a strong sense of connection with those clients and a sense of joining with them in mutually supportive partnerships. These types of experiences nourish and sustain practitioners and motivate and inspire them in their work (Rosa & Hasselkus, 1996). Interestingly, findings from this same research suggest that not being able to work collaboratively with clients can be associated with a drain on practitioners' emotional resources and feelings of guilt, rejection, and even failure.

THE CHALLENGES OF CLIENT-CENTERED COLLABORATION

In view of the ethical mandate to be client-centered and the documented benefits to clients and practitioners alike, it is important to point out that being client-centered has been troublingly elusive for occupational therapy practitioners. Studies have shown, for example, that practitioners do not always attempt to collaborate with clients; do less than they could to ensure clients' participation in problem identification, goal setting, and intervention planning; and employ communication styles that inhibit client participation and information sharing (Allison & Strong, 1994; Clark, Corcoran, & Gitlin, 1995; Hasselkus & Dickie, 1990, 1994; Helm & Dickerson, 1995; Levine & Gitlin, 1993; Neistadt, 1995; Northen, Rust, Nelson, & Watts, 1995; Rosa & Hasselkus, 1996). The reasons for these behaviors can be complex. Challenges include institutional barriers associated with therapy settings and personal factors related to both therapists and clients.

Contextual Influences on Client-Centered Collaboration

Occupational therapy practitioners have traditionally worked in hospitals and other medical settings where the medical or expert model tends to be the dominant model of service delivery. Historically, the medical model has included the beliefs that power and control over medical decisions rightly reside primarily with professionals because of their superior knowledge and authority. In this model, clients have a corresponding duty to comply with the expert advice that medical professionals offer. The expert model continues to exert a strong influence in some settings (Fearing & Ferguson-Pare, 2000; Kyler, 2005; Lawlor & Mattingly, 1998; Wilkins, Pollock, Rochon, & Law, 2001). Being client-centered in such contexts challenges practitioners to advocate for clients whose voices might not otherwise be heard and to provide leadership in promoting change within the institution (Fearing & Ferguson-Pare, 2000).

In rehabilitation settings, the goals and expectations of therapy emphasize independence, hard work, and having clients do as much as possible for themselves. Because these goals are so universal in rehabilitation and so strongly advocated, at times without a determination of whether they are in line with what clients want for themselves, some have suggested that they constitute a rehabilitation ideology (Hasselkus, Dickie, & Gregory, 1997; Lawlor & Mattingly, 1998). Indeed, occupational therapy practitioners working in rehabilitation settings have described ways in which they persisted in pushing such a rehabilitation agenda even in the face of strong resistance from clients (Rosa and Hasselkus, 2005). The challenge for practitioners working in rehabilitation is to understand clients' values and concerns and reflect on the extent to which these may differ from any taken-for-granted goals and expectations that might be imposed on clients as the result of a rehabilitation ideology.

Personal Influences on Client-Centered Collaboration

In addition to institutional barriers, personal factors associated with both clients and therapists can present barriers to the process of information sharing and negotiation necessary to practicing in a collaborative, client-centered way. If clients are either unable or unwilling to express themselves, voice their concerns, or otherwise take an active part in the process or if practitioners do not listen carefully for clients' concerns or do not have the skills or patience necessary to work around the many difficulties that can arise, the process can break down.

Among the reasons why clients might be unable or unwilling to be effective partners with therapists are language differences, aphasia, hearing loss and other barriers to basic communication, physical or cognitive deficits, psychological issues, and cultural differences. Clients might simply be too sick or too tired to identify goals or make decisions about their care. Cognitive limitations, level of education, and mental illness can interfere with a client's ability to think clearly or comprehend issues involved. Distrust of others, anger, anxiety, depression, and disorganized and delusional thinking can limit the ability to engage in effective partnerships. Clients might have cultural beliefs that cause them to be uncomfortable making decisions about their own care. Practitioners are called on to overcome the barriers that are present to the extent possible in an effort to understand clients as fully as they can and share the power and responsibility of decision making (Precin, 2002; Sumsion, 1999).

The above examples make clear that collaborative, client-centered care can require high-level communication and sophisticated personal interaction skills. Thomson (2000) has suggested, in fact, that clients who present some of the kinds of difficulties referred to above should perhaps be considered "specialist cases" (p. 11) because of the level of advanced skill Thomson believes is necessary to collaborate with them effectively.

In addition to skill, practitioners must be open to exploring differences regarding therapy goals and expectations with clients whose goals, culture, and life experiences might be very different from their own (Sumsion & Smyth, 2000). The range of individual differences within cultures and the potential for vastly different world views between cultures can offer new challenges with each patient. When differences are present, effective communication demands an openness to exploring these differences with clients in addition to skill and patience in negotiating them.

Findings from a recent study reveal that occupational therapists do not always display this kind of openness to exploring differences with clients (Rosa & Hasselkus, 2005). Rather, agreement on therapy goals and expectations seemed to be based on compatibility with clients rather than on negotiating differences with them. The occupational therapists who participated in the study collaborated readily with clients with whom they felt considerable rapport, clients who were "on the same wavelength" when it came to therapy goals and expectations and with whom they felt a strong connection. Conversely, therapists found themselves at odds with clients with whom this was not the case and experienced conflict and tension surrounding therapy goals and expectations when working with these clients.

Social psychologists tell us that it is natural for each of us to be more open to some people than others. For example, we are more likely to help someone to whom we are attracted, we are attracted to people with whom we feel some measure of compatibility, and we communicate most readily with those with whom we have positive interactions (Schroeder, Penner, Dovidio, & Piliavin, 1995). These behaviors are a spontaneous expression of our feelings toward those to whom we feel attracted and with whom we feel some connection. Correspondingly, it might be only natural for us to be less open to helping clients who are angry, demanding, or unpleasant or who present us with other tough behavioral or communication challenges. It is easy to understand, then, that it might be harder for us to find the motivation to understand clients like these.

In professional-client relationships, the professional has the responsibility to try to understand all clients, even those with whom they feel they have little or nothing in common, who are unpleasant, or with whom they feel little or no attraction or rapport. If occupational therapy practitioners are to accept the responsibility to face these challenges, to bridge differences, and to resolve conflicts, they, like all professionals, must get beyond what simply comes naturally to them. This is the point that Montgomery (1993), a nurse scholar and researcher, stresses:

> This natural state of responsiveness and commitment is not adequate by itself to ensure effective caring on a professional level. Clients who have contact with helping professionals expect more than good intentions. Therefore, helping professionals not only must be competent in the skills and science of their profession, but also must possess sophisticated relational and communication abilities to handle a variety of interpersonal and relational challenges and demands. In other words, making a commitment to care is not easy. Caregivers need to develop communication abilities that will allow them to continue to stay involved and continue to be therapeutic in the face of these demands and challenges. (p. 14)

Because of the many challenges that may be present, engaging in the kind of dialogue necessary to achieve effective collaboration and meaningful exchange of information with all clients can be inordinately difficult. The importance of developing strong communication and interpersonal skills cannot be emphasized enough.

CONCLUSION

Occupational therapy practitioners have an ethical responsibility to include clients in discussions regarding their own care and to provide them with the opportunity to share in the decisions that affect them. But as we have seen, multiple factors present a host of difficult challenges to uphold-

ing our profession's ideal of client-centered collaboration. To be successful, occupational therapy practitioners must work against the institutional factors that can negatively influence decision-making processes, commit themselves to developing the requisite communication skills, and strive for the kind of openness to difference with others over values and beliefs that is necessary to overcome gaps in understanding. Only then will occupational therapy professionals be able to nurture greater health and well-being for the clients they so want to help and for themselves.

PROVOCATIVE QUESTIONS

1. Should all clients be considered "autonomous moral agents"? Might there be some individuals who are not capable of serving as their own moral agents?
2. Penny Kyler (2005) has advocated that occupational and physical therapists go beyond a client-centered or family-centered model to a relationship-centered approach, which takes into consideration the individual client and his or her relationships to others and to all of the external environments that may exert influence the therapist-client interaction. These external environments include the social, political, economic, physical, and cultural contexts in which the client-therapist interaction takes place. To what extent do you agree with Kyler? Does the model of client-centered collaboration described here fit with Kyler's notion of a relationship-centered approach?
3. How do you feel about the relative importance of clients' personal knowledge of their illness experiences and the evidence-based, technical knowledge that therapists have? To what extent do you agree that the first may be more important that the second?

REFERENCES

Allison, H., & Strong, J. (1994). Verbal strategies used by occupational therapists in direct client encounters. *Occupational Therapy Journal of Research, 14,* 112–129.

American Occupational Therapy Association. (1998). Standards of practice for occupational therapy. *American Journal of Occupational Therapy, 52,* 866–869.

American Occupational Therapy Association. (2002). Occupational therapy practice framework: Domain and process. *American Journal of Occupational Therapy, 56,* 609–639.

American Occupational Therapy Association. (2005). Occupational therapy code of ethics—2005. *American Journal of Occupational Therapy, 59,* 639–642.

Bartholome, W. G. (1992). A revolution in understanding: How ethics has transformed health care decision making. *Quality Review Bulletin, 18,* 6–11.

Case-Smith, J. (2003). Outcomes in hand rehabilitation using occupational therapy services. *American Journal of Occupational Therapy, 57,* 499–506.

Clark, C. A., Corcoran, M., & Gitlin, L. N. (1995). An exploratory study of how occupational therapists develop therapeutic relationships with family caregivers. *The American Journal of Occupational Therapy, 49,* 587–594.

Corcoran, M. A. (1993). Collaboration: An ethical approach to effective therapeutic relationships. *Topics in Geriatric Rehabilitation, 9*(1), 21–29.

Corring, D., & Cook, J. (1999). Client-centered care means that I am a valued human being. *Canadian Journal of Occupational Therapy, 66,* 71–82.

Darragh, A. R., Sample, P. L., & Krieger, S. R. (2001). "Tears in my eyes 'cause somebody finally understood": Client perceptions of practitioners following brain injury. *American Journal of Occupational Therapy, 55,* 191–199.

Fearing, V. G., & Ferguson-Pare, M. (2000). Leadership in daily practice. In V. G. Fearing & J. Clark (Eds.), *Individuals in context: A practical guide to client-centered practice* (pp. 3–14). Thorofare, NJ: Slack.

Hasselkus, B. R., & Dickie, V. (1990). Themes of meaning: Occupational therapists' perspectives on practice. *Occupational Therapy Journal of Research, 10,* 195–207.

Hasselkus, B. R., & Dickie, V. (1994). Doing occupational therapy: Dimensions of satisfaction and dissatisfaction. *American Journal of Occupational Therapy, 48,* 145–154.

Hasselkus, B. R., Dickie, V. A., & Gregory, C. (1997). Geriatric occupational therapy: The uncertain ideology of long-term care. *American Journal of Occupational Therapy, 51,* 132–139.

Helm, T., & Dickerson, A. E. (1995). The effect of hand therapy on a patient with a Colles' fracture: A phenomenological study. *Occupational Therapy in Health, 9,* 69–77.

Horowitz, B. P. (2002). Occupational therapy home assessments: Supporting community living through client-centered practice. *Occupational Therapy in Mental Health, 18,* 1–17.

Kyler, P. L. (2005). The ethics of client-centered models. In R. B. Purtillo, G. M. Jensen, & C. B. Royeen (Eds.), *Educating for moral action: A sourcebook in health and rehabilitation ethics* (pp. 159–167). Philadelphia: F. A. Davis.

Law, M. (1998). Does client-centered practice make a difference? In M. Law (Ed.), *Client-centered occupational therapy* (pp. 19–27). Thorofare, NJ: Slack.

Law, M., Baptiste, S., & Mills, J. (1995). Client-centered practice: What does it mean and does it make a difference? *Canadian Journal of Occupational Therapy, 62,* 250–257.

Law, M., & Mills, J. (1998). Client-centered occupational therapy, In M. Law (Ed.), *Client-centered occupational therapy* (pp. 1–18). Thorofare, NJ: Slack.

Lawlor, M. C., & Mattingly, C. C. (1998). The complexities embedded in family-centered care. *American Journal of Occupational Therapy, 52,* 259–267.

Levine, R. E., & Gitlin, L. N. (1993). A model to promote activity competence in elders. *American Journal of Occupational Therapy, 47,* 147–153.

McKinnon, A. L. (2000). Client values and satisfaction with occupational therapy. *Scandinavian Journal of Occupational Therapy, 7,* 99–106.

Montgomery, C. L. (1993). *Healing through communication: The practice of caring.* Newbury Park, CA: Sage.

Neistadt, M. E. (1995). Methods of assessing clients' priorities: A survey of adult physical dysfunction settings. *American Journal of Occupational Therapy, 49,* 428–436.

Northen, J. G., Rust, D. M., Nelson, C. E., & Watts, J. H. (1995). Involvement of adult rehabilitation patients in setting occupational therapy goals. *American Journal of Occupational Therapy, 49,* 214–220.

Palmadottir, G. (2003). Client perspectives in occupational therapy in rehabilitation services. *Scandinavian Journal of Occupational Therapy, 10,* 157–166.

Precin, P. (2002). *Client-centered reasoning.* Boston: Butterworth Heinemann.

Rosa, S. A., & Hasselkus, B. R. (1996). Connecting with patients: The personal experience of professional helping. *Occupational Therapy Journal of Research, 16,* 245–260.

Rosa, S. A., & Hasselkus, B. R. (2005). Finding common ground with patients: The centrality of compatibility. *American Journal of Occupational Therapy, 59,* 198–208.

Schroeder, D. A., Penner, L. A., Dovidio, J. F., & Piliavin, J. A. (1995). *The psychology of helping and altruism: Problems and puzzles.* New York: McGraw-Hill.

Sumsion, T. (1999). The client-centered approach. In T. Sumsion (Ed.), *Client-centered practice in occupational therapy* (pp. 15–20). Edinburgh: Churchill Livingstone.

Sumsion, T. (2005). Facilitating client-centered practice: Insights from clients. *Canadian Journal of Occupational Therapy, 72,* 13–20.

Sumsion, T., & Smyth, G. (2000). Barriers to client-centeredness and their resolution. *Canadian Journal of Occupational Therapy, 67,* 15–21.

Thomson, D. (2000). "Problem" patients as experienced by senior physiotherapists in the context of their working lives. *Advances in Physiotherapy, 2,* 2–13.

Van Leit, B., & Crowe, T. K. (2002). Outcomes of an occupational therapy program for mothers of children with disabilities: Impact on satisfaction with time use and occupational performance. *American Journal of Occupational Therapy, 56,* 402–410.

Wilkins, S, Pollock, N, Rochon, S., & Law, M. (2001). Implementing client-centered practice: Why is it so difficult to do? *Canadian Journal of Occupational Therapy, 68,* 70–79.

Wressle, E., Eeg-Olofsson, A., Marcusson, J., & Henriksson, C. (2002). Improved client structure: Participation in the rehabilitation process using a client-centered formulation. *Journal of Rehabilitation Medicine, 34,* 5–11.

Evidence-Based Practice

Using Available Evidence to Inform Practice

LINDA TICKLE-DEGNEN

30

Learning Objectives

After completing this chapter, you will be able to:

1. Describe how research evidence provides central tendency, or generality, information about individuals as well as individual variation among individuals.
2. Describe the clinical tasks for which to use evidence.
3. Name the basic steps of using evidence.
4. Write answerable clinical questions.
5. Identify key terms for searching research literature effectively.
6. Describe how to appraise the clinical relevance and trustworthiness of a research report.
7. Describe qualities of effective communication about evidence.
8. Describe how evidence-based practice can be client-centered.

INTRODUCTION

Imagine that you are going to work with a new client tomorrow. What do you do? How do you decide what this client needs and how you might help the client to achieve occupational goals? You might do what an occupational therapy student, Rebecca Reis (1994), did as she prepared to meet a new client. Rebecca's fieldwork supervisor assigned her to work with Wanda, a middle-aged woman with a Colles' fracture, who up until then had been receiving occupational therapy from the supervisor. Wanda would be not only a new client to Rebecca, but also her first client in a busy, fast-paced outpatient clinic and one with an unfamiliar diagnosis.

In preparation, Rebecca discussed Wanda with her supervisor to receive expert guidance and then looked over Wanda's medical chart to orient herself to the nature of Wanda's medical problem and current interventions. During their initial session together, Rebecca asked Wanda directly how she was managing at home, to understand Wanda's personal experience of daily life activities with this type of fracture, and examined her wrist to assess directly the nature of Wanda's wrist functioning. Wanda reported minor problems at home, and Rebecca implemented a supervised protocol of modalities and exercises directed at maximizing Wanda's wrist function.

Over five or six sessions, Rebecca found Wanda to be pleasant and courteous but relatively indifferent to questions about how she was managing at home with regard to her wrist. They passed their therapy sessions in light conversation until their very last session together. At that time, Wanda opened up and told her personal details about her life, including sexual abuse as a child and lengthy rehabilitation for her own substance abuse. She talked about how a girlfriend had always told her she should write a book about all that she had experienced and how she had once started to write it all down. Rebecca was "stunned" (Reis, 1994, p. 351) and moved. Rebecca ended the therapy sessions believing the Colles' fracture to be insignificant in the scheme of Wanda's life. Rebecca did not know what to do with the information that Wanda had given her in that last session, although she recognized that the information was quite significant.

We, like Rebecca, cannot know whether or not the information that she learned in that last session could have been used or could have been helpful if known earlier or whether, if known earlier, it would have changed the direction of therapy or its outcome. However, for the purposes of this chapter, I use Rebecca's vivid story (Reis, 1994), as reported to Mattingly and Fleming (1994) for their research study on clinical reasoning, to illuminate how **evidence-based practice** might create a different scenario for working with a client like Wanda. In fact, Rebecca and Wanda worked together before the movement of **evidence-based practice** had taken hold in healthcare (Sackett et al., 2000). Rebecca did everything correctly, given her student role and the standards of occupational therapy and other health care professions in the 1980s and into more recent times. She recognized that she needed information, or evidence, for providing occupational therapy that would ben-

efit Wanda. The forms of evidence that she used to inform her work with Wanda were expert opinion, medical records about tests and interventions conducted with Wanda, information from Wanda herself, and direct observation of Wanda's wrist function.

Because it was not common practice to do so at the time, there is a form of evidence that Rebecca did not seek out or use. She did not use evidence from research studies to inform her practice with Wanda, the type of evidence meant in the term *evidence-based practice*. It is only now, approximately 20 years later, that occupational therapy practitioners are starting to use this type of evidence in their practice, though not yet consistently. This chapter describes how evidence from research studies can be put into practice consistently and in a manner that enriches the contributions of occupational therapy and the outcomes of clients.

CLINICAL REASONING ABOUT HUMAN BEINGS IN RELATION TO RESEARCH EVIDENCE

> Central tendency is an abstraction, variation the reality. . . . I am not a measure of central tendency, either mean or median. I am one single human being with mesothelioma. . . . I must not simply assume that my personal fate will correspond to some measure of central tendency. (Gould, 1996, pp. 48–49)

My suggestions for evidence-based practice are informed by Gould's (1996) insights about research findings and personal outcomes as applied to his own experience with mesothelioma. He was told that his postdiagnosis survival would be eight months, based on research findings. Instead, he lived for more than 20 years postdiagnosis, having a prolific scientific and writing career as an evolutionary paleontologist. I use the concepts that Gould represents in the above quote as the basis for describing clinical reasoning about evidence that balances an understanding of the **central tendency**, or generality, of individuals' attributes, with an understanding of the **individual variation** of these attributes (Tickle-Degnen, 2001). This perspective is consistent with Mattingly and Fleming's (1994) concept of conditional reasoning.

One of the strengths underlying the use of research findings to guide practice with an individual client is that human beings share many similar attributes by virtue of sharing genes and the ecosystem of the earth. As a result, there is a degree of **central tendency** or generality in human behavior and outcomes that can be gleaned from research studies of humans. It is possible that an individual client will respond to assessment and intervention procedures in the same manner in which participants in research studies responded. On the other hand, every individual is unique, having a pattern of life experiences, thoughts, and perceptions in different contexts that matches no other's exactly. In applying research evidence to individuals, we must be

PRACTICE DILEMMA

WHAT COULD REBECCA HAVE DONE?

As an occupational therapy practitioner in an outpatient clinic, what could Rebecca have done with the information about Wanda's background and life? More important, what if Rebecca had heard this information earlier in her sessions with Wanda? Would therapy have been different? Would Rebecca have felt that she had had a more meaningful intervention with Wanda?

highly cognizant of this **individual variation**, assessing at all decision points how this particular client may vary from the others. Understanding this dynamic of generality and variation is the key to using evidence-based practice effectively with all clients, including Wanda.

THE EVIDENCE-BASED PRACTITIONER

Imagine yourself, in the present, as an evidence-based practitioner who is just about to meet the Wanda of Rebecca's clinical experience. As an evidence-based practitioner, you would use scientific reasoning along with the current and best evidence from research studies to support central clinical tasks, such as the selection of appropriate and valid assessment procedures, interventions, and procedures for monitoring clinical progress (Law, 2002; Sackett et al., 2000). It is important to understand that in evidence-based practice, scientific reasoning does not replace reasoning that is informed by clinical experience, theory, core values of practice, and ethics. Nor does the use of research evidence replace the clinical use of information derived from observing clients and talking with their family members or from consulting with experts and peers. Evidence-based clinical reasoning involves the use of all forms of evidence in the pursuit of optimal client outcomes. It is the integration of scientific reasoning with reasoning that has been matured by clinical experience, validated practice theory, and client-centered values and ethics (Egan,

Dubouloz, von Zweck, & Vallerand, 1998; Lee & Miller, 2003; Rappolt, 2003).

ORGANIZING EVIDENCE AROUND CENTRAL CLINICAL TASKS

Table 30.1 shows how, you, the evidence-based practitioner, could organize the search for and interpretation of evidence around central clinical tasks, in general, and, specifically, with respect to Wanda. One of the first clinical tasks that the practitioner faces in working with a client is that of *getting to know the client* with respect to occupational needs and status, to ensure that services are relevant and beneficial specifically for that person. Research evidence that would be relevant to this task includes findings about (1) typical occupational experiences and needs of individuals with personal characteristics or health care conditions similar to the client and (2) the quality of occupational assessment procedures with respect to identifying the unique clinical needs of these types of individuals.

With respect to Wanda, descriptions of the occupational lives of women with Colles' fractures or similar injuries could enhance your understanding of possible issues that Wanda might face in her own life and could generate a discussion with Wanda about her own life. Such a discussion might identify what specific types of in-depth information about Wanda you want to learn in the assessment procedures. After targeting key areas to assess, you could go back to the research literature to find evidence

TABLE 30.1   ORGANIZING EVIDENCE AROUND CLINICAL TASKS WITH WANDA

Central Clinical Task	Research Evidence	Use of Evidence for Wanda's Specific Case
I. Get to know a client	A. Typical occupational experiences and needs of clients from populations who can be compared to Wanda B. Quality (e.g., reliability, validity, trustworthiness, usefulness) of occupational assessment procedures for these populations	Generate a discussion with Wanda about her own occupational experiences and needs in comparison with the research samples Select the best assessment method to identify Wanda's unique occupational experiences and needs
II. Choose an effective intervention	Relative effectiveness of different types of interventions designed for these populations	Select, ideally in collaboration with Wanda, a potentially beneficial intervention
III. Monitor response to intervention	Quality of occupational assessment procedures for monitoring changes in clients from these populations with respect to achieving intervention goals	Select the best assessment method for monitoring change in Wanda

about the reliability, validity, trustworthiness, or clinical usefulness of methods to select the most valuable methods for assessing those areas.

A second central clinical task is that of *choosing an effective intervention* approach and procedure for addressing the client's specific needs and goals. The research evidence that would be relevant to this task includes findings about the relative effectiveness of different types of interventions designed for individuals with a particular type of personal characteristic or health care condition. With respect to Wanda, you could use **effectiveness evidence** about interventions designed for individuals with Colles' fractures and similar injuries to select an appropriate intervention. In a client-centered approach, this selection would involve collaboration with Wanda (Tickle-Degnen, 2002a).

A third central clinical task is that of *monitoring response to intervention*. Once an intervention has been chosen and then implemented with the client, its effectiveness for that particular client must be monitored, documented, and revised if necessary. The research evidence that would be relevant to this task includes findings about the quality of occupational assessment procedures with respect to monitoring changes in the client related to progress toward intervention goals. Notice how this task is different from the initial getting-to-know task in which assessment procedures are selected for initial identification of a client's needs and for developing therapeutic goals that are uniquely relevant for the client. Assessment procedures that are valid for that initial assessment might or might not be valid for assessing change. With respect to Wanda, you could use information about the reliability, validity, trustworthiness, or clinical usefulness of methods for evaluating change in Wanda with respect to the goals established for her occupational therapy.

In addition to the three central clinical tasks discussed here—getting to know the client, choosing an effective intervention, and monitoring response to intervention—there are other important clinical tasks that occupational therapy practitioners undertake with their clients, such as designing and implementing a discharge plan. Regardless of which tasks are central to a particular practitioner's practice or setting, the procedures of evidence-based practice are the same with respect to an emphasis on using *systematic and reflective analysis of evidence* to guide decision making and clinical procedures toward beneficial outcomes with clients.

THE STEPS OF EVIDENCE-BASED PRACTICE

The evidence-based practitioner systematically integrates research evidence into practice by carrying out a series of steps around each clinical task (Law, 2002; Sackett et al., 2000; Tickle-Degnen, 1999):

1. Writing down an answerable clinical question
2. Gathering current published evidence that might answer the question
3. Appraising the gathered evidence to determine what is the "best" evidence for answering the question
4. Communicating with clients and colleagues about the evidence for decision making

Step 1: Writing an Answerable Clinical Question

The first systematic step, writing down a question, helps the practitioner to focus on the specific type of evidence that would help a clinical task. The question must be written by using key words and terminology that tap into a general body of research literature that may hold an answer to the question and that locate evidence that is relevant to performing a particular clinical task with a specific client. An *answerable* question, therefore, must be neither too broad nor too narrow in its focus (Sackett et al., 2000). For occupational therapy, this type of question is composed of three elements (Tickle-Degnen, 1999): (1) the *type of evidence* that is needed to address the particular clinical task; (2) a *variable* or attribute that is related to occupational experience, behavior, the occupational therapy process, or outcomes; and (3) a description of the *client's population*.

Type of Evidence

The clinical task dictates what type of evidence is needed. To be able to find the evidence successfully, the practitioner must have a basic working knowledge of the terminology of research designs and methods or use a research methods textbook as a reference manual (e.g., Domholdt, 2005; Portney & Watkins, 2000). The task of getting to know a client involves gathering evidence that is descriptive of the experiences and needs of clients in general (i.e., clients who have been research participants in published studies) and evidence that tests the quality of assessment procedures for determining an individual client's unique experiences and needs. **Descriptive evidence** is published in studies that used a descriptive research design or procedure, including correlational studies, qualitative interview studies, and participant-observation studies. **Assessment evidence** is published in studies that use a methodological design to study the reliability, validity, or trustworthiness of an assessment procedure.

The task of choosing an effective intervention for a client involves gathering evidence that evaluates the effectiveness or efficacy of a type of intervention in comparison to alternative interventions or no intervention at all. **Effectiveness evidence** is published in studies that used an intervention or treatment research design or procedure, including randomized controlled trials and other forms of experiments, or quasi-experimental and other nonexperimental intervention studies.

The task of monitoring response to intervention involves gathering evidence that tests the responsiveness of tests and procedures to clinical change in clients. **Responsiveness evidence** is published in studies that use a repeated measures design across time periods to evaluate the reliability, validity, or trustworthiness of an assessment procedure with respect to monitoring change in clients.

Occupational Variable

In addition to writing an answerable question in language that shows what type of evidence is being sought, the question must be written in language that shows what type of occupational variable or variables are of interest. Variables of interest are attributes of clients that are addressed in occupational therapy, such as their physical or psychosocial functioning, occupational performance, or satisfaction with outcomes. Models and theories of occupation and occupational therapy, such as the Person-Environment-Occupation Model (Law, Cooper, Strong, Stewart, Rigby, & Letts, 1996), as well as more general models of health that encompass an occupational therapy perspective, such as the International Classification of Functioning, Disability & Health (World Health Organization, 2005), provide the language needed to identify occupational variables. The evidence-based practitioner uses reference resources, such as this current edition of *Willard & Spackman's Occupational Therapy*, as a tool for identifying and naming these variables.

Client Population

A final element found in the wording of an answerable clinical question identifies features of the client population of interest, such as the client's clinical condition or diagnosis, gender, ethnicity, age group, and socioeconomic status. The evidence-based practitioner uses clinical knowledge, clinical textbooks, and other practice resources to identify which features of the client's population are important for guiding clinical reasoning and decision making. Important features are those that identify populations or subpopulations of which the client is a member, ensuring that retrieved evidence will be relevant to the client.

Step 2: Gathering Current Published Evidence

Once a clinical question has been written, the practitioner draws on the elements of the written question to search for and gather evidence for finding possible answers to the question. Relevant research is published in a variety of fields: occupational therapy, medicine, nursing, physical therapy, education, psychology, sociology, anthropology, and so on. Consequently, search strategies should tap into the research literature of different disciplines.

Each element of an answerable clinical question contains one or more *key terms* for searching the literature. A whole body of literature can be excluded inadvertently simply because the key terms that are used in the search do not match terminology used by the researchers or the cataloguers of the research literature. Some of the important terms that occupational therapy practitioners use to identify clinical conditions (e.g., sensory integrative disorder) or occupational variables (e.g., occupational performance) are not the most typical terms used to describe or catalogue research studies in the broader literature. Therefore, it is important to generate a list of synonyms for each key term in each element of the question before beginning the search. Fortunately, electronic databases are becoming increasingly flexible in linking terminology across different disciplines. Literature search services such as PubMed (U.S. National Library of Medicine, 2005) provide online tutorials so that evidence-based practitioners can learn how to effectively search the literature with key terms.

Table 30.2 shows examples of questions that you could write with respect to Wanda for the clinical task of getting

TABLE 30.2 CLINICAL QUESTIONS, KEY TERMS, AND ALTERNATIVE TERMS (IN PARENTHESES) FOR GUIDING THE SEARCH FOR EVIDENCE ABOUT GETTING TO KNOW CLIENTS LIKE WANDA

Clinical Question	Type of Evidence	Occupational Variable	Clinical Population
		Elements of the Question	
A. What are the daily life roles of women with a Colles' fracture?	Descriptive (correlational) (client report)	Daily life roles (activities of daily living) (quality of life)	Women with Colles' fracture (middle-age) (wrist)
B. What is a valid method for assessing the occupational goals of clients with hand dysfunction?	Validity (assessment) (methodological)	Occupational goals (goals) (aspirations)	Hand dysfunction (women) (wrist fracture)

to know her. Possible key terms and alternatives that are synonyms, or are broader or more specific terms are listed. With respect to Question A in Table 30.2 ("What are the daily life roles of women with a Colles' fracture?"), the combination of the three terms *descriptive, daily life roles,* and *women with Colles' fracture* returned 0 abstracts from PubMed. Replacing the term *daily life roles* with *activities of daily living* also returned 0 abstracts. The combination of the terms *descriptive, quality of life,* and *women with Colles' fracture* returned a single abstract (Dolan, Torgerson, & Kakarlapudi, 1999). Replacing the term *women with Colles' fracture* with *middle-aged women* returned far too many abstracts to be useful (466), and replacing the term with *wrist* returned one abstract about spinal cord injury.

With respect to Question B ("What is a valid method for assessing the occupational goals of clients with hand dysfunction?"), the terms *validity, occupational goals,* and *hand dysfunction* returned 0 abstracts. The terms *validity, occupational goals,* and *women* returned six abstracts, including one published in the *American Journal of Occupational Therapy* (Melville, Baltic, Bettcher, & Nelson, 2002).

Perhaps after performing an occupational therapy assessment with Wanda, you learned about her interest in writing about her life. If the Colles' fracture had affected her ability to write or type, you might have the following question: "What is an effective intervention for improving writing ability in women with a Colles' fracture?" This and other intervention effectiveness questions are useful for choosing an intervention after the practitioner has gotten to know the client's needs and goals. One search service that is particularly designed to find citations of research related to intervention questions is OTseeker (Bennett et al., 2003, link found at www.otseeker.com). Many searchable databases are helpful (e.g., ProQuest at www.proquest.com or Ovid at www.ovid.com) if you have access to them through library resources.

Finally, you could write a question designed to help you find an assessment for monitoring Wanda's response to intervention, such as "What is a responsive method for assessing recovery of writing ability in women with a Colles' fracture?" Search procedures are similar to those used for the descriptive and assessment questions listed in Table 30.2.

Experience will show you that different combinations of key terms return abstracts with varying success. There is no fail-safe method for returning the most relevant abstracts for answering the questions. An electronic search on key terms is only a partial strategy for retrieval of research evidence. Once a single relevant study is located, the reference list of the study should be examined for other relevant studies. Also you can search the *Related Links* associated with the electronic abstract. Obviously, these searching strategies require time to produce evidence that is useful and comprehensive.

Efficient Gathering of Evidence

Occupational therapy practitioners are very busy and rarely have enough time to complete a reflective, systematic, and thorough review of the literature to guide their clinical tasks with a single client. It must be remembered that the knowledge gained through gathering evidence is cumulative; that is, knowledge of the research literature accrues steadily as more and more clients are seen. Because there is at least a small (sometimes larger) degree, of generality, or central tendency, across clients (e.g., sharing of age, gender, or socioeconomic status), information found with respect to one client or one client group typically can be at least minimally useful for informing your practice with all clients in general. As a result, practitioners can develop routines for collecting and cataloguing evidence for efficient use with future clients. These routines can include the following ones (Tickle-Degnen, 2000a):

1. Periodically search for and retrieve research synthesis articles or practice guidelines that are relevant to your area of practice. These syntheses give a large amount of evidence in a concise and rigorous format.
2. Maintain an up-to-date library of texts that compile current evidence, such as this text and others (e.g., Law, Baum, & Dunn, 2005).
3. Collect and file bibliographies and reference lists from practice conferences and journals.
4. Participate in a journal group or electronic mailing list that discusses relevant evidence.
5. Write down a clinical question every time one is stimulated by a clinical dilemma or need, and then categorize and prioritize the ones most relevant to your practice. This simple exercise will keep you alert to evidence as it arises in your professional life.

The Importance of Gathering Disconfirming Evidence

One goal of gathering research evidence is to determine under which conditions and with which populations occupational therapy assessments are most valid and occupational therapy interventions are most effective. Naturally, there will be some situations in which assessments are less valid and interventions less effective. To provide the best services to clients, the evidence-based practitioner must go beyond one goal, that of the *confirmation* of the value of occupational therapy assessments and interventions, toward a second goal, that of the *disconfirmation* of their value. Having this balanced view about evidence promotes a search that is complete, open-minded, and critical, as opposed to incomplete, closed-minded, and unreflective. Cherished or entrenched practice beliefs and expectations might be disconfirmed or revised, but client outcomes are likely to be maximized. For example, in the case of Wanda, you might find that focusing occupational therapy on her wrist function alone, to the exclusion of her psychosocial needs, will not be as helpful as you thought it would be (e.g., Chan & Spencer, 2004).

Step 3: Appraising the Evidence

The goal of the search for evidence is to find the *best* possible answer to the clinical question, not a single *correct* answer (Sackett et al., 2000; Tickle-Degnen, 2000b). The evidence may be useful and valuable for guiding work with a client even though it cannot give a definitive prescription of practice. It offers hypotheses to test and possibilities to try out. Before you can use the evidence, however, you must determine systematically just how useful and valuable it is for providing a possible answer to your question.

The Basics of Appraising the Relevance and Trustworthiness of Research Evidence

Evidence that is clinically useful and valuable is both relevant to the clinical task and trustworthy (Domholdt, 2005). There are many excellent resources for guiding the appraisal of research evidence (e.g., Law, 2002; Sackett et al., 2000). Therefore, the presentation here is on the general systematic reasoning that underlies the appraisal process.

APPRAISING THE RELEVANCE OF A RESEARCH STUDY. The **relevance** of a research study is determined by the degree to which it answers the clinical question and by the degree to which its methods fit within the constraints and resources of the practitioner's context of practice (Tickle-Degnen, 2001, 2002b). Rarely will the search for evidence locate a study or set of studies that directly answers the clinical question. The studies were designed to answer the authors' research questions, not your clinical question. The most relevant research study is one that (1) provides the type of evidence that is needed for the clinical task, (2) investigates a variable that is the occupational variable of interest or one highly related to that variable, (3) includes research participants who are members of your client's population, and (4) offers clinical methods that are suitable to your context of practice.

To illustrate the process of examining relevance, we return to the citations retrieved in response to Question B in Table 30.2, "What is a valid method for assessing the occupational goals of clients with hand dysfunction?" One citation was for a paper by Melville and colleagues (2002) that can be retrieved in full text from the American Occupational Therapy Association's Website (www. aota.org). Full text retrieval for papers published in the *American Journal of Occupational Therapy* is available to all members.

The purpose of Melville and colleagues' (2002) research study was to investigate patient perspectives of the validity of the Self-Identified Goal Assessment (SIGA). Patients were interviewed about the usefulness of the

instrument with respect to identifying their own goals. This purpose signifies that the study provides **assessment evidence** about occupational goals and thus is relevant with respect to the type of evidence and occupational variable elements of the clinical question. Remember, however, that the key term *women* was used to retrieve this citation after the term *hand dysfunction* failed to retrieve any citations with the relevant type of evidence and occupational variable. As a result, the study is less relevant with respect to the clinical population element of the question. With respect to Wanda, the sample consisted primarily of women; however, they were older and frail, on the average, rather than middle-aged and relatively robust. More important, they were inpatients in a subacute rehabilitation inpatient unit, not outpatients. Items contained in the SIGA were worded around identifying tasks "you would like to work on or improve on in therapy before you go back home" (p. 653). Therefore, although the assessment is relevant for assessing the occupational goals of inpatients, it is not relevant, as worded, for assessing the goals of outpatients.

Although the SIGA might not be the most relevant assessment for Wanda because of some of its wording, its structure is highly practical for your busy outpatient practice. The authors (Melville et al., 2002) found that the mean administration time of the SIGA was 5.6 minutes, compared to 18.8 minutes for administering another possibly relevant goal assessment measure, the Canadian Occupational Performance Measure (COPM; Law et al., 2005). Since the SIGA generally is relevant to your purposes, you should continue with your appraisal of the trustworthiness of the findings of the study.

APPRAISING THE TRUSTWORTHINESS OF A RESEARCH STUDY. Whereas the relevance of a research study is assessed primarily as a degree of fit between your clinical need, as represented in the clinical question, and the methods of the study, the **trustworthiness** of a research study is assessed primarily as a degree of fit between the researcher's research question, or purpose, and the methods of a study. A trustworthy study is one for which the conclusions are defensible with respect to the methods of the study, and there are few if any alternative plausible, scientific explanations for the findings beyond the conclusions drawn from the study and its researchers (Domholdt, 2005). Trustworthiness is enhanced when the researcher carefully and rigorously maintains standards of discovery, description, and explanation (Carpenter & Hammell, 2000).

The most trustworthy research study is one that (1) gathers the type of evidence that achieves the stated purpose, (2) investigates trustworthiness using a variety of methods, and (3) clearly identifies the study's methods, strengths, and limitations with respect to standards of science. The evidence-based practitioner attempts to evaluate the degree to which a descriptive study provides a defensible description of a client or clinical population;

the degree to which an assessment study provides a strong test of the reliability, validity, or usefulness of an assessment procedure; or the degree to which an intervention effectiveness study supports the conclusion that client outcomes were caused by the intervention and not by other factors.

In general, studies that are of interest to occupational therapy practitioners, that is, studies of clinically relevant human performance, behavior, motives, and interests, have limitations in their ability to meet their purposes. For example, individuals from a given clinical population might be rare or have difficulty participating in research procedures. Or the variable of interest might be complex and difficult to describe or assess. Or factors that are not anticipated or understood by the researchers might contribute to the findings, such as unexpected cold weather affecting an individual's response to exercise. Nonetheless, some studies provide stronger evidence with respect to trustworthiness than others because they have attempted to carefully and rigorously address these and other potential limitations (Domholdt, 2005).

With respect to the study of the SIGA by Melville and colleagues (2002), the stated purpose of the study was to investigate patient perspectives of the validity of the SIGA. Clearly, the purpose was to collect **assessment evidence**. To accomplish this purpose, the investigators modeled their design and procedures after those used for validation studies of the COPM. Occupational therapy practitioners administered the SIGA to 20 women and 10 men close to admission in a subacute rehabilitation unit and then once again before discharge. Following each administration, an investigator conducted a structured interview of each patient to gather patient perspectives related to the usefulness of the SIGA in identifying personal therapy-related goals. Data analysis consisted of descriptively analyzing the results of the SIGA administration to clients (e.g., numbers and types of goals identified) and summarizing, quantitatively and qualitatively, the clients' responses to the structured interviews about the usefulness of the SIGA. The investigators compared their results with the results of a previous study of the SIGA as well as results from studies of the COPM, finding results to be similar. They also discussed clearly the strengths and limitations of the study methods and the SIGA and provided suggestions for future validation studies.

From your reading of the SIGA assessment study, you might conclude the following:

1. The study gathered data from a relatively small sample in a manner that used interview procedures that were rigorous for measuring subacute rehabilitation patient perspectives about the SIGA. The investigators were careful to have the SIGA administered by the patient's occupational therapy practitioner and to have an impartial researcher carry out the interviews to gather patient perspectives. The items in the inter- view were designed to gather evidence that would elicit patient perspectives that were both positive (i.e., confirming) and negative (i.e., disconfirming) with respect to the usefulness of the SIGA.

2. The study compared their findings with the results of a previous study of the SIGA and published studies of the COPM. This comparison was used to determine whether the results of the SIGA study converged toward or diverged from the results of the other studies, enabling an additional test of the trustworthiness of the study findings.

3. The report of the study included clear information about the study's strengths and limitations, including a listing of other validation studies that were needed to provide a stronger test of the validity of the SIGA. In addition, the authors refer the reader to a Website where the reader can download the SIGA and its administration protocol. This access enables the reader to inspect the measure closely and evaluate strengths and weaknesses further.

Although the study was small and limited in scope for testing validity, the research methods were rigorous and generally conformed to standards of sound scientific practice with respect to gathering preliminary evidence on a new measure. It is reasonable to trust the study's findings for the small sample that it tested. Yet it is also reasonable to be cautious in concluding that the findings would be similar for other patients in subacute rehabilitation settings and to be more cautious about conclusions with respect to other clinical populations, such as clients in outpatient settings.

Interpretation of the Results of a Study

Now that you have completed a basic evaluation of the relevance and trustworthiness of the evidence from the study, it is time to examine the results in terms of how they can help answer the clinical question. The general results of the Melville and colleagues' (2002) study were favorable to the validity of the SIGA. Generally, the findings were convergent with other studies on client goal assessments, lending credibility to the usefulness of goal assessments with clients in general. For example, the SIGA identified goals that almost all of the patients tended to remember within 48 hours after administration and to view as their own goals as opposed to goals that others wanted for them. The SIGA was more valid for identifying one's immediately current goals and less valid for identifying goals that were consistently held by the patients. One third of the participants said that they would like to modify their goals 48 hours after administration. The researchers make a defensible argument that the SIGA may be useful as a means for monitoring changing goals and for revising goals as clients engage in therapy over time.

Central tendency research findings, such as averages and majority responses, are helpful for understanding how clients will respond in general, and individual variation research findings are helpful for anticipating the range of possibilities of how a single client might respond (Glasziou et al., 1998; Tickle-Degnen, 2001). For example, although the majority of clients (29 out of 30) saw the SIGA as useful, there was one individual who found it to be not very useful. And although the SIGA identified goals with which 70% of participants continued to be satisfied 48 hours later, 30% were ready to change their goals at that follow-up period. Melville and colleagues (2002) conducted open-ended interviews and described qualitatively individual responses in a manner that individualizes the quantitative responses. This description helps the reader to understand how participants arrived at their views of the SIGA. In studies with larger sample sizes than that of Melville and colleagues, individual variation information is found in descriptive statistics, such as the ranges and standard deviations (Tickle-Degnen, 2003), and in the results of analyses for different subgroups of research participants, such as separate findings reported for females and males (Tickle-Degnen, 2001).

On the basis of both central tendency and individual variation findings as well as your evaluation of the relevance and trustworthiness of the results, you may interpret the results as indicating that it is possible that a goal assessment procedure similar to the SIGA would be a valid means for getting to know Wanda better. Your reading of Melville and colleagues (2002) points you to the possibility of using the COPM. It would be ideal for you to go through the same evaluation process as outlined here for a study of the SIGA with a study of the COPM. Your new assessment question might be "Is the Canadian Occupational Performance Measure a valid method for assessing the occupational goals of clients with hand dysfunction?" A search using the PubMed database on the key terms *Canadian Occupational Performance Measure* and *hand dysfunction* returns five abstracts, including one that specifically addresses use of the COPM in an intervention effectiveness study of occupational therapy with women who have Colles' fractures (Dekkers & Soballe, 2004). Although the study was designed to collect intervention effectiveness evidence, it provides assessment evidence as well. The *Related Articles* link in PubMed attached to this article links to 102 references that are relevant to the rehabilitation of Colles' fractures. It might be helpful to look over some of these abstracts to gain a better understanding of what Wanda faces with respect to her Colles' fracture.

If there is time, or at a later date, you should evaluate the body of evidence as a whole with respect to answering the clinical question, giving extra weight to the single studies with the strongest evidence. The "best" evidence is the best that can be found, not "best" in the sense of meeting all of the standards. The possible answer this best evidence delivers may be one about which you can feel a high, moderate, or low degree of confidence. You might not have enough time to gather and evaluate enough evidence to form a confident opinion, which is very likely, given, in this scenario, how busy you are as a practitioner in an outpatient clinic. Even with little research evidence about which you feel a modicum of confidence, you may go to the next step of evidence-based practice: communication about the evidence with the client, in this case Wanda, and other individuals who are important to the client.

Step 4: Communicating About the Evidence for Decision Making

The primary purpose of communication about evidence is making wise decisions about therapeutic goals and procedures (Tickle-Degnen, 2000b, 2002c). Wise decisions are ones that are likely to benefit the client and family members and are embraced by client, family members, you (the occupational therapy practitioner), and others of importance to the client, such as other practitioners. Communication that achieves these types of decisions (1) has content that accurately represents the research evidence, including its strengths and weaknesses related to relevance and trustworthiness, (2) involves language that is mutually understandable to all participants, and (3) encourages an open and mutual discussion of information and ideas rather than a closed-ended or unidirectional delivery of information from one individual to another. Even a small amount of evidence in which you have a small degree of confidence can be helpful in decision making if it is presented with these qualities in mind.

Accurate Content About the Evidence

Accurate communication content is balanced in its description of central tendency findings about average or majority responses of research participants, and variation findings about the degree to these participants differ in their responses. Communication with an overfocus on central tendency findings implies that the client surely has the same occupational issues, goals, and outcomes as the majority of research participants or the ones with an average response. For example, a statement that is overfocused on central tendency findings might be the following: "Clients find satisfaction in forming their own goals for therapy" (or, if the evidence pointed in this direction, replacing *satisfaction* with wording associated with dissatisfaction). This example implies that all participants in the research studies were satisfied, which was not the case. On the other hand, communication with an overfocus on variation findings implies that the client surely will have different occupational issues, goals, and outcomes than will the majority or average research participant. For example, consider the statement "Some clients are satisfied and some are not with making their own goals for therapy, because everyone is different and unique." This example fails to inform Wanda about majority or average responses, which she might find helpful in orienting her own response.

An example of a communication that balances central tendency findings with a variation perspective, and therefore is more accurate than the statements in the previous paragraph, would be "Generally, clients have found satisfaction in forming their own goals for therapy. However, some have been more satisfied than others in participating in forming their own goals. Would you like to be involved in forming some of the goals that you and I work toward in therapy?" In this communication, the findings are accurately portrayed, in the past rather than present tense, and the pertinent relevance issue is addressed, enabling Wanda to assess the evidence herself.

Balance in central tendency and variation findings is the basis of communication for all types of evidence. When the evidence is about descriptive, intervention, or **responsiveness evidence**, the same wording issues apply. Wording such as "You must do this intervention because it has been found to work for other clients" is inaccurate, misleading, and contrary to client-centered practice.

Mutually Understandable Language

Information that is understandable is communicated with words and grammar that fit the client's background and comprehension ability. The point is to provide information that supports the client's active participation in clinical decisions. The use of professional terminology (e.g., *functional performance*) or jargon (e.g., *ADL*) should be avoided or explicitly taught to the client. Similarly, scientific, research, and statistical terminology should not be used unless it is of interest to the client. As was shown in the previous sections, findings can be discussed without going into a complex description or explanation.

The main goal of communicating about evidence is to inform the process of decision making, not to elaborate on detailed points that are not necessary for this goal. Information that is understandable and usable is brief and to the point. Pictures and graphs may be used depending on the client's preferred learning style (Redman, 1997).

Encouraging an Open and Mutual Discussion of Information and Ideas

In her review of research on client-centered practice, Law (1998) demonstrated that respect and collaboration elements of the therapeutic relationship were important predictors of rehabilitation outcome, just as they are in all health care relationships (Martin, Garske, & Davis, 2000). Practitioners and clients come to an understanding of one another's perspectives through communication and the therapeutic activities they do with one another (Crepeau, 1991; Mattingly & Fleming, 1994). When the practitioner begins a discussion about evidence, the wording should reflect that the discussion will be about open-ended probabilities and possibilities, rather than about closed-ended certainties.

In communicating with Wanda about the possibility of performing an assessment of her occupational goals,

building on the communication qualities described previously, you might say, "Wanda, there are some questions I could ask you about your goals for therapy that might be helpful for me getting to know more about what is important to you, so that we can focus on those things in therapy. In a research study, most patients were satisfied with these questions for identifying their goals, although some were not satisfied. It was a fairly small study of people who were older than you and staying in a hospital, but the general method seems useful for our needs right now. Do you have any thoughts about me asking questions about your goals for therapy?" Later, if the two of you try out the assessment methods, modified for Wanda's situation, you could suggest to Wanda that you repeat similar questions at each session, since the research study by Melville and colleagues (2002) suggested that people may change their goals quickly.

ETHICS, PRACTICE VALUES, AND EVIDENCE-BASED PRACTICE

As has been put forward in this chapter, evidence-based practice emerges from the core values and ethics of occupational therapy (American Occupational Therapy Association, 2000; Christiansen & Lou, 2001; Kanny, 1993). Evidence-based practice occurs in a respectful, truthful, and collaborative relationship with the client and with those acting on the client's behalf. Clients are viewed as active contributors to the planning and intervention process of therapy rather than as passive recipients of information or services (Law, Baptiste, & Mills, 1995). To be active rather than passive, that is, to act with as much autonomy as possible and the least amount of dependency, clients and those acting on their behalf must be informed rather than uninformed or misinformed. To be an informed client means to know the meaning of one's occupational status in relationship to one's quality of life, to know the nature and quality of possible occupational therapy assessments to be undertaken, to know the quality and probable outcomes of relevant interventions, and to have the means to assess one's own progress toward meaningful outcomes. Once informed, clients and those acting on their behalf can reason and act with the degree of autonomy of which they are capable.

One implication of autonomous reasoning and action is that clients can choose to participate or not participate in occupational therapy assessments and interventions. Likewise, family members or other health practitioners may decide to encourage or discourage client participation. Evidence-based practice is not about the imposition of the will of one individual on the will of the other, but rather is a mutual search for and discussion about information that will aid informed, wise decision making. The practitioner's responsibility is to provide information in such a manner that reasoned decision making is maximized.

EMBRACING AN IDEOLOGY OF CHANGE IN OCCUPATIONAL THERAPY KNOWLEDGE AND PRACTICE

Perhaps one of the greatest challenges of evidence-based practice is that what is considered to be the best evidence to answer a clinical question can change as more research is conducted. What might be the best information for working with Wanda today might be substandard a year from now. That there is no fixed answer to how to work with people like Wanda requires an approach to occupational therapy education, practice, and theory development that embraces an ideology of change and development. We certainly embrace this ideology for our clients, expecting them to be open to, and changing with, the new circumstances of their lives, to losses, and to gains.

How can we embrace this ideology of change? First, we must recognize that knowledge is not static and closed, but rather dynamic and open (Kaplan, 1964/1998). Strategies for using dynamic and open evidence begin with recognizing that knowing how to learn on a daily basis is a fundamental skill of an occupational therapy practitioner. Expertise is not knowing facts but rather knowing how to find out probabilistic answers to complex questions in a manner that can help us to make practical decisions (Mattingly & Fleming, 1994; Tickle-Degnen & Bedell, 2003).

Second, we must advocate for resources to do evidence-based practice. Using an ever-changing pool of evidence requires time and institutional, organizational, and government support in the form of policy, training, and infrastructure. Without this time and support at a systemic level, it is very difficult for individual practitioners to be evidence-based (Illott, 2003).

By adapting to changing circumstances and changing evidence, occupational therapy will continue to be a vibrant, healthy, and important force in the health of individuals with occupational needs. The tools and strategies of evidence-based practice harness this change to the benefit of our clients and our own professional development.

PROVOCATIVE QUESTIONS

1. What is the evidence that hand injury or hand therapy is interrelated with psychosocial aspects of clients' lives and experiences?
2. What should Rebecca do with the information that Wanda disclosed to her during therapy?
3. Imagine that you have a new client with a diagnosis of adrenoleukodystrophy, a diagnosis that is unfamiliar to you. What steps would you take to find evidence that would provide you with a better understanding of the needs of clients from this population?
4. As you are developing an intervention plan, you can find no evidence specifically about the effectiveness of occupational therapy on outcomes for individuals with adrenoleukodystrophy. What should you do as an evidence-based practitioner?
5. In a clinical setting that does not provide organizational support for evidence-based practice, what strategies would you develop to support your evidence-based practice?

REFERENCES

American Occupational Therapy Association. (2000). Occupational therapy code of ethics. Retrieved June, 6, 2005, from http://www.aota.org/general/coe.asp

Bennett, S., Hoffmann, T., McCluskey, A, McKenna, K., Strong, J., & Tooth, L. (2003). Introducing OTseeker (Occupational Therapy Systematic Evaluation of Evidence): A new evidence database for occupational therapists. *American Journal of Occupational Therapy, 57,* 635–638.

Carpenter, C., & Hammell, K. (2000). Evaluating qualitative research. In K. W. Hammell, C. Carpenter, & I. Dyck (Eds.), *Using qualitative research: A practical introduction for occupational and physical therapists.* Edinburgh: Churchill Livingstone.

Chan, J., & Spencer, J. (2004). Adaptation to hand injury: An evolving experience. *American Journal of Occupational Therapy, 58,* 128–139.

Christiansen, C., & Lou, J. Q. (2001). Ethical considerations related to evidence-based practice. *American Journal of Occupational Therapy, 55,* 230–232.

Crepeau, E. B. (1991). Achieving intersubjective understanding: Examples from an occupational therapy treatment session. *American Journal of Occupational Therapy, 45,* 1016–1025.

Dekkers, M., & Soballe, K. (2004). Activities and impairments in the early stage of rehabilitation after Colles' fracture. *Disability & Rehabilitation, 26,* 662–668. Abstract retrieved October 1, 2005, from PubMed database.

Dolan, P., Torgerson, D., & Kakarlapudi, T. K. (1999). Health-related quality of life of Colles' fracture patients. *Osteoporosis International, 9,* 196–199. Abstract retrieved October 1, 2005, from PubMed database.

Domholdt, E. (2005). *Rehabilitation research: Principles and applications* (3rd ed.). St. Louis: Elsevier Saunders.

Egan, M., Dubouloz, C.-J., von Zweck, C., & Vallerand, J. (1998). The client-centered evidence-based practice of occupational therapy. *Canadian Journal of Occupational Therapy, 65,* 136–143.

Glasziou, P., Guyatt, G. H., Dans, A. L., Dans, L. F., Straus, S., & Sackett, D. L. (1998). Editorial: Applying the results of trials and systematic reviews to individual patients. *ACP Journal Club, 129,* A15–16.

Gould, S. J. (1996). *Full house: The spread of excellence from Plato to Darwin.* New York: Three Rivers Press.

Illott, I. (2003). Challenging the rhetoric and reality: Only an individual and systemic approach will work for evidence-based occupational therapy. *American Journal of Occupational Therapy, 57,* 351–354.

Kanny, E. (1993). Core values and attitudes of occupational therapy practice. Retrieved June 6, 2005, from http://www.aota.org/members/area2/links/link05.asp

Kaplan, A. (1964/1998). *The conduct of inquiry: Methodology for behavioral science.* New Brunswick, NJ: Transaction.

Law, M. (1998). Does client-centered practice make a difference? In M. Law (Ed.), *Client-centered occupational therapy* (pp. 19–27). Thorofare, NJ: Slack.

Law, M. (Ed.) (2002). *Evidence-based rehabilitation: A guide to practice.* Thorofare, NJ: Slack.

Law, M., Baptiste, S., Carswell, A., McColl, M.A., Polatajko, H., & Pollock, N. (2005). *Canadian Occupational Performance Measure* (4th ed.). Ottawa: Canadian Association of Occupational Therapists.

Law, M., Baptiste, S., & Mills, J. (1995). Client-centered practice: What does it mean and does it make a difference? *Canadian Journal of Occupational Therapy, 62,* 250–257.

Law, M., Baum, C., & Dunn, W. (Eds.). (2005). *Measuring occupational performance: Supporting best practice in occupational therapy* (2nd ed.). Thorofare, NJ: Slack.

Law, M., Cooper, B., Strong, S., Stewart, D., Rigby, P., & Letts, L. (1996). The Person-Environment-Occupation Model: A transactive approach to occupational performance. *Canadian Journal of Occupational Therapy, 63,* 9–23.

Lee, C. J. & Miller, L. T. (2003). The process of evidence-based clinical decision-making in occupational therapy. *American Journal of Occupational Therapy, 57,* 473–477.

Martin, D. J., Garske, J. P., & Davis, M. K. (2000). Relation of the therapeutic alliance with outcome and other variables: A meta-analytic review. *Journal of Consulting & Clinical Psychology, 68,* 438–450.

Mattingly, C., & Fleming, M. H. (1994). *Clinical reasoning: Forms of inquiry in a therapeutic practice.* Philadelphia: Davis.

Melville, L. L., Baltic, T. A., Bettcher, T. W., & Nelson, D. L. (2002). Patients' perspectives on the self-identified goals assessment. *American Journal of Occupational Therapy, 56,* 650–659.

Portney, L. G., & Watkins, M. P. (2000). *Foundations of clinical research* (2nd ed.). Upper Saddle River, NJ: Prentice Hall Health.

Rappolt, S. (2003). The role of professional expertise in evidence-based occupational therapy. *American Journal of Occupational Therapy, 57,* 589–593.

Redman, B. K. (1997). *The practice of patient education* (8th ed.). St. Louis: Mosby.

Reis, R. (1994). Wanda. In C. Mattingly & M. H. Fleming, *Clinical reasoning: Forms of inquiry in a therapeutic practice* (pp. 349–351). Philadelphia: Davis.

Sackett, D. L., Straus, S. E., Richardson, W. S., Rosenberg, W., & Haynes, R. B. (2000). *Evidence-based medicine* (2nd ed.). Edinburgh: Churchill Livingstone.

Tickle-Degnen, L. (1999). Organizing, evaluating, and using evidence in occupational therapy practice. *American Journal Occupational Therapy, 53,* 537–539.

Tickle-Degnen, L. (2000a). Gathering current research evidence to enhance clinical reasoning. *American Journal Occupational Therapy, 54,* 102–105.

Tickle-Degnen, L. (2000b). Communicating with clients, family members, and colleagues about research evidence. *American Journal of Occupational Therapy, 54,* 341–343.

Tickle-Degnen, L. (2000c). Monitoring and documenting evidence during assessment and intervention. *American Journal of Occupational Therapy, 54,* 434–436.

Tickle-Degnen, L. (2001). From the general to the specific: Using meta-analytic reports in clinical decision-making. *Evaluation & the Health Professions, 24,* 308–326.

Tickle-Degnen, L. (2002a). Client-centered practice, therapeutic relationship, and the use of research evidence. *American Journal of Occupational Therapy, 56,* 470–474.

Tickle-Degnen, L. (2002b). Communicating evidence to clients, managers, and funders. In M. Law (Ed.), *Evidence-based rehabilitation: A guide to practice* (pp. 221–254). Thorofare, NJ: Slack.

Tickle-Degnen, L. (2003). Where is the individual in statistics? *American Journal of Occupational Therapy, 57,* 112–115.

Tickle-Degnen, L., & Bedell, G. (2003). Heterarchy and hierarchy: A critical appraisal of "levels of evidence" as a tool for clinical decision-making. *American Journal of Occupational Therapy, 57,* 234–237.

U.S. National Library of Medicine. (2005). PubMed database. Retrieved October 1, 2005, from http://www.ncbi.nlm.nih.gov/entrez/query.fcgi

World Health Organization. (2005). *International classification of functioning, disability, and health.* Online browser. Retrieved October 1, 2005, from http://www3.who.int/icf/onlinebrowser/icf.cfm

Protecting Vulnerable Clients

31

Preventing and Responding to Client Maltreatment Through Direct Service, Case Management, and Advocacy

DEBORA A. DAVIDSON

> I am only one. But I am still one. I cannot do everything, but still can do something. I will not refuse to do the something I can do.
>
> —EDWARD EVERETT HALL (1822–1909)

> The moment you have protected the individual you have protected society.
>
> —KENNETH KANUDA (B. 1924)

Learning Objectives

After reading this chapter, you will be able to:

1. Define the terms *abuse*, *neglect*, and *exploitation*, and give examples of each of these as they relate to people with disabilities across the life course.
2. Recognize the main risk factors that contribute to clients' vulnerability and know ways to identify these in individuals' lives.
3. Identify ways in which abuse and neglect may be prevented through occupational therapy.
4. Understand the law and the American Occupational Therapy Association's standards of practice regarding an occupational therapy practitioner's role in responding to suspected abuse or neglect.

INTRODUCTION

Occupational therapy's domain of practice and primary mission is the promotion of individuals' engagement in meaningful activities and roles within their homes and communities (American Occupational Therapy Association, 2002). Preventing the abuse, neglect, and exploitation of occupational therapy clients fulfills two central missions of the profession: helping people to pursue occupational goals and protecting them from harm. A sense of physical and emotional safety is needed for clients to work toward the achievement of many occupational performance goals (Christiansen & Townsend, 2004). The Occupational Therapy Code of Ethics—2005 cites beneficence, or the demonstration of concern for clients' well-being, as its first principle (American Occupational Therapy Association, 2005). Clearly, occupational therapy practitioners have a mandate to understand the dynamics that result in harm to clients and to join with colleagues from other helping disciplines to strive to eliminate this public health problem. The purpose of this chapter is to assist the reader in understanding why and how abuse occurs, to help prevent such situations from developing, and to recognize and respond to abusive situations affecting a variety of client populations.

MALTREATMENT AND OCCUPATIONAL PERFORMANCE

For many individuals with disabilities, experiences of maltreatment by family members or paid caregivers result in long-term reductions in their occupational opportunities. Maltreatment includes economic exploitation, neglect, and various forms of abuse (see Box 31.1.) Research has shown links between maltreatment early in life and lifelong neurological, developmental, and psychiatric problems (Egeland, Sroufe & Erickson, 1983; Haskett & Kistner, 1991; Hoffman-Plotkin & Twentyman, 1984; Jaudes & Diamond, 1985; Manly, Kim, Rogosh, & Cicchetti, 2001; Pears & Fisher, 2005; Putnam, 2003). Individuals with disabilities who are enduring maltreatment might avoid opportunities to participate in occupational roles because of fear of punishment, or they might have restricted access to resources and contexts requisite to many activities (Milberger et al., 2003; Ryan, Salenblatt, Schiappacasse, & Maly, 2001; Stancliff, 1997).

DISABILITY: A RISK FACTOR FOR ABUSE ACROSS THE LIFE COURSE

People of all ages with disabilities are at significantly increased risk of neglect, abuse, and exploitation when compared with those whose abilities are typical (McAllister, 2000; Milberger et al., 2003; Spencer et al., 2005; Strand, Benzein & Saveman, 2004). A study comparing the prevalence of maltreatment in school children found a rate of 11% among nondisabled children and a rate of 31% in the disabled group (Sullivan & Knutson, 2000). In 47% of the cases, the child's disability was thought to have been a causative factor in the abuse; in over 14% of the cases, disabilities were the result of abuse. In a survey of agencies serving survivors of sexual abuse and assault, Sobsey (as cited by Lumley & Miltenberger, 1997) found that 54% of the clients had cognitive impairment. A study of women with mild mental retardation found that 71% of the sample had experienced forced or coerced sexual contact (Stroms-

---

BOX 31.1 DEFINITIONS OF TERMS

- **Economic exploitation** is the unethical use or taking of another person's money or property, either without their knowledge or through the use of undue influence. Theft and coercion to "give" gifts or loans are examples of this.
- **Neglect** is the withholding of nutrition, shelter, clothing, or medical care, such that a dependent person's health is endangered. Undersupervision and abandonment are included in this category.
- **Self-neglect** occurs when an older person engages in behavior that places his or her safety or health in danger without the cognitive capacity or judgment to anticipate consequences.

- **Physical abuse** includes punching, shaking, kicking, biting, throwing, burning, and other forms of injurious punishment.
- **Sexual abuse** is any seduction, coercion, or forcing of a person to observe or participate in sexual activity for the sexual gratification of a more powerful individual.
- **Psychological abuse** involves coercion and punishment through threats of harm to the individual or those he or she cares about, humiliation, or otherwise deliberately undermining a person's self-esteem and well-being.

ness, 1993). Research involving 177 women with physical disabilities, most of whom lived independently, found that 56% of the sample had experienced some form of abuse (Milberger et al., 2003). Results of a national study indicated that at least 450,000 elderly Americans experienced abuse, neglect and/or exploitation in 1996 (National Center on Elder Abuse, 1998). The National Center on Elder Abuse (1998) estimated that for every case of elder abuse, neglect, or financial exploitation reported to state authorities, about five others have gone unreported.

Studies have shown that abuse occurs in many settings: homes, schools, work settings, group homes, and residential care facilities (Lumley & Miltenberger, 1997; Marchetti & McCartney, 1990). The home is the most common site of maltreatment, although abuse in institutional settings is also well documented (Bonner, Crow, & Hensley, 1997; National Center on Elder Abuse, 1998). Data regarding the incidence of abuse and neglect are not complete or entirely accurate, due to significant underreporting and limitations in data collection (Bonner et al., 1997; Kenny, 2001; Oktay & Tompkins, 2004). It is very likely that the actual numbers of people suffering mistreatment are much greater than can be established through current methods of data collection (National Center on Elder Abuse, 1998).

CAUSES OF ABUSE AND NEGLECT

Abuse, neglect, and exploitation are the outcomes of a dynamic interplay of factors that involve the environment, the perpetrator, and the victim (Hoffman-Plotkin & Twentyman, 1984; McAllister, 2000). Only by understanding each of these domains and how they interact can problems of mistreatment be prevented and methods of dealing with mistreatment be improved.

Environmental Risk Factors

Prevailing societal, community, and family attitudes about how to resolve conflict and the value of persons with disabilities influence individuals' behaviors. In the dominant culture of the United States, individualism is generally valued over collectivism (Kondo, 2004). Individuals and families are encouraged to take responsibility for themselves, and privacy is highly valued. Self-reliance and achievement through independent effort are also prized. These values have helped the United States to become the greatest economic power the world has ever known. These values might also have contributed to the isolation and disparagement of people who have needs that require a more interdependent way of life. Additionally, contemporary American culture promotes violence as an acceptable solution for conflict, a means of establishing power, and even a source of entertainment (Noguera, 2001; Prothrow-Stith, 1991). The prevailing cultural conditions

result in an environment that supports the use of aggression in American homes and institutions.

The more immediate community culture can have a greater impact on individuals' behavior than the culture that is found at the national level. Some neighborhoods and towns are cohesive and interactive, resulting in available positive support and social scrutiny, a combination that tends to reduce antisocial behavior (Sampson & Groves, 1989). In other communities, neighbors might not know one another at all or might harbor mistrust and dislike of each other. In such communities, there might be no one to turn to in times of crisis and no sense of mutual concern or interest. In communities where people commonly verbally and/or physically batter one another or where neighbors rarely interact, all people are at increased risk of victimization (Vondra, 1990).

Poverty is a risk factor for many public health problems, including domestic violence and neglect. It correlates positively with increased rates of child abuse and neglect (Coulton, Korbin, Su, & Chow, 1995; Sedlak & Broadhurst, 1996; U.S. Department of Health and Human Services, 2000). Additionally, unemployment (Milberger et al., 2003) and lower income (Oktay & Tompkins, 2004) are positively correlated with maltreatment of adults with disabilities. Although poverty is linked to increased levels of abuse, high levels of social integration and community morale appear to be mitigating factors that can reduce levels of child abuse even in low-income neighborhoods (Garbarino & Kostelny, 1992).

Risk Factors Related to Caregivers

People who perpetrate abuse range from the overwhelmed parent or caregiver who occasionally reacts harshly out of exhaustion and despair to the calculating sociopath who deliberately seeks and systematically hurts victims (Mac-Namara, 1992). Some caregivers are neglectful out of ignorance of the medical or daily care needs of the individual in their care or because of a lack of resources. Sometimes family caregivers have health or life complications of their own and are unable to manage the demands of juggling a complex array of responsibilities (McAllister, 2000). Some caregivers harbor feelings of anger and resentment based on a history of conflict with a spouse or parent who is now in their care.

Social isolation, a critical risk factor in maltreatment, can be a function of the person as well as the environment. Many caregivers, both family members and paid staff, work alone for long hours, resulting in increased stress and a lack of oversight by outsiders. If a caregiver has limited contact with others who are emotionally and functionally supportive, the risk of abuse increases (Windham, 2000). Caregivers who seek and utilize social supports within the family or community are reducing the risk of maltreatment as well as increasing their job satisfaction (Gerits, Derksen, & Verbruggen, 2004).

Caregivers who have little sensitivity to others' feelings or perspectives, limited capacity for putting others' needs before their own, and/or a low tolerance for frustration are at increased risk of acting abusively. People who abuse alcohol or drugs or who have other mental health problems such as depression or borderline personality disorder are more prone to act abusively than is the typical caregiver. An adolescent mother is at increased risk of mistreating her child, just by virtue of being young, both psychologically and neurologically (Strauch, 2003). As with all risk factors, these personal characteristics are not reliable predictors. However, they are factors that, when combined with other features of the situation, can influence outcomes.

Risk Factors Related to the Client

A trait that is shared by people who become victims of domestic or institutional abuse or neglect is dependence on others for meeting basic needs, such as shelter, food, clothing, medical care, or social contact. This group includes all infants and children, with or without typical development, as well as adolescents and adults with significant disabilities and the elderly. The longer the duration of a person's dependency, the longer is the duration of increased risk of maltreatment.

The more fragile an individual's health, the greater are the chances of long-term harm from maltreatment. Infants and young children are at higher risk for life-threatening injuries than are older children and adolescents (Sedlak & Broadhurst, 1996). Of all elders, those aged 80 years and older were abused at two to three times the rate of younger respondents in a national sample (National Center on Elder Abuse, 1998).

People who are unable to report or resist mistreatment are at increased risk of abuse and neglect for multiple reasons (Lumley & Miltenberger, 1997; Vondra, 1990). Individuals with cognitive disabilities are often acculturated to be passive and compliant (Tharinger, Horton, & Millea, 1990). They are expected to trust and obey a wide array of caregivers and are often rewarded for being "good" (Lumley & Miltenberger, 1997). Assertive disagreement or resistance to following directives may be construed as problematic or even symptomatic and may be treated accordingly. In addition to issues of acculturation, many people with limited independence have severely restricted social lives and are eager to please their caregivers, whom they may construe as potential friends.

If an abusive or exploitative caregiver provides essential assistance, the care recipient might be unable or unwilling to risk the loss of services, even if it means enduring mistreatment (Milberger et al., 2003). In some cases, even if victimized individuals would like to have help, their disabilities and social isolation prevent effective communication of the problem.

In addition to prolonged dependence, some individuals have inherent and learned traits or behaviors that may trigger aggression by a susceptible caregiver. Depen-

dent individuals who resist attempts to provide care and those who are more active, for example, may elicit aggressive reactions more often than do passive individuals (Strand et al., 2003). Clients who have cognitive deficits might strike or otherwise hurt caregivers, who might then retaliate (Oktay & Tomkins, 2004; Strand et al., 2004).

However, current evidence indicates that caregiver characteristics are more important in predicting abuse than are the level of dependence and the severity of impairment of the care recipient. One recent study of characteristics of children who were abused concluded that parental attitudes toward the children were more predictive of abuse than was the type or severity of the child's health problems (Sidebotham & Heron, 2003). Personal care assistants of adults with disabilities are more likely to abuse if they are male, are inexperienced, work long hours, or have a low income (Oktay & Tompkins, 2004). An exception to this trend may be women with hearing impairment, which may be a type of disability that, in and of itself, increases the risk of abuse, regardless of caregiver characteristics (Milberger et al., 2003).

PREVENTING MISTREATMENT

MacNamara (1992, p. 4) states, "One reason for the persistence of the problem [of abuse] is that it tends to be treated episodically and not systematically." Occupational therapy practitioners can influence the environment, including the caregivers, and the client. Helping clients to develop skills that reduce dependency in activities of daily living reduces caregivers' stress and necessary intrusion. The routine involvement of people with disabilities in community functions also reduces the risk of victimization. Not only is social isolation reduced, but the disabled individual has opportunities to develop social and decision-making skills that are antithetical to acting like a victim.

Most abuse is caused by someone familiar with access to the victim (Sobsey & Doe, 1991). Caregivers can benefit from a supportive educational approach that includes hands-on training and performance evaluation, which facilitates a sense of empowerment along with needed skills. Helping family caregivers to develop a schedule of family, friends, or community members who can regularly visit with, assist, or provide respite to the caregiver eases isolation and reduces the risk of abuse at home. Connecting families with consumer support groups and social service agencies that provide professional respite, day programs, supervised group living, transportation, or other services to disabled individuals is another way of reducing the risk of abuse and neglect.

When clients enter institutional care, their likelihood of experiencing sexual abuse increases significantly (Lumley & Miltenberger, 1997). Occupational therapy practitioners can provide needed support and information to institutional workers via regular consultative visits and during direct intervention (Marchetti & McCartney, 1990). An even more sustaining approach is to advise managers on ways to maximize the quality of staffing. Establishing shifts that are predictable and of reasonable duration, providing frequent and regular supervision, and requiring staff development and training help to reduce the risk of abuse in institutional settings (MacNamara, 1992).

Another level of preventive intervention lies in the larger environment. Occupational therapy practitioners are positioned to help facilities to develop programs that bring community members into the facility and take people with disabilities out into the community. Occupational therapy practitioners can educate members of community agencies and businesses regarding opportunities to include people with developmental disabilities and their caregivers. Such groups include churches, Junior League, Lions Club, Rotary Club, Boy and Girl Scouts, Small Business Associations, groups of artists and musicians, and Junior Achievement. Institutions that invite the public in via volunteer opportunities and open social events and that establish a high profile in the community provide a healthier environment for both staff members and residents.

Assertiveness training that specifically teaches individuals to recognize and respond to dangerous or exploitative situations can help clients to avoid victimization (Khemka & Hickson, 2000; Lumley & Miltenberger, 1997). Sexuality education is a necessary and often overlooked intervention for people with developmental disabilities (Lumley & Miltenberger, 1997; Tharinger, Horton & Millea, 1990). It is impossible for clients and caregivers to make good choices without adequate information. Occupational therapy practitioners who have completed appropriate educational preparation can make important contributions here,

either independently or in conjunction with other professionals on the intervention team.

IDENTIFYING AND RESPONDING TO MISTREATMENT

Unfortunately, it is not always possible to prevent abuse from occurring. Occupational therapy practitioners can play an effective role in identifying and intervening in existing cases of abuse. The presence of practitioners in institutional, community, and home settings allows them to continuously evaluate clients' interactions with paid and family caregivers, friends, and work associates during routine activities. Often, the signs of ongoing physical or sexual abuse are subtle and indirect, especially if the client has limited language, is intimidated, or is habitually compliant. Practitioners must be sensitive to changes in demeanor and nonverbal communications to evaluate the possibility of abuse (Tharinger et al., 1990). Client behaviors that may indicate abuse include acting anxious or out of character in the presence of a particular individual. Occupational therapy practitioners should be vigilant for physical evidence of abuse, such as bruises or other types of injury that are not logically explained. Interactions between the caregiver and client may indicate patterns of domination, intimidation, or neglect. Caregivers should be evaluated by interview and observation for signs of distress and burnout, anger, or lack of preparedness for the tasks for which they are responsible. The caregivers' work-related social supports and resources that they can access in emergencies are part of the evaluation as well.

PRACTICE DILEMMA: Iris and the "Teasing" Co-Worker

Iris was a 23-year-old woman with Down syndrome who was in her second month of a competitive employment position in a discount retail store, where she stocked shelves and swept the floor. Iris received weekly job coaching by an occupational therapy practitioner, who was impressed by Iris's developing work habits and social skills. One week, the practitioner noticed that Iris appeared subdued and preoccupied. When she asked Iris how things were going and how she was feeling, Iris characteristically answered, "Fine." During the following visit, the practitioner learned that Iris had missed two days of work in the previous week. The occupational therapy practitioner observed Iris and a male coworker, Bob, as they stocked shelves. Bob teased Iris by "accidentally" knocking items off the shelves so that she would then

bend over to pick them up as he watched. He called her "hot stuff," which made Iris blush and look uncomfortable. When asked privately how she felt about working with Bob, Iris replied, "He bugs me!"

Questions for Reflection and Discussion

◆ What are three signs that there is risk of abuse in this situation?

◆ What is the occupational therapy practitioner's responsibility in this situation?

◆ How could the occupational therapy practitioner intervene by facilitating changes in the environment?

◆ How could the occupational therapy practitioner intervene by facilitating changes in the client's behavior?

Practitioners in all 50 states are legally mandated to refer cases of suspected abuse or neglect to the appropriate agency and to know their state's regulations and procedures for reporting suspected abuse (Child Welfare Information Gateway, 2005; Schauer, 1995; Tharinger et al., 1990). In many cases, a decision to refer a family to Child or Adult Protective Services is made by a team, and the team's leader makes the report. However, in the absence of a team decision, an individual practitioner who has reason to suspect maltreatment is legally and ethically responsible for making a referral independently. People who report reasonable concerns to protective services are legally protected from prosecution, and their identity will be held confidential. If abuse, neglect, or exploitation is suspected, the occupational therapy practitioner should call the local branch of the appropriate state agency. Contact information for this is available in the telephone book in the government agencies and emergency numbers sections and via the Internet.

All reports that are made in good faith are acceptable, even if it becomes apparent that maltreatment has not occurred. Referrals involve making a telephone call followed by a letter that outlines the client's name, age, and address and a summary of the reasons for concern. Reports are categorized by severity and type, and investigations are scheduled accordingly. The occupational therapy practitioner should submit repeated reports if continued observations of the problem behaviors occur; multiple referrals are sometimes needed before a case qualifies for an in-depth Protective Services evaluation or a legal intervention. The average time period between referral and the initiation of intervention services is 29 days (U.S. Department of Health and Human Services, 2000).

Approximately 21% of reported child abuse and neglect cases reach the courts (U.S. Department of Health and Human Services, 2000). Available figures indicate that 7% of cases of elder abuse are resolved in court (National Center on Elder Abuse, 1998). Judges rely on professionals' notes and reports to make decisions about cases of alleged abuse. For documentation to serve as credible evidence in court, it must be deemed reliable and valid (Barth & Sullivan, 1985; Kreitzer, 1981). Reliable evidence is documented close to the event's occurrence and, when possible, by more than one observer. Repeated observations or measures taken over a period of time strengthen the report. Valid evidence employs a variety of direct measures, involves standardized tests as much as possible, and is based on objective information rather than the practitioner's interpretation.

Involving Protective Services in a case adds another facet to the work of the treatment team. The role of Protective Services is to screen cases for possible abuse or neglect; evaluate those whose problems meet intake criteria; and intervene in identified cases of abuse, neglect, or exploitation. Protective Services agencies offer or arrange for an array of services to families who are admitted to the caseload. Services may include case management, mental health counseling, drug and alcohol treatment, in-home assistance, respite care, and assistance with housing and medical care (National Center on Elder Abuse, 1998; U.S. Department of Health and Human Services, 2000).

Protective Services agencies are frequently criticized by the media and the community at large. They are typically overburdened and underfunded (Faller, 1985; Roche et al., 2000). Protective Services caseworkers are typically paraprofessionals who carry large, emotionally stressful caseloads and find limited resources to meet clients' complex needs. They earn relatively low wages for long hours of stressful and often dangerous work. Occupational practitioners whose clients are involved with Child or Adult Protective Services should strive to initiate and maintain regular contact with their clients' caseworkers to share information and form a positive working relationship. Protective Services workers can in turn support therapeutic efforts by encouraging clients and their caregivers to attend appointments and work with the practitioner.

Occupational therapy practitioners are strategically positioned, have the knowledge and skills, and are ethically and legally mandated to address this public health concern at every level. For society to reach the goal of full inclusion, it is essential to create and maintain environments that are free of abuse and exploitation. All occupational therapy practitioners should be proficient in preventing, identifying, and intervening in cases of suspected or actual abuse.

OCCUPATIONAL THERAPY INTERVENTION FOR ABUSED CHILDREN AND THEIR CAREGIVERS

Effective intervention with victimized clients and their families or caregivers requires an interdisciplinary team approach that addresses the needs of the system as well as the needs of individual family members. In many settings, the team includes social workers, teachers, psychologists, physicians, nurses, speech therapists, and/or physical therapists.

Intervention for the Caregivers or Parents

The occupational therapy practitioner can assist caregivers by helping them to identify and build on their family's strengths, teaching concepts and skills that may be lacking, and assisting with building a natural social support system. The development of a support system begins with the caregiver-practitioner relationship, which is facilitated via the practitioner's communication of caring and respect. When the caregiver views the practitioner as someone in whom to trust and confide and as someone who will try to help, a milestone has been reached. Educational and support groups for parents or other caregivers help participants to learn that they are not uniquely troubled, and they often discover helpful solutions to commonly experienced problems. Even more enduring forms of support can be developed by helping parents or other caregivers to develop mutual relationships with reliable friends, family, and community resources.

Caregiver education must be customized to fit the developmental, cognitive, physical, social, and emotional abilities of the client and the context of his or her life. Bearing this in mind, caregiver education could include behavior management techniques such as praising approximations of desirable behaviors, sticker charting, and gentle time-out. Information related about the client's developmental needs and capacities for self-regulation and safety can reduce frustration and danger caused by caregivers' unrealistic expectations. Role-playing and practicing new skills in client-caregiver activity-based sessions help to consolidate new knowledge and skills. Assertiveness training can help parents and other caregivers to improve general communication abilities and facilitate empowerment. Education and practice of crisis prevention techniques (i.e. list making; financial budgeting; planning work, leisure, and health care obligations around daily care and transportation resource availability) is often useful. Carefully timed and tactful referral for further help such as that afforded by psychotherapists, day care programs, adult educational or vocational training programs, and financial advisors can also significantly influence family functioning.

Intervention for the Child

Emotional bonding with a caring adult is requisite to healthy personality development (Bowlby, 1988; Feeny, 1996; Hazan & Zeifman, 1999; Waters & Stroufe, 1983) and subsequent social relationships (Schneider, Atkinson & Tardif, 2001). Ideally, this type of relationship should be developed with a caregiver who is a permanent member of the child's world. Sometimes the practitioner must assist the child in establishing initial trust in therapy and then transferring this new ability to a caregiver in the larger world. The practitioner may facilitate a child's ability to form relationships through activities found in healthy parent-child interactions, including cuddling and holding, feeding, grooming, and teaching developmentally appropriate skills. Reliability, gentleness, and communication of caring are essential features in this kind of therapy. Approaches for addressing the abused child's psychosocial needs may be combined with occupational therapy techniques used in treating other developmental needs, such as motor skills, dressing, and eating. Therapeutic activities based on sensory integration theory, neurodevelopmental treatment, and behavioral approaches are easily performed with attention to the nature and quality of the therapeutic relationship.

Intervention for the Parent-Child Relationship

The most desirable outcome for troubled families is reunification of children and parents, given that a safe and caring environment has been established. As the parent and child become better able to receive and respond to support from the practitioner, the likelihood of facilitating their own positive interactions increases. The occupational therapy practitioner can select activities to elicit appropriate caregiving behaviors by grading the amount of interaction and external structure required. Activities should be selected for appropriateness in terms of the parent's and the child's developmental levels and should be presented in a supportive mode. The practitioner might need to demonstrate and teach some of the activities initially. In all activities, gentle physical contact, pleasant conversation, and mutual enjoyment are the main goals. The occupational therapy practitioner can also use parent-child sessions to teach concepts of child development. Parent-child sessions can also allow parents to observe and practice behavior management skills, such as praising and correcting behaviors.

OCCUPATIONAL THERAPY INTERVENTION FOR ADULT CLIENTS

Occupational therapy intervention with adult clients who have experienced abuse or neglect is focused largely on securing an appropriate environment and, when possible, helping the client to achieve knowledge and skills to reduce future risk. The occupational therapy practitioner can be instrumental in determining the appropriate levels of support needed by an adult with cognitive or physical disabilities and can work with the intervention team to help locate or design a safe living situation that maximizes opportunities for participation. Many clients benefit from occupational therapy assistance in establishing a durable and accessible network of friends, thereby reducing social isolation. This may be achieved by connecting clients and caregivers with groups who share the client's interests, such as social clubs and activity groups. Communication skills training and practice can also be useful for improving clients' ability to express wants, set limits, and ask for help. Occupational therapy practitioners working in home and residential settings can help to prevent abuse by educating and supporting the primary caregivers. People in these roles are at risk for caregiver burnout, a problem that can be decreased through improved working conditions, predictable scheduling, appropriate knowledge and skills, and the empathy and respect of others (Marchetti & McCartney, 1990). Clients or caregivers who demonstrate severe or chronic emotional distress should be referred for mental health evaluation by appropriate professionals.

CASE STUDY: *Hannah's "Evil Temper"*

Two-year-old Hannah was referred by her pediatrician for an occupational therapy evaluation to determine her developmental status, which was monitored annually at an outpatient clinic for prematurely born infants and toddlers. During the preassessment interview, Hannah's mother, Joyce, commented that her daughter had "an evil temper, just like her dad." Joyce was especially distressed because Hannah's attendance at day care was in jeopardy due to her having bitten other toddlers. "If I don't have day care, I'll lose my job. Her dad doesn't even help with child support. I'll end up on the street!" lamented Joyce.

As part of the developmental evaluation, the practitioner asked Joyce to entice Hannah to play with a toy box with multiple buttons and levers that released pop-up toy figures. Joyce showed the box to Hannah, who became excited and reached for the toy. Joyce quickly became frustrated by Hannah's inability to immediately use the levers and buttons and abruptly pulled the toy out of Hannah's reach to play with the box herself. Hannah then hit her mother and collapsed in anguish as Joyce rolled her eyes and said, "See what I mean? She's violent!"

Results of the developmental evaluation indicated that Hannah's gross motor development was appropriate but her fine motor, language and cognitive-adaptive skills were below expected levels. Added to these concerns were observed risk factors for child abuse or neglect. Joyce had demonstrated a limited understanding of Hannah's developmental level and needs, was feeling frustrated, and negatively associated Hannah's behavior with that of the child's father. Joyce interacted with Hannah in an insensitive manner and seemed preoccupied by her own needs. Money was a concern, and a financial crisis was possible. Hannah's day care providers had assessed her aggressive behavior as beyond that of typical children in severity and frequency. Hannah had trouble communicating, causing her frustration and increased dependence on others' ability to discern her needs and wants.

The occupational therapist was pleased that this child and mother had come into care at this time, before more serious problems had developed. At the occupational therapist's recommendation, the medical team agreed to refer Joyce to an outpatient social worker who would work with her to evaluate her needs and resources related to finances and housing and who could connect Joyce with legal advice regarding child support. Joyce was receptive to this and to a referral to state-funded early childhood services that would provide needed developmental services and parental education. The occupational therapist obtained Joyce's written permission to contact Hannah's day care providers and offered them up to two hours of consultation related to helping Hannah participate successfully and safely in day care.

CASE STUDY: *Mrs. Nash's Missing Money*

Jonita was an occupational therapy practitioner working in home health. Mrs. Nash, her client, was recovering from a cerebrovascular accident. Mrs. Nash lived alone, with the occasional assistance of her son and his family and twice-weekly personal care assistance from a local agency. During one session, Jonita and Mrs. Nash were working on money management, cognitive skills, and fine motor skills by balancing Mrs. Nash's checkbook together. After helping Mrs. Nash to assemble and arrange the needed materials for the task and then problem solving how to open the envelopes from three months of unopened bank receipts, they began the process of reviewing the bank statements and comparing entries with those in the checkbook. It soon became evident that the balance shown in the checkbook did not remotely match that from the bank. Several hundred-dollar withdrawals had been made, reducing Mrs. Nash's funds dramatically. Mrs. Nash was agitated by this discovery and could not recall having made the transactions. She expressed concern that she was "losing her mind."

After carefully looking at the dates of the withdrawals, Jonita and Mrs. Nash realized that the withdrawals had occurred on days when Mrs. Nash was driven to hair salon appointments by the personal care assistant. Jonita learned that Mrs. Nash had given her debit card to the caregiver to withdraw cash from the ATM while driving to the appointments. It was likely that extra cash had been stolen from the account at those times.

Jonita and Mrs. Nash worked together to make a plan of action that included (1) terminating the offending caregiver's employment and recruiting a replacement, (2) going to the bank to change her debit card and checking account numbers, (3) agreeing that Mrs. Nash would henceforth balance her checkbook within two days of receiving a statement, (4) involving Mrs. Nash's son in helping to screen potential paid caregivers and taking Mrs. Nash to the bank weekly, and (5) obtaining and reviewing educational materials from the bank and online resources to learn about financial exploitation of elders and ways to prevent this.

CONCLUSION

Occupational therapy practitioners establish helping relationships with clients in settings that range from institutions of care to the community and home. In addition to working directly with individual clients, contemporary occupational therapy practitioners interact with caregivers, administrators, and colleagues in other disciplines to create environments that support individuals' optimal occupational performance. Such a wide span of influence allows occupational therapy practitioners to initiate and guide systemic improvements that are essential to preventing and ameliorating victimization.

PROVOCATIVE QUESTIONS

1. Occasionally, colleagues from other disciplines are surprised and dismayed that the team occupational therapy practitioner is raising concerns about potential abuse of a client. What would you say if someone asked "Why are you so concerned about this? Isn't that the social worker's role?"
2. What is the potential impact of abuse or neglect on an elderly individual's occupational performance?

REFERENCES

American Occupational Therapy Association. (2002). Occupational therapy practice framework: Domain and process. *American Journal of Occupational Therapy, 56*(6), 609–639.

American Occupational Therapy Association. (2005). Occupational therapy code of ethics—2005. *American Journal of Occupational Therapy, 59*(6), 639–642.

Barth, R., & Sullivan R. (1985, March–April). Collecting competent evidence in behalf of children. *Social Work,* 130–136.

Bowlby, J. (1988). *A secure base: Parent-child attachment and health.* New York: Basic Books.

Bonner, B., Crow, S., & Hensley, L. (1997). State efforts to identify maltreated children with disabilities: A follow-up study. *Child Maltreatment, 2,* 52–60.

Child Welfare Information Gateway. (2005). Mandatory reporters of child abuse and neglect: State statutes series. Retrieved March, 2007 from http://www.childwelfare.gov/systemwide/laws_policies/statutes/manda.cfm

Christiansen, C., & Townsend, E. (2004). *Introduction to occupation: The art and science of living.* Upper Saddle River, NJ: Prentice Hall.

Coulton, C., Korbin, J., Su, M. & Chow, J. (1995). Community level factors and child maltretment rates. *Child Development, 66,* 1262–1276.

Egeland, B., Sroufe, A., & Erickson, M. (1983). The developmental consequences of different patterns of maltreatment. *Child Abuse and Neglect, 7,* 459–469.

Faller, K. C. (1985). Unanticipated problems in the United States child protection system. *Child Abuse and Neglect, 9,* 63–69.

Feeny, J. A. (1996). Attachment, caregiving, and marital satisfaction. *Personal Relationships, 3,* 401–416.

Garbarino, J., & Kostelny, K. (1992). Child maltreatment as a community problem. *Child Abuse and Neglect, 16,* 455–464.

Gerits, L., Derksen, J., & Verbruggen, A. (2004). Emotional intelligence and adaptive success of nurses caring for people with mental retardation and severe behavior problems. *Mental Retardation, 42,* 106–121.

Haskett, M., & Kistner, J. (1991). Social interactions and peer perceptions of young physically abused children. *Child Development, 62,* 979–990.

Hazan, C., & Zeifman, D. (1999). Pair bonds as attachments. In J. Cassidy & P. Shaver (Eds.), *Handbook of attachment: Theory, research, and clinical applications* (pp. 336–354). New York: Guilford Press.

Hoffman-Plotkin, D., & Twentyman, C. (1984). A multi-modal assessment of behavioral and cognitive deficits in abused and neglected preschoolers. *Child Development, 55,* 794–802.

Jaudes, P. K., & Diamond, L. J. (1985). The handicapped child and child abuse. *Child Abuse and Neglect, 9,* 341–347.

Kenny, M. (2001). Child abuse reporting: teachers' perceived deterrents. *Child Abuse and Neglect, 25,* 81–92.

Khemka, I., & Hickson, L. (2000). Decision-making by adults with mental retardation in simulated situations of abuse. *Mental Retardation, 38,* 15–26.

Kondo, T. (2004). Cultural tensions in occupational therapy practice: Considerations from a Japanese vantagepoint. *American Journal of Occupational Therapy, 58,* 174–184.

Kreitzer, M. (1981). Legal aspects of child abuse: Guidelines for the nurse. *Nursing Clinics of North America, 16,* 149–160.

Lumley, V., & Miltenberger, R. (1997). Sexual abuse prevention for persons with mental retardation. *American Journal on Mental Retardation, 101,* 459–472.

MacNamara, R. D. (1992). *Creating abuse-free caregiving environments for children, the disabled, and the elderly: Preparing, supervising, and managing caregivers for the emotional impact of their responsibilities.* Springfield, IL: Charles Thomas.

Manly, J. T., Kim, J. E., Rogosh, F. A. & Cicchetti, D. (2001). Dimensions of child maltreatment and children's adjustment: Contributions of developmental timing and subtype. *Development and Psychopathology, 13,* 759–782.

Marchetti, A., & McCartney, J. (1990). Abuse of persons with mental retardation: Characteristics of the abused, the abusers, and the informers. *Mental Retardation, 28,* 367–371.

McAllister, M. (2000). Domestic violence: A life-span approach to assessment and intervention. *Lippincott's Primary Care Practice, 4,* 174–189.

Milberger, S., Israel, N. LeRoy, B., Martin, A., Potter, L., & Patchak-Schuster, P. (2003). Brief report: Violence against women with disabilities. *Violence and Victims, 18,* 581–591.

National Center on Elder Abuse. (1998). *National elder abuse incidence study: Final report.* Retrieved December 2005 from http://www.elderabusecenter.org

Noguera, P. (2001). *Youth perspectives on violence and the implications for public policy: Coming to terms with violence in America.* Retrieved December 2005 from http://www.inmotionmagazine.com/er/pnyp1.html

Oktay, J., & Tompkins, C. (2004). Personal assistance providers' mistreatment of disabled adults. *Health and Social Work, 29,* 177–188.

Pears, K. & Fisher, P. A. (2005). Developmental, cognitive, and neuropsychological functioning in preschool-aged foster children: Associations with prior maltreatment and placement history. *Journal of Behavioral and Developmental Pediatrics, 26,* 112–123.

Prothrow-Stith, D. (1991). *Deadly consequences: How violence is destroying our teenage population and a plan to begin solving the problem.* New York: HarperCollins.

Putnam, F. W. (2003). Ten-year research review update: Child sexual abuse. *Journal of the American Academy of Child and Adolescent Psychiatry, 42,* 269–278.

Roche, T., with August, M. Grace, J, Harrington, M., Hylton, H. Monroe, S., & Willwerth, J. (2000, November). The crisis of foster care. *Time Canada, 156*(20), 52.

Ryan, R., Salenblatt, J., Schiappacasse, J., & Maly, B. (2001). Physician unwitting participation in abuse and neglect of persons with developmental disabilities. *Community Mental Health Journal, 37,* 499–509.

Sampson, R. J., & Groves, W. B. (1989). Community structure and crime: Testing social-disorganization theory. *American Journal of Sociology, 94,* 775–802.

Schauer, C. (1995). Special report: Protection and advocacy: What nurses need to know. *Archives of Psychiatric Nursing, 9,* 233–239.

Schneider, B. H, Atkinson, L. & Tardif, C. (2001). Child-parent attachment and children's peer relations: A quantitative review. *Developmental Psychology, 37,* 86–100.

Sedlak, A. J., & Broadhurst, D. D. (1996). *Executive summary of the third national incidence study of child abuse and neglect.* Washington, DC: U.S. Department of Health and Human Services, National Center on Child Abuse and Neglect.

Sidebotham, P., & Heron, J. (2003). Child maltreatment in the "children of the nineties": The role of the child. *Child Abuse and Neglect, 27,* 337–352.

Sobsey, D., & Doe, T. (1991). Patterns of sexual abuse and assault. *Sexuality and Disability, 9,* 243–259.

Spencer, N., Devereux, E., Wallace, A., Sundrum, R., Shenoy, M., Bacchus, C., & Logan, S. (2005). Disabling conditions and registration for child abuse and neglect: A population-based study. *Pediatrics, 116,* 609–614.

Stancliff, B. (1997, October). Invisible victims: Alert practitioners can help identify domestic abuse. *OT Practice,* 18–28.

Strand, M., Benzein, E., & Saveman, B. ((2004). Violence in the care of adult persons with intellectual disabilities. *Journal of Clinical Nursing, 13,* 506–514.

Strauch, B. (2003). *The primal teen: What the new discoveries about the teenage brain tells us about our kids.* New York: Anchor Press.

Stromsness, M. M. (1993). Sexually abused women with mental retardation: Hidden victims, absent resources. *Women and Therapy, 14,* 139–152.

Sullivan, P. M., & Knutson, J. F. (2000). Maltreatment and disabilities: A population-based epidemiological study. *Child Abuse and Neglect, 24*(10), 1257–1273.

Tharinger, D., Horton, C., & Millea, S. (1990). Sexual abuse and exploitation of children and adults with mental retardation and other handicaps. *Child Abuse and Neglect, 14,* 301–312.

U.S. Department of Health and Human Services. (2000). *Child maltreatment 1998: Reports from the states to the National Child Abuse and Neglect Data System.* Washington, DC: U.S. Government Printing Office.

Vondra, J. (1990). Sociological and ecological factors. In R. E. Helfer & R. S. Kempe (Eds.), *The battered child* (3rd ed., pp. 49–85). Chicago: University of Chicago Press.

Waters, E., & Stroufe, A. (1983). Social competence as a developmental construct. *Developmental Review, 3,* 79–97.

Windham, D. (2000). The millennial challenge: Elder abuse. *Journal of Emergency Nursing, 26,* 444–447.

OTHER RESOURCES

Child Abuse Prevention Network:
    <http://child-abuse.com>
Disability, Abuse and Personal Rights Project:
    <http://www.disability-abuse.com/about.htm>
Elder Abuse Law Center:
    <http://www.elder-abuse.com>
National Center on Elder Abuse:
    <http://www.elderabusecenter.org/>
National Coalition Against Domestic Violence:
    <http://www.ncadv.org/gemeric>

VI

THE THERAPEUTIC PROCESS

"Therapists work to create significant experiences for their patients because if therapy is to be effective, the therapeutic process must matter to the patient."

Cheryl Mattingly

Professional Reasoning in Practice

BARBARA A. BOYT SCHELL

Learning Objectives

1. Describe important aspects of reasoning in occupational therapy practice
2. Identify the different facets of professional reasoning based on personal reflection, practitioners' descriptions, and case studies.
3. Describe the process of developing expertise and discuss characteristic reasoning processes along a continuum of expertise.

INTRODUCTION

Professional reasoning is the process that practitioners use to plan, direct, perform, and reflect on client care. It is typically performed quickly because the practitioner has to act on that reasoning right away. It is a complex and multifaceted process, and it has been called by several different names. In the past, many authors referred to it as **clinical reasoning** (Mattingly & Fleming, 1994; Rogers, 1983; Schell, 2003), but more recently, terms such as **professional reasoning** (Schell & Schell, 2008) and *therapeutic reasoning* (Kielhofner & Forsyth, 2002) have surfaced in an attempt to find a word that is not so closely aligned with medicine, since occupational therapy practices not only in medical settings, but in many educational and community settings as well. When using these labels, authors are talking about how therapists *actually think* when they actually are engaged in practice. This requires **metacognitive** analysis or, in simple terms, *thinking about thinking.* This is important because newcomers to the field might incorrectly understand professional reasoning as something that practitioners "choose to do" or confuse it with the many occupational therapy intervention theories. It is neither of those things. Whenever you are thinking about or doing occupational therapy for an identified individual or group, you are engaged in professional reasoning. It is not a question of whether you are doing it, only a question of how well. Furthermore, many practice theories are discussed throughout this text that will inform your reasoning and help you to think about your clients. However, the theories about reasoning that are discussed in this chapter are theories about how you as an occupational therapy practitioner are likely to think as you engage in therapy. Thus, the focus is on the therapist, not on the client, although obviously, therapists do this thinking in the service of client care. Keep in mind these important distinctions as you become mindful of your own reasoning processes.

This chapter examines professional reasoning from several perspectives. To help you see real examples of the material discussed, the following Case Study, which is adapted, with name changes, from an actual situation, provides an example of an encounter between an occupational therapist, Terry, and her client, Mrs. Munro. Read this case study before continuing with the text, paying special attention to the different kinds of issues and problems that the occupational therapy practitioner has to address. Then keep referring back to it as you read about the nature of professional reasoning.

CASE STUDY: *Terry and Mrs. Munro: Determining Appropriate Recommendations*

Terry, an occupational therapist, goes up to a client's room in the neurology unit of a regional medical center. Along the way, she shares her thoughts with Barb, a researcher who is observing Terry's practice. Terry fills Barb in on the client they are about to see. The client, Mrs. Munro, is a widow who lives alone in a house in town. A couple of days earlier, she suffered a stroke—a right cerebrovascular accident—and was brought by a neighbor to the hospital. Mrs. Munro has made a rapid recovery and demonstrates good return of her motor skills. She still has some left-side weakness and incoordination, along with some cognitive problems. She is a delightful, pleasant older woman and is anxious to return home.

Terry is seeing this client for the third time, and her primary concern is to assess whether Mrs. Munro has any cognitive residual effects from her stroke that would put her at serious risk if she returned home alone. Terry plans to do some more in-depth activities of daily living with Mrs. Munro to see how well she demonstrates safety awareness. Terry thinks that she will probably have Mrs. Munro get out of bed, obtain her clothing and hygiene supplies, perform her morning hygiene routines at the sink, and then get dressed. Terry wants to see the degree to which Mrs. Munro is spontaneously able to manage these tasks as well has how good her judgment appears to be. Terry's thought is that if she can engage Mrs. Munro in several multistep activities that also require her to perform in different positions, Terry should be able to detect any cognitive and motor problems that pose a serious safety threat.

When Terry arrives at the room, she greets Mrs. Munro, who says, "I am so excited. The doctor says I can go home tomorrow."

Terry turns to Barb and raises her eyebrows as if to say, "I told you so." On the way to the room, Terry had told Barb that she was worried that the physician who was managing Mrs. Munro's case tended to think that as soon as clients could physically get up, they could go home. Terry went on to defend the physician by saying that in today's cost-conscious environment, doctors were under a lot of pressure not to keep clients in the hospital.

As Terry converses with Mrs. Munro about generalities, she notices that Mrs. Munro is already dressed in her housecoat. When she talks to Mrs. Munro about doing some self-care activities, it becomes apparent that Mrs. Munro has already completed her bathing and dressing routines, with help from a nurse. When Terry suggests that she perhaps brush her teeth and comb her hair, Mrs. Munro is happy to get up out of bed but notes that her neighbor never did bring in her dentures. Mrs. Munro sits on the edge of the bed and, after a reminder from Terry, puts on her slippers. She then stands and walks to the nearby sink, finds her comb, and combs her hair. While she is doing this, Terry looks around for some other ideas about what to do, since Mrs. Munro has already completed the self-care tasks Terry had planned to do with her.

Terry's eyes light on some wilted flowers by the bed. She suggests to Mrs. Munro that she might want to dispose of the flowers and clean the vase so that it will be ready to pack when it is time to go home. Mrs. Munro agrees and proceeds to walk somewhat unsteadily over to the vase. Picking it up, she carries it to the sink, where she pulls out the dead flowers. Terry follows her, staying slightly behind and within reach of Mrs. Munro. When Mrs. Munro stops after removing the flowers, Terry suggests that she rinse out the vase, which she does. She then dries it and returns the vase to the bedside table. Terry reminds her to throw out the dead flowers. While Mrs. Munro does this, they talk some more about her plans to return home.

Mrs. Munro tells Terry that she has lived in her home for 40 years, and even though her husband died over 10 years ago, she still feels his presence there. He used to love her cooking, and she still cooks three meals a day for herself. Mrs. Munro starts to cry when they talk about cooking but then cheers up. Terry tells her that it might be safer if she had someone around the house for a few weeks, until she recovers a bit more from her stroke. Mrs. Munro thinks that she can get some help from her neighbor. Terry says she is also going to suggest some home-care therapy, just to make sure Mrs. Munro is safe in the kitchen, bathroom, and so on, noting, "We sure don't want to see you have a bad fall just when you are doing so well after your stroke."

Continued

CASE STUDY: *Terry and Mrs. Munro: Determining Appropriate Recommendations* *Continued*

After reviewing some coordination exercises for Mrs. Munro's left hand, Terry says good-bye. Terry and Barb leave the room. Terry stops at the nurses' station to note in the chart that Mrs. Munro demonstrated good safety awareness in familiar tasks at her bedside but did require cueing to complete multistep tasks. Terry also notes some motor instability in task performance during ambulation. Terry recommends a referral to a home health occupational therapy practitioner "to assess safety and equipment needs during bathroom activities, meal preparation, and routine homemaking tasks." Terry comments to Barb, as they walk off the unit, that she thinks Mrs. Munro did pretty well, but Terry remains concerned about the risks once Mrs. Munro goes home, particularly when she is tired. Terry wants someone to monitor Mrs. Munro in a familiar setting to see whether she handles her daily routines adequately. Terry would really like to see Mrs. Munro go to a rehab center, but the client has no insurance funding to support that. Terry believes that she might at least be able to get some home care, because there are a few programs around that provide some services to indigent elderly. Staying in her own home seems to be Mrs. Munro's major goal, and Terry is going to do what she can to try to help her attain that goal. Terry will catch up with the social worker later to discuss the need for Mrs. Munro to have good support from any neighbors, friends, or relatives.

Questions and Exercises

1. How did Terry develop her concerns about Mrs. Munro?
2. How did Terry know what to do when her initial plans did not work out?
3. What factors seem to guide Terry's recommendations at the end?

REASONING IN PRACTICE: A WHOLE-BODY PROCESS

With the case study in mind, let's explore the nature of reasoning during practice. Perhaps one of the first things to note is that professional reasoning is a *whole-body* process. That is one reason why it is a different experience to read a case study than to be the practitioner in the situation. Some professional reasoning involves straightforward thinking processes that the practitioner can easily describe. Examples include assessing occupational performance, such as daily living skills and work behaviors. Occupational therapy practitioners use their observations and theoretical knowledge to identify relevant client factors that contribute to occupational performance problems. Practitioners also attend to the contextual factors that affect performance. For instance, Terry was able to describe her concerns about Mrs. Munro's safety in returning home. In particular, Terry was addressing self-care and homemaking activities. She had analyzed relevant contextual factors about the home setting and Mrs. Munro's social and financial situation. Terry had identified some impairments in cognition and motor control that were affecting her client's occupational performance skills. This was all information that Terry could readily share with Barb. However, there was more knowledge from the therapy session that Terry either did not or could not put into words.

Part of Terry's professional reasoning involved body-based knowledge that she gained from her senses. For instance, Terry used her sense of touch to feel the muscle tension (or lack of tension) in Mrs. Munro's affected arm when she was doing an activity. During her evaluation, Terry did some quick stretches to Mrs. Munro's elbow and wrist to determine whether she could feel evidence of spasticity, an abnormal reflex response that is commonly found in individuals who are recovering from a stroke. When Mrs. Munro stood up, Terry carefully gauged the distance she stood from Mrs. Munro, because Mrs. Munro was at some risk of falling. Terry was careful to stand not so close that she crowded or overprotected Mrs. Munro but close enough to protect her should she lose her balance. While close to Mrs. Munro, Terry could smell her, gaining a quick sense of possible hygiene or continence problems. Terry used her voice quality to display encouragement and support. Terry watched and listened carefully for clues about the nature of Mrs. Munro's emotional state. In particular, she watched facial expressions and listened for evidence of fear or insecurity during Mrs. Munro's performance of activities. All of these sensations contributed to an image of Mrs. Munro that influenced Terry's practice.

There are other aspects of reasoning during therapy that are even harder to describe. Fleming (1994a) described this as "knowing more than we can tell" (p. 24). She explained that much of the profession's knowledge is practical knowledge, which is "seldom discussed and rarely described" (p. 25). This tacit knowledge, combined with the rich sensory aspects of actual practice, helps to explain why reading about therapy and doing therapy are such different experiences. In fact, recent work (Harris, 2005) suggests that each therapist's individual bodily differences and preferences may subtly shape therapy, in that some therapists might avoid situations that they find physically uncomfortable (e.g., if they are intolerant of certain smells) and others might engage in therapy practices that they themselves find comforting (e.g., applying deep pressure, much like what one gets when being hugged). Hooper (1997, 2007) has also noted the importance of how our own values, beliefs, and assumptions underpin each practitioner's grasp of the therapy process. So keep in mind that therapy always happens in the real world with real people, and you will see variations because each therapist is different.

THEORY AND PRACTICE

There has been a long-standing discussion in many professions about the role of theory in professional practice (Kessels & Korthagen, 1996). Theories help practitioners to make decisions, although Cohn (1989) noted that the problems of practice rarely present themselves in the straightforward manner described in textbook theories. Professional reasoning involves the naming and framing of problems on the basis of a personal understanding of the client's situation (Schön, 1983). In problem identification and problem solution, practitioners blend theories with their own personal and practice experiences to guide their actions. Theoretical knowledge helps the practitioner to avoid unjustified assumptions or the use of ineffective therapy techniques and to reflect on how his or her own experiences in therapy are similar to or different from theoretical understandings (Parham, 1987). In Chapter 42, you will find more information about how theories inform practice. The point here is that although practice can (and should) be informed by theories, it is ultimately a result of how each therapist interprets each therapy situation and then acts on that understanding.

COGNITIVE PROCESSES UNDERLYING PROFESSIONAL REASONING

In the case study, Terry had to remember, obtain, and manage a great deal of information quickly to provide effective and efficient intervention. How did she do it? Research findings from the field of cognitive psychology help to explain how practitioners think and how experience combined with reflection fosters increasing expertise. Individuals receive, store, and organize information in *frames* or *scripts*, which are complex representations of phenomena (Bruning, Schraw, & Ronning, 1999; Carr & Shotwell, 2007). This process involves both working memory and long-term memory. Working memory can hold very few thoughts at a time, which is one reason that one sometimes has to look at the phone book two or three times in order to correctly recall a number one is dialing. Similarly, students and new practitioners find it challenging to try to keep all the important considerations in mind

when dealing with a client. Practitioners with extensive experience have this information organized and stored in their long-term memories and thus do not have to actively juggle all the details. For example, in school, Terry probably learned many of the common problems associated with someone who has had a stroke. She also has seen perhaps 100 people with strokes over the past several years. She has built up a general representation in her mind of what to expect when she receives a referral for someone who has had a stroke. She anticipates that many of these individuals will have thick medical charts, because they almost always have prior medical problems, such as diabetes and high blood pressure. She will not be surprised if the person is overweight. She expects to see impairments in cognition that often affect the person's ability to do everyday tasks, such as dressing, cooking, and driving. As part of her frame, Terry has built-in mental rules that help her to categorize and detect differences. For instance, although she knows that many people who have strokes have movement impairments, she knows that not all do. Furthermore, when movement is impaired, she expects individuals with a left cerebrovascular accident (CVA) to have right-side weakness and those with a right CVA to have left-side weakness. Additionally, she knows that a person's social support system is critical for promoting an adaptive response to disability. She may use certain cues, such as the presence or absence of frequent family visits, to prompt her to categorize a family as supportive or nonsupportive.

In addition to framing or "chunking" information, Terry also creates and uses scripts or procedural rules that guide her thinking (Bruning et al., 1999; Carr & Shotwell, 2007). Just as her mental frames help her to organize and retrieve her knowledge about common aspects of stroke, scripts help her to organize common occurrences or events. For instance, she understands that her role involves responding to the referral by seeing the client, writing her findings on the correct form, providing interventions, communicating verbally with the other team members, and developing discharge plans. Terry likely has scripts about the implications for clients with supportive families and those without. In her experience, a supportive family cares for its family member at home, regardless of the family's financial resources. Alternatively, clients with little family support are more likely to face institutional care. Again, these scripts are formed by Terry's observations and experiences over time and serve the purpose of helping her to anticipate likely events.

The mind appears to use frames and scripts to support effective processing of information by providing efficient mental frameworks for handling complex information. Each person individually constructs them. It is no surprise that students and new practitioners often struggle to retain and effectively use their therapy knowledge. It takes time and repetition of experiences to develop effective reasoning based on efficient storage in long-term memory allowing for targeted use of short-term memory as therapy happens. Important aspects of the process are as follows (Bruning et al., 1999; Roberts, 1996; Robertson, 1996):

♦ *Cue acquisition:* Searching for the helpful and targeted information through observation and questioning.
♦ *Pattern recognition:* Noticing similarities and differences among situations.
♦ *Limiting the problem space:* Using patterns to help focus cue acquisition and knowledge application on the most fruitful areas.
♦ *Problem formulation:* Developing an explanation of what is going on, why it is going on, and what a better situation or outcome might be.
♦ *Problem solution:* Identifying courses of action based on the problem formulation.

These cognitive processes are interactive and rarely occur in a linear fashion. Rather, the mind jumps around between the information at hand and that which has been stored up from prior learning while attempting to make sense of the situation.

ASPECTS OF PROFESSIONAL REASONING

Although there appear to be common processes underlying reasoning in practice, the focus of that mental activity appears to vary with the demands of the problems to be addressed. Fleming (1991) was the first within occupational therapy to describe how occupational therapists seemed to use different thinking approaches, depending on the nature of the clinical problem they were addressing. She referred to this process as the "therapist with the three-track mind" (p. 1007). Since that time, others have examined the different aspects of occupational therapy professional reasoning. The vast majority of this research has been done with occupational therapists, although at least one case study (Lyons & Crepeau, 2001) suggests there is some application for occupational therapy assistants as well. These aspects of professional reasoning are listed in Table 32.1, along with the typical focus and clues for recognizing when that sort of reasoning is occurring.

Scientific Reasoning

Scientific reasoning is used to understand the condition that is affecting an individual and to decide on interventions that are in the client's best interest. It is a logical process that parallels scientific inquiry. Forms of scientific reasoning that are described in occupational therapy are diagnostic reasoning (Rogers & Holm, 1991) and procedural reasoning (Fleming, 1991, 1994b) in addition to the general use of hypothetical-deductive reasoning (Tomlin, 2008). Scientific reasoning is also referred to as treatment

planning (Pelland, 1987), in which the therapist uses selected theories both to identify problems and to guide decision making.

Diagnostic reasoning is concerned with clinical problem sensing and problem definition. The process starts in advance of seeing a client. Occupational therapy practitioners, because of their domains of concern, look primarily for occupational performance problems. Furthermore, the nature of the problems they expect to find is influenced by the information in the requests for services. Some of Terry's diagnostic reasoning, described earlier, included information about the typical symptoms associated with having a stroke.

Procedural reasoning occurs when practitioners are "thinking about the disease or disability and deciding which intervention activities (procedures) they might employ to remediate the person's functional performance problems" (Fleming, 1991, p. 1008). This may involve an interview, an observation of the person engaged in a task, or formal evaluations using standardized measures. Although one hopes that procedural reasoning is science-based, Tomlin makes the important observation that procedural reasoning can become an unquestioned implementation of therapy protocols, in which case it becomes less scientific in nature (Tomlin, 2008). That is why there is such an emphasis on evidence-based practice, which challenges the practitioner to routinely evaluate customary therapy approaches based on of the best information currently available (Holm, 2001; Law, 2002; Tickle-Degnen, 1998).

In the case study, Terry used a combination of interview and observation, both of which were guided by her working hypothesis that Mrs. Munro had cognitive problems that might affect her safe performance at home. She was likely operating on the basis of her understanding of cognitive theories (such as those described in Chapter 57), as well as her own experience with similar clients. As intervention begins, more data are collected, and the occupational therapy practitioner gains a sharper clinical image. This clinical image is the result of the interplay between what the occupational therapy practitioner expects to see (such as the usual course of the disease) and the client's actual performance. In the case study, there was congruence between Mrs. Munro's abilities and problems in performing activities of daily living and Terry's expectations of someone making a good recovery from a stroke.

Mattingly (1994a) made the point that occupational therapists have a "two-body practice" (p. 37). By that, she meant that occupational therapy practitioners view a person in two ways: the body as a machine, in which parts may be broken, and the person as a life, filled with personal meanings and hopes. Much of the procedural reasoning in occupational therapy addresses issues related to the body as machine. The next form of reasoning, narrative reasoning, provides the occupational therapy practitioner with a way to understand a person's illness experience.

TABLE 32.1 DIFFERENT ASPECTS OF REASONING IN OCCUPATIONAL THERAPY

Aspect of Reasoning	Description and Focus	Clues for Recognizing in Therapist Discussions
Scientific reasoning	Reasoning involving the use of applied logical and scientific methods, such as hypothesis testing, pattern recognition, theory-based decision making and statistical evidence.	Impersonal, focused on the diagnosis, condition, guiding theory, evidence from research or what "typically" happens with clients like the one being considered.
Diagnostic reasoning	Investigative reasoning and analysis of cause or nature of conditions requiring occupational therapy intervention. Can be considered one component of scientific reasoning.	Uses both personal and impersonal information. Therapists attempt to explain why client is experiencing problems using a blend of science-based and client-based information.
Procedural reasoning	Reasoning in which therapist considers and uses intervention routines for identified conditions. May be science-based or may reflect the habits and culture of the intervention setting.	Characterized by therapist using therapy regimes or routines thought to be effective with problems identified and that are typically used with clients in that setting. Tends to be more impersonal and diagnostically driven.
Narrative reasoning	Reasoning process used to make sense of people's particular circumstances, prospectively imagine the effect of illness, disability, or occupational performance problems on their daily lives, and create a collaborative story that is enacted with clients and families through intervention.	Personal, focused on the client, including past, present, and anticipated future. Involves an appreciation of client culture as the basis for understanding client narrative. Relates to the "so what" of the condition for the person's life.
Pragmatic reasoning	Practical reasoning which is used to fit therapy possibilities into the current realities of service delivery, such as scheduling options, payment for services, equipment availability, therapists' skills, management directives, and the personal situation of the therapist.	Generally not focused on client or client's condition, but rather on all the physical and social "stuff" that surrounds the therapy encounter, as well as the therapist's internal sense of what he or she is capable of and has the time and energy to complete.
Ethical reasoning	Reasoning directed toward analyzing an ethical dilemma, generating alternative solutions, and determining actions to be taken. Systematic approach to moral conflict.	Tension is often evident as therapist attempts to determine what is the "right" thing to do, particularly when faced with dilemmas in therapy, competing principles, risks, and benefits.
Interactive reasoning	Thinking directed toward building positive interpersonal relationships with clients, permitting collaborative problem identification and problem solving.	Therapist is concerned with what client likes or does not like. Use of praise, empathetic comments, and nonverbal behaviors to encourage and support client's cooperation.
Conditional reasoning	A blending of all forms of reasoning for the purposes of flexibly responding to changing conditions or predicting possible client futures.	Typically found with more experienced therapists who can "see" multiple futures, based on therapists past experiences and current information.

Used with permission from Schell & Schell (Eds.), (2008), and based on writings by Tomlin, Hamilton, Schell, Kanny, and Slater in Schell & Schell (2008); Rogers & Holm (1991); and Mattingly & Fleming (1994).

Narrative Reasoning

Understanding the meaning that a disease, illness, or disability has to an individual is a task that goes beyond the scientific understanding of disease processes and organ systems. Rather, it requires that practitioners find a way to understand the meaning of this experience from the client's perspective. Mattingly (1994b) suggested that practitioners do this through a form of reasoning called narrative reasoning. Narrative reasoning is so named because it involves thinking in story form. It is not uncommon for an occupational therapy practitioner who is preparing to substitute for another with a client to ask the other practitioner, "So what is the client's story?" As Kielhofner (1997) noted, narrative reasoning "becomes particularly important for considering how the person's disrupted life story can be constituted or reconstituted" (p. 316). Box 32.1 explains how narrative reasoning relates to scientific reasoning.

In the case study, part of Terry's reasoning was concerned with making decisions in light of what was important to Mrs. Munro. This process of collaboration and empathy has been described as "building a communal horizon of understanding" (Clark, Ennevor, & Richardson,

1996, p. 376). Terry gained understanding by listening attentively to Mrs. Munro's stories about her husband and how he loved her cooking. It is apparent from this session that Mrs. Munro's home is more than just a house. It is the place in which she lived with her husband, where he died, and where she still felt his presence. Part of Mrs. Munro's story is that going home is going back to her husband. If this stroke were to prevent that, Mrs. Munro would lose more than her independence; she would lose symbolic connections to her husband. Although a logical case might be made that Mrs. Munro should start considering a more supportive living environment, Terry understands that for Mrs. Munro, this would not be an acceptable ending. Consequently, Terry worked hard to obtain the support systems that would be necessary for Mrs. Munro to function in her chosen environment, where she will continue her life story.

Often, occupational therapy practitioners work with individuals whose life stories are so severely disrupted that they cannot imagine what their future will look like. Mattingly (1994b) believes that in these situations, skillful practitioners help their clients to invent new life stories. To some degree, these stories become visible as the occupational therapy practitioner and the client develop goals together. The use of life stories is also apparent when activities are selected for both their healing potential and their particular significance to the person. To do this, one must first solicit occupational stories from the individual (Clark et al., 1996). With an understanding of clients' past occupational stories, practitioners can help individuals to create new stories and new futures for themselves. If Mrs. Munro's symptoms were more severe and she was in a more extended therapy process, Terry might explore Mrs. Munro's interest in cooking as an activity that she liked and that would offer many therapeutic opportunities. Further, Mrs. Munro might find that she could express her pleasure in cooking for others by making special treats, first for other clients and then perhaps for neighbors in exchange for their help with chores. During this process, Mrs. Munro would not only be regaining coordination and dexterity, she would also be regaining her sense of self as a productive person. This narrative aspect of clinical reasoning, which ultimately focuses on the person as an occupational being, provides a link between the founding values of the profession and current practice demands (Gray, 1998).

Pragmatic Reasoning

Pragmatic reasoning is yet another strand of reasoning that goes beyond the practitioner-client relationship and addresses the world in which therapy occurs (Schell, 2008; Schell & Cervero, 1993 This world is considered from two perspectives: the practice context and the personal context. Because reasoning during therapy is a practical activity, a number of everyday issues have been identified over the years that affect the therapy process. These include resources for intervention, organizational

---

BOX 32.1

SCIENTIFIC AND NARRATIVE THINKING: TWO SIDES OF A COIN

Narrative thinking deals in subjective, personalized particulars and specifics of lived experience, human intention, and action that connects events across time and defines possibilities. The use of personal experience and concern for the human condition defines its characteristic subjective and personalized position. A frequent and inaccurate assumption is that scientific thinking and narrative thinking are opposed to each other or that one is has more validity or utility than the other does. . . . We can illustrate this by examining a coin. We notice that each side contributes different aspects to the coin that we label the "head" and the "tail." Regardless of the side showing, we recognize the object as a coin. Similarly, when using a coin to make a purchase, it does not matter how we insert the coin in the vending slot or hand it to the cashier. The coin's validity is apparent regardless of which side of the coin shows. . . . Together scientific and narrative thinking and reasoning help us form perspectives on a single reality and truth, just as the head and tail of a coin show different sides of one coin.

Hamilton (2008).

culture, power relationships among team members, reimbursement practices, and practice trends in the profession (Barris, 1987; Howard, 1991; Neuhaus, 1988; Rogers & Holm, 1991). Studies examining clinical reasoning have confirmed that occupational therapy practitioners both actively consider and are influenced by their practice contexts (Creighton, Dijkers, Bennett, & Brown, 1995; Schell, 1994; Strong, Gilbert, Cassidy, & Bennett, 1995). An example of pragmatic reasoning in the case study was Terry's use of immediate resources (the flower vase) in Mrs. Munro's room as a therapy tool. Although Terry had thought of appropriate activities related to self-care, she had to identify practical alternatives quickly when it turned out that Mrs. Munro was already dressed. Practical constraints for Terry included (1) the time it would take to move Mrs. Munro to the clinic, where there might be more resources; (2) the need to get the required information on that day, since Mrs. Munro was going home; and (3) the physical constraints of what was available within the room. Terry's invention of a feasible alternative was a product of both her therapeutic imagination and the cues that were provided within her practice setting.

Terry's attention to the influence of team members demonstrates pragmatic reasoning directed to interpersonal and group issues. She knew that the physician had the power to make discharge decisions. She was aware of the pressures on the physician by third-party payers to discharge clients as quickly as possible. Practice requires that practitioners reason about negotiating their clients' interests within the practice culture.

The practitioner's personal situation also is part of the pragmatic reasoning process. A person's clinical competencies, preferences, commitment to the profession, and life role demands outside of work all affect the therapy choices that are considered and thus enter into the reasoning process. For instance, if a practitioner does not feel safe helping a client stand or transfer to a bed, the therapist is more likely to use tabletop activities, in which the client can participate from a wheelchair. Another occupational therapy practitioner might feel uncomfortable interacting with individuals who have depression and therefore might be quick to suggest that such clients are not motivated for therapy. A practitioner who has a young family to go home to might opt not to schedule clients late in the day, so as to get home as early as possible. These simple personal issues result in clinical decisions that affect the scope and timing of therapy services. Hooper (1997, 2008) suggested that fundamental issues, such as a practitioner's values and general worldview, strongly affect the way in which an individual constructs his or her reasoning. Such worldviews play an important role in the next kind of reasoning: ethical reasoning.

Ethical Reasoning

All of the forms of reasoning that have been described so far help the practitioner to respond to the following questions: What is this person's current occupational situation? What can be done to enhance the person's situation? Ethical reasoning goes one step further and asks: What should be done? Rogers (1983) framed these three questions (here paraphrased) in her Eleanor Clark Slagle Lecture and went on to state, "The clinical reasoning process terminates in an ethical decision, rather than a scientific one, and the ethical nature of the goal of clinical reasoning projects itself over the entire sequence" (p. 602). In the case study, Terry's ethical dilemma is to understand Mrs. Munro's personal wishes and to honor them when developing a therapy plan that realistically addresses Mrs. Munro's limitations. This can be particularly challenging when the pressures of financial realities (such as Mrs. Munro's lack of insurance) affect available options. A number of occupational therapy authors have addressed the ethical aspect of professional reasoning (Fondiller, Rosage, & Neuhaus; 1990; Howard, 1991; Neuhaus, 1988; Peloquin, 1993), and Chapter 28 of this text is devoted to the issue of the ethics of the profession. The purpose here is to introduce ethical reasoning as yet another of the components of professional reasoning in occupational therapy.

Interactive Reasoning

The provision of therapy is inherently a communicative process (Schwartzberg, 2002). In occupational therapy, practitioners must gain the trust of their clients and of people who are important in the clients' world. This is because occupational therapy involves "doing with" as opposed to "doing to" clients (Mattingly & Fleming, 1994, p. 178). A therapist gains this trust by entering the client's life world (Crepeau, 1991) and by using a number of interpersonal strategies that are designed to motivate clients, such as those discussed in Chapter 33. Once they are in the client's life world, occupational therapy practitioners can better understand how to help the individual resolve performance problems.

It is likely that some reasoning focused on interaction is conscious, as when a practitioner remembers that "I need to be sure to praise the client often, because he gets discouraged so easily." Other interpersonal acts might be quite automatic, such as when a therapist touches a person's arm to convey sympathy. It is sometimes easiest to detect the importance of effective interactive reasoning when the therapist makes a mistake or gets an unexpected reaction and is forced to regroup and rebuild the therapy relationship.

PROFESSIONAL REASONING: A PROCESS OF SYNTHESIS

The preceding section described the aspects of professional reasoning separately to illustrate the different parts of the process. Table 32.2 provides a summary of the kinds of

TABLE 32.2   ASPECTS AND EXAMPLES OF THE CLINICAL REASONING PROCESS

Primary Clinical Reasoning Concerns

What are the person's occupational performance concerns?

What are the person's occupational performance status and potential?

What will be done to improve occupational performance?

How are effective are interventions?

When and how should interventions stop?

Scientific	Narrative	Pragmatic	Ethical	Interactive
Used to understand the nature of the condition	Used to understand the meaning of the condition to the person	Used to understand the practical issues affecting clinical action	Used to choose morally defensible actions, given competing interests	Used to develop and promote positive interpersonal relationships with the client
What is the nature of the illness, injury, or development problem?	What is this person's life story?	Who referred this person and why?	What are the benefits and risks to the person related to service provision and do the benefits warrant the risks?	How can I best relate to this person?
What are the common disabilities resulting from this condition?	What is the nature of this person as an occupational being?	Who is paying for services, and what are the expectations?	In the face of limited time and resources, what is the fairest way to prioritize care?	How can I put this person at ease?
What are the typical impairments associated with this condition?	How has the health condition affected the person's life story or ability to continue his or her life story?	What family or caregiver resources are there to support intervention?	How can I balance the goals of the person receiving services with those of the caregiver when they don't agree?	What is the best way for me to encourage this person?
What are the typical contextual factors that affect performance?	What occupational activities are most important to this person?	What are the expectations of my supervisor and workplace?	To what degree should I customize documentation of services to improve reimbursement?	What nonverbal strategies should I use in this situation?
What theories and research are available to guide assessment and intervention?	What occupational activities are both meaningful to this person and useful for meeting therapy goals?	How much time is there to see this person? What therapy space and equipment are available?	What should I do when other members of the treatment team are operating in ways that I feel conflict with the goals of the person receiving services?	Where should I place myself relative to this person so that I support him or her but do not "invade" the person?
What intervention protocols are applicable to this person's condition?		What are my practice competencies?		What cultural factors do I need to consider as I engage with the person?

questions that practitioners seek to answer with the different aspects of professional reasoning. However, these facets of reasoning are not separate or parallel processes; rather, the opposite appears to be the case. Virtually all the research about reasoning in practice suggests that these different forms interact with each other.

Reasoning to Solve Problems

Scientific, narrative, pragmatic, ethical, and interactive reasoning processes are intertwined throughout the therapy process. Indeed, each perspective informs the other. In the case study, Terry's understanding of medical science helped her to know what might be potential impairments and performance problems, but her narrative reasoning helped her to understand the importance for Mrs. Munro of returning home. Put together, these two forms of reasoning help Terry to reach an unspoken understanding that there would be a high risk for depression (which could worsen her client's medical condition) if Mrs. Munro did not return to her home, which means so much to her. Furthermore, the practical constraints associated with the setting and Mrs. Munro's reimbursement prompted Terry to reason about the ethics of referring Mrs. Munro to a rehabilitation center (which she could not afford), of allowing her to return home alone (where she might not be safe), and finally of allowing her to return home with the support of home health care and neighbors.

Conditional Process

Not only must practitioners blend different aspects of reasoning in order to interact effectively with their clients, but they must also flexibly modify interventions in response to changing conditions. Terry showed her flexibility by inventing an activity with the flower vase when her plan to work with Mrs. Munro on bathing and dressing did not pan out. Creighton and colleagues (1995) noticed that occupational therapy practitioners preplanned interventions in a hierarchical manner. They observed that practitioners typically brought several sets of supplies to an intervention session. One set would be directed to the expected level of performance, the others to a stage higher and a stage lower than the expected performance. As an example, one practitioner, in preparation for a writing activity with a client who had a spinal cord injury, brought a short writing splint and unlined paper. This practitioner also brought a longer splint to provide wrist support (in case the client's hand control was worse than expected) and lined paper, which required more precision (in case the hand control was better than expected). This practitioner blended scientific and pragmatic concerns in a way that anticipated several possible situations that might occur.

On a larger scale, Fleming (1994c) described the ability of skilled occupational therapy practitioners to "form an image of future life possibilities for the person" (p. 234). The ability to form these images (or schemata, to use a cognitive terms) seems to require a blend of all the forms of clinical reasoning, along with sufficient clinical experience to have seen a variety of different outcomes with former clients. These images help practitioners to select therapeutic activities on a day-to-day basis. For instance, the writing activity for the client who had a spinal cord injury not only is a good activity for increasing coordination, but also presages occupations that will enable the client to regain control of his life through writing his own checks, signing his name on legal documents, and using various forms of technology for work and play. If this client were an accountant, these would be powerful images. Conversely, if the client were a professional athlete, the occupational therapy practitioner might have to create different activities to allow the client to develop a vision of himself as a future coach or teacher. The activities that are used in occupational therapy can help to meet specific short-term goals and shape long-term expectations. It is in this way that practitioners help individuals to reengage in their lives through the use of meaningful occupations.

ECOLOGICAL VIEW OF PROFESSIONAL REASONING

In Unit I, a number of chapters discussed how occupational performance is the result of a complex transaction among a person's inherent capacities, the person's prior experiences, and the demands of the performance context. Similarly, the professional reasoning process and the resulting therapy actions represent transactions that occur among the practitioner, the client, and the therapy context (Schell, Unsworth, & Schell, 2008) as illustrated in Figure 32.1.

The practitioner's reasoning is shaped by both personal and professional perspectives. Each practitioner brings to the therapy situation knowledge and skills that are grounded in life experiences, including personal characteristics such as physical capacities, personality, values, and beliefs. These form a *personal self.* These personal factors shape each person's perception and interpretation of all life activities and thus act as a lens through which each practitioner views all life events. Layered over or entwined with this personal self is the *professional self,* which includes the therapist's professional knowledge from education, experiences from prior clients, and beliefs about what is important to do in therapy, along with knowledge of specific technical skills and therapy routines available for use in the practice context. The personal and professional selves act in concert to respond to various problems of practice.

Similarly, the client comes to therapy with his or her own life experiences and personal characteristics, life

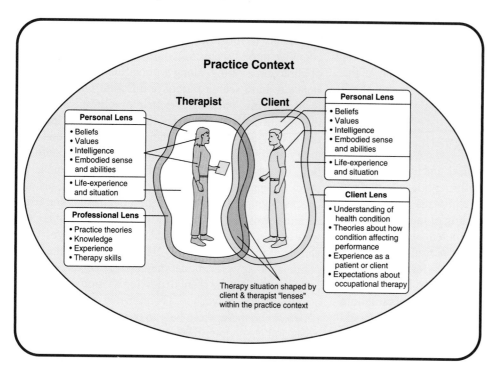

FIGURE 32.1 Schell's ecological model of professional reasoning. [Adapted from Schell, B. A. B., Unsworth, C., & Schell, J. (2008).]

situation, and performance problems that prompted the need for therapy. The client also comes with his or her own theories about what is causing performance problems and what to expect from the therapy process. The therapist and the client function within a community of practice that shapes the nature, scope, and trajectory of the therapy process.

DEVELOPING AND IMPROVING PROFESSIONAL REASONING

Understanding the complexity of professional reasoning helps students and practitioners alike to appreciate why it takes so long to truly become an excellent practitioner. Research shows that it typically takes a minimum of 10 years for individuals to gain expertise within a given field (Boshuizen & Schmidt, 2000). Although experience is necessary, experience alone is not sufficient to ensure advancement in clinical reasoning skills. Therapists must reflect on that experience in order to gain expertise.

Reflection in Practice

Schön (1983) proffered the term *reflective practitioner* to describe how experts think critically about their own experience. Reflection happens in two ways. First, practitioners "reflect-in-action" (p. 49). This involves the practitioner's ability to think in the midst of action and adapt to meet the demands of the situation. Reflection in action most often occurs when the usual approaches are not working. "Reflection-on-action" (p. 61) is the

term Schön uses for critical thinking that occurs after the fact. Reflection about practice, identifying what worked and what did not, and being open to alternative conceptions are necessary to support the learning associated with advancing expertise. The use of research evidence to support practice and the application of formal theories, along with systematic observation and data collection, can be invaluable aides to the reflection process (Gambrill, 2005; Tickle-Degnen, 2000).

Expertise Continuum

Although there is a growing body of evidence about the nature of professional reasoning in occupational therapy, there is still little empirical research that directly examines its development beyond entry level into the profession. Dreyfus and Dreyfus's (1986) conceptualization of professional expertise has been applied to occupational therapy (Slater & Cohn, 1991). This conceptualization, summarized in Table 32.3, describes changes in the reasoning of occupational therapists as they develop expertise. Although the changes that are listed in Table 32.3 are presented as a hierarchy tied to years of experience, it is important to recognize that development is dynamic and influenced by many factors beyond just the years of experience. Both professional and personal experiences, along with active reflection about those experiences, are critical to becoming an expert (Benner, 1984; Gambrill, 2005; Slater & Cohn, 1991). Furthermore, expertise is a function of how the person performs within a given context. Someone who demonstrates expertise at providing services in a school setting might be just minimally competent in a nursing

TABLE 32.3 PROFESSIONAL REASONING CONTINUUM AND CHARACTERISTICS

Category	Years of Reflective Practice	Characteristics
Novice	0	◆ No experience in situation of practice; depends on theory to guide practice ◆ Uses rule-based procedural reasoning to guide actions but does not recognize contextual cues; not skillful in adapting rules to fit situation ◆ Narrative reasoning is used to establish social relationships but does not significantly inform practice ◆ Pragmatic reasoning is stressed in terms of job survival skills ◆ Recognizes overt ethical issues
Advanced beginner	< 1	◆ Begins to incorporate contextual information into rule-based thinking ◆ Recognizes differences between theoretical expectations and presenting problems ◆ Limited experience impedes recognition of patterns and identification of salient cues; does not prioritize well ◆ Gaining skill in pragmatic and narrative reasoning ◆ Begins to recognize more subtle ethical issues
Competent	3	◆ Automatically performs more therapeutic skills and attends to more issues ◆ Is able to develop communal horizon with people receiving service ◆ Is able to sort relevant data and prioritize intervention goals related to desired outcomes ◆ Planning is deliberate, efficient, and responsive to contextual issues ◆ Uses conditional reasoning to modify intervention but lacks flexibility of more advanced practitioners ◆ Recognizes ethical dilemmas posed by practice setting but may be less sensitive to justifiably different ethical responses
Proficient	5	◆ Perceives situations as wholes ◆ Reflects on expanded range of experiences, permitting more focused evaluation and more flexibility in intervention ◆ Creatively combines different diagnostic and procedural approaches ◆ More attentive to occupational stories and relevance for intervention ◆ More skillful in negotiating resources to meet patient/client needs ◆ Increased sophistication in recognizing situational nature of ethical reasoning
Expert	10	◆ Clinical reasoning becomes a quick intuitive process, which is deeply internalized and embedded in an extensive range of case experiences, permitting practice with less routine analysis, except when confronted with situations in which approach is not working ◆ Highly skillful use of occupational story making during intervention to promote long-term occupational performance satisfaction

Modified from Dreyfus and Dreyfus (1986) to include information from Benner (1984); Clark, Ennevor, and Richardson (1996); Creighton, Dijkers, Bennett, and Brown (1995); Mattingly and Fleming (1994); Slater and Cohn (1991); and Strong, Gilbert, Cassidy, and Bennett (1995).

home setting. Refer to Chapter 25 for a discussion of competence and practice context.

CONCLUSION

Professional reasoning is the process that practitioners use to plan, direct, perform, and reflect on client care. It is a whole-body and multisensory process that requires complex cognitive activity. Practitioners develop cognitive frames and scripts as they gain experience, forming the basis of professional knowledge and action. Professional reasoning is multifaceted and enables practitioners to understand client issues from different perspectives. Practitioners use the logical processes associated with scientific reasoning to understand the client's impairments, disabilities, and performance contexts and to predict the impact these have on occupational performance. Narrative reasoning helps practitioners to appreciate the meaning of occupational performance limitations to the client, thus supporting client-centered care. Practitioners use pragmatic reasoning when they address the practical realities associated with service delivery. All of these forms of reasoning lead to an ethical reasoning process by which practitioners select the best therapy action to respond to the client's occupational performance needs. The process of professional reasoning involves a transaction among the practitioner's personal and professional perspectives, the client's perspectives, and the demands of the practice context. Expertise develops as the practitioner gains experience and reflects on that experience for deeper understanding.

PROVOCATIVE QUESTIONS

1. What are some of the personal factors in your life that you think will influence the way in which you practice occupational therapy?

2. How do you think you might deal with research evidence that is in conflict with your own experience or personal beliefs? What are some appropriate responses?

REFERENCES

Barris, R. (1987). Clinical reasoning in psychosocial occupational therapy: The evaluation process. *Occupational Therapy Journal of Research, 7,* 147–162.

Benner, P. (1984). *From novice to expert.* Menlo Park, CA: Addison-Wesley.

Boshuizen, H. P. A., & Schmidt, H. G. (2000). The development of clinical reasoning expertise. In J. Higgs & M. Jones (Eds.), *Clinical reasoning in the health professions* (2nd ed., pp. 15–22). Boston: Butterworth Heinemann.

Bruning, R. H., Schraw, G. J., & Ronning, R. R. (1999). *Cognitive psychology and instruction* (3rd ed.). Upper Saddle River, NJ: Merrill.

Carr, M., & Shotwell, M. (2007). Information processing and clinical reasoning. In B. A. B. Schell & J. W. Schell (Eds.), *Clinical and professional reasoning in occupational therapy.* Baltimore: Lippincott Williams, & Wilkins.

Clark, F., Ennevor, B. L., & Richardson, P. L. (1996). A grounded theory of techniques for occupational storytelling and occupational story making. In R. Zemke & F. Clark (Eds.), *Occupational science: The evolving discipline* (pp. 373–392). Philadelphia: F. A. Davis.

Cohn, E. S. (1989). Fieldwork education: Shaping a foundation for clinical reasoning. *American Journal of Occupational Therapy, 43,* 240–244.

Creighton, C., Dijkers, M., Bennett, N., & Brown, K. (1995). Reasoning and the art of therapy for spinal cord injury. *American Journal of Occupational Therapy, 49,* 311–317.

Crepeau, E. B. (1991). Achieving intersubjective understanding: Examples from an occupational therapy treatment session. *American Journal of Occupational Therapy, 44,* 1016–1024.

Dreyfus, H. L., & Dreyfus, S. E. (1986). *Mind over machine: The power of human intuition and expertise in the era of the computer.* New York: Free Press.

Fleming, M. H. (1991). The therapist with the three-track mind. *American Journal of Occupational Therapy, 45,* 1007–1014.

Fleming, M. H. (1994a). The search for tacit knowledge. In C. Mattingly & M. H. Fleming (Eds.), *Clinical reasoning: Forms of inquiry in a therapeutic practice* (pp. 22–33). Philadelphia: F. A. Davis.

Fleming, M. H. (1994b). Procedural reasoning: Addressing functional limitations. In C. Mattingly & M. H. Fleming (Eds.), *Clinical reasoning: Forms of inquiry in a therapeutic practice* (pp. 137–177). Philadelphia: F. A. Davis.

Fleming, M. H. (1994c). Conditional reasoning: Creating meaningful experiences. In C. Mattingly & M. H. Fleming (Eds.), *Clinical reasoning-forms of inquiry in a therapeutic practice* (pp. 197–235). Philadelphia: F. A. Davis.

Fondiller, E. D., Rosage, L. J., & Neuhaus, B. E. (1990). Values influencing clinical reasoning in occupational therapy: An exploratory study. *Occupational Therapy Journal of Research, 10,* 41–55.

Gambrill, E. (2005). *Critical thinking in clinical practice: Improving the quality of judgments and decisions* (2nd ed.). Hoboken, NJ: John Wiley & Sons.

Gray, J. M. (1998). Putting occupation in practice: Occupation as ends, occupation as means. *American Journal of Occupational Therapy, 52,* 354–364.

Hamilton, T. B. (2007). Narrative reasoning. In B. A. B. Schell & J. W. Schell (Eds.), *Clinical and professional reasoning in occupational therapy.* Baltimore: Lippincott Williams & Wilkins.

Harris, D. L. (2005). *Therapist's sensory processing and its influence upon occupational therapy interventions in children with autism.* Unpublished master's thesis, Brenau University, Gainesville, GA.

Holm, M. B. (2001). Our mandate for the new millennium: Evidence-based practice. The 2000 Eleanor Clarke Slagle Lecture. *American Journal of Occupational Therapy,* (6), CE-1–CE12.

Hooper, B. (1997). The relationship between pretheoretical assumptions and clinical reasoning. *American Journal of Occupational Therapy, 51,* 328–338.

Hooper, B. (2007). Therapists' assumptions as a dimension of professional reasoning. In B. A. B. Schell & J. W. Schell (Eds.), *Clinical and professional reasoning in occupational therapy.* Baltimore: Lippincott Williams, & Wilkins.

Howard, B. S. (1991). How high do we jump?: The effect of reimbursement on occupational therapy. *American Journal of Occupational Therapy, 45,* 875–881.

Kessels, J. P. A. M., & Korthagen, F. A. (1996). The relationship between theory and practice: Back to the classics. *Educational Researcher, 25*(32), 17–22.

Kielhofner, G. (1997). *Conceptual foundations of occupational therapy* (2nd ed.). Philadelphia: F. A. Davis.

Kielhofner, G., & Forsyth, K. (2002). Thinking with theory: A framework for therapeutic reasoning. In G. Kielhofner (Ed.), *A model of human occupation: Theory and application* (3rd ed., pp. 162–178). Baltimore: Lippincott Williams & Wilkins.

Law, M. (Ed.). (2002). *Evidence-based rehabilitation: A guide to practice.* Thorofare, NJ: Slack.

Lyons, K. D., & Crepeau, E. B. (2001). Case report: The clinical reasoning of a certified occupational therapy assistant. *American Journal of Occupational Therapy, 55,* 577–581.

Mattingly, C. (1994a). Occupational therapy as a two body practice: Body as machine. In C. Mattingly & M. H. Fleming (Eds.), *Clinical reasoning: Forms of inquiry in a therapeutic practice* (pp. 37–63). Philadelphia: F. A. Davis.

Mattingly, C. (1994b). The narrative nature of clinical reasoning. In C. Mattingly & M. H. Fleming (Eds.), *Clinical reasoning: Forms of inquiry in a therapeutic practice* (pp. 239–269). Philadelphia: F. A. Davis.

Mattingly, C., & Fleming, M. H. (1994). Interactive reasoning: Collaborating with the person. In C. Mattingly & M. H. Fleming (Eds.), *Clinical reasoning: Forms of inquiry in a therapeutic practice* (pp. 178–196). Philadelphia: F. A. Davis.

Neuhaus, B. E. (1988). Ethical considerations in clinical reasoning: The impact of technology and cost containment. *American Journal of Occupational Therapy, 42,* 288–294.

Parham, D. (1987). Nationally speaking—toward professionalism: The reflective occupational therapy practitioner. *American Journal of Occupational Therapy, 41,* 555–561.

Pelland, M. J. (1987). A conceptual model for the instruction and supervision of treatment planning. *American Journal of Occupational Therapy, 41,* 351–359.

Peloquin, S. M. (1993). The depersonalization of patients: A profile gleaned from narratives. *American Journal of Occupational Therapy, 49,* 830–837.

Roberts, A. E. (1996). Clinical reasoning in occupational therapy: Idiosyncrasies in content and process. *British Journal of Occupational Therapy, 59,* 372–376.

Robertson, L. J. (1996). Clinical reasoning, part 2: Novice/expert differences. *British Journal of Occupational Therapy, 59,* 212–216.

Rogers, J. C. (1983). Clinical reasoning: The ethics, science, and art. *American Journal of Occupational Therapy, 37,* 601–616.

Rogers, J. C., & Holm, M. B. (1991). Occupational therapy diagnostic reasoning: A component of clinical reasoning. *American Journal of Occupational Therapy, 45,* 1045–1053.

Schell, B. A. B. (1994). The effect of practice context on occupational therapy practitioner's clinical reasoning (Doctoral dissertation, University of Georgia, 1994). *Dissertation Abstracts International,* AAT 9507243.

Schell, B. A. B. (2003). Clinical reasoning: The basis of practice. In E. B. Crepeau, E. S. Cohn, & Schell, B. A. B. (Eds.), *Willard and Spackman's Occupational Therapy* (10th ed., pp. 131–139). Philadelphia: Lippincott Williams & Wilkins.

Schell, B. A. B. (2007). Pragmatic reasoning. In B. A. B. Schell & J. W. Schell (Eds.), *Clinical and professional reasoning in occupational therapy.* Baltimore: Lippincott Williams and Wilkins.

Schell, B. A., & Cervero, R. M. (1993). Clinical reasoning in occupational therapy: An integrative review. *The American Journal of Occupational Therapy, 47,* 605–610.

Schell, B. A. B., & Schell, J. W. (2007). *Clinical and professional reasoning in occupational therapy.* Baltimore: Lippincott Williams and Wilkins.

Schell, B. A. B., Unsworth, C., & Schell, J. (2008). Theory and practice: New directions for research in professional reasoning. In B. A. B. Schell & J. W. Schell (Eds.), *Clinical and professional reasoning in occupational therapy.* Baltimore: Lippincott Williams and Wilkins.

Schön, D. A. (1983). *The reflective practitioner: How professionals think in action.* New York: Basic.

Schwartzberg, S. (2002). *Interactive reasoning in the practice of occupational therapy.* Upper Saddle River, NJ: Prentice Hall.

Slater, D. Y., & Cohn, E. S. (1991). Staff development through analysis of practice. *American Journal of Occupational Therapy, 45,* 1038–1044.

Strong, J., Gilbert, J., Cassidy, S., & Bennett, S. (1995). Expert clinicians and student view on clinical reasoning in occupational therapy. *British Journal of Occupational Therapy, 58,* 119–123.

Tickle-Degnen, L. (1998). Using research evidence in planning treatment for the individual client. *Canadian Journal of Occupational Therapy, 65,* 152–159.

Tickle-Degnen, L. (2000). Evidence-based practice forum: Gathering current research evidence to enhance clinical reasoning. *American Journal of Occupational Therapy, 54,* 102–105.

Tomlin, G. (2007). Scientific reasoning. In B. A. B. Schell & J. W. Schell (Eds.), *Clinical and professional reasoning in occupational therapy.* Baltimore: Lippincott Williams and Wilkins.

The Therapeutic Relationship

33

POLLIE PRICE

Learning Objectives

After reading this chapter, you will be able to:

1. Identify the phases of the therapeutic relationship and stages of the therapeutic process.
2. Describe strategies to establish a therapeutic relationship with clients.
3. Describe strategies to move a therapy process toward desired outcomes.

WHY IS THE THERAPEUTIC RELATIONSHIP IMPORTANT IN OCCUPATIONAL THERAPY?

All professionals who provide services enter into relationships of some sort with people seeking services. In some service fields, the relationship is secondary, superficial, and based on exchange of information. However, occupational therapy practitioners often meet people at points of significant transition, requiring more intimate exchanges. Practitioners may meet parents when they are first told that their 3-year-old child has autism, when a man wakes up in the intensive care unit to find that he has had a stroke and is paralyzed on one side of his body, when a woman arrives at a shelter with her two young children to take refuge from an abusive husband, or when a young adult has a confusing and frightening experience of schizophrenia. Occupational therapists who enter individuals' lives at such times are called on to quickly create therapeutic relationships that convey empathy and a consistent willingness to both "be there" and "do with" clients through a process that the clients did not bargain for and might not be able to work through alone (Lawlor, 2003; Peloquin, 1995).

In occupational therapy, therapeutic relationships are not just a byproduct of working with human beings. Rather, the therapeutic relationship is the central aspect of the therapeutic process of occupational therapy and one catalyst for change (Devereaux, 1984; Peloquin, 1990; Price, 2003; Schwartzberg, 1993; Yerxa, 1967). Occupational therapists understand that to take action on their own behalf, clients need hope as well as professional guidance (Fleming, 1994). An individual's process of recovery and adaptation requires professional expertise but also an empathic partner who is willing to feel the individual's fear, uncertainty, or despair and to provide support, encouragement, and hope. The degree to which the occupational therapist is able to understand the fears, hopes, priorities, and desires of the client and family will influence collaborative goal setting, intervention plans and activities, and the entire therapy process (Van Amburg, 1997).

> **The therapeutic relationship is the central aspect of the therapeutic process of occupational therapy and one catalyst for change.**

The relationship aspect of the therapy process has often been called "the art of practice." The process of establishing a relationship with another person is a creative and interdependent act and requires that two people come to understand, trust, and respect one another and create shared meanings about what the therapy process means for the person's life and future (Clark, 1993; Clark, Ennevor, & Richardson, 1996). The interactive qualities that enable two people to build a therapeutic relationship are not instinctive or automatic but require mutual willingness, vigilance, attention, and responsiveness (Tickle-Degnen, 2003). The interactive aspects of the therapeutic relationship require interpersonal and communicative skills that an occupational therapist can learn and develop through reflective practice. In a recent study, Gahnström-Strandqvist, Tham, Josephsson, and Borell (2000) called these skills **"empathic competence"** (p. 23), which is defined as the therapist's emotional ability to accurately perceive and respond to clients and their experiences in order to fine-tune the therapy process. The researchers provided empirical evidence that empathic competence is an important feature of professional competence and professional knowledge (Gahnström-Strandqvist et al., 2000). These interactive, interpersonal, and communication skills cannot be learned and applied in practice as a list of procedures and techniques; rather, therapeutic relationships emerge out of real care, from dynamic and responsive interactions, and from both tacit and explicit reasoning as the therapist and client work together toward a common desired outcome. Therefore, truly understanding and caring about clients and their experiences, hopes, and dreams are essential to this emotional aspect of practice and require a personal commitment to self-awareness, reflection, and development of interactive, interpersonal, and communication skills.

For a variety of reasons, occupational therapists frequently get "stuck" in their work with clients, and the therapeutic process stalls. At these stuck points, therapists must reflect on their approaches and determine how to improve them in order to move the therapy process forward or to work more effectively with subsequent clients (Spencer, Davidson, & White, 1996). Consequently, experienced therapists who have reflected on their processes are likely to have more highly developed interactive skills than are novice therapists (Mattingly & Fleming, 1994). Occupational therapy students and new practitioners are encouraged to focus on developing their interactive, interpersonal, and communicative skills as much as they would focus on developing their manual muscle testing skills (Neistadt, 1995).

The therapeutic relationship provides the foundation for collaborative partnerships to develop between clients and therapists. Two important predictors of rehabilitation outcomes are the respect and collaboration that develop between clients and their therapists (Law, 1998). Collaborative goal setting leads to shorter inpatient stays, better goal attainment, and increased client satisfaction (Neistadt, 1995). Occupational therapists feel most competent when both they and their clients are satisfied with the therapy outcomes they achieve (Gahnström-Strandqvist et al., 2000). By blending professional and empathic competence, therapists can help clients to envision a course of action that is both attainable and worth working toward (Gahnström-Strandqvist et al., 2000; Mattingly, 1994; Peloquin, 1990). Understanding that it is not enough to present clients with a set of procedures and techniques that will optimize physical, emotional, or medical outcomes, occupational therapists embark on a spiritual or existential journey with clients by collaborating and helping to create possibilities.

Collaboration and collaborative relationship have been used interchangeably in the literature and are closely related in meaning to "client-centered practice" (Law, Baptiste, & Mills, 1995). **Client-centered occupational therapy** has been described as a philosophy of service committed to "respect for and partnership with people receiving services" (Law et al., 1995, p. 253). **Collaboration** has been described as the process through which therapists and clients discuss priorities, set goals, and make decisions about intervention and postintervention options (Cipriani et al., 1999; Spencer, 1993) and work together in mutual effort toward goals (Neistadt, 1995). However, clients have different needs and desires related to the degree and type of collaboration in therapeutic relationships. Some clients want the therapist to be "the expert" in making clinical decisions, while others want to take the lead in their therapy process. When therapists meet clients' needs, clients experience positive relationships with their therapists and satisfaction with therapy outcomes (Cipriani et al., 1999).

HOW DO THERAPISTS AND CLIENTS DEVELOP A THERAPEUTIC RELATIONSHIP?

In occupational therapy, the therapeutic relationship requires a degree of intimacy that develops along a continuum depending on the nature of the individual's condition, the degree of disruption to his or her life and identity, the extent of recovery expected, and the length and complexity of the recovery and adaptation process, including the occupational therapy process. Several authors have theorized that the therapeutic relationship develops in phases and that the developing relationship both shapes and is shaped by the therapist and client's engagement in and experience of the therapy process (see Table 33.1) (Paddy,

TABLE 33.1 HOW THE THERAPEUTIC RELATIONSHIP INTERSECTS WITH THE THERAPEUTIC PROCESS

Phases of Relationship Development	Strategies	Stages of Therapeutic Process	Strategies
Phase 1: Develop rapport	◆ Honor the client's dignity. ◆ Demonstrate willingness to experience the client's grief, despair, and hope. ◆ Meet the client's desired level of intimacy.	**Stage 1: Being there and understanding the client**	◆ *Be with* socially. ◆ Ask about habits, roles, interests, priorities, and resources. ◆ Generate past and present narrative images of the client. ◆ Observe the client's responses, abilities, and adaptive style.
Phase 2: Establish trust	◆ Create trust by spending time, giving information, and ensuring client choice. ◆ Convey best practice options within an understanding of the client's priorities.	**Stage 2: Engaging the client in therapy**	◆ Get the client to self-appraise through doing, using a functional measurement scale, videotapes, and other clients to increase awareness. ◆ Offer meaningful options and explore possibilities. ◆ Explain the purpose of therapy activities.
Phase 3: Develop a collaborative partnership	◆ In the role of covenanter (Peloquin, 1990), share the difficult path to knowledge and competence.	**Stage 3: Working together**	◆ The therapist and client take on active and equal roles and effort. ◆ The therapist brings professional expertise; the client brings expertise about his or her own life. ◆ Support the client to set goals and make decisions about therapy activities. ◆ Convey trust in the client's abilities. ◆ Uncover and activate the client's resources and problem solving. ◆ Have the client perform to explore limitations and solutions.
Phase 4: Sustain a therapeutic relationship	◆ As trust and confidence deepen, therapeutic roles, strategies, and activities change. ◆ The client fluctuates between need for affiliation and need for autonomy.	**Stage 4: Enabling occupational performance**	◆ Pool resources and persevere in creating solutions. ◆ Point out disabilities and accomplishments. ◆ Adjust therapeutic strategies. ◆ Teach problem solving and convey confidence through taking risks; create opportunities to practice in real situations. ◆ Go with the client's time rhythm. ◆ Change roles from director to follower.
Phase 5: Relationship endures	◆ The relationship endures after therapy ends. ◆ The client is "held in mind" (Paddy et al., 2002); "they would always be there for you" (Mitchell, Price, & Ward, 2006).	**Stage 5: Outcomes**	◆ Clients reach *their* goals. ◆ Clients live fulfilling lives doing their occupations. ◆ Therapy results are satisfying to both client and therapist. ◆ The client has a sense of control and autonomy over managing his or her life.

Wright-Sinclair, & Smythe, 2002; Peloquin, 1993, 2003; Tickle-Degnen, 2002).

Phase One: Development of Rapport: Entering the Life World of Another

When developing rapport, the therapist and client exchange information in order to understand each other's desires and motives. To establish rapport, the therapist must honor the client's dignity or worthiness (Devereaux, 1984; Peloquin, 1990, 1995, 2003) and convey professional competence and empathy (Figure 33.1). "**Empathy**, in health care practice, is the enactment of the conviction that, empowered by someone else's willingness to understand, a person will gather courage" (Peloquin, 2003, p. 159). Becoming a part of a client's life requires a deep knowingness that comes from concern, openness, listening and responding, and relating as a fellow human being (Paddy et al., 2002; Peloquin, 1995). When therapists convey genuine interest in understanding the client's life world, the client may be more likely to embark in a collaborative and mutually created therapeutic process.

The occupational therapy process begins with an occupational profile, which consists of a formal interview with the client and/or important others (e.g., spouse, parent, teacher, caregiver), using, for example, the Canadian Occupational Performance Measure (Law et al., 1990), or the Occupational Performance History Interview (Kielhofner et al., 1997). These measures help occupational therapists begin to explore a client's life world, occupational history, and priorities.

In addition to using formal interview measures, therapists use informal narrative strategies, including storytelling (Clark, 1993; Jackson, 1998; Mattingly, 1994; 1998; Spencer, Krefting, & Mattingly, 1993). Enabling clients to tell stories about their lives and their hopes for the future is a skill therapists can develop (Clark, 1993; Mattingly, 1994, 1998). Therapists use several strategies to enable clients to tell and make stories, such as sharing personal experiences, talking about shared interests, and asking questions such as "What do you most look forward to resuming?" or "What would you be doing if you were home and feeling well? (Price-Lackey & Kennedy, unpublished data)." Such simple gestures convey humanity and offer clients an opportunity to tell therapists what they care about and may also allow the discovery or creation of adaptive strategies (Clark, Ennevor, & Larsen, 1996).

Phase Two: Establishing Trust

A therapist engenders trust by spending time with the client, giving undivided attention to the client, and eliciting and listening to stories. Conveying interest and verbalizing an understanding of the client's life world, fears, and priorities will provide a narrative context for considering and offering the best intervention options. A therapist demonstrates both professional and empathic competence when offering clients a choice of evidence-based options that address their priorities (Gahnström-Strandqvist et al., 2000; Peloquin, 1990, 2003). This blend of competencies creates the foundation for trust and confidence to be established between therapists and clients and will launch collaborative partnerships.

Phase Three: Developing a Collaborative Partnership

Based on a foundation of mutual respect and trust that is developed between clients and therapists in the first few interactions, a working alliance can then be developed (Tickle-Degnen, 2002). Therapist and client together discuss what is important to the client, identify desired outcomes, develop goals and therapy plans, and commit to work together toward those goals. The therapist and client discuss and make decisions about treatment options based on current research evidence (Cipriani et al., 1999;

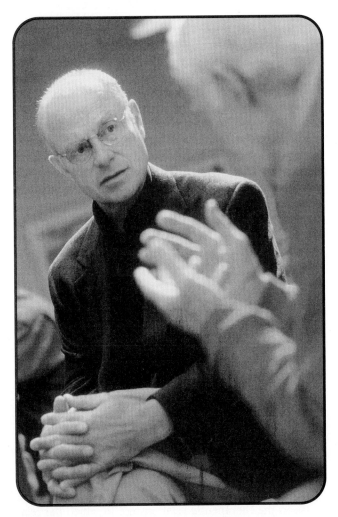

FIGURE 33.1 Therapist listening to client to establish rapport.

Tickle-Degnen, 2002). As therapy begins, there may be a period of trial and error and a revision of plans, activities, and approaches (Mattingly & Fleming, 1994). The therapist may take on different roles, taking more of a lead at first and then hanging back to let clients explore their abilities, limitations, and potential solutions, all the while conveying to the client that the therapist will continue to be there for professional guidance, personal support and encouragement, and accurate feedback about the client's abilities and potential (Gahnström-Strandqvist et al., 2000; Guidetti & Tham, 2002). This "doing with" conveys the quality of being a "covenanter" who will be with the client until the client can do on his or her own (Peloquin, 1990). As trust deepens, the therapist may place increased demands on the client and let the client take more risks and possibly experience failure to help the client develop more awareness, problem solving, and effective solutions (Guidetti & Tham, 2002). The therapeutic relationship changes as a shared understanding of what is important and at stake grows. This increased understanding shapes the therapeutic process, enabling the therapist to fine-tune and individualize the therapy to address the outcomes in which the client is most invested (Crepeau, 1991). These developments strengthen the relationship as the client and therapist continually re-evaluate the therapy goals and therapy process until goals are reached and the formal relationship is dissolved.

The therapist and client continue to disclose important information through interactions that are interwoven within the actions of therapy, including storytelling and storymaking (Clark, 1993; Jackson, 1998; Mattingly, 1994). Through mutual engagement in the process of therapy and the creation of narrative stories, shared meaning is created between therapist and client about the relationship of the therapy to the client's goals for the future (Mattingly, 1991, 1994, 1998; Price, 2003). For example, one of the therapists in Gahnström-Strandqvist and colleagues' (2000) study encouraged her client to fix a dripping tap:

> I encouraged him to fix a dripping tap, which was so annoying to him. "If I were well, I would do it," he said. "But, you can still do this," I said, "do it now." He was very thorough and it took a long, long time, but he did it." (p. 21)

From a narrative standpoint, the therapy activity, fixing a dripping tap, was loaded with symbolic meaning. It conveyed the therapist's trust in the client's ability to complete the task competently and drew on the client's trust in the therapist's professional competence to choose a task that he was capable of doing. Finally, by picking a task that was essentially occupational in nature, the therapist provided an opportunity for the client to experience his "self" doing an old occupation in a new way.

Storytelling can help therapists to understand the meanings and motives underlying their clients' decisions,

actions, and inactions; storymaking can help therapists and clients to generate narrative meaning about what might be possible in the future and may enable clients to take actions based on hope and new possibilities (Clark, 1993; Mattingly, 1994; Polkinghorne, 1996).

In summary, establishing a collaborative relationship requires that clients be willing to actively engage as partners in the therapy process and that therapists be willing to offer and finely adjust therapy activities on the basis of clients' priorities and a careful reading of their desires, motives, and experiences of therapy.

Phase Four: Sustaining the Therapeutic Partnership

Once a collaborative partnership has been established and the client and therapist are mutually engaged in the therapeutic process, the communication between therapist and client must continue in regard to the client's experiences, the need for revision of goals and plans, and the fluctuations in need for affiliation and relationship or autonomy and privacy (Tickle-Degnen, 2002). As the relationship grows more comfortable, the client and therapist may take more risks in communication, or they may become less attentive. In all phases of the therapeutic relationship, communication errors or misunderstandings can occur that threaten the relationship and require attention, sensitivity, responsiveness, and correction (Tickle-Degnen, 2002). Therapist and client continue to explore additional intervention options and make decisions about outcome goals, needed community resources and supports, and termination of therapy when therapist and client are satisfied with outcomes that have been achieved (Tickle-Degnen, 2002).

Several scholars have theorized that the therapeutic relationship and roles within the relationship change as the client acquires competence, confidence, and independence in problem solving and in managing and directing his or her own life (Peloquin, 1990; Price, 2003). For example, therapists are often quite directive at the beginning of therapy in teaching strategies, physically assisting or *doing with* clients to encourage them and ensure success. However, research has shown that as clients demonstrate emerging abilities, therapists' roles change to that of corrector; and as clients achieve competence in skills, therapists' roles change to that of follower or coach (Clark, 1993; Gahnström-Strandqvist et al., 2000; Guidetti & Tham, 2002; Price, 2003).

Phase Five: Enduring Relationships

Paddy and colleagues (2002) suggested that there is a fifth phase to the therapeutic relationship, in which the relationship endures after the formal process of therapy is terminated. The following client's description of her ongoing relationship with her therapist illustrates what Paddy and colleagues called "being held in mind":

> I feel like she has me in her mind when she's doing things. I may not have talked to her for quite a few months . . . when there's been a long gap, I can just ring her up when I need to. . . . It seems that when she comes across something that is suitable she thinks of me and that's really brilliant. . . . I feel that I'm always with her. (p. 17)

This client's reflections demonstrate that the quality of the therapeutic relationship has an enduring impact on both therapist and client.

THERAPEUTIC PROCESS IS INTERTWINED WITH AND PROPELLED BY THE THERAPEUTIC RELATIONSHIP

The therapeutic relationship and the intervention process are dynamic, intertwined, and interdependent as they influence each other (Gahnström-Strandqvist et al., 2000; Guidetti & Tham, 2002; Price, 2003; Rosa & Hasselkus, 1996). As therapist and client deepen their understanding of what is important to the client and the resources and adaptive skills the client has to draw on, the therapist adjusts and individualizes intervention. As the client begins to experience progress, the trust the client feels for the therapist deepens. If the client and therapist feel that the client is ready, they may increase the complexity, demands, or risk of the therapy, with the therapist close by if the client needs assistance.

> **The therapeutic relationship and the intervention process are dynamic, intertwined, and interdependent as they influence each other.**

The therapeutic process includes all of the multiple actions, interactions, activities, and strategies that occur among therapist, client, and family that help the client and family move toward the desired outcomes. In studies of the practices of experienced therapists, therapists work from the tacit knowledge they have developed through practical experience, continuously improvising, creating, negotiating, and directing the therapeutic conditions toward the mutually desired goal (Crepeau, 1991; Mattingly & Fleming, 1994; Price, 2003). Using a blend of professional and empathetic competence (Guidetti & Tham, 2002; Peloquin, 1990) and scientific and narrative understandings (Mattingly, 1994), the therapist employs numerous strategies (Price, 2003) to keep the therapy process moving toward the outcome and to develop and maintain the therapeutic relationship (see Table 33.1).

Five stages of the therapy process parallel and intersect with the process of relationship development described above. The stages of the therapy process are (1) being there and understanding the client, (2) engaging the client, (3) working together, (4) enabling occupational performance, and (5) achieving outcomes. These stages do not occur in a discrete, linear manner; rather, the roles the therapist and client assume and the strategies the therapist uses shift and blend throughout the therapy process.

The outcome toward which a therapist and client work will have a significant influence on what they decide to do in therapy and how. Achieving outcomes that are valued and satisfying to both the client and the therapist is the overarching theme and the hallmark of a strong interpersonal connection between the therapist and the client (Gahnström-Strandqvist et al., 2000; Rosa & Hasselkus, 1996). In a study of therapeutic strategies used by occupational therapists to conduct self-care training in rehabilitation settings, Guidetti and Tham (2002) concluded that the therapists used various strategies to enable clients to achieve independence and adaptation in managing themselves in a "new body in a new everyday world" (p. 273). Through the process of self-care training, therapists helped clients to confront their disabilities, acknowledge their abilities, and develop their capacities for problem solving and adaptation, which ultimately helped them to regain a sense of control, autonomy, and independence in their lives. As clients move from a more or less dependent and therapist-directed position to a more independent and self-directed position, the therapeutic relationship changes and mirrors the therapeutic process as it evolves. The strategies that a therapist uses also change as the client becomes more competent and self-directed.

Stage One: Being There and Understanding the Client

The first stage of the therapeutic process, *being there*, includes all of the actions a therapist takes to express the desire to deeply understand the client and his or her experiences, desires, motivations, fears, and hopes (Peloquin, 1990; Rosa & Hasselkus, 1996). These actions parallel the process of *developing rapport*. In developing rapport, the therapist conveys that he or she honors the client's dignity, respects the client's personhood, and empathizes with the client's situation.

Therapists build rapport through their actions. To convey respect, therapists begin by introducing themselves and explaining the role and objectives of occupational therapy. To maximize the client's privacy, therapists might close a door or curtain before providing information about the evaluation and therapy process. Therapists convey interest by maintaining appropriate and respectful eye contact, leaning slightly toward the client, and maintaining an open posture. It is important to discern the depth of sharing the client is ready to engage in and to engage at that level of intimacy. To encourage and assist the client to express emotions and thoughts, therapists use a similar tone to reflect back their understanding of what the client may be feeling (Tickle-Degnen, 2003). The therapist can then ask the client to elaborate on or confirm what was conveyed. Showing care can help the client to feel more at ease and be more willing to engage in the therapy process.

To understand a person's occupational profile, therapists ask about the client's life, fears, concerns, priorities and previous occupations, including hobbies and interests, and try to understand the meaning these hold for the client (McAndrew, McDermott, Vitzakovitch, & Holm, 1999). Therapists might start by using a formal interview tool, such as the Canadian Occupational Performance Measure (Law et al., 1990) to begin a dialogue with the client about occupational priorities. Following a formal interview, therapists might ask more informal questions such as "What do you enjoy about [occupation]?" that will provide clients with an opportunity to express what they care about. To help with envisioning potential outcomes, therapists then ask about the client's resources and supports in the community (McAndrew et al., 1999).

Clients' desire for collaboration may vary (Cipriani et al., 1999). Some clients want to be involved in making all decisions about their care, while other clients want the "expert" to tell them what to do. A client might have cognitive limitations that make it difficult to process information and make decisions. In this case, consulting with a person close to the client helps to understand the client's needs and desires. Ultimately, the goal is to support the client to be involved in making plans and goals; however, this might not be possible with all clients (Cipriani et al., 1999).

On the basis of an understanding of the client's life, resources, priorities, and concerns, therapists assess the client's ability to perform meaningful tasks and occupations in the most natural context possible within the parameters of the setting (Price, 2005). Therapists share the results and implications of the evaluation and provide intervention options that are informed by evidence and address the client's goals, priorities, and adaptive style (Spencer, 1993; Tickle-Degnen, 2002).

Stage Two: Engaging the Client in the Therapy Process

The second stage of the therapy process is *engaging the client in the therapy process.* Because the outcomes of occupational therapy often require transformation and adaptation, clients must take an active role in their own recovery. A client might be open and willing to engage in a therapy process if he or she feels that therapy will help. Another client might have difficulty engaging in occupational therapy. Clients might resist occupational therapy, be suspicious of therapy, or fail to see the relevance or opportunity for help. Therapists use several strategies and subtle negotiations to help the client generate meaning and motive for participating in therapy (Gahnström-Strandqvist et al., 2000; Mattingly, 1994, 1998; Price, 2003). Some options include "planting a seed" (Gahnström-Strandqvist et al., 2000, p. 20) by spending time with the client, providing information and options, and ensuring that the client has control in decision making, including the decision to participate in therapy.

In hospital settings in which clients must receive a certain amount of therapy each day to remain on the unit, the need to *engage the client in the therapy process* is more urgent. The therapist must be careful not to manipulate or coerce the client by threatening, as this approach will certainly preclude the development of rapport and collaboration. Giving information, options, and control over the decision to participate in therapy within a certain time frame puts the client and family at the center of decision making and will potentially strengthen the relationship.

Therapists use their professional knowledge to explain the disability or disease process, help clients to envision possible outcomes, and identify goals and therapy activities that are substantiated by research evidence (Mattingly, 1994, 1998; Spencer, 1993; Tickle-Degnen, 2003). Explaining the purpose of the therapy activities in relation to the client's life or asking a client to engage in challenging tasks to help the client self-appraise strengths and limitations can generate meaning and desire for participating in therapy. Therapists might use a scale such as the Functional Independence Measure (Center for Functional Assessment Research, 1996), a videotape, or another client to help the client understand the therapy process and to generate intentionality to engage in the hard work of therapy.

Engaging the client in the therapy process parallels and intersects with the second phase of the relationship: *establishing trust.* By providing the client with an opportunity to engage in meaningful activities, the client can better experience and appreciate his or her abilities and limits and begin to trust the therapist and the therapy process, even if tentatively (Figure 33.2).

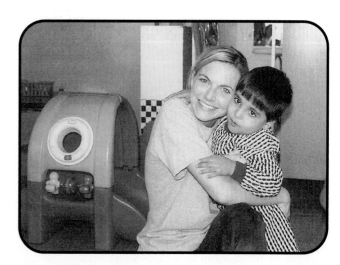

FIGURE 33.2 Child and therapist develop a trusting relationship.

Stage Three: Working Together

Working together corresponds with the third phase of relationship development: *developing a collaborative relationship.* The most satisfying therapy experiences are those in which the client and therapist are equally invested and engaged in the therapy process, each bringing his or her own expertise. Therapists bring their professional knowledge and experience, and clients bring expertise about their lives, roles, occupations, and adaptive styles. Therapists provide information about the evaluation process and results and offer best treatment options based on both evidence and an understanding of the client's priorities. Together, the client and therapist establish goals and outcomes of therapy and embark on a sometimes difficult road to develop the knowledge and competence the client will need to live a satisfying life (Gahnström-Strandqvist et al., 2000).

The following excerpt from an observation of an occupational therapist as he conducts an initial evaluation in the home of a woman who had sustained multiple injuries in a bicycle accident illustrates the goal-setting process (Price, unpublished data).

> The therapist asks her about her hours, responsibilities, organizational strategies, and other activities outside of work. After he does several physical and cognitive assessments with her, he asks, ". . . What things do you want to accomplish? What are some of the expectations you have for yourself as far as personal goals . . . ?" She replied . . . "I want to be able to get back to work . . ." At the end of the session, he summed up his understanding of her priority for therapy, "We're gonna [help you] to return to work . . ."

Stage Four: Enabling Occupational Performance

The initial stages of intervention are marked by trial and error in identifying intervention activities, mutual problem solving regarding approaches, and revisions in plans and outcomes. Therapists use various strategies to engage in a collaborative relationship based on mutual effort and joint problem solving that will enhance the client's occupational performance.

Provide Options and Choices of Therapy Activities

Therapists ask clients whether they want to do certain therapy activities; the client may decline or offer alternatives. For example, a client-informant in a study by Cipriani and colleagues (1999) mused, "she'll ask if I want to do it . . . if I don't feel like it I'll tell her so" (p. 51). Another patient, Mary, said her therapist gave her the opportunity to make decisions about therapy activities, "If I want to do certain things, she lets me do them" (Cipriani et al., p. 51).

Therapists use a variety of strategies to help the client fully engage in and improve occupational performance through the therapy process (Gahnström-Strandqvist et al., 2000; Guidetti & Tham, 2002). These strategies emphasize the client doing occupations to get a feel for limitations and abilities. Therapists grade the difficulty of the activities, change the physical and social demands in the environment, and provide more or less support, depending on the client's needs. Often, therapists help clients to generate adaptations or teach clients to problem-solve and generate their own solutions.

Developing the Client's Capacity for Generating His or Her Own Solutions

To help a client problem-solve, therapists need to convey trust in the client's abilities to perceive, through experiencing himself or herself doing occupational activities, the skills the client needs to develop personal solutions. Therapists often wait, let the client attempt to work out the problem, and intervene when the client needs support. Sometimes, therapists encourage the client to engage in an occupational activity that the therapist believes the client is capable of performing, even when the client is unsure of the outcome. This approach conveys the therapist's confidence in the client but also elicits the client's trust in the therapist's professional judgment and expertise in assessing the client's ability and potential. Mutual respect, confidence, and joint effort reinforce the collaborative relationship.

Adjusting the Task and Environmental Conditions

Therapists fine-tune the demands and opportunities of the therapy conditions to provide the right amount of challenge for clients. This approach is easiest to implement when intervention occurs in natural settings such as home, school, community, and work (Dunn, Brown, & McGuigan, 1994; Hocking, 2001; Pierce, 2001, 2003). However, when this is precluded by the intervention setting, such as in acute rehabilitation settings, asking about the client's previous and current habits, patterns, and routines and conducting a visit to home, community, school, or work help therapist and client to visualize the client's physical and social environments and create therapy conditions that are closer to real life for the client. While observing the client perform desired activities, therapists adjust the difficulty of the tasks by breaking tasks down into smaller steps, adding adaptive equipment, teaching an adaptive technique, or instructing in energy conservation techniques. Encouraging the client to try different solutions based on the therapist's experiences of what has worked for others can enable the client to develop strategies that optimize occupational performance (Unsworth, 2005). Teaching the client to problem-solve her or his own solutions can enhance problem solving, autonomy, and control in unfamiliar and challenging situations in the client's future life (Mattingly & Fleming, 1994; Mitchell, Ward, & Price, 2006). Therapists provide opportunities for the client to generalize his or her problem-solving skills and strengthen a sense of personhood by having the client practice in a variety of social settings that are not adapted. Community outings often provide potent experiences for both clients and therapists to give clients confidence to forge ahead in their social worlds (Jackson, 1998).

Using Time Strategically

Occupational therapists take the time to let clients work at their own pace (Gahnström-Strandqvist et al., 2000; Guidetti & Tham, 2002). Therapists use professional judgment to discern when to let the client continue and when to step in. Stepping in too early or rushing through an activity just to get tasks done stifles the adaptation process and diminishes the client's opportunity to engage in problem-solving his or her own situations.

Another way in which therapists and clients use time strategically is by using time as markers for progress (Guidetti & Tham, 2002). Efficiency in completing one's morning self-care routine, crossing at a street light, or completing grocery shopping can be an important goal for a client and may make a difference in whether the client can live and function independently or with assistance.

Adjust the Therapist's Role According to the Client's Need

Therapists use themselves as therapeutic agents when they shift their roles in relation to the client's needs and abilities. Therapists shift among multiple roles such as director, coach, supporter, and follower, fluidly responding and using multiple strategies (Gahnström-Strandqvist et al., 2000; Guidetti & Tham, 2002, p. 257; Price, 2003, 2006). Therapists are often in the leader role at the beginning of a therapy process, focusing the client's attention, teaching and demonstrating techniques, generating ideas, and offering solutions. As the client engages in and begins to experience success in problem-solving occupational performance problems, therapists assume a more corrective, supporting, or coaching role (Hasselkus, 2002; Price, 2003). As the client acquires competence in problem solving and occupational performance, therapists become followers, even distancing themselves from the clients by staying quiet, moving away, or leaving the room (Guidetti & Tham, p. 268). These strategies convey confidence in the client and help to engender a sense of competence, one desired outcome of occupational therapy.

As clients develop their own problem-solving skills and competence in occupational performance, therapists' roles and strategies change in response. The therapeutic relationship is embedded and intertwined in this forward-moving process. As the client experiences success, more trust is built between therapist and client. The client trusts the therapist's professional expertise, and the therapist trusts the client's emerging capacities for autonomy. This enables the therapist and client to decide when to increase the complexity and difficulty of the therapy demands and when the client is ready to take more risks. Often, as therapy progresses, the client's needs will shift between interdependence with the therapist and the need for autonomy (Tickle-Degnen, 2002). Sustaining the therapeutic relationship through this dynamic process takes vigilance and a keen perception of what the client is experiencing, good communication, and a responsiveness to finely adjust the therapy demands and opportunities.

Stage Five: Outcomes

Finally and ideally, the outcomes of therapy have set the client on a trajectory that will enable him or her to reach desired goals; live a fulfilling life engaging in desired occupations; have control, autonomy, and confidence in managing life; and be optimistic about the future (Gahnström-Strandqvist et al., 2000; Guidetti & Tham, 2002; Rosa & Hasselkus, 1996). The therapeutic relationship between therapist and client, whether positive or negative, often endures long after formal therapy ends (Paddy et al., 2002). Therapists hold a narrative vision of successful clients as having "an expanded and enriched life world" (Gahnström-Strandqvist et al., 2000, p. 17). Clients who have had a good therapeutic relationship with their therapists feel that they are "held in mind" (Paddy et al., 2002, p. 17), that is, clients could call the therapist at any time and the relationship and partnership would still be intact. While reflecting on the experience of occupational therapy, one client said, ". . . it will be the occupational therapist that will spend, you know, the rest of your life . . . they would always be there for you" (Mitchell, Ward, & Price, 2006). Clients often come back months after therapy ends to thank therapists and to share stories of the significance of the therapy and the therapist in helping them resume their lives.

The therapeutic relationship is central to the occupational therapy process (Devereaux, 1984; Peloquin, 1990; Schwartzberg, 1993; Yerxa, 1967). The therapeutic process proceeds in stages and is intertwined with and propelled by the therapeutic relationship. Evidence shows that therapists use multiple personal strategies (therapeutic use of self) to make therapy meaningful and relevant. Once clients are engaged in therapy, therapists use multiple personal strategies to adjust and individualize intervention. Through providing the right amount of challenge and support, clients experience success, which increases the trust and confidence clients and therapists have in each other. The strengthened relationship sustains and boosts the therapeutic process toward mutually satisfying outcomes and endures long after therapy ends.

AN EXAMPLE FROM PRACTICE

Data from observations and interviews (Price, 2003) illustrate the numerous strategies and negotiations that one therapist used to develop a therapeutic relationship. The example shows that the therapeutic relationship is embedded in and drives the therapeutic process.

The data is from one observation conducted with a therapist, Nancy, as she worked with Hannah toward Hannah's goal of going to school and being a friend. The data demonstrate that Nancy used numerous personal strategies with Hannah, such as storytelling and pushing Hannah to stay engaged, to keep her moving toward their mutually desired goal (Clark, 1993; Mattingly, 1994; Price, 2006). Their relationship—specifically, the trust and confidence they had in each other—kept them mutually engaged and moved the therapeutic process forward.

Nancy and Hannah began working together when Hannah was two and a half. Hannah's mother explained that from the time Hannah was a very young child, she was afraid of anyone other than her mother. Hannah screamed and cried when Nancy first began to see her for therapy. Hannah, now four, was still very stilted and quiet around other children; however, during sessions without other children, she was spontaneous, playful, and talkative with Nancy. Throughout therapy, Hannah and Nancy maintained a therapeutic relationship that enabled occupational performance. Nancy sustained the relationship by finding a balance between supporting and pushing Hannah to increase her performance and competence in a more expansive play repertoire and in becoming a member of a social group. Table 33.2 provides an abbreviated overview of the observation and interpretations of the phases and stages of the therapeutic relationship and process to illustrate the strategies Nancy used to move the process forward. The example illustrates the blending of professional and empathic competence in the process of therapy between Nancy and Hannah (Gahnström-Strandqvist et al., 2000; Peloquin, 1990). Hannah trusted Nancy to provide her with the right amount of challenge. Nancy's confidence in Hannah's emerging abilities enabled Hannah to embark on a transformation that she and her mother could not have made happen on their own (Lawlor, 2003). Hannah's mother, Susan, talked about the progress she observed in Hannah's comfort and ability to engage with family, neighbors, and friends because of seeing Nancy. Then she talked about their relationship:

> Hannah adores Nancy. I think, for Hannah, Nancy was the first person who she felt loved her and challenged her at the same time. I think Hannah, she has such a respect, she has such a different relationship with Nancy . . . it's almost like she wants to like show Nancy what she's accomplished. But at the same time, I think she feels like equal with Nancy; like there's like a trust level there, of that she knows that if she tries something and it doesn't work, it's okay too.

Susan's description of Nancy and Hannah's relationship illustrates that the therapeutic relationship, based on mutual respect and confidence, is embedded in the therapeutic process and that the therapeutic process is a blend of empathic and professional competence (Gahnström-Strandqvist et al., 2000; Peloquin, 1990).

CONCLUSION

Occupational therapists often enter clients' lives as they face significant life challenges that preclude them from participating in "life as usual." Therapists are compelled to quickly create therapeutic relationships that convey respect, empathy, and a willingness to "be there" and "do with"; these actions and attitudes engender trust and establish rapport. Because achieving outcomes that are both achievable and desirable can be a complex and difficult process, clients need therapists who are both professionally and empathically competent (Gahnström-Strandqvist et al., 2000; Peloquin, 1990, 2003). The degree to which therapists are willing and able to enter the life worlds of clients and listen deeply to and experience their hopes and fears will determine the degree of collaboration clients and therapists can undertake to develop meaningful interventions (Van Amburg, 1997).

Therapeutic relationships develop in phases: *developing rapport, establishing trust, developing a collaborative partnership, sustaining the therapeutic relationship,* and *holding enduring relationships* after formal therapy has ended. Therapists use multiple personal strategies, such as asking clients to tell stories about their lives, concerns, and priorities. Therapists carefully and intently listen and reflect back empathy and understanding. Therapists *do with* clients until they can do on their own; even then, therapists "hold in mind" their patients and relationships (Paddy et al., 2002).

The therapeutic process is intertwined with and propelled by the therapeutic relationship. The therapeutic process also evolves in stages: *being there and understanding the client, engaging the client in therapy, working together, enabling occupational performance,* and *achieving outcomes.* Therapists use multiple strategies to help clients experience their abilities, limitations, and adaptive capacities through engagement in therapy activities. Therapists adjust the therapy demands to provide the right amount of physical, social, and emotional challenge while also adjusting their roles and levels of support. Through a complex synthesis of professional and empathic competence, therapists enable clients to take up or resume lives of possibility (Gahnström-Strandqvist et al., 2000; Peloquin, 1990).

TABLE 33.2   ANALYSIS OF HANNAH AND NANCY'S THERAPY PROCESS AND RELATIONSHIP

Observation and Interview Data	Phases and Stages of Therapeutic Relationship Development and Process and Strategies Used
Hannah: My legs got bigger. **Nancy** (*gestured growing up with her hand as it moved higher*): Oh, my gosh, you are bigger! Do you think maybe you'll be ready for school pretty soon? **Hannah:** Um hm (*yes*), my school's not open yet. **Nancy:** You know, a lot of other kids are waiting too, to go to school. **Hannah:** Hm. **Nancy:** And those might be good friends, huh? **Hannah:** Hm, cause I'm growing real real up. **Nancy:** You are. You know, you're gonna be ready for school. You're gonna be fine. **Hannah:** Hm.	**Phase 3 of relationship development:** sustaining their relationship **Stage 4 of therapeutic process:** enabling occupational performance **Strategies:** ♦ Conveying trust and confidence in Hannah's abilities and potential to reach her goal ♦ Occupational storytelling and storymaking (Clark, 1993; Mattingly, 1994, 1998): Hannah's long legs mean that she is getting ready for school and to become a friend
Nancy: You know, Hannah, I'm kind of hungry for spaghetti. **Hannah:** (*No response*) **Nancy:** You know what, we're just pretending. This is my little plate (*the lid to the play dough container*). I'm so hungry. **Hannah:** Hm, I'm making it. (*She began cutting the thin strips into pieces.*) **Nancy:** Are you the cook? **Hannah:** Um hm (*yes*). (*Hannah put two chunks of play dough on Nancy's "plate."*) **Nancy:** Oooh! Are those the meatballs? **Hannah:** Um hm (*no*). **Nancy:** What are those? **Hannah:** Play dough. **Nancy:** Well, we have to pretend. What is it? I can't eat play dough. **Hannah:** Hm hm (*no*). **Nancy:** What is it? **Hannah:** That's a pretend. **Nancy:** What should I pretend this is? **Hannah:** Hm. Chewy. **Nancy:** It's chewy. Uh, is it a piece of bread? **Hannah:** Hm hm (*yes*). (*Hannah put clumps of play dough on the "plate."*) **Hannah:** Here's the food. **Nancy:** Is it ready to eat? **Hannah:** Hm. **Nancy:** Yes? **Hannah:** Now it's white. **Nancy:** Wait. I want to eat first. . . . better see if I like it. Want a bite? **Hannah:** Um hm (*no*). **Nancy:** Here. Have a pretend (*held the dough up to Hannah's mouth*). Look at my lips. You don't have to really eat it. (*Nancy put the dough up to her mouth and smacked her lips.*) You just pretend and it makes a sound.	**Stage 3 of therapeutic process:** creating a social situation in which they would work together to explore Hannah's limitations and activate her resources **Strategies:** ♦ Adjusting therapy strategies to use Hannah's resources, strong cognitive skills, to teach Hannah what other children would learn tacitly Hannah tries to escape from the pretend play by declaring that it is time to play with the white play dough. **Strategies:** ♦ Pushing Hannah to stay with the demands ♦ Conveying trust that she could do it ♦ Drawing on Hannah's trust that Nancy would not demand more than she could handle ♦ Providing opportunities for Hannah to explore her limits, create strategies, and draw upon her resources

TABLE 33.2   ANALYSIS OF HANNAH AND NANCY'S THERAPY PROCESS AND RELATIONSHIP   *Continued*

Observation and Interview Data	Phases and Stages of Therapeutic Relationship Development and Process and Strategies Used
Hannah *(watched)*: hm. Nancy: Okay, you try. Look, Hannah. *(Nancy held the dough up to her mouth, smacking, then held the dough up to Hannah's mouth, who reluctantly smacked.)* Here, have another bite. Hannah: Okay. *(Nancy smacked, and then Hannah smacked.)* Nancy: It's delicious. Give me five; you're a great chef!	**Strategies:** ♦ Praising Hannah, a narrative strategy that conveys confidence in Hannah that she is moving toward her goal
Nancy: Why don't you like to pretend to eat those things? Why do you think? Is it too silly *(Hannah: hm)* or you just don't like it? Hannah: I don't like it. Nancy: You don't like it. *(whispered)* But you know what? Hannah: hm? Nancy: Sometimes, if you're at school, you might have to pretend with the kids. Hannah: Okay. Nancy: You know that? So, even if you don't like it. Hannah: Can I get white? *(Nancy tried to get Hannah to pretend to eat some spaghetti, and Hannah was very reluctant.)* Nancy *(acquiescing)*: I'll get white. *(whispered to Hannah)*: You know what? Sometimes, little girls like to pretend. Did you know that? Hannah: (unclear). Nancy: Let's take some deep breaths, okay?	**Strategies:** ♦ Engaging Hannah in problem solving and self-appraisal ♦ Conveying respect for Hannah's experience ♦ Drawing on Hannah's resources, strong cognitive skills, to teach her what other kids would learn tacitly ♦ Going with Hannah's time rhythm, knowing when to give her a break ♦ Storymaking (Clark, 1993; Mattingly, 1994) to increase the demands of therapy and to expand Hannah's play repertoire, to enable her to make and keep friends in preschool ♦ Drawing on Hannah's personal resources (Kielhofner, 2002): breathing is a strategy that Nancy taught Hannah to use and that Hannah could use to calm herself
Nancy: *(Hannah resumed cutting dough)* Do you know what I think? Maybe you'll make some food for me. But you know, I don't have any plate. I have to make one. Hannah: With play dough, like pretend. Nancy *(softly)*: Like pretend, that's right, sweetie. *(Nancy made a small bowl out of play dough as Hannah continued cutting.)* Nancy: Hannah? Hannah: hm? Nancy: Do you think you could give me some play dough soup? Hannah: All right. *(Hannah pretended to fill the bowl.)* Nancy: Oh, thank you! It's very good. What did you put in it? Hannah: Hm. Hm. Rice. Nancy: Nancy: Hmm. *(pretend slurp)* You want a taste? *(Nancy put the spoon up to Hannah's mouth, and Hannah pretended to taste.)* Nancy: Oh, that was a good taste.	**Relationship development:** Nancy conveys confidence in Hannah by asking her to reengage; Hannah conveys trust in Nancy by reengaging **Therapy process:** Hannah demonstrated her learning by pretending; **Strategy:** ♦ Praising Hannah softly. A breakthrough; Hannah demonstrates that she can pretend, even if she does not like it; a highly narrative moment (Mattingly, 1998) that symbolizes Hannah's ability to engage in play that would help her to make and keep friends

Source: Adapted from Price (2003).

PROVOCATIVE QUESTIONS

1. Reflect on Nancy and Hannah's interactions: How do you think the therapy process and outcomes would be influenced if emphasis on the therapeutic relationship was minimized?

2. How would you feel and what would you do if your therapy process with a client was not effective?

REFERENCES

Center for Functional Assessment. (1996). *Functional independence measure (FIM).* Buffalo: State University of New York at Buffalo.

Cipriani, J., Hess, S., Higgins, H., Resavy, D., Sheon, S., Szychowski, M., & Holm, M. (1999). Collaboration in the therapeutic process: Older adult's perspectives. *Physical and Occupational Therapy in Geriatrics, 17*(1), 43–54.

Clark, F. (1993). Interweaving occupational science and occupational therapy. 1993 Eleanor Clark Slagle Lecture. *American Journal of Occupational Therapy, 47,* 1067–1078.

Clark, F., Ennevor, B. L., & Richardson, P. L. (1996). In R. Zemke & F. Clark (Eds.), *Occupational science: The evolving discipline* (pp. 373–392). Philadelphia: F. A. Davis.

Crepeau, E. B. (1991). Achieving intersubjective understanding: Examples from an occupational therapy treatment session. *American Journal of Occupational Therapy, 45*(11), 1016–1025.

Devereaux, E. B. (1984). Occupational therapy's challenge: The caring relationship. *American Journal of Occupational Therapy, 38,* 791–798.

Dunn, W., Brown, C., & McGuigan, A. (1994). The ecology of human performance: A framework for considering the effect of context. *American Journal of Occupational Therapy, 48,* 595–607.

Fleming, M. H. (1994). Conditional reasoning: Creating meaningful experiences. In C. Mattingly & M. H. Fleming (Eds.), *Clinical reasoning: Forms of inquiry in a therapeutic practice* (pp. 197–236). Philadelphia: F. A. Davis.

Gahnström-Strandqvist, K., Tham, K., Josephsson, S., & Borell, L. (2000). Actions of competence in occupational therapy practice. *Scandinavian Journal of Occupational Therapy, 7*(15), 15–25.

Guidetti, S., & Tham, K. (2002). Therapeutic strategies used by occupational therapists in self-care training: A qualitative study. *Occupational Therapy International, 9*(4), 257–276.

Hasselkus, B. R. (2002). *The meaning of everyday occupation.* Thorofare, NJ: Slack.

Hocking, C. (2001). The issue is: Implementing occupation-based assessment. *American Journal of Occupational Therapy, 55,* 463–469.

Jackson, J. (1998). The value of occupation as the core of treatment: Sandy's experience. *American Journal of Occupational Therapy, 52,* 466–473.

Kielhofner, G. (2002). *A model of human occupation: Theory and application* (3rd ed). Philadelphia: Lippincott Williams & Wilkins.

Kielhofner, G., Mallinson, T., Crawford, C., Nowak, M., Rigby, M., Henry, A., & Wallens, D. (1997). *A user's guide to the occupational performance history interview-II (OPHI-II) (Version 2.0).* Chicago: Model of Human Occupation Clearinghouse, Department of Occupational Therapy, University of Illinois.

Law, M. (1998). Does client-centered practice make a difference? In M. Law (Ed.), *Client-centered occupational therapy* (pp. 19–27). Thorofare, NJ: Slack.

Law, M., Baptiste, S., McColl, M., Opzoomer, A. Polatajko, H., & Pollock, N. (1990). The Canadian occupational performance measure; An outcome measure for occupational therapy. *Canadian Journal of Occupational Therapy 57,* 82–87.

Law, M., Baptiste, S., & Mills, J. (1995). Client-centered practice: What does it mean and does it make a difference? *Canadian Journal of Occupational Therapy, 62,* 250–257.

Lawlor, M. (2003). The significance of being occupied: The social construction of childhood occupation. *American Journal of Occupational Therapy, 57,* 424–434.

Mattingly, C. (1991). The narrative nature of clinical reasoning. *American Journal of Occupational Therapy, 45*(11), 998–1005.

Mattingly, C. (1994). The narrative nature of clinical reasoning. In C. Mattingly & M. H. Fleming (Eds.), *Clinical reasoning: Forms of inquiry in a therapeutic practice* (pp. 239–269). Philadelphia: F. A. Davis.

Mattingly, C. (1998). *Healing dramas and clinical plots: The narrative structure of experience.* Cambridge, UK: Cambridge University Press.

Mattingly, C., & Fleming, M. H. (1994). *Clinical reasoning: Forms of inquiry in a therapeutic practice.* Philadelphia: F. A. Davis Company.

McAndrew, E., McDermott, S., Vitzakovitch, S., & Holm, M. (1999). Therapist and patient perceptions of the occupational therapy goal-setting process: A pilot study. *Physical and Occupational Therapy in Geriatrics, 17*(1), 55–63.

Mitchell, J., Ward, K., & Price, P. (in press). Occupation-based practice and its relationship to social and occupational participation in adults with spinal cord injury. *Occupational Therapy Journal of Research.*

Neistadt, M. (1995). Methods of assessing clients' priorities: A survey of adult physical dysfunction settings. *American Journal of Occupational Therapy, 49,* 428–436.

Paddy, A., Wright-Sinclair, V., & Smythe, L. (2002). Aspects of the relationship following face-to-face encounters in occupational therapy practice. *New Zealand Journal of Occupational Therapy, 49*(2), 14–20.

Peloquin, S. M. (1990). The patient-therapist relationship in occupational therapy: Understanding visions and images. *American Journal of Occupational Therapy, 44,* 13–22.

Peloquin, S. M. (1993). The depersonalization of patients: A profile gleaned from narratives. *American Journal of Occupational Therapy, 47,* 830–836.

Peloquin, S. M. (1995). The fullness of empathy: Reflections and illustrations. *American Journal of Occupational Therapy, 49,* 24–39.

Peloquin, S. M. (2003). The therapeutic relationship: Manifestations and challenges in occupational therapy. In E. B. Crepeau, E. S. Cohn, & B. A. B. Schell (Eds.), *Willard and Spackman's occupational therapy* (10th ed., pp. 157–170). Philadelphia: Lippincott Williams & Wilkins.

Polkinghorne, D. (1996). Transformative narratives: From victimic to agenic life. *American Journal of Occupational Therapy, 50,* 299–305.

Pierce, D. (2001). Occupation by design: Dimensions, therapeutic power, and creative process. *American Journal of Occupational Therapy, 55,* 249–259.

Pierce, D. (2003). *Occupation by design: Building therapeutic power.* Philadelphia: F. A. Davis.

Price, P. (2003). Occupation-centered practice: Providing opportunities for becoming and belonging. *Dissertation Abstracts International, 65*(05), 2382B. (UMI No. 3133327)

Price, P. (2005). Measuring occupational performance within a socio-cultural context. In M. Law, C. Baum, & W. Dunn (Eds.), *Measuring occupational performance: Supporting best practice in occupational therapy* (pp. 347–367). Philadelphia: Slack.

Price, P., Miner S. (2007). Occupation emerges in the process of therapy. *American Journal of Occupational Therapy, 51,* 441–450.

Rosa, S. A., & Hasselkus, B. R. (1996). Connecting with patients: The personal experience of professional helping. *Occupational Therapy Journal of Research, 16*(4), 245–260.

Schwartzberg, S. L. (1993). Tools of practice: Therapeutic use of self. In H. L. Hopkins & H. D. Smith (Eds.), *Willard & Spackman's occupational therapy* (8th ed., pp. 269–274). Philadelphia: Lippincott.

Spencer, E. A. (1993). Preliminary concepts and planning. In H. L. Hopkins & H. D. Smith (Eds.), *Willard & Spackman's occupational therapy* (8th ed., pp. 269–274). Philadelphia: Lippincott.

Spencer, J. C., Davidson, H., & White, V. (1996). Continuity and change: Past experience as adaptive repertoire in occupational adaptation. *American Journal of Occupational Therapy, 47,* 303–309.

Spencer, J. C., Krefting, L. & Mattingly, C. (1993). Incorporation of ethnographic methods in occupational therapy assessment. *American Journal of Occupational Therapy, 47,* 303–309.

Tickle-Degnen, L. (2002). Client-centered practice, therapeutic relationship, and the use of research evidence. *American Journal of Occupational Therapy, 56,* 470–474.

Tickle-Degnen, L. (2003). Therapeutic rapport. In C. A. Trombly & M. V. Radomski (Eds.), *Occupational therapy for physical dysfunction* (5th ed., pp. 299–311). Philadelphia: Lippincott Williams & Wilkins.

Unsworth, C. (2005). Using a head-mounted video camera to explore current conceptualizations of clinical reasoning in occupational therapy. *American Journal of Occupational Therapy, 59,* 31–40.

Van Amburg, R. (1997). A Copernican revolution in clinical ethics: Engagement versus disengagement. *American Journal of Occupational Therapy, 51,* 186–190.

Yerxa, E. J. (1967). Authentic occupational therapy. The 1966 Eleanor Clark Slagle Lecture. *American Journal of Occupational Therapy, 21,* 1–9.

The Interview Process in Occupational Therapy

34

ALEXIS D. HENRY AND
JESSICA M. KRAMER

> " I interview because I am interested in other people's stories. . . stories are a way of knowing. "
>
> —IRVING SEIDMAN (1991)

Learning Objectives

After reading this chapter, you will be able to:

1. Describe the use of interviewing as an evaluation procedure in occupational therapy.
2. Identify features of an effective interview.
3. Identify available standardized interviews and self reports designed to identify clients' occupational needs and desires.

After reviewing preliminary information about a client, interviewing is the first step in conducting a client-centered evaluation and developing an occupational profile (American Occupational Therapy Association, 2002). Interviewing is an essential skill for one of the most common assessment procedures used by occupational therapy practitioners. The goals of interviewing are both product and process. Beyond gathering information (product), interviews are useful because they help to develop a therapeutic alliance with the client (process).

WHAT IS INTERVIEWING?

Interviewing has been defined as a shared verbal experience, jointly constructed by the interviewer and the interviewee, organized around the asking and answering of questions (Mishler, 1986). While your "job," as the interviewer, is primarily to ask the questions and the client's "job," as the interviewee, is primarily to answer, effective interviewing does not proceed in a stilted, "stimulus-response" manner. Rather, you and the client are attempting to achieve some shared understanding of a particular reality. That reality is the client's story.

When you first meet a client, the information that you are most likely to have is a label that identifies the client as having a particular type of problem. Most often, this label takes the form of a diagnosis; for example, the client might have a diagnosis of schizophrenia or arthritis or a learning disability. The diagnosis is likely to lead you to make certain assumptions about the occupational performance problems this client might have, based on either your past experience with other people who had that same diagnosis or your textbook knowledge of the diagnostic condition. But in reality, information such as a client's diagnosis has limited usefulness in influencing the course of intervention. To develop a meaningful intervention plan, you need to know the particulars of the client's situation, and you need to know them from the client's perspective. In other words, you need to understand the client's story.

When a practitioner considers how the client's present situation fits into the client's larger life story, the practitioner is thinking narratively about the client (Clark, 1993; Franits, 2005; Frank, 1996; Helfrich & Kielhofner, 1994; Mattingly, 1991). A narrative or life story approach involves considering the particular set of circumstances that describe a client's life before he or she came for intervention, how the client views his or her life now, and where the client sees that life going after intervention. When thinking narratively, the practitioner strives to understand the client's values and motives in order to make interventions meaningful.

Interviews are strategies that can help you to think about the client in narrative terms. The client's story, goals, concerns, and aspirations are essential for determining the course of intervention. When there is a mismatch between your perception and the client's perception of what is needed, interventions are likely to become stalled (Mattingly, 1991). A shared perception of what is needed can best be achieved through a dialogue between you and the client.

Interviews are structured strategies for engaging the client in a dialogue, although interviews function best when they proceed as normal conversation rather than as a formal question-and-answer session. An interview should always take place at the beginning of the intervention process. At the beginning of intervention, one important goal of an interview is to gather specific information about the client. In this way, an interview is one of many procedures that might be used in a comprehensive evaluation of a client. However, because it is an interaction between you and the client, an interview is also an intervention that can have therapeutic value in its own right. In the context of an interview, you and the client can together begin to construct a new life story for the client (Mattingly & Fleming, 1994).

WHEN AND WHOM TO INTERVIEW

The Initial Interview: Interview as Assessment

Because interviewing is an integral part of a comprehensive evaluation of a client's occupational functioning, it most frequently occurs at the beginning of your work with a client. During this initial interaction, your goal is to begin to understand the client's story (see Box 34.1). The second, but not unrelated, goal is to begin to form a collaborative relationship with the client. These and other goals of interviewing will be discussed later in this section.

BOX 34.1   **PRACTICE NOTES**

In my own practice, when I worked on an inpatient psychiatry unit, an interview was almost always my first significant interaction with a new patient. Before administering any other assessment, I would sit down with the patient to talk. Who is this person? What brought the person here? What does the person care about? Where does the person hope to go from here? The answers to these questions were important in shaping the recommendations that I would make for the work we could do together in the time we had. *AH*

During the Course of Therapy: Interview as Intervention

Although interviewing is virtually always done at the beginning of an intervention process, the beginning is not the only time an interview may be appropriate. An interview that occurs after your work with a client has begun can be both a form of reevaluation and an intervention. Such interviews are usually less structured than the data-gathering process used during the formal initial evaluation phase. This more informal kind of interaction can involve you and the client in reviewing what has happened thus far and anticipating and planning for the future. This discussion can help the client to construct an image of a future self who is able to do more than the client can do now. Such images are important in making the intervention something the client can commit to and invest in (Helfrich & Kielhofner, 1994; Polkinghorne, 1996). In addition, reviewing your work together can be a useful strategy when you seem to be at a "stuck" point, when it seems that the intervention is not progressing. Together, you and the client can ask, "Why is this not working?" and "What can we do to make things better?" In these ways, interviewing is a collaborative tool that is used repeatedly throughout the intervention process.

Interviewing Older Adolescents and Adults

Most older adolescents and adults that you will encounter in practice are appropriate candidates for interviewing. The techniques for interviewing that are discussed later in this section apply, for the most part, to interviewing individuals of these ages. However, some people are not appropriate candidates for interviews or should be interviewed only in highly structured situations. For example, individuals with severe depression might have difficulty concentrating on and responding to interview questions; people with mania might be too distracted by external stimuli to attend to an interview. People with psychosis might have such disorganized thinking that their answers to questions are difficult to understand. People with expressive or receptive language deficits (e.g., aphasia) might either not comprehend questions or not be able to respond even if they understand. If an interview is approached as a conversation, a time when you and the client are going to "talk," rather than as a formal evaluation of the client, then either continuing or discontinuing the interview (if that seems necessary) can be done without making the client feel that he or she has failed the evaluation.

Interviewing Children and Younger Adolescents

Although pediatrics is one of the largest practice areas in occupational therapy, until recently, few interview procedures had been developed to gather data on children's occupational behavior directly from children. Some advances have been made in developing interview and other self-report procedures for use with children; some of these procedures will be discussed later in the chapter.

Children pose a unique challenge for the interviewer. The ability of children to describe their experiences and their feelings depends on their acquisition of the requisite cognitive, linguistic, and social skills (Krahenbuhl & Blades, 2006; Stone & Lemanek, 1990). Before the age of 7 or 8 years, most children describe themselves only in terms of observable characteristics and behaviors and make differentiations between themselves and others on the basis of these observable traits rather than on internal states. For example, a young child may be able to describe herself in terms of the physical attributes (e.g., "I have blue eyes."), possessions (e.g., "I have a cat."), or preferred activities (e.g. "I like to ride my bike."). However, these notions about the self are not integrated into a global self-concept (Stone & Lemanek, 1990). In addition, young children may have difficulty labeling or verbally communicating their subjective emotional state (LaGreca, 1990). Young children also have difficulty relating events in a temporal order, especially if the events happened in the (relatively) distant past.

At around age 8 years, children acquire a more global sense of the self. After this age, children are better able to report on their thoughts and feelings and to provide more accurate information on diverse experiences and situations. During adolescence, the capacity for self-reflection increases further. Adolescents have the capacity to describe themselves in abstract psychological and interpersonal terms rather than the concrete, physical terms used by younger children. In addition, adolescents begin to evaluate their own thoughts and behaviors critically and to analyze others' reactions to their behavior (Stone & Lemanek, 1990). Thus, as self-awareness increases, older children and younger adolescents are able to respond to interview questions with increasing sophistication. However, the increased use of social comparisons and greater psychological awareness that come as children age may contribute to a tendency to respond to interview questions in a socially desirable manner (Stone & Lemanek, 1990).

Other factors can influence the way in which children and adolescents respond during interview situations. One of the most important to consider is the inherent power imbalance in the relationship between a child and an adult interviewer (Cohn, 1994). Adults generally have greater social power than children do; children are, for the most part, socialized to respond to adults in ways they think adults want to hear. Because of the power imbalance, whether real or merely perceived, children may unintentionally fabricate answers to questions to please an adult interviewer (Cohn, 1994; Krahenbuhl & Blades, 2006).

Establishing rapport and a sense of trust is critical to the successful interview. With children, engaging the child in a play activity or a discussion about a favorite book or movie before the interview can help to establish rapport (see Box 34.2). With adolescents, honest communication about the reasons for the interview and the confidential nature of the interview can help to instill

<table>
<tr><td>

BOX 34.2   ## PRACTICE NOTES

Instead of immediately focusing on what a child or adolescent is having a hard time doing, start by asked the child what he or she likes and what he or she is good at doing. This lets the child know that you are equally interested in the child's abilities as well as his or her challenges and creates a safe and positive therapeutic interaction. When talking about the challenges, instead of asking children to report what they have a hard time doing, ask children what makes it difficult for them to perform to the best of their ability. This allows the child to focus on the environment in addition to his or her abilities. *JK*

</td></tr>
</table>

trust. Age-appropriate communication is another key to a successful interview. With young children, the use of simple vocabulary, short sentences, and concrete, direct questions (e.g., "What do you do during school?") can be effective. Adolescents can usually answer more complex, open-ended questions (e.g., "Tell me about how school has been going for you.").

Finally, the process of gathering information concerning children's occupations should involve other people in the child's environment, including parents and teachers (LaGreca, 1990). Because children are under the social control of others, their behavior in one environment might not be the same as their behavior in another environment. Therefore, it is important to gather information from the multiple contexts within which the child functions (see Box 34.3). Moreover, because children are referred for intervention by others, usually a parent, it is important to understand and respect the perspective of the people who may be distressed by the child's behavior (LaGreca, 1990).

<table>
<tr><td>

BOX 34.3   ## PRACTICE NOTES

When I was a school-based occupational therapist, interviewing parents and teachers was an essential part of my job. However, fitting an interview into a busy IEP meeting was difficult. By breaking questions down into smaller chunks that could be answered during a quick phone call, through e-mail, or in a short discussion in the hallway, classroom, or front office, I could gather enough information to complete an assessment. *JK*

</td></tr>
</table>

WHY INTERVIEW

Understanding the Client's Story

The single most important reason to interview the client is so that you can better understand how the client sees things. As was previously discussed, an interview is an opportunity for the client to tell you his or her story. Mattingly (1991) has noted, "a disability is something that interrupts and irreversibly changes a person's life story"; "therapy can be seen as a short story within the patient's longer life story" (p. 1000). During the course of the interview, you are trying to uncover the "plot" of the client's story. Before the interview, you might have some general information about the client. During the interview, you want to fill in the particulars of the story. So your main questions should be as follows:

♦ What happened to you?
♦ How did you get to occupational therapy?
♦ What was a typical day like for you before you came here (hospital, clinic, etc.)?
♦ What was and is important to you?
♦ Where do you hope to go after you leave here?

Asking and valuing the answers to these questions are what it means to be "client-centered" (Law, 1998). Client-centered occupational therapy is "an approach to service which embraces a philosophy of respect for, and partnership with, people receiving services" (Law, Baptiste, & Mills, 1995, p. 253). Client-centered occupational therapy interventions are individualized and developed in collaboration with the client. An interview can be an effective fist step in individualizing and prioritizing service with a particular client.

Building the Therapeutic Alliance

Because an interview is an interaction between two people, a relationship begins to develop during the course of the interview. During the interview, you want to establish a relationship with the client that will help you together to set and attain the goals of intervention. The manner in which you conduct the interview will either foster or inhibit the development of that relationship (Haidet & Paterniti, 2003). As you talk with a client, your ability to communicate a sense of concern and respect for the individual and the information being shared and your ability to be real and genuine in the interaction will go a long way toward establishing this relationship. The client has come to you for help. For the client to feel that you are someone who can be of help, a sense of safety, trust, and collaboration must develop between the two of you (Okun, 1997). An interview can enhance a sense of collaboration between you and the client, because it gives you an opportunity to communicate that you care about what is important to the client. To the extent to which you have a collaborative relationship with the client, you will be much more likely to achieve intervention goals (Neistadt, 1995; Tickle-Degnen, 1995).

Gathering Information and Developing the Occupational Profile

Occupational therapy interviews are used to gather information about the client's functioning in occupations. Most interviews consider the client's current or recent functioning; some also take a historical perspective and seek to understand the client's functioning over time. Although the specific questions vary across different interviews, in general, interviews solicit information about the client's performance patterns, such as daily use of time, past and current role involvement (e.g., worker, student, homemaker, parent), play and leisure participation, and the client's values, goals, and sense of competence relative to occupations. Some interviews also ask questions about the client's current environment (human and nonhuman), to evaluate whether the environment supports or constrains the person's functioning. This information forms the occupational profile (AOTA, 2002).

It is important to gather information about the client's functioning in the past, because past functioning often is one of the best predictors of future functioning (Figure 34.1). The impairments, limitations, and restrictions associated with a particular health condition may predict a client's future to some extent (World Health Organization, 2001). But the successes a person has had in the past, particularly the recent past, are often resources on which he or she can draw. A person's goals and sense of competence are indicators of the person's desire and motivation to return to his or her prior life.

Observing Behavior

During the course of an interview, you have an opportunity to observe the client's behavior. The client's ability to participate in an interview can reveal much about his or her current functioning. You will be able to make observations about the client's energy level, stamina, affect, comprehension, memory, concentration, thought organization, physical appearance, and interpersonal behavior.

- Is the client able to actively engage with you through a 45-minute interview without fatiguing?
- Does the client appear depressed or elated?
- Does the client's memory seem intact? For example, is the client able to remember the dates of his or her last few jobs and relate them to you in chronological order?
- Does the person comprehend the questions being asked?
- Is the client able to convey his or her history in a manner that you can understand and follow?
- Is the client's thinking organized and goal-directed, or is the thinking tangential (i.e., "off track")?
- Is the client appropriately dressed and groomed for the situation, or does the client appear unkempt?
- Is the client friendly and forthcoming with information, or does the client seem angry, hostile, or resistant to being interviewed?

When you make these kinds of behavioral observations, an interview can serve as a kind of screening procedure and give you an indication of whether it might be appropriate to administer any additional assessment of performance skills. In addition, the extent to which the client engages with you during an interview may be some

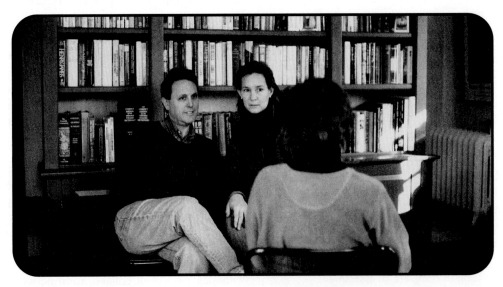

FIGURE 34.1   An occupational therapist interviewing parents about their 4-year-old child.

indication of the extent to which he or she will engage in interventions. Of course, if the client appears to be defensive or resistant during the interview, it is important to ask yourself whether there is something that you are doing to make the client feel defensive.

Identifying Client Strengths and Potential Problem Areas

As the interview progresses and you begin to achieve a deeper understanding of the person's story and observe his or her behavior, you should begin to formulate an initial sense of the client's strengths or assets as well as problems that might be addressed by occupational therapy interventions. All clients, regardless of disability, bring certain strengths (current competencies, past experiences, and environmental supports and resources) to their work with you. It is important to identify these early on, as the client will be able to draw on these assets over the course of the intervention.

A set of problems will also begin to take shape from the things the client tells you and the things you observe. It is important to remember, however, that this initial idea about the problems is tentative and subject to revision as you and the client begin to work together. Moreover, your perspective of the problems the client faces might not be the same as the client's perspective. You must share your initial impression with the client to confirm the extent to which you are seeing things in the same way. This involves both restating what you have perceived as the client's major concerns and sharing your impressions and observations during the interview regarding the client's strengths and potential problems. By engaging in mutual problem setting, you lay the groundwork for a client-centered, collaborative relationship. Toward the end of an interview, you might say to the client, "Well, from what you've told me, it sound like you are concerned about . . . , and it seems to me that you are also having some difficulty with. . . ." The goal is for the two of you to arrive at an agreement about the problems the client faces.

Clarifying Your Role in the Setting

You can also use the end of an interview to elaborate on and clarify your role in the setting and the work you and the client may do together. Do not be surprised if the client does not know what occupational therapists do. At this point, you can explain what services occupational therapy offers, what options might be available to the client, whether you and another provider (e.g., a physical therapist, nurse or social worker) might be working with the client together, or whether you might refer the client to another provider for a service that occupational therapy does not offer. It is at this point that you can make initial recommendations about the possible interventions.

Establishing Priorities for Intervention

Once you and the client agree on the work to be done, you have explained your role and the services that occupational therapy can offer, and you have made some initial recommendations for intervention, then you and the client can work collaboratively to establish intervention priorities. Being client-centered means that the client's priorities should be your priorities. However, it is important to recognize other factors that might influence the recommendations you make. For example, you might be influenced by the services that are most easily provided in your setting, your own interests and competencies, and funding and reimbursement, among other things. The client's goals and priorities are central in determining the course of intervention. Engaging the client in goal setting and prioritizing is a good way to finish up an interview.

HOW TO INTERVIEW

It might seem that interviewing should come naturally; after all, you talk to people every day. But much of our day-to-day communication with other people is quite superficial. When you conduct an interview with a client, you are engaging in a dialogue with the express purpose of trying to understand that other person so that you can be helpful (Coulehan et al., 2001; Okun, 1997). Thus, "therapeutic communication" differs from day-to-day conversation in fundamental ways. Developing the communication skills that are needed to become an effective interviewer takes time and experience. The skills of effective interviewing and ways to structure a therapeutic interview are discussed below.

The Skills of Effective Interviewing

Preparing

Preparing for the interview is an important first step. Before conducting an interview, you should prepare yourself, the client, and the environment. In preparing yourself, you should have some notion of the questions you want to ask the client. Several different occupational therapy interview procedures have been published in the past several years, and these will be discussed later in this section. It is preferable to use one of the existing interviews rather than developing your own, as these procedures have generally been subjected to examinations of reliability and validity. If you are a novice interviewer, you will need to practice before interviewing your first client. Observing experienced interviewers, noting how they structure the interview, ask questions, and respond to information the client shares, is a good way to begin to develop a sense of how an interview flows. You might also practice administering the interview to a colleague or supervisor and have that person give you feedback. Videotaping and critiquing your practice interviews can also help you to hone your interviewing skills.

Before conducting an interview with a client, you should read whatever preliminary information might be available on the client. This information can give you some initial ideas about areas on which you might focus during the interview. Moreover, information about the client's diagnosis or presenting problem can help you to anticipate how actively the client can participate in the interview, whether the client might tolerate only a short interview, or whether interviewing the client might not be appropriate at this time. In settings such as hospitals, nursing homes, or day programs, nursing staff or others who are in close contact with the client might have useful information about how the client was doing that day.

In addition to preparing yourself, you should prepare the client for the interview. When meeting a new client for the first time, make sure to introduce yourself and briefly tell the client about your role in the setting. Ask permission to do the interview, telling the client briefly about the content and purpose of the interview. Depending on the setting and time constraints, you might conduct the interview "on the spot," or you might schedule an appointment for a later time. Scheduling an appointment (even if just for later that same day) can give your client a degree of control; the client then has some choice about when he or she will see you. Some times of the day are better than others for many people. For example, many people with depression feel worse in the morning and experience improvements in their mood and energy level as the day progresses. By allowing the client to have some degree of control in a situation in which he or she might feel out of control, you help to set the tone for a collaborative relationship. Finally, you need to pay some attention to the environment in which you will conduct the interview. Obviously, a private space is the most desirable. Some of the questions you will be asking are highly personal, and a private space will make you both feel more comfortable. You should not make assumptions about what might and might not be a personal or difficult question for the client. A client might have an emotional response to a particular question that you had not anticipated. Chairs should be an appropriate distance apart (three or four feet). The room should be at a temperature that is comfortable for both of you and should be well lighted. Have tissues and water available. If it is not possible to have a private space, then creating some sense of privacy in a more open space by arranging the chairs in a corner of the room would be suitable. There might be times when you need to conduct an interview in a setting where privacy is very limited; for example, on a medical inpatient unit, you might need to interview a client in a semiprivate room who cannot leave the bed. In a situation such as this, you will want to make sure that the client feels comfortable answering your questions when others might be able to hear your conversation.

Questioning

Interviewing involves the asking of questions. The way you pose questions will influence the quality and amount of information you obtain and thus the level of understanding of the client's story you can achieve. How you ask questions will also influence how you are perceived by the client and will influence the development of your relationship with the client (Coulehan et al., 2001). In general, open-ended questions encourage the client to tell his or her story and are more likely to yield meaningful information from a client than are closed questions that require only a yes or no answer or a very brief response. For example, the question "Did you like your job?" can be answered "yes" or "no." "Tell me what you liked about your job" is a question that will likely result in a more detailed response. In addition, the use of probes and follow-up questions (e.g., "Tell me more about that") encourages the client to relate his or her story and helps to establish empathy (Coulehan et al., 2001). During the course of an interview, it is likely that you will ask two types of questions: those that are factual or descriptive in nature (e.g., "What do you do for work?"), and those that are intended to elicit more narrative data. Narrative questions yield data on events in the client's life and the client's perceptions and motives concerning events (e.g., "Tell me about a time when work was going very well for you"). Kielhofner and Mallinson (1995) suggest that effective interviewing involves a weaving of these two ways of questioning. There might be certain clients for whom a more structured, factual approach to questioning is appropriate. For example, a client whose thinking is disorganized might have difficulty answering more open-ended or narrative questions in a coherent manner but can respond to a more structured question such as "Where do you live?" It will usually be apparent when you need to use a more structured approach to the interview.

During the interview, you want to be conscious of whether the questions you are asking are making the client anxious or uncomfortable. Your intention is to put the client at ease. To do this, it is best if your questions are open, clear, singular (i.e., you ask only one question at a time), and nonjudgmental and you encourage the client to tell his or her story. You want to avoid putting the client on the defensive. Sometimes, questions that begin with "why" (e.g., "Why did you do that?") can have the unintended effect of making clients feel that they owe you an explanation about their feelings or behavior (Okun, 1997). Particularly during the initial interview, it is more useful to assume a neutral, nonjudgmental stance.

Responding

An interview needs to be more than a series of questions on your part, interspersed with answers from the client. You will need to respond to the information that the client is sharing with you. There are many ways in which you might respond. Often, because of a desire to help, our impulse is to respond with advice or suggestions. However, particularly during an initial interview, you want to resist this impulse, at least until you have come to the end of the interview (Coulehan et al., 2001). Before that, it is doubtful that you will have sufficient information on which to base advice. So even though you want to resist giving advice until you have achieved some understanding of the client's story, you still need to respond. During the course of the interview, your responses should primarily be attempts to paraphrase what the client has just said. Paraphrasing is more than just repeating what the client has said. It involves trying to capture the essence of what the client has said and restating it in your own words to communicate your desire to understand (Coulehan et al., 2001). Paraphrasing helps you to communicate to the client that you have listened to, heard, understood, and valued the information being shared with you. Paraphrasing also allows you to confirm that you have, in fact, clearly understood the client.

There are two general types of responses that you can use during an interview: content responses and affective responses. Content responses are used when you want to clarify the facts or communicate that you have understood what the client means. A content response might begin "So, you're saying that. . . ." Content responses serve the purpose of clarifying information and meaning. Affective responses are used when you want to reflect the underlying affect or feeling tone that the client is communicating. An affective response might begin "It seems like you're feeling . . ." or "I might have felt very . . . in that situation." An affective response should be phrased somewhat tentatively until you have confirmed that the client feels this way. Affective responses serve the purpose of communicating that you are trying to understand and are concerned about how the client feels.

Attending and Observing

Attending involves the use of both nonverbal and verbal behaviors that help to communicate your interest in the client and can facilitate the development of therapeutic rapport. Nonverbal behaviors include positions and movements of the face and body, as well as qualities of the voice, such as tone, intensity, and speed (Sommers-Flanagan & Sommers-Flanagan, 2003; Tickle-Degnen, 1995). Having your chair and the client's chair either facing each other or slightly angled, about three feet apart, allows you to see the client fully and the client to see you. You can communicate your interest in the client by making frequent eye contact. Other nonverbal behaviors that communicate interest include head-nodding, smiling, and leaning forward. Verbal behaviors, such as saying, "uh-huh," "humm," "yes," or "go on," let the client know that you are listening and encourage the client to continue with his or her story. Tickle-Degnen (1995) notes that tone of voice is

an important attribute to attend to. A cheerful tone of voice is not always the most appropriate to use. Rather, a tone of voice that is genuine and conveys concern about the client may be more effective. Effective interviewers often accommodate their bodies, movements, and tone of voice to be "in sync" with the client's (Bradburn, 1992; Tickle-Degnen, 1995).

Attending also involves observing how the client seems to be feeling as the interview progresses. Does the client seem to be fatiguing? Does the interview content seem to be emotionally difficult for the client? If you sense that the client is finding the interview difficult, you should ask to verify this. For example, questions such as "How are you doing?" and "Are you getting tired?" communicate that you are concerned about the client. A common side effect of psychiatric medications is dry mouth; offering a glass of water is another way of showing that you are attending. Effective observation involves noting the client's behavior as the interview progresses.

Effective Listening

Finally, although it seems obvious to say so, throughout the interview, you need to listen to the client. Listening effectively allows you to respond effectively. Paying close attention to both the content and the underlying feeling or affect takes energy (Sommers-Flanagan & Sommers-Flanagan, 2003). Listening is more difficult than it sounds, because there are many distractions to effective listening. There can be external distractions, such as activity in the environment, or internal distractions, such as your thoughts about a meeting you just came from or your next client. Even when your attention is focused on the client, there can be distractions. Denton (1987) has identified certain blocks to effective listening to the client; she calls these *thinking about the person, thinking for the person,* and *thinking ahead of the person.*

Thinking about the person involves making judgments about the client's lifestyle, morals, and motives; such judgments can create distance between you and the client and interfere with your being able to understand the client's perspective. When you think for the person, you prematurely think about solutions to the client's problems. Because one aim of the interview is to facilitate a collaborative relationship with the client, prematurely offering solutions diminishes the client's role in the relationship and can reinforce the client's sense of helplessness. Thinking ahead of the person involves rushing the client through his or her story just to get the facts. This can happen when you feel that you already know the story, when the client is relating too much or seemingly irrelevant details, or when you feel pressed for time (Denton, 1987; Haidet & Paterniti, 2003). The reality is that you never already know the story; each person's story is unique. However, if the client is giving you more detail than you need at the moment and you begin to run out of time, you can respectfully redirect the client by saying, "I can hear that this topic is very important to you. Perhaps we should set another time to really talk about this. Right now, I need to ask you some questions about something else."

Finally, particularly if you are a novice interviewer, you can be distracted from listening because you are thinking about what you should say next. If you are thinking about what you should say next, then you are not listening to the client. One way to improve your listening skills is to learn to use silence effectively. Most of us feel uncomfortable with silence and feel a need to fill a silent space as soon as it occurs. However, if you can feel comfortable taking a brief silent pause to think about what the client has just said and about what you might say next, then you will not need to prepare your next question while the client is talking. You can even say to the client, "I'm just taking a moment to think about what you've said." Rarely will you need more than 10 seconds to do this.

Structuring the Interview

Regardless of the type of interview you use, there are three phases to an interview: the opening, the body of the interview, and closure (Sommers-Flanagan & Sommers-Flanagan, 2003).

Opening

At the opening of the interview, you let the client know the purpose of the interview. Even though you probably did so when you made the appointment for the interview, you might want to reintroduce yourself, to say again that you are an occupational therapist, and to briefly describe your role in the setting. You should then explain the purpose of the interview and the types of questions that you will be asking.

Body

The body is the exploration and development phase of the interview, the time when you and the client are actively constructing the client's story. Although specific interview procedures often provide a recommended sequence of questions, it is a good idea to enter into this phase of the interview with relatively general and neutral questions that allow you to begin to sketch the background of the story. Because you are interested in a client's occupations, you might begin by asking how the client spends his or her time on a typical day. Such a broad question tends to be nonthreatening but allows you to begin to develop a picture of the client's roles. Subsequent questions serve to fill in the details. Some clients are very forthcoming and are able to relate their stories easily; others will need much support and structure. It is during this phase that you will call on your skills in listening, attending, responding, and questioning.

Closure

Toward the end of the interview, you will need to begin to put closure on the session. It is important not to end the interview abruptly. Make sure that you allow sufficient time to summarize information, identify important themes in the client's story, and address how you and the client will work together. This will often be the time when you and the client mutually begin to set goals for intervention. As the interview comes to an end, you should let the client know what the next steps will be and when you will see the client again. You might set a time for your next appointment. You should also thank the client for sharing his or her story with you.

OCCUPATIONAL THERAPY INTERVIEWS

Over the past two decades, a variety of interviews have been developed for use with both children and adults. The interviews that are briefly reviewed next all provide methods of collecting information directly from the intended service recipient or client. There are also interviews that allow you to collect data from other informants, often caregivers or parents. For example, the Play History (Behnke & Fetkovich, 1984) collects information from a parent on a child's participation in play. Interviews that collect data from informants other than the intended service recipient are not described here but are reviewed elsewhere throughout the book. All of the interviews reviewed here can assist you in developing an occupational profile of the client and have demonstrated at least preliminary evidence of reliability and validity.

Interviews for Use with Children and Adolescents

The School Setting Interview

The School Setting Interview (SSI) (Hemmingsson, Egilson, Hoffman & Kielhofner, 2005) is a collaborative interview that allows children and adolescents with disabilities (including physical, developmental, and emotional/behavioral disabilities) to describe the impact of the environment on their functioning in multiple school settings (e.g., classroom, playground, gymnasium, corridors) and to identify any needs for accommodations. Appropriate for students from about age 9 years through high school, the SSI requires about 40 minutes to administer. The SSI was originally developed in Sweden and has been translated into English. Studies indicate that the SSI has good test-retest reliability (Hemmingsson & Borrell, 1996), demonstrates construct validity (Hemmingsson, Kottorp, & Bernspång, 2004), effectively measures the unmet needs for school environment accommodations of students with disabilities (Borg & Nålsén, 2003), and can be used to examine student-environment fit in school settings (Hemmingsson & Borrell, 1996, 2000).

Adolescent Role Assessment

The Adolescent Role Assessment (ARA) (Black, 1976) is an occupational therapy interview that is specifically targeted for adolescents. The ARA is a semistructured interview procedure that gathers information on the adolescent's occupational role involvement over time and across domains. The 21 questions of the ARA cover six areas: childhood play, socialization within the family, school functioning, socialization with peers, occupational choice, and anticipated adult work. Early research found that the ARA had acceptable test-retest reliability, and scores on the ARA were found to discriminate between psychiatrically hospitalized adolescents and nonhospitalized adolescents (Black, 1982). A recent study that sought to explore the ARA's usefulness as a measure of adolescent career adaptability (Huebner, Emery, & Shordike, 2002) found that the internal consistency of the ARA was low. However, factors that were identified through factor analysis (developing aspirations, self-efficacy, interpersonal competencies, and autonomy) were consistent with career adaptability literature, and these factors were found to differentiate between low- and high-scoring adolescents. Given the paucity of interview procedures specifically targeted for adolescents, further development and refinement of the ARA and similar interviews should be a priority.

Interviews for Use with Adolescents and Adults

The Occupational Circumstances Assessment Interview and Rating Scale

The newest version of the Occupational Circumstances Assessment Interview and Rating Scale (OCAIRS) (Forsyth, Deshpande et al., 2005), a revision of the original OCAIRS developed by Kaplan and Kielhofner (1989), provides therapists with a method for gathering data on a client's occupational adaptation. Three semistructured interview formats targeted to the needs of different client groups (physical disability, mental health, and forensic mental health) are administered and clients are then rated on 12 items using a four-point rating scale. The items cover the client's personal causation, values and goals, interests, roles, habits, skills, physical and social environments, and readiness for change. The OCAIRS can be used with adolescent and adult clients with a variety of disabilities and requires about an hour to administer and rate.

Studies have shown the revised OCAIRS to have acceptable internal consistency and excellent interrater reliability (Haglund, Thorell & Walinder, 1998a; Lai, Haglund, & Kielhofner, 1999). OCAIRS scores also have been shown to discriminate between clients who need occupational therapy intervention and those who do not and between those with different severities of psychiatric disorder (Haglund et al., 1998a, 1998b).

The Occupational Performance History Interview— Second Version

The Occupational Performance History Interview— Second Version (OPHI-II) (Kielhofner, Mallinson, et al., 2004) is a historical interview that gathers information about a client's occupational adaptation over time and can be used with adolescents and adults in a variety of settings. The OPHI-II consists of three parts: (1) a semistructured interview concerning a client's occupational life history; (2) three rating scales that quantify a client's occupational identity, occupational competence, and the impact of environment; and (3) a life history narrative with a narrative slope. The flexible interview format is designed to gather information in five thematic areas: (1) activity/occupational choices, (2) critical life events, (3) daily routines, (4) occupational roles, and (5) the environment. The three ratings scales provide a measure of (1) a client's interests, values, and confidence; (2) a client's ability to sustain satisfying occupational participation; and (3) the impact of the environment on a client's occupational life. The life history narrative and slope provide both a qualitative and visual description of the client's history. The OPHI-II can be administered in about an hour.

Validity of the original OPHI was examined in studies of individuals with physical and psychiatric disabilities (Henry, 1994; Lynch & Bridle, 1993; Mauras-Nelson & Oakley, 1996). An international study of the OPHI-II (using six different language versions) provided evidence of the internal consistency and construct validity of the three rating scales of the OPHI-II (Kielhofner, Mallinson, Forsyth, & Lai, 2001). Therapists can also use the client's ratings to obtain instantaneous interval client measures using a paper-and-pencil keyform as a way to document client function, monitor progress, and track change for outcome evaluation (Kielhofner, Dobria, Forsyth, & Basu, 2005).

The OPHI-II has been used in many settings with many types of clients, including clients transitioning to powered mobility (Buning, Angelo, & Schmeler, 2001), people with chronic fatigue syndrome (Gray & Fossey, 2003), clients in forensic psychiatric placements (Farnworth, Nikitin, & Fossey, 2004), homeless adolescent mothers (Levin & Helfrich, 2004), and people with HIV/AIDS (Braveman & Helfrich, 2001; Kielhofner, Braveman, et al., 2004). Therapists and clients report that the OPHI-II interview is a good opportunity to build rapport and is helpful when setting goals and planning the intervention, and clients often use the narrative slope as a motivational tool (Apte, Kielhofner, Paul-Ward, & Braveman, 2005).

The Worker Role Interview

The Worker Role Interview (WRI) is a semistructured interview that gathers data on psychosocial and environmental factors related to work and is appropriate to use with any individual whose disability has had an impact on their participation in work (Braveman et al., 2005). The WRI includes a set of recommended questions (including an interview format for clients with chronic disabilities, an interview format for those with recent injuries or disabilities, and an interview that combines WRI and OCAIRS questions) that are used to gather information in order to rate clients on 16-items using a four-point rating scale. The items form six subscales that reflect the worker's sense of personal causation, values, interests, roles, and habits related to work, as well as the influence of the environment. Studies indicate that therapists use the WRI in a consistent manner (good interrater reliability) and items represent the construct of ability to return to work (construct validity) (Biernacki, 1993; Forsyth et al., 2006; Velozo et al., 1999). Research conducted on WRI translations in other languages demonstrates the instrument's validity across other cultures (Fenger & Kramer, 2007; Haglund, Karlsson, Kielhofner, & Shei Lai, 1997), and one study using the Swedish translation found that certain items on the WRI predicted success for return to work (Ekbladh, Haglund, & Thorell, 2004).

The Work Environment Impact Scale

The Work Environment Impact Scale (WEIS) (Corner, Kielhofner, & Olson, 1998) is a semistructured interview and rating scale designed to examine how individuals with disabilities experience the work environment. The WEIS is intended for use with individuals who are currently working or are actively anticipating returning to a specific job or type of work. The WEIS asks questions regarding work environment factors such as space, social supports, temporal demands, objects used, and job functions, and the scale items reflect the extent to which environmental factors affect performance, satisfaction, and physical, social, and emotional well-being of the worker. Studies of the WEIS provide evidence of its construct validity and internal consistency (Corner, Kielhofner, & Lin, 1997; Kielhofner, et al., 1999).

The Canadian Occupational Performance Measure

The Canadian Occupational Performance Measure (COPM) (Law et al., 1998) is a client-centered semi-structured interview procedure designed to measure a client's perceptions of his occupational performance over time. During an initial evaluation, the therapist interviews the client about his or her functioning in the areas of self-care, productivity, and leisure. The client is asked to identify any activities that are difficult to do in each area and to indicate how important it is to be able to do those activities. Finally, the client is asked to identify his or her five most important problems and to rate his or her performance and level of satisfaction in these activities. The client rates the importance of the activity to the client, the quality of the client's performance, and the client's level of satisfaction using similar 10-point scales. The specific focus of the COPM on client-identified problems is intended to facilitate collaborative goal setting between the therapist and client. The COPM can also be used for reevaluation and to detect changes in the client's perceptions over time; thus, it has utility as an outcome measure (Law et al., 1998).

Across multiple studies, the COPM has been shown to have good test-retest reliability (Carswell et al., 2004; Law et al., 1998). Other studies have provided evidence of concurrent and construct validity of the COPM (Carpenter, Baker & Tyldesley, 2001; McColl, Paterson, Davies, Doubt, & Law, 2000). Studies that use the COPM as an outcome measure indicate that the COPM is sensitive to change following rehabilitation interventions (Corr & Wilmer, 2003; Lewis & Jones, 2001) while also being clinically useful and meaningful (Carswell et al., 2004).

ADJUNCTS TO INTERVIEWS: PAPER-AND-PENCIL SELF-REPORT MEASURES

In addition to interviewing, paper-and-pencil self-report measures can be a useful method of obtaining information from the client. Self-report measures include surveys, forms, and checklists that the client completes. Sometimes, a client can complete the form or checklist on his or her own, making this a convenient way to obtain information. More often, however, you should be present when the client is completing the measure, to ensure that the client comprehends what is being asked and is responding appropriately. Just as with interviews, self-report measures might not be appropriate for all clients.

In practice, self-report measures should not be used to substitute for a face-to-face interview with the client. They can be a helpful adjunct, however, because they tend to gather detailed information on a specific topic, such as time use or interest patterns. They are most useful when used in conjunction with an interview. Once a client has completed a self-report measure, the client and therapist should review the form together. Self-report measures help to focus the discussion around a particular topic or issue.

Self-Report Measures for Children and Adolescents

The Pediatric Interest Profiles

The Pediatric Interest Profiles (PIPs) (Henry, 2000) are paper-and-pencil surveys of play and leisure interests that are designed to be used with children and adolescents.

The three versions of the PIPs include the Kid Play Profile (KPP), for children ages 6 to 9 years; the Preteen Play Profile (PPP), for children 9 to 12 years; and the Adolescent Leisure Interest Profile (ALIP), for adolescents ages 12 to 21 years. Each version asked the youth to report his or her interest and/or participation in a variety of age-appropriate leisure activities and to indicate his or her feelings of enjoyment and competence in the activities. The PIPs also asked whether the youth does the activities alone or with others. The Kid and Preteen versions of the PIPs use pictorial representations of play activities. Total scores for the three versions of the PIPs have acceptable test-retest reliability (Henry, 2000). In addition, scores on the ALIP have been found to discriminate between adolescents with and without disabilities (Henry, 1998).

The Children's Assessment of Participation and Enjoyment and the Preferences for Activities of Children

The Children's Assessment of Participation and Enjoyment (CAPE) (King, et al., 2004) is a two-part self-report measure that gathers information on children's participation in everyday activities outside of mandated school activities. The CAPE is intended for children ages 6 years and up. In Phase 1, the child (or child and parent) indicates how often he or she has done a variety of activities in the past four months. In Phase 2, a practitioner interviews the child about the activities in which the child participates, regarding enjoyment in the activities and where and with whom activities are done. As in the PIPs, activity items are represented pictorially. The Preferences for Activities of Children (PAC) (King et al., 2004) examines a child's preferences for activities. The child sorts 50 activity cards, indicating whether she would "really like to," "sort of like to," or "not like to" do each activity. The PAC and the CAPE can be used together or separately. The CAPE/PAC manual reports evidence of the test-retest reliability, internal consistency, and correlations among the CAPE participation intensity scores and among the PAC preference scores (King et al., 2004). In one study, the CAPE was completed with 427 children between the ages of 6 and 14 years with physical disabilities to assess participation in nonschool activities (Law et al., 2004). Low to moderate, but significant, correlations were found between a child's sense of competence and the types of activities the child both prefers and enjoys, and boys and girls were found to have significantly different levels of participation intensity, preference, and enjoyment for certain activities (e.g., social activities versus active physical activities) (King et al., 2007).

Child Occupational Self-Assessment

Modeled after the Occupational Self-Assessment (see the section entitled "Self-Report Measures for Adults"), the 25 items of the Child Occupational Self-Assessment (COSA) (Keller, Kafkes, Basu, Federico, & Kielhofner,

2005) cover a range of everyday activities, including self-care, school tasks, social activities, and family-related activities, that children and youths rate through self-report. Young clients reflect on how competent they feel doing each activity and how important each activity is to them (Figure 34.2). Targeted to children ages 8–12 years, the COSA has also been used successfully with youth up to age 17 years (Keller, Kafkes, & Kielhofner, 2005; Keller & Kielhofner, 2005). Visual cues such as smile faces and stars support children and youths in completing the self-assessment, and a variety of modifications can be made without affecting the reliability of the rating scales (Keller & Kielhofner, 2005). Research has demonstrated that the COSA's two rating scales (competence and value) can be used in a consistent and valid manner and that the items represent a valid construct of children's and youth's occupational competence and value (importance) for occupations (Keller et al., 2005; Keller & Kielhofner, 2005).

Perceived Efficacy and Goal Setting System

The Perceived Efficacy and Goal Setting System (PEGS) (Missiuna, Pollock, & Law, 2004) provides young children

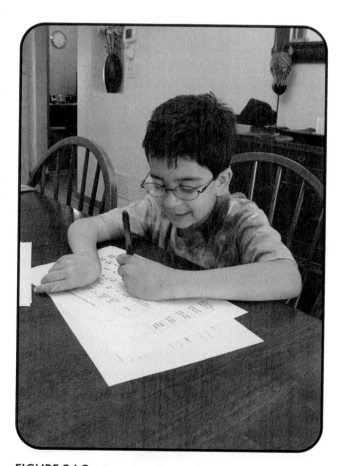

FIGURE 34.2   By completing a self-report assessment, a young client has an opportunity to talk about the things he likes doing and identify any trouble he is having doing activities that are important to him.

with an opportunity to report their efficacy for performing occupations that involve gross and fine motor tasks. Based on the All About Me scale (Missiuna, 1998), the PEGS includes pictures representing 24 activities, 12 in each subscale of fine motor and gross motor activities (such as "bicycle" and "doing up buttons"). Two related pictures represent each task, the images depicting a child performing an activity in a more competent or less competent manner. Children indicate which image is more like them and whether that image is a lot or a little like their performance. Then, to identify goals for therapy, the child then prioritizes tasks that he or she has reported having difficulty performing.

The PEGS items were found to discriminate between children with motor difficulties and those without and was moderately correlated with other standardized motor assessments (Missiuna, 1998), indicating that the instrument has discriminative and construct validity. Parent and teacher PEGS ratings were significantly correlated with the School Functional Assessment (Coster, Deeney, Haltiwanger, & Haley, 1998), but children's scores were not (Missiuna, Pollock, Law, Walter, & Cavey, 2006). Internal consistency was acceptable (Missiuna et al., 2006), subscale reliability was good for both subscales, and test-retest reliability over two weeks for one group of children was also good (Missiuna, 1998). While children using the PEGS rated themselves as more competent compared to parent or teacher ratings, parents, teachers, and children often agreed which tasks were more or less difficult for each child (Missiuna & Pollock, 2000; Missiuna et al., 2006). Children were also found to use the goal-setting processes effectively over time; after two weeks, 92% of children selected between two and four of the same goals (Missiuna et al., 2006).

Play Skills Self Report Questionnaire

The Play Skills Self Report Questionnaire (PSSRQ) (Sturgess, 2007) initially developed and reported as the Playform (Sturgess & Ziviani, 1995, 1996), is designed for children aged from 5 to 10 years and includes a Parent Version. Continued research on the Playform (Sturgess, 1997, 2003), some yet to be published, has resulted in modifications. The PSSRQ now consists of a booklet containing a question and a supporting line drawing on each page. The child rates himself or herself on 30 play skills that incorporate play alone, play in a dyad, play in a group, pretend play, rough and tumble play, games with rules, collecting things, and others. Children respond to questions such as "Are you good at making up ideas for pretend games?" and "Are you good at running and climbing and moving when you play?" using four different size stars that symbolize "not good," "OK," "good," and "very good." Parent and child versions have the same graphic to assist in ensuring that both are referring to a similar stimulus and enhance reliability of answers.

Content validity for the items and validity for the structure was established through a series of pilot studies with expert clinicians, parents, and children. Data have been analyzed from the responses of 176 typically developing children and their parents, which provide preliminary normative and comparative data (Sturgess, 2007). No total score is generated, as each item is unique, and no factor structure was found. The PSSRQ is designed to be used with one child over time; can be used to develop goals for intervention; and may also be valuable in health promotion, parent education, and other situations in which play is recognized as having a positive influence on healthy behaviors.

Self-Reports for Use with Parents of Children and Adolescents

Children Helping Out: Responsibilities, Expectations, and Supports (CHORES) (Dunn, 2004) is a parent self-report that was developed to assess children's participation in household tasks and changes in the amount of assistance needed to participate. The CHORES consists of 34 items that represent typical household tasks; 13 items form a self-care subscale (such as "picks up own bedroom" and "makes self a snack"), and 21 items form a family care subscale (such as "sets or clears the table," "cares for younger siblings," and "feeds pet(s)"). For each item, parents indicate whether the child participates in the household task and describes that participation using a two-part scale. If the parent reports that the child does not do the task, the parent indicates whether the child is not expected to do the task or the child cannot perform the task. If the parent reports that the child engages in the task, a five-point scale is used to report the level of assistance and supervision the child needs. At the end of the survey, parents rate how important their child's involvement in household tasks is to them and their level of satisfaction with their child's participation.

CHORES has been used with children and adolescents with and without disabilities who have a variety of cultural backgrounds (Dunn, 2004). The CHORES performance and assistance scores show adequate variance to identify differences in participation in household tasks, and parent's reports were found to remain stable from test to retest (Dunn, 2004). There is evidence for discriminate and face validity (Dunn, 2004).

Self-Report Measures for Adults

Interest Checklists

Interest checklists are among the most commonly used self-report measures. Interest checklists are used to tap a client's level of interest in a range of activities, most often leisure activities. Age-targeted measures of interest in activities are likely to yield more relevant data than a general measure, because leisure interests vary widely across the age span. Interest checklists are useful in identifying problems related to leisure and for identifying potential activities to use in treatment.

One of the oldest checklists is the NPI interest checklist (Matsutsuyu, 1969). The NPI interest checklist contains 80 activity items, grouped into five categories: activities of daily living, manual skills, cultural and educational activities, physical sports, and social and recreational activities. In completing the checklist, the client indicates strong, casual, or no interest in the activity (Rogers, 1988). The original NPI interest checklist was found to have acceptable test-retest reliability and to show evidence of construct and predictive validity (Barris et al., 1986; Ebb, Coster, & Duncombe, 1989; Henry, 1994; Weinstein, 1979). Kielhofner and Neville (1983) modified the NPI interest checklist to include questions concerning changes in activity preferences over time and the desire to participate in interests in the future.

Gregory (1983) described two self-report measures of activity involvement that are specifically designed for older adults. Total scores on both the Activity Index, which taps activity interest and participation, and the Meaningfulness of Activity Scale, which taps feelings of enjoyment, autonomy, and competence relative to activities, demonstrated good test-retest reliability with small pilot samples. Scores on both measures were also correlated positively with a measure of life satisfaction.

The Role Checklist

The Role Checklist (RC) (Oakley, Kielhofner, Barris, & Reichler, 1986) is a two-part, paper-and-pencil inventory of ten occupational roles, including worker, student, family member, homemaker, caregiver, volunteer, and hobbyist. The first part of the RC examines a client's past, present, and future intentions related to performance of each role. The second part examines the value assigned to each role by the client. The RC has been translated into 10 languages, and a Spanish translation has been determined to have content validity (Colon & Haertlein, 2002). Studies have indicated that the RC has good test-retest reliability (Barris, Oakley, & Kielhofer, 1988), is sensitive to role changes (Hallett, Zasler, Maurer, & Cash, 1994), and discriminates between adults without disabilities and those with psychiatric or physical disabilities (Dickerson, 1999). The RC has also been successfully used as an outcome assessment tool in studying the efficacy of occupational therapy interventions (Corr, Phillips & Walker, 2004; Corr & Wilmer, 2003; Schindler, Laguardia, Melchiorre, & Bailey, 2004).

Occupational Self-Assessment

The Occupational Self-Assessment (OSA) (Baron, Kielhofner, Iyenger, Goldhammer, & Wolenski, 2002) is a self-report measure designed to gather data on a client's perception of his or her occupational competence (21 items) and the impact of the environment on her functioning (eight items). The OSA also asks clients to indicate the importance of specific areas of functioning and to identify priorities for change, making it particularly useful to use in conjunction with an interview. The OSA can be used as an initial assessment and as a follow-up or outcome measure that captures client-reported change in functioning. A series of studies, involving 1,000 international clients, have been conducted on the OSA to refine the rating scales, increase the sensitivity of the instrument, and confirm the validity of the items on the assessment (Kielhofner & Forsyth, 2001; Kielhofner, Forsyth, Kramer & Iyenger, 2007). An analysis of OSA time 1 and time 2 assessment results confirmed that items on the competence scale, the competence rating scale, and the values rating scale remained stable over time, allowing the creation of the OSA paper keyforms (Kielhofner, Forsyth, Dobria, & Kramer, 2007). Similar to the OPHI-II keyforms, the OSA keyforms allow therapists to generate instantaneous client measures that can be used to document change.

CONCLUSION

In addition to providing information about a client's functioning in specific occupations, interviews are among the most useful strategies available to practitioners both to better understand the client's perspective of his or her situation and to enhance the working relationship with the client. Each of the interviews and self-report measures discussed in this chapter has unique characteristics. Practitioners should choose the combination of interview and other assessments that best fits the needs of their clients and setting.

REFERENCES

American Occupational Therapy Association. (2002). Occupational therapy practice framework: Domain and process. *American Journal of Occupational Therapy, 56,* 609–639.

Apte, A., Kielhofner, G., Paul-Ward, A., & Braveman, B. (2005). Therapists' and clients' perceptions of the Occupational Performance History Interview. *Occupational Therapy in Health Care, 19,* 173–192.

Barris, R., Kielhofner, G., Burch, R. M., Gelinas, I., Klement, M., & Schultz, B. (1986). Occupational function and dysfunction in three groups of adolescents. *Occupational Therapy Journal of Research, 6,* 301–317.

Barris, R., Oakley, F., & Kielhofner, G. (1988). The role checklist. In B. Hemphill (Ed.), *Mental health assessment in occupational therapy: An integrative approach to the evaluation process* (pp. 73–91). Thorofare, NJ: Slack.

Baron, K., Kielhofner, G., Iyenger, A., Goldhammer, V., & Wolenski, J. (2002). *The Occupational Self Assessment (Version 2.1).* Chicago: Model of Human Occupation Clearinghouse, Department of Occupational Therapy, College of Applied Health Sciences, University of Illinois at Chicago.

Behnke, C. J., & Fetkovich, M. M. (1984). Examining the reliability and validity of the Play History. *American Journal of Occupational Therapy, 38,* 94–100.

Biernacki, S. D. (1993). Reliability of the worker role interview. *American Journal of Occupational Therapy, 47,* 797–803.

Black, M. M. (1976). Adolescent role assessment. *American Journal of Occupational Therapy, 30,* 73–79.

Black, M. M. (1982). Adolescent role assessment. In B. Hemphill (Ed.), *The evaluative process in psychiatric occupational therapy* (pp. 49–53). Thorofare, NJ: Slack.

Bradburn, S. L. (1992). *Psychiatric occupational therapists' strategies for engaging patients in treatment during the initial interview.* Unpublished masters thesis, Tufts University, Medford, MA.

Braveman, B., & Helfrich, C. A. (2001). Occupational identity: Exploring the narratives of three men living with AIDS. *Journal of Occupational Science, 8,* 25–31.

Braveman, B., Robson, M., Velozo, C., Kielhofner, G., Fisher, G., Forsyth, K., et al. (2005). *The Worker Role Interview (version 10.0).* Chicago: Model of Human Occupation Clearinghouse, Department of Occupational Therapy, College of Applied Health Sciences, University of Illinois at Chicago.

Borg, G., & Nålsén, H. (2003). *Validitetsprövning av instrumentet Bedömning av anpassningar i skolmiljön (BAS). Mäter BAS behovet av anpassningar i skolmiljön?* [Validation of the School Setting Interview. Does the SSI measure the need for adjustments in the school setting?] Stockholm: Neurotec, Karolinska Institutet.

Buning, M. E., Angelo, J. A., & Schmeler, M. R. (2001). Occupational performance and the transition to powered mobility: A pilot study. *American Journal of Occupational Therapy, 55,* 339–344.

Carpenter, L., Baker, G. A., & Tyldesley, B. (2001). The use of the Canadian Occupational Performance Measure as an outcome of a pain management program. *Canadian Journal of Occupational Therapy, 68,* 16–22.

Carswell, A., McColl, M. A., Baptiste, S., Law, M., Polatajko, H., & Pollock., N. (2004). The Canadian Occupational Performance Measure: A research and clinical literature review. *Canadian Journal of Occupational Therapy, 71*(4), 210–222.

Clark, F. (1993). Eleanor Clarke Slagle Lectureship, 1993. Occupation embedded in a real life: Interweaving occupational science and occupational therapy. *American Journal of Occupational Therapy, 47,* 1067–1078.

Cohn, E. (1994). *Interviewing children.* Unpublished manuscript, Boston University.

Colon, H., & Haertlein, C. (2002). Spanish translation of the Role Checklist. *American Journal of Occupational Therapy, 56,* 586–589.

Corner, R. A., Kielhofner, G., & Lin, F.-L. (1997). Construct validity of a work environment impact scale. *Work: A Journal of Prevention, Assessment and Rehabilitation, 9,* 21–34.

Corner, R., Kielhofner, G., & Olson, L. (1998). *Work Environment Impact Scale (WEIS) (Version 2.0).* Chicago: Model of Human Occupation Clearinghouse, Department of Occupational Therapy, College of Applied Health Sciences, University of Illinois at Chicago.

Corr, S., Phillips, C. J., & Walker, M. (2004). Evaluation of a pilot service designed to provide support following a stroke: A randomized cross-over design study. *Clinical Rehabilitation, 18*(1), 69–75.

Corr, S., & Wilmer, S. (2003). Returning to work after a stroke: An important but neglected area. *British Journal of Occupational Therapy, 66,* 186–192.

Coster, W. J., Deeney, T., Haltiwanger, J., & Haley, S. M. (1998). *School Function Assessment.* San Antonio, TX: Psychological Corporation.

Coulehan, J. L., Platt, F. W., Egener, B., Frankel R., Lin, C. T., Lown, B., et al. (2001). "Let me see if I have this right . . .": Words that help build empathy. *Annals of Internal Medicine, 135,* 221–227.

Denton, P. L. (1987). *Psychiatric occupational therapy: A workbook of practical skills.* Boston: Little, Brown.

Dickerson, A. E. (1999). The Role Checklist. In B. J. Hemphill-Pearson (Ed.), *Assessments in occupational therapy in mental health: An integrative approach.* (pp. 175–191). Throrofare, NJ: Slack.

Dunn, L. (2004). Validation of the CHORES: A measure of school-ages children's participation in household tasks. *Scandinavian Journal of Occupational Therapy, 11,* 179–190.

Ebb, E. W., Coster, W., & Duncombe, L. (1989). Comparison of normal and psychosocially dysfunctional male adolescents. *Occupational Therapy in Mental Health, 9,* 53–74.

Ekbladh, E., Haglund, L., & Thorell, L. H. (2004). The Worker Role Interview: Preliminary data on the predictive validity of return to work of clients after an insurance medicine investigation. *Journal of Occupational Rehabilitation, 14,* 131–141.

Farnworth, L., Nikitin, L., & Fossey, E. (2004). Being in a secure forensic psychiatric unit: Every day is the same, killing time or making the most of it. *British Journal of Occupational Therapy, 67,* 430–438.

Fenger, K., & Kramer, J. M. (2004). Worker Role Interview: Testing the psychometric properties of the Icelandic version. *Scandinavian Journal of Occupational Therapy, 14,* 160–172.

Forsyth, K., Braveman, B., Kielhofner, G., Ekbladh, E., Haglund, L., Fenger, K., & Keller, J. (2006). Psychometric properties of the Worker Role Interview. *Work: A Journal of Prevention, Assessment, & Rehabilitation, 27,* 313–318.

Forsyth, K., Deshpande, S., Kielhofner, G., Chris Henriksson, C., Haglund, L., Olson, L., et al. (2005). *The Occupational Circumstances Assessment Interview and Rating Scale (version 4.0).* Chicago: Model of Human Occupation Clearinghouse, Department of Occupational Therapy, College of Applied Health Sciences, University of Illinois at Chicago.

Franits, L. E. (2005). Nothing about us without us: Searching for the narrative of disability. *American Journal of Occupational Therapy, 59,* 577–579.

Frank, G. (1996). Life histories in occupational therapy clinical practice. *American Journal of Occupational Therapy, 50,* 251–264.

Gray, M. L., & Fossey, E. M. (2003). Illness experience and occupations of people with chronic fatigue syndrome. *Australian Occupational Therapy Journal, 50*(3), 127–136.

Gregory, M. (1983). Occupational behavior and life satisfaction among retirees. *American Journal of Occupational Therapy, 37,* 548–552.

Haglund, L., Karlsson, G., Kielhofner, G., & Shei Lai, J. (1997). Validity of the Swedish version of the Worker Role Interview. *Scandinavian Journal of Occupational Therapy, 4,* 23–29.

Haglund, L., Thorell, L., & Walinder, J. (1998a). Assessment of occupational functioning for screening of patients to occupational therapy in general psychiatric care. *Occupational Therapy Journal of Research, 4,* 193–206.

Haglund, L., Thorell, L., & Walinder, J. (1998b). Occupational functioning in relation to psychiatric diagnoses: Schizophrenia and mood disorders. *Nordic Journal of Psychiatry, 52,* 223–229.

Haidet, P., & Paterniti, D. A. (2003). "Building" a history rather than "taking" one. *Archives of Internal Medicine, 163,* 1134–1140.

Hallett, J. D., Zasler, N. D., Maurer, P., & Cash, S. (1994). Role change after traumatic brain injury. *American Journal of Occupational Therapy, 48,* 241–246.

Helfrich, C., & Kielhofner, G. (1994). Volitional narratives and the meaning of therapy. *American Journal of Occupational Therapy, 48,* 319–326.

Hemmingsson, H., & Borell, L. (1996). The development of an assessment of adjustment needs in the school setting for use with physically disabled students. *Scandinavian Journal of Occupational Therapy, 3,* 156–162.

Hemmingsson, H., & Borell, L. (2000). Accommodation needs and student-environment fit in upper secondary school for students with severe physical disabilities. *Canadian Journal of Occupational Therapy, 67,* 162–173.

Hemmingsson, H., Egilson, S., Hoffman, O., & Kielhofner, G. (2005). *The School Setting Interview (version 3.0).* Chicago: Models of Human Occupation Clearinghouse, Department of Occupational Therapy, College of Applied Health Sciences, University of Illinois at Chicago, and Swedish Association of Occupational Therapists.

Hemmingsson, H., Kottorp, A., & Bernspång, B. (2004). Validity of the school setting interview: an assessment of the student-environment fit. *Scandinavian Journal of Occupational Therapy, 11,* 171–178.

Henry, A. D. (1994). *Predicting psychosocial functioning and symptomatic recovery of adolescents and young adults with a first psychotic episode: A six-month follow-up study.* Unpublished doctoral dissertation, Boston University.

Henry, A. D. (1998). Development of a measure of adolescent leisure interests. *American Journal of Occupational Therapy, 52,* 531–539.

Henry, A. D. (2000). *The Pediatric Interest Profiles: Surveys of play for children and adolescents.* San Antonio, TX: Therapy Skill Builders.

Huebner, R. A., Emery, L. J., & Shordike, A. (2002). The adolescent role assessment: psychometric properties and theoretical usefulness. *American Journal of Occupational Therapy, 56*(2), 202–209.

Kaplan, K., & Kielhofner, G. (1989). *Occupational case analysis interview and rating scale.* Thorofare, NJ: Slack.

Keller, J., Kafkes, A., Basu, S., Federico, J., & Kielhofner, G. (2005). *The Child Occupational Self Assessment (version 2.1).* Chicago: Models of Human Occupation Clearinghouse, Department of Occupational Therapy, College of Applied Health Sciences, University of Illinois at Chicago.

Keller, J., Kafkes, A., & Kielhofner, G. (2005). Psychometric Characteristics of the Child Occupational Self Assessment (COSA). I: An initial examination of psychometric properties. *Scandinavian Journal of Occupational Therapy, 12*(3), 118–127.

Keller, J., & Kielhofner, G. (2005). Psychometric Characteristics of the Child Occupational Self Assessment (COSA): II. Refining the psychometric properties. *Scandinavian Journal of Occupational Therapy, 12,* 147–158.

Kielhofner, G., Braveman, B., Finlayson, M., Paul-Ward, A., Goldbaum, L., & Goldstein, K. (2004). Outcomes of a vocational program for persons with AIDS. *American Journal of Occupational Therapy, 58,* 64–72.

Kielhofner, G., Dobria, L., Forsyth, K., & Basu, S. (2005). The construction of keyforms for obtaining instantaneous measures from the Occupational Performance History Interview Rating Scales. *OTJR: Occupation, Participation & Health, 25,* 23–32.

Kielhofner, G., & Forsyth, K. (2001). Measurement properties of a client self report for treatment planning and documenting therapy outcomes. *Scandinavian Journal of Occupational Therapy, 8,* 131–139.

Kielhofner, G., Forsyth, K., Kramer, J., & Iyenger, A. (2007). *Developing a client self-report measure: Assuring internal validity and sensitivity.* Manuscript submitted for publication.

Kielhofner, G., Forsyth, K., Dobria, L., & Kramer, J. (2007). *Developing a client self report measure: Determining stability, ability to detect change, and achieving instantaneous measurement.* Unpublished manuscript. University of Illinois at Chicaga. Chicago, Illinois.

Kielhofner, G., Lai, J. S., Olson, L., Haglund, L., Ekbadh, E., & Edlund, M. (1999). Psychometric properties of the work environment impact scale: A cross-cultural study. *Work: A Journal of Prevention, Assessment and Rehabilitation, 12,* 17–77.

Kielhofner, G., & Mallinson, T. (1995). Gathering narrative data through interviews: Empirical observations and suggested guidelines. *Scandinavian Journal of Occupational Therapy, 2,* 63–68.

Kielhofner, G., Mallinson, T., Crawford, C., Nowak, M., Rigby, M., Henry, A., et al. (2004). *The Occupational Performance History Interview—II (version 2.1).* Chicago: Model of Human Occupation Clearinghouse, Department of Occupational Therapy, College of Applied Health Sciences, University of Illinois at Chicago.

Kielhofner, G., Mallinson, T., Forsyth, K., & Lai, J.-S. (2001). Psychometric properties of the second version of the Occupational Performance History Interview. *American Journal of Occupational Therapy, 55,* 260–267.

Kielhofner, G., & Neville, A. (1983). *The modified interest checklist.* Unpublished manuscript, University of Illinois at Chicago.

King, G., Law, M., King, S., Hanna, S., Kertoy, M., Rosenbaum, P., et al: (2004). *Children's Assessment of Participation and Enjoyment (CAPE) and Preferences for Activities of Children (PAC).* San Antonio, TX: Harcourt Assessment.

King, G., Law, M., King, S., Hurley, P., Hanna, S., Kertoy, M., et al: (2007). Measuring Children's Participation in Recreation and Leisure Activities: Construct Validation of the CAPE and PAC. *Child: Care, Health, and Development, 33,* 28–39.

Krahenbuhl, S., & Blades, M. (2006). The effect of interviewing techniques on young children's responses to questions. *Child: Care, Health and Development, 32,* 321–331.

LaGreca, A. M. (Ed.). (1990). *Through the eyes of the child. Obtaining self-reports from children and adolescents.* Boston: Allyn and Bacon.

Lai, J.-S., Haglund, L., & Kielhofner, G. (1999). The Occupational Case Analysis Interview and Rating Scale: Construct validity and directions for future development. *Scandinavian Journal of Caring Sciences, 13,* 267–273.

Law, M. (Ed.). (1998). *Client-centered occupational therapy.* Thorofare, NJ: Slack.

Law, M., Baptiste, S., Carswell, A., McColl, M. A., Polatajko, H., & Pollock, N. (1998). *Canadian occupational performance measure* (3rd ed.). Toronto: Canadian Association of Occupational Therapists.

Law, M., Baptiste, S., & Mills, J. (1995). Client-centred practice: What does it mean and does it make a difference? *Canadian Journal of Occupational Therapy, 62,* 250–257.

Law, M., Finkelman, S., Hurley, P., Rosenbaum, P., King, S., King G., et al. (2004). Participation of children with physical disabilities: Relationships with diagnosis, physical function, and demographic variables. *Scandinavian Journal of Occupational Therapy, 11,* 156–162.

Lewis, J., & Jones, P. (2001). Measuring handicap in rheumatic disease: Evaluation of the Canadian Occupational Performance Measure. *ARHP Annual Meeting, 45*(6), S90.

Levin, M., & Helfrich, C. (2004). Mothering role identity and competence among parenting and pregnant homeless adolescents. *Journal of Occupational Science, 11,* 95–104.

Lynch, K. B., & Bridle, M. J. (1993). Construct validity of the occupational performance history interview. *Occupational Therapy Journal of Research, 13,* 231–240.

Matsutsuyu, J. (1969). The interest checklist. *American Journal of Occupational Therapy, 23,* 323–328.

Mattingly, C. (1991). The narrative nature of clinical reasoning. *American Journal of Occupational Therapy, 45,* 998–1005.

Mattingly, C., & Fleming, M. H. (1994). *Clinical reasoning: Forms of inquiry in a therapeutic practice.* Philadelphia: F. A. Davis.

Mauras-Nelson, E., & Oakley, F. (1996, April). *Bone marrow transplantation: Implications on function.* Poster presentation at the American Occupational Therapy Association Annual Conference, Chicago, IL.

McColl, M. A., Paterson, M., Davies, D., Doubt, L., & Law, M. (2000). Validity and community utility of the Canadian Occupational Performance Measure. *Canadian Journal of Occupational Therapy, 67,* 22–30.

Mishler, E. G. (1986). *Research interviewing: Context and narrative.* Cambridge, MA: Harvard University Press.

Missiuna, C. (1998). Development of "All About Me," a scale that measures children's perceived motor competence. *Occupational Therapy Journal of Research, 18,* 85–108.

Missiuna, C., & Pollock, N. (2000). Perceived efficacy and goal setting in young children. *Canadian Journal of Occupational Therapy, 67,* 101–109.

Missiuna, C., Pollock, N., & Law, M. (2004). *Perceived Efficacy and Goal Setting System (PEGS).* San Antonio, TX: Psychological Corporation.

Missiuna, C., Pollock, N., Law, M., Walter, S., & Cavey, N. (2006). Examination of the Perceived Efficacy and Goal Setting System (PEGS) with children with disabilities, their

parents, and teachers. *American Journal of Occupational Therapy, 60,* 204–214.

Neistadt, M. E. (1995). Methods of assessing clients' priorities: A survey of adult physical dysfunction settings. *American Journal of Occupational Therapy, 49,* 428–436.

Oakley, F., Kielhofner, G., Barris, R., & Reichler, R. (1986). The role checklist: Development and empirical assessment of reliability. *Occupational Therapy Journal of Research, 6,* 157–170.

Okun, B. F. (1997). *Effective helping: Interviewing and counseling techniques.* Pacific Grove, CA: Brooks/Cole.

Polkinghorne, D. E. (1996). Transformative narratives: From victimic to agentic life plots. *American Journal of Occupational Therapy, 50,* 299–305.

Rogers, J. C. (1988). The NPI Interest Checklist. In B. J. Hemphill (Ed.), *Mental health assessment in occupational therapy: An integrative approach to the evaluation process.* Thorofare, NJ: Slack.

Schindler, V., Laguardia, R., Melchiorre, S., & Bailey, H. (2004). An evidence-based intervention to develop roles and skills in clients with mental illness. *OT Practice, 9,* 16–20.

Sommers-Flanagan, J. & Sommers-Flanagan, R. (2003). *Clinical interviewing.* Hoboken, NJ: John Wiley & Sons.

Stone, W. L., & Lemanek, K. L. (1990). Developmental issues in children's self-reports. In A. M. LaGreca (Ed.), *Through the eyes of the child: Obtaining self-reports from children and adolescents.* (pp. 18–55). Boston: Allyn and Bacon.

Sturgess, J. L. (1997). Current trends in assessing children's play. *British Journal of Occupational Therapy, 60,* 410–413.

Sturgess, J. (2007). *The development of a play skills self-report questionnaire (PSSRQ) for 5–10 year old children and their parents/carers.* Unpublished doctoral dissertation, University of Queensland, Queensland, Australia.

Sturgess, J. (2003). A model describing play as a child-chosen activity: Is this still valid in contemporary Australia? *Australian Occupational Therapy Journal, 50,* 104–108.

Sturgess, J., & Ziviani, J. (1995). Development of a self-report play questionnaire for children aged 5 to 7 years: A preliminary report. *Australian Occupational Therapy Journal, 42,* 107–117.

Sturgess, J., & Ziviani, J. (1996). A self-report play skills questionnaire: technical development. *Australian Occupational Therapy Journal, 43,* 142–154.

Tickle-Degnen, L. (1995). Therapeutic rapport. In C. A. Trombly (Ed.), *Occupational therapy for physical dysfunction* (4th ed., pp. 277–285). Baltimore: Williams & Wilkins.

Velozo, C., Kielhofner, G., Gern, A., Lin, F., Azhar, F., Lai, J., et al. (1999). Worker Role Interview: Toward validation of a psychosocial work-related measure. *Journal of Occupational Rehabilitation, 9,* 153–168.

Weinstein, J. (1979). *The generation of profiles of adolescent interests.* Unpublished master's thesis, University of Southern California, Los Angeles.

World Health Organization. (2001). *International classification of functioning, disability and health.* Geneva: Author.

Analyzing Occupations and Activity

**ELIZABETH BLESEDELL CREPEAU
AND BARBARA A. BOYT SCHELL**

35

Learning Objectives

After reading this chapter, you will be able to:

1. Describe approaches to analyzing occupations and activities in occupational therapy.
2. Describe the similarities and difference between activity analysis and occupational analysis.
3. Understand how occupational performance is the result of skilled transactions between the person and the performance context.
4. Define occupational orchestration.
5. Analyze activity in general and as experienced by an individual.
6. Describe how grading and adapting activities can be used to meet the needs of clients.

Think about all the things you have or will do today, as you go about your daily rounds. Perhaps you started your day with a bath or shower. Did you do that? Or do you prefer to bathe at night? Or, are you someone who prefers to bathe every other day? If you did bathe or shower, did you wash your hair? If you washed your hair, did you shampoo it once or twice? Did you apply a conditioner? Did you wash your hair before you washed the rest of your body or after? Were you standing in a shower, sitting in a tub, or leaning over a sink? How hot was the water? Did your arms get tired? Did you dry your hair with a towel or just comb it and let it dry itself? Or did you style your hair with a hair dryer? Did you use a pick, comb, or brush? What physical functions would you say are critical to doing your hair? What mental functions? What features of the setting or context are important to you? Do you think the same things are important for all people? Answering questions such as these are part of the daily thinking processes that occupational therapy practitioners consider when they go about planning and implementing care for their patients and clients. Whether the attention is on self-maintenance activities, such as bathing and hair care, or on work activities, such as driving a bull-dozer, practitioners require systematic frameworks to understand exactly what each person wants or needs to do. Application of these systematic frameworks is called **occupational analysis and activity analysis**.

Occupational therapy practitioners analyze activities to understand their component parts, their possible meaning to clients, and their therapeutic potential. Practitioners analyze the occupations of clients to gain an appreciation of specific performance strengths and potential problems clients are encountering. The analysis is used to design therapeutic intervention to enable clients to engage or re-engage in those occupations that have particular meaning and value. Practitioners also analyze how clients orchestrate their occupations across a day, week, and longer periods of time. **Occupational orchestration** reflects the capacity of individuals to enact their occupations on a daily basis to meet both their own needs and those in their social world. Orchestration, a musical term, implies a rhythmic, harmonious composition of daily life that has habitual or routine components but is also responsive to changes in demands from day-to-day (Larson, 2000). Occupational therapy intervention is based on engaging clients in meaningful occupations to enable or improve their ability to meet their goals and participate in daily life. The occupations may be seemingly minor, such as the morning shower, or the orchestration of the complex array of daily occupations necessary to live a full and satisfying life, such as managing the pastoral care committee of the church while working full time and caring for the family. Consequently, the analytic processes practitioners bring to their work are at the core of occupational therapy practice. This chapter describes these processes and links them to professional reasoning as it occurs throughout the therapeutic process.

TWO PERSPECTIVES ON ANALYSIS: OCCUPATION AND ACTIVITY

Occupational therapy practitioners approach the process of activity analysis from two different perspectives, occupational analysis and activity analysis. In the first approach, practitioners are concerned with understanding the specific situation of the client, and therefore must understand the specific **occupation**s the person wants or needs to do in the actual context in which these occupations are performed. We refer to this as occupational analysis, because the term occupation connotes personally experienced performance (Pierce, 2001). As discussed in the AOTA Practice Framework, 2nd Ed. (AOTA, 2007) this is a customized approach that is embedded in the entire occupational therapy process. Occupational analysis attends carefully to the specific details of the person's occupations within his or her own context. Indeed, it is this customized approach that differentiates the occupational therapy perspective from that of many other professions who do activity analysis, such as vocational educators and industrial engineers. In the bathing example provided in the opening paragraph, your answers to how you specifically performed the process of bathing represents part of an occupational analysis, in

that it helps describe the way that you actually do a particular occupation in your own life. See Box 35.1 for the rationale for the specific terms we are using in this chapter.

The second approach is commonly called activity analysis. In activity analysis, the practitioner considers an activity in the abstract, as it might typically be done within a given culture (Pierce, 2001). Practitioners do this sort of activity analysis for at least two reasons. First, the practitioner may wish to anticipate possible areas of concern in working with clients with different kinds of health conditions or concerns. Secondly, practitioners often need to generate **purposeful activities**, goal-directed behaviors leading to an occupation, (AOTA, 2007) which can be usefully designed or graded to help a client develop, recover from an impairment, or learn an adaptive approach. For instance, if a practitioner thinks about what is typically involved in bathing or showering for many people in the United States, then he or she might be able to anticipate possible problems for someone with a partial paralysis or difficulty remembering how to sequence activities. Alternatively, while at a toy store or hardware store, the practitioner might notice toys or objects that lend themselves to helping individuals develop or improve in various skills or bodily capacities, or which require particular kinds of problem solving. Having these ideas in the practitioner mental "toolbox" makes it easier to generate therapy possibilities for working with clients. Such consideration of activity possibilities is a *decontextualized approach,* because it is an abstract idea of what the practitioner thinks typically occurs. It is not what any one particular person actually experiences.

To summarize, the term **activity** is used in this chapter to represent an *abstract idea* about kinds of things individuals do and the way they typically do them in a given culture (Pierce, 2001). The term occupation(s) is used to denote the *personal activities* that individuals choose to engage in, and the ways in which each individual actually experiences them. Practitioners must be able to analyze both the abstract idea of an activity within a culture, as well as the actual occupations as they are performed by particular individuals. These perspectives can also be applied to groups of people (such as members of a choir or workers in a plant), organizations (such as the local recreation center), and populations (such as middle school students or elders in a community). This chapter will focus primarily on analysis of activity and occupation at the individual level, as the application to groups builds on these core analytic approaches. Other chapters later in the text provide illustrations of how occupational analysis can be used in relation to groups, organizations and populations.

PERFORMANCE CONTEXTS AND ENVIRONMENTS

Occupational performance is by nature embedded within a social and physical environment, situated in a performance context (AOTA, 2007; Dunn, Brown, & Youngstrom,

BOX 35.1 WORDS MATTER: DEFINING ACTIVITY AND OCCUPATION

Words matter because they shape the way we think and the meanings we ascribe to their underlying concepts (Hymes, 1972). Occupational therapy, like many other professions and disciplines, engages in ongoing debates about the meaning of specific terms as they relate to the profession. This debate can become confusing, as professional jargon may or may not parallel the way that the same words are used in everyday speech (Reed, 2005). Occupation and activity are two such words with everyday meanings and specialized professional meanings. Because these terms are so central to our field, many scholars have attempted to articulate precise meanings. The abundance of these definitions can be confusing, especially to occupational therapy students who are new to the field and seeking to understand it.

Definitions of *occupation* typically include a combination of the following concepts[a]:

- Personally experienced and goal directed
- Reflects culture and cultural values
- Provides meaning
- Involves multiple tasks
- Provides organization and structure to living
- Meets needs of the individual and others in the social world
- Fills time
- Uses abilities and skills
- May have a physical and/or mental component
- Is recognized by the culture
- Provides pleasure and enjoyment
- Contributes to family and broader community
- Contributes to health and well-being
- Aligns with development of the individual

Definitions of *activity* typically share a mix of the core concepts listed below. Activity is frequently modified with terms such as *purposeful, occupational,* or *functional* to give it more specific meaning. In these cases the term activity itself is not defined but assumed to be common knowledge. The core concepts[b] for most definitions of activity include the following:

- Small units of behavior
- Use of objects
- Action
- May or may not produce an object
- Goal directed
- Required for development, maturation and use of sensory-perceptual, motor, social, psychological, and intellectual functions

In contrast, Pierce has defined activity as

. . . an idea held in the minds of persons and in their shared cultural language. An activity is a culturally defined and general class of human actions . . . An activity is not experienced by a specific person; is not observable as an occurrence; and is not located in a fully existent temporal, spatial, and socio-cultural context. (Pierce, 2001, p. 139)

For the purpose of this chapter we have chosen to adopt Pierce's definition of activity because this definition enables us to make the distinction between the abstract ideas we have about a particular activity for activity analysis, for example swimming, versus the engagement in swimming as an occupation that is dependent on the way or ways a particular person swims and the meaning he or she ascribes to it. Consequently, throughout the chapter when you read *activity* you should remember that this reflects the abstract, decontextualized concept and *occupation* is the way a particular person enacts this activity in a specific context. In other chapters in this book you will find terminology used differently. You need to look behind the terminology to understand the intent of the authors in their word choice.

[a]Compiled from: Christiansen, Baum, Bass-Haugen, 2005; Spear & Crepeau, 2003; Hinojosa & Kramer, 1997; Law, Polatakjo, Baptiste, & Townsend, 1997; Nelson & Jebson-Thomas, 2003; Clarke et al., 1991.
[b]Compiled from: Allen, 1987; 2007; Cynkin, 1995; Hinojosa & Kramer, 1997; Llorens, 1986; Mosey, 1981; Reed, 2005; Trombly, 1995.

2003; Pierce, 2001). *Environment* includes the physical and social environments in which the client performs their occupations. *Context* includes the external physical, social, and cultural environments in which people function, as well as the internal or personal aspects, such as age, gender, motivation of the person. Additionally, occupations are located in a temporal context, both in terms of the specific amount of time involved, as well as the history and projected future related to occupation. Finally, some occupations occur on virtual contexts, such as web-based blogs and spaces. Paralleling the distinction just made between activity and occupation, many aspects of the environment and context can be considered in abstract or as the client actually experiences them.

Arenas and Settings

Lave (1988), an anthropologist, makes a distinction between the potential uses of environmental contexts and the ways people actually interact with them. She used the term **arena** to describe the places in which activities occur, such as a library, school, or hospital. In contrast, she used the word **setting** to describe those aspects of the arena to which the person attends. This distinction is useful in that it, once again, illustrates the twin ideas of actual experience versus abstract conceptualizations. For example, a library is an arena, and many of us conjure up an idea of what a library is. In fact, we may even think of a particular library. However, each individual will use the library in different ways and to construct different meanings from their experiences. A man entering the library with his young child will most likely go to the children's section to look at colorful picture or chapter books. He is likely to sit on a small chair or a pillow while reading to his child. Later, he may help the child select books to take home. In contrast, another person may go to the audio section to check out an audio-book to listen to while commuting to work. Thus, while the library as an arena remains the same, the library as a setting differs from person to person. Consequently, the distinction Lave makes between arena and setting is similar to the distinction made earlier between activity and occupation. Like activity, arena is an abstract idea, whereas settings are where occupational activities are actually done.

Roles: Social Constructions versus Personally Enacted

Role theory has had an influence on the development of theory within the profession. For instance, the Model of Human Occupation described in Chapter 44 uses role as a way of articulating how individuals see themselves and the multiple aspects of a person's life. The concept of role filters down into assessments such as the Role Checklist and Worker Role Interview (see Unit XVI for information on these and other examples). In sociological and psychological theories, roles are seen as social positions (Jackson, 1998a, Hagendorn, 2000). As Fisher noted in her Slagle lecture, "the role dimension pertains to the relationship between one's roles and the related collection of task performances that must unfold in a logical, timely, and socially appropriate manner. We must understand the person's perceived roles and any incongruities between his or her role behavior and the role behavior that is expected by society or desired by the person" (1998, p. 544). Thus roles can be thought of as normative models shaped by the culture. They help articulate expectations for what constitutes being a "good" mother, father, student, etc. and what people in these positions are supposed to do. Individuals within

roles may adopt these normative expectations or may interpret the expectations to fit their own values and beliefs.

Jackson (1998a, 1998b) argued that our concern should be on the occupations individuals engage in, not their roles because the concept of role is problematic from several perspectives. First, roles may overlap. For example, it is often impossible to distinguish a child's "student" role from their "friend" role. When someone is cooking, is it in their role as mother or father, church volunteer, or chef? In both instances, our concern is in the occupation, the person's ability to engage in the occupation, and the meaning they ascribe to it, not the role to which the occupation connects. Second, while the concept of role provides a shorthand way of understanding the occupational world of an individual, Jackson (1998a) argued that this approach is risky because inherent in the concept of role are the power issues embedded in many cultural models. For example, who decides what a "good mother" is? Who says the mother is the one to do the cooking for the family?

Still, role is not easy to ignore because it is such a widely held concept. For example, Trombly Latham (1995; 2008) uses role as an organizing construct, however she cautions that when considering role it should be from the definitional perspective of the individual, rather than the normative expectations of society. But how does one get to this definitional perspective except through understanding the occupations the individual attaches to a particular role? By focusing on occupations people engage in, we can see what they do, what the occupation means to them, how they feel about their performance, and how they organize their occupations to meet their needs and those of the people around them. Our analysis begins with occupation and may result, if needed, in clustering these occupations into the individual's personal definition of the occupations associated with their roles. Once again, we see the contrast between the abstract notion of role and the personally experienced situation of the individual, sometimes called **occupational role**.

Jackson's (1998a, 1998b) cautions about the use of role are important because it is easy to unconsciously slip into normative expectations or use one's personal experience to frame the expectations for others. As discussed earlier in Chapter 32, practitioners bring unarticulated personal assumptions to the therapy process. Consequently, we have chosen not to use role as an organizational construct for this chapter because we want to focus on those occupations that are most important to an individual regardless of what role or roles to which they might be assigned. Instead, we look at the orchestration of occupations as they are enfolded, and integrated in the course of daily life.

OCCUPATIONAL ANALYSIS AND MEANING

Over and over again practitioners need to remind themselves that meaning is individually constructed and interpreted and is central to human existence (Bruner, 1990; Frankl, 1959; Hasselkus, 2002; Peloquin, 2005, 2007). A practitioner is obligated to understand the meaning of occupations from the client's perspective. Using the library example discussed previously, it is possible if you talked to the father about the meaning of going to the library with his child that he might mention the pleasure he derives from instilling in his child the value and enjoyment of reading and the quiet time they share together. He might recall his childhood and the times he went to the library with one of his parents. Alternatively, he might explain that he never had the opportunity to go to the library with his father because his father had abandoned the family. The latter experience would create an entirely different meaning and motivational structure for this father–child dyad as they engage in this **co-occupation**.

As this example illustrates, the different experiences, values, and beliefs of clients make the interpretation of meaning a particularly complex aspect of practice. This challenge is exacerbated by potential cultural and socio-economic differences between practitioners and their clients making it more challenging for practitioners to fully understand the experiences of their clients and the meanings they ascribe to their occupations (Crepeau, 1991; Kielhofner & Barrett, 1998; Payne, DeVol, & Smith, 2001) (See also Chapters 6 through 9 in this text which address culture, socioeconomics, place, and spirituality). It is the practitioner's responsibility to develop the therapeutic relationships that foster an understanding of clients and their world (Crepeau, 1991; Peloquin, 1995; see also Chapter 29 which addresses client-centered collaboration and Chapter 33 which addresses the therapeutic relationship). Activity analysis and occupational analysis are part of the tools that practitioners can use to achieve this understanding. Table 35.1 provides a quick reference to remind readers as to what concepts are tied to the person's subjective experience versus what terms are more related to practitioners' abstract understanding of typical demands.

ACTIVITY AND OCCUPATIONAL ANALYSIS IN PRACTICE

Occupational therapy practitioners draw on their education, knowledge of activities, and professional experience when analyzing activities (Neistadt, McAuley, Zecha, & Shannon, 1993). This analysis is so automatic that it is often ignored or unappreciated, becoming another aspect of the tacit nature of the reasoning process used by practitioners (Mattingly & Fleming, 1994; Schell & Cervero, 1993). Practitioners analyze activities from the perspective of practice theories to understand problems in performance and intervention strategies appropriate from that theoretical perspective. Their analysis is also based on access to particular activities and the degree to which they are willing to engage in trial and error or experimentation to understand activities more fully (Schell, 2007).

Studies that have attempted to make activity analysis an objective process have demonstrated that the number of variables is so great that the goal of objectivity would be exceedingly difficult to achieve (Llorens, 1986; Neistadt et al., 1993; Trombly, 1995). Adopting the distinction between activity analysis and occupational analysis renders this concern moot. If the outcome of activity analysis is to understand the *potential* demands of an activity, objectivity is not the goal. Rather, identifying the multiple skills typically required and the potential meanings the activity may have enables practitioners to have a deeper understanding of this activity in general.

In contrast to the abstract consideration of activities for their therapeutic implications, occupational analysis is a highly individualized process because it is embedded in the particular perspective of the person, the person's occupational performance, and the performance context. Occupational analysis occurs when attempting understand the person as an occupational being in concert with identifying occupational performance and barriers to effective performance (Coster, 1998; Fisher, 2001; Hocking, 2001; Polatajko, Mandich, & Martini, 2000; Trombly, 1995; Trombly Latham, 2008). Client-centered evaluation models examine the ability of a person to engage in a valued occupation and the transaction among actual performance, activity demands, and context (Law, 1998). Box 35.2 provides examples of the various degrees of focus that practitioner's use to consider occupations.

Both occupational and activity analysis are required for effective practice. By blending these analytic models, practitioners can gain an understanding of the particular ways in which clients relate to their occupations and can

TABLE 35.1   TERMS: FROM THE ABSTRACT TO THE PARTICULAR

	Abstract Concept	Real Experience
What is done	Activity	Occupation
Where and with whom	Arena	Setting
How it is organized	Social role	Occupational orchestration

BOX 35.2 OCCUPATIONAL SCALE: A QUESTION OF FOCUS

Just as there is little agreement in the field about the definition of activity, there is little agreement about the scope or scale of what actually constitutes an occupation. Hinojosa captured this dilemma eloquently when he shared his personal reflections about occupation:

> I am uncomfortable with the current trend in the profession to call everything we do as occupation. I personally cannot believe that brushing my teeth or being able to effectively use toilet paper in the bathroom is an occupation. I do believe that they

are important purposeful activities. I have come to realize that the combination of these two activities is fundamental to complete personal hygiene occupations (Hinojosa, Kramer, Royeen & Luebben, 2003, p. 8).

Hinojosa's question could be restated as follows:

Is an occupation a collection of tasks within a broad scope of one's life (cooking) or some of the sub-tasks within this category (making a meal) or even smaller units (preparing vegetables for the salad)?

Lens	Example: Cooking	Analytical Questions
Panoramic (Zoom Out)	Making a meal 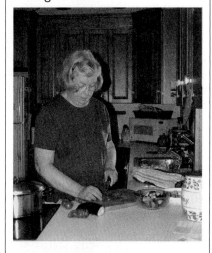	What does this person cook and why? In what settings do they cook (ie, home, community center, homeless shelter kitchen?) How often does the person cook? How does it overlap or enfold within other occupations (ie, is it important in their job, to their duties to their spouse or partner?) Can the person do the planning and organization necessary? Does the person have skills to prepare the food? Does the person get each part of the meal done in a timely manner? Is the quality of the result satisfactory to the person and significant others?
	Preparing a salad 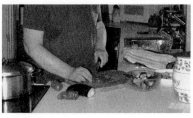	Can the person get the salad ingredients from the refrigerator? Does the person rernember to get all they need? Can the person use a knife safely with different ingredients? Can the person use a knife effectively with all the ingredients? Can the person get the salad to the table? Does the person season it to their own standards and that of those sharing the salad?
Close-Up (Zoom In)	Slicing a tomato 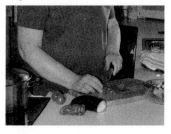	Can the person grasp the tomato? Does the person hold it too tightly or too loosely? Can the person hold the knife by the handle? Does the person know to hold the handle as opposed to the blade? Does the person position the knife relative to the tomato? Is the person at risk of being cut? Does the person cut the tomato in the desired shape? Do the tomato slices meet the person's own standards and that of others eating the salad?

BOX 35.2 OCCUPATIONAL SCALE: A QUESTION OF FOCUS *Continued*

There is little agreement in the field on this issue with scholars proposing a variety of ways to nest the sub-units of occupations within the broader category. These include the following:

◆ Trombly Latham nests activities within tasks which constitute life roles (1995, 2008).
◆ Polatajko, Mandich, and Martini (2000) break down occupations into tasks which contain segments, units, and sub-units
◆ Baum and Christiansen (2005) start with roles, tasks, and actions
◆ Fisher considers the role dimensions of an individual's occupations and places tasks (what the person does)

within this category (1998), but notes the importance of starting with a person's goals

Our purpose here is to point out the lack of agreement and say that we have no solution to the problem. We just want you to recognize that there are varying ways to consider analyzing occupations. We borrow Crabtree's (1998) metaphor comparing the occupational therapy reasoning process to a camera lens. Sometimes we zoom out to see the big picture and sometimes we zoom in to capture the fine details. The depth and scope of analysis is directly related to the goals by the client for intervention and the reasoning process of the practitioner in responding to these goals.

---

then use their knowledge of activity and practice theories to harness those occupational activities for therapeutic purposes. This understanding is achieved through both forms of analysis. Table 35.2 on page 367 summarizes the questions addressed in both activity and occupational analysis. Box 35.3 shows how practitioners weave analysis of occupational performance throughout the therapy process. Box 35.4 lists some of ways that these analyses inform practice decisions.

ACTIVITY ANALYSIS

Activity analysis is a way of thinking about activities. Practitioners must perform quick analyses while working with clients. In addition, occupational therapy practitioners may also think about activities for their therapeutic potential, for instance by sizing up new games, cooking gadgets, and other objects or activities. Activity analysis addresses the typical demands of an

BOX 35.3 ANALYSIS OF OCCUPATIONAL PERFORMANCE

Occupational performance is the accomplishment of the selected occupation or activity resulting from the dynamic transaction among the client, the context and environment, and the activity. Evaluation of occupational performance involves

◆ Synthesizing information from the occupational profile to focus on specific areas of occupation and contexts that need to be addressed.
◆ Observing the client's performance in desired occupations and activities, noting effectiveness of the performance skills and performance patterns.
◆ Selecting and using specific assessments to measure performance skills and patterns as appropriate.

(AOTA, 2007, p. 21).

◆ Selecting assessments, as needed, to identify and measure more specifically contexts or environments, activity demands, and client factors that are influencing performance skills and performance patterns.
◆ Interpreting the assessment data to identify what supports performance and what hinders performance.
◆ Developing and refining hypotheses about the client's occupational performance strengths and limitations.
◆ Creating goals in collaboration with the client that address the desired outcomes.
◆ Determining procedures to measure the outcomes of intervention.
◆ Delineating potential intervention approach or approaches based on best practice and available evidence.

BOX 35.4 WAYS ACTIVITY AND OCCUPATIONAL ANALYSIS INFORM PRACTICE

Practitioners analyze activity in the abstract for the following reasons:

◆ Understand the therapeutic potential of a wide range of activities
◆ Identify activities which lend themselves to
  a. Improving client performance through acquiring new skills or learning adaptive strategies
  b. Restoring a skill or client factor which impacts performance skills
  c. Prevention of future problems by changing or adapting activity demands or performance context

Practitioners analyze the occupations of their clients to

◆ Evaluate quality of current performance in valued occupations and the effectiveness of their capacity to orchestrate their occupations.
◆ Determine impact of personal factors (including health condition) on current performance.
◆ Determine impact of contextual factors on current performance
◆ Prognosticate future performance in identified contexts
◆ Identify ways to grade or adapt occupations for foster improved performance

---

activity, the range of skills involved in its performance, and the various cultural meanings that might be ascribed to it. The goal of activity analysis is to understand as much as possible about an activity, including the particular skills required to do it competently and its relation to participation in the world at large (Cynkin, 1995). It is this knowledge of activities, their properties, and their potential cultural meanings that sensitizes practitioners to the occupations of their clients and helps practitioners know which particular activities to suggest to their clients. Through activity analysis practitioners gain an understanding of the therapeutic potential of a wide range of activities. Because practitioners are constantly analyzing activities, they develop the capacity to quickly analyze a wide range of activities for their therapeutic or evaluation potential. For example, in the vignette that opens Chapter 32, Terry, the occupational therapist, had to very quickly identify alternate ways to evaluate Mrs. Munro's safety. The therapist had planned to use observation of self-care to check out how safely Mrs. Munro moved and if she remembered and sequenced appropriately. Since Mrs. Munro had already done her self-care, Terry quickly found a relevant cleaning task that would essentially demand similar skills based on cognition and mobility.

Activity Analysis Format

The activity analysis format is based on the organization of the *Occupational Therapy Practice Framework* (AOTA, 2002) and the subsequent edition (AOTA, 2007) as well as information from various chapters within this text. The *Occupational Therapy Practice Framework* is designed to reflect the current practice of occupational therapy and its concern for occupational engagement to support health and participation of people in our society. Activity analy-

sis focuses on the identification of activity demands and performance skills. Activity demands include aspects of the activity such as the objects typically used, the space and social demands of the activity. The analysis format also includes consideration of the typically required body structures and functions as they relate to the skills often used in the activity. Also included in the analysis are the expected skills which represent the interface between the person and the performance setting.

As part of activity analysis, practitioners may consider the utility of the activity as viewed through different theoretical lenses. For instance, a therapist who is working with a population of people with biomechanically related impairments (i.e., hand injuries, back injuries) may analyze activities in terms of the typical strength, range of motion, and endurance required to complete them. Alternatively, someone who is concerned about supporting interpersonal skills in clients with mental illness may look primarily at the complexity of social interactions which the activity typically demands (Davidson, 2003). By using the principles of a particular practice theory, occupational therapy practitioners analyze activities as they think about performance strengths and problems addressed by the particular theory. The potential therapeutic intervention should be consistent with the theory and will likely entail the grading and adaptation of the occupations chosen by the client. Table 35.2 presents a format for analysis of activities.

OCCUPATIONAL ANALYSIS

In contrast to activity analysis, occupational analysis *places the person in the foreground* by taking into account the particular person's life experiences, values, interests, goals. Occupational analysis attends to their actual body functions and structures and considers the actual performance arena, including physical and social contexts along with the demands of the occupation itself. These considerations shape the practitioner's efforts to help the person reach his or her goals through carefully designed evaluation and intervention. Practitioners vary the scope of the occupational analysis depending on the nature of the client concerns, health problem and the nature of the intervention setting.

As discussed earlier, occupational analysis may be focused on a particular occupation, such as using a keyboard on the computer or brushing one's teeth, or it may be focused on a broader scope of how individuals orchestrate numerous aspects of occupational performance into daily life, such as being an effective worker. We illustrate two approaches to analyzing occupations, which vary by the scope of the client's concerns.

- **Occupational analysis:** Analysis of occupations parallels activity analysis, with the important difference that it is examining an actual occupation that the person does in his or her own unique way. Questions used for occupational analysis are found in the last column of Table 35.2.
- **Analysis of occupational orchestration:** Table 35.3 illustrates ways to consider how individuals engage and manage their multiple occupations.

OCCUPATION AS THERAPY

The careful use of occupations for therapeutic change is what makes occupational therapy unique. Intervention strategies typically involve changing occupations in ways that either facilitate development or improvement in desired performance or allow for participation in spite of limitations. Inherent in these approaches is attention to developing and maintaining the client's motivation for change. Common approaches are **grading**, **scaffolding**, **fading**, **coaching**, and **adaptation** or **modification**. The ability to use these approaches for a wide variety of activities/occupations and from various theoretical perspectives is a core skill for occupational therapy practitioners.

Grading

The grading of an occupation involves sequentially increasing its demands to stimulate the person's function or conversely, reducing the occupational demands to respond to client difficulties in performance. Often, practitioners grade occupations to improve the client's underlying capacities and skills (Fisher, 2001). Depending on the nature of the client's performance problems and the practice theory or theories selected by the prac-

titioner to address these problems, the particular way of grading will vary. For example, a practitioner may grade the occupation from a sensory integrative theory perspective when working with a child who wants to ride a two-wheeled bicycle but who is unsuccessful at balancing sufficiently. The practitioner may provide intervention for the child a sensory-enriched environment (suspended equipment, large therapy balls, climbing equipment) designed to evoke active exploration on the part of the child. The available sensory equipment provides a variety of vestibular, tactile, and proprioceptive stimuli for creating sensory experiences that require postural control, including balance. The child initiates the desired occupation within the sensory enriched environment and, based on careful observation of the child's reaction, the practitioner may reduce or increase the balance demands of the occupation to provide the "just right challenge" for the child. The child can learn to use his or her body in new and novel ways so that increasingly complex possibilities for physical engagement emerge (see Chapter 59). The practitioner sets up the structure and possibilities in which the child's interests and ability to cope with the sensory, motor, and organization demands dictate the level of challenge and intensity of the activities. The practitioner may then use a motor learning perspective (see Chapter 55) to have the same child practicing posture and balance skills directly on a bicycle with training wheels, varying the demands of the terrain (i.e., turning corners, going up a slope) and eventually carefully removing supports such as training wheels to allow for greater balance demands, until the child was ready to ride a bicycle without supervision or physical assistance.

Scaffolding, Fading, and Coaching

Practitioners observe clients' occupational performance and adjust their grading to create the level of demand at the appropriate level to stimulate therapeutic growth or change but not so difficult as to frustrate the person, that is, to create the "just right challenge" (Ayres, 1973). Scaffolding (Rogoff, 2003; Rogoff, Goodman Turkanis, & Bartlett, 2001) is a term used when the practitioner helps the client by doing parts of the task that are too hard, but then has the client do the rest, so that a task may be completed. Much like the scaffold on a building supports the building until it is built, practitioners using this approach help clients stay motivated by seeing that they can substantially complete a task. As clients develop or improve their skills, practitioners fade or systematically withdraw supports, so that the task demands increase until the person is doing the whole task or occupation independently. For larger scale changes in constellations of occupational activities, practitioners may engage in coaching. Coaching involves providing verbal expectations and support designed to help the

TABLE 35.2   ANALYSIS FORMAT FOR ACTIVITIES AND OCCUPATIONS

	Activity Analysis	Occupational Analysis
Description	Describe the activity in one to two sentences.	Briefly describe the occupation. How does the person usually do this occupation and in what settings.
Objects used and their properties	Describe the tools, materials, and equipment typically used. Note the potential symbolism/meaning of the objects in the relevant culture.	Describe the tools, materials, and equipment actually used. Note the symbolism/meaning of the objects to this person.
Space demands	Describe the physical environment in which the activity is being analyzed. Include key aspects, such as the following: ◆ Does this occur in a natural or built environment? ◆ What are the major natural or built structures? ◆ Describe the placement of any furnishings and equipment. ◆ What is the light level? Does is change or is it constant? ◆ Describe the kind and level of noise. How might it impact the activity to be performed? ◆ Describe any other features which may impact the senses (ie, smell, texture, temperature) and affect performance. ◆ Is this the typical context for this activity? If not, what other contexts might be appropriate? Briefly describe them, with emphasis on how the other contexts are different.	Describe the actual physical environment in which the occupation will be performed. Consider how the physical environment supports or impedes performance. Include key aspects, such as the following: ◆ Does this occur in a natural or built environment? ◆ What are the major natural or built structures? ◆ How do structures, furnishings and equipment affect the person's performance? ◆ What is the light level and does it change? How does lighting affect performance? ◆ Describe the kind and level of noise, and how it affects performance. ◆ Describe any other features which affect the person's performance (ie, smell, texture, temperature). ◆ In addition to the context just described, where else does this person engage in this occupation? Briefly describe all additional contexts, with emphasis on how they are different from the first one described.
Social demands	Describe the social and cultural demands or the range of demands that may be required by this activity or elicited by engagement in this activity, using the categories listed below. ◆ Describe other people involved in the activity. What is their relationship to each other? What do they expect from each other? ◆ Describe the typical rules, norms, and expectations involved in doing this activity. ◆ Describe the cultural and symbolic meanings typically ascribed to this activity. ◆ Speculate about other social contexts in which the activity might be performed. How might the rules, expectations, and meanings vary from this setting?	Describe the social and cultural demands as the person engages in this occupation, using the categories listed below. ◆ Describe other people involved in the occupation. What is their relationship to each other? What do they expect from each other? ◆ Describe the rules, norms, and expectations of this person as he or she engages in this occupation. ◆ Describe the cultural and symbolic meanings that this person and his or her significant others ascribe to this occupation. ◆ Consider all the other social contexts in which the occupation might be performed. How do the rules, expectations, and meanings vary from this setting?

TABLE 35.2   ANALYSIS FORMAT FOR ACTIVITIES AND OCCUPATIONS   *Continued*

	Activity Analysis	Occupational Analysis
Sequence, timing & patterns	List the sequential steps (no more than 15) of the activity. Include any timing requirements, such as waiting for glue to dry, bread to rise, etc. ◆ How much flexibility exists in the sequence and timing of the steps of this activity? ◆ Does this activity typically occur or reoccur at a specific time of day? With what frequency? (ie, daily, weekly, monthly?)	List the sequential steps (no more than 15) of the occupation as the person does it. Include any timing requirements, such as waiting for glue to dry, bread to rise, etc. ◆ How much flexibility exists in the sequence and timing of the steps of this occupation? ◆ Does this occupation typically occur or reoccur at a specific time of day? When and with what frequency? (ie, daily, weekly, monthly?)
Required skills (observable actions)	Using the OT Practice Framework, or other published list of skills, identify 5-10 skills critical to activity performance. ◆ Consider skills which demand from the person movement, cognition, sensory and emotional perception, as well as communicative and social actions. ◆ Consider skills typically demanded from the applicable environment (physical, social and virtual).	Using the OT Practice Framework, or other published list of skills, identify 5–10 skills critical to this person's occupational performance. ◆ Consider skills which demand from the person movement, cognition, sensory and emotional perception, as well as communicative and social actions. ◆ Consider skills typically demanded from the applicable environment (physical, social and virtual).
Required body structures and functions	Consider the underlying capacities of the person which are typically required when doing this activity ◆ Briefly list the body structures (anatomical parts of the body) typically used. ◆ Briefly list the essential body functions (physiological and psychological).	Consider the underlying capacities of the person which are required when doing this occupation in the contexts just identified ◆ Briefly list the body structures (anatomical parts of the body) the person uses. ◆ Briefly list the essential body functions (physiological and psychological).
Safety hazards	List potential safety hazards for this activity. Think especially of children, people with cognitive and judgment problems, people with diminished sensation, etc.	List potential safety hazards for this person as he or she performs this occupation. Consider cognitive and judgment problems, diminished sensation, etc.
Adaptability to promote participation	How much flexibility exists for people to do this activity in different ways? Consider: ◆ Person-based variables (ie, personal context, impairments) ◆ External contextual variables (physical, social, temporal, virtual, cultural)	How much flexibility exists for this person to do this occupation in different ways? How willing is the person and key stakeholders to consider doing it differently? Consider: ◆ Person-based variables (ie, personal context, impairments) ◆ External contextual variables (physical, social, temporal, virtual, cultural)
Grading	List three ways to make the task easier in relation to an identified personal or contextual variable. List three ways to make the task more challenging in relation to an identified personal or contextual variable.	List three ways to make the occupation easier in relation to an identified personal or contextual variable. List three ways to make the occupation more challenging in relation to an identified personal or contextual variable.

[a]Adapted from AOTA (2002; 2007).

TABLE 35.3 ANALYSIS OF ORCHESTRATION OF OCCUPATIONS

	Analysis of Orchestration of Occupations
Occupations	Identify the occupations that are central to the person's identity. List these occupations.
Meaning	◆ How meaningful are these occupations to the individual? ◆ How central are the occupations to the person's identity? ◆ How important are the occupations to the individual? ◆ How important is the occupation to others in the person's social world (family, friends, co-workers, etc.)?
Purpose	What purpose(s) does each occupation play in the individual's life, e.g. self-maintenance, health, support to family, support to friends or others, contribution to community, play or leisure, work.
Level of Skill and Efficiency	For each occupation, does the individual feel that he or she is able to do this occupation at an appropriate level of skill within the expected time lines? ◆ If not what are the problems/concerns from the individual's perspective? ◆ If not, what are the problems/concerns from the perspective of people in the individual's social world?
Routines	Identify the pattern in which the individual engages in these occupations. ◆ What occupations occur daily? ◆ What occupations occur weekly? ◆ What occupations occur monthly and annually? ◆ Describe a typical day? ◆ Describe a typical week?
Organization of Routines	To what extent is the daily and weekly pattern of occupations routinized? (patterns of behavior that are observable, regular, repetitive, and provide structure for daily life. Routines, occupations with established sequences. ◆ Is the individual satisfied with this level of organization? If not, why not? ◆ To what extent do these routines meet the expectations of family, friends, co-workers ◆ Are these expectations reasonable given the person's family, physical and emotional capacities, expectations from the context, family, friends, employers? ◆ Describe the degree to which these routines are disorganized, stable, or hyperstable.
Adaptability to Promote Participation	To what extent are the occupations and/or routines flexible based on ◆ Individual-based variables: personal context, impairments, openness to change? ◆ Expectations from social environment (family, friends, co-workers) ◆ Environmental (potential to change physical environment to promote increased participation)
Needs	Describe the extent to which the occupational routine is sufficient to meet the person's needs and the needs of those in his/her social world? Describe the changes required to meet the individual's needs ◆ Changes in the individual (skill development) ◆ Changes in the social environment (expectations for performance) ◆ Changes in the occupation (adapting or grading to promote more effective performance)

individual engage in and sustain growth or changes (Clark, Ennevor, & Richardson, 1996).

Adaptation and Modification

The goal of adaptation or modification is to allow the person involvement in a valued occupation. Rather than striving to improve or change the functional capacity of the individual, adaptation focuses on changing the demands of the occupation so they are congruent with the person's ability level. These adaptations may involve the modification of the occupation itself by reducing its demands, the use of assistive devices, or changes in the physical or social environment (Dunn, McLain, Brown, & Youngstrom, 2003; Fisher, 2001, 2006). Changing the demands of the occupation may involve making it simpler cognitively or reducing the physical skills required to do it. Adaptive equipment, such as reachers or holders, may be used to enable dressing or a ramp may be used to enable access to the playground for a child who uses a wheelchair. Voice-

Lauro is a 14-year-old junior high student At a recent educational-planning meeting Lauro stated that he would like to go with his friends to a nearby sports complex on Wednesdays after school. He doesn't want his mom to drive him, but would rather go on the subway with his bud- dies. Lauro has never used public transportation and has lit- tle understanding of how to manage money. As a first step, Lauro and his OT decide to go to the subway and purchase a fare card for him to use.

Skills Selected	Behavior Observed	Performance Quality	Personal Factors Affecting Performance	Contextual Factor Affecting Performance
Three skills done well				
1. Inquires	Asked attendant where to get fare cards	Required minimal ver- bal cuing, and was generally socially appropriate	Appropriate awareness and thought func- tions needed for task, good regula- tion of emotions	Signage in subway entrance clearly indicates avail- ability of atten- dant for help
2. Manipulates	Placed coins in the machine and is able to pick up card from machine.	Required little physi- cal effort, was done efficiently and independently	Good sensation, joint range and muscle strength in UE	Coin slot within easy reach, as is card that comes out
3. Conforms	Waited patiently in line to ask atten- dant questions	Required no cuing, seemed to do automatically	Cognitively aware of implicit social rules, place of body in space, need for calm emotional response	Line was short, only had to wait about 3 minutes
Three "problem" skills				
1. Gathers	Pulled all his money out of pocket and just stood there with it in hands	Required verbal and physical cues in the form of point- ing out different coins to gather needed coins	Cognitive/knowledge limitations-Not sure he knows value of coins? Can he discriminate among coins by size and design?	No wallet to organize money Few visual cues on machine as to appearance of money required
2. Chooses	As noted above, did not attempt to select coins	Needed maximum verbal assistance to select correct coins at each phase of process	Same as above	No auditory cues from machine to support performance
3. Heeds	When putting money in machine, did not change amounts he was putting in (quarters) after message told him he only needed 10 cents more	Needed verbal cues to read and interpret message, change kind of coin	Attention to visual cues, ability to match written amount (10 cents) to coin (dime).	No system for sorting change by value in his pocket Visual cues from machine placed below eye level

(Format adapted from Fisher, 2005).

Questions

1. Using the occupational analysis format, what might you do to help Lauro become better able to do the key tasks required?

2. What modifications might you make to the task or the performance setting to help Lauro perform more effectively?

3. What would you like to know about Lauro in order to make a more customized (i.e., occupational) plan?

recognition software may be used for someone who can no longer use a keyboard. Adaptation may also involve changing the social world through the provision of assistance by another person, such as a personal-care attendant or family member, to help someone with chronic mental illness to function more effectively in society (Davidson, 2003). For people with degenerative conditions, these adaptations may need to be made repeatedly as the individual's skills diminish. People with AIDS, cancer, arthritis, bipolar disorder, and other chronic illnesses may require daily adaptation because of the fluctuating levels of function typical of these conditions.

ANALYSIS OF OCCUPATIONAL PERFORMANCE SKILLS

Occupational therapy practitioners apply the analytic processes just described when observing individuals as they engage in their desired occupations. This may range from observing a student in the classroom or on the playground, a person working in an office or factory, an older adult at an assisted living facility, or a homeless person at a shelter. In all these situations the practitioner's attention is on the dynamic transaction of the person's occupational performance within the performance environment and context. Although the practitioner must be concerned with the quality of the results, the major focus is on the process of engagement. Thus, practitioners become adept at carefully observing skills associated with occupational performance. These skills represent small units of occupation, in that they are instances of the transaction among the person, occupation, and the environment in a goal-directed manner. See the Case Study for an example of how careful observations lead to intervention options using activity and occupational analysis.

CONCLUSION

This chapter describes two types of analyses: activity analysis, occupational analysis. Use of these analyses requires practitioners to understand the following:

* The general properties and demands of activities as they are customarily performed in given settings and cultures.
* How to select activities that are occupationally relevant to clients.
* How to select, grade, and adapt activities/occupations based on theoretical knowledge to foster development, bring about therapeutic change, or to improve performance.
* How to use occupations valued by clients to achieve their goals as occupational beings

These core skills are critical for effective occupational therapy evaluation and intervention. Both processes ultimately center on occupation and its capacity to motivate people to act and to create meaning in their lives. Brockelman (1980), a philosopher, recognized the importance of occupation in the following statement: "The tools of our minds and the tools of our hands are of meaningless use without deep and personal reasons of the heart to set their purpose and guide their use" (p. 24). It is through practitioners' deep understanding of people as occupational beings that effective occupational therapy intervention occurs.

ACKNOWLEDGEMENTS

We thank Anne Fisher and Ellen Cohn for their multiple conversations which contributed to the development of this chapter. Anne James and Ellen's reviews assisted in clarifying the concepts and text.

REFERENCES

Allen, C. A. (1987). Activity, occupational therapy's treatment method. Eleanor Clarke Slagle Lecture. *American Journal of Occupational Therapy, 41,* 563–575.

American Occupational Therapy Association. (2002). Occupational therapy practice framework: Domain and process. *American Journal of Occupational Therapy, 56,* 609–639.

American Occupational Therapy Association. (2007, June). Occupational therapy practice framework: Domain and process, 2nd ed. (Draft). Author.

Ayres, A. J. (1973). *Sensory integration and learning disorders.* Los Angeles: Western Psychological.

Baum, C. M., & Christiansen, C. H. (2005) Person-environment-occupation-performance: An occupation-based framework for practice. In C. H. Christiansen, C. M. Baum, & J. Bass-Haugen (Eds.). *Occupational therapy: Performance, participation, and well-being* (3rd ed., pp. 243–266). Thorofare, NJ: SLACK.

Brockelman, P. T. (1980). *Existential phenomenology and the world of ordinary experience: An introduction.* Lanham, MD: University of America Press.

Bruner, J. (1990). *Acts of meaning.* Cambridge, MA: Harvard University Press.

Christiansen, C. H., & Baum, C. M. (2005). The complexity of human occupation. In C. H. Christiansen, C. M. Baum, & J. Bass-Haugen (Eds.). *Occupational therapy: Performance, participation, and well-being* (3rd ed., pp. 4–23). Thorofare, NJ: SLACK.

Clark F., Ennevor, B. L., & Richarson, P. L. (1996). A grounded theory of techniques for occupational storytelling and occupational story making. In R. Zemke, & F. Clark (Eds.), *Occupational science: The evolving discipline* (pp. 373–392). Philadelphia: F. A. Davis.

Clarke, F., Parham, D., Carlson, M., Frank, G., Jackson, J., Pierce, D., Wolfe, R. J., & Zemke, R. (1991). Occupational science: Academic innovation in the service of occupational therapy's future. *American Journal of Occupational Therapy, 45,* 300–310.

Coster, W. (1998). Occupation-centered assessment of children. *American Journal of Occupational Therapy, 52*, 337–344.

Crabtree, M. (1998). Images of reasoning: A literature review. *Australian Occupational Therapy Journal, 45*, 113–123.

Crepeau, E. B. (1991). Achieving intersubjective understanding: Examples from an occupational therapy treatment session. *American Journal of Occupational Therapy, 44*, 311–317.

Cynkin, S. (1995). Activities. In C. B. Royeen (Ed.). *The practice of the future: Putting occupation back into therapy: AOTA self-study series* (Module 7; pp. 1–52). Rockville, MD: American Occupational Therapy Association.

Davidson, L. (2003). *Living outside mental illness: Qualitative studies of recovery in schizophrenia.* New York: New York University Press.

Dunn, W., Brown, C., & Youngstrom, M. J. (2003). Ecological model of occupation. In P. Kramer, J. Hinojosa, & C. B. Royeen (Eds). *Perspectives in human occupation* (pp. 1–17). Philadelphia, PA: Lippincott Williams & Wilkins.

Dunn, W., McClain, L. H., Brown, C., & Youngstrom, M. J. (2003). The ecology of human performance. In E. B. Crepeau, E. S. Cohn, & B. A. B. Schell (Eds.), *Willard and Spackman's occupational therapy* (10th ed., pp. 223–227). Philadelphia: Lippincott.

Fisher, A. G. (1998). Uniting practice and theory in an occupational framework. Eleanor Clarke Slagle Lecture. *American Journal of Occupational Therapy, 52*, 509–521.

Fisher, A. G. (2001). *Assessment of Motor and Process Skills: Vol. 1. Development, standardization, and administration manual* (4th ed.). Fort Collins, CO: Three Stars Press.

Fisher. A. G. (2005). *Occupational Therapy Intervention Process model* (unpublished manual).

Frankl, V. E. (1959). *Man's search for meaning: An introduction to logotherapy.* New York: Pocket Books.

Hagendorn, R. (2000). Glossary. In R. Hagendorn (Ed.), *Tools for practice in occupational therapy: A structured approach to core skills and processes,* (pp. 307–312). Edinburgh, UK: Churchill Livingstone.

Hasselkus, B. R. (2002). *The meaning of everyday occupation.* Thorofare, NJ: SLACK.

Hinojosa, J., & Kramer, P. (1997). Fundamental concepts of occupational therapy: Occupation, purposeful activity, and function [Statement]. *American Journal of Occupational Therapy, 51*, 864–866.

Hinojosa, J., Kramer; P., Royeen, C. B, & Luebben, A. (2003). Core concepts of occupation. In P. Kramer, J. Hinojosa, & C. B. Royeen (Eds). *Perspectives in human occupation* (pp. 1–17). Philadelphia, PA: Lippincott Williams & Wilkins.

Hocking, C. (2001). Implementing occupation-based assessment. *American Journal of Occupational Therapy, 55*, 463–469.

Hymes, D. (1972). Toward ethnographies of communication: The analysis of communicative events. In P. P. Giglioli (Ed.) *Language and social context* (pp. 21–44). New York: Pelican.

Jackson, J. (1998a). Contemporary criticisms of role theory. *Journal of Occupational Science, 5*, 49–55.

Jackson, J. (1998b). Is there a place for role theory in occupational science? *Journal of Occupational Science, 5*, 56–65.

Kielhofner, G., & Barrett, L. (1998). Meaning and misunderstanding in occupational forms: A study of therapeutic goal setting. *American Journal of Occupational Therapy, 52*, 345–353.

Larson, E. A. (2000). The orchestration of occupation: The dance of mothers. *American Journal of Occupational Therapy, 54*, 269–280.

Lave, J. (1988). *Cognition in practice: Mind, mathematics and culture in everyday life.* Cambridge, UK: Cambridge University Press.

Law, M. (Ed.). (1998). *Client-centered occupational therapy.* Thorofare, NJ: Slack.

Law, M., Polatakjo, H., Baptiste, W., & Townsend, E. (1997). Core concepts in occupational therapy. In E. Townsend (Ed.), *Enabling occupation: An occupational therapy perspective* (pp. 29–56). Ottawa, ON: Canadian Association of Occupational Therapists.

Llorens, L. A. (1986). Activity analysis: Agreement among factors in a sensory processing model. *American Journal of Occupational Therapy, 40*, 103–110.

Mattingly, C., & Fleming, M. H. (1994). *Clinical reasoning: Forms of inquiry in a therapeutic practice.* Philadelphia: Davis.

Mosey, A. C. (1981). *Occupational therapy: Configuration of a profession.* New York: Raven.

Neistadt, M. E., McAuley, D., Zecha, D., & Shannon, R. (1993). An analysis of a board game as a treatment activity. *American Journal of Occupational Therapy, 47*, 154–160.

Nelson, D., & Jebson-Thomas, J. (2003). Occupational form, occupational performance, and a conceptual framework for therapeutic occupation. In P. Kramer, J. Hinojosa, & C. Brasic Royeen (Eds), *Perspectives in human occupation: Participation in life.* (pp. 87–155). Philadelphia: Lippincott Williams & Wilkins.

Payne, R. K., DeVol, P., & Smith, T. D. (2001). *Bridges out of poverty: Strategies for Professionals and Communities* (revised edition). Highland, TX: Aha Process Inc.

Peloquin, S. M. (1995). The fullness of empathy: Reflections and illustrations. *American Journal of Occupational Therapy, 49*, 24–31.

Peloquin, S. M. (2005). Embracing our ethos: Reclaiming our heart. The 2005 Eleanor Clarke Slagle Lecture. *American Journal of Occupational Therapy, 59*, 611–625.

Peloquin, S. M. (2007). A reconsideration of occupational therapy's core values: The issue is. *American Journal of Occupational Therapy, 61*, 474–478.

Pierce, D. (2001). Untangling occupation and activity. *American Journal of Occupational Therapy, 55*, 138–146.

Polatajko, H. J., Mandich, A., & Martini, R. (2000). Dynamic performance analysis: A framework for understanding occupational performance. *American Journal of Occupational Therapy, 54*, 65–72.

Reed, K. L. (2005). An annotated history of the concepts used in occupational therapy. In C. H. Christiansen, C. M. Baum, and J. Bass-Haugen (Eds.), *Occupational therapy: Performance, participation, and well-being* (3rd ed., pp. 571–626). Thorofare, NJ: SLACK.

Rogoff, B. (2003). *The cultural nature of human development.* New York: Oxford University Press.

Rogoff, B., Goodman Turkanis, C., & Bartlett, L. (Eds.), (2001). *Learning together: Children and adults in a school community.* New York: Oxford University Press.

Schell, B. A., & Cervero, R. M. (1993). Clinical reasoning in occupational therapy: An integrative review. *American Journal of Occupational Therapy, 47*, 605–610.

Schell, B. A. (2008). Pragmatic reasoning. In B. A. B. Schell & J. W. Schell (Eds). *Clinical and professional reasoning in occupational therapy.* (pp. 169–187). Philadelphia, PA: Wolters Kluwer/Lippincott Williams & Wilkins.

Spear, P. S., & Crepeau, E. B. (2003). Glossary. In E. B. Crepeau, E. S. Cohn, & B. A. B. Schell, (Eds.). *Willard & Spackman's occupational therapy* (10th ed.; pp. 1025–1035). Philadelphia: Lippincott Williams & Wilkins

Trombly Latham, C. A. (2008). Conceptual foundations for practice. In M. V. Radomski & C. A. Trombly Latham (Eds.) *Occupational therapy for physical dysfunction* (6th ed., pp. 1–20). Baltimore: Lippincott Williams & Wilkins.

Trombly, C. A. (1995). Occupation, purposefulness and meaningfulness as therapeutic mechanisms. [Eleanor Clarke Slagle Lecture]. *American Journal of Occupational Therapy, 49,* 960–972.

Principles of Learning and Behavior Change

PERRI STERN

36

Learning Objectives

After reading this chapter, you will be able to:

1. Identify and describe five theories of learning: behaviorist, social cognitive, constructivist, self–efficacy, and motivational
2. Compare the essential elements and assumptions of each theory of learning
3. Explain how different theories of learning contribute to occupational therapy intervention

INTRODUCTION

♦ Julia, an inquisitive 4-year-old girl, attends the Plymouth Community Preschool. She is very talkative, friendly, and interested in most activities. However, Julia frequently takes toys from other children during free play activities. Julia's behavior causes the other children great distress, and Julia gets a lot of negative attention for her actions.

♦ Jake is a 14-year-old boy who struggles with school. For many years, he had poor school performance and was constantly told by his teachers and parents, "If you would only try harder, you'd do fine" and "We know you are smart. Why don't you work to your potential?" Over the years, Jake developed a sense of his school performance and his mental abilities as "not good enough."

♦ John, a 37-year-old man, attends a community independent living center in Boston. He has several goals, one of which is to improve his ability to organize and structure his daily self-care, productivity, and leisure occupations. A solitary person by nature, John is somewhat anxious about his ability to be successful in the program.

In addition to the situations described above, think of the many things you may have taught to different people. Perhaps you taught a younger sibling how to share toys; a friend how to navigate a bus or subway system; grandparents how to keep track of their medicines; a classmate how to organize information and prepare for an important test; a son or daughter how to overcome a fear or anxiety; yourself a new art, craft, or leisure activity. How did you decide *how* to teach the person? Why did you teach the skill or behavior *in a particular way?* What *strategies* did you use? *What beliefs about how people learn guided you in your selection of strategies?* In your efforts to teach others, you have most likely developed a beginning set of beliefs about how people learn best.

This chapter presents an overview of selected *theories of learning.* In general, "learning theories" explain a perspective on what is "knowing" and how a person "comes to know" (Fosnot, 1996, p. ix). Five different overall ways of thinking about and conceptualizing theories of learning are reviewed in this chapter: behaviorist, social cognitive, constructivist, self–efficacy, and motivational. There are many other theories of learning, but these five are all relevant to occupational therapy.

> Learning theories explain a perspective on what is "knowing" and how a person "comes to know."

WHY SHOULD OCCUPATIONAL THERAPISTS STUDY THEORIES OF LEARNING?

Suinicki (2004) identified several reasons to study theories of learning. Many of these are relevant to occupational therapists. Box 36.1 summarizes six important reasons for occupational therapy practitioners to study theories of learning.

- Theory provides an overall *foundation for practice* in all areas of practice. People often come to occupational therapy because they want to learn new ways of doing what is important to them, and occupational therapy practitioners help people to change behaviors so that they can engage in meaningful occupations. Theory provides the basis for designing specific interventions to address client issues.
- Theory *guides* and *informs* practice. Theory provides us with a conceptual framework related to observations of

human behavior. Theories offer guidance about what to observe and answer questions about how best to facilitate behavior change.

- Theory presents an organizing framework of ideas about how people learn that leads to questions that can be tested in practice—in other words, *research.* Asking and answering questions about occupational therapy practice through research is a core responsibility for all occupational therapy practitioners.
- The primary goal of occupational therapy is to help people function in their daily occupations. Interventions may be designed, suggested, and implemented in many different ways. Practitioners who understand different perspectives on how people learn are likely to be more *effective* at presenting a range of interventions that match their clients' learning needs and learning styles. And when problems do arise, it is important to be able to analyze why the intervention may not be working. Understanding theories of learning will help you to *solve problems* that emerge during intervention and generate new approaches when an intervention strategy is not effective.
- Each client with whom you work will have different values, interests, needs, abilities, and preferred ways of learning. Understanding theories of learning will help you to design *individualized* and *creative* interventions that respond to each client's unique strengths and limitations.
- Occupational therapy practice should always be moving forward; it is not static. Neither is theory. Ongoing exploration of theory and theory development is a *professional responsibility* of all occupational therapy practitioners.

Theories of learning serve several other purposes. At perhaps the most basic level, they provide us with a way to organize vast amounts of knowledge that is used in practice. Theory helps us to put our knowledge together, to organize otherwise random knowledge into a cohesive set of ideas that explains some phenomenon—in this case, learning. Theories of learning enable us to see how interesting and complex even the most seemingly simple things can be. This does not mean that theory makes things more *complicated.* Rather, theory helps you to see that there is usually more to any teaching-learning situation than meets the eye. Learning theories can explain how people gather and interpret information and then determine how, if at all, information is meaningful, relevant, and memorable to their life circumstances. Theories of learning reflect beliefs about how people think and how they store and use information (Suinicki, 2004). And "since most human behavior is learned, investigating the principles of learning will help us understand why we behave as we do. An awareness of the learning process will not only allow greater understanding of normal and adaptive behavior, but will also allow greater understand-

---

BOX 36.1	**REASONS TO STUDY THEORIES OF LEARNING**

1. Provides a foundation for practice
2. Guides and informs practice
3. Leads to researchable questions
4. Enhances practitioners' effectiveness and ability to solve problems
5. Promotes individualized and creative interventions
6. Core professional responsibility

ing of the circumstances that produce maladaptive and abnormal behavior" (Hergenhahn, 1976, p. 12). In any intervention situation, practitioners need to understand the reason or reasons that contribute to problematic behavior.

WHERE TO BEGIN?

What is learning? How do we know when someone is learning? Under what conditions does learning occur? Why does learning occur? What does the learner do to cause the learning? What are the outcomes of learning? The answer to all of these questions is "it depends." It depends because different learning theories attribute different causes, reasons, actions, and circumstances to learning.

BEHAVIORIST THEORY

Behaviorist theory focuses on how observable, tangible behaviors are learned in response to some environmental stimulation (Ormrod, 1990). Behaviorist theorists focus on observable events rather than mental processes. For example, how does a child learn to take turns while playing a game with friends, how might a person with a developmental disability learn to respond appropriately in a conversation, and how would a person learn to propel and navigate a wheelchair in an urban community? In these examples, the observable events are the child waiting for and taking his or her turn during a game of kickball, a person waiting for a conversation partner to finish speaking before providing new information, and a person successfully navigating the urban community in a wheelchair. The overall emphasis in behavioral theories of learning is on the relationship between an environmental stimulus and a behavioral response and on how learning is indicated by an observed change in behavior.

What Are the Essential Elements and Assumptions of Behaviorist Learning Theory?

Behaviorists use the term *conditioning* to explain changes in behavior rather than learning, as behaviorist theory assert that a person's behavior is conditioned by events in the environment. A behavior is gradually shaped, changed, and molded as it reflects the environment's response to the behavior. There are several key terms that you will notice in most types of behavioral theory: **conditioning** (designing situations that increase or decrease the likelihood of a behavior being performed), **stimulus** (something that prompts a behavior), **response** (the reaction to the stimulus), **shaping** (a strategy to develop closer and closer approximations of a behavior), **punishment** (response to an undesired behavior), and **reinforce-**

ment (something that causes a behavior to be strengthened and performed again).

Many well-known theorists have contributed to the development of the behavioral perspective, such as Ivan Pavlov (1849–1936), Edward Thorndike (1874–1949), John Watson (1878–1958), and Burrhus Frederic (B. F.) Skinner (1904–1990). Although their theories are slightly different from each other, they do share common assumptions about the nature of learning, chiefly the need to focus on external, observable events as evidence of learning (Ormrod, 1990).

Ivan Pavlov developed the theory of *classical conditioning*, which resulted from his initial studies of a dog's salivation response to a *neutral stimulus*, then to a neutral stimulus plus an *unconditioned stimulus*, and finally to a *conditioned stimulus*. As a result of his experiments and observations, Pavlov concluded that changes in behavior (learning) are due to *experience*.

Thorndike's perspective is known as *connectionism*, whereby learning is seen as a process of making connections between things, understanding the relationship of a stimulus to a response. Thorndike studied how people established those connections and therefore how people developed and maintained behaviors. He emphasized the role of practice and experience in strengthening or weakening the connections between a stimulus and a response. Through a series of experiments, Thorndike concluded that the learning of a behavior is elicited by the consequences of the behavior. So responses to a behavior that were followed by a satisfying experience would be rewarded, thus strengthening the connection, the neural bond between the stimulus and the response, and increasing the likelihood that the behavior would be produced again. He originally thought that responses that were followed by discomfort or dissatisfying experiences would be weakened and eventually stop; but he revised that and deemphasized the role of punishment. Instead, Thorndike believed that punishment would have an indirect effect on learning—that as a result of some dissatisfying response from the environment, an organism would engage in some other behavior.

Watson introduced the term *behaviorism*. He emphasized the importance of focusing on observable behaviors. Watson was greatly influenced by the work of Pavlov. As he expanded on Pavlov's work, Watson proposed two "laws" that explained the relationship between stimulus and response and ultimately how behavior is learned. Watson proposed that "the more frequently a stimulus and response occur in association with each other, the stronger that Stimulus-Response habit will become" (Ormrod, 1990, p. 20). This was termed the *Law of Frequency*. Watson also proposed that "the response that has most recently occurred after a particular stimulus is the response most likely to be associated with that stimulus" (Ormrod, 1990, p. 20). This was termed the *Law of Recency*.

B. F. Skinner was influenced by both Pavlov and Watson. He coined the term **operant conditioning**. Skinner's basic principle was that a response followed by some reinforcement is likely to be strengthened. And since a response is a change in behavior, then from a behaviorist perspective, this indicates learning. Any behavior, positive or negative, can be reinforced.

Skinner used the term *reinforcement* rather than *reward* for two reasons. First, he believed that the term *reward* implies something pleasant or desirable, but sometimes people intentionally do things to produce an unpleasant consequence (e.g., a person might do something to make another person angry because the first person enjoys watching the second person get angry). Second, the terms *reward, pleasant,* and *desirable* are highly subjective terms. Behaviorists such as Skinner preferred to keep things objective and scientific.

There are three important conditions for operant conditioning. First, the reinforcement must follow, not precede the response. Second, the reinforcement should immediately follow the behavior. Otherwise, the reinforcement will have less effect. Third, the reinforcement must be contingent on the response; it should not be given for an unintended or unrelated response.

How is operant conditioning different from classical conditioning? In classical conditioning, there is an unconditioned stimulus and a conditioned stimulus. The conditioned stimulus brings about the conditioned response. The response is automatic and involuntary. In operant conditioning, a response is *followed by* a reinforcing stimulus. The response is *voluntary.* The organism has control over whether it emits the response. For example, operant conditioning would be illustrated when John, the 37-year-old man attending a community independent living center, receives praise and enthusiasm when he attends the center. As a result, John attends the center much more regularly.

Occupational Therapy and Behaviorist Theory

Occupational therapy practitioners using behaviorist theory to understand human learning and guide their intervention would analyze a complex behavior that needs to be learned (e.g., Julia's need to take turns when she plays) and sequence that behavior from simple to complex. Intervention would consist of opportunities for the person to participate in increasingly complex behaviors, using behaviorist principles such as reinforcement, shaping, and reward. Progress would be measured by clients' observed occupational performance and their ability to complete increasingly complex behaviors necessary for occupational performance.

Occupational therapy practitioners have used the behavioral theory of learning in several ways to guide their interventions with clients. For example, Giles and Wilson (1988) and Giles, Ridley, Dill, and Frye (1997) described

programs to help retrain people who had sustained severe brain injuries. The clients had severe physical and cognitive impairments and needed help with washing and dressing, basic self-care behaviors. The practitioners designed and implemented a program that consisted of individualized plans to break down each larger activity (getting dressed) into its smaller elements. Practitioners used a specific set of instructions to gradually add skills to each person's repertoire and eventually teach the entire behavior.

Katzmann and Mix (1994) presented a case report of a 34-year-old woman with viral encephalitis. The woman had difficulty processing written and verbal information and had great difficulty with various complex self-care tasks. The practitioners' intervention was influenced by behavioral theories, using such techniques as prompting with step-by-step instructions, shaping, and verbal or physical cues. The practitioners identified and sequenced all of the steps required for the woman to complete her washing, dressing, and grooming routine, which began with getting out of bed and ended with going to breakfast in the rehabilitation facility. A series of step-by-step instructions, gradual and consistent shaping of behavior, verbal cues, and physical assistance helped the woman to improve her overall ADL functioning. The practitioners cued the woman with directions or provided physical assistance for a step that needed to be completed and gradually removed the cues as she initiated and completed the task independently.

Behaviorist theories emphasize observable behavior, rewarding and reinforcing desirable behavior and reducing problematic behaviors. Clients who might benefit from intervention approaches that are grounded in behaviorist theories of learning include people who have difficulty planning and organizing activities, those who have problems with memory and/or attention, those who have deficits in sequencing activities, and those who demonstrate inappropriate social behaviors. Some strategies that could help Julia to develop sharing and turn-taking skill include praising appropriate behavior (to provide reinforcement for sharing), not giving attention every time she takes toys from others (to decrease the reinforcement for the undesired behavior), using a sticker chart to document sharing (to gradually shape appropriate behavior), and providing rewards to Julia for good sharing, such as letting her stand first in line to go to the playground.

SOCIAL LEARNING AND SOCIAL COGNITIVE THEORY

The social learning and social cognitive theory of learning are an outgrowth of behaviorist theories. Theorists such as Piaget (1970) and Bandura (1977a) were dissatisfied with the limits of behaviorist theory, because they believed that there was more to learning than just the interaction of a person with the environment. They developed theories of learning that integrated behavioral, social, and cognitive processes. Although there are individual variations and areas of focus, in general social cognitive theory explains learning as occurring in a social context, that is, the "where, what, when, with whom, how often, and under what circumstances" aspects of our lives. Humans learn by observing others, cognitively processing observations, storing those observations and thoughts, and then using them, sometimes at a much later time. This is an important contrast with behaviorists, who view learning as an observable change in behavior. Social learning/social cognitive theorists disagree and say that *learning can occur even in the absence of an observable change in behavior.* Social and cognitive processes such as observation, storing observations in memory, self–assessment, and appraisal promote learning. The interactions between a person, behavior, and the environment are emphasized.

Five major assumptions are inherent to social learning/social cognitive theory (Ormrod, 2006). First, *people can learn by observing others.* Second, *learning is an internal process.* Learning itself might or might not lead to an observable change in behavior. For example, people might observe various social skills, such as how to introduce themselves to someone they meet, how to end a conversation politely, and how to maintain an appropriate social distance during a conversation. These skills might be stored in memory for future use and not be immediately demonstrated. Third, people are generally *motivated to achieve goals* for themselves, and their behavior is typically directed toward those goals. Fourth, social cognitive theories assert that instead of learning being a direct response to and dependent on environmental stimuli, learning occurs as *people regulate and adjust their own behavior.* This means that people would observe others, determine their own individual standard, and then work to behave according to those standards. Fifth, feedback via reinforcement and punishment affect learning and behavior *indirectly* (not directly, as the behaviorists believe). This means that people can adjust their behavior on the basis of the *anticipated* (positive or negative) consequences. Or people might observe the outcomes of a behavior that is demonstrated by others and adjust their behaviors on the basis of that observation. (Ormrod, 2006). Box 36.2 summarizes these major assumptions.

It is important for a person to observe skills and behaviors via models and to note the reinforcement that models receive for behaviors. Models can be *live,* that is, a person with whom the learner has actual contact, or *symbolic,* some pictorial or abstract representation of behavior, such as through television or other media. Whatever the source, the modeled behavior serves as information to the observer/learner. A person can also learn *vicariously,* increasing or decreasing a given behavior on the basis of the reinforcement that the person observes someone else receiving. If a behavior is positively reinforced, the observer might increase that behavior. If the behavior is negatively rein-

> ### BOX 36.2 MAJOR ASSUMPTIONS OF SOCIAL COGNITIVE THEORY OF LEARNING
>
> - People can learn by observing others.
> - Learning is an internal process.
> - People are motivated to achieve goals.
> - People regulate and adjust their own behavior.
> - Reinforcement and punishment may have an indirect effect on behavior.

forced, the observer might decrease that behavior. Other determining factors include how much attention gets paid to the model, how credible or prestigious the model is, and how the model is rewarded (Ormrod, 2006).

Because people can learn by observing others, *attention* is a very important factor. A learner is more likely to remember information when the learner consciously attends to the behavior, rehearses it in his or her own mind, and develops personal verbal or visual ways to represent the information for future use (Ormrod, 1990). A person should be able to describe the behavior or have a picture of that behavior in his or her mind, stored for future use.

People develop expectations about what they think will happen as a result of different behaviors. Thus, *incentive* is an important consideration. Incentive is the anticipation that something will happen (reinforcement) if a particular behavior is performed or not performed. This is another difference from behaviorist theory. According to operant conditioning theory, the reinforcement comes after the behavior has been performed. In social cognitive theory, an anticipated outcome might precede the behavior being performed (or not performed).

An occupational therapy practitioner working with Jake, the 14-year-old who is having difficulty at school, might have Jake *identify* specific problem situations (e.g., being distracted in class, using minimal effort to complete projects, or becoming bored in class) and then identify specific strategies to address these difficulties (e.g., sitting at the front of the classroom, setting "effort goals" for himself, identifying at least one interesting aspect of any project), *set* manageable and measurable goals, and then *develop* a mechanism to determine how well he had achieved his goals. The occupational therapy practitioner might also encourage Jake's teacher to pair him with classmates who demonstrate good study habits and who are highly motivated for learning. Or the practitioner might role-play conversations that Jake is likely to have with his parents or teachers about his feelings and attitudes toward schoolwork. The role-play conversations could help Jake to articulate his concerns and then work to support his learning.

A variety of occupational therapy intervention programs have incorporated aspects of social learning theories.

Jao and Lu (1999) studied the effects of a problem-solving intervention on the interpersonal skills of people with chronic schizophrenia. They found that helping people with schizophrenia to recognize and define problems, think of alternative solutions, and determine the best course of action facilitated the development of interpersonal problem-solving skills.

Stern (1991) described a psychoeducation treatment program on a research unit for people with schizophrenia. Here, clients participated in a series of weekly intervention groups that were based on the assumption that behavior that departs from social norms is the result of a person's unsuccessful attempts to cope with environmental demands and that skill deficits are primarily a result of insufficient or unavailable opportunities for social learning. Clients attended groups to help them develop skills for managing time, stress, money, and their own personal care.

Most of these programs emphasize the importance of learning in a social context, providing numerous opportunities for clients to develop or relearn essential skills for living, and employ activities such as role-play, observation, problem solving, and practice in real-life situations.

CONSTRUCTIVIST THEORY

Suppose you are an occupational therapy practitioner working in a community independent living center. Your clients are typically recovering from substance abuse or might have chronic mental illness. Part of your intervention includes a series of Life Skills sessions that are designed to help people learn or relearn different instrumental activities of daily living. A new session will begin next week with five new clients. One segment of your program focuses on time use and leisure planning. Will all of the five clients come to the course with the same life experiences? Will all of the five people have the same outlook on life? How might you understand the teaching-learning process, given these individual differences and experiences?

A constructivist would assert that individual differences are to be expected, that "everyone's construction of the world is unique even though we share a great many concepts" (Suinicki, 2004, p. 14). Although there are several "traditional" methods of providing information, such as through imparting information or finding information in books or on the Internet, this does not necessarily indicate or result in learning, according to constructivism. For constructivists, the learner must *access* information, use this information to *alter* or modify existing knowledge and understanding, and *integrate* the new information with previous information to *create* a new understanding that is relevant to himself or herself (Marlowe & Page, 1998). For the Life Skills challenge posed above, a constructivist would embrace the members' different perspectives and perceive them as essential to individual learning.

There are some basic assumptions about the teaching-learning process that are common to constructivism: First, learners must be *active participants* in their learning. Second, the learner is capable of *creating* his or her own *knowledge* through interaction with the human and non-human environment. Third, when learners participate in this type of learning environment, they develop the *ability to think critically* to solve problems. Fourth, when actively engaged in constructing their own knowledge, people *gather information and develop strategies* at the same time (Marlowe & Page, 1998).

Bruner (1961) has had a major influence in the development of constructivism or "discovery" learning. According to Bruner (1961), a constructivist approach fosters *intellectual potency,* meaning that when people seek and find information for themselves, that information is more meaningful, relevant, and powerful for them. Furthermore, people organize information they find for themselves so that it is more efficiently and effectively retrieved for future use. Second, since the learners "own" the information, this approach fosters *intrinsic motivation.* Rather than settling into a pattern in which learners conform to what the instructor wants them to learn, learners *discover* for themselves. This promotes motivation to learn. Third, the only way to improve one's ability to think, question, and discover is to do it, actively and repeatedly; to engage in the process. Constructivism fosters people's learning the *process of discovery.* Finally, when people learn and discover for themselves, they also organize, categorize, and store that information in ways that are personally meaningful. Such information is more easily accessed when needed. Constructivists call this a *conservation of memory.* Box 36.3 summarizes the major assumptions of constructivism.

A practitioner who utilizes a constructivist approach in the teaching-learning process emphasizes skills and activities such as asking questions, independent exploration, identifying problems, brainstorming, and generating individual solutions to problems. The practitioner emphasizes the *client's essential role in the process* and sees his or her own role as facilitating clients' progress. The practitioner views the therapy process as recognizing, embracing, respecting, and encouraging people to develop individual meanings, to promote and enhance the client's knowledge and skill.

In this perspective, clients are expected to actively direct what needs to be learned and how the learning will occur. Clients help to determine the resources that will enhance their learning. Independent thinking, collaborative problem solving, and using past experience to reframe and revise new learning are all important. The practitioner's knowledge and expertise are still very important; however, in this perspective, the practitioner uses his or her knowledge and expertise as a point of reference. In many ways, the practitioner takes a "back seat" as the client pursues learning; the practitioner's role is to address problems that arise. The practitioner facilitates the process, using himself or herself to promote the client's ability to identify, address, and solve problems.

BOX 36.3

MAJOR ASSUMPTIONS OF CONSTRUCTIVIST THEORY OF LEARNING

- Learners must be active participants in their learning.
- Learners are capable of discovering and creating their own knowledge.
- Active participation in the learning environment enhances critical thinking and problem-solving abilities.
- Active participation in the learning environment enhances the meaning and relevance of the learning experience and motivation for learning.
- In learning, people gather information and develop problem-solving strategies simultaneously.

Constructivism "allows for multiple perspectives to emerge and new solutions to arise synergistically. The role of teacher shifts from one of directing and controlling learning to that of facilitating change" (Lederer, 2000, p. 84). Rather than being viewed as the expert and the person who will recommend a particular intervention or plan of action, the practitioner facilitates discovery and meaning, discussion, and problem solving. The occupational therapy practitioner does not provide "the intervention" but instead works to facilitate the person's developing his or her own strategies to deal with his or her own issues. The practitioner is alert to major issues but is neither prescriptive nor directive.

PRACTICE DILEMMA

CONSTRUCTIVIST PERSPECTIVE ON LEARNING

If each person constructs his or her own learning and therefore there is no "objective reality," what challenges does that present to an occupational therapy practitioner who advocates a constructivist perspective on learning? What opportunities does it provide to the practitioner and/or to the person with whom the practitioner is working? What are some strategies that you could implement to address clients' time use and leisure skill development in the Life Skills program described earlier?

SELF-EFFICACY THEORY

The self-efficacy theory of learning focuses on a person's individual beliefs about how effective he or she is or will be at learning or completing a new skill or behavior. Albert Bandura (1977b) first articulated a theory of self-efficacy. His perspective on how behaviors are learned and changed involved behavioral *and* cognitive processes. His central thesis is that a person's **efficacy expectations**, the person's beliefs about how successful or unsuccessful he or she will be at performing a skill or occupation, will greatly influence their execution of that skill or occupation. The emphasis here is on the *person's beliefs* and *how those beliefs influence their performance.* For example, a person might believe that a particular action performed or executed by a person *in general* will produce a certain outcome. However this is different from the person's belief that he or she has the ability to perform the action and that it will result in a successful outcome. A person's efficacy expectations also influence the person's *persistence* with different occupations. "Efficacy expectations determine how much effort people will expend and how long they will persist in the face of obstacles and aversive experiences. The stronger the perceived self efficacy, the more active the efforts" (Bandura, 1997b, p. 194).

Efficacy expectations have three important dimensions: magnitude, generality, and strength (Bandura, 1977b). *Magnitude* involves the level of difficulty for a task—for example, making a sandwich versus making an elaborate dinner or writing an outline versus writing a lengthy research paper. *Generality* involves the degree to which a person's perceived self-efficacy for one task transfers to another—for example, maneuvering a wheelchair around the occupational therapy clinic versus maneuvering a wheelchair in a busy urban community or making a sandwich at the occupational therapy clinic versus making a sandwich at home. *Strength* refers to the degree to which people believe they can be successful—for example, being very, very confident and having strong beliefs about one's success versus being only slightly confident or uncertain about the likelihood of success.

Typically, a person's self-efficacy is developed over time and through four sources of information: outcomes that were generated by the person's own *personal accomplishments;* through *vicarious experience,* that is, seeing others perform a skill and through that vicarious experience believing that "if the other person can accomplish the skill so can I"; by being *persuaded* by others that the person can be successful; and by *feeling calm and relaxed* when performing a skill (Bandura, 1997b). Which of those four elements has the strongest effect? Personal accomplishment. Although a person might perform a task successfully as observed by an outsider or through feedback from the environment, the person's *own cognitive appraisal* of how successful or unsuccessful he or she was will greatly affect the person's efficacy expectation. Vicarious experience, persuasion, and a calm feeling are all helpful, but none are as strong as a person's actual success in performing a skill (Bandura, 1997b).

The power of a person's beliefs about his or her skills and abilities is an important point. As Gage and Polatajko (1994) noted,

> Therapists often try to convince clients that they are able to go home and live independently, or return to work, only to be confronted with a barrage of reasons why the client is not yet ready. These patients are labeled as fearful or, worse yet, as malingerers. Perhaps it is simply their perceived self efficacy for home management or work activities that has not yet reached the level necessary to engage the activity independently. If one accepts that persuasion is the least influential method of raising efficacy expectations, then the therapist must devise new intervention techniques. (p. 460)

Although the two concepts are related, perceived self-efficacy is not the same as self-esteem. Perceived self-efficacy is what you believe you can do with your skill. Self-esteem refers to a person's negative or positive sense of self. So a person might feel that he or she is competent and successful in completing a variety of occupations but might have an overall negative feeling about himself or herself. Certainly, perceived self-efficacy might contribute to a person's self-esteem, but they are two separate concepts (Gage and Polatajko, 1994).

According to Bandura (1997a), self-efficacy relates to behavior change very directly. If a person has only weak expectations for his or her success, it is likely that unsuccessful experiences will quickly result in the person's not performing the skill or behavior. If the person's beliefs about his or her success are strong, then it is likely that the person will persist, even through negative or unsuccessful experiences.

PRACTICE DILEMMA

PROMOTING SELF-EFFICACY

Core principles of occupational therapy, such as using strengths to overcome limitations, and person-centered intervention, are very consistent with developing and promoting self-efficacy. And according to Gage & Polatajko (1994), "the most effective means of enhancing perceived self-efficacy is deemed to be through performance based procedures" (p. 452). At the beginning of this chapter, you read about Jake and his difficulties at school. How might you understand his situation from the perspective of self-efficacy theories? What are some strategies that might be helpful to Jake?

MOTIVATIONAL THEORY

Prochaska, Norcross, and DiClemente (1992) propose a *transtheoretical stage theory* of how people learn to change behaviors. The term *transtheoretical* refers to the integration of several different theories from the disciplines of psychology and psychotherapy. Prochaska and his colleagues have applied their transtheoretical theory of change to a variety of health behaviors and systems issues, such as smoking cessation (Prochaska & DiClemente, 1983), addressing health risk behaviors (Nigg et al., 1999), arthritis self-management (Keefe et al., 2000), organizational change (Prochaska, Prochaska, & Levesque, 2001), and weight control (Sarkin, Johnson, Prochaska, & Prochaska, 2001). This model has two essential elements: the five integrated *stages* of change and the various *processes* that can facilitate a person's moving from one stage to the next.

The stages of change begin with *precontemplation*. Here, a person might have a behavior that is perceived by others to be harmful or destructive (e.g., a substance use or addiction, poorly controlled anger or stress, or general health and wellness issues). The person might be unaware or minimally aware of his or her problem, or the person might be aware of the problem but resistant to fully acknowledging or addressing it. A person who has progressed to the second stage, *contemplation,* is likely to be aware of his or her problem and is thinking about overcoming it but is not quite ready to take action. When a person begins to make some small changes in his or her behavior, the person has progressed to the third stage, *preparation.* The fourth stage is *action.* This is when the most substantive change occurs. The person is putting forth great energy to modify behaviors, the environment, or his or her experiences to effect serious change. The fifth stage is *maintenance.* Here, the person works to sustain accomplishments and prevent relapse (Prochaska, Norcross, & DiClemente, 1992).

These stages might appear to be linear, occurring in a step-by-step progression from one stage to the next. However, Prochaska, Norcross, and DiClemente (1992) explain change as occurring in a spiral fashion, because most people experience relapses or other setbacks as they work to change behaviors. Have you or a friend set out to change a certain behavior and achieved stage three (preparation) or stage four (action) only to experience some setback and spiral back down to an earlier stage? According to Prochaska's theory, this is common and to be expected.

The *processes* of change, the second part of Prochaska's theory, explain *how* to promote the shifts. According to Prochaska, Norcross, and DiClemente, (1992), people who have reached the contemplation stage are ready to understand the processes that can contribute to behavioral change. Their research indicates that people who are in the precontemplation stage lack the awareness to engage in or benefit from the processes of change. People who have progressed to the contemplation stage may benefit from *consciousness-raising* strategies that help them to get information about their problem and themselves, by being encouraged to express their feelings about their problems through various *dramatic relief* strategies such as role-playing, and by *environmental reevaluation* to assess how their behavior affects their physical and social surroundings (e.g., perhaps a person's smoking deters family or friends from visiting or there are stains and cigarette burns on the person's furnishings). Strategies such as values clarification exercises to enhance *self-reevaluation,* or how one thinks and feels about himself or herself, can be helpful as one moves to the preparation stage. Making a real commitment to change, believing in one's ability to change, and using techniques such as personal goal setting to enhance *self-liberation* or will power can be helpful during the action stage. Several processes are important in the maintenance stage, such as fostering *helping relationships* and social supports that encourage the person to be open and honest about his or her problems, avoiding things that elicit the problem behavior and substituting alternatives (*stimulus control* and *counterconditioning*), and *reinforcement management,* rewarding oneself for making changes. *Social liberation* helps to promote change across various stages through advocacy, empowerment, and social change mechanisms (Prochaska, Norcross, & DiClemente, 1992).

The key to success for this model is the careful, systematic, and close fit between the person, the stage, and the process. According to Prochaska, Norcross, and DiClemente, (1992), "efficient self-change depends on doing the right things (processes) at the right time (stages)" (p. 1110). Table 36.1 summarizes Prochaska, Norcross, & DiClemente's (1992) stages and processes of change.

OCCUPATIONAL THERAPY, SELF–EFFICACY THEORY, AND MOTIVATIONAL THEORY

Both self-efficacy theories and motivational theories have great relevance for occupational therapy. Often, a person's self-perceptions and beliefs about his or her ability to be successful with an occupation influence the person's decision about whether to participate in that occupation. For example, a person who believes that he or she has good interview skills will be more likely to respond to a job advertisement even though he or she might not have direct experience with the type of work that needs to be done. A person who did not have that sense of effectiveness might be less likely to pursue the job. Intervention strategies to promote a person's perceived self-efficacy in the job interview situation described here would include determining with the person that he or she had all the requisite skills to be successful, using peer role models so that the person could practice or "try on" the essential skills and behaviors, having the person practice interview skills, providing feedback on specific successes, and encouraging the person to evaluate his or her skills in a personal way rather than comparing these skills to someone else's. These theories all emphasize the importance of an individual's participation in *meaningful* occupations as both the foundation and result of motivation and self-efficacy.

Gage, Noh, Polatajko, and Kaspar (1994) developed an assessment that could be helpful to occupational therapists. Their assessment, the Perceived Self Efficacy Gauge, evaluates perceived self-efficacy of adults who have physical disabilities and identifies changes in a person's perceived self-efficacy over time. It promotes the belief that "clients with greater confidence in their ability to regain their usual level of competence for daily activities are less likely to develop hopeless feelings" (Gage, Noh, Polatajko, & Kaspar 1994, p. 785).

Ehrenberg, Cox, and Koopman (1991) studied the relationship between perceived self-efficacy and depression in adolescents. "Perception of self-efficacy can be critical to adolescent development, especially in regard to academic performance, social competence, career choice and physical confidence" (p. 363). Ehrenberg, Cox, and Koopman (1991) learned that adolescents with higher levels of perceived self-efficacy had less depression than did adolescents who had lower levels of perceived self-efficacy.

TABLE 36.1   STAGES AND PROCESSES OF CHANGE

Stage	Process (How to Promote Change)
Precontemplation	Strategies are not effective, as the person lacks awareness to engage in or benefit from change
Contemplation	Consciousness-raising strategies to learn about problem, role-play strategies to express feelings, assessment of how behavior affects physical and social environment
Preparation	Values clarification exercises to promote reevaluation of feelings or self-perception
Action	Goal-setting strategies and techniques
Maintenance	Development of social supports, substitution of alternatives to problem behavior, avoidance of experiences that elicit the problem behavior, rewarding oneself for making changes

CASE STUDY: *Olivia: Behavior Change*

Olivia, a 55-year-old woman has always been severely overweight. Over the years, she has tried many different diets and has joined (and quit) numerous exercise programs and groups. After a recent episode of chest pain, Olivia's health care provider strongly recommended that she participate in organized nutrition, exercise, and overall health-promotion activities.

> How might you help Olivia to understand and reflect on her challenges with health and wellness issues over the years through the transtheoretical perspective?
>
> What stage might she be at currently?
>
> How might you help her move from one stage to the next?
>
> How might you work to minimize any setbacks to the process and remedy those setbacks when they occur?

Strategies might include the following:

> The occupational therapy practitioner would work with Olivia to help her understand the processes of change. Their work together would include helping Olivia to understand how change occurs, the spiraling nature of change, and the natural, to-be-expected gains and setbacks that occur.
>
> The occupational therapy practitioner would use counseling and discussion to encourage Olivia's conscious reflection on her behavior and recognition of the different stages of change. Olivia's current stage could be seen as preparation.
>
> A variety of intervention strategies, such as personal goal setting, developing social supports, creating a self-reward system for positive change or progress, and evaluation and reevaluation of progress, could be suggested.
>
> Olivia would also be encouraged to view earlier obstacles or setbacks to change as typical and predictable. When setbacks do occur, the occupational therapy practitioner would reinforce the importance of conscious understanding of the spiraling nature of progress, the success of identifying setbacks when they occur, the opportunity to prevent any setback from spiraling too far down, and a return to strategies that were successful in the past or continuing to develop new strategies. The occupational therapy practitioner would reinforce the ongoing nature of change and progress.

CONCLUSION

Behaviorist, social cognitive, constructivist, self-efficacy, and motivational theories of learning have great relevance and utility for occupational therapy practitioners. Table 36.2 summarizes the five different theories of learning that were presented in this chapter and highlights their relevance to occupational therapy practice. The information presented in this chapter can be used to influence how you think about the learning needs of patients and clients, to reinforce the importance of designing optimal learning environments, to contribute to your ongoing professional development, and to promote your clients' abilities to achieve their goals.

TABLE 36.2   SUMMARY TABLE

Theory	Major Emphases	Relevance to Occupational Therapy Practice
Behaviorist	◆ Learned behavior as an observable event (not a mental process) ◆ Behavior is conditioned by the environment ◆ Environmental response alters subsequent behaviors	◆ Analyze and sequence behaviors from simple to complex ◆ Measure progress as the person completes increasingly complex behaviors ◆ Use strategies including reinforcement, shaping, and rewards

TABLE 36.2   SUMMARY TABLE   *Continued*

Theory	Major Emphases	Relevance to Occupational Therapy Practice
Social learning/social cognitive	◆ Integrates behavior, social, and cognitive processes ◆ Learning occurs in a social context ◆ Learning may occur without observable behavior change ◆ Person regulates and adjusts his or her own behavior	◆ Emphasize client learning essential skills for living ◆ Use role-play, peer observation, role modeling, problem solving, and real-life practice activities to promote learning ◆ Encourage the client to identify the problem, set goals, develop a plan, evaluate outcomes
Constructivist	◆ Learner is an active participant in his or her own learning ◆ Learner creates/constructs knowledge through past experience and interaction with the environment ◆ Self-constructed knowledge has great meaning and relevance for the learner ◆ Self-constructed knowledge promotes the learner's motivation for learning	◆ Client actively directs what is to be learned and how learning will occur ◆ Use strategies including brainstorming, individual problem-solving, independent exploration, asking questions. ◆ Occupational therapist facilitates but does not direct the learning process
Self-efficacy	◆ Emphasize a person's beliefs about how effective he or she is or will be ◆ Efficacy expectations influence a person's persistence with an activity ◆ Efficacy expectations are influenced by the difficulty of the task, how well completing a task transfers to other situations, and the degree to which a person believes that he or she will be successful ◆ Self-efficacy is developed over time and through experience	◆ Personal accomplishment has the greatest effect ◆ Self-evaluation, personal appraisal are important ◆ Tasks should be challenging but not overwhelming, should be transferable to other situations ◆ Vicarious, observation experiences and/or persuasion to enhance the person's beliefs that he or she can be successful are less effective
Motivational	◆ Learning and change occurs in a spiral fashion. It is not linear. ◆ A person's readiness for change will influence the outcomes ◆ Relapses are common and to be expected	◆ Intervention processes must match behavior stage ◆ Intervention processes become increasingly active, self-directed and self-monitored

REFERENCES

Bandura, A. (1977a). *Social learning theory.* Upper Saddle River, NJ: Prentice Hall.

Bandura, A. (1977b). Self-efficacy: Toward a unifying theory of behavioral change. *Psychological Review, 84*(2), 191–215.

Bruner, J. S. (1961). The act of discovery. *Harvard Educational Review, 31*(1), 21–32.

Ehrenberg, M. F., Cox, D. N., & Koopman, R. F. (1991). The relationship between self-efficacy and depression in adolescents. *Adolescence, 26*(192), 361–374.

Fosnot, C. T. (Ed.). (1996) *Constructivism: Theory, perspectives and practice.* New York: Teachers College Press.

Gage, M., Noh, S., Polatajko, H. J., & Kaspar, V. (1994). Measuring perceived self-efficacy in occupational therapy. *American Journal of Occupational Therapy, 48,* 783–790.

Gage, M., & Polatajko, H. J. (1994). Enhancing occupational performance through an understanding of perceived self efficacy. *American Journal of Occupational Therapy, 48,* 452–461.

Giles, G. M., & Wilson, J. C. (1988). The use of behavioral techniques in functional skills training after severe brain injury. *American Journal of Occupational Therapy, 42,* 658–665.

Giles, G. M., Ridley, J. E., Dill, A., & Frye, S. C. (1997). A consecutive series of adults with brain injury treated with a washing and dressing retraining program. *American Journal of Occupational Therapy, 51,* 256–266.

Hergenhahn, B. R. (1976). *An introduction to theories of learning.* Englewood Cliffs, NJ: Prentice Hall.

Jao, H.-P. I., & Lu, S.-J. (1999). The acquisition of problem-solving skills through instruction in Siegel and Spivack's problem solving therapy for the chronic schizophrenic. *Occupational Therapy in Mental Health, 14*(4), 47–63.

Katzmann, S., & Mix, S. (1994). Improving functional independence in a patient with encephalitis through behavior modification shaping techniques. *American Journal of Occupational Therapy, 48,* 259–262.

Keefe, F. J., Lefebvre, J. C., Kerns, R. D., Rosenberg, R., Beaupre, P., Prochaska, J., Prochaska, J. O., & Caldwell, D. S. (2000). Understanding the adoption of arthritis self-management: Stages of change profiles among arthritis patients. *Pain, 87*(3), 303–313.

Lederer, J. M. (2000). The application of constructivism to concepts of occupation using a group process approach. *Occupational Therapy in Health Care, 13*(1), 81–93.

Marlowe, B. A., & Page, M. L. (1998). *Creating and sustaining the constructivist classroom.* Thousand Oaks, CA: Corwin Press/Sage.

Nigg, C. R., Burbank, P. M., Padula, C., Dufresne, R. Rossi, J. S., Velicer, W. F., LaForge, R. G., & Prochaska, J. O. (1999). Stages of change across ten health risk behaviors for older adults. *Gerontologist, 39*(4), 473–482.

Ormrod, J. E. (1990). *Human learning: Principles, theories and educational applications* (2nd ed.). New York: Macmillan.

Ormrod, J. E. (2006). *Educational psychology: Developing learners* (5th ed.). Upper Saddle River, NJ: Prentice Hall.

Piaget, J. (1970). Piaget's theory. In P. H. Mussen (Ed.), *Carmichael's Manual of Psychology.* New York: Wiley.

Prochaska, J. O., & DiClemente, C. C. (1983). Stages and processes of self change of smoking: Toward an integrative model of change. *Journal of Consulting and Clinical Psychology, 51*(3), 390–395.

Prochaska, J. O., Norcross, J. C., & DiClemente, C. C. (1992). In search of how people change: Applications to addictive behaviors. *American Psychologist, 47,* 1102–1113.

Prochaska, J. M., Prochaska, J. O., & Levesque, D. A. (2001). A transtheoretical approach to changing organizations. *Administration & Policy in Mental Health, 28*(4), 247–261.

Sarkin, J. A., Johnson, S. S., Prochaska, J. O., & Prochaska, J. M. (2001). Applying the transtheoretical model to regulate moderate exercise in an overweight population: Validation of a stages of change measure. *Preventive Medicine, 33*(5), 462–469.

Stern, P. (1991). Patient education in a research/clinical setting: The schizophrenia research unit. *Occupational Therapy Practice, 2*(3), 21–30.

Suinicki, M. D. (2004). *Learning and motivation in the postsecondary classroom.* Bolton, MA: Anker.

Group Process

SHARAN L. SCHWARTZBERG

Learning Objectives

After reading this chapter, you will be able to:

1. Appreciate the complexity and value of small groups in occupational therapy.
2. Understand factors influencing small group development and leadership.
3. Analyze the influence of intrapersonal, interpersonal, and intersubjective aspects of group process and dynamics.
4. Identify the impact of task, leader, and member responses on group processes and the effect of group dynamics and processes on individuals, subgroups, and the group as a whole.

INTRODUCTION

Occupational therapists work in groups in a variety of settings. These settings include natural groups such as staff meetings and intervention groups for the purpose of therapy. Occupational therapy groups include energy conservation groups, psychoeducation groups, social skills groups, activities of daily living groups, reminiscence groups, and sensory stimulation groups, among others. The age range of members of these groups is very broad, from children to older adults, and settings include all areas of practice. There are sets of dynamics that operate in small groups regardless of setting. The interrelationships between members, leaders, and the group as a whole are called **group process**. The purpose of this chapter is to define group process and the dynamics that influence **group cohesiveness** and the dissolution of a small group. Factors such as cohesiveness, hope, and interpersonal learning are what make therapeutic groups beneficial (Falk-Kessler, Momich, & Perel, 1991; Yalom, 1985; Yalom & Leszcz, 2005).

DEFINING GROUP PROCESS

Group process "is the **here-and-now** experience in the group that describes how the group is functioning, the quality of relationships between and among group members and with the leader, the emotional experiences and reactions of the group, and the group's strongest desires and fears" (Brown, 2003, p. 228). According to Brown, "the proposed definition has the following components and assumptions: (1) process occurs in the here-and-now; (2) process includes present relationships and interactions among group members and with the leader; (3) reactions, responses, and feelings provide access to and meaning for process; and (4) process exists at both the micro and macro levels" (2003, p. 228). Each of these components will be explained in terms of processes relevant to occupational therapy (Figure 37.1).

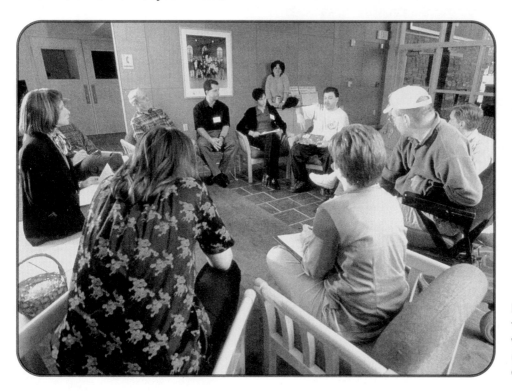

FIGURE 37.1 Occupational therapy often occurs within a group format. (Photo courtesy of Kinda Clinetf.)

Here-and-Now Process

The moment-to-moment interaction between leaders and members makes up the here-and-now process of a group. At a minimum, as an interdependent system, interaction operates simultaneously in six ways: (1) member to member, (2) leader to member and member to leader, (3) subgroups, (4) group as a whole, (5) engagement in occupation, and (6) the culture or environment. In a **functional group** (Howe & Schwartzberg, 2001; Schwartzberg, Howe, & Barnes, 2008), purposeful action promotes adaptation through engagement in occupation. The actions that are characteristic of a functional group, described by Howe and Schwartzberg (2001), include four types of group action: (1) purposeful action, (2) self-initiated action, (3) spontaneous action or here-and-now action, and (4) group-centered action. A snapshot example of group-centered action is a group of people making a decision together to do something of value to the group. The members act spontaneously in offering suggestions and supporting each other emotionally. There is a balance between getting the decision made and feeling satisfied (Box 37.1).

Relationships and Interactions Among Members and with the Leader

Factors that influence the group process include the role of the group leader, the group format, and the functional level of the members. Leadership can be highly structured and autocratic (leader-centered), centered on the needs of the group, or open-ended. Groups can be closed, with no

new members added, or open with changing membership. Members can be selected to be like one another or heterogeneous. Small groups can range in size from three members to ten or even twelve members. Group size influences group methods, leader strategies, and outcomes (Howe & Schwartzberg, 2001).

Group membership roles have been categorized into three types of roles that are social-emotional positive or negative and task area neutral (Bales, 1950): (1) group maintenance and building roles, such as "encourager," "harmonizer," and "compromiser;" (2) group task roles, such as "initiator-contributor," "information seeker," and "information giver"; and (3) individual member roles, such as, "aggressor," "blocker," and "recognition seeker"

BOX 37.1 HOWE AND SCHWARTZBERG'S (2001) FUNCTIONAL GROUP ACTIONS

- **Purposeful action:** Meaning for individuals and group as a whole
- **Self-initiated action:** Member takes initiative verbally or nonverbally
- **Spontaneous action:** Action occurs in the here and now
- **Group-centered action:** Member actions are interdependent

BOX 37.2 — GROUP MEMBERSHIP ROLES (BENNE & SHEATS, 1978)

- **Group maintenance-building roles:** Social-emotional roles that support group processes
- **Group task roles:** Member roles that support group task goals
- **Individual member roles:** Individual roles that detract from group processes

(Box 37.2) (Benne & Sheats, 1978). People take on these various roles in task-oriented groups. There may be a mismatch between the roles members take on and the demands of a situation. If everyone offers emotional support and no one carries out actions such as offering suggestions, the group falters. Conversely, if the group focuses only on getting the job done, the members will feel emotionally dissatisfied and isolated. Group cohesion results when the member roles are congruent with the task.

The developmental level of the group can be viewed in relation to the member function, complexity of task, and leader role. Mosey (1970) categorized developmental group interaction levels as parallel, project, egocentric cooperative level, cooperative, and mature. In a developmental hierarchy, from more directive to group-centered, a more mature group is able to direct itself and support its needs (Box 37.3). The members' flexibility in meeting the demands of the task and setting demonstrates its adaptability, maturity, and ability to function. A parallel, less mature group is less able to carry out the task and support emotional needs. At times, a group task demands different levels of interaction.

The task of selecting activities and materials is an important leader function that relates to the symbolic meanings of group processes. When activities are selected that lack meaning for the group members, interest and motivation dwindle. As a leader, operating from one's own cultural orientation alone is ethnocentric rather than group-centered or client-centered. Such ethnocentrism is illustrated when a group leader plans holiday activities around Christian holidays and no one takes initiative in the group. Conversely, an example of a culturally responsive

CASE STUDY: *Silence and Competition*

A task-oriented process group focuses on helping members learn more adaptive ways of socially participating in a group through analysis of the relationships between process, product, and interaction. Suppose that in a task-oriented process group, a subgroup of three people initiated the planning of group games for subsequent sessions. No one in the larger group disagreed with the plan until two members expressed apathy and boredom after three weeks of parallel "ice-breaker" question-and-answer-type activities with no group interaction required. The subgroup members expressed shock and anger that no one had spoken up earlier. "Well if you felt that way, why didn't you say so?" one member of the subgroup said. There was silence in the room.

What does the silence symbolize for the group and its members? It is possible that members had not voiced their disagreement for fear of rejection. They might have been acting out, or acting in, because feelings of competition with the more active members had been aroused. The choice of a parallel activity was also of importance. In a parallel activity, there is no competition. Members work side by side in an activity that is structured to guarantee a win-win situation for all. Again, it is likely that the group was avoiding competition. By suggesting the parallel activity, the active members were in **collusion** with the silent members to avoid competition. Only when the two members who expressed apathy and boredom gave voice to their concerns did competition emerge in an overt manner.

When the factors that are operating for the group to so fiercely avoid competition with each other and with the leaders are examined at level of process, this yields a lot of information about the group. At the structural level of group process, one might find an imbalance of group membership roles. Member role taking in the social-emotional realm, such as encouraging, compromising, gatekeeping, and harmonizing, would help the group to explore likes, dislikes, and conflicts. In this group, the members are leaning toward task-oriented roles such as information giving, coordinating, and energizing the group into action. Psychodynamic aspects of group process call attention to underlying or latent issues. **Antigroup** forces (Nitsun, 1996, 2002), psychodynamic in nature, suggest that feelings of rivalry and envy toward other group members or the leaders as well as fear of rejection are possible factors contributing to the group reaction.

The gender of members is also relevant to the group's process around competition. In the scenario described above, all the members are female. There might be a strong positive bias toward win-win in a task versus win-over. If men were introduced into the process, it is possible that the group would experience different scenarios, such as more comfort with overt competition. Furthermore, there is the possibility that in the mixed group, the role balance would shift toward gender stereotypes. The latent potential for women to assume more social-emotional caretaking roles and the men to assume more task roles deserves examination.

BOX 37.3 · MOSEY'S DEVELOPMENTAL GROUP LEVELS (DONOHUE, 2003; MOSEY, 1970)

- **Parallel:** Minimal sharing of task; leader emotionally supports and structures task
- **Project:** Short-term sharable task; leader helps with task selection and cooperation
- **Egocentric cooperative:** Joint interaction with self-interest; leader role model; leader assumes missing roles and acts as resource person
- **Cooperative:** Members able to assume social-emotional roles and mutual need satisfaction; leader acts as consultant
- **Mature:** Members able to balance roles to support and maintain task without supervision; leadership is shared; therapist is peer

activity selection is adolescents in a cooking group selecting and sharing foods that are representative of their culture or cultures.

THE MEANING OF PROCESS

Whether they are short-term or long-term, groups change over time. A variety of interpersonal concerns emerge as groups evolve. The **phases of group development** provide a conceptual model of the evolution of a group issues. Bion (1959) proposed that tensions emerge in a group and their resolution forms the basis and process of group development. He identified three stages and processes of coping with tension: (1) fight or flight, (2) dependence and counterdependence on the leader, and (3) pairing (Box 37.4). The group becomes a working group as members resolve the tensions inherent in the task of operating as a group. Similarly, Tuckman (1965) identified four

BOX 37.4 · TENSION COPING BEHAVIORS (BION, 1959)

- **Fight or flight:** Hostile and hierarchical; time spent selecting enemies and attacking them
- **Dependency:** Insists leader protect and expresses dissatisfaction with adequacy for task
- **Pairing:** Failure to develop group cohesiveness; pairs dominate

BOX 37.5 · TUCKMAN'S (1965) STAGES OF GROUP DEVELOPMENT

- **Forming:** Uncertainty of role in group, purpose, and procedures of group
- **Storming:** Conflict and rebellion in group as members resist group influence
- **Norming:** Group discovers ways to work together, set norms to enable cohesiveness
- **Performing:** Group is flexible in ways of working together to achieve aims

stages of group development: (1) forming, (2) storming, (3) norming, and (4) performing (Box 37.5). The group progresses as members resolve and adjust to underlying emotional issues in relation to each other and the leader. Progress waxes and wanes as stresses emerge in the group, such as those occurring with the addition of a new member or loss of a long-standing member. Although the notion of schemes of group development has been an issue of debate, there is substantial empirical evidence to support the emergence of phases in a group (MacKenzie, 1994). The phases are supported by a systems-centered model (Agazarian & Gantt, 2003) and have relevance to the leader function and intervention strategies in facilitating functional group action (Howe & Schwartzberg, 2001). In a system-centered model, the group is viewed as an organized body of mutually dependent ingredient parts. "It is the interactive system that changes through the developmental stages, not the individual group members" (Howe & Schwartzberg, 2001, p. 22). In spite of verification, the empirical evidence has not quieted the debate over whether or not distinct phases of group development truly exist.

MICRO AND MACRO LEVELS OF PROCESS

Micro Level

Interpersonal difficulties can emerge between individuals at the structural or micro level of process. It is inevitable that all occupation-focused groups lack cohesiveness at one time or another, depending on the group's maturity. The members might be unable to make a group decision or carry out a plan. In groups that are structured for the purpose of self-examination and evaluating performance, such as a task-oriented process group, part of the work of the group is to identify structural problems in the group. Members' fear of ridicule, for example, might lead to premature decision making or sole reliance on the leader for ideas. Lippitt (1961) long ago identified factors that facilitate group decision making. These include clear definition of the problem,

CASE STUDY: *Late or Absent Members*

Week after week, a member arrives late. No one in the group says anything to the late member. The member gives excuses such as the traffic and the weather. It is in the group contract, a written agreement, that members attend group regularly and arrive on time. The leader confronts the group member about being late. Members express anger at the leader for being too harsh, for singling out the chronically late member, and for embarrassing the person.

In this scenario, it is important to ask about the group's phase of development. Are the late member's behavior and the group's reaction evidence of storming and the beginning of pulls toward independence? Are members avoiding a direct confrontation with the leader about limits being imposed? As members solidify around a peer, the leader, by keeping to boundaries, helps the group to become cohesive and self-directing. Trust is more likely to be established when limits are reasonable and consistently upheld by the leader and group. When boundaries are not maintained, the behavior is explored and examined. Such exploration involves discovering conscious and unconscious motives for behavior, including following and not following expectations. At times, a member might be asked to leave a group if the behavior is detrimental to the process and to the individual and/or the group. Such a situation is bound to test the leader's vulnerability to rejection and desire to be helpful.

---

clear understanding of who is responsible for the decision, effective communication for producing ideas, appropriate group size for decision making, means for testing different alternative decisions, commitment to the decision, commitment of the leader to the decision-making process, and agreement on the procedures and methods for decision making before deliberations on the issue (Lippitt, 1961). Lippitt's factors set forth clear structural parameters and can assist in decision making in task-oriented groups.

Macro Level

At the macro or psychodynamic level, the member's covert or latent conflicts, wishes, and unknown fantasies emerge in the form of behaviors. Underlying the behavior are negative attitudes toward the group that have been characterized as **antigroup** forces (Nitsun, 1996). If these forces are not recognized or contained, they can interfere with the group's process.

According to Nitsun (2002), antigroup processes that emerge include threat to privacy of self and psychic survival; idealization of the one-to-one relationship; communication failures, particularly empathy and attunement in groups; fears around sexual exposure or rejection; arousal of feelings of rivalry and envy with the therapist and between members; attacks on connectedness of thoughts, feelings, and actions; and projective identification. These group processes can be expected to surface in psychotherapy groups, and when explored, they can form a basis for development. Antigroup forces occur at the level of the individual, the subgroup, and the group as a whole. These forces can be destructive or challenging and are widespread in larger groups such as institutions and organizations (Nitsun, 2002).

In occupational therapy groups, the antigroup forces often take the form of subgrouping, scapegoating, role lock, anger, withdrawal or silence, and competition. **Subgroups** are clusters or dyads of members that subconsciously band together to avoid something displeasing. They emerge when the emotional task is anxiety-provoking (Bion, 1959). The scapegoat receives the projection of unwanted parts of individuals in the group or operates through **projective identification**. "Projective identification is an unconscious interpersonal transaction in which one person or subgroup finds a willing container for unwanted projections; the recipient then identifies with these projections, that is, the disowned parts of the projector" (Weber & Gans, 2003, p. 408). **Scapegoating** is putting the unwanted and disavowed feelings of group members into one member (Weber & Gans, 2003). **Role lock** is the group's confining a member's participation to a restricted part of that individual (Weber & Gans, 2003). For example, in an occupational therapy group, the members might rely solely on one member to bring supplies and to start the activity or a discussion. The initiator who is cast into this role misses opportunities to be on the receiving end, and the other members are locked into passive, dependent behaviors. Ultimately, such role lock leads to dissatisfaction for all the members and a breakdown in the group process and task completion.

LEADER RESPONSES

"Countertransference responses in therapists vitally need to be understood and managed. The Anti-Group tends to arouse feelings of incompetence, failure, helplessness, and anger in the group therapist, and it is crucial in such a situation that the therapist has a professional support system and access to regular supervision" (Nitsun, 2002, p. 464). These responses are both subjective and objective reactions to group members.

The leader response might be one of shame (Weber & Gans, 2003) or the coconstruction of the difficult patient (Gans & Alonso, 1998). "Usually when people refer to the difficult patients, they speak of how such patients: (a) promote or impede group work; (b) accept or fail to accept

CASE STUDY: *Subgroup Meetings Outside of Group*

To promote group unity, group members are told that as part of the group contract, it is preferred that discussions about the group not occur outside of scheduled sessions. If members do have contact outside the group, it is expected that the events and discussion be brought back to the group. For example, a member casually mentions having invited another member to her home and says that her mother was so glad to meet a group member. A silence ensues. The event occurs during one of the earlier group sessions of this time-limited group.

Many issues can be underlying the group's process. Consider reasons for the subgroup formation. Were the two members expressing something on behalf of the other members of the group? By having the outside contact and bringing it back to the group, were the two members testing the group's and leader's reactions? Fears of being forced out of the group and the wish to be held and contained by the group are stirred. The leader is challenged to bridge the emotional concerns to discourage a split in the group. Such an encounter forces the leader to avoid taking sides or acting out through the subgroups.

feedback from other group members and/or the leader(s), (c) come to symbolize and amplify the most problematic parts of each member, (d) and challenge the members' and the leader's trustworthiness, empathic capacity, and competence" (Gans & Alonso, 1998, p. 314).

Therapist examination of **countertransference** yields understanding of the subjective and objective. In the case of subjective countertransference, the therapist's unexamined projections of himself or herself are seen in the patient. The therapist's reaction is based on his or her own response (Ormont, 1991). In objective countertransference, the patient elicits a common induced emotional response across individuals that is not an idiosyncratic reaction of the therapist. Weber and Gans (2003) note that "four common challenges that can evoke countertransference difficulties and produce therapist shame include (1) collusion with role lock or scapegoating, (2) containing and detoxifying noxious projective identifications, (3) negative transference, and (4) idealization of the therapist" (p. 407). **Transference** can be negative or positive. The group leader experiences the projected or unwanted parts of the members at the level of the group or individuals.

A violation of confidentiality calls into question trust of the leader and fellow members. Furthermore, one can ask what role the "violator" plays for the group. There is a risk that he or she will become the scapegoat or target for hostility and distrust. Should the leader not address the member's breach, the boundaries of the group are weakened, trust is unlikely to be established, and the group is likely to dissolve. Examination of member transference

relative to past violations as well as leader self-reflection of countertransference could bolster the group and shore up the boundaries necessary for emotional safety.

It is important for leaders to examine their own behaviors so that interventions are fully centered on the member rather than in fulfilling the leader's own needs. Weber and Gans (2003) describe the ego ideal as being all knowing, all loving, and all powerful. Because therapists can never achieve that perfection, they are bound at times to feel inadequate. These feelings can be particularly acute in the new therapist and may be unconscious. By unconsciously acting out through their own behaviors, leaders can contribute to problems in group process by the construction of difficult members (Gans & Alonso, 1998). Gans and Alonso describe leader actions that can result in the creation of problematical group members. "These include (a) faulty patient selection; (b) inept or harmful handling of boundary violations, scapegoating, and group norms; (c) inability or unwillingness to acknowledge mistakes; (d) refusal to be a lightning rod for negative feelings; (e) failure to set limits on members' expression of sado-masochism; and (f) failure to accept one's own limits as they affect clinical practice during the inevitable, painful vicissitudes that punctuate one's professional career and personal life" (1998, pp. 316–317).

Occupational therapy practitioners may participate in or lead many types of groups. Group processes such as phases of group development, group member roles, and covert interpersonal and intrapersonal dynamics affect all groups. When understood, the leader's countertransference

CASE STUDY: *Breach of Confidentiality*

In the first meeting of a group, the leader explains that material in the group stays in the group and is not to be shared outside of the session. Immediately afterward, a member comments, "Remember in the last group, one of the girls, what was her name, Mary Smith, broke up with

her boyfriend and cried all the time?" The group begins to question the member about circumstances and presses to know more about the incident. The leader is appalled and angry with the group member for revealing the name and circumstances of another member.

CASE STUDY: *Coleader Colludes with Group*

In an occupational therapy student supervision group, during one leader's absence, the coleader brings a game for the group to play rather than planning process with the group, which involves discussing alternatives for the use of the group time. When the absent leader returns, she expresses confusion about the group's agenda. The group members are silent and play the game until the "colluding coleader" expresses exasperation at not knowing how to follow the rules of the group.

The change in direction suggests competition between the leaders and unconscious acting out. Is the coleader changing the process to gain favor or approval from the group? Is the division symbolic of subgroups within the group or expressed anger in the group? Perhaps the introduction of more structure through the use of the game is an attempt to ease the group's and coleader's anxieties about the absence of the other leader. The group might be using the structure of the game as a means to avoid feelings of loss.

CASE STUDY: *Group Member Refuses to Participate in Activity*

A group member will participate only when working by the leader's side. As soon as the leader attempts to help someone else, this person leaves the room or sits in a corner and sulks.

The member's behavior raises questions about the suitability of the group for this individual. The member's group interaction skills might not be at a developmental level at which he or she can share attention. The group task might also be faulty, as the member is unable to successfully engage in the activity without one-on-one support. The reasons for faulty patient or activity selection need examination. Such a mismatch can stem from within the leader as well as from agency pressures for member inclusion in group programs.

COMMENTARY ON THE EVIDENCE

Group Process

Evidence suggests that occupational therapy–related intervention in groups is effective in addressing outcomes in body function (e.g., mental functions) and occupational performance areas and skills such as social participation and communication/interaction skills (Howe & Schwartzberg, 2001). Evidence-based techniques vary depending on the desired outcomes and client problem. Intervention for performance areas and skills conducted in a group setting may result in greater client satisfaction and compliance with intervention regimes (Howe & Schwartzberg, 2001). Because the range of skills addressed is so varied, it is best to examine the literature specific to the client factor and outcome in question.

The range of concerns related to group process is very broad and also dependent on group context, setting, and population. Studies of interest to support practice include the emergence of phases of group development (Agazarian & Gantt, 2003), group size and its influence on group accomplishment (Howe & Schwartzberg, 2001; Yalom & Leszcz, 2005), and the importance of self-initiated and purposeful action in a group. There is a need to expand the evidence in all areas of occupational therapy intervention in which group process is applied to specific client problems or as a means to enhance problem-specific methodologies.

A good example of such needed research is a randomized controlled trial that was conducted to evaluate the efficacy of an eight-session, group-based program designed to reduce fear of falling and increase activity levels among older adults (Peterson, 2003; Tennstedt et al., 1998). "Data collected over 12 months showed that compared with control subjects, intervention subjects experiences increased social participation and community mobility" (Peterson, 2003, p. 12).

reactions can influence strategies that are used to enhance group effectiveness. These group processes are important consideration for facilitating effective groups. Understanding the dynamics that influence group cohesiveness can lead to more successful leadership of small groups in occupational therapy.

PROVOCATIVE QUESTIONS

1. Recall a time when you were in a task group and experienced strong emotions. What was happening in the group at the time? What feelings did you experience—for example, anger, frustration, sadness, jealousy, envy? Consider the range of feelings that might have been hidden or covert and those that were overt or known to yourself and others.

2. In the situation you recalled in question 1, how did you respond to others in the group? What feelings might have been in conflict? Consider analogous feelings, such as anger and sadness, anxiety, and calmness. What group membership roles do you tend to assume? What is the underlying psychological or social gain? For example, do you tend to be a mediator in a group to avoid conflict or competition?

3. Return to your situation described in question 1. Alter the circumstance in the group. For example, you might change the number of people in the group, the gender of the members, the task, the rewards, and the leaders. How might the group process and role in the group change? Consider the following illustration. It is the first day of class, and your professor asks students to decide when they would like to present their final project to the class. A student whom you regard as typically aggressive and self-centered picks all the dates that work best for you. By the time you have the courage to say what date you prefer, the only dates left conflict with a fieldwork assignment. You feel angry and helpless. Rather than sulking, you could alter the process by suggesting that students rank order their preferences and trade dates with each other, for example.

REFERENCES

Agazarian, Y., & Gantt, S. (2003). Phases of group development: Systems-centered hypotheses and their implications for research and practice. *Group dynamics: Theory, Research, and Practice, 7*(3), 238–252.

Bales, R. (1950). *Interaction process analysis.* Reading, MA: Addison Wesley.

Benne, K., & Sheats, P. (1978). Functional roles of group members. In L. Bradford, (Ed.), *Group development* (2nd ed., pp. 52–61). La Jolla, CA: University Associates.

Bion, W. R. (1959). *Experiences in groups and other papers.* New York: Basic Books.

Brown, N. W. (2003). Conceptualizing process. *International Journal of Group Psychotherapy, 53*(2), 225–244.

Donohue, M. (2003). Group profile studies with children: Validity measures and item analysis. *Occupational Therapy in Mental Health, 19*(1), 1–23.

Falk-Kessler, J., Momich, C., & Perel, S. (1991). Therapeutic factors in occupational therapy groups. *American Journal of Occupational Therapy, 45*(1), 59–66.

Gans, J. S., & Alonso, A. (1998). Difficult patients: Their construction in group therapy. *International Journal of Group Psychotherapy, 48*(3), 311–326.

Howe, M. C., & Schwartzberg, S. L. (2001). *A functional approach to group work in occupational therapy* (3rd ed.). Philadelphia: Lippincott Williams and Wilkins.

Lippitt, G. L. (1961). How to get results from a group. In L. P. Bradford (Ed.), *Group development.* Washington, DC: National Training Laboratories, National Education Association.

MacKenzie, K. R. (1994). Group development. In A. Fuhriman & G. M. Burlingame (Es.), *Handbook of group psychotherapy* (pp 223–268). New York: Wiley.

Mosey, A. C. (1970). The concept and use of developmental groups. *American Journal of Occupational Therapy, 24*(4), 272–275.

Nitsun, M. (1996). *The anti-group: Destructive forces in the group and their creative potential.* New York: Routledge.

Nitsun, M. (2002). The future of the group. *International Journal of Group Psychotherapy, 50*(4), 455–472.

Ormont, L. R. (1991). Use of the group in resolving the subjective countertransference. *International Journal of Group Psychotherapy, 41*(4), 433–447.

Peterson, E. W. (2003). Evidence-based practice: Case example: A matter of balance. *OT Practice,* February 10, 2003, *8*(3), 12–14.

Schwartzberg, S. L., Howe, M., & Barnes, M. (2008). Groups: Applying the functional group model. Philadelphia: FA Davis.

Tennstedt, S., Howland, J., Lachman, M. E., Peterson, E., Kasten, L., & Jette, A. (1998). A randomized, controlled trial of a group intervention to reduce fear of falling and associated activity restriction in older adults. *Journals of Gerontology Series B: Psychological Sciences, 53,* 383–394.

Tuckman, B. W. (1965). Developmental sequence in small groups. *Psychological Bulletin, 63,* 384–399.

Weber, R., L., & Gans, J. S. (2003). The group therapist's shame: A much undiscussed topic. *International Journal of Group Psychotherapy, 53*(4), 395–416.

Yalom, I. D. (1985). *The theory and practice of group psychotherapy* (3rd ed.). New York: Basic Books.

Yalom, I. D., & Leszcz, M. (2005). The theory and practice of group psychotherapy, (5th ed). New York: Basic Books.

VII

COMMUNICATION IN OCCUPATIONAL THERAPY

" Say what you mean and mean what you say. "

George S. Patton

Team Interaction Models and Team Communication

ELLEN S. COHN

" The path to greatness is along with others. "

—BALTASAR GRACION, SPANISH PRIEST (1637)

Learning Objectives

After reading this chapter, you will be able to:

1. Describe the benefits of a team approach to intervention.
2. Describe the roles of medical, rehabilitation, and educational professionals.
3. Describe the communication dynamics of team process.

TEAMS AND TEAMWORK

In the often-cited poem about Hinduism, "The Blind Men and the Elephant," John Godfrey Saxe described the plight of six men, all blind, who happened on an elephant. The first man, feeling the elephant's side, reported that the animal was like a wall. The second, feeling the tusk, interpreted the creature to be like a spear. The third, finding its trunk, declared it to be like a snake, and so on. Thus, when each observer stated his opinion of the elephant, "each was partly in the right, and all were in the wrong!" (Saxe, 1871, p. 260). Herein lies the concept underlying the use of team communication. Although each member, representing a different perspective, is hardly blind, a single way of observing limits the ability to comprehend the whole.

It is the combined vision, evaluation, and coordinated intervention plan that provides a complete picture of the whole client receiving intervention.

For most areas of practice, interdisciplinary team interactions are the norm. Successful intervention involves a collaborative and mutual process during which practitioners and clients develop the care plan together (Golin & Duncanis, 1981; Humphry, Gonzalez, & Taylor, 1993; Leff & Walizer, 1992). According to Parham (1987), occupational therapists are "concerned with understanding the occupations of human beings, the ways in which people organize the activities that fill their lives and give their lives meaning" (p. 555). To understand how a particular client experiences illness or disability in the context of his or her occupations and daily life, the occupational therapy practitioner needs to collaborate with other members of the team involved in providing care for that client.

The team comprises a variety of different specialists who have different backgrounds, training, values, and worldviews and sometimes different goals. These specialists work together in different configurations, depending on the client's needs, the type of setting in which the intervention is provided, and available resources. The intervention team for a child with traumatic brain injury returning to elementary school after two months in a rehabilitation hospital might include the child and his or her parents, a special educator, a speech-language pathologist, an occupational therapist, an adapted physical education teacher, and a school nurse. An older adult who recently had a mild stroke affecting her vision and who lives in low-income housing might receive intervention services from an occupational therapist, an optometrist, a physical therapist, and a social worker. Practitioners providing intervention to communities might work with teams of people representing local businesses, voluntary citizen's organizations, or local government officials. Each team member addresses the client's concerns from a unique perspective, and all perspectives are then coordinated to structure the client care plan. It is assumed that this coordinated perspective will make a difference in the ultimate outcome for the recipient of the care plan (Crepeau, 1994a, 1994b; Unsworth, Thomas, & Greenwood, 1995).

Ideally, interdisciplinary team members share a common concept of the client's concerns and a common philosophy of intervention. They synthesize the diverse information gathered from their own evaluations and those of outside consultants, and they work together to formulate and implement a comprehensive care plan based on the available data. Most important, the team should act as a functional unit whose members are willing to learn from each other and modify their own opinions, when appropriate, on the basis of the combined observations and expertise of the entire group (Perlmutter, Bailey, & Netting, 2001). The advantages of a team approach are a more holistic approach to client care, integrated interventions, the reduction or elimination of duplicated services and fragmentation or gaps in care, and quicker and better-informed decisions for client plans (Stancliff, 1995).

Historically, health care teams have generated a client's care plan behind closed doors, without the client's input, and then shared their plans with the client. In current practice, however, additional voices are influencing the team process. Health professionals now espouse incorporation of the client as a member of the team and view this as crucial to the eventual success of the care plan (Baum, 1998; Crepeau, 1994a, 1994b). Moreover, the Individuals with Disabilities Education Improvement Act, IDEA 2004 (P.L. 108-446), federal legislation outlining the educational requirement for children with special needs, clearly specifies that students and their parents or caregivers must be involved in team decisions regarding the student's needs. In the managed care environment, which focuses on both cost containment and quality of care, the third-party payer's perspective is increasingly considered to be another crucial factor in the team's decision-making process.

An understanding of the potential contributions of the various people and professionals involved in the client's life enables the practitioner to develop a more meaningful plan for each client (Figure 38.1). The members of the team have interrelated functions. Depending on the practice environment, the occupational therapy practitioner's interactions with other professionals and with the important people in the client's life vary. In a medical setting, such as an acute care hospital or a rehabilitation unit, the team members might operate under a physician's order, and practitioners might interact with team members numerous times a day. Alternatively, a practitioner who is in private practice or employed by a home-care agency might not have frequent contact with other specialists but might have more repeated contact with family members or other significant people in the client's life.

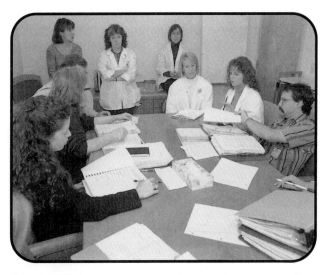

FIGURE 38.1 Team meetings foster collaboration and integrated intervention planning.

Regardless of the environment, occupational therapy practitioners need to be aware of the roles of the other members of the team in order to be clear about the contributions that occupational therapy can make and how everyone can work together for the client's benefit. Therefore, occupational therapy practitioners need to interpret their role and contribution to the intervention team, for it is never safe to assume that other members of any particular team have a full understanding of the potential contributions of occupational therapy. Consider, for example, Rose's story in the following case study.

TEAM INTERACTION MODELS

Each client usually has an identified case manager or team leader. The case manager is the designated person on whom clients and their family members can consistently rely to explain, clarify, or acquire necessary information. This case manager may also serve as the client's ombudsman. The leadership of the team or the case management may change over time, according to the identified concerns of a particular client, the members of the team, the nature of the task, and the structure of the organization. In a traditional medical model, the physician is often the leader of the team. Today, especially in rehabilitative, long-term care, community-based, or educational settings, a therapist, social worker, nurse, special service coordinator, or teacher may lead or coordinate the team and simultaneously serve as the case manager.

Teams may be organized according to a multidisciplinary, interdisciplinary, or transdisciplinary model. Often, however, a team moves from one model to another and functions in its own unique variation of the classic models. In the multidisciplinary team approach, team members work side by side. Each member has a clearly defined role with specific areas of responsibility; team members understand each others' professional scope of practice and rely on each team member to address their area of concern. Although evaluation, planning, and therapy take place independently, the team members may communicate with each other on a regular basis or through the client's record or chart. Generally, families and clients meet with the team members of each discipline separately. Examples of this type of team interaction might be seen in an outpatient situation when a person is receiving intervention services from a home health aide, occupational therapy, and physical therapy.

In an interdisciplinary team approach, team members share responsibility for providing services, often supporting the goals of other team members. They conduct separate evaluations but share the results to develop an integrated and coordinated care plan. The team members have substantial knowledge of each other's discipline and begin to understand the perspective of others. Clients and families or other significant people in clients' lives meet with the team or a representative of the team, such as the team leader or case manager. Effective interdisciplinary teams communicate to resolve conflicts and make shared decisions. Common examples of interdisciplinary teams are found in rehabilitation hospitals, where professionals from numerous disciplines (the client and caregivers, occupational therapy, speech-language pathology, physical therapy, nutrition, social work, therapeutic recreation, nursing, and medicine) meet to share perspectives and develop a coordinated intervention plan.

CASE STUDY: *Rose: An Interdisciplinary Approach to Planning for Transition to Home for a Woman with Multiple Traumas*

Rose is a 72-year-old who was recently hospitalized after experiencing multiple traumas from an automobile accident. She is now receiving occupational therapy services in her home. Although her husband is devoted to her, he is unable to help her maintain the home. A social worker is available to consult with the intervention team. Together, the occupational therapist, the client, her husband, and their adult children, along with the social worker, determined that seeking the services of a Meals-on-Wheels program would alleviate the pressure of preparing major meals. Additionally, Rose's adult children, all of whom live at a distance, have offered to pay for a house cleaning service for three months while she recovers. This team decision-making process helped the occupational therapist to determine the focus of occupational therapy intervention. With Rose's most strenuous homemaking duties alleviated, the occupational therapist was able to focus on helping Rose to regain and monitor her strength and endurance so that she could completely manage her self-care and prepare light meals, as well as joining her husband at their weekly singing group. With the assistance of the intervention team, occupational therapy focused on meaningful activities for Rose and her husband.

Although practically every medical, health, or educational professional may be called on to provide services to address the range of client conditions seen by occupational therapy practitioners, the professionals listed in Table 38.1 may be especially relevant to occupational therapy intervention (Wachtel & Compart, 1996). The Websites of professional associations provide overviews of the qualifications of various professionals with whom occupational therapy practitioners are likely to work.

TABLE 38.1   MEDICAL, REHABILITATION, AND EDUCATIONAL PROFESSIONALS AND PROFESSIONAL ASSOCIATIONS

Professionals	Associations
Adapted physical educator: Adapts sporting equipment and games for individuals with special needs.	National Consortium for Physical Education and Recreation for Individuals with Disabilities (NCPERID): http://www.uwlax.edu/sah/ncperid
Administrator: Applies and enforces federal, state, and local laws that regulate finances, standards, and environments for most health and educational programs; has valuable expertise in management of personnel, space, and finances.	*School administrator:* American Association of School Administrators (ASA): http://www.aasa.org *Hospital administrator:* American Hospital Association (AHA): http://www.aha.org
Audiologist: Specializes in diagnosis and treatment of hearing impairments; administers a variety of tests to determine hearing level and site of damage to the auditory system; recommends hearing aids and other assistive devices to enhance residual hearing loss or the need for special training.	American Academy of Audiology (AAA): http://www.audiology.org
Biomedical engineer: Specializes in the application of scientific theory and technology to the development of devices and techniques for medical treatment, rehabilitation, and research; provides technical expertise in recommendation of commercial products and the modifications of existing devices or the design and fabrication of custom equipment or adjusted environments.	Biomedical Engineering Society (BES) http://www.bmes.org
Chaplain: Focuses on religious and spiritual needs of clients; provides nondenominational individual and family counseling; offers special services.	Association of Professional Chaplains (APC): http://www.professionalchaplains.org
Optometrist: Examines, diagnoses, treats, and manages diseases, injuries, and disorders of the visual system, the eye, and associated structures and identifies related systemic conditions affecting the eye.	American Optometric Association (AOA): http://www.aoa.org
Orthotist and prosthetist: Orthotist makes and fits braces to support or correct body parts weakened by disease, injury, or congenital deformity or to help prevent deformities. Prosthetist designs and fabricates artificial limbs, with special attention to enhancing fit, function, and appearance.	American Orthotic & Prosthetic Association (AOPA): www.ama-assn.org
Nurse: Provides goal-directed, personalized care that encompasses preventive, maintenance, and restorative aspects of nursing; administers medication and instructs client and significant others in care management and health maintenance programs.	American Nurses Association (ANA): http://www.nursingworld.org
Nutritionist: Plans food and nutrition programs and supervises the preparation and serving of meals; helps to prevent and treat illnesses by promoting healthy eating habits and recommending dietary modifications, such as the use of less salt for those with high blood pressure or the reduction of fat and sugar intake for those who are overweight.	American Dietetic Association (ADA): http://www.eatright.org
Physical therapist: Evaluates physical capacities and limitations; administers treatment designed to alleviate pain, correct or minimize deformity, increase strength and mobility, and improve general health.	American Physical Therapy Association (APTA): http://www.apta.org

Continued

TABLE 38.1 MEDICAL, REHABILITATION, AND EDUCATIONAL PROFESSIONALS AND PROFESSIONAL ASSOCIATIONS *Continued*

Professionals	Associations
Physicians (specialists): Usually specialists to whom a client has been referred by the primary-care physician (e.g., orthopedists, ophthalmologists, neurologists, cardiologists, physiatrists, psychiatrists).	American Medical Association (AMA): www.ama-assn.org
Psychologist: Provides psychological, projective, and behavioral assessments; provides individual, couple, family, and group psychotherapy related to behavioral or adjustment issues.	American Psychological Association (APA): http://www.apa.org/
Rehabilitation counselor: Assists individuals with physical, mental, cognitive, or sensory disabilities to become or remain self-sufficient, productive citizens; helps clients to cope with societal and personal problems, plan careers, and find and keep satisfying jobs.	National Rehabilitation Counseling Association (NRCA): http://nrca-net.org
Respiratory therapist (inhalation therapist): Administers oxygen and mists for medical purposes; provides oxygen assessment programs and client education.	American Association of Respiratory Care (AARC): http://www.aarc.org
Social worker: Assists client, family, or other important people in the client's life to achieve a maximal level of social and emotional functioning; provides client and family counseling, discharge planning, and education on entitlements and other available resources; assists in identifying transportation and attendant care resources.	National Association of Social Workers (NASW): http://www.socialworkers.org
Special educator: Serves as a teacher of children with unusually high intellectual potential or children who live with mental illness, learning disabilities, or developmental deviations; may have advanced skills in teaching children who are blind, deaf, emotionally disturbed, developmentally delayed, or have physical disabilities.	National Association of Special Education Teachers (NASET): http://www.naset.org
Speech-language pathologist: Specializes in speech disorders, the development of language and speech production, the physiology of speech, theories, and measurement of hearing and phonetics.	American Speech-Language-Hearing Association (ASHA): http://www.asha.org
Teacher: Certified to provide education at the early childhood, kindergarten, elementary, secondary, or high school level.	National Education Association (NEA): http://www.nea.org
Therapeutic recreation specialist (recreation therapist): Facilitates the enjoyable use of leisure time to promote mental and physical well-being; uses social and recreational activities to aid in adjustment to disability and participation in community activities.	American Therapeutic Recreation Association: http://www.atra-tr.org

Practitioners working in schools also work in interdisciplinary teams, often with teachers, school administrators, and perhaps an adapted physical educator, speech-language pathologist, psychologist, or classroom aide.

In a transdisciplinary team approach, team members commit to teaching, learning, and working across disciplinary boundaries to plan and provide integrated services. The evaluation is planned, implemented, and summarized by the team as a whole. The team assimilates the perspectives of the various team members to make joint decisions. Traditional role boundaries are crossed, and the skills of other disciplines are integrated into a total care plan. This approach requires that professionals share discipline-related information. The client typically interacts with one professional, who consults with other professionals on the team to communicate a shared perspective to the client and carries out the recommendations and interventions of the entire team. Transdisciplinary teams are sometimes found in early intervention settings in which all team members evaluate a child in an arena model. One team member interacts with the child, while other team members observe the child and interact with the parents, seeking help and interpretation of the child's behavior. After such an evaluation, the entire team synthesizes the evaluation results to identify expected outcomes and develop specific interventions that are implemented by one of the team members. This approach reduces duplication and potential fragmentation of services.

CREATING SHARED MEANING AND A COMMON LANGUAGE

Professionals and clients may have different viewpoints or priorities for intervention, or they may have the same goals yet differ in the meaning of the goals or the approach to take for reaching goals. Therefore, it is essential for the team members to develop shared meaning about the client's entire condition. For the intervention to be effective, the team must understand each client's (Crepeau, 1994a; Salisbury, 1992):

- Beliefs
- Attitudes
- Ways of making meaning of his or her life world
- Knowledge of his or her condition
- Expectancies for the future
- Expectancies about treatment

The constructionist process, as described by Buckholdt and Gubrium (1979) and Crepeau (1994a, 1994b), involves the individual reasoning of the team members and the collective reasoning of the group. Formal lines of communication and methods for sharing these interpretations often develop through team meetings, collaborative intervention sessions, written evaluations, and progress notes. Each team member makes his or her own interpretation of the client's lived experience and then articulates this interpretation to the other team members. The team collectively reconstructs the interpretation to create a unified image from the diversity of their individual perspectives. Through this constructionist process, team members discover, interpret, and negotiate their understanding of the client by "sorting out conflicting data to arrive at a common definition of the problems faced by the patient" (Crepeau, 1994b, p. 161).

To develop a cohesive treatment team that uses a constructionist process, the team must focus its energy and creativity to establish a shared mission. Only in a climate of mutual trust and respect can a group of people with diverse perspectives develop into a cohesive team (Zenger, Musselwhite, Hurson, & Perrin, 1994). Thus, it is important to acknowledge that team building is a developmental process; it takes time and energy to learn about each member's values, goals, and communication style (Blechert, Christiansen, & Kari, 1987).

Although teams may have different needs at different times, Blechert and colleagues (1987) found that team development can be described in terms of life stages. In the first stage, team members explore and define their roles within the context of the team and work setting. Each team member identifies his or her area of expertise and interest, thereby defining each member's unique contribution. Once the team has worked together, adjustment and rearrangement of roles might be necessary to progress to the next stage. Finally, as team members redefine their roles and learn to value each other, they begin to think about issues from multiple points of view. When functioning well, the team members are able to see the issues as a whole. Similar to the blind men with the elephant, the image that the team develops is broader and richer when multiple perspectives are shared to construct a unified image.

CASE STUDY: *Interdisciplinary Communication in a Community Residence*

Coordinating an interdisciplinary approach to provide intervention within a community residence for young adults with persistent mental illness requires ongoing communication among all the members and staff in the community residence. The occupational therapist, nutritionist, and clients of the group home designed an intervention to help the clients establish healthy habits related to eating and increasing physical exercise in their daily lives. The clients and therapist designed a daily walking program for the clients, but the staff at the residence repeatedly served high-calorie snacks or invited the clients to join them in watching a favorite television program during the designated walking time.

The occupational therapist realized that for the intervention to be implemented successfully, the entire staff needed to collaborate in the program design. To build consensus among all the staff and clients in the residence, the therapist scheduled a meeting with the entire residential community to set group goals and explore everyone's ideas for program success. Collectively, the members of the residential community, staff and clients, generated a list of potential problems and barriers to the success of the program. With the barriers made explicit, the group was then able to identify strategies to promote the program. The staff decided to post a chart in the communal living room to document the amount of time and distance covered in daily walks. The clients decided to plan a special outing to a favorite water slide park for all clients who reached the goal of walking 10 miles by the end of the month. Two staff member who were interested in exercise volunteered to be the "Exercise Group" leaders, and the entire community voted on a new name for the group: "Step in Time." The trip to the water slide park required use of the agency van, and the director of the residence had to complete the paperwork for approval to use the van. The intervention would be successful only if everyone shared the common goal.

PRACTICE DILEMMA

COMMUNICATING THE ROLE OF OCCUPATIONAL THERAPY

Carmen, a registered occupational therapist, has worked in a local early childhood program for the last five years. During this time, Carmen and the psychologist collaborated to colead a social skills group for children with autism spectrum disorders. During a recent reorganization of the program, the psychologist was reassigned to another program in the district. The new psychologist has never worked with an occupational therapist and does not understand Carmen's con-tribution to the group. The new psychologist and Carmen do not agree about a particular child's readiness to participate in the social skills group.

Questions

1. How might Carmen communicate the role of occupational therapy to the new psychologist?
2. How might Carmen and the psychologist develop a "common language" to communicate?

PROVOCATIVE QUESTIONS

1. Why is it essential for an intervention team to develop consensus about a client's needs?
2. What strategies might you use if the intervention team you were working with did not value each team member's expertise?
3. Some would argue that a transdisciplinary team is effective because the client has to work with only one person. Others argue that it is inappropriate for a professional to provide services "outside" of his or her professional discipline. What are your thoughts about using a transdisciplinary approach in an early-intervention setting?

REFERENCES

Baum, C. (1998). Client-centered practice in a changing health care system. In M. Law (Ed.), *Client-centered occupational therapy* (pp. 29–45). Thorofare, NJ: Slack.

Blechert, T. F., Christiansen, M. F., & Kari, N. (1987). Intra-professional team building. *American Journal of Occupational Therapy, 41,* 576–582.

Buckholdt, D. R., & Gubrium, J. F. (1979). Doing staffing. *Human Organization, 38,* 255–264.

Crepeau, E. B. (1994a). Three images of interdisciplinary team meetings. *American Journal of Occupational Therapy, 48,* 717–722.

Crepeau, E. B. (1994b). Uneasy alliances: Belief and action on a geropsychiatric team. (Doctoral dissertation, University of New Hampshire, 1994). *Dissertation Abstracts International,* 9506410.

Golin, A. K., & Duncanis, A. J. (1981). *The interdisciplinary team.* Bethesda, MD: Aspen.

Humphry, R., Gonzalez, S., & Taylor, E. (1993). Family involvement in practice: Issues and attitudes. *American Journal of Occupational Therapy, 47,* 587–593.

Individuals With Disabilities Education Improvement Act. (2004). P.L. 108-446, 20 U.S.C. §1400 *et seq.*

Leff, P. T., & Walizer, E. H. (1992). *Building the healing partnership: Parents, professionals, and children with chronic illnesses and disabilities.* Cambridge, MA.: Brookline.

Parham, D. (1987). Toward professionalism: The reflective therapist. *American Journal of Occupational Therapy, 41,* 555–561.

Perlmutter, F. D., Bailey, D., & Netting, F. E. (2001). *Managing human resources in the human service.* New York: Oxford University Press.

Salisbury, C. (1992). Parents as team members: Inclusive teams, collaborative outcomes. In B. Rainforth, J. York, & C. MacDonald (Eds.), *Collaborative teams for students with severe disabilities* (pp. 43–68). Baltimore: Brookes.

Saxe, J. G. (1871). *The poems of John Godfrey Saxe.* Boston: Fields, Osgood.

Stancliff, B. L. (1995, November). Rehabilitation teams versus individual departments. *OT Practice,* 21–22.

Unsworth, C. A., Thomas, S. A., & Greenwood, K. M. (1995). Rehabilitation team decisions on discharge housing for stroke patients. *Archives of Physical Medicine and Rehabilitation, 76,* 331–340.

Wachtel, R. C., & Compart, P. J. (1996). Preparing pediatricians. In D. Bricker & A. Widerstrom (Eds.), *Preparing personnel to work with infants and young children and their families: A team approach* (pp. 181–198). Baltimore: Brookes.

Zenger, J. H., Musselwhite, E., Hurson, K., & Perrin, C. (1994). *Leading teams: Mastering the new role.* Homewood, IL: Business One Irwin.

Documentation in Practice

KAREN M. SAMES

> ❝ It's not what you tell them . . . it's what they hear. ❞
>
> —RED AUERBACH

Learning Objectives

After reading this chapter, you will be able to:

1. Identify the primary reasons for documentation of occupational therapy services
2. Describe the types of clinical, educational, and administrative documentation used in occupational therapy practice
3. Identify the key features of occupational therapy documentations in clinical and educational settings

INTRODUCTION

Occupational therapy practitioners communicate with many different types of people on a daily basis. They provide instructions for home programs to clients and their caregivers. They inform other professionals on the care team about the client's progress in occupational therapy. They write letters to foundations seeking funding for new programs. This chapter will address the various audiences and types of documentation that occupational therapy practitioners may use at some point during their careers.

AUDIENCE

How one documents depends greatly on who will receive the communication—one's audience. Writers must understand the reader's background and motives (Oliu, Brausaw, & Alred, 1995). How a letter to an insurance company is worded might be very different from the way a letter to a parent or physician is worded. Documentation that is read by a physical therapist might use more precise anatomical and technical words than would an Individual Family Service Plan that is shared with the parents of a 2-year-old. Knowing who will read what is being communicated is an important aspect of effective documentation.

The potential audiences for occupational therapy documentation include the following:

- Medical professionals (medical doctors, nurses, psychologists, physical therapists, speech-language pathologists, social workers, case managers, quality management staff, etc.)
- Education professionals (teachers, principals, etc.)
- Lawyers, judges, and juries
- Accreditation agencies (JCAHO, CARF, Department of Education, etc.)
- Payers (HMOs, Medicare intermediaries, Medicaid reviewers, etc.) and
- The client or the client's guardian

Each audience reads documentation through a different lens, depending on practice setting, educational level, and cultural background (Sames, 2005).

When one is communicating with medical professionals, one needs to be very precise. A physician, for example, would not be satisfied with a diagnosis of "stroke" for a client with whom the occupational therapist is working. The physician might want to know whether the stroke was affecting the right or left side, whether it was mild or severe, and how long it has been since the stroke. Nurses need to know more than that the patient needs assistance with dressing; they need to know how much assistance and the nature of the assistance.

When one is communicating in a school setting, there is a need to focus on the educational relevance of the information. The entire team working with the child might not understand medical jargon, so educational terms are more appropriate.

Occupational therapy practitioners need to communicate with each other and with other professionals and may do so by using formal letters, memos, e-mails, or phone calls. The word choices and the tone of the writing or speech used in professional, or formal, communication are very different from those used in informal communication between friends. Professional communication requires a level of respect and formality that is not required in informal communication.

Professional communication uses complete sentences and avoids slang or emotionally charged words. Informal communication often uses slang and emotionally charged words, may use phrases, and is usually directed toward someone known by the speaker or writer. When writing appeal letters, official memos, or plans of care, the writer might or might not know the person on the receiving end of the communication. Professional titles, rather than first names, are used in professional communication. This is where first impressions count.

Formal documentation often requires compliance with specific standards. For example, the **Individuals with Disabilities Act (IDEA)** requires that specific items be included on the Individualized Education Program, and Medicare requires specific documentation elements for outpatient therapy reimbursement. The Joint Commission on Accreditation of Health Care Organizations (JCAHO) requires that certain abbreviations be avoided to minimize the likelihood of medical errors due to abbreviations that are remarkably close in appearance (JCAHO, 2004). In addition, employers might have policies or procedures that further direct the method (electronic or paper and pen), timing, placement, and word choices of the documentation. Box 39.1 contains some documentation tips that apply to all documentation.

Two points are important considerations for all documentation (Sames, 2005):

1. People form an impression of your professionalism and intelligence by reading what you write.
2. What you write can be used as evidence in a court proceeding, whether you are on trial or not.

LEGAL AND ETHICAL CONSIDERATIONS

Medical records are legal documents. Medical records can be entered as evidence in any type of legal proceeding involving **malpractice**, **fraud**, **negligence**, or **incompetence**. The occupational therapy documentation can be called into court, with or without the occupational therapist being there to explain the documentation, even years after the services were provided. What was written at or near the actual time the event or events in question occurred is stronger evidence than what a person can recall months or years after the event. To remain mindful that all documentation is legal evidence, some people mentally preface their documentation by saying to themselves "Ladies and gentlemen of the jury . . ." before putting pen to paper (Sames, 2005).

BOX 39.1 DOCUMENTATION TIPS

- Use correct
  - Grammar
  - Spelling
  - Syntax
  - Word choice
  - Literacy level for the reader(s)
- Read spell-checker and grammar-checker recommendations carefully; sometimes it is better to click "Ignore" than to use what they recommend.
- Proofread carefully.
- Follow directions carefully.
- Have a dictionary and a writing manual handy.
- Write legibly (Sames, 2005).

Medicare and other government payers can review clinical documentation and client charge (billing) records at any time to determine whether fraud has been committed. If documentation is not adequate to support the charges, Medicare (and other payers) can refuse to pay for the services, and the occupational therapist responsible for documenting the services could face both civil and criminal penalties, as well as loss of certification and licensure (American Occupational Therapy Association [AOTA], 2000; Fremgen, 2002; Kornblau and Starling, 2000; Liang, 2000).

In addition to legal issues of documentation, there are ethical concerns. The AOTA Code of Ethics (2005) states in Principle 6.C that the "use of any form of communication that contains false, fraudulent, deceptive, or unfair statements or claims" is unethical. This is further clarified in the AOTA *Guidelines to the Code of Ethics:* "Occupational therapy personnel do not make deceptive, fraudulent, or misleading statements about the nature of the services they provide or the outcomes that can be expected" (AOTA, 2006, 2.1).

DOCUMENTATION IN CLINICAL SETTINGS

In hospitals, rehabilitation facilities, outpatient clinics, long-term care, mental health centers, home health, and related settings, similar types of documentation are used, although the frequency of documentation may vary. Clinical documentation generally involves reporting and interpreting the clients' responses on assessments and to interventions in a medical record. Clinical documentation is important for the following reasons:

◆ Continuity of care within the department
◆ Communication across shifts, disciplines
◆ Chronological record of care
◆ Legal record
◆ Reimbursement requirements (Sames, 2005)

It is critical that the objective information reported in the documentation be clearly differentiated from the subjective information. If a practitioner states that a client appeared depressed, that is a subjective statement. It is a conclusion drawn from the practitioner's observations. To make an objective statement, the practitioner should describe what was seen or heard that would logically lead to the conclusion that the client appeared depressed. For example, the practitioner could say, "Client stared at the floor for the entire session. She slouched forward in her chair, responded to questions with one syllable words, and did not initiate any conversations with peers."

All clinical documentation must be done in compliance with the standards of the setting as well as standards set by the profession. For example, every entry in the clinical record must be dated (AOTA, 2003). With electronic documentation, the date is automatically recorded by the sys-

tem. If the documentation is handwritten, the date must be put either at the top of the documentation or at the bottom, by the signature, whichever is the standard at the facility (AOTA, 2003). The essential features of all clinical documentation are as follows:

◆ Date of completion of report
◆ Full signature and credentials
◆ Type of document
◆ Client name and case number
◆ Acceptable abbreviations as determined by the facility
◆ Acceptable terminology as determined by the facility
◆ Corrections made with a single line through the error and initials of person who made the error are written above
◆ No use of an eraser or correction tape or fluid
◆ Record storage and disposal that complies with federal and state laws and facility procedures
◆ Protections of confidentiality
◆ Black or blue ink, never pencil (Sames, 2005)

The occupational therapy practitioner's rationale—the reasons behind the intervention—should be made clear in the documentation. For example, clients with mental health challenges might have problems in living that are not as visible as physical challenges. While people who uses wheelchairs might have difficulty with grocery shopping because they cannot reach all the shelves or push the cart while seated in a wheelchair, people with bipolar disorder might have difficulty shopping because of an inability to control impulses to buy everything and talk to everyone in the store.

Documentation of the Initiation of Occupational Therapy Services

The first type of clinical documentation reflects the first steps in the clinician-client interaction. In some settings, such as in a long-term care facility, the first step is a **screening** of all new admissions to the facility. In other settings, the first step might be an introduction, or it might be the beginning of the evaluation process.

If the client is seen for a screening or introduction prior to an **evaluation**, a short note is usually written in the medical record summarizing the conversation and/or results of the screening. The occupational therapist or occupational therapy assistant writes a short summary and indicates the next step in the intervention process.

Evaluation reports are written by occupational therapists to document the starting point of occupational therapy intervention. Evaluation reports contain factual data collected during the evaluation process and an interpretation of the evaluation findings. The need for occupational therapy services must be documented before interventions can be implemented. The report must show which occupations are limited or at risk of being limited. Typically, there will be an initial **plan of care** (care plan, treatment plan or intervention plan). This plan includes measurable, functional, and time-limited goals for the client (Borcherding, 2000; Sames, 2005).

The AOTA (2003) guidelines for documentation identify content needs for an evaluation report. The evaluation report content is based on the *Occupational Therapy Practice Framework* (AOTA, 2002). In an acute care setting, especially for short-stay clients, a complete evaluation might not be conducted. Although AOTA recommends that a complete evaluation be conducted and documented for each client, the time constraints of certain settings might require that the occupational therapist abbreviate the evaluation process and documentation.

Because payers often make decisions about whether or not to pay for occupational therapy on the basis of the evaluation report, it must show the need for skilled occupational therapy intervention (Lemke, 2004). The documentation must contain enough information to communicate that occupational therapy is the appropriate discipline to provide the needed intervention, that it meets a medical need, and that intervention will result in change in the client's function (Lemke, 2004).

Typically, the evaluation report contains the following (AOTA, 2003; Sames, 2005):

- Identifying information and background information (e.g., client's name, age, diagnosis or condition, date of referral, date of report, **precautions**, and **contraindications**)
- Referral information (date, who referred the client, and why)
- Evaluation procedures and/or tests used
- **Occupational profile** (client's perception of the need for occupational therapy, contexts that support or hinder occupational performance, brief occupational history)
- Findings or results of the evaluation process
- An interpretation of the meaning of the findings or results that reflects the occupational needs of the client
- A plan, including goals, frequency, duration, and location of intervention
- Signature and **credentials** of the occupational therapist

Documentation of Continuing Occupational Therapy Services

In clinical settings, **progress notes**, or clinical notes, are usually written after each intervention session. These may be written in a narrative or SOAP format or on a flow sheet (Sames, 2005). Regardless of the format, this documentation must show what the client did in occupational therapy and describe the client's reaction to the intervention that was provided. The progress note should include more than a list of the activities the client engaged in during the session. A reader will want to know how client's performance has changed since the last intervention session, any functional improvements, adaptive equipment provided, and client or caregiver understanding of any instructions (Lemke, 2004; Sames, 2005).

One of the most common forms of documenting the client's progress is called a **SOAP note**. This note-writing format is used by many medical disciplines, a practice that strengthens communication among professionals. Lawrence Weed, M.D., developed the SOAP note format in the 1960s as part of a Problem-Oriented Medical Record (Borcherding, 2000; Sames, 2005). Each letter of the word SOAP represents a different component of the note (Borcherding, 2000; Sames, 2005):

S = Subjective: the subjective experience of the client, what the client says
O = Objective: the clinician's objective observations and measurements
A = Assessment: the clinician's interpretation of the meaning of the "O" section
P = Plan: description of what will happen next (frequency, duration, location)

The most difficult part of writing a SOAP note is separating the objective information from the interpretation of it (assessment). Box 39.2 shows an example of a SOAP note.

BOX 39.2

SOAP NOTE

S: "It hurts to reach items on the second shelf. No way could I reach the top shelf. I can't even put my hair in a ponytail. It just hurts too much."

O: Client reached items on the second shelf of the kitchen cabinet with her right hand, expressing discomfort throughout the range. Client did not attempt to reach items on the top shelf. Client pointed to the anterior aspect of the glenoid fossa when asked where it hurt. Scapular elevation and trunk rotation substituted for part of shoulder flexion and abduction; she never raised her arm above 80°. Client used internal rotation to place items retrieved from the shelf on the counter with no complaints. Client did not use external rotation in replacing objects on shelf, reporting severe pain using that kind of motion. She rated her pain a 9 on a 0–10 point scale.

A: Right shoulder range of motion is severely limited and very painful. Limited range of motion interferes with meal preparation, dressing, hygiene, and grooming.

P: OT 2×/wk, for 30 min outpatient sessions to instruct client in use of reacher, discuss environmental adaptation principles related to placement of objects within comfort zone, and develop a home program to facilitate regaining pain-free range of motion.

In settings in which clients are seen for an extended period of time (over 30 calendar days), an updated plan of care is written. A plan of care shows what progress has occurred since the last plan of care was written (or an explanation for lack of progress); updates goals and sets new ones; and verifies the frequency, duration, and location of continued intervention (AOTA, 2003; Sames 2005).

Documentation of Termination of Occupational Therapy Services

Once clients have met their goals or other circumstance require that occupational therapy services end, a **discontinuation summary** (discharge summary) is written (AOTA, 2003; Sames 2005). This summary includes the following:

- Identifying and background information
- Summary of the client's functional status at the initiation of occupational therapy services
- Summary of change in functional status at the close of occupational therapy services
- Recommendations for follow-up
- Signature, credentials, and date

DOCUMENTATION IN SCHOOL SETTINGS

Documentation in educational settings can be very different from clinical documentation, but the same documentation principles apply. Documentation in school systems can be divided into three main categories: notice and consent forms, **Individualized Family Service Plans (IFSPs)**, and **Individualized Education Programs (IEPs)** (AOTA, 1999; Sames, 2005).

Documentation of Notice and Consent

According to the Individuals with Disabilities Education Act (IDEA), notice and consent forms are required to communicate with parents or guardians of children being served by the school district. Documents may include notices of team meetings, notice and consent for evaluation or reevaluation, referral for an initial evaluation, procedural safeguards, and a report of an IFSP or IEP meeting (Sames, 2005).

Documentation of Services from Birth Through Age 2 Years

Services for infants and toddlers are described in Part C of IDEA (AOTA, 1999). IFSPs are written to address these services. Each state designates a lead agency (education, health, or human services) to serve the needs of infants and toddlers with special needs to help ready them for school. The lead agency is responsible for creating an IFSP for each child served that is tailored to the specific needs of the child and the child's family. Occupational therapists can serve as **service coordinators** (case managers) for IFSPs. The service coordinator is responsible for ensuring that the proper documentation is completed and scheduling team meetings as needed or required by IDEA. An IFSP includes the following:

- A summary of the child's present level of performance (physical, cognitive, communicative, social or emotional, and adaptive development)
- Identification of the family's concerns, priorities, and resources
- A summary of expected outcomes (measurable goals)
- Identification of early intervention services needed, including frequency, intensity, and service delivery method
- Identification of the child's natural environment (where services will be delivered)
- Date services will start and the anticipated length of services
- Identification of a service coordinator for the child and
- Identification of the steps that will be taken to help the toddler transition to the preschool setting (20 U.S.C., Chapter 33, Subchapter III, Sect. 1436 [d] [1–8]).

Documentation of Services from Age 3 to 21 Years

The IEP is the document that guides services for a child with disabilities between the ages of 3 and 21 years. The requirements for IEPs are described in Part B of IDEA. IEP services may include both **special education** and **related services**. For the purposes of the IEP, occupational therapy services are considered related services. As a related service provider, the occupational therapist would not serve as a service coordinator for children with IEPs but would contribute to the process of writing and revising the IEP. The IEP is written every year and reviewed every six months.

An IEP must contain the following elements:

- Present level of educational performance
- Annual goals
- Special education and related services
- Participation with nondisabled children
- Participation in statewide and districtwide tests
- Starting date and location of services
- Transition services (for children age 14 years and older transitioning to adult programs or work settings)
- Measurement of progress (20 U.S.C. Chapter 33, Subchapter III, Sect. 1414)

The fundamental difference between the IFSP and the IEP is that the IFSP is more holistic; it can address a broader range of needs (AOTA, 1999). An IEP must be educationally related. Each state or each school district within a state may establish its own forms for these documents; the federal regulations do not require use of specific forms. The federal regulations mandate the timetables for completing the documents and the content of the documents (Sames, 2005).

DOCUMENTATION IN EMERGING PRACTICE SETTINGS

Occupational therapy practitioners are now working in community-based programs such as homeless shelters, prisons, Welfare to Work programs, home hospice, and summer camps. In some cases, occupational therapy programs are new to these settings. The clinical approach to documentation might not be appropriate, especially if there is no medical record. If the occupational therapy practitioner is working with individuals in the new program, it is advisable to develop evaluation, intervention plan, progress, and discontinuation reports that are consistent with the AOTA documentation guidelines (2003) to the greatest extent possible. However, if the occupational therapy practitioners are providing services at a community or population level, they may simply provide the agency with periodic consultation reports with a less structured format.

Most consultation reports are narrative descriptions of the needs assessment, plan, implementation, and/or outcomes of the occupational therapy program.

Since occupational therapy practitioners in emerging practice settings are demonstrating the value of occupational therapy in new ways, they may use their documentation as a mechanism to demonstrate successful outcomes and benefits of occupational therapy services.

ADMINISTRATIVE DOCUMENTATION

Occupational therapists in any setting may have to write an incident report, a letter of appeal to a payer source, a grant proposal, or **policies** and **procedures**. These types of documentation are administrative because they are necessary for the ongoing administration of occupational therapy services. For example, to be paid for delivering occupational therapy services, occupational therapy providers may need to write letters to request funding or to respond to a denial of a payment. Policies and procedures must be written clearly so that all employees of the department understand and follow the departmental standards, ensuring that the

BOX 39.3 WRITING FOR AN EVALUATION REPORT COMPARED TO A PRIOR AUTHORIZATION REQUEST LETTER

Tatiana is a 16-month-old girl from a large Midwestern city. Three weeks ago, while under the care of her mother's boyfriend, she was allegedly shaken violently. Her mother brought her to the hospital two days later because the baby was sleepier than normal, did not seem to want to eat or drink, did not hold her head up, and did not engage in any play activities or smile at her mother.

Excerpt from Evaluation Report:

Tatiana did not focus on or visually track any objects in any direction. She did not reach for any toys that were quietly placed in front of her, but she did turn her head to localize sounds and flailed her hands in reaction to sound. Her fingers closed around a rattle placed in the palm of her hand. Passive range of motion was within normal limits in all extremities. Muscle tone was generally low. She rubbed her face or arm in response to light touch. When placed on her stomach, she rolled her head from side to side but did not lift her head. When placed in a sitting position, she was unable to hold her head up or maintain sitting unassisted. Tatiana made no attempts to roll over or bear weight on her arms. She is fed through an N-G tube; therefore chewing and swallowing were not evaluated at this time. She cried and made other noises but did not

form any words. Tatiana will need adaptive seating with head support and occupational therapy intervention to maximize her abilities to actively interact with people and her environment.

Excerpt from Prior Authorization Letter:

This 16-month-old girl was diagnosed with Shaken Baby Syndrome resulting in severe head trauma. She has low muscle tone and cannot assume or maintain a seated position unassisted. This child will need adaptive seating and positioning devices to ensure proper positioning of her trunk and limbs and to prevent deformities. Proper positioning is also important for her cognitive, social, and physical development. Her vision is severely limited; she is functionally blind. In a seated position, she will better be able to localize sound, use her arms and hands, and begin to engage in social interactions. Please refer to attached list of recommended adaptive positioning devices and their respective costs. In addition, I recommend occupational therapy intervention twice a week for three months (24 visits) to work on developing the movement, social, and cognitive skills needed to enable participation in daily life activities of typical toddlers. A list of measurable goals is included. . . .

department functions well. To effectively do their jobs, aides, who are high school graduates with some on-the-job training, as well as professional staff must understand policies and procedures.

Administrative documentation requires the use of terminology that anyone can understand; people who have limited understanding of occupational therapy jargon or medical terms may read these documents. Often, the first person who reads an appeal letter will be someone who is trained to interpret insurance company standards but who might not have a medical background.

Box 39.3 shows an example of a section of an evaluation report written for a medical record, and how it might be translated in a letter to an insurance company requesting authorization for services.

ELECTRONIC DOCUMENTATION

As more facilities move to electronic medical records, it is becoming more common to use a keyboard to enter data and comments than to pick up a pen and write on a form. Each electronic documentation system has its quirks, strengths, and weaknesses. Some systems are highly specialized for occupational therapy practitioners, which makes it more likely that all the required information will

TABLE 39.1 ADVANTAGES AND DISADVANTAGES OF ELECTRONIC DOCUMENTATION SYSTEMS	
Advantages	**Disadvantages**
Legibility	Less flexibility in content
Speed (one click may enter a full sentence)	Investment in time and money
Automatic entry of client information	Learning curve required to develop proficiency in the system
Instant availability to anyone on the team	

Source: Sullivan (2001).

be included in the documentation. Others are more generic and might not have adequate space to add vital information. It is critical that the system be set up so that documentation will be in compliance with facility accreditation standards and payer requirements. Table 39.1 lists the pros and cons of electronic documentation systems.

ETHICAL DILEMMA

Documentation Standards

You work for a company that provides on-call occupational therapy personnel to hospitals and long-term care facilities in a large metropolitan area. You have been asked to work at a large long-term care facility that normally has a part-time occupational therapist and a full-time occupational therapy assistant. The occupational therapist went into labor early, and the temporary person who was hired to take her place during her maternity leave cannot start for at least three weeks. You have never worked in this facility before, but you have worked in other long-term care facilities and are familiar with the documentation requirements for Medicare and Medicaid.

On your first day there, you open the file for your patients and see that a few patients should have had 30-day intervention plans (renewals) written last week, but you can find no evidence that this was done. You ask the occupational therapy assistant whether the documentation could be somewhere else, and he says no. You find some progress notes on these patients, but they are irregular and inconsistent. Mostly, they just list some activities the patients worked on and say that the patients continue to progress toward their goals. Ten minutes later, you get a call from the medical records director saying that there are five patients for whom she cannot find a discontinuation summary and that the discontinuation summaries are needed for reimbursement. She asks you to write them, even though you have never seen the patients and the patients were discharged from the facility over a week ago. You know that the documentation must be done in order for the facility to get paid, but you feel uncomfortable documenting the care of patients you have never seen. The occupational therapy assistant says that he cannot help you because he is too busy with his own patients and he did not pay a lot of attention to the patients the occupational therapist was working with. What do you do?

PROVOCATIVE QUESTIONS

1. Can my documentation be used in a trial, even if I am not the one being sued?
2. If I am not a member of AOTA, do I have to follow AOTA standards for documentation?
3. What do I do if the electronic documentation system at my hospital does not offer a prewritten statement that accurately reflects my client's status?

REFERENCES

American Occupational Therapy Association. (1999). *Occupational therapy services for children and youth under IDEA* (2nd ed.). Bethesda, MD: Author.

American Occupational Therapy Association. (2000). *Final civil fraud and abuse penalties rule.* Retrieved May 12, 2002, from http://www.aota.org/members/area5/links/link56.asp

American Occupational Therapy Association. (2002). Occupational therapy practice framework: Domain and process. *American Journal of Occupational Therapy, 56,* 609–639.

American Occupational Therapy Association. (2003). Guidelines for documentation of occupational therapy. *American Journal of Occupational Therapy, 57,* 646–649.

American Occupational Therapy Association. (2005). Occupational therapy code of ethics. *American Journal of Occupational Therapy, 59,* 639–642.

American Occupational Therapy Association. (2006). Guidelines to the occupational therapy code of ethics. *American Journal of Occupational Therapy, 60,* 652–658.

Borcherding, S. (2000). *Documentation manual for writing SOAP notes in occupational therapy.* Thorofare, NJ: Slack.

Fremgen, B. F. (2002). *Medical law and ethics.* Upper Saddle River, NJ: Prentice Hall.

Joint Commission on Accreditation of Health Care Organizations. (2004). *Questions about Goal #2 (Communications) and the official "do not use" list.* Retrieved July 26, 2005, from http://www.jcaho.org/accredited+organizations/06_goal2_faqs.pdf

Kornblau, B. L., & Starling, S. P. (2000). *Ethics in rehabilitation.* Thorofare, NJ: Slack.

Lemke, L. (2004). Defensive documentation: Managing Medicare denials. *OT Practice, 9*(16), 8–12.

Liang, B. A. (2000). *Health law & policy: A survival guide to medicolegal issues for practitioners.* Woburn, MA: Butterworth-Heinemann.

Oliu, W. E., Brusaw, C. T., & Alred, G. J. (1995). *Writing that works: How to write effectively on the job* (5th ed.). New York: St. Martins.

Sames, K. M. (2005). *Documenting occupational therapy practice.* Upper Saddle River, NJ: Prentice Hall.

Sullivan, C. (2001). Electronic documentation: The process of facility-wide implementation. *Administration and Management Special Interest Section Quarterly, 17*(3), 1–3.

20 U.S.C., Chapter 33, Subchapter III, Sect.1436 [d] [1–8]. Retrieved March 29, 2006, from http://uscode.house.gov/download/pls/20C33.txt

20 U.S.C. Chapter 33, Subchapter III, Sect. 1414. Retrieved March 29, 2006, from http://uscode.house.gov/download/pls/20C33.txt

Professional Presentations and Publications

KAREN JACOBS

The greatest problem in communication is the illusion that it has been accomplished.

—DANIEL W. DAVENPORT

Learning Objectives

After reading this chapter, you will be able to:

1. Describe the seven aspects to an effective professional presentation.
2. List four nonverbal factors in the delivery of a professional presentation
3. Describe the difference between a peer-reviewed and a non-peer-reviewed publication.
4. Describe aspects of an effective professional publication

PROFESSIONAL PRESENTATIONS

Occupational therapy practitioners frequently provide professional presentations to a variety of audiences. We have listened to professional presentations—some great, some that put us to sleep. Thinking back to professional presentations that you liked (or did not like), you could easily come up with lists of what to do and what not to do (Merchant 2005). Payne names seven factors that are important to an effective professional presentation: purpose, audience, speaker, message, language and delivery, audiovisual aids, and feedback (Payne, 2002, p. 142).

Purpose

The first step in the process of developing a professional presentation is to decide on its purpose. Why are you presenting? Is it to inform, instruct, define, demonstrate, or teach? For example, you might be asked to provide a professional presentation at a weekly staff meeting during your Level II fieldwork on the effectiveness of assistive technology for clients who have low-vision impairments. The purpose in this situation might be to inform your colleagues of the most recent evidence-based research on the topic. Perhaps the purpose of your professional presentation is to persuade, influence, convince, or market a product or service. For instance, you might have the opportunity to provide a professional presentation on energy conservation strategies to a consumer group, such as the National Multiple Sclerosis Society. The purpose here might be to market occupational therapy services available at your workplace. Perhaps the purpose of your presentation might be to inspire or entertain your audience. One example of an inspirational professional presentation is the yearly presidential keynote address at the American Occupational Therapy Association (AOTA) national conference. Once you have decided on the purpose of your professional presentation, the next step is to conduct an audience analysis.

Audience

Who is your audience? Before preparing your professional presentation, it is important to analyze the background, demographics, interests, attitudes, and expectations of your audience. Having information about your audience, such as its preexisting knowledge, beliefs, and attitudes about your topic will help you better match your message and its delivery to the needs and expectations of the group (Payne, 2002). At the very least, determine the expected size of the audience. Presenting to a small group of colleagues at your Level II fieldwork site would be quite different from presenting to an audience of 50 to 100 occupational therapy practitioners at a state or national conference.

Speaker

Important, but sometimes overlooked, is how the audience's interest and potential knowledge gain from a presentation may be directly influenced by the speaker himself or herself. A speaker who has perceived expertise, such as career success (e.g., a Fellow of the American Occupational Therapy Association), work experience (e.g., 20 years of practice in the area of ergonomics), or job responsibility (e.g., Director of Rehabilitation Services); one who conveys trustworthiness, reliability, or sincerity; one with whom the audience has a degree of identification; or one who is charismatic has the right characteristics to make a professional presentation great (Payne, 2002) (Figure 40.1).

Message

The message of a presentation has three parts: the introduction, the body, and the conclusion.

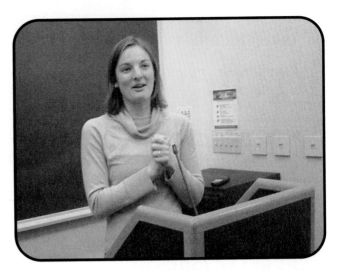

FIGURE 40.1 A charismatic speaker inspires the audience with her enthusiasm and hand gestures.

Introduction

The introduction should always begin with a simple greeting, such as "good morning," or a thank you to the host (e.g., "Thank you, Dr. Jacobs, for inviting me to speak today"). One then continues with a brief preview of the presentation. A relevant joke, short story, or quote can also make an impressive starting statement. Whatever technique is used, it should arouse the audience's curiosity about your presentation and capture the audience's attention.

Body

The body of the presentation should contain at least 75% of your key points. The rule of three major points is always good to follow:

1. Preview your points.
2. Describe and substantiate them in a logical order.
3. Summarize your points (Payne, 2002, p. 145).

Use natural transitions between each point; transitions "form a bridge between parts of your presentation" (Milan, 2002, p. 2). Be sure to include references when invoking evidence-based research or supporting materials.

Conclusion

You have made it to the conclusion of your presentation. Now is your chance to tell the audience what you expect them to remember. Keep the conclusion brief, review salient points, and include a final statement that will leave a lasting impact. One could use a memorable quotation or reinforce a point from the story with which your introduction began. Always finish your presentation with a pause and then a "thank you," which gives the audience a sense of closure, and be sure to leave some extra time for

BOX 40.1 | **EXAMPLE OF AN OUTLINE FOR A PERSUASIVE SPEECH**

Purpose

To persuade an audience that consists primarily of university graduate students of the importance of sitting properly at the computer, taking breaks, and using computer equipment.

Introduction

◆ Open with a greeting that refers to the group, such as "Good morning, Boston University graduate students. I am Dr. Karen Jacobs, a professor in occupational therapy at Sargent College."

◆ Introduce the topic by using a rhetorical question (e.g., "How many of you enjoy having aches and pains from using your computer?"), wait for a show of hands, and continue: "University students are spending more and more time sitting at a computer workstation to do homework, surf the Internet, and play video games. How you position yourselves in a chair, and how you use the computer equipment can affect not only your comfort, but also your health" (quote from AOTA).

◆ State that "Today I am here to talk to you about the importance of healthy computing and what you can do to stay healthy."

◆ Preview the points to be covered: (1) proper posture, (2) computer workstation arrangements, and (3) frequent stretch breaks.

Body

Begin with an attention-getting statement, and then focus on the three points with examples:

1. Proper posture: Encourage proper posture of the head, forearms, back, and feet: The head should be level with the monitor and the top of the screen at eye level. The forearms should be parallel to the keyboard and held only slightly above it. The lower back should be supported while sitting in front of a computer. Place a small pillow or rolled up towel between the back of the chair and the lower back to provide back support. The feet should rest flat on the floor or on a footstep.

2. Computer workstation arrangements: Arrange the computer desk and equipment so as to avoid glare from sunlight. Set the monitor 18 to 30 inches away from the person. Adjust the chair to an appropriate height for the person.

3. Frequent stretch breaks: Every 30 minutes, take a stretch break from the computer.

References to evidence-based literature are included.

Conclusion

◆ End the presentation by highlighting the responsibility each student has to his or her health.

◆ Briefly review the three points covered: proper posture, computer workstation arrangements, and frequent stretch breaks.

End with a quote or refer back to the rhetorical question in the introduction.

◆ Thank the audience for the opportunity to speak to them.

◆ Pass out your business cards so that interested listeners can contact you if they have any questions.

Sources: Some of the content related to computing was taken from the AOTA consumer brochures: Healthy computing for adults *(2002)* and Healthy computing for today's kids *(2001). Copyright American Occupational Therapy Association, Inc. All Rights Reserved. Information from the fact sheet may be reproduced and distributed without prior written consent (www.aota.org). See also Payne, G. (2002). Oral presentations. In D. Nelson, R. Brownson, P. Remington, & C. Parvanta (Eds.),* Communicating public health information effectively: A guide for practitioners *(pp. 141–154). Washington, DC: American Public Health Association.*

responding to the audience's questions. Box 40.1 provides an example of an outline for a persuasive professional presentation.

Language and Delivery

Language

The language you use will depend on your audience analysis. If you are presenting to occupational therapy practi-tioners, you want to make sure that the language you use conforms with the American Occupational Therapy Association's (AOTA) Framework. For an audience of people who are not occupational therapists, minimize the use of highly technical language or jargon. In general, use conventional words and phrases, use links and transitions, and try to use similes and metaphors to paint pictures in the minds of the audience. "The guiding principle is that language be suitable for the speaker, the subject, and the occasion." (Payne, 2002, p. 147).

BOX 40.2 RECOMMENDATIONS FOR THE DELIVERY OF PROFESSIONAL PRESENTATIONS

Verbal Factors

◆ Vary your voice pitch or melody; avoid speaking in a monotone.

◆ Pronounce and articulate your words and syllables.

◆ Speak slowly; an optimal range is 150–185 words per minute.

◆ Avoid filler sounds and words (e.g., "er," "uh," "you know," "okay").

◆ Project your voice; if your voice is soft, use a microphone.

◆ Use pauses or changes in your voice level to stress key points.

◆ Make sure your sentences are grammatically correct.

◆ Always stay within your allotted time.

Nonverbal Factors

◆ Dress conservatively, and avoid excessive jewelry; your appearance directly affects your credibility.

◆ Look at your audience.

◆ Make sure your facial expressions agree with your message.

◆ Interact with your visual aids, but do not read from them.

◆ Involve your audience; ask questions and wait for responses; call on individuals.

◆ Avoid clutching or leaning on the podium.

◆ Use gestures and movements appropriately.

◆ Avoid distracting mannerisms (e.g., drinking water, chewing gum, hands in pockets, twirling or clicking a pen).

Source: Adapted from Payne, G. (2002). Oral presentations. In D. Nelson, R. Brownson, P. Remington, & C. Parvanta (Eds.), Communicating public health information effectively: A guide for Practitioners (pp. 141–154). Washington, DC: American Public Health Association.

Delivery

Avoid using filler sounds and words, such as "er," "uh," "you know," and "okay" in the delivery of your presentation. These fillers are distracting and can reduce a speaker's credibility. "A speaker's delivery plays a vital role in enabling audiences to receive and respond to the message, and consists of both verbal and non-verbal aspects" (Payne, 2002, p. 147). Box 40.2 provides examples of recommendations for the delivery of professional presentations.

Now that you understand the need for effective language and delivery, practice, practice, practice your presentation! Rehearsing the presentation can help you to raise your confidence and sense of preparedness and develop a "can-do" attitude. Practice in front of friends and family, and ideally, videotape your presentation and review it to critically analyze your message, language, delivery, and use of audiovisual aids.

Audiovisual Aids

Audiovisual aids used in professional presentations include flip charts, posters, blackboards, overheads, slides, computer graphics, audio and video clips, and direct use of Internet sites. To be effective, audiovisual aids should help one to clarify, enhance, and support the message while holding the interest of one's audience (Payne, 2002). If you are using a visual aid, such as Microsoft Office PowerPoint®, apply the guidelines in Box 40.3.

BOX 40.3 GUIDELINES FOR SLIDES

◆ Slides should be an outline of the presentation.

◆ Use no more than six lines per slide, with six words to a line maximum.

◆ Font sizes should be 32 point minimum for titles.

◆ Font sizes should be 20 point minimum for text.

◆ Use no more than one slide per minute.

◆ Illustrate concepts with images or other visuals.

◆ Credit the author, date, title of article, and journal title on the slide in small print (18 point) at the bottom.

◆ References should be on the last slide in American Psychological Association (APA) format. Prepare backup materials, that is, print slides on overhead transparencies or bring handouts, just in case the computer or projector decides to be uncooperative.

◆ Rehearse and view visual aids ahead of time in the room where you will use them.

◆ Arrive at least 30 minutes before your presentation time, set up your audiovisuals. and stand in the back of the room to make sure they are visible.

◆ In a room with ambient light, it is best to use high-contrast colors; a dark background (e.g., blue) with light letters (e.g., yellow) is typically visually appealing.

ETHICAL DILEMMA

How Can an Occupational Therapy Student Meet Time Demands and Still Provide a Professional Evidence-Based Presentation?

Ariel, an occupational therapy graduate student, is anxious about presenting her first professional presentation at a local Parents-Teachers Association meeting. She has been invited to speak briefly on the importance of junior high school students' proper use of backpacks and has been instructed to limit her presentation to 10 minutes and 10 slides. She has so much information to put on the slides that she has decided not to include any citations or references on the slides. She will be providing her slides as handouts to the meeting's participants.

Questions

1. Does Ariel have an ethical responsibility to include citations or references on the slides?
2. What conflicts are present between not including citations or references on the slides and giving slides as a handout to the meeting's participants?

Feedback

You are now almost finished with your first professional presentation. Suppose you have noticed throughout that members of your audience have been nodding their heads as you speak, others have spontaneously laughed at your jokes, and still others are smiling when you make eye contact with them. This nonverbal feedback from your audience communicates that your presentation has been a success. Feedback is the final aspect of a professional presentation, and it is typically nonverbal. With experience, you can easily identify the nonverbal cues that audiences convey when a presentation is not a success: arched eyebrows, yawning, restlessness, talking, or even walking out of the presentation. It is your responsibility as a speaker to be constantly aware of your audience's nonverbal communication and to make necessary adjustments to your message or its delivery to better meet their needs and expectations.

PROFESSIONAL PUBLICATIONS

In the first part of this chapter, you learned about professional presentations. Now let us look at another important aspect of professional communication: professional publications. There are a variety of professional publications. Among them are books, journals, chapters in books, trade and magazine journals, newsletters, conference proceedings, and films or videos. There are also various media types. These include print, CD-ROM, audio, video, web, and software. In the hierarchy of professional publications are the following:

- Peer-reviewed journals
- Peer-reviewed conference proceedings
- Non-peer-reviewed books
- Non-peer-reviewed chapters in books
- Other non-peer reviewed materials

Peer-reviewed documents are those that are reviewed by "expert readers." Non-peer-reviewed documents typically have less demanding standards for screening prior to publication. Examples of these two kinds of publications include feature-length articles, briefs, reviews, case reports, letters to the editor, practice forums, and technical notes. The focus of the remainder of this chapter will be on peer-reviewed and non-peer-reviewed documents in occupational therapy.

Peer-Reviewed Journals

The peer review process is a form of assessment that is designed to provide constructive feedback to authors about their potential publication. Typically, submissions are evaluated by at least two reviewers, without their knowing the identity of the authors ("blind"). Reviewers are typically members of the journal's editorial board and are experts in their specific areas of practice. Depending on the scope of the journal, manuscripts are evaluated as to their relevance and contribution to the knowledge and practice of occupational therapy, aspects of methodology, statistical analyses, theoretical contributions, clarity, and style of writing. A typical review process is outlined in Box 40.4.

The most widely read peer-reviewed occupational therapy journal is the *American Journal of Occupational Therapy* (AJOT). It "is the official publication of the

BOX 40.4   TYPICAL MANUSCRIPT REVIEW PROCESS FOR PEER-REVIEWED JOURNALS

◆ Submission of original manuscript and editor assignment (~1 week).

A manuscript is submitted by its authors to the editor of the journal. The editor evaluates whether the manuscript is within the scope of the journal and whether it fulfills the journal's scientific and technical standards.

◆ Manuscript is provided to peer reviewers for blind review (~4–8 weeks).

Manuscripts, without any identification of authorship, are reviewed by at least two peer reviewers. Each journal has specific criteria for its review of a manuscript, but in general, the article is evaluated is on the basis of its contribution to the knowledge and practice of occupational therapy, methodology, statistical analyses, theoretical and empirical contributions, and clarity and style of writing. Typically, peer reviewers have four possible options for each manuscript:

1. Accept the manuscript without revision
2. Accept the manuscript after revision
3. Neither accept nor reject until the author(s) make revisions and resubmit the manuscript
4. Reject the manuscript

◆ Editor reads peer reviews and compiles correspondence to the contact author (~1–3 weeks).

The editor compiles the peer reviews and communicates the status of the manuscript to the contact author.

◆ Publication of manuscript

1. If the manuscript is accepted without revision, it is placed in the queue for publication. The manuscript is submitted to the publisher, who will send proofs of the manuscript to be reviewed by author(s) (~ **3–12 months**, depending on the journal's publication schedule).
2. If the manuscript is accepted after it is revised, the manuscript is placed in the queue for publication once the revision has been reviewed and accepted. The manuscript is submitted to the publisher, who will send proofs of the manuscript to be reviewed by author(s) (~ **5–14 months**, depending on the journal's publication schedule).
3. If the manuscript is neither accepted nor rejected, the resubmitted revised manuscript will be sent out for review; typically by the original peer reviewers.

American Occupational Therapy Association, Inc. and is published 6 times per year. This peer reviewed journal focuses on research, practice, and health care issues in the field of occupational therapy" (AOTA, 2007). "The journal publishes articles that are theoretical and conceptual and that represent theory-based research, research reviews and applied research related to innovative program approaches, educational activities and professional trends" (AOTA, 2007).

Another peer-reviewed occupational therapy journal is the *Occupational Therapy Journal of Research: Occupation, Participation and Health* (OTJR). In contrast to AJOT, OTJR focuses on research articles and systematic review papers that advance the knowledge of occupation or focus on improving the lives of people who are at risk for restrictions to their participation in meaningful activities (American Occupational Therapy Foundation, 2007).

In the area of occupational science, the premier journal is *The Journal of Occupational Science* (JOS). The stated aim of this journal is to "give voice to the unique experiences, concerns and perspectives of the study of humans as occupational beings." It is "designed to provide opportunities to publish articles of interest to many

disciplines such as: anthropologists, ethnologists, ethologists, human geographers, philosophers, psychologists, occupational therapists, sociologists and social biologists" (Association of Occupational Science, 2007).

Box 40.5 contains a listing of the major international peer-reviewed journals with a primary focus on occupational therapy.

Non-Peer-Reviewed Documents

Some examples of non-peer-reviewed materials are books, chapters in books, trade journals, magazines, and newsletters. The best-known non-peer-reviewed magazines and newsletters in occupational therapy are *OT Practice,* the SIS *Quarterly* newsletters, and *1-Minute Update E-Newsletter,* published by AOTA, and *ADVANCE for Occupational Therapy Practitioners,* published by Merion Publications, Inc. These magazines and newsletters typically have less demanding screening standards before publication than do peer-reviewed journals but may include scholarly materials and newsy articles. Specifically, *OT Practice* "covers professional information in all aspects of occupational therapy practice today. Features include

BOX 40.5 PEER-REVIEWED OCCUPATIONAL THERAPY JOURNALS

American Journal of Occupational Therapy
Australian Journal of Occupational Therapy
British Journal of Occupational Therapy
Canadian Journal of Occupational Therapy
Israel Journal of Occupational Therapy
Journal of the New Zealand Association of Occupational Therapists
Journal of Occupational Therapy Science Australia
Journal of Occupational Therapy Students

Occupational Therapy in Health Care
Occupational Therapy in Mental Health
Occupational Therapy Journal of Research
OTJR: Occupation, Participation and Health
Physical & Occupational Therapy in Geriatrics
Physical & Occupational Therapy in Pediatrics
Scandinavian Journal of Occupational Therapy
The Journal of Occupational Science
Work: A Journal of Prevention, Assessment & Rehabilitation

everything from hands-on techniques to continuing education, legislative issues to career advice and job opportunities, to the latest professional news" (AOTA, 2007).

AOTA publishes 11 different SIS *Quarterly* newsletters, each of which focuses on a specific practice area, such as work, gerontology, school-based practice, or technology. These newsletters are published four times per year. The *1-Minute Update E-Newsletter* is a biweekly e-mail newsletter that features important news about occupational therapy, trends, ideas, and products. These publications are free to those with AOTA membership, or they may be purchased separately

ADVANCE for Occupational Therapy Practitioners is a biweekly news magazine that contains "stories on the newest treatment arenas, protocols and products, therapy equipment and modalities along with regular columns" (ADVANCE for Occupational Therapy Practitioners, 2005). There is no charge for subscriptions to *ADVANCE for Occupational Therapy Practitioners.*

CONCLUSION

As you finish this chapter on professional presentations and professional publications, think about setting these goals for yourself:

1. To follow the strategies described in the chapter for your next and all future professional presentations.

2. To keep up with the expanding body of knowledge in occupational therapy by reading at least three peer-reviewed articles a month.
3. To develop your skills to write articles/manuscripts for a professional publication.

REFERENCES

ADVANCE for Occupational Therapy Practitioners. (2005). Retrieved June 29, 2005, from http://occupational-therapy.advanceweb.com/common/editorial/editorial.aspx?CTID=23

American Occupational Therapy Association. (2007?). Retrieved January 13, 2007, from http://www.aota.org/ajot/about ajot.asp

American Occupational Therapy Association. (2007). Publications. Retrieved January 13, 2007, from http://www.aota.org/nonmembers/area7/index.asp

American Occupational Therapy Foundation. (2007). Retrieved January 13, 2007, from http://www.aotf.org

Association of Occupational Science. *Aim and scope.* (2007). Retrieved January 13, 2007, from http://www.jos.org.au/aim.asp

Merchant, S. (2005) *Oral communication.* Retrieved June 28, 2005, from http://planet.tvi.cc.nm.us/merchant/classesi.htm

Milan, S. (2002). *Public speaking.* Boca Raton, FL: Bar Chart.

Payne, G. (2002). Oral presentations. In D. Nelson, R. Brownson, P. Remington, & C. Parvanta (Eds.), *Communicating public health information effectively: A guide for practitioners* (pp. 141–154). Washington, DC: American Public Health Association.

Client Education

SUE BERGER

Learning Objectives

After reading this chapter, you will be able to:

1. Understand key factors that contribute to effective client communication
2. Understand the importance of health literacy throughout all types of client education
3. Choose and/or develop appropriate written client education materials

INTRODUCTION

As health care professionals, occupational therapy practitioners are educators. We teach our clients knowledge and skills they need to enhance well-being and live as safely as possible. Yet our own education focuses more on intervention skills and less on the strategies we need to be effective teachers. Chapter 36 provides the theoretical background related to learning; this chapter focuses on specific education strategies and how to effectively use them.

Rankin, Stallings, and London (2005) emphasize that client education is a partnership, involving both listening and sharing. Osborne (2001) identifies five key strategies to enhance communication in a client–health care professional partnership:

- Creating a positive environment
- Limiting the objectives of the communication
- Conveying the information clearly and slowly
- Using multiple strategies to communicate the message
- Verifying understanding

When possible, these five strategies should be used in all types of communication.

COMMUNICATING VERBALLY

We are constantly teaching our clients. We teach them how to perform one-handed dressing after they have had a stroke. Practitioners educate classroom teachers about appropriate environments to facilitate learning for students with special needs. We teach individuals about strategies for safely using community transportation. Often, the teaching occurs verbally. Whom one speaks with (characteristics of the client), how it is said (organization of the information), what is said (information included), and when it is said (environment and timing) all affect how the information is received, learned, and used.

Characteristics of the Client

As with all intervention, knowing the client and his or her strengths, limitations, culture, values, interests, age, and education level is fundamental. In communicating orally, knowing the client's literacy skills, native language, and auditory ability is also important. Though the definition of literacy refers to reading and writing, it also affects one's ability to comprehend oral information (American Medical Association [AMA], 1999). In communicating with someone with low literacy skills, it is helpful to be consistent with word choice. During a session on feeding skills, for example, the word *silverware* should be used throughout instead of alternating with *utensil*. Unusual or challenging words used in conversation should be defined, and acronyms should be explained (Centers for Disease Control and Prevention [CDC], 1999). Words such as *assessment* or *intervention* should be defined, or more common words should be used. Acronyms such as *ROM* and *ADL* should be used only after they are fully explained. If you are unsure of word choice, ask the client what word he or she uses to describe an item, and use that word consistently. For example, you might ask a girl or woman whether she refers to her top as her *shirt* or *blouse*.

Communicating with clients who are hard of hearing poses other challenges. It is helpful to choose an environment that is quiet and free of distractions, get the client's attention before speaking, and position oneself directly in front of the client (Osborne, 2001). Often, a client hears better from one side than the other, so it is important to take the time to find this out and position oneself on the stronger side. If the person wears hearing aids, make sure they are in place and working. If hearing is severely impaired, use other methods of communication along with, or instead of, speaking. When entering an environment in which there are distractions, ask the client whether you can move to another location, turn the television off, or find a better time that might be more beneficial for instruction.

Organization of the Information

Organization of information to be presented helps clients to understand and apply information. Though this is especially true for individuals with low literacy, all people, especially those who are in a new environment, are learning new information, are in pain, or are anxious, will benefit when material is presented clearly and in an organized manner. Therefore, plan the information to be conveyed before talking and speak in sequence (Osborne, 2001). For example, if you are working with a group of children to help them lighten their backpacks, begin by stating, "First decide what needs to go in; second, put heavy books at the back of the pack; and third, put lighter objects in the front of the pack."

Using demonstrations, models, and pictures along with oral communication also helps people to understand information (AMC Cancer Research Center, 1994). When teaching clients about the importance of eliminating clutter for safety, show before-and-after pictures of a kitchen and point out safety hazards and ways they were resolved. When teaching use of adaptive equipment, explain and demonstrate. Use multiple teaching methods, especially when working with groups of individuals, because different people learn differently. Even when working with one client, multiple teaching methods help to emphasize key information and facilitate comprehension and memory.

Finally, one must verify understanding. The practitioner might believe that he or she was clear, organized, and consistent, but if the client did not understand the message, the practitioner was not successful. There are many ways to verify understanding, including asking the client to demonstrate, to repeat in his or her own words, or to explain a concept using a different example (Doak, Doak, & Root, 1996). The individual who is passive or constantly nodding in agreement might not fully understand or adhere to the recommendations. Therefore, it is helpful to encourage questions, input, and ideas, all of which lead toward involvement and more potential for follow-through (DiMatteo, 1995). When possible, ask one client to demonstrate or to teach other clients. Clients are more likely to ask questions and admit lack of understanding with a peer than with a therapist.

Information Included

Several studies have found large discrepancies between what clients wanted to know and what health professionals believed was most important. Davis, Fredrickson and colleagues (1998) found that low-income, low-literacy, minority women were most interested in learning about cost of procedures, something that was rarely addressed. Reid and colleagues (1995) learned that many people wanted information about treatment and prognosis, yet this was often not addressed. To facilitate comprehension and recall, it is important to understand what information the client wants and needs to know and to communicate this information clearly (AMA, 1999).

Recall of information depends on two factors: the type of information and how the information is presented. Bradshaw, Ley, and Kincey (1975) studied participants' recall about how to develop healthy eating habits. The participants remembered information when it was perceived as important. Also, information that was given as specific suggestions was recalled more often than general suggestions were. For example, "Walk briskly for 30 minutes three times a week" would be recalled more often than "Exercise several times a week."

Cultural sensitivity is a critical factor for effective client education. Terminology, topics, and ideas should all be relevant to the intended audience. When possible, communication should be in the person's native language. Professional interpreters are best to prevent miscommunication and ensure privacy (Rankin et al., 2005). However, this is not always possible, and family members might be the only available interpreters. Caution should be used in this situation, as family members' own opinions and reactions are often conveyed as well or instead of the client's (CDC, 1999). The best interpreters are those who have been trained to interpret, not just someone who speaks the same language.

Being culturally sensitive involves more than speaking in the client's native language. One should use culturally relevant examples, consider the meaning of personal space and time within the client's culture, and be careful about making judgments or interpretations without checking this out with the person (Purtilo & Haddad, 2002). Being cognizant of cultural differences and beliefs in health and wellness is the first step toward effective communication with individuals of cultures other than one's own. See Huff, and Kline (1999), Rankin and colleagues (2005), or World Education (2000) for more in depth information on culturally competent client education.

Environment and Timing

The environment in which client education occurs can influence comprehension and recall. It is important for information to be shared in a shame-free environment (Osborne, 2005), a setting in which the client feels free to ask questions, admit lack of understanding, or ask for repetition. Internal distractions such as pain, anxiety, hunger, or need to use the bathroom also affect one's ability to absorb and understand information. And because some people are "morning people" and others are more alert (and receptive to information) in the evening, timing of all client education is important.

When working in schools, schedule evening hours to provide parent education. Parents who need to take time off from work to attend a meeting may arrive frustrated and angry and will be less open to hearing new information.

COMMUNICATING IN WRITING

Kessels (2003) showed that most people forget up to 80% of what they are told during a patient-physician interaction and that almost half of what they believe they remember, they remember incorrectly. Reinforcing oral communication with print material can help recall and comprehension. Written forms of communication reinforce what is said, provide a record of what is said, and provide reminders of what is conveyed. If it is worth the time to write down information, it is important to ensure that the reader can use the material.

The main considerations for effective written communication include the characteristics of the user of the material; the information the therapist wants to covey or, more important, the information the client needs and wants to know; the **reading level** of the material; the presentation of the material; and the cultural relevance of the material (Butow, Brindle, McConnell, Boakes, & Tattersall, 1998; National Cancer Institute, 2003).

Characteristics of the Client

In all occupational therapy practice, it is important for the practitioner to know the client and his or her strengths, limitations, culture, values, interests, age, and education level. For written communication, knowing someone's general reading ability is also important. Reading levels may be impaired for individuals with disabilities, those who are reading material that is not in their native language, and, of course, those who never learned to read. When giving any written material to a client, one should note whether the client states something similar to "I'll read this later so I can discuss it with my husband," "I left my glasses at home," or "I'll remember what you say—no need to write it down." Does the client appear to read something but then is unable to follow the instructions? Good observation skills can provide a great deal of information about reading level. Knowing that a client struggles with reading will guide a practitioner to use some of the strategies discussed below. Though there are standardized reading level assessments, more research is needed to determine whether formally assessing a client for reading level affects practitioner-client relationship or improves outcomes (AMA, 1999). Reading literacy also does not imply reading comprehension.

Just asking, "Do you read much?" can guide intervention. If the answer is no, that can be a cue to use strategies other than written materials to reinforce information.

Information Included

As with oral communication, it is important to focus on material that the client wants or needs to know when developing or choosing print materials. Though something that is "nice to know" might seem valuable to include, more is often not better (CDC, 1999; Osborne, 2001). In considering what material to include in written pamphlets, brochures, or home programs, prioritize the information and focus on a few key, relevant objectives. Remember to prioritize information by what is important to the client, not what you believe is important for the client to know.

Reading Level of the Material

Much public information, such as newspapers, is written at the tenth-grade level or higher. However, the 2003 National Adult Literacy Survey (NALS) found that approximately one out of three Americans is functionally illiterate, defined as reading below the fifth-grade level, and this number increases to one in two people who struggle with reading when those with only marginally better reading skills are included (Kutner, Greenberg, Jin, & Paulsen, 2006). Though about 20% of these people either have learning disabilities or were born outside the United States, the majority of those who cannot read are white, native-born Americans (AMA, 1999). Butow and colleagues (1998) looked at preferences for brochures about cancer. Participants showed a clear preference for the brochure that was written at an eighth-grade level as compared to those at the eleventh-grade level. In a large randomized controlled study about polio immunization information, Davis, Fredrickson, and colleagues (1998) found that comprehension increased with written material at a fourth- to sixth-grade level for all individuals. The study also showed that the simpler form did not insult those with higher education and higher income. Use of a low reading level in written materials meets the needs of a large number of people.

Though there are numerous assessments to determine the reading level of written material, in general using short sentences and one- or two-syllable words is a simple strategy that will keep the reading level low (AMC Cancer Research Center, 1994). Though it is often impossible, and sometimes not desirable, to eliminate all words of three or more syllables, it is a good idea to use a simpler, common word when feasible. Using the word *doctor* instead of *physician* or using the term *thinking skills* instead of *cognition* is sometimes appropriate. One must be careful when using this strategy, however. Short, choppy sentences are not always easier to read, and some three-syllable words that are commonly used in conversation can facilitate readability (Reid et al., 1995). Shorter sentences and use of primarily one- or two-syllable words should be used as a guideline only. If the reader wants to learn more about standardized readability formulas or computer generated formulas, the book by Doak and colleagues (1996) or the help feature in Microsoft Word 2007 are recommended.

In addition to reading level, other factors influence the readability of printed material. For example, the use of all capital letters is more challenging to read than is a combination of uppercase and lowercase letters, because readers use the shapes of words to help read. For example, when typed in all capitals, "AND" looks like a rectangle and is visually very similar to "FOR," "THE," or any other three-letter word. If typed with lowercase letters, "and," "for," and "the" all have different shapes, and it is therefore easier to quickly determine the word (Doak et al., 1996). Box 41.1 provides examples of easy and difficult to use layouts and fonts.

The use of common words makes reading easier as well (CDC, 1999; Executive Secretariat, 2003; Osborne, 2005). Most people understand the term *high blood pressure* better than they do *hypertension.* If it is important to use the term *hypertension,* it is suggested to define it and use it consistently. Use of descriptions that are simple to

BOX 41.1 — EXAMPLES OF FONTS AND LAYOUT THAT ARE EASY VERSUS DIFFICULT TO READ

1. It is easier to read material that is written using a combination of uppercase and lowercase letters THAN MATERIAL WRITTEN IN ALL CAPITALS.
2. It is easier to read print in Times New Roman, a font with serifs, than to read material printed in Arial, a sans serif font.
3. It is easier to read material that uses a 12-point font than material that uses a 9-point font.
4. It is easier to read the material written above that is single-spaced than what you are reading right now, which is less than single space. Remember that spacing and allowing for white space are important.

visualize is another helpful strategy. In encouraging someone to lift only small items, the commonly used expression "no bigger than a bread box" is easier to understand than "no bigger than 2 feet by 1 foot by 1 foot."

To make written information readable, use active rather than passive wording and use positive terminology (CDC, 1999; Executive Secretariat, 2003; Osborne, 2001). For example, write, "Put your right arm in first when getting dressed" instead of "Your right arm should be put in first when getting dressed," and state, "Raise your arm slowly" instead of "Do not raise your arm quickly." Use acronyms, such as ADL or ROM, only after they have been clearly explained; even then, be sure to verify comprehension.

Presentation of the Material

The overall presentation of any written communication is important. Presentation includes, but is not limited to, the type of paper used, the color of paper and print, font size and style, visuals, and organization. These factors affect one's ability to see the material, read the material, and understand the material and one's motivation to read the material.

Font and Paper

To ensure that the majority of people can see the written material, it should be typed in a font with serifs (the small lines at the end of characters) and a font size between 12 and 14 points (CDC, 1999) or a font size of 14 points or greater for readers with low vision (Osborne, 2001) (see Box 41.2). The CDC (1999) also recommends limiting the use of fancy fonts or italics. In general, the same font style should be used throughout a document.

BOX 41.2   EXAMPLES OF DIFFICULT-TO-READ VERSUS EASY-TO-READ FORMATS

Difficult to Read	Easy to Read
Bedroom	◆ **Bedroom**
–Put a light on the bed table	–Put a light on the bed table
–Keep a telephone next to the bed	–Keep a telephone next to the bed
Bathroom	
–Keep a nightlight on at night	◆ **Bathroom**
–Put nonskid decals in the tub	–Keep a nightlight on at night
	–Put nonskid decals in the tub

Matte paper should be used, as glossy paper can cause glare and make reading difficult. Black print on white paper is often most effective for contrast (Osborne, 2001). However, if color is desired, it is important to use opposing colors from the color wheel. For example, if yellow paper is to be used, the font should be blue (opposite yellow) rather than orange (next to yellow). Finally, to ensure that the written material can be seen, the reader should read it in an area with adequate lighting.

Organization

The organization of the material affects readability. Highlighting key information by making it bold or underlining it adds focus to important information. Headings are helpful to group information. Including white space, rather than filling up all the paper with words and pictures, facilitates self-efficacy (Osborne, 2001). Looking at a brochure that is unappealing and crammed with information will be discouraging for clients, regardless of the information in the brochure. Include key information first or last, as readers remember this information best (CDC, 1999; National Cancer Institute, 2003).

Spacing is important for visual cues. Leave more space above headings and subheadings than below. This ties information together at a quick visual glance. Consider using simple questions as headers, such as "What is energy conservation?" and "What are the key principles of energy conservation?" Chunking information into five or fewer categories facilitates recall. Information can be divided by rooms in a house (for a handout on environmental adaptations), by principles (for a handout on energy conservation), or according to any categorization that is appropriate for the topic. Box 41.2 provides examples of formatting that are easy and difficult to use.

When possible, the material should be personalized. This can be done simply by writing the user's name at the top of the material or by leaving blank space for individualizing exercises or adding suggestions. Using terminology such as "your exercise program" rather than "the exercise program" has been shown to make a difference in both

recall and satisfaction with the material (Wagner, Davis, & Handelsman, 1998).

Visuals

The old saying "A picture is worth a thousand words" is true only if the picture is clear and appropriate. Several studies have shown that written materials that used both text and visuals were better received than were materials with text alone (Bernardini, Ambrogi, Rardella, Perioli, & Grandolini, 2001; Davis, Bocchini, et al., 1996; Michielutte, Bahnson, Dignan, & Schroeder, 1992). Health literacy literature emphasizes the importance of visuals that are culturally appropriate, simple to understand, and used with simple captions (CDC, 1999; National Cancer Institute, 2003). Use shapes with simple words that are often universally recognized. For example, use a picture of a stop sign to reinforce the importance of stopping activity before pain occurs. Visuals, like words, should convey the positive. For example, include pictures of healthy foods rather than a picture of chips and cookies with a line through it. Some visuals can be confusing rather than helpful. For example, pictures with many arrows or bus schedules with small font and many columns are difficult to use. The purpose of using visuals is to facilitate comprehension. Pictures as decorations can detract from the message. All pictures that are included should convey an idea, enhancing the message in the text (AMC Cancer Research Center, 1994; CDC, 1999).

Cultural Relevance

It is important to be culturally sensitive in all written material, both words and visuals. Terminology, topics, and ideas should be relevant to the intended audience. The most effective way to ensure cultural relevance is to get input from the intended user (CDC, 1999) both in the development of the material and for feedback and suggestions once the material is in final draft form and during revisions. As with oral communication, print material, whenever possible, should be available in the client's native language, with particular emphasis on the use of culturally relevant terminology. Though there are Websites and computer programs that translate material, they translate word for word and are not as effective as having a person translate.

Assessing Print Material

Table 41.1 provides a quick checklist to consider in developing or choosing print material to use with clients. There are several published assessments to use to ensure that

TABLE 41.1   GUIDELINE TO CONSIDER WHEN DEVELOPING OR CHOOSING PRINTED MATERIALS

Characteristics of the user

1. Was the age of the user considered?
2. Was the education and/or reading level of the user considered?
3. Were the values, beliefs, and interests of the user considered?

Information included

1. Is the information what the user might want to know?
2. Is the information what the user might need to know?
3. Is only key information included?

Reading level of the material

1. Are there a limited number of long and/or compound sentences?
2. Are the majority of words that are three or more syllables common, everyday words?
3. Are unusual words defined? When possible, are common words used?
4. Is the same term used consistently?
5. Are common descriptions used to assist with visualization?
6. Is active terminology used?
7. Is terminology phrased in the positive?

Presentation of the material

1. Is a font style with serif used?
2. Is the font size at least 12 points (greater for people with low vision)?
3. Is there a strong contrast between color of print and color of paper?
4. Is matte paper used?
5. Is bold or underlining used for emphasis?
6. Are headings and subheadings used to chunk information and for layout?
7. Is adequate white space used?
8. Is key information included first or last?
9. Is information personalized?

Visuals

1. Are visuals culturally appropriate?
2. Are simple captions included for each visual?
3. Are visuals conveyed in the positive?
4. Do the visuals convey information (not just for decoration)?
5. Are the visuals clearly sequenced?

Cultural relevance

1. Is the material relevant to the intended audience?
2. Is the terminology culturally appropriate?
4. Was the material reviewed with the intended audience prior to distribution?
5. Is the material available in the user's native language?

written materials are developed well. The Suitability Assessment of Materials is commonly used and was developed and validated by Doak and colleagues (1996). It takes approximately 30 minutes, and the result is a numerical score, with a higher score indicating better suitability of the material for a given audience. The best way to assess printed material is to ask potential users for feedback.

COMMUNICATING WITH MEDIA

Audio, video, and **multimedia** communications are other strategies that can be used to communicate information to clients. These modes of communication can be effective if developed well. Individuals with low literacy skills may benefit from listening to and viewing information if it is developed in a fun, interactive, and appropriate way. However, videos are not a panacea for those with low literacy skills. While possibly having average or above-average intelligence, individuals who struggle to read often process information differently and might have limited vocabulary and a limited attention span (Doak et al., 1996). Everyone has a different learning style. Some learn best by reading, others by listening, and others by seeing. For many, learning information in multiple forms reinforces the information and assists with recall.

In choosing or developing audio or video materials, similar considerations should be used as for written materials. For instance, limiting objectives is important for all client education., The message should be five minutes or less for audio and eight minutes or less for video unless breaks are incorporated (Doak et al., 1996). While for printed material, information included at the beginning and the end of the material is most often remembered, with audio and video, the information presented at the end is recalled most often (Doak et al., 1996). For audio, when possible, use voices of people like the intended audience, and for video, be sure that images are of people like the intended audience. Whenever possible, these tools should be used in an interactive format.

Multimedia is still new technology, and research on its use is limited, though there is some evidence to support it. Computer games and software that require touch screen interaction (with the response generating the next question) are often fun, motivating and effective in conveying information (AMC Cancer Research Center, 1994; Rankin et al., 2005).

Video, audio, and multimedia are effective methods of communication, but they are more expensive to produce and more time consuming to develop than are written materials (AMC Cancer Research Center, 1994). Though there are numerous ways, as discussed earlier, to make written material user-friendly and increase readability, many people cannot understand print materials alone no matter how well developed they are (Atkinson, 2003). For the client who struggles to read, the use of video, audio, or multimedia might be worth the expense and time (Rankin et al., 2005).

CONCLUSION

Numerous studies have shown that no one method of client education is effective for all individuals (Friedrich, Cermak, and Maderbacher, 1996; Moore et al., 2002). Some material and learning are better suited for certain methods of teaching, and some individuals learn best via certain teaching strategies. "One size fits all" is not an effective motto for client education. Though more research is needed to determine the best ways to provide

---

PRACTICE DILEMMA

COMMUNICATING WITH CLIENTS

You work in an outpatient clinic with an 85-year-old client who comes twice a week to therapy secondary to a stroke three weeks ago. He has aphasia and struggles to read, though he can read single words. He understands most of what is being said. He achieved a sixth-grade education. His goal is to be able to do his own self-care, as his wife's emphysema is getting worse and she needs to cut down on the assistance she provides for him. Currently, he is working on one-handed dressing. Though he can don his sweater in the clinic with visual and verbal cues,

you want to send home instructions for reminders so that he can practice in between sessions, when dressing at home.

1. What are some strategies to use to make this handout user-friendly for this client?

2. Develop a one-page handout focusing on donning a shirt.

3. Are there other strategies you could use besides print material to reinforce at home what is learned in the clinic?

client education, considering multiple modes of communication and the specific needs of the individual or groups of individuals will help to convey valuable information to clients.

PROVOCATIVE QUESTION

What are some of the many ways in which low literacy skills affect clients' abilities to participate in meaningful occupations?

REFERENCES

AMC Cancer Research Center. (1994). *Beyond the brochure: Alternative approaches to effective health communication.* Retrieved on April 11, 2005, from http://www.cdc.gov/cancer/publica.htm

American Medical Association. (1999). Health literacy: Report of the council on scientific affairs. *Journal of the American Medical Association, 281*(6), 552–557.

Atkinson, T. (2003). Plain language and patient education: A summary of current research. *Research Briefs on Health Communication.* The Centre for Literacy, 1. Retrieved on March 8, 2005, from http://www.centreforliteracy.qc.ca/health/briefs/no1/no1.pdf

Bernardini, C., Ambrogi, V., Rardella, G., Perioli, L., & Grandolini, G. (2001). How to improve the readability of the patient package leaflet: A survey on the use of colour, print size, and layout. *Pharmacological Research, 43*(5), 437–444.

Bradshaw, P. W., Ley, P., & Kincey, J. A. (1975). Recall of medical advice: Comprehensibility and specificity. *Journal of Social Clinical Psychology, 14,* 55–62.

Butow, P., Brindle, E., McConnell, D., Boakes, R., & Tattersall, M. (1998). Information booklets about cancer: Factors influencing patient satisfaction and utilization. *Patient Education and Counseling, 33,* 129–141.

Centers for Disease Control and Prevention. (1999). *Scientific and technical information: Simply put* [Brochure]. Atlanta: Author.

Davis, T. C., Bocchini, J. A., Fredrickson, D., Arnold, C., Mayeaux, E. J., Murphy, P. W., Jackson, R. H., Hanna, N., & Paterson, M. (1996). Parent comprehension of polio vaccine information pamphlets. *Pediatrics, 97*(6), 804–810.

Davis, T. C., Fredrickson, D. D., Arnold, C., Murphy, P. W., Herbst, M., & Bocchini, J. A. (1998). A polio immunization pamphlet with increased appeal and simplified language does not improve comprehension to an acceptable level. *Patient and Education Counseling, 33,* 24–37.

DiMatteo, R. (1995). Patient adherence to pharmacotherapy: The importance of effective communication. *Formulary, 30*(10), 596–602.

Doak, C. C., Doak, L. G., & Root, J. H. (1996). *Teaching patients with low literacy skills* (2nd ed.). Philadelphia: J. B. Lippincott.

Executive Secretariat. (2003). *The plain language initiative.* Retrieved June 22, 2005, from http://execsec.od.nih.gov/plainlang/guidelines/index.html

Friedrich, M., Cermak, T., & Maderbacher, P. (1996). The effect of brochure use versus therapist teaching on patients performing therapeutic exercise and on changes in impairment status. *Physical Therapy, 76*(10), 1082–1088.

Huff, R. M., & Kline, M. V. (Eds.). (1999). *Promoting health in multicultural populations: A handbook for practitioners.* Thousand Oaks, CA: Sage.

Kessels, R. P. C. (2003). Patients' memory for medical information. *Journal of the Royal Society of Medicine, 96,* 219–222.

Kutner, M., Greenberg, E., Jin, Y. & Paulsen, C. (2006). *The Health Literacy of America's Adults: Results from the 2003 National Assessment of Adult Literacy* (NCES 2006-483). U.S. Department of Education. Washington, DC: National Center for Education Statistics.

Michielutte, R., Bahnson, J., Dignan, M. B., & Schroeder, E. M. (1992). The use of illustrations and narrative text style to improve readability of a health education brochure. *Journal of Cancer Education, 7*(3), 251–260.

Moore, L., Campbell, R., Whelan, A., Mills, N., Lupton, P., Misselbrook, E., & Frohlich, J. (2002). Self help smoking cessation in pregnancy: Cluster randomized controlled trial. *British Medical Journal, 325,* 1383–1389.

National Cancer Institute. (2003). *Clear and simple: Developing effective print materials for low-literate readers.* Retrieved February 3, 2005, from http://cancer.gov/aboutnci/oc/clear-and-simple/allpages/print

Osborne, H. (2001). *Overcoming communication barriers in patient education.* Gaithersburg, MD: Aspen.

Osborne, H. (2005). *Health literacy from A to Z: Practical ways to communicate your health message.* Sudbury, MA: Jones and Bartlett.

Purtilo, R., & Haddad, A. (2002). *Health professional and patient interaction.* Philadelphia: W. B. Saunders.

Rankin, S. H., Stallings, K. D., & London, F. (2005). *Patient education: Issues, principles, and practices* (5th ed.). Philadelphia: Lippincott.

Reid, J. C., Klachko, D. M., Kardash, C. A. M., Robinson, R. D., Scholes, R., & Howard, D. (1995). Why people don't learn from diabetes literature: Influence of text and reader characteristics. *Patient Education and Counseling, 25,* 31–38.

Wagner, L., Davis, S., & Handelsman, M. M. (1998). In search of the abominable consent form: The impact of readability and personalization. *Journal of Clinical Psychology, 54*(1), 115–120.

World Education. (2000). *Culture, health and literacy.* Retrieved June 9, 2005, from http://www.worlded.org/us/health/docs/culture/matl_websites.html

VIII

CONCEPTUAL BASIS
FOR PRACTICE

" A theory is a good theory if it satisfies two requirements: it must accurately describe a large class
of observations on the basis of a model that contains only a few arbitrary elements, and it
must make definite predictions about the results of a future observation. "

Stephen W. Hawking

Theory and Practice in Occupational Therapy

42

ELIZABETH BLESEDELL CREPEAU, BARBARA A. BOYT SCHELL, AND ELLEN S. COHN

Learning Objectives

After reading this chapter, you will be able to:

1. Discuss the importance of theory in shaping knowledge in the field.
2. Describe the relationship between theory and practice.
3. Discuss how assumptions, personal theory and more formal theory. shapes the clinical reasoning of occupational therapy practitioners.
4. Discuss how to evaluate theory and why this is important.

Becoming an occupational therapy practitioner involves learning the knowledge, skills, and values of the field. An important part of this process is the ability to understand and use theoretical knowledge (Parham, 1987). Theoretical knowledge or ideas, when combined with the practitioners' personal and professional experiences, form the basis for professional action. As described in Chapter 32, the combination of all these factors results in the development of individual professional paradigms or mental models that practitioners use to guide their actions (see also Cervero, 1988; Griswold, 1995; Hooper, 1997, 2007, Törnebohm, 1991). An individual's professional paradigm involves an integration of the following elements:

- The practitioner's underlying beliefs, values and commitments
- The practitioner's occupational therapy knowledge, abilities, and skills including theories, evaluation, and intervention strategies
- The practitioner's professional values as expressed in a commitment to the field and to people who seek his or her care.

Practitioners draw on their professional paradigms as they work to enhance their clients' abilities to engage in valued occupations. Through experience, professional paradigms become more highly developed and provide a greater resource for practitioners to reflect about their practice and the problems encountered by their clients (Griswold, 1995; Schön, 1983; Törnebohm, 1991). Refer to Chapter 32 to learn more about these clinical reasoning processes and how they are developed. Of particular interest for this current section is to explore theoretical knowledge and why it is important for effective occupational therapy practice.

WHY IS THEORY IMPORTANT?

The inability of experienced practitioners to explain their actions based on underlying assumptions and theories is one of the most perplexing issues for occupational therapy students as they enter the field. Such experiences can lead students to wonder why learning theory is important if practitioners aren't even using it in their daily work with their clients. In fact, practitioners do "use" theory all the time, they just can't always easily identify all the theories which inform their practice. This chapter explains how practitioners use theory and why theory is important.

Theory Shapes Profession's Practices

Theory is important because it is part the knowledge base of the field and an important aspect of each practitioner's professional paradigm (Argyris & Schön, 1974). However, practitioners do not necessarily retain the sources of the knowledge that form their professional paradigm. For instance, practitioners are generally very ethical in their practice, but few would be able to list all the specific terms associated with their ethical knowledge. With increased experience, practitioners tend to integrate knowledge in such a way that it becomes automatic (Argyris & Schön, 1974; Schön, 1983, 1987). Think about how little experienced drivers pay attention to the mechanics of operating a car. In the same way, practitioners become more automatic in their use of theoretical knowledge and just "do therapy." So, although theoretical knowledge may be embedded in the professional paradigm, it is part of the data practitioners bring to the therapeutic encounter (Rogers, 1983, 1986). It helps practitioners to "name and frame" the problems they encounter (Parham, 1987, Schön, 1983, 1987).

Use of Theories Varies with Experience

Theory may be particularly important for new practitioners who have little experience to draw upon. It can be seen as borrowed experience, a thinking frame (Neistadt, 1998), or metaphor (Parham, 1987) to assist new practitioners in their professional reasoning. For experienced practitioners, theory helps their reflective processes as they work to articulate reasons for their actions, and evaluate the effectiveness of these actions against existing theory and the responses of their clients. The current emphasis on evidence-based practice in health care is an attempt to have all practitioners be

more systematic in understanding the sources and validity of knowledge they use in practice. In order for practice to improve, it is practitioners' ethical responsibility to routinely and systematically check their professional paradigms against emerging theory and research.

WHAT IS THEORY?

In the broadest sense, a theory is a set of ideas or concepts that people use to guide their actions (Morse, 1997). A theory reflects an image or explanation of why or how a phenomenon occurs. When fully developed a theory defines concepts and states relationships between them (Morse, 1997) giving people the tools to understand, explain, or predict phenomenon (McColl et al., 2003). Theory in occupational therapy concerns occupation, how occupation influences health and well-being, and how occupation can be used therapeutically to enable people to engage in those occupations they value most. Types of theories range from **personal theories**, which are private understandings about the issue of concern, to **formal theories**, which are publicly articulated, published, and validated to varying degrees by scientific study. For example, one occupational therapy student indicated that she had learned to suspect a violent or abusive cause whenever a woman came to the clinic with tendon and nerve injuries from lacerations to the palms of her hands. She had noticed, while working as an aide, that such women described using their hands to protect their faces when attacked by abusers with knives, and hence, would get knife wounds on the palms of their hands. This would be an example of a personal theory, because this student had never really even talked about her observations, much less researched or published her impressions. However, her personal theory did serve to guide her thinking to some degree. Alternately, another student might find that she was able to use information from both cognitive and occupational behavior theories to understand why a client in the nursing home did not seem motivated to dress herself or take her medications. In this case, the student would be using one or more formal theories to support her professional reasoning.

Scope of Theories

Formal theory can be considered in terms of the breadth or scope of the theory as it relates to professional practice. For instance, there are theories that address occupation from a broad perspective. These theories include theories from occupational science about the nature of humans as occupational beings, which shape how members of the profession view human activity. Information from occupational science and related disciplines formed the basis for chapters in Unit I. Occupational theories tend to be over-arching theories which are broad in scope and help translate our understanding of the occupational nature of humans (McColl, et al., 2003). The remaining chapters in this unit

CASE STUDY: *Thinking Behind the Therapy: George Shows Mrs. Rivera a Bathtub Transfer*

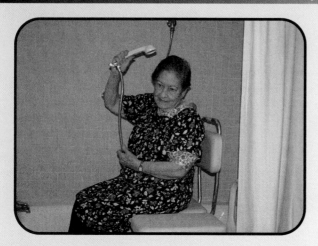

Look at this picture of Mrs. Rivera, a fully clothed older woman of Hispanic descent, sitting on a shower seat in a bathtub holding a hand-held showerhead. Outsiders to the health care field might have difficulty making sense of this picture. Why would a fully dressed, well-groomed, dignified older woman be sitting on a shower stool holding the shower over her head in a completely dry (thankfully!) bathtub? The answer for us is obvious; she is receiving occupational therapy following a mild cerebrovascular accident. George, the occupational therapy practitioner, acted on his own assumptions and theoretical perspectives to use a "practice" shower such as this rather than having Mrs. Rivera actually take a shower in her current living environment.

What Do You See?

What assumptions guided George, Mrs. Rivera's OT practitioner, to have her "take" a shower in this way? Based on what you see in the picture, can you articulate the assumptions the practitioner might have made about

- Autonomy, independence, interdependence?
- The importance of daily hygiene?
- Transfer of learning?
- Motivation?
- Cultural values?
- Occupation-based practice?
- Therapeutic change?

What Theories Might Have Shaped George's Thinking?

What theories might have shaped George's thinking? Probably there are some overarching theories about the importance of engaging in occupation that provide general guidance to the therapy process. An example in this case is the Model of Human Occupation or the Person-Environment-Occupation model, which direct the therapist to attend to Mrs. Rivera's desire to perform her self-care activities at home. The Theory of Occupational Adaptation might provide insight as to the ways Mrs. Rivera responds, as well as her own evaluation how satisfactory this approach to bathing is likely to be. There are also likely some other theories obtained from other professions, such as education and psychology, which form the basis for assumptions about how people learn, and the best way to teach them. One can presume from this picture that the therapist believes that this experience in the clinic learning to use a bath bench will enable Mrs. Rivera to use one at home to bathe more safely. Other theories, both within and outside of occupational therapy help inform the practitioner about more focused aspects of the therapy process. For instance, biomechanical theories and principles drawn from kinesiological theories would help the practitioner safely help Mrs. Rivera to position herself as she transfers in and out of the tub. The mechanisms of change are embedded in all of these theories

Theoretical Approaches and Mechanisms of Change

George, the occupational therapy practitioner, was probably using several theoretical perspectives when he asked Mrs. Rivera to "take a shower." Even though they may not be able to readily articulate their theoretical perspective (see Chapter 32 for an explanation of professional and clinical reasoning) practitioners should understand the mechanisms of change embedded in the theoretical perspectives they have adopted so that the intervention strategies are aligned with this perspective.

- What caused Mrs. Rivera's problem?
- Select a theory or theories that would be appropriate for this problem.
- Based on your theoretical perspective(s) what do you expect to change and why?
- Where do the ideas about change come from?
- What does the theory or model suggest will bring about change?
- Is there evidence to support the theory's assumptions about change?

After you have read through the theories in this unit, as well as learned more about the many theories informing practice, you may want to revisit this case to see the many theories which may inform a simple OT intervention like teaching someone a tub transfer.

address these overarching theories. Narrowly focused theories tend to focus on more specific aspects of occupational therapy evaluation and intervention. For example, biomechanical theory is concerned with the mechanics of body movement, such as joint mobility and posture, while motor control theories speak to the neuromuscular processes involved in performing skilled movements necessary in responding to daily life demands. Theories concerned with cognitive skills such as executive functions and problem solving provide guidance for practitioners working with individuals with brain injury and persistent mental illnesses. Such theories may include tested strategies to help individuals to improve their capacity to plan and sequence their daily tasks and activities. These more focused theories are discussed in the chapters in Units XI and XII, which address evaluation and intervention for personal factors and the environment. Practitioners have access to an increasing number of formal theories that they can use to guide their practice. Refer to Table 42.1 for examples of both broad and focused theories used in occupational therapy.

TABLE 42.1   DEFINITIONS OF COMMONLY USED TERMS

Term	Definition	Function	Examples
Paradigm	A paradigm provides a conceptual structure for understanding the world. A professional paradigm provides an accepted orienting structure for the profession, its values, beliefs, and knowledge.	Supports field's identity by providing common focus	Through engagement in occupations, people find meaning, health, and well being.
Professional Model	A professional model delineates and defines the scope or area of concern for a profession. It articulates the overall beliefs and knowledge of the profession. A professional model is derived from the profession's paradigm.	Defines the scope of practice.	Canadian Model of Occupational Performance
Theory	A general term that describes an image or provides an explanation of why or how a phenomenon occurs and how that phenomenon can be controlled	Organizes observations and understandings for easier use	See below for both formal and informal examples
Formal Theory	Explains observable events or relationships by stating a series of abstract propositions or principles. These theories are based on systematic research with carefully defined concepts and explanations of relationships between these concepts.	Systematically explains predicts, or describes phenomena	◆ Model of Human Occupation ◆ Ecology of Human Performance ◆ Occupational Adaptation ◆ Person Environment Occupation Model
Personal Theory	Private understandings based on experience	Helps individuals articulate their experience.	◆ A practitioner's theory that her female client's hand wounds were the result of protecting themselves from physical abuse.
Frame of Reference	Frames of reference guide practice by delineating the beliefs, assumptions, definitions, and concepts within a specific area of practice. A frame of reference is drawn from a theoretical base and has a particular view of the function/dysfunction continuum. A frame of reference delineates evaluation processes and intervention strategies that are consistent with the theoretical base.	Guide a specific area of practice	◆ Motor control ◆ Self-Advocacy ◆ Rehabilitation ◆ AOTA Practice Guidelines

(Kielhofner, 1997; McColl et al., 2003; Morse, 1997; Mosey, 1992; Turner, 1986)

Terms Used for Different Levels of Theory

Readers may also come across other terms related to theories, such as practice models, or frames of reference. Generally such terms are used to describe the level of development or complexity of a theory or as a way of differentiating practice guidelines from more formal theory (Mosey, 1992). Although helpful for scholars, for purposes of this chapter, these distinctions are less important. Examples of these terms are found in Table 42.1. More critical for new practitioners is the ability to understand the differing purposes or scopes of major theories used in the profession, their components, and how well these theories have been validated by research and found useful in practice.

SCOPE OF PRACTICE AND THE PROFESSION'S THEORIES

Broadly accepted professional knowledge about occupational therapy is often articulated in major documents approved and published by professional organizations, such as the American Occupational Therapy Association or the Canadian Occupational Therapy Association. The Canadian Model of Occupational Performance (Townsend, 1997) serves as a general guide to the profession and defines its scope of practice and the expertise and knowledge of occupational therapy practice. It provides a framework that delimits the profession's range of interest and focuses attention to those aspects of human functioning that are of greatest concern to occupational therapy practitioners (Moyers, 1999). Such documents often attempt to distill the assumptions, knowledge, values and beliefs commonly accepted throughout the profession (Mosey, 1981) and evolve to reflect the changing nature of professional practice. The knowledge base is derived from research and theories in occupational therapy, occupational science, and disciplines beyond the field.

Although such documents are useful in helping to frame the general concerns of the profession, and as such serve as good starting points for students, they rarely reflect the detailed information provided in various formal theories. Formal theories explain observable events or relationships by stating a series of abstract propositions or principles. These theories are based on systematic research with carefully defined concepts and explanations of relationships between these concepts (Turner, 1986). Formal theories are publicly shared through presentations at professional meetings, and publications in research journals or texts. This public sharing promotes critical analysis of theoretical assumptions, which in turn serves to gradually refine theories in response to continued analysis and research. For example, the Model of Human Occupation is a broad theory of occupational behavior that has evolved over nearly thirty years and been continually revised in response to criticisms from the field, research directed to testing aspects of the theory, and evolving theories from fields outside of occupational therapy (see Chapter 44 for a discussion of some of this evolution). Similarly, theories of about sensory processing, cognition, etc. (see Chapters 57 and 58) have been developed, revised, and improved through the scholarly process. Other theories are newer to the field, and thus have had less time to develop such as the Theory of Occupational Adaptation. Finally, there are some theories that have not been researched significantly since they were introduced into the field. This leads to the importance for practitioners to stay abreast of knowledge development in the field.

RELATIONSHIP BETWEEN THEORY AND PRACTICE

Theories, whether they are formal, informal, personal, process, or content, can help practitioners reason about what to observe, how to understand the occupational problems faced by clients, and how to intervene to address particular kinds of problems in practice. By explaining factors that affect a person's occupational performance, many theories provide practitioners with a map for thinking about the mechanism of change. The term *mechanism of change* refers to how an action or a set of actions result in desired changes. For example, motor learning theories suggest that motor learning results from experience and practice, which produces permanent changes in behavior. Motor learning theories also postulate that verbal feedback from the practitioner about the quality of movement helps the person know whether modification is needed for the next movement attempt (see Chapter 55 for a further review of motor learning theory).

EVALUATING KNOWLEDGE AND REFLECTIVE INQUIRY

It is essential to view theory as evolving knowledge. It is not a fixed, objective truth. Because theory involves the evolution of knowledge—whether it is formal theory or personal theory derived from professional experience and reflective inquiry—it needs constant examination and testing. This can involve continued research about the theory, critical examination of the research supporting the theory, or the reflective inquiry described by Schön (1983) and summarized earlier in Chapter 25 as it relates to competence and Chapter 32 as it relates to professional reasoning. Table 42.2 lists six questions that practitioners can use to guide the process of examining theoretical knowledge. These questions can be used to promote examination of published research and theories as well as to guide practitioner reflections on specific practice situations.

TABLE 42.2   EVALUATING THEORETICAL KNOWLEDGE FOR ACTION

What theory or theories are embedded in your practice?	◆ What theoretical knowledge do you use? ◆ Which theories are personal and which public?
What is the theory's focus?	◆ Who developed the theory? ◆ What is it trying to explain? ◆ What kind of clients or settings was it intended for? ◆ How well does it match your therapy needs?
How do you know?	◆ Upon what data is this knowledge based? ◆ What literature relates to this knowledge? ◆ How relevant is the literature to your needs?
How well do you know?	◆ How was the knowledge developed? ◆ How were the data collected? ◆ How were data analyzed and interpreted? ◆ What were the research circumstances? ◆ Where is the theory published? Is the venue of high quality? ◆ What were the qualifications of the authors of the theory?
How will your understanding shape your practice decisions?	◆ To what extent is this theory unique and offer a new way of considering your practice? ◆ How does the theory enhance your understanding? ◆ What are its strengths and limitations? ◆ How does this information affirm your current approaches? ◆ How does it contradict your current approaches? ◆ What different approaches will you use based on your understanding?
What additional information do you need?	◆ What further questions do you have? ◆ What sources can help answer these questions? ◆ How will you access this information?

Adapted from McColl et al., 2003; Watson, 2000

CONCLUSION

It is essential for a profession to have a base of knowledge grounded in well-articulated and specified theories that, in turn, provide scientific support for practice and test the effectiveness of occupational therapy interventions.

The following chapters in this unit provide an introduction to the occupation-based theories in our field. These are broad-based theories which form the knowledge base of the profession and provide important constructs of practitioners' professional paradigm. Units X through XII provide many examples of more focused theories, as well as how to blend the overarching perspectives of occupational theories with more focused theories and frames of reference guiding evaluation and intervention. One of the challenges of professional practice is the need to bridge the gap between current theoretical knowledge and practitioners' use of such knowledge within their professional paradigm. Taking a reflective stance toward practice assists practitioners to understand their professional reasoning and to explore the theoretical underpinnings of this process.

REFERENCES

Argyris, C., & Schön, D. A. (1974). *Theory in practice: Increasing professional effectiveness.* San Francisco, CA: Jossey-Bass.

Cervero, R. M. (1988). *Effective continuing education for professionals.* San Francisco, CA: Jossey.

Griswold, L. A. (1995). *Professionalization of occupational therapists: A study of emergent identities.* Unpublished doctoral dissertation, University of New Hampshire, Durham.

Hawking, S. W. (1988). *A brief history of time* (p. 10). Toronto: Bantam Books.

Hooper, B. (2007). Therapists' assumptions as a dimension of professional reasoning. In B. A. B. Schell & J. W. Schell (Eds.), *Clinical and professional reasoning in occupational therapy* (pp. 13–35). Baltimore: Lippincott Williams, & Wilkins.

Hooper, B. (1997). The relationship between pretheoretical assumptions and clinical reasoning. *American Journal of Occupational Therapy, 51,* 328–338.

Kielhofner, G. (1997). *Conceptual foundations of occupational therapy* (2nd. ed.). Philadelphia: F. A. Davis.

McColl, M. A., Law, M., Stewart, D., Doubt, L., Pollock, N. & Krupa, T. (2003). *Theoretical basis of occupational therapy* (2nd ed.). Thorofare, NJ: SLACK.

Morse, J. M. (1997). Considering theory derived from qualitative research. In J. M. Morse (Ed.), *Completing a qualitative project: Details and dialogue* (pp. 163–188). Thousand Oaks, CA: Sage.

Mosey, A. C. (1981). *Occupational therapy: Configuration of a profession.* New York: Raven.

Mosey, A. C. (1992). *Applied scientific inquiry in the health professions: An epistemological orientation.* Rockville, MD: American Occupational Therapy Association.

Neistadt, M. E. (1998). Teaching clinical reasoning as a thinking frame. *American Journal of Occupational Therapy, 52,* 221–229.

Parham, D. (1987). Nationally speaking—toward professionalism: the reflective therapist. *American Journal of Occupational Therapy, 41,* 555–561.

Rogers, J. C. (1983). Clinical reasoning: The ethics, science, and art. *American Journal of Occupational Therapy, 37,* 601–616.

Rogers, J. C. (1986). Clinical judgment: The bridge between theory and practice. In American Occupational Therapy Association (Ed.), *Target 2000: occupational therapy education* [Proceedings]. Rockville, MD: Author.

Schön, D. A. (1983). *The reflective practitioner: How professionals think in action.* USA: Basic Books.

Schön, D. A. (1987). *Educating the reflective practitioner.* San Francisco: Jossey-Bass.

Törnebohm, H. (1991). What is worth knowing in occupational therapy. *American Journal of Occupational Therapy, 45,* 451–454.

Townsend, E. (Ed.). (1997). *Enabling occupation: An occupational therapy perspective.* Ottawa, Canada: CAOT Publications.

Turner, J. H. (1986). *The structure of sociological theory* (4th ed.). Belmont, CA: Wadsworth.

Watson, G. H. (2000). Oh no! Its theory O! *Quality Progress, 33*(10), 16.

Ecological Models in Occupational Therapy

CATANA E. BROWN

Chapter Objectives

After reading this chapter, you will be able to:

1. Explain how an understanding of the environment is essential to understanding occupational performance.
2. Describe the ecological models (Ecology of Human Performance, Person Environment Occupation, and Person Environment Occupation Performance) and their concepts.
3. Describe and distinguish the five intervention strategies: establish/restore, adapt/modify, alter, prevent, and create.

In the 1990s, three groups of occupational therapists working independently created three separate models that emphasized the importance of considering the environment in occupational therapy practice. The three models, the Ecology of Human Performance model (EHP) (Dunn, Brown, & McGuigan, 1994), the Person Environment Occupational Performance model (PEOP) (Christiansen & Baum, 1997), and the Person Environment Occupation model (PEO) (Law et al., 1996) share many similarities and a few distinctions. The three dynamic models consider occupational (task) performance as the primary outcome of interest to occupational therapists. In addition, all of the models indicate that occupational performance is determined by the person, environment (context), and occupation (task). However, of the constructs of person, environment, and occupation, the developers of the models were most intent on promoting the significance of the environment. Occupational therapists tend to focus on person factors and neglect the influence of the environment on occupational performance. Therefore, the ecological models were developed so that along with consideration for the person and occupation, occupational therapy practice includes assessments and interventions that focus on the environment. When the distinct characteristics of the person, environment, and task are taken together, the uniqueness of each situation is fully appreciated. The differences in the models lie primarily in the definitions, components, and structures of the models, which will be discussed further in the sections that follow.

INTELLECTUAL HERITAGE

The ecological models were built on social science theory, earlier occupational therapy models, and the disability movement. Each of the ecological models draws heavily on social science theories that describe person-environment interactions. Bronfenbrenner (1979) developed an ecological model that explored the influence of social factors on development. This nested model has the individual at the center of a system that is influenced by family, friends, communities, and institutions. These interactions can either enhance or inhibit development. For example, changes in economic systems have had a major influence on the family in terms of the increased numbers of women who are working. This in turn affects the development of the child. Gibson's (1979) concept of affordances is applied primarily to the physical environment. People perceive objects in the environment as having specific characteristics that result in action or meaning. People do not consciously think about affordances, but people's perceptions determine how they interact with objects. For example, the flat surface of a table affords such activities as eating a meal or writing a letter. Lawton (1986) developed the concept of environmental press. *Press* is described as the demands of the environment. A good fit occurs when the person's adaptive behavior and affect match the environmental press; a poor fit occurs when the person cannot meet the demands of the environment. When curb cuts are available, the environmental press is more adaptive for a wheelchair user; however, other environmental features, such as a sidewalk with a steep grade or snow, can create demands that make performance impossible. Csikszentmihalyi (1990) created another goodness-of-fit model based on the concept of flow. A flow experience occurs when the person's skills and abilities match the challenges of the activity. Even more, when in flow, the person is at one with the occupation and so completely absorbed that the passage of time goes unnoticed. The EHP, PEO, and PEOP models are also based on the idea of goodness of fit. Occupational performance is optimal when the environment and the person's skills and abilities match the demands of the occupation (task). A disruption in any area, person, environment, or occupation will interfere with performance.

Earlier models of occupational therapy do take account of the environment and contributed to the conceptualization of EHP, PEO, and PEOP. In the Model of Human Occupation (Kielhofner, 2004), environmental impact refers to the unique influence of the environment on the person. Environments are a source of opportunities and resources as well as demands and constraints. David Nelson (1988) makes a distinction between the terms *occupational performance* and *occupational form. Performance* is the doing of an occupation. *Form* is the context in which the doing takes place and includes the physical and sociocultural circumstances that are external to the person. Occupational form contributes to the personal meaning and purpose that the individual attributes to an occupation. Occupational Adaptation (Schkade & Schultz, 1992) proposes that the person desires mastery and the occupational environment demands mastery. Therefore, the interaction of the person and environment combine in a press for mastery that results in an adaptive response.

Finally, the ecological models in occupational therapy were influenced by civil rights movements that arose from disability groups. Health care practice is dominated by a focus on impairment in the person and interventions that are designed to fix that impairment. Individuals with disabilities have challenged this perspective. People in the independent living movement have pointed out that environmental barriers are typically the greatest impediment to a successful and satisfying life (DeJong, 1979; Shapiro, 1994). Furthermore, individuals with psychiatric disabilities have revealed that the power of stigma and the subsequent discrimination interfere with full participation in community life (Chamberlin, 1990; Deegan, 1993). The disability movements have pushed for civil rights for individuals with disabilities and promote self-determination and empowerment. The ecological models have embraced the values of the disability movement. This is reflected in both the emphasis on the environment as a significant barrier and facilitator of occupational performance and the adoption of principles of client-centered practice. In the ecological models, the first step in the occupational therapy process involves identifying the areas of occupational performance that are important to the individual. Moreover, the service recipient remains the primary decision maker in all steps of the process.

DEFINITIONS

Person

EHP, PEO, and PEOP have similar definitions of the person. A unique and holistic view of the person acknowledges the mind, body, and spirit. Variables associated with the person include values and interests, skills and abilities, and life experience. Values and interests help to determine what is important, meaningful, and enjoyable to the person. Skills and abilities include cognitive, social, emotional, and sensorimotor skills as well as abilities such as reading and knowing how to balance a checkbook. Life experiences form the person's history and personal narrative. The person influences and is influenced by the environment. For example, a person's family and friends contribute to the development of particular values and interests and vice versa. A child might develop a love of reading because of the availability of books in the home and parents who read to the child, while having a child in the home might cause the parents to be more concerned about having healthy foods at home and creating a safe physical environment.

Environment

The environment is also described similarly across the three models. The environment is where occupational performance takes place and consists of physical, cultural, and social components. The EHP model also includes the temporal environment. The physical environment is the most tangible. It includes built and natural features, large elements such as the terrain or buildings, and small objects such as tools. The cultural environment is based on shared experiences that determine values, beliefs, and customs. The cultural environment includes but is not limited by ethnicity, religion, and national identity. For example, individuals may also adopt values and beliefs from the culture of their family, professional identity, organizations or clubs, and peer group. The social environment is made up of many layers. It includes close interpersonal relationships such as family and friends. The next layer includes social groups such as work groups or social organizations to which the individual belongs. The social environment is also made up of large political and economic systems, which can have a profound effect on the daily life of people with disabilities. These systems make decisions related to the rights of people with disabilities, availability of services, and financial benefits such as social security disability insurance. The temporal environment is made up of time-oriented factors associated with the person (developmental and life stage) and the task (when it takes place, how often and how long). Occupational performance cannot be understood outside of the context or environment. The environment can both create barriers to performance and enhance occupational performance. For example, a well-organized and familiar grocery store that provides foods that are culturally familiar and consistent with the person's likes might be described as an adaptive environment. The grocery store might also be a barrier if the person is overwhelmed by many choices, cannot find the items he or she is looking for, and is anxious when there are too many people around.

Occupation/Task

The biggest difference in the three models is found in the concepts related to occupations or tasks. PEO and PEOP use the term *occupation*, whereas EHP uses *task*. The developers of EHP were intentional about the selection of the term *task* because a primary purpose of the model was to facilitate interdisciplinary collaboration. It was felt that the term *task* would be more accessible to other disciplines. Tasks are defined as objective representations of all possible activities available in the universe. Although this was not explicitly expressed in the early writings of EHP, occupations exist when the person and context factors come together to give meaning to tasks (Dunn, McClain, Brown, & Youngstrom, 2003). The PEO and PEOP models describe a series of nested concepts that make up occupations. In PEO, activities are the basic units of tasks. Tasks are purposeful activities, and occupations are self-directed tasks that a person engages in over the life course. The PEOP model involves actions, which are observable behaviors; tasks, which are combinations of actions with a common purpose; and occupations, which are goal-directed, meaningful pursuits that typically extend over time. For example, chopping vegetables might be the observable behavior or activity, embedded within the task of preparing soup, which falls under the larger occupation of cooking dinner for the family. See Table 43.1 for a comparison of definitions of the ecological models.

TABLE 43.1 DEFINITIONS OF TASK, ACTIVITY, AND OCCUPATION USED BY ECOLOGICAL MODELS

	PEO	PEOP	EHP	Example
Activity	Recognizable and observable behavior	Basic units of tasks	Tasks and activities are not differentiated. Tasks are an objective set of behaviors necessary to achieve a goal.	Chopping vegetables
Task	Purposeful activities recognized by the task performer	Combinations of actions with a common purpose		Cooking a meal
Occupation	Self-directed tasks that a person engages in over the life course	Goal-directed meaningful pursuits that extend over time	Tasks that acquire meaning through the person-environment interaction	Making dinner for the family

Occupational Performance

Occupational performance is the outcome that is associated with the confluence of the person, environment, and occupation factors. The degree to which occupational performance is possible depends on the goodness of fit of these factors. The structures of the models are depicted in slightly different ways. In PEO, a Venn diagram is used to illustrate the meeting of person, environment, and occupation variables (Figure 43.1). The space in which the three circles come together is occupational performance. PEOP is similar however instead of three circles there are four (Figure 43.2). Person and environment touch but do not overlap. Occupation and performance are two separate circles that overlay person and environment. These circles come together to form occupational performance and participation. In EHP, the person is embedded inside the context, with tasks floating all around (Figure 43.3). The performance range includes the tasks that are available to the person because of the existing environment supports and his or her own skills, abilities and experiences. In all of the models, the performance range or occupational performance area is constantly changing as the other variables change. The area of occupational performance increases or the performance range expands when the person acquires new skills. Likewise, expansion occurs when stigma is decreased, physical barriers are removed, additional social supports are acquired, or schedules are accommodating. Unfortunately, many people with disabilities are often faced with limited personal capacities and multiple environmental barriers. The role of the occupational therapist is to change this dynamic so that more occupations are available to the person.

Intervention Strategies

Additional terms that are included in the EHP model are five different intervention strategies: (1) establish/restore, (2) adapt/modify, (3) alter, (4) prevent, and (5) create. These interventions were spelled out so that occupational therapists would consider the full range of options. In particular, the enumeration of intervention choices was designed to encourage occupational therapists to use more interventions directed at the environment.

- **Establish/restore interventions** target the person and are aimed at developing and improving skills and abilities so that the person can perform tasks (occupations) in context. Increasing range of motion so that an individual can better manage self-care tasks and teaching someone how to use a microwave oven for meal preparation involve establish/restore strategies.
- **Adapt/modify interventions** change the environment or task to increase the individual's performance range. Using assistive devices such as an adapted car for driving or a built-up handled spoon for eating are interventions that change the typical environment. Changes to the physical environments are most common in occupational therapy; however, it is important to consider interventions that target the social and cultural environment as well. Adapt/modify strategies can include providing education about disabilities to students in an elementary school classroom so that the special needs child will be more accepted. This is an adapt/modify

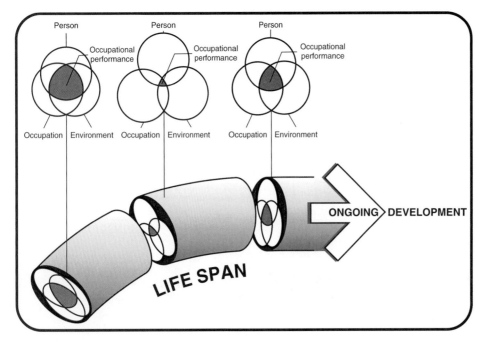

FIGURE 43.1 Person Environment Occupation model. (Reprinted with permission from Law et al., 1996.)

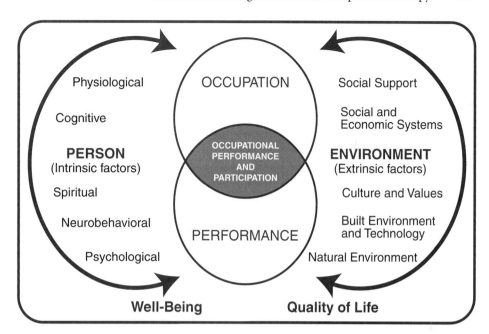

FIGURE 43.2 Person Environment Occupation Performance model. (Reprinted with permission from Christiansen, Baum & Bass-Haugen, 2005.)

strategy because the social environment is being changed. Other adapt/modify interventions could include providing social support for someone who is fearful of riding the bus or changing the schedule for someone with endurance problems so that physically demanding tasks are spread throughout the day.

♦ **Alter interventions** do not change the person, task, or environment but are designed to make a better fit. Occupational therapists might be reluctant to consider alter interventions because it does not appear that they are "doing" anything. However, alter interventions can

be some of the most effective because they take advantage of what is already naturally occurring. Making a good match requires that the occupational therapist have strong skills in activity analysis and environmental assessment. Moving from a two-story house with stairs to a ranch home would be an alter intervention for someone with limited endurance. Helping an individual to find a club or organization to join based on his or her values and beliefs would also utilize alter strategies. Matching the person's skills with a job match is another example of an alter intervention.

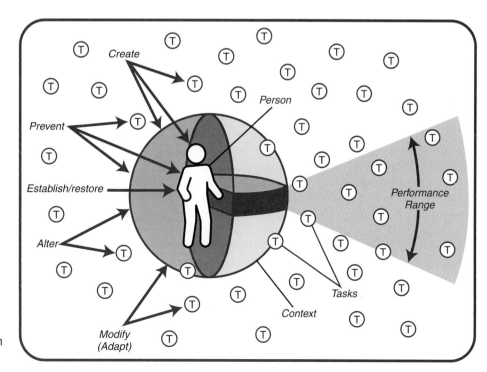

FIGURE 43.3 Ecology of Human Performance model. (Reprinted with permission from Dunn et al., 2003.)

◆ **Prevent interventions** are implemented to change the course of events when a negative outcome is predicted. Prevention can utilize interventions that change the person (establish/restore), change the environment (adapt/modify), or make a better match (alter) but occur before the problem develops. Teaching at-risk parents skills in facilitating developmentally appropriate play is an example of a prevent strategy, as is using a special cushion in a wheelchair to prevent decubitus ulcers.

◆ **Create interventions** do not assume that a problem has occurred or will occur but are designed to promote performance in context. These interventions enrich occupational performance in context. Like the prevent strategies, create interventions can utilize establish/restore, adapt, or alter approaches. Setting up a study space within a quiet area with adequate lighting is a create strategy. Finding a good roommate match is another create strategy, and so is practicing interviewing skills before going out on an actual job interview.

ASSUMPTIONS OF THE ECOLOGICAL MODELS

◆ The relationships between people, environments, and occupations are dynamic and unique. They interact continually and across time and space. Therefore, occupational therapists should approach each situation as ever changing and distinct.

◆ The environment is a major factor in the prediction of successful and satisfying occupational performance. Environments can either facilitate or inhibit occupational performance. All aspects of the environment (physical, social, cultural, and temporal) should be evaluated to determine relevant environmental influences.

◆ Rather than exclusively using interventions that change the person, it is often more efficient and effective to change the environment or find a person-environment match.

◆ Occupational performance is determined by the confluence of person, environment, and occupation factors. People, environments, and occupations are constantly changing, and as these factors change, so does occupational performance.

◆ Occupation therapy practice begins by identifying what occupations the person wants or needs to perform. Using a top-down approach, the targeted area of occupational performance is identified first by the client or family. This is followed by an assessment of barriers and facilitators within the person, environment, and occupation that affect occupational performance.

◆ Occupational therapy practice involves promoting self-determination and the inclusion of people with disabilities in all environments. The person or system that is the service recipient is the primary decision maker in the occupational therapy process. Occupational therapists should act as advocates for people with disabilities and should support their clients in self-advocacy.

APPLICATION TO PRACTICE

The ecological models provide a framework for thinking about occupational therapy practice but do not delineate specific assessments or techniques. Using an ecological model requires an intentional effort on the part of the occupational therapist to consider the environment as extensively as he or she considers the person. An overarching value of the ecological models is a client-centered approach to practice. The person and occupational therapist collaborate throughout all stages of the occupational therapy process, and the process begins by identifying what the person wants or needs to do in his or her life (see Box 43.1). Consequently, the stage is set so that assessment and intervention are not driven by the therapist but are framed in terms of what is most important to the person. The person is not viewed in isolation but instead is considered in terms of the environment in which occupational performance takes place. The dynamic interrelationships of person, environment, and occupation compel the therapist to appreciate the uniqueness of each situation. This means that practice is not an unyielding protocol applied to everyone with the same diagnosis but a thoughtful, reasoned, and collaborative process of assessment and intervention.

Once the person identifies the relevant area(s) of occupational performance, the assessment process is directed at determining what features of the person, environment, and occupation support and interfere with occupational performance. Therefore, occupational therapy assessment must be comprehensive and include measures that consider the person, environment, and occupation. Occupational therapists are most familiar with measures of person factors and are skilled at complex task analysis. Environmental assessment is an area that has received less attention, though there are several good resources describing numerous environmental measures (Cooper, Letts, Rigby, Stewart, & Strong, 2001; Letts et al., 1994; Letts, Rigby, & Stewart, 2003). Occupational therapists should choose assessments that evaluate the environment in which the chosen occupation takes place. They should also conduct a skilled observation of the relevant environment. Observing the person performing the occupation in the natural environment is a powerful and informative assessment strategy. Therapists will need to bring in more specific practice models to guide the selection of assessments and later the inter-

CLINICAL QUESTIONS RELATED TO CONSTRUCTS OF THE ECOLOGICAL MODELS

BOX 43.1

Person

Skills (cognitive, social, psychological, sensory, motor)
- What are the person's inherent strengths?
- What are potential areas of cognitive, social, or sensorimotor impairment?

Life skills
- What life skills has the person learned and what skills has the person not learned?
- What life skills has the person mastered and what skills are problematic?

Interests
- What does the person like to do?

Experiences
- What are the life experiences that contribute to or interfere with occupational performance?
- What are the major life events for the person?
- What are themes in the person's life story?

Environment/Context

Culture
- What cultural groups does the person identify with?
- What values does the person derive from these cultural groups?
- Are the beliefs and expectations of these cultural groups accepting of the person?

Social
- Are friends and family available to provide support?
- What providers are involved?
- How does public policy influence the person's ability to engage in tasks or occupations?

Physical
- Does the built environment or the natural environment create barriers to performance?
- Does the person have access to objects that facilitate performance?

Temporal
- Is the person able to engage in occupations that are consistent with the person's developmental or life phases?
- Does the person have too much time or not enough time to perform important tasks or occupations?

Occupation/Tasks

- What does the person want or need to do?
- What occupations or tasks come together to create roles or identity for the person?
- What occupations or tasks give meaning to the person's life?

Performance/Performance Range

- Which tasks or occupations fall inside out outside of the performance range?
- Are there factors related to the person, environment/context, or occupation that interfere with performance?

Therapeutic Intervention

- What intervention approach would be the most efficient and have the most desirable outcomes?
- Is there evidence to support the intervention approach?
- Which intervention approach does the service recipient want?

---

vention plan. Ecological models provide a framework for practice but do not provide specific guidelines or theory about specific assessments or intervention techniques. However, the selection of practice models should be faithful to the values of the ecological models. Mostly, this means that the practice models that are used to guide assessment and intervention cannot be limited to person and occupational factors but most address the environment as well. The dynamic nature of the ecological models indicates that situations are constantly changing. Taking this change into account means that regular reevaluation should occur.

The five intervention options proposed by the EHP model require occupational therapists to utilize a wide range of intervention approaches. Intervention can take many directions, and those interventions that target the environment should always be considered as one option. Furthermore, occupational therapy practice is not limited to existing problems but includes enhancing occupational performance and prevention of occupational performance problems. The association of ecological models with disability rights means that occupational therapists should also be involved at the systems level, supporting policy that promotes full participation in all aspects of community life.

CASE STUDY: *The Asbury Café*

The Asbury Café is an employment program developed by the author. The Asbury Café operates every Wednesday night at a local church. Five individuals with serious mental illness are employees of the café. A meal is served at a reasonable cost for church members, neighbors, and friends. An occupational therapist oversees the running of the café, assisted by volunteers and college students. It is an example of a program that utilizes the principles of the ecological models to promote work performance for people with psychiatric disabilities. However, that is just one of the aims of the program, which on a larger scale aspires to make changes in social and cultural environments to reduce the stigma associated with serious mental illness. People with serious mental illness are frequently depicted in the media as dangerous, peculiar, and in need of care and protection.

Although serious mental illness is common, many people do not disclose their diagnosis because of the associated stigma. The Asbury Café provides an opportunity for people with and without mental illness to come together and interact in a positive environment (Figure 43.4).

The first aim of the program is to provide employment to individuals with psychiatric disabilities. Individuals who are referred by the vocational team to this work site are typically individuals who have less work experience, have more overt symptomatology, and need more extensive adaptations to the work environment. No formal assessments are completed; however, extensive skilled observation and task analysis are used to match employees with tasks and to make adaptations to the task and environment.

TARGET AREA OF OCCUPATIONAL PERFORMANCE: WORK

Ecological Model Components	Interventions
Person Factors	
Individuals with serious mental illness often have cognitive impairments that slow information processing and interfere with learning of the job tasks.	Establish/restore: Provide simple instructions with demonstration, models, and regular feedback. Alter: Match worker with café task that best meets the person's interests and abilities. Adapt: Pair workers so that one with stronger skills can model, help focus, and provide feedback to the worker with developing skills.
Psychiatric symptoms such as anxiety and auditory hallucinations can make it more challenging to focus work tasks.	Establish/restore: Teach the worker individual strategies to use when feeling anxious (e.g., deep breathing) or experiencing hallucinations (e.g., talk aloud to others). Adapt: Allow for frequent breaks, set up an environment of acceptance and support, use the environment to create distractions from hallucinations or worries.
Environmental Factors	
Fewer job opportunities are available to the employees the café in the neighborhoods where they live, and typical work sites do not offer the limited schedule needed and desired by current employees.	Adapt: The full Asbury Café program is an adapt strategy. Supervisors and volunteers have experience in mental health services. Employees at the café are individuals who need more extensive supports for successful work performance.
Employees at the café do not have cars, and no public transportation is available to the work location.	Adapt: Although this is not ideal, the mental health center provides transportation.
Occupation	
The major occupation is work is in the area of meal preparation, serving, and cleanup. Each task has many subcomponents.	Adapt: The tasks are often adapted so that there are fewer steps, or one task is done by two or three people so that the full task is not too difficult for an individual. Alter: Over time, the best matches become known, and individual workers assume responsibility for their tasks. They are able to perform these tasks without assistance or oversight.

CASE STUDY: *The Asbury Café* *Continued*

The second purpose of the Asbury Café is to reduce the stigma associated with serious mental illness by promoting positive social interactions between people with and without mental illness.

TARGET AREA OF OCCUPATIONAL PERFORMANCE: SOCIAL INTERACTION

Ecological Model Components	Interventions
Person Factors	
Many of the customers at the café have limited exposure to individuals with serious mental illness.	Alter: Employees with mental illness are assigned work tasks so that they have opportunities to interact directly with the café customers (taking money, serving meals). Employees with mental illness are also assigned work tasks that require regular contact with church staff. This provides an opportunity for real work relationships to develop.
Environmental Factors	
Our culture tends to portray individuals with serious mental illness as dangerous, unpredictable, and in need of protection. Yet the church is an environment that is open to accepting diverse individuals and welcomes the program.	Establish/restore: Educational opportunities are provided through the church in the form of lectures, articles in the newsletter, and presentations by consumers of the mental health center to provide accurate information to potential café customers about serious mental illness. Adapt: The program director and volunteers create an environment that models positive interactions with individuals with serious mental illness (e.g., avoiding distinguishing between those who do and do not have mental illness; in addition to working alongside one another, also socializing together during breaks)
Occupation	
Eating together socially	Alter: The Asbury Café provides a naturally occurring opportunity for people to socialize in a natural setting. The café workers, supervisor, and volunteers eat during the time when the customers are eating so that there are more times for interaction.

The Asbury Café demonstrates how occupational therapy can have an impact outside of a traditional service setting. The café is true to the values of the ecological models, which emphasize client-centered practice and full participation in community life. The program enhances occupational performance in the areas of work and social interaction by providing interventions targeting the person, environment, and occupation. The program itself is designed to change the stigmatizing social and cultural environment that is currently so pervasive for people with serious mental illness.

EVIDENCE SUPPORTING THE ECOLOGICAL MODELS

Studies indicating a relationship between environment and occupational performance provide support for the ecological models. Occupational therapists are conducting more and more research in this area. For example, children with disabilities and their families identified physical, social, cultural, and institutional barriers as limiting transition to adulthood (Law et al., 1999). In a study of independence and employment for people with AIDS, environmental factors presented significant barriers to occupational performance (Paul-Ward, Kielhofner, Braveman, & Levin, 2005). One of the greatest barriers to independent living was the lack of low-income housing. Barriers to employment included procedures related

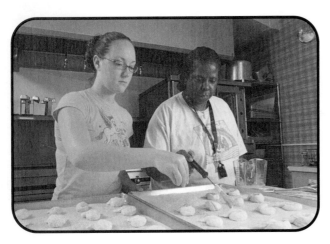

FIGURE 43.4   Jess and Janet at the Asbury Café. (Courtesy of C. Brown)

to social security benefits and stigma by employers. A qualitative study of the home environment for people with physical disabilities found that social support was a major factor in overcoming impairments and inaccessibility in the home (Lund & Nygard, 2004). Time use was affected by the availability of support from others, and these individuals often spend much time waiting for others before they can engage in a desired occupation. Another study found that the home can present physical environmental barriers for stroke survivors (Reid, 2004). For the most part, the stroke survivors were able to engage in desired occupations; however, getting through doorways and up and down stairs was difficult. Uneven ground outside the home was also a problem.

There are several examples of research that support the efficacy of occupational therapy interventions with an ecological basis. Some of these interventions were intentionally designed by using one of the ecological models, while others utilize the environment in the intervention approach. Brown, Rempfer, and Hamera (2002) used the EHP model as a conceptual framework to develop a grocery shopping intervention for people with schizophrenia. In the intervention, participants were taught strategies to better use the naturally occurring environmental features of the grocery store (e.g., overhead signs, generic products). The intervention was effective in improving grocery shopping accuracy and efficiency. The PEO model was used to develop a peer mentorship program for adolescents and young adults with physical disabilities (Stewart, 2003). The peer support of the mentorship program resulted in greater exploration of the self and the environment. This included an increased desire to try new things, socialize with others, and get out in the community. The Environmental Skill Building Program (ESP) (Corcoran et al., 2002), based on environmental press theory, incorporates environmental strategies to promote adaptive behavior in individuals with dementia. In ESP, the therapist works with a caregiver to adapt the home environment and teach inter-

action strategies. In a randomized controlled trial, caregivers who received the intervention were less upset with disruptive behaviors, had better affect, and had better overall well-being (Gitlin et al., 2003). Another study considered the social environment as a factor in play skill development (Tanta, Deitz, White, & Billingsley, 2005). Using a single subject design, preschool children with delayed play skills were paired with children who had a lower developmental play skills and a peer with a higher development play skills. The children with delayed play skills were more likely to initiate play and respond to the peer when paired with the child with higher play skills.

This growing body of research provides support for the impact of the environment on occupational performance. In particular, the research provides information about which specific environmental factors are the most important for a specific occupational performance for a specific group of people, again emphasizing the uniqueness of each situation. Therefore, as research provides occupational therapists with more specific information about environments, occupational therapists can design more relevant interventions.

CONCLUSION

Occupational therapy practice is aimed at promoting occupational performance. Ecological models provide a framework for understanding the multiplicity of factors that must be taken into account in assessing and providing interventions to enhance occupational performance. These models require that the occupational therapist use a client-centered approach and always consider the importance of the environment in the occupational therapy process.

PROVOCATIVE QUESTIONS

1. What are additional examples of interventions an occupational therapist might make to help support the goals of the Asbury Café? Do the interventions that you selected most often target changes in the person, changes in the environment, or making a person-environment match?

2. Can you think of ways in which the Asbury Café might interfere with its own goals? For example, might the Asbury Café interfere with its employees' future employment goals? Could the Asbury Café reinforce existing prejudices?

3. What are the features of this intervention that demonstrate the strengths of using an ecological approach?

4. If you wanted to duplicate the Asbury Café in your community, what affordances and barriers would you need to consider. How would you use the affordances? How would you address the barriers?

5. Using the Asbury Café as a model, apply EHP to describe another intervention that would address the needs of clients with mental illness and aim to reduce stigma in your community.

REFERENCES

Bronfenbrenner, U. (1979). *The ecology of human development: Experiments by nature and design.* Cambridge, MA: Harvard University Press.

Brown, C., Rempfer, M., & Hamera, E. (2002). Teaching grocery shopping skills to people with schizophrenia. *Occupational Therapy Journal of Research, 22*(Suppl. 1), 90S–91S.

Chamberlin, J. (1990). The ex-patients' movement: Where we've been and where we're going. *Journal of Mind and Behavior, 11*(3 & 4), 323–336.

Christiansen, C., & Baum C. (Eds.). (1997). *Occupational therapy: Enabling function and well-being.* (2nd ed.). Thorofare, NJ: Slack.

Christiansen, C., Baum, C., & Bass-Haugen. J. (Eds.). (2005). *Occupational therapy: Performance, participation and well-being* (3rd ed.). Thorofare, NJ: Slack.

Cooper, B., Letts, L., Rigby, P., Stewart, D., & Strong, S. (2001). Measuring environmental factors. In M. Law, C. Baum, & W. Dunn (Eds.), *Measuring occupational performance: Supporting best practice in occupational therapy* (pp. 229–256). Thorofare, NJ: Slack.

Corcoran, M. A., Gitlin, L. N., Levy, L., Eckhardt, S., Earland, T. V., Shaw, G., et al. (2002). An occupational therapy home-based intervention to address dementia-related problems identified by family caregivers. *Alzheimer's Care Quarterly, 3*(1), 82–90.

Csikszentmihalyi, M. (1990). *Flow: The psychology of optimal experience.* New York: Harper & Row.

Deegan, P. E. (1993). Recovering our self of value after being labeled. *Journal of Psychosocial Nursing, 31*(4), 7–11.

DeJong, G. (1979). Independent living: From social movement to analytic paradigm. *Archives of Physical Medicine and Rehabilitation, 60,* 435–446.

Dunn, W., McClain, L. H., Brown, C., & Youngstrom, M. J. (2003). The ecology of human performance. In E. B. Crepeau, E. S. Cohn, & B. A. B. Schell (Eds.), *Willard & Spackman's occupational therapy* (10th ed., pp. 223–226). Philadelphia: Lippincott, William & Wilkins.

Dunn, W., Brown, C., & McGuigan, A. (1994). The ecology of human performance: A framework for considering the impact of context. *American Journal of Occupational Therapy, 48,* 595–607.

Gibson, J. J. (1979). *The ecological approach to visual perception.* Boston, MA: Houghton Mifflin.

Gitlin, L. N., Winter, L., Corcoran, M., Dennis, M. P., Schinfeld, S., & Hauck, W. W. (2003). Effects of the home environmental skills building program on the caregiver-care recipient dyad: 6-month outcomes from the Philadelphia REACH initiative. *Gerontologist, 43,* 532–546.

Kielhofner, G. (2004). *Conceptual foundations of occupational therapy* (3rd ed.). Philadelphia: F. A. Davis.

Law, M., Cooper, B., Strong, S., Stewart, D., Rigby, P., & Letts, L. (1996). The person-environment-occupation model: A transactive approach to occupational performance. *Canadian Journal of Occupational Therapy, 63,* 9–23.

Law, M., Haight, M., Milroy, B., Willms, D., Stewart, D., & Rosenbaum, P. (1999). Environmental factors affecting the occupations of children with physical disabilities. *Journal of Occupational Science, 6,* 102–1220.

Lawton, M. P. (1986). *Environment and aging* (2nd ed.). Albany, NY: Plenum.

Letts, L., Law, M., Rigby, P., Cooper, B., Stewart, D., & Strong, S. (1994). Person-environment assessments in occupational therapy. *American Journal of Occupational Therapy, 48,* 608–618.

Letts, L., Rigby, P., & Stewart, D. (Eds.). (2003). *Using environments to enable occupational performance.* Thorofare, NJ: Slack.

Lund, M. L., & Nygard, L. (2004). Occupational life in the home environment: The experience of people with disabilities. *Canadian Journal of Occupational Therapy, 71,* 243–252.

Nelson, D. L. (1988). Occupation: Form and performance. *American Journal of Occupational Therapy, 42,* 633–641.

Paul-Ward, A., Kielhofner, G., Braveman, B., & Levin, M. (2005). Resident and staff perceptions of barriers to independence and employment in supportive living settings for persons with AIDS. *American Journal of Occupational Therapy, 59,* 540–545.

Reid, D. (2004). Accessibility and usability of the physical housing environment of seniors with stroke. *International Journal of Rehabilitation Research, 27,* 203–208.

Schkade, J. K., & Schultz, S. (1992). Occupational adaptation: Toward a holistic approach to contemporary practice, Part I. *American Journal of Occupational Therapy, 46,* 829–837.

Shapiro, J. P., (1994). *No pity: People with disabilities forging a new civil rights movement.* New York: Three Rivers Press.

Stewart, D. (2003). Peer mentorship as an environmental support for adolescents and young adults with disabilities. In L. Letts, P. Rigby, & D. Stewart (Eds.), *Using environments to enable occupational performance* (pp. 197–206). Thorofare, NJ: Slack.

Tanta, K. J., Deitz, J. C., White, O., & Billingsley, F. (2005). The effects of peer-lay level on initiations and responses of preschool children with delayed play skills. *American Journal of Occupational Therapy, 59,* 437–445.

The Model of Human Occupation

GARY KIELHOFNER, KIRSTY FORSYTH,
JESSICA M. KRAMER, JANE MELTON,
AND EMMA DOBSON

Learning Objectives

After reading this chapter, you will be able to:

1. Describe the major personal factors addressed by the Model of Human Occupation and articulate how each concept affects occupational life.
2. Describe the major environmental factors that are addressed by the Model of Human Occupation and articulate how each concept affects occupational life.
3. Identify the three levels that the Model of Human Occupation uses to describe and examine what a person does.
4. Describe the six steps of therapeutic reasoning in the Model of Human Occupation.
5. Articulate how change occurs in occupational therapy and identify client actions and therapeutic strategies that lead to change.
6. Describe how the Model of Human Occupation can be applied to clients with a variety of diagnoses across the life course in different practice contexts.

Betty is 82 years old. She was admitted to the hospital following a fall at home in which she fractured the neck of her femur. After surgery and two days in acute care, she was transferred to a skilled nursing facility (SNF), where she was to receive occupational therapy.

Lin is a 3-year, 6-month-old boy with a seizure disorder/epilepsy, hydrocephalus, hypotonia, and profound mental retardation. He has several seizures a day, eats a restricted pureed food diet in addition to receiving nutrition through a g-tube, and fatigues easily. During a special education interdisciplinary educational placement meeting, Lin's parents identified that their main goal was that Lin be able to accept food more easily.

Each of these clients' occupational therapy practitioners chose to use the Model of Human Occupation (MOHO) to guide their intervention. In the course of the chapter, these cases will be used to illustrate the theory and application of this model.

INTRODUCTION

MOHO was introduced nearly three decades ago by three practitioners seeking to articulate an approach to occupation-based intervention. They described MOHO as a theory to guide thinking about clients and the therapy process (Kielhofner, 1980a, 1980b; Kielhofner & Burke, 1980; Kielhofner, Burke, & Heard, 1980). Evidence indicates that MOHO is now the most widely used occupation-based model in practice worldwide (Haglund, Ekbladh, Thorell, & Hallberg, 2000; Law & McColl, 1989; National Board for Certification in Occupational Therapy, 2004; Wilkeby, Pierre, & Archenholtz, 2006). A national study of occupational therapists in the United States (Lee, Taylor, Kielhofner, & Fisher, in press) indi-

cated that 75.7% of therapists make use of MOHO in their practice. These therapists reported that MOHO allows them to have an occupation-focused practice and a clearer professional identity. They also reported that MOHO provides a holistic view of clients, supports client-centered practice, and provides a useful structure for intervention planning.

MOHO has been developed through the efforts of an international community of scholars and practitioners. It is supported by a substantial evidence base of well over 400 articles and chapters that present theoretical, applied, or research aspects of MOHO. A current bibliography of this literature is maintained on the Website www.moho.uic. edu. The most comprehensive and authoritative discussion of MOHO is the book *A Model of Human Occupation: Theory and Application,* which is now in its fourth edition (Kielhofner, 2007). This chapter provides a brief overview of this model's focus, theory, and resources for application in practice.

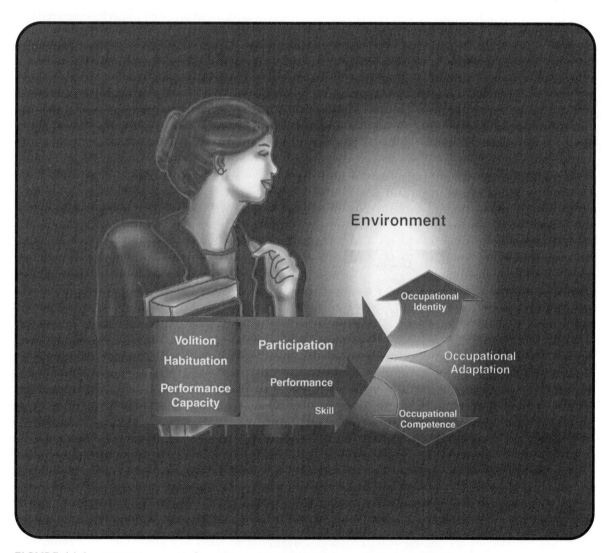

FIGURE 44.1   MOHO concepts. (Reprinted with permission from Kielhofner, 2007.)

THE FOCUS OF THE MODEL OF HUMAN OCCUPATION

This model emerged at a time when the field was just beginning to rediscover the importance of occupation as an outcome and means of intervention. In the 1970s, when MOHO was being formulated as an approach to practice, most occupational therapy theory and practice focused on understanding and reducing impairment. The impetus for developing MOHO was the recognition that many factors beyond motor, cognitive, and sensory impairments contribute to difficulties in everyday occupation. These include barriers posed by the physical and social environment, difficulties in choosing and finding meaning in occupations, and the challenge of maintaining positive involvement in life roles and routines. MOHO was developed to address these factors.

Consequently, the concepts that make up the theory of this model address the motivation for occupation, the routine patterning of occupations, the nature of skilled performance, and the influence of environment on occupation. These concepts seek not only to offer explanations of these factors, but also to provide a framework for gathering data about a client's circumstances, generating an understanding of the client's occupational strengths and limitations, and selecting and implementing a course of occupational therapy. A wide range of assessments and intervention strategies that correspond to the concepts of this model have also been developed to support practice. MOHO can be applied to clients with a wide range of impairments (physical, mental, cognitive, and sensory) throughout the life course. MOHO can also used in many types of intervention settings.

THE MODEL OF HUMAN OCCUPATION CONCEPTS

The Model of Human Occupation is ultimately concerned with the extent to which individuals can participate in life occupations and achieve a state of positive adaptation (Figure 44.1). The model begins with the idea that a person's inner characteristics and external environment are linked together into a dynamic whole. Moreover, the model asserts that inner capacities, motives, and patterns of performance are maintained and changed through engagement in occupations. MOHO conceptualizes occupational therapy as a process in which practitioners support client engagement in occupations in order to shape the clients' abilities, their routine ways of doing things, and their thoughts and feelings about themselves.

MOHO Concepts Related to the Person

To explain how occupations are chosen, patterned, and performed, MOHO conceptualizes people as composed of three interacting elements: volition, habituation, and performance capacity. The sections that follow will discuss these elements.

Volition

Volition refers to the process by which people are motivated toward and choose what activities they do. The concept of volition asserts that all humans have a desire to engage in occupations and that this desire is shaped by previous experiences. Volition consists of thoughts and feelings that occur in a cycle of anticipating possibilities for doing, choosing what to do, experiencing what one does, and subsequent interpretation of the experience. These thoughts and feelings are concerned with three issues: how capable and effective one feels, what one holds as important, and what one finds enjoyable and satisfying. They are referred to as personal causation, values, and **interests**.

Personal causation refers to thoughts and feelings about one's capacities and effectiveness that people have as they do everyday activities. These include, for example, recognizing one's strengths and weaknesses, feeling confident or anxious when faced with a task, and reflecting on how well one did after doing something.

Values are beliefs and commitments about what is good, right, and important to do. They include thoughts and feelings about activities that are worth doing, beliefs about the proper way to complete those activities, and the meanings that are ascribed to things one does. Values specify what is worth doing, how to perform, and what goals or aspirations deserve commitment. People experience a sense of correctness and belonging when they engage in activities that enact their values.

Interests are generated through the experience of pleasure and satisfaction in occupation. Interests begin with natural dispositions (e.g., the tendency to enjoy physical or intellectual activity). They further develop through the experience of pleasure and satisfaction derived from occupational engagement (Matsutsuyu, 1969). Therefore, the development of interests depends on available opportunities to engage in occupations.

Volition has a pervasive influence on occupational life. It shapes how people see the world and the opportunities and challenges it presents. Volition guides choices of what to do and determines the experience of doing. It shapes how people make sense of what they have done. To a large extent, how people experience life and how they regard themselves and their world have to do with volition. Volition is also central to the occupational therapy process. All therapy requires that clients make choices to do things; therefore, it must engage clients' volition. Moreover, how clients experience what they do in therapy (a function of volition) to a large extent determines therapy outcomes.

Habituation

Habituation refers to a process whereby people organize their actions into patterns and routines. Through repeated action within specific contexts, people establish habituated patterns of doing. These patterns of action are governed by **habits** and roles. Together, they shape how people go about the routine aspects of their lives. Because of roles and habits, most routines of daily life unfold automatically and predictably.

Habits involve learned ways of doing things that unfold automatically. Habits operate in cooperation with context, using and incorporating the environment as a resource for doing familiar things. They influence how people perform routine activities, use time, and behave. For instance, habits shape how people intuitively go about self-care each morning, organize the weekly routine, and complete a familiar task.

Roles give people an identity and a sense of the obligations that go with that identity. People see themselves as students, workers, and parents and recognize that they should behave in certain ways to fulfill these roles. Much of what people do is done as a spouse, parent, worker, student, and so on. The expectations that others hold for a role and the nature of the social system in which each role is located serve as guides for learning how to behave within most roles. Thus, through interaction with others, people internalize an identity, an outlook, and a way of behaving that belong to each role they have internalized.

The habits and **internalized roles** that make up habituation guide how people interact with their physical, temporal, and social environments. When habituation is challenged by impairments and/or environmental circumstances, people can lose a great deal of what has given life familiarity, consistency, and relative ease. One of the major tasks of therapy is to reconstruct habits and roles so that the person can more readily participate in life occupations within the everyday environment.

Performance Capacity

Performance capacity refers to underlying mental and physical abilities and how they are used and experienced in performance. The capacity for performance is affected by the status of musculoskeletal, neurological, cardiopulmonary, and other bodily systems that are called on when a person does things. Performance also calls on mental or cognitive abilities such as memory. Biomechanical, motor control, cognitive, and sensory integration approaches to practice address this aspect of performance capacity from an objective point of view by focusing on physical and mental capacities as phenomena that can be observed, measured, and modified (Ayres, 1979; Trombly & Radomski, 2001).

MOHO recognizes the importance of approaches that address physical and mental capacities for performance and is typically used in conjunction with such models. MOHO stresses the importance of also paying attention to the experience of performance and, in particular, the experience of having limitations in performance. It asserts that by paying careful attention to how people experience impairments, practitioners can be more helpful to clients. This includes, for instance, paying attention to how people's bodies feel to them and how they perceive the world when they have impairments. For example, research based on this approach has shown that people with a variety of physical impairments are often alienated from or do not feel at one with their bodies. Therapy can support people to "reclaim" their bodies or parts of their bodies and to integrate their bodies into a new way of doing things.

MOHO Concepts Concerning the Environment

MOHO stresses that all occupation results from an interaction of the inner characteristics of the person (volition, habituation, and performance capacity) with the characteristics of the physical and social environment. The **environment** can be defined as the particular physical, social, cultural, economic, and political features within a person's context that influence the motivation, organization, and performance of occupation. There are several dimensions of the environment that may have an impact on an individual's occupational life. For example, people encounter different physical spaces, objects, and people, as well as expectations and opportunities for doing things. At the same time, the larger culture, economic conditions, and political factors also exert an influence. Accordingly, the environment includes the following dimensions: the objects that people use when they do things; the spaces within which people do things; the occupational forms or tasks that are available, expected, and/or required of people in a given context; the social groups (e.g., family, friends, coworkers, neighbors) that make up the context; and the surrounding culture, political, and economic forces.

The things that people do and how they think and feel about these things reflect a complex interplay of motives, habits and roles, and abilities with the dimensions of the environment noted above. Political and economic conditions determine what resources people have for doing things and what occupational roles are available to them. Culture shapes the formation of ideas about how one should perform and what is worth doing. The demands of a task can determine the extent to which a person feels confident or anxious. The match of objects and spaces to the capacity of the individual influence how the person performs. In these and a myriad of other ways, the environment has an impact on what people do and how they think and feel about their doing. In turn, people also choose and modify their environments. For instance, people select environments that match and allow them to realize their values and interests.

Dimensions of Doing

As Figure 44.1 shows, MOHO identifies three levels at which we can examine what a person does: occupational participation, occupational performance, and occupational skill.

Occupational participation refers to engaging in work, play, or activities of daily living that are part of one's sociocultural context and that are desired and/or necessary to one's well-being. Examples of occupational participation are volunteering for an organization, working in a full- or part-time job, regularly getting together with friends, doing self-care, maintaining one's living space, and attending school. Each area of occupational participation involves a cluster of related things that one does. For example, maintaining one's living space may include paying the rent, doing repairs, and cleaning. Doing a task related to participation in a major life area is referred to as **occupational performance**.

During occupational performance, we carry out discrete purposeful actions. For example, making coffee is a culturally recognizable occupational form or task in many Western cultures. To do so, one *gathers* together coffee, coffeemaker, and a cup; *handles* these materials and objects; and *sequences* the steps necessary to brew and pour the coffee. These actions that make up occupational performance are referred to as **skills.** Skills are goal-directed actions that a person uses while performing (Fisher, 1998; Fisher & Kielhofner, 1995; Forsyth, Salamy, Simon, & Kielhofner, 1998). In contrast to *performance capacity*, which refers to underlying ability (e.g., range of motion and strength), *skill* refers to the actions within an occupational performance such as reaching or sequencing. There are three types of skills: motor skills, process skills, and communication and interaction skills. Detailed taxonomies of each of the three types of skills have been developed (Bernspang & Fisher, 1995; Doble, 1991; Fisher, 1995; Forsyth, Lai & Kielhofner, 1999; Forsyth, Salamy, Simon, & Kielhofner, 1998).

Occupational Identity, Competence, and Adaptation

Over time, what people do creates their **occupational identity.** This identity, generated from experience, is the cumulative sense of who people are and who they wish to become as occupational beings. The degree to which people are able to sustain a pattern of doing that enacts their occupational identity is referred to as **occupational competence.** These two essential elements of **occupational adaptation** entail the creation of an occupational identity and the ability to enact this identity in a variety of circumstances. As Figure 44.1 shows, people's occupational adaptation is reflected in the extent to which they can create and enact a positive occupational identity.

THE PROCESS OF CHANGE AND THERAPY

A basic premise of MOHO is that all change in occupational therapy is driven by clients' occupational engagement. The term **occupational engagement** refers to clients'

doing, thinking, and feeling under certain environmental conditions in the midst of therapy or as a planned consequence of therapy.

When clients engage in occupational forms or tasks in therapy or as a result of therapy, volitional, habituation, and performance capacity are all involved in some way. For example, in any moment of therapy, a client may be (1) drawing on performance capacity to exercise skill in occupational performance, (2) evoking old habits that shape how the occupational performance is done, (3) enacting or working toward acquiring a role, (4) experiencing a level of satisfaction and enjoyment (or dissatisfaction and displeasure) with occupational performance, (5) assigning meaning and significance to what is done (i.e., what this means for the client's life), or (6) feeling able (or unable) in doing the occupational form/task.

Each of these aspects of what the client does, thinks, and feels shapes the change process. For this reason, practitioners using MOHO are mindful of their clients' volition, habituation, performance capacity, and environmental conditions in the midst of therapy and how these elements are interacting as the therapy unfolds. To help practitioners think about the process of occupational engagement, MOHO identifies the nine dimensions of occupational engagement shown in Table 44.1. These identified dimensions of occupational engagement do not exhaust the possibilities for what clients do to achieve change. Nonetheless, they provide a basic structure for thinking about how clients achieve change and for planning how therapy goals will be achieved. This process is discussed in the next section.

USING MOHO IN PRACTICE: THE SIX STEPS OF THERAPEUTIC REASONING

Using MOHO in practice involves thinking with its theoretical concepts, a process referred to as *therapeutic reasoning.* Therapeutic reasoning refers specifically to the use of MOHO concepts in thinking about clients' needs throughout the occupational therapy process (American Occupational Therapy Association, 2002). The therapeutic reasoning process has six steps: (1) generating questions about the client, (2) gathering information on and with the client, (3) using the information gathered to create an explanation of the client's situation, (4) generating goals and strategies for therapy, (5) implementing and monitoring therapy, and (6) determining outcomes of therapy. Practitioners generally move back and forth between these steps over the course of therapy. Each step is briefly discussed below.

Generating Questions

Practitioners must come to understand their clients in order to plan and implement therapy. This understand-

TABLE 44.1   DIMENSIONS OF CLIENT OCCUPATIONAL ENGAGEMENT

Dimensions of Occupational Engagement	Definition
Choose/Decide	Anticipate and select from alternatives for action.
Commit	Decide to undertake a course of action to accomplish a goal or personal project, fulfill a role, or establish a new habit.
Explore	Investigate new objects, spaces, social groups, and/or occupational forms/tasks; do things with altered performance capacity; try out new ways of doing things; examine possibilities for occupational participation in one's context.
Identify	Locate novel information, alternatives for action, and new feelings that provide solutions for and/or give meaning to occupational performance and participation.
Negotiate	Engage in a give-and-take with others that creates mutually agreed-upon perspectives and/or finds a middle ground between different expectations, plans, or desires.
Plan	Establish an action agenda for performance or participation.
Practice	Repeat a certain performance or consistently participate in an occupation with the intent of increasing skill, ease, and effectiveness of performance.
Reexamine	Critically appraise and consider alternatives to previously held beliefs, attitudes, feelings, habits, or roles.
Sustain	Persist in occupational performance or participation despite uncertainty or difficulty.

ing begins with asking questions about their clients. MOHO theory allows a practitioner to generate these questions systematically. That is, the major concepts of the theory (environmental impact, volition, habituation, performance capacity, participation, performance, skills, occupational identity, and occupational competence) orient the practitioner to be concerned about certain things when learning about a client. For example, practitioners using MOHO would ask what their clients' thoughts and feelings are in relation to personal causation, values, and interests. Moreover, they would ask about their clients' roles and habits and how these affect the clients' routines. These questions would, of course, be tailed to the clients' circumstances.

Gathering Information

To answer the questions generated in the first step, practitioners must gather information on and with the client. Practitioners may take advantage of naturally occurring opportunities to gather information. For example, a practitioner might learn about a client's personal causation by observing the client's emotional reaction when attempting to learn a challenging new task or by engaging in informal conversation about the client's fears about the future. Practitioners also use structured assessments that have been developed to generate information that is relevant to MOHO con-

cepts. Some MOHO assessments gather specific information on such factors as interests and roles. Other assessments attempt to capture more in-depth information on one aspect of MOHO, such as assessments that focus on volition. Still other MOHO assessments will capture comprehensive information on several aspects of the person and the environment. A wide range of MOHO-based assessments have been developed; they are summarized in Table 44.2. See Unit XVII for additional information about these assessments. Thus, practitioners using MOHO have a range of choices when they decide which assessment(s) to use.

Creating a Theory-Based Understanding of the Client

The information that the practitioner gathers to answer questions about a client is used to create a theory-based understanding of that client. In this step, the practitioner uses MOHO theory as a framework for creating a conceptualization or explanation of that particular client's situation. As will be demonstrated in the cases of Betty and Lin, the therapists use MOHO to create a conceptualization of each of these client's occupational circumstances to guide the next step of generating goals and strategies for therapy.

As part of creating a conceptualization of clients' circumstances, practitioners identify problems or challenges

TABLE 44.2 MOHO ASSESSMENT SUMMARY TABLE

MOHO Assessment	Method of Administration	Description
Assessment of Communication and Interaction Skills (ACIS)	Observation	Gathers information about the communication and interaction skills that a person displays while engaged in an occupation across the domains of physicality, information exchange, and relations. Used to generate goals for therapy related to communication/interaction skills and to assess outcomes/changes in skill.
Assessment of Motor and Process Skills (AMPS)	Observation	Gathers information about the motor and process skills that a person displays while engaged in an occupation. Used to generate goals for therapy related to motor and process skills and to assess outcomes/changes in skill.
Assessment of Occupational Functioning-Collaborative version (AOF-CV)	Interview and/or client self-report	Yields qualitative information and a quantitative profile of the impact of a client's personal causation, values, roles, habits, and skills on occupational participation. Used to inform intervention.
Child Occupational Self Assessment (COSA)	Client self-report	Children and youths rate their occupational competence for engaging in 25 everyday activities in the home, school, and community and the importance of those activities. Used to generate goals and assess outcomes/change in competence and values.
Interest Checklist	Client self-report	Checklist that indicates strength of interest and past, present, and future engagement in 68 activities. Used to inform intervention.
Model of Human Occupational Screening Tool (MOHOST)	Observation, interview(s), and/or chart review	Information gathered assesses impact of volition, habituation, skills, and environment on client's occupational participation. Used to generate goals and assess outcomes/changes in participation.
NIH Activity Record	Client self-report	Self-report "log" records information in half-hour intervals throughout the day on perceptions of competence, value, enjoyment, difficulty, and pain experienced when engaging in various occupations in that time period. Used to inform intervention and assess outcomes/change in participation.
Occupational Circumstances Assessment-Interview and Rating Scale (OCAIRS)	Interview	Interview yields information to assess values, goals, personal causation, interests, habits, roles, skills, readiness for change, and environmental impact on participation. Used to generate goals and assess outcomes/changes in participation.
Occupational Performance History Interview-II (OPHI-II)	Interview	Detailed life history interview that yields (a) scales measuring competence, identity, and environmental impact and (b) a narrative representation/analysis of the life history. Used as an in-depth, comprehensive assessment to generate goals, inform intervention, and build the therapeutic relationship.
Occupational Questionnaire (OQ)	Client self-report	Self-report "log" records information in half-hour intervals throughout the day on perceptions of competence, value, and enjoyment experienced when engaging in various occupations in that time period. Used to inform intervention and assess outcomes/change in participation.

TABLE 44.2 MOHO ASSESSMENT SUMMARY TABLE *Continued*

MOHO Assessment	Method of Administration	Description
Occupational Self Assessment (OSA)	Client self-report	Clients rate their occupational competence for engaging in 21 everyday activities and the importance of those activities. Allows clients to set priorities for change. Used to generate goals and assess outcomes/change in competence and values.
Pediatric Interest Profiles (PIP)	Client self-report	Assessment includes three age-appropriate scales (some with line drawings) for children and adolescents to indicate participation, interest, and perceived competence in a variety of play and leisure activities. Used to generate goals and assess outcomes/changes in participation.
Pediatric Volitional Questionnaire (PVQ)	Observation	Guides a systematic observation of a child across multiple environments to assess volition and the impact of the environment on volition. Used as an in-depth assessment of volition to generate goals and assess outcomes/change in volition.
Role Checklist	Client self-report	Checklist provides information on past, present, and future role participation and the perceived value of those roles. Used to inform intervention and assess outcomes/changes in role performance.
Short Child Occupational Profile (SCOPE)	Observation, interview(s), and/or chart review	Information gathered assesses impact of volition, habituation, skills, and environment on child's/adolescent's occupational participation. Used to generate goals and assess outcomes/changes in participation.
School Setting Interview (SSI)	Interview	Interview works with students to gather information on student-environment fit and identify need for accommodations. Used to generate goals, inform intervention, and assess outcomes/changes in student-environment fit.
Volitional Questionnaire (VQ)	Observation	Guides a systematic observation of a client across multiple environments to assess volition and the impact of the environment on volition. Used as an in-depth assessment of volition to generate goals and assess outcomes/change in volition.
Worker Role Interview (WRI)	Interview	Interview yields information to rate the impact that volition, habitation, and perceptions of the environment have on psychosocial readiness for the worker role/return to work. Used to generate goals and assess outcomes/changes in psychosocial readiness for work.
Work Environment Impact Scale (WEIS)	Interview	Interview works with client to assess environmental impact on participation in the worker role and to identify needed accommodations. Used to generate goals and inform intervention.

that need to be addressed in therapy as well as strengths that can be drawn on in therapy. Problems and challenges may be a function of volition, habituation, performance capacity, or the environment.

Generating Therapy Goals and Strategies

This step involves creating therapy goals (i.e., identifying what will change as a result of therapy), deciding what kinds of occupational engagement will enable the client to change, and determining what kind of therapeutic strategies will be needed to support the client to change.

Goals indicate the kinds of changes that therapy will aim to achieve. Change is required when the client's characteristics and/or environment are contributing to occupational problems or challenges. For instance, if a client feels ineffective, therapy would seek to enable the client to feel more effective, or if a client has too few roles, therapy would seek to enable the client to choose and enact new roles, or if the environment was affecting the client's performance in a negative way, therapy would seek to modify that environment. In this way, identifying challenges or problems in the third step allows one to select the goals in the fourth step.

The next element in this step is to identify how the goals will be achieved. This involves indicating what occupational engagement on the part of the client will contribute to achieving these goals and how the practitioner will support the client. The previous section on change offered nine dimensions of occupational engagement, and these serve as a framework for thinking in this step. MOHO also identifies key therapeutic strategies that practitioners will use; these are listed in Box 44.1.

The text *The Model of Human Occupation: Theory and Application* (Kielhofner, 2007) provides a comprehensive resource, the Therapeutic Reasoning Table, for this component of the therapeutic reasoning process. It identifies a wide range of problems and challenges that correspond to the concepts of MOHO along with types of changes that would be warranted. The table also indicates what types of occupational engagement could contribute to achieving those changes and what type of support from the practitioner could facilitate change. Table 44.3 shows one small section from this Therapeutic Reasoning Table related to personal causation.

Implementing and Monitoring Therapy

To implement therapy means not only following the plan of action that was set out in the previous step, but also monitoring how the therapy process unfolds. This monitoring process might confirm the practitioner's conceptualization of the client's situation or require the practitioner to reconceptualize the client's situation. The monitoring process also can confirm the utility of the

> ## BOX 44.1 THERAPEUTIC STRATEGIES IDENTIFIED BY MOHO
>
> - **Validating:** Attending to and acknowledging the client's experience.
> - **Identifying:** Locating and sharing a range of personal, procedural, and/or environmental factors that can facilitate occupational performance.
> - **Giving feedback:** Sharing your understanding of the client's situation or ongoing action.
> - **Advising:** Recommending intervention goals/strategies.
> - **Negotiating:** Engaging in a give-and-take with the client.
> - **Structuring:** Establishing parameters for choice and performance by offering a client alternatives, setting limits, establishing ground rules.
> - **Coaching:** Instructing, demonstrating, guiding, verbally and/or physically prompting.
> - **Encouraging:** Providing emotional support and reassurance in relation to engagement in an occupation.
> - **Physical support:** Using one's body to provide support for a client to complete an occupational form/task.

planned client occupational engagement and therapist strategies or require the practitioner to change the goals and/or planned client occupational engagement and therapist strategies. When things do not turn out as expected, the practitioner returns to earlier steps of generating questions, selecting methods to gather information, conceptualizing the client's situation, setting goals, and establishing plans.

Collecting Information to Assess Outcomes

Determining therapy outcomes is an important final step in the therapy process. Typically, therapy outcomes are documented by examining the extent to which goals have been achieved and readministering structured assessments that were administered initially. Both these approaches are valuable in documenting outcomes. Assessing outcomes by examining goal attainment is helpful in reflecting on the extent to which the therapeutic reasoning process resulted in good decisions for therapy. Using structured assessments also allows one to compare change across different clients or when different strategies are used. In this way, they can contribute to evidence-based therapy.

TABLE 44.3 EXCERPT FROM THE THERAPEUTIC REASONING TABLE SHOWING A PROBLEM/CHALLENGE RELATED TO PERSONAL CAUSATION, AND CORRESPONDING INTERVENTION GOALS AND STRATEGIES

Problem/Challenge	Goal	Client Occupational Engagement	Therapeutic Strategies to Support the Client
♦ Feelings of lack of control over occupational performance leading to anxiety (fear of failure) within occupations.	♦ Reduce client's anxiety and fear of failure in occupational performance (e.g., "The client will complete a simple 3-step meal in 20 minutes without verbalizing anxiety or concern."). ♦ Build up confidence to face occupational performance demands (e.g., "The client will identify and participate in 3 new leisure activities with minimal support in 1 week").	♦ *Reexamine* anxieties and fears in the light of new performance experiences. ♦ *Choose* to do relevant and meaningful things that are within performance capacity. ♦ *Sustain* performance in occupational forms tasks despite anxiety.	♦ *Validate* how difficult it can be to do things that provoke anxiety. ♦ *Identify* client's strengths and weaknesses in occupational performance. ♦ Give *feedback* to client about match/mismatch between choice of occupational forms/tasks and performance capacity. ♦ Give *feedback* to support a positive reinterpretation of their experience of engaging in an occupation. ♦ *Advise* client to do relevant and meaningful things that match performance capacity.

Source: Kielhofner (2007).

	Roles	Habits	Personal Causation	Values	Interests	Skills	Short-term Goals	Long-term Goals	Interpretation of Past Experiences	Physical Environment	Social Environment	Readiness for Change
	F	F	F	(F)	(F)	F	F	F	(F)	F	(F)	(F)
	A	(A)	A	A	A	A	(A)	(A)	A	A	A	A
	(I)	I	I	I	I	(I)	I	I	I	(I)	I	I
	R	R	(R)	R	R	R	R	R	R	R	R	R

F	Facilitates	Facilitates Participation in Occupation
A	Allows	Allows Participation in Occupation
I	Inhibits	Inhibits Participation in Occupation
R	Restricts	Restricts Participation in Occupation

FIGURE 44.2 Betty's OCAIRS Ratings (see case study p. 456)

CASE STUDY: *Betty: An 82-Year-Old Woman with a Hip Fracture*

Collecting Information and Creating a Theory-Based Understanding of Betty

On arrival in the rehabilitation ward, Betty required physical assistance with all activities owing to limited mobility. She was using a walker and required physical assistance to ambulate. Betty clearly lacked a sense of efficacy and was anxious when engaging in activities of daily living. The therapist's major questions about Betty were as follows:

1. What had been her major life roles and routines before the injury?
2. How was her volition affected by her injury and subsequent impairment?
3. What was her functional capacity?
4. Was her functional capacity likely to improve to the level necessary to meet her goals?

In addition to a functional evaluation, the therapist elected to use the Occupational Circumstance Assessment Interview and Rating Scale (OCAIRS) (Forsyth et al., 2005) in order to gain a comprehensive understanding of Betty's occupational life. The therapist selected this semistructured interview as the method of assessment because Betty had the cognitive and emotional ability to engage in an interview and related well through conversation. The OCAIRS interview was completed in one session. The interview was conducted informally to encourage Betty to share her experiences, thoughts, and feelings about her occupational participation before the fall, currently, and in the future. Betty responded well to the interview and thanked the therapist for the opportunity to share her experiences and her concerns about the future.

The results of the OCAIRS interview were summarized in a rating scale (shown in Figure 44.2). As the OCAIRS ratings show, Betty has values and interests that facilitate her participation; the major factor restricting her participation is her personal causation. The pattern shown in the OCAIRS scale is reflected in the following conceptualization that the therapist wrote concerning Betty's occupational circumstances:

At the time of her fall, Betty lived alone since her husband passed away four years ago. She lives in her family home in the same small town where she spent her whole life. Betty has a daughter and two grandsons, whom she sees on weekends since they live in another town. She talks with her daughter daily on the phone.

Betty worked in a shop before she was married, but once married, remained at home to raise her daughter. She still highly values her homemaker role. Prior to admission, she was independent with all household tasks, including self-care, cooking, and shopping. Betty spends much of her time in leisure pursuits of knitting, baking, and listening to country music on the radio. She attends community groups at a local church on a weekly basis and attends the weekly church service. She has good friends from the church who provide social support.

Betty reports feeling that she has lost family roles, particularly since her husband died and her daughter moved away.

Her daughter and grandsons are very important to her and she looks forward to their weekly visits. She very much wants to regain her role of homemaker and churchgoer, as these roles structured her daily and weekly activities.

Returning home is the most important thing to her, and she is highly motivated to regain her previous daily routine and roles, though she is unclear on how she is going to achieve this, given her current situation. Betty does not have a good sense of what her physical capacity will be. She very much values her independence and is unhappy about requiring assistance from staff. She feels unsure about her current abilities and her future. Overall, Betty feels that she had lost control of her life and is anxious about her situation. At the same time, she has clear interests and goals as well as intentions for reinstating her previous habits and roles.

Therapy Goals and Strategies

Following the interview, the therapist validated Betty's feelings and concerns and advised her that the goal of returning home was achievable. Together, they identified the following goals for therapy:

◆ With modifications, independently complete all personal self-care ADLs in two weeks,
◆ With modifications, independently complete home I-ADLs, including making a bed, sweeping, and preparing a three-step meal in two weeks,
◆ Demonstrate improved confidence while completing ADLs and I-ADLS in two weeks, and
◆ Identify ways to resume three leisure activities with modifications in preparation for return home.

Implementing and Monitoring Therapy

The therapist collaborated with Betty to identify daily goals and to review Betty's progress daily with feedback from the therapist. Therapy first consisted of Betty's engaging in activities of daily living. The therapist provided advice, encouragement, and physical assistance as required. As Betty practiced self-care tasks with modifications and sustained engagement when the tasks were difficult, she gained a greater sense of efficacy. She then began engaging in leisure activities as well as I-ADLs in the SNF's model apartment, such as cooking and household chores. Throughout this time, the therapist and Betty monitored her progress and discussed its implications for her ability to return home safely and independently.

Outcomes

After two weeks, Betty had achieved independence with ADLs and I-ADLs within the SNF environment. She was spontaneously engaging in leisure, homemaker, and self-care activities and displayed confidence and a sense of capacity of her abilities within the SNF. Betty's discharge plan confirmed that Betty was ready to return home.

CASE STUDY: *Lin: A Preschooler with Seizure Disorder and Other Developmental Problems*

Collecting Information and Creating a Theory-Based Understanding of Lin

Because the therapist knew that attaining the parents' desired goal and Lin's success in school depended on arousing his motivation, the therapist asked the following questions:

1. What volitional factors might motivate Lin in the educational environment?
2. What aspects of the environment would best support Lin's participation in school activities?

The therapist first informally observed Lin in the classroom. Lin did not seem interested in any of the activities in the room and refused hand-over-hand support to participate in play or educational activities. He rarely smiled or made eye contact.

The therapist decided to use the Pediatric Volitional Questionnaire (PVQ) (Basu, Kafkes, Geist, & Kielhofner, 2002) in order to better understand Lin's volition and the environmental factors that that might support it. The therapist also decided to use the Short Child Occupational Profile (SCOPE) (Bowyer, Ross, Schwartz, Kielhofner, & Kramer, 2006) to document how various personal and environment factors influenced Lin's level of participation in the classroom. Both assessments can be administered from observation and do not require specific task performance, so they were suitable for Lin. The therapist supplemented her observation with parent and teacher interviews to complete the SCOPE.

The therapist asked Lin's parents about the things he enjoyed, the family routine at home, and Lin's engagement in activities. Lin's mother shared that Lin was a pleasant and easygoing child who enjoyed listening to music and singing and being held. Lin's father said that Lin was compliant during bathing, dressing, diaper changes, g-tube feedings, and other routines. However, he had problems with oral feedings. Lin's parents' concern for his health and well-being led them to protect him and limit his fatigue. As a result, they did not expect Lin to actively engage in any activity. Mealtime, however, was one occupation that demanded Lin's active engagement.

The next day, the therapist attempted to engage Lin in play, using a toy his mother reported to be his favorite (a crib toy that featured different music and a projected light display) as well as other toys and objects. When placed on his stomach with the light next to his head, Lin turned his head toward the toy, but he did not raise his head up against gravity or reach toward the toy. When the music stopped, Lin would softly whine until the therapist pressed the small button to start the music. Lin also showed interest in a similar toy that also vibrated and was activated by

a large, soft touch pad. The therapist attempted to use hand-over-hand assistance to have Lin reach, press the pad, and start the music and vibration again. Lin showed no inclination or interest in being able to turn on the toy by himself. The therapist conducted a second observation during mealtime. The therapist encouraged Lin to hold his spoon and bring it to his mouth with hand-over-hand support, but Lin resisted. When the therapist put a spoonful of food in his mouth, Lin dropped his head, and the pureed mixture fell onto his bib. The therapist used this information from the interview and observations to rate the PVQ and the SCOPE (see Figures 44.3 and 44.4). As the SCOPE shows, Lin's skills mainly restrict his participation and his volition and habituation mostly interfere with his participation. His main resources for participation are his vocal expressions and his environment. The therapist rated the PVQ twice on the basis of the floor play and lunch observations. Lin's scores indicate that he is passive or hesitant in demonstrating volitional behaviors in both contexts. His scores are indicative of a child with very limited volition.

On the basis of the PVQ and SCOPE scores, the therapist arrived at the following conceptualization of Lin's occupational circumstances:

Lin's low tone, poor coordination, limited endurance, and unstable health have led to a pattern of his passive involvement in his environment. His parents provide him with his basic needs as well as pleasurable experiences. He has had limited demands and opportunities to test his abilities. As a result, Lin's sense of capacity to affect the environment is mainly limited to his ability to affect others' actions through vocalizations. His interests are based on passive sensory stimulation such as music, light, and vestibular input. At this point, Lin's volition is a major barrier, since he tolerates and enjoys only passive involvement in learning, play, and self-care activities. While Lin's impairments contribute to his limited skill set, his lack of interest in exploring his environment has also limited the development of skills necessary for learning and participating in the educational environment.

Lin is able to comply with routines related to his care as long as he is expected only to be passive. When there are expectations for performance, he withdraws or becomes resistive. He does not have an awareness of role behaviors and routines associated with being a student.

Goals and Strategies for Therapy

The therapist established the following goals for school occupational therapy:

◆ Lin will develop the volition to actively explore educational toys and activities by reaching, looking, and interacting with toys for 10 minutes with verbal cues and environmental modifications,

Continued

FIGURE 44.3 Lin's SCOPE Ratings

Category	Item	F	A	I	R
Volition	Exploration	F	A	(I)	R
Volition	Enjoyment	F	A	(I)	R
Volition	Preferences	F	A	(I)	R
Volition	Response to Challenge	F	A	—	(R)
Habituation	Daily Activities	F	A	(I)	R
Habituation	Response to Transitions	F	A	(I)	R
Habituation	Routine	F	A	(I)	R
Habituation	Roles	F	A	(I)	R
Communication & Interaction Skills	Nonverbal Communication	F	A	—	(R)
Communication & Interaction Skills	Verbal/Vocal Expression	F	(A)	—	R
Communication & Interaction Skills	Conversation	F	A	—	(R)
Communication & Interaction Skills	Relationships	F	A	—	(R)
Process Skills	Understands & Uses Objects	F	A	—	(R)
Process Skills	Orientation to Environment	F	A	(I)	R
Process Skills	Makes Decisions	F	A	—	(R)
Process Skills	Problem Solving	F	A	—	(R)
Motor Skills	Posture & Mobility	F	A	(I)	R
Motor Skills	Coordination	F	A	—	(R)
Motor Skills	Strength	F	A	—	(R)
Motor Skills	Energy/Endurance	F	A	—	(R)
Environment: School	Physical Space	F	(A)	—	R
Environment: School	Physical Resources	F	(A)	—	R
Environment: School	Social Groups	F	(A)	—	R
Environment: School	Occupational Demands	F	A	(I)	R
Environment: School	Family Routine	F	(A)	—	R

F	Facilitates	Facilitates Participation in Occupation
A	Allows	Allows Participation in Occupation
I	Inhibits	Inhibits Participation in Occupation
R	Restricts	Restricts Participation in Occupation

458

Pediatric Volitional Questionnaire

Session I Comments:	Session I — Date: 09/12/07 — Setting: Floor Play				Items	Session II — Date: 09/13/07 — Setting: Lunch				Session II Comments
Turned head toward new toy but did not look at therapist/playmate.	P	(H)	I	S	Shows Curiosity	(P)	H	I	S	*Lin was not interested in feeding or related activities.*
Turned head toward toys, minimally tolerated reaching to activate preferred toy.	P	(H)	I	S	Initiates Actions	(P)	H	I	S	*Did not observe Lin initiating any interactions with his environment.*
Did not attempt to reach for switch toy even with support.	(P)	H	I	S	Task-directed	(P)	H	I	S	
Likes noninteractive music toys.	P	H	I	(S)	Shows Preferences	P	H	(I)	S	*Lin communicated his disinterest in eating by crying and putting head down.*
Quiet and usually attentive to new toy.	P	(H)	I	S	Tries New Things	(P)	H	I	S	*Resistive to holding and using spoon.*
Quiet and usually attentive to toy.	P	H	(I)	S	Stays Engaged	(P)	H	I	S	
	(P)	H	I	S	Expresses Mastery Pleasure	(P)	H	I	S	
	(P)	H	I	S	Tries to Solve Problems	(P)	H	I	S	
To have music continue, Lin whined to the therapist when it stopped.	P	(H)	I	S	Tries to Produce Effects	P	H	(I)	S	*Lin placed head down so he would not have to work at moving bolus in his mouth.*
Required significant physical and verbal support to practice reaching to activate toy.	P	(H)	I	S	Practices Skill	(P)	H	I	S	*Was not interested in holding, using spoon, even in a play fashion, with support from therapist.*
	(P)	H	I	S	Seeks Challenges	(P)	H	I	S	
	(P)	H	I	S	Organizes/Modifies Environment	(P)	H	I	S	
	(P)	H	I	S	Pursues Activity to Completion	(P)	H	I	S	
Not goal directed.	(P)	H	I	S	Uses Imagination/Symbolism	(P)	H	I	S	

Key:
P = Passive (Does not show behavior even with support, structure, and encouragement)
H = Hesitant (Shows behavior with maximal amount of support, structure, and encouragement)
I = Involved (Shows behavior with minimal amount of support, structure, and encouragement)
S = Spontaneous (Shows behavior without support, structure, and encouragement)

FIGURE 44.4 Lin's Initial PVQ Ratings

459

- Lin will participate in classroom activities and interact with teachers and peers using environmental supports and modifications implemented by educational staff (i.e., positioning, modified switches),
- Lin will actively participate in feeding at lunchtime by bringing his spoon to his mouth and keeping his head up with minimal assistance.

The therapist recognized that it was first necessary to address Lin's limited volition, since he would not choose to explore, engage in school activities, or more actively cooperate with daily routines and, in fact, resisted these types of occupations. Therefore, the therapist planned to structure the environment so that Lin could explore new interests and experience a sense of efficacy and success when trying new things. In addition, the therapist planned to work with the classroom teacher to ensure that expectations for performance in the classroom would be aligned with Lin's current abilities and interests.

Implementing and Monitoring Therapy

The therapist began attending Lin's classroom during floor time and worked with the teaching assistant to develop a positioning schedule to facilitate Lin's interaction with the environment. When Lin was positioned in a corner seat, standing in a supine stander, or lying prone on a wedge, the therapist or teaching assistant encouraged and physically assisted Lin to lift his head, reach, and touch toys and switches. The therapist ensured that Lin's attempts to affect the environment were pleasurable and successful.

This experience increased Lin's sense of capacity for play. After four weeks, Lin was able to actively explore for 10 minutes during floor time.

During oral feeding, the therapist graded her expectations and began by increasing Lin's head control. In addition to providing physical assistance and verbal encouragement, the therapist played a tape of Lin's favorite music as long as he kept his head up. This interest was enough to encourage Lin to cooperate with the therapist and keep his head up. With his head upright, Lin was better able to manage the bolus during feeding.

Outcomes

The therapist used specific PVQ items as indicators to track Lin's volitional progress halfway through the fall school term. At this point, Lin showed curiosity and visually attended to four new toys while positioned. He demonstrated his preferences by lifting his head against gravity when the therapist or teaching assistant brought out a favorite toy. Lin showed that he had an increased sense of capacity by initiating a reach with his right arm to interact with an educational toy. During lunch, Lin could keep his head upright and engage in the lunch routine for the five minutes. He was unable to hold the spoon on his own, even with adaptations such as a built-up handle, and did not tolerate a hand strap. However, he demonstrated an increased awareness of and cooperation with this self-care routine. Overall, Lin demonstrated an increased sense of personal causation to engage in play and feeding.

CONCLUSION

This chapter provided an overview of the theory and practice resources of MOHO. Two cases were used to demonstrate how MOHO concepts are used to guide the process of therapeutic reasoning. As the cases illustrate, therapists can use MOHO to support a client-centered and occupationally focused practice. This chapter was able to demonstrate only a small fraction of the theoretical, empirical, and practical resources that are available under this model. Anyone who wishes to use MOHO is encouraged to take advantage of those resources.

PROVOCATIVE QUESTIONS

1. Think of an occupation that you participate in. Identify how your volition (including personal causation, values, and interest), habituation (including habits and roles), performance capacity, and various environments (including spaces, objects, social groups, and occupational forms/tasks) influence your occupational participation. Imagine that your performance capacity has changed because of an illness or impairment. How would your volition, habituation, performance capacity, and the environment now impact your occupational participation?

2. Read the following mini-case about Joseph. When you have finished, use the therapeutic reasoning process to generate MOHO based questions about Joseph's current occupational circumstances. Create a conceptualization of Joseph's current occupational circumstances using MOHO terms to describe the factors impacting his occupational participation.

   Joseph, a 30-year old African-Caribbean, was referred to occupational therapy during admission to a mental health inpatient unit. He had recently been experiencing psychotic symptoms. His neighbors sought help from the police when Joseph was observed pacing the street and wearing no shoes on a cold wet day.

Observation of Joseph on the unit indicated that he was mainly withdrawn and inactive during the day, wary of others, and did not engage in self care. His personal belongings were shoved under his bed. Joseph was frail and refused many of his meals on the ward. He often dozed off while sitting and watching television. Nonetheless, when certain music was being played on the ward radio, Joseph quietly sang along to the music or tapped the rhythm with his hands and became more visibly relaxed. During occupational therapy group, he expressed interest in painting, but then refused to engage in the activity because "he would not do a good enough job." When touring the OT kitchen area, Joseph mentioned that he was known for his home-cooked vegetarian meals, but didn't think he could remember any of his recipes.

During her brief conversations with Joseph, the practitioner learned that he lived alone in a small apartment. Since the age of 16, when he left school, Joseph had drifted in and out of employment as an unskilled laborer working in restaurants and hotels. For the past few years, he played drums in a band, and spent his leisure time listening to music, practicing alone, rehearsing or performing with the band. Joseph had a long term relationship with a woman who was part of the band. Recently, this relationship ended and Joseph chose not to continue with the band.

ON THE WEB

♦ Therapeutic Reasoning Form to use with Provocative Question 2.

REFERENCES

American Occupational Therapy Association. (2002). Occupational therapy practice framework: Domain and process. *American Journal of Occupational Therapy, 56,* 609–639.

Ayres, A. J. (1979). *Sensory integration and the child.* Los Angeles: Western Psychological Services.

Basu, B., Kafkes, A., Geist, R., & Kielhofner, G. (2002). *The Pediatric Volitional Questionnaire (PVQ)* (version 2.0). Chicago, IL: University of Illinois at Chicago, College of Applied Health Sciences, Department of Occupational Therapy, Model of Human Occupation Clearinghouse.

Bernspang, B., & Fisher, A. (1995). Differences between persons with a right or left cerebral vascular accident on the assessment of motor and process skills. *Archives of Physical Medicine and Rehabilitation, 75,* 1144–1151.

Bowyer, P., Ross, M., Schwartz, O., Kielhofner, G., & Kramer, J. (2006). *The Short Child Occupational Profile (SCOPE)* (version 2.1). Chicago, IL: University of Illinois at Chicago, College of Applied Health Sciences, Department of Occupational Therapy, Model of Human Occupation Clearinghouse.

Doble, S. (1991). Test-retest and interrater reliability of a process skills assessment. *Occupational Therapy Journal of Research, 11,* 8–23.

Fisher, A. (1998). Uniting practice and theory in an occupational framework. *American Journal of Occupational Therapy, 52,* 509–520.

Fisher, A, & Kielhofner, G. (1995). Skill in occupational performance. In Kielhofner, G. (Ed.), *A model of human occupation: Theory and application* (2nd ed., pp. 113–137). Baltimore: Lippincott Williams & Wilkins.

Forsyth, K., Deshpande, S., Kielhofner, G., Henriksson, C., Haglund, L., Olson, L., et al. (2005). *The Occupational Circumstances Assessment Interview and Rating Scale* (version 4.0). Chicago, IL: University of Illinois at Chicago, College of Applied Health Sciences, Department of Occupational Therapy, Model of Human Occupation Clearinghouse.

Forsyth, K., Lai, J., & Kielhofner, G. (1999). The assessment of communication and interaction skills (ACIS): Measurement properties. *British Journal of Occupational Therapy, 62*(2), 69–74.

Forsyth, K., Salamy, M., Simon, S., & Kielhofner, G. (1998). *Assessment of Communication and Interaction Skills* (version 4.0). Chicago, IL: University of Illinois at Chicago, College of Applied Health Sciences, Department of Occupational Therapy, Model of Human Occupation Clearinghouse.

Haglund, L., Ekbladh, E., Thorell, L., & Hallberg, I. R. (2000). Practice models in Swedish psychiatric occupational therapy. *Scandinavian Journal of Occupational Therapy, 7*(3), 107–113.

Kielhofner, G. (1980a). A model of human occupation: 2. Ontogenesis from the perspective of temporal adaptation. *American Journal of Occupational Therapy, 34,* 657–663.

Kielhofner, G. (1980b). A model of human occupation: 3. Benign and vicious cycles. *American Journal of Occupational Therapy, 34,* 731–737.

Kielhofner, G. (2007). *A model of human occupation: Theory and application* (4th ed.). Baltimore: Lippincott Williams & Wilkins.

Kielhofner, G., & Burke, J. (1980). A model of human occupation: 1. Conceptual framework and content. *American Journal of Occupational Therapy, 34,* 572–581.

Kielhofner, G., Burke, J., & Heard, I. C. (1980). A model of human occupation: 4. Assessment and intervention. *American Journal of Occupational Therapy, 34,* 777–788.

Law, M., & McColl, M. A. (1989). Knowledge and use of theory among occupational therapists: A Canadian survey. *Canadian Journal of Occupational Therapy, 56*(4), 198–204.

Lee, S. W., Taylor, R., Kielhofner, G., & Fisher, G. (in press). A national survey of therapists who use the model of human occupation. *American Journal of Occupational Therapy.*

Matsutsuyu, J. (1969). The Interest checklist. *American Journal of Occupational Therapy, 23,* 323–328.

National Board for the Certification in Occupational Therapy. (2004). A practice analysis study of entry-level occupational therapists registered and certifies occupational therapy assistant practice. *OTJR: Occupation, Participation and Health, 24*(Suppl. 1), s1–s31.

Trombly, C. A., & Radomski, M. V. (2001) *Occupational Therapy for Physical Dysfunction* (5th ed.). Baltimore: Lippincott Williams and Wilkins.

Wilkeby, M., Pierre, B. L., & Archenholtz, B. (2006) Occupational therapists' reflection on practice within psychiatric care: A Delphi Study. *Scandinavian Journal of Occupational Therapy, 13,* 151–159.

Theory of Occupational Adaptation

SALLY SCHULTZ

Learning Objectives

After reading this chapter, you will be able to:

1. State the features of occupational adaptation (OA) that most distinguish it from other occupation-based theories of practice.
2. Describe the necessity of using the Guide to Therapeutic Reasoning for an OA-based treatment program.
3. Describe key aspects of the OA Guide to Evaluation and Intervention.
4. Explain why the therapeutic use of self is one of the most powerful therapeutic tools.
5. Explain why it is necessary for therapists to use an articulated theory to develop an authentic occupation-based practice.

A lfonso is an 11-year-old boy attending public school in the fifth grade. He was referred to occupational therapy for help with attention deficit disorder, reading problems, and behavioral problems both in the classroom and at recess. His occupational therapist, Claudette, plans to include Alfonso in a therapy group with other boys who are having similar difficulties. This group is based on the theory of occupational adaptation. Some of Claudette's work with Alfonso, is described in the case study later in the chapter.

INTELLECTUAL HERITAGE

In 1987, a group of Texas Woman's University occupational therapy faculty was charged by Dr. Grace Gilkeson (Dean of the School of Occupational Therapy at the university) to develop a Ph.D. program in occupational therapy. One of the group's challenges was to name and frame how the program would contribute to the discipline and practice of occupational therapy. After lengthy study and debate, the committee reached agreement that there were two concepts that were unquestionably fundamental to occupational therapy and should be emphasized throughout the doctoral program. These two concepts were occupation and adaptation. The committee saw occupation and adaptation as integral to the profession's beginnings, central to its philosophy, and essential for the integrity of its future. The research focus for the new doctoral program was thus identified as occupational adaptation (OA).

The design of the doctoral program progressed, and responsibilities were divided among the committee members. Sally Schultz and Janette Schkade were asked to develop the group's conceptualization of occupational adaptation into the perspective that would be the core of the doctoral program. Drs. Anne Henderson, Lela Llorens, and Kathlyn Reed, noted occupational therapy scholars, provided ongoing consultation in the development of the Ph.D. program and the research focus on occupational adaptation. The program was established in 1994. By 2007, there were more than 30 graduates of the program. Schkade and Schultz expanded on the initial concept of **occupational adaptation**. They introduced OA as a frame of reference (Schkade & Schultz, 1992; Schultz & Schkade, 1992) and most recently (Schkade & Schultz 2003) as an overarching theory for occupational therapy practice and research.

The theory of occupational adaptation describes the integration of two global concepts that have long been present in occupational therapy thinking: **occupation** and **adaptation**. The intellectual heritage of this theory dates back to the writings of William Dunton (1913) and Adolph Meyer (1922). Schkade and Schultz were also significantly influenced by the writings of several contemporary theorists both within and outside the field of occupational therapy (i.e., Gilfoyle, Grady, & Moore, 1990, King, 1978; Llorens, 1970; Selye, 1956). OA interventions for specific populations were first published in 1992 (Schkade & Schultz, 1992). A model outlining home health interventions appeared in 1994 (Schultz & Schkade, 1994). Numerous population-specific OA applications have appeared over the years (e.g., Ford, 1995; Garrett & Schkade, 1995; Pasek & Schkade, 1996; Ross, 1994; Schkade, 1999; Schkade & McClung, 2001; Schkade & Schultz, 2003; Schultz, 1997, 2000, 2003; Schultz & Schkade, 1994; Werner, 2000).

GUIDING ASSUMPTIONS OF OA THEORY

All theories are based on assumptions. Most occupational therapy is driven by the assumption that as clients become more functional, they will be more adaptive. The theory of occupational adaptation takes the opposite point of view. Practice based on occupational adaptation is driven by the assumption that if clients become more adaptive, they will become more functional.

The founders of the theory of occupational adaptation (Schkade & Schultz, 1992) proposed six guiding assumptions about the relationship between occupational performance and human adaptation. The assumptions are presumed to be normative and applicable across the lifespan. These six assumptions are as follows:

1. Competence in occupation is a lifelong process of adaptation to internal and external demands to perform.
2. Demands to perform occur naturally as part of the person's occupational roles and the context (person–occupational environment interactions) in which they occur.
3. Dysfunction occurs because the person's ability to adapt has been challenged to the point at which the demands for performance are not met satisfactorily.
4. The person's **adaptive capacity** can be overwhelmed by impairment, physical or emotional disabilities, and stressful life events.
5. The greater the level of dysfunction, the greater is the demand for changes in the person's adaptive processes.
6. Success in occupational performance is a direct result of the person's ability to adapt with sufficient mastery to satisfy the self and others.

These six assumptions are not about occupational therapy. They are about the normative relationship between occupational performance and human adaptation. The assumptions are relevant to occupational therapy because they provide the practitioner with a way of viewing the client and the problems that are presented in therapy. The most common viewpoint the occupational therapy practitioner experiences is the medical model and its underlying assumptions. In medicine, patients are generally viewed in terms of their body systems. Treatment is focused on correcting the breakdown within the identified system(s). Medicine's underlying assumptions about illness and treatment shape the view and the interventions that are used. For example, a nurse reviews the chart's lab results, vital signs, and progress. The nurse visits the 68-year-old white male and asks, "How are you doing today?" The patient answers, "Pretty good, but I'm still having a lot of pain, and I get tired so easily." The nurse asks the physician to write an order for more pain medication and increased activity.

A practitioner whose practice is based on OA will view the client through the filter of the six assumptions that ground the theory. The OA constructs, models, and intervention methods are all based on these assumptions. They form the core of the theory of occupational adaptation. The OA-based practitioner visits the same 68-year-old client. The practitioner is aware that the man is a retired bus driver, that he is married to the mother of his four children, and that they have nine grandchildren. The practitioner wonders aloud to the client, "What would you be doing today if you hadn't broken your hip?" The client responds, "Oh, I don't know, the only thing that matters now is getting me back on my feet." The practitioner replies, "Yes, we'll focus on that. You had a pretty bad break, and you might need to do some things differently when you go home. I will help with that. Let's talk about what matters the most to you."

INTRODUCTION TO THE THEORY OF OCCUPATIONAL ADAPTATION

The first publication on the theory of occupational adaptation was presented in two parts (Schkade & Schultz, 1992; Schultz & Schkade, 1992). Part 1 presents the theory's assumptions about the relationship between human adaptation and the performance of everyday occupations. A normative model, the **occupational adaptation process**, was proposed to describe the interaction of the person, the environment, and the internal adaptive processes that occur when individuals engage in their occupations of daily living (Schkade & Schultz, 1992). The model is presented in a linear format. However, the author recognizes that the actual process of occupational adaptation is characterized by complexity, randomness, and nonlinearity (e.g., Davies, 1988; Gleick, 1987; Prigogine & Stengers, 1984). Such

human processes are inherently not describable in two-dimensional models. On the other hand, the benefit of a linear model is that it provides a rudimentary organization of highly interactive and complex phenomena. Such organization is necessary to engage in a systematic examination. In sum, the occupational adaptation process is a highly interactive, complex, and self-organizing process that has the goal of achieving mastery over the environment. The linear model provides a basis for scholarly dialogue. The objective in dynamic self-organizing processes is not to achieve a determined balance or equilibrium. The theory of occupational adaptation proposes that equilibrium or homeostasis can actually result in a state of dysadaptation. Personal adaptation is proposed in the theory as a human phenomenon that is in a continuous process of order and disorder and reorganization. Figure 45.1 presents a modified version of the original 1992 model. The revised model is somewhat simplified from the one that was presented in 1992. It is also a linear model that was created to serve as a vehicle for examining these very complex processes. Although dynamic models are often more inclusive of the multiple phenomena,

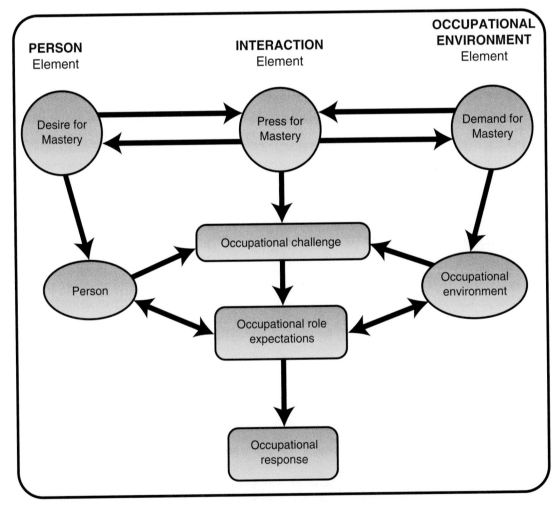

FIGURE 45.1   Model of the Occupational Adaptation Process. Adapted from the OA Process Model (Schkade & Schultz, 1992).

an identifiable process is often elusive. The model of the OA process (Figure 45.1) is based on three overarching elements: the person, the **occupational environment**, and their interaction. Each is a dynamic, ever-changing state that influences the other. The following discussion elaborates on Figure 45.1. Terminology that is specific to the theory and/or model is initially presented in italics.

Person: Internal Factors of the OA Process

The left side of the model is devoted to the internal factors: those that occur within the *person*. The process begins with a *desire for mastery*. The desire for mastery is proposed in OA theory as a constant factor in the OA process; it is ever present. Even at the cellular level, there is constant demand for adaptation and mastery (Reilly, 1962). Seeking mastery over the environment is understood to be an innate human condition. The second factor, the person, is made up of the individual's unique sensorimotor, cognitive, and psychosocial systems. These person systems are unique to the individual, with specific attributes and deficits. They are also uniquely affected by the individual's genetic, biological, and phenomenological influences. The theory of occupational adaptation posits that all occupations are holistic. That is, all occupations involve the sensorimotor, cognitive, and psychosocial systems. The relative contribution of each system shifts on the basis of the circumstances surrounding the occupation.

Occupational Environment: External Factors of the OA Process

The right side of the model is devoted to external factors that affect the *person* (see Figure 45.1). Correspondingly, the external process also begins with a constant factor: the *demand for mastery*. OA theory proposes that any circumstance presents itself with at least a minimal degree of demand for mastery. The second external factor is the *occupational environment*. The term was coined by the founding authors with the intent to capture the dynamic meaning that they ascribed to the complexity of factors that are external to the person in the OA process. The occupational environment is highly significant in that it not only has an expectation of the person, but also has a direct impact on the person. The occupational environment represents the overall context within which the person engages in the particular occupation and *occupational role*. There are three broad types of occupational environment: work, play/leisure, and self-care. Each type of occupational environment is affected by the physical, social, and cultural influences that are part of the individual's experiential context. The physical influence consists of the actual setting in which the occupation occurs. The social influence is made up of the individuals who are participants within the occupational environment. The cultural influence presents the habits, mores, and traditions and rituals that exist in the

occupational environment. The occupational environment is also a continuously dynamic and experiential context.

The OA Process: Interaction of Internal and External Factors

The internal and external factors are continuously interacting with each other through the modality of occupation. The ongoing interaction of the person's desire for mastery and the occupational environment's demand for mastery creates a third constant: the *press for mastery*. This constant forms the middle of the OA process model. The press for mastery yields the *occupational challenge*. The *occupational role expectations* of the person and of the occupational environment intersect in response to the unique occupational challenge that the individual experiences. A demand for adaptation occurs. The person makes an internal adaptive response to the situation and then produces an *occupational response*. The *occupational response* is the outcome—the observable by-product of the adaptive response. It is the action or behavior the individual carries out in response to the occupational challenge. The occupational adaptation process begins at the top of both the left and right sides of the model at the same time.

The OA Process: Adaptive Response Subprocesses

Within the broad occupational adaptation process, there are three subprocesses that are internal to the person. They are proposed to provide an explanation of the adaptive processes that the individual activates in response to an occupational challenge. The OA subprocesses enable the individual to plan the adaptive response, evaluate the outcome, and integrate the evaluation into the person as adaptation. The three subprocesses are identified as the generation subprocess, the evaluation subprocess, and the integration subprocess.

The *adaptive response generation subprocess* is the anticipatory portion of human adaptation (see Figure 45.2). The generation subprocess is activated by a mechanism that explains how an adaptive response is created. The *adaptive response mechanism* consists of *adaptation energy, adaptive response modes* and *adaptive response behaviors*. The mechanism and the three components are interactive; they are neither liner nor hierarchical. These components provide the resources that the individual draws from to generate an adaptive response to an occupational challenge. The adaptive response mechanism is best understood as a dynamic system (e.g., Davies, 1988; Gleick, 1987; Prigogine & Stengers, 1984).

OA theory proposes that the individual uses adaptation energy at either a primary or a secondary level of cognitive awareness. If the individual is at a high level of cognitive awareness when attempting to generate an adaptive response: the *primary* level of adaptation energy is being used.

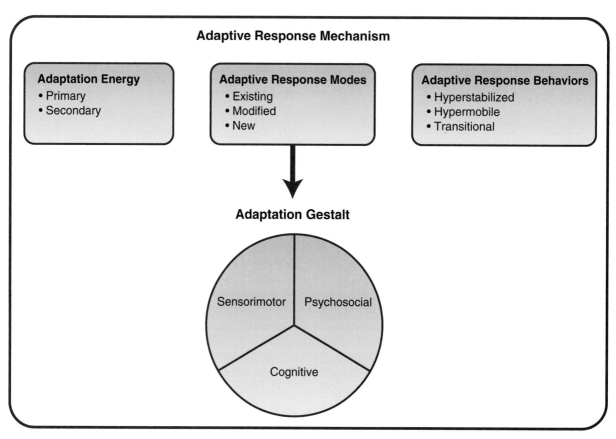

FIGURE 45.2   The *Adaptive Response Generation Subprocesses* are internal to the person (see Figure 45.1)

If the individual is not highly engaged in creating an adaptive response, a *secondary* level of adaptation energy is being used. To illustrate, an individual may work and work on a problem (using primary energy). When a solution is not forthcoming, the individual might decide to mow the lawn or cook dinner (such routine activities allow secondary energy to continue to process and work on the problem). Often, when the individual returns to the original problem, a "light comes on," and the individual has a new idea—a solution that was elusive while the individual was focused on the problem. In some cases, the solution appears even sooner while the individual is still engaged in the routine activity. The common explanation for this occurrence is something like "I just had to get it off my mind." However, OA theory proposes that the problem was not off the individual's mind; rather, the problem was still being processed at another level, that is, with secondary energy. The following paragraph provides a more thorough discussion on this phenomenon.

The notion of adaptation energy is based on Selye's (1956) research on stress and its effect on adrenal glands in laboratory animals. Selye concluded that unremitting stress led to excessively high use of the adaptive capacity of the animals' endocrinological systems and led to premature death. He posited a general adaptation syndrome to describe this process, and he extrapolated the presence

of a similar process in humans. On the basis of Selye's work and that of Posner (1973), OA theory posits that the above example illustrates the use of adaptation energy, which occurs at both primary and secondary levels of cognitive attention. Posner's notion of information processing at simultaneous or parallel levels was a major influence on this assumption. A second influence was the literature on creative problem solving (Whetton & Cameron, 1984). Creative problem solving involves methods for seeking alternatives to existing approaches ("breaking set") when other attempts have failed to produce solutions.

In the first part of the above scenario, the individual used adaptation energy at the primary level of cognitive awareness. When engaged in the routine activity, the individual had not "gotten it off his or her mind." As the individual changed to other activities, the problem was shunted to the secondary level of awareness. The secondary level is not inferior to the primary level. The secondary level of awareness continues to work on the problem (using adaptation energy) at a more efficient and sophisticated manner than that of the primary level. The idea of a secondary level of cognitive attention bears some conceptual similarities to Ayres's (1972) concept of subcortical processing. However, in the theory of occupational adaptation, the secondary level of cognitive processing is understood to remain within the cortical area of the brain.

The second component of the adaptive response mechanism is identified as the adaptive response modes. This set of modes contains the adaptive patterns or strategies that the individual has established through life experiences. They are classified as existing, modified, or new. Adaptive response modes begin as reflexive or random actions in the infant. They are reinforced as they are generalized to new challenges with successful outcomes. When first confronted with an occupational challenge, the individual usually selects an existing adaptive response mode and acts on it. If the outcome is unsuccessful, the individual may modify the mode and then achieve a successful outcome. The individual develops a new mode when the challenge is a significant departure from those previously experienced. However, the degree of challenge can exceed the individual's experiences and *adaptive capacity.*

The third component is identified as the adaptive response behaviors. According to OA theory, there are three general classes of such behaviors: hyperstable, hypermobile, and transitional. This classification system was drawn from that of Gilfoyle, Grady, and Moore's theory of spatiotemporal adaptation (1990). As with the other two components of the adaptive response mechanism, these behaviors exist within the person's repertoire of experience. When faced with an occupational challenge, the individual selects one of the behaviors to use in response to the challenge. Hyperstable behaviors are those in which the individual either continues to attempt the same solution or becomes "stuck" (e.g., the individual who sits and stares at the computer screen waiting for ideas to come). The individual who selects a hypermobile behavior will move rapidly from one solution to another with a great deal of activity but no resulting product. Transitional behavior is a blending of hyperstable and hypermobile that allows for greater opportunity for a positive outcome.

In summary, when an individual is faced with an occupational challenge, the adaptive response mechanism is activated. The individual will draw from prior experience that is available within the adaptive response mechanism. The individual selects a level of adaptation energy, an adaptive response mode, and an adaptive response behavior to use in adapting to the challenge. At this point, the plan of action has been created. This completes the first stage of generating an adaptive response.

The second stage is equally significant. The individual configures his or her person systems (sensorimotor, cognitive, and psychosocial) to carry out the plan. The configuration results in what is termed an **adaptation gestalt** of the individual's idiosyncratic sensorimotor, cognitive, and psychosocial functioning. Figure 45.2 presents the systems as equally balanced within the gestalt of the whole. However, in real-world situations, the relative balance of the person systems will adjust according to the occupational challenge and the individual's personal functioning. As with the adaptive response mechanism, the adaptation gestalt is also drawn from the individual's previous experience. Gestalts that the individual previously found effective might prove ineffective for future needs. Depending on circumstances, the individual might produce a gestalt that is destined to fail. For example, the challenge might demand a high level of cognitive activity and calm emotions; but because of anxiety, the person's gestalt might be overloaded in the psychosocial and sensorimotor realms and thereby compromise the remaining gestalt available for cognitive processing.

The adaptive response mechanism and the adaptation gestalt produce the internal adaptive response to the occupational challenge. The occupational response is the product of the individual's internal adaptive response. Although the adaptive response is not directly observable, it does become operationalized within the occupational response. The nature of the internal adaptive response can be readily gleaned from careful observation and analysis of the individual's approach to the task, his or her problem-solving methods, and the resulting outcome.

The *adaptive response evaluation subprocess* is activated when the individual assesses the quality of the occupational response (see Figure 45.3). The individual assesses the quality by evaluating his or her experience of mastery. Because this is a personal assessment, the evaluation is relative to the individual—hence the term *relative mastery.* There are four measures within **relative mastery**: efficiency (use of time, energy, resources); effectiveness (the extent to which the desired goal was achieved); satisfaction to self; and satisfaction to society. Relative mastery is inherently phenomenological. If the individual's assessment of the occupational response is positive overall, there is probably little need for further adaptation. If the result is negative, the *adaptive response integration subprocess* (see

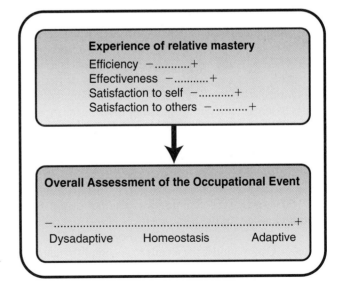

FIGURE 45.3 Adaptive Response Evaluation Subprocess: The *Adaptive Response Subprocesses* are internal to the Person (see Figure 45.1)

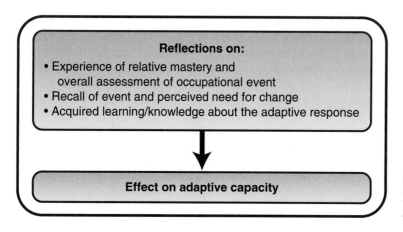

FIGURE 45.4 Adaptive Response Integration Subprocess: The Adaptive Response Subprocesses are internal to the Person (see Figure 45.1)

Figure 45.4) communicates this information to the person. The individual may then generate a modified or new adaptive response in order to better reach the desired level of mastery in any one or all of the measures of relative mastery. The above describes the normative adaptive response generation, evaluation, and integration subprocess.

INTRODUCTION TO PRACTICE BASED ON THE THEORY OF OCCUPATIONAL ADAPTATION

It is often difficult to distinguish between prominent theories of occupational therapy. Students and practitioners have often stated, "There's so much overlap, and it seems like there are only slight differences between the various theories." What is the uniqueness of occupational adaptation for practice? The following provides a reply to this question.

The theory of occupational adaptation directs practice to be focused on the therapeutic use of occupation to promote adaptation. Occupation is the tool. It is the medium that the practitioner uses to improve the client's **adaptiveness**. Therefore, the foremost intervention goal is to maximize the client's effectiveness in using his or her own ability to be adaptive. The theory of occupational adaptation is based on a unique core assumption: that as the individual becomes more adaptive, he or she will become more able to be an active participant in daily life. This is a departure from other prominent occupation-based theories of practice, which emphasize increased function and/or occupational performance as the goal of therapy. All therapy is driven by core assumptions, whether or not these assumptions are in the consciousness of the practitioner. OA theory focuses on developing the individual's adaptiveness. Occupation is the means to accomplish that goal. An OA-based practitioner selects interventions that are congruent with the theory's most basic assumption. The practitioner accomplishes the overarching therapy goal by presenting interventions that will activate and improve the individual's internal adaptation process. The practitioner guides the individual to select an occupational role on

which he or she wants to focus. Individuals will readily identify activities that they want to be able to do. However, it is important for the practitioner to help clients tease out a life role in which they have a significant investment. OA theory posits that activities take on meaning only within the context of a role.

The theory asserts that it is the client's adaptiveness that determines occupational performance. Some individuals are characteristically very adaptive and will respond effectively whether they face a divorce, the birth of a child, a stroke, depression, or a major move to a new city. They take charge of their lives and adapt. They are adaptive people. Others are, by nature, more easily overwhelmed by life's challenges. Their adaptive capacity (ability to generate effective adaptive responses) is limited.

Each occupational therapy client presents with his or her own unique pattern of personal adaptation. Adaptiveness is relative to the individual. Each client also presents with a variety of cognitive, sensorimotor, and psychosocial factors that may impair or facilitate the client's ability to be adaptive. With each added complication, including internal and external role expectations, the demand on the individual to adapt becomes greater and greater.

In an OA-driven practice, the practitioner's focus must be on increasing the client's ability to adapt. The goal is not to help the client adapt. The goal is to help the client become adaptive. In the beginning stage of therapy, the practitioner might teach the client adaptive methods and might introduce assistive devices or teach specific skills (**occupational readiness**). However, the therapy must progress as quickly as possible to **occupational activities** that the client finds meaningful (Frankl, 1984). The OA Clinical and Professional Reasoning Process provides a systematic progression of questions that the practitioner uses to frame his or her overall thinking and therapeutic program (see Figure 45.5). Figure 45.6 presents the OA Guide to Assessment and Intervention.

Clients are most inclined to discover their own ability to adapt when they are challenged within occupational activities, that is, activities that are meaningful, have a beginning and an end, are process-oriented, and have an end product (Schkade & Schultz, 1992). It is human

Data Gathering and Evaluation

What are the client's *occupational environments and occupational roles (OE/OR)*?
- Which role is of primary concern to client and family?
- What occupational performance is expected in the primary OE/OR?

What are the *physical, social, cultural* features of the primary OE/OR?
What is the client's *sensorimotor, cognitive, and psychosocial* status?
What is the client's level of *relative mastery* in the primary OE/OR?
What is facilitating or limiting *relative mastery* in the primary OE/OR?

Planning and Intervention

What combination of occupational readiness and occupational activity is needed to promote the client's *occupational adaptation process*?
What help will the client need to assess his or her *occupational responses* and use the results to increase his or her adaptiveness?
What is the best method to engage the patient in the intervention process?

Evaluating Intervention Outcomes

How well is the program affecting the client's *occupational adaptation process*?
- Which *adaptation energy* level is used most often *(primary or secondary)*?
- What changes are occurring in the *adaptive response mode (existing, modified, or new)*?
- What is the most common *adaptive response behavior (hyper-stable, hyper-mobile, or transitional)*?

What outcomes does the client show that reflect positive change in overall adaptiveness?
- Self-initiated adaptations?
- Enhanced *relative mastery*?
- Generalization to novel activities?

What changes are needed in the program to help the client maximize his or her adaptiveness?

FIGURE 45.5   Occupational Adaptation: Therapeutic Reasoning Process

nature to be motivated to participate enthusiastically if the activity is personally meaningful. The individual's attraction to the activity fuels the desire to adapt. The client's *adaptive capacity* is triggered by meaning. Meaningful activity gives the practitioner a powerful tool to observe the client's internal adaptation process. Adaptation patterns that interfere with the client's ability to adapt can be readily observed. The practitioner intervenes when opportunities are presented during the client's engagement in the activity. Such opportunities are typically inherent in the activity and call for the client to make an adaptive response. The practitioner seizes this window of opportunity to facilitate the client's adaptiveness. The intervention may focus on the client's overall approach to the problem, difficulty generating an adaptive response or evaluating the effectiveness of responses, repetition of ineffective techniques, diminished adaptive capacity, depression, frustration, and so on. These are common roadblocks that interfere with the client's *adaptive response processes*. The practitioner intervenes through a progressive system of posing questions and making observations to the client. The framing of questions and observations is tailored to the client's cognitive and psychosocial functioning. The practitioner guides the client, through questions and observations, to assume the role of decision maker and problem solver. The practitioner provides no more direction than is absolutely essential. It is better to err on the side of too little direction than too much. The more the practitioner directs, solves, and teaches, the less adaptive the client will become.

The therapeutic relationship is of critical significance in the theory of occupational adaptation. The relationship evolves into an artful dance between the client and practitioner. It is a partnership in which the client takes the lead. The practitioner becomes the facilitator. That is, the practitioner's function is to help the client discover his or her own ability to be adaptive. The practitioner is the agent of the occupational environment. The client is the agent of change (Schkade & Schultz, 1993).

INTERRUPTION IN THE OA PROCESS

Although the theory of occupational adaptation is not about mastery, per se, it is the constant presence of the desire, demand, and press for mastery that provide the impetus for the individual to adapt. In other words, these constants are pervasive and ongoing influences. As long as the individual can reach a mutually satisfactory balance between the desire and demand for mastery, the normative occupational adaptation process (see Figure 45.1) is working effectively and occurs with little fanfare. Day-to-day challenges occur, and adaptive responses are generated, evaluated,

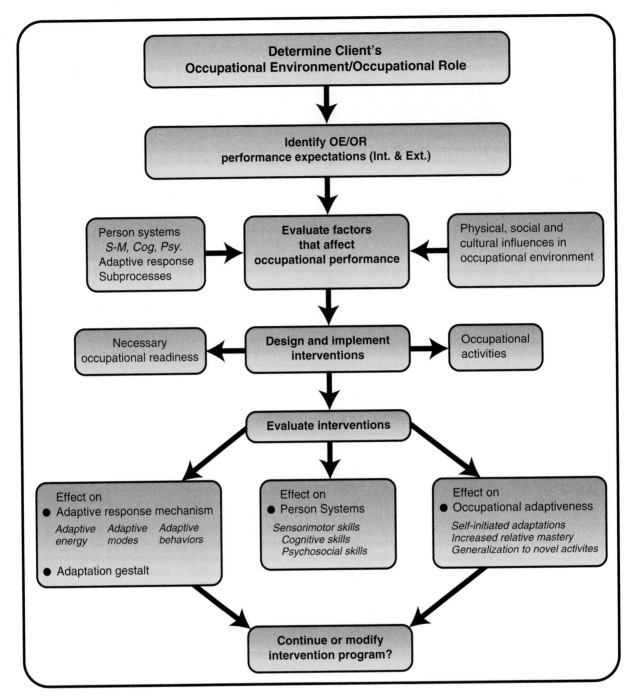

FIGURE 45.6 Occupational Adaptation: Guide to Evaluation and Intervention

and integrated. The individual is able to draw from the existing person systems and repertoire of adaptive responses in order to produce a satisfactory outcome.

When the normative OA process is seriously disrupted, the person's adaptive responses are often inadequate. Impairments in person systems place significant limits on the individual's ability to effectively use former or existing adaptive responses. Cognitive issues often further limit the ability to adapt. Depression emerges, and the person's relative mastery becomes lower and lower. This sce-

nario is a common occurrence for clients who are referred to occupational therapy. The challenges exceed the client's ability to adapt.

The case study depicts a school-based situation. However, the approach will be the same whether the client is a hospital patient with a stroke or a mother with a fragile premature baby. OA-based therapy is focused on working with the client to develop his or her ability to respond more adaptively to occupational challenges. At times, occupational readiness needs may supplant those for increased

CASE STUDY: *Alfonso Learns a New Response to Frustration*

Claudette greets Alfonso at the door as he enters the classroom. "Hello, Alfonso, my name is Ms. Murphy. Welcome to the group. Why don't you look around for a while . . . we can talk some later." As Alfonso begins to find his way into the occupational environment, there is a notable hum of activity—talking and doing. The group members (six altogether) notice Alfonso. Some greet him; others don't. He hesitantly observes a couple of the boys working on their individual projects. Claudette notices that Alfonso is waiting for her to take control. He is reluctant to touch any of the materials. He glances toward Claudette for direction. She slowly nods and turns her attention to another student. Claudette's manner of including the student in the group is integrally related to her intervention approach.

The group is grounded by the theory of occupational adaptation. This is reflected in the therapeutic tools that Claudette uses (see Box 45.1). One tool is her management, or agency, of the therapeutic occupational environment (OE). The second is Claudette's management of herself, that is, her ability to incorporate "therapeutic use of self" in the therapy sessions. This skill is intrinsically interwoven throughout the case study. The reader is referred to the early classical work of Gail Fidler (1963) for elaboration on specific methods and techniques. The third tool is Claudette's understanding of how occupation can be used to help an individual become more adaptive and respond more effectively to occupational challenges. The fourth and most powerful tool is her unwavering acceptance of the student as the agent of change.

Occupational activities (arts and crafts that are meaningful to the students) are the chosen intervention modality. The media are selected for their range of occupational challenge and attractiveness to the students. Some of the media are inherently structured; others are very openended. Claudette has very carefully created the nature and substance of the therapeutic OE; that is, she arranged the physical space, selected the media, and established the social climate and cultural standards for the therapy group.

Claudette follows the clinical and professional reasoning process identified in Figure 45.5. The practitioner must engage in the reasoning process to design appropriate OA-based interventions. The format in Figure 45.5 prompts the practitioner on what questions he or she must ask throughout the course of therapy. Figure 44.6 presents a model of intervention that puts into action the reasoning presented in Figure 45.5. Claudette's methods and interventions are consistent with both Figures 45.5 and 45.6.

In school-based therapy, the OE and related occupational role are predetermined. The overarching OE focuses on education-related work and play. (Each has its own physical, social, and cultural influences.) The occupational role is, by definition, that of being a student. The OE has a specific demand for mastery and occupational role expec-

tations (see Figure 45.1) of the student. These include a demand for a minimal level of performance in learning and behavior. Before meeting Alfonso, Claudette completed her assessment of the general OE in which Alfonso is a participant. She also assessed the OE's occupational role expectations for Alfonso. She found that school personnel expect Alfonso to cause trouble and to drop out of school when he is old enough. These are the actual occupational role expectations that Alfonso experiences, day in and day out.

As is shown in the OA process model (Figure 45.1), an individual's occupational role expectations are affected by those of the OE. After the initial therapy sessions, Claudette deduces that Alfonso has been strongly affected by the school's expectations. In fact, he has integrated them as his own. His innate desire for mastery has become one of a power struggle with the OE. He and the school are enmeshed in a no-win situation.

Claudette has also reviewed the school's records on Alfonso's person system deficits. His attention deficit disorder, hyperactivity, and difficulty with reading are clearly documented. She could incorporate occupational readiness interventions with the goal of increasing his ability to stay on task and help him learn how to better regulate his hyperactivity. Claudette has also observed during the therapy groups that Alfonso has a severe developmental delay in his adaptive response subprocesses. See Figures 45.2, 45.3, and 45.4 for further clarification. (These subprocesses are internal to the person.) Claudette has observed that whenever Alfonso has difficulty with projects, he tends to generate the same adaptive response mode repeatedly: He experiences himself as a failure. He routinely acts out this mode by tearing up the project or work. making a joke out of his work. or causing trouble with another student in the group. Alfonso's teacher reports that this situation is also a frequent occurrence in the classroom.

As a result of his adaptive response mode, Alfonso's adaptation gestalt (Figure 45.2) is composed largely of angry emotion and sensorimotor agitation. Very little cognitive activity is present within the adaptation gestalt. As a result, the next step in his adaptive subprocesses, the evaluation of outcome, does not occur (see Figure 45.3). His adaptation gestalt doesn't allow room for very much cognitive reasoning. Claudette concludes that it is very unlikely that Alfonso will respond more effectively to occupational challenges unless he acquires new or modified adaptive response modes. His current sense of himself as a failure (the adaptive response mode) leads to an occupational response (behavior that is observed) that is neither efficient, effective, nor satisfying to himself or others. His relative mastery is very low.

Claudette completes her assessment of the factors that are affecting his occupational performance (see Figure 45.6)

Continued

CASE STUDY: *Alfonso Learns a New Response to Frustration*   *Continued*

and concludes that her interventions should be focused on increasing Alfonso's ability to generate a more effective adaptive response mode. Because Claudette's practice is OA-based, she will not focus therapy on changing Alfonso's behavior; this would be incongruent with the theory. Claudette's interventions will be designed to expand his adaptive response repertoire with a new mode, such as "When I have trouble with a project, I can stop and figure out what the problem is." This will be an entirely new response mode for Alfonso. As he begins to acquire the new mode, it will affect his adaptation gestalt by decreasing the negative emotion and agitation that is present and freeing up space in the gestalt for cognitive processing. With his current adaptive response mode, Alfonso is at the mercy of his emotions. They are in control. As he experiences an adaptive response mode in which he has a greater sense of mastery, he will have the potential not only to control his emotions, but also to control his behavior.

Claudette plans to work with Alfonso using occupational activities that he self-selects. Most occupational therapy is driven by the assumption that if the client becomes more functional, he or she will be able to adapt. The theory of occupational adaptation takes the exact opposite point of view. Practice based on occupational adaptation is driven by the assumption that if the client becomes more adaptive, he or she will be able to function.

Through activities that Alfonso enjoys and finds meaningful, Claudette can more closely observe his adaptive processes and begin to intervene as appropriate. On the basis of OA theory, Claudette believes that Alfonso must develop the wherewithal to respond to occupational challenges in new ways. Her method will be to facilitate this through the four core intervention tools listed in Box 45.1. Claudette's challenge is to seize the opportunities for intervention that Alfonso presents during occupational activities. Intervention in the adaptive response generation subprocess cannot occur after the occupational response (observed behavior). The intervention must occur at the same time that the client is beginning to generate an adaptive response. This is a brief "window" that tends to open and close very quickly. Catching the window is an artful skill that requires a great deal of practice. To accomplish the goal, Claudette realizes that she must use each of the four therapeutic tools. The following presents an example of how the four tools may actually play out in a practice situation.

As she continues to observe Alfonso's adaptive response patterns and resulting occupational responses, Claudette begins to recognize the cues for when the opportunity for intervention might present itself. She sits next to Alfonso, makes a general matter-of-fact comment, and begins to watch and wait. He has started a project, a soapbox derby–type wooden car. This is his second attempt. Claudette

believes that his desire for mastery in the activity is beginning to emerge. The first car ended up in the trash after he tried to hammer the axle into the tire rather than sanding the axle. Soon, he faces the same challenge as he had with the first wooden car. He starts to pick up the hammer. The window for intervention has presented itself. Claudette believes that the most direct route to Alfonso's adaptive response mode will be through his adaptation gestalt. His adaptation gestalt is so overweighted with emotion and tension that the adaptive response mode is not readily available for therapeutic access. Claudette's therapy begins with a technique that she believes will have the desired positive effect on his gestalt. She will accomplish this through her role as agent of the OE. Claudette initiates the intervention by slowly stating to the student (as she reaches for the axle and wheel), "I wonder why this thing is so hard to get in here?" It is a rhetorical statement, not really a question to Alfonso. It is an observation that she is making aloud for the student to hear. It is as if she is giving a voice to the adaptive response mode ("I can stop and figure this out") that Alfonso lacks. She is not teaching it to him; she is showing it. As she quietly and slowly manipulates the objects, Claudette notices that Alfonso has sat back some in his chair; his adaptation gestalt appears to be changing. He relaxes somewhat; his affect softens. Claudette has used her agency of the OE to affect his adaptation gestalt. With calmness and curiosity, she has assumed physical control of the derby car. Her action reduces the sensorimotor demands that Alfonso was experiencing. The change in his OE allows him to distance himself from the emotions that he was experiencing as well. Through her management of the OE, Claudette has promoted a powerful shift in Alfonso's adaptation gestalt. Shortly, he exhales loudly, "Whew!" After a few moments, Claudette responds to his verbalized self-awareness. She comments, "It's frustrating when things don't work!" (The fewer the words, the more powerful the impact.) Again, her comment is not being made directly to Alfonso. It is an observation that is presented for him to hear and perhaps use, allowing him to gain some control over his emotions by turning feelings into a cognitive thought.

As a result of the intervention, Alfonso experienced a new adaptation gestalt. Claudette now directs the intervention toward his first experience with the new adaptive response mode ("I can stop and figure things out") by presenting him with another observation. "Well," she says, "You tried hammering it in before, and that didn't work, so. . . ." Claudette's observation is the first step in helping Alfonso to develop the new mode. She is prompting him to experience himself in the new mode—that is, to experience himself as a problem solver. The key to the interventions being described is that they are not artificial. They are not

CASE STUDY: *Alfonso Learns a New Response to Frustration*   *Continued*

contrived or role-played; they occur in vivo. Alfonso interjects with excitement, "Maybe it's just a crummy kit. I'll get another one." Alfonso retrieves another car and soon discovers the same problem. His enthusiasm drains away. Claudette does not become enmeshed with his disappointment. She maintains her therapeutic focus and again initiates an intervention to affect his adaptation gestalt by managing the OE. She states aloud, "Hmm, I wonder if the directions say anything about how to put the axle in the wheel." She has again made a statement that prompts Alfonso to be in the problem solver role. Alfonso replies, "I don't know, I don't like directions." This is a pivotal point in the intervention. Because it is the first direct intervention with Alfonso, Claudette knows that she needs to provide enough support but no more than is absolutely necessary. Claudette also believes that Alfonso finds the project very meaningful and might be willing to risk trying to read the instructions. (The instructions are consistent with his read-

ing potential.) As may be anticipated, he attempts to replay his typical battle with the OE by stating to Claudette, "Why don't you show me what to do? Isn't that your job?" Claudette matter-of-factly replies, "It's not my project . . . it's yours." She is careful to offer this statement with the same delivery as her others. It is presented merely as an observation. Through such a comment, she communicates her commitment to Alfonso that he is the agent of change. His comment was a test of her authenticity. Claudette will continue to work with Alfonso, following the principles of OA and using the four core therapeutic tools. Each intervention will be focused on helping him to acquire a new adaptive response mode ("I can stop and figure things out"). As he begins to assume the new mode, Claudette will shift her focus to the second subprocess: his ability to evaluate the outcome of his adaptive response. Figures 45.5 and 45.6 provide the reader with a more in-depth explanation of the complete process of evaluation and intervention.

adaptiveness. This is a judgment that the practitioner makes. Many times, both can be addressed during therapy. The greater the severity of impairment or limitation, the greater is the need for the client to become as adaptive as possible.

STRENGTHS AND LIMITATIONS

The theory of occupational adaptation presents practitioners with a theoretical orientation that is holistic. Its assumptions adhere to the ideas of occupation and adaptation that are inherent in the profession's history and philosophy (Schultz & Schkade, 1997). It provides an organized way to think and communicate about occupational therapy intervention that is occupation-based, process-oriented, and client-focused. Another strength is OA's compatibility with terminology from the World Health Organization

BOX 45.1

OCCUPATIONAL ADAPTATION: CORE THERAPEUTIC TOOLS

1. Practitioner is the agent of the occupational environment.
2. Practitioner incorporates principles of therapeutic use of self.
3. Practitioner uses occupation to promote adaptiveness.
4. Client is the agent of change.

(2004) and its concern with the ability of individuals and groups of individuals to participate fully in society. From an OA standpoint, occupation plays a significant role as a facilitator of social participation. Likewise, dysfunction in occupation becomes a significant factor in limiting social participation. The theory of occupational adaptation provides practitioners with one way to think about, describe, and plan occupation-based intervention.

Practitioners often question whether the theory of occupational adaptation is applicable to people with an impaired cognitive system. This is an unfortunate misunderstanding of the theory. The theory of occupational adaptation is as applicable to people with cognitive deficits as to those with sensorimotor or psychosocial deficits. The demand to adapt is as great for someone with a severe cerebral vascular accident (CVA) as it is for someone with a hand injury. The practitioner must adjust communication and methods of intervention to suit the person's ability to process information. The goal remains to help the person become as adaptive as possible. The more the individual is unable to manage his or her person systems, the more the practitioner must manage the occupational environment to facilitate the person's potential to experience the highest possible level of relative mastery.

At times, the primary avenue for communication with the person might be limited to the sensorimotor system. The effectiveness of such intervention was borne out in the author's consultation with a state hospital for adults with severe and profound mental retardation. The direct care staff used a reward system with the patients. When the clients were "good," that is, compliant with care routines and not yelling out, they were rewarded with the desired stuffed animal, music, or video. The staff was attempting to stop the patient's negative behavior. Change was externally driven. I worked with the staff to redesign the rehabilitation program to reflect the residents' occupational interests. A daily schedule of occupational activities was created for each person. Routine care was reframed from that of tasks that the staff must do for the patients to tasks that will help the patients to do what they found meaningful. The new objective was to increase the residents' experience of mastery over their environment. The necessity of turning the patient to prevent bedsores became one of positioning with purpose—for example, in order to watch the preferred video or to better hold the stuffed animal. For a patient who hated bath time, the preferred music helped her to relax. The occupational environment was managed so that residents had the potential to increase their experience of mastery over situations that they disliked. In the OA approach, change was driven by the patient's preferences. As a result of the patients' increased sense of relative mastery, they demonstrated less spasticity and fewer emotional outbursts. Although unable to communicate their relative mastery through words, they expressed it very clearly through their sensorimotor system.

Another limitation of this intervention approach lies within those practitioners who are willing to stay enmeshed in intervention practices and settings of the past 50 years. Such practitioners believe that intervention based on meaning is not practical in the everyday world of practice. These providers appear indifferent to the wide variety of modalities that a practitioner may use in practice. Outcomes are the issue at hand for practice. Research based on occupational adaptation interventions supports the notion that clients whose therapy has been based on meaningful activity and the development of adaptiveness will outperform those whose therapy has concentrated on activities of daily living that might have little meaning for the clients (e.g., 1999; Buddenberg & Schkade, 1998; Dolecheck, & Schkade, Ford, 1995; Jackson & Schkade, 2001; Johnson & Schkade, 2001).

Another frequently mentioned limitation is the lack of an OA assessment tool. I have been reluctant to encourage development of such a tool for several reasons. From my point of view, the most significant deficit that the profession faces is that the majority of practice is not theory driven. It appears that assessment tools are driving practice. Practitioners seem to prefer to use a static measure, rather than a theory, to guide their thinking process. This affects the nature of practice and the quality of research that can be carried out. A theory-driven practice is mandatory for occupational therapy to become clearly differentiated in health care. OA assessment is inherent in the Therapeutic Reasoning Process (see Figure 45.5). The new OA Guide to Evaluation and Intervention (Figure 45.6) was developed to provide additional direction for the therapist. It appears there are some dynamic systems process-oriented approaches to assessment that may be compatible with the theory of occupational adaptation and are worthy of exploration.

RESEARCH

Research on the effectiveness of OA intervention has included various methods. Most have been quasi-experimental with random assignment to treatment and control groups. There have been two main OA assumptions and related outcomes under study. The first assumption is that OA-based interventions will have a greater effect on functional independence than therapy based on traditional activities of daily living. The second OA assumption is that OA-based interventions will result in greater generalization of skills learned in therapy than traditional occupational therapy rehabilitation methods. The Functional Independence Measure (FIM) was used to test the first assumption. Performance on a patient selected novel activity was used to test the second assumption. In Gibson and Schkade (1997), the FIM scores of CVA inpatients were significantly higher on eight of the FIM scores than those of the control group. Jackson and Schkade (2001) conducted a similar study with hip fracture in-patients and found comparable FIM results. Buddenberg and Schkade (1998) researched generalization of skills learned in therapy to novel activities with hip fracture inpatients. The OA-based group performed significantly better on tasks on which they had not been previously trained than the control group. Dolecheck & Schkade (1999) studied the affects of an OA-based program with CVA in-patients. They served as their own control group over a period of six weeks. The patients were able to stand longer when engaged in personally meaningful occupation than when engaged in the facility's traditional occupational therapy. Johnson & Schkade (2001) conducted a single subject study with three CVA patients who had been discharged from home health because of insufficient progress in mobility. At the conclusion of the OA-based intervention, each of the patients made significant gains in mobility, self-care, and overall level of activity level. This description represents a portion of the research efforts to evaluate the effectiveness of OA-based interventions in practical applications.

CONCLUSION

The theory of occupational adaptation is presented as an overarching theory for practice. Traditional interventions such as neurodevelopmental approaches, sensory integration, and biomechanics are readily interfaced as part of the occupational readiness portion of intervention planning. Occupational readiness interventions are limited to addressing deficits in the person systems. The focus in such interventions is on improved performance. However, OA embraces a broader perspective. Intervention is focused on increasing the patient's adaptiveness.

ACKNOWLEDGMENT

This chapter is a direct extension of the author's many years of scholarly work in collaboration with Janette Schkade, Ph.D., OTR, FAOTA, Professor Emeritus, Texas Woman's University. The benefit of such a mutually rewarding relationship eludes description. I, along with so many of her students, became a more mature thinker and learned to embrace the pure pleasure of energetic and impassioned scholarly exchange through our work together.

REFERENCES

Ayres, A. J. (1972). *Sensory integration and learning disorders.* Los Angeles: Western Psychological Services.

Buddenberg, L. A., & Schkade, J. K. (1998). A comparison of occupational therapy intervention approaches for older patients after hip fracture. *Topics in Geriatric Rehabilitation, 13*(4), 52–68.

Davies, P. (1988). *The cosmic blueprint.* New York: Simon & Schuster.

Dolecheck, J. R., & Schkade, J. K. (1999) Effects on dynamic standing endurance when persons with CVA perform personally meaningful activities rather than non-meaningful tasks. *Occupational Therapy Journal of Research. 19*(1), 40–53.

Dunton, W. (1913). Occupation as a therapeutic measure. *Medical Record, 3,* 388–389.

Fidler, G., & Fidler, J. (1963). *Occupational therapy: A communication process in psychiatry.* Macmillan Company: New York.

Ford, K. (1995). Occupational adaptation in home health: A therapist's viewpoint. *Home Health and Community Special Interest Section Newsletter, 2*(1), 2–4.

Frankl, V. (1984). *Man's search for meaning* (3rd ed.). New York: Simon & Schuster.

Garrett, S., & Schkade, J. K. (1995). The occupational adaptation model of professional development as applied to level II fieldwork in occupational therapy. *American Journal of Occupational Therapy, 49,* 119–126.

Gibson, J., & Schkade, J. K. (1997). Effects of occupational adaptation treatment with CVA. *American Journal of Occupational Therapy, 51,* 523–529.

Gilfoyle, E., Grady, A., & Moore, J. (1990). *Children adapt.* Thorofare, NJ: Slack

Gleick, J. (1987). *Chaos: Making a new science.* New York: Penguin Books.

Jackson, J. P., & Schkade, J. K. (2001). Occupational adaptation model vs. biomechanical/rehabilitation models in the treatment of patients with hip fractures. *American Journal of Occupational Therapy, 55*(5), 531–537.

Johnson, J., & Schkade, J. K. (2001). Effects of occupation-based intervention on mobility problems following a cerebral vascular accident. *Journal of Applied Gerontology, 20*(1), 91–110.

King, L. (l978). Toward a science of adaptive responses. 1978 Eleanor Clarke Slagle Lecture. *American Journal of Occupational Therapy, 32*(7), 429–437.

Llorens, L. (1970). Facilitating growth and development: The promise of occupational therapy. *American Journal of Occupational Therapy, 24,* 93–101.

Meyer, A. (1922). The philosophy of occupational therapy. *Archives of Occupational Therapy, 1,* 1–10.

Pasek, P. B., & Schkade, J. K. (1996). Effects of a skiing experience on adolescents with limb deficiencies: An occupational adaptation perspective. *American Journal of Occupational Therapy, 50,* 24–31.

Posner, M. I. (1973) *Cognition: An introduction.* Glenview, IL: Scott, Foresman.

Prigogine, I., & Stengers, I. (1984). *Order out of chaos: Man's new dialogue with nature.* New York: Bantam Books.

Reilly, M. (1962). Occupational therapy can be one of the great ideas of 20th century medicine. Eleanor Clarke Slagle Lecture. *American Journal of Occupational Therapy, 16,* 1–9.

Ross, M. M. (1994, August 11). Applying theory to practice. *OT Week,* 16–17.

Schkade, J. K. (1999). Student to practitioner: The adaptive transition. *Innovations in Occupational Therapy Education, 1,* 147–156.

Schkade, J. K., & McClung, M. (2001). *Occupational adaptation in practice: Concepts and cases.* Thorofare, NJ: Slack.

Schkade, J. K., & Schultz, S. (1992). Occupational adaptation: Toward a holistic approach to contemporary practice, Part 1. *American Journal of Occupational Therapy, 46,* 829–837.

Schkade, J. K., & Schultz, S. (1993). Occupational adaptation: An integrative frame of reference. In H. Hopkins & H. Smith, (Eds.), *Willard and Spackman's occupational therapy* (8th ed., pp. 87–91). Philadelphia: Lippincott.

Schkade, J. K., & Schultz, S. (2003). Occupational adaptation. In P. Kramer, J. Hinojosa, & C. Royeen (Eds.), *Perspectives in human occupation* (pp. 181–221). Philadelphia: Lippincott Williams & Wilkins.

Schultz, S. (1997, April). *Treating students with behavior disorder.* An Institute presented at the American Occupational Therapy Association Convention, Orlando, FL.

Schultz, S. (2000). Occupational adaptation. In P. A. Crist, C. B. Royeen, & J. K. Schkade (Eds.), *Infusing occupation into practice* (2nd ed.) Bethesda MD: AOTA.

Schultz, S. (2003, September). Psychosocial interventions for students with behavior disorders: Identify challenges and clarify the role of occupational therapy in promoting adaptive functioning. *OT Practice, 8* (16), CE-1-CE-8.

Schultz, S., & Schkade, J. K. (1992). Occupational adaptation: Toward a holistic approach to contemporary practice, Part 2. *American Journal of Occupational Therapy, 46,* 917–926.

Schultz, S., & Schkade, J. K. (1994). Home health care: A window of opportunity to synthesize practice. *Home & Community Health, Special Interest Section Newsletter, 1*(3), 1–4.

Schultz, S. & Schkade, J. (1997). Adaptation. In C. Christiansen & C. Baum (Eds.), *Occupational therapy: Enabling function and well being* (2nd ed., pp. 458–481). Thorofare, N.J.: Slack.

Selye, H. (1956). *The stress of life.* New York: McGraw-Hill.

Werner, E. (2000). *Families, children with autism and everyday occupations.* Unpublished doctoral dissertation. Nova Southeastern University, Fort Lauderdale, FL.

Whetton, D. A., & Cameron, K. S. (1984). *Developing management skills.* Glenview, IL: Scott, Foresman.

World Health Organization (2004). *International classification of functioning, disability, and health (ICF).* Geneva: Author. Retrieved July 24, 2007, from http://www.who.int/classifications/en/

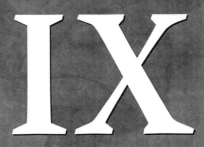

IX

OCCUPATIONAL THERAPY PRACTICE

"A client-centered intervention in which the occupational therapy practitioner and client collaboratively select and design activities that have specific relevance or meaning to the client and support that client's interests, need, health, and participation in daily life."

Occupational Therapy Practice Framework, American Occupational Therapy Association

The Occupational Therapy Process

JOAN C. ROGERS AND
MARGO B. HOLM

Learning Objectives

After reading this chapter, you will be able to:

1. Explain the occupational therapy process and discuss the importance of each of its components.
2. Apply the Person-Task-Environment transaction to client cases.
3. Discuss the advantages and disadvantages of three approaches to implementing the occupational therapy process: bottom-up, top-down, client-in-context.
4. Develop a structured problem statement to guide intervention and explain its usefulness for guiding intervention.

This chapter focuses on the occupational therapy process and consists of eight major sections. In the first section, we present an overview of the occupational therapy process and its major components: theory, evaluation, problem definition, intervention planning, intervention implementation, and re-evaluation. In the second and third sections, the salience of theory in explaining occupational performance—the transaction of the person, task, and environment—is traced historically and then each of the three factors is elaborated on in detail. This discussion provides the background for understanding the complexity of the behavior that occupational therapy practitioners evaluate and treat. In the fourth through seventh sections, the remaining components of the occupational therapy process are discussed in turn—evaluation, problem definition, intervention planning and implementation, and re-evaluation. Section eight revisits the entire occupational therapy process to emphasize its integrative nature. The chapter ends with a conclusion.

OVERVIEW OF THE OCCUPATIONAL THERAPY PROCESS

The **occupational therapy process** is the therapeutic problem-solving method used by practitioners to help clients improve their occupational performance. It consists of six major components—theory, evaluation, problem definition, intervention planning, intervention implementation, and re-evaluation (Figure 46.1) (Line, 1969; Rogers & Holm, 1989). During evaluation, practitioners systematically collect and organize data about occupational performance. During problem definition, these data are synthesized to formulate a profile of the client's abilities and disabilities in occupational performance, and to delineate problems that are to be targeted through occupational therapy interventions. During intervention planning, specific occupational therapy strategies and modalities for alleviating targeted problems are proposed. Simultaneously, **outcomes** are established to mark the endpoints of therapy and serve as markers of the effectiveness of the intervention plan. During implementation, the intervention plan is operationalized, that is, actions are initiated to achieve the stated outcomes. During re-evaluation, the same data that were collected during the evaluation that led to problem definition are re-collected. Initial data are matched to re-evaluation data to determine if the anticipated, stated outcomes were met. If intervention outcomes are met, new outcomes, appropriate for the client's improved performance, are added or occupational therapy services are discontinued, because they are no longer needed. If the outcomes are not met, the outcomes or the intervention plan are modified, or occupational therapy services are discontinued, because maximum benefit has been achieved. At any point in the process, occupational therapy practitioners may refer clients for other occupational therapy (e.g. special services, such as a driving or a home safety evaluation), medical, educational, or social services.

The occupational therapy process is theory-based and data-driven. (In this chapter, our use of the term *theory* is synonymous with that of frame of reference, conceptual model, theoretic framework, conceptual framework, or framework as discussed in Chapter 42). In Figure 46.1, the theory component of the process is represented by the oval at the top of the diagram. Each component of the occupational therapy process is influenced by the theory the practitioner uses to explain occupational performance in a particular client. The underlying theory determines the data that are to be collected, the meaning of that data and its organization into problem statements, the selection of interventions to manage identified problems, the timing and duration of interventions that are implemented, and the choice of outcomes to be used to evaluate whether the interventions achieved the intended purpose.

Like many helping professions, occupational therapy is a multitheory profession. This means that practitioners adhere to several theories (e.g., neurodevelopment, Model of Human Occupation, biomechanical frame of reference, rehabilitation frame of reference) to explain occupational performance on not just one theory. These theories have been generated by occupational therapists (e.g., Model of Human Occupation), other rehabilitation practitioners (e.g., rehabilitation theory), and other professionals (e.g., developmental model). Different theories may be applied to achieve different outcomes. For example, the Model of Human Occupation may be used to revitalize daily living habits, while the biomechanical frame of reference may be applied to restore transfer skills. Different theories may also be applied to the same performance problem to achieve the same outcome. For example, in a client with upper extremity weakness, independence in feeding (outcome) may be achieved using the biomechanical approach, through functional resistive activities to increase upper extremity strength. However, in the same client, feeding independence may also be accomplished using a compensatory approach—using eating utensils with enlarged handles that substitute for reduced hand grip strength. Accordingly, if a stated functional outcome is not well managed by one theory, another theory may be tried. When one theory replaces another theory, the entire occupational therapy process is repeated.

As the science underlying occupational therapy progresses, more data about the effectiveness of occupational therapy interventions will be available, and the occupational therapy process will become more precise. Information on

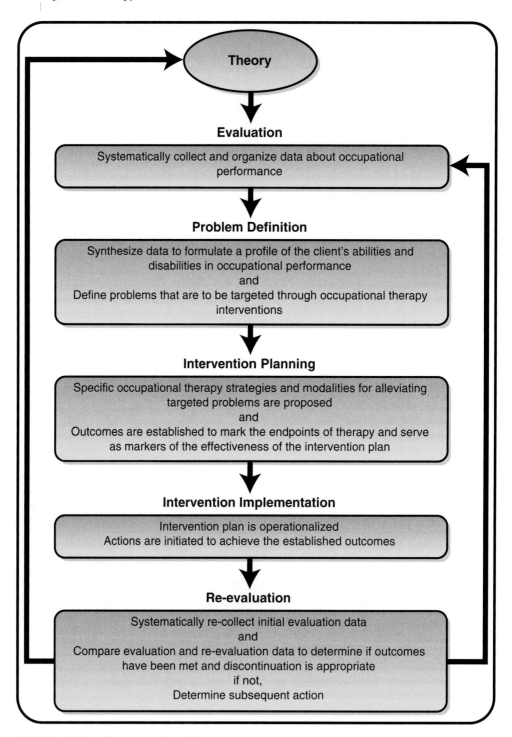

FIGURE 46.1 The occupational therapy process.

specific occupational therapy theories is addressed in other chapters in this book (see Units VIII, X, XI, and XII). What is important to realize in this chapter is the pivotal role that theory plays in directing the occupational therapy process.

Several characteristics of the occupational therapy process warrant highlighting in addition to its reliance on theory.

1. First, the occupational therapy process of evaluation, problem definition, planning, implementation, and re-evaluation is generic. Its basic structure is neither condition (disease, trauma etc.) nor age specific and is culturally sensitive. It supports all therapeutic reasoning, regardless of occupational construct (e.g., occupational area, performance skills or patterns) or theory

(e.g., sensory integration, occupational behavior). It can be applied in any practice setting—hospital, outpatient clinic, client's home, school, or workplace. The process becomes specific in the practice situation depending on a client's condition; the practitioner's skill, knowledge, and experience; and, the client's reason for seeking occupational therapy services.

2. Second, the occupational therapy process is dynamic. In introducing the occupational therapy process, the five major components were presented as though they occurred in a linear sequence, with evaluation followed by problem definition followed by intervention planning and so on. However, in the practice situation, the components are highly interactive. For example, practitioners formulate and refine problem statements in "real time" as data are collected, rather than waiting until all evaluation data are gathered (Elstein, Shulman, & Sprafka, 1978).

3. Third, in addition to being dynamic, the process is cyclical. For example, when re-evaluation data indicate that the intervention plan is not achieving desired results, the plan is revised, thus there is movement from component 5 (re-evaluation) to component 3 (plan). Similarly, as some performance problems are resolved (e.g., sitting balance), other problems may be targeted (e.g., dressing or computer usage). Thus, having completed the process for one problem the practitioner may begin the process anew for other problems.

4. Fourth, the occupational therapy process is accomplished collaboratively between clients and their advocates and practitioners (Cipriani et al., 2000; McAndrew, McDermott, Vitzakovich, Warunek, & Holm, 2000). The validity of evaluation and re-evaluation data rests on clients' willingness to respond openly and truthfully when interviewed or on questionnaires and to put forth the needed effort during performance testing. Problem definition takes into account clients' preferences and priorities. Stated outcomes center on activities that are meaningful to clients in their living, working, and playing environments. Occupational therapy interventions require the active participation of clients in developing the skills and habits required in daily living.

5. Fifth, the occupational therapy process is problem-focused. The statement of the problem or 'occupational diagnosis' is pivotal for intervention planning (Rogers & Holm 1989; Rogers & Holm, 1991). An accurate description of the problem (what is dysfunctional and why) is critical for selecting the most efficacious intervention (solution) for achieving specific outcomes (desired results). With the advent of occupational therapy practice in preventive, health promotion, and wellness settings, the definition of problem needs to be broadened to include potential problems as well as existing problems. Problems may potentially develop in the near (e.g., prediction of upper extrem-

ity musculoskeletal pain with prolonged typing) or distant (prediction of diabetes and related sensory problem in clients who are presently obese) future. Awareness of potential problems reflects a proactive approach that does not wait until problems develop but rather recognizes conditions that portend problems and seeks to manage them before they cause harm.

6. Sixth, the occupational therapy process is results-oriented. The entire process is intended to achieve an outcome (Evans, Small, & Ling, 1995). Occupational performance is expected to change, in a positive direction, as a result of intervention.

7. Lastly, the occupational therapy process provides the foundation for therapeutic reasoning but it is distinct from it. It outlines the building blocks for thinking but it does not explain how practitioners move from one component to another or how they integrate information efficiently and effectively to make therapeutic decisions.

OCCUPATION PERFORMANCE: HISTORICAL PERSPECTIVE

Because occupational performance drives the entire occupational therapy process, it is critical for practitioners to understand its nature and appreciate its complexity. Occupational performance is hypothesized to be a function of the **transaction** between factors internal (person) and external (task and task environment) to humans. The operative word in this equation is transaction, which requires that the person, task, and environment be viewed as a single, integrated unit as opposed to three separate units, with the task and environment being viewed in isolation from the person (Wachs, 1999). Transaction implies negotiation for the purpose of reaching agreement, that is, a balance or equilibrium among person (client) and task and environment factors that optimally supports occupational performance. If occupational therapy practitioners are to understand occupational performance, and evaluate it with the goal of improving performance, the client must be perceived as connected to the task and the environment or environments in which the task usually occurs.

Thus, incorporating the transactional perspective into the occupational therapy process requires not only that client, task, and environmental factors be considered, it requires that the three factors be considered *together*. When *evaluating* bathing performance, for example, it is not sufficient to evaluate client factors, (e.g., upper and lower musculoskeletal capacities) in isolation from the demands of bathing (e.g., reach feet, reach faucet) and of the bathing area (e.g., bathing equipment, wet tub, caregiver support for independent bathing). Similarly, when *intervening* to improve bathing (task) safety, recommending a safety device, such as a bathtub rail would be useless unless the recommendation was accompanied by client (person) and caregiver (environment) training in using the device for bathtub transfers.

Just as juggling three balls increases the difficulty of juggling, so too evaluating three distinct but integrated factors and intervening to change one, two, or three of these factors to achieve optimal performance is extremely complex. Early leaders in occupational therapy acknowledged the contribution of the environment to occupational performance, with Slagle (1922), Meyer (1922), and Haas (1944) suggesting adapting the environment to improve clients' performance. However, serious attempts to elucidate this complexity and translate early occupational therapy philosophy into practice models date from the 1980s. Since then a series of ecological models concerned with interactions between people and their environments have been developed by occupational therapy and rehabilitation theorists to assist practitioners in understanding the person-task-environment transaction. A brief review of these models in occupational therapy and rehabilitation and healthcare is instructive for fostering understanding of occupational performance.

Person-Environment Models in Occupational Therapy

In 1982, Rogers borrowed concepts from the behavioral sciences to modernize and enrich the fundamental premises about the link between functional independence and the environment. Independent behavior was viewed as a result of the interaction between the competence of the person and the demands of the physical, social, and temporal environments. Normally, habits of daily living enable humans to respond automatically and appropriately to a variety of environmental demands. The balance achieved between personal competence and environmental demands may be disrupted by physical, cognitive, and affective impairments related to disease, accident, developmental disorders, or advanced age. A fundamental therapeutic strategy for increasing functional independence reduced by these impairments is to initially lower environmental demands, and then raise them gradually as competence improves. Kiernat (1982) further articulated the concept of the environment as a therapeutic modality.

Barris (1982) developed the concept of environment proposed by Kielhofner and Burke (1980) in the Model of Human Occupation. Accordingly, individuals choose environments to become involved with based on environmental properties such as novelty, complexity, and compatibility with interests and values. Environmental demands for performance, which are associated with the people and objects in the environment, strongly influence the development of roles, habits, and skills. The development of competence involves the ability to interact successfully with an increasingly broader range of environments. Thus, Barris clarified three aspects of person-environment interrelationships and the ways in which choice, objects, and settings can be used therapeutically.

Howe and Briggs (1982) formulated the Ecological Systems Model in which humans and their environments shape each other. People are at the center of the ecosystem and are surrounded by three interacting environmental layers—the immediate setting, social networks and institutions, and ideology. These layers make up the life space for the performance of life tasks and roles. Behavior is functional when person-environment interactions enable individuals to achieve goals that are consonant with their view of quality of life. Goal achievement involves adaptation to changing environments and by changing a client's relationship to the environment the adaptive process may be called forth therapeutically.

When defining occupation, Nelson (1988) distinguished between occupational form and occupational performance. He argued that occupational performance, or action, can be understood only in the context of occupational form—that is, "an objective set of circumstances, independent of and external to a person" (p.633). One dimension of occupational form involves the physical stimuli present in the environment, including the materials used, the surrounding environment, the human context, and temporal relationships. A second dimension of occupational form is the sociocultural. The first dimension focuses on the doing aspect of performance, while the second dimension emphasizes the symbolic aspect (e.g., values and norms). According to Nelson, occupational performance, then, is the "action elicited, guided, or structured" by an occupational form (p.633).

Holm and Rogers (1989) described the person-task-environment (PTE) transaction as a relationship between the capabilities required of a task performer and the inherent properties, procedures, equipment, and materials involved in functional activities. Emphasis was placed on the natural setting, as opposed to the clinical setting, as a means of eliminating contrived environmental influences. Subsequently, Rogers and Holm (1991) adapted Lawton's (1982) ecological model of aging to explicate further the PTE transaction. Lawton described behavior as resulting from the interaction of person capabilities and environmental demands or press. As a person's capabilities become impaired, the influence of the environment on behavior increases. By implication, then, occupational performance depends on the match between the capabilities of the person and the demands the environment places on these capabilities. To highlight the role of the nonhuman environment on performance, and as a resource for resolving or alleviating performance problems, Rogers and Holm (1991) expanded the definition of the environment to include assistive technology devices, objects in the environment, and the structural environment.

The Person-Environment-Performance Model introduced by Christiansen (1991) viewed person factors (e.g., motivation, experience, beliefs, abilities, and skills) as intrinsic enablers of performance. Performance includes activities, tasks, and roles of occupations, and the environment includes physical, social, and cultural factors. A unique contribution of this model is the emphasis on person capabilities as enablers of performance.

The Occupational Adaptation frame of reference detailed by Schkade and Schulz includes the person, the occupational environment, and the interaction of the person and occupational environment during occupation (Schkade & Schulz, 1992; Schultz & Schkade, 1992). It focuses on the client's experience of self in relevant occupational contexts and the use of meaningful occupations to affect the client's internal adaptation process rather than outward measures of performance (Dolecheck & Schkade, 1999; Gibson & Schkade, 1997). Desired outcomes of the occupational adaptation framework are effective, efficient, and satisfying responses to the demands posed by the environment.

The Ecology of Human Performance (EHP) framework (Dunn, Brown, & McGuigan, 1994) builds on the premise that "interaction between person and the environment, affects human behavior and performance, and that performance cannot be understood outside of context" (p.598). Context is the viewpoint from which persons perceive their work and encompasses temporal, physical, social, and cultural factors. The EHP defines person, task, performance, and context, using the "Uniform Terminology for Occupational Therapy—Third Edition" (American Occupational Therapy Association (AOTA), 1994), and describes possible relationships among the four components. In addition, five collaborative approaches to intervention (establish/restore, alter, adapt, prevent, and create) that incorporate all four components of the EHP framework are described.

In a further theoretical development of the Model of Human Occupation, Kielhofner (1995) identified the environment as influencing occupational behavior through affording and pressing. The environment affords opportunities for performance, and presses for certain types of behavior. The physical environment was conceptualized as being composed of natural and built environments and objects. The social environment consists of social groups and occupational forms—that is, rule-bound action sequences. The physical and social environments intertwine to create occupational behavior settings, or meaningful contexts for occupational performance.

A primary intent of the Person-Environment-Occupational (PEO) model (Law et al., 1996; Strong et al., 1999) was to explicate use of the environment in practice. Occupational therapy's unique view of occupational performance encompasses the intersection of person, occupation, and environment. The environment consists of cultural, socioeconomic, institutional, physical, and social domains, all of which are constantly changing. The environment can have a positive or negative influence on occupational performance, enabling or constraining it, and is more readily changed than the person.

Task analysis, which is essential to occupational therapy practice, merits recognition as an ecological framework. Task analysis defines the relationship between the person and the environment as an action (e.g., reaches) oriented toward an object (e.g., into the cupboard). As a conceptual approach, task analysis has been highly developed in human factors engineering (Militello & Hutton, 1998a, b; Pelland & McKinley, 2001; Schaafstal, Schraagen, & van Berlo, 2000; Yu, Hwang, & Huang, 1999). A human factors approach to capacity-demand models uses task analysis to divide tasks into discrete sequential steps and then defines the physiological (e.g., actions, postures, grasps), sensory (e.g., feels, sees), and cognitive (e.g., searches, scans) requirements for successful task completion (Faletti, 1984). The occupational therapy practitioner then compares the demands of each step of the task and the ambient environment (e.g., heat, light), with the capacities of the person. When the task-environmental demands are greater than the person's capacities, the specific area for intervention is targeted (Clark, Czaja, & Weber, 1990; Czaja, Weber, & Nair, 1993).

Most recently, the Occupational Therapy Practice Framework (OTPF) was introduced (AOTA, 2002) for use within the profession, with a second edition in process (AOTA, in press). The OTPF defines occupational performance as "resulting from the dynamic transaction among client, the context and the activity" (2002, p. 632). Client factors support the development of performance skills (for example, motor, process and communication) necessary for everyday occupations, and as routines are developed in the performance of those skills, performance habits emerge. As people fulfill the social roles that are expected, required, or desired by them, they combine the performance skills and habits of occupations into broader engagement in everyday life situations, known as social participation. Engagement takes place in seven areas of occupation: activities of daily living (ADL), instrumental activities of daily living (IADL), education, work, play, leisure, social participation. Within occupational areas, each activity has unique demands, associated with its complexity, properties, and use (e.g., social demands, sequencing and timing). The performance of any activity is influenced by the various contexts in which it occurs. By definition, context includes seven interrelated conditions: cultural, physical, social, personal, spiritual, temporal, and virtual. Spirituality, along with values and beliefs may be listed as a client factor in the OTPF 2nd Edition (AOTA, in press), illustrating that there is no clear distinction between client and context and that these conditions are conceptualized as within and surrounding clients. Similarly, the demand character of activity spans aspects intrinsic (e.g., required body functions and structures and actions) and extrinsic (e.g., objects, space, social demands, sequencing or timing) to clients.

Person-Environment Models in Rehabilitation and Health Care

Although occupational therapy has historically acknowledged the person-task-environment transaction, this triad emerged to the forefront of theory and practice in rehabilitation and health care in recent years in part because of disability rights advocates, who emphasized the role of the environment in causing performance problems. Hence, over the past two decades, a major shift has occurred in the way in which health policy groups have defined disability, or limitations in socially defined activities and roles. In the Institute of Medicine's (1991) initial presentation of the enabling-disabling process, the environment was named as one of three disability risk factors. However, in a subsequent expansion of the model, the environment became a key feature, with the level of support provided by the physical and social environment responsible for the severity of disability experienced by the person (Institute of Medicine, 1997).

An increased emphasis on external versus internal disability factors is also evident in the sequence of models developed by the World Health Organization. The International Classification of Impairments, Disabilities, and Handicaps (World Health Organization, 1980), which was designed to describe the functional consequences of medical conditions, did not acknowledge the environment. Nonetheless, the environment emerged into prominence in the latest model, the International Classification of Functioning, Disability and Health (ICF) (World Health Organization, 2001). The ICF portrays health as having two parts: Part 1 concerns functioning and disability, while Part 2 emphasizes contextual factors. Functioning indicates nonproblematic health states, identified as body structures and functions, activity, and participation. In the ICF, functioning is built on a foundation of health, manifested in the "functional and structural integrity" of body functions and body structures. In the health condition, activities (i.e., tasks and actions executed by a person) are not limited. When activities are carried out in a standardized environment, such as an occupational therapy clinic, it is referred to as *activity capacity*. When activities are carried out in the real-life environment, such as a client's home or workplace, it is known as *activity performance*. When discrete activities are combined to enact social roles in real-life situations, it is referred to as *participation*. Activities and participation can occur in nine categories: learning and applying knowledge, general tasks and demands, communication, mobility, self-care, domestic life, interpersonal interactions and relationships, major life areas, and social and civic life. Each component of functioning can be expressed in negative terms, resulting in a disability continuum comprised of impairments of body structures and functions, activity limitations, and participation restrictions.

In Part 2 of the ICF, contextual factors are divided into two major groups—environmental and personal. Environmental factors are classified into five categories: products and technology; natural environment and human-made changes to the environment; support and relationships; attitudes; and services, systems and policies. Factors such as gender, race, age, fitness, lifestyle, and habits are grouped under the personal label. Environmental factors account for external influences on functioning and disability, while personal factors account for internal influences.

The OTPF and the ICF

Because of the salience of the Occupational Therapy Practice Framework (OTPF; AOTA, 2002) in occupational therapy, and the International Classification of Functioning, Disability and Health (ICF; WHO, 2001) in rehabilitation and healthcare, we juxtaposed the two frameworks in Figure 46.2 to illustrate concept relationships. Although neither the OTPF nor the ICF order concepts in a hierarchy, we created a hierarchy based on increasing complexity of person-task-environment interaction, to facilitate concept comparison. Figure 46.2 is designed to illustrate concept similarity not equivalence.

In the ICF model, disability arises from disease or disorder. Disease and disorder represent two opposing explanations of disability—namely, the medical model and the social model. The medical model views disability as a consequence of factors within the person, whereas the social model views disability as a consequence of factors extrinsic to the person. Thus, disease and disorder were deliberately used in the ICF to blend the perspectives of both models into a biopsychosocial approach. When disease or disorder negatively affects a person, change or loss of body functions and structures can occur, leading to impairment. In turn, impairment can negatively influence activity capacity and performance, yielding activity limitations. When one or more discrete activities are limited, this can lead to reduced involvement in everyday life situations, or participation restrictions. Neither functioning nor disability occurs in a vacuum. Both are influenced by contextual factors. Factors internal to people with disabilities, such as low self-esteem or self-efficacy, and factors external to them, such as buildings that are not wheelchair accessible or prejudicial attitudes toward people with disabilities, can negatively influence activity and participation, and thus accentuate disability.

Because the OTPF is silent on disease and disorder, we incorporated the ICF biopsychosocial approach as the lowest level on the OTPF hierarchical scheme. Wellness has a positive influence, while disease or disorder (further specified as trauma, developmental delay, age-associated declines, psychological maladaptation, environmental deprivation), can have a negative effect on a client's performance capacities (e.g., mental, sensory, neuromuscular). Consequently, performance skills and habits used to carry out everyday occupations (e.g., ADL, IADL, leisure) can also be negatively affected. In turn, social participation

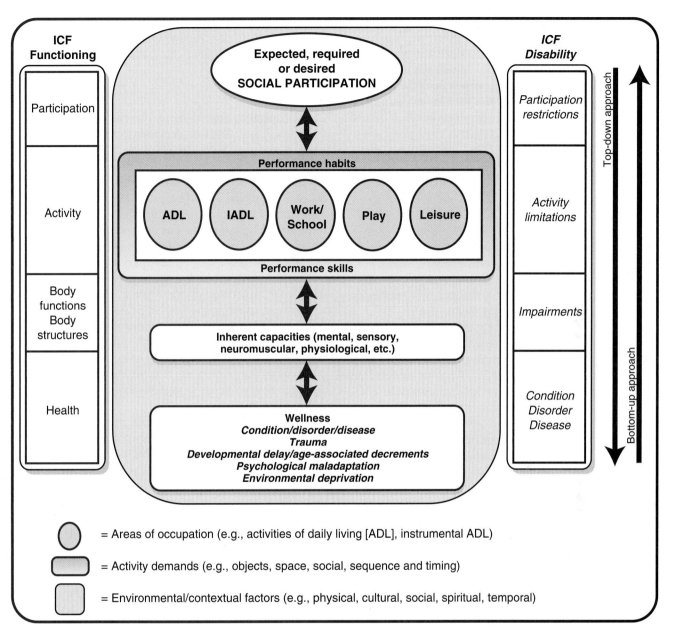

FIGURE 46.2   The relationship of concepts from the ICF and the OTPF.

roles may not be fulfilled adequately or at all. As part of an occupational profile, practitioners routinely evaluate clients for capacities unaffected by disease and disorder as well as unaffected skills and habits. Unaffected skills and habits constitute a client's strengths and can compensate for or replace those capacities that are dysfunctional.

Unlike the ICF, the OTPF not only recognizes the influence of context on occupational performance but also recognizes that each occupation has unique activity demands (e.g., objects, space, sequence of steps). In both models, the person-task-environment transaction becomes particularly salient at the third level of the hierarchy (i.e., activities and activity limitations, occupations), and maintains significance at the fourth level of the hierarchy

(i.e., participation and participation restriction, social participation). Hence, factors that are essential to the transaction, although external to clients, must be taken into account when intervening for disability (i.e., activity limitations, participation restriction).

Summary

This brief review of ecological models indicates that the person-task-environment transaction has been described from numerous perspectives, within and outside of occupational therapy, and with different emphases on the various factors. A common theme emerging from them is that people use their capacities to accomplish a task at a given time, using the objects available, in a specific place. Hence, the **outcomes** of a person's performance, in terms of parameters such as task independence, safety, and adequacy, depend on the transactions between and among the capacities of the person; the demands of the task; and the cumulative demands of the various environments (e.g., cultural, physical, social, temporal) in which the task takes place.

OCCUPATIONAL THERAPY PROCESS: THEORY

The components of the occupational therapy process—evaluation, problem definition (diagnosing), intervention planning and implementation, and re-evaluation—are common to all professions as well as common to the application of all occupational therapy theories. What makes the application of these components unique to a profession is the profession's overarching view of the phenomenon that it treats or services. The phenomenon that makes occupational therapy unique is occupational performance, which is why it is essential for occupational therapy students and practitioners to understand its fundamental nature and complexity. To facilitate this understanding, we present a perspective of occupational performance that is sufficiently general that it can inform any theory.

Our perspective of occupational performance builds on the construct of the person-task-environment transaction (PTE). A performance transaction, the PTE, implies a negotiation or arrangement among three factors: person capacities (P), task demands (T), and environmental demands (E). The task, whether it is dressing, writing, driving a car, cooking a meal, or playing golf, is pivotal to the PTE. It is the task and the various environments in which it takes place that require clients to perform in defined ways to accomplish an outcome. After defining and describing each of the three factors separately, we view them in concert in the discussions of the transaction (PTE) and of performance discrepancy.

Person (Client) Capacities

Person (client) capacities include inherent generic abilities and task-specific skills. Numerous mental, sensory, and neuromuscular abilities and other bodily functions and structures underlie, support, and enable the performance of multiple tasks (AOTA, 2002). Examples of generic abilities are attention, proprioception, and joint mobility. Generic abilities coalesce into unique combinations to form task-specific performance skills and habits. Task-specific skills and habits emerge to affect performance and participation in real-life occupations, such as dressing, meal preparation, website designing, and playing wheelchair basketball. Task-specific skills are developed through training and practice—that is, through the learning and

repetition of the PTE transaction in standardized and real-life situations (Giles, Ridley, Dill, & Frye, 1997; Ma & Trombly, 1999; Mathiowetz & Wade, 1995; WHO, 2001)

Task Demands

Client capacities are challenged by the requirements of tasks, which are called **task demands** (Johnson, 2000; Seki, Ishiai, Koyama, & Sato, 1999; Steptoe, Cropley, & Joekes, 2000). Task demands are identified through **task analysis**, which is the analytic process of breaking tasks down into discrete, sequential steps (Creighton, 1992; Cynkin, 1979). Task analysis identifies the actions that clients are to perform in relation to objects. For example, to make a cup of tea, clients must perform six actions (see Table 46.1).

The actions making up task performance are highly influenced by the objects used to perform them, which include the task materials, tools, and equipment. Task objects have inherent properties that influence task demands. For instance, pancake batter presents less resistance than stiff cookie dough when stirred, a plastic garbage bag placed on a car seat provides less resistance than cloth seat covers when transferring into and out of a car, and, an overhead knit shirt stretches more easily than one with a cotton weave when donned.

When calculating the demand properties of a task, the properties of task objects must be analyzed. One method practitioners use to analyze the properties of task objects is to consider the effect the properties have on the senses. When touched, lifted, carried, pushed, or pulled, task objects can be slick, sticky, wet, dry, greasy, crumbly, hard, soft, warm, cold, sharp, scratchy, smooth, heavy, or light. When visualized, they can be large, small, colorful, bright, dull, far, or near and have distinct shapes and patterns. When listened to they can produce loud, soft, irritating, soothing, or inaudible sounds. Task objects can taste sweet, sour, salty, or bitter and emanate odors that are pleasant, noxious, or unnoticeable. The properties of objects can also be hazardous to health, such as certain chemicals, solvents, heavy metals, and radiation materials

---

TABLE 46.1   SIX STEP TASK ANALYSIS FOR MAKING TEA

Action	Object
1. Locate	Tea bag and drinking container
2. Place	Tea bag in drinking container
3. Obtain	Container for water
4. Obtain and heat	Water
5. Pour	Water over tea bag
6. Remove	Tea bag

(Brigham, Engelberg, & Richling, 1996). Task materials (e.g., bread, shirt, shampoo bottle), tools (e.g., fork, drill, ice-cream scoop), and equipment (e.g., computer, stove, work bench) vary based on their function, design, size, and shape (Cynkin, 1979; Demore-Taber, 1995; Hagedorn, 1995; Levine & Brayley, 1991; Rogers & Holm, 1991).

The properties of task objects can increase or decrease the demand quality of tasks for clients. For example, the task demands for making a cup of tea can vary greatly depending on the method of heating, the type of tea, and the drinking container. Heating water for a cup of tea can be accomplished by placing a pan or teapot on the stove-top, heating a cup of water in a microwave oven, plugging in an electric kettle, or inserting an electric heating element into the cup. The tea leaves can be loose in a can, contained in a tea bag, or ground into powder for instant tea. The tea can be served in a ceramic mug, a plastic mug, a china cup, or the lid of a Thermos™. Thus, the task steps, and the inherent properties and design of specific task objects used to perform a task, have a strong influence on the task demands and performance outcomes.

In the example of making tea, task demands exerted their influence through the client's manipulation of task objects. However, the demands of tasks may also be brought to bear on clients when they perform in relation to objects. When executing transfers, for example, clients perform in relation to chairs, commodes, beds, and cars and the specific features of these objects have a direct influence on task performance.

Environmental Demands

In addition to the demands inherent in tasks, task performance is also influenced by the environment surrounding the task (AOTA, 2002; Christiansen, 1991; Dunn et al., 1994; Iwarsson, Isacsson, & Lanke, 1998; Law et al., 1996; Letts et al., 1994; Rogers, 1982). This influence is called **environmental demands**. Although environment is a multi-faceted construct (e.g., physical, social, cultural, temporal), for the purposes of illustration, we will discuss only its physical and social features.

The properties of the physical environment usually include space, arrangement of equipment and objects, equipment controls, surface heights, lighting, temperature, noise, humidity, vibration, and ventilation (Demore-Tabor, 1995; Hagedorn, 1995; Jacobs, 1999; Raschko, 1991). Each of these properties has been further delineated in architectural (Raschko, 1991; Stamps, 2000), anthropometric (Baker, 1999; Diffrient, Tilley, & Bardagjy, 1974; Pheasant, 1998), ergonomic (Jacobs, 1999; Kroemer & Grandjean, 1997; Rice, 1998), or occupational health and safety literature (Brigham et al., 1996; Carson, 1994; Kroemer & Grandjean, 1997; Moore & Garg, 1995). Not only are there static aspects of the physical environment to consider but there are also dynamic aspects: machines that have moving parts, temperatures that fluctuate, noise levels that rise and fall, humidity that rises and falls, and ventilation that fluctuates.

The demands of the physical environment may compound those of the task. If a toilet is on the second floor of a two-story house and a client cannot climb stairs, the client will not be able to get to the toilet to use it. A portable toilet may need to be purchased or rented and installed in a first-floor bedroom or closet to reduce the demands of physical structures. Furthermore, if space in the bedroom is restricted, or if there is no lighting in the closet, the safety of toilet transfers may be compromised, and adaptations may need to be made to reduce the negative effect of environmental demand.

Often environmental demand is viewed solely in terms of the physical environment. However, task performance is also surrounded by a social environment (Woodward, Hales, Litidamu, Phillips, & Martin, 2000). The social environment includes more than the mere number of people in the home, school, or workplace. The knowledge, skills, habits, expectations, values, attitudes, and motivations of these people create a social climate that fosters or hinders task performance (MacDonald, Karasek, Punnett, & Scharf, 2001; Seki et al., 1999; Walker, Goodwin, & Warren, 1995). Cultural beliefs, norms, customs, and practices also influence the social environment (Hagedorn, 1995). Moreover, people arrange their temporal environment as well as their physical and social environments. For example, they establish daily schedules and the pacing of tasks (MacDonald et al., 2001), in addition to selecting and placing task objects, and organizing and governing social groups. In so doing, people set the overall level of stimulation (e.g., too much, just right, too little) surrounding them during task performance (Christiansen, 1991; Gerdner, Hall, & Buckwalter, 1996; Keuter, Byrne, Voell, & Larson, 2000). At any given time, a person can have numerous roles (e.g., worker, parent, husband, grandparent, co-worker, volunteer, client, and social activist), each of which has unique task demands that occur in separate or overlapping physical and social contexts.

The Transaction

Clients are not passive recipients of the effects of their environments. Rather, they act on, as well as are acted on, by task and environmental forces. This creates a trans-actional relationship that is characterized as an interdependence between person capacities, task demands and environmental demands (Dunn et al., 1994; Law et al., 1996; Lawton, 1982; Rogers, 1982). For example, a client who is unable to get up the stairs to the bathtub may build a shower on the first floor of the home, install a stair lift to the second level, or bathe at the kitchen sink. Each of these decisions changes the task objects and the task environment, and, in turn, these environmental changes alter the PTE transaction.

Performance Discrepancy: Demands Exceed Capacities

When the capacities of a client are sufficient to manage the demands of the task and the surrounding environment, the client's performance and the level of performance that is expected, required, or desired are congruent. However, when demands (task and/or environmental) exceed capacities, task performance is compromised, and there is a **performance discrepancy** between actual performance and the performance skills or habits that are expected, required, or desired (Lawton, 1982; Mager & Pipe, 1984; Mangino, 2000). The performance discrepancy can be reduced, eliminated, or prevented by establishing or restoring capacities, reducing task demands, reducing environmental demands, or by using a combination of these three methods (Holm, Santangelo, Fromuth, Brown, & Walter, 2000; Law et al., 1996; Mathiowetz & Matuska, 1998; Rogers et al., 1999; Rogers et al., 2000; van Heugten et al., 1998). With the diminishment of their capacities through impairment, trauma, developmental delay, age-related decrements, psychological maladaptation, or environmental deprivation, clients become more susceptible to environmental influences. They have fewer internal resources and less energy to resist external forces or to devise adaptive strategies to counteract them (Lawton, 1982). By designing a therapeutic environment to accommodate diminished capacity, practitioners may be able to improve task performance (Close et al., 1999; Cummings et al., 1999; Mee & Sumsion, 2001; Rogers et al., 1999, 2000).

OT PROCESS: EVALUATION

The theory of occupational performance selected by the occupational therapy practitioner permeates the entire occupational therapy process, but is initially applied to **evaluation**. Evaluate means to examine and form an opinion about. Examination involves the systematic gathering of information about a client's occupational performance. Opinion formation involves combining the information gathered with professional knowledge and judgment to: describe the client's occupational profile, define client's performance problems (discrepancies), hypothesize about the causes of these problems, establish the occupational outcome(s) to be achieved through intervention, and, determine the "best" intervention to bring about the stated outcomes.

Evaluation Protocols: What Combination Is Appropriate—PTE, PT, P?

Practitioners use one of three person-task-environment (PTE) protocols, alone or in combination, to evaluate the transaction. Recognizing the combined influence of task and environmental demands on clients' capacities, the optimal protocol (PTE) is to evaluate all three components directly and simultaneously in the actual, real-life task situation. Accordingly, clients perform targeted tasks in their usual manner, with familiar task objects and equipment, in the setting or settings in which they typically perform these tasks. When performance discrepancies emerge, the relative contribution of person capacities, task demands, and environmental demands to their development can be readily determined. Practitioners working in home care, long-term care facilities, school systems, or work environments have the opportunity to implement the optimal PTE protocol, because evaluation and intervention occur in the real-life situation.

In most other practice settings, such as hospitals, rehabilitation facilities, and outpatient clinics, evaluations are conducted in clinic environments. Clients' performance capacities are evaluated under laboratory rather than real-life conditions. Laboratory conditions may place very different demands on clients' capacities because task objects and equipment are usually not identical to those in the real-life situation. Executing bed transfers may be easier in the clinic than in a client's home because the bed is lower in the clinic. The clinic (task objects and environment) may facilitate performance, because of its enabling, prosthetic features that reduce disability (e.g., wheelchair accessibility) or it may hinder performance, because task objects and equipment are unfamiliar (e.g., cooking with an electric rather than a gas range). In the second PTE protocol (PT), unless clients bring in their own task materials to use during the evaluation (e.g., clothing, medications), their capacities are evaluated with unfamiliar task materials and equipment. The extent to which unfamiliarity has a positive, neutral, or negative influence on task performance is largely unknown. Research suggests that this influence is task dependent (Raina, Rogers, & Holm, 2007). When clients' performance is tested in clinic environments, every effort should be made to approximate the real-life situation to elicit a "true" baseline performance profile. Under the laboratory conditions of clinics, the influence of the environment can be known only indirectly through client or proxy report. Hence, practitioners must use their therapeutic judgment to infer real-life performance from laboratory performance to identify appropriate performance problems, interventions, and outcomes.

While the first PTE protocol accounts directly for person, task, and environment (PTE), and the second protocol accounts for the person and the task (PT), the third protocol (P) accounts only for the person. Hence, it requires an even greater reliance on therapeutic judgment than the person-task (PT) protocol because only person capacities are directly evaluated. Data gleaned from the evaluation are matched to the practitioner's knowledge of task and environmental demands and a judgment is made about tasks clients will and will not be able to performance based on this match. For example, knowing that shoulder

COMMENTARY ON THE EVIDENCE

Occupational Therapy and Evidence Related to the Occupational Therapy Process

Evidence related to the occupational therapy process can be found in the literature on problem-solving/information processing, clinical reasoning, therapeutic reasoning and evidence-based practice. One thrust of the problem-solving/information processing and clinical reasoning literature has been the differences between novices and experts, or students and experienced practitioners. Most occupational therapy literature on this topic has been position papers, reviews of related literature, books, and studies with small samples (Higgs & Jones, 2000; Line, 1969; Robertson, 1996, Rogers, 1983). Research evidence from quasi-experimental, pre-post designs has shown that using a structure, such as the occupational therapy process, provides novices with a way to organize current knowledge (client evaluation data; didactic knowledge) and it also provides experts with a way to organize and use both current knowledge and prior knowledge (previous experience) (Griffin, 1975; Neistadt, 1987, 1992, 1998, Rogers & Masagatani, 1982).

More recently, research has shifted from the teaching of therapeutic reasoning to using research evidence in critical thinking and making well-reasoned decisions by practitioners (Gambrill, 2005). Although the research literature confirming the effectiveness and efficacy of occupational therapy interventions has increased exponentially in the last ten years (see Commentaries on the Evidence throughout this text), unfortunately, evidence on the use of that research by practitioners is not encouraging at this time. Surveys, reviews, interviews, and pre-post evidence-based practice interventions primarily revealed a focus on barriers that impeded use of research evidence, including time, knowledge of research methods, access to research literature, and feelings of inadequacy associated with not understanding research (Dubouloz, Egan, Vallerand, & Von Zweck, 1999; Dysart, & Tomlin, 2002; Koch, Cook, Tankersley, & Rumrill, 2006; McKenna, Bennett, Dierselhuis, Hoffmann, Tooth, & McCluskey, 2005). Of even greater concern, however, are the findings of a moderately robust pre-post evidence-based practice intervention study which found that although practitioners' knowledge of evidence-based practice improved significantly, even with continuous support their use of research evidence in practice did not change (McKluskey & Lovarini, 2005).

Moreover, in a study examining the use of research evidence by a sample of 131 registered therapists and members of the American Occupational Therapy Association, the findings indicated that as the educational level of the respondents increased the view of the importance of research decreased, and as the years of practice increased, the use of evidence for therapeutic decision-making decreased (Cameron et al., 2005).

ETHICAL DILEMMA

Ethics, Education, and Intervention

Although the current AOTA Code of Ethics (AOTA, 2005) specifically addresses intervention, a major component of the occupational therapy process, it is silent in regard to evaluation, another major component of the occupational therapy process. Because intervention is based on evaluation, does this present an ethical dilemma?

external rotation is needed to brush hair on the back of the head, and having ascertained that a client is unable to perform this action, the practitioner may infer from this range of motion restriction that the client is dependent in hair combing. Hair combing is not "tested," only the range of motion needed to comb hair. Research has shown that this protocol is most discrepant from the PTE protocol and often leads to inaccurate inferences about occupational performance (Rogers et al., 2003).

Regardless of the specific conceptualization or theory of occupational performance, data collection is systematic, that is, it is guided by that conceptualization or theory and follows a logical sequence. Just as the primary care physician methodically reviews body systems during the annual physical, so too the occupational therapy practitioner systematically evaluates the PTE transaction and its components. The advantage of collecting data systematically was demonstrated by Edwards and colleagues (2006) in a study of post-stroke patients. Two methods were used to identify cognitive and sensory impairments in 53 patients hospitalized for acute stroke. The first method applied a research protocol that followed the Clinical Practice Guidelines for Post-Stroke Rehabilitation recommended by the Agency for Healthcare Research and Quality, while the second method obtained data from a review of the patient's medical chart. The first method, that is, the research protocol, identified significantly more impairments than the chart review regarding memory, visuospatial neglect, and depression. These results suggest that without structured evaluation procedures numerous impairments may not be identified, and therefore may go untreated.

Methods of PTE Evaluation: How Should Data Be Gathered?

There are three primary methods for practitioners to obtain data about clients' occupational performance:

1. Asking questions about performance using structured or open-ended interviews or questionnaires.
2. Observing performance, in a laboratory (i.e., clinical) or natural (i.e., home, school, workplace) context, using structured or unstructured assessments.
3. Testing performance, using norm-referenced or criterion-referenced assessments.

Practitioners may also obtain data from medical records or case conferences, however, data obtained from these sources were initially collected through questioning, observing, or testing.

Each data-gathering method has advantages and disadvantages. The questioning method is more subjective than observing or testing, and this subjectivity may reduce reliability. Questioning is also less expensive and labor intensive. Interviews and questionnaires can be administered by less costly personnel than observational instruments and tests, because they require less skilled judgment.

Moreover, clients are not placed at physical risk for injury when they talk about their occupational performance, as they may be when they actually perform tasks. Hence, performance observation requires skilled personnel to manage risk during evaluation.

Through observation and testing, practitioners objectively rate task performance. Questioning yields subjective ratings of task performance. When observation is structured, reliability is improved because task items must be operationalized to be performed. Thus, the ambiguity associated with questioning (e.g., Can you perform heavy housework?) is removed (i.e., heavy housework is operationalized as using an upright vacuum cleaner to vacuum a room). Increased reliability, in turn, facilitates detecting changes in performance, which is an essential psychometric property for evaluating the effectiveness of an intervention (Guralnik, Branch, Cummings, & Curb, 1989). Structured observation and testing are similar in their standardization, but testing allows practitioners to compare their clients' performance outcomes to that of peer reference groups (norm-referenced testing) or performance standards (criterion-referenced testing). Practitioners may use a norm-referenced test, for example, when they want to know how a child's social skills compare to those of children the same age or if an older adult is able to react as quickly as a younger person. In contrast, they may use a criterion-referenced test to ascertain if an adolescent can perform all essential functions of a short-order cook or an older adult, who is legally blind, can perform the tasks required to live independently and safely in the community. The disadvantages of observation and testing over questioning are that they are more costly in terms of personnel skill and time, as well as space, and equipment (Rogers et al., 2003).

Although no data-gathering method is intrinsically superior, one method may be preferred over others for some evaluative purposes. For example, questioning is preferred for evaluating how often a task is performed, or performance habits, because observing or testing habits would require repeated evaluation over time and would be extremely costly. Similarly, questioning is the method of choice for evaluating occupational role, that is, the unique configuration of tasks that comprise various roles (personal care, worker, parent, etc.) for a client, because "role" is an abstract construct that needs to be operationalized to be observed. Conversely, observation or testing is preferred for evaluating the reason(s) for a performance discrepancy because clients may not be aware of why they are having a performance problem or these methods may be needed to provide precise measurement (e.g., degrees of range of motion restriction).

The selection of a data-gathering method, or combination of methods, is largely determined by the overall purpose for conducting the evaluation in conjunction with practicalities, such as the time allowed for the evaluation and the equipment available. Some instruments, the Handicap Assessment and Resource Tool (HART) (Vertesi, Darzins, Lowe, McEvoy, & Edwards, 2000) being an example, permit collecting data from several sources. Practitioners need to be aware, however, that different data-gathering methods do not necessarily yield the same findings in regard to the same task. Clients may perceive themselves as independent in bathing, while practitioners may rate their performance as partially dependent because of their need for physical support while entering and exiting the bathtub (Rogers & Holm, 2000; Rogers et al., 2003; Sager et al., 1992).

PTE Content: What Occupational Areas Should Be Evaluated?

When planning an evaluation, decisions must be made about the areas of occupations and the specific tasks to be evaluated as well as the parameters of tasks to be evaluated. What tasks are of concern to the client? Dressing? Computer use? Getting to work? The occupational therapy process should revolve around tasks that have meaning to clients. Decisions about the tasks to evaluate are based on the client's values. Clients' problems may occur in one or several areas of occupation—activities of daily living (ADL), instrumental activities of daily living (IADL), education, work, play, leisure, or social participation. Each of these seven occupational areas contains an array of individual tasks (AOTA, 2002). Education, for example, consists of formal educational participation, exploration of informal personal educational needs or interests, and informal personal education participation and, in turn, each of these activities consists of individual tasks. Early in the occupational therapy process the tasks that clients need to perform or want to perform or are problematic to perform or are becoming problematic to perform are identified. Typically, priorities and problems are initially identified through structured or unstructured interviews or questionnaires administered to clients or their advocates, if clients are not able to respond on their own behalf. Assessments such as the Role Checklist (Oakley, Kielhofner, Barris, & Reichler, 1986) and the Canadian Occupational Performance Measure (COPM) (Law et al., 2005) are examples of tools that serve this purpose.

Value reflects the relative importance that various occupational areas and tasks have for clients. When energy is limited, humans typically establish priorities for how they want to use their energy. Hence, clients may choose to have a spouse dress them, rather than dress themselves, so that they can save the energy that they would expend dressing to go to a theater or restaurant. Because motivation for occupational engagement is influenced by personal values, ascertaining the relative value that various occupational areas and tasks have for clients is useful for establishing intervention priorities.

Individual tasks are sequenced together to form personalized daily living routines and habits as well as socially defined roles. One person's daily living routine, for example, moves from arising from sleep in the morning, showering, dressing and simultaneously eating cold cereal and reading the newspaper, while another person's routine calls for arising, cooking and eating breakfast and then dressing, leaving bathing for the evening. These daily living routines are incorporated into the "personal care role" which requires adults to perform the occupations necessary to fill their need for food, clothing, and shelter. The personal care role, in turn, supports other roles such as those of student, worker, homemaker, and spouse. Appraising the extent to which problems in valued tasks disrupt the performance of routines, habits, and roles places these problems in the context of normal living, and thus provides an essential facet of the client's emerging occupational profile.

PTE Parameters: What Do We Want to Know about Occupational Performance?

In addition to ascertaining the occupational areas and specific tasks to be evaluated, practitioners need to decide what they want to know about occupational performance. Key questions about occupational performance to be answered through the evaluation are: Can clients perform the task by themselves? Can they perform it safely and can they do it adequately? What explains or accounts for the performance discrepancy? Each question requires practitioners to use a different measurement parameter or yardstick (see Box 46.1).

Independence

The most common parameter used to measure occupational performance is the level of **independence** clients exhibit when performing a task. Ratings of independent or able mean that clients can perform a task, without assistance from another person, although they may use assistive technology. Conversely, dependent or unable implies that help from another person is required. When performance is not totally dependent, it may be rated using the percentage of the task completed independently (e.g., 75%, 50%, 25%) or the quantity of help needed (e.g., no, minimal, moderate, maximal).

When assistance is required to complete a task, the type of assistance may also be added to the rating scale. Three general types of assistance are recognized and are rank ordered from least to most assistive as: assistive technology, nonphysical assistance, and physical assistance (see Box 46.1). Assistive technology qualifies as the least assistive type of assistance when it enables task performance to be adaptive but independent. The performance of clients feeding themselves using utensils with enlarged or elongated handles fits this definition.

A client who requires nonphysical assistance is considered to be less dependent than one who needs physical, hands-on help. Nonphysical assistance takes into account multiple techniques, including task setup, supervision,

BOX 46.1

PTE EVALUATION PARAMETERS

INDEPENDENCE

Independent _____ Dependent
Able _____ Unable
100% Independent _____ 0% Independent
No assistance _____ Maximal assistance
☐ from 1 person
☐ from 2 persons

Type of Assistance

☐ No assistance

☐ Assistive technology
1. _____
2. _____
3. _____
4. _____

Non-physical
☐ Setup
☐ Supervision
☐ Standby assist
☐ Verbal cues
☐ Nonverbal cues

Physical
☐ Physical guidance
☐ Physical assistance

Self-efficacy for Independence

I believe I can _____ I believe I cannot

SAFETY

Safe _____ Unsafe
No risk   At risk
☐   Person risk   ☐
☐   Environmental risk   ☐

ADEQUACY OF OUTCOMES

Efficiency of Action

No difficulty _____ Severe difficulty
Without difficulty _____ Unable to do
No pain _____ Severe pain
Pain does not interfere   Pain prevents
with performance _____ performance
Fatigue does not interfere   Fatigue prevents
with performance _____ performance
Within normal limits for time _____ Exceeds normal limits for time

Acceptability of Outcomes

Within norms _____ Non-normative
Meets standards _____ Does not meet standards
Satisfied _____ Not satisfied
100% Satisfied _____ 0% Satisfied
Absence of aberrant   Presence of aberrant
activity behaviors _____ activity behaviors

EXPLANATORY FACTORS RELATED TO PERFORMANCE DISCREPANCIES

Yes ☐   Person factors   ☐ No
Yes ☐   Task factors   ☐ No
Yes ☐   Environmental factors   ☐ No
Yes ☐   Task Experience   ☐ No
Yes ☐   Resources   ☐ No

standby assistance, and verbal and nonverbal cues to give encouragement or instruction. Examples of task setup are opening milk cartons and arranging clothing on a chair in the sequence in which items are to be donned. Supervision means that the caregiver may not be consistently present, but is available to monitor task performance and to intervene if problems arise. Standby assistance requires the caregiver to be physically present and near the client at all times. A caregiver who checks to see if the fried eggs are sufficiently cooked is an example of supervision; one who walks alongside a client who is climbing stairs is an example of standby assistance. Verbal cuing means using spoken or written words to motivate or instruct clients about task performance. Putting a sign saying "toilet" on a bathroom door to aid the wayfinding of a client with dementia is an example of a verbal cue. In nonverbal cuing, communication is accomplished through demonstration or gestures.

Physical assistance involves physically guiding clients to do a task or part of a task and doing the task for them. With physical guidance, clients are expected to participate actively in the task, whereas with physical assistance, clients are expected to cooperate with caregiving. Positioning a client's hands on a walker illustrates physical guidance, while lifting a client from a chair illustrates physical assistance.

The Functional Independence Measure (FIM) (UDSMR, 1997) and the Inpatient Rehabilitation Facility Patient Assessment Instrument (IRF-PAI) (www.resdac.umn.edu/IRF-PAI; accessed August 13, 2007) are examples of measures using independence as the measurement parameter.

Perceived self-efficacy, or clients' beliefs about their ability to perform tasks independently, is another facet of task independence. If the distance between the bed and the wheelchair looks like the Grand Canyon to clients and they believe that they do not have the ability to perform the transfer, it is unlikely that they will perform the transfer. Self-perceptions of performance ability influence performance as significantly as actual abilities (Gage, Noh, Polatajko, & Kaspar, 1994). Perceived self-efficacy is specific to individual tasks. Thus, clients do not perceive themselves as able or unable but rather as being able to do some tasks but not others. The Perceived Self-Efficacy Scale for People with Arthritis (Lorig, Chastain, Ung, Shoor, & Holman, 1989) and the Self-Efficacy Gauge (Gage, Noh, Polatajko, & Kaspar, 1994) are examples of self-efficacy measures.

Safety

Safety is the risk incurred by clients or to the environment when clients perform tasks. Safety is not a quality of the environment per se, but rather is a characteristic of the person-task-environment transaction. Although a bathtub safety rail is a safety feature, its presence in the bathroom will not improve clients' safety unless it is actually used, and used correctly, when bathtub transfers are executed.

However, unsafe features of a home may indicate unsafe task performance or increased risk. A can of bacon grease on the stove or an electrical cord traversing a sink suggests that the client, or someone else in the home, has unsafe daily living habits.

Commonly, risk connotes physical risk as occurs when there is concern that clients may cut themselves while preparing food or may sustain a fracture if they trip over an uneven carpet. Safety risks may also involve poor judgment, for example, forgetting to extinguish a burning candle, taking too much or too little prescribed medication, or flashing $50 bills around the bus station. Safety is rated by the absence, presence, or extent of risk.

Although safety has always been recognized as a critical evaluation parameter in occupational therapy, it has usually been rated as a part of task independence. However, humans can perform independently but unsafely and instruments such as the Performance Assessment of Self-Care Skills (PASS) (Rogers & Holm, 1994b) and the Safety Assessment of Function and the Environment for Rehabilitation—Health Outcome Measurement and Evaluation (SAFER-HOME) (Letts & Marshall, 1995) account for this in their scoring. When working with clients, it is often difficult to know where the line between safe and unsafe performance should be drawn and to determine when task performance is sufficiently unsafe that independence should be restricted. As occupational therapy moves more into clients' homes; interfaces more with the legal system for the purposes of guardianship, conservatorship, and involuntary commitment; and, becomes more oriented toward prevention and health promotion, safety will increasingly shift to the forefront of evaluation technology.

Adequacy

Adequacy refers to the *efficiency* of performing tasks as well as the *acceptability* of the outcome of performance. For example, when dressing, movement may be fluid or uneven (efficiency) and when dressing is completed, the person may look neat or disheveled (acceptability). Similarly, when clients with essential tremor write checks, their hands may shake and their signature may be readable or unreadable.

EFFICIENCY.   Efficiency of task performance implies a minimum of unnecessary effort. Common parameters emphasizing the efficiency of action or process are: difficulty, pain, fatigue and dyspnea, and duration.

DIFFICULTY.   Difficulty is the perceived ease with which a task is accomplished. Rehabilitation theorist Verbrugge (1990) argued that difficulty is the most appropriate way to measure activity limitations because ratings of difficulty come from clients, whereas ratings of the amount of assistance required to complete tasks come from clients' caregivers. Caregiver ratings of assistance may be more reflective of the assistance given than of the assistance that is actually needed. The Functional Status Index (FSI), an activity limitation measure designed for use with adults with arthritis, uses a four-point scale of no, mild, moderate, and severe difficulty (Jette, 1980). The Health Assessment Questionnaire (HAQ), another activity instrument designed for clients with arthritis, also employs a four-point scale. The HAQ scale considers without any difficulty, with some difficulty, with much difficulty, and unable to do (Fries, Spitz, Kraines, & Holman, 1980).

The level of difficulty experienced during task performance is increasingly being viewed as a marker of preclinical disability—that is, as a symptom that indicates that the individual is at risk for decline in function even though the decline is not yet apparent (Fried, Herdman, Kuhn, Rubin, & Turano, 1991). Unless the onset of pathology is sudden, such as that arising from a car accident or stroke, it is likely that clients will find it harder to perform tasks before they are unable to perform them at all. Along similar lines, an increase in perceived difficulty or the spread of difficulty from more difficult (e.g., heavy housework) to easier (e.g., oral hygiene) tasks may signal the progression of occult disability.

PAIN.   Pain is the discomfort or sensation of hurting that is experienced during task performance and may continue after performance has stopped (Jette, 1980). In relation to task performance, the component of pain that is of most concern is the extent to which it interferes with performance. Interference may be ascertained in relation to specific tasks, such as walking or cooking a meal, or may be gauged more globally in reference to clients' overall activity level (McDowell & Newell, 1996). Because of pain, tasks may be modified, done at a slower pace, done less often or less adequately, or eliminated from one's daily routine. In addition to interference with tasks, it may be useful to note the presence or absence of pain, the location and distribution of pain, the intensity of pain (none, mild, moderate, severe), and/or the character of the pain experienced (shooting, burning, dull). The Functional Status Index (Jette, 1980) examines pain in relation to activity performance.

FATIGUE AND DYSPNEA.   Fatigue is the discomfort or sensation of tiredness, weariness, or exhaustion that is experienced during or after task performance (Hart & Freel, 1982; Tack, 1991). When fatigued, clients describe themselves as tired and needing to rest (Freal, Kraft, & Coryell, 1984). Fatigue and dyspnea often occur together. Dyspnea is a sensation of difficult or labored breathing (Gift, 1987). Clients describe their symptoms of dyspnea as feeling short of breathe, not getting enough air, chest tightness, and finding it hard to move air (Janson-Bjerklie, Carrieri, & Hudes, 1986). Fatigue and dyspnea may interfere with the ability to do tasks and may be exacerbated by physical activity. Similar to pain, they may lead to modifications in the manner in which tasks are done, including a slower pace, decreases in participation, and the transfer of responsibility to others. An interesting aspect of fatigue and dyspnea is that they can result from too much (e.g., strenuous housework) as well as too little (e.g., sedentary lifestyle) physical activity (Gift & Pugh, 1993). They may be a component of both physical (e.g., chronic lung disease) and mental (e.g., anxiety) illness. As with pain, the fatigue/dyspnea–activity limitation relationship is generally approached by ascertaining the extent of interference with specific tasks and usual activity level. Scales may also record the presence or absence, the amount (none, a lot), and the severity (mild, severe) of the fatigue or dyspnea (McDowell & Newell, 1996). A subscale of the Multidimensional Assessment of Fatigue (MAF) (Tack, 1991) asks respondents to rate the degree to which fatigue has interfered with their ability to engage in routine activities. The Multidimensional Assessment of Fatigue (MAF) (Tack, 1991) and the London Chest Activity of Daily Living Scale (LCADL) (Garrod, Bestall, Paul, Wedzicha, & Jones, 2000) are examples of instrument that rate activity interference secondary to fatigue and shortness of breathe, respectively.

DURATION.   The duration of task performance—that is, the time needed to complete a task—is often used as a measure of efficiency. Less time is interpreted as increased efficiency. In essence, time gives a measure of the speed of performance. Some functional assessment instruments include a time criterion in the definition of independence. The Functional Independence Measure™ specifies, for example, that activities must be completed in "reasonable time" (UDSMR, 1997). Practitioners often comment on tasks being completed "within normal limits." It is interesting that neither the average length of time adults take nor the minimum time they need to perform various daily living tasks has been calculated.

Although time to task completion provides a ratio scale for measuring task performance, it is cumbersome data to collect in the therapeutic situation, because it requires the use of a stopwatch and the designation of precise beginning and ending points for each task. Furthermore, the time needed to complete tasks depends on the reason for engaging in the task. Dressing to do housecleaning is likely to take less time than dressing to go out to work. Time is also a poor marker of efficiency for clients who are impulsive or manic, because they may rush through tasks with little consideration for safety or adequacy. Although such individuals may prepare a meal in record time, for example, the food may be unappetizing and the kitchen cluttered with pots and cooking utensils when they are finished.

ACCEPTABILITY.   Regardless of the efficiency with which a task is performed, the acceptability of the outcome of that performance is a critical criterion of occupational performance. To evaluate acceptability, however, a performance standard is required. Measurement parameters emphasizing the acceptability of the outcome or product of the action are: societal standards, satisfaction, experience, aberrant activity.

SOCIETAL STANDARDS.   One approach to evaluating the acceptability of task outcomes or products is to evaluate those results against the normative expectations of society. The degree of difference or deviation from the 'normal' is the performance standard. For example, humans are expected to maintain personal cleanliness and not to overdraw their checking accounts. Although there may be a wide, rather than a narrow, line between what is acceptable and unacceptable, task performance that consistently goes outside the line will be labeled unacceptable, inappropriate, or inadequate according to societal standards. In applying normative standards, practitioners must be careful to make allowance for cultural diversity as this is expressed in occupational performance (Purnell & Paulanka, 2005).

SATISFACTION.   A second parameter of acceptability of task outcomes or products is satisfaction. Satisfaction refers to the experience of pleasure and contentment with one's performance (Yerxa, Burnett-Beaulieu, Stocking, & Azen, 1988; Pincus, Summey, Soraci, Wallston, & Hummon, 1983). As a parameter of performance, it is likely that satisfaction interacts with an individual's willingness to engage in a task or embrace a role. If clients fail to derive satisfaction from their performance, they may restrict their participation. In relating satisfaction to performance, a dichotomous scale may be used consisting of satisfied or dissatisfied. Alternatively, satisfaction may be rated according to the proportion of time that clients experienced satisfaction (e.g., 100%, 75%, and so on) as is done on the Satisfaction with Performance Scaled Questionnaire (SPSQ) (Yerxa et al., 1988) or on a Likert-type scale (e.g., not at all satisfied to extremely satisfied) as is done on the Canadian Occupational Performance Measure (COPM) (Law et al., 2005). Caregivers of clients may also be asked to rate the extent to which they are satisfied with the care recipient's task performance. This procedure has the potential for providing practitioners with information about the normative expectations for task performance within a social unit (e.g., family, cultural group), as previously discussed under societal standards.

ABERRANT TASK BEHAVIORS.   The task analyses used on measures are based on the way in which tasks are normally performed—that is, the way in which they are usually performed by individuals without disabilities. However, individuals with cognitive impairments, such as those associated with dementia, traumatic brain injury, schizophrenia, and mental retardation, may exhibit behaviors that are aberrant or abnormal. For example, they may pocket food in their cheeks or spit food out. Clothing items may be put on the wrong body parts. In contrast to the subtasks derived from task analyses, which are to be encouraged during intervention, aberrant behaviors are to be extinguished or reduced in frequency. These behaviors are not well represented on available instruments measuring activities of daily living, with the exception of the Routine Task Inventory, an instrument specifically devised for use with a psychiatric population (Allen, 1985).

PTE Explanatory Factors for Performance Discrepancies

When performance is problematic, whether performance is dependent, unsafe, inefficient or unacceptable, practitioners seek to identify factors that contribute to the loss of performance ability. In other words, they seek to explain what accounts for the performance discrepancy. Salient explanations for a performance discrepancy are: a deficit in one or more of the components of the PTE transaction and a lack of experience.

PTE Deficit

Breakdown of the PTE transaction may account for a performance discrepancy. When performing any task, clients must have the affective capacity to motivate them to perform the task; the cognitive capability to plan, execute, monitor, and terminate the task; the motoric capacity to perform the task; a task consonant with their competence level, and, lastly, an environment that supports performance. If any of the required affective, cognitive, motoric, task, or environmental factors is lacking or deficient, task performance will be dysfunctional. Ascertaining the most likely explanation for a performance discrepancy provides critical information for planning interventions. If the hypothesized explanation for a dressing dysfunction is a deficit in active range of motion (e.g., stiff joints), the intervention will be different than if the explanation is apraxia (e.g., problems in executing planned movement), apathy (e.g., lack of responsiveness or initiative), a task that is too complex (e.g., buying stocks and bonds for someone with dementia), or, environmental (e.g., a closet that is not wheelchair accessible). Similarly, the appropriate intervention for a skill deficit would be different from that for a habit deficit. A skill deficit would be approached by practicing the skill under supervised conditions to prompt improvement. However, if clients possess the needed skill but fail to use it routinely—that is have a habit deficit—a motivational intervention plan, to increase the frequency of using the skill, would be in order.

When a performance discrepancy is identified, practitioners may reason that it can be explained by one or more of the transactional components—person, task, and/or environment. Hence, they may undertake a more thorough or detailed evaluation of one or more of these factors *in isolation* to shed insight on the performance discrepancy.

PERSON CAPACITIES. In reference to the person, affective, cognitive, and motoric capacities are measured with capacity-specific assessments. For affective function, a depression assessment might be used; for cognitive capacity, a mental status examination; and for motoric capacity, an active range of motion measure. Measurement parameters previously discussed, such as pain or discomfort, fatigue, and dyspnea, may also explain dependent, unsafe and inadequate behavior. Data from capacity assessments typically indicate the extent of deviation from a standard. For example, a client may obtain a score of 6 of 30 on the Mini-Mental State Examination (Folstein, Folstein, & McHugh, 1975). On this test, 24 or above is interpreted as within normal limits. The client's score of 6 deviates 18 points from 24 (normalcy), and is indicative of severe cognitive impairment.

TASK DEMANDS. To enhance understanding of task demands, a detailed analysis is done of task requirements. For example, the action of entering and exiting a bathtub might be expanded to 5 steps: enter tub; lower self to a seated position on tub bottom; sit on tub bottom; raise self from tub bottom; and exit tub. Measurement of task demands would account for the number of steps clients could complete independently, safely, and adequately. By observing clients perform each step, practitioners learn the point of task breakdown, which is one explanation of a performance discrepancy. Assessments based on task analysis include the Performance Assessment of Self-Care Skills (PASS) (Rogers & Holm, 1994b) and the Klein-Bell Activities of Daily Living Scale (Klein & Bell, 1982).

PHYSICAL ENVIRONMENT. Recent attention to the environment as an explanatory factor for performance discrepancies is slowly filtering into assessment technologies. The physical environment figures most prominently, with assessment focused on functionality and safety demands. However, facilitating function and safety is interpreted differently for different impairment groups. Curb cuts, for example, assist those in wheelchairs, but pose a hazard for those who are blind or have low vision. Thus, environmental assessments tend to be impairment group specific. They center on accommodations in space and equipment for people in wheelchairs; the use of textures and sound to promote wayfinding for those with visual impairment; the absence of tripping hazards, for those who fall; and, the presence of barriers to prevent access to spaces and objects that may be used in a harmful way (e.g., put excess salt on a tomato), for those who are cognitively impaired. Historically, environmental assessments have been of the "garden variety," with each occupational therapy setting devising its own assessments. "Scoring" has been qualitative with the recording of factors that facilitate and hinder function. These setting specific instruments became more standardized and universal over time. The Checklist for Readily Achievable Barrier Removal (http://

www.usdoj.gov/crt/ada/checkweb.htm; accessed August 13, 2007) and Safety for Older Consumers Home Safety Checklist (http://www.cpsc.gov/CPSCPUB/PREREL/prhtml87/87026.html; accessed August 13, 2007) are illustrative of this trend. More recently, rather than assessing environments in isolation from the person and using descriptive recording, newer instruments favor assessing the person-in-environments, using numerical recording, and establishing the psychometric properties of instruments. The Functioning Everyday with a Wheelchair (FEW; previously titled Functional Evaluation in a Wheelchair) is an example of a person-task-environment instrument (Mills et al., 2002).

SOCIAL ENVIRONMENT. People and their perspectives expressed in the attitudes that they express and the policies and procedures that they formulate can cause performance discrepancies as readily as the physical barriers that they construct! For instance, if nursing home regulations specify that residents cannot bathe themselves, residents become dependent in bathing. Historically, assessment of social environments has been limited to recording who (people) and what (services) are available to clients. Clients' resources must be taken into account in addition to their capacities and skills when determining the severity of performance discrepancies. Consider, for example, Ms. Cross and Ms. Lum, who are unable to use the range and oven safely to prepare hot food. Ms. Cross has a niece who lives on the same city block as she does and is willing to assist her in preparing hot meals. Ms. Lum lives in a rural community, which does not have a Meals-on-Wheels program, and her neighbors are elderly themselves and unable to assist her. Although the meal preparation skills of both of these clients are the same, Ms. Lum is at greater risk for adverse outcomes than Ms. Cross because she has less supportive living resources available to her. Thus, the evaluation of occupational performance becomes meaningful only when deficits are linked to resources and this linkage is particularly important when evaluation is a part of discharge planning. The Assessment of Living Skills and Resources (ALSAR) links person capacities with environmental resources—resources that are available and those that are needed (Williams et al., 1991).

Experience

One reason that clients may not be able to perform a task is because they never learned how to do it at all or how to do it adequately. Experience is the direct participation in a task that a person has accumulated. Experience provides the opportunity for practice and for perfecting performance and outcomes. All humans generally learn functional mobility and personal care tasks during childhood and adolescence. As tasks basic to and essential for daily living, they are practiced regularly over adulthood. Possible exceptions to this norm include hair care that is done by beauticians, fingernail care that is done by manicurists, and toenail care that is done by podiatrists. Nonetheless, the societal expectation is that all adults have a wide range of experience with these tasks and perform them adequately. However, a similar expectation does not hold for other types of tasks, for which humans have more options. Some clients may have no experience in preparing meals, doing the laundry, or managing finances. Similarly, work and leisure tasks are very individualized. Clients' task performance history is essential for understanding their current performance level.

In addition to past experience, recent or current experience must also be evaluated. When tasks are not performed regularly, the proficiency needed to do them can fall into disuse or become obsolete with technological advances. Inquiries about recency and frequency of task experience are generally approached by ascertaining clients' skills and habits (Rogers & Holm, 1991). Skill refers to the capability to do a task, whereas habit refers to usual or routine task performance. In their repertoires, all humans have tasks that they usually do not perform but that they could perform if situations arise where they have to do them or want to do them. For example, you may know how to cook but prefer to let your spouse cook on a daily basis. However, if your spouse goes away on a business trip, you are able to cook dinner for yourself. When using questioning to evaluate task skills and habits, inquiries about task skills are generally phrased as, "Can you [name the task]?," while those referring to habits use "Do you [name the task]?"

OCCUPATIONAL THERAPY PROCESS: PROBLEM DEFINITION

Data about clients, their task priorities, and environments obtained through evaluation are synthesized. In addition to a profile of clients' abilities and disabilities, the synthesis yields a **problem definition** or several definitions—the occupational diagnosis (Rogers & Holm, 1989; Rogers, 2004). The problem statement has four distinct

but related parts. Each part will be illustrated through Mr. Martin, an older client with Alzheimer's type dementia (see Table 46.2).

The first part of the problem statement is a descriptive phrase that identifies the problematic task and the measurement parameter defining the problem. In Table 46.2, for example, "unable to get out of the bathtub" is the problematic task and independence is the measurement parameter that defines the problem. In this case task independence was measured in terms of caregiver assistance. As depicted in Box 46.1, there are options in the ways in which performance independence, safety, and adequacy can be measured. However, practitioners typically evaluate these parameters regardless of the specific tasks evaluated. These performance characteristics are essential to competent occupational performance. Performance that is not independent indicates a need for assistance from technology or humans. Performance that is independent but unsafe places clients at risk. Performance that is independent but inadequate restricts clients' role performance and may also place them at risk. As is also apparent from Box 46.1, there is more variability in the measurement parameters for task adequacy than there is for independence and safety. For each client, practitioners select the adequacy parameters that are most applicable for the client's condition or task environment. The extent to which pain interferes with performance, for instance, would be appropriate to rate in clients with fibromyalgia or rheumatoid arthritis, but would likely not be appropriate for those with Parkinson's disease or bipolar disorder (decision based on condition). Similarly, inadequate hygiene may be admissible at home but may be offensive in the classroom or workplace (decision based on task environment).

The second part of the problem statement is the explanatory phrase, which indicates the practitioner's explanation for the identified problem. The explanatory phrase is followed by the cue phrase which records the data, obtained through observing, questioning, or testing, that the practitioner used to identify the problem. For Mr. Martin, the practitioner hypothesized that the bathtub transfer problem was related to apraxia, which was exhibited in several observable cues: ineffective positioning for

TABLE 46.2.   STRUCTURE OF THE PROBLEM STATEMENT

Descriptive Phrase	Explanatory Phrase	Cue Phrase	Pathologic Phrase
Unable to get out of the bathtub (problematic tasks) without physical assistance (parameter of concern)	*Related to* apraxia	*As evidenced by* client placing himself in positions that prevent desired motion; required instructional cues for task completion; does not integrate upper and lower extremity motions for task accomplishment	*Due to* Alzheimer's dementia

action, incoordination of upper and lower extremities, and the need for instruction. The selection of the explanatory factor or factors to evaluate emanates from the practitioner's hypothesis about the reason for the performance problem, and this in turn, is guided by the theory the practitioner has applied to the occupational therapy process.

The last part of the problem statement identifies the medical condition or health problem, that is the secondary or remote explanation for the performance problem. Although Mr. Martin's need for assistance in transferring can be explained by dementia, apraxia is given as the primary reason and dementia as the secondary reason. Occupational therapy practitioners treat the consequences of disease (apraxia), while physicians treat the disease (dementia).

Hence, apraxia is the primary explanation for the problem that is the object of occupational therapy interventions. Nonetheless, recognizing that the apraxia is secondary to Alzheimer's dementia—a progressive, degenerative disease—informs the practitioner of the likely etiology of apraxia and limits the theoretic options available for occupational therapy interventions (e.g. a curative approach would be inappropriate).

Defining a performance discrepancy involves more than merely 'finding' a problem. A well formulated problem statement clarifies the performance problem as well as provides information useful for guiding problem solution, that is, intervention. As we have seen, problem definition embodies two levels of evaluation: evaluation of the performance problem and of the etiology of the performance problem. Problem definition stands at the interface between evaluation and intervention.

OT PROCESS: INTERVENTION PLANNING AND IMPLEMENTATION

Once an occupational performance problem has been defined, practitioners search for a solution to the problem, decide on a plan, and implement the plan. Evaluative data are blended with occupational therapy knowledge to create a future profile of the client—a profile that will be achieved through occupational therapy intervention(s).

Performance discrepancies occur because of a misfit between a client's performance capacities, the task demands, and the environmental demands. To achieve a better or optimal person-task-environment fit, person capacities may be changed, task demands may be modified, or environmental demands may be modified. Several types of outcomes may emerge from occupational therapy interventions (Rogers & Holm, 1994a).

1. One possible outcome is the *development* of a capacity, task skill, or habit that did not previously exist. Development is typically the therapeutic goal for infants and young children who are not developing normally, but it is also appropriate for adults who need to or want to learn new skills or healthy lifestyle habits. For example, the development of crawling might be appropriate for a developmentally delayed, non-ambulatory child. Similarly, a widower, who never learned to cook, may need to develop cooking skills following the death of his wife. An adolescent, who uses a wheelchair for mobility and is obese, may wish to develop healthier leisure time habits to promote weight control.

2. Another possible outcome is the *restoration* of occupational performance. Restoration interventions are directed at person capacities that were lost or became impaired as a result of a health condition. They may be curative or compensatory. Constraint induced movement therapy for clients with stroke is a curative intervention intended to cure paralysis of the upper extremity so that the extremity returns to its pre-morbid, non-paralyzed state and functions normally again (Taub et al., 1993). In the same clients, use of the non-paralyzed upper extremity to perform actions and skills previously done with the paralyzed upper extremity, is an example of a compensatory intervention.

3. A third possible outcome is the *stabilization* of occupational performance. When the overall course of a medical condition is downward, for example with Alzheimer disease or multiple sclerosis, intervention to stabilize or maintain a function for as long as possible is appropriate. By delaying the onset or slowing the rate of functional decline, clients continue a higher level of functioning for a longer time.

4. A fourth possible outcome is *prevention*. To prevent a performance problem from occurring, practitioners must predict the occurrence of a negative event from the present situation. We know, for example, that in clients with C5-C6 spinal cord injury, pressure ulcers will likely develop on the ischial tuberosities unless pressure on the buttocks is relieved. To prevent the occurrence of pressure ulcers, risk reduction interventions would be instituted. These might include a Roho™ seat cushion, and training clients to perform periodic pressure relief push ups to relieve pressure on the tissue over the ischial tuberosities.

5. Lastly, the therapeutic outcome may be *palliation*. When clients' health status is progressively deteriorating, interventions directed toward support and comfort are appropriate. Occupational therapy practitioners working in hospice or end-of-life-care, for example, may assist caregivers to manage effectively clients' personal care. Using ergonomically correct postures for feeding care recipients or procedures for transfers might be critical skills for caregivers to master.

In addition to stipulating the desired outcomes of intervention, practitioners make a functional prognosis, that is, a judgment of the chances that the desired outcome will be achieved. In the case of clients with spinal cord injury, for example, the prognosis for preventing pressure ulcers depends on clients' willingness to perform periodic push-ups during each hour of sitting. Clients who develop this habit would have a good prognosis, while those who do not would have a poor prognosis.

Simultaneous with deciding the specific kind of intervention(s) to administer, practitioners also need to make decisions about the duration (e.g., how long will occupational therapy be needed?), frequency (e.g., How often does intervention need to occur?), and intensity (e.g., How long will each occupational therapy session be?). Should the intervention be administered for 1 hour, 3 times per week for 4 weeks? Or, is it preferable to administer it for ½ hour, 5 times per week for 2 weeks? In inpatient settings, these decisions may be established through clinical guidelines, whereas in other settings practitioners may need to exercise more judgment. In either case, decisions should be based on scientific evidence about the best schedule for eliciting change in occupational performance.

These decisions involve prognostic judgment. In other words, taking into account the client's medical diagnosis (or other health condition) as it is manifested in 'this' client, in concert with occupational therapy knowledge of the likely functional course of the condition, practitioners foretell (prognosticate) clients' future occupational profile with the proposed course of occupational therapy. As occupational therapy science accumulates, more knowledge will become available to practitioners to aid in making these decisions.

Case Scenarios for Intervention

In the following discussion, intervention strategies directed toward person capacities, task demands or environmental demands are defined and then illustrated with case scenarios involving skill and habit deficits. Although we present each intervention strategy separately, they are typically used in combination. Thus, for a client who has had a stroke, a practitioner may simultaneously or sequentially apply a person-oriented strategy (e.g., restore an extremity affected by stroke), a task-oriented strategy (e.g., provide an enlarged handled spoon to enhance grip) and an environmentally-oriented strategy [install ramps for a wheelchair (e.g., physical environment); educate the spouse (social environment)].

Change Person Capacities

When implementing the develop or restore intervention strategy, occupational therapy practitioners focus on the person component of the PTE transaction with the goal of establishing, (initially developing), or restoring (returning to its former state) a specific capacity or several capacities (Dunn et al., 1994). Following the establishment or restoration of capacities, it is assumed that performance discrepancies in tasks that require these capacities will be resolved and performance will be normalized. The four

case scenarios for skill deficits illustrate *developing* coordination and strength through functional activities (Chelsea) and coping skills through training in daily problem-solving (Mrs. Vocelli) and *restoring* upper extremity function through functional activities (Merilee) and hearing through adaptive technology (Reverend Tengesdal). Two cases highlight habit *development* and employ a cognitive prosthesis (checklist) as a reminding aid (Mrs. Vocelli) and splinting and exercise routines to alleviate the symptoms of sensory impairment in the hands (Cara).

CASE EXAMPLES: DEVELOP/RESTORE PERSON SKILL FOR PERFORMANCE IN ANY ENVIRONMENT

- Chelsea is a 5-year-old female with cerebral palsy and upper limb spasticity. Prior to beginning kindergarten, her physician suggested Botulinum Toxin A injections in the biceps, pronator teres, flexor carpi radialis, flexor carpi ulnaris, and thenar muscles. In addition, she was referred to occupational therapy to improve upper extremity function in preparation for handwriting and other fine motor skills associated with school (Friedman, Diamond, Johnston, & Daffner, 2000). Her occupational therapy program focused on using everyday activities to improve strength and coordination, and to establish a functional hand grasp for handwriting. After 1 month, Chelsea achieved improved range and strength at the wrist, and a functional hand grasp.
- Mrs. Vocelli is a 72-year-old female with osteoarthritis who was widowed one year ago. Although her family believed initially that her apathy and withdrawal from her favorite activities over the past year was due to grief, her primary care physician referred her to a geriatric psychiatrist, who diagnosed her with major depression. In addition to anti-depressant medication, Mrs. Vocelli was referred to outpatient occupational therapy. According to the occupational therapy referral, Mrs. Vocelli was accustomed to having her husband make all decisions and do everyday problem-solving. He also "lifted, carried, pushed and pulled" when Mrs. Vocelli's arthritis was painful. Consequently, Mrs. Vocelli felt ill-equipped for surviving by herself, which in turn contributed to her depressed mood. Mrs. Vocelli joined the functional problem-solving therapy (PST) group run by an occupational therapy practitioner. Each week, group members, including Mrs. Vocelli, brought examples of recent problems that "got them down." At the beginning of each session the occupational therapy practitioner reviewed the seven PST steps, namely, define the problem, choose realistic goals for resolving the problem, generate multiple solutions, implement decision-making guidelines, evaluate and choose preferred solution(s), implement preferred solutions, and evaluate the outcome (Jang, Haley, Small, & Mortimer, 2002; Oxman & Hull, 2001). The group then applied the PST steps to the problems previously vocalized by its members. Solutions were tried out over the following week. With repetition

of the PST process, and assistance from the group, Mrs. Vocelli established problem-solving skills that helped equip her for solving everyday functional problems (Lin et al., 2003).

♦ Merilee is a 46-year-old female who sustained a right hemisphere ischemic stroke 3 months ago. She completed a 2-week rehabilitation program, and is now seen as an outpatient twice a week. Although she has made significant gains, she still has difficulty with right-sided upper extremity forward flexion, wrist extension, and grasp. Merilee's occupational therapy practitioner suggested that Merilee put her plastic glasses into the sink and practice picking them up and placing them on the counter 3 times per day. The practitioner made the suggestion based on the evidence indicating that the use of functional objects for practicing reach and grasp to restore function yields significantly better outcomes than just practicing reach and grasp in isolation (Dromerick, Edwards & Hahn, 2000; Platz et al., 2001; Wu, Trombly, Lin, & Tickle-Degnen, 1998, 2000).

♦ The Reverend Tengesdal is 83 years old and has profound deafness, which is corrected slightly with a hearing aid. He is the visiting pastor of a large church and is having difficulty hearing his wife and some of the frail home-bound parishioners he routinely visits. Recently, he began removing himself from conversations with more than one person because he could no longer hear. His daughter, an occupational therapy practitioner, recommended a Pocket Talker with a magnetic loop to enhance his hearing aids and an attached microphone (Fig. 46.3). The Pocket Talker allows him to hear clearly the voice of his bride of 50 years, as well as those of his parishioners—individually or in groups.

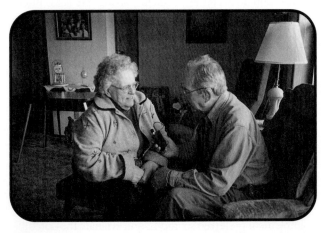

FIGURE 46.3 The Pocket Talker has a magnetic loop that the user wears around the neck to enhance the magnification of the sound in the hearing aid, which allows easier communication with those in the social environment.

CASE EXAMPLES: DEVELOP/RESTORE PERSON HABITS FOR PERFORMANCE IN ANY ENVIRONMENT

♦ Mrs. Vocelli is a 72-year-old female with osteoarthritis who was widowed one year ago. One year after her husband's death, she was diagnosed with major depression, and referred to outpatient occupational therapy. In occupational therapy, she joined a functional problem solving therapy (PST) group to develop skills in everyday problem-solving. As her depression resolved and she began to re-engage in some of her former activities, she developed anxiety attacks. She was prescribed an anti-anxiety medication and again referred to the outpatient problem solving therapy (PST) group. Mrs. Vocelli reported that the more she went out into the community, the more she worried about whether she left the stove or iron on, the water running, or the space heater too near the drapes. After reviewing the seven steps in the PST process, the solution arrived at by the group was for Mrs. Vocelli to make a checklist of the items she needed to check before she went out. She was encouraged to make a habit of going through the checklist before she left her house, dating it, and then putting it in her purse so that she could refer to the list if she became anxious. The group suggested that she also make a habit of making checklists for other activities that made her anxious, for example, taking the bus. The bus checklist could include: bringing the bus schedule, checking to make sure she had her Senior Citizen Pass, asking for a transfer, and telling the bus driver where she wants to get off the bus. Mrs. Vocelli was seen once a month for the next 6 months to maintain the habits that she had begun to put into place. She reported that the checklists worked and her anxiety was under control.

♦ Cara is a 24-year-old doctoral student who was referred to an occupational therapy practitioner with expertise in hand therapy because of numbness and tingling in her hands. She reported that she used a computer for her doctoral work in history as well as in her part-time job as a research assistant. In addition to bilateral neutral wrist splints to be worn at night (Burke, Burke, Stewart, & Cambre, 1994; Sevim et al., 2004), the occupational therapy practitioner emphasized the necessity of developing habits to interrupt static postures, promote motion, and increase blood flow to the wrist and hands. The practitioner taught Cara exercises (stretching and relaxation) for the hand, wrist and shoulders that she needed to implement routinely, provided her with handouts illustrating these exercises, and suggested that Cara make a habit of setting a timer each hour to carry out the exercises. Three months later Cara reported that her "healthy hand habits" were in place. She no longer had numbness or tingling and she continued to wear her splints at night.

Modify Task Demands to Enable or Improve Performance

When modifying a task, practitioners alter the properties of the task to achieve a desired outcome, which may be to facilitate performance that is functional or hinder performance that is dysfunctional. (Dunn et al., 1994). One task modification strategy involves adapting equipment to compensate for impairments, for example, replacing foot controls with hand controls (Keenan). A second strategy involves enhancing task properties to facilitate function, as was accomplished for Mrs. Rogers when lighting was improved to facilitate seeing. A third strategy relies on assistive technology, which ranges from low 'tech' assistive devices (e.g., a raised toilet seat) to high end products (Mr. Ibrahim's bathtub bench; Mr. Jakke's adapted car). When adaptive equipment is not commercially available, practitioners may fabricate it (Matt). Under habits, the case of Ms. Desai illustrates the use of an audiocassette player to replace a disturbing habit (screaming) with a nondisturbing one (listening to music), while that of Gary emphasizes use of the same equipment to develop a habit (sitting upright). Gary's case also exemplifies the value of task breakdown for adapting tasks (use of nails for sorting). Unlike Mrs. Vocelli, who was able to internalize a reminding strategy by using checklists, Mark was unable to do this and hence an automatic reminding system was prescribed.

CASE EXAMPLES: MODIFY TASK DEMANDS FOR SKILL DEFICIT

◆ Keenan is a 3-year-old boy with a closed head injury, seizures, and lower extremity paralysis. His occupational therapy practitioner adapted Bigfoot (a motorized ride-on vehicle) with hand controls, to replace the foot controls. This modification allows him to move around his yard and neighborhood (Fig. 46.4).

◆ Mrs. Rogers is an 83-year-old female with a 5-year history of macular degeneration, resulting in loss of central vision and fluctuating acuity in her peripheral vision. She has always enjoyed sewing items for craft fairs, but she can no longer see to thread the needle on her sewing machine, even when she uses a wire needle threader. She also cannot see the tension and stitch settings on the machine, and therefore leaves them on the same settings, which is not always appropriate for what she wants to sew. Without assistance, she is unable to pursue her hobby. The occupational therapy practitioner suggested a lighted magnifier, which enables Mrs. Rogers to use her sewing machine and continue a meaningful pastime (Fig. 46.5).

◆ Mr. Ibrahim is a 72-year-old male with a 30-year history of rheumatoid arthritis and a 10-year history of type 2 diabetes who has incurred a mild, right cerebral vascular accident. His wife is concerned about how she

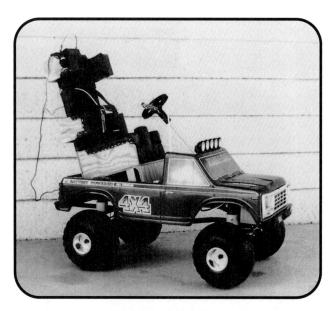

FIGURE 46.4 Adapted motorized vehicles, such as this Bigfoot, enable functional mobility and exploration capacities for children with motor impairments (Vehicles adapted by S. Shores, Good Samaritan Hospital, Puyallup, WA.).

will manage him during bathtub transfers. Mr. Ibrahim likes to soak twice a day in the bathtub to relieve his arthritis pain. The home health occupational therapy practitioner recommended a spring-loaded mechanical bathtub seat that allows Mr. Ibrahim to transfer safely into the bathtub, move down to and up from the bottom of the bathtub, and transfer out of the bathtub, thus preventing falls (Fig. 46.6).

◆ Mr. Jakke is a 48-year-old male with a 10-year history of multiple sclerosis, resulting in bilateral lower extremity weakness and numbness, decreased balance,

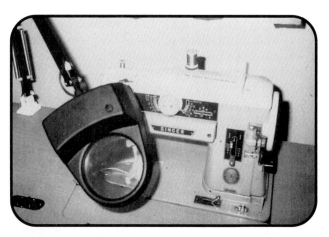

FIGURE 46.5 A lighted magnifier used to adapt a sewing task.

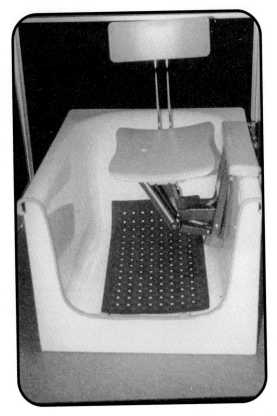

FIGURE 46.6 The mechanical tub seat is spring loaded and raises from the tub bottom with a weight shift and a simultaneous pushing up on the tub edges.

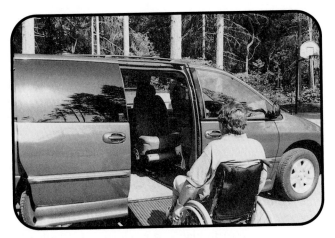

FIGURE 46.7 This adapted van allows the driver to open the door with a remote control and then enter the van via a ramp. The ramp folds into the door when it closes, and the driver transfers into the bucket seat and engages the hand controls.

CASE EXAMPLES: MODIFY TASK DEMANDS FOR HABIT DEFICIT

◆ Ms. Desai is a 26-year-old female who is confined to bed and has an organic brain disorder secondary to a brain tumor. Unable to communicate her wants and needs, she learned to scream to get assistance from the nursing home staff. Eventually, she began to scream all the time when left alone. Because of her screaming, other residents avoided her and the staff placed her in her room with the door shut to reduce the disturbance to others. The occupational therapy practitioner suggested using an audiocassette tape player and headset

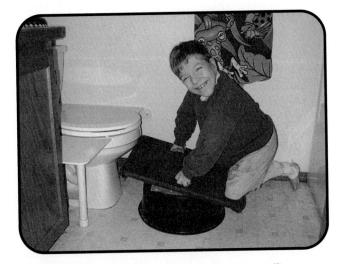

FIGURE 46.8 A custom ramp mounted on a rolling library stool enables access to the toilet as well as the couch, bed, tub, and chairs. (Built by S. Shores, Good Samaritan Hospital, Puyallup, WA.).

and decreased sensation in his hands. Since the last exacerbation of symptoms, Mr. Jakke has been unable to transfer independently into his car, and decided to invest in a car that will suit his needs. The occupational therapy practitioner recommended a van with a remote control and hand controls and referred him to a company that specializes in adapting vehicles. The remote control operates the van door and positions the driver's seat, thus enabling Mr. Jakke to transfer easily in and out of the van (Fig. 46.7). The hand controls provide him with better vehicle control of his lower extremity spasticity. These adaptations enable Mr. Jakke to transport his children to and from school and social activities. He can also take himself to therapy and support groups, while his wife is at work.

◆ Matt is a 7-year-old boy with multiple pterygium syndrome and arthrogryposis. These medical conditions have resulted in severe limitations in all joints and contractures and deformities. He was referred to occupational therapy because his ability to perform transfers is restricted. The occupational therapy practitioner designed a custom ramp (mounted on a rolling library stool) that allows him to access areas that he cannot get up to, such as the couch, bed, tub, dining room chair, or toilet (Fig. 46.8).

and playing tapes of her favorite music to engage her attention (Casby & Holm, 1994). Her family brought in her tape collection, and within 1 week, Ms. Desai's screaming habit was reduced to only one or two cycles a day.

◆ Gary is a 17-year-old male with cerebral palsy (hemiplegia) and moderate mental retardation. As part of his individualized vocational plan, he spends 3 hours each day in a work program. He is assigned to the lawn decorations assembly crew to develop work habits. The special education teacher notified the occupational therapy practitioner that Gary does not maintain a good posture while working and that he has difficulty assembling the pinwheel pieces in the correct order. The occupational therapy practitioner modified the assembly task by breaking it down into several additional steps that Gary can manage. She put nails in a board so that Gary can sort the pinwheel pieces in the basket by color in the correct sequence for assembly, then pick up the pieces from the nail board in correct sequence and assemble them onto a jig for the next student to continue the assembly. In regard to posture, the occupational therapy practitioner observed that once Gary becomes engaged in his tasks, he forgets about his posture. To solve this problem, a tape player with one of Gary's favorite tapes was attached to a switch plate (Fig. 46.9). To trigger the switch plate, Gary has to have most of his hand on the switch. To achieve this position, he must develop the habit of sitting upright instead of listing to the left with his shoulder protracted, elbow flexed, and wrist flexed.

◆ Mark is an 18-year-old male whose diagnosis is undifferentiated schizophrenia. An occupational therapy practitioner has seen him as an outpatient as part of a supported employment program. Mark is being placed in a fast-food restaurant and is assigned to work in the supply room and on the grill. To develop appropriate work habits, Mark is supplied with a NeuroPage System (Hersh & Treadgold, 1994) that is programmed to activate to cue him to: wake up in the morning, gather items needed for work (e.g., lunch), and take his medications as prescribed (e.g., time, name). The target outcome is to decrease Mark's reliance on the paging system.

Modify the Environment to Enable or Improve Performance

The environment can be visualized as a series of increasingly larger concentric circles with clients at the center. The client's immediate environment consists of the people (e.g. immediate family) and physical structures (e.g., private homes or apartments, workstations) surrounding the task. Broader circles encompass extended family members, friends, co-workers, peers, politicians, policies and procedures, cultures, private and public buildings, neighborhoods and communities and so on. Although all levels exert an influence on task performance, this chapter deals with the occupational therapy process as it is applied at the individual level. Hence, discussion of the environment is confined to the immediate environment.

Occupational therapy practitioners implement two basic strategies for modifying environmental demands. The first strategy is to modify the present environment. As demonstrated in the case of Mrs. Hill, the installation of a ladder was a relatively minor home modification but it allowed her to meet her goal of staying at home by herself. In contrast, major modifications were required in Mr. Jakke's blueprints for his new home to accommodate wheeled mobility as well as in his yard for him to continue his leisure activity of gardening. Interventions to promote safe mobility and wayfinding are exemplified in the cases of Ms. Yi-Sun and Mrs. Kochinski, respectively. Modifications targeted at the social environment are key in effective management of Mrs. Prescott's skill deficits secondary to her dementia.

The second environmental strategy practitioners employ is to recommend a different environment. For Mr. Bitner, for example, the practitioner recommended enrollment in adult day care, which provided a limited change of environment. For Andrew, the characteristics of his study space were dramatically altered to create an environment to reduce distraction and facilitate studying.

CASE EXAMPLES: MODIFY ENVIRONMENTAL DEMANDS FOR SKILL DEFICITS

◆ Mrs. Hill is a 63-year-old female with a 20-year history of multiple sclerosis that resulted in bilateral numbness and weakness below the hips, decreased sensation in the hands, and low back pain with prolonged sitting. Because of several recent falls from her wheelchair when transferring, her family members want her to have an attendant while her husband is at work. She adamantly rejects their suggestion. Because Mrs. Hill used a ladder successfully in the physical therapy clinic to get

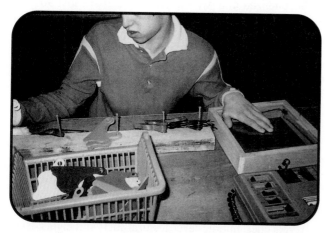

FIGURE 46.9 A switch plate adapted to trigger a tape player when the student's hand is placed firmly on the switch.

back into her chair, the occupational therapy practitioner recommended that a similar ladder be installed in the home. A suitable site for the ladder was located, and when Mrs. Hill slips to the floor during a transfer from bed to wheelchair, she is able to crawl to the ladder, pushing her wheelchair ahead of her, and use the ladder to get back in her chair (Fig. 46.10).

♦ Before Mr. Jakke and his family moved into their new home, several alterations were made to accommodate a wheelchair. Mr. Jakke (a contractor) reviewed the relevant dimensions (Fig. 46.11). and made several alterations to the physical structure. The plumbing was recessed under the bathroom sink to allow Mr. Jakke to roll under the sink without worrying about burning his insensate lower extremities on the pipes, and two drawers were made into one deep drawer so that items could be obtained and stored easily from a seated position (Fig. 46.12). The standard 15-in. high toilet was replaced with an 18-in. high toilet for easier transfers. Oak grab bars were installed next to the toilet and doubled as an assistive device for standing pivot transfers and as a towel rack (Fig. 46.13). In the kitchen, static shelves were replaced with pull-out drawers for easier

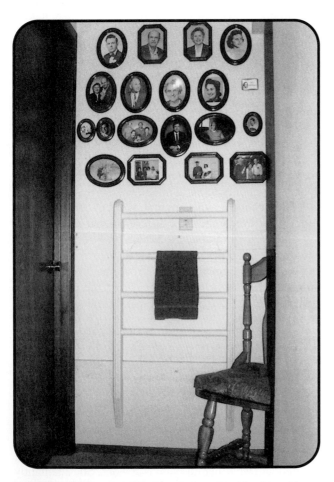

FIGURE 46.10 A wall ladder designed to blend in with the decor of the home environment.

access to items (Fig. 46.14). The microwave oven was positioned by the cutting board to facilitate transferring hot dishes to the table (Fig. 46.15). This setup allows Mr. Jakke, who has weakness and some loss of sensation in his hands, to move a hot dish from the microwave to the counter, reposition it, move it from the counter to the cutting board, reposition it, and then move it from the cutting board to the table. Finally, a counter was built in the laundry room to enable Mr. Jakke to fold laundry while seated in his wheelchair (Fig. 46.16).

♦ Ms. Yi-Sun is the occupational therapy practitioner at Vintage Long Term Care Facility. She is asked by the administration to create an environment that will be safe for residents with dementia to wander and pace when they become anxious (Hall & Buckwalter, 1987). With the assistance of students from the nearby educational program for occupational therapy assistants, she designs stations in a hallway where residents can stop and wind pocket watches, fold towels, sort and stack heavy plastic dishes, watch fish in an eye-level aquarium, and pick up finger foods. Outside, in the fenced-in patio area, they build raised plant boxes that can be tended without bending and place fencing around areas where the ground is uneven or there are tripping hazards that could place residents at risk for falls (Fig. 46.17). All the staff and residents enjoy the patio on nice days, creating a positive environment for everyone.

♦ Mrs. Kochinski is an 86-year-old female with multi-infarct dementia, who currently resides in an assisted living center. Because she is having difficulty locating her room after meals and other activities, the occupational therapy practitioner helped her put some favorite pictures of herself and her husband (circa 1940) on her door and then cued her to find the door with her pictures after each meal and activity session (Fig 46.18). In 3 days, her way-finding skills were established in her new environment.

♦ Mrs. Prescott is 51-years old and has a rapidly progressing dementing illness of unknown origin. She was hospitalized in a psychiatric unit after she lost 30 lb in 2 months, exhibited apraxia during everyday tasks, and became extremely labile. At discharge, she is unable to dress herself, cannot remember how to use silverware, and is incontinent. Her family wants to care for her at home and has hired a live-in attendant. The occupational therapy practitioner met with the family and the attendant to demonstrate a hierarchy of assists that are available to them to maintain the skills Mrs. Prescott retains and provide the necessary support as her capacities decline. The occupational therapy practitioner showed the caregivers a videotape made while Mrs. Prescott prepared a meal during therapy. As they watched the tape, the practitioner identified lower-level verbal cues, middle-level gestural cues, and higher-level physical assists (physical guidance and total assistance) as each was given. Using lower-level assists before

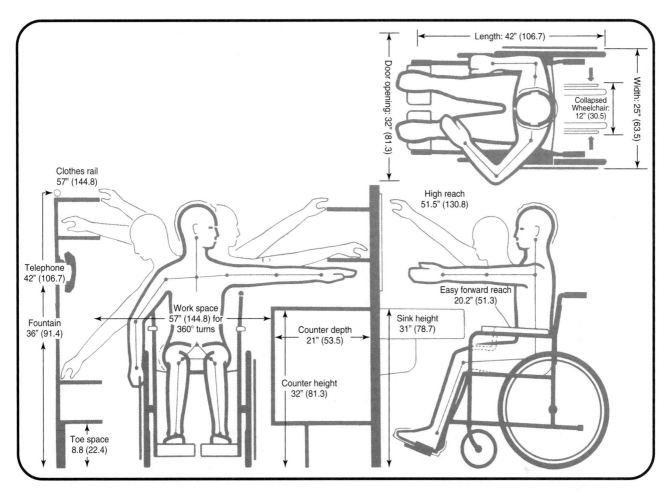

FIGURE 46.11 Basic measurements and proportions can be used when planning home modifications. Measurements are given in inches and centimeters. (Adapted from Diffrient, Tilley, & Bardagly, 1974).

higher-level assists, varying the type of assists from day-to-day as Mrs. Prescott's performance fluctuates, and increasing the use of high-level assists as dementia progresses were discussed with the caregivers. The practitioner gave each caregiver a list of the types of assists that Mrs. Prescott required for personal care tasks, explaining each one and then responding to questions. Although Mrs. Prescott's progressive deterioration cannot be prevented, the appropriate level of assists from the social environment can prevent a faster rate of skill deterioration (Rogers et al., 2000).

CASE EXAMPLES: MODIFY ENVIRONMENTAL DEMANDS FOR HABIT DEFICITS

◆ Mr. Bitner is a 68-year-old male with dementia of the Alzheimer type. He is a retired pharmaceutical company executive, and he and his wife, Anne, enjoy entertaining family and friends in their home. Mr. Bitner's current stage of dementia is manifested in continuous repetitive questioning of Mrs. Bitner, difficulty concentrating, loss of interest in activities, withdrawal from social activities, and constant pacing. Even though Mrs. Bitner had

rearranged furniture to accommodate her husband's new habit of pacing, 2 weeks ago Mr. Bitner sustained bilateral Colles' fractures, when he tripped over a coffee table in the family room. After assisting Mrs. Bitner with suggestions for her husband's personal care, the occupational therapy practitioner gave her information about adult day-care programs for persons with dementia. Adult day care has benefits for both the care recipient and the caregiver, with Mr. Bitner receiving needed stimulation and appropriate supervision and Mrs. Bitner receiving respite from Mr. Bitner's repetitive question and pacing habits.

◆ Andrew is a 13-year old male who has a diagnosis of attention deficit disorder. He has his own room with a desk for studying, but he becomes distracted and rarely completes his homework. Andrew's psychologist works with an occupational therapy practitioner consultant, whom he asked to evaluate Andrew and make recommendations. The therapist recommended the following: *Organize all items on Andrew's desk so that there is a clear system for accessing materials. Move posters from the walls surrounding his desk to another place in his*

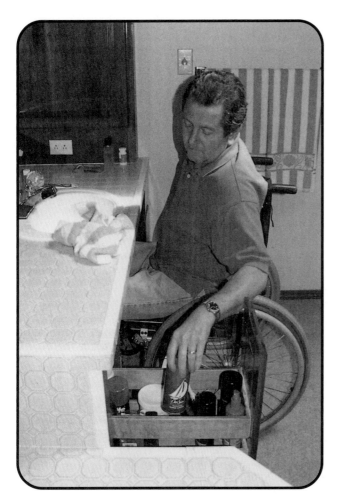

FIGURE 46.12 Recessed plumbing and double-deep drawers allow easy access to the sink area from a seated position.

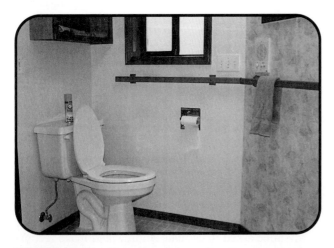

FIGURE 46.13 The oak grab bars also serve as a towel rack and the extra-high toilet enables an easy side-to-side transfer from a wheelchair.

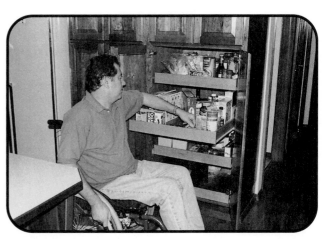

FIGURE 46.14 Shallow drawers on gliders make all goods accessible from a seated position.

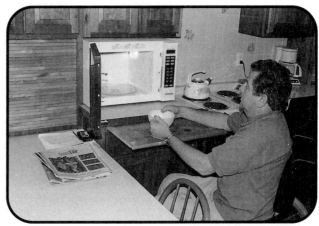

FIGURE 46.15 The placement of the microwave enables hot items to be stepped down to the cutting board and then transferred to the table with ease.

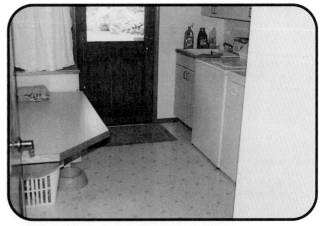

FIGURE 46.16 The laundry table is angled to allow a clear pathway for the wheelchair, and the counter height is 32 in. for ease of use when seated, with clear access underneath.

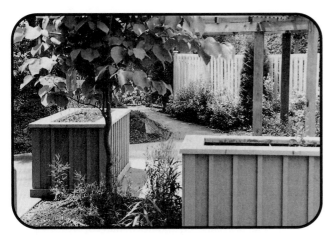

FIGURE 46.17   The wandering paths and built-up planter enable nursing home residents to pace and wander in a safe and attractive environment.

room. When he gets ready to study, have Andrew pull only items necessary for a particular assignment onto his desk. To decrease visual stimuli, the only light in Andrew's room should be his desk lamp. In addition, have Andrew take frequent study breaks. Andrew should study at the same time every evening, and go through the same routines to set up his study area until habit patterns are established and maintained.

The intervention was successful.

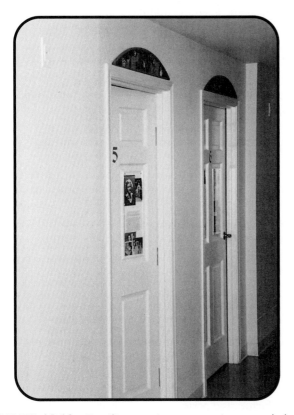

FIGURE 46.18   Familiar cues in a new environment help assisted living center residents find their way home.

♦ Mr. Jakke has always liked being outdoors. Several years ago he took up gardening and his daily routine involved spending about 2 hours each morning tending his vegetables, flowers, and bonsai trees. Previously, he used a portable kneeler/bench to support kneeling or sitting. However, he is no longer able to use this device because of increased lower extremity spasticity. Hence, his morning gardening routine has come to a halt. The occupational therapy practitioner suggested raised gardens for his vegetables and flowers (Fig. 46.19) and a fence with shelves to tend and display his bonsai trees. The modifications enabled Mr. Jakke to resume his morning gardening routine.

OT PROCESS: RE-EVALUATION

The fifth component of the occupational therapy process is re-evaluation. During re-evaluation, the predicted outcomes are evaluated using the same measures as during the evaluation. The purpose of re-evaluation is to ascertain if occupational therapy interventions achieved the intended outcomes. Hence, the criteria for re-evaluation are the stated outcomes. If the stated outcome was to restore independence in feeding, at re-revaluation clients' ability to feed themselves independently would be tested under various conditions. The conditions would involve eating liquids (beverages) and solids (meat, mash potatoes), using various eating utensils. If the practitioner had hypothesized that the feeding discrepancy was related to inadequate grip strength for holding feeding utensils, and the intervention implemented to achieve feeding independence was graded functional activities to strengthen grip, the practitioner may also wish to re-test grip strength. If the desired outcome was achieved (independence in feeding) and grip strength was increased, the practitioner's hypothesis explaining the performance discrepancy would be confirmed. However, if grip strength was increased but the outcome was not achieved, the practitioner would need

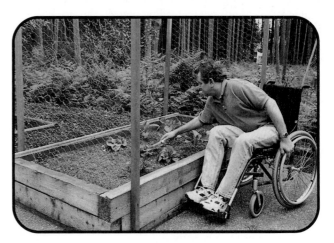

FIGURE 46.19   The raised gardens enable clients to tend plants from a seated position.

to decide to: (1) continue the graded functional activities intervention (e.g., longer duration is needed to achieve change); (2) change the intervention, for example, to try an adaptive device (e.g., compensate for reduced grip strength), (3) continue the graded functional activities intervention but add another modality, or (4) revise the outcome (e.g., increased independence vs. independence). To make these decisions, practitioners draw on their book knowledge, hands-on knowledge, and their experience with "this" particular client.

The timing of re-evaluation is based on the practitioner's prediction (prognostic judgment) of how long it will take the intervention to have an effect. The following question must be addressed: Given Xx occupational therapy intervention, at Aa intensity, with Bb frequency, for Cc duration, how long will it take for the targeted outcome to be achieved? For example, given graded functional activities (intervention) for 1 hour (intensity), 3 times per week (frequency) for 4 weeks (duration), how long will it take the client to move from being dependent in feeding to being independent in feeding. Intensity, frequency, and duration of rehabilitation interventions have risen to the forefront of discussion with constraint induced movement therapy (CIMT). The original treatment protocol called for a massed practice schedule of 6 hours per day for 5 days per week for 2 weeks (Ostendorf & Wolf, 1981). The positive results seen over 2 weeks with CIMT have spurred practitioners to inquire if greater benefit would be derived from protocol variations by increasing the intensity, frequency, or duration. Significantly, a meta-analysis of studies involving different intensities of stroke rehabilitation found a statistically significant effect for activities of daily living (Kwakkel, Wagenaar, Koelman, Lankhorst, & Koetsier, 1997).

Re-evaluation then should be scheduled to coincide with the estimated time needed for change in the outcome variables to occur. Modifying the task or the environment often results in immediate improvement in occupational performance, whereas the effects of changing client capacities may take longer. For example, clients with spinal cord injury, who cannot hold a feeding utensil, can usually feed themselves immediately following application of a universal cuff to the hand with a spoon inserted into the cuff pocket. Restoring sufficient grip strength to hold the spoon may take months or may not be feasible. Practitioners often combine person-task-environment strategies in the overall intervention plan to take advantage of the 'almost' immediate results obtained when task and environmental demands are manipulated as well as the 'delayed' changes obtained with person-oriented interventions. The 'immediate' results following task and environmental interventions often motivate clients to participate fully in person-oriented interventions that require more effort. Nonetheless, the specific combination of interventions influences how soon functional outcomes can be achieved.

The risk in re-evaluating before change has had the opportunity to develop is that a successful intervention may be deemed unsuccessful. The timing of re-evaluations is often addressed in practice guidelines and by third party insurance carriers. Although practice guidelines and insurance regulations are increasingly being formulated based on evidence, this is not always the case and practitioners need to be aware of this possibility.

In addition to judging the success of occupational therapy interventions on clients' occupational performance, re-evaluation provides practitioners with the opportunity to assess their own performance. The accuracy of their therapeutic judgments about the definition and nature of performance discrepancies and the intensity, frequency, and duration of interventions can be evaluated against stated outcomes that are achieved and not achieved. Reflecting on one's therapeutic decisions and discussing them with more experienced practitioners is an excellent way of improving one's therapeutic reasoning skills (Rogers, 1983; Rogers & Holm, 1989).

The Hierarchy of Occupational Performance: Implications for Evaluation and Intervention

The hierarchy of occupational performance provides a useful perspective for delineating the major evaluation and intervention approaches for performance discrepancies used in occupational therapy. Occupational performance may be envisioned as a three-layer phenomenon—the top layer represents occupational role performance (e.g., student, home maker); the middle layer represents task performance (e.g., dressing, meal preparation, school work); the bottom layer represents capabilities (e.g., range of motion, short-term memory, motivation). These layers are arranged in a hierarchy as capabilities coalesce to make up task-performance skills, and tasks coalesce to make up occupational roles. Thus, it is salient to ask, at what level should the occupational therapy evaluation begin and how should it move forward. Similarly, at what level should occupational therapy interventions be targeted?

Trombly (1993, 1995) labeled the approach that begins with capabilities as the bottom-up approach and the approach that begins with role performance as the top-down approach. The top-down approach reflects the position delineated in the Occupational Therapy Practice Framework (AOTA, 2002). A third approach, that initially focuses on the client-in-context was delineated by Hinojosa and Kramer (1998).

Bottom-Up Approach to Performance Discrepancy

When using a *bottom-up approach,* occupational therapy practitioners focus evaluation and intervention on the client's generic abilities (i.e., body functions and structures and related impairments according to the ICF model; or client factors and performance skills using the OTPF). For Mrs. Fisher, a 63-year-old client who sustained a right cerebrovascular accident (CVA), the practitioner might focus the evaluation on muscle tone, reflexes, postural control, visual motor integration, and short-term memory. Interventions are restorative in nature with the intent of normalizing body functions and structures lost secondary to stroke.

The rationale underlying the bottom-up approach is that body structures and functions support task performance in all occupational areas and that by restoring these abilities to their normal state, task performance, which was previously dysfunctional, automatically becomes functional, because the skills and habits needed to perform these tasks are once again intact. Once generic abilities are revitalized, some restorative interventions may be devised for task performance to reintegrate newly restored generic abilities into everyday performance of the client's personal care, home management, work, and play or leisure activities. This intervention would not need to be extensive, however, because the "cure" of impairments re-establishes the client's capacities, and task reactivation occurs rapidly, particularly for well-learned and well-practiced everyday skills. Hence, the bottom-up approach to performance discrepancy is efficient because the restoration of task abilities returns clients to their premorbid (pre-disease, pre-disorder) condition, and tasks and role participation are resumed at their prior level.

The bottom-up approach permits the occupational therapy practitioner to focus the evaluation and intervention on discrete client capacities without initially having to consider task or environmental demands. Mrs. Fisher's muscle tone, reflexes, and postural control can be evaluated on a mat table and her visual-motor integration and short-term memory can be evaluated through tests as she sits in her wheelchair. Interventions to normalize tone, and improve postural control can also be implemented with Mrs. Fisher on the mat table. Interventions to resolve problems in form constancy, visual closure, figure-ground perception, and short-term memory can be implemented through paper-and-pencil exercises done on a lapboard. For the most part, environmental interactions are limited to test and intervention objects and instructions.

The demands of real-life situations are introduced into the intervention plan once generic abilities have been restored or their improvement has stabilized. For example, because Mrs. Fisher has not achieved full voluntary control of her affected left extremities and cannot perform transfers in a typical manner, her occupational therapy practitioner practices bed and toilet transfers with her to help her integrate postural control techniques and manage abnormal tone during these procedures.

Top-Down Approach to Performance Discrepancy

The second major approach to occupational therapy evaluation and intervention—the *top-down approach*—begins by establishing performance discrepancies at the highest level—that is, the level of social role. It then moves to the tasks necessary to sustain valued social roles—that is, to the ICF level of activities/activity limitations or to the OTPF level of occupations and related performance skills and patterns. Finally, the focus is transferred to generic abilities that support activities and social role performance, or to the OTPF level of inherent client factors or the ICF level of body functions and structures/impairments. The fundamental rationale underlying the top-down approach is that even though impairments cannot always be cured, activities and social participation can be improved through adapted performance of tasks and actions associated with these activities and social roles. The following logic undergirds this rationale (Mathiowetz, 1993; Trombly, 1993, 1995):

♦ Evaluation and intervention begin with tasks that are of value to clients (i.e., necessary for carrying out valued activities and social roles).

♦ Factors external to clients that contribute to performance discrepancies can be identified during task performance.

♦ Inferences about probable external causes of performance discrepancies can be verified by changing the task or environmental demands during task performance, thereby reducing or resolving the performance discrepancy.

♦ The contribution of capacities and impairments can be observed as they interact synergistically in the performance of real-life activities and social roles.

♦ A more focused evaluation of impairments can occur in the context of task performance to formulate appropriate intervention strategies to establish, restore, or prevent loss of generic capacities.

For Mrs. Fisher, who sustained a right CVA, the occupational therapy practitioner begins by evaluating Mrs. Fisher's participation in the social roles that would most likely be restricted after a stroke. Mrs. Fisher values most her roles as a wife and homemaker. She enjoys cooking for her husband and baking for her grandchildren, who visit her every Tuesday. She is also concerned about her role as a self-carer. In addition to walking, feeding, bathing, toileting, dressing, and hygiene, Mrs. Fisher expresses concern about medication management and emergency communication when her husband is not home.

Once the most salient tasks comprising each social role have been identified, performance-based evaluation is initiated to identify task performance that is unaffected as well as task limitations. In-depth evaluations are needed to identify the specific point in a task sequence where breakdown occurs, as well as the task demands, and to develop therapeutic hypotheses about the impairments responsible for this breakdown. Intervention strategies to reduce task and environmental demands involving compensatory methods of task performance, the use of adaptive equipment, and modification of the ambient physical and social environmental may be implemented. These compensatory strategies may resolve performance discrepancies relatively quickly, and they may be temporary or permanent solutions to performance discrepancies. If temporary solutions, they are usually implemented to enable adapted task performance while capacity (impairment)-oriented interventions are instituted later to restore person abilities.

The top-down approach to performance discrepancies permits the occupational therapy practitioner initially to focus evaluation and intervention on the social roles and responsibilities that define a client's participation in the home and community. Knowledge of task demands and the physical and social environment are integral to the occupational therapy process from the beginning.

Mrs. Fisher, for example, indicated that her present concerns center on her roles as self-carer, wife, grandparent, and homemaker. She is anxious about her ability to carry out these roles since her stroke. Ideally, evaluation of the critical tasks that constitute her homemaker role (e.g., meal preparation, household maintenance, clothing care) and her self-carer role (e.g., bathing, toileting, dressing) would be carried out in her home so that information obtained about the PTE transaction is accurate and valid. Under less-than-ideal conditions, these tasks are evaluated in an occupational therapy clinic. Accuracy and validity of information are increased under clinical conditions by simulating as much as possible the task and environmental demands that Mrs. Fisher will face in her home at discharge. For example, because the bathroom in the Fisher home is too narrow to allow Mrs. Fisher to turn her wheelchair around in the bathroom while she is sitting in it, the occupational therapy practitioner trained Mrs. Fisher to back her wheelchair This procedure enabled Mrs. Fisher to practice transfers to the bathtub bench as well as the toilet, toward the stronger, unaffected right side of her body. She then learned to collapse the wheelchair and reposition it in the opposite direction before transferring out of the bathtub. Turning the chair allowed her to again transfer toward her stronger, unaffected side. The space needed to turn the chair is less when she is not in the chair because her thigh length does not need to be taken into account. In addition to the compensatory approaches, neurodevelopmental interventions (i.e., restorative) to improve postural control by normalizing muscle tone and inhibiting abnormal reflex patterns would be incorporated into transfer practice exercises.

The Client-in-Context Approach to Performance Discrepancy

Unlike the bottom-up and top-down approaches, the third approach to performance discrepancies does not prescribe a specific starting point or sequence. Rather, the occupational therapy process begins with a screening evaluation, which is structured to ascertain the client's area of greatest need (Weinstock-Zlotnick & Hinojosa, 2004). The practitioner seeks to understand why the client came or was referred to occupational therapy. Data from the screening

evaluation directs the subsequent comprehensive evaluation. If the problem is situated in a body structure or function, this structure or function is then evaluated more comprehensively. If the problem resides in the task or environment, the task or environment is examined in detail. The client's presenting problem is the trigger for future actions.

During the screening evaluation, Mrs. Fisher clarifies that her greatest concerns are her ability to transfer to the toilet, manage her medications, and communicate in an emergency when her husband is at work or away from the home. Therefore, during the comprehensive evaluation, the practitioner observes Mrs. Fisher perform a toilet transfer, sort several medications onto a daily schedule according to the directions on the prescription containers, and make a 911 call from the floor (as if she had fallen) by pulling the telephone to the floor using the cord. Additionally, she assessed Mrs. Fisher's motor control after observing the toilet transfer and floor mobility. Intervention focused on management and use of the wheelchair during toilet transfers, sorting medications for the next week by day and time, and subscription to a medical alert system for assistance in case of a fall or an emergency. Mrs. Fisher was also scheduled for outpatient rehabilitation to focus on normalizing the tone in her affected side, as well as improving postural control.

Advantages and Disadvantages of the Approaches to PTE Transaction Discrepancies

The Bottom-Up Approach

An advantage of the bottom-up approach to PTE discrepancies is that intervention aimed at developing or restoring generic abilities may benefit many tasks. For example, increasing muscle strength or range of motion in the upper extremities will facilitate all tasks for which these abilities were deficient. Similarly, reducing apathy will foster reengagement in previously neglected occupational areas. Likewise, correcting visual-sequencing deficits will enhance the performance of all tasks negatively affected by this impairment. Thus, potentially, by remediating neuromuscular, mental, or psychological impairments, multiple task disabilities can be treated simultaneously.

Because the bottom-up approach emphasizes performance factors that are internal to clients, consideration of external, environmental factors is extremely limited. Therefore, the approach is economical to administer because occupational therapy practitioners do not need to assess or manage the demands of tasks and the surrounding physical and social environment, or how they impinge on the client's abilities.

Nonetheless, an inherent disadvantage of the bottom-up approach is that improvements in generic abilities may not generalize to specific tasks (e.g., dressing, medication management) or actions (e.g., buttoning, sorting medications). Generalization may not occur for several reasons. First, abilities-oriented interventions concentrate on the body functions and structures that are common to many tasks. However, task performance requires the application of these abilities to the unique demands of specific tasks. Improvements in visual figure-ground perception demonstrated on paper-and-pencil tests, using black-and-white stimulus materials, may not enable clients to identify hazards, such as water spills, on a multicolored and patterned vinyl floor surface. Second, when abilities are exercised in isolation from tasks, they are not integrated with the other abilities that are also needed to perform these tasks (Ma & Trombly, 1999; Trombly & Wu, 1999). In other words, discrete abilities-oriented interventions do not acknowledge either the interaction between task-related abilities or their coalescence in the PTE transaction in which the discrete abilities will be used. Perceiving a water spill on the floor must be accompanied by the cognitive capacity to motor plan to avoid the spill and the neuromuscular strength and endurance to execute walking around it. Finally, generalization may not occur because although abilities may be improved, they may not be improved sufficiently to meet task demands. An increase in range of motion of 10° at the shoulder joint is still inadequate for grooming if 25° more motion is needed to comb the hair on the back of the head.

The bottom-up approach may also result in the identification and treatment of impairments that may not actually be causing performance dysfunctions. A deficit score on a test of visual figure-ground perception may not translate into performance deficits on well-learned daily living skills. Without assessing the PTE transaction during tasks, the meaning of impairments for performance is vague.

The bottom-up approach is generally initiated with the intent to switch to the top-down approach if full recovery does not occur or once maximum benefit is obtained from restorative interventions. The danger in this tactic is that too much intervention time may be spent on remediating impairments. At the outset of intervention, it is difficult to predict if full recovery will be achieved, and occupational therapy practitioners are prone to persist in restorative interventions as long as gains are being made. Unfortunately, if full recovery is not achieved, there may be little 'reimbursable' intervention time left for addressing activity limitations or participation restrictions. Clients may then be deprived of independent, safe, and adequate task performance that could have been achieved—or achieved more readily— through compensatory interventions. The risk of clients being discharged from therapy before maximum improvement in task performance has been achieved has been intensified by managed care and reduced time allocations for rehabilitation (Angelelli, Wilber, & Myrtle, 2000; Banja & DeJong, 2000; Cope & Sundance, 1995; Eastwood, 1999).

Another disadvantage of the bottom-up approach is that clients may not see the connection between interventions aimed at discrete impairments (e.g., motor control exercises, visual-scanning programs on a computer, stacking cones) and improvement of their daily living activities and social participation. Hence, they may be less motivated to participate in occupational therapy. However, by educating clients and their families about the connection between impairment reduction and task improvement, this disadvantage may be overcome or minimized.

Top-Down Approach

A primary advantage of the top-down approach is that evaluation and intervention center on social role participation and task performance that are meaningful to clients, yet are discrepant with the levels of performance that are expected, required, or desired (Trombly, 1993). Consistent with this advantage are two additional benefits. First, because the occupational therapy process focuses on social role participation and activity performance that are meaningful to clients, the relevance of therapy for improving daily life is readily apparent to clients (Trombly, 1993). Thus motivation to participate in therapy is heightened. Second, social role and task performance are influenced directly by the intervention. Real-life performance is both the medium and the outcome of therapy (Dirette & Hinojosa, 1999; Dolecheck & Schkade, 1999; van Heugten et al., 1998).

The top-down approach also has the advantage of reinforcing and expediting an approach that people often implement naturally when problems are experienced in task performance (Fried, Herdman, Kuhn, Rubin, & Turano, 1991; Yakobina, Yakobina, & Tallant, 1997). When difficulties are encountered in doing tasks, people tend to seek the assistance of others, use a tool to help themselves, or try a different way of performing the task. These compensatory procedures foster task completion. Because the top-down approach enhances processes that people turn to naturally when problems are encountered, it is familiar to clients, and hence it is likely to be accepted by them.

The top-down approach provides a further advantage at the point at which intervention switches from a social role participation or task focus to an impairment orientation. The top-down approach facilitates the identification of impairments in the context of social roles and the tasks embodied in these roles; consequently, the relevance of impairments for social roles and their tasks is clear to clients. In contrast, in the bottom-up approach, by which impairments are evaluated in isolation, their relevance for social roles and tasks can only be inferred. The visual-perceptual impairments identified through a paper-and-pencil test may or may not impair social roles and activities. The identification of role and task-related impairments, in turn, enables a more targeted evaluation of impairments as well as more precisely directed restorative interventions.

The disadvantage of the top-down approach is that evaluation and intervention are social role and task specific, and there may be little transfer from one task to another. Moreover, for intervention to be maximally effective, it must occur in the occupational context in which the client lives, works, or plays, which may be difficult to arrange and may not be reimbursable. Thus the approach requires the occupational therapy practitioner to take into account the complexity of environmental factors that impinge on performance.

Rogers and Holm stressed the salience of the top-down approach as well as compensatory interventions for maximizing performance gains (Holm & Rogers, 1989, 1991; Rogers & Holm, 1989; Rogers et al., 1997). Research shows that the correlation between task abilities and task performance although positive is low. Mathiowetz (1993), in a discussion of neuromuscular capacity evaluation and intervention for function, noted that it is possible for some clients to have grip or pinch strength within normal limits but not be able to accomplish necessary functional tasks and for others to have grip or pinch strength below normal limits and yet be able to accomplish all their functional tasks. He further pointed out that the kinesiology literature suggests that motor learning is task specific, with little carryover to other tasks, and thus the best way to improve motor function is to practice the task for which it is required. According to Trombly (1993), "we have no definitive study in occupational therapy that indicates that a person's occupational functioning is better as a result of restorative therapy rather than adaptive therapy" (p. 255), and Wood (1996) summarized concerns about a singular use of the bottom-up approach to PTE transaction discrepancies (Humphrey, Jewell, & Rosenberger, 1995; Neistadt, 1994a, 1994b; Trombly, 1995) by noting that there "has been increasing evidence that improvements in performance components do not necessarily translate into competent functioning in everyday life" (p. 631).

Additional compelling arguments for the top-down approach have come from health insurance companies because they define acceptable outcomes of therapy through their reimbursement practices. For example, Blue Cross of California defined a meaningful outcome of therapy as "one in which the activity level achieved by the patient . . . is that level necessary for the patient to function most effectively at home or at work" (Stewart & Abeln, 1993, p. 213). Another parameter of acceptability, a utilitarian outcome of therapy, is defined as a functional outcome that is economically and efficiently achieved (Eastwood, 1999; Stewart & Abeln, 1993).

Finally, the disability rights movement has also promoted the top-down approach and compensatory interventions by focusing on task and environmental adaptations. When using compensatory interventions, practitioners probe to identify how task and environmental demands affect role and task performance and then seek to work around problems or capitalize on assets (Dunn et al., 1994; Verbrugge, 1990). Thus, compensatory interventions do not assume that there is something wrong with the person with a disability that needs to be fixed or changed. It is the task or the environment that needs to be changed to accommodate the person's abilities. As Verbrugge (1990) noted, the request of advocacy groups for persons with disabilities is: "Change the milieu, not me" (p. 68).

The Client-in-Context Approach

The client is the pivotal point in the client-in-context approach. A major advantage of this approach is that the territory of inquiry for evaluation is immediately and efficiently narrowed. Furthermore, it is narrowed to a primary concern of the client, thus peaking the client's interest in therapy and facilitating cooperation. A client presents with a diagnosis of carpel tunnel syndrome of moderate severity reporting pain and weakness that interfere with daily living tasks. The practitioner responds by fabricating a night splint that keeps the wrist and metacarpophalangeal joints in a neutral position and teaching tendon and nerve gliding exercises (Brininger et al., 2007). The pain and weakness resolve over 3 weeks and the performance of daily activities is no longer problematic.

The advantages provided by an occupational therapy process that is highly focused and efficient and that builds on problems identified by clients are offset by several disadvantages. First, for clients to identify problems amenable to occupational therapy interventions, they must have a clear understanding of occupational therapy. Unfortunately, occupational therapy is poorly understood by the public and health care professionals alike (Ahlstrand, 1989; Chakravorty, 1993; Jamnadas, Burns, & Paul, 2001; Kane, Robinson, & Leicht, 2005; McAvoy, 1999; Patel & Shriber, 2000; Royeen, Zardetto-Smith, Duncan, & Mu, 2001). Hence, clients may need to be coached about occupational therapy before they are able to articulate performance problems.

Second, clients with cognitive impairments may not be able to identify their performance problems. Clients with dementia, for example, may deny that they have problems in caring for themselves or their homes. Similarly, those with mental retardation may want to live in a group home but may not be aware of the daily living skills required by these residences. Clients may also be unaware of their problems, may refuse to report them, or may exaggerate them, as often occurs for clients with mental health diagnoses (e.g., schizophrenia, depression, bipolar disorder) (Branch & Meyers, 1987; Pearson, 2000).

Third, clients may be reluctant to state their problems. Older adults, for example, may hesitate to acknowledge dependencies fearing that this may be interpreted as an inability to continue to reside independently in the community.

THE OCCUPATIONAL THERAPY PROCESS REVISITED

Occupational performance is the human behavior addressed by occupational therapy practitioners. Performance—'doing'—is one of the defining characteristics of our profession and in the therapeutic situation practitioners are often anxious to move quickly to the 'doing.' The six components of the occupational therapy process serve as a cognitive assistive device to remind practitioners to 'think before they act.' Although we have discussed theory, evaluation, problem definition, intervention planning and implementation, and re-evaluation separately, in the practice situation, the process shuffles back and forth among components. Practitioners do not collect 'all' evaluative data and then organize it to define problems. Rather, they move back and forth between theory, evaluation, and problem definition almost simultaneously theorizing, evaluating, defining, and intervening.

Some occupational therapy interventions particularly lend themselves to an 'evaluation-intervention-re-evaluation' mode of operation. For instance, suppose that a practitioner ascertains, through performance <u>evaluation</u>, that a client is dependent in transferring out of the bathtub. Further, suppose that the practitioner reasons that this dependency is secondary to apraxia—an inability to problem solve how to get out of the tub. Because the client cannot be left seated in the tub, the practitioner initiates interventions to facilitate exiting the tub. The client is instructed (<u>intervention</u>) to position the feet under the body to rise from the tub bottom and then exit the tub. The intervention is successful and the client exits the tub (<u>re-evaluation</u>). Hence, the practitioner's hypothesis about the reasons for the performance deficiency is at least partially confirmed, and the practitioner has gained new information about the client's capacity (e.g., the client can follow verbal instructions) that can be used in therapy. The 'evaluation-intervention-re-evaluation' mode is referred to as a dynamic or interactive assessment process (Rogers, Holm, & Stone, 1997) and it encapsulates all components of the occupational therapy process.

Evaluation plays a key role in understanding the performance problems experienced by clients. However, to be optimally serviceable, evaluation must yield data useful for selecting interventions and outcomes as well as defining problems. Outcomes stipulate the results that are to be achieved through occupational therapy interventions (Rogers & Holm, 1994a). As pointed out by the wisdom of the Cheshire Cat, in the following dialogue, outcomes determine methods.

> *Alice: Oh, no, no. I was just wondering if you could help me find my way*
> *Cheshire Cat: Well that depends on where you want to get to.*
> *Alice: Oh, it really doesn't matter, as long as...*
> *Cheshire Cat: Then it really doesn't matter which way you go.*

Practitioners plan interventions with an outcome in mind, thus forging the link between re-evaluation and intervention.

CONCLUSION

The occupational therapy process is theory-based and data-driven. It is the therapeutic problem solving process used by practitioners to respond to their clients' occupational performance needs. The occupational therapy process is first driven by theory, and then consists of five additional major components—evaluation, problem definition, intervention planning, intervention implementation, and re-evaluation. Each component was presented and its therapeutic utility discussed. In this chapter, we chose to elucidate the occupational therapy process using the construct of the person-task-environment transaction (PTE), rather than choosing a specific theoretical approach. The PTE transaction implies a negotiation or arrangement among three factors: person capacities (P), task demands (T), and environmental demands (E). Finally, we provided numerous case examples that combined aspects of the occupational therapy process, and the PTE transaction.

PROVOCATIVE QUESTIONS

1. When all factors of the Person-Task-Environment transaction are not taken into consideration during an evaluation, what possible impacts could this have on intervention choices and client outcomes?
2. Structuring a problem statement stands at the interface between evaluation and intervention, and provides information useful for guiding problem solution. For Mrs. Rogers, found under "Case Examples: Modify Task Demands for Skill Deficit," structure a problem statement. Also try to structure problem statements for other Case Examples.

REFERENCES

Ahlstrand, S. S. (1989). *Awareness and image study.* Unpublished report by The Gallup Organization. Lincoln, Nebraska.

Allen, C. K. (1985). *Occupational therapy for psychiatric diseases: Measurement and management of cognitive disabilities.* Boston: Little, Brown.

Angelelli, J., Wilber, K., & Myrtle, R. (2000). A comparison of skilled nursing facility rehabilitation treatment and outcomes under Medicare managed care and Medicare fee-for-service reimbursement. *Gerontologist, 40,* 646–653.

American Occupational Therapy Association [AOTA] (1994). Uniform terminology for occupational therapy (3rd ed.). *American Journal of Occupational Therapy, 48,* 1046–1054.

American Occupational Therapy Association [AOTA] (2002). *Occupational therapy practice framework: Domain & Process.* Bethesda, MD: AOTA Press.

American Occupational Therapy Association [AOTA]. (2005). Occupational therapy code of ethics (2005). *American Journal of Occupational Therapy, 59,* 639–642.

American Occupational Therapy Association [AOTA] (in press). *Occupational therapy practice framework: Domain & Process* (2nd ed.). Bethesda, MD: AOTA Press.

Baker, N. A. (1999). Anthropometry. In K. Jacobs (Ed.). *Ergonomics for therapists* (2nd ed., pp. 49–84). Boston: Butterworth-Heinemann.

Banja, J., & DeJong, G. (2000). The rehabilitation marketplace: Economics, values, and proposals for reform. *Archives of Physical Medicine and Rehabilitation, 81,* 233–240.

Barris, R., (1982). Environmental interactions: An extension of the model of human occupation. *American Journal of Occupational Therapy, 36,* 637–644.

Branch, L. G., & Meyers, A. R. (1987). Assessing physical function in the elderly. *Clinics in Geriatric Medicine, 3,* 29–51.

Brigham, C., Engelberg, A. L., & Richling, D. E. (1996, February 16). The changing role of rehab: Focus on function. *Patient Care,* 144–184.

Brininger, T. L., Rogers, J. C., Holm, M. B., Baker, N. B., Li, Z-M., & Goitz, R. J. (2007). Efficacy of a fabricated customized splint and tendon and nerve gliding exercises for the treatment of carpal tunnel syndrome: A randomized controlled clinical trial. *Archives of Physical Medicine and Rehabilitation, 88,* 1429–1435.

Burke, D., Burke, M., Stewart, G., & Cambre, A. (1994). Splinting for carpal tunnel syndrome: In search of the optimal angle. *Archives of Physical Medicine and Rehabilitation, 75,* 1241–1244.

Cameron, K., Ballantyne, S., Kulbitsky, A., Margolis-Gal, M., Daugherty, T., & Ludwig, F. (2005). Utilization of evidence-based practice by registered occupational therapists. *Occupational Therapy International, 12*(3), 123–136.

Carson, R. (1994). Reducing cumulative trauma disorders: Use of proper workplace design. *AAOHN Journal, 42,* 270–276.

Casby, J., & Holm, M. B. (1994). The effect of music on repetitive disruptive vocalizations of persons with dementia. *American Journal of Occupational Therapy, 48,* 883–889.

Chakravorty, B. G. (1993). Occupational therapy services: Awareness among hospital consultants and general practitioners. *British Journal of Occupational Therapy, 56,* 283–286.

Christiansen, C. (1991). Occupational therapy intervention for life performance. In C. Christiansen & C. Baum (Eds.). *Occupational therapy: Overcoming human performance deficits* (pp. 3–43). Thorofare, NJ: Slack.

Cipriani, J., Hess, S., Higgins, H., Resavy, D., Sheon, S., Szychowski, M., & Holm, M. B. (2000). Collaboration in the therapeutic process: Older adults' perspectives. *Physical & Occupational Therapy in Geriatrics, 17*(1), 43–54.

Clark, M. C., Czaja, S. J., & Weber, R. A. (1990). Older adults and daily living task profiles. *Human Factors, 32,* 537–549.

Close, J., Ellis, M. Hooper, R., Glucksman, E., Jackson., S., & Swift, C. (1999). Prevention of falls in the elderly trial (PROFET): A randomised controlled trial. *Lancet, 353,* 93–97

Cope, D. N., & Sundance, P. (1995). Conceptualizing clinical outcomes. In P. K. Landrum, N. D. Schmidt, & A. McLean (Eds.). *Outcome-oriented rehabilitation* (pp. 43–56). Gaithersburg, MD: Aspen.

Creighton, C. (1992). The origin and evolution of activity analysis. *American Journal of Occupational Therapy, 46,* 45–48.

Cummings, R. G., Thomas, M., Szonyi, G., Salkeld, G., O'Neill, E., Westbury, C., & Frampton, G. (1999). Home visits by an occupational therapist for assessment and modification of environmental hazards: A randomized trial of falls prevention. *Journal of the American Geriatrics Society, 46,* 1397–1402.

Cynkin, S. (1979). *Occupational therapy: Toward health through activities.* Boston: Little, Brown.

Czaja, S., Weber, R. A., & Nair, S. N. (1993). A human factors analysis of ADL activities: A capability-demand approach. *Journals of Gerontology, 48,* 44–48.

Demore-Taber, M. (1995). Americans with Disabilities Act work site assessment. In K. Jacobs & C. Bettencourt (Eds.). *Ergonomics for therapists* (pp. 229–244). Boston: Butterworth-Heinemann.

Diffrient, N., Tilley, A., & Bardagjy, F. (1974). *Humanscale 1/2/3.* Cambridge, MA: MIT Press.

Dirette, D., & Hinojosa, J. (1999). The effects of a compensatory intervention on processing deficits of adults with acquired brain injuries. *Occupational Therapy Journal of Research, 19,* 223–240.

Dolecheck, J. R. & Schkade, J. K. (1999). The extent dynamic standing endurance is effected when CVA subjects perform personally meaningful activities rather than nonmeaningful tasks. *Occupational Therapy Journal of Research, 19,* 40–54.

Dromerick, A. W., Edwards, D. F., & Hahn, M. (2000). Does the application of constraint-induced movement therapy during acute rehabilitation reduce arm impairment after ischemic stroke? *Stroke, 31,* 2984–2988.

Dubouloz, C., Egan, M., Vallerand, J., & Von Zweck, C. (1999). Occupational therapists' perceptions of evidence-based practice. *American Journal of Occupational Therapy, 53,* 445–453.

Dunn, W., Brown, C., & McGuigan, M. (1994). The ecology of human performance: A framework for considering the effect of context. *American Journal of Occupational Therapy, 48,* 595–607.

Dysart, A., & Tomlin, G. (2002). Factors related to evidence-based practice among U.S. occupational therapy clinicians. *American Journal of Occupational Therapy, 56,* 275–284.

Eastwood, E. A. (1999). Functional status and its uses in rehabilitation medicine. *Mt. Sinai Journal of Medicine, 66,* 179–187.

Edwards, D. F., Hahn, M. G., Baum, C. M., Perlmutter, M. S., Sheedy, C., Dromerick, A. W. (2006). Screening patients with stroke for rehabilitation needs: Validation of the post-stroke rehabilitation guidelines. *Neurorehabilitation & Neural Repair, 20*(1), 42–48.

Elstein, A. S., Shulman, L. S., & Sprafka, S. A. (1978). *Medical problem solving: An analysis of clinical reasoning.* Cambridge: Harvard University Press.

Evans, R. W., Small, L., & Ling, J. S. (1995). Independence in the home and community. In P. K. Landrum, N. D. Schmidt, & A. McLean (Eds.). *Outcome-oriented rehabilitation* (pp. 95–124). Gaithersburg, MD: Aspen.

Faletti, M. V. (1984). Human factors research and functional environments for the aged. In I. Altman, M. P. Lawton, & J. F. Wohlwill (Eds.). *Elderly people and the environment* (pp. 191–237). New York: Plenum.

Folstein, M. F., Folstein, S., & McHugh, P. R. (1975). Mini-Mental State: A practical method for grading the cognitive state of patients for the clinician. *Journal of Psychiatric Research, 12,* 189–198.

Freal, J., Kraft, G., & Coryell, J. (1984). Symptomatic fatigue in multiple sclerosis. *Archives of Physical Medicine and Rehabilitation, 65,* 135–138.

Fried, L. P., Herdman, S. J., Kuhn, K. E., Rubin, G., & Turano, K. (1991). Preclinical disability. *Journal of Aging and Health, 3,* 285–300.

Fries, J. F., Spitz, P., Kraines, R. G., & Holman, H. R. (1980). Measurement of patient outcomes in arthritis. *Arthritis & Rheumatism, 23,* 146–152.

Friedman, A., Diamond, M., Johnston, M., & Daffner, C. (2000). Effects of botulinum toxin A on upper limb spasticity in children with cerebral palsy. *American Journal of Physical Medicine & Rehabilitation 79,* 53–59.

Gage, M., Noh, S., Polatajko, H. J., & Kaspar, V. (1994). Measuring perceived self-efficacy in occupational therapy. *American Journal of Occupational Therapy, 48,* 783–790.

Gambrill, E. (2005). Clinical thinking in clinical practice: Improving the quality of judgments and decisions (2nd ed.). Hoboken: John Wiley & Sons.

Garrod, R., Bestall, J. C., Paul, E. A., Wedzicha, J. A., & Jones, P. W. (2000). Development and validation of a standardized measure of activity of daily living in patients with severe COPD: the London Chest Activity of Daily Living Scale (LCADL). *Respiratory Medicine, 94,* 589–596.

Gerdner, L. A., Hall, G. R., & Buckwalter, K. C. (1996). Caregiver training for people with Alzheimer's based on a stress threshold model. *Image: Journal of Nursing Scholarship, 28,* 241–246.

Gibson, J., & Schkade, J. (1997). Occupational adaptation intervention with patients with cerebrovascular accident: A clinical study. *American Journal of Occupational Therapy, 51,* 523–529.

Gift, A. G. (1987). Dyspnea: A clinical perspective. *Scholarly Inquiry in Nursing Practice, 1,* 73–85.

Gift, A. G., & Pugh, L. C. (1993). Dyspnea and fatigue. *Nursing Clinics of North American, 28,* 373–384.

Giles, G., Ridley, J., Dill, A., & Frye, S. (1997). A consecutive series of adults with brain injury treated with a washing and dressing retraining program. *American Journal of Occupational Therapy, 51,* 256–266.

Griffin, N. L. (1975). Four models in imparting decision-making information. *American Journal of Occupational Therapy, 29,* 349–351.

Guralnik, J. M., Branch, L. G., Cummings, S. R., & Curb, J. D. (1989). Physical performance measures in aging research. *Journals of Gerontology: MEDICAL SCIENCES, 44A,* M141–146.

Haas, L. (1944). *Practical occupational therapy.* Milwaukee: Bruce.

Hagedorn, R. (1995). Environmental analysis and adaptation. In R. Hagedorn (Ed.). *Occupational therapy: Perspectives and processes* (pp. 239–257). Melbourne, Australia: Churchill Livingstone.

Hall, G. R., & Buckwalter, K. C. (1987). Progressively lowered stress threshold: A conceptual model for care of adults with Alzheimer's disease. *Archives of Psychiatric Nursing, 1,* 399–406.

Hart, L., & Freel, M. (1982). Fatigue. In C. Norris (Ed.). *Concept clarification in nursing* (pp. 251–262). Rockville, MD: Aspen.

Hersh, N., & Treadgold, L. (1994). Neuropage: The rehabilitation of memory dysfunction by prosthetic memory and cuing. *NeuroRehabilitation, 4,* 187–197.

Higgs, J., & Jones, M. (2000). *Clinical reasoning in the health professions.* Oxford: Butterworth Heinemann.

Hinojosa, J., & Kramer, P. (1998). Evaluation—Where do we begin? In J. Hinojosa & P. Kramer (Eds.), *Occupational therapy evaluation: Obtaining and interpreting data* (pp. 1–15). Bethesda, MD: American Occupational Therapy Association.

Holm, M. B., & Rogers, J. C. (1989). The therapist's thinking behind functional assessment, II. In C. Royeen (Ed.). *Assessment of function: An action guide* (pp. 1–34). Rockville, MD: American Occupational Therapy Association.

Holm, M. B., & Rogers, J. C. (1991). High, low, or no assistive technology devices for older adults undergoing rehabilitation. *International Journal of Technology and Aging, 4,* 153–162.

Holm, M. B., Santangelo, M., Fromuth, D., Brown, S., & Walter, H. (2000). Effectiveness of everyday occupations for changing client behaviors in a community living arrangement. *American Journal of Occupational Therapy, 54,* 361–371.

Howe, M. C., & Briggs, A. K. (1982). Ecological systems model for occupational therapy. *American Journal of Occupational Therapy, 36,* 322–327.

Humphrey, R., Jewell, K., & Rosenberger, R. C. (1995). Development of in-hand manipulation and relationship with activities. *American Journal of Occupational Therapy, 49,* 763–771.

Institute of Medicine (U.S.) (1991). *Disability in America: Toward a national agenda for prevention.* Washington, D. C.: National Academy Press.

Institute of Medicine (U.S.) (1997). *Enabling America: Assessing the role of rehabilitation science and engineering.* Washington, D.C.: National Academy Press.

Iwarsson, S., Isacsson, A., & Lanke, J. (1998). ADL dependence in the elderly population living in the community: The influence of functional limitations and physical environmental demand. *Occupational Therapy International, 5,* 173–193.

Jacobs, K. (Ed.). (1999). *Ergonomics for therapists* (2nd ed.). Boston: Butterworth-Heinemann.

Jamnadas, B., Burns, J., & Paul, S. (2001). Understanding occupational therapy: nursing and physician assistant students' knowledge about occupational therapy. *Occupational Therapy in Health Care, 14*(1), 13–25

Jang, Y., Haley, W., Small, B., & Mortimer, J. (2002). The role of mastery and social resources in the associations between disability and depression in later life. *Gerontologist 42,* 807–813.

Janson-Bjerklie, S., Carrieri, V. K., & Hudes, M. (1986). The sensations of pulmonary dyspnea. *Nursing Research, 35,* 154–159.

Jette, A. M. (1980). Functional Status Index: Reliability of a chronic disease evaluation instrument. *Archives of Physical Medicine and Rehabilitation, 61,* 395–401.

Johnson, D. N. (2000). Task demands and representation in long-term repetition priming. *Memory and Cognition, 28,* 1303–1309.

Kane, M., Robinson, A., Leicht, S. (2005). Psychologists' perceptions of occupational therapy in the treatment of eating disorders. *Occupational Therapy in Mental Health, 21* (2), 39–53.

Keuter, K., Byrne, E., Voell, J., & Larson, E. (2000). Nurses' job satisfaction and organizational climate in a dynamic work environment. *Applied Nursing Research, 13* (1), 46–49.

Kielhofner, G. (1995). Environmental influences on occupational behavior. In G. Kielhofner (Ed.). *A model of human occupation: Theory and application* (2nd ed., pp. 91–111). Baltimore: Williams & Wilkins.

Kielhofner, G., & Burke, J. P. (1980). A model of human occupation, Part I. Conceptual framework and content. *American Journal of Occupational Therapy, 34,* 572–581.

Kiernat, J. M. (1982). Environment: The hidden modality. *Physical and Occupational Therapy in Geriatrics, 2* (1), 3–12.

Klein, R. M., & Bell, B. (1982). Self-care skills: Behavior measurements with the Klein-Bell ADL Scale. *Archives of Physical Medicine and Rehabilitation, 63,* 335–338.

Koch, L., Cook, B., Tankersley, M., & Rumrill, P. (2006). Utilizing research in professional practice. *Work, 26,* 327–331.

Kroemer, K. H., & Grandjean, E. (1997). *Fitting the task to the human: A textbook of occupational ergonomics* (5th ed.). London: Taylor & Francis.

Kwakkel, G., Wagenaar, R. C., Koelman, T., Lankhorst, G., & Koetsier, J. (1997). Effects of intensity of rehabilitation after stroke: A research synthesis, 28, 1550–1556.

Law, M., Cooper, B., Strong, S., Stewart, D., Rigby, P., & Letts, L. (1996). The person-environment-occupational model: A transactive approach to occupational performance. *Canadian Journal of Occupational Therapy, 63,* 9–23.

Law, M., Baptiste, S., Carswell, A., McColl, M. A., Polatajko, H., & Pollock, N. (2005). Canadian Occupational Performance Measure (4th Edition). *Toronto, CAOT Publications ACE.*

Lawton, M. P. (1982). Competence, environmental press, and the adaptation of older people. In M. P. Lawton, P. G. Windley, & T. O. Byerts (Eds.). *Aging and the environment: Theoretical approaches* (pp. 33–59). New York: Springer.

Letts, L, Law, M., Rigby, P., Cooper, B., Stewart, D., & Strong, S. (1994). Person-environment assessments in occupational therapy. *American Journal of Occupational Therapy, 48,* 608–618.

Letts, L., & Marshall, L. (1995). Evaluating the validity and consistency of the SAFER tool. *Physical & Occupational Therapy in Geriatrics, 13* (4), 49–66.

Levine, R. E., & Brayley, C. R. (1991). Occupation as a therapeutic medium. In C. Christiansen & C. Baum (Eds.). *Occupational therapy: Overcoming human performance deficits* (pp. 591–631). Thorofare, NJ: Slack.

Lin, E., Katon, W., VonKorff, M., Tang, L., Williams, J., Kroenke, K., et al. (2003). Effect of Improving depression care on pain and functional outcomes among older adults with arthritis: a randomized controlled trial. *JAMA, 290,* 2428–2429.

Line, J. (1969). Case method: As a scientific form of clinical thinking. *American Journal of Occupational Therapy, 23,* 308–313.

Lorig, K., Chastain, R., Ung, E., Shoor, S., & Holman, H. R. (1980). Development and evaluation of a scale to measure perceived self-efficacy in people with arthritis. *Arthritis & Rheumatism, 32,* 37–44.

Ma, H., & Trombly, C. (1999). The effect of context on skill acquisition and transfer. *American Journal of Occupational Therapy, 53,* 138–144.

MacDonald, L., Karasek, R., Punnett, L., & Scharf, T. (2001). Covariation between workplace physical and psychosocial stressors: Evidence and implications for occupational health research and prevention. *Ergonomics, 10,* 696–718.

Mager, R. F., & Pipe, P. (1984). *Analyzing performance problems* (2nd ed.). Belmont, CA: Lake.

Mangino, M. (2000). The aging employee: The Impact on occupational health. *AAOHN Journal, 48,* 349–357.

Mathiowetz, V. (1993). Role of physical performance component evaluations in occupational therapy functional assessment. *American Journal of Occupational Therapy, 46,* 225–230.

Mathiowetz, V., & Matuska, K. (1998). Effectiveness of inpatient rehabilitation on self-care abilities of individuals with multiple sclerosis. *NeuroRehabilitation, 11,* 141–151.

Mathiowetz, V., & Wade, M. (1995). Task constraints and functional motor performance of individuals with and without multiple sclerosis. *Ecological Psychology, 7* (2), 99–123.

McAndrew, E., McDermott, S., Vitzakovich, S., Warunek, M., & Holm, M. B. (2000). Therapist and patient perceptions of the occupational therapy goal setting process: A pilot study. *Physical & Occupational Therapy in Geriatrics, 17* (1), 55–63.

McAvoy, E. (1999). Occupational who? Never head of them! An audit of patient awareness of occupational therapists. *British Journal of Occupational Therapy, 55,* 229–232.

McDowell, I., & Newell, C. (1996). *Measuring health: A guide to rating scales and questionnaires* (2nd ed.). New York: Oxford University Press.

McKenna, K., Bennett, S., Dierselhuis, Z., Hoffmann, T., Tooth, L., & McCluskey, A. (2005). Australian occupational therapists' use of an online evidence-based practice database (OTseeker). *Health Information & Libraries Journal, 22,* 205–214.

McCluskey, A., & Lovarini, M. (2005). Providing education on evidence-based practice improved knowledge but did not change behaviour: A before and after study. *BMC Medical Education, 5,* 40.

Mee, J., & Sumsion, T. (2001). Mental health clients confirm the motivating power of occupation. *British Journal of Occupational Therapy, 64* (3), 121–128.

Meyer, A. (1922). The philosophy of occupational therapy. *Archives of Occupational Therapy, 1,* 1–10.

Militello, L. G., & Hutton, R. J. (1998a). Applied cognitive task analysis (ACTA): A practitioner's toolkit for understanding cognitive task demands. *Ergonomics, 41,* 1618–1641.

Militello, L. G., & Hutton, R. J. (1998b). Learning to think like a user: Using cognitive task analysis to meet today's health care design challenges. *Biomedical Instrumentation and Technology, 32,* 535–540.

Mills, T., Holm, M. B., Trefler, E., Schmeler, M., Fitzgerald, S. & Boninger, M. (2002). Development and consumer validation of the Functional Evaluation in a Wheelchair (FEW) instrument. *Disability and Rehabilitation, 24,* 38–46.

Moore, J. S., & Garg, A. (1995). The strain index: A proposed method to analyze jobs for risk of distal upper extremity disorder. *American Industrial Hygiene Journal, 56,* 443–456.

Neistadt, M. (1987). Classroom as clinic: A model for teaching clinical reasoning in occupational therapy education. *American Journal of Occupational Therapy, 41,* 631–637.

Neistadt, M. (1992). The classroom as clinic: Applications for a method of teaching clinical reasoning. *American Journal of Occupational Therapy, 46,* 814–819.

Neistadt, M. E. (1994a). Perceptual retraining for adults with diffuse brain injury. *American Journal of Occupational Therapy, 48,* 225–233.

Neistadt, M. E. (1994b). The effects of different treatment activities on functional fine motor coordination in adults with brain injury. *American Journal of Occupational Therapy, 48,* 877–882.

Neistadt, M. (1998). Teaching clinical reasoning as a thinking frame. *American Journal of Occupational Therapy, 52,* 221–229.

Nelson, D. L. (1988). Occupation: Form and performance. *American Journal of Occupational Therapy, 42,* 633–641.

Oakley, F., Kielhofner, G., Barris, R., & Reichler, R. K. (1986). The Role Checklist: Development and empirical assessment of reliability. *Occupational Therapy Journal of Research, 6,* 157–169.

Ostendorf, C. G., & Wolf, S. L. (1981). Effect of forced use of the upper extremity of a hemiplegic patient on changes in function. *Physical Therapy, 7,* 1022–1025.

Oxman, T. E., & Hull, J. G. (2001). Social support and treatment response in older depressed primary care patients. *Journals of Gerontology: PSYCHOLOGICAL SCIENCES and SOCIAL SCIENCES, 56B,* 35–45.

Patel, A., & Shriber, L. (2000). Nurse practitioners' knowledge of occupational therapy. *Occupational Therapy in Health Care, 13*(2), 53–71.

Pearson, V. I. (2000). Assessment of function in older adults. In R. L. Kane & R. A. Kane (Eds.), Assessing older persons: Measures, meaning, and practical application (pp. 17–48). New York, NY: Oxford University Press.

Pelland, L, & McKinley, P. (2001). The Montreal Rehabilitation Performance Profile: A task-analysis approach to quantify stair descent performance in children with intellectual disability. *Archives of Physical Medicine and Rehabilitation, 82,* 1106–1114.

Pheasant, S. (1998). *Bodyspace: Anthropometry, ergonomics, and the design of work* (2nd ed.). London: Taylor & Francis.

Pincus, T., Summey, J. A., Soraci, S. A., Wallston, K. A., & Hummon, N. P. (1983). Assessment of patient satisfaction in activities of daily living using a modified Stanford Health Assessment Questionnaire. *Arthritis & Rheumatism, 26,* 1346–1353.

Platz, P., Winter, T., Müller, N., Pinkowski, C., Eikhof, C., & Mauritz, K. (2001). Arm ability training for stroke and traumatic brain injury patients with mild arm paresis: a single-blink, randomized, controlled trial. *Archives of Physical Medicine and Rehabilitation, 82,* 961–968.

Purnell, L. D., & Paulanka, B. J. (2005). *Guide to culturally competent health care.* Philadelphia: F. A. Davis Company.

Raina, K. D., Rogers, J. C., & Holm, M. B. (2007). Influence of the environment on activity performance in older women with heart failure. *Disability and Rehabilitation, 29,* 545–557.

Raschko, B. B. (1991). *Housing interiors for the disabled and elderly.* New York: Von Nostrand Reinhold.

Rice, V. (Ed.). (1998). *Ergonomics in health care and rehabilitation.* Boston: Butterworth-Heinemann.

Robertson, L. (1996). Clinical reasoning, Part 1: the nature of problem solving, a literature review. *British Journal of Occupational Therapy, 59,* 178–182.

Rogers, J. C. (1982). The spirit of independence: The evolution of a philosophy. *American Journal of Occupational Therapy, 36,* 709–715.

Rogers, J. C. (1983). The Eleanor Clarke Slagle Lecture: Clinical reasoning: The ethics, science, and art. *American Journal of Occupational Therapy, 37,* 601–616.

Rogers, J. C. (2004). Occupational diagnosis. In M. Molineux (Ed.). *Occupation for occupational therapists* (pp. 17–31). Oxford, UK: Blackwell.

Rogers, J. C., & Holm, M. B. (1989). The therapist's thinking behind functional assessment, I. In C. Royeen (Ed.). *Assessment of function: An action guide* (pp. 1–29). Rockville, MD: American Occupational Therapy Association.

Rogers, J. C., & Holm, M. B. (1991). Task performance of older adults and low assistive technology devices. *International Journal of Technology and Aging, 4,* 93–106.

Rogers, J. C. & Holm, M. B. (1994a). Accepting the challenge of outcome research: Examining the effectiveness of occupational practice. American Journal of Occupational Therapy, 48, 871–876.

Rogers, J. C., & Holm, M. B. (1994b). *Performance Assessment of Self-Care Skills, Version 3.1.* Unpublished instrument, University of Pittsburgh, Pittsburgh.

Rogers, J. C., Holm, M. B., & Stone, R. G. (1997). Evaluation of daily living tasks: The home care advantage. *American Journal of Occupational Therapy, 51,* 410–422.

Rogers, J. C., Holm, M. B., Burgio, L. D., Granieri, E., Hsu, C., Hardin, J. M., & McDowell, B. J. (1999). Improving morning care routines of nursing home residents with dementia. *Journal of the American Geriatrics Society, 46,* 1049–1057.

Rogers, J. C., & Holm, M. B. (2000). Daily living skills and habits of older women with depression. *The Occupational Therapy Journal of Research, 20,* 68S–85S.

Rogers, J. C., Holm, M. B., Burgio, L. D., Hsu, C., Hardin, J. M., & McDowell, B. (2000). Excess disability during morning care in nursing home residents with dementia. *International Psychogeriatrics, 12,* 267–282.

Rogers, J. C., Holm, M. B., Beach, S., Schulz, R., Cipriani, J., Fox, A., & Starz, T. W. (2003). Concordance of four methods of disability assessment using performance in the home as the criterion method. *Arthritis & Rheumatism (Arthritis Care & Research), 49,* 640–646.

Rogers, J. C., & Masagatani, G: (1982). Clinical reasoning of occupational therapists during the initial assessment of physically disabled patients: A pilot study. *Occupational Therapy Journal of Research, 2,* 195–219.

Royeen, C. B., Zardetto-Smith, A. M., Duncan, M., & Mu, K. (2001). What do young school-age children know about occupational therapy? An evaluation study. *Occupational Therapy International, 8,* 263–272.

Sager, M. A., Dunham, N. C., Schwantes, A., Mecum, L., Halverson, K., & Harlowe, D. (1992). Measurement of activities of daily living in hospitalized elderly: A comparison of self-report and performance-based methods. *Journal of the American Geriatric Society, 40,* 457–462.

Schaafstal, A., Schraagen, J., & van Berlo. (2000). Cognitive task analysis and innovation of training: The case of structured troubleshooting. *Human Factors, 42*(1), 75–86.

Schkade, J. K., & Schultz, S. (1992). Occupational adaptation: Toward a holistic approach for contemporary practice, part 1. *American Journal of Occupational Therapy, 46,* 829–837.

Schultz, S. & Schkade, J. K. (1992). Occupational adaptation: Toward a holistic approach for contemporary practice, part 2. *American Journal of Occupational Therapy, 46,* 917–925.

Seki, K., Ishiai, S., Koyama, Y., & Sato, S. (1999). Unassociated responses to two related task demands: A negative factor for improvement of unilateral spatial neglect. *Neuropsychologia, 37*(1), 75–82.

Sevim, S., Dogu, O., Camdeviren, H., Kaleagasi, H., Aral, M., Arslan, E., et al. (2004). Long-term effectiveness of steroid injections and splinting in mild and moderate carpal tunnel syndrome. *Neurology Science, 25,* 48–52.

Slagle, E. C. (1922). Training aides for mental patients. *Archives of Occupational Therapy, 1,* 11–17.

Stamps, A. E. (2000). Evaluating architectural design review. *Perceptual & Motor Skills, 90,* 265–271.

Steptoe, A., Cropley, M., & Joekes, K. (2000). Task demands and the pressures of everyday life: Associations between cardiovascular reactivity and work blood pressure and heart rate. *Health Psychology, 19*(1), 46–54.

Stewart, D. L., & Abeln, S. H. (1993). *Documenting functional outcomes in physical therapy.* St. Louis: Mosby.

Strong, S., Rigby, P., Stewart, D., Law, M., Letts, L., & Cooper, B. (1999). Application of the person-environment-occupation model. *Canadian Journal of Occupational Therapy, 66,* 122–133.

Tack, B. B. (1991). *Dimensions and correlates of fatigue in older adults with rheumatoid arthritis.* Unpublished doctoral dissertation, University of California at San Francisco, San Francisco.

Taub, E., Miller, N. E., Novack, T. A., Cook, E. W., Fleming, W. C., Nepomucena, C. S., Connell, J. S., & Crago, J. E. (1993). Technique to improve chronic motor deficit after stroke. *Archives of Physical Medicine and Rehabilitation, 74,* 346–354.

Trombly, C. (1993). Anticipating the future: Assessment of occupational function. *American Journal of Occupational Therapy, 46,* 253–257.

Trombly, C. (1995). Occupation: Purposefulness and meaningfulness as therapeutic mechanisms. [Eleanor Clarke Slagle Lecture]. *American Journal of Occupational Therapy, 49,* 960–972.

Trombly, C., & Wu, C. (1999). Effect of rehabilitation tasks on organization of movement after stroke. *American Journal of Occupational Therapy, 53,* 333–344.

Uniform Data System for Medical Rehabilitation [UDSMR]. (1997). *Guide for the Uniform Data Set for Medical Rehabilitation (including the FIM instrument (Version 5.1).* Buffalo: State University of New York.

van Heugten, D., Dekker, J., Deelman, B., van Dijk, A., Stehmann-Saris, J., & Kinebanian, A. (1998). Outcome of strategy training in stroke patients with apraxia: A phase II study. *Clinical Rehabilitation, 12,* 294–303.

Verbrugge, L. M. (1990). The iceberg of disability. In S. M. Stahl (Ed.). *The legacy of longevity: Health and health care in later life* (pp. 55–75). Newbury Park, CA: Sage.

Vertesi, A., Darzins, P., Lowe, S., McEvoy, E., & Edwards, M. (2000). Development of the Handicap Assessment and Resource Tool (HART). *Canadian Journal of Occupational Therapy, 67,* 120–127.

Wachs, T. D. (1999). Celebrating complexity: Conceptualization and assessment of the environment. In S. L. Freidman & T. D. Wachs (Eds.), *Measuring environments across the lifespan: Emerging methods and concepts* (pp. 357–392). Washington, DC: American Psychological Association.

Walker, B. Jr., Goodwin, N., & Warren, R. C. (1995). Environmental health and African Americans: Challenges and opportunities. *Journal of the National Medical Association, 87*(2), 123–129.

Weinstock-Zlotnick, G., & Hinojosa, J. (2004). Bottom-up or top-down evaluation: Is one better than the other? *American Journal of Occupational Therapy, 58,* 594–599.

Williams, J. H., Drinka, T. J. K., Greenberg, J. R., Farrel-Holtan, J., Euhardy, R., & Schram, M. (1991). Development and testing of the Assessment of Living Skills and Resources (ALSAR) in elderly community-dwelling veterans. *Gerontologist, 31,* 84–91.

Wood, W. (1996). Legitimizing occupational therapy's knowledge. *American Journal of Occupational Therapy, 50,* 626–634.

Woodward, A., Hales, S., Litidamu, N., Phillips, D., & Martin, J. (2000). Protecting human health in a changing world: The role of social and economic development. *Bulletin of the World Health Organization, 78,* 1148–1155.

World Health Organization. (1980). *International classification of impairments, disabilities, and handicaps: A manual of classification relating to the consequences of disease.* Geneva: Author.

World Health Organization [WHO]. (2001). *International classification of functioning, disability and health (ICF).* Geneva: Author.

Wu, C., Trombly, C. A., Lin, K., & Tickle-Degnen, L. (1998). Effects of object affordances on reaching performance in persons with and without cerebrovascular accident. *American Journal of Occupational Therapy, 52,* 446–456.

Wu, C., Trombly, C. A., Lin, K., & Tickle-Degnen, L. (2000). A kinematic study of contextual effects on reaching performance in persons with and without stroke: influences of object availability. *Archives of Physical Medicine and Rehabilitation, 81,* 95–101.

Yakobina, Y., Yakobina, S., & Tallant, B. K. (1997). I came, I thought, I conquered: Cognitive behavior approach applied in occupational therapy for the treatment of depressed (dysthymic) females. *Occupational Therapy in Mental Health, 13*(4), 59–73.

Yerxa, E. J., Burnett-Beaulieu, S., Stocking, S., & Azen, S. P. (1988). Development of the Satisfaction with Scaled Performance Questionnaire (SPSQ). *American Journal of Occupational Therapy, 42,* 215–222.

Yu, F., Hwang, S., & Huang, Y. (1999). Task analysis for industrial work process from aspects of human reliability and system safety. *Risk Analysis, 19,* 401–415.

Critiquing Assessments

JANICE MILLER POLGAR

Learning Objectives

After reading this chapter, you will be able to:

1. Describe a format for critiquing assessments in occupational therapy and apply it in practice
2. Describe the process of construction of a standardized test
3. Describe five benefits of a standardized test over a nonstandardized test
4. Define reliability and critique evidence of reliability relevant to a specific assessment
5. Define validity and critique evidence for it relevant to a specific assessment
6. Describe issues related to fair testing practices and apply them in practice

Evaluation has two main purposes in the practice of occupational therapy: as part of the therapy process to aid the determination of occupational performance issues (Townsend et al., 2002) and to provide support for the evidence base of our profession (Hamer & Collinson, 1999; Sackett, Straus, Richardson, Rosenberg, & Haynes, 2000). When a standardized assessment is used, it is crucial that the occupational therapist has critiqued it to determine its appropriateness for the individual or group to be evaluated as well as the purpose of the evaluation. As part of an occupational therapy practice process, it is important to review the underlying theoretical construct of the test to establish its congruence with the frame of reference that is guiding intervention (Townsend et al., 2002). The occupational therapist must ensure that the method of test development, standardization, development of norms, and **psychometric properties** meet an acceptable standard when determining the test's **clinical utility**. This chapter provides an understanding of why it is important to critically appraise these assessments and discuss each component of a thorough appraisal.

The primary purpose of this chapter is to inform occupational therapists of the purposes of **evaluation** and the necessity of critiquing the assessments we use in our practice. A framework will be presented to organize the critique. Issues of test development and standardization, reliability and validity, and the influence of age, culture, and disabilities on test use will be presented. This chapter is meant to provide sufficient information to enable an adequate appraisal of assessments used in occupational therapy. It is not meant to provide a detailed discussion of the various statistical analyses that are involved in test development or establishment of psychometric properties. Sources for more detailed information are identified at the end of the chapter. In the literature, various labels are used to identify a measurement tool, including *test, instrument, evaluation, measurement,* and *assessment.* Either *assessment, instrument,* or *test* will be used in this chapter. *Evaluation* in this chapter refers not to a test instrument but to the whole process of assessing a client.

MEASUREMENT

Measurement is the process of assigning numbers to represent quantities of a trait, attribute, or characteristic, or to classify objects (Nunnally & Bernstein, 1994). It enables therapists to understand aspects of clients' function, abilities, or personal characteristics. An important distinction here is that measurement enables therapists to quantify attributes of individuals but not individuals themselves (Nunnally & Bernstein). It provides a means to operationally define behaviors and, by quantifying these behaviors, to make comparisons between individuals or to compare the same person at two different times (Dunn, 2001).

Some fundamental assumptions of measurement are critical to an understanding of the properties of psychometrically sound instruments (Dunn, 2001). The definition of measurement presented in the foregoing paragraph assumes that psychological, sociological, and biological functions are observable and thus measurable. A second assumption is that what is observable and quantifiable corresponds to aspects of human behavior. Third, it is assumed that these attributes have a normal distribution in the population, a concept that will be discussed later. Finally, it is assumed that some traits are relatively stable across time while others are expected to change.

PURPOSES OF EVALUATION IN OCCUPATIONAL THERAPY

Tests are used in different ways, depending on the purpose of a given evaluation. Three main purposes have been identified for evaluation (Jackowski & Guyatt, 2003). The first purpose is discriminative. When the occupational therapist's intent is to describe individuals within a group or to discriminate between members of a group, an instrument should be chosen that measures the desired attribute comprehensively (Law, 1987). For example, if an occupational therapist is interested in describing a child's ability to operate a powered wheelchair, the instrument should measure all components that are considered necessary for this task.

A second purpose is to predict either future function or function in a related area (Jackowski & Guyatt, 2003). The occupational therapist might be interested in understanding the relationship between performance on a measure of motor skills in infancy and subsequent performance

on a test of fine motor skills at the age of 5 years. Alternatively, the therapist might be interested in determining the relationship between achievement of a certain score on a vocational test and function on the job site.

Finally, occupational therapists use measurement to evaluate outcomes of therapeutic intervention. In this instance, it is important to use an instrument that will detect change that has occurred (Jackowski & Guyatt, 2003). Two situations are important here. In the first, evaluation of intervention with a single client helps to determine the client's response to treatment. In the second, cumulative evidence of the outcome of intervention provides support for occupational therapy practice.

Whether an instrument is used for discriminative purposes, to predict function, or to evaluate outcome, the results of testing are used to guide decisions (Dunn, 2001). For example, we determine a person's suitability for returning to work or to his or her community, whether a person should receive assistive technology, or whether a person is safe to continue to drive or not. We also make decisions about the efficacy of our practice. These decisions have important implications for the lives of our clients and our practice. Because of the importance of our decisions, it is crucial that occupational therapists critique assessments to confirm that they are selecting an appropriate test.

CRITIQUING ASSESSMENTS

An outline to guide the critique of an instrument can be seen in Box 47.1.

Theoretical Context of Assessment

Some theoretical perspective guides each occupational therapist's approach to intervention, whether it is explicit or tacit. In selecting an assessment, it is important to consider whether the theoretical foundation of the assessment is congruent with that of the therapist. Subsequent sections will describe the process of test development in which one step is to describe the construct to be measured by the test and the related domain of concern. This information provides the user with an understanding of the test developer's theoretical perspective.

Why is it important to determine a test's underlying construct and the evidence that the scores are indeed reflective of that construct? Let's consider a situation in which a therapist is assessing a child with a motor problem. The therapist's frame of reference views motor planning, an executive function, as the foundation of the motor problem. An available test of motor function is based on the premise that motor difficulties are due to a lack of opportunity to engage in physical activities, including factors such as parental involvement in sport and the existence of organized activity programs within the community, to choose an extreme example. The resulting scores on the

BOX 47.1 A FRAMEWORK FOR CRITIQUING ASSESSMENTS

1. Is the purpose of the assessment to:
   - Describe the client's current level of function?
   - Evaluate the client's response to service delivery?
   - Predict future function?
   - Evaluate an intervention program?
2. Theoretical frame of reference
   - Is the underlying construct of the test congruent with the clinician's frame of reference?
   - What information does it provide?
   - Is the information obtained meaningful and relevant to the client population?
3. Clinical utility
   - Is the test readily available and easy to use?
   - Are specific qualifications required to administer the test?
   - Can the test be administered in a reasonable amount of time?
   - Is the test difficult to learn to use?
   - What is the test format?
   - What are the test procedures?
   - What is the response format (e.g., motor or verbal response)?
   - Is the test easy to score?
4. Technical considerations
   a. Norms
      - What type of score is obtained (e.g., percentile rank, standard score)?
   - What are the characteristics of the standardization sample?
   - What were the standardization procedures?
   Reliability: What evidence exists to support?
   - Test-retest reliability?
   - Interrater reliability?
   - Alternative form reliability?
   - Internal consistency of the test?
   b. Validity: What evidence exists to support the construct relative to:
      - Content?
      - Internal structure?
      - Response processes?
      - Relationship to external variables?
5. Fair testing issues: How did the test developers address potential bias issues related to:
   - Culture?
   - Language?
   - Age?
   - Disability?
6. External review comments
   - What information is available from published evaluations of the test?
7. Summary of strengths and weaknesses of the test

test might lead the therapist to recommend that the parents become more involved in sport with their child or lobby for more organized physical activity programs within their community. While these outcomes are not necessarily bad, they illustrate the point that if the test does not provide information that is relevant to the frame of reference that guides the therapist, the intervention that follows will not be specific to the identified occupational performance issues, which may then lead to an unsatisfactory outcome.

Clinical Utility

Occupational therapy service delivery faces increasing demands for efficiency and economy of time management. Realistically, only tests that help the clinician to meet these demands will be used in practice. **Clinical utility** is defined as ease, efficiency, and use of a test and the clinical relevance and meaning of the information that it provides (Law,

King, & Russell, 2001; Letts et al., 1999). A framework was described to evaluate the clinical utility of a test (Barlow & Miller Polgar, 2002). It proposed six areas that should be considered with respect to clinical utility. The framework was modified for this chapter to include (1) availability of test and ease of use, (2) administration time, (3) clinician's qualifications, (4) aspects related to learning the test, (5) format, (6) test procedures, (7) response format, and (8) scoring. With the exception of the first point, all of this information should be in the test manual. It can also be found in published reviews of the test (see the end of the chapter for sources of these reviews), and a brief description should also be available from the test publisher. Discussion of each element follows.

Test Construction

The test manual should describe the manner in which the test was constructed. It should give sufficient information for the individual who is evaluating the test to be able to determine whether it was developed in a logical, systematic, and stringent fashion.

Defining the Construct

The current *Standards for Psychological and Educational Measurement* (American Educational Research Association [AERA], American Psychological Association [APA], & National Council on Measurement in Education [NCME], 1999) define a *construct* as the concept, characteristic, or behavior that a test is designed to measure. Because there are many ways of understanding a construct, the test developers must articulate their understanding of the construct and its content domain. Furthermore, they should articulate some theoretical structure to the construct that is grounded in relevant literature (Wilson, 2005).

Item Development

Development of the test items is an involved process, detailed discussion of which is beyond the scope of this chapter. For our purposes, it is important to start with the definition of the construct, as defined by the test developer. The process of developing and selecting test items and the response format (e.g., rating scale, forced-choice response) can then be reviewed. The following should be considered: (1) item definition and selection process, (2) the process of determining the response format, (3) the method of establishing congruence of items with total test (e.g., factor analysis or investigation of internal consistency), and (4) the design of the research process for making revisions to test structure, items, and response format. These issues will be described further in subsequent sections of this chapter.

Scales of Measurement

There are four scales of measurement: nominal, ordinal, interval, and ratio (Pedhazur & Schmelkin, 1991; Portney & Watkins, 2000). The *nominal scale* involves mutually exclusive categories (e.g., female versus male, geographic location). This scale simply identifies differences with no attempt to quantify or order those differences.

A second level is the *ordinal scale.* This scale involves rank-ordering scores. The order indicates greater (or better) than, but no inference can be made about the magnitude of the difference between scores. *Interval scales* are a third level. This type of scale is the most common in measures found in occupational therapy. The intervals between scores are equal so that comparisons can be made between individuals (Pedhazur & Schmelkin, 1991). However, 0 is not an absolute point on these scales. Because 0 is arbitrary, ratio comparisons between scores cannot be made (Pedhazur & Schmelkin; Portney & Watkins, 2000). For example, if person A scores 20 on a test of self-esteem and person B scores 40 on the same test, it is not meaningful to

say that person B has twice as much self-esteem as person A. To make this comparison meaningfully, 0 would have to be a fixed point.

On *ratio scales,* 0 does have a fixed point, and ratio comparisons can be made (Pedhazur & Schmelkin, 1991). To use these scales, absence of the attribute being measured must be meaningful. In measuring volume, a score of 0 indicates the absence of liquid. In occupational therapy, range of motion can be understood as a ratio scale, as there can be absence of measurable movement around a joint, and it is meaningful to indicate that a person has gained twice as much movement between measurements.

Development of Norms

Many of the tests that occupational therapists use are norm-referenced (Anastasi & Urbina, 1997; Murphy & Davidshofer, 1998). Norms are statistics that are generated from a well-defined group that has been evaluated using the test in a standardized manner (Bolton, 2001; Salvia & Ysseldyke, 2004). Usually, but not necessarily, norms are measures of the average performance of this reference group. These statistics are used to make comparisons between the individual who is being tested and this reference group (i.e., the norms provide a point of reference for comparison of the individual's score).

It is crucial to understand that the norms provided in the manual are not *the* definitive norms (Murphy & Davidshofer, 1998). They represent the performance of the individuals who were tested for the development of the norms. The usefulness of the norms for making a meaningful interpretation of an individual's score is dependent on the information that is given about the characteristics of the **sample** used to create the norms, the method of recruiting the sample, and the degree to which the sample represents the test's target **population**.

At some point in the development of the test, a target population is identified (Murphy & Davidshofer, 1998; Salvia & Ysseldyke, 2004). The population defines the group for whom the test is intended. The test manual should clearly state the intended target population. Before using a test, the therapist must determine that it is intended to evaluate people with characteristics similar to those of the client.

Salvia and Ysseldyke (2004) describe three main issues that are relevant in determining the usefulness of the norms related to the target population: They should be representative, relevant, and recent. The sample *represents* the target population when the distribution of critical characteristics of the population is reflected in the sample. A test that is targeted for national (or international) use must demonstrate that the norms were developed to represent the distribution of region, urban or rural living, gender, ethnicity, and any other relevant characteristics of the national or international population (Murphy & Davidshofer, 1998; Salvia & Ysseldyke, 2004). A test that is intended to provide information about performance at different ages must use a sample including individuals of each age.

The test manual should include clear information about the selection of the normative sample (AERA, APA, & NCME, 1999). Random-sampling procedures should be used that involve selection based on the distribution of the characteristics of the population identified, not convenience (Salvia & Ysseldyke, 2004). The sample size should be sufficient to minimize measurement errors and to maximize the confidence the test user has in the norms provided.

The normative sample should be *relevant* to the target population (Salvia & Ysseldyke, 2004). It should have characteristics similar to the population. For example, norms that have been developed from the motor performance of adults are of little use in providing a meaningful interpretation of the motor performance of preschoolers.

Finally, norms should be *recent* (Salvia & Ysseldyke, 2004). Test material can become dated. For example, consider a picture vocabulary test. It is unlikely that children today will correctly identify a picture of a typewriter—not because they do not have the vocabulary to give a correct response but because a typewriter is no longer a common object and it is not within the children's experience to recognize it. Over time, performance or attributes may change in the population. Twenty years ago, many executives had little or no keyboarding skills and so would have performed poorly on tests measuring this ability. Now, with the pervasive use of computers, the ability to input keystrokes is a more universal skill.

Standardized Scores

Raw scores are usually converted into another form to facilitate comparison and a meaningful interpretation. These forms include percentiles, *z*-scores, *t*-scores, stanines, and age- or grade-equivalent scores (Murphy & Davidshofer, 1998; Salvia & Ysseldyke, 2004). These will be discussed below, but first, some basic statistical concepts related to test scores will be reviewed briefly. There are three measures of central tendency: mean, median, and mode. The *mean* is the arithmetic average of the cumulative measures (Murphy & Davidshofer, 1998; Portney & Watkins, 2000). The *median* is the point in the distribution of the scores that divides the scores in half (i.e., 50% are above the median and 50% are below it). The *mode* is the most frequently occurring score (Portney & Watkins, 2000). It is important to know which of these measures of central tendency is being reported.

For a given population, scores are considered to be distributed normally. In the *normal distribution,* the bulk of the scores are at the center of the range, with fewer scores found at the extremes of the range (Portney & Watkins, 2000). The *range* of the distribution is the span between the lowest score and the highest score (Portney & Watkins, 2000). The *variance* indicates the dispersion of the scores

(Portney & Watkins, 2000). *Standard deviation* (SD) is the square root of the variance and is the most common method of dividing the normal distribution. It represents the spread of the scores in the same units as the test score (Salvia & Ysseldyke, 2004). Approximately 68% of the scores fall within −1.0 and +1.0 SD, 95% fall within −2.0 and +2.0 SD, and 99% fall within −3.0 and +3.0 SD (Portney & Watkins, 2000).

Standard scores use the standard deviation to obtain a scale with equal intervals. There are several forms of standard scores. A *z*-score has a mean of 0 and a standard deviation of 1 and is used to plot the area under the curve of the normal distribution (Hogan, 2003); *t*-scores are standardized scores with a mean of 50 and a standard deviation of 10 (Hogan, 2003). The *percentile rank* is expressed as a whole number between 1 and 99. The number represents the percentage of test takers who scored at or below a given score (Portney & Watkins, 2000; Salvia & Ysseldyke, 2004). An individual whose score is at the 75th percentile performed as well as or better than 75% of those tested. Percentile rank is an ordinal scale so the intervals between the ranks are not equal (Salvia & Ysseldyke, 2004). It is considered to have a normal distribution, with the majority of the scores falling around the 50th percentile (Portney & Watkins, 2000).

Stanine is an abbreviated form of the term *standardnine* (Salvia & Ysseldyke, 2004). This method of standardizing scores divides the normal distribution into nine components, each making up one half of a standard deviation to provide equal units of measure. It minimizes a tendency to overinterpret small differences in scores, but it might not be sufficiently sensitive to detect small changes (Salvia & Ysseldyke, 2004).

Age- or grade-equivalent scores relate the individual's performance on the test to that of the typical individual of a particular age or grade (Murphy & Davidshofer, 1998). It is crucial that the sample that is used to create the norms has sufficient representation of the comparison grades or ages.

Standardized Tests

In clinical practice, both standardized and nonstandardized tests are used. **Standardized tests** are assumed to have undergone a rigorous development process and are administered and scored in a prescribed manner. Of course, review of the rigor of the standardization process is critical. Nunnally and Bernstein (1994) identify five advantages of standardized tests: (1) They provide an objective means of measuring a specific construct; (2) the construct is operationally defined and can be quantified; (3) communication among professionals who use the test is enabled by a common understanding of the construct; (4) when appropriate, a therapy aide can administer a standardized assessment, reducing the cost of the administration; and (5) generalization of the results is facilitated by a well-constructed standardized test. Without standardization, there is no assurance that it measures the construct it is intended to measure, that the scores are reliable, or that sources of variation in the derived scores are minimized.

Test Standardization

Because of the effect that decisions from test scores have on people's lives, it is important that as many extraneous factors as possible are eliminated from the method of administering, scoring, and interpreting the scores (Murphy & Davidshofer, 1998). Test standardization procedures are used to ensure the maximum level of consistency in testing situations.

The test manual should clearly describe the arrangement of the testing environment, the presentation of materials, standardized instructions, and time limits (AERA, APA, & NCME, 1999). When the test developers have made modifications to any of these areas to accommodate individuals with different abilities, these modifications should be clearly indicated so that they can be replicated in appropriate situations. Moreover, the manual should include clear guidelines for scoring the test and interpreting the scores (AERA, APA, & NCME, 1999).

It is not possible to standardize all aspects of test administration. Aspects of the environment, such as noise, or individual factors such as the examinee's mood at the time of testing are not controllable. Because of these uncontrollable factors, which can affect the reliability of the test score, it is important to follow the standardized instructions of the test exactly. Failure to do so will influence the reliability of the test scores (AERA, APA, & NCME, 1999). It is also important to ensure that the test user is adequately trained or prepared to administer the test. Many tests indicate the type of training that is necessary for administration. Indeed, some tests are not available except to people who hold the necessary qualifications.

RELIABILITY

Definition of Reliability

First, let's consider the general definition of reliability. A standardized test used to evaluate the performance of an individual or to measure the existence of a specified trait yields a score. It is important to demonstrate that the score resulting from the use of a test is consistent and repeatable. Consistency and repeatability are aspects of **reliability**, defined as "the consistency of . . . measurements when the testing procedure is repeated on a population of individuals or groups" (AERA, APA, & NCME, 1999, p. 25). Reliability is based on the correlation coefficient and referred to as a reliability coefficient. The reliability coefficient can range from 0 to +1, with 0 indicating no consistency and +1 indicating perfect consistency.

Theoretical Perspectives of Reliability

Two theoretical perspectives concerning reliability will be considered here: classical test theory and generalizability theory (Thompson, 2003). Classical test theory suggests that a test score has two components—the true score and measurement error—and that while there are many sources of error, only one is estimated with any given study. Generalizability theory also recognizes different sources of error and attempts to quantify the error from those various sources. A third perspective, item response theory, is not considered in this chapter.

Both generalizability theory and classical test theory assume that each person has a true score (Hogan, 2003). In classical test theory, this true score is assumed to be stable across various situations; that is, the true score is independent of the testing context (Portney & Watkins, 2000). In contrast, generalizability theory assumes that the true score and testing conditions are not independent and that certain factors (called *facets*) influence the true score. In other words, the variation across test administrations is not considered to be solely random error from a generalizability perspective.

Classical Test Theory

A test score is considered to be reliable when similar results are achieved under various situations, such as repeated administrations, different raters, and when there is consistency among the items on a test. Classical test theory assumes that a test score consists of three components: (1) the obtained scored; (2) the true score variance, considered to be a hypothetical, unobservable quantity of the specific attribute under consideration (Portney & Watkins, 2000); and (3) random error. The relationship between these components is expressed as follows:

$$\text{obtained score} = \text{true score variance} + \text{random error}$$

In other words, every obtained score is made up of two components: a portion of the score that reflects the "true" quantity of an attribute and random errors that contribute to inconsistency in the measurement (Murphy & Davidshofer, 1998). It is assumed that no relationship exists between true scores and the error component (Murphy & Davidshofer, 1998). Reliability is high when the proportion of the obtained score due to measurement error is low.

Generalizability Theory

Cronbach, Gleser, Nanda, and Rajaratnum (1972) introduced generalizability theory, which recognizes a variety of sources of error variance and provides a means to estimate these in a single study. Generalizability theory assumes that the derived test score is one of a number of possibilities within a universe of scores obtained under equivalent testing conditions and specifies these testing conditions.

Interclass correlation (ICC) is used to estimate the variance from a variety of sources with a single administration using analysis of variance. With this analysis, it is possible to calculate variance due to specified facets as well as the interaction between these facets. Identification of the facet of interest is crucial when conducting this analysis. Different models are used to determine the ICC, and it is important to understand the structure of these models and to determine whether they were applied appropriately in a reliability study. A full discussion of ICC is beyond the scope of this chapter; however, Portney and Watkins (2000) provide an excellent discussion of this topic.

Sources of Error Variance

Thorndike (2001) identified six sources of variation that can contribute to measurement error. *Lasting general characteristics* are individual characteristics that are expected to be stable over a time that are not specific to the construct being measured, such as literacy or fluency. *Lasting specific characteristics* are personal attributes, stable over a long period of time, that are specific to the construct being measured, such as previously acquired knowledge or skills such as ability to respond to multiple choice items (Murphy & Davidshofer, 1998). These affect performance on the test as a whole or on specific subsets of a test. *Temporary general characteristics* are nonspecific personal aspects that are present in the short term, such as fatigue or emotional state (Murphy & Davidshofer, 1998; Thorndike, 2001). *Temporary specific characteristics* are short-term qualities that are specific to a test, such as recognition of a pattern of correct responses or response to unintentional clues in the test format (Thorndike, 2001).

Administration and appraisal of test performance sources stem from issues related to the assessor, such as familiarity or training and adherence to test standardization; issues related to the testing environment, such as distractions, time limits, or length of assessment; and issues related to the standardization and construction of the test. *Chance variance* derives from factors that are not systematic, such as incorrectly recording the examinee's response on a data collection form (Murphy & Davidshofer, 1998; Thorndike, 2001).

Types of Reliability

The reliability of a test score is important in three different situations: when the test is administered on more than one occasion, when comparable tasks are involved, and when the test is administered and scored by different raters. These forms of reliability are test-retest, alternative forms, and interrater reliability, respectively. A further form of reliability is referred to as *internal consistency,* which examines the structure or consistency of the items that compose a test.

Test-Retest Reliability

Test-retest reliability is a measure of the consistency of an assessment over time. It has also been termed *stability* (Salvia & Ysseldyke, 2004), as it estimates the stability of the measurement over time. This form of reliability is determined by administering an evaluation on two occasions separated by a time interval. Nunnally and Bernstein (1994) suggest that a desirable separation is two weeks. With a shorter time period, the examinee might remember the test items; with a longer time period, actual changes might occur (Hogan, 2003). A correlation approaching +1.0 suggests that a test is stable across time.

Test-retest reliability or stability is meaningful only when the trait that is being measured is expected to be stable over the testing interval (AERA, APA, & NCME, 1999). An evaluation of mood, for example, is not expected to yield consistent results over a period of weeks, for mood is considered to fluctuate. Alternatively, a trait such as height is stable and should yield little variability in the obtained scores over repeated measurements. Many attributes that are measured in occupational therapy are not as clearly consistent or inconsistent as the examples just given. In each case, individuals considering the test must compare their understanding of the construct or attribute being measured with that described in the test manual to assess whether that attribute is stable and whether an indication of stability is essential.

Alternative Form Reliability

The establishment of reliability using alternative forms has some similarities to test-retest reliability, since it is estimated by testing the same group of people on two separate occasions (Hogan, 2003). However, it differs from test-retest reliability estimation with its use of two distinct but parallel forms of a test (Hogan, 2003). When estimating alternative form reliability, the test administration should occur about two weeks apart to account for day-to-day fluctuations in performance (Nunnally & Bernstein, 1994).

Occasionally, in occupational therapy treatment, a client's performance in a specific area must be evaluated repeatedly. Repeated administrations of the same instrument causes problems because the person might remember test items or practice them. Thus, repeated exposure to the same test might artificially inflate the obtained score. The use of parallel forms minimizes the influence that memory or practice can have on inflating the estimated reliability. These two forms should not differ in a substantive manner (Hogan, 2003).

Interrater Reliability

This form of reliability can be considered to be the consistency between scores assigned by different raters when using the same assessment at the same time or when observing the same behavior (Auerbach, Heft La Porte, &

Caputo, 2004). It is important to have confidence in the consistency between raters for both assessment and outcome evaluation of clinical practice.

The method of estimating interrater reliability is an important consideration in choosing a specific assessment. Simply calculating the correlation between scores assigned by different raters might overestimate reliability if the raters differ in a consistent manner (Auerbach et al., 2004). Cohen's kappa and the ICC are more appropriate statistical analyses (Portney & Watkins, 2000). Cohen's kappa measures the degree of agreement between raters by comparing the number of items for which agreement is found between raters with the number of items for which agreement is expected (Auerbach et al., 2004). Cohen's Kappa ranges from –1 to 1, with 1 indicating perfect agreement and 0 indicating agreement that occurs at the chance level. Application of the ICC here would specify "rater" as the facet of interest.

Internal Consistency

Internal consistency is an estimation of the homogeneity of the structure of a test. One that is intended to measure a single construct should have a high degree of internal consistency; that is, all test items should be highly correlated to each other. The simplest and crudest type of internal consistency is split-half reliability (Nunnally & Bernstein, 1994; Pedhazur & Schmelkin, 1991), in which reliability is determined by dividing the test items in half and obtaining the correlation between these two halves. The split-half method of estimating reliability is limited by the variety of ways of dividing the items that can result in different reliability coefficients (Hogan, 2003).

More sophisticated methods of estimating internal consistency take into account the correlation of each item with every other item as well as with the total score (Hogan, 2003; Nunnally & Bernstein, 1994; Pedhazur & Schmelkin, 1991). These inter-item and item-total correlations provide an estimate of how consistent the items are with each other. Items that do not correlate highly with other items or with the total test might measure a different construct.

The most common ways to estimate the internal consistency are through the use of Cronbach's alpha (Cronbach, 1951) or the Kuder-Richardson formulas (Kuder & Richardson, 1937). Cronbach's alpha is computed when the items are scored in a nondichotomous manner. When the scoring is dichotomous, the Kuder-Richardson formulas are used. For further information on the theory and calculations of internal consistency, refer to one of the books marked with an asterisk in the references at the end of this chapter.

Standard Error of Measurement

In instances when the therapist would like to understand how close the obtained score is to the true score for an individual, the estimates from group data can be used to calculate the standard error of measurement (SEM). The SEM indicates how much variability in the test scores can be attributed to error (Murphy & Davidshofer, 1998). As can be seen from the following equation, as reliability increases, the standard error of measurement decreases:

$$SEM = SD\sqrt{1 - r_{xx}}$$

In this equation, SD refers to the standard deviation of the group from which the reliability is calculated.

Once the SEM has been calculated, a confidence interval can be constructed around the obtained score. A *confidence interval* is defined as the range into which it can be stated with a specified degree of confidence that a certain score would fall (Portney & Watkins, 2000). The degree of confidence is determined from the properties of the normal distribution. To calculate a confidence interval, the precise SD that corresponds to 95% of the distribution, for example, must be used. Thus, from the normal distribution, 95% of the scores fall within –1.96 and +1.96 SD from the mean, and 99% fall within –2.54 to +2.54 SD from the mean (Anastasi & Urbina, 1997). To construct a 95% confidence interval, the SEM is multiplied by 1.96 (Murphy & Davidshofer, 1998). Thus, the true score is known, with 95% confidence, to fall between [obtained score –1.96(SEM)] and [obtained score +1.96(SEM)].

How High Should the Reliability Coefficient Be?

The question "How high should the reliability coefficient be?" does not have a ready answer. The purpose of the test should be considered when deciding whether the reliability reported is acceptable (Salvia & Ysseldyke, 2004). Tests that are used to make decisions about a person, such as determining whether he or she is capable of returning to work, should have a higher level of reliability than tests that are intended to serve as screening or descriptive instruments (Hogan, 2003; Murphy & Davidshofer, 1998; Salvia & Ysseldyke, 2004). Similarly, the instruments that attempt to categorize people, such as a test that is used to assign cognitive levels, should have a high degree of reliability (Murphy & Davidshofer, 1998).

The following minimal levels of reliability should be considered as guidelines. Generally, a reliability coefficient of .90 is considered to be high, 0.80 moderate, 0.70 low, and 0.60 generally unacceptable for clinical use (Murphy & Davidshofer, 1998). It is recommended that when a test score is to be used to make significant decisions about an individual, such as placement decisions, a minimum level of reliability of 0.90 should be reported (Salvia & Ysseldyke, 2004); Nunnally and Bernstein (1994) suggest .95 as desirable. If the test has been administered to a group and the data are reported for the group as a whole, a minimum level of 0.60 has been suggested (Salvia & Ysseldyke, 2004).

It should be clear from this discussion that reliability estimates are not fixed entities. When examining reliability during the decision to use a particular assessment, it is important to remember that the reliability reported reflects the specific situation and the sample used to collect the data. The potential test users must ensure that they understand the type of reliability that has been reported, the appropriate means of establishing that specific reliability, and its applicability for the purpose of the test. Table 47.1 summarizes this information.

VALIDITY

Definition of Validity

Contemporary understanding of validity is that it is a unitary concept and that the establishment of validity is the process of accumulating evidence to support the underlying construct that an evaluation is considered to measure (Cronbach, 1988; Messick, 1988, 1989, 1995). This notion is relevant not only to the interpretation of the test score but also to the social consequences of that interpretation. The current edition of *Standards for Educational and Psychological Testing* (AERA, APA, & NCME, 1999) defines **validity** as "the degree to which evidence and theory support the interpretations of test scores entailed by proposed uses of tests" (p. 9). Messick adds that validity is the "appropriateness, meaningfulness, and useful-

ness of inferences and actions based on test scores" (Messick, 1988, p. 33). Further, evidence for validity is concerned with the relevance and utility of scores for particular persons or groups and the significance of the value attributed to the score or underlying construct as they relate to the social consequences for the individual or group (Messick, 1988).

What conclusions can we draw from these defining statements? First, let's consider the ideas of appropriateness, meaningfulness, and usefulness, which are relevant to how the test is used and the consequences of the inferences made from interpretation of the scores. Appropriateness refers to the question of whether the construct and elements of the test are suitable for the target population and the context and purpose of the evaluation. Meaningfulness is associated with the articulation of the underlying construct and how it explains or describes the trait being measured. Finally, usefulness is concerned with the utility of the test in terms of the information that is gained from the test results in consideration of the effort required to undertake the test. Evidence of validity, as it provides support for the underlying construct, is necessary to justify a particular test with a specific population in a given context.

These statements are very clear that it is not the test that has validity. Rather, validity relates to the interpretations and actions derived from the resulting scores (Messick, 1988, 1989, 1995). Both empirical and theoretical evidence of validity are required to provide support for these interpretations and actions. Thus, an assessment must be based on a well-founded or articulated theoreti-

TABLE 47.1 A SUMMARY OF THE TYPES OF RELIABILITY, THEIR APPLICATION, AND SOURCES OF VARIABILITY RELATED TO EACH

Type of Reliability	Provides Evidence For	Sources of Variability
Test-retest	Stability	Length of time between testing stability of trait measured Memory of test items Actual change in trait measured
Alternative form	Equivalence of parallel forms (equivalence and stability if forms are administered at two times)	Ability to generate parallel forms
Interrater	Consistency across raters	Adherence of tester to scoring Adequacy of description of scoring criteria
Internal Consistency: Split-half	Homogeneity of items	Method of splitting items Length of test Consistency of content of test
Cronbach's alpha Kuder-Richardson	Homogeneity of items	Consistency of content of test

cal construct, and there should be empirical evidence to support the hypotheses derived from the theory. Otherwise, the inferences made from the test scores are without meaning and are not justifiable.

Further, these definitions suggest a variety of uses of the test results. Consequently, evidence of validity must be provided for each of the intended uses. When first using an assessment, the occupational therapist must be very clear on its intended use. How will the test score be interpreted and how will that interpretation affect the client's life? Is the therapist's intended use of the assessment congruent with that articulated by the test developers? Is the therapist's theoretical approach to intervention congruent with the theoretical foundation of the test? The answers to these questions will influence the appropriateness, meaningfulness, and usefulness of inferences made from the test scores.

Before a discussion of sources of validity evidence, two threats to validity will be described. These are construct underrepresentation and construct irrelevance (AERA, APA, & NCME, 1999: Messick, 1989, 1995). *Construct underrepresentation* refers to an inadequate sampling of the construct domain in the test items; that is, content is missing (AERA, APA, & NCME, 1999; Messick, 1989, 1995). The resulting interpretation of the score is not comprehensive, because the test did not tap some content, underlying processes, or response means that are important to the understanding of the construct.

Construct irrelevance is present when test scores are influenced by processes or abilities that are not pertinent to the construct (AERA, APA, & NCME, 1999; Messick, 1988, 1995). Here, the person who is being evaluated must have a certain level of ability, skill, or knowledge, extraneous to the construct being measured, in order to make a response or achieve a satisfactory score. A valid interpretation of a low score cannot be made because it cannot be determined whether the score reflects performance on the construct or some other ability. An example of this type of variance is a test of arithmetic ability that requires reading comprehension to complete the problems satisfactorily.

Evidence of validity comes from examination of different aspects of the test and performance in different situations. Synthesis and analysis of available studies related to each of the following dimensions helps the test user to construct an argument concerning relevant validity.

Evidence of Validity

Evidence of Validity Derived from Content

The current *Standards for Educational and Psychological Testing* refer to content as themes, wording, item format, response method, and guidelines for procedures for administration and scoring (AERA, APA, & NCME, 1999). In other words, not only does the actual content of the test items provide important evidence, but so do the processes that underlie the respondent's interpretation of the items

and the response format. Construct representativeness is interpreted here as how well the content of the evaluation represents the hypothesized content domain and structure. Construct relevancy considers how relevant the content, means of interpretation, and response format are to the construct.

Validation of the content of a test begins at the test development stage. As was described previously, the initial stages of test construction begin with a clear articulation of the theory underlying the construct. Theoretical ideas operationally define the construct, that is, what behaviors are considered to be indicators of the construct (Pedhazur & Schmelkin, 1991), and hypothesize the structure and elements of the construct and the relationship among them (Messick, 1988, 1989). From here, a table of specifications is developed to guide the content, the item difficulty, and the proportions of the test that represent particular dimensions of the theoretical construct to be represented on the test.

Validation of the content is derived from consideration of the sampling of the construct domain, that is, that all aspects of the domain are adequately covered, content is relevant to the construct, and the underlying processes necessary for satisfactory interpretation of test items and response are also relevant (AERA, APA, & NCME, 1999; Messick, 1988, 1989). One means of gathering this evidence is through the examination of the content by a panel of experts to determine relevance and representativeness. For example, consider an instrument that is designed to measure performance in activities of daily living (ADL). The test developers articulate their understanding of the construct of ADL, create items that are considered to measure ADL performance, and assemble these in an assessment. A panel of occupational therapists who are considered experts review the assessment. Their analysis provides evidence for content representativeness and relevance.

When a test is used with a population that is different from the one for which it was originally intended or for a different purpose, the test user must examine the content to determine that it is appropriate for that population or purpose. In particular here, issues of relevance are important. The test user must determine whether any aspects of test administration, item interpretation, or response format are a source of bias for their purpose or population (AERA, APA, & NCME, 1999; Messick, 1988, 1989, 1995).

Inferences of low scores that are based on content can only suggest that the respondent was not competent in taking the test. The interpretation that the individual is incompetent on the underlying skill or has inadequate knowledge cannot be made. Other sources of variance might have contributed to this low score (Messick, 1989).

Evidence from Test Structure

To compile evidence from the structure of the test, it is necessary to examine the relationship of the hypothesized structure of the construct to the structure of the assessment (AERA, APA, & NCME, 1999; Messick, 1989). This examination is completed through empirical analysis of the relationship between the items (interitem) and to the total score (AERA, APA, & NCME, 1999). If the conceptual framework suggests that the underlying construct is unidimensional, then analysis of the relationship between the items should reveal a single dimension. Alternatively, if a multidimensional structure is hypothesized, then analysis should support this structure with multiple dimensions of content that are distinct from each other and congruent with the structure that was hypothesized from the theory. More simply put, if the construct is hypothesized to have three dimensions, analysis should reveal three factors. Items that load on those factors should have content that is congruent to articulation of the construct. Additionally, the scoring structure should reflect the theorized dimensionality of the construct (Messick, 1989).

Evidence from Response Processes

Part of the hypotheses of the construct includes the underlying processes that are necessary for indicating the intended response (AERA, APA, & NCME, 1999). Examination of how respondents arrive at a response provides evidence for this element of the validity argument. For example, a professional certification examination might be hypothesized to require clinical reasoning to achieve a correct response. It is only through examination of an individual's approach to answering questions on this examination that evidence is provided to support or refute this hypothesis.

The issue of construct irrelevance is important here. As was indicated previously, evidence must be provided that the means of deriving an answer and indicating a response are relevant to the construct. This evidence is important during test construction, but, more important for occupational therapists, it is necessary when considering a test that was not developed for the population or purpose for which the therapist intends. Evidence must be provided that these elements of validity are not a source of bias for our clients.

Evidence from the Relationship to External Variables

When examining the relationship to other variables, we are considering the "extent to which the test's relationship with other tests and nontest behavior reflects the expected high, low and interactive relations implied in the theory of the construct being assessed" (Messick, 1989, p. 45). Here, we are looking for convergent evidence (i.e., the test is highly related to other tests or nontest behavior that is theoretically related to the construct) or divergent evidence (i.e., the test is not related to other tests or nontest behavior that is theoretically not related to the construct). Both convergent and divergent evidence provide necessary information for our understanding of the theoretical construct and our ability to measure it. This evidence is derived from empirical studies.

Historically, there are two types of studies that are important here (AERA, APA, & NCME, 1999): predictor and concurrent studies. Predictor studies provide evidence that performance on the test predicts performance on a criterion later in time. Clinically, such evidence is useful to guide decisions on who will benefit from a given intervention. Concurrent studies provide evidence of the relationship between the test and a given criterion at the same point in time. Such studies are useful when examining different methods for measuring the same construct or when analyzing a client's behavior or abilities (AERA, APA, & NCME, 1999).

Examination of the relationship to other variables provides information about group differences. It may support predicted differences between groups with different characteristics, suggesting that the meaning of the score is different for members of different groups (AERA, APA, & NCME, 1999). It is important to provide evidence that the differences are congruent with hypotheses derived from the construct and not due to some source of construct irrelevance.

Another construct that is important when considering evidence of validity is responsiveness. When a measure is used to evaluate outcomes, either individually or cumulatively, evidence of responsiveness is important (Guyatt, Walter, & Norman, 1987). *Responsiveness* is defined as the ability of a test to detect a change that is considered to be clinically meaningful and important relative to a client's function following intervention (Guyatt et al., 1987; Jackowski & Guyatt, 2003; Liang, 2000; Patrick & Chiang, 2000). What specifically constitutes a clinically meaningful and important change can be difficult to determine. Liang (2000) suggested that gathering the perspectives of the client, significant others, and the clinician is important in the determination of a clinically meaningful change.

Social Consequences

There is some debate as to whether consideration of the social consequences of inferences and actions based on a test score are relevant to the validity argument (Lees-Haley, 1996; Messick, 1988, 1989, 1995; Zimiles, 1996). However, both Messick (1988, 1989, 1995) and the current *Standards for Educational and Psychological Testing* (AERA, APA, & NCME, 1999) make a compelling argument that these consequences need to be considered in the evaluation process, although they do not, in and of themselves, provide evidence for the validity argument. Social consequences refer to the implications that inferences that are made and actions that are taken from the test score have for the life of the individual who is being tested. High-stakes testing (Haertel, 1999) involves assessment in which the results have significant implications for the life of the individual, such as access to education, treatment, or a career; the value associated with a labeling derived from the score; and costs that result from actions based on the score. How are these important for occupational therapists?

When we assess a client, we do so from a particular theoretical framework, tacit or otherwise. This framework guides what we measure, the meaning given to a score, and the interpretation. Furthermore, it influences the label that results; for example, performance on certain measures of motor performance result in the child being labeled as having developmental coordination disorder. It is important to recognize the value associated with a label and whether the value has positive or negative connotations in the lives of our clients.

Results of our assessment guide who will receive intervention and the theoretical ideas of change resulting from therapy guide indicators of when therapy should cease. There are implications here for costs, both actual and in time and effort, for the therapist and client. Given the economic state of many health care systems, the evidence to support decisions related to where therapy efforts will be directed, in what manner, and for how long is crucial.

Constructing the Validity Argument

The preceding discussion of various sources of evidence concerning the validity of inferences and actions based on test scores suggests a dynamic and continuing process. An initial argument to support the use and interpretation of test scores is constructed from the available evidence. However, subsequent studies could provide information that weakens the initial argument when hypothesized relationships are not supported or new sources of construct irrelevance are uncovered. This fluidity underscores the importance for occupational therapists of examining evidence to determine that the proposed use of the test is appropriate and that the interpretation of the scores can be made with some degree of confidence. Table 47.2 identifies different elements that contribute to the validity argument, the information they provide and methods used to build evidence for statements about validity.

FAIR TESTING PRACTICES

It is the responsibility of the test user to take whatever measures are possible to minimize bias in testing for particular groups. Because the outcome of occupational therapy evaluation has implications not only for the lives of our clients but also for the distribution of scarce health care dollars, we must seriously consider whether an assessment is fair for our clients and what extraneous variables might influence their scores. The *Standards for Educational and Psychological Testing* (AERA, APA, & NCME, 1999) describes four aspects of **fair testing**, reflecting the idea that testing does not need to be identical for all groups but that there should be evidence that interpretation of the score is valid, without undue influence of construct underrepresentation or irrelevance (AERA, APA, & NCME, 1999). Sources of bias should be identified and eliminated, where feasible, so that they do not alter the meaning of scores obtained by our clients. When bias cannot be removed satisfactorily, the assessment should not be used. All clients should be treated in an equitable manner with respect to the context and purpose of the test and the way in which the test scores are used and should have a reasonable opportunity or means to demonstrate their competence on

---

TABLE 47.2   SUMMARY OF THE EVIDENCE FOR VALIDITY RELATED TO DIFFERENT ASPECTS OF TEST CONTENT, RESPONSE PROCESSES, STRUCTURE, AND RELATIONSHIP TO EXTERNAL VARIABLES

Evidence	Information	Method of Determination
Content	Content adequately samples the domains of the construct and reflects the hypothesized structure	Support for content is found in the literature and expert opinion
Response processes	The means of deriving and indicating a response are congruent with construct hypotheses	Examination of how the respondent forms and indicates a response
Test structure	Structure of the test, e.g., dimensions or scores congruent with that of underlying construct	Examination of relationship of items to each other and with total test
Relationship to external variables	Test scores relate to other measures or nontest behaviors as predicted by theoretical construct	Empirical studies of hypothesized relationships

the construct measured. Differences in outcomes across groups do not necessarily mean that one group is disadvantaged relative to another. However, such differences need to be examined to determine whether such a situation is present. Finally, all groups should have a similar opportunity to learn or practice knowledge or behaviors measured by the test (AERA, APA, & NCME, 1999). For our purposes, three specific instances of fair testing practices will be considered: culture, seniors, and people with disabilities.

When discussing changes to a test that are intended to enhance fair testing practice, a distinction is made in some sources concerning accommodation versus modification of assessments (Education Accountability Act, 2000; Individuals with Disabilities Education Act Amendments, 1997). Accommodations are considered to be changes that enable a person to participate in an assessment but do not alter content, performance requirements, response method, reliability, or validity (Ministry of Education, 2000). Modifications, by contrast, are more significant changes to the assessment and do have implications for reliability, validity, and subsequent inferences made from obtained scores.

Culturally Fair Evaluation

In many countries, cultural diversity is increasing. Occupational therapists may be required to assess an individual whose first language is not the official language of the country. There are two main issues here: the influence of a native language other than English on interpretation of and response to test items and the influence of cultural expectations, behaviors, and values on test performance (AERA, APA, & NCME, 1999; Padilla, 2001).

Even within North America, among people whose first language is English, there is a disparity of culture (Padilla, 2001). The life experience of people living in remote areas of the Arctic is vastly different from that of individuals living in urban areas, and both are different from the experiences of many people of color.

Language can significantly confound the results that are obtained on an assessment. When the assessment requires a verbal response or when the test items contain a substantial verbal component, the test may measure language ability more than the underlying construct (AERA, APA, & NCME, 1999). The intelligibility of the test items and instructions for individuals whose first language is not English must be determined (Springer, Abell, & Hudson, 2002).

One seemingly obvious means to minimize the language issue is to directly translate the test. However, this approach is not as useful as it would appear, as language is dynamic, filled with cultural and historical context (Hambleton & Patsula, 1998). Many words or phrases do not have the same meaning when translated from one language to another. For example, in French, *poser un lapin à quelqu'un* means "to stand someone up." This phrase translates in English as "to lay a rabbit on someone," which

creates quite a different visual image than the French meaning. The naming of common objects differs, even among English-speaking cultures. For example, in Britain, *nappy, petrol,* and *bonnet* refer to a diaper, gasoline, and the hood of a car, respectively. Similarly, concepts may differ between cultures.

Behavioral expectations vary from one culture to another (AERA, APA, & NCME, 1999). Children in one culture might be discouraged from responding directly to an adult or from engaging in a detailed conversation, as it is considered rude (Salvia & Ysseldyke, 2004). If the assessment requires expression of ideas, children of this culture are likely to perform poorly, not because their ideas are ill-formed but because of their cultural expectations.

People from cultures in which speed is not emphasized, as it is in North America, will not perform as well on a timed test. The actual test situation might be unfamiliar for people from some cultures (Hambleton & Patsula, 1998). The very act of placing people into a testing situation can put them at a disadvantage. Similarly, some people might not be familiar with completion of computer-marked response cards, so the means of indicating a response in this situation requires skills or exposure to media that are not universal.

The foregoing discussion illustrates the complexity of the issue of performing assessments with individuals of a culture different from the one for which the instrument was standardized. The *Standards for Educational and Psychological Testing* (AERA, APA, & NCME, 1999) present several standards to minimize the potential disadvantage to individuals of a diverse culture. These standards and the recommendations from other writers that follow recognize that it is not generally feasible to create a test that can be considered free of cultural bias. It is the ethical responsibility of the examiner to ensure that measures have been taken to minimize the cultural bias (AERA, APA, & NCME, 1999).

The *Standards for Educational and Psychological Testing* recommend that tests and their use for non-English speakers or for people who speak certain English dialects "should be designed to reduce threats to the reliability and validity of test score inferences that may arise from language differences" (AERA, APA, & NCME, 1999, p. 97). The ability of non-English speakers to understand the test items or instructions should be ascertained, perhaps through the administration of practice items (Hambleton & Patsula, 1998). When language or other modifications have been made to tests that were originally developed in English, information should be provided in the test manual to document those modifications and their influence on the psychometric properties of the test.

Critiquing Assessments for Older Adults

Little attention has been paid in the psychometric literature to the issues related to assessment of older adults. Yet this group is a growing segment of our population, with estimates suggesting that over 21% of Canadians will be over the age of 65 years by 2026 (Statistics Canada, 2001) and 78 million Americans will be over this age by 2050 (Rosenbloom, 2004). This group represents a significant proportion of the clients for whom occupational therapists provide service.

First, let's consider some of the personal issues that will influence an older adult's performance on a standardized test. Many of these issues are well documented in the literature, so they will simply be identified here. Changes in physical function and the incidence of physical disabilities increase with age. A survey of physical limitations identified that people 75 years of age and older were the most likely to report the presence of three or more disabilities (Statistics Canada, 2002). Vision changes include difficulty in low-light situations, loss of visual acuity, and slowed visual scanning, along with impairments such as cataracts, glaucoma, and macular degeneration (Owsley, 2004). Cognitive issues include loss of memory, attentional difficulties, and dementia. Affective concerns include anxiety related to the testing situation and depression.

World views, life experiences, and goals may differ between the client and the clinician or test developer (Mouton & Esparza, 2003). These have the potential to affect the client's interpretation of the purpose of the test and the specific items that make up the test. Issues that were identified previously about response to testing and interpretation of test items, based on culture and life experience, are relevant to this discussion.

A final personal issue is one that is perhaps less recognized. The issue of social consequences was discussed earlier in reference to validity. With older adults, social consequences refer to decisions that significantly affect their lifestyle. Two situations illustrate this point. The outcome of a driving assessment might be the loss of the legal right to drive, leading to negative consequences for the driver and family (Suen & Sen, 2004). Similarly, results of a functional or competency assessment may influence whether a senior can remain in his or her own home or must give up that independence and enter supported living. It is very obvious, then, that seniors facing assessment might bring fears to the situation about the consequences to their lifestyle and the meaning of those consequences to their self-concept.

Issues related to the test itself can be inferred from the previous discussion. When selecting an assessment to use with a senior, the clinician should appraise its appropriateness for this age group (e.g., did the normative sample include seniors?). The content should be examined for bias related to expected knowledge and literacy level. Consideration of the response format should include whether it is reasonable to expect that the client will have sufficient recent experience to provide an answer. Cultural issues also need to be examined. Physical issues of test such as font and layout can affect performance. Time constraints may be a source of anxiety.

The testing situation can also be a source of bias. It is important to ensure that sufficient lighting is available and that the client is comfortably positioned. The test administrator should ensure that the testing environment is as supportive as possible.

Issues in the Evaluation of People with Disabilities

Because of the nature of our profession, the clients whom we assess typically have some form of disability. As with the use of tests with people of diverse cultures and older adults, the issues here are complex, and the solutions are often incomplete. Individuals with disabilities may have impairments that affect their ability to perceive test instructions or materials, process information related to formation of a response, or indicate a response through verbal or motor means (Hacker & Porter, 1987; Salvia & Ysseldyke, 2004; Taylor, Sternberg, & Richards, 1995). Further, a mental health issue might limit the client's ability to engage in the testing situation (Taylor et al., 1995).

The *Standards for Educational and Psychological Testing* (AERA, APA, & NCME, 1999), recommend that people who modify any test for use with an individual with a disability do so with the assistance of an individual who is an expert in psychometrics. Furthermore, the test user should have knowledge about the manner in which the disability might affect the reliability and validity of the inferences of the test score. As always, these changes should be reported in the test manual.

When conducting assessments with children with disabilities in the school system, occupational therapists must know the regulations that govern such assessment. Two examples of these regulations will be described: Individuals with Disabilities Education Act Amendment of 1997 (P.L. 105-17) and the Education Accountability Act in the province of Ontario, Canada. Both pieces of legislation require that students with disabilities be afforded the opportunity to participate in provincial or state standardized testing. Assessment must be conducted in such a way that the score can be meaningfully interpreted to reflect the child's performance on the underlying construct and not be biased by some variable, irrelevant to the construct, such as language or motor ability (Education Accountability Act, 2000; IDEA, 1997).

Both IDEA (1997) and the Education Accountability Act (2000) indicate that modifications or accommodations are to be used as appropriate, provided that there is evidence of reliability and validity with the specific modifications. Specific modifications include changes to time requirements, format of administration or response, language, setting, and individual or group administration. Specific accommodations include alteration of test administration (e.g., large print, Braille translation, interpreter for the hearing impaired, multiple sessions) response method (e.g., oral response, use of computer access devices), and setting (e.g., segregated area) (*Federal Register*, 1999; Ministry of Education, 2000).

This discussion of the challenges of evaluating clients in a fair manner underlines the responsibility of the therapist. Satisfactory validity evidence must be present to support the intended purpose of the test, interpretation of the scores, and actions that arise from that interpretation. Particularly when the outcome of the evaluation has the potential to influence education, employment, or living situation, the therapist must be able to demonstrate the validity of the inferences that are made from the score.

SOURCES OF INFORMATION ON PUBLISHED TESTS

This chapter has provided an overview of issues with which an occupational therapist must be familiar to critique an assessment. A number of sources are available that provide reviews of published tests. The *Mental Measurements Yearbooks* provide reviews of most commercially available tests. Test reviews are available online at http://burros.unl.edu/buros/jsp/search.jsp. *Tests in Print* (e.g., Murphy, Plake, Impara, & Spies, 2002) provides descriptive information and bibliographies. An excellent source of test information that is specific to occupational therapy is *Measuring Occupational Performance: Supporting Best Practice in Occupational Therapy* (Law, Baum, & Dunn, 2001)

This chapter was meant to be an overview of the critical concerns in the critique of assessments. It was not intended to include a detailed discussion of the various aspects, formulas, or calculations of test construction, item analysis, reliability, and validity. For further information, the books on the reference list marked with asterisks (*) provide more detailed information and, frequently, reviews of assessments commonly used in occupational therapy.

CASE STUDY: *Application of Critiquing Assessments Framework to the FIM™ Instrument*

Note: This review of the FIM™ instrument is for illustrative purposes only and is not intended to be an exhaustive review of the literature related to this test.

Purpose of the Test

The FIM™ instrument is a measure of function and disability based on the concept of burden of care (Hamilton, Granger, Sherwin, Zielezny, & Tashman 1987). It is used to describe current function, predict future function and discharge destination, and evaluate a client's response to intervention (Timbeck & Spaulding, 2003). It is part of the Uniform Data System for Medical Rehabilitation (USDMR) (Deutsch, Fiedler, Granger, & Russell, 2002).

Theoretical Frame of Reference

The FIM™ instrument is based on the concept of burden of care. Disability is rated according to how much assistance a person requires to perform daily activities (Hamilton et al., 1987). It is intended for an adult rehabilitation population and provides information on motor and social aspects of function.

Clinical Utility

Information: Information about the FIM™ instrument is available from the Uniform Data System for Medical Rehabilitation: www.udsmr.org.
Qualifications: Facilities that wish to be part of the (USDMR) must be accredited. Clinicians who administer the FIM™ instrument within an accredited facility must take a training course and pass a test.
Support for learning: Workshops are available for clinicians who will administer the test within an accredited facility. For others, training materials, including videos, are available.
Test format: The FIM™ instrument has 18 items in six areas: self-care, sphincter control, mobility, locomotion, communication, and social cognition. Individual items are rated from 1 (total dependence) to 7 (full independence) with a total score range of 18–126. The first four areas form the motor subscale, and the last two form the cognitive subscale.
Test procedures: Information is obtained through direct observation, interview, or chart review.
Administration time: The FIM™ instrument takes approximately 30 minutes to administer.
Response format: Both motor and verbal responses are required.
Scoring: Score derived from observation of performance, interview, or chart review. Guidelines, case studies, and decision trees are available to support determination of rating.

Technical Considerations

Norms: No norms are available, but performance profiles can be obtained (Letts & Bosch, 2001)

Continued

CASE STUDY: *Application of Critiquing Assessments Framework to the FIM™ Instrument* *Continued*

Reliability: Analysis of 11 studies investigating reliability found high interrater reliability with stronger correlations for motor subscales than for cognitive subscales. Correlations were strong for test-retest and equivalent forms reliability (Ottenbacher, Hsu, Granger, & Fiedler, 1996). Examination of internal consistency supports the structure of the FIM™ instrument (Hobart et al., 2001; Hsueh, Lin, Jeng, & Hsieh, 2002).

Validity: Research consistently supports a strong relationship with the Barthel Index (Deutsch et al., 2002; Hobart et al., 2001; Hsueh et al., 2002). The FIM™ instrument is consistently found to be responsive to change in functional status for a CVA in-patient rehabilitation population (Desrosier et al., 2003; Dromerick, Edwards, & Diringer, 2003; Hseuh et al., 2002). The admission FIM™ instrument score was found to be a strong predictor of discharge FIM™ instrument score, disability rating, dis-charge rating, and discharge location (MacNeill & Lichtenberg, 1998; Timbeck & Spaulding, 2003).

Fair-Testing Issues

Observation of required activities can occur in a variety of settings or conditions, allowing for administration of the FIM™ instrument in an environment that is supportive for the client. The instrument can be administered to any rehabilitation client regardless of age or disability. Individuals who use assistive technology to complete daily activities cannot receive a maximum score whether they require assistance from another person or not (Minkel, 2002).

Reviewer's Comments

The FIM™ instrument is a widely used tool that is excellent for program evaluation in a rehabilitation setting. The psychometric properties are strong, making it a good first choice as an outcome measure in a variety of settings (Letts & Bosch, 2001)

ACKNOWLEDGMENTS

A special thank you to Jill Jacobson, School of Occupational Therapy, The University of Western Ontario, who provided meticulous editing and endless support in the preparation of the current version of this chapter. Jennifer Landry, Ph.D. student, University of Toronto, and Linda Miller, School of Occupational Therapy, The University of Western Ontario, provided valuable feedback on an earlier draft of this chapter. Joseph Hansen, Detroit Country Day School, provided French language consultation.

REFERENCES

American Educational Research Association, American Psychological Association, & National Council on Measurement in Education. (1999). *Standards for educational and psychological testing.* Washington, DC: American Psychological Association.

Anastasi, A., & Urbina, S. (1997). *Psychological testing* (7th ed.). Upper Saddle River, NJ: Prentice Hall.

Auerbach, C., Heft La Porte, H., & Caputo, R. K. (2004). Statistical methods for estimate of interrater reliability. In A. R. Roberts & K. R. Yaeger (Eds.), *Evidence-based practice manual: Research and outcome measures in health and human services* (pp. 444–448). New York: Oxford Press.

Barlow, I., & Miller Polgar, J. (2002). Measuring clinical utility of an assessment: The example of the Canadian Occupational Performance Measure. *Proceedings of the International Seating Symposium, 18,* 53–57.

Bolton, B. F. (2001). *Handbook of measurement and evaluation in rehabilitation* (3rd ed.). Gaithersburg, MD: Aspen.

Cronbach, L. J. (1951). Coefficient alpha and the internal structure of tests. *Psychometrika, 16,* 297–334.

Cronbach, L. J. (1988). Five perspectives on validity. In H. Wainer & H. Braun (Eds.), *Test validity* (pp. 3–17). Hillsdale, NJ: Lawrence Erlbaum Associates.

Cronbach, L. J., Gleser, G. C., Nanda, H., & Rajaratnum, N. (1972). *The dependability of behavioral measurements: Theory of generalizability for scores and profiles.* New York: John Wiley.

Desrosier, J., Rochette, A., Noreau, L., Bravo, G., Hébert, R., & Boutin, C. (2003). Comparison of two functional independence scales with a participation measure in post-stroke rehabilitation. *Archives of Gerontology and Geriatrics, 37,* 157–172.

Deutsch, A., Fiedler, R. C., Granger, C. V., & Russell, C. F. (2002). The Uniform Data System for Medical Rehabilitation report of patients discharged from comprehensive medical rehabilitation programs in 1999. *American Journal of Physical Medicine and Rehabilitation, 81,* 133–142.

Dromerick, A. W., Edwards, D. F., & Diringer, M. N. (2003). Sensitivity to changes in disability after stroke: A comparison of four scales useful in clinical trials. *Journal of Rehabilitation Research and Development, 40,* 1–8.

Dunn, W. (2001). Measurement issues and practices. In M. Law, C. Baum, & W. Dunn (Eds.), *Measuring occupational performance: Supporting best practice in occupational therapy* (pp. 43–56). Thorofare, NJ: Slack.

Education Accountability Act. (2000). Toronto, ON: Queen's Printer for Ontario.

Federal Register. (1999). C.F.R.34, Parts 300, 303.

Guyatt, G., Walter, S., & Norman, G. (1987). Measuring change over time: Assessing the usefulness of evaluative instruments. *Journal of Chronic Diseases, 40,* 171–178.

Hacker, B. J., & Porter, P. B. (1987). Use of standardized tests with the physically handicapped. In L. King-Thomas & B. J. Hacker (Eds.), *A therapist's guide to pediatric assessment* (pp. 35–40). Boston: Little, Brown.

Haertel, E. (1999). Validity arguments for high-stakes testing: In search of evidence. *Educational Measurement, 18,* 5–9.

Hambleton, R. K., & Patsula, L. (1998). Adapting tests for use in multiple languages and cultures. *Social Indicators Research, 45,* 153–171.

Hamer, S., & Collinson, G. (1999). *Achieving evidence-based practice: A handbook for practitioners.* Edinburgh: Baillère Tindall.

Hamilton, B. B., Granger, C. V., Sherwin, F. S., Zielezny, M., & Tashman, J. S. (1987). A uniform national data system for medical rehabilitation. In M. J. Fuhrer (Ed.), *Rehabilitation outcomes: Analysis and measurement* (pp. 137–147). Baltimore: Brookes.

Hobart, J. C., Lamping, D. L., Freeman, J. A., Langdon, D. W., McLellan, D. L., Greenwood, R. J., et al. (2001). Evidenced-based measurement: Which disability scale for neurologic rehabilitation? *Neurology, 57,* 639–644.

Hogan, T. P. (2003). *Psychological testing: A practical introduction.* New York: John Wiley and Sons.

Hsueh, I. P., Lin, J. H., Jeng, J. S., & Hsieh, C. L. (2002). Comparison of the psychometric characteristics of the Functional Independence Measure, 5 item Barthel Index and 10 item Barthel Index in patients with stroke. *Journal of Neurology, Neurosurgery & Psychiatry, 73,* 188–190.

Individuals with Disabilities Education Act Amendments of 1997. U.S.C.A. §600 et seq.

Jackowski, D., & Guyatt, G. (2003). A guide to health measurement. *Clinical Orthopaedics and Related Research, 413,* 80–89.

Kuder, G. F., & Richardson, M. (1937). The theory of the estimation test reliability. *Psychometrika, 2,* 151–160.

Law, M. (1987). Measurement in occupational therapy: Scientific criteria for evaluation. *Canadian Journal of Occupational Therapy, 54,* 133–138.

Law, M., Baum, C., & Dunn, W. (2001). *Measuring occupational performance: Supporting best practice in occupational therapy.* Thorofare, NJ: Slack.

Law, M., King, G., & Russell, D. (2001). Guiding decisions about measuring outcomes in occupational therapy. In M. Law, C. Baum, & W. Dunn (Eds.), *Measuring occupational performance: Supporting best practice in occupational therapy* (pp. 31–40). Thorofare, NJ: Slack.

Lees-Haley, P. R. (1996). Alice in validityland, or the dangerous consequences of consequential validity. *American Psychologist, 51,* 981–983.

Letts, L., & Bosch, J. (2001). Measuring occupational performance in basic activities of daily living. In M. Law, C. Baum, & W. Dunn (Eds.), *Measuring occupational performance: Supporting best practice in occupational therapy* (pp. 121–159). Thorofare, NJ: Slack.

Letts, L., Law, M., Pollock, N., Stewart, D., Westmoreland, M., Philpot, A., et al. (1999). *A programme evaluation workbook for occupational therapists: An evidence-based practice tool.* Ottawa, ON: CAOT Publications.

Liang, M. H. (2000). Longitudinal construct validity: Establishment of clinical meaning in patient evaluative instruments. *Medical Care, 38*(Suppl. II), II-84–II-90.

MacNeill, S. E., & Lichtenberg, P. A. (1998). Predictors for functional outcome in older rehabilitation patients. *Rehabilitation Psychology, 43,* 246–257.

Messick, S. (1988). The once and future issues of validity: Assessing the meaning and consequences of measurement. In H. Wainer, & H. Braun, (Eds.), *Test validity* (pp. 33–45). Hillsdale, NJ: Lawrence Erlbaum Associates.

Messick, S. (1989). Validity. In R. L. Linn (Ed.), *Educational measurement* (pp. 13–103). New York: Macmillan.

Messick, S. (1995). Validity of psychological assessment: Validation inferences from person's responses and performances as scientific inquiry into score meaning. *American Psychologist, 50,* 741–749.

Ministry of Education. (2000). *Individual education plans: Standards for development, program planning, and implementation.* Toronto, ON: Author.

Minkel, J. L. (2002). A controlled environment study of functional mobility skills. *Proceedings of the International Seating Symposium, 18,* 117–120.

Mouton, C. P., & Esparza, Y. B. (2003). Ethnicity and geriatric assessment. In J. J. Gallo, T. Fulmer, G. J. Paveza, & W. Reichel (Eds.), *Handbook of geriatric assessment* (3rd ed., pp. 13–27). Sudbury, MA: Jones & Bartlett.

Murphy, K. R., & Davidshofer, C. O. (1998). *Psychological testing: Principles and applications* (4th ed.). Upper Saddle River, NJ: Prentice Hall.

Murphy, L. L., Plake, B. S., Impara, J. C., & Spies, R. A. (Eds.). (2002). *Tests in print VI: An index to test, test reviews, and the literature on specific tests.* Lincoln, NE: Buros Institute of Mental Measurements.

Nunnally, J. C., & Bernstein, I. H. (1994). *Psychometric theory* (3rd ed.). Toronto, ON: McGraw-Hill.

Ottenbacher, K. J., Hsu, Y., Granger, C. V., & Fiedler, R. C. (1996). The reliability of the Functional Independence Measure: A quantitative review. *Archives of Physical Medicine and Rehabilitation, 77,* 1226–1232.

Owsley, C. (2004). Driver capabilities. *Proceedings of the Transportation Research Board of the National Academies, 27,* 44–55.

Padilla, A. M. (2001). Issues in culturally appropriate assessment. In L. A. Suzuki, J. G. Ponterotto, & P. J. Meller (Eds.), *Handbook of multicultural assessment: Clinical, psychological, and educational applications* (2nd ed., pp. 5–27). San Francisco: Jossey-Bass.

Patrick, D. L., & Chiang, Y. (2000). Measurement of health outcomes in treatment effectiveness evaluations: Conceptual and methodological challenges. *Medical Care, 38*(Suppl. II), II-14–II-25.

Pedhazur, E. J., & Schmelkin, L. P. (1991). *Measurement, design and analysis: An integrated approach.* Hillsdale, NJ: Lawrence Erlbaum Associates.

Portney, L. G., & Watkins, M. P. (2000). *Foundations of clinical research: Applications in practice* (2nd ed.). Upper Saddle River, NJ: Prentice Hall.

Rosenbloom, S. (2004). Mobility of the elderly: Good and bad news. *Proceedings of the Transportation Research Board of the National Academies, 27,* 44–55.

Sackett, D. L., Straus, S. E., Richardson, W. S., Rosenberg, W., & Haynes, R. B. (2000). *Evidence-based medicine: How to practice and teach EBM* (2nd ed.). Edinburgh: Churchill Livingstone.

Salvia, J., & Ysseldyke, J. E. (2004). *Assessment in special and inclusive education* (9th ed.). Boston: Houghton Mifflin.

Springer, D. W., Abell, N., & Hudson, W. W. (2002). Creating and validating rapid assessment instruments for practice and research: Part 1. *Research on Social Work Practice, 12,* 408–439.

Statistics Canada. (2001). *The 2001 census: CANSIM, Table 052-0001* [Electronic version]. Retrieved June 21, 2004, from http://www.statcan.ca/english/Pgdb/demo23a.htm

Statistics Canada. (2002). *A profile of disability in Canada, 2001: Tables.* Retrieved April 7, 2003, from http://www.statcan.ca/english/Ottawa/PS/Data

Suen, S. L., & Sen, L. (2004). Mobility options for seniors. *Proceedings of the Transportation Research Board of the National Academies, 27,* 97–113.

Taylor, R. L., Sternberg, L., & Richards, S. B. (1995). *Exceptional children: Integrating research and teaching* (2nd ed.). San Diego, CA: Singular Publishing Group.

Thompson, B. (Ed.). (2003). *Score reliability: Contemporary thinking on reliability issues.* Thousand Oaks, CA: Sage.

Thorndike, R. M. (2001). Reliability. In B. F. Boulton (Ed.), *Handbook of measurement and evaluation in rehabilitation* (3rd ed., pp. 29–48). Gaithersburg, MD: Aspen.

Timbeck, R., & Spaulding, S. (2003). Ability of the Functional Independence Measure to predict rehabilitation outcomes after stroke: A review of the literature. *Physical and Occupational Therapy in Geriatrics, 22,* 63–76.

Townsend, E., Stanton, S., Law, M., Polatajko, H., Baptiste, S., Thompson-Franson, T., et al. (2002). *Enabling occupation: An occupational therapy perspective* (2nd ed.). Ottawa, ON: CAOT Publications.

Wilson, M. (2005). *Constructing measures: An item response modeling approach.* Mahwah, NJ: Lawrence Erlbaum Associates.

Zimiles, H. (1996). Rethinking the validity of psychological assessment. *American Psychologist, 51,* 980–981.

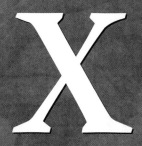

X

OT EVALUATION AND INTERVENTION: OCCUPATIONS

" ... the small experiences of everyday life and everyday occupation have complexity; beauty, meaningfulness, and relevance to health and well-being that belie their aura of ordinariness and routine. "

Betty Risteen Hasslekus

Activities of Daily Living and Instrumental Activities of Daily Living

48

ANNE BIRGE JAMES

Learning Objectives

After reading this chapter, you will be able to:

1. Describe the purposes of an occupational therapy ADL and IADL evaluation.
2. Given a client case, identify client and contextual factors that would influence the evaluation plan.
3. Develop individualized client goals that will drive the intervention process.
4. Describe contextual considerations that influence goal development.
5. Explain the most common approaches to ADL and IADL intervention.
6. Describe the role of client and caregiver education in treatment of ADL and IADL deficits.
7. Grade treatment activities to progress clients toward increased participation in ADLs and IADLs.

This section focuses on the evaluation and treatment of areas of occupation that are classified as activities of daily living (ADLs) and instrumental activities of daily living (IADLs) in the Occupational Therapy Practice Framework (OTPF) (American Occupational Therapy Association, 2002). Dysfunctions in ADLs and IADLs are termed *activity limitations* in the International Classification of Functioning, Disability, and Health (World Health Organization, 2001) framework. Evaluation and treatment of ADL and IADL dysfunction are central to individuals' participation in meaningful occupation. Individuals may value ADLs and IADLs as meaningful in and of themselves and as prerequisite tasks to meaningful engagement in education, work, play, leisure, and social participation.

DEFINITION OF ADL AND IADL

Conceptually, the term *activities of daily living* (ADLs) could apply to all activities that individuals perform routinely. In the OTPF, however, ADLs are defined more narrowly as "activities that are oriented toward taking care of one's own body" (AOTA, 2002, p. 620), which include 11 activity categories: bathing/showering, bowel and bladder management, dressing, eating, feeding, functional mobility, personal device care, personal hygiene and grooming, sexual activity, sleep/rest, and toilet hygiene. IADLs are defined as "activities that are oriented toward interacting with the environment and that are often complex in nature" (AOTA, 2002, p. 620). IADLs also include 11 activity categories: care of others, care of pets, child rearing, communication device use, community mobility, financial management, health and maintenance, home establishment and management, meal preparation and clean up, safety procedures and emergency responses, and shopping. Although both ADLs and IADLs include essential occupational performance tasks, IADLs are typically easier to delegate to another person (AOTA, 2002).

The OTPF (AOTA, 2002) provides a nomenclature and organizational scheme for occupational therapy practitioners in the United States. The OTPF's definitions of ADLs and IADLs are consistent with those of the National Center for Health Statistics (2007); however, other health care and social services practitioners or occupational therapists outside the United States might use other terms to refer to these same ADL and IADL concepts or use the same terms but define them differently. The term *ADL* is typically restricted to activities involving functional mobility (ambulation, wheelchair mobility, bed mobility, and transfers) and personal care (feeding, hygiene, toileting, bathing, and dressing), consistent with the OTPF, although some practitioners define *ADL* more broadly, referring to all activities that are performed in daily life. Other terms that are used to refer specifically to functional mobility and personal care are *basic ADL* and *personal ADL* respectively (AOTA, 2002). The term *IADL* appears outside the occupational therapy literature in a less consistent way. Measures of IADL vary considerably according to the activities that are included in the scales (Chong, 1995); for example, the Nottingham Extended Activities of Daily Living Scale includes leisure activities and feeding (Nouri & Lincoln, 1987), tasks that fall outside the OTPF definition of *IADL*. Synonyms for *IADL* are *independent living skills* and *extended ADL* (Nouri & Lincoln, 1987). More recently, the acronym AADL—for advanced activities of daily living—has come into use. The term AADL has also been used in different ways by various authors, for example, to capture activities that are more physically strenuous than IADLs (Reuben, Laliberte, Hiris, & Mor, 1990) or to refer to activities that are "volitional" rather than essential (Ashworth, Reuben, & Benton, 1994), such

as hobbies, recreation, and volunteer work (Moore, Endo, & Carter, 2003); these definitions are more in line with the OTPF concept of play or leisure. The crucial point is to understand that terms that refer to daily activities are used in variable ways, so it is important, in referring to written work, to look for operational definitions of terms used by authors and, in a clinical setting, to find out the conventional language used by practitioners. Occupational therapy practitioners need to be aware of the differences in terminology and use commonly accepted terms for the context when communicating with other professionals and when selecting assessment instruments.

This chapter focuses on the evaluation and treatment of occupational performance limitations specifically related to ADLs and IADLs as defined by the OTPF. It is essential to have a fundamental understanding of the occupational therapy process before reading this chapter; the process is described in Chapter 46. The reader should be aware that ADLs and IADLs, while often a primary focus of occupational therapy practice, do not typically represent the full complement of occupational performance tasks needed for satisfying and meaningful participation in individual and societal roles. Evaluation and treatment should always begin with a comprehensive occupational profile (AOTA, 2002). Treatment should address all of the client's priorities, which will typically extend beyond ADLs and IADLs, although the rest of this chapter will focus exclusively on ADLs and IADLs.

EVALUATION OF ADLS AND IADLS

Evaluation refers to the overall process of gathering and interpreting data needed to plan intervention, including developing an evaluation plan, implementing the data collection, interpreting the data, and documenting the evaluation results (AOTA, 1995). **Assessment** refers to the specific method that is used to collect data, which is one component of the evaluation process (AOTA, 1995). Standardized assessment methods are referred to as *assessment tools* or *instruments*. The evaluation is carried out by an occupational therapist; an occupational therapy assistant may participate in selected assessments under the supervision of an occupational therapist, who is responsible for interpreting assessment data for use in intervention planning.

The ADL/IADL evaluation is discussed in two stages in this chapter: (1) planning the evaluation, which includes selecting specific assessment methods, and (2) implementing the evaluation, which includes gathering assessment data, making critical observations, hypothesis generation, and ongoing revision of the evaluation plan until adequate data have been collected. Keep in mind that ADL and IADL evaluation is only one part of a more comprehensive occupational therapy evaluation, which should address all areas of occupation that are relevant to each client.

Evaluation Planning: Selecting the Appropriate ADL and IADL Assessments

Occupational therapists can choose from a variety of ADL and IADL assessments, designed to meet the varied needs of clients and treatment settings. Selecting an appropriate assessment will facilitate optimal treatment planning and can be initiated by following these steps:

1. Identify the overall purpose(s) of the evaluation.
2. Have clients identify their needs, interests, and perceived difficulties with ADLs and/or IADLs as part of the occupational profile.
3. Further explore the client's relevant activities so that the activities are operationally defined.
4. Estimate the client factors that affect occupational performance and/or the assessment process.
5. Identify contextual features that affect assessment.
6. Consider features of assessment tools.
7. Integrate the information from steps 1–6 to select the optimal ADL and IADL assessment tools.

In practice, the experienced occupational therapist completes this process quickly, so much of the ADL and IADL evaluation is completed in the first occupational therapy session. Also, although these steps appear to follow a linear progression, in practice the steps become integrated as the occupational therapist continually blends knowledge and experience with information from and about the client. For the developing therapist, however, it is helpful to explore each step independently to examine critical factors that contribute to the complex clinical reasoning process that is employed in planning an evaluation.

Step 1: Identify the Purpose of the ADL/IADL Evaluation

ADLs and IADLs may be evaluated for different purposes. At the level of individual client care, evaluation may be done to assess activity limitations to plan occupational therapy intervention or to facilitate decision making concerning discharge environment, competency, conservatorship, and/or involuntary commitment. At the programmatic level, evaluation may be done to document the need for program development and to appraise outcomes. Before starting an evaluation, the practitioner must determine how the information will be used so that appropriate and sufficient data are obtained. The extent of data gathering depends on the specific purpose for which the evaluation is being conducted.

EVALUATION TO PLAN AND MONITOR OCCUPATIONAL THERAPY INTERVENTIONS.   Before practitioners intervene to improve performance of ADLs or IADLs, they must evaluate clients' baseline performance. When an evaluation is conducted to plan occupational therapy intervention, certain types of data are needed (Rogers, Holm, & Stone, 1997). First, activities in which performance is deficient need to be identified so that intervention can focus on components that are dysfunctional while simultaneously maintaining and enhancing those that are functional. Second, data are needed about the cause or causes of the activity limitation. For example, a limitation in cooking might be caused by low vision, a wheelchair-inaccessible kitchen, or poor motivation to cook. Occupational therapy intervention for a limitation in cooking is different for each of these causes. To understand the etiology of an activity limitation, data about occupational areas (ADLs, IADLs) need to be supplemented with data about the client's performance patterns and skills, client factors, activity demands, and contexts. Third, the occupational therapy evaluation should provide data about the possibilities for modifying the client's activity performance. Information about the activity demands and context should include consideration of which aspects might be modifiable to support performance and which features cannot be changed. The potential to change performance patterns and skills or client factors must also be assessed. Interventions that involve skill acquisition are feasible for some clients, depending on the factors that are interfering with task performance. For example, a child with balance deficits secondary to cerebral palsy might have the potential to increase balance skills to support participation across several ADLs and IADLs, while a person with similar deficits from Parkinson's disease might not because the disorder is progressive. All three types of data are needed to devise adequate intervention plans.

EVALUATION TO FACILITATE DECISION MAKING ABOUT ELIGIBILITY OR DISCHARGE ENVIRONMENT.   Clients may also be referred for evaluation of ADLs and IADLs to facilitate decision making about eligibility or discharge environment. The ability to care for oneself and one's home can make the difference between independent and supported or assisted living. Supported living represents a continuum of options that includes in-home services (e.g., chore services), personal care assistants, assisted living centers, foster homes, group homes, independent living centers, supervised apartments, transitional apartments, and long-term care facilities. Varied levels of support are offered within these settings to maintain or enhance daily living skills. When ADLs and IADLs are evaluated to serve eligibility or discharge decisions, the evaluation may be less comprehensive and detailed than when it is done to plan individual interventions. The primary question to be answered through the evaluation is "Does the client meet the functional criteria?" This question can generally be answered by identifying activities in which limitations are present.

A somewhat similar evaluation objective occurs when occupational therapy practitioners are asked to make recommendations regarding legal competence for independent living. This usually involves competence in caring for oneself or competence in managing one's property. Difficulties with the first type of competence lead to legal proceedings called *guardianship,* whereas difficulties with the second type of competence involve *conservatorship.* Evaluation may also be requested in conjunction with involuntary commitments to psychiatric facilities to appraise the influence of psychiatric status on daily living. When competence is used in the legal sense, the capacity to make judicious or responsible decisions usually takes precedence over the capacity to perform activities. Individuals who have the ability to procure services and supervise caregivers in managing their personal care and living situation are viewed as competent, even though they might not be able to perform these activities themselves. Thus, occupational therapy evaluations that are conducted with guardianship, conservatorship, or involuntary commitment in mind must take into account the decisional capacities and supervisory skills needed by clients.

EVALUATION FOR PROGRAMMATIC USES. Although this chapter emphasizes evaluation for individual client care, it is important to recognize that data gathered about clients may be aggregated for programmatic purposes. For example, data about the ADL and IADL characteristics of clients who are served in an occupational therapy clinic can be used to document the extent of particular activity limitations and to support the development of new or expanded programs to manage them. In the current health care climate of cost-effectiveness and cost containment, group data are increasingly being used to evaluate the outcomes of occupational therapy programs and occupational therapy interventions. Occupational practitioners are often expected to measure and document ADL and IADL data consistently across clients so that they can be used effectively for program evaluation (Robertson & Colburn, 2000).

Step 2: Have Clients Identify Their Needs, Interests, and Perceived Difficulties with ADLs and/or IADLs

Once the purpose of the ADL/IADL evaluation has been determined, the occupational therapist must identify the specific activities to be evaluated. This is *one* component of the occupational profile, which will also encompass other aspects of occupational performance, including education, play, leisure, work, and social participation (AOTA, 2002). Developing the client's occupational profile is a crucial step in a client-centered evaluation, which enhances both the process and outcomes of occupational therapy (Law, 1998). A client-centered approach to ADL and IADL evaluation requires practitioners to begin by discovering the ADL and IADL problems of concern to the *client* (Law & Baum, 2005). Practitioners can expect the activities of concern to vary significantly for a 10-year-old elementary school student, a 29-year-old homemaker caring for three young children, and a 49-year-old business executive; and

the evaluations of these clients need to be tailored to take the clients' lifestyle differences into account. It is easy to make assumptions about a client's priorities, based on both clinical and personal experience and values; however, it is important to remember that unique circumstances may affect clients' selection of the ADLs or IADLs that they wish to address in treatment. Clients' perception of their ADL and IADL problems, needs, and goals can be gathered through a semistructured interview process or through a more formal assessment, such as the Canadian Occupational Performance Measure (COPM) (Law et al., 2005). The relative value of activities can be quantified by having clients rate the activities on a Likert scale on which, for example, 1 = "not at all important to perform effectively" and 10 = "crucial to perform." Alternatively, clients can be asked to rank a list of ADLs and IADLs in order of importance to identify priorities.

Step 3: Further Explore Clients' Relevant Activities So that the Activities Are Operationally Defined

The meanings of terms that are used for selected ADLs and IADLs can vary among individuals. Before activities can be evaluated, they must have an **operational definition**; that is, the occupational therapy practitioner and client must be clear on the precise meaning of each term. For example, meal preparation for a middle school student might consist of making cereal for breakfast and packing a lunch, whereas meal preparation for a homemaker feeding a family of five involves a much wider range of food preparation tasks and a very different set of skills. Because different assessment tools define activities differently, it is important to select an instrument that is congruent with the activities as defined by the client. For example, in using the Barthel Index to assess feeding, clients are rated "independent" if they can feed themselves, which includes cutting up food and spreading butter on bread (Mahoney & Barthel, 1965). Clients are rated as "needing assistance" if they can get food from the plate to the mouth but need help cutting food into bite-sized pieces. The Katz Index of ADLs, however, does not include preparation of food on the plate (e.g., cutting and spreading butter on bread) in the operational definition of feeding, so clients are rated independent if they can get food from the plate to the mouth, even if they cannot cut food or butter bread (Katz, Ford, Moskowitz, Jackson, & Jaffe, 1963). Many adolescents and adults would be dissatisfied with their feeding performance if their food had to be cut or their bread buttered by another person, so the Katz Index of ADL would not be an appropriate measure for individuals who consider cutting and buttering to be essential components of feeding.

The operational definitions of IADLs are more varied than those for ADLs because of their greater complexity. Consider the task of meal preparation. On the Instrumental Activities of Daily Living Scale (IADL Scale), which is generally considered to be the prototype assessment instrument for IADLs, the highest level of competence is described as "plans, prepares, and serves adequate meals independently" (Lawton, 1972, p. 133). Comparable items on the Nottingham Extended ADL Index examine the ability to make a hot drink and hot snack alone and easily (Nouri & Lincoln, 1987). Thus, a rating of independence in cooking achieved on the Nottingham Extended ADL Index implies a lower level of competence than does a rating of independence on the IADL Scale.

Occupational therapy practitioners also need to consider relevant performance parameters when planning an evaluation. **Performance parameters**, which are described in detail in Chapter 46, include independence, safety, and adequacy. Operational definitions of acceptable ADL and IADL performance should include attention to all relevant parameters in order to establish appropriate baseline data and intervention outcomes.

LEVEL OF INDEPENDENCE. Although clients often wish to be independent in ADLs and IADLs, practitioners should not make this assumption, as some level of assistance, either verbal or physical, might be acceptable. For example, a client who has had a total hip replacement may not don shoes and socks independently without adaptive equipment for two months postoperatively while movement restrictions are in place. Some clients who live with others might prefer to have assistance with this task rather than purchasing and using the required adaptive equipment. As long as the context supports this, that is, as long as they have someone who is willing and able to assist, a goal for assisted lower extremity dressing is perfectly appropriate, and treatment may focus on making sure that the patient and caregiver can complete the task together while adhering to total hip precautions. Independence is the performance parameter that is the focus of most assessment tools, so occupational therapists can select from a variety of assessment tools that measure independence. Several other considerations, discussed later in this chapter, can help the occupational therapist to identify which of the many assessment tools is best for the situation.

SAFETY. Many assessment tools address safety indirectly by specifying that performance be completed in a safe manner in order to be rated as independent (e.g., the FIM™; U.B. Foundations Activities, 2004). Some tools do not address safety directly (e.g., the Katz Index of ADL; Katz et al., 1963), and a few rate safety separately from independence (e.g., the Performance Assessment of Self-Care Skills; Holm & Rogers, 1999; Rogers & Holm, 1994). When safety is a particular concern, for example, with clients who have cognitive deficits that impair judgment, a separate measure of safety can be more effective for documenting progress toward treatment goals. A separate safety measure also makes it clear in the occupational therapy documentation that safety has been addressed.

ADEQUACY. Clients may have criteria regarding the efficiency of task performance and the acceptability of the outcome of the performance, and these should be considered in selecting assessment tools. For example, a client might be safe and independent in lower body dressing but deem her performance inefficient because it takes her over an hour to complete the task and she is too physically exhausted after dressing to attend to work duties. Or a client might be independent and safe in feeding himself but find his performance outcome unacceptable if he drops food onto his clothing during each meal. If an assessment tool measured only independence and safety, it would be hard to justify intervention in either of the above examples because both clients were safe and independent. There are, however, occupational performance problems in both cases that might be addressed effectively through treatment, that is, reducing the time needed to complete lower body dressing or reducing the amount of food spilled on clothing during eating. Adequacy parameters that warrant consideration in the context of ADL and IADL performance include perceived difficulty, pain, fatigue, **dyspnea**, societal standards, satisfaction, aberrant behaviors, and past experience with the activity. Specific options for measuring adequacy parameters are described in Chapter 46. Practitioners must keep in mind that independence might not be the only important performance parameter to assess in the occupational therapy evaluation.

Step 4: Estimate the Client Factors That Affect ADLs/IADLs and the Assessment Process

One purpose of the ADL/IADL evaluation is to provide insight into the problems underlying occupational performance deficits. However, some estimate of these deficits prior to the assessment can help the occupational therapist to select the assessment tools that will be most effective in identifying and documenting occupational performance problems and the underlying deficits. Occupational therapists use their knowledge of pathology and how it affects occupational performance when selecting assessment tools. For example, some instruments rely on self-report, which is a very efficient way to gather information about a wide range of activities. However, if the client has significant cognitive deficits (e.g., a person with Alzheimer's disease), distorted thought functions (e.g., a person with schizophrenia), or little experience with the disorder (e.g., a teenager who sustained a spinal cord injury with quadriplegia just five days earlier), self-reported measures could be inaccurate. For many types of deficits, insight into clients' underlying problems will be enhanced by actually seeing the client attempt to perform tasks rather than relying on a description of the problem. For example, a client who has had a stroke might report that he is unable to reach items stored above chest height with his affected hand, but the occupational therapy practitioner can gain additional information needed for treatment by observing the client while he is reaching by looking for clues as to whether the movement problem is due to limitations in movement of the scapula, glenohumeral joint, or elbow or some combination of the three. Knowledge of underlying pathology and anticipated impairments also enables occupational therapists to select appropriate assessment tools that are designed for specific diagnostic groups, focusing on activities that are more commonly problematic for that population. For example, the Arthritis Impact Measurement Scale was developed for adults with rheumatic diseases and includes not only measures of ADL and IADL performance, but also symptoms that are commonly experienced by people with arthritis during or following activities, such as pain and fatigue (Meenan, Mason, Anderson, Guccione, & Kazis, 1992).

Step 5: Identify Contextual Features That Affect Assessment

In this step, the occupational practitioner considers the intervention context and its impact on the evaluation of ADLs and IADLs. These include physical context, social context, safety, the client's experience, time constraints, the practitioner's training and experience, availability of resources, and mandates from facilities or **third-party payers**.

PHYSICAL CONTEXT.   Practitioners may observe activity performance under natural or clinical conditions. Under natural conditions, performance is observed within the context in which it usually takes place or is expected to take place, including the location (e.g., home), the objects that are usually used for activities (e.g., bathtub, soap), and the routine time when activities take place, when possible. These conditions, which can often be met in long term-care settings and home-based care, provide the most accurate assessment of clients' performance (Rogers et al., 2003). When clients are seen in the hospital or outpatient clinics, observation of activity performance takes places under clinical conditions. Regardless of where an assessment takes place, the influence of the physical context on activity performance must be taken into account so that valid conclusions about performance can be drawn. Occupational therapy clinics are designed to promote function and have numerous adaptive features to compensate for impairments. These features can make it easier for clients to perform activities in the clinic than in their own homes. Conversely, performance might be more difficult for some tasks because clients are unfamiliar with the clinic setting. When an evaluation is done in the home, clients have the advantage of using their own activity objects in the confines of familiar architecture. Research in this area is limited but demonstrates the variable impact of context on performance. For example, Brown, Moore, Hemman, and Yunek (1996) found that clients with mental illness performed

similarly on a simulated purchasing task in the clinic and an actual purchasing task in a store, whereas Park, Fisher, and Velozo (1994) found that older adults' process skills during IADLs were higher in their homes than in clinic settings. More research is needed to identify the relationships among different types of client impairments and varied evaluation contexts.

SOCIAL CONTEXT.   The occupational therapy evaluation also occurs in a social context. Practitioners must oversee activity performance during assessment, and their very presence can affect the manner and adequacy of the activities performed. The practitioner's presence especially affects the client's ability to initiate participation in ADLs or IADLs, since the structure of the assessment process itself prompts clients to engage in the tasks. If initiation of task performance is impaired, the practitioner must supplement performance measures from a structured therapy session. For example, the Independent Living Scale includes a subscale for initiation (Ashley, Persel, & Clark, 2001). Alternatively, family members might be asked to keep track of the number of days the client completed pet care responsibilities without being asked, for example. Clients' occupational performance might be also be impaired or enhanced in the natural environment compared to the clinic, depending on their needs and the differences in social context between clinic and natural environments. For example, a client with a spinal cord injury who must be skilled in directing a personal care attendant during ADLs might give directions effectively to a rehabilitation aide who is familiar with caring for people with similar needs but might not give detailed enough instructions for an employee in the home who has less experience. Conversely, a client who requires setup to feed herself will be more independent at home than in the clinic if she lives in a family where meals are routinely set up for the entire family by a parent who does all the cooking.

SAFETY.   Occupational therapists must assess risks associated with ADLs or IADLs that have been identified as priorities by clients and might need to defer assessment of a task that they believe could be unsafe. Identifying the potential risk of a given assessment is based on occupational therapists' expertise in determining activity demands combined with their estimate of client problems, outlined in step 4 above. For example, a client who suffered a recent stroke resulting in very poor sitting balance might identify showering as an important goal; however, getting the client onto a shower chair in a wet and slippery environment for an assessment might be unsafe, given the level of assistance she needs for maintaining balance so soon after the stroke. Instead, the occupational therapist might suggest beginning with an assessment of bathing skills that can be completed at bedside and defer a shower assessment until sitting balance is improved.

THE CLIENT'S EXPERIENCE. Clients will come with varied experience with ADLs and IADLs based on personal context. Typically, ADL practice begins in childhood, and the societal expectation is that adolescents and adults have a wide range of experience with these activities and can perform them adequately. However, a similar expectation does not hold for IADLs, for which people have more options. Therefore, clients might not have developed proficiency in all IADL activities. Some might have no experience in planning and preparing meals, doing the laundry, or managing finances. Children with developmental disabilities often experience delays in the acquisition of ADL and IADL skills and might lack experience that a typically developing child would have at a given age. Clients' activity performance history is essential for understanding their current performance level. An activity limitation is interpreted differently for a client who has had no or little prior experience performing the activity than for one who had been doing it immediately premorbidly.

TIME CONSTRAINTS. The time that is available for occupational therapy intervention is often limited by a number of factors, including reimbursement policies, so the evaluation process must be done efficiently. For clients with a long list of ADL and IADL goals, selecting key activities could be necessary so that the intervention designed to enhance occupational performance can be initiated in a timely manner. As goals are met, additional assessments may be initiated to document baseline performance of other ADLs or IADLs and to justify additional occupational therapy goals and treatment.

THE OCCUPATIONAL THERAPY PRACTITIONER'S TRAINING AND EXPERIENCE. An occupational therapy practitioner's experience can also affect the selection of assessment tools. Familiarity with an instrument can increase efficiency of use and effectiveness of interpreting assessment results. Some assessment tools require specialized training, so they are not options for therapists who lack the training. For example, the Assessment of Motor and Process Skills (AMPS) (Fisher, 2006a, 2006b) relies on software that can be accessed only by practitioners who have completed the training course and calibration process (Gitlin, 2005).

AVAILABILITY OF RESOURCES. The materials that are required for ADL and IADL assessments vary, and the occupational therapist must make sure that the necessary materials are readily available. Completing a cooking assessment using a client's favorite cookie recipe might be excellent for examining the client's performance, but because of the logistics and cost of procuring the ingredients, this activity is not likely to be practical for an occupational therapy practitioner in a hospital setting, whereas a client who is being seen in home-based therapy might have the required resources readily available in the home. Some assessments require special test kits, which can be costly, and facilities might have only a few such tools available for use.

MANDATES FROM FACILITIES OR THIRD-PARTY PAYERS. Many facilities or third-party payers have assessment forms or procedures that must be completed for all clients. For example, rehabilitation facilities must use the Inpatient Rehabilitation Facilities–Patient Assessment Instrument (IRF-PAI), which includes the Functional Independence Measure (FIM™) for measuring ADLs (U.B. Foundation Activities, 2004). If a client's description of a selected ADL differs from that of the FIM™ or if the client would like to address adequacy parameters in addition to independence and safety, then the occupational therapist must use a supplemental assessment, since documentation of the FIM™ scores is required.

Step 6: Consider Features of Assessment Tools

The occupational therapist must be familiar with available assessments and consider what tasks are included in the assessment, how tasks are defined, the psychometric properties, the type of data to be collected, and the method of data collection.

TASKS ASSESSED. Tasks that are included in an ADL or IADL assessment should be consistent with clients' priorities, and the operational definition of effective performance should fit clients' needs and address all parameters of importance. For example, many assessment instruments measure independence, but if clients would also like to complete tasks independently without experiencing shortness of breath or pain, occupational therapists might want to use a dyspnea or pain scale in conjunction with the independence measure.

STANDARDIZED VERSUS NONSTANDARDIZED ASSESSMENTS. Some assessments are not standardized; that is, the individual therapist designs the assessment and decides the type of information to gather, or practitioners in a clinic might develop their own instrument for assessment. Nonstandardized assessments lack testing of psychometric properties, such as reliability, validity, or sensitivity to change in a client's status (Lorch & Herge, 2007). Standardized assessments rely on a well-described, uniform approach. There is a lot of variability in the extent to which the psychometric properties of standardized assessments have been established. Some assessments have been extensively studied and include a wide range of psychometric statistics to support the reliability and validity of the tool. The psychometric properties of test instruments may be published in the test manual or through peer-reviewed publications, such as the *American Journal of Occupational Therapy* (AJOT). When possible, it is best to use an assessment with established psychometric properties (Lorch & Herge, 2007).

There are different types of standardized assessments, including norm-referenced tests and criterion-referenced tests. Types of evaluations are described in more detail in Chapter 47. The purpose of norm-referenced testing is to compare a client's performance on a test to that of other people on the same test (Benson & Schell, 1997). ADL and IADL assessments are not usually norm-referenced tests, which tend to be used to assess developmental levels, performance skills, or client factors, such as visual perception, grip strength, or coordination. ADL and IADL assessments are typically criterion-based, that is, tests that compare a client's performance to a performance standard (Benson & Schell, 1997). Criterion-referenced tests stress activity mastery and address questions such as "Can clients perform all activities, or procure the services, needed to live in the community on their own?" Criterion-referenced tests often incorporate activity analyses, and the degree of structure that is imposed on testing is usually more flexible than those for norm-referenced testing, allowing therapists to tailor tests appropriately. For example, a dressing assessment is typically done with clothes that the client needs to and wants to wear, which can have an impact on performance. If a patient needs to be able to manage buttoning, that should be incorporated into the assessment even if it is difficult for the patient; however, if the patient has not worn garments with buttons for many years, there is no reason to assess buttoning ability.

DESCRIPTIVE VERSUS QUANTITATIVE DATA. Some non-standardized assessments use a descriptive approach, that is, the salient characteristics of clients' activity performance are observed or obtained through client or caregiver descriptions. Clients' status is documented by simply describing their performance. Quantitative ADL and IADL measures use a scale that converts observed or reported behavior into a number. Standardized quantitative measures include instructions for the person who is completing the assessment, which makes the assessment more reliable when the tool is used for reassessment or when there are multiple therapists in a facility. For example, the term *moderate assistance* could be interpreted in a number of ways, but if it is specifically described as "The patient requires more help than touching, or expends between 50 and 74% of the effort" (U.B. Foundation, 2004, p. III-7), there is likely to be better agreement among therapists using the instrument. Reducing observed behavior to a number also makes it efficient for reporting data in documentation. However, loss of descriptive data can make it difficult for the reader to get a clear understanding of the client's limitations. Often, documentation includes quantitative assessment data that are accompanied by some descriptive data to provide a more comprehensive picture of client performance. A brief case, presented in Table 48.1, compares descriptive and quantitative data from two cases.

It is possible to use descriptive data to document a client's baseline status, which is needed to determine whether or not progress is made in treatment; however, this can be difficult and time-consuming. For example, if Melinda and David's occupational therapist had to document the status of *all* ADLs and IADLs as in Table 48.1, the evaluation report would take a great deal of time to write and to read. Additionally, the occupational therapy practitioner who is documenting descriptive data should be very careful to distinguish between *observations* and *clinical judgments* (subjective interpretations about the observations). The statements listed in Table 48.1 are observations. A statement of clinical judgment is interpretive, and several plausible interpretations could be made from the more objective observations. For example, the occupational therapy practitioner could conclude that David has weak trunk muscles that interfere with balance. This conclusion should be presented as a hypothesis, not as an observation, because David's inability to maintain balance while dressing could be due to other factors, such as impaired vestibular and proprioceptive input that interferes with his ability to detect when he is starting to fall to one side.

Quantitative methods provide a more efficient way to document progress, although it might not provide the reader with adequate information. For example, although Melinda and David have the same quantitative score on the Wee FIM™, the descriptive information enables readers to see that there are very different underlying problems. Occupational therapists can document some key descriptive data to support their evaluation and treatment plan, but most descriptive observations are simply used by therapists for planning treatment, while quantitative data are recorded in documentation. Many quantitative ADL scales are available; however, it can be difficult for occupational therapy practitioners to find standardized assessments for some IADLs, so a descriptive approach also provides a reasonable option for the assessment of selected tasks for which no quantitative measure exists.

REPORTED VERSUS OBSERVED PERFORMANCE. Data about ADL and IADL performance can be gathered by report or through direct observation. Reported data about the client's abilities and limitations in performance can be gathered from the client, the caregiver, and/or another health professional. The occupational therapy practitioner poses questions about ADL and IADL performance. The questioning method may be implemented in an oral or a written format, using interviews or questionnaires, respectively. Although the questioning is frequently done face to face, either format can be done without physical interaction. Interviews may be conducted over the telephone. Questionnaires may be completed while the client is waiting for an appointment or can be mailed out in advance of a session. Gathering data via report can be done

TABLE 48.1   COMPARISON OF DESCRIPTIVE AND QUANTITATIVE DATA FROM A DRESSING ASSESSMENT OF TWO CHILDREN

Client Description	Melinda is an 8-year-old child who sustained a traumatic brain injury. Before her injury, she was a typically developing child who dressed herself independently.	David is an 8-year-old child with cerebral palsy affecting the right side of his body. His mother has been dressing him before this assessment.
Descriptive Data	◆ Well-coordinated and smooth movements of both upper extremities when manipulating clothing. ◆ Maintenance of appropriate posture (unsupported, sitting on the bed) for the task. ◆ Able to reach all areas of her body (reach behind, overhead, and to feet) without loss of balance or any apparent instability in maintaining her position on the bed. ◆ Frequently stopped midtask to verbally express thoughts to the occupational therapy practitioner, which were disjointed and difficult to follow. ◆ Made repeated (total of 5) attempts to get her left arm in a sleeve that was turned inside out without attempts to correct the orientation of the garment. Did not respond to verbal directions to turn the sleeve right side out. The practitioner turned the sleeve right side out for Melinda after 3 attempts at giving verbal cues and gesturing toward the sleeve. ◆ Melinda left the dressing task to go look out the window when she heard a plane passing overhead and continued to talk about the plane when asked by the practitioner to return to the dressing task. ◆ Melinda returned to the task when the practitioner physically guided her to the bed and placed one of Melinda's arms in the sleeve. Melinda then completed putting the shirt on her other arm without physical assistance or cues. ◆ When asked to button her shirt, Melinda completed 2 of 6 buttons, which were misaligned. When asked how well her shirt was buttoned, she looked down at herself and said, "It's perfect," then skipped out of the room saying that she wanted to go to the TV room.	◆ Started to put left (stronger) arm in his shirtsleeve first. Responded immediately to verbal cue to dress the right side of the body first. ◆ Wavering of trunk when both upper extremities were being used to position the shirt. Therapist steadied David's trunk to prevent him from falling forward when he pulled the shirt across his back. He could not get the shirt far enough around to reach the sleeve, and the practitioner moved the shirt so he could reach it with the left upper extremity. ◆ Left upper extremity movements were smooth and well-coordinated when manipulating clothes and fasteners. ◆ Right upper extremity movements were slower and ineffective for fine tasks, such as buttoning. Several attempts were required to complete the bottom 3 buttons, and the occupational therapy practitioner had to complete the top 3. ◆ Dressing the upper body required 25 minutes, and David reported that he felt "pretty tired" at the end of the session. Throughout the session, David worked consistently, even when his little brother ran into and out of the room several times. ◆ David followed instructions consistently and made 4 or 5 attempts to help solve problems he encountered along the way, for example, suggesting that he wear pullover shirts that do not have buttons. ◆ When asked at the end of the session which arm he will dress first when he tries the task tomorrow, David responded, "My right arm."
Quantitative Data Based on the Wee FIM™	Upper Body Dressing = 4	Upper Body Dressing = 4

informally; that is, the practitioner develops the questions to be asked and the actual data that are gathered, or through the use of a standardized instrument such as the COPM (Law et al., 2005), the Occupational Self Assessment (Baron, Kielhofner, Iyenger, Goldhammer, & Wolenski, 2002), or the Child Occupational Self Assessment (Federico & Kielhofner, 2002). Although self-report is an efficient way to measure ADLs and IADLs, it is not always consistent with actual performance (Brown et al., 1996; Hilton, Fricke, & Unsworth, 2001; Rogers et al., 2003), and the occupational therapist should do selected performance-based assessments when the client's accuracy is in question.

In some situations, clients might be unable to respond on their own behalf. For example, they might be too physically ill or depressed to participate in questioning, or they might lack insight into their problems because of cognitive deficits. In these situations, caregivers or other proxies can be asked to respond on behalf of clients. The usefulness of the information that is obtained from caregivers or proxies depends on their familiarity with the client's ADLs and IADLs. For example, if the caregiver or proxy has not actually observed a client bathing or has not done this for some time, the information that this person gives about bathing might be based more on opinion than on concrete knowledge of performance. In addition, there are known biases in the reporting tendencies of caregivers and proxies. Family proxies are prone to perceiving clients as being more disabled than clients perceive themselves to be and to perceiving clients as more disabled than do professional caregivers (Rubenstein, Schairer, Wieland, & Kane, 1984). Caregivers and proxies can readily observe evaluation parameters such as independence, safety, and aberrant activity behaviors. For some evaluation parameters, however, clients are the only appropriate respondents. For example, values, satisfaction with performance, and activity-related pain are subjective, and indices of these parameters are difficult for others to observe.

Assessments that rely on self-report or caregiver's report are particularly useful for screening for activity limitations, because a large number of activities can be queried in a short amount of time. Questioning is also the data-gathering method of choice when information is needed about daily living *habits*—that is, about what clients usually do on a daily basis—or to learn about clients' ADL and IADL experience. However, reporting is less useful in evaluating limitations for the purposes of intervention because clients might not be able to describe their limitations in sufficient detail to target the components of activities that are problematic.

Assessment data can also be gathered through direct observation of ADLs and IADLs, which gives the practitioner more information about how the client performs a task. Observation of performance, however, requires more time and material resources and is therefore more costly.

Direct observation of performance can also be done in a nonstandardized way or through use of a standardized assessment. The constraints of practice settings, often imposed by third-party payers or limited funding, can place restrictions on the time an occupational therapist has available for evaluation. Occupational therapists must be strategic in selecting ADL and IADL assessments that will provide information that is relevant to the client and can be generalized to other tasks so that the practitioner does not have to observe all meaningful ADLs and IADLs that may be addressed in treatment. For example, if a client requires assistance with cooking because of an inability to transport food and cooking equipment safely while using a walker, the occupational therapist can reasonably project, without having to observe performance, that the same client will require assistance in doing laundry, since laundry also requires the transportation of task objects.

Selected standardized ADL and IADL assessments are listed in Table 48.2. The ADL assessments that are included in Table 48.2 are readily available and either are commonly used in practice (e.g., the FIM™) or provide a unique approach to assessment. For example, the Independent Living Scale measures task initiation (Ashley et al., 2001). Information for learning to use each assessment is also provided. The IADL instruments that were selected include a range of activities. More ADL and IADL assessments can be found in the resources listed in Box 48.1, and a more comprehensive list of assessments can be found in Unit XVI.

Step 7: Integrate the Information from Steps 1–6 to Select the Optimal ADL and IADL Assessment Tools

After establishing the purpose of the evaluation and the client's priorities and gathering some preliminary information about the client and relevant contextual features, assessment instruments can be selected that are client-centered, yield appropriate data, are reliable and valid, and are feasible to administer. Occupational therapists should engage in best practice by considering the evidence regarding the selection and use of assessments, for example, the reliability of instruments and the validity for a given clinical situation. Additional considerations for evidence-based evaluation are discussed in the Commentary on the Evidence box. Perhaps the best data-gathering strategy is to use a combination of methods and sources, relying on the convergence of data for the best profile of clients' activity abilities and limitations.

It is often most effective to begin the evaluation with a questioning approach to provide an overall profile of the client's abilities and limitations, to understand clients' priorities, and to target activities that require in-depth evaluation. Questioning is then followed by observational

TABLE 48.2   SUMMARY OF SELECTED ADL AND IADL INSTRUMENTS

Title	Areas Addressed	Population	Method/Rating	Learning to Use the Assessment
Assessment of Living Skills and Resources (ALSAR)	11 IADL skills	Adults	Interview with guiding questions; uses a three-point ordinal scale	Self-study using published references, including Williams et al. (1991) and Hilton, Fricke, & Unsworth (2001).
Assessment of Motor and Process Skills (AMPS)	85 calibrated ADL and IADL activities; client and therapist select 2 or 3 for assessment	Children and adults	Interview to identify 2 or 3 tasks for performance testing; activities rated on 16 motor skills (e.g., reaches, lifts) and 20 process skills (e.g., initiates, searches); uses a four-point ordinal scale	Training required. Software for scoring and required rater calibration available only through course. Course information and extensive reference list are available from AMPS Project International: http://www.ampsintl.com
Canadian Occupational Performance Measure (COPM)	Activities classified into three areas: self-care (ADLs and some IADLs), productive (some IADLs and work), and leisure	Children and adults	Self-report using a semi-structured interview; problems identified by client are rated for importance (scale of 1–10); the five most important problems are rated for both performance and satisfaction (also scales of 1–10).	Self-guided training available through the manual (Law et al., 2005) and on DVD or video from the Canadian Occupational Therapy Association: www.caot.org
Functional Independence Measure (FIM™)	18 activities: 13 ADL tasks and 5 tasks involving communication and social cognition (no IADL tasks)	Adolescents and adults	Observation by a trained observer; uses a seven-point ordinal scale, grading amount of assistance needed by clients to complete activity.	Training recommended for interrater reliability. Training often provided by employer. Also available from the Uniform Data System for Medical Rehabilitation: http://www.udsmr.org/fim2_services.php

TABLE 48.2   SUMMARY OF SELECTED ADL AND IADL INSTRUMENTS   *Continued*

Title	Areas Addressed	Population	Method/Rating	Learning to Use the Assessment
Independent Living Scale	6 ADL tasks and 10 IADL tasks. Also rates behaviors in the context of tasks, including initiation and aberrant task behaviors.	Adolescents and adults with traumatic brain injury	Observation over the course of a week (needed for measuring initiation and aberrant task behaviors). Data may be supplemented by other team members.	Instructions for the test are available in Ashley et al. (2001). The ILS form and general information can be downloaded for free at http://www.neuroskills.com/cns/ilsmenu.shtml. The Ashley et al. article can be ordered for a nominal fee.
Kohlman Evaluation of Living Skills (KELS)	17 activities grouped into categories: ADLs, safety and health, selected IADLs, work, and leisure. Tends to emphasize knowledge component of activities.	Adults with cognitive impairments.	Combination of interview and performance; uses a three-point ordinal scale.	Manual included in test kit describes testing procedures. The KELS can be purchased from AOTA: www.aota.org
Melville-Nelson Self-Care Assessment	7 ADLs that are consistent with the Minimum Data Set	Adults in skilled nursing facilities	Performance-based. Tasks are rated on two scales: how much the client does and how much/what type of assistance is given. Client performance ratings are made for subtasks and sub-subtasks to help with planning intervention	Protocol describes standardized administration procedures. The form and protocol are available at http://hsc.utoledo.edu/allh/ot/melville/sca.html
Minimum Data Set— Section G. Physical Functioning and Structural Problems Scale (MDS)	10 ADL tasks activities	Residents in long-term care.	Performance, ascertained from multiple health care professionals, over all shifts during past 7 days; activities rated for self-performance and support provided	The Health Care Quality Improvement & Evaluation System (QIES) has manuals and self-help guides at https://www.qtso.com/mdsdownload.html#RAI Recorded training sessions are available at https://www.yourvirtualconference.com/qiesclasses.php

Continued

TABLE 48.2   SUMMARY OF SELECTED ADL AND IADL INSTRUMENTS *Continued*

Title	Areas Addressed	Population	Method/Rating	Learning to Use the Assessment
Milwaukee Evaluation of Daily Living Skills (MEDLS)	20 ADL and IADL tasks	Adults with chronic mental health problems	Screening, based on information from clients, clients' families, health care team, and medical record to determine items to be examined; in examination, activities are performed, simulated, or described	Information on testing procedures in Leonardelli (1988) and Haertlein (1999)
Outcome and Assessment Information Set (OASIS)	8 ADL tasks and 8 IADL tasks	Clients in home care	Data may be obtained through various methods (observation, client or proxy report); ratings are differentiated by task characteristics; scale varies from item to item	The Health Care Quality Improvement and Evaluation System (QIES) has manuals and self-help guides at: https://www.qtso.com/mds download.html#RAI Recorded training sessions are available at https://www.yourvirtualconfer ence.com/qiesclasse s.php
Pediatric Evaluation of Disability Inventory (PEDI)	ADLs, including mobility, social function. Has broad IADL tasks (household chores and community function)	Children 6 months to 7½ years (or older if development is delayed)	Report of clinicians or educators who are familiar with the child or through parental interview. The PEDI is a normed test.	Manual includes detailed instructions and cases to practice scoring the PEDI. Ordering instructions can be found at www.bu.edu/hdr/products/pedi/order.html
Performance Assessment of Self-Care Skills (PASS)	26 tasks, including ADL and home management IADL tasks; there are different protocols for use in the client's home and in an occupational therapy clinic.	Adults,	Performance-based observational tool that yields summary scores of activity independence, safety, and adequacy; uses a four-point ordinal scale	Standardized procedures described in the manual. The PASS is available from Dr. Margo Holm at the University of Pittsburgh, School of Health and Rehabilitation Sciences, Pittsburgh, PA (mbholm@ pitt.edu). Manual includes detailed instruction and

TABLE 48.2   SUMMARY OF SELECTED ADL AND IADL INSTRUMENTS *Continued*

Title	Areas Addressed	Population	Method/Rating	Learning to Use the Assessment
				users can arrange to go to the University of Pittsburgh to establish interrater reliability with experienced PASS users.
Wee FIM II^SM	Measures disability severity related to physical impairment, across health, development, educational, and community settings. 0-3 Module measures precursors to function.	Children from 6 months to 7 years	Observation, interview, or both; uses same rating system as FIM™; scores range from 18 (total dependence) to 126 (complete independence)	At least 80% of clinicians at subscribing facilities must be credentialed. Training may be provided by employer or several training options available through UDSMR. Training information at http://www.udsmr.org/wee_training.php

---

BOX 48.1   **RESOURCES FOR ADL AND IADL ASSESSMENTS**

Asher, I. A. (2007). *Occupational therapy assessment tools: An annotated index* (3rd ed.). Bethesda, MD: American Occupational Therapy Association.

Bolton, B. F. (2001). *Handbook of measurement and evaluation in rehabilitation* (3rd ed.). Austin, TX: Pro-Ed.

Finch, E., Brooks, D., Stratford, P. W., & Mayo, N. E. (2002). *Physical rehabilitation outcome measures* (2nd ed.). Philadelphia: Lippincott Williams & Wilkins.

Dittmar, S. S., & Gresham, G. E. (1997). *Functional assessment and outcome measures for the rehabilitation health professional*. Austin, TX: Pro-Ed.

Gallo, J., Reichel, W., & Andersen, L. (2003). *Handbook of geriatric assessment* (3rd ed.). Boston: Jones & Bartlett.

Hemphill-Pearson, B. J. (Ed.). (2008). *Assessments in occupational therapy mental health: An integrative approach* (2nd ed.). Thorofare, NJ: Slack.

Kane, R. L., & Kane, R. A. (Eds.). (2000). *Assessing older persons: Measures, meaning, and practical applications*. Oxford, UK: Oxford University Press.

Law, M., Baum, C., & Dunn, W. (Eds.). (2005). *Measuring occupational performance: Supporting best practice in occupational therapy* (2nd ed.). Thorofare, NJ: Slack.

Law, M., King, G., Russell, D., Stewart, D., Hurley, P., & Bosch, E. (1999). *All about outcomes: An educational program to help you understand, evaluate, and choose pediatric outcome measures* [software]. Thorofare, NJ: Slack.

Law, M., King, G., Russell, D., Stewart, D., Hurley, P., & Bosch, E. (2000). *All about outcomes: An educational program to help you understand, evaluate, and choose adult outcome measures* [software]. Thorofare, NJ: Slack.

McColl, M. A., Carswell, A., Law, M., Pollock, N., Baptiste, S., & Polatajko, H. (2006). *Research on the Canadian Occupational Performance Measure (COPM): An annotated resource*. Toronto, ON: CAOT Publications.

McDowell, I., & Newell, C. (2006). *Measuring health: A guide to rating scales and questionnaires* (3rd ed.). New York: Oxford University Press.

Osterweil, D., Brummel-Smith, K., & Beck, J. C. (2000). *Comprehensive geriatric assessment*. New York: McGraw-Hill.

COMMENTARY ON THE EVIDENCE

Putting Evidence into Practice Through the Use of Standardized Assessments

Best practice in occupational therapy indicates that standardized ADL and IADL assessments should be used because they provide objective measures that are both reliable and valid (Dunn, 2005; Fasoli, 2008; Lorch & Herge, 2007). Reliable assessments enable practitioners to trust that differences in scores measured at different times represent true changes in ADL or IADL status and that reassessments done by another clinician can be reliably compared to a client's prior scores (Fasoli, 2008). Third-party payers also prefer documentation that describes clients' status and progress toward goals with standardized assessments. In spite of this, many clinicians continue to rely on nonstandardized assessments in clinical practice, often citing time constraints as a significant barrier to their use (Lorch & Herge, 2007). Many standardized ADL and IADL assessments, however, do not require much, if any, additional time or effort to conduct once practitioners are familiar with assessment protocols and scoring. For example, clinicians frequently begin their assessment with an interview to establish an occupational profile and clients' priorities (Radomski, 2008; Stewart, 2005). Practitioners can use the Canadian Occupational Performance Measure (COPM) to gather the same data in approximately the same amount of time. The COPM gathers descriptive data, as an informal interview does, but also includes reliable and valid quantitative measures of clients' self-reported performance ability and satisfaction on client-selected occupational performance tasks (Law et al., 2005). Clients' initial COPM scores serve as an objective baseline measure, and reassessment of clients' perceived progress can be quickly done by asking clients to rerate their performance and satisfaction on previously rated tasks. Standardized tests that do not require extensive additional time can also be selected when practitioners need to observe clients' actual performance. For example, the Performance of Self-Care Skills (PASS) uses a standardized approach to assessing a number of ADLs and IADLs, often by structuring observations of key elements of a task, such as sweeping up cereal placed on the floor by the therapist rather then having to observe the client sweep the entire kitchen (Holm & Rogers, 1999; Rogers & Holm, 1994). Practitioners must first become familiarized with the PASS scoring system, but once the practitioner is experienced, the assessment can be scored quickly and yields measures of three different parameters: independence, safety, and adequacy. Any or all of these performance parameters can be tracked and reported to document clients' progress toward goals.

Many standardized assessments are available for measuring ADL performance (Letts & Bosch, 2005). Why, then, do many practitioners continue to use informal ADL assessments in clinical practice? A search of the literature failed to reveal substantial research that answers this question. Research should be conducted to examine barriers that interfere with occupational therapy practitioners' use of standardized ADL assessments to enhance best practice during the evaluation process. Appropriate assessment tools for IADLs are more difficult to find. Standardized assessment of IADLs is more challenging because of the variability and complexity of IADL tasks.

One potential limitation to using standardized assessments for IADLs is that many IADL assessments that examine a range of IADL tasks (rather than a single skill, such as cooking) rely on self-report or proxy report; examples are the Extended Activities of Daily Living (Nouri & Lincoln, 1987), COPM (Law et al., 2005), Assessment of Living Skills and Resources (Williams et al., 1991), and some parts of the Kohlman Evaluation of Living Skills (Kohlman Thomson, 1992). The limitations of using reported performance were addressed earlier in this chapter. The development of reliable and valid IADL assessments that enable occupational therapy practitioners to objectively measure observed performance across many IADL tasks would increase their ability to engage in evidence-based evaluation.

assessments. If observational assessments raise additional questions about the client's activity performance abilities, the evaluation plan can be modified to gather more or different data.

Planning an effective ADL and IADL evaluation is best illustrated by a case example, following the steps described above.

Implementing the Evaluation: Gathering Data, Critical Observation, and Hypothesis Generation

Gathering Data and Critical Observation

Once occupational therapists develop an evaluation plan, they must carry it out. The thoughtful and deliberate

---

CASE STUDY: *Evaluation of a Client with Morbid Obesity and Respiratory Failure*

Mrs. Howard is a 59-year-old woman with a history of morbid obesity (she is 5'1" tall and weighs 376 pounds). She was admitted to a hospital with difficulty breathing secondary to an allergic reaction to an over-the-counter medication. She subsequently went into respiratory arrest and required a tracheostomy and mechanical ventilation. She was weaned from the ventilator six weeks later and placed on supplemental oxygen. She developed a right foot drop, secondary to peroneal nerve compression that occurred during her prolonged bedrest. After two months in acute care, Mrs. Howard was transferred to a rehabilitation hospital, where she participated in occupational therapy (OT) for ADL and IADL training and physical therapy (PT) for mobility training. She was dependent in all areas of ADL and IADL on admission and made considerable gains in function before her discharge home, six months after her initial hospitalization. At discharge, she was ambulating short distances (up to 50 feet) independently with a rolling walker and a brace on the right foot (the brace was attached to her shoe). She had an extra-wide wheelchair for limited community outings (e.g., doctor's appointments), but the chair did not fit in her home. She continued to require supplemental oxygen and was independent in tracheostomy care and suctioning. Mrs. Howard was referred for home-based services, including skilled nursing, nutritional counseling, home health aide (three days a week, two hours each day), PT, and OT.

Occupational Profile

Mrs. Howard lived with her husband of 30+ years. He worked full time but was physically able and willing to assist his wife when he was home. Mr. and Mrs. Howard had two grown children and two school-aged grandchildren who lived in the area. Before hospitalization, Mrs. Howard was independent in ADLs and IADLs. She had primary responsibility for cooking, light housekeeping, and laundry. She worked 20 hours a week at the local public library. Mrs. Howard had several close friends she enjoyed meeting for lunch or shopping, especially bargain hunting at flea markets. She and her husband also frequently attended their grandchildren's sports events in a nearby town. The following considerations were used to select appropriate ADL and IADL assessments for Mrs. Howard:

1. **Identify the overall purpose(s) of the evaluation.** The primary purpose was to plan and monitor OT intervention, so baseline data needed to be effective for determining progress toward goals.
2. **Have clients identify their needs, interests, and perceived difficulties with ADLs and/or IADLs.** Mrs. Howard's primary goal was to regain her independence in ADLs and IADLs and leisure. She identified ADLs and IADLs, including driving, as priorities because she was concerned about being a burden on her husband. She reported that her biggest difficulties were with lower body ADLs (unable to reach) and with all IADLs (fatigue, shortness of breath, limited reach and mobility). She had frequent medical appointments and lived in a rural area, and she hated relying on others for getting to and from appointments.
3. **Further explore the client's relevant activities so that the activities are operationally defined.** The "problem activities" that Mrs. Howard had were briefly discussed for more detail. ADLs were completed in the typical fashion, except for the brace that she wore on the right foot. She reported that sexual activity was not currently a priority but that she would like to address it later, once she had sufficient energy for and independence in ADLs. IADL priorities for Mrs. Howard included the following:
   - Transporting laundry from the bedroom to the kitchen (top-loading washer) and out to the clothesline to dry (no dryer).
   - Cooking complete dinners, including accessing the refrigerator, oven, stovetop, cooking utensils, dishwasher, and sink. A sample dinner would include fish, baked potatoes, steamed green beans, and a salad.
   - Driving and riding in her minivan.
   - Accessing all areas of her one-story home except the basement, (home office for doing finances and using the computer, linen closets, etc.).

Additionally, Mrs. Howard reported adequacy parameters, including the ability to complete ADLs and IADLs in a timely manner and regain the ability

Continued

to sustain activity without fatigue or shortness of breath.

4. **Estimate the client factors that affect occupational performance and/or the assessment process.** Mrs. Howard's primary problems limiting function were caused by her obesity, which limited her reach and ability to move and caused fatigue and dyspnea. Cognition and perception did not appear to be factors that interfered with function on initial review of her rehabilitation records and the initial interview.

5. **Identify contextual features that affect assessment.** Contextual features that supported the evaluation process included the following:
   - The assessment occurred in Mrs. Howard's home, providing the advantage of a natural environment.
   - There was a ramp into the home, providing access to the yard and driveway.
   - Mrs. Howard had years of experience with all of the tasks she wished to return to, which would support performance of tasks.

   Contextual features that were barriers to the evaluation process included the following:
   - Clutter in the home that presented a potential safety issue.
   - Mrs. Howard was on oxygen, with the unit in the bedroom and a very long tube that connected to her nasal cannula, so she had to manage the tubing as she moved around the house.
   - The evaluation occurred during the week, and the therapist was alone with a client whose weight presented a potential safety problem to the therapist, who had no assistance for guarding Mrs. Howard when trying a new task.
   - Mrs. Howard had private insurance, which required that the OT evaluation be completed in one visit.

6. **Consider features of assessment tools.** This step is included in the discussion of step 7.

7. **Integrate the information from steps 1–6 to select the optimal ADL and IADL assessment tools.** The time limit of one visit (approximately 60–75 minutes) had a significant impact on which assessments were selected. The occupational therapist decided to start with the COPM based on the following considerations:
   - The COPM had well-established psychometric properties and assessed both ADLs and IADLs (Law et al., 2005).
   - The COPM relied on self-report; however, Mrs. Howard was cognitively intact and had been learning to live with her disability for the past four

months. One advantage of the self-report format is that it did not pose any safety hazards. For example, the occupational therapist got a baseline performance and satisfaction rating on riding in a car (including getting in and out) without having to attempt the task alone with Mrs. Howard.
   - Mrs. Howard indicated that she felt stress about burdening her husband. The COPM would help Mrs. Howard and the occupational therapist to prioritize the ADLs and IADLs that would reduce caregiver burden.
   - The COPM included a satisfaction measure, which reflected some of the adequacy parameters that Mrs. Howard identified (e.g., if she could dress independently but it took her 45 minutes, she would give that a low satisfaction score).
   - The COPM could be completed in about 20 minutes.

After the COPM, the occupational therapist selected the FIM™ subtests of transfers, lower body dressing, and grooming. Other subtests were not observed because they were activities that Mrs. Howard reported no difficulty with (including feeding, toileting, and upper body dressing) or because of time constraints (e.g., bathing). The FIM™ was identified as an appropriate measure for the following reasons:
   - Mrs. Howard reported that she required physical assistance for lower body dressing and getting out of bed (on the FIM™, transfers start from supine and end in standing for people who do not use a wheelchair), and the scale was believed to have adequate sensitivity in levels of physical assistance to document progress.
   - The FIM™ included client appliances in the lower body dressing measure, and Mrs. Howard reported that her brace was one thing she was not able to master while in the rehabilitation center.
   - The occupational therapist had discharge FIM™ scores from the rehabilitation center, so performance in the clinic could be compared to performance in the home with the same tool to examine the impact of the home context on performance and aid in problem-solving for intervention.
   - These tasks could be completed in 25 minutes.

Two additional parameter measures were used to supplement the FIM™. Lower body dressing and grooming were timed, which required no additional assessment time. Dyspnea was measured after each of the three subtasks, using a 100-mm visual analogue scale, where 0 = "no shortness of breath," 50 mm = "moderate shortness of breath,"

CASE STUDY: *Evaluation of a Client with Morbid Obesity and Respiratory Failure*   *Continued*

and 100 mm = "severe shortness of breath" (Lansing, Moosavi, & Banzett, 2003). Mrs. Howard was asked to place a mark on the line that best represented her dyspnea. Completion of the dyspnea scales required little additional time, fitting into the 25 minutes allowed for the FIM™.

At this point, Mrs. Howard needed a rest, although the occupational therapist wanted to include some observation of IADLs in the evaluation. While Mrs. Howard took a rest, the therapist used the walker to do an informal accessibility assessment for several key areas in the home, including Mrs. Howard's dresser, closet, personal computer, kitchen appliances, and cabinets. Although standardized assessments are available, the occupational therapist used a nonstandardized approach because Mrs. Howard's walker required additional room for accessibility and the therapist needed to focus on a few key areas, since time was limited. The occupa-

tional therapist could also begin some immediate treatment by making a list of suggestions that would make Mrs. Howard's environment more accessible. The therapist could review the recommendations with Mrs. Howard so that she could enlist a friend or family member in modifying the context, making treatment sessions more effective. The informal assessment of context and review with Mrs. Howard could be completed in 15 minutes.

Finally, the evaluation was concluded with a nonstandardized assessment of a kitchen task. Mrs. Howard made a cup of tea. The kettle was placed in a low cabinet to assess her ability to retrieve it. The tea was in an over-counter cabinet. The therapist gathered descriptive data and also timed the task and used the visual analogue scale to measure dyspnea on completion. The task took less than 10 minutes. After the assessment, Mrs. Howard settled into her favorite chair to enjoy her cup of tea.

---

selection of appropriate assessments, described above, is key in making the actual data gathering run smoothly. A few additional considerations about the actual implementation of the evaluation warrant discussion. The occupational therapy practitioner who is doing an assessment should do the following:

- Collect all equipment and supplies needed for carrying out the evaluation plans, making sure test kits are complete and organized and that necessary equipment and supplies are available, including clients' personal items (e.g., clothing from home). Novice practitioners might find it helpful to create a list of needed items to make sure that everything is available and in working order.
- Schedule assessment sessions in the best environment available. For example, a client in an inpatient rehabilitation center would find it more comfortable to dress in his or her room than in a curtained-off area in a busy clinic.
- Be sensitive to individual needs for modesty, which can vary greatly among clients. Many ADLs are personal tasks that are typically done alone, including dressing, bathing, and toileting. Assessment for potential impairment in sexual activity should be included in ADL assessments but must be handled with sensitivity.
- Structure the optimal social context. For example, the practitioner might wish to have family members present during an interview to gain their perspectives about a client's abilities or needs, whereas having several family members observing a performance-based assessment of

cooking might be distracting to the client and interfere with the evaluation process.

- Bring appropriate tools to record data. A well-planned evaluation session will reveal a lot of information about a client. Standardized tests often come with forms for recording data. Facilities may also have forms for recording data using assessments typically performed in that setting. The practitioner might also want to jot down relevant observations, for example, noting that a client complained of shoulder pain when putting a shirt on overhead or that a client's grocery list included primarily nonnutritious foods. If possible, practitioners should record directly on facility-based documentation forms to reduce the time needed for completing the evaluation report later on.

During the evaluation, the practitioner should engage in critical observation, which can be framed by questions the practitioners ask themselves throughout the process, such as the following:

- What are some of the possible underlying causes of the occupational performance deficits that are being observed or reported? For example, a client who is unable to reach the clothes in his or her closet might may be limited by a variety different factors, including upper extremity weakness, impaired range of motion, poor coordination, diminished standing balance, or a clothes rod that is out of reach for the client's height. Observations that are made as the client tries to get clothes from the closet can provide clues to the underlying causes that

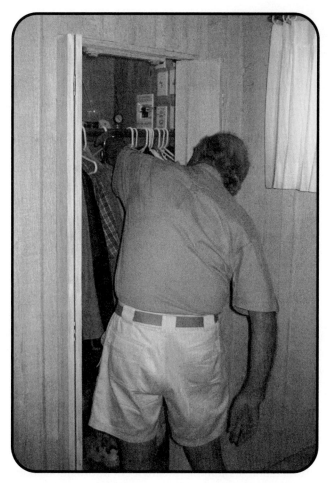

FIGURE 48.1   Observations made during reach: Lateral flexion of the trunk suggests that the client is compensating for an inability to raise the arm, which could be from limited passive range of motion or decreased strength. The height of the closet rod relative to the client's size should require only about 50% of typical shoulder flexion. Balance does not appear to be an issue, as the client appears stable even while shifting his center of gravity toward the left as he reaches.

will aid the occupational therapist in making sound treatment decisions, as shown in Figure 48.1.

♦ What changes might need to be made in the initial evaluation plan on the basis of data from the first assessments? For example, a cooking assessment might reveal mild cognitive deficits that were not apparent during initial interactions with a client, so the occupational therapist would add a cognitive assessment to the evaluation plan.

♦ Are there discrepancies in the evaluation data that were collected? Discrepancies need to be clarified and reconciled and can provide valuable insight into the nature of the client's ADL and IADL limitations. For example, a practitioner might ascertain through performance testing that a client can execute bed-to-wheelchair transfers, yet the client might insist that he cannot. The inconsistency might arise because, although the client

performs the transfer independently with the practitioner present, he feels insecure about his abilities and will not transfer on his own. In this example, the use of different data sources identified a performance discrepancy between skill and habit that would not have been apparent from the use of one source alone.

Hypothesis Generation

The evaluation data that are obtained through questioning, observing, and testing methods must be analyzed, synthesized, and integrated into a cohesive problem statement. This integration of data is accomplished through diagnostic reasoning, which is a component of clinical reasoning (Rogers, 1983; Rogers & Holm, 1991). The clinical reasoning of practitioners occurs as a kind of internal dialogue about the interpretation of the data. Evidence supporting one interpretation is weighed against evidence rejecting that interpretation, and the interpretation that has the most supporting or compelling evidence is selected. If the evidence fails to sufficiently support one interpretation over another, more evaluative data are collected to supplement the reasoning process. This process is best illustrated through an example, based on the cases presented in Table 48.1. Melinda and David had the same dressing scores on the FIM™, a quantitative ADL assessment, but the occupational therapist's clinical interpretation of the descriptive data will lead to very different assumptions about the problems that are causing dressing impairments for the two children. Before reading on, take a minute to reflect on the different observations reported in Table 48.1, and consider the following:

♦ What are the underlying factors that interfere with Melinda's ability to dress independently? What are Melinda's strengths, that is, what skills support her dressing performance? What observed behaviors led to your conclusions about Melinda's strengths and limitations?

♦ What are the underlying factors that interfere with David's ability to dress independently? What are David's strengths, that is, what skills support his dressing performance? What observed behaviors led to your conclusions about David's strengths and limitations?

For Melinda, limited attention, impaired awareness of occupational performance deficits, and inconsistent response to feedback seemed to be underlying problems that limited her ability to dress independently. This is a hypothesis or clinical judgment rather than an objective observation, because constructs such as attention and awareness of deficits cannot be directly observed and must be inferred from specific behaviors. At the same time, Melinda's physical capabilities seemed to be an asset and supported performance in many ways. Compare the observations and clinical judgments made by the occupational therapist about Melinda to those made about David. In both cases, the children required verbal cueing and occasional physical assistance; however, descriptive data led the occupational therapist to a very different hypothesis about David's dressing limitations. The underlying problems for David were physical impairments, for example, diminished sitting balance, incoordination of the right upper extremity, and decreased endurance. Behaviors that supported performance included attention to task, follow-through with feedback, the ability to recall adaptive strategies, and engagement in active problem solving. Generating hypotheses about the nature of the occupational performance deficit is crucial for selecting effective intervention, which must address the underlying problem. For example, adaptive equipment could be provided to help David reach his feet independently or to compensate for poor right hand coordination during buttoning; however, this equipment would be of no help to Melinda and would likely impede performance by distracting her from the task.

Through this process, the practitioner arrives at a cohesive understanding of the ADL and IADL performance of the client, factors that are interfering with performance, and appropriate therapeutic actions given the nature of the client's deficits. This understanding is presented to clients or their proxies for verification and collaborative decision making concerning the therapeutic action to be implemented.

ESTABLISHING CLIENTS' GOALS: THE BRIDGE BETWEEN EVALUATION AND INTERVENTION

The OTPF includes the establishment of clients' goals as the final step in the evaluation process and as the first component of the intervention plan (AOTA, 2002), so this important step really serves as a transition from evaluation to intervention. Synthesizing evaluation results into a meaningful, individualized intervention plan is a complex cognitive task and can be overwhelming for the student or new occupational therapy practitioner. The process of planning and implementing interventions is much easier for practitioners who have reasonable, attainable, and measurable goals. The following section is focused on the multiple factors that influence outcomes to help guide novice practitioners in the clinical reasoning for establishing effective client goals and to structure the problem-solving process for more experienced practitioners, especially when they are managing particularly complex or challenging clients.

Establishing goals requires analysis of the evaluation results in conjunction with additional factors that influence outcome, namely, the client's ability to learn, the client's prognosis, the time allocated for intervention, the client's discharge disposition, and the client's ability to follow through with new routines or techniques. The next section focuses on using performance parameters to

establish meaningful goals for clients that have a clearly identified behavior and an appropriate degree of performance, that is, a characteristic of the behavior that is measurable (e.g., "independently" or "without pain") (Sames, 2005). Goal behaviors may be aimed at underlying skills, for example, increasing strength or range of motion to support participation in ADLs. However, examples in this chapter will focus on establishing goals with occupational performance behaviors, such as bathing or doing laundry.

Identifying Appropriate Goal Behaviors

A comprehensive evaluation examines ADL and IADL performance across relevant performance parameters, described earlier in this chapter and in Chapter 46. Three of these performance parameters—value, level of difficulty, and fatigue and dyspnea—can be used to establish goals for intervention that target appropriate client behaviors.

Value

Occupational therapists should select goal behaviors, that is, ADL and IADL tasks, that reflect the values that the client defined during the evaluation. The value that clients place on given activities influences their motivation for participation in any intervention aimed at improving performance for that activity. Because many occupational therapy interventions require the acquisition of new skills through practice, motivation can greatly influence the ultimate functional outcome. Clients who put little value on the activity that is being addressed during an intervention might appear to be uncooperative in treatment and are unlikely to follow through with programs outside of direct treatment that are necessary for improving skill in that activities.

ADLs and IADLs are often highly valued by both children and adults because of the dependency on others that accompanies role dysfunction (Robinson-Smith, Johnston, & Allen, 2000). However, occupational therapy practitioners should be careful not to assume that ADLs and IADLs are immediate priorities. Some people, especially those with severe activity limitations, might need or want to accept assistance from others in ADLs so that they can conserve energy to perform other activities. This was the case with Mr. Fritz, a 32-year-old with a recently sustained spinal cord injury that resulted in C6 quadriplegia. He was married, had three small children, and was self-employed as a tax accountant. His wife worked part-time as a nurse and took care of their children before and after school. The family depended on Mr. Fritz's income, and he had no disability insurance coverage. Although outcomes in ADLs were initially established for Mr. Fritz, it soon became apparent that attempts at self-care retraining were being met with resistance and frustration. Further discussion of the targeted intervention outcomes revealed that Mr. Fritz was anxious to return to work and that he could do this if he could use the computer in his home office. Although he expressed an interest in becoming independent in self-care, he felt that the best option for him was to return to work as quickly as possible to minimize the financial burden on his family from his current inability to work. His wife was able and willing to help him with self-care tasks at home. The couple felt that self-care retraining could be delayed until the family business was again operational. With intervention outcomes refocused on activities most valued by Mr. Fritz—namely, computer access and home mobility—he became highly motivated to participate in therapy.

Clients' values should drive long-term goals, but occupational therapy practitioners may help clients focus on ADLs initially when they establish priorities in more complex occupational performance areas (e.g., IADLs, work, or leisure) that make the intervention process inefficient and potentially ineffective (Cipriani et al., 2000). Self-care training often helps clients to develop capacities and problem-solving skills that can later be applied to activities that are more complex than self-care, particularly when dealing with severe disorders of sudden onset (e.g., stroke, traumatic injury). For example, suppose Mr. Fritz could not work from a home office and wanted to focus on driving in order to get to work, which is a realistic ultimate goal for someone with C6 quadriplegia. Initiating intervention with driver training, however, would be impractical because Mr. Fritz lacked the prerequisite functional mobility skills early in his rehabilitation. ADL training—involving bathing, dressing, transferring, and wheelchair mobility—can facilitate the development of functional mobility skills. Such training, therefore, would logically precede driver training. In this situation, Mr. Fritz's needs could be met by referring him to social services for assistance with financial planning to help the family manage until he could return to work. The occupational therapy practitioner should also educate Mr. Fritz about the commonalities among skills needed for both self-care and driving. This plan recognizes Mr. Fritz's valued roles and progresses him to the desired outcome in the most efficient way possible.

When the most valued activities and roles are beyond the client's potential skill level, the occupational therapy practitioner helps the client to refocus priorities so that goals are realistic and achievable. If Mr. Fritz were the owner and cook of a small restaurant, for example, it is unlikely that he would meet the essential job requirements of a short-order cook even if the kitchen were adapted for wheelchair accessibility, because the activities require bilateral hand function and must be done quickly. It is possible, however, that he could perform the activities of restaurant owner. For example, he could manage personnel, handle the finances, operate the cash register, and seat customers. In this and similar situations, occupational therapy practitioners assist clients in establishing goals that reflect realistic behaviors by using their expertise in activity analysis and functional adaptation (Liddle & McKenna, 2000).

Difficulty

The perceived ease with which a client completes an activity and the projected difficulty that will remain after intervention are important considerations in selecting goal behaviors (Thornsson & Grimby, 2001). The occupational therapy practitioner, who is skilled in activity analysis and has knowledge of pathology and impairment, must determine the prognosis for functional difficulty. This prognosis must then be communicated to clients so that decisions about acceptable levels of difficulty can be made collaboratively. Clients set intervention priorities, in part, by weighing the projected level of difficulty within the context of value—that is, how much difficulty they are willing to tolerate to be independent in an activity. The frequency with which an activity is performed should also be considered in establishing goals for ADLs and IADLs that are likely to remain difficult for a client to perform. In general, a higher level of proficiency or ease of performance is needed for activities that need to be done routinely, whereas a lower level of proficiency or ease of performance may be acceptable for activities that are done only occasionally.

For example, James is a seven-year-old boy with spina bifida, which damaged his spinal cord at T4. He has a neurogenic bladder and requires routine intermittent catheterization. He identified self-catheterization as a critical task for fulfilling his roles as self-carer and student, because he would prefer not to have help with this personal task from family or school personnel. James will need to be able to self-catheterize independently and efficiently for this task to fit into his school day. The occupational therapist believes that James will be capable of achieving independence with little difficulty after a period of practice. The goal is agreed upon, and treatment begins. Another client, Amy, also has spina bifida, which resulted in incomplete spinal cord damage at C7. She can typically get adequate emptying of her bladder without self-catheterization. On rare occasions, however, she has episodes of urinary retention, requiring catheterization within about one hour of experiencing symptoms. Amy would also like to be independent so that when she must be catheterized at school, she does not need help. The occupational therapist thinks that independent self-catheterization using safe and clean technique is a reasonable goal for Amy, but it will always be difficult because she has impaired hand function and positioning herself so that she can see and reach to insert the catheter is challenging. Amy will need to go to the nurse's office to transfer to a bed. Despite the difficulty, Amy opts to work on this goal. Because she has to catheterize herself so infrequently, she believes that her skill level will be adequate for meeting her needs.

Fatigue and Dyspnea

Fatigue, the sensation of tiredness that is experienced during or following an activity, and dyspnea, difficult or labored breathing, can interfere with activity performance (Fuchs-Climent et al., 2001; Liao & Ferrell, 2000; Vanage, Gilbertson, & Mathiowetz, 2003). Both fatigue and dyspnea are likely to be exacerbated by activity performance. The occupational therapist uses activity analysis to take into account the effort that is required to perform a task and its typical duration. In addition, the client's entire daily routine must be examined so that the energy demands of one activity can be weighed in relation to the client's other activities (Mathiowetz, Matuska, & Murphy, 2001). Assisting clients to examine the physical demands of their preferred activities can help them to prioritize activities so that appropriate goals can be established. Similar to budgeting money, clients must be encouraged to look at their "energy dollars" and decide how they wish to spend them. The occupational therapy practitioner contributes to this decision-making process by bringing valuable information about options for activity adaptation that can reduce the energy demands of activities, thereby saving clients' energy for other tasks.

For example, Mrs. Hernandez lived alone in an apartment in a retirement community. Her sister and brother-in-law also resided in the community, and she had many close friends there. She has had multiple sclerosis for many years, with some weakness and spasticity, but she remained independent in her ADLs until a recent exacerbation, which required hospitalization. An increase in fatigue and decrease in strength resulted in the need for physical assistance with ADLs and the use of a wheelchair for mobility. The retirement community required residents to manage their own ADLs and prepare breakfast and a light evening snack. A hot meal was provided at midday. Mrs. Hernandez reported that she could not afford to hire an aide to help her daily with these tasks. The occupational therapy practitioner explained to Mrs. Hernandez that although independence in ADLs and simple meal preparation were reasonable goals, completing her ADL would likely be time-consuming and fatiguing, leaving her little energy for other activities. Mrs. Hernandez was enthusiastic about beginning therapy, indicating that she was willing to engage in fewer IADLs and leisure activities in order to be independent in ADLs and simple meal preparation because it would enable her to remain in the retirement community with family and friends.

A different scenario played out with Mrs. McKay, who also had multiple sclerosis. Like Mrs. Hernandez, she had a recent exacerbation that caused a functional decline, and achieving independence in ADLs was likely to expend much of her daily energy. Mrs. McKay had been working full-time as a programmer for a local radio station and was the mother of two young children. She perceived her role as a self-carer to be important, along with those of worker and mother. However, when it became apparent that independence in ADLs would leave her with little energy for performing work and parenting roles, she decided not to establish goals for independence in ADLs, opting instead

to hire a personal care attendant for assistance so she could focus on work and parenting goals.

Identifying Appropriate Goal Levels

Treatment goals must include a measurable outcome that indicates how well or at what level the identified behavior will be done, sometimes referred to as the *degree of performance* (Kettenbach, 2004). Independence is the most common degree of performance; however, several performance parameters can also provide effective goals, especially when the client is independent but occupational performance deficits remain that warrant treatment. For example, this would be the case when a client can open jars independently, but it is painful and results in deforming forces to the hand joints.

Independence

The performance parameter that is most commonly focused on in occupational therapy interventions is independence in activity performance, which becomes the degree or measurable part of the goal (Sames, 2005). Across all ages and disabilities, the goal is generally to increase the level of independence (Croser, Garrett, Seeger, & Davies, 2001; Ford et al., 2000; Healy & Rigby, 1999; Nyland et al., 2000). Independence in activity performance may be divided into three phases: initiation of a task, continuation of a task, and completion of a task. The most common occupational therapy goals focus on the completion of the task, which implies that initiation and continuation of the task occurred; for example, a goal might be *"Client will be independent in feeding her cats by December 12, 2007"* or *"Client will require moderate assistance for bed to/from wheelchair transfers in one week."* Occupational therapy practitioners might also want to focus an independence goal on initiation of task performance when that is particularly difficult for a client.

Initiation is an aspect of activity performance that is frequently overlooked when goals are established, in part because it is difficult to evaluate and treat. The very presence of the occupational therapy practitioner may be a cue to initiate a task, and certainly a greeting, such as "Good morning, Mrs. Smith, today we will work on dressing," serves as a prompt for action. Adults are typically expected to initiate ADLs and IADLs independently. Expectations for children also exist, depending on the children's ages and skills and the division of task responsibilities among family members. Impairments in activity initiation may occur as a result of many diseases and disorders, such as attention deficit disorder, dementia, depression, schizophrenia, brain injury from trauma or stroke, multiple sclerosis, and Parkinson's disease. Family members generally find it frustrating to have to cue ("constantly nag") a client who has an initiation impairment for each aspect of a daily routine. The occupational therapist may write an independence goal that includes initiation, such as *"Client will initiate and complete bathing independently three to seven times a week by November 30, 2007."* In this example, measuring progress toward the goal would require the client or a proxy to record the number of times in a week that the client initiated bathing without cueing or assistance from another person.

Safety

Safety is a quality of the person–task–environment transaction, so it cannot be observed or treated in isolation from independence (Letts, Scott, Burtney, Marshall, & McKean, 1998; Russell, Fitzgerald, Williamson, Manor, & Whybrow, 2002). Goals related to safety are typically linked to independence outcomes; that is, independent performance is assumed to be safe, since an occupational therapist could not ethically create a goal for independent performance that was not deemed to be safe. Although occupational therapy practitioners agree that safety is an intervention priority, there is less consensus about specific activity behaviors that are safe or unsafe. Many behaviors fall into a questionable zone, where some would rate them as safe while others perceive them as unsafe. In determining acceptable risk for setting independence goals, it is useful to consider clients' comfort level with risk, their ability to analyze the risks associated with a particular activity and devise a plan for managing them, and, most important, their ability to implement the plan expeditiously despite impairments. At times, the goal for level of independence in activity performance might need to be sacrificed for safety. A comparison of two clients with bilateral lower extremity fractures sustained in car accidents who are learning independent transfers illustrates this point.

Ted and Ryan were both recently injured, are non-weight-bearing on both lower extremities, and are learning sliding board transfers. Ted demonstrates good judgment and a realistic perception of his skills. The occupational therapist has determined that the following goal is realistic: *"Client will be independent in sliding board transfers from wheelchair to/from bed within three therapy sessions."* Through training, Ted learns to transfer safely with a sliding board by following specific guidelines (e.g., position wheelchair at a 45-degree angle to the bed; secure brakes on wheelchair; ascertain that bed height is level with the wheelchair). After a couple of sessions, he is able to follow these guidelines consistently; therefore, his goal of independence in transferring wheelchair to and from bed is met. Ryan's injuries are similar to Ted's, but he also incurred a mild brain injury. Although Ryan's motor skills are comparable to Ted's, Ryan has difficulty recalling the guidelines for transfers and is at risk for bearing weight on his lower extremities during transfers, which could interfere with fracture healing. Therefore, the occupational therapist believes that independent transfers could be unsafe because Ryan's memory deficits place him at risk for violat-

ing weight-bearing precautions. The occupational therapist incorporates safety considerations by setting a goal for Ryan that is aimed at a lower level of independence, for example, *"Client will require supervision and occasional verbal cues for sliding board transfers from wheelchair to/from bed while adhering to weight-bearing precautions within six therapy sessions."* The degree of independence in Ryan's goal was adjusted to realistically reflect his capacity for safe transfer performance.

In some situations, it may be better to establish client goals in which the goal behavior is directly related to safety rather than being assumed in the degree of independence indicated. Goals can be aimed at the occupational performance level, that is, the IADL "safety procedures and emergency responses" (AOTA, 2002); for example, the goal might be *"Client will verbally describe correct responses to a minimum of 10 potential home emergencies with 100% accuracy within three weeks."* Safety goals may also be aimed at developing safe habits, for example, *"Client will pause when entering a room and scan for obstacles on the floor 100% of the time to reduce fall risk during functional mobility by December 1, 2007."* or *"Client will report 100% compliance with condom use to reduce the risk of sexually transmitted diseases within three weeks."*

Adequacy

Several aspects of activity performance contribute to the adequacy or quality of the behavior stated in the goal, which can also be reflected in the goal as the degree to which the behavior is expected to be done. In addition to independence, these performance parameters may be crucial components of meaningful goals, especially for clients who are independent and safe with their performance but who feel dissatisfied with the process or some other aspect of the outcome. Goals with measurable adequacy parameters can be used to justify treatment even if clients are independent in tasks. Six adequacy parameters can be used as measurable outcomes: pain, fatigue and dyspnea, duration, societal standards, satisfaction, and aberrant task behaviors. Some of these parameters may be interdependent within a single client. For instance, pain might lead to changes in duration of activity performance (e.g., the activity takes longer) as well as the ability to meet normative standards and personal satisfaction. A goal should include only one measurable parameter so that it is clear what has changed in documenting progress toward goals.

PAIN.   Pain, either during or following an activity, can negatively influence engagement in ADLs or IADLs even if the activity is completed independently (Birkholtz & Blair, 2001a, 2001b; Dudgeon, Tyler, Rhodes, & Jensen, 2006; Mullersdorf, 2000). The source of pain and the prognosis for it must be carefully considered in establishing goals and selecting an intervention approach. Both the evaluation and the goals must include an index of pain so that intervention remains focused on achieving the projected level of independence while simultaneously reducing the presence of pain. Often, the pain assessment can be incorporated into the goal as an indicator of the degree of pain; for example, the goal might be *"Client will prepare a simple meal (soup, sandwich, and beverage) independently with a maximum pain level of 2 cm on a 10-cm visual analogue scale within 2 weeks."*

FATIGUE AND DYSPNEA. Fatigue and dyspnea can influence the actual task behaviors that are selected for client goals, as was described earlier in this section, but when fatigue or dyspnea can be reduced through task adaptation or conditioning, goals can be established that use these performance parameters as performance outcomes. The initial evaluation should include baseline data for comparison. For example, a goal might be *"Client will complete morning care routine (shower, grooming, dressing) with a maximum score of 6 on the Borg Reported Perceived Exertion Scale* (Borg, 1998) *by November 28, 2007."* As long as the Borg Scale was used during the initial evaluation, a lower number (meaning less exertion) can be used in a goal to indicate progress toward becoming less fatigued during ADL or IADL tasks. Dyspnea can be monitored in a similar way, using a visual analogue scale or numerical rating scale (Gift & Narsavage, 1998). Diagnosis is important to consider when goals are formulated relative to fatigue and dyspnea. Overexertion can exacerbate symptoms or even the disease process itself for conditions such as cardiac disease and multiple sclerosis. Prognosis is another important diagnostic consideration in setting goals that measure fatigue or dyspnea. Clients with chronic obstructive pulmonary disease are likely to become worse; therefore, goals must be reasonable to achieve through activity adaptations and might need to accommodate a decline in function. A client with paraplegia secondary to spinal cord injury, by contrast, experiences fatigue from having to use the smaller muscles of the upper extremity for wheelchair mobility to compensate for the larger lower extremity muscles previously used for walking. Endurance is likely to improve significantly as upper extremity strength increases with use, and more ambitious goals for reducing fatigue could be appropriate.

DURATION. The length of time that is required to complete activities is typically thought of as a reflection of efficiency, which may be affected by many different impairments, including poor endurance, impaired coordination, and cognitive deficits such as difficulty sustaining attention for tasks, which is common in people with a variety of mental health disorders. Although measuring performance time may be relatively simple, interpreting time data in a meaningful way is often difficult. The duration of daily living activities depends highly on the nature of the activity and the task objects that people choose to use in performing the activity. It takes longer to prepare dinner than it does to fix a light snack. Most of us spend more time dressing when we are going out to dine in an elegant restaurant than we do we when we are going to a fast-food establishment. Therefore, it is difficult to establish meaningful norms for ADLs and IADLs, but duration is often a parameter that clients wish to incorporate into their occupational therapy goals when they are frustrated by slow performance.

Establishing acceptable time frames for ADL goals must be done collaboratively with clients and their significant others. Occupational therapists should consider safety and independence parameters simultaneously. Clients may be at increased risk when they rush through activities or even when they attempt them at a typical pace. For example, clients with swallowing deficits might need to eat more slowly than people without such deficits to avoid choking. People with poor fine motor coordination or sensory deficits might need to slow down when using sharp knives to improve control of the knives and prevent injury. In these examples, setting goals to decrease the duration of performance would be inappropriate because it could result in unsafe performance.

Societal and cultural standards also need to be taken into consideration in establishing outcomes for activity duration. In the United States, timeliness is highly valued, and efficient performance in community skills is expected. Shoppers might become irritated when they are standing in a checkout line behind a customer who takes five minutes to identify and count currency, though in other cultures, this delay might go unnoticed. An American with cognitive or visual impairments that interfere with the ability to count currency might wish to decrease the time required for this activity to reduce embarrassment when shopping. The goal, then, needs to include an efficiency measure to reflect this performance parameter, for example, *"Client will independently complete a simple cash transaction (select appropriate currency and count change) in less than one minute within three weeks to support participation in shopping."*

SOCIETAL STANDARDS. Performance standards, determined by the society and culture in which the client lives, are likely to exist in terms of both the end result and the process through which it is achieved. As is discussed in Chapter 46, the line between acceptable and unacceptable performance is likely to be thick rather than narrow and may vary considerably, depending on characteristics such as age, gender, and cohort (generation) membership.

Societal standards exist, for example, for neatness. A client might dress safely and independently, but if the colors of clothing clash or the client's appearance is disheveled (the end product), this client's dressing might not meet societal standards. If the client is a teenager, such an appearance might be considered acceptable. However, if the client is a public relations manager going to work, it is likely to be labeled unacceptable and could well put the client's job in jeopardy. Occupational therapists and clients may identify relevant societal standards for inclusion in goals. Identifying societal standards might seem subjective and difficult, but the use of measurable indicators of societal standards is critical for effective goals and can justify intervention. A goal for a client who eats rapidly, putting food in his mouth when it is still full, might include a measure of societal standard, such as *"When eating during a social event, the client will demonstrate appropriate pacing as evidenced by completing a meal in no less than 15 minutes, swallowing each bite before putting additional food in his mouth, and conversing between bites of food by December 10, 2007."*

SATISFACTION. In addition to societal standards, clients have their own standards of acceptable performance, which also need to be incorporated into goals (Natterlund & Ahlstrom, 1999). Setting goals with satisfaction measures requires collaboration with clients, as personal standards will vary greatly from person to person. Mr. Balouris, for example, is always losing things. He never seems to know where his wallet and keys are, and he is always searching for something. Nonetheless, items seem to turn up, and he sees no reason to go to the trouble of organizing his apartment better to help him keep track of his belongings. Mr. Johns, however, has always been meticulously neat and could put his hands on items the minute he wanted them. Recently, he sought medical attention for memory problems. He complained that he needed to search for items because he failed to put them in their usual places. He was particularly concerned about his memory problem because of a family history of Alzheimer's disease. He was referred to occupational therapy to learn strategies to help him remember where items are placed. Objectively, Mr. Johns is not performing any worse than Mr. Balouris; however, Mr. Johns interprets his performance as impaired; furthermore, he is dissatisfied with his performance.

Clients must rate their own level of satisfaction with a task, since it is a subjective experience. Client satisfaction can be measured quickly and easily with a visual analogue scale or numerical scale, such as the ten-point scale that is used in the COPM (Law et al., 2005). Satisfaction measures are easily incorporated into goals to reflect the degree of performance, for example, *"Client will be independent in locating items needed for ADLs and IADLs in the home with a satisfaction rating of at least 8/10 within 3 weeks to support participation in ADLs and IADLs."*

ABERRANT TASK BEHAVIORS. Goals and interventions may also address any aberrant task behaviors that interfere with activity performance (Ashley et al., 2001; Rogers et al., 2000). Aberrant task behaviors vary widely and include unwanted motor behavior, such as athetoid or ballistic movements, and behavioral problems, such as self-stimulation or hitting caregivers. Exploration of the underlying cause of the aberrant task behavior facilitates the establishment of realistic goals and the selection of effective intervention strategies. Goals are aimed at eliminating or diminishing aberrant task behavior in the context of ADL and IADL tasks, for example, *"Client will decrease tongue-thrusting behaviors during feeding to a maximum of 3 episodes a meal within two months to support oral feeding that meets the client's nutritional needs."*

Additional Considerations for Setting Realistic Client Goals

The occupational therapist uses performance parameters to identify goal behaviors and degrees of performance, but a number of additional factors that can affect goal achievement must also be considered. Most of these are contextual, such as physical and social environment, financial resources, time available for intervention, and the client's past experience and learning ability. The prognosis for impairments, given the client's disability, can also affect goal achievement.

Prognosis for Impairments

The client's potential for improvement of performance skills and patterns and client factors must be examined within the context of any existing disease or disorder and resulting impairments (Hansen & Atchison, 1999; Ostchega, Harris, Hirsch, Parsons, & Kington, 2000). First, the practitioner must consider any precautions or contraindications pursuant to the diagnosis that could preclude the use of certain intervention strategies. Compare, for example, two clients whose endurance significantly limits their performance. Mrs. Tanaka has chronic fatigue syndrome, a disorder that may worsen if she becomes overfatigued. An aggressive program to increase endurance is contraindicated for her, so alternative intervention strategies should be explored, and goals for increasing endurance for ADLs must be reasonable, given Mrs. Tanaka's potential for exacerbation of her disease. Conversely, Mr. Krull is very deconditioned from inactivity resulting from major depressive illness and would like to increase his endurance to support participation in heavy home maintenance tasks, such as mowing the lawn and finishing an addition on his house. An activity program to increase endurance is not contraindicated and would help to increase Mr. Krull's participation in IADLs.

Second, the prognosis for improvement of impairments, given the client's diagnosis (i.e., disease, disorder, or condition), must be considered. Increasing impairment is expected in progressive disorders, such as muscular dystrophy, Alzheimer's disease, and rheumatoid arthritis (both adult and juvenile). Goals must be established with these potential declines in mind so that the goals are realistic. Occupational therapy practitioners must evaluate impairments separately, however, because progressive diseases might not affect all bodily structures and functions directly. Jorge, a teenager who has muscular dystrophy, illustrates this point. He has significant muscle weakness in the trunk and all four extremities and has developed some limitations in pelvic and ankle range of motion (ROM) that preclude maintaining an optimal position for functioning from his wheelchair. His muscle strength is expected to decline, even with intervention. His ROM restrictions, however, are secondary to the muscle weakness, not a direct result of the muscular dystrophy. Intervention gains can be expected in ROM with treatment, despite the overall prognosis. In turn, increased ROM can enhance function by increasing the options available for positioning Jorge in his wheelchair.

Stable or diminishing impairments may be anticipated in many disorders and after injury. Pharmacological intervention, for example, may improve the impairments associated with depression so that occupational therapy intervention can be focused on transferring gains made in mental and psychological capacities into ADL and IADL performance. Typically, clients of all ages who have had brain injuries from trauma or strokes can expect some spontaneous return of motor function in the early stages of recovery. Projected intervention goals should take into account the typical improvements for this diagnosis. Accuracy in predicting "typical improvements" takes time and experience to develop, and the novice practitioner might find it helpful to consult with more experienced clinicians to facilitate the ability to set realistic goals.

Experience

Information gathered in the evaluation about a client's past and recent experience with an activity is important to consider so that relevant and attainable goals can be established. Recent experience may facilitate progress in reestablishing independence in an activity because the client is learning a new way to do the activity rather than developing a new skill. For example, Mrs. McCarthy needs to relearn cooking skills following a stroke. She uses a wheelchair for mobility and has minimal use of her right (dominant) hand. Her cognitive skills are intact, and she can easily follow a recipe. Furthermore, she demonstrates good problem-solving skills in adapting cooking activities to improve her performance. Miranda, a 19-year-old with spastic hemiplegia secondary to cerebral palsy, has limited use of one hand and uses a wheelchair for mobility, like Mrs. McCarthy. She wants to cook simple meals and bake cookies. Her intervention is likely to require more time and guidance than Mrs. McCarthy's intervention, because Miranda has to learn basic cooking skills along with the activity adaptations that are required to compensate for her impairments.

At times, adults are also confronted with needing to learn new activities. Some of these activities relate to skills that are needed to manage new impairments, such as performing self-catheterization, donning pressure garments, or learning to operate an environmental control unit. New learning may also be needed when new roles are assumed,

for example, when a spouse becomes disabled or dies and the partner has to take on new responsibilities. Whenever a skill is unfamiliar to a client, additional intervention time and education from the occupational therapy practitioner might be needed for basic skill acquisition and should be incorporated into the goal and the intervention plan.

Client's Capacity for Learning and Openness to Alternative Methods

The client's capacity for learning and openness to using alternative methods for task completion must be evaluated, because intervention often requires learning new methods of completing activities (Flinn & Radomski, 2008; Fuhrer & Keith, 1998). Fewer intervention options exist for clients with limited learning capacity, and the duration of the intervention might need to be longer. Some clients who do not want to use a special device to do a task that most people do without a device might resist treatment that incorporates adaptive equipment (Lund & Nygård, 2003). Clients with a good capacity for learning and openness to alternative methods often are able to address more task deficits because of increased intervention options and the reduced time required for learning. It is important to view capacity for learning on a continuum; clients can fall between the extremes, and capacity might be better for some tasks than for others. A client might be capable of learning the relatively simple task adaptation of using a joystick to drive a wheelchair but be unable to master a more complex electronic aid to daily living, even one that relies on the same movements that are used to control the joystick.

Projected Follow-Through with Program Outside of Treatment

Efforts to contain health care costs have led to increasingly shorter lengths of stay in hospitals and rehabilitation centers and a reduction in outpatient and home-health visits. Clients are expected to take a more active role in their therapy programs and to supplement formal interventions with self-directed intervention (e.g., home programs). Goals therefore need to be established with some estimate of the client's capacity to follow through with a self-directed program, as this will greatly influence the success of any intervention (Cope & Sundance, 1995).

Several of the performance parameters that were previously delineated can give the occupational therapy practitioner guidance in this area. Clients have more motivation for programs that are aimed at activities that they highly value than at those that they do not value, making a client-centered approach critical for success. In addition, performance parameters such as difficulty, fatigue, pain, and satisfaction must be graded so that self-directed programs are manageable within the context of the client's daily routines. The meaning of *manageable* must be established by clients in consultation with the occupational therapy practitioner and should take into consideration clients' daily activities and responsibilities, tolerance for frustration, and perseverance.

Many clients require some assistance to practice activities, and the occupational therapy practitioner must be sure that these resources are available. This assistance may include setting up an activity, providing assistance for specific activity steps, and allowing ample time (as prescribed) for effective practice. It is important to remember that impairments can affect the client's ability to initiate or persevere with everyday activities. For these clients, assistance is needed for initiation and follow-through in the home program. This responsibility often falls on family members, and occupational therapy practitioners need to interact with and educate family members about their critical role.

Time for Intervention

The projected timeline for occupational therapy may be influenced by multiple factors, including the functional prognosis, the client's motivation for improvement, and the client's finances. In managed health care, it is becoming common for health insurance carriers to set the number of visits or length of stay (Kramer et al., 2000). The occupational therapy goals must be tailored to meet the client's

needs as much as possible within the time allotted. Nonetheless, it must also be recognized that best practice takes into account *all* the client's needs. Often, with clear and complete documentation of adequate progress toward established goals, third-party payers will approve additional occupational therapy visits. Occupational therapy practitioners need to be aware of their professional responsibility to clients to request intervention extensions and to support these requests through detailed documentation.

Resources and the Expected Discharge Context

Established functional goals must be achievable within the client's available resources, including social and financial resources (Seigley, 1998). Clients' expected discharge environments must be considered in establishing goals and selecting interventions that will be relevant to the environment in which clients will ultimately perform tasks (Cox, 1996; Dunn, 1993; Dunn, Brown, & McGuigan, 1994; Law et al., 1996). The social context is critical for clients who require assistance from others after discharge; that is, it is important to determine whether there are people who are willing and able to provide needed assistance. Clients' needs vary broadly in terms of the type and dura-

ETHICAL DILEMMA

Can Client-Centered Care Conflict with the Needs of an Organization?

Jessica is an occupational therapist working in a subacute rehabilitation unit in a skilled nursing facility. She completed an evaluation on Mrs. Cabrini, an 82-year-old woman with multiple medical problems, including a recent total hip replacement secondary to a fracture, cardiovascular disease, and rheumatoid arthritis. Mrs. Cabrini would like to be independent in transfers, indoor mobility, and toileting, which would enable her to return to her home in an assisted living facility. She reported that she could get daily help with dressing and bathing and would prefer to do that because she fatigues quickly and wants to save her energy for the daily morning craft group. During the evaluation, Mrs. Cabrini tolerated about 30 minutes of therapy in the morning and 30 minutes in the afternoon, divided between occupational therapy and physical therapy. Jessica established client-centered goals collaboratively with Mrs. Cabrini. The physical therapist agreed that the client could work productively for only two 30-minute treatments a day, and they opted to split the time, so Jessica

documented that the intensity of occupational therapy would be 30 minutes daily, seven days a week.

Jessica's supervisor approached Jessica and asked her to increase Mrs. Cabrini to 45 minutes a day so that Mrs. Cabrini would qualify for a higher Resource Utilization Group (RUG) under the Medicare prospective payment system. The supervisor told Jessica that if the facility cannot increase reimbursement rates by having more clients in higher RUGs, they might need to lay off staff, which would have a negative impact on client care. Jessica's supervisor also suggested that it would be easy to justify the increased treatment if Jessica added more ADL goals, such as independence in dressing and bathing, to Mrs. Cabrini's care plan.

1. What should Jessica do in this situation?
2. How might client-centered care influence Jessica's actions?
3. How can Jessica balance the needs and wishes of her client with the needs of the facility?

tion of assistance required. Some clients need only supportive services, such as help with shopping or housecleaning. Those with significant activity limitations and intact cognition might require considerable physical assistance but can be left alone once ADLs have been completed, they have eaten, and they are mobile in their wheelchairs. Clients with cognitive impairments do not always need physical assistance but might need verbal cueing to maintain activity performance, and this assistance might need to be constant. Inadequate support in the client's expected environment can necessitate a change in the discharge plan. Some families or friends might be able to provide the level and type of assistance needed, whereas other families might be unable or unwilling to do this.

The physical environment must also be considered in setting realistic goals (Gitlin, Corcoran, Winter, Boyce, & Hauck, 2001). For example, Mr. Feng has reached his goal of independence in bathing during his hospital-based rehabilitation. He requires a transfer tub seat, a hand-held shower hose, and a grab bar to bathe safely without help. The occupational therapy practitioner wants to order this equipment for him. However, Mr. Feng reports that he must shower in a 4 by 4 foot shower stall because the only bathtub is on the second floor and he cannot manage stairs. His shower will not accommodate the transfer tub bench that he requires for safe transfers and balance during showering. An alternative bathing goal should have been established at the beginning of intervention so that Mr. Feng's program focused on developing skills he could use at home, such as sponge bathing at the sink.

The adaptability of the discharge environment must also be explored before setting goals. A house that is high above the street on a small lot with 21 steps to the front door makes the installation of a properly graded ramp impossible. Wall grab bars cannot be installed on fiberglass tub surrounds, making a safety rail placed on the side of the bathtub the only feasible option, regardless of where the client really needs the most support. Clients living in rental units might be unable to make structural alterations as desired because they do not own the unit.

Last, the client's expected discharge environments must be explored if activities are likely to be performed in more than one place. Clients in a hospital-based setting may be focused primarily on returning home, but most people do not confine themselves to a single environment. Adaptations for toilets, such as raised toilet seats and toilet armrests, are commonly used for people with limited mobility. Home adaptations are easily made, but clients are often in environments that have not been adapted, such as public buildings, friends' homes, airplanes, hotels, and portable toilets at the local fair. If clients are likely to be in these environments, their goals should address their ability to perform tasks in varied settings.

PRACTICE DILEMMA

HOW DOES ONE PROVIDE OPTIMAL CARE WITH LIMITED RESOURCES?

Jon is an occupational therapist in a large rehabilitation hospital in major city. The occupational therapy department recently installed the latest **electronic aids to independent living (EADLs)** in an on-site apartment that they use for treatment. Henry is a 16-year-old who has muscular dystrophy. He has a reclining power wheelchair that he can drive independently with a head switch. He has very limited use of his upper extremities. Henry lives alone with his mother, who works in a low-wage job. He receives Medicaid.

Henry's disease has progressed such that he is no longer able to get into and out of his home without assistance or operate common electronic devices, including the television, telephone, and lights. Because his mother works during the day, Henry must attend an after-school program, which is primarily for small children. Henry has told his occupational therapist that his most important goal is to be able to go home from school and access his home. The occupational therapist is sure that this could be an achievable goal for Henry with an EADL system that would enable him to be independent in unlocking and opening the door, turning lights and electronic devices on and off, and using the telephone and computer. The therapist is also aware, however, that Medicaid will not pay for an EADL in his state.

1. How should Jon proceed? Should he train Henry in the use of the EADL, even if it will not be possible for him to purchase it?
2. What team members might the occupational therapist consult with to help him progress Henry toward his goal?
3. Does the diagnosis of muscular dystrophy, a progressive disorder, affect the approach that Jon would take to solve this problem?
4. How can Jon help Henry to achieve his goal?

INTERVENTIONS FOR ADL AND IADL DEFICITS

Interventions for ADL and IADL deficits are based on clients' goals and involve selecting treatment approaches and activities, carrying out the treatment, and reviewing the intervention to ensure that it is effective in progressing clients toward their goals.

Planning and Implementing Intervention

Five intervention approaches are described in the OTPF: create/promote, prevent, maintain, modify/adapt, and establish/restore (AOTA, 2002). While any of these approaches can be used to support ADL and IADL performance, modify/adapt and establish/restore are the most commonly used in practice and will be the focus of intervention discussed in this chapter. Both the adaptive and restorative approaches need to be combined with client and/or caregiver education to ensure carryover of the program to function in everyday life (Flinn & Radomski, 2008). The selection of specific treatment activities is guided in large part by the frame(s) of reference selected by the occupational therapy practitioner for each client. Specific frames of reference are beyond the scope of this chapter but can be found in Unit VIII. The following subsection focuses on broader intervention approaches and their related strategies. It includes a discussion of client and caregiver education, grading activities to progress clients to the established goals.

Selecting an Intervention Approach

The occupational therapy practitioner considers a number of variables when deciding whether it is more appropriate to focus on compensating for a client's deficits through adaptation or restoring underlying skills needed to reach goals. These considerations are addressed in the sections that follow.

MODIFY.   Activity performance can be enhanced through compensation for activity limitations rather than restoration of previous capacities. This is often necessary when restoration is not an option. For example, at this time, a client with a complete C5 quadriplegia will not regain previous hand function, regardless of the restorative approach used. Compensation for impairments is needed for successful participation in ADLs and IADLs. Even for clients for whom restoration is possible, a compensatory approach might be more appropriate if time limitations or client motivation would lead to less than optimal outcomes. Compensatory strategies may also be warranted when some but not full restoration of function is achieved. Generally, compensatory strategies require less intervention time for achieving functional outcomes compared with restorative strategies.

Intervention for limitations in safe activity performance is often aimed at adapting the activity or the environment so that performance can be improved as soon as possible (Close et al., 1999; Cummings et al., 1999). In contrast, improvement in independence can occur over time, as long as adequate assistance is available. Intervention for safety should include an educational component for clients and their caregivers when clients are relearning familiar activities with reduced capacities or within new and unfamiliar performance environments.

Three general intervention strategies may be employed under the compensatory approach. The activity or task method may be altered, the task objects may be adapted, or the environment may be modified. Combinations of these methods may be used to maximize client performance. Examples of these three intervention strategies for selected ADLs and IADLs are included in Table 48.3.

ALTER THE TASK METHOD.   When the task method is altered, the task objects and contexts are unchanged, but the method of performing the task is altered to make the task feasible given the client's impairments. Many one-handed techniques for tasks that are normally done with two hands use this strategy, including one-handed dressing, one-handed shoe-tying (Figure 48.2), and one-handed typing techniques. To master an altered task method successfully, clients require the capacity to learn. The necessary level of learning capacity depends on the complexity of the method that is to be learned. People often rely on automatic processing for well-learned ADLs and IADLs so that they require little direct attention. Automatic processing of routine tasks frees the individual for other things, such as planning one's workday while getting ready in the morning or chatting with a child while grocery shopping. Practice is a necessary component of all learning and is especially crucial for clients who wish to develop or return to automatic performance of ADLs (Flinn & Radomski, 2008). Clients benefit from good follow-through with a training program to meet adequacy parameters, such as reducing difficulty and duration of performance and increasing satisfaction.

ADAPT THE TASK OBJECTS OR PRESCRIBE ASSISTIVE DEVICES. The objects that are used for the task may be altered to facilitate performance. For example, handles can be built up on utensils for clients with decreased finger ROM or training in the use of memory aids (e.g., memory notebooks, checklists, cue cards, and electronic cueing devices) may help clients who have difficulty initiating tasks (Knoke, Taylor, & Saint-Cyr, 1998; Schwartz, 1995). For some task adaptations, the task objects do not significantly alter the task method, so the need for learning is less than it is when the method is altered. When this is the case, the need for practice is also reduced, and performance can improve quickly. Examples of simple adaptations include utensils with enlarged or extended handles, a cutting

TABLE 48.3		EXAMPLES OF THE THREE APPROACHES TO MODIFYING TASKS TO COMPENSATE FOR IMPAIRMENTS	

Task	Alter the Method	Alter the Task Objects	Modify the Task Environment
Bathing	Substitute washing at the sink for someone who is unable to get into and out of the tub safely even with adaptive equipment.	Use a bath mitt and soap on a rope so that objects are not dropped by someone who cannot bend down to retrieve them.	Install grab bars and a transfer tub seat to enable the client to remain seated during bathing.
Grooming	Client learns to stabilize small containers with the ulnar digits while unscrewing lids with the radial digits to compensate for loss of the use of one hand.	An extended handle is added to a razor so that a woman can shave her legs without bending forward.	An extendable, wall-mounted mirror is mounted at an appropriate height for a wheelchair user.
Toileting	Use an alarm watch to encourage regular emptying of the bladder.	Use a toilet aid to extend the range of reach for toilet hygiene.	Install a bidet on the toilet to eliminate the need for manipulating toilet paper for hygiene.
Dressing	Learn to dress the affected side first to compensate for loss of use of one side of the body.	Use a sock aid to put socks on without having to reach the feet.	Lower clothing racks or replace a high dresser with a low one to increase access to clothes.
Feeding	Serve different food items (e.g., meat, starch, vegetable) in consistent places on the plate for someone who is blind.	Use a built-up handled utensil to compensate for diminished prehension in the hand.	Have an elementary school child eat with a few friends in a small room rather than the cafeteria, which is too busy and distracting.
Transfers	Sit first in the car seat before swinging the legs in rather than entering the car by leading with the leg.	Use a sliding board to eliminate the need for the lower extremities to support body weight.	Rearrange furniture to allow the wheelchair to be positioned near to the bed or a favorite chair.
Cooking	Sit at the kitchen table to chop vegetables to conserve energy.	Use a cutting board with aluminum nails to hold vegetables for cutting or peeling.	Install a mirror above the stove to enable a wheelchair user to see items cooking.
Paying bills	Round check entries to the nearest dollar to simplify the math for a client with cognitive impairment.	Use large checks, a dark pen, and a writing guide to compensate for low vision.	Install four plastic wall pockets to sort bills due each week of the month for a client with poor attention or memory.
Shopping	Shift to online and catalogue shopping to reduce the need for community mobility.	Purchase a walker basket for carrying items.	Request assistance from a grocery store employee to help reach items.

board with nails to stabilize food while cutting, and elastic shoelaces.

The prescription of assistive devices must take into account the client's capabilities and willingness to use the device, as well as the features of the device, a process that is frequently oversimplified. For example, a sock aid can help a client with poor sitting balance to reach her feet without leaning forward, which could throw her off balance. However, if the client's balance deficit is secondary to hemiple-

gia and she also has poor use of one hand, it will be very difficult or impossible for her to get the sock onto the sock aid, which typically requires both hands (Figure 48.3). Figure 48.4 depicts the number of decisions that an occupational therapy practitioner makes when selecting an adapted spoon, a very simple type of adaptive equipment. Although many assistive devices that occupational therapy practitioners prescribe are quite simple mechanically, some are sophisticated and include complex electronics, circuits, and

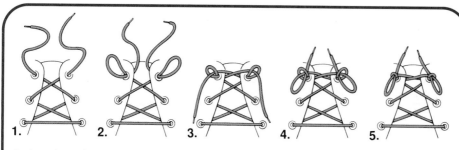

1. Lace laces in usual way.
2. Put both lace ends back through the holes they exited until the loops formed are small.
3. Put the lace ends through the opposite loops and pull to tighten loops, allowing just enough room to put the lace end back through the loop.
4. Put lace ends back through the loops, forming another loop.
5. Pull on these loops alternately to tighten.

FIGURE 48.2 One-handed shoe-tying method.

microprocessors, such as electronic aids to daily living that interact with smart houses.

One disadvantage of adapting task objects is that the adaptive equipment must be available to clients whenever and wherever they engage in the task. This might or might not pose a problem, depending on the task and the adaptation. Clients who use memory books at work to compensate for cognitive impairments can incorporate the structure and cues needed into a daily planner or a hand-held personal data assistant, a tool that was used habitually before the impairment. If a client requires built-up utensils for eating, however, and wishes to eat at a restaurant, the utensils must be taken along. This is cumbersome, and some clients find it embarrassing.

Finally, some clients find that the use of adaptive equipment reduces satisfaction with task performance. To enhance personal satisfaction with task performance, they might be willing to cope with the increased

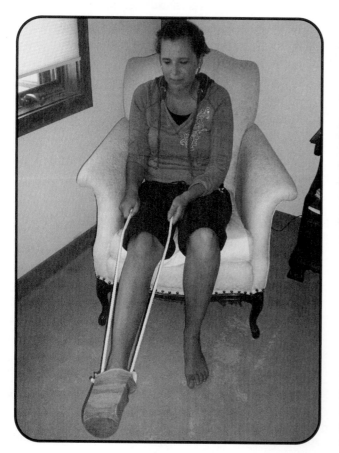

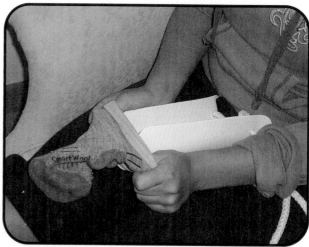

FIGURE 48.3 A sock-aid is useful for people with limited reach, for example, from limited balance or range of motion. However, the client needs to have the use of both hands to get the sock onto the device, which could make it impractical for some clients.

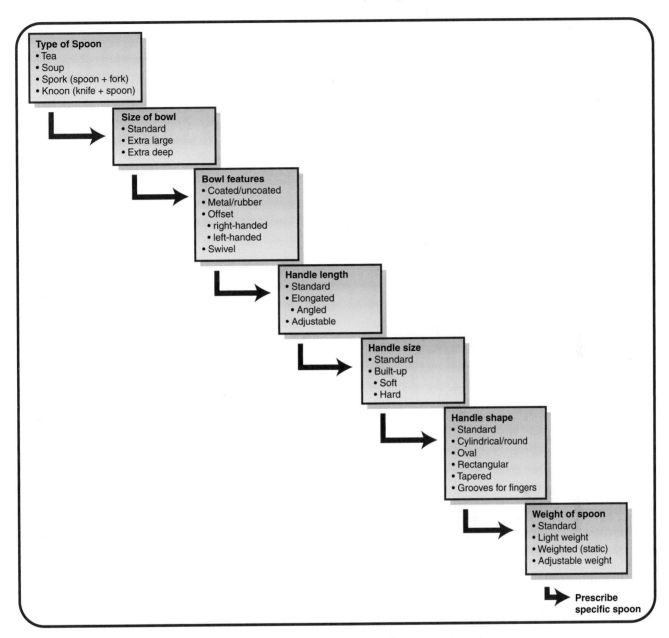

FIGURE 48.4   Potential decisions for the prescription of one assistive device, an adapted spoon.

difficulty of doing a task without adapted tools. For example, Ms. Lindstrom, a woman with multiple sclerosis, found that her mobility was safer and easier in a wheelchair, but she preferred to walk when out in the community. Her dissatisfaction with the wheelchair overrode other considerations.

MODIFY THE TASK ENVIRONMENT.   Modification of the environment itself may be used to facilitate task performance (Dunn et al., 1994). Typically, when the environment is modified, the demand for learning and practice is less than that required for learning an alternative method or using adapted task objects. Environmental modifica-

tions are often fixed in place so that clients do not need to remember to bring along the necessary adaptations and the adaptations cannot be easily displaced (e.g., they cannot be dropped out of reach). Usually, the task method is unchanged, or only minimally changed, so that clients can rely on previous experience. Examples include installing a wheelchair ramp, installing a floor-to-ceiling pole in the bathroom (Figure 48.5), recessing plumbing under the sink to accommodate a wheelchair user, increasing available light, labeling cupboard doors to compensate for cognitive deficits, and installing a toilet seat frame.

The biggest drawback of environmental modifications is that clients might become limited in terms of performance

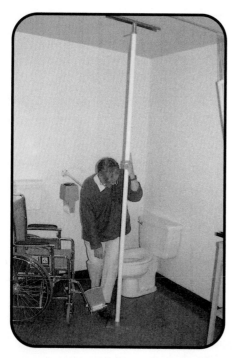

FIGURE 48.5   A floor-to-ceiling pole that can be used to facilitate stability during transfers.

context. They must do the task in the modified environment or in one that has been similarly modified, because the modifications are not easily transportable and might be custom designed for a specific setting.

ESTABLISH/RESTORE.   A restorative approach typically focuses intervention at the impairment level with the aim of restoring or establishing the capacities that are needed for functional tasks (AOTA, 2002). Intervention may be used to restore capacities such as strength, endurance, ROM, short-term memory, visual scanning, and interests. More information about specific techniques can be found in the chapters in Unit XI. Regardless of the specific frame of reference or techniques used, however, one must always establish the link between the impairment and the resulting activity limitations. Careful documentation of the evaluation assists other health professionals and third-party payers to understand the connection between the intervention and the established functional outcomes. Clients must also be educated about the relationship between their inherent capacities and the everyday tasks that they pursue so that they understand how the intervention will ultimately lead to improved task performance.

All intervention programs that are designed to restore or establish inherent capacities must provide clients with a structured opportunity to transfer the gains made in these capacities to relevant functional tasks (Latham, 2008a). This ensures that the intervention outcome is functional and helps to maintain gains made through increasing capacity and reducing impairment by providing an oppor-

tunity for practice within the daily routine. For example, stretching exercises that result in increased right shoulder flexion active motion should be accompanied by functional tasks that require movement into the newly acquired range, such as using the right upper extremity to reach up to pin pictures on a bulletin board or dusting bookshelves. Other examples can be found in Table 48.4.

Intervention that is aimed at restoration is often most efficient for clients for whom a few impairments affect many tasks and for whom diminished capacities can be expected to improve. For example, Mr. Stapinski had circumferential second-degree burns to both upper extremities. The resulting bilateral restrictions in elbow flexion prevented him from completing most ADLs owing to an inability to reach his face, head, or trunk. Tasks could be easily adapted by using long-handled devices, but extended tools would have been needed for many ADL tasks (e.g., eating utensils, toothbrush, comb, brush, bath sponge). Because clients with burns can be expected to increase ROM with passive stretching, scar management, and exercise, intervention was most efficient when it was aimed at increasing Mr. Stapinski's elbow flexion. Adapting selected task objects improved his ADL performance in the short-term; however, the long-term goal of restoring Mr. Stapinski's capacity to flex his elbows enhanced function across many different tasks.

A restorative approach may be appropriate for some clients with progressive disorders even though their capacities are expected to deteriorate, given the typical course of the condition. The focus, however, becomes slowing the decline of specific capacities and skills. For example, clients with Parkinson's disease may reduce bradykinesia with the use of a movement exercise program (Curtis, Bassile, Cote, & Gentile, 2001).

For clients with some types of impairments, carefully structured everyday activities can restore or establish capacities while simultaneously permitting the practice of the activities. Clients who are severely deconditioned might find their activity level limited by poor endurance. Intervention could rely on aerobic exercise to increase cardiopulmonary endurance, with the goal of participating in functional activities when an adequate increase in cardiopulmonary capacity was achieved. Instead, an intervention that graded the intensity and duration of daily activities could be as effective in increasing cardiovascular fitness while enabling the client to participate in desired tasks. In addition, gains that are made in endurance are immediately transferred into functional activities. Children and adults may engage more effectively in play activities that incorporate the necessary repetitive movements compared to a rote exercise (Melchert-McKearnan, Deitz, Engel, & White, 2000). Practice and participation in ADL and IADL programs also give clients with a new disability an opportunity to become familiar with their new bodies (Guidetti, Asaba, & Tham, 2007)

TABLE 48.4 INTEGRATING TREATMENT GAINS FROM AN ESTABLISH OR RESTORE APPROACH INTO FUNCTIONAL TASKS

Impairment	Task to Reduce Impairment	Task to Integrate Gains Made into ADL/IADL	Functional Outcomes
Impaired grip strength	Theraputty exercises	Cooking task that begins with light resistance (e.g. stirring Jello) and progress (e.g., stirring brownie mix)	Increased ability to grasp task objects firmly (e.g. opening containers, doors, pulling up pants)
Decreased upper extremity muscle endurance	Using an arm ergometer	Wheelchair mobility, increasing time and difficulty (e.g., progress from flat surfaces to ramps)	Increased ability to engage in sustained upper extremity work (e.g., propelling a wheelchair, shampooing hair, washing windows)
Hyperresponsiveness to tactile stimuli	Brushing skin	Progress from bathing in a tub to a shower, which provides a stronger stimulus	Ability to tolerate tactile stimuli in everyday tasks, including dressing, brushing teeth, and interacting with others
Poor visual scanning	Paper-and-pencil cancellation tasks (e.g., cross out all the M's on a sheet of letters)	Find items in a kitchen cupboard or grocery store shelf	Ability to use a more organized scanning process for locating objects (e.g., finding a blouse in the closet, a brush on a cluttered dresser, the milk in the refrigerator)

Depending on the nature of the performance discrepancy and the degree of impairment, the intervention time that is needed in establishing or restoring underlying skills can be longer than that required for compensatory approaches. This increased time must be taken into consideration, particularly in managed care settings. In addition, clients must recognize that the rehabilitation period might be longer and that follow-through with a home program is vital if gains are to be made.

INTEGRATING INTERVENTION FOR IMPAIRMENTS AND ACTIVITY LIMITATIONS. At first glance, it might seem that the modify/adapt and establish/restore approaches are mutually exclusive—that is, that the outcome is either to establish/restore the impaired capacity or to compensate for it. Using both approaches simultaneously might seem a bit like using a belt and suspenders. However, a carefully crafted program enables clients to be more functional through the use of compensatory strategies while at the same time working to restore functional capacities. It is critical that the occupational therapy practitioner reduce the use of compensatory strategies as clients make gains in skill performance when using the two approaches.

For example, Mr. Stapinski, whose burns resulted in bilateral limitations in elbow flexion, might benefit from using utensils with extended handles. With the extended handles on the utensils, he can feed himself independently during the two to three weeks that it takes to increase his elbow flexion sufficiently for him to feed himself without these utensils. The extended handles should be fabricated to require him to flex fully within his available range and should be shortened as gains in ROM are made, so that the new range is incorporated into the feeding task.

Whenever task or environmental adaptations are anticipated to be temporary, it is necessary to consider cost in relationship to the anticipated time the equipment will be needed, and the potential benefit to clients. Thermoplastic or wood extensions can be added temporarily to the handles of regular utensils rather than prescribing the more costly commercially available utensils with elongated handles. For some tasks, safety concerns supersede cost considerations. Using a collapsible lawn chair in the shower would be an inexpensive alternative to a shower chair, but it would not provide adequate stability.

Education of the Client or Caregiver

Caregiver training may be implemented to maximize a client's functional outcome while minimizing the efforts of the caregiver (Bogardus et al., 2001; Dooley & Hinojosa,

2004; Hepburn, Tornatore, Center, & Ostwald, 2001; Miller & Butin, 2000). For example, Mr. Ford sustained a left cerebrovascular accident and required minimal physical assistance with verbal cueing from the occupational therapy practitioner for wheelchair transfers. Mrs. Ford was physically able to help her husband but had no prior experience in transferring a person with hemiparesis. One day, she decided to help her husband move from his hospital bed to the chair. Because she did not block his right knee or tell him to wait for her cue before standing, they both fell onto the bed while attempting to execute the transfer. Fortunately, no one was hurt. As a consequence of this experience, Mrs. Ford was convinced that she could not care for her husband at home. At the same time, she was distressed by the thought of having to admit him to a long-term care facility. She was receptive to receiving transfer training from the occupational therapy practitioner and was delighted to find that by using the proper physical and verbal techniques, she could easily and safely assist her husband. In this example, caregiver training increased the client's level of independence and the probability that he could go home at discharge.

INSTRUCTIONAL METHODS. A variety of instructional methods are available for client and caregiver education (Fuhrer & Keith, 1998), and methods should be selected that best meet the person's needs. When a facility has a homogeneous client population, group instruction can be an efficient and effective method for providing basic education. Many arthritis centers provide group instruction in joint-protection techniques. Teaching a group is cost-effective and, when well structured, can facilitate learning through peer interaction. For caregiver groups, the contact with others who are experiencing similar problems in their caregiving roles can provide valuable emotional support and an opportunity for constructive group problem solving.

Some type of individualized instruction is typically needed to complement group instruction so that information can be tailored to meet the specific and unique needs of each person. If group instruction has preceded the individualized instruction, the client-specific sessions can be relatively short and focused on application of the information learned in the group to the client's particular circumstances. For example, clients would be taught how to apply proper lifting techniques to the weights and dimensions of objects in their own homes.

Individualized instruction is more appropriate for many clients and caregivers because the personal nature of the tasks that need to be learned does not lend itself to group instruction (e.g., bathing). Furthermore, in intervention settings that serve a diverse case mix, the opportunity for group instruction rarely occurs. One-to-one client or caregiver education and training enables the occupational therapy practitioner to obtain immediate feedback from the person as the session progresses and to alter the amount and focus of learning accordingly.

A vast array of media are available to occupational therapy practitioners to facilitate the client's or caregiver's learning process. Written materials may be developed specifically for a client or caregiver, or published materials can be used if appropriate ones are available. Video-cassette or digital recorders are widely available, even in clients' homes, and custom or commercially made video-tapes or DVDs can be effective teaching tools. Audiotapes can also be effective, particularly when visual input would be distracting. For example, an audiotape may be used to facilitate visual imagery for relaxation or stress reduction. The Internet is accessible to the general population, and many occupational therapy clinics have Internet access. A wealth of information about a variety of disorders is available that is specifically geared toward clients and caregivers. Clients can also find peer support groups through chat rooms, Web forums, or e-mail lists.

CAREGIVER TRAINING. In addition to evaluating clients' learning capacity, the learning capacity of their caregivers needs to be appraised. Like clients, caregivers have varied learning styles, capacities, and experience. In many situations, the caregiver is a family member who is still coping with the emotional impact of having a family member with a disability, whether it is a new parent with a child with cerebral palsy or the spouse of a someone who has had a stroke. People who are under emotional stress often need more time and repetition to process information accurately (Blake & Lincoln, 2000). In other cases, caregivers have been providing care for years and bring a wealth of caring expertise to the treatment session. The occupational therapy practitioner should work collaboratively with all caregivers but may move into a more consultative role with experienced caregivers who can articulate problems and engage actively in problem solving based on prior learning (Toth-Cohen, 2000). When caregivers are expected to assist clients physically, their physical capacity for providing this assistance also warrants evaluation.

Caregivers have varied learning styles, and instruction that caters to their preferred style is likely to be the most efficient and effective (Banford et al., 2001). Some people, for example, are kinesthetic learners. They learn most quickly through doing. Visual learners might prefer to watch a demonstration of the activity several times before attempting it themselves. Others might prefer written instructions. All learners benefit from the opportunity to ask questions to clarify instructions. Media that support teaching by a practitioner can be a great asset. Videotapes or DVDs, for example, provide caregivers with an excellent visual image of how an exercise or activity is to be done. Often, home- or clinic-made videotapes can be made of a client's activity performance. These productions add little time to the intervention session, because they are recorded as activities are practiced during regular therapy. They have the advantage of providing richer and more detailed information than is feasible in oral or written instructions.

When caregivers are helping to carry out an intervention program, the goals and general intervention strategies should be made clear to them. For restoration programs, clients might need assistance with implementing specific exercises or grading of activities in a way that will help to restore skills. Caregivers need to learn specific cueing strategies so that home programs are carried out accurately, whether in clients' homes, group homes, or long-term care settings. Caregivers are often pivotal in motivating clients. Motivating clients who have disorders that impair motivation, such as depression, can be particularly challenging. Helping caregivers to understand that disinterest and lack of motivation are a part of the disorder and providing concrete strategies for managing the "getting going" phase of the home program will foster its success (Resnick, 1998). For clients with behavior problems, such as the reactions that may accompany autism or Alzheimer's disease, teaching caregivers behavior management strategies that defuse potentially volatile situations can be invaluable to their success as caregivers.

Caregiver training for assisting clients with functional activities should focus first on safety for clients and caregivers. The occupational therapy practitioner should emphasize components of the activity that promote safety, such as locking the wheelchair brakes or blocking the client's knee to prevent buckling when transferring to and from the wheelchair. As intervention progresses, the occupational therapy practitioner should inform caregivers of the activities that are safe and unsafe to perform outside of the therapy situation. For example, although a client might be working on bathtub transfers during therapy, skilled facilitation to get into and out of the tub safely might be required, making it premature for the client to practice these transfers at home.

When caregivers need to provide physical assistance, they should be trained in using proper body mechanics, especially during transfers or bed mobility and also for wheelchair positioning. Assisting a client in a wheelchair with ADLs, such as brushing teeth or feeding, while the caregiver is standing can fatigue the caregiver's lower back muscles. Taking care of the caregiver is frequently overlooked in occupational therapy interventions, but it is an essential component of the person–task–environment transaction, particularly when it is anticipated that the client will require assistance over a long period of time.

COMMENTARY ON THE EVIDENCE

Finding the Best Educational Strategies for Client Learning

As individual treatment time has been reduced by third-party reimbursement plans, client and caregiver education has played a more important role in treatment. Many studies have demonstrated the effectiveness of different and varied educational programs. For example, patient education programs have been effective in improving self-management and reducing pain and disability for people with rheumatoid arthritis (Hammond, 2004), reducing the impact of fatigue on occupational performance in people with multiple sclerosis (Vanage et al., 2003), and increasing confidence and activity participation in older adults who have a fear of falling (Cheal & Clemson, 2001). Eklund, Sonn, and Dahlin-Ivanoff (2004) compared a health education program for people who have visual impairment with traditional individualized intervention and reported that participants in the health education program had higher perceived security for a number of ADLs and IADLs, supporting the need for structured client education programs. Researchers typically describe the educational programs that were used in their studies, and the educational methods reported vary significantly. Although there is ample research to support the efficacy of patient education programs on client outcomes, no studies were found that compared varied educational approaches for clients to identify best practice in this area. Learning is a complex process, and factors such as motivation and self-efficacy should be addressed in planning learning experiences (Edelstein, 2005). Clients must be ready to learn, so the timing of education can also affect its effectiveness (Hammond, 2004) and should be further explored. Many educational programs are aimed at changing clients' habits, such as engaging in home exercise programs or incorporating energy conservation techniques into daily activities, which may require behavioral approaches for supporting the development of new habits (Hammond, 2004). Future research should also examine the impact of varied impairments on the effectiveness of education, for example, problems with initiation, attention, or executive function. Gathering additional evidence will enable practitioners to become even more effective in helping clients to reach their goals.

Grading the Intervention Program

Intervention programs should never be static. It is important to progress the client continually toward the established intervention goals. The specific means of grading intervention when a restoration approach is being implemented depends on the impairments and the intervention strategies that are being used (Latham, 2008b). (The chapters on restoration of impairments in this text provide more specific guidance.) If the intervention plan uses both restoration and compensation, the program can be graded by reducing the amount of task and environmental adaptations as clients' capacities are restored. Intervention for activity limitations can be graded by modifying many of the performance parameters that were described earlier in the chapter. Clients may increase their level of independence in task performance, take more responsibility for safety, feel more personal satisfaction from a task, reduce the level of difficulty or required exertion, or decrease the duration or the occurrence of aberrant task behaviors.

GRADING TASK PROGRESSION FROM EASIER TO HARDER. One means of grading an intervention program is to begin with easier tasks and progress to more difficult ones. Task difficulty will be relative to a client's activity limitations and underlying impairments. For example, paying bills might be relatively easy for a client with quadriplegia to perform once the use of a writing tool is mastered, whereas lower extremity dressing is much more difficult. Conversely, a client with a head injury that resulted in significant cognitive impairment with relatively preserved motor skills is likely to find lower extremity dressing to be relatively easy but money management extremely difficult.

INCREASING COMPLEXITY WITHIN THE TASK. Rather than progressing only from easier to harder activities, intervention may also be graded by increasing the complexity within an activity or by progressing from simple to more complex ways of doing it. Cooking skills might extend from simple preparations such as cold sandwiches to more complex, multiple-course dinners. Even seemingly simple tasks can often be graded. A sock-donning intervention, for example, might be scaled from using looser ankle socks to tighter knee socks and finally to tight antiembolus hose.

SAME TASK IN VARIED PERFORMANCE ENVIRONMENTS. A critical part of a graded intervention program involves progression from the intervention environment to the real-life environment in which the activity will actually be performed. This can involve transfer from a clinic to a home setting or the more subtle dynamics associated with the transfer of help from the occupational therapy practitioner to the natural caregiver. The client who is independent in donning a jacket while sitting on a mat table in the clinic might be unable to do so when sitting on a chair with a back or when standing (the way a jacket is typically donned by people who are able to walk). Providing practice in increasingly demanding performance environments can facilitate the generalization of skills, thereby enhancing the client's functional flexibility.

Intervention Review

ADLs and IADLs are evaluated on entry to occupational therapy to provide a measure of the client's baseline performance status. Regardless of the extent and length of the intervention, reevaluation of ADL and IADL performance is needed to ascertain whether the intervention is resulting in improvement, whether the intervention should be continued or changed, or whether maximal benefit from occupational therapy has been achieved and activity performance has reached a plateau. Occupational therapy practitioners routinely engage in informal review of interventions by observing clients' performance during treatment and considering the actual or potential impact of their performance on established goals.

Periodically, a more formal intervention review or reevaluation is needed to objectively measure clients' progress toward goals and for documenting their progress in clinical records. The best strategy for reevaluation is to readminister the evaluations that were done at entry. Using the same ADL and IADL content, the same measurement parameters, and the same data-gathering methods enhances the possibility of detecting change in the client's performance that is attributable to intervention. If the reevaluation varies from a prior evaluation, the potential for detecting change is reduced. For example, if ADL performance is evaluated in the occupational therapy clinic by using observation immediately before discharge and by using a telephone survey sometime after discharge, it is not possible to determine whether increased performance is reflecting the client's actual improvement or is the result of the change in data-gathering method (observation versus questioning).

CONCLUSION

This chapter described the complex practice of evaluating and treating clients with ADL and IADL deficits. Performance parameters of value, independence, safety, and adequacy were reviewed, and their relevance to the selection of specific assessment tools was described. Occupational therapists should establish objective baseline measures through the use of standardized ADL and IADL assessments whenever possible; however, the realities of the treatment setting may also require the use of nonstandardized assessments. Developing objective goals that address all relevant performance parameters is a crucial first step in implementing treatment by providing a "road map" for guiding client care. General treatment approaches that occupational therapists use to increase participation in ADLs and IADLs include modifying the task or environment, establishing or restoring underlying impairments, and client and caregiver education. Grading activities effectively will maximize clients' progress toward goals. Specific treatment activities vary significantly according to the clients' ages and disabilities and are beyond the scope of this chapter. Readers should use this chapter to guide them in the overall process of ADL and IADL intervention and refer to sources that focus on specific client populations and service delivery models when selecting specific treatment activities.

ACKNOWLEDGMENTS

I would like to thank Dr. Margo B. Holm and Dr. Joan Rogers for inviting me to coauthor two prior editions of the ADL/IADL treatment chapters for *Willard & Spackman's Occupational Therapy*, which ultimately led to the opportunity to author this evaluation and treatment chapter. Dr. Holm and Dr. Rogers have an ability to conceptualize and articulate occupational therapy practice that is both scholarly and practical. Their contributions from prior editions continue to shine brightly through in this chapter.

PROVOCATIVE QUESTIONS

1. The only occupational therapist at a small community hospital happens to be male. He receives a referral on a female client who sustained a lumbar fracture and must wear a back brace at all times. The client cannot reach her perianal area for hygiene and bathing and needs to be able to manage these tasks, as well as dressing, when she returns home. The client comes from a culture in which it is unacceptable for women to be seen unclothed by men. She has requested a female occupational therapist, but the hospital does not employ any. How should the occupational therapist handle this situation?

2. How would intervention differ for clients who wish to be autonomous (i.e., able to direct their own care) but plan to have assistance with ADLs and/or IADLs on a long-term basis?

3. What do you do when clients and their caregivers have different opinions about treatment priorities? For example, the mother of a 12-year-old boy with cerebral palsy would like her son to become independent in getting ready for school in the morning, but he thinks that it would take too long and would require him to get up too early. Or a 73-year-old woman who has had a stroke with resulting left hemiparesis and a moderate left neglect would like to cook again, but her husband thinks that she would be unsafe and would rather do the cooking himself. He says that it would be much more efficient, and it is very frustrating for him to have to cue her all the time.

REFERENCES

American Occupational Therapy Association. (1995). Clarification of the use of terms assessment and evaluation. *American Journal of Occupational Therapy, 49,* 1072–1073.

American Occupational Therapy Association. (2002). Occupational therapy practice framework: Domain & process. *American Journal of Occupational Therapy, 56,* 609–639.

Ashley, M. J., Persel, C. S., & Clark, M. C. (2001). Validation of an Independent Living Scale for post-acute rehabilitation applications. *Brain Injury, 15,* 435–442.

Ashworth, J. B., Reuben, D. B., & Benton, L. A. (1994). Functional profiles of healthy older persons. *Age and Ageing, 23,* 34–39.

Banford, M., Kratz, M., Brown, R., Emick, K., Ranck, J., Wilkins, R., et al. (2001). Stroke survivor caregiver education: Methods and effectiveness. *Physical and Occupational Therapy in Geriatrics, 19*(1), 37–51.

Baron, K., Kielhofner, G., Iyenger, A., Goldhammer, V., & Wolenski, J. (2002). *The Occupational Self Assessment* (Version 2.0). Chicago: University of Illinois at Chicago, College of Applied Health Sciences, Department of Occupational Therapy, Model of Human Occupation Clearinghouse.

Benson, J., & Schell, B. A. (1997). Measurement theory: Application to occupational and physical therapy. In J. Van Deusen & D. Brund (Eds.), *Assessment in occupational and physical therapy* (pp. 3–24). Philadelphia: W. B. Saunders.

Birkholtz, M., & Blair, S. (2001a). Chronic pain—The need for an eclectic approach: Part 1. *British Journal of Therapy and Rehabilitation, 8*(2), 68–73.

Birkholtz, M., & Blair, S. (2001b). Chronic pain—The need for an eclectic approach: Part 2. *British Journal of Therapy and Rehabilitation, 8*(3), 96–99.

Blake, H., & Lincoln, N. B. (2000). Factors associated with strain in co-resident spouses of patients following stroke. *Clinical Rehabilitation, 14,* 307–314.

Bogardus, S., Bradley, E., Williams, C., Jaciejewski, P, van Doorn, C., & Inouye, S. (2001). Goals for the care of frail older adults: Do caregivers and clinicians agree? *American Journal of Medicine, 110,* 97–102.

Borg, G. (1998). *Borg's perceived exertion and pain scales.* Champagne, IL: Human Kinetics.

Brown, C., Moore, W. P., Hemman, D., & Yunek, A. (1996). Influence of instrumental activities of daily living assessment method on judgments of independence. *American Journal of Occupational Therapy, 50,* 202–206.

Cheal, B., & Clemson, L. (2001). Older people enhancing self-efficacy in fall-risk situations. *Australian Occupational Therapy Journal, 48,* 80–91.

Chong, D. K.-H. (1995). Measurement of instrumental activities of daily living in stroke. *Stroke, 26,* 1119–1122. Retrieved January 4, 2007, from http://stroke.ahajournals.org/content/vol26/issue6/

Cipriani, J., Hess, S., Higgins, H., Resavy, D., Sheon, S., Szychowski, M., et al. (2000). Collaboration in the therapeutic process: Older adults' perspectives. *Physical and Occupational Therapy in Geriatrics, 17*(1), 43–54.

Close, J., Ellis, M., Hooper, R., Glucksman, E., Jackson, S., & Swift, C. (1999). Prevention of falls in the elderly trial (PROFET): A randomised controlled trial. *Lancet, 353,* 93–97.

Cope, D. N., & Sundance, P. (1995). Conceptualizing clinical outcomes. In P. K. Landrum, N. D. Schmidt, & A. McLean (Eds.), *Outcome-oriented rehabilitation* (pp. 43–56). Gaithersburg, MD: Aspen.

Cox, C. (1996). Discharge planning for dementia patients: Factors influencing caregiver decisions and satisfaction. *Health and Social Work, 21*(2), 97–104.

Croser, R., Garrett, R., Seeger, B., & Davies, P. (2001). Effectiveness of electronic aids to daily living: Increased independence and decreased frustration. *Australian Occupational Therapy Journal, 48,* 35–44.

Cummings, R., Thomas, M., Szonyi, G., Salkeld, G., O'Neill, E., Westbury, C., et al. (1999). Home visits by an occupational therapist for assessment and modification of environmental hazards: A randomized trial of falls prevention. *Journal of the American Geriatrics Society, 47,* 1397–1402.

Curtis, C. L., Bassile, C. C., Cote, L. J., & Gentile, A. M. (2001). Effects of exercise on the motor control of individuals with Parkinson's disease: Case studies. *Neurology Report, 25,* 2–11.

Dooley, N. R., & Hinojosa, J. (2004). Improving quality of life for persons with Alzheimer's disease and their family caregivers: Brief occupational therapy intervention. *American Journal of Occupational Therapy, 58,* 561–569.

Dudgeon, B. J., Tyler, E. J., Rhodes, L. A., & Jensen, M. P. (2006). Managing usual and unexpected pain with physical disability: A qualitative analysis. *American Journal of Occupational Therapy, 60,* 92–103.

Dunn, W. (1993). Measurement of function: Actions for the future. *American Journal of Occupational Therapy, 47,* 357–359.

Dunn, W. (2005). Measurement issues and practices. In M. Law, C. Baum, & W. Dunn (Eds.), *Measuring occupational performance: Supporting best practice in occupational therapy* (2nd ed., pp. 21–32). Thorofare, NJ: Slack.

Dunn, W., Brown, C., & McGuigan, A. (1994). The ecology of human performance: A framework for considering the effect of context. *American Journal of Occupational Therapy, 48,* 595–607.

Edelstein, J. E. (2005). Motivating elderly patients with recent amputations. *Topics in Geriatric Rehabilitation, 21,* 116–122.

Eklund, K., Sonn, U., & Dahlin-Ivanoff, S. (2004). Long-term evaluation of a health education programme for elderly persons with visual impairment. A randomized study. *Disability and Rehabilitation, 26,* 401–409.

Fasoli, S. E. (2008). Assessing roles and competence. In M. V. Radomski & C. A. T. Latham (Eds.), *Occupational therapy for physical dysfunction* (6th ed., pp. 65–90). Philadelphia: Wolters Kluwer Lippincott Williams & Wilkins.

Federico, L., & Kielhofner, G. (2002). *The Child Occupational Self Assessment* (Version 1.0). Chicago: University of Illinois at Chicago, College of Applied Health Sciences, Department of Occupational Therapy, Model of Human Occupation Clearinghouse.

Fisher, A. G. (2006a). *Assessment of Motor and Process Skills. Vol. 1: Development, standardization, and administration manual* (6th ed.). Fort Collins, CO: Three Star Press.

Fisher, A. G. (2006b). *Assessment of Motor and Process Skills. Vol. 2: User manual* (6th ed.). Fort Collins, CO: Three Star Press.

Flinn, N. A., & Radomski, M. V. (2008). Learning. In M. V. Radomski & C. A. T. Latham (Eds.), *Occupational therapy for physical dysfunction* (6th ed., pp. 382–401). Philadelphia: Wolters Kluwer Lippincott Williams & Wilkins.

Ford, A. B., Haug, M. R., Stange, K. C., Gaines, A. D., Noekler, L. S., & Jones, P. K. (2000). Sustained personal autonomy: A measure of successful aging. *Journal of Aging and Health, 12,* 470–489.

Fuchs-Climent, D., Le Gallais, D., Varray, A., Desplan, J., Cadopi, M., & Prefaut, C. G. (2001). Factor analysis of quality of life, dyspnea, and physiological variables in patients with chronic obstructive pulmonary disease before and after rehabilitation. *American Journal of Physical Medicine and Rehabilitation, 80,* 113–120.

Fuhrer, M., & Keith, R. (1998). Facilitating patient learning during medical rehabilitation: A research agenda. *American Journal of Physical Medicine and Rehabilitation, 77,* 557–561.

Gift, A. G., & Narsavage, G. (1998). Validity of the numeric rating scale as a measure of dyspnea. *American Journal of Critical Care, 7,* 200–204.

Gitlin, L. N. (2005). Measuring performance in instrumental activities of daily living. In M. Law, C. Baum, & W. Dunn (Eds.), *Measuring occupational performance: Supporting best practice in occupational therapy* (2nd ed., pp. 227–247). Thorofare, NJ: Slack.

Gitlin, L. N., Corcoran, M., Winter, L., Boyce, A., & Hauck, W. W. (2001). A randomized, controlled trial of a home environmental intervention: Effect on efficacy and upset in caregivers and on daily function of persons with dementia. *Gerontologist, 41,* 4–14.

Guidetti, S., Asaba, E., & Tham, K. (2007). The lived experience of recapturing self-care. *American Journal of Occupational Therapy, 61,* 303–310.

Haertlein, C. L. (1999). The Milwaukee Evaluation of Daily Living Skills. In B. J. Hemphill-Pearson (Ed.), *Assessments in occupational therapy mental health: An integrative approach* (pp. 245–257). Thorofare, NJ: Slack.

Hammond, A. (2004). Rehabilitation in rheumatoid arthritis: A critical review. *Musculoskeletal Care, 2,* 135–151.

Hansen, R. A., & Atchison, B. (1999). *Conditions in occupational therapy: Effect on occupational performance* (2nd ed.). Philadelphia: Lippincott Williams & Wilkins.

Healy, H., & Rigby, P. (1999). Promoting independence for teens and young adults with physical disabilities. *Canadian Journal of Occupational Therapy, 66,* 240–249.

Hepburn, K., Tornatore, J., Center, B., & Ostwald, W. (2001). Dementia family caregiver training: Affecting beliefs about caregiving and caregiver outcomes. *Journal of the American Geriatrics Society, 49,* 450–457.

Hilton, K., Fricke, J., & Unsworth, C. (2001). A comparison of self-report versus observation of performance using the Assessment of Living Skills and Resources (ALSAR) with an older population. *British Journal of Occupational Therapy, 64,* 135–143.

Holm, M. B., & Rogers, J. C. (1999). Performance Assessment of Self-care Skills. In B. J. Hemphill-Pearson (Ed.), *Assessments in occupational therapy mental health: An integrative approach* (pp. 117–124). Thorofare, NJ: Slack.

Katz, S., Ford, A. B., Moskowitz, R. W., Jackson, B. A., & Jaffe, M. A. (1963). Studies of illness in the aged: The Index of

ADL. *Journal of the American Medical Association, 185,* 914–919.

Kettenbach, G. (2004). *Writing SOAP notes* (3rd ed.). Philadelphia: F. A. Davis.

Kohlman Thomson, L. (1992). *Kohlman Evaluation of Living Skills* (3rd ed.). Bethesda, MD: American Occupational Therapy Association.

Knoke, D., Taylor, A. E., & Saint-Cyr, J. A. (1998). The differential effects of cueing on recall in Parkinson's disease and normal subjects. *Brain and Cognition, 38,* 261–274.

Kramer, A. M., Kowalsky, J. C., Lin, M., Grigsby, J., Hughes, R., & Steiner, J. F. (2000). Outcome and utilization differences for older persons with stroke in HMO and fee-for-service systems. *Journal of the American Geriatrics Society, 48,* 726–734.

Lansing, R. W., Moosavi, S. H., Banzett, R. B. (2003). Measurement of dyspnea: Word labeled visual analog scale vs. verbal ordinal scale. *Respiratory Physiology & Neurobiology, 3,* 77–83.

Latham, C. A. T. (2008a). Conceptual foundations for practice. In M. V. Radomski & C. A. T. Latham (Eds.), *Occupational therapy for physical dysfunction* (6th ed., pp. 1–20). Philadelphia: Wolters Kluwer Lippincott Williams & Wilkins.

Latham, C. A. T. (2008b). Occupation as therapy: Selection, gradation, analysis, and adaptation. In M. V. Radomski & C. A. T. Latham (Eds.), *Occupational therapy for physical dysfunction* (6th ed., pp. 358–381). Philadelphia: Wolters Kluwer Lippincott Williams & Wilkins.

Law, M. C. (1998). *Client-centered occupational therapy.* Thorofare, NJ: Slack.

Law, M., Baptiste, S., Carswell, A., McColl, M. A., Polatajko, H., & Pollock, N. (2005). *The Canadian Occupational Performance Measure* (4th ed.). Toronto, ON: CAOT Publications.

Law, M., & Baum, C. (2005). Measurement in occupational therapy. In M. Law, C. Baum, & W. Dunn (Eds.), *Measuring occupational performance: Supporting best practice in occupational therapy* (2nd ed., pp. 3–20). Thorofare, NJ: Slack.

Law, M., Cooper, B., Strong, S., Stewart, D., Rigby, P., & Letts, L. (1996). The person–environment–occupation model: A transactive approach to occupational performance. *Canadian Journal of Occupational Therapy, 63,* 9–23.

Lawton, M. P. (1972). Assessing the competence of older people. In D. P. Kent, R. Kastenbaum, & S. Sherwood (Eds.), *Research planning and action for the elderly: The power and potential of social science* (pp. 122–143). New York: Behavioral Publications.

Leonardelli, C. A. (1988). *The Milwaukee Evaluation of Daily Living Skills.* Thorofare, NJ: Slack.

Letts, L., & Bosch, J. (2005). Measuring occupational performance in basic activities of daily living. In M. Law, C. Baum, & W. Dunn (Eds.), *Measuring occupational performance: Supporting best practice in occupational therapy* (2nd ed., pp. 179–225). Thorofare, NJ: Slack.

Letts, L., Scott, S., Burtney, J., Marshall, L., & McKean, M. (1998). The reliability and validity of the safety assessment of function and the environment for rehabilitation (SAFER Tool). *British Journal of Occupational Therapy, 61,* 127–132.

Liao, S., & Ferrell, B. (2000). Fatigue in an older population. *Journal of the American Geriatrics Society, 48,* 426–430.

Liddle, J., & McKenna, K. (2000). Quality of life: An overview of issues for use in occupational therapy outcome measurement. *Australian Occupational Therapy Journal, 47,* 77–85.

Lorch, A., & Herge, E. A. (2007, May 28). Using standardized assessments in practice. *OT Practice,* 17–22.

Lund, M. L., & Nygård, L. (2003). Incorporating or resisting assistive devices: Different approaches to achieving a desired occupational self-image. *OTJR: Occupation, Participation, and Health, 23,* 67–75.

Mahoney, F. I., & Barthel, D. W. (1965). Functional evaluation: The Barthel Index. *Maryland State Medical Journal, 14,* 61–65.

Mathiowetz, V., Matuska, K. M., & Murphy, M. E. (2001). Efficacy of an energy conservation course for persons with multiple sclerosis. *Archives of Physical Medicine and Rehabilitation, 82,* 449–456.

Meenan, R. F., Mason, J. H., Anderson, J. J., Guccione, & A. A., Kazis, L. E. (1992). AIMS2: The content and properties of a revised and expanded Arthritis Impact Measurement Scales Health Status Questionnaire. *Arthritis and Rheumatism, 35,* 1–10.

Melchert-McKearnan, K., Deitz, J., Engel, J. M., & White, O. (2000). Children with burn injuries: Purposeful versus rote exercise. *American Journal of Occupational Therapy, 54,* 381–390.

Miller, P. A., & Butin, D. (2000). The role of occupational therapy in dementia: COPE (Caregiver options for practical experiences). *International Journal of Geriatric Psychiatry, 15,* 86–89.

Moore, A. A., Endo, J. O., & Carter, M. K. (2003). Is there a relationship between excessive drinking and functional impairment in older persons? *Journal of the American Geriatric Society, 51,* 44–49.

Mullersdorf, M. (2000). Factors indicating need of rehabilitation: Occupational therapy needs among persons with long-term and/or recurrent pain. *International Journal of Rehabilitation Research, 23,* 281–294.

National Center for Health Statistics. (2007, January). *NCHS Definitions.* Retrieved May 29, 2007, from http://0-www.cdc.gov.mill1.sjlibrary.org/nchs/datawh/nchsdefs/list.htm

Natterlund, B., & Ahlstrom, G. (1999). Problem-focused coping and satisfaction with activities of daily living in individuals with muscular dystrophy and postpolio syndrome. *Scandinavian Journal of Caring Sciences, 13*(1), 26–32.

Nouri, F. M., & Lincoln, N. B. (1987). An extended activities of daily living scale for stroke patients. *Clinical Rehabilitation, 1,* 301–305.

Nyland, J., Quigley, P., Huang, C., Lloyd, J., Harrow, J., & Nelson, A. (2000). Preserving transfer independence among individuals with spinal cord injury. *Spinal Cord, 38,* 649–657.

Ostchega, Y., Harris, T. B., Hirsch, R., Parsons, V. L., & Kington, R. (2000). The prevalence of functional limitations and disability in older persons in the United States: Data from the National Health and Nutrition Examination Survey III. *Journal of the American Geriatrics Society, 48,* 1132–1135.

Park, S., Fisher, A. G., & Velozo, C. A. (1994). Using the Assessment of Motor and Process Skills to compare occupational performance between clinic and home settings. *American Journal of Occupational Therapy, 48,* 697–709.

Radomski, M. V. (2008). Planning, guiding, and documenting practice. In M. V. Radomski & C. A. T. Latham (Eds.), *Occupational therapy for physical dysfunction* (6th ed., pp. 40–64). Philadelphia: Wolters Kluwer Lippincott Williams & Wilkins.

Resnick, B. (1998). Motivating older adults to perform functional activities. *Journal of Gerontological Nursing, 24*(11), 23–30.

Reuben, D. B., Laliberte, L., Hiris, J., & Mor, V. (1990). A hierarchical exercise scale to measure function at the advanced activities of daily living (AADL) level. *Journal of the American Geriatrics Society, 38,* 855–861.

Robertson, S. C., & Colburn, A. P. (2000). Can we improve outcomes research by expanding research methods? *American Journal of Occupational Therapy, 54,* 541–543.

Robinson-Smith, G., Johnston, M. V., & Allen, J. (2000). Self-care self-efficacy, quality of life, and depression after stroke. *Archives of Physical Medicine and Rehabilitation, 81,* 460–464.

Rogers, J. C. (1983). Clinical reasoning: The ethics, science, and art. Eleanor Clarke Slagle Lecture. *American Journal of Occupational Therapy, 37,* 601–616.

Rogers, J. C., & Holm, M. B. (1991). Occupational therapy diagnostic reasoning: A component of clinical reasoning. *American Journal of Occupational Therapy, 45,* 1045–1053.

Rogers, J. C., & Holm, M. B. (1994). *Performance Assessment of Self-Care Skills (PASS)* (Version 3.1). Unpublished manuscript, University of Pittsburgh at Pittsburgh.

Rogers, J. C., Holm, M. B., Beach, S., Schulz, R., Cipriani, J., Fox, A., et al. (2003). Concordance of four methods of disability assessment using performance in the home as the criterion method. *Arthritis Care & Research, 49,* 640–647.

Rogers, J. C., Holm, M. B., Burgio, L. D., Hsu, C., Hardin, J. M., & McDowell, B. (2000). Excess disability during morning care in nursing home residents with dementia. *International Psychogeriatrics, 12,* 267–282.

Rogers, J. C., Holm, M. B., & Stone, R. G. (1997). Assessment of daily living activities: The home care advantage. *American Journal of Occupational Therapy, 51,* 410–422.

Rubenstein, L. A., Schairer, C., Wieland, G. D., & Kane, R. (1984). Systematic biases in functional status assessment of elderly adults. *Journal of Gerontology, 39,* 686–691.

Russell, C., Fitzgerald, M. H., Williamson, P., Manor, D., & Whybrow, S. (2002). Independence as a practice issue in occupational therapy: The safety clause. *American Journal of Occupational Therapy, 56,* 369–379.

Sames, K. M. (2005). *Documenting occupational therapy practice.* Upper Saddle River, NJ: Pearson Prentice Hall.

Schwartz, S. M. (1995). Adults with traumatic brain injury: Three case studies of cognitive rehabilitation in the home setting. *American Journal of Occupational Therapy, 49,* 655–657.

Seigley, L. (1998). The effects of personal and environmental factors on health behaviors of older adults. *Nursingconnections, 11*(4), 47–58.

Stewart, K. B. (2005). Purposes, processes, and methods of evaluation. In J. Case-Smith (Ed.), *Occupational therapy for children* (5th ed., pp. 219–240). St. Louis: Elsevier Mosby.

Thornsson, A., & Grimby, G. (2001). Ability and perceived difficulty in daily activities in people with poliomyelitis sequelae. *Journal of Rehabilitation Medicine, 33,* 4–11.

Toth-Cohen, S. (2000). Role perceptions of occupational therapists providing support and education for caregivers of persons with dementia. *American Journal of Occupational Therapy, 54,* 509–515.

U.B. Foundation Activities. (2004). *The Inpatient Rehabilitation Facility-Patient Assessment Instrument (IRF-PAI) training manual: Effective 4/01/04.* Buffalo, NY: U.B. Foundation Activities, Inc. Retrieved May 30, 2007, from http://www.cms.hhs.gov/InpatientRehabFacPPS/04_IRFPAI.asp

Vanage, S. M., Gilbertson, K. K., & Mathiowetz, V. (2003). Effects of an energy conservation course on fatigue impact for persons with progressive multiple sclerosis. *American Journal of Occupational Therapy, 57,* 315–323.

Williams, J. H., Drinka, T. J. K., Greenberg, J. R., Farrel-Holtan, J., Euhardy, R., et al. (1991). Development and testing of the Assessment of Living Skills and Resources (ALSAR) in elderly community-dwelling veterans. *Gerontologist, 31,* 84–91.

World Health Organization. (2001). *International classification of functioning, disability, and health (ICF).* Geneva, Switzerland: Author.

Caregiving and Childrearing

ELLEN S. COHN AND ALEXIS D. HENRY

49

❝One person caring about another represents life's greatest value❞

—JIM ROHN

Learning Objectives

After reading this chapter, you will be able to:

1. Describe an ecological, developmental, and occupation-centered perspective of caregiving and childrearing.
2. Discuss the process for evaluating caregiving and childrearing needs.
3. Choose interventions based on clients values and occupational performance relative to caregiving and childrearing.

Caregiving and childrearing, which are essential to the continuity of life, are common yet highly complex occupations. Both public and private, these occupations are deeply significant, intensely personal, openly shared, and socially constructed. In this chapter, the terms caregiving and childrearing are used interchangeably to describe the occupation of nurturing the well-being of others. Understanding the meaning, ideals, and values of caregiving and childrearing from societal and individual perspectives is essential to occupational therapy practice. Historically, intervention focused primarily on parents whose child had a disability. Interventions were typically designed to help parents support the development of their child with disabilities, and limited attention was given to helping parents create sustainable routines to enhance family priorities and lifestyles. Also overlooked by occupational therapy are caregivers who have a disability themselves. Accordingly, this chapter presents an overview of childrearing and caregiving occupations, followed by evaluation and intervention approaches for those who are caring for individuals with disabilities across the life course and those who are caregivers with a disability.

Historically, childrearing and caregiving were most often provided by women, with men having limited participation in caretaking of others. Today, males are more often active participants in childrearing and caregiving (Lamb, 2000). Therefore, in this chapter, childrearing and caregiving are viewed as gender-neutral occupations.

CHILDREARING AND CAREGIVING OCCUPATIONS

Childrearing and caregiving take place in multiple environments and can be conceptualized by using ecological (Bronfenbrenner, 1979), developmental (Olson et al., 1983), and occupation-centered (Jackson, 1998) perspectives. Ecological perspectives support the view that childrearing and caregiving are influenced by the interaction between the person, the occupation, and the environment. These interactions are reciprocal and dynamic. People generally interpret experiences through their own customized world view. The ecological perspective reminds practitioners to consider the numerous factors that influence caregivers' ideals, decisions, and actions. The **family**, defined, as "a group of people living together or in close contact to take care of each other and provide guidance for their dependent members," is the center of the ecological system, supporting the growth of family members (Wood, 1995). Personal factors such as family member characteristics (e.g., age, education, socioeconomic status) and characteristics of the care recipient (e.g., age, type of disability) influence how a family conceptualizes parenting, disability, and the role of services (Luster & Okagaki, 1993).

On the basis of an ecological perspective, Harkness and Super (1994) proposed a theoretical framework, the "developmental niche," for understanding how cultural settings influence children's lives, including their daily activities. In this framework, the cultural constructed environment of the child is conceptualized as including three interrelated operational subsystems: (1) the physical and social setting where the child lives, (2) culturally regulated customs of child care and childrearing, and (3) the psychology of the caretakers. The physical and social setting shapes a person's activity through the kinds of activities available and through the defining activities of the people who are present. Customs, as defined by Harkness and Super (1994), refer to techniques of protecting, teaching, and socializing that are so commonly used by members of the community and are so thoroughly integrated into the larger culture that caretakers do not need to give them conscious consideration. That is, customs are often viewed as the natural way to do things. The caretakers' psychology, including their beliefs and values, organize their behavior toward others and many larger decisions, such as the appropriateness of certain behaviors. These subsystems operate in a coordinated manner, interact differentially with other features of the larger environment, and are mutually adapted. The concept of a developmental niche provides a useful framework for identifying and collecting relevant information related to factors that affect caregiving and childrearing occupations.

For example, cultural and societal factors influence caregiving actions. In Asian cultures, elderly people are cared for within the family; therefore, alternative living situations outside the family home might not be acceptable options for older adults in Asian cultures (Spector, 1996). In the Hmong culture, epilepsy is seen as a gift that is possessed only by the respected shaman. This cultural belief is contradictory to the medical model in Western societies, which considers epilepsy a disease to be treated with medication. Such clashing worldviews can have major implications for practitioners who are striving to support people in their childrearing and caregiving occupations (Fadiman, 1997). Only when the influence of cultural beliefs is examined is it possible to understand caregivers' actions and goals for intervention.

Extended family, neighborhoods, coworkers, and other parents may be integral components of a caregiver's personal social network, therefore influencing the attitudes and beliefs of caregivers (Dyck, 1990). This social network can provide childrearing assistance and support for caregivers. Although social networks are typically a source of support for caregivers, extended family members can in some cases undermine the confidence of a struggling parent or caregiver.

Another factor that influences caregivers and families is the developmental concept of the family life cycle. Olson and colleagues (1983) proposed a model to conceptualize and describe the family life cycle that includes specific phases or life events and challenges to be confronted during each phase in the family life cycle. For example, families make a transition when a child is old enough to be launched from the immediate family system and live on his or her own or in a new setting. Developmental trajectories intersect with other family dynamics, and over time, changes occur in both the structure and function of the family. Practitioners need to understand and consider the impact of the major events that families might be experiencing at a given time.

Along with ecological and developmental perspectives, scholars in occupational science advocate for an occupation-centered perspective (see Chapter 1). Rather than focusing on specific tasks or activities in isolation, separate from an understanding of the meaning of tasks, an occupation-centered analysis focuses on the overarching occupation itself. Ruddick's (1995) analysis of mothering helps us to understand the meaning associated with childrearing across cultures and countries. Although Ruddick focuses on mothering, her analysis is applicable to fathers as well. According to Ruddick, the "work" of parenting includes protection, nurturance, and training. Protection requires scrutiny of the child and the environment, coupled with an acceptance that a child will inevitably be subjected to minor or major mishaps that parents cannot control. Parents must accept their own limits as protector and still continue with the intent of keeping their child safe. Protection falls on a continuum from a lack of protection to overbearing. Nurturance or fostering of growth refers to developing a child's body and spirit. Fostering growth requires the ability to change as the child grows. A caregiver provides the conditions for growth; these conditions vary among cultures, socioeconomic levels, and other environmental factors. Training involves teaching the child behaviors and values that are necessary to achieve acceptance by family and society. Along with protection, nurturance, and training, parents of children with disabilities identify advocacy and obtaining appropriate resources as a critical aspect of parenting (Landsman, 1998).

Jackson (1998) addresses the "enfolded nature of occupations," a term that acknowledges the multiple factors that influence occupations (pg. 58). Jackson cites DeVault's (1991) research, which suggests that parents are often not delineating their childrearing and caregiving tasks; rather, they are folding them into one another. De Vault's example of "feeding the family" illustrates that parents provide sustenance to the child while simultaneously fostering social communication skills for acceptance into society. Dyck's (1990) analysis of working parents offers another example of enfolded occupations. Dyck proposed that women develop strategies to remain a "good mother" while participating in the labor force. Strategies might involve hiring an after-school babysitter to drive a child to activities so that the parent can work while the child engages in developmentally stimulating programs. An occupation-centered analysis directs practitioners to consider the social, symbolic, and interpersonal meaning associated with childrearing and caregiving (Jackson, 1998).

Caring for individuals with disability, whose needs may extend indefinitely into the future, poses potential benefits and burdens. The demands of long-term caregiving have been associated with depression, grief, physical health problems such as fatigue, and occupational imbalance, which can lead to social isolation for the caregiver (Pearlin, Mullan, Semple, & Skaff, 1990). Donovan VanLeit, Crowe, and Keefe (2005) interviewed mothers of children with disabilities and found that the mothers were most concerned about taking care of their own health and well-being; expanding their social life; improving their child's quality of life; managing their household (including time and resources); balancing work, home, and community responsibilities; and sharing the work load. Similar concerns have been expressed by caregivers of individuals with other diagnostic conditions and ages (Hasselkus & Murray, 2007).

Caregiving does not always result in long-term negative effects on family members. Rather, the lives of many parents, across socioeconomic classes and in families with children with various disabilities, are positively changed as a result of the birth of a child with a disability (Scorgie & Sobsey, 2000). Some parents reexamine their expectations, with a transformation of values, resulting in a new sense of "what really matters." Chen and Greenberg (2004) noted that family members of relatives with schizophrenia report greater sensitivity to others and awareness of themselves and view the family member with schizophrenia as an active and valued member of their family. Parents of younger children with disabilities report acquiring new life-enriching roles such as being a parent-group leader, writer, or speaker at conferences. Some parents learned better communication skills and used these skills to foster open, supportive family relationships (Scorgie & Sobsey, 2000).

EVALUATING CAREGIVING

The first step in developing interventions for parents and family caregivers is to gain an understanding of the daily experiences and responsibilities of the individuals who are engaged in these occupations. The evaluation process should be family-centered and collaborative, with a goal of identifying family strengths, priorities, and values as well as challenges associated with caregiving. It is best to begin with an open-ended conversation or interview, initially focusing on the daily routines associated with caregiving and family life, which can help the practitioner to gain an understanding of the daily challenges a parent or caregiver might face. This process can also help to develop trust and rapport between the practitioner and the caregiver (Orsmond, 2005). The practitioner might begin by asking a parent to describe a typical day, from morning to night. Who in the family is responsible for the daily tasks of caregiving, and how and when are these tasks accomplished? How do weekdays differ from weekend days? What makes a typical day go well or not so well? What are the typical stressors, and how or when do they occur? In addition to the parent or primary caregiver, other family members can be asked about their daily routines.

In the context of a conversation about a typical day, the practitioner can explore how the family's customs, beliefs, and attitudes affect the daily routines of caregiving. It is also important for the practitioner to gain an understanding of the person's sense of competence as a parent or caregiver, as well as in other important occupations. What does the individual feel that she or he does well, and what does the family do well? What things are difficult? What are the strengths or assets of the children or other family members? What aspects of caregiving are most important to the individual and other family members? In what areas are changes needed?

In addition to exploring the daily routines and challenges of parenting and caregiving, the practitioner can use an interview to understand whether and how the individual is able to meet his or her own needs while caring for other family members. For those with the responsibility of caring for other family members, participation in other occupations is largely dependent on their ability to adequately meet the demands of their caregiving occupation. It is important for the practitioner to explore how caregivers balance the demands of caring for others with the demands of school, work, homemaking, and self-care.

The supports and resources that are available to the family and caregiver should also be explored. During the interview, the practitioner can determine the extent to which other people, such as friends, neighbors, and extended family members, are a source of support for the caregiver and family. Beyond social supports, what other resources are available to the caregiver and family? Does the family have adequate financial and other material resources to meet their needs in terms of housing, food, transportation, health care, and recreation?

No occupational therapy interviews have been developed that specifically focus on the occupations of child-rearing or caregiving. However, questions about these occupations can easily be incorporated into existing broad occupational performance interviews, such as the Occupational Performance History Interview II (OPHI-II) (Kielhofner et al., 2004) or the Canadian Occupational Performance Measure (COPM) (Law et al., 1998). The Importance, Satisfaction, and Performance scales of the COPM could be used to rate the tasks associated with the caregiving occupations. These two interviews are discussed in greater detail in Chapter 34. Whether a practitioner uses one of these formal interviews or a more informal approach, the practitioner should be mindful that he or she might be interviewing vulnerable families, with either children or adults at risk. Interviews should be conducted in an honest, sensitive, and respectful manner that avoids judgment but seeks to identify the strengths and needs of the caregiver and other family members (Orsmond, 2005). An important goal of an occupational therapy interview is to develop a positive partnership with the parent or caretaker so that occupational therapy interventions can empower caregivers and enhance their ability to meet their caregiving obligations. Guidelines for effective interviewing are discussed in Chapter 34.

Following an interview, the practitioner might elect to conduct further evaluations of specific occupational performance skills and patterns, such as hands-on child-care or homemaking activities. For example, because these activities often involve both physical and cognitive tasks, a practitioner might elect to evaluate biomechanical capacities related to lifting, transferring, carrying, bending, and squatting while caring for others (Sanders & Morse, 2005) or might evaluate cognitive capacities related to money and household management or meal planning (see Chapters 54 and 57).

Numerous rating scales have been developed to assess various aspects of parenting and caregiving. Although such rating scales should never substitute for a face-to-face conversation with a client about his or her parenting or caregiving occupations, practitioners might find one or more of these measures to be useful adjuncts to an interview and/or performance skills assessments in planning interventions. Additionally, these types of scales can be appropriate to use as outcome measures to assess the impact of supports and services for families. Basic information on a sampling of existing parenting and caregiver assessments is presented in Table 49.1.

A family-centered, collaborative evaluation process leads to goal setting and intervention planning that is directed by the parent or caregiver's values, beliefs, goals, experiences, and needs. Approaches to goal setting and intervention are discussed below.

Parenting a Child with a Disability

When parents learn that their child has a disability, there may be feelings of anger and a process of mourning the loss of the "perfect child." Initially, parents may have feelings of shock and denial, followed by anger and depression. Parents may repeat the process of mourning as they encounter unexpected discrepancies between reality and their hopes and expectations. Among and within families, there may be great variability in reactions to and perceptions of the family member with a disability. Mothers of children with disabilities report more stress than fathers do, while fathers report more trouble forming bonds with their children (Beckman, et al., 1998). Services need to be tailored to meet the different needs of each family member. Scorgie and Sobsey recommend that practitioners avoid catastrophizing the effects disability can have on a family. Rather, parents should be made aware that initial feelings of grief are common but that many families adapt to disability in the family. Connecting parents in the initial stages of coping with parents who have adapted positively to life with a child with a disability can aid families in forming a positive outlook for the future (Scorgie & Sobsey, 2000).

Within the last decade, research on parenting children with disabilities has focused on adaptation and adjustment with an emphasis on what families do to sustain daily routines that consider families realities, interests, and values (Fiese et al., 2002; Gallimore, Bernheimer, & Weisner, 1999; Segal, 2004; Summers et al., 2006). Bedell, Cohn, and Dumas (2005) note that families typically have intimate and firsthand expertise and knowledge related to their family members, family life, and the illness or disability of their family member and know best which intervention recommendations can most likely be implemented in the home and community. In their exploration of the strategies that parents use to promote social participation for their children with acquired brain injury, Bedell, Cohn, and Dumas observed that parents need time to allow the recovery process to unfold for themselves and their children. To develop effective interventions based on collaborative partnership with families that honor families' knowledge and expertise, Bedell and colleagues advocate asking parents about the strategies that parents already use and whether they perceive the strategies to be effective rather than reinventing the wheel.

Caring for an Adult with a Disability

Parents of a child with disabilities often continue parenting throughout the child's life into adulthood (Hodapp,

TABLE 49.1   PARENTING AND CAREGIVING ASSESSMENTS

Title	Authors (Date)	Major Domains Assessed	Method of Administration
		Parenting and Family Life Scales	
Parenting Stress Index	Abidin (1995)	Parent characteristics such as competence, isolation, attachment, health, role restriction; child characteristics such as distractibility/hyperactivity, adaptability, demandingness; overall family stress	Self-report
Parenting Sense of Competence Scale	Johnston & Marsh (1989)	Parenting self-esteem, parenting efficacy, and parenting satisfaction	Self-report
Family Environment Scale	Moos & Moos (1983)	Dimensions of family environment, including quality of relationships within the family, opportunities for personal growth, and degree of organization/control within family	Self-report
Family Support Scale	Dunst, Trivette, & Deal (1988)	Perceived helpfulness of partner/spouse support, informal kinship support, formal kinship support, social organizations and professional services, total number of sources of support, and overall social support	Self-report
Home Observation for Measurement of the Environment Inventory	Caldwell & Bradley (1984, 2001)	Quality and quantity of psychological stimulation and cognitive support available in the home; four versions for children from ages 0–3, 3–6, 6–10, and 10–15 years are available	Observations and rating of parent/child interaction; parent interview
Beach Center Family Quality of Life Scale	Park, Hoffman, Marquis, Turnbull, Poston, Mannan, Wang, & Nelson (2003) Hoffman, Marquis, Poston, Summers, & Turnbull (2006)	Perceived importance of and satisfaction with family interaction, parenting, emotional well-being, physical/material well-being, and disability-related supports	Self-report

Continued

583

TABLE 49.1 PARENTING AND CAREGIVING ASSESSMENTS *Continued*

Title	Authors (Date)	Major Domains Assessed	Method of Administration
		Adult Caregiving Scales	
Caregiver Strain Index	Robinson (1983)	Perceived strain related to caregiving and impact on caregiver's employment, finances, physical and social well-being, and time use	Self-report
Caregiver Well-Being Scale	Berg-Weger, Rubio, & Tebb (2000)	Caregiver well-being from a strengths-based perspective, assesses caregivers' basic human needs and satisfaction with activities of daily living	Self-report
Zarit Burden Interview	Zarit, Reever, & Bach-Peterson (1980) Zarit, Todd, & Zarit (1986)	Perceived burden among family caregivers of older adults with dementia	Interview or self-report
Perceived Change Index	Gitlin, Winter, Dennis, & Hauck (2006)	Brief, 13 items, perceived change in well-being in affect, somatic, and ability to manage	Self-report
Caregiver Well-Being Scale	Tebb (1995) Berg-Weger, Rubio, & Tebb (2000)	Extent to which caregiver's basic human and activity of daily living needs are met	Self-report
Bakas Caregiver Outcome Scale	Bakas & Champion (1999)	Changes in caregiver's social functioning, subjective well-being, and physical health as a result of caregiving	Interview or self-report
Task Management Strategy Index	Gitlin, Winter, Dennis, Corcoran, Schinfeld, & Hauck (2002)	Caregiver's use of strategies to simplify everyday self-care tasks for people with Alzheimer's disease and related disorders	Self-report

Dykens, Evans, & Merighi, 1992). Adolescence is often a time when caregivers realize the permanence of the child's disabilities and begin to worry about the future. The features of the disability may change as the child ages and the child's size increases (Seltzer, Krauss, Orsmond, & Vestal, 1997). As the caregiver ages, his or her health needs may change. Aging can have an effect on community involvement, leading to increased social isolation and stress for both the person with a disability and the caregiver. Practitioners can address the caregiver's physical and psychological well-being by providing additional supports in the home and community, making referrals for respite services, and, if appropriate, providing strategies to minimize behavioral difficulties (Biegel, Sales, & Schultz, 1991).

Middle-aged adults, often described as the "sandwich generation," may face the simultaneous demands of parenting adolescents or young adults and caring for their elderly parents (Sorensen & Zarit, 1996). Family caregivers are the primary source of support for frail older people, and 80% of all family caregivers for the elderly provide unpaid help seven days a week (Hasselkus, 1989). Hasselkus's (1989) research on family caregivers for frail older people living in the community suggests that caregivers are focused on getting things done to sustain the family system, achieving a sense of well-being for the care receiver, and achieving a sense of well-being for themselves. The caregiver's quality of life is linked to the quality of life for care recipients; therefore, both the caregiver and recipients will benefit from supportive intervention. Caregivers of older adults, either their spouse or parent, often require support to address the emotional stress of experiencing a loved one decline in function. Hasselkus and Murray (2007) recommend collaborative intervention in which the practitioner strives to understand the meaning caregivers attach to their role and supports the caregiver to balance daily occupations.

BEING A CAREGIVER WITH A DISABILITY

Adults with disabilities experience the same desires to form intimate relationships and to have and raise children as do adults without disabilities. Estimates of the prevalence of disability suggest that there are millions of families in the United States in which one or both parents have a disability (LaPlante, Carlson, Kaye, & Bradsher, 1996; Nicholson, Biebel, Williams, & Katz-Leavy, 2004). Moreover, families in which an adult has a disability have an increased likelihood of having at least one child with a disability (LaPlante et al., 1996). Caregivers with disabilities and/or persistent illness have not historically received services from occupational therapy practitioners or other rehabilitation providers. Despite a functional approach, few rehabilitation providers have been responsive to an individual's

needs as a parent. One cancer survivor stated, "Nobody ever asked me if I had children" (Tannen, 2000).

Caregivers with disabilities face the same daily responsibilities and stresses associated with childrearing as do those without disabilities. Having a disability adds additional challenges, and limitations associated with a disability can affect a caregiver's ability to perform daily occupations. Caregivers may have physical, cognitive, or psychiatric challenges. Other factors that can put an individual at risk for difficulty in caregiving include being a teen parent, having a history of substance abuse, having been abused in childhood, domestic violence, and divorce (Huxley & Warner, 1993; Kowal et al., 1989; Panzarine, 1988). Moreover, to the extent to which disability and other risk factors are associated with poverty, a lack of knowledge of and access to supports and resources, lack of education, lack of skills, and limited life experience, parents with disabilities may face even more daunting challenges (Whitman & Accardo, 1993).

Current research on the effects of disability and persistent illness on parenting is limited. Disability or illness is often viewed as the predominant characteristic of the individual. Emerging from this perception of disability are numerous stereotypes concerning parents with disabilities and illness. These stereotypes include the ideas that parents with disabilities are too immersed in their own self-care to adequately care for their children, that children are used to satisfy the personal needs of parents with disabilities, that parental tasks cannot be performed effectively by parents with disabilities, and that parents with disabilities pass on a negative self-image to their children. These stereotypes can be challenged with interventions to support parents (Tannen, 2000).

Parents with Physical Disabilities

Parents with physical disabilities may have compromised mobility, movement, and/or stamina, which present challenges to the physical demands of parenting. A national survey of parents with disabilities that was conducted in the late 1990s indicates that parents with physical disabilities encounter multiple barriers to parenting and have service needs across multiple areas (Toms Barker & Maralani, 1997). Many parents reported needing adapted baby- and child-care equipment; barriers to obtaining equipment included lack of availability and cost. A majority of parents reported using personal assistance services for help with caregiving, yet many felt that these services interfered with their role as parents. Parents also reported having difficulty in obtaining affordable accessible housing, needing assistance in recreation with their children, and encountering problems with transportation that interfered with or prevented routine child-care activities (Kirshbaum & Olkin, 2002; Toms Barker & Maralani, 1997).

Thus, parents with physical disabilities can be helped by environmental modifications that allow them to participate fully in their role as parents (Farber, 2000). Occupational therapists at Through the Looking Glass, a community-based nonprofit organization in Berkeley, California, that provides services to parents with disabilities, have developed resources and training materials on adaptive baby-care equipment for parents with physical disabilities (Vensand, Rogers, Tuleja, & DeMoss, 2000). Parents with conditions that are characterized by periods of symptom exacerbation and diminution, such as multiple sclerosis or rheumatoid arthritis, might need assistance in planning for these periods and in accessing community support services that will be useful during exacerbations (Crist, 1993). Women with physical disabilities who are planning pregnancy might need to consider the possible medical complications that can occur with disability. Prospective mothers need practitioners who have positive attitudes and expertise in managing pregnancy in women with physical disabilities (Toms Barker & Maralani, 1997).

Parents with Cognitive Disabilities

Parents with cognitive disabilities might lack knowledge and skill in specific areas of parenting, such as providing for a child's safety, nutrition, or daily routine care. These parents can have difficulty with problem solving, social skills and advocacy for family needs. For example, a woman with a traumatic brain injury, which can cause cognitive and social skill deficits, might have a difficult time assisting her 12-year-old daughter in solving social problems between friends at school (Uysal, Hibbard, Robillard, Pappadopulos, & Jaffe, 1998).

Parents with cognitive disabilities might have difficulty following directions or learning new skills. They might tend to overgeneralize skills and problem-solving strategies to contexts that require different or more complex skills. Individuals with cognitive disabilities have greater success in learning when strategies are broken down into steps; are demonstrated, modeled, and practiced; and are paired with rewards. Because of difficulties with generalization, skills-training services to parents with cognitive disabilities should be provided in naturally occurring environments, such as the home and community (Bakken, Miltenberger, & Schauss, 1993).

Parents with Psychiatric Disabilities

The stigma associated with mental illness is probably the most pervasive factor affecting access to and participation in services among parents with psychiatric disabilities. Because of the presumption that people with psychiatric disabilities are compromised in their ability to parent, many parents do not seek support services because they fear the loss of custody of their children. Parents with psychiatric disabilities (and those with developmental dis-

abilities) are at an increased risk of custody loss, yet many parents with psychiatric disabilities are raising or helping to raise their children (Hemmens, Miller, Burton, & Milner, 2002; Nicholson, Biebel, Hinden, Henry, & Stier, 2001; Wong, 1995).

The needs of a family in which a parent has a psychiatric disability are often not addressed until the child is in need of services. When services are provided, they are often child-centered and provided by clinicians who are not trained to work with adults. Moreover, services have tended to be problem-focused and deficit-based rather than preventive or strengths-based (Nicholson, Geller, Fisher, & Dion, 1993). Across the country, strengths-based, family-centered services that are specifically targeted to the needs of parents with psychiatric disabilities and their children are rare, but their numbers appear to be growing. Recent efforts by Nicholson and colleagues have focused on articulating the needs of parents with psychiatric disabilities and their families and on identifying emerging practices to build an evidence base for services for these families (Hinden, Biebel, Nicholson, Henry, & Katz-Leavy, 2006; Nicholson & Henry, 2003a; Nicholson, Hinden, Biebel, Henry, & Katz-Leavy, in press).

Parents with psychiatric disabilities may benefit from parenting skills training and from training in strategies to cope with exacerbations in symptoms. For example, parents might need help in planning for care for their children during times when the parent need to be hospitalized. Parents can also benefit from training in ways to advocate for services for themselves and their children (Henry & Nicholson, 2005). Peer support groups can provide opportunities to build social networks and decrease isolation. A strong social support network can act as a mediator of stress, increasing the parent's functioning during stressful times. Extended family members can be an important source of support for parents with psychiatric disabilities. However, in instances when parents with psychiatric disabilities have strained or disrupted relationships with their families of origin, extended family members might not offer support or might even undermine the individual's role as parent. Many parents worry about their children's understanding of mental illness; practitioners can help parents to develop ways of talking with children about mental illness that are age-appropriate (Nicholson, Henry, Clayfield, & Phillips, 2001).

Nicholson and Henry (2003b) developed a collaborative goal-setting checklist, the *ParentingWell® Strengths and Goals* form (Box 49.1), which practitioners can use together with parents to help parents identify things that they do well, to determine the things that parents would like to do better, and to set priorities for change. Although developed for use with parents with psychiatric disabilities, the form lists typical parenting responsibilities and concerns and so can be appropriate to use

---

BOX 49.1 **PARENTINGWELL® STRENGTHS & GOALS**

Here is a list of things you may need to do as a parent. For each one that applies to you, *circle* the answer that describes you best.

	This is a strength of mine.	I do this okay.	I'd like to do this better.	Does not apply.	Check items to work on.
1. Manage everyday household tasks	Strength	Okay	Better	DNA	
2. Plan and make healthy meals	Strength	Okay	Better	DNA	
3. Understand the relationship between my feelings and my actions	Strength	Okay	Better	DNA	
4. Manage my family's money	Strength	Okay	Better	DNA	
5. Set limits with my child	Strength	Okay	Better	DNA	
6. Have positive interactions/visits with my child	Strength	Okay	Better	DNA	
7. Have a pleasant routine with my child	Strength	Okay	Better	DNA	
8. Find fun things to do with my child	Strength	Okay	Better	DNA	
9. Get adequate child care for my child	Strength	Okay	Better	DNA	
10. Balance work or school, and parenting	Strength	Okay	Better	DNA	
11. Know what to do when my child has problems	Strength	Okay	Better	DNA	
12. Identify my child's strengths	Strength	Okay	Better	DNA	
13. Have positive "family time"	Strength	Okay	Better	DNA	
14. Know my legal options as a parent	Strength	Okay	Better	DNA	
15. Get help for myself, if I need it	Strength	Okay	Better	DNA	
16. Talk with my child about my situation or worries	Strength	Okay	Better	DNA	
17. Keep in touch with my child who is not living with me	Strength	Okay	Better	DNA	
18. Live a substance free lifestyle	Strength	Okay	Better	DNA	
19. Communicate well with my child	Strength	Okay	Better	DNA	
20. Have good relationships with my child's caregivers/helpers	Strength	Okay	Better	DNA	
21. Express anger without hurting anyone	Strength	Okay	Better	DNA	
22. Keep my child and myself safe	Strength	Okay	Better	DNA	
23. Make time to take care of myself	Strength	Okay	Better	DNA	
24. Manage stress and worries in healthy ways	Strength	Okay	Better	DNA	
25. Cope with bad things that have happened to me in my life	Strength	Okay	Better	DNA	
26. Get special services and supports for my child	Strength	Okay	Better	DNA	
27. Other:	Strength	Okay	Better	DNA	

Used with permission ©2003 J. Nicholson, PhD & A. Henry, ScD, OTR/L. ParentingWell® is a trademark of Strengths Based Solutions, LLC. www.parentingwell.org

---

with a variety of parents served by occupational therapy practitioners.

INTERVENTIONS FOR CAREGIVERS

Occupational therapy can involve the provision of direct or indirect services. In partnership with parents and caregivers, practitioners can provide direct services in skills training, environmental adaptations, or support services.

Areas of skills training may include the following:

◆ Helping the caregiver to organize daily and weekly schedules to support the well-being of the caregiver and recipient, including engagement in meaningful occupations and physical well-being
◆ Teaching the caregiver biomechanical principles to promote proper alignment of the body and safety for both caregiver and recipient

CASE STUDY: *A Mother with Depression*

Missy, a mother of two who has coped with depression for many years, talks about the importance of connecting with others:

*I can't possibly overstate the importance of my support network in getting me through rough times. My family, my friends, my doctor, my minister—they have all been my scaffolding during bad times and good. There is nothing like experiencing a mental illness (or any other, for that matter) to teach you the strength of those bonds. Something my minister said to me once had a huge impact on me. I was in the midst of a terrible depression, and, as happens with a depressed mind, I kept thinking that eventually everybody would get tired of my dark mood and not want to be around me anymore. I felt like I was sucking all the good energy out of these people I love so much and giving nothing back but darkness and despair. On a particularly bad day, my minis-*ter said to me, "You need to know that you are still a blessing to other people, even during your darkest moments." It was a lesson in what it means to love and be loved—that good relationships can endure the ups and downs. I can't think of a lesson more relevant to the job of parenting, which is all about unconditional love. Parenting is the world's hardest job, with or without a chronic illness. As much as I would prefer not to have this illness, it has taught my children early on in their lives about the need for compassion and that nobody, not even Mom, is without challenges in life. And they have benefited from the care of so many people who have been there to help. If it truly "takes a village to raise a child," and I think it does, it means you have to push back against the tendency to isolate yourself in your own home, to be willing to ask for help and then be willing to accept it when it is offered.*

- Teaching parenting skills such as home maintenance, time and money management, child behavior management, and advocacy for services
- Teaching parents to support their child's development and to nurture their relationship with their child
- Helping caregivers to communicate with recipient about disability

Environmental adaptations may include the following:

- Creating living spaces in the home that are accessible for family members with disabilities

- Helping caregivers to access human and other resources
- Designing or choosing adapted caregiving equipment with design features that promote safety and proper body alignment
- Designing environments to minimize fatigue

Support services may include the following:

- Providing support groups for family caregivers or parents with disabilities
- Accessing naturally occurring resources such as friends, neighbors, and community services

---

COMMENTARY ON THE EVIDENCE

Intervention for Caregivers

A meta-analysis of the research on caregiver intervention has shown that such intervention can result in positive outcomes for families (Sorensen, Pinquart, & Duberstein, 2002). One impressive example is an occupational therapy intervention designed by Laura Gitlin and her colleagues. They conducted a randomized controlled study of the effectiveness of their Home Environmental Skill-Building Program, a skills training intervention to help families manage dementia care problems at home. The program, consisting of home visits and telephone sessions, focused on education, problem solving, communication, environ-mental and task simplification techniques, and home modifications (Gitlin & Corcoran, 2005). The recipients of intervention reported less upset with memory-related behaviors, less need for assistance from others, and better affect. Their spouses reported less upset with disruptive behaviors. Men reported spending less time in daily oversight, and women reported less need for help from others, better affect, and enhanced management ability, overall well-being, and mastery relative to control group counterparts (Gitlin et al., 2003). These findings provide valuable support for the benefits of occupational therapy interventions for caregivers.

In addition to direct services, practitioners can provide indirect services, such as advocacy for the needs of families in which a member has a disability or referral to a range of community-based services that may be available for parents and caregivers. These can include formal services such as mental health and substance abuse services, Early Intervention and Head Start programs, school-based services, and respite services. In addition, there are a variety of informal services that may benefit parents and caregivers. These can include national self-help and support groups such as Children and Adults with Attention Deficient/Hyperactivity Disorder (CHADD), the National Depressive and Manic Depressive Association, and the Alzheimer's Association. Many of these national groups have local chapters. Finally, there are many community supports, such as faith-based institutions, community centers, and libraries, that provide assistance to parents and caregivers.

SUMMARY

Childrearing and caregiving are complex lifelong occupations. Across the life course, individuals are likely to engage in parenting and or caring for other family members. People who are engaged in these occupations might benefit from direct or indirect interventions to support their nurturing role. Engaging caregivers in meaningful occupations has the potential to contribute to the well-being of both caregivers and care receivers.

REFERENCES

Abidin, R. R. (1995). *Parenting stress index* (3rd ed.). Odessa, FL: Psychological Assessment Resources.

Bakas, T., & Champion, V. (1999). Development and psychometric testing of the Bakas Caregiving Outcomes Scale. *Nursing Research, 48,* 250–259.

Bakken, J., Miltenberger, R. G., & Schauss, S. (1993). Teaching parents with mental retardation: Knowledge versus skills. *American Journal of Mental Retardation, 97,* 405–417.

Beckman, P. J., Barnwell, D., Horn, E., Hanson, M. J., Gutierrez, S., & Leiber, J. (1998). Communities, families, and inclusion. *Early Childhood Research Quarterly, 13,* 125–150.

Bedell, G. M., Cohn, E. S., & Dumas, H. M. (2005). Exploring parents' use of strategies to promote social participation of school-age children with acquired brain injuries. *American Journal of Occupational Therapy, 59,* 273–284.

Berg-Weger, M., Rubio, D. M., & Tebb, S. S. (2000). The Caregiver Well-Being Scale revisited. *Health & Social Work, 25,* 255–263.

Biegel, D. E., Sales, E., & Schulz, R. (1991). Common factors affecting family caregivers. In D. E. Biegel & R. Schulz (Series Eds.), *Family caregiver application series: Vol. 1. Family caregiving in chronic illness* (pp. 199–214). London: Sage.

Bronfenbrenner, U. (1979). *The ecology of human development: Experiments by nature and design.* Cambridge, MA: Harvard University Press.

Caldwell, B. M., & Bradley, R. H. (1984). *HOME Inventory for Measurement of the Environment.* Little Rock, AR: University of Arkansas at Little Rock.

Caldwell, B. M., & Bradley, R. H. (2001). *HOME Inventory administration manual: Learning to use the HOME.* Little Rock, AR: University of Arkansas at Little Rock.

Chen, F. P., & Greenberg, J. S. (2004). A positive aspect of caregiving: The influence of social support on caregiving gains for family members of relatives with schizophrenia. *Community Mental Health Journal, 40,* 423–435.

Crist, P. (1993). Contingent interaction during work and play tasks for mothers with multiple sclerosis and their daughters. *American Journal of Occupational Therapy, 47,* 121–131.

DeVault, M. (1991). *Feeding the family.* Chicago, IL: University of Chicago Press.

Donovan, J. M., VanLeit, B. J., Crowe, T. K., & Keefe, E. B. (2005). Occupational goals of mothers of children with disabilities: Influence of temporal, social, and emotional contexts. *American Journal of Occupational Therapy, 59,* 249–261.

Dunst, C. J., Trivette, C. M., & Deal, A. G. (1988). *Enabling and empowering families: Principles and guidelines for practice.* Cambridge, MA: Brookline Books.

Dyck, L. (1990). Space, time, and renegotiating motherhood: An exploration of the domestic workplace. *Environment and Planning D: Society and Space, 8,* 459–483.

Fadiman, A. (1997). *The spirit catches you and you fall down.* New York: Noonday Press.

Farber, R. S. (2000). Mothers with disabilities: In their own voice. *American Journal of Occupational Therapy, 54,* 260–268.

Fiese, B. H., Tomcho, T. J., Douglas, M., Josephs, K., Poltrock, S. & Baker, T. (2002). A review of 50 years of research on naturally occurring families routines and rituals: Cause for celebration? *Journal of Family Psychology, 16,* 4, 381–390.

Gallimore, R., Bernheimer, L. P., & Weisner, T. S. (1999). Family life is more than managing crisis: Broadening the agenda of research on family adapting to childhood disability. In R. Gallimore, L. P. Bernheimer, D. L. MacMillan, D. L. Speece, & S. Vaughn (Eds.), (1999). *Developmental perspectives on children with high-incidence disabilities* (pp. 55–80). Mahwah, NJ: LEA Press.

Gitlin, L. N., & Corcoran, M. (2005). *Occupational therapy and dementia care: The Home Environmental Skill-Building Program for Individuals and Families.* Bethesda, MD: American Occupational Therapy Association.

Gitlin, L. N., Winter, L., Corcoran, M., Dennis, M. P., Schinfeld, S., & Hauck, W. W. (2003). Effects of the home environmental skill-building program on the caregiver-care recipient dyad: 6-month outcomes from the Philadelphia REACH initiative. *Gerontologist, 43,* 532–546.

Gitlin, L. N., Winter, L., Dennis, M. P., Corcoran, M., Schinfeld, S., & Hauck, W. W. (2002). Strategies used by families to simplify tasks for individuals with Alzheimer's disease and related disorders: Psychometric analysis of the Task Management Strategy Index. *Gerontologist, 42,* 61–69.

Gitlin, L. N., Winter, L., Dennis, M. P., & Hauck, W. W. (2006). Assessing perceived change in the well-being of family caregivers: Psychometric properties of the perceived change index and response patterns. *American Journal of Alzheimer's Disease & Other Dementias, 21,* 304–311.

Harkness, S., & Super, C. M. (1994). The "developmental niche": A theoretical framework for analyzing the household production of health. *Social Science and Medicine, 38,* 217–226.

Hasselkus, B. R. (1989). The meaning of daily activity in family caregiving for the elderly. *American Journal of Occupational Therapy, 43,* 649–656.

Hasselkus, B. R., & Murray, B. J. (2007). Everyday occupation, well-being, and identity: The experience of caregivers in families with dementia. *American Journal of Occupational Therapy, 61,* 9–20.

Hemmens, C., Miller, M., Burton, V. S., & Milner, S. (2002). The consequences of official labels: An examination of the rights lost by the mentally ill and mentally incompetent ten years later. *Community Mental Health Journal, 38,* 129–140.

Henry, A. D., & Nicholson, J. (2005). Helping mothers with serious mental illness. In *Directions in Rehabilitation Counseling* (Vol. 16, Lesson 3, pp. 19–32). Long Island City, NY: Hatherleigh.

Hinden, B. R., Biebel, K., Nicholson, J., Henry, A., & Katz-Leavy, J. (2006). A survey of programs for parents with mental illness and their families: Identifying common elements to build the evidence base. *Journal of Behavioral Health Services and Research, 33,* 21–38.

Hodapp, R. M., Dykens, E. M., Evans, D. W., & Merighi, J. R. (1992). Maternal emotional reactions to young children with different types of handicaps. *Developmental and Behavioral Pediatrics, 13,* 118–123.

Hoffman, L., Marquis, J. G., Poston, D. J., Summers, J. A. S., & Turnbull, A. P. (2006). Assessing family outcomes: Psychometric evaluation of the Beach Center Family Quality of Life Scale. *Journal of Marriage and Family, 68,* 1069–1083.

Huxley, P., & Warner, R. (1993). Primary prevention of parenting dysfunction in high-risk cases. *American Journal of Orthopsychiatry, 63,* 582–587.

Jackson, J. (1998). Is there a place for role theory in occupational science? *Journal of Occupational Science, 5,* 56–65.

Johnston, C., & Marsh, E. J. (1989). A measure of parenting satisfaction and efficacy. *Journal of Clinical Child Psychology, 18,* 167–175.

Kielhofner, G., Mallinson, T., Crawford, C., Nowak, M., Rigby, M., Henry, A., et al. (2004). *The Occupational Performance History Interview—II (version 2.1).* Chicago: University of Illinois at Chicago, College of Applied Health Sciences, Department of Occupational Therapy, Model of Human Occupation Clearinghouse.

Kirshbaum, M., & Olkin, R. (2002). Parents with physical, systemic or visual disabilities. *Sexuality and Disability, 20,* 65–80.

Kowal, L. W., Kottmeier, C. P., Ayoub, C. C., Komives, J. A., Robinson, D. S., & Allen, J. P. (1989). Characteristics of families at risk of problems in parenting: Findings from a home-based secondary prevention program. *Child Welfare, 68,* 549–538.

Lamb, M. (2000). The history of research on father involvement: An overview. In H. E. Peters, G. W. Peterson, S. K. Steinmetz, & R. D. Day (Eds.), *Fatherhood: Research, Interventions, and Policies* (pp. 23–41). New York: Haworth.

Landsman, G. H. (1998). Reconstructing motherhood in the age of "perfect" babies: Mothers of infants and toddlers with disabilities. *Signs: Journal of Women in Culture and Society, 24,* 69–99.

LaPlante, M. P., Carlson, D., Kaye, H. S., & Bradsher, J. E. (1996*). Families with disabilities in the United States* (Report 8). San Francisco: University of California at San Francisco, Disability Statistics Center.

Law, M., Baptiste, S., Carswell, A., McColl, M. A., Polatajko, H., & Pollock, N. (1998). *Canadian Occupational Performance Measure* (3rd ed.). Toronto: Canadian Association of Occupational Therapists.

Luster, T., & Okagaki, L. (1993). *Parenting: An ecological perspective.* Hillsdale, NJ: Lawrence Erlbaum Associates.

Moos, R., & Moos, B. (1983). Clinical applications of the Family Environment Scale. In E. Filsinger (Ed.), *A sourcebook of marriage and family assessment* (pp. 253–273). Beverly Hills, CA: Sage.

Nicholson, J., Biebel, K., Hinden, B., Henry, A., & Stier, L. (2001). *Critical issues for parents with mental illness and their families.* Report prepared for the Center for Mental Health Service of the Substance Abuse and Mental Health Services Administration. Washington: D.C.: U.S. Department of Health and Human Services.

Nicholson, J., Biebel, K., Williams, V. F., & Katz-Leavy, J. (2004). Prevalence of parenthood in adults with mental illness: Implications for state and federal policymakers, programs, and providers. In R. W. Manderscheid & J. J. Henderson (Eds.), *Mental health, United States, 2002* (pp. 12–137). DHHS Pub No. (SMA) 3938. Rockville, MD: Substance Abuse and Mental Health Services Administration.

Nicholson, J., Geller, J. L., Fisher, W. H., & Dion, G. L. (1993). State policies and programs that address the needs of mentally ill mothers in the public sector. *Hospital and Community Psychiatry, 44,* 484–489.

Nicholson, J., & Henry, A. D. (2003a). Achieving the goal of evidence-based psychiatric rehabilitation practices for mothers with mental illness. *Psychiatric Rehabilitation Journal, 27,* 122–130.

Nicholson, J., & Henry, A. D. (2003b). *ParentingWell® Strengths and Goals.* Strengths Based Solutions, LLC. Available at: www.parentingwell.org

Nicholson, J., Henry, A. D., Clayfield, J., & Phillips, S. (2001). *Parenting well when you're depressed: A complete resource for maintaining a healthy family.* Oakland, CA: New Harbinger Press.

Nicholson, J., Hinden, B. R., Biebel, K., Henry A. D., & Katz-Leavy, J. (in press). A qualitative study of programs for parents with serious mental illness and their children: Building practice-based evidence. *Journal of Behavioral Health Services & Research.*

Olson, D. H., McCubbin, H. I., Barnes, H., Larson, A., Muxen, M., & Wilson, M. (1983). *Families: What Makes Them Work.* Beverly Hills, CA: Sage.

Orsmond, G. I. (2005). Assessing interpersonal and family distress and threats to confident parenting in the context of early intervention. In M. J. Guralnick (Ed.), *The developmental systems approach to early intervention,* (pp. 185–213). Baltimore, MD: Paul H. Brookes.

Panzarine, S. (1988). Teen mothering. *Journal of Adolescent Health Care, 9,* 443–448.

Park, J., Hoffman, L., Marquis, J., Turnbull, A. P., Poston, D., Mannan, H., et al. (2003). Toward assessing family outcomes of service delivery: Validation of a family quality of life survey. *Journal of Intellectual Disability Research, 47*(4–5), 367–384.

Pearlin, L. I., Mullan, J. T., Semple, S. J., & Skaff, M. M. (1990). Caregiving and the stress process: an overview of concepts and their measures. *The Gerontologist, 30,* 583–594.

Robinson, B. (1983). Validation of a caregiver strain index. *Journal of Gerontology, 38,* 344–348.

Ruddick, S. (1989). *Maternal thinking: Toward a politics of peace.* Boston: Beacon Press.

Sanders, M. J., & Morse, T. (2005). The ergonomics of caring for children: An exploratory study. *American Journal of Occupational Therapy, 59,* 285–295.

Scorgie, K., & Sobsey, D. (2000). Transformational outcomes associated with parenting children who have disabilities. *Mental Retardation, 38,* 195–206.

Segal, R. (2004). Family routines and rituals: A context for occupational therapy interventions. *American Journal of Occupational Therapy, 58,* 499–508.

Seltzer, M. M., Krauss, M. W., Orsmond, G. I., & Vestal, C. (1997). Families of adolescents and adults with autism: Uncharted territory. *International Review of Research in Mental Retardation, 20,* 267–294.

Sorensen, S., Pinquart, M., & Duberstein, P. (2002). How effective are interventions with caregivers?: An updated meta-analysis. *Gerontologist, 42,* 589–602.

Sorenson, S., & Zarit, S. H. (1996). Preparation for care giving: A study of multigeneration families. *International Journal of Aging and Human Development, 42,* 43–64.

Spector, R. E. (1996). *Cultural diversity in health and illness* (4th ed.), Stamford, CT: Appleton & Lange.

Summers, J., Poston, D., Turnbull, A., Marquis, J., Hoffman, L., Manna, H., et al. (2005). Conceptualizing and measuring family quality of life. *Journal of Intellectual Disability Research, 49,* 777–783.

Tannen, N. (2000). *The impact of parental illness on the child and family: Implications for system change.* Monograph produced by The National Technical Assistance Center for Children's Mental Health, The Georgetown University Child Development Center. (FAM04).

Tebb, S. S. (1995). An aid to empowerment: A caregiver well-being scale. *Health & Social Work, 20,* 87–92.

Toms Barker, L. T. & Maralani, V. (1997). *Challenges and strategies of disabled parents: Findings from a national survey of parents with disabilities.* Oakland, CA: Berkeley Planning Associates.

Uysal, S., Hibbard, M. R., Robillard, D., Pappadopulos, E., & Jaffe, M. (1998). The effect of parental traumatic brain injury on parenting and child behavior. *Journal of Head Trauma Rehabilitation, 13*(6), 57–71.

Vensand, K., Rogers, J., Tuleja, C., & DeMoss, A. (2000). *Adaptive baby care equipment: Guidelines, prototypes and resources.* Berkeley, CA: Through the Looking Glass.

Whitman, B. Y., & Accardo, P. J. (1993). The parent with mental retardation: Rights, responsibilities, and issues. *Journal of Social Work and Human Sexuality, 8,* 123–136.

Wood, B. L. (1995). A developmental biopsychosocial approach to treatment of chronic illness in children and adolescents. In R. H. Midesell & P. Lusterman (Eds.), *Integrating family therapy: Handbook of family psychology and systems theory* (pp. 437–455). Washington, DC: American Psychological Association.

Wong, K. (1995, March–April). Dependency proceedings show biases against mentally disabled parents. *Youth Law News,* 13–16.

Zarit, S. H., Reever, K. E., & Bach-Peterson, J. (1980). Relatives of the impaired elderly: correlates of feelings of burden. *Gerontologist, 20,* 649–655.

Zarit, S. H., Todd, P. A., & Zarit, J. M. (1986). Subjective burden of husbands and wives as caregivers. *Gerontologist, 26,* 260–266.

Occupational Therapy Evaluation and Intervention Related to Education

YVONNE L. SWINTH

Learning Objectives

After reading this chapter, you will be able to:

1. Identify different educational settings in which an occupational therapist may provide services.
2. Describe the OT process within an educational setting.
3. Recognize key requirements of occupational therapy services under the Individuals with Disabilities Education Improvement Act.
4. Describe how a disability may affect the occupation of student.

OCCUPATIONAL THERAPY IN EDUCATIONAL SETTINGS

Occupational therapy practitioners work in a variety of educational settings. These may include public schools, charter schools, private schools, alternative schools, vocational schools, and university settings (Case-Smith, Rogers, & Johnson, 2001). Across these settings, practitioners work with students in a variety of age groups across the age span. For example, an occupational therapy practitioner might work with young children in a preschool or elementary-age children in public schools or adolescents in an alternative high school. Occupational therapists might also work with an older adult client who is returning to school to learn a new skill after an injury (e.g., work hardening, job retraining) or for personal enhancement (i.e., leisure activity). Public schools are the most common work setting for occupational therapy practitioners; more than 30% of all practitioners who are members of the American Occupational Therapy Association (AOTA) identify public school as their primary work setting (AOTA, 2003). According to the Bureau of Labor Statistics (2006), "employment growth [for occupational therapy practitioners] in schools will result from the expansion of the school-age population, the extension of services for disabled students, and an increasing prevalence of sensory disorders in children. Therapists will be needed to help children with disabilities prepare to enter **special education** programs." It also is anticipated that the niche for occupational therapists working in other educational settings (e.g., colleges, universities, community colleges, and continuing education venues) will grow as these children become young adults and desire to continue their education.

The primary focus of this chapter is on the evaluation and intervention of occupational performance within early intervention and public schools, since this is the most common educational setting that employs occupational therapy practitioners. However, the reader is encouraged to consider the wide variety of educational settings that may benefit from the skills and expertise of an occupational therapist. These types of occupational therapy services may be innovative and preventive and may increase the occupational performance of individuals in ways that historically have not been explored or considered. For example, occupational therapy practitioners might develop a health promotion program for an entire school system to increase students' engagement in physical activity. Colleges or universities may benefit from an occupational therapist's expertise in addressing universal design, access to curricular materials for students with disabilities, or ergonomic needs of staff and students. Many of the principles that are discussed in this chapter can be generalized to any educational setting.

A variety of legislative and funding sources support occupational therapy services in different educational settings. While the Individuals with Disabilities Education Improvement Act (IDEA, 2004) specifically addresses services in early intervention and schools, every educational setting must meet the requirements of Section 504 of the Rehabilitation Act (1973) as well as the Americans with Disabilities Act of 1990 (ADA) (P.L. 101-336). Thus, occupational therapy services in settings such as universities and continuing education venues can be provided under Section 504 and the ADA. Section 504 supports reasonable accommodations for individuals with a disability, a history of a disability, or a perceived disability if accommodations are needed to allow the individual to participate in educational settings. The ADA is a civil rights act and provides protection to individuals with disabilities similar to those provided to individuals on the basis of race, color, sex, national origin, age, and religion. The ADA

supports the right of individuals with disabilities to have equal opportunities to live, work, and play within society (including educational settings).

Additionally, an occupational therapy practitioner may work in a hospital or private clinic as the primary work setting and contract services to an educational setting. In some instances, a public school district may hire occupational therapy practitioners to provide services to any student that needs their support (special education or general education). Table 50.1 provides an overview of legislation and funding that support occupational therapy services in educational settings.

Practice within the public schools is guided by federal legislation, with a focus on the occupation of education and the role of the student. Occupational therapists began working in the schools after 1935, when federal grants to the states created Crippled Children's Services under a special section of the Social Securities Act. Initially, these services were provided in segregated settings or special schools and primarily to children with orthopedic and neurological impairments (Hanft & Place, 1996). In 1975, the Education for All Handicapped Children Act (EHA) (P.L. 94-142) was enacted. This act required states to provide special education and **related services**, including occupational therapy, to all eligible children ages 6 through 21. Amendments to the EHA in 1986 (P.L. 99-457), added services for preschoolers (ages 3 to 5 years), and provided incentives for states to develop statewide systems for providing early intervention services to infants, toddlers, and their families. In 1990, the EHA was renamed the Individuals with Disabilities Education Act, or IDEA (P.L. 101-476), and additional services were added. These included assistive technology devices and services, transition services, and increased focus, funds, and programs for children with emotional disturbances. Further amendments were made to the IDEA in 1997 (P.L. 105-117), which mostly fine-tuned the original intent of the law (AOTA, 1999) and included increased emphasis on access to the general education curriculum for students with disabilities (see Box 50.1).

The latest amendments were completed in December 2004, and the name was changed to the Individuals with Disabilities in Education Improvement Act—IDEA 2004 (P.L. 108-446) or "the new IDEA." These amendments continued the trend toward increased access to the general education curriculum and increased the emphasis on pre-referral intervention or **early intervening services** (commonly referred to as *response to intervention* or RtI) by bringing more of the IDEA 2004 in line with the No Child Left Behind Act of 2001. The amendments also place an emphasis on the use of scientifically based (research-based, evidence-based) practices, high-quality preservice training and professional education, dispute resolution without going to court, increased representation of minorities in fields such as teaching and occupational therapy, and the use and development of appropriate technology (including

TABLE 50.1   OCCUPATIONAL THERAPY SERVICES IN EDUCATIONAL SETTINGS

Legislation/Sources of Funding	Population Served	Role of Occupational Therapist
Individuals with Disabilities Education Improvement Act of 2004 (IDEA, 2004)	Students who are eligible for special education and require the related service of occupational therapy in order to receive FAPE in the LRE (IDEA 2004 is applicable only for students (age 0 to 21) who receive special education services through their public school setting.)	To collaborate with the IEP team to determine the student's needs and then to provide services as outlined in the IEP in order to support student performance relevant to the educational environment.
Section 504 of the Rehabilitation Act	Students who have a disability, a history of a disability, or a perceived disability that affects their performance in school. (In the public schools, these are generally students who are not eligible for special education.) Students who meet the definition of "individual with a disability" are defined as those individuals who have a physical or mental impairment that substantially limits one or more major life activities.	To collaborate with the 504 team to provide the accommodations and adaptations that the student needs to access the school environment and services.
Americans with Disabilities Act (ADA)	The ADA ensures equal opportunity for individuals with disabilities in employment, state and local government services, public accommodations, commercial facilities, and transportation. Thus, it is a civil rights legislation that supports participation in the educational setting by students who have a disability.	To provide support through consultation and monitoring to ensure that students with disabilities have access to and can participate in the educational setting. Often involves working with environmental adaptations, accommodations, and the use of assistive devices.
Other funding sources ◆ General education funds (for public schools) ◆ Private insurance ◆ Private agencies (e.g., United Cerebral Palsy) ◆ State agencies (e.g., Division of Vocational Rehabilitation)	Any student who needs the support of an occupational therapy practitioner.	To support student performance in occupations relevant to the educational environment.

Adapted from Swinth, Y., Chandler, B., Hanft, B., Jackson, L., & Shepherd, J. (2003, April). *Personnel issues in school-based occupational therapy: Supply and demand, preparation, and certification and licensure.* Gainesville, FL: Center on Personnel Studies in Special Education. Retrieved July 15, 2003, from http://www.coe.ufl.edu/copsse

assistive technology). It should be noted that this emphasis on the use of research to inform practice is applicable across all educational settings, not just the public schools, owing to both policy priorities and the priorities of the AOTA.

Since 1975, the key goals of the IDEA 2004 (originally the EHA) have remained the same (see Box 50.2), with an increasing shift from the old paradigm of "if we cannot fix them, we exclude them" to a new paradigm of "disability as a natural and normal part of the human experience" (Silverstein, 2000, p. 1761). Thus, the role of occupational therapy under the IDEA 2004 has shifted to include a focus on contextual factors such as access to the environment so

BOX 50.1

KEY CHANGES IN THE IDEA OF 1997

1. Participation of children and youths with disabilities in state and districtwide assessment programs
2. Expanded parent participation in any decisions made about their child
3. Addition of transition planning starting at age 14, and younger if needed
4. Supporting professional development to ensure that all school personnel have the needed knowledge and skills to educate children with disabilities

NICHY (1998)

that individuals with disabilities can participate in their environments rather than on "fixing" the disability.

The IDEA 2004 has four parts, A through D; however, this chapter will primarily address parts B and C. (Part A addresses the general provisions of the IDEA, and Part D addresses research and training.) A positive addition to the 2004 amendments is the inclusion of related service providers, including occupational therapists, as a priority for monies and support, under Part D, related to research and training. Under Part C of the IDEA 2004, occupational therapy can be a primary service for infants and toddlers from birth through 2 years of age who are eligible for early intervention services (AOTA, 1999). Part B of the IDEA 2004 identifies occupational therapy, as a related service, for children ages 3 through 21 years for whom the team determines the service is necessary in order for students to benefit from their special education program. Two key concepts of Part B of the IDEA 2004 are **free appropriate public education** (**FAPE**) in the **least restrictive environment** (**LRE**). (See Box 50.3 for definition of key terms found within the IDEA 2004.) The IDEA 2004 allows each state and local education agency some latitude in how the federal legislation will be imple-

BOX 50.2

KEY ASSUMPTIONS OF THE IDEA

1. Equality of opportunity for all individuals
2. Full participation (empowerment)
3. Independent living
4. Economic self-sufficiency

Silverstein (2000)

BOX 50.3

COMMON TERMS IN THE IDEA 2004

Early intervening services: Academic and behavior support to succeed in general education but is not part of special education.

Free Appropriate Public Education (FAPE): Special education and related services provided at public expense that meets the standards of the state education agency (SEA).

General education: The environment, curriculum, and activities that are available to all students.

General education curriculum: The same curriculum as for nondisabled children.

Individualized Education Program (IEP): A commitment of services that ensures that an appropriate program is developed that meets the unique educational needs of children ages 3–21.

Individualized Family Services Plan (IFSP): A commitment of services that ensures that an appropriate program is developed that meets the unique developmental and preeducational needs of children 0–3 and their families.

Least Restrictive Environment (LRE): The environment that provides maximum interaction with nondisabled peers and is consistent with the needs of the child/student.

No Child Left Behind: P.L. 107-110, aimed at improving the educational performance of all students by increasing accountability for student achievement. Emphasizes standards-based education reform with the belief that high expectations will result in success for all students.

Related services: Transportation and such developmental, corrective and other supportive services (including speech-language, audiology, psychological, and physical and occupational therapy services) needed to help the child benefit from special education.

Response To Intervention (REI): An integrated approach to service delivery that includes both general and special education and includes high-quality instruction, interventions matched to student need, frequent progress monitoring and data-based decision making.

Special education: Specially designed instruction at no cost to parents to meet the unique needs of a child with a disability.

Source: Adapted from National Council on Disabilities. (2000). *Back to school on civil rights: Advancing the federal commitment to leave no child behind.* Washington DC: National Council on Disabilities

mented as long as the FAPE and LRE provisions are not compromised. Thus, there are differences across states and local programs regarding the specifics of how services are provided under the IDEA 2004.

The purpose of the IDEA 2004 is "to ensure that all children with disabilities have available to them a free appropriate public education that emphasizes special education and related services designed to meet their unique needs and prepare them for further education, employment and independent living" (Section 300.1). Occupational therapy practitioners in the public school setting provide services within this structure and are generally a related (supportive) service to the educational program (specially designed instruction). Students come to school to get an education, and in the schools, occupational therapy serves this priority. Thus, occupational therapy services in an educational setting are different from services in a clinical setting.

FACTORS THAT INFLUENCE THE OCCUPATIONAL THERAPY PROCESS IN EDUCATIONAL SETTINGS

A variety of factors affect the occupational therapy process in educational environments. Two key factors are the composition of the educational team and how decisions are made. Regardless of the educational setting in which an occupational therapist works, typically, a team of professionals typically influence the occupational therapy process.

Educational Teams

The concept of teaming, or collaborating as a team, to make decisions about the program and services to be provided has been a guiding principle of occupational therapy services in public schools since the inception of federal law. With the reauthorization in 1997, the IDEA became more explicit regarding the emphasis on teaming and collaboration among professionals and families to make effective decisions about student need(s). The IDEA 1997 clearly specified that whenever decisions are made about a student, the parents or caregivers must be involved. Two types of teams are involved in a student's program: the evaluation team and the Individualized Education Program (IEP) team. Both teams must include qualified professionals who are knowledgeable about the student and his or her need(s). If a decision is being made about occupational therapy involvement in a student's program, then an occupational therapist must be involved in the teaming process. The IDEA 2004 has maintained these tenets regarding decision-making and teams, although according to IDEA 2004, a team member may not attend a meeting, if there is written permission from the parent and the absent team member sends relevant data to the meeting.

In the public schools, the specific composition of each team is driven by the student's needs and may include general and special education teachers, therapists (physical, occupational, and speech), psychologists, counselors, parents, the student, and different community members. The focus of the team decision-making process must be on student outcomes and performance with an emphasis on participation in the general education environment whenever possible.

Team Decision Making

Effective and efficient delivery of services in the school environment requires a systematic process for team decision making and problem solving. There is a tendency by professionals to identify a need and immediately start proposing and implementing solutions without first identifying the necessary outcomes needed for the student to participate in the educational environment. Educational teams employ a variety of tools that support a systematic process of decision making and team problem solving (e.g., McGill Action Planning System, Choosing Outcomes and Accommodations for Children). For example, the McGill Action Planning System (MAPS) consists of seven specific questions that support the planning process and identification of team generated outcomes for students with disabilities (O'Brien, Forest, Snow, Pearpoint, & Hasbury, 1989). The questions include the following:

1. What is the student's history?
2. What are your dreams for the student?
3. What are your fears for the student?
4. Who is the student? (one-word statements that describe the student)
5. What are the student's strengths, gifts, and abilities?
6. What are the student's needs?
7. What would the student's ideal day at school look like and what must be done to make it happen?

A typical MAPS planning session can take up to two hours. The entire team (parents, students, therapists, and teachers) as well as other invited members (siblings, other family members, or community members) provide input in answer to each question. The questions are not quick or easy to answer, but the result of a good planning session is a strong foundation from which to develop the student's program, including any occupational therapy services. The process focuses on the value of integrating the student in neighborhood schools and in general education classes in order to develop friendships and to ensure a high-quality education for the child (Vandercook & York, 1988). By the time the team members are addressing question 6 ("What are the student's needs?"), they have the background to be able to establish both short-term and long-term outcomes. These outcome goals are then used to guide a discussion regarding the student's ideal day and how to get there.

One primary role of the occupational therapy practitioner in the school setting is to contribute to the evaluation process. Ideally, this is done in a collaborative manner with other team members. The practitioner's contribution might be to help the educational team determine eligibility for special education and/or related services and/or collaborate to determine the need for occupational therapy. Several key assumptions underlie the evaluation process in schools under the IDEA 2004 that occupational therapy practitioners do not have to address in other settings. These assumptions are briefly discussed below.

ASSUMPTIONS ABOUT THE EVALUATION PROCESS IN THE SCHOOLS

As with other occupational therapy practice areas, the **evaluation** process in the schools is dynamic and ongoing and often continues during intervention (Stewart, 2005). According to the IDEA 2004, the evaluation determines whether a child has a disability and the nature and extent of the special education and related services that the child needs (Section 300.15). The IDEA 2004 does not require use of a specific type of **assessment** method or tool. Rather, it requires that a variety of tools and strategies be used to gather relevant "functional and developmental information" related to enabling the child to "be involved in and progress in the general education curriculum" (Section 300.304(1)). In addition, the evaluation should help to determine the child's educational needs and how the disability affects the child's participation in school activities. A child does not "qualify" for occupational therapy on the basis of testing under the IDEA 2004. Instead, occupational therapy services should be recommended and provided for a child if necessary for the child to "benefit from their special education program." Even though the evaluation process in the schools is guided by federal law, occupation remains the core of the occupational therapy practitioner's theoretical perspective. Within the educational setting, therapy practitioners draw on the appropriate frames of reference to guide the evaluation process.

In the public schools, a team of qualified individuals, which may include an occupational therapist, school psychologist, special education and general education teachers, physical therapist, speech-language pathologist, and others, is responsible for conducting the evaluation. The purpose of the evaluation process is not only to determine the student's needs in order to have access to the educational environment to the maximum extent possible, but also to determine the student's needs in order to perform within the school setting. Additionally, the IDEA 2004 requires that the evaluation help to determine services that will support a student's ability to demonstrate outcomes with a focus on the general education curriculum.

Therefore, the evaluation process is driven by contextual factors (the school environment) and student (client) needs (Dunn, Brown, & McGuigan, 1994). In other educational settings, although the IDEA 2004 requirement to have a "team of qualified professionals" is not mandated, it is consistent with best practice. In most other settings, the team will be smaller, but seldom does an occupational therapy practitioner make decisions in isolation. Regardless of the setting, the emphasis of the evaluation is on the occupational performance area of *education*. However, other areas of occupation such as social participation might need to be addressed if participation in these areas is affecting educational performance.

The evaluation process should be individualized (student-centered) and should use a top-down approach (Coster, 1998). This means that the occupational therapy evaluation should start by looking at student performance within context versus evaluating specific client factors out of context. As with any occupational therapy evaluation, a broad view of the student (client) must be considered. Thus, the emphasis is on the educational context, including physical, temporal, social, and cultural considerations. Within the educational setting, the focus of special education and related services is on student outcomes. If the educational staff and/or parents require services (e.g., specialized training) for the student to reach his or her outcomes, then the practitioner is responsible for addressing these needs (Primeau & Ferguson, 1999) as well as broader systems issues (e.g., curriculum, environmental adaptations) that might require occupational therapy input and support (Muhlenhaupt, 2003). Under the IDEA 2004, occupational therapy services are supportive in nature in order to help the child be successful in school as well as in after-school activities (Giangreco, 2001). Additionally, services can be provided "on behalf of" the child and "to the parents, teachers and other staff" so that these individuals can better support the child's learning (see Table 50.2).

THE EVALUATION PROCESS

The occupational therapist in the school setting focuses his or her evaluation on what is needed for the student to engage in meaningful and purposeful school occupations. The occupational therapy evaluation addresses the student's areas of strengths and concerns in areas of occupation, including activities of daily living, education/work, play/leisure, and social participation. In each of these areas, the occupational therapist addresses the performance skills and the student's physical, sensory, neurological, and cognitive/mental function. First, an occupational profile is developed in collaboration with the team, including the family and student, as appropriate. This profile is followed by an analysis of the student's occupational performance within the educational setting.

TABLE 50.2 CLIENTS TO CONSIDER DURING THE OCCUPATIONAL THERAPY EVALUATION PROCESS	
Client	**Evaluation Consideration(s)**
Student	Gather data regarding the occupational profile and occupational performance
Parents/educational staff	On the basis of the student's occupational profile and occupational performance, determine whether there is any need for specific training, support, and/or dissemination of information.
System	On the basis of the student's occupational profile and occupational performance, determine whether any system supports (e.g., environmental modifications, curriculum development) are needed.

Following is a brief description of the occupational therapy evaluation process. The specific role of the occupational therapist during the evaluation process for any given student will depend on the expertise and skills of all the team members as well as the referral concerns. There may be overlap across professional disciplines regarding specific skills accessed (e.g., gross motor skills with physical therapy, feeding with speech therapy, or psychosocial issues with psychology), but the input of an occupational therapist is needed because of the unique emphasis of occupational therapy on occupation and context/environmental factors that affect occupational performance (see Fig. 50.1).

As in all other settings in which occupational therapy practitioners work, the occupational therapist is responsible for the administration of the evaluation methods and measures, the interpretation and documentation of results, and the communication of evaluation results with other team members. However, if an occupational therapy assistant is part of the team, he or she may contribute to any part of the process under the direct supervision of the occupational therapist.

Referral

Generally, the process of referral within the school setting is different from that in a clinical setting. As with any procedures within special education, specific steps can vary from state to state or from setting to setting. However, in most public school situations, if there is a concern about student performance, a team of professionals will discuss and implement different strategies within the general education classroom before referring the student for special education. If these strategies are not successful, then the student is referred for a special education evaluation to determine eligibility for services. Occupational therapy might or might not be involved in this step of the process. If the occupational therapist is not involved in the initial evaluation process, then the team may request an occupational therapy evaluation at any time after determining that the student is eligible for special education. If the occupational therapist is working in a state where the occupational therapy practice act requires a physician referral for services, then such a referral may be necessary before the implementation of services. If a physician refers a student for an occupational therapy evaluation, this referral does not guarantee services in a school setting. The occupational therapist in the public school must first ensure that the student is eligible for special education and then determine whether services are necessary for the student to benefit from his or her education program.

In other educational settings, the referral process may be less formal. For example, in some university settings, a referral might come through the center for disability access (e.g., a student access concern) or human resources (e.g., a staff ergonomic concern). Therapists who provide services in these types of settings might need to develop a referral system to ensure that the process meets the needs of the client(s). If a physician referral is required by a state

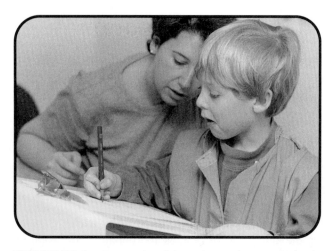

FIGURE 50.1 Occupational therapists evaluate a student's occupational performance within the educational context.

practice act, then the occupational therapist must comply with this requirement regardless of the setting.

Early Intervening Services

Over the years, educators and others have recognized the importance of providing appropriate support, when needed, as early as possible to students who are struggling. However, the current special education system requires that a student fail before being able to receive services. Over the past few years, some districts have explored providing services as early as possible. Because of the positive outcomes (e.g., many of these students never require special education services) of these services, the IDEA 2004 supports the option for a small amount of special education funds to be used for early intervening services or response to intervention (RtI). Within the IDEA 2004, RtI is defined as services that are provided for students, not in special education, who need "additional academic and behavioral support to succeed in a general education environment" (Section 300.226). Thus, in the public schools, when a classroom teacher is concerned about a student, initial interventions can be developed and implemented through a collaborative team process before the student is referred to special education. Increasingly, occupational therapy practitioners are involved with the planning and implementation of such prereferral or early intervening services. In some cases, effective prereferral interventions, such as the use of a move-and-sit cushion for a fidgety student or the development and implementation of a handwriting curriculum, may successfully support the student within the educational environment, and further intervention might not be needed.

Increasingly, research is suggesting that students need effective support when they first start having difficulty in school. Thus, IDEA 2004 has included early intervening services within the statutes. At this time, these services are not mandated, but part of special education funds (up to 15%) can be used by systems that wish to implement early intervening services. These services are for students "kindergarten through 12th grade (with particular emphasis on kindergarten through grade 3) who are not currently identified as needing special education or related services, but who need additional academic and behavioral support to succeed in a general education environment" (CFR, Section 300.226(a)). These supports are often referred to as *prereferral interventions* or *whole-school approaches*. Many districts are now implementing the RtI model to address this need (National Association of State Directors of Special Education, 2005).

RtI, which is based on research evidence and student outcome data, is an integrated approach to service delivery that includes both general and special education and includes high-quality instruction, interventions matched to student need, frequent progress monitoring, and data-based decision making (NASDSE, 2005). It is a whole-school approach to services that are specifically directed at student need. RtI is based on a problem-solving model in which the team defines the problem, analyzes what is happening, develops a plan, and evaluates the effectiveness of the plan. This model generally uses a three-tiered approach to support (see Figure 50.2). The first tier involves screening and group intervention; this approach will generally address about 80% of the problems. The second tier is targeted, short-term interventions, addressing another 15% of the student needs. The final tier is intensive instruction, which is required by about 5% of the students. The role of occupational therapy at each tier varies across school districts. Some districts feel that the first tier should be addressed by the immediate team, whereas others include the occupational therapist early in the process. If the underlying concern is within the domain of occupational therapy, a therapist may be involved in the second or third tier of interventions. The following case study provides an illustration of how occupational therapy may be involved in early intervening services.

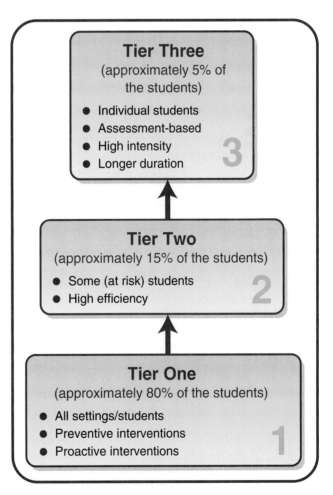

FIGURE 50.2   RtI three-tiered model. Adapted from NASDSE (2005).

CASE STUDY: *Early Intervening Services to Support Devon's Educational Program*

Background

Devon is 7 years old and in first grade. He has been having difficulty with literacy activities in the classroom since the beginning of the school year. His kindergarten teacher reports that Devon struggled the previous year as well but always "just made it." His first grade teacher is concerned that if Devon continues to struggle, he will eventually fall too far behind his peers to catch up. The elementary school that he attends has just started implementing prereferral interventions using a RtI model.

Tier One

Devon's student response team discusses his case with his first grade teacher. His teacher reports that he has difficulty copying and writing more than one or two words during any writing assignment. He often refuses to participate in reading activities as well. She reports that during literacy activities, Devon is fidgety and easily distracted and at times has behavioral outbursts. Using a problem-solving model, they determine that because it is November, they need to provide some proactive support to prevent future difficulties. The team decides to put Devon in a specialized literacy group that is explicitly designed to target first grade literacy outcomes. Occupational therapy was not involved during this first meeting because the team did not feel that there were concerns about Devon's performance that required the skills and expertise of an occupational therapist.

Tier Two

For three months, Devon participated in the specialized literacy group, and data were systematically recorded to track the interventions that were used and Devon's progress. Devon's reading and writing skills improved, but he continued to be fidgety and easily distracted and to exhibit behavior problems during literacy activities. The team invites an occupational therapist to the second team meeting, wondering whether sensory processing might be affecting Devon's performance. The occupational therapist recommends strategies to the classroom teacher that can support Devon's sensory processing (e.g., use of a move-and-sit cushion, allowing Devon to hold small objects in his hand to fidget, use of a water bottle) during literacy activities. Devon's parents also agree to try these strategies at home. The teacher introduced the strategies to the entire group and allowed anyone to use them. Data were recorded to help Devon and the team determine the best strategies for him. The combination of the targeted instruction by the teacher and sensory strategies recommended by the occupational therapist resulted in improved performance, and Devon did not need to receive Tier Three intervention. One year later, he was still doing well.

In the public schools, if the early intervening services are not effective, the student is then referred to a special education evaluation team. The evaluation team determines whether the special education process, as outlined in the IDEA 2004, should be initiated or whether the student should be referred for some other type of support. Such support is provided under Section 504 of the Rehabilitation Act. For example, if a student requires additional accommodations or adaptations but does not require specially designed instruction to meet educational outcomes, then the evaluation team might not recommend a full special education evaluation. They would then refer the student to the school's 504 team. If the evaluation team feels that the student might need specially designed instruction (special education) in order to receive FAPE in the LRE, then the special education evaluation process would be initiated. Ideally, the occupational therapist should be involved throughout the decision-making process if the evaluation team feels that the student might require the services of an occupational therapy practitioner or that the student has needs that might require the expertise of an occupational therapist. Once the student is referred to special education and it is determined that the referral is appropriate, a team of qualified professionals design and initiate the evaluation.

The team should be knowledgeable about the student and the suspected areas of disability. The purpose of the evaluation is to determine whether the student has a disability, whether the disability adversely affects the student's educational performance in the general education curriculum, and the nature and extent of the student's need for specially designed instruction and any necessary related services.

THE OCCUPATIONAL THERAPY PROCESS

When occupational therapy is involved in the evaluation process, the occupational therapist can use the Occupational Therapy Practice Framework (AOTA, 2002a) as a guide to the process. As described below, the special education process closely parallels the occupational therapy process described in the Framework. A description of this process follows.

Occupational Profile

The occupational profile is developed by gathering data from the student, family, and educational staff (AOTA,

2002a). The occupational therapy assistant, community providers, and others who know the student also may contribute to this process. Often, the development of the occupational profile occurs over time. Several assessments and procedures that have been designed for use in the educational setting may be used to develop the occupational profile. Table 50.3 lists some of the assessments and procedures that are used in educational settings.

Most of these assessments are process oriented and must be completed with input from all team members, including the student and family. Many of the assessments have a problem-solving focus that addresses the student's strengths and concerns as well as contextual factors that may affect student performance and outcomes. The assessments also will help the occupational therapy practitioner to identify performance patterns and activity demands. By

TABLE 50.3   COMMON EVALUATION METHODS AND TOOLS USED IN EDUCATIONAL SETTINGS

Assessment	Participation		Areas of Occupation					Client Factors	
	Characteristics	Contextual Factors	Activity Interests	Activity Choices	Subjective Experience	Personal Meaning	Satisfaction	Performance Skills	Abilities
Part I: Process-Oriented Assessment Tools: support gathering data for the occupational profile and analysis of occupational performance									
Assessment of Motor and Process Skills (School Version (AMPS)	◆	◆	◆	◆	◆	◆	◆	◆	◆
Children's Assessment of Participation and Enjoyment (CAPE)/ Preferences fro Activities of Children (PAC)	◆	◆	◆	◆	◆	◆	◆	◆	◆
Choosing Outcomes and Accommodations for Children(COACH)	◆	◆	◆	◆	◆	◆	◆	◆	◆
Canadian Occupational Performance Measure (COPM)	◆	◆	◆	◆	◆	◆	◆	◆	◆
Making Action Plans (MAPs)	◆	◆	◆	◆	◆	◆	◆	◆	◆
Miller Fun scales			◆	◆		◆	◆	◆	◆
Planning Alternative Tomorrows with Hope (PATH)	◆	◆	◆	◆	◆	◆	◆	◆	◆
Perceived Efficacy and Goal Setting Scale(PEGS)	◆	◆	◆	◆	◆	◆	◆	◆	◆
Interview with the student, educational staff, parents, and others	◆	◆	◆	◆	◆	◆	◆	◆	◆
School Function Assessment (SFA)	◆	◆			◆			◆	◆
Skilled observation	◆	◆	◆	◆	◆	◆	◆	◆	◆
Vermont Interdependent Services Team Approach (VISTA)	◆	◆	◆	◆	◆	◆	◆	◆	◆

Continued

TABLE 50.3 COMMON EVALUATION METHODS AND TOOLS USED IN EDUCATIONAL SETTINGS *Continued*

	Participation		Areas of Occupation					Client Factors	
	Characteristics	Contextual Factors	Activity			Experience		Performance Skills	Abilities
			Activity Interests	Activity Choices	Subjective Experience	Personal Meaning	Satisfaction		
Part II: Assessments of Client Factors: supports analysis of occupational performance with specific performance skills, patterns, and tasks									
Beery Developmental Test of Visual Motor Skills (Beery VMI)								♦	♦
Bruininks-Oseretsky Test of Motor Proficiency-2 (BOT-2)								♦	♦
Children's Handwriting Evaluation Scale (CHES)								♦	♦
DeGangi-Berk Test of Sensory Integration								♦	♦
Development Test of Visual Perception (DVPT)								♦	♦
Evaluation Tool of Children's Handwriting (ETCH)								♦	♦
Gross Motor Function Measure (GMFM)	♦					♦		♦	
Knox Preschool Play Scale				♦				♦	
Interest Checklist			♦						
Leisure Diagnostic Battery	♦	♦		♦	♦				
Minnesota Handwriting Assessment								♦	♦
Motor Free Visual Perception Test (MVPT)								♦	♦
Peabody Developmental Motor Scales -2 (PDMs-2)								♦	♦
Pediatric Evaluation of Disability Inventory (PEDI)	♦	♦						♦	♦
Sensory Integration and Praxis Test (SIPT)	♦	♦						♦	♦
Sensory Profile (Infant/Toddler) Sensory Profile (Adolescent/Adult)	♦							♦	♦
Social Skills Rating System	♦					♦	♦	♦	
Test of Handwriting Skills								♦	♦
Test of Visual Perceptual Skills (TVPS)								♦	♦
Test of Visual Motor Skills (TVMS)								♦	♦

OCCUPATIONAL PROFILE QUESTIONS FROM THE OCCUPATIONAL THERAPY PRACTICE FRAMEWORK (Adapted for the Educational Setting)

1. Who is the student?
2. Why was the student referred to special education and/or for an occupational therapy evaluation in the schools?
3. In what areas of educational occupations (ADLs, education, work, play/leisure, and/or social participation) is the student successful, and what areas are causing problems or risks?
4. What contexts support engagement in desired educational occupations, and what contexts are inhibiting engagement?
5. What is the student's occupational history?
6. What are the student's, family's, and educational staff's priorities and desired target outcomes?

Adapted from AOTA (2002a).

completing one or more of these process-oriented assessments, the occupational therapy practitioner will have addressed most of the occupational profile questions that are outlined within the Occupational Therapy Practice Framework (see Box 50.4).

Analysis of Occupational Performance

Once the occupational profile has been developed, the occupational therapist works with the team to determine whether more specific assessments are needed to help further determine a student's needs. Within the educational setting, the occupational therapist addresses performance in all areas of occupation as it relates to the child's educational needs (see Table 50.4). Often the process-oriented tools not only help with the development of the occupational profile, but also help the occupational therapist better understand contextual factors, potential "whole-school approaches," and curricular and extracurricular issues. These tools help the occupational therapist to communicate observations of the person-activity-environment fit as it relates to the student's occupational performance in school.

TABLE 50.4   OCCUPATIONAL PERFORMANCE AREAS ADDRESSED FROM THE OCCUPATIONAL THERAPY PRACTICE FRAMEWORK (Adapted for the Educational Setting)

Occupational Performance Area	How Addressed in the Educational Setting
Activities of daily living (basic and instrumental)	Cares for basic self needs in school (e.g., eating, toileting, managing shoes and coats, dressing up and down for PE); uses transportation system and uses communication devices to interact with others
Education	Participates and performs in the educational environment including academic (e.g., math, reading, writing), nonacademic (e.g., lunch, recess, after-school activities), prevocational, and vocational activities
Work	Develops interests, aptitudes, and skills necessary for engaging in work or volunteer activities for transition to community life on graduation from school
Play/leisure	Identifies and engages in age-appropriate toys, games, and leisure experiences; participates in art, music, sports, and after-school activities
Social participation	Interactions with peers, teachers, and other educational personnel during academic and nonacademic educational activities including extracurricular and preparation for work activities

Adapted from Swinth, Y., Chandler, B., Hanft, B., Jackson, L., & Shepherd, J. (2003, April). *Personnel issues in school-based occupational therapy: Supply and demand, preparation, and certification and licensure.* Gainesville, FL: Center on Personnel Studies in Special Education. Retrieved July 15, 2003, from http://www.coe.ufl.edu/copsse

CASE STUDY: *Process for Developing an Occupational Profile for Kristi, A 13-Year-Old Student with Cerebral Palsy*

Background

Kristi is a 13-year-old student with tetraplegia cerebral palsy. She has received occupational therapy in the past in both clinical and school-based settings. Kristi and her family had recently moved, and the education team in her new school district decided to complete an evaluation to determine her educational needs.

Occupational Profile

The occupational therapist started gathering data for the occupational profile by talking to Kristi and her family and reviewing Kristi's past records. Through this process, the occupational therapist began to develop a summary of Kristi's occupational history and her strengths and concerns in the areas of occupation related to Kristi's educational program. The therapist then observed Kristi in her academic courses, physical education class, lunch, and transitional periods (e.g., on and off the bus, between

classes). The team also met with Kristi and her parents to complete a MAPS.

Analysis of Occupational Performance

On the basis of the data that had been gathered, the occupational therapist summarized Kristi's occupational performance (strengths and concerns) related to most of Kristi's physical, sensory, neurological, and/or mental functions. Because Kristi had some difficulty with handwriting, the therapist also completed a Test of Visual Perceptual Skills and a Test of Visual Motor Skills to assess potential underlying client factors affecting Kristi's handwriting performance. The therapist also completed a manual muscle test to determine Kristi's strength and range of motion.

Summary

The occupational therapist summarized the following findings and recommendations to the educational team:

Occupational Performance Area	Strengths and Concerns
Activities of daily living (basic and instrumental)	Kristi is able to take care of her basic self-care needs within her school environment at this time. However, she has difficulty with some dressing activities that could affect her ability to participate in PE activities when she moves to the junior high and high school settings. Kristi and her mother also want Kristi to take a cooking class as soon as possible to determine Kristi's need for adaptive equipment for cooking. Kristi uses a school bus with a lift to get to and from school. She is able to communicate with her peers and teachers without any difficulty.
Education	Kristi is able to participate and complete assignments in her general education classes with accommodations and adaptations. She requires additional time to complete written assignments and utilizes a computer for longer papers. She needs to develop the self-determination skills necessary to independently problem-solve and implement accommodations/adaptations.
Work	Kristi states that she would like to be a lawyer or special education teacher. At age 14, the team will collaborate with Kristi and her parents to begin to develop her transition plan. This plan will support the assessment and address her needs for future environments.
Play/leisure	Kristi rides horses, swims at the YMCA, and enjoys playing computer games and watching TV.
Social participation	Kristi tends to keep to herself at school. Her mother states that Kristi is very social when at home with her family but that she has minimal interaction with other students her age. Kristi reports that she enjoys sports and that even though she cannot play, she would like to be involved by keeping scores or helping in some other way.

If it is determined that additional information about occupational performance related to physical, sensory, neurological, and/or mental functions of the student is needed, the occupational therapist may use standardized or nonstandardized assessments that focus on client factors (see Table 51.3). These assessments can help to determine specific information about occupational performance but should not be used without one or more of the process-oriented assessments. Additionally, the occupational therapist may use observation, parent or teacher interviews, and file review to support the analysis of a student's performance. The following case study describes the process of developing an occupational profile for Kristi, a junior high school student with cerebral palsy, as well as other steps of the occupational therapy process.

These findings and recommendations were included in the special education evaluation report, and the team used them to develop Kristi's special education program. Once her program was developed, the team discussed Kristi's need for occupational therapy support to meet her educational goals and objectives.

INTERVENTION

Occupational therapy service may address a student's performance in education, work, play/leisure, and social skills, with outcomes that are directed toward improving the student's participation in the curriculum, access to the school environment, and participation in extracurricular activities (see Fig 50.3 and 50.4). Within educational settings, occupational therapy practitioners need to be famil-

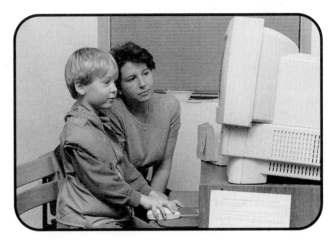

FIGURE 50.4 Occupational therapy facilitates student's use of a computer for written communication.

iar with and understand the educational environment in which they work as well the legislation and/or funding source(s) that support their involvement in the particular education setting.

Factors That Influence Occupational Therapy Interventions in Educational Environments

In addition to the setting and legislation, a variety of factors affect the planning and implementation of intervention by occupational therapy practitioners within educational environments. These include the unique characteristics of the system, the range of services provided, and the research evidence supporting intervention.

Unique Characteristics of the System

Each educational setting has unique characteristics that must be considered in planning and implementing intervention. Even within the same school district, different schools have unique strengths and barriers. Many occupational therapists who work in educational settings are itinerant and work among three or more schools. Variability can make it challenging for therapists to keep track of the uniqueness of different settings. Additionally, the different legislation (e.g., 504, ADA) and different emphasis (e.g., public schools, universities, continuing education, virtual classroom) also affect the uniqueness of the system. Therapists in educational settings need to attend to systemic issues, changes, and challenges in order to provide the most effective services. The reader is referred to Chapter 63 for an example of the reasoning of a school-based occupational therapist.

Range of Services

Occupational therapy practitioners provide a range of services in educational settings. Intervention may include

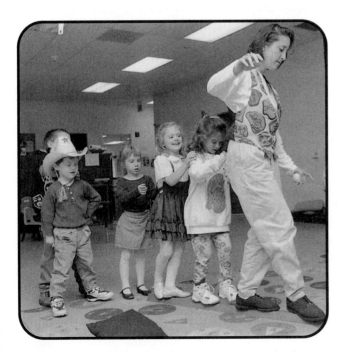

FIGURE 50.3 Occupational therapy in a group facilitates social and motor skills.

hands-on services (such as one-on-one or group activities) or team supports to identify and implement environmental adaptations and modifications to the physical layout of the school campus or the classroom. Finally, services may include system supports, which are activities such as working with the curriculum committee of a district to establish a handwriting curriculum or working with an elementary school principal to help design an accessible play area to be used during recess. Regardless of how services are provided, practitioners working in public schools must be aware of curricular issues such as education reform, standards-based assessment, and the requirements of general education. The IDEA 2004 requires that students with disabilities be considered for and have access to the general education curriculum whenever possible and be included in education reform and statewide assessments. Therefore, occupational therapy services may address the requirements of general education as well. For example, in some states, occupational therapists are being asked to address alternative assessments for students who have severe disabilities, or occupational therapists are involved in making decisions about reasonable testing accommodations for students with learning disabilities. To fully participate in these discussions and to support the implementation of the recommendations, the occupational therapist must have a basic understanding of the identified educational outcomes and testing requirements within the education system.

Additionally, occupational therapists need to understand the difference between accommodations and modifications and how these affect learning outcomes. Often these terms are used interchangeably, but in educational settings, the same strategies may be used in both categories, yet they have very different outcomes. *Accommodations* are adaptations or strategies that support student learning but require the same learning outcome as other students. *Modifications* are adaptations or strategies that change the learning outcome by requiring the student to learn something different or to learn less (Nolet & McLaughlin, 2000). Table 50.5 provides some examples of accommodations and modifications to illustrate these differences.

In educational systems such as universities or continuing education settings, a range of occupational therapy services may be provided as well. However, at this time, most occupational therapy services in these settings tend to be more collaborative/consultative or focus on accommodations rather than direct hands-on therapy services. For example, an occupational therapist might consult to a university computing center to recommend appropriate ergonomic arrangements or provide resources related to healthy computing.

Development of the Individualized Family Service Plan (IFSP) or Individualized Education Program (IEP)

Once the evaluation has been completed, the IFSP or IEP team collaborates to design the child or student's program (Giangreco, 2001). IFSPs are plans that include the child and family needs and are used in early intervention (0–3 services) programs. IEPs are programs that address the needs of students in preschool through high school. When developing the IFSP or IEP, the team, which includes the parents and student (if old enough), first reviews the evaluation results and writes a summary of the student's educational performance, called ***present levels of academic achievement and functional performance***. The present levels describe the student's strengths and areas of concern in relation to the expectations of the general education curriculum. The IEP team then develops the student's *goals and objectives* on the basis of the data summarized in the present levels and the agreed-upon outcomes that the team has identified.

TABLE 50.5 EXAMPLES OF ACCOMMODATIONS AND MODIFICATIONS	
Accommodations	**Modifications**
Alternative acquisition modes ◆ Sign-language interpreters ◆ Voice-output computers ◆ Tape-recorded books	Teaching less content ◆ Discriminating between animals and plants versus telling the distinguishing characteristics of animal and plant cells
Content enhancements ◆ Advance organizers ◆ Visual displays ◆ Study guides ◆ Peer-mediated instruction	Teaching different content ◆ Identifying different animals versus learning the human anatomy
Alternative response modes ◆ Scribe ◆ Untimed response situations	

COMMENTARY ON THE EVIDENCE

School-Based Practice

The IDEA 2004 requires that therapists utilize "scientifically based instructional practices, to the maximum extent possible" (Section 601(c)(5)(E)). This requirement is congruent with occupational therapy in any setting and is applicable to all professionals who provide services in public schools. Occupational therapy practitioners can use research evidence to examine the assumptions that guide their practice. For example, the value of consultation and education approaches and providing intervention within natural performance contexts is well documented in the research literature and serves as a guideline for best practice (Spencer, Turkett, Vaughan, & Koenig, 2006).

Although some research evidence is available, rigorous studies supporting effective practice in schools are still emerging. Swinth, Spencer, and Jackson (2007), in a paper developed for the Center on Personnel Studies in Special Education (COPSSE), summarized the current state of research supporting effective practices in the schools. (The reader is referred to the full report for specifics and in-depth information.) Since the mandate of IDEA is for services to be provided within the natural context as much as possible, Swinth and colleagues recommend that "occupational therapists working within the schools must consider outcomes within the context of the environment as well as the expectations in which their services are provided" (p. 8). Considering outcomes within the educational setting creates a challenge for therapy practitioners because some intervention strategies that have a strong research base in a clinical setting might not be as appropriate or as effective in educational settings. For example, rather than working on sensory processing in a one-on-one setting down the hall from the classroom in an environment that simulates a clinical setting, therapists in the schools might work with the teacher and student to implement sensory processing strategies in the classroom. The school-based therapist might work with the teacher to integrate tools such as move-and-sit cushions, a ball chair, and fidgets into the classroom routine (Schilling, Washington, Billingsley, & Deitz, 2003). Additionally, the therapist might work with the teacher to adjust the classroom environment, such as playing low music, decreasing the lights or using natural lighting, or developing a "quiet corner" where students can go to decrease the amount of sensory input they are receiving.

The COPSSE review of the evidence specific to school-based practice revealed a lack of high-level research-based evidence due to the few randomized controlled trails or meta-analyses of such trials related to school-based occupational therapy services. Despite this finding, a growing body of descriptive research does exist. "Thus, currently occupational therapists must rely more on effective or promising practices, clinical expertise and client values as well as systematically collected data when delivering effective practices" (Swinth et al., 2007, p. 34). To increase the breadth and depth of the evidence, a culture of inquiry needs to be established among school-based practitioners. Within this culture of inquiry, a strong research agenda should be established to help inform and shape school-based practice. This research agenda should study current practice strategies (e.g., the use of sensory principles in the classroom, the best use of the skills and expertise of an occupational therapist to address handwriting) as well as the current assumptions of school-based occupational therapy service delivery (e.g., therapy in a therapy room versus in the classroom, the effectiveness of collaborative service delivery). It should be noted that several studies support the idea that intervention in natural contexts is effective (Dunn, 1991; Palisano, 1989; Friend & Cook, 2003; Snell & Janney, 2005; Walther-Thomas, Korinek, McLaughlin & Williams, 2002; Thousand & Villa, 2000) However, many systems and school-based therapists continue to struggle with how and when to effectively move services out of a direct approach in a pull-out environment. Research is needed to help inform occupational therapy practitioners and others about how direct services can be provided effectively within natural contexts as well as how other approaches to service delivery (such as team supports or system supports) can be provided efficiently and effectively to improve student outcomes. Finally, high-level experimental and quasi-experimental studies that address the effectiveness of specific occupational therapy practices on students' educational access, participation, and performance (outcome measures) are needed.

Evidence reviews related to school-based practice are available from AOTA; one review addresses the psychosocial needs of children in the schools, and one review address school-based practice (Jackson & Arbesman, 2005;

Continued

COMMENTARY ON THE EVIDENCE *Continued*

AOTA, 2002b). Although these two reviews are not specific to occupational therapy services under the IDEA 2004, some of the summaries and data that are contained in the reviews can help to inform occupational therapy services in the schools.

School-based occupational therapy practitioners must balance the current state of the research with the need to make the best decisions possible to support student outcomes. Ilott (2004) has noted that occupational therapy is a "research emergent" profession. At times, the profession, including practitioners working in the schools, lacks a sufficient evidence base to fully determine which practices and interventions are most effective. "As a result, the competent school-based occupational therapist must think about 'effective practice' and engage in systematic data collection related to desired student outcomes. At all times, the therapist must utilize student/client evaluation and intervention activities to collect and document student performance (outcomes) which justify on-going decisions [related to] OT service continuation, modification, or discontinuation" (Swinth et al., 2007, p. 35). The following table provides an example of how school-based therapists can use research evidence to support their reasoning about intervention.

Intervention Question	Evidence Reviewed	Implications for Intervention Outcomes
Should school-based occupational therapists provide hands-on direct services in a one-on-one setting to address the handwriting needs of students?	♦ Case-Smith (2000) ♦ Case-Smith (2002) ♦ Denton, Cope, & Moser (2006) ♦ Cooley (2004)	Occupational therapy practitioners should consider the following when determining the type(s) of intervention provided to support a student's handwriting performance: ♦ While the research supports direct intervention to improve handwriting, it might not be the best use of the skills and expertise of an occupational therapist to address this need ♦ The implementation of a sensorimotor aspect to handwriting instruction may not be as effective as therapeutic practice ♦ Use of play with younger children may support improved fine motor skills ♦ Occupational therapy may help to improve letter legibility but might not affect speed or numerical legibility ♦ The dynamic tripod grasp is not the only functional pencil grip utilized in handwriting activities

Conclusion: On the basis of the evidence review, the occupational therapist determined that a greater emphasis on team and system support might better support the handwriting needs of the students in his district. The therapist felt that intervention for each student who is referred to occupational therapy could be best served through collaboration with teachers to develop handwriting clubs, implement adaptations in the classroom (e.g., pencil grasps, writing templates, assistive technology), promote fine motor practice and activities within the natural context of the classroom, and implement a comprehensive handwriting curriculum across the district. Direct occupational therapy services through one-on-one or group intervention would be provided only if it was determined through an occupational therapy evaluation that a student had underlying client factors (e.g., biomechanical, visual-motor, fine motor) affecting handwriting performance that could be improved through such direct intervention. The therapist hypothesized that by providing services through a team or system support approach, more children would benefit from occupational therapy, albeit indirectly, and that the number of referrals to occupational therapy would decrease so that the therapist would be evaluating only those children with handwriting concerns that had underlying client factors.

Different settings have different requirements for how goals and objectives are written. Under the IDEA 2004, the ideal is that goals and objectives are developed as a team. Thus, there might not be an "occupational therapy goal page." This is particularly common in some early intervention settings and is becoming increasingly common across all settings. Generally, it is expected that goals and objectives will identify a functional outcome (Fig 50.5), will state what the student will do and under what conditions the skill or behavior will be performed, and will include a timeline for completion (Borcherding, 2005).

As was discussed previously, collaborating with the team is an important aspect of occupational therapy service delivery in the schools. This collaboration sets the stage for focusing intervention strategies on specific student outcomes. Because parents (and older students) are involved in the team planning and decision-making process, their perspectives are well represented in the occupational profile that the occupational therapist develops. Throughout the collaborative process, the occupational therapist identifies where she or he may be able to support the student's occupational performance in the educational environment. The following case study provides an example of the goal-setting documentation for Shanna, a sixth grade middle school student with spina bifida.

After the goals and objectives have been developed, the team discusses which professional(s) should address particular goals (e.g., teacher and occupational therapist or maybe occupational therapist and speech-language pathologist), when they will be addressed (e.g., during physical education, during art, when walking in the hall), and where they will be addressed (e.g., in the general education classroom, in the cafeteria, on the playground). Each of these decisions is made on the basis of the student's need, not the personal preferences of professionals. Thus,

if needed, the occupational therapist designs the OT intervention plan on the basis of the outcomes that the entire educational team has identified.

The Occupational Therapy Intervention Plan

Once the team has developed the program and determines that a student would benefit from receiving occupational therapy as a related service, in order to reach anticipated outcomes, the occupational therapy practitioner develops a specific OT intervention plan. The intervention plan addresses the occupational performance areas as well as the performance skill or student factor that is affecting the student's ability to fully participate in the educational environment.

As in other settings, the occupational therapy practitioner considers student factors such as motor skills, process skills, and communication/interaction skills when determining student needs. Additionally, the practitioner considers performance patterns, such as habits and routines, the activity demands in the school setting, and the entire school context when determining student needs. With occupational performance as the core, a variety of conceptual frameworks for practice and frames of references guide occupational therapy interventions in educational settings. The primary perspectives may include occupational behavior, developmental, neurodevelopmental, learning, biomechanical, sensory integration, and coping perspectives (Kramer & Hinojosa, 1999). However, there are limited randomized controlled trials supporting or refuting specific occupational therapy interventions. Therefore, as much as possible, intervention needs to relate to the student's response to the intervention based on the occupational therapy and teacher data. Throughout occupational therapy intervention, the occupational therapy practitioner utilizes systematic data collection to inform intervention decisions, ensure the effectiveness of the intervention for the specific student, and help to support the best outcomes for the student.

SERVICE DELIVERY

Planning Intervention

When planning the intervention implementation, occupational therapists must consider the least restrictive environment requirement of the IDEA 2004: "to the maximum extent appropriate, children with disabilities are to be educated with children who are not disabled . . . removal of these children from the general educational environment occurs only when the nature or severity of the disability is such that education in regular classes with the use of supplementary aids and services cannot be achieved satisfactorily (Least Restrictive Environment)" (Section 300.114(a)(2)(i)). Thus, occupational therapy is provided in the student's typical environment to the extent possible. Such environments may include the classroom, lunchroom, bathroom, or playground.

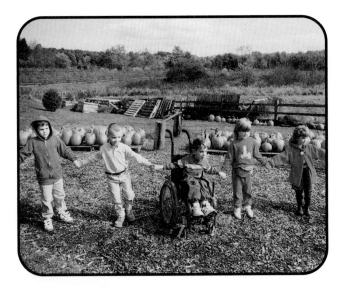

FIGURE 50.5 A functional outcome for a child in a preschool setting is participation with classmates during a field trip to pick pumpkins.

CASE STUDY: *Goal-Setting Documentation for Shanna*

Shanna is in the sixth grade at the Norwood Middle School. She has spina bifida and some cognitive delays. The school psychologist, Shanna's teacher, the occupational therapist, the physical therapist, and the speech therapist each completed an individualized evaluation. The occupational therapy evaluation included an occupational profile and an analysis of Shanna's occupational performance in her educational setting. As a result of the individual assessments, an evaluation report was written, and the following are some of the strengths and concerns identified:

Strengths

- Able to independently move about the school in her wheelchair
- Social skills with peers
- Verbal expressive language
- Creativity

Concerns

- Easily distracted in the classroom
- Cannot transfer in and out of her wheelchair independently
- Receptive language
- Written language
- Fine and gross motor skills

(This is not an inclusive list of strengths and concerns.)

Excerpts from Shanna's Present Levels of Academic Achievement and Functional Performance

(Note: These excerpts and goal examples were developed and written as a team, not solely by the occupational therapist.)

Shanna currently participates in her general education classroom throughout her day. Her assignments are modified so that she can complete them in the same amount of time as her peers. Noise and visual stimuli can easily distract Shanna within her classroom environment. She goes to the resource room for assistance with math and written language when she cannot complete the assignment independently in her general education classroom.

Shanna can move about her school environment without assistance, using her manual wheelchair. In the classroom, she requires physical assistance to transfer from her wheelchair to desk chair and back. She has difficulty with fine motor skills. She is unable to control a writing utensil for a sustained period (more than five minutes). Her difficulty with writing affects her ability to complete written assignments and art projects with her peers. Her delays in gross motor skills affect her ability to participate in physical education and recess activities.

Shanna demonstrates good adaptive skills during social interactions with her peers. However, she is becoming increasingly aware of her disability and limitations. This awareness has caused some episodes of depression and has resulted in extended absences from school. Shanna demonstrates emerging self-determination skills in other areas as well. She can describe potential accommodations and adaptations that she would like to her parents and other familiar adults, but she does not advocate for herself during school.

Goal Examples

- **To address psychosocial skills:** Shanna will demonstrate improved self-determination and self-advocacy by collaborating with her therapists and teachers to identify and implement any needed modifications and adaptations into her educational program from less than 50% of the time to 90% of the time as measured by therapist and teacher data by June.
- **To address written language:** Shanna will use identified accommodations/adaptations and/or assistive technology (e.g., word processor, spell checker, adapted writing utensil) in order to complete her classroom assignments within the general education setting within the same amount of time as her peers from 75% of the time to 100% of the time as measured by therapist and teacher data by June.

Outline of OT Intervention Plan

Using the team-identified goals and objectives as a guide, Shanna's occupational therapist developed an intervention plan. This plan included some direct therapy to identify and to teach Shanna how to implement any needed accommodations or adaptations and how to use any assistive technology. The occupational therapist also worked with Shanna to teach other school district personnel about her accommodations and adaptations and assistive technology. Ongoing consultation and monitoring were included to ensure that Shanna was able to participate within her educational environment. Finally, because Shanna also received therapy from a community-based occupational therapist, the school therapist contacted the community therapist at least every six months to discuss Shanna's program. The therapist did not directly address written language or work on improving handwriting. This was part of the teacher's lesson plan. The occupational therapist collaborated with the teacher to address the underlying concerns affecting handwriting performance, including the implementation of accommodations and adaptations.

Service Delivery Models

Many different service delivery models are used within the educational setting. The IDEA 2004 defines four different categories for service delivery:

♦ Specially designed instruction
♦ Related services
♦ Supplemental aids and services
♦ Services on behalf of the child

In most educational settings, occupational therapists provide related services, supplemental aids and services, and services on behalf of the child. Depending on the rules and regulations in a particular state, an occupational therapist might provide the specially designed instruction. Generally, it would be rare that an occupational therapist would be the only professional providing special education services to a student with a disability. However, a student with normal cognition but significant motor delays (e.g., muscular dystrophy, spina bifida, cerebral palsy) might require more support than just accommodations or adaptations in order to participate within his or her educational setting.

Occupational therapists may choose to use a variety of service models specified in IDEA 2004. However, student need is the driving factor in deciding how services should be provided. The three most commonly described models in the occupational therapy literature are direct services, consultation, and monitoring (Case-Smith et al., 2001; Dunn, 1988; Hanft & Place, 1996). Direct service, often the most common model, occurs when the practitioner meets directly with the student or group of students on a regular basis. Monitoring occurs when the practitioner identifies the student's needs and designs appropriate interventions but another person implements the plan. The practitioner meets with the student regularly to monitor progress. Consultation uses the specialized expertise of the practitioner to improve the educational environment and train the teacher and parents to implement interventions for the student. The practitioner does not work directly with the student. The consultative therapy model is increasing in popularity as practitioners, parents, and teachers are becoming more educated and are recognizing the importance of communication among all team members in achieving desired outcomes (Sandler, 1997). However, the term *collaboration,* rather than *consultation,* reflects the interactive communication among team members (Friend & Cook, 2003; Snell & Janney, 2005; Thousand & Villa, 2000; Villa, Thousand, Nevin, & Malgeri, 1996; Walther-Thomas, Korinek, McLaughlin, & Williams, 2002). Terms such as *collaboration* might better describe the continuum of occupational therapy services and may be better understood by all team members. Finally, newer publications (Hanft & Shepherd, in press) are using terms such as *hands-on* (includes one-on-one, small group services, and the like in pull-out or natural contexts), *team supports,* and *system supports* to describe

services in the schools. The terms to describe services in the schools continue to be refined and could be somewhat different depending on the setting, state, or system in which the therapist works.

Regardless of the terms that are used to describe services, it is not uncommon for service delivery models to be presented as a continuum and in a linear fashion. As a result, the assumption is made that services that are more collaborative are less restrictive than are direct services, and the goal is therefore to move toward a consultative or monitoring type of service delivery. However, for some students, the opposite might be true. Therefore, it could be more appropriate to view all the service delivery models as integrated features of an entire service delivery approach. Each service delivery model is important and valuable. To meet a student's identified need(s), therapy practitioners working in the schools may use a variety of service delivery models concurrently (e.g., some one-on-one, some small group, and some collaborative services) (Fig 50.6).

In addition to providing services on behalf of a specific student, some occupational therapy practitioners also provide services to the educational staff, parents, and/or the educational system. If the services are provided on behalf of a specific student, they are documented on that student's IEP. However, if occupational therapy practitioners are providing general services, then the recipient of services (or "client") may actually be the educational staff/parents or the system. Table 50.6 provides example of the range of interventions provided by an occupational therapy practitioner in the school setting.

Interagency Collaboration

Another important aspect of occupational therapy service delivery in educational settings includes collaboration between school personnel and staff from any clinic a child might be attending, as well as collaboration with other agencies. Interagency collaboration is particularly neces-

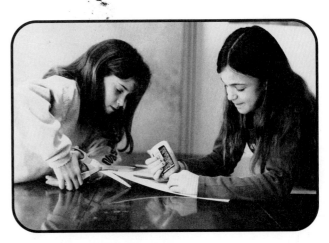

FIGURE 50.6 School-age children share materials in an occupational therapy group.

TABLE 50.6   OT INTERVENTIONS IN SCHOOL SETTINGS*

Performance Skill	Student Interventions	Educational Staff Interventions	Systems Intervention
Process skills ◆ Energy ◆ Knowledge ◆ Temporal orientation ◆ Organizing space and objects ◆ Adaptation	◆ Learning about self-regulation/levels of arousal and attention ◆ Use of sensory media during intervention ◆ Sensory integrative techniques ◆ Initiates activities and sustains attention to complete them ◆ Organization of desk and other work areas ◆ Accommodates/adapts to changes in the routine ◆ Work on visual perceptual skills ◆ Orientation to time and place ◆ Problem-solving ◆ Self-determination ◆ Behavior management	◆ Teach staff how to use sensory processing techniques in the classroom ◆ Provide in-services on programs such as the Alert Program (Williams & Shellenberger, 1994) to help students learn to recognize how alert they are feeling and to identify sensorimotor experiences that can be used to change the level of alertness ◆ Training and collaborative program development	◆ Participate on curriculum committees ◆ Educate the system about specific environmental factors that support self-regulation and arousal in the school ◆ Environmental modifications
Motor skills ◆ Posture ◆ Mobility ◆ Coordination ◆ Strength and effort ◆ Energy	◆ Participation in physical education and recess activities ◆ Participation in classroom activities such as written work ◆ Posture/body alignment during school activities ◆ Mobility within the school environment ◆ Accessing assistive technology ◆ Teach energy conservation techniques	◆ Training on use of adaptive equipment and accommodations and modifications ◆ Training on positioning, lifting, and transferring	◆ Work with the school system to adopt a handwriting curriculum ◆ Application of universal design to physical environment and the curriculum ◆ Ordering appropriate adaptive equipment (e.g. lifts) for staff safety ◆ Campaign for proper use of backpacks ◆ Adapted equipment (e.g., weight training machines)
Communication/ interaction skills ◆ Physicality ◆ Information exchange ◆ Relations	◆ Social skill development ◆ Psychosocial skill development ◆ Peer interactions ◆ Development of self-determination skills	◆ Training and collaborative program development	◆ Staff development activities ◆ Participation on curriculum committees

*This is not an inclusive list of interventions; rather, it is an outline of some possibilities. Specific needs of the student, staff, and system would help to define the specific interventions to be used.

sary if the occupational therapy practitioner is providing services for students who use assistive technology or during transition planning for older students. Interagency collaboration is important for any educational setting. For example, if a student with a disability who is attending a university needs specialized adaptive equipment in order to fully participate in the setting, the Department of Vocational Rehabilitation might help with the procurement of such device. Or if an occupational therapist is providing a continuing education course and one of the attendees is deaf, a sign-language interpreter might be needed.

Periodic Review

Inherent in service delivery in any setting is the documentation of services. Documentation serves as a communication tool to the students and families regarding the individualized program. Additionally, all decision making about occupational therapy intervention in the schools should be based on data, including research to the maximum extent possible. IDEA 2004 requires that the IFSP or IEP be reviewed at least annually, with regular updates to the family regarding the student's progress. (The IDEA 2004 requires that updates regarding student progress on IEPs be at least at the same intervals as general education report cards.) However, the occupational therapist should consistently (more often than quarterly) reevaluate the intervention plan to ensure that the student is moving toward achieving targeted outcomes. If necessary, the occupational therapy intervention plan or even the IFSP or IEP might need to be modified before the annual review.

OUTCOMES

Outcomes in any educational setting are determined by increased ability of the client (child, student, other professional(s), family, etc.) to participate (or support participation) in the occupation of student. With the emphasis in today's educational settings on evidence-based practices, it is important that occupational therapists working in these settings use strategies and techniques that are supported by research or effective or promising practices (Swinth et al., 2007). The challenge for most therapists in these settings is that there is limited research and the research that exists tends to be descriptive. However, in the public schools, the federal government has recognized this dearth in research and therefore supports promising practices. Occupational therapy practitioners working in educational settings can respond to this challenge by systematically collecting data when working with their clients and then using these data to support or change intervention. It is important that occupational therapists use research-based reasoning to inform their practice but that they not allow the lack of more experimental research to limit the scope of their practice in education settings.

SUMMARY

Occupational therapy intervention in the schools is guided by the IDEA 2004. Practitioners working in the schools collaborate with the IEP team to determine student needs and targeted outcomes. Once these needs and outcomes have been defined in the IEP and the team determines that occupational therapy services are needed, then the occupational therapist designs the specific OT intervention plan. Occupational therapy intervention in the schools focuses on the occupational performance of the student within the educational environment. Practitioners may also provide services that are directed to the needs of the educational staff, parents, or system. Specific intervention strategies and approaches should be based on research to the maximum extent possible. When research is not available but preliminary data indicate that a particular intervention or service delivery could be effective (promising), then the occupational therapy practitioner should utilize systematic data-based decision making to inform decisions about intervention for individual students.

PROVOCATIVE QUESTIONS

1. A school district administrator has asked you to design a specialized therapy room for the elementary schools. On the basis of current evidence, legislation, and what you know about school-based practice, what would you do?
2. The first grade teacher calls the occupational therapist "the handwriting teacher." What might you do to broaden the teacher's perspective on the role of occupational therapy in the schools?

REFERENCES

American Occupational Therapy Association. (1999). *Occupational therapy services for children and youth under the Individuals with Disabilities Education Act* (2nd ed). Bethesda, MD: AOTA.

American Occupational Therapy Association. (2002a). *Occupational therapy practice framework* Bethesda, MD: Author.

American Occupational Therapy Association. (2002b). *AOTA evidence briefs: School-based interventions.* Retrieved April 23, 2006, from www.aota.org/members/area15/links/link07.asp?PLACE=/members/area15/links/link07.asp

American Occupational Therapy Association. (2003). *AOTA member compensation survey.* Bethesda, MD: Author

Americans with Disabilities Act of 1990, 42 U.S.C. Section 12134.

Borcherding, S. (2005). *Documentation manual for writing SOAP notes in occupational therapy* (2nd ed.). Thorofare, NJ: Slack.

Bureau of Labor Statistics, U.S. Department of Labor. Occupational therapists. In *Occupational outlook handbook* (2006–07 ed.). Retrieved September 10, 2006, from http://www.bls.gov/oco/ocos078.htm

Case-Smith, J. (2000). Effects of occupational therapy services on fine motor and functional performance in preschool children. *American Journal of Occupational Therapy, 54,* 372–380.

Case-Smith, J. (2002). Effectiveness of school-based occupational therapy intervention on handwriting. *American Journal of Occupational Therapy, 56*, 17–25.

Case-Smith, J., Rogers, J., & Johnson, J. H. (2001). School-based occupational therapy. In J. Case-Smith (Ed.), *Occupational therapy for children* (4th ed., pp. 757–779). Philadelphia: Mosby.

Cooley, C. (2004). *Is the dynamic tripod grasp the most functional grip for handwriting?* UPS Evidence-Based Practice Symposium. Retrieved April, 6, 2006, from www.ups.edu/~ot

Coster, W. (1998). Occupation-centered assessment of children. *American Journal of Occupational Therapy, 52*(5), 337–344.

Denton P. L., Cope, S., & Moser, C. (2006). The effects of sensorimotor-based intervention versus therapeutic practice on improving handwriting performance in 6- to 11-year-old children. *American Journal of Occupational Therapy, 60*, 16–27

Dunn, W. (1988). Models of occupational therapy service provision in the school system. *American Journal of Occupational Therapy, 42*(11), 718–723.

Dunn, W. (1991). A comparison of service provision models in school-based occupational therapy services: A pilot study. *The Occupational Therapy Journal of Research, 10*, 300–320.

Dunn, W., Brown, C., & McGuigan, M. (1994). The ecology of human performance: A framework for considering the effect of context. *American Journal of Occupational Therapy, 48*, 595–607.

Education for All Handicapped Children Act of 1975. P.L. 94-142, 20 U.S.C. §1401, Part H, Section 677.

Friend, M., & Cook, L. (2003). *Interactions: Collaboration skills for school professionals.* Boston: Allyn & Bacon.

Giangreco, M. (2001). Interactions among program, placement, and services in educational planning for students with disabilities. *Mental Retardation, 39*(5), 341–350.

Hanft, B. E., & Place, P. A. (1996). *The consulting therapist: A guide for OTs and PTs in schools.* San Antonio, TX: Therapy Skill Builders.

Hanft, B., & Shepherd, J. (in press) *Collaboration and teamwork: Essential to school-based occupational therapy.* Bethesda: AOTA.

Ilott, I. (2004). Evidence-based practice forum: Challenges and strategic solutions for a research emergent profession. *American Journal of Occupational Therapy, 58*, 347–352.

Individuals with Disabilities Education Act Amendments of 1990. P.L. 101-476, 20 U.S.C. §1400–1485.

Individuals with Disabilities Education Improvement Act. (2004). P.L. 108-446, 20 U.S.C. §1400 *et seq.*

Jackson, L., & Arbesman, M. (2005). *Children with behavioral and psychosocial needs: Occupational therapy practice guidelines.* Bethesda, MD: American Occupational Therapy Association.

Kramer, P., & Hinojosa, J. (1999). *Frames of reference for pediatric occupational therapy* (2nd ed.). Philadelphia: Lippincott Williams & Wilkins

Muhlenhaupt, M. (2003). Enabling student participation through occupational therapy services in the schools. In L. Letts & D. Stewart (Eds.), *Using environments to enable occupational performance* (pp. 177–196), Thorofare, NJ: Slack.

National Association of State Directors of Special Education. (2005). *Response to intervention: Policy considerations and implementation* Alexandria, VA: Author

National Information Center for Children and Youth with Disabilities. (1998). The IDEA amendments of 1997. *NICHY New Digest, 26* (rev. ed.).

No Child Left Behind Act of 2001. P.L. 107-110, 115 Stat. 1425 (2002).

Nolet, V., & McLaughlin, M. J. (2000). *Accessing the general curriculum: Including students with disabilities in standards-based reform.* Thousand Oaks, CA: Corwin Press.

O'Brien, J., Forest, M., Snow, J., Pearpoint, J., & Hasbury, D. (1989). *Action for inclusion: How to improve schools by welcoming children with special needs into regular classrooms.* Toronto: Inclusion Press.

Palisano, R. J. (1989). Comparison of two methods of service delivery for students with learning disabilities. *Physical and Occupational Therapy in Pediatrics, 9*, 79–100.

Primeau, L. A., & Ferguson, J. M. (1999) Occupational frame of reference. In P. Kramer & J. Hinojosa (Eds.), *Frames of reference for pediatric occupational therapy* (2nd ed., pp. 469–516). Philadelphia: Williams & Wilkins.

Reauthorization of the Individuals with Disabilities Education Act of 1990 (1997). Pub. L. 105-17, 20 U.S.C.

Rehabilitation Act of 1973, 29 U.S.C. Section 504 (1973).

Sandler, A. G. (1997). Physical and occupational therapy services: Use of a consultative therapy model in the schools. *Preventing School Failure, 41*, 164–167.

Schilling, D. L., Washington, K., Billingsley, F. F., & Deitz, J. (2003). Classroom seating for children with attention deficit hyperactivity disorder. *American Journal of Occupational Therapy, 57*, 534–541.

Silverstein, R. (2000). An overview of the emerging disability policy framework: A guidepost for analyzing public policy. *Iowa Law Review 85*, 1757–1802.

Snell, M., & Janney, R. (2005). *Collaborative teaming* (2nd ed). Baltimore: Paul H. Brookes.

Spencer, K. C., Turkett, A., Vaughan, R., & Koenig, S. (2006). School-based practice patterns: A survey of occupational therapists in Colorado. *American Journal of Occupational Therapy, 60*, 81–91.

Stewart, K. (2005). Purposes, processes, and methods of evaluation. In J. Case-Smith (Ed.), *Occupational therapy for children* (5th ed., pp, 218–245). St. Louis: Elsevier.

Swinth, Y. L, Spencer, K. C., & Jackson, L. (2007). *Occupational therapy: A report on effective school-based practices within a policy context.* Gainesville, FL: Center on Personnel Studies in Special Education.

Thousand, J., & Villa, R. (2000). Collaborative teaming: A powerful tool in school restructuring. In R. Villa & J. Thousand (Eds.), *Restructuring for caring and effective education* (pp. 254–291). Baltimore: Paul H. Brookes.

Villa, R., Thousand, J., Nevin, A., & Malgeri, C. (1996). Instilling collaboration for inclusive schooling as a way of doing business in public education. *Remedial and Special Education, 1793*, 169–181.

Vandercook, T., & York, J. (1988, Winter). Integrated education: MAPS to get you there. IMPACT: Feature issue on integral education. Minneapolis: University of Minnesota, Institute on Community Integration, p. 17.

Walther-Thomas, C., Korinek, L., McLaughlin, V., & Williams, B. (2002). *Collaboration for inclusive education: Developing successful programs.* Boston: Allyn & Bacon.

Williams, M. S., & Shellenberger, S. (1994). *How does your engine run?: A leader's guide to the Alert Program for Self-regulation.* Albuquerque, NM: TherapyWorks.

Work

PHYLLIS M. KING AND DARCIE L. OLSON

Learning Objectives

After reading this chapter, you will be able to:

1. Explain the definitions and meanings of the terms *work* and *occupation* in occupational therapy practice.
2. Understand work practice in occupational therapy as it applies to populations described across the life course and by physical, mental, and social conditions.
3. Identify services offered by occupational therapy in work practice.
4. Understand the various types of practice settings in which occupational therapy provides work evaluation and interventions.

Occupational therapists and occupational therapy assistants strive to promote optimal levels of work performance for all individuals to promote a sense of well-being. The profession of occupational therapy supports the use of work as an evaluation and treatment medium, essential to providing a sense of meaning and productivity that is vital to health.

DEFINITION OF WORK

Work and work-related treatments have always been at the core of occupational therapy. *Webster's Universal College Dictionary* (1997) defines work as "exertion or effort directed to produce or accomplish something" (p. 906). In occupational therapy, the focus is directed more to the intrinsic value of work as "meaningful occupation." The profession defines *occupation* as a meaningful, purposeful activity (Primeau, 1996). In other words, occupational therapy considers work to be an occupation. Work is "any activity that contributes to the goods and services of society, whether paid or unpaid" (p. 57). It is one of the major human performance areas that encompasses life roles such as wage earner, homemaker, volunteer, and student.

ROLE OF WORK

Work plays an important role in an individual's life, contributing to the development of self-esteem, volition, a sense of belonging, and a sense of competence (Westmorland, Williams, Strong, & Arnold, 2002). "Work can offer a sense of mastery over the environment, as well as a sense of accomplishment and competence leading to an improved quality of life" (Siporin, 1999, p. 23). It provides structure for a person's life; fulfills the

Outline *Continued*

work ethic; and improves an individual's morale, discipline, self-worth, and dignity (Harvey-Krefting, 1985). Engagement in meaningful occupations, including work, is known to promote good health and occupational balance (Wilcox, 1998). For many people, an interruption in work can disrupt that balance and have a significant impact on health.

ROLE OF OCCUPATIONAL THERAPY

Work performance can be influenced by physical, cognitive, perceptual, psychological, social, and/or developmental factors. Occupational therapists receive a comprehensive education in all of these areas as they relate to evaluation, treatment, and prevention programs. Work performance is just one of many areas to consider. The occupational therapist or the occupational therapy assistant (under the supervision of the occupational therapist) collaborates with the individual, other team members (e.g., employers, case managers), or agencies (e.g., educational, local/state mental health, vocational rehabilitation) to develop intervention strategies. These strategies are based on the individual's interests, abilities, and needs and are designed to explore and expand work options, to enhance or develop work-related capabilities, and to obtain or retain employment (Commission on Practice, 1999).

HISTORICAL CONTEXT

The precursors of occupational therapy and work programs date back to the 1800s, when "work programs" were formed to promote sanity and good morale in people with mental illness (Paterson, 1997). Soon afterward, work-related therapy was also used for people with physical disabilities to promote good health. Adolph Meyer (1977), one of the founders of occupational therapy, provided the first philosophy of the profession when he wrote that healthy living involved a "blending of work and pleasure" (p. 640). The use of occupation soon gained a reputation as being therapeutic. In the early 1900s, the "work cure" was incorporated into workshops where clients received profits from producing marketable goods. Therapeutic occupations, habit training, handiwork occupa-

tions, and preindustrial shops as curative work became more common (Jacobs & Baker, 2000).

Today, occupational therapy continues to be committed to work and work-related activities, with a greater focus and expansion on injury prevention services (e.g., ergonomics, preplacement screenings, joint protection education, and postural awareness) and engagement in partnerships to serve industry. Therapists increasingly practice outside of the medically based facilities and more in the workplace, engaging with employees and employers.

OCCUPATIONAL THERAPY THEORY AND FRAME OF REFERENCE

Occupational therapy theory, practice, and research have always approached performance from a holistic perspective. One model, the Person-Environment-Occupation Model emphasizes the complex, dynamic relationships among the person, the environment, and the occupation. It describes occupational performance as the outcome of a dynamic, interwoven relationship that exists among individuals, their roles and occupations, and the environments in which they live, work, and interact. According to this model, occupational therapy intervention seeks to enable optimal performance in occupations that the client defines as important (Kornblau, Lou, Weeder, & Werner, 2002). For example, Lori, an occupational therapist, assisting Jim, a 42-year-old husband and father of two children who seeks to return to his job as an office manager following a T12–L1 spinal cord injury, must consider Jim's personal strengths and limitations in the performance of self-cares, his psychological and social adjustment to his disability, and mobility skills in preparation for return to work. Variables in the home and office environment must be assessed and modified to optimize independence in functioning. Doorways might need to be widened, and a ramp might need to be installed for entry and exit to both environments. Transportation issues will need to be addressed with adaptation of Jim's motor vehicle to incorporate hand controls. An analysis of his office job will need to be conducted to identify work accommodations that will enable him to perform his job independently. Such accommodations might include a larger office space, a desk that accommodates a wheelchair, and relocating office equipment for ease in reach.

Occupational adaptation suggests competence in a person's occupational response. To obtain competence, the person must interact with the occupational challenges within the environmental context. A person's performance is largely dependent on the level of desire for mastery, the environment's demand for mastery, and the resulting press for mastery (Schkade & Schultz, 1992). How a person responds adaptively determines whether the person will experience relative mastery in his or her occupations. The strength of this desire influences the achievement of mastery. The occupational environment presents challenges to an individual's performance. Physical, social, and cultural aspects of the environment can either facilitate or impede performance based on the individuals' aptitudes and adaptive capacity. Occupational therapists can act as facilitators of the environment. They can address both the person-system deficits and the environmental demands to facilitate a person's mastery in his or her preferred work occupation (Kornblau et al., 2002).

According to the occupational adaptation frame of reference, Lori will need to consider Jim's level of motivation to return to work and the tasks that his job requires. He might need to return to his job to financially support his family. In this case, Jim's desire for mastery is probably high. The office setting might present physical challenges for him, with limitations in space in the office and bathroom to accommodate a wheelchair. Adaptation and relocation of office equipment such as a computer, telephone, desk, and file cabinets will need to be considered to optimize his ability to perform his job.

POPULATIONS

"Occupational therapists and occupational therapy assistants provide services to individuals or populations with deficits or problems in the area of work performance" (American Occupational Therapy Association, 2005, p. 676). Work-related services can be provided to individuals of all ages. Throughout the life course, participation in work provides social, developmental, and economic benefits. E. A. Larson (2004) suggested that children benefit from culturally acceptable work roles such as cleaning up after oneself or participating in household chores. Early exposure to self-care and chores can affect the child's relationships with family members and provide the foundation for other work skills in the future. Studies of adults with disabilities have shown that quality of life is improved through participation in competitive employment and meaningful occupations (Bond, 2004; Dickie, 2003). Working with older adults to promote participation in work is an emerging practice area for occupational therapists. As the proportion of older adults in the population grows, the role of the occupational therapist will be expanded to accommodate the needs of the older worker. Occupational therapy services are not limited to individuals with physical and developmental disabilities. Work participation is a part of occupational therapy programs for all individuals, including those with mental and behavioral disabilities.

School Programs

In 1997, the Individuals with Disabilities Education Act (IDEA, 1997, P.L. 105-17) mandated that along with the Individualized Education Plan, each adolescent who participates in special education would have an Individualized Transition Plan before reaching the age of 14. Transition is the process in which the members of the education and rehabilitation team prepare the student to leave the school setting and enter into employment and community living (Kardos & White, 2005). **Transition planning** includes four primary areas: postsecondary education, community participation, postsecondary employment needs, and residential outcomes (K. C. Spencer, 2000).

Occupational therapists offer a unique role in the transition process by promoting movement from school to postschool activities through occupation-based evaluation and interventions (J. E. Spencer, Emery, & Schneck, 2003). Career interest inventories and job exploration may be conducted. Interventions such as the use of adaptive equipment or assistive technologies might be considered to maximize function in chosen postschool activities. Occupational therapists incorporate daily living skills, work readiness, and community involvement into the students' therapy programs to prepare for eventual employment and community living.

Occupational therapists participate in achieving transition outcomes for each student by addressing their specific needs. Working with the student ensures that his or her preferences and interests provide the foundation for transition planning. Along with the students, their families, and the transition team, the occupational therapist may develop and provide prevocational programs, facilitate functional living skill development, modify environments, facilitate inclusion in community experiences, and provide education to parents and other staff. Occupational therapy in transition planning uses functional, real-life tasks and task analysis to help students develop functional living skills.

Work as a Focus with the Aging Population

Having a work identity is central to being an adult in the United States. "In contemporary American society, a sense of being something (at minimum, being a productive person) seems critical to perceptions of belonging and status as well as one's sense of personal worth" (Dickie, 2003, p. 251). According to the Bureau of Labor Statistics (1999), the median age of the American workforce is rising sharply and is expected to continue to rise through 2015 as the baby boomers (individuals born between 1946 and 1964) approach retirement age. The average American worker is projected to be over 40 years old in 2012, constituting more than 40 percent of the labor force. The increased age of the American worker is affected by both the aging of the baby boomers and the projected increased participation rates of workers over age 55 (BLS, 1999). As the workforce continues to age, significant challenges face employers and rehabilitation providers. Age-related neurological, cognitive, physical, and psychological changes need to be considered in working with older adults (Gupta & Stoffel, 2001). Older workers have been found to require more days off work to recover from injuries than their younger counterparts do (BLS, 2005). This is suggested to be due to slower recovery and comorbid conditions.

Kornblau (2000) viewed the changing workforce as a trend to be embraced by occupational therapists. "Occupational therapists can play a big role in designing and adapting the workplace for the changing workforce" (p. 1). Occupational therapists provide services to facilitate successful aging in the workplace. They help older workers and employers to understand occupational performance issues and strategies that are specific to older employees (Gupta & Stoffel, 2001). Occupational therapists help older workers and their employers to optimize the fit between a person's abilities and the demands imposed by the occupation and the environment (Sterns and Miklos 1995).

CONDITIONS

Problems in work performance can arise from aging, physical or mental illness or injury, and/or developmental or behavioral impairments. Occupational therapists provide services to individuals with a wide variety of conditions who have a particular goal of enhancing participation in work. The practice settings often, but not always, define the age and conditions of the population that is being served. School systems serve youths with learning and developmental disabilities as they transition to adult life and employment opportunities. Individuals with mental or behavioral illness are served in a variety of settings, including hospitals, community clinics, and homeless shelters. Work-focused interventions for individuals with these conditions include assessment, education and training in key areas to enhance successful integration into competitive employment. Occupational therapists working in hospitals, clinics, and on-site in industry provide services for adults with a wide array of medical conditions. Physical injuries and illnesses related to employment such as musculoskeletal disorders and traumatic workplace injuries benefit from integrated services that involve the worker, the employer, health care providers, and others involved in safe return-to-work planning. Non-work-related medical conditions such as traumatic injuries or illnesses also require integrated planning to enhance the opportunities for participation in

work. Individuals with disabilities benefit from the education that occupational therapists provide regarding services and programs that promote safe employment. Legislation and federal and community agencies provide incentives to work, although many individuals lack awareness of the programs or are fearful that working will affect their benefits from Medicare, welfare, disability, insurance or workers' compensation (Fiedler, Indermuehle, Drobac, & Laud, 2002). Work-focused assessments, education, and interventions and the integration of services are apparent in all practice areas of occupational therapy for individuals of all ages and conditions.

SERVICES

Wellness, Health Promotion, and Injury Prevention

Wellness integrates fitness, nutrition, healthy relationships, a positive self-image, and the ability to take personal responsibility for self-care; it is the process of taking responsibility for realizing one's maximum health potential (Rothman, 1998). **Health promotion** is the movement toward optimal health and high-level wellness. These concepts are the basic tenets of occupational therapy. Rehabilitation programs commonly include strategies for empowering the client to gain or regain responsibility for optimal health and function. Community education programs, including topics such as energy conservation and work simplification, have long been part of occupational therapy's health promotion campaign. More recently, occupational therapists have conducted on-site educational programs in industries to encourage personal responsibility for wellness through prevention programs (Mungai, 1985). These prevention programs include stretching, fitness, safe work practices, and early recognition, reporting, and management of physical problems associated with work (Olson, 1999). Prevention, an important dimension of wellness, is defined as taking steps to avert the development of disease or illness (Rothman, 1998).

Wellness and prevention programs positively influence health and prevent injury (Massy-Westropp and Rose, 2004; Yassi, Gilbert, and Cvitkovich, 2005). Two major factors that motivate companies to initiate wellness programs are the resulting reduction of work-related injuries and the associated costs savings of a healthier workforce (Melnik, 2000; Naso, 2003; Rothman, 1998). Occupational therapists can incorporate wellness and health promotion into any practice setting. Siporin, (1999) emphasized the importance of training programs for individuals who have mental or behavioral disabilities in areas such as social skills, proper hygiene, and dressing for work. In this context, health promotion involves training in areas that prepare for more successful integration into community environments. Health promotion programs can include the assessment of health risk factors, such as problem assessments, workforce symptom surveys or hazard checklists, education and training in lifestyle improvements, safety precautions, safe working techniques, and fitness programs (Olson, 1999; Rothman, 1998). In industry, on-site wellness programs result in decreased absenteeism, reduced health care costs, protection from lower back problems and musculoskeletal injuries, and improved productivity (Carrivick, Lee, Yau, & Stevenson, 2005; Melnik, 2000; Naso, 2003; Rothman, 1998).

Ergonomics

Ergonomics is a relatively new profession that focuses on the use of a **systems approach** for improving safety and productivity through the design of work systems and environments. The practice of ergonomics has been evident through documents dating back to the 1800s; however, the term *ergonomics* was not coined until 1949 (Dahl, 2000; Vitalis, Walker and Legg, 2001). The most recent definition of the term was established in 2000 by the International Ergonomics Association (IEA, 2005) as "the scientific discipline concerned with the understanding of interactions among humans and other elements of a system, and the profession that applies theory, principles, data and methods to design in order to optimize human well-being and overall system performance" (Marshall, 2000, p. 1). In short, ergonomics has been defined as considering the whole system in the process of "fitting the job to the man" (Vitalis et al., p.1295).

A systems approach views the properties of the whole, or system, as arising from interactions and relationships among the parts. In this framework, the practitioner integrates the biological, psychological, and social factors of human performance within the environmental context (Dahl, 2000). Occupational therapists provide ergonomic services for individuals and populations in a variety of systems and settings. They use the principles of ergonomics to design safe and efficient living environments, workplaces, and products. The role of the occupational therapist in ergonomics is informed by knowledge of human performance and potential and the legislation that mandates safe accessible workplaces.

Workplace environments or systems include the organizational structure, environmental factors, tools and equipment, job tasks, and the workers (Dahl, 2000). All aspects of the system are considered in ergonomics. The occupational therapist assesses and analyzes the system to identify the presence of ergonomic risk factors. Workplace surveys, hazard assessments, and job task analyses are tools that are available to the practitioner. Collaboration with others within the system is necessary for an accurate and thorough assessment and intervention. The other members of the system include the workers, supervisors, engineers, and administration.

The occupational therapist benefits from good communication skills as well as comprehensive knowledge in the field of ergonomics.

Ergonomic interventions generally fit within three primary categories: administrative, engineering, and individual. **Administrative controls** or interventions include changes in the nature of work, such as scheduling, worker rotation, or the assignment of work tasks. **Engineering controls** include equipment and workplace designs or changes that reduce the human efforts that are needed. **Individual controls** include the physical, cognitive, and social skills and performance of the workers. Safe, efficient job design depends on coordination of all aspects of the system. Matoushek (2005) used the term *work integration programs* to refer to the incorporation of the clinical features of the injured worker into the organizational and ergonomic aspects of the system. Occupational therapists address both the accessibility of the workplace for all workers and the reasonable placement of individuals who have physical, psychological, or behavioral issues. Awareness of ergonomic principles provides a foundation for safely integrating workers into work.

Job Analysis

"Work performance supports participation and productivity, which are essential to the health and well-being of each individual" (AOTA, 2005, p. 676). The role of the occupational therapist in enhancing participation in occupation may include an analysis of work settings. A job analysis provides an objective basis for hiring, evaluating, training, accommodating, and supervising people with disabilities (U.S. Department of Labor, 1994). Regardless of the practice setting, the principles of job analysis are beneficial tools for the occupational therapist. Occupational therapists use these tools when planning the school-to-work transition for school-aged students and participation in supported employment or sheltered workshops by individuals with physical and/or mental disabilities. A job analysis also benefits clients who are preparing for their first experience with competitive employment or who are returning to employment after illness or injury. In addition, therapists who are employed in industrial programs may be called on to assist employers in describing jobs and/or determining the safety of the workplace. The occupational therapist may be engaged in assessing the job site with a thorough investigation of all aspects of the work environment or perhaps simply to explore discrete components of the job. "Approaches and techniques are intended to provide a foundation for analysis that can be applied to reducing the likelihood of injury, interrupting or minimizing the progression of an illness, or reducing the resultant disability of an injured worker" (Bohr, 1998, p. 229). Job analysis is a dynamic process that is appropriate to all practice settings that considers the worker, work environment, and work demands.

Job Description

A **job description** defines the essential functions of the job and how the job relates to other jobs and to the workplace (Bohr, 1998; Ellexson, 2000). An accurate and functional job description must define the essential work tasks, the physical and mental requirements of the worker, the necessary tools and equipment, and a description of the work space and environmental conditions of the job.

Essential tasks are the basic job duties that all employees must be able to perform with or without reasonable accommodation (Ellexson, 2000). The Americans with Disabilities Act (1990) mandated that job descriptions include the essential job functions. The essential duties are the reason that the position exists and the degree of expertise or skill that is necessary to perform the task. The job description also includes the **marginal functions** of a job. These are tasks that are not essential to the specific job or tasks that could, if necessary, be completed by another worker. Identification of marginal tasks assists the therapist in determining job placement and provides guidelines for training the worker for work.

Task Analysis

The terms *job analysis* and *job task analysis* refer to a thorough assessment of the physical, cognitive, and psychological demands of the job. **Job analysis** includes a formal methodology that details the interaction between the worker and the equipment of a system. It defines the performance requirements of the worker by a detailed description of the human task requirements. Job **task analysis** is the specific assessment of a particular task or procedure. A thorough job analysis includes employer and worker interviews; observation of multiple workers performing the task (if possible); measurement of the forces, frequencies, and durations of work tasks; postural requirements such as reaching and leaning; and the environmental and psychosocial conditions that are present in the workplace.

Methods

Before conducting a job analysis, it is imperative to discuss with management or the supervisor several issues regarding the assessment process. The employer will be able to provide information on the least disruptive methods for conducting the evaluation and the necessary safety precautions for the evaluator. Personal protective equipment, such as safety glasses, steel-toed shoes, hearing protection, or special clothing might be required while on the job site. There might be restrictions on interviewing workers while they are performing their work. Interviews might need to occur during the worker's lunch or break periods. In addition, the therapist should discuss and receive permission in advance for use of any audio, photographic, or video equipment.

Detailed, organized documentation of the information that is gained during the job analysis will be the most useful. Many checklists or forms are available to use as a starting point, allowing the therapist to highlight specific areas to target for more thorough analysis (Occupational Safety and Health Administration, 2002; Washington State Department of Labor and Industries, 2005). It is also helpful to use audiotape, photographic, or video equipment to record the worker or workers performing the job, allowing a more thorough analysis at a later time. Other common supplies that are helpful in job analysis are a tape measure, a force pressure gauge, a stopwatch, and a goniometer. In addition, specific tools can be investigated for measuring noise, heat, and vibration, as shown in Figures 51.1 and 51.2.

Supervisor and worker interviews provide valuable insight into all aspects of the job. According to OSHA (2002), "involving employees will help minimize oversights and ensure a quality analysis" (p. 9). The interviews can be a method of learning about routine and infrequent tasks and about flow patterns and sequences and to obtain workers' perspectives of physical and mental work stresses (Bohr, 1998; OSHA, 2002).

Formal Measurements

Job analysis involves measurements of many of the aspects of the job (Ellexson, 2000). This includes the dimensions of the workspace and the materials that are handled. Measuring the workspace includes measuring the dimensions of reach required for the various tasks, the distances required to transport items, and the heights of work surfaces. The weight of objects that are lifted or lowered is documented, as are the frequency, duration, distance, and quality of the task, such as the handholds, or the stability of the load. Other forces that the worker encounters are also measured, such as pushing and pulling, and use of tools, gloves, and other personal protective equipment is assessed. The body positions of the worker, such as leaning, reaching, or other postures, should be measured or

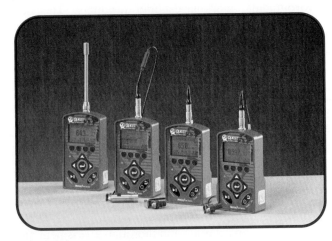

FIGURE 51.1 Instruments for measurement of noise levels. (Photograph provided by Quest Technologies.)

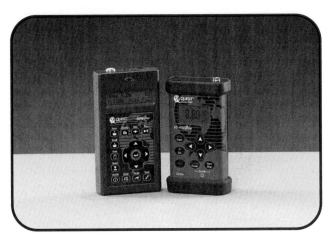

FIGURE 51.2 Instruments for measuring vibration. (Photograph provided by Quest Technologies.)

estimated, and the duration and frequency should be recorded. It might be possible to record only the initial and terminal postures for dynamic motions. Video recordings or photographic equipment aid in the assessment of body postures by allowing the evaluator to assess angles, frequency, duration, or other variables later (Bohr, 1998). Finally, the conditions of the workspace and environmental considerations such as the ambient temperature, surface temperatures, humidity, noise level, illumination, and vibration are also documented and measured. To assist the therapist in identifying the safe working levels, databases of acceptable working conditions are available. These are based on epidemiological, biomechanical, psychophysical, and physiological approaches (Eastman Kodak Company, 1983; Snook and Cirello, 1991; Washington State Department of Labor and Industries, 2005; Waters, Putz-Anderson, Garg, & Fine, 1993).

The job analysis is completed by preparing a summary that is specifically developed for the customer. Generally, the report will include an overview of the data that have been collected, the problems that have been identified, and recommendations for addressing the problems. "It is often a good idea to offer staged solutions for addressing the problems" (Bohr, 1998, p. 244). The therapist should prioritize solutions that will be the most effective in the short term to assist the employer in analyzing the cost-benefit ratio. The emphasis of the report will vary depending on the customer. When the customers are concerned about job placement for a client, the focus of the report will be on the individual. The report will highlight the necessary physical demands and rehabilitation needs such as strengthening, endurance and/or flexibility. When the focus is on workplace safety, the report will highlight hazardous conditions, with recommendations for safety, efficiency, and productivity. Regardless of the purpose of the assessment, the job analysis will identify factors that will either enhance or restrict participation in the occupation of work with

recommendations for the client, the rehabilitation team, and/or the employer. "Through observation, demonstration, participation, documentation and analysis, the skilled occupational therapist can develop a clear and concise picture of a specific job" (Ellexson, 2000, p. 6). Box 51.1 lists some resources that relate to job analysis.

Functional Capacity Evaluation

The **functional capacity evaluation** (FCE) is an integral assessment tool that is used for work injury prevention and rehabilitation. FCEs define an individual's functional abilities and/or limitations in the context of safe, productive work tasks. An FCE itself involves a process of systematically gathering and testing information and making and testing hypotheses about performance, often in relation to an occupation in context. The therapist begins by reviewing referral information related to a client's medical and work history. A series of test activities are then administered to measure whether the person has the abilities to meet the required job demands, to determine a level of disability, or to demonstrate the need for, and progress in, rehabilitation (Harwood, 2004). Physicians, employers, insurers, and benefits adjudicators often rely on FCEs to provide definitive answers in a variety of situations involving work. Results of these evaluations have significant implications for further rehabilitation efforts, employment, compensability determinations, and cash benefits.

FCEs include a wide range of evaluation activities. The simplest evaluations involve a series of standardized tasks with measured weights and distances and a trained observer; these are available for upper extremity as well as back and lower extremity activities. Other approaches use machines to measure average and peak forces, velocity, and range of motion in several different planes. In these situations, workers are generally asked to exert a maximal effort. Job simulation, using tasks and equipment that are specific to a particular job, has recently become more popular, in part because of the Americans With Disabilities Act (ADA) requirement that valid testing should be job-specific and focus on a comparison of capacity to actual job demands (Lechner, 1998).

The concept of matching job or workplace demands to the capabilities and limitations of a worker is a fundamental assumption underlying FCE application. One of the most important aspects of an FCE is that the measurement of capacity is specific to the demands that the job poses. The estimates of job demands are inexact generalizations that have not been scientifically validated. A formal job analysis is desirable for FCEs that are intended to measure the ability to work at a specific job. Discussions with employees and written company job descriptions are also helpful in obtaining accurate assessments of job demands.

FCE5 are usually performed in the clinic and may range from 2 to 4 hours in duration over the course of a

BOX 51.1 REFERENCES AND RESOURCES FOR CONDUCTING A JOB ANALYSIS

General Assessments

- http://www.osha.gov/SLTC/ergonomics/analysis_tools.html
- http://www.lni.wa.gov/

Rapid Entire Body Assessment (REBA)

- Hignett, & McAtamney, L. (2000) *Applied Ergonomics, 31*, 201–205.

Rapid Upper Limb Assessment RULA

- McAtamney, L., & Corlett, N. E. (1993). RULA: A survey method for the investigation of work-related upper limb disorders. *Applied Ergonomics, 24*(2), 91–99.
- http://ergo.human.cornell.edu/ahRULA.html

Lifting Assessments

- Waters, T. R., Putz-Anderson, V., Garg, A., & Fine, L. (1993). Revised NIOSH equation for the design and evaluation of manual lifting tasks. *Ergonomics, 36*(7), 749–776.
- http://www.cdc.gov/niosh/94-110.html
- http://www.lni.wa.gov/Safety/Topics/Ergonomics/Services Resources/Tools/default.asp

Force Measurement

- Chatillon Force Pressure Gauge
- http://www.chatillon.com/Contact%20Us/contactus.html

Vibration

- http://www.lni.wa.gov/
- American Conference of Governmental Industrial Hygienists, ACGIF: www.acgif.org
- Whole-Body Vibration: TLV® Physical Agents 7th Edition Documentation, ACGIH® Publication #7DOC-648 (Copyright © 2001)
- Hand-Arm Vibration: TLV® Physical Agents 7th Edition Documentation, ACGIH®

Illumination

- Recommended lighting levels by the Illuminating Engineering Society of North America, http://www.iesna.org/

Noise

- OSHA Noise standard, 29, DFR 1910.95(a) and (b)

Repetition

- www.acgih.org: Hand Activity Level (HAL): Threshold Limit Value (TLV®) Physical Agents 7th Edition Documentation, ACGIH®, Publication #7DOC-646 (Copyright © 2001)

---

two-day period. Protocols often extrapolate from tasks that are stereotypical or performed at near-maximal levels for a short period of time to predict ability to sustain job activities for a full workday and workweek. Performance on FCE tasks are often compared with population or coworker norms, as actual job force requirements are not often estimated during this process. It is important for therapists to use good observational skills throughout the assessment to ensure a client's safe performance (King, 2004).

FCEs are generally classified into two broad categories: comprehensive and job-specific (Frings-Dresen & Sluiter, 2003; King, Tuckwell, & Barrett, 1998). When administering the comprehensive FCE, most evaluators use a complete battery of tasks that cover all 20 physical demands listed in the *Dictionary of Occupational Titles* (U.S. Department of Labor, 1977).

In job-specific testing, the evaluator tests only those tasks that are directly related to the job. The job-specific testing is more cost effective and is often used for disability determination. However, if the client cannot return to the former job, then additional testing might be required.

FCE reporting formats vary in length from one page to 35 pages or more. The primary objective is to describe the client's safe level of overall exertion ranging from sedentary to very heavy. A summary cover page is usually attached to the FCE data collection forms when FCE information is submitted to referral sources.

In these times of unprecedented workers' compensation costs and disability costs, there is a pressing need to return workers to gainful employment if possible and to make appropriate disability decisions for those who are unable to work. A well-designed FCE can provide objective information on a wide range of functional activities for clinical decision making (Isernhagen, 1988; Lechner, Jackson, Roth, & Straaton, 1994; Lechner, Roth, & Straaton, 1991).

Preplacement Assessment

Preplacement assessments (PPAs) are used by employers to determine whether an individual is capable of performing the job. The results of these assessments help employers to make appropriate decisions related to the placement of individuals in jobs without hazards to the safety of themselves or others. Proper PPAs can reduce the number and costs of employee injuries as well as absenteeism attributed to ill health (Nachreiner et al., 1999).

Before passage of the ADA in 1990, prework screening was performed for the purpose of excluding individuals from employment if they presented an increased risk of any type of illness or injury (Andstadt, 1990). These screenings are no longer legal; PPAs have taken their place. Applicants must now be given a conditional offer of hire based on successful completion of the PPA. The preplacement screen is viewed as an injury prevention strategy, not as a means to screen out applicants. The employer's decision to withdraw a job offer must be based on the applicant's inability to perform the essential functions of the job with or without accommodations. A prospective employee can be denied the job only if he or she is at definite risk of specific injury or illness while performing the essential functions of the job. Employers are required to provide reasonable accommodation to mitigate these risks as much as possible (Nachreiner et al., 1999).

Occupational therapists design and administer preplacement screenings. The screening occurs after a conditional offer of hire, and it must apply to all applicants for a specific job position. First, the therapist requests a job description to ascertain the essential functions of the job. If a job description is not available, the therapist must perform a job analysis to determine the physical demands of the job. This entails observing job tasks, videotaping employees performing the job, and collecting workstation measurements to obtain accurate information to design an appropriate preplacement screen. Once the job description has been developed, the therapist develops a standardized test of the physical demands of the job. To verify that the preplacement screen tests what it is intended to test, a sample of current employees performing the particular job are selected to validate the job description and pilot the test. The therapist rates the performance of the individual according to the validated physical demands of the job. The applicant receives the scoring information. The evaluator does not make hiring interpretations. The ultimate decision to hire is in the hands of the employer.

Work Hardening and Work Conditioning Programs

The term *work hardening* came into being in the late 1970s as professionals used work as a treatment or evaluation modality. Other terms that are used synonymously are *work conditioning, work readiness,* and *work capabilities* (Isernhagen, 1988). In 1988, the Commission on Accreditation of Rehabilitation Facilities (CARF) officially defined **work hardening** as "a highly structured, goal-oriented, individualized treatment program designed to maximize the individual's ability to return to work" (CARF, 1988, p. 69). The guidelines recommended that work hardening programs be interdisciplinary and capable of addressing the functional, physical, behavioral, and vocational needs of the person who is being served. CARF suggested the use of real or simulated work activities in conjunction with conditioning activities to improve biomechanical, neuromuscular, cardiovascular/metabolic, behavioral, and vocational functioning (King, 1998). Work hardening programs usually employ exercise equipment, a work simulation area, and a quiet, private area for testing and evaluation.

Work conditioning programs emphasize physical conditioning, which addresses issues of strength, endurance, flexibility, motor control, and cardiopulmonary function (Helm-Williams, 1993). They are shorter in duration than work hardening programs; use exercise, aerobic conditioning, education, and limited work task simulation; and require less physical space than work hardening programs. Work conditioning programs usually involve only one or two disciplines and are usually half-day programs. Work hardening and work conditioning programs are increasingly being located in nonmedical settings such as industrial parks, strip shopping malls, and office complexes and at the worksite. Programs that are implemented at the worksite provide a more realistic environment and place the employee back at work and in close communication with the employer.

The work hardening and work conditioning evaluation and treatment process consists of entrance criteria whereby clients are unable to return to work due to pain or dysfunction following injury and the clients agree to participate in the program. The clients must also have a reasonably good prognosis for improvement of employment capacity and a job-oriented goal (King, 1998). The occupational therapist initially interviews the client to gather valuable information related to his or her medical and work history. Insight into what procedures have worked or failed in the past, as well as the client's beliefs or misperceptions about his or her condition, can be ascertained. Job history, before and after the injury, and how long the client has been off work or on light duty are important pieces of information to have in designing a work rehabilitation program. An evaluation of a client's functional capabilities is performed before performance of any conditioning and/or work-related activities. The purpose of this evaluation is to become familiar with the client's current functional status, behaviors associated with work activity, potential latent symptom responses after activity, and body mechanics techniques. This information is compared with the client's job demands and goals for progress.

The client's length of time in work hardening and work conditioning programs depends on his or her individualized treatment needs and the treatment protocols that have been established by the program. Typically, clients are started in programs for two hours per day, eventually progressing to four hours as tolerated. This requires highly focused and well-managed treatment plans. Most programs start with warm-up exercises, followed by strengthening and job simulation activities. Education on risk factors to injury and prevention of injuries with use of proper body mechanics and work methods is woven into the program. Clients are discharged when (1) they meet their goals, (2) progress has stopped or slowed to an imperceptible level, (3) the client has medical complications, or (4) the client is noncompliant with the program.

Case Management

An increasing number of occupational therapists are assuming case management roles. Case management is not a profession; it is an area of practice within a profession. Therapists, nurses, social workers, and rehabilitation counselors may all serve as case managers. Their goal is to achieve a successful, cost-effective method of returning clients to work.

The nonprofit organization Case Management Society of America (CMSA) was established in 1989. Its *Standards of Practice for Case Management* defines **case management** as "a collaborative process which assesses, plans, implements, coordinates, monitors, and evaluates options and services to meet an individual's health needs through communication and available resources to promote quality cost effective outcomes" (CMSA, 1995, p. 8). A certification process was established to monitor professional conduct and provide standards of practice to those who perform case management functions. Certified or not, a successful case manager must be skilled in communication, diplomacy, and relationship building. He or she must demonstrate skill in identifying cost-effective resources and make appropriate referrals to promote case closure.

In a work injury case, in which workers' compensation is involved, the case manager will usually interact with several players: the injured employee, the employer, the insurance carrier, and the physician. Each player has a different perspective on the injury. Case management services are not restricted to workers' compensation cases, however. Case management services are just as important in other areas of work rehabilitation, such as those that involve individuals who have mental illness and developmental disabilities. The primary difference in case management practice with different populations is the team of players and the

resources that are investigated to facilitate a successful outcome. Regardless of the population that is being served, case management requires the ability to coordinate a complex mix of resources and services. These skills are dependent, at least in part, on clinical experience.

SETTINGS

Work programs in occupational therapy are evident in a variety of different settings. Traditional settings include hospitals, clinics, schools. Nontraditional occupational therapy settings include on-site programs in industry, fitness centers, and community rehabilitation programs. Regardless of the setting, the focus on the therapeutic value of work is a key aspect of occupational therapy.

On-Site Rehabilitation and Injury Management

The industrial rehabilitation movement in the 1980s provided the impetus for the development of on-site rehabilitation programs in industry. Although therapists working on-site in industry represent only a fraction of those who are involved in occupational rehabilitation, the many benefits of these programs foster their continued growth (Jundt & King, 1999; Tramposh, 1998). Occupational therapists working on-site or consulting with industry have many roles that include prevention, assessment, and rehabilitation programming. The benefits of on-site programming are decreased overall costs and improved quality care (B. A. Larson, 2000; Melnik, 2000). Therapists working on-site in industry enjoy improved communication with the employer, increased autonomy, and the ability to assess and intervene from an informed perspective, consistent with the holistic philosophy of occupational therapy. The clients benefit from on-site programs in several ways. On-site programs can reduce the waiting time for appointments, enhancing recovery through immediate care. The integration of the on-site therapist into the culture of the industrial setting can improve reasonable restricted duty placement and progression toward full-duty work. Awareness of the job demands and the worker's physical capacity can prevent re-injury while allowing the worker to safely continue in productive employment.

The employer also benefits from on-site programming. Successful programs allow the employer to oversee an employee's path through rehabilitation. Communication is improved through on-site interactions between the employee, the supervisor, and the practitioner. Improved communication speeds the rehabilitation process, reducing overall workers' compensation costs (Tramposh, 1998). The costs that are associated with travel to and from off-site clinics are also reduced by keeping the workers on-site for their therapy visits.

On-site therapists enjoy immersion in the culture of the industry, enhancing their realistic programming for the client and adding the benefits of early rehabilitation. Therapists who work on-site often work autonomously and require a thorough understanding of work injury assessment, rehabilitation, prevention, and the psychosocial aspects of disability (B. A. Larson, 2000; Tramposh, 1998). In addition, knowledge of the rehabilitation system, the ability to analyze tasks and the ability to creatively adapt the physical environment are all important skills. The setting requires skills in decision making and in dealing with people from various socioeconomic and cultural backgrounds. The therapist's role is often that of an intermediary between the injured worker, the employer, and the workers' compensation carrier, each bringing forth their own perspectives and issues.

On-site prevention programs include educational offerings such as back schools, stretching programs, fitness programs, and other health promotion or wellness activities (Melnik, 2000). Prevention can also include worker symptom surveys, hazard assessments, ergonomic assessments, writing job descriptions, and participation in safety teams and committees (Rothman, 1998). Prevention programs must be continually adapted to the constantly changing industrial environment. Successful programs require management support, supervisor buy-in, employee participation, and ongoing support and reinforcement (Melnik, 2000).

Assessment and rehabilitation of injured workers in on-site clinics include a vast array of services. Early intervention assessments may involve screening, education, and prevention activities for workers who have experienced mild symptoms or discomfort (Olson, 1999). Comprehensive assessments include worker evaluations for specific injuries as well as functional capacity evaluations. Rehabilitation programming can include the management of a specific injury, such as carpal tunnel syndrome, or more intensive work hardening and work conditioning programs. On-site therapists have the advantage of integrating services within the context of the worker's physical job demands. On-site therapists may also be involved in job analysis, ergonomic analysis, job placement, and the design of restricted duty programs (see Figure 51.3). The occupational therapist's role on-site in industry is to provide prevention, assessment, and intervention services to enhance a safe, efficient, and productive work environment for the worker and the employer.

Work Clinics

Throughout the history of occupational therapy, participation in valued occupations, including work, has provided the foundation of rehabilitation (Lysaght & Wright, 2005). In the late 1970s and 1980s, many industrial rehabilitation clinics emerged, providing services that focused on return to work as the outcome of intensive rehabilitation programs. (Jacobs & Baker, 2000; Tramposh, 1998)

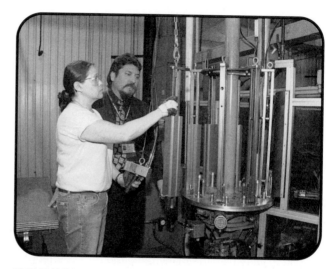

FIGURE 51.3   A therapist conducting a worksite job analysis.

The individualized therapy programs included functional capacity evaluations and progressive strengthening based on simulating the critical aspects of the client's work. Rehabilitation included creating workstations that represented the client's actual work tasks. The integrated services were designed to safely identify a client's tolerance for work tasks and to progress toward returning the client to productive employment. Although the primary focus of work has been obvious in these "end-of-rehabilitation programs," it has been no less evident in other rehabilitation settings. Safe, productive return to work has been included to some extent in all contexts of occupational therapy.

Hospital-Based and Freestanding Clinics

Traditional occupational therapy programs exist in hospitals and clinics providing inpatient and outpatient services to individuals with illnesses or injuries. Work, as a focus of rehabilitation, can be enhanced by the occupational therapist who analyzes the multidimensional issues faced by these individuals. Standardized rehabilitation assessment tools are available and can be customized to assess the physical, cognitive, and behavioral abilities of the individual in relation to the demands of the workplace. These skills are measured within the framework of productivity, interpersonal skills, and safety (Chappell, Higham, & McLean, 2003; Jackson, Harkess, & Ellis, 2004). Treatment programs address the identified deficit areas in performance and simulate the unpredictable nature of actual workplace demands. Studies have shown that use of a formal tool for addressing work abilities improved the decisiveness and clear recommendations by the therapist and provided a clear standard for formatting reports, and the clients expressed satisfaction that alternatives

---

CASE STUDY: *An Injured Sheet Metal Worker*

Thomas is 42 years old and employed as a sheet metal worker. He is married and has two sons, and he is the primary source of income for his family. Two months ago, a machine malfunctioned and crushed his right hand. He has had multiple surgeries to structurally restore the hand. He continues to experience problems in sensation, muscle strength, and coordination in his hand. Workers' compensation is providing him financial assistance in the form of income and medical expense coverage, but he is concerned about his job and when and whether he will be able to return to work. His physician has referred him to a work rehabilitation program. His occupational therapist, Sandy, addresses the many dimensions that affect his rehabilitation.

Questions

1. What is the occupational therapy process for Thomas's rehabilitation?
2. How does Sandy determine Thomas's functional abilities to return to work?

Discussion

Sandy should review Thomas's work, social, and medical history. Sandy's intake interview information will likely reveal Thomas's desire to return to his previous job. A job description from the employer should be obtained, and Sandy should ask Thomas to describe his usual work duties by talking through a usual day at work. If needed, a job analysis or job task analysis will provide objective information about the essential duties Thomas will need to perform to return to his previous job. Sandy will need to conduct an initial musculoskeletal assessment to determine the extent of Thomas's impairments. Sandy can then establish a work rehabilitation program to address the identified impairments. This program should include job simulation tasks to address the functional capabilities needed to perform his job. Sandy will need to communicate with the employer and/or case manager to promote an early return-to-work plan. The employer might be willing to accept Thomas back sooner if the employer understands Thomas's abilities and Sandy articulates job accommodation measures.

---

were suggested that included alternative work, further education, and voluntary work options (Jackson et al., 2004). Also, use of a standardized assessment resulted in increased client participation in hobbies and leisure pursuits.

Occupational therapists must consider barriers to employment when designing rehabilitation programs. Awareness of problem areas can guide assessment, training, and intervention. Lack of transportation, concerns about loss of financial benefits, and lack of awareness of social and federal programs have been cited as barriers to employment among the disabled (Fiedler et al., 2002). Occupational therapy interventions focus on overcoming barriers through specifically designed rehabilitation programs and education that is presented in a timely fashion. In a study of individuals with spinal cord injuries who were discharged from an inpatient rehabilitation unit, Fiedler and colleagues (2002) found that information on vocational services was presented too early in the rehabilitation process, limiting retention and usefulness. Although provision of the vocational information was a standard aspect of care, the majority of the study participants were unaware of federal vocational programs that were available to them.

The rehabilitation phase provides multiple opportunities for occupational therapists to explore issues and barriers to participation in work activities. The comprehensive occupational therapy program for individuals who receive services in hospital or clinic settings should include a work-focused standardized assessment, individualized intervention guided by the assessment, and education and training in areas that are informed by awareness of the barriers to employment.

Community Work Programs

Occupational therapy practitioners play major roles in using and developing the social context for vocational exploration and placement of people who have mental illness and developmental delays. Therapists are instrumental in developing community programs that are built on strong support networks and relationships with employers and other community job service agencies and health personnel. To influence the social context, practitioners use various management skills: needs evaluation, program development, worksite development, evaluation and monitoring of placements, and advocacy at the community level (Ramsey, Starnes, & Robertson, 2000).

Occupational therapy practitioners who are involved in vocational programming must be knowledgeable about work incentive issues that help people to make the transition to work. Supplemental Security Income, Social Security Disability Insurance, Welfare-to-Work incentives, and other public assistance programs must be well understood in order to adhere to the policies that qualify recipients to continue receipt of benefits while making the transition to gainful employment.

Many different program models exist to address vocational needs of individuals with serious mental illness and developmental delays. Overall, program models fall into two categories: programs that train and programs that both train and place.

Training Programs

Both simulated and actual work settings are used in training programs that are designed to train the client for general work habits and specific work skills. These programs encourage clients to obtain employment that pays at least minimum wage. Integrated environments provide for additional learning opportunities with individuals without mental illnesses or developmental disabilities.

Place and Train Programs

Place and train programs put clients into actual work environments that require them to learn to solve problems and adapt to work styles in a real work environment. Initially, the occupational therapist will evaluate the client's vocational potential by assessing medical and work history, work skills, social skills, specific job stresses, transportation needs, and the like to determine an appropriate job placement. No best way exists for designing work programs that meet all clients' needs. Instead, occupational therapy programs that offer a range of services best respond to client and employer needs.

Vocational programs require a continuum of services. The developer of these programs must help clients to build work habits and skills at one end of the continuum and locate independent part-time or full-time paid employment at the other end of the continuum.

Sheltered Workshops

Sheltered workshops are noncompetitive employment settings intended to provide many of the positive benefits of a work atmosphere for individuals with disabilities. A longstanding model of vocational rehabilitation, sheltered workshops strive to provide a protected work environment while developing vocational competency and providing behavioral interventions if needed (Siporin, 1999). Some individuals with physical or mental disabilities struggle with many issues in competitive employment settings, such as social skills, personal hygiene, and appearance. Difficulties in these areas can further isolate individuals rather than foster inclusion (Krupa, Lagarde, & Carmichael, 2003). Siporin suggested that the occupational therapist is ideally suited to work in the sheltered workshop setting by assisting clients to build on existing skills or train for new skills aimed at successful employment. The occupational therapists' role in sheltered workshop settings includes assessment and training in activities of daily living, sensorimotor skills, cognitive abilities and social skills. Although the protected environment of the sheltered workshop remains a successful option for some individuals with disabilities, studies have indicated that supported employment has proved to be a better option for many to enhance quality of life while allowing clients to earn competitive wages in the community (Bond, 2004; Siporin & Lysack, 2004).

Supported Employment

Supported employment is competitive work in an integrated work environment that is consistent with the strengths, resources, priorities, concerns, abilities, capabilities, interests, and informed choice of the individual (Rehabilitation Act Amendments, 1998). The Rehabilitation Act Amendments of 1986 provided the initial springboard for the transition from sheltered workshops into supported employment programs. These amendments were intended to foster inclusion and integration of people with disabilities into the economic, political, social, cultural, and educational mainstream of American society. They were based on the premise that work is a valued activity for everyone, including people who have disabilities. They stated that work fulfills the individual's need to be productive, promoted independence, enhanced self-esteem, and allowed for participation in the mainstream of life in the United States, which included earning competitive wages. The three essential characteristics of supported employment are paid work, employment in an integrated work setting, and ongoing support services that are available to meet continuous or periodic training needs. The ongoing services may include a job coach, a job trainer, a work-study coordinator, and/or an employment counselor. Studies have shown that participation in supported employment improved the quality of life for people with disabilities (Bond, 2004; Siporin & Lysack, 2004). Greater benefits were realized by consumers who held their competitive jobs for sustained periods of time, when they worked in jobs that reflected their choices, and when clients were placed directly into the work environment rather than undergoing training prior to placement. Strong evidence supports the integration of rehabilitation and vocational services (Bond, 2004). The occupational therapist in many different practice settings can play an integral role in preparing a client for supported employment, such as the client shown in Figure 51.4. School systems, mental health settings, and rehabilitation units all promote work as a valued outcome of occupational therapy intervention. The occupational therapist is ideally positioned to include motor skills function, cognitive function, social skills, activities of daily living, and adaptive equipment as part of the comprehensive treatment program. "Occupational

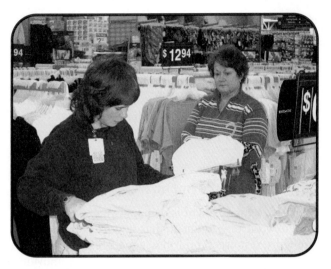

FIGURE 51.4 Courtney's supported employment began with several hours per week with a job coach who was provided by the local school system. Courtney has progressed to needing less than one hour with the coach every other week. Courtney plans to work full-time after high school and eventually to live independently in the community.

therapists can contribute to closing the gap between the impairments of individuals with developmental disabilities and the complex demands of supported employment and even the competitive workplace" (Siporin & Lysack, 2004, p. 463).

PRACTICE DILEMMA

ISSUES IN WORK PRACTICE

Imagine that you are an occupational therapist in the following practice settings, and describe the assessments and interventions that you would pursue for your clients.

♦ You are a school-based therapist working with a 16-year-old boy who has spasticity of the upper extremities due to cerebral palsy.
♦ The factory where you provide on-site services employs many workers over the age of 50.
♦ You are working in a homeless shelter with a 27-year-old single mother who has two small children and an eighth-grade education.
♦ The inpatient rehabilitation unit is well known for treatment of individuals with spinal cord injuries. Your caseload includes individuals between 16 and 35 years of age.

FUNDING AND LEGAL ISSUES

There are specific laws that govern and influence practice in work programs. Therapists should become familiar with this legislation and how it affects practice and the various populations they serve.

Workers' Compensation

The workers' compensation law is actually a system of individual state workers' compensation laws. These laws were designed to (1) cover the medical expenses and wage loss of workers who are injured or develop illnesses on the job and (2) shield employers from costly negligence lawsuits. Most states require employers to carry workers' compensation insurance. The states differ in respect to employers' insurance arrangements and the benefits that are offered to employees. However, most states cover medical expenses (including rehabilitation), disabilities (partial, total, temporary, permanent), and survivors' benefits (Business and Legal Reports, 1997).

Virtually all workers' compensations systems are fundamentally a no-fault mechanism through which employees who incur work-related injuries and illnesses are compensated with monetary and medical benefits (Box 51.2). Either party's potential negligence is usually not an issue as long as there is an employer-employee relationship. Employees are guaranteed a percentage of wages (usually two thirds) and full payment for their medical costs when they are injured on the job. Employers are guaranteed a reduced monetary cost for these injuries or illnesses and are provided with protection from additional or future legal action by the employee for the injury.

Americans With Disabilities Act

The ADA was passed in 1990 to prohibit discrimination against qualified individuals with physical or mental disabilities in all employment settings. The ADA is divided into five titles. Table 51.1 provides an outline of the areas of coverage.

Rehabilitation Act of 1973

Many of the concepts that the ADA contains have as their origin the Rehabilitation Act of 1973. By its terms, the Rehabilitation Act of 1973 was limited in scope. It prohibited discrimination only by federal agencies, entities that have contracts with the federal government, and recipients of federal financial assistance. Three major classes of recipients of federal funds are public school systems; colleges and other institutions of higher learning; and health, welfare, and social service providers (Domer, 1998).

In 1992, the Rehabilitation Act of 1973 was amended so that its terms would conform to those set forth in the ADA. State plans were developed that allowed each state

BOX 51.2 FEATURES OF WORKERS' COMPENSATION SYSTEMS

- Coverage of workers' compensation is limited to employees who are injured on the job.
- Workers' compensation is automatic.
- Employees' injuries and illnesses that arise out of the course of employment are usually considered compensable.
- Most workers' compensation systems include wage-loss benefits, which are usually between one half and three fourths of the employee's average weekly wage.
- Most workers' compensation systems require payment of all medical expenses, including such expenses as hospital, rehabilitation, and prosthesis expenses.
- Administration of workers' compensation is usually assigned to a commission or board within each state.

- In accepting workers' compensation, injured employees waive the right to take any common law action to sue the employer.
- When an injury is of a permanent nature, a dollar value for the percentage of loss to the injured employee is assigned and known as permanent partial disability or permanent total disability.
- In most states, employers with one or more employees are normally required to possess workers' compensation.
- Workers' compensation benefits are generally separate from the employment status of the injured employee.
- The workers' compensation commission or board in each state normally develops administrative rules and regulations for the administration and hearing procedures (Schneid & Schumann, 1997).

to submit to the commissioner of the Rehabilitation Services Administration a plan for vocational rehabilitation and assign a state agency to administer or supervise the plan. The 1992 amendments to the act emphasized individual written rehabilitation programs that were designed to achieve an employment objective consistent with the individual's unique strengths, resources, priorities, concerns, abilities, and capabilities and include a statement of the long-term rehabilitation goals. The term *disability* was substituted for *handicap* in the statute.

TABLE 51.1 THE FIVE TITLES OF THE AMERICANS WITH DISABILITIES ACT

Title	Area	Description
I	Employee provisions	Protects employees with disabilities from discrimination with regard to job applications, hiring, advancement, discharge, compensation, training, and other terms, conditions, and privileges of employment.
II	Public services	Prohibits discrimination against people with disabilities by public entities. This covers all governmental programs, services, activities, and employment but not the private sector. Requires that public transportation entities make a good faith effort to obtain or make vehicles accessible to people with disabilities.
III	Public accommodations	Extends the requirements in Title II to private sector public facilities. Requires that all goods, services, privileges, advantages, or facilities of any public place be offered to people with disabilities.
IV	Telecommunications	Requires telecommunication services to provide individuals with speech-related disabilities with the ability to communicate with hearing individuals through the use of telecommunication devices for the deaf.
V	Miscellaneous provisions	Addresses insurance related issues, such as allowing insurance providers to continue to use the preexisting condition clause, but prohibits denial of health insurance coverage to individuals on the basis of their disability. Does not limit or invalidate other federal or state laws that provide equal or greater protection to persons with disabilities.

The act provided for training and community rehabilitation programs. It authorizes grants and contracts to ensure that skilled personnel are available to provide rehabilitation services to individuals with disabilities through vocational, medical, social, and psychological rehabilitation programs and through supported employment programs, independent living services programs, and client assistant programs (Domer, 1998). The grants and contracts exist to provide training and information to individuals with disabilities and to their parents, families, guardians, advocates, and authorized representatives.

Social Security Disability

In the mid-1950s, the Social Security Act (SSA) established a social insurance program that was designed to provide guaranteed income to individuals with disabilities when they are found to be generally incapable of gainful employment. Its purpose is to provide a basic level of financial support for people who cannot support themselves because of disability. The SSA provides for disability benefit programs administered by the SSA, including Social Security Disability Insurance (SSDI) and Supplemental Security Income (SSI) programs. The SSDI program provides benefits to disabled workers, dependents, and widows and widowers if the worker is insured under the provisions of the program. The SSI program provides benefits to disabled individuals whose incomes and assets fall below a specified level (Domer, 1998).

SUMMARY

Occupational therapists address work issues for clients as young as 14 years old in school-based transition programs and across the life course to older adults who continue to benefit from work activities. The practice settings are varied including both traditional and nontraditional environments. Work-related assessments and interventions require the occupational therapist to integrate medical, psychological, behavioral, and philosophical dimensions to address the specific needs of the client, the population, the setting, and the system. Communication and collaboration with the clients, their families, and the team members enhance the success of work programs in all settings. The basic premise of work as a meaningful occupation provides the foundation for occupational therapy in work programs.

PROVOCATIVE QUESTIONS

1. What assessment and intervention activities would you design for a 23-year-old man who is considered to have moderate to severe mental retardation, is living in a group home, and wants to work?
2. If you were hired as an on-site therapist in a manufacturing plant and knew that the majority of the workers in the plant are over age 45, what types of services could you provide as a benefit to the employer and employees?

REFERENCES

American Occupational Therapy Association. (2005). Occupational therapy services in facilitation work performance. *American Journal of Occupational Therapy, 59*(6), 676–679.

Americans With Disabilities Act of 1990. P.L. 101-336. July 26, 1990. 42 U.S.C. § 12101 *et seq.*

Andstadt, G. (1990). Occupational medicine forum. *Journal of Occupational Medicine, 32*(4), 295–296.

Bohr, P. C. (1998). Work analysis. In: P. M. King (Ed.), *Sourcebook of occupational rehabilitation* (pp. 229–245). New York: Plenum Press.

Bond, G. R. (2004). Supported employment: Evidence for an evidence-based practice. *Psychiatric Rehabilitation Journal, 27*(4), 345–360.

Bureau of Labor Statistics. (1999). *The "grayby" boom ages the labor force.* Retrieved November 19, 2005, from http://www.bls.gov/opub/ted/1999/Dec/wk3/art01.htm

Bureau of Labor Statistics. (2005). *Older workers and severity of occupational injuries and illnesses involving days away from work.* Retrieved November 19, 2005, from http://www.bls.gov/opub/cwc/sh20050713ch01.htm

Business and Legal Reports. (1997). *Encyclopedia of workers' compensation.* Madison, CT: Author.

Carrivick, P. J. W., Lee, A. H., Yau, K. W., & Stevenson, M. R. (2005). Evaluating the effectiveness of a participatory ergonomics approach in reducing the risk and severity of injuries from manual handling. *Ergonomics, 48*(8), 907–914.

Case Management Society of America. (1995). *CMSA standards of practice for case management guidebook.* Rolling Meadows, IL: Author.

Chappell, I., Higham, J., & McLean, A. M. (2003). An occupational therapy work skills assessment for individuals with head injury. *The Canadian Journal of Occupational Therapy, 70*(3), 163–169.

Commission on Accreditation of Rehabilitation Facilities. (1988). *1988 standards manual for organizations serving people with disabilities.* Tucson, AZ: Author.

Commission on Practice. (1999). *Work practice statement: Occupational therapy services in facilitating work performance.* Bethesda, MD: AOTA.

Dahl, R. (2000). Ergonomics. In B. L. Kornblau & K. Jacobs (Eds.), *Work: Principles and practice—A self-paced course from AOTA* (Lesson 12) (pp. 1–50). Bethesda, MD: American Occupational Therapy Association.

Dickie, V. A. (2003). Establishing worker identity: A study of people in craft work. *American Journal of Occupational Therapy, 57,* 250–261.

Domer, T. (1998). Regulatory agencies and legislation. In P. King (Ed.), *Sourcebook of occupational rehabilitation* (pp. 43–68). New York: Plenum.

Eastman Kodak Company. (1983). *Ergonomic design for people at work: A sourcebook for human factors practitioners in industry including safety, design, and industrial engineers, medical, industrial hygiene, and industrial relations personnel, and management.* Belmont, CA: Lifetime Learning Publications.

Ellexson, M. T. (2000). Job analysis. In B. L. Kornblau & K. Jacobs (Eds.), *Work: Principles and practice—A self-paced course from AOTA* (Lesson 5) (pp. 1–14). Bethesda, MD: American Occupational Therapy Association.

Fiedler, I. G., Indermuehle, D. L., Drobac, W., & Laud, P. (2002). Perceived barriers to employment in individuals with spinal cord injury. *Topics in Spinal Cord Injury Rehabilitation, 7*(3), 73–82.

Frings-Dresen, M. H. W., & Sluiter, J. (2003). Development of a job-specific FCE protocol: The work demands of hospital nurses as an example. *Journal of Occupational Medicine, 13*(4), 233–248.

Gupta, J., & Stoffel, S. (2001). Take action: OT and older workers. *American Occupational Therapy Association: Gerontology, Special Interest Section Quarterly, 24*(1), 1–2.

Harvey-Krefting, L. (1985). The concept of work in occupational therapy: An historical review. *American Journal of Occupational Therapy, 39*, 301–317.

Harwood, K. (2004). A review of clinical practice guidelines for functional capacity evaluations. *Journal of Forensic Vocational Analysis, 7*, 67–74.

Helm-Williams, P. (1993, March). Industrial rehabilitation: Developing guidelines. *Magazine of PT,* 65–68.

International Ergonomics Association. (2005). *The discipline of ergonomics.* Retrieved October 29, 2005, from http://www.iea.cc/ergonomics/.

Isernhagen, S. (1988). *Work injury: Management and prevention.* Gaithersburg, MD: Aspen.

Jackson, M., Harkess, J., & Ellis, J. (2004). Reporting patients' work abilities: How the use of standardized work assessments improved clinical practice in Fife. *British Journal of Occupational Therapy 67*(3), 129–132.

Jacobs, K., & Baker, N. A. (2000). The history of work-related therapy in occupational therapy. In B. L. Kornblau & K. Jacobs (Eds.), *Work: Principles and practice—A self-paced course from AOTA* (Lesson 1) (pp. 1–11). Bethesda, MD: American Occupational Therapy Association.

Jundt, J., & King, P. M. (1999). Work rehabilitation programs: A 1997 survey. *Work: A Journal of Prevention, Assessment & Rehabilitation, 12,* 139–144.

Kardos, M., & White, B. P. (2005). The role of the school-based occupational therapist in secondary education transition planning: A pilot survey study. *American Journal of Occupational Therapy 59*(2), 173–180.

King, P. M. (1998). Sourcebook of occupational rehabilitation. New York: Plenum.

King, P. M. (2004). Analysis of the reliability and validity supporting functional capacity evaluations. *Journal of Forensic Vocational Analysis, 7*(2), 75–82.

King, P., Tuckwell, N., & Barrett, T. (1998). A critical review of functional capacity evaluations. *Physical Therapy, 78*(8), 852–866.

Kornblau, B. L. (2000). The future of OT work practice. *Work programs: Special Interest Section Quarterly, 14*(4), 1–2.

Kornblau, B. L., Lou, J. Q., Weeder, T. C., & Werner, B. (2002). Occupational therapy and theories of career choice and vocational development. In B. L. Kornblau & K. Jacobs (Eds.), *Work: Principles and practice—A self-paced course from AOTA* (Lesson 2) (pp. 1–23). Bethesda, MD: American Occupational Therapy Association.

Krupa, T., Lagarde, M., & Carmichael, K. (2003). Transforming sheltered workshops into affirmative businesses: An outcome evaluation. *Psychiatric Rehabilitation Journal, 26*(4), 359–367.

Larson, B. A. (2000). On-site work programs. In B. L. Kornblau & K. Jacobs (Eds.), *Work: Principles and practice—A self-paced course from AOTA* (Lesson 8) (pp. 1–12). Bethesda, MD: American Occupational Therapy Association.

Larson, E. A. (2004). Children's work: The less considered childhood occupation. *American Journal of Occupational Therapy, 58*(4), 369–379.

Lechner, D. (1998). Functional capacity evaluation. In P. King (Ed.), *Sourcebook of occupational rehabilitation* (pp. 209–227). New York: Plenum.

Lechner, D., Jackson, J., Roth, D., & Straaton, K. (1994). Reliability and validity of a newly developed test of physical work performance. *Journal of Occupational Medicine, 36,* 997–1004.

Lechner, D., Roth, D. & Straaton, K. (1991). Functional capacity evaluation in work disability, *Work, 1,* 37–47.

Lysaght, R., & Wright, J. (2005). Professional strategies in work-related practice: An exploration of occupational and physical therapy roles and approaches. *American Journal of Occupational Therapy, 59*(2), 209–217.

Marshall, A. (2000, August 1), IEA Executive council defines ergonomics. *Congress Current,* 1.

Massy-Westropp, M., & Rose, D. (2004). The impact of manual handling training on work place injuries: A 14 year audit. *Australian Health Review, 27*(2), 80–87.

Matoushek, N. (2005). Work integration programs: Improving return to work. *Advance for Occupational Therapy, November 14,* 15–16.

Melnik, M. S. (2000). Injury prevention. In B. L. Kornblau & K. Jacobs (Eds.), *Work: Principles and practice—A self-paced course from AOTA* (Lesson 11) (pp. 1–14). Bethesda, MD: American Occupational Therapy Association.

Meyer, A. (1977). The philosophy of occupation therapy. *American Journal of Occupational Therapy, 31,* 639–642.

Mungai, A. (1985). The occupational therapist's role in employee health promotion programs. In F. S. Cromwell (Ed.), *Work-related programs in occupational therapy* (pp. 67–77). Binghamton, NY: The Haworth Press.

Nachreiner, N., McGovern, P., Kochevar, L. K., Lohman, W. H., Cato, C. & Ayers, E. (1999). Preplacement assessments: Impact on injury outcomes. *AAOHN Journal, 47*(6), 245–253.

Naso, M. (2003, May). Stretching the limits. *Safety and Health,* 48–50.

Occupational Safety and Health Administration. (2002). *Job hazard analysis: OSHA 3071.* Retrieved November 17, 2005, from http://www.osha.gov/Publications/osha3071.pdf#search='job%20analysis'

Olson, D. L. (1999). An on-site ergonomic program: A model for industry. *Work: A Journal of Prevention, Assessment & Rehabilitation, 13*(3), 229–238.

Paterson, C. (1997). An historical perspective of work practice services. In J. Pratt & K. Jacobs (Eds.), *Work practice: International perspectives* (pp. 25–38). Boston: Butterworth-Heinemann.

Primeau, L. A. (1996). Work versus non-work the case of housework. In R. C. Zemke & F. Clark (Eds.), *Occupa-*

tional science: The evolving discipline (pp. 57–69). Philadelphia: F. A. Davis.

Ramsey, D. L., Starnes, W., & Robertson, S. C. (2000). Work programs for persons with serious and chronic mental illnesses. In B. L. Kornblau & K. Jacobs (Eds.), *Work: Principles and practice—A self-paced course from AOTA* (Lesson 9) (pp. 1–22). Bethesda, MD: American Occupational Therapy Association.

Rehabilitation Act Amendments of 1986. P.L. 99-506, Title IV, 39.

Rehabilitation Act Amendments of 1998. Title IV of the Workforce Investment Act of 1998, P.L. 105-220, 112 Stat. 936. Retrieved on November 20, 2005, from http://www.nationalrehab.org/website/history/rehabact1998%"20full.pdf

Rothman, J. (1998). Wellness and fitness programs. In: P. M. King (Ed.), *Sourcebook of occupational rehabilitation* (pp. 127–144). New York: Plenum Press.

Schkade, J. K., & Schultz, S. (1992). Occupational adaptation: Toward a holistic approach for contemporary practice, Part 1. *American Journal of Occupational Therapy, 46*(9), 829–837.

Schneid, T., & Schumann, M. (1997). *Legal liability: A guide for safety and loss prevention professionals.* Gaithersburg, MD: Aspen.

Siporin, S. (1999, October). Help wanted: Supporting workers with developmental disabilities. *OT Practice,* 19–24.

Siporin, S., & Lysack, C. (2004). Quality of life and supported employment: A case study of three women with developmental disabilities. *American Journal of Occupational Therapy, 58,* 455–465.

Snook, S. H., & Cirello, V. M. (1991). The design of manual handling tasks: Revised tables of maximum acceptable weights and forces. *Ergonomics, 34*(9), 1197–1213.

Spencer, J. E., Emery, L. J., & Schneck, C. M. (2003). Occupational therapy in transitioning adolescents to post-secondary activities. *American Journal of Occupational Therapy 57,* 435–441.

Spencer, K. C. (2000). Transition from school to adult life. In B. L. Kornblau & K. Jacobs (Eds.), *Work: Principles and practice—A self-paced course from AOTA* (Lesson 3) (pp. 1–24). Bethesda, MD: American Occupational Therapy Association.

Sterns, H. L., & Miklos, S. M. (1995). The aging worker in a changing environment; Organizational and individual issues. *Journal of Vocational Behavior, 47*(3), 248–268.

Tramposh, A. K. (1998). On-site therapy programs. In P. M. King (Ed.), *Sourcebook of occupational rehabilitation* (pp. 275–286). New York: Plenum Press.

U.S. Department of Labor, Employment and Training Administration. (1977). *Dictionary of occupational titles* (4th ed.). Washington, DC: U.S. Government Printing Office.

U.S. Department of Labor, Office of Disability Employment Policy. (1994). *Job analysis: An important employment tool.* Retrieved November 17, 2005, from http://www.dol.gov/odep/pubs/fact/analysis.htm

Vitalis, A., Walker, R., & Legg, S. (2001). Unfocused ergonomics. *Ergonomics, 44*(14), 1290–1301.

Washington State Department of Labor and Industries. (2005). *Evaluation tools.* Retrieved November 17, 2005, from http://www.lni.wa.gov/Safety/Topics/Ergonomics/ServicesResources/Tools/default.asp

Waters, T. R., Putz-Anderson, V., Garg, A., & Fine, L. J. (1993). Revised NIOSH equation for the design and evaluation of manual lifting tasks. *Ergonomics, 36*(7), 749–776.

Webster's universal college dictionary. (1997). New York: Random House.

Westmorland, M., Williams, R., Strong, S., & Arnold, E. (2002). Perspectives on work (re)entry for persons with disabilities: Implications for clinicians. *Work: A Journal of Prevention Assessment & Rehabilitation, 18*(1), 29–40.

Wilcox, A. A. (1998). *An occupational perspective of health.* Thorofare, NJ: Slack.

Yassi, A., Gilbert, M., & Cvitkovich, Y. (2005). Trends in injuries, illnesses, and policies in Canadian healthcare workplaces. *Canadian Journal of Public Health, 96*(5), 333–339.

Play and Leisure

LOREE A. PRIMEAU

52

Learning Objectives

After reading this chapter, you will be able to:

1. Describe four definitions of play and leisure.
2. Describe guidelines and parameters for evaluation of play and leisure.
3. Identify selected assessments that can be used to develop an occupational profile and to evaluate play and leisure.
4. Describe three purposes of play and leisure in intervention.
5. Define play and leisure as lures or rewards, as means, and as ends.
6. Explain how play and leisure as means can be used for intervention.
7. Describe three types of occupational therapy intervention to facilitate play and leisure as ends.

WHAT ARE PLAY AND LEISURE?

Occupational therapy practitioners have a long tradition of considering play and leisure in the lives of people with whom they work (Parham & Primeau, 1997). In the founding years of the profession, the "play spirit" was seen as essential for living a worthwhile life (E. B. Saunders, 1922; Slagle, 1922; Ziegler, 1924). Over time, as occupational therapy practitioners became increasingly concerned with scientific and technical aspects of intervention, play and leisure were thought to be unscientific and inappropriate for use in practice. Late in the 20th century, scholars in occupational therapy and occupational science reclaimed play and leisure (Bundy, 1993; Canadian Association of Occupational Therapists [CAOT], 1996; Parham, 1996; Parham & Fazio, 1997; Primeau, 1996; Reilly, 1974; Suto, 1998).

Although multiple definitions of *play* and *leisure* have been proposed in the literature, consensus has not been reached on how to define these terms. Lack of definitional clarity for these terms, however, should not prevent occupational therapy practitioners' consideration of their clients' performance in these areas of occupation. From a pragmatic point of view, play and leisure are powerful tools for practice, but single, precise, and all-purpose definitions that are responsive to the needs of an entire profession might not be required or desired, even if they were possible (Parham & Primeau, 1997). Nevertheless, definitions of play and leisure in the literature tend to converge into four major categories: (1) play and leisure as discretionary time, (2) play and leisure as context, (3) play and leisure as observable behavior or activity, and (4) play and leisure as disposition or experience (Gunter & Stanley, 1985; Rubin, Fein, & Vandenberg, 1983).

Play and Leisure as Time

The category of play and leisure as discretionary time views them as leftover or residual time after obligatory activities, such as paid or unpaid work and self-maintenance tasks, have been completed (Gunter & Stanley, 1985; Tinsley & Tinsley, 1982). Play and leisure are defined by what they are not: They are not work or school activities; they are not activities of daily living or instrumental activities of daily living. By definition, play and leisure are quantified as the time that is spent by the individual who is engaged in them. This view of play and leisure lends itself easily to measurement and is often the focus of evaluation in occupational therapy through the use of activity configurations as an assessment tool (Suto, 1998). Although practitioners need to know about their clients' use of time and its relationship to their health and well-being, equally important for evaluation of play and leisure are the contexts in which they occur, the clients' activities, and their experience of those activities.

Play and Leisure as Context

The category of play and leisure as context identifies and describes them in terms of the conditions under which they occur. Contexts that are friendly, safe, and comfortable with a variety of materials, objects, people, and activities and that also denote cultural sanctions for play and leisure are more likely to elicit them (Figure 52.1). Freedom of choice to engage or not to engage in play and leisure and freedom from hunger, fatigue, illness, or other stressors are also identified as conditions that are conducive to play and leisure (Rubin et al., 1983). Beliefs held by people in a specific culture will determine what is and is not considered to be play and leisure and the con-

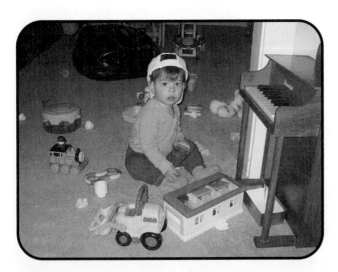

FIGURE 52.1 The definition of play as context can be seen in this boy's enjoyment of conditions that support his engagement in play.

ditions under which they will occur. Practitioners often draw from this category when they evaluate supports and barriers in their clients' contexts that facilitate or hinder their engagement in play and leisure. One problem with the view of play and leisure as context is that although the conditions described above are necessary for play and leisure, they are not sufficient, meaning that producing such a context does not ensure that play and leisure will emerge in it (Rubin et al., 1983). Because play and leisure are transactions between clients and their contexts (Bundy, 2001b), clients' play and leisure activities and their experience of them must also be considered.

Play and Leisure as Activity

The category of play and leisure as activity views them as behaviors or activities that can be observed and named. Taxonomies are used to identify and describe types of play and leisure activities. For example, Primeau and Ferguson (1999) named children's play using the following taxonomy: sensorimotor play, object play, social play, motor play, imaginative play, and game play. Such taxonomies are useful because they provide descriptive criteria for observation and evaluation of clients' play and leisure behaviors (Rubin et al., 1983), including their interests (Primeau, 1996). This view of play and leisure as activity is also easily quantified and measurable. It is familiar to practitioners in the form of many assessments, including checklists used to identify interests as well as strengths and problem areas in performance of play and leisure activities (Suto, 1998). A drawback to the view of play and leisure as activity is lack of consideration of the experience of the activities themselves (Primeau, 1996; Suto, 1998).

Play and Leisure as Experience

The category of play and leisure as experience views them as the overall experience of a client's engagement in play and leisure. Disposition, attitude, or state of mind while participating in play and leisure are of primary importance (Iso-Ahola, 1979; Tinsley & Tinsley, 1982). Personal meanings of play and leisure arise from these subjective experiences (Primeau, 1996). Several qualities of play and leisure as experience have been identified in the literature, including freedom from obligation or constraint, freedom of choice, enjoyment, fun, intrinsic motivation, low work-relation, flow, self-expression, active engagement, aesthetic appreciation, relaxation, internal locus of control, and suspension of reality (Bundy, 1997; Csikszentmihalyi, 1975; Iso-Ahola, 1979; Rubin et al., 1983; Samdahl, 1988; Shaw, 1985; Tinsley, Hinson, Tinsley, & Holt, 1993). Of all these qualities, freedom from constraint and freedom of choice are most often identified as defining characteristics of play and leisure as experience (Henderson, Bialeschki, Shaw, & Freysinger, 1996). Practitioners recognize the importance of evaluation of play and leisure as experience by gathering data on clients' experiences through interviews, participant observations, and specific formal assessments.

The view of play and leisure as experience holds the most promise for occupational therapy practice (Bundy, 1993; Primeau, 1996; Suto, 1998). Although evaluation of play and leisure as time, context, and activity are necessary, they are not sufficient to understand clients' participation in play and leisure. Best practice dictates that evaluation of play and leisure as experience must also be conducted to obtain the clearest picture of clients' engagement in play and leisure.

EVALUATION OF PLAY AND LEISURE

Guidelines for Evaluation of Play and Leisure

Evaluation of play and leisure should be client-centered and should follow a top-down approach. Client-centered evaluation is a collaborative process that combines the perspectives, expertise, and experiences of clients and practitioners to determine what is evaluated, how it is evaluated, and what will be the focus of intervention. To be truly client-centered, evaluation of play and leisure should occur in clients' natural settings (home, school, work, and community) whenever possible (Townsend, 1997). For practitioners who work with children, clients can "include the child, parents, siblings, other family members, peers, teachers, and other adults who are responsible for the child" (Primeau & Ferguson, 1999, p. 470). As the practitioner considers the child in each setting, a new group of individuals may become central to the collaborative process.

A top-down approach to evaluation begins with the client's occupational profile, including the client's participation in play and leisure in home, school, work, and community settings (American Occupational Therapy Association [AOTA], 2002; Trombly, 1993). The client and the practitioner collaboratively identify what the client wants to do, needs to do, or is expected to do (Law et al., 1990) and the extent to which the client is able to engage in play and leisure in these settings (Coster, 1998). Analysis of the client's occupational performance follows, with a specific focus on performance in the areas of occupation that were identified in the occupational profile (AOTA, 2002). Evaluation of play and leisure addresses the following issues: (1) how the client's contexts facilitate or inhibit his or her engagement in play and leisure, (2) how the client's performance in the areas of occupation of play and leisure is enhanced or limited by the types of play and leisure activities in which he or she engages and his or her experience of these activities, and (3) how limitations or impairments in performance skills and client factors affect the client's ability to engage in play and leisure activities.

Parameters for Evaluation of Play and Leisure

Client-centered and top-down approaches to evaluation guide practitioners in the process of evaluation, or *how* to evaluate play and leisure. The client's overall pattern of participation in play and leisure across home, school, work, and community settings is the content, or *what* needs to be evaluated. The four definitions of play and leisure described above provide parameters for evaluation that are aligned with the two substeps of the evaluation process: occupational profile and analysis of occupational performance (AOTA, 2002). Play and leisure as time aligns with the substep of the occupational profile, whereas play and leisure as context, as activity, and as experience are addressed in the substep of analysis of occupational performance. Specifically, play and leisure as context aligns with the domain area of contexts, and play and leisure as activity and as experience align with the domain area of performance in areas of occupation (AOTA, 2002). Also evaluated during the analysis of occupational performance are the domain areas of performance skills and client factors; however, parameters for evaluation of these areas are drawn from general occupational therapy assessments used to evaluate clients in these areas and are not necessarily specific to play and leisure assessments. Table 52.1 lists assessments that can be used to develop the client's occupational profile and to evaluate play and leisure in the areas of contexts, performance in areas of occupation, performance skills, and client factors.

Occupational Profile: Play and Leisure

When developing an occupational profile, occupational therapy practitioners gather information about the client's past and current play and leisure participation (AOTA, 2002). **Play and leisure participation** is defined as the client's engagement in play and leisure occupations that are typically expected of and available to a person of the same age and culture in home, school, work, and community settings (Coster, 1998; Primeau & Ferguson, 1999). This profile is used to determine clients' **characteristics of play and leisure participation** (nature, quality, frequency, and duration) in these settings.

Play and leisure participation may be restricted in nature, quality, frequency, or duration. Restrictions are relative to typical participation in each setting. Practitioners compare their clients' participation to that of individuals without participation restrictions to determine the clients' degree of participation or participation restriction (World Health Organization, 2001). They draw from their knowledge base about play and leisure as it occurs naturally in home, school, work, and community settings and from their observations of a typical person engaged in play and leisure in a particular setting to understand the play and leisure of people without restrictions in that setting (Dunn, 1998). Then they may interview their clients

TABLE 52.1 ASSESSMENTS OF PLAY AND LEISURE

Assessment[a]	Occupational Profile		Analysis of Occupational Performance						
	Characteristics	Contexts	Performance in Areas of Occupation					Performance Skills	Client Factors
		Contextual Features	Activity		Subjective Experience	Experience			
			Activity Interests	Activity Choices		Personal Meaning	Satisfaction		
Activity Card Sort	◆		◆	◆					
Activity Index & Meaningfulness of Activity Scale	◆		◆	◆					
Adult Playfulness Scale			◆		◆			◆	◆
Assessment of Ludic Behaviors (ALB)	◆		◆	◆	◆				
CAPE/PAC				◆	◆				
Child Behaviors Inventory of Playfulness									
Interest Checklist			◆	◆					
Knox Preschool Play Scale							◆	◆	
Leisure Boredom Scale					◆		◆		
Leisure Competence Measure	◆		◆	◆	◆	◆		◆	
Leisure Diagnostic Battery		◆	◆	◆	◆			◆	
Leisure Interest Profile for Adults	◆		◆	◆	◆				
Leisure Interest Profile for Seniors	◆		◆	◆	◆	◆	◆		
Leisure Satisfaction Scale	◆				◆				
Pediatric Interest Profiles				◆	◆				
Playform	◆	◆		◆	◆			◆	
Play History	◆	◆	◆	◆	◆	◆	◆	◆	◆
Qualitative Methods[b] (Interview, Observation)	◆	◆	◆	◆	◆				
Self Directed Search—The Leisure Activities Finder		◆	◆						
Test of Environmental Supportiveness (TOES)		◆							
Test of Playfulness (ToP)					◆			◆	
The Experience of Leisure Scale (TELS)					◆			◆	

a See Unit XVI: Assessments for author, source, and descriptions of assessments.

b See Bundy (1993, p. 220), Burke & Scaaf (1997, pp. 75–77), and Florey & Greene (1997, p. 137) for samples of interview and observation guides.

and/or observe them to gather data on their participation in play and leisure, including their personal preferences, and compare this information to that of a person without participation restrictions.

The focus of evaluation is on the nature, quality, frequency, and duration of clients' play and leisure participation. The nature and quality of participation can be addressed by answering the following questions (Coster, 1998): Is the client's participation in play and leisure positive? Does it support the client's physical, cognitive, and psychosocial growth? Is it personally satisfying? Does the client have access to the same opportunities for play and leisure as others of the same age and culture do? Is the client's participation in play and leisure acceptable to others in his or her settings? Frequency and duration of participation are related to definitions of play and leisure as time. Does the client participate in play and leisure to the same extent as others in that setting? One study that asked this question found that boys with developmental dyspraxia participated in games on school playgrounds less often and for shorter time periods than did boys without developmental dyspraxia (Primeau, 1989), indicating a gap between typical participation and that of children with developmental dyspraxia. When gaps in nature, quality, frequency, or duration of participation are found, practitioners must evaluate the client's play and leisure contexts to identify ways to bridge these gaps (Dunn, 1998).

Analysis of Occupational Performance: Play and Leisure

EVALUATION OF PLAY AND LEISURE CONTEXTS.   Evaluation of play and leisure contexts is related to definitions of play and leisure as context. Contexts may be cultural (customs, beliefs, values), physical (built and natural environments, objects), social (individuals, groups, organizations, systems), personal (age, gender, socioeconomic status), spiritual (greater or higher purpose, meaning), temporal (time of day/year, stage of life), and virtual (chat rooms, simulated environments) (AOTA, 2002). Practitioners identify **contextual features** in their clients' settings of interest and then determine whether these features facilitate or hinder participation in play and leisure in those settings. Gathering objective data on contextual features is not sufficient; practitioners must assess the impact of these features on their clients' engagement in play and leisure (Dunn, 1998). Interviewing and observing clients in natural settings are optimal methods for doing this. For example, physical accessibility to a restaurant does not ensure that a client living with severe physical disabilities will dine out with friends. Cultural and social features can affect the client's comfort level in that setting, thereby restricting his or her participation. The practitioner would need to ask questions to discover the source of this client's restriction.

EVALUATION OF PERFORMANCE IN AREAS OF OCCUPATION: PLAY AND LEISURE.   Definitions of play and leisure as activity and as experience are central to evaluation of performance in these areas of occupation. Evaluation focuses on clients' play and leisure performance (what they actually do and their experience while doing it). Practitioners assess clients' play and leisure activities and their experience while engaged in these activities to identify performance limitations and determine how to enhance performance. Evaluation of **play and leisure activity** considers **activity interests** and **activity choices**, whereas evaluation of **play and leisure experience** explores **subjective experience**, **personal meaning**, and **satisfaction with experience**.

EVALUATION OF PLAY AND LEISURE ACTIVITY.

- **Activity interests.** *Interests* are defined as "dispositions to find pleasure and satisfaction in occupations and the self-knowledge of enjoyment of occupations" (Kielhofner, Borell, Burke, Helfrich, & Nygard, 1995, p. 47). When this definition of interests is applied to play and leisure activities, it addresses clients' affective responses to play and leisure activities (often expressed as preferences or as likes, dislikes, and indifferences) and their perceptions and awareness of themselves and their environments (Matsutsuyu, 1969). Assessments of play and leisure activity interests provide information in two areas: preferences and self-knowledge as they relate to play and leisure activities. Clients are asked to identify their preferences for a variety of play and leisure activities. On the basis of their responses, practitioners can determine the extent and quality of clients' self-knowledge and awareness of these interests. For example, a client living in a cold, landlocked area who identifies scuba diving, surfing, and snorkeling as leisure interests displays limited preferences (he identifies only three) and a lack of awareness of the leisure activities that his environment offers him, indicating that he will most likely encounter limitations in his performance of leisure activities.

- **Activity choices.** Activity choices consist of the activities in which the client engages during play and leisure. Assessments in this area examine what clients do, with whom, and how often. Play and leisure activities are characterized as general categories (e.g., object play, games, hobbies, sports) or specific activities (e.g., play with blocks, board games, woodworking, soccer). Other areas to explore include whether the activity is done alone or with others, including friends, family, or coworkers, and how often a particular play and leisure activity is performed. This indicator of frequency differs from that evaluated in the occupational profile because practitioners are concerned here with the client's individual performance of a specific play and leisure activity, regardless of the setting in which it occurs, as an indicator of the client's history and familiarity with it. Recall the example of the boys with developmental dyspraxia who exhibited decreased frequency and duration of participation in games on the school playground.

Evaluation of their activity choices would focus on their history and familiarity with games (whether they had played games before and, if so, what types, with whom, and how often) rather than on their overall participation in play on the school playground.

EVALUATION OF PLAY AND LEISURE EXPERIENCE.

◆ **Subjective experience.** Subjective experience refers to two aspects of engagement in play and leisure activities: state of mind with which these activities are approached and the affective experience of engagement in them. State of mind, often termed playfulness, is characterized by freedom from constraint, freedom of choice, intrinsic motivation, internal control, active engagement, and freedom to suspend reality (Bundy, 1997; Henderson et al., 1996). The affective experience of engagement in play and leisure is a positive one, marked by feelings of fun, enjoyment, happiness, satisfaction, and pleasure (Csikszentmihalyi, 1988). Assessments of subjective experience explore these two areas: playfulness and affective experience. Practitioners must remember that the subjective experience of play and leisure transcends cultural definitions of play, leisure, work, and activities of daily of living (Primeau, 1996). For example, a mother describing her experience of playing with her children while doing housework as "play-work" stated, "It's like work with an *attitude*. It's my way to get things done in a *fun way*. . . . No, [it] isn't exactly what I want to do right now, . . . but I'm getting it done and *we're all enjoying it* at the same time." (Primeau, 1995). Although she recognizes that she is restricted in her choice of activity, her use of the words "attitude" and "fun way" demonstrate a playful approach, and her statement that "we're all enjoying it" refers to a positive affective experience, suggesting that her subjective experience is one of play and leisure.

◆ **Personal meaning.** Personal meaning derives from the subjective experience of play and leisure performance. Satisfaction of conscious or unconscious needs and benefits attributed to this experience create personal meanings, which often become motivation for clients' future engagement in play and leisure activities. Personal meanings can be categorized as physiological (e.g., physical fitness, stress reduction and recovery), educational/cognitive (e.g., learning, intellectual stimulation), social (e.g., social interaction, companionship), psychological (e.g., self-identity, self-expression), aesthetic (e.g., appreciation of beauty, arts, and symbolic systems of meaning), and spiritual (e.g., heightened awareness, transcendent experiences) (Beard & Ragheb, 1980; Driver, Brown, & Peterson, 1991). Evaluation of personal meaning becomes particularly important when practitioners want to increase their clients' repertoire of play and leisure activities (Bundy, 2001b) or substitute a new activity for one that is no longer viable (Bundy, 1993). Clients' identified personal meanings can be matched with play and leisure activities that provide those meanings in the form of benefits derived from them, offering new play and leisure options. For example, a study found that bingo, bowling, ceramics, dancing, and volunteer activities were all rated as providing high levels of the benefit of companionship by elderly adults living in the community (Driver, Tinsley, & Manfredo, 1991). Practitioners could suggest these activities, or others that provide a similar benefit, for their elderly clients who have expressed a desire for companionship.

◆ **Satisfaction with experience.** Satisfaction with experience refers to clients' overall feelings and perceptions related to their play and leisure experiences. Feelings and perceptions can be positive (contentment and satisfaction) (Beard & Ragheb, 1980) or negative (boredom and dissatisfaction) (Iso-Ahola & Weissinger, 1990). Satisfaction with play and leisure experience is thought to have powerful consequences for clients' physical health, mental health, life satisfaction, and personal growth (Driver, Tinsley, & Manfredo, 1991). Evaluation must capture clients' range of feelings and perceptions about their play and leisure satisfaction across all activities and settings in which they participate (Figure 52.2). For example, elderly clients' decreased participation in and access to leisure activities did not translate into dissatisfaction with their leisure experience, suggesting that, although their range of activity choices were restricted, even infrequent participation in valued activities added meaning and satisfaction to their lives (Griffin & McKenna, 1998).

EVALUATION OF PERFORMANCE SKILLS AND CLIENT FACTORS. Practitioners can choose from many general occupational therapy assessments and some specific play and leisure assessments that are designed to assess performance

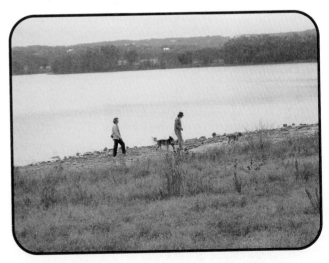

FIGURE 52.2 Participation in valued leisure activities, even if it is infrequent, adds meaning and satisfaction to people's lives.

skills and client factors. Practitioners can also make informal observations during clients' engagement in play and leisure activities. Specific assessments and observations ensure that practitioners are examining clients' performance skills and body functions and structures that are actually used in play and leisure activities (Bundy, 2001b), thereby increasing the likelihood that their intervention will be focused on outcomes related to clients' participation in play and leisure. For example, practitioners often observe children at play with their peers to assess how the children's motor, process, and communication/interaction skills as well as their physical, cognitive, and psychosocial abilities affect their play with others.

Summary of Evaluation of Play and Leisure

Evaluation of play and leisure is guided by client-centered and top-down approaches and is focused on clients' overall patterns of participation in play and leisure across home, school, work, and community settings. The occupational profile gathers information related to clients' play and leisure participation, specifically characteristics of their participation (nature, quality, frequency, and duration). Analysis of occupational performance of clients' play and leisure consists of evaluation of their play and leisure contexts and their performance in the areas of occupation of play and leisure, including play and leisure activity (activity interests, activity choices), and play and leisure experience (subjective experience, personal meaning, satisfaction with experience). Evaluation of performance skills and client factors related to play and leisure is conducted by using general occupational therapy assessments, specific play and leisure assessments, and observation. Practitioners who use this conceptual framework to evaluate play and leisure will be able to design and implement interventions that are directly related to their clients' participation in play and leisure in home, school, work, and community settings.

PLAY AND LEISURE INTERVENTION

To understand play and leisure in intervention, a conceptual framework based on the work of Blanche (1997) and Pierce (1997) is presented. Play and leisure in intervention may be (1) lures or rewards, (2) means to achieve intervention goals, and (3) ends or intervention outcomes. This conceptual framework guides how occupational therapy practitioners use play and leisure in intervention. The occupational therapy intervention approaches (create/promote, establish/restore, maintain, modify, and prevent) within the Occupational Therapy Practice Framework (AOTA, 2002) direct the use of play and leisure toward specific intervention outcomes. Examples below highlight their application.

Play and Leisure as Lures or Rewards

Practitioners use **play and leisure as lures or rewards** to motivate clients to participate in therapeutic activities or to reward them for their participation in intervention (Blanche, 1997; Pierce, 1997). The use of play and leisure in this manner corresponds to the therapeutic use of self (personality, attitude, tone of voice, body language) as a type of occupational therapy intervention (AOTA, 2002). A survey of 222 occupational therapists working with preschool-aged children indicated that all respondents regarded play as important in motivating children to participate in intervention; 91% reported that it was very important (Couch, Deitz, & Kanny, 1998). Pierce (1997) describes the use of play with a toy as a therapy lure when it is presented out of reach of a child. The child is then encouraged to move toward the toy and, when successful, is allowed to play with it. Another example of play and leisure as lures is practitioners' frequent use of a playful attitude in their interactions with clients in order to draw them into intervention activities. Practitioners have historically attended to this affective aspect of therapy by creating intervention settings that are infused with feelings of cheerfulness, an esprit de corps, and hope (Kielhofner & Burke, 1983). Of 77 occupational therapists who reported using leisure assessments to plan their intervention, 32% reported using leisure activity to motivate their clients and facilitate their interest and participation in intervention (Turner, Chapman, McSherry, Krishnagiri, & Watts, 2000).

Play and leisure as rewards are also frequently employed in intervention. Of 203 occupational therapists working with preschool-aged children, 99% reported their use of play as a reinforcer; 40% indicated this use in over 50% of their caseload (Couch et al., 1998). Play as reinforcer is typically used when practitioners provide an opportunity for children to engage in free-play activities during, or at the conclusion of, an intervention session. Blanche (1997) urges those who use play to reinforce children's specific actions to allow time for play consistently throughout a session, rather than banishing it to the end of a session. The common practice of timing opportunities for free play at the end of a session leaves it open to interruption or postponement, suggesting that it is less important than other intervention activities and disregards children's view of play as one of primary importance (Blanche, 1997). Leisure is also used as a reinforcer, particularly when participation in specific leisure activities is the culmination of intervention sessions in which clients planned and organized these activities.

Play and Leisure as Means

Play and leisure as means refers to their use as a type of occupational therapy intervention (therapeutic use of occupations and activities) to achieve specific intervention goals (AOTA, 2002). Clients' engagement in play and

COMMENTARY ON THE EVIDENCE

Play and Leisure in Evaluation and Intervention

The occupational therapy literature provides numerous rationales for the use of play and leisure in evaluation and intervention in occupational therapy practice; however, few studies exist that provide direct evidence of their use and effectiveness in practice. Rationales for use of play and leisure in occupational therapy include descriptions of their general use in practice (Bundy, 1993; CAOT, 1996; Di Bona, 2000; Parham & Primeau, 1997; Primeau, 1996; Read, 1996; Rigby & Huggins, 2003; Stagnitti, 2004; Stagnitti & Unsworth, 2000; Sturgess, 1997; Suto, 1998) as well as their use with specific populations, such as children with autistic spectrum disorder (Desha, Ziviani, & Rodger, 2003; Ziviani, Boyle, & Rodger, 2001), juvenile idiopathic arthritis (Hackett, 2003), and other special needs (Segal, Mandich, Polatajko, & Cook, 2002); adolescents (Passmore & French, 2003); adults with mental illness (Ivarsson, Carlsson, & Sidenvall, 2004; Pieris & Craik, 2004), dual diagnoses (Hodgson, Lloyd, & Schmid, 2001), and physical disabilities (Sandqvist, Akesson, & Eklund, 2005; Specht, King, Brown, & Foris, 2002) and those in forensic settings (Gooch & Living, 2004); and elder adults living in extended care facilities (Atwal, Owen, & Davies, 2003). The majority of these papers are either review articles (Gooch & Living, 2004; Segal et al., 2002; Ziviani et al., 2001) or qualitative studies (Atwal et al., 2003; Hackett, 2003; Hodgson et al., 2001; Passmore & French, 2003; Pieris & Craik, 2004; Specht et al., 2002) that describe play and leisure participation of specific population groups (in some cases, including environmental facilitators and barriers) and make recommendations for use of play and leisure in occupational therapy practice. The remaining three studies use combinations of interviews, observations, questionnaires, and formal assessments to describe population-specific play behaviors and preferences (Desha et al., 2003) or levels of low satisfaction with leisure performance and/or leisure participation (Ivarsson et al., 2004; Sandqvist et al., 2005), leading to recommendations for occupational therapy practice.

Studies that provide direct evidence of the use and effectiveness of play and leisure in occupational therapy practice can be organized according to their focus: (1) play and leisure evaluation in specific populations and (2) support for use of play and leisure as means or ends in intervention. Four studies found in the literature evaluated play behaviors in children using specific play assessments, including the Test of Playfulness (Leipold & Bundy, 2000; Okimoto, Bundy, & Hanzlik, 2000) and the Child-Initiated-Pretend Play Assessment (Stagnitti, Unsworth, & Rodger, 2000), or other structured, formal play observations conducted in clinical settings (Ziviani, Rodger, & Peters, 2005). Each study had small sample sizes ($n \leq 82$), used a control group of typically developing children, and found differences in play behaviors between the control groups and children with autistic spectrum disorder (Ziviani et al., 2005), those with attention deficit/hyperactivity disorder (Leipold & Bundy, 2000), those with cerebral palsy and developmental delays (Okimoto et al., 2000), and those experiencing preacademic problems (Stagnitti et al., 2000). In all cases, the children with disabilities exhibited problematic play behaviors when compared to the control groups.

Seven studies supporting the use of play as means to address client factors and performance skills were found in the literature. Four studies examined the use of games to enhance prone extension (Sakemiller & Nelson, 1998), promote arm reach (Sietsema, Nelson, Mulder, Mervau-Scheidel, & White, 1993), increase standing tolerance (Hoppes, 1997), and enhance motivation (Harris & Reid, 2005). Although sample sizes were small ($n \leq 20$), these studies indicated that play in the form of games had positive effects on these client factors. Additionally, a systematic review of eight studies that investigated the effect of leisure activity on depression or self-esteem in elder adults suggested that leisure activity does have a positive effect on depression and self-esteem (Fine, 2000). Finally, two correlational studies found significant relationships between playfulness and coping skills in both preschool children and adolescents, suggesting that the use of play as means can positively affect coping skills in these groups (Hess & Bundy, 2003; I. Saunders, Sayer, & Goodale, 1999).

Only two studies were found in the literature that investigated play and leisure as ends in occupational therapy

Continued

(O'Brien et al., 2000; Okimoto et al., 2000). One study (*n* = 8) used play as means to examine the effects of intervention on playfulness in children with developmental disorders; no differences were found between the play as means group and the control group that received a home program to promote playfulness (O'Brien et al., 2000). The second study (*n* = 38) compared the effects of the consultation process to improve mother-child interactions with a neurodevelopmental treatment (NDT) session on playfulness of children with cerebral palsy and developmental delays (Okimoto et al., 2000). Although the ToP scores of the children whose mothers received the consultation were higher after the intervention than before, they were not significantly higher than those of the children who received direct NDT.

The state of the evidence in the literature for the use of play and leisure in occupational therapy practice is problematic. While numerous rationales are provided for their use, direct evidence of their use and effectiveness is lacking because too few studies have been reported in the literature, and those that have been reported are limited by methodological weaknesses and small sample sizes. The evidence indicates an urgent need for systematic and methodologically rigorous studies that examine the use of play and leisure in evaluation and intervention in occupational therapy.

leisure is the method or process through which change occurs (Gray, 1998; Trombly, 1995). Practitioners employ play and leisure as means to target change in client factors and performance skills (underlying all areas of occupation) and performance in two specific areas of occupation (play and leisure).

Means to Address Client Factors and Performance Skills

Play and leisure as means are frequently used to address impairments in clients' body functions and structures and limitations in their performance skills. Using the intervention approach of *establish/restore* (AOTA, 2002), practitioners engage their clients in play and leisure activities that are designed to facilitate their achievement of intervention goals related to these impairments and limitations. Survey results indicated that 100% of 212 occupational therapists working with preschool-aged children used play as a therapeutic modality to enhance motor, sensory, or psychosocial outcomes; 92% indicated this use in over 50% of their caseload (Couch et al., 1998). These results resonate with occupational therapy literature in which play is typically described as means to facilitate children's development of their physical, cognitive, and psychosocial abilities and their acquisition of motor, process, communication, and interaction skills (Blanche, 1997; CAOT, 1996; Morrison & Metzger, 2001; Parham & Primeau, 1997; Pierce, 1997).

Although descriptions of leisure as means in the occupational therapy literature are limited (Bundy, 1993;

Suto, 1998), other literature indicates that it is used to achieve physical, cognitive, psychological, social, and spiritual benefits (Driver, Brown, & Peterson, 1991). Occupational therapy practitioners often employ leisure activities, such as games or crafts, as means to improve their clients' manual dexterity, increase their attention to task, develop their social skills, or enhance their feelings of self-efficacy and self-esteem. Of 77 occupational therapists who reported using leisure assessments to guide their intervention, 38% said that they used their clients' leisure interests to address their clients' development of skills (Turner et al., 2000).

Means to Enhance Performance in Areas of Occupation: Play and Leisure

Play and leisure as means can target change in performance in two specific areas of occupation: play and leisure. They are used to address limitations in clients' play and leisure performance (what they actually do and their experience while doing it). Practitioners engage their clients in play and leisure activities to achieve intervention goals related to their competence in and experience of these activities. Intervention provides opportunities for clients to practice specific play and leisure activities, explore new ones, or enhance their experience while engaged in them (Bundy, 2001a; Gray, 1998; Morrison & Metzger, 2001). For example, a Saturday morning group called Kids' Club, an occupational therapy intervention focusing on play and social participation, uses play as means in the form of games with rules to provide opportunities for children with developmental disorders to practice playing familiar games with their peers, explore games that are new to them, and experience fun and enjoyment during their participation in these games (Box 52.1).

When clients demonstrate problems with competence in their chosen play and leisure activities, practitioners can provide opportunities for them to practice play and leisure activities in a positive and safe environment or to explore alternate play and leisure activities in which they can experience higher levels of competence. For example, intervention for a boy with developmental dyspraxia who has difficulty playing soccer with his peers can include therapy sessions in which he and the occupational therapy practitioner actually play soccer so that he can

practice the skills and tasks required for success in a safe and positive environment with no serious consequences for failure (Morrison & Metzger, 2001). In addition, on the basis of evaluation of this boy's activity interests and activity choices, the practitioner can address the mismatch between his interest in and choice of soccer and his limited competence in it by engaging him in other sport activities that might provide a better match. Here, the practitioner uses the intervention approach of *prevent* to mitigate the effects of the boy's feelings of incompetence in soccer, thereby enhancing his performance in sports activities and reducing his risk for restricted participation in play and leisure activities.

When clients report problems with their experience of play and leisure, practitioners can design and adapt play and leisure activities and the environments in which they occur (Bundy, 2001a; Morrison & Metzger, 2001) to facilitate their clients' experience of playfulness, positive affect, personal meaning, and overall satisfaction with their play and leisure experience. For example, an elderly woman reported that the leisure experience she had previously obtained through cooking was no longer satisfying and personally meaningful because of her physical impairments related to a cerebrovascular accident (Bundy, 2001a). Using the intervention approach of *modify*, the practitioner adapted the leisure activity of cooking to facilitate the client's performance in such a way that her leisure experience during cooking was enhanced. Specifically, the practitioner demonstrated and taught the client adapted procedures that she could use to compensate for the mild weakness and abnormal muscle tone in her affected arm, such as sliding pans onto and off the cooktop rather than lifting and carrying them. Instead of focusing intervention on her body functions and structures and performance skills in the context of remediation of motor control, the practitioner used the client's leisure activity of cooking as means to enable her to regain the experience of leisure.

Play and Leisure as Ends

Play and leisure as ends refers to clients' participation in play and leisure as the goal or outcome of intervention (Gray, 1998; Trombly, 1995). Intervention focuses on their ability to engage in play and leisure occupations that are typically expected of and available to people of the same age and culture in home, school, work, and community settings (Box 52.2) (Coster, 1998; Primeau & Ferguson, 1999). Practitioners who address clients' play and leisure as ends promote clients' play and leisure participation for its own sake, not as a means to some other end (Blanche, 1997; Bundy, 1993; Parham & Primeau, 1997).

Although occupational therapy claims to value play and leisure as ends, the literature does not support this claim. Practitioners who address play as ends are rare (Pierce, 1997), as indicated by a survey finding that only 2% of 205 occupational therapists focused on preschool-aged

---

◆ **BOX 52.1** **CRAIG AND THOMAS**

The occupational therapist uses play as means in the form of a game with rules in an intervention session with Craig and Thomas (Figure 52.3). Client factors (e.g., orientation, attention, motivation, and muscle power) and motor, process, and communication/interaction performance skills (e.g., stabilizes, aligns, coordinates, calibrates, grips, attends, handles, heeds, gazes, orients, shares, sustains, focuses, and responds) are all addressed through their engagement in this game. Additionally, the boys' performance in the area of occupation of play is enhanced by the opportunity to play this game in a safe environment and by their positive and enjoyable experience of it.

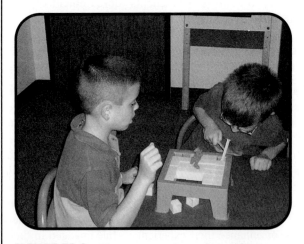

FIGURE 52.3   Play as means is used to address these boys' client factors and performance skills and to enhance their performance in the area of occupation of play.

<table>
<tr><td>

KIDS' CLUB

An occupational therapist in private practice offers a Saturday morning program called Kids' Club, a group intervention for children with developmental disorders focusing on play as ends, that is, the children's engagement in play and social participation as the outcome of intervention. She uses play as means, in the form of games with rules, to address client factors, performance skills, performance in the area of occupation of play, and play as ends. The power of the use of occupation of play as means to facilitate play as ends is demonstrated by two children's stories as told by their mothers.

Fredrick, a 6-year-old boy who was adopted from an Eastern European country, is nonverbal and demonstrates physical and social delays. He had been coming to Kids' Club for a few weeks. His mother called the therapist one night during the week to tell her excitedly about Fredrick's behavior that night in the waiting area outside his sister's karate class. She stated that Fredrick had, for the first time ever, approached a peer (who was also waiting for a sibling) and took his hand to lead him over to the area where Fredrick had been playing. His mother was very happy to see Fredrick initiate play with a peer in this everyday setting, and she attributed it directly to his participation in Kids' Club.

Daryll, a 6-year-old boy diagnosed with pervasive developmental disorder (NOS), had been coming to Kids' Club for about six months when his mother told the therapist that she and her husband had gotten up that Saturday morning to find that Daryll was out of bed and fully dressed. He had also already gotten himself his breakfast of cold cereal and milk. He was ready to leave for Kids' Club, and he was waiting for them to get up and take him there. She said that he had never before shown this kind of motivation to go anywhere. Clearly, Daryll's experience in Kids' Club was more than a means to an ends. His behavior suggested that he enjoyed his participation in Kids' Club as an ends and for its own sake.

</td></tr>
</table>

back to the 1970s, demonstrates a high correlational relationship between leisure satisfaction and overall life satisfaction (Parker, Gladman, & Drummond, 1997). Even though issues of causality in these studies are inconclusive (Headey, Veenhoven, & Wearing, 1991), they indicate that leisure participation can have significant repercussions on overall life satisfaction and quality of life (Brown & Frankel, 1993; Lloyd, 1996; Marans & Mohai, 1991), leading some authors to suggest that participation in play and leisure has a direct role in prevention, health promotion, and population health initiatives (Caldwell & Smith, 1988; Coleman & Iso-Ahola, 1993). Practitioners promote clients' play and leisure as ends through their use of the following types of occupational therapy intervention: therapeutic use of occupations and activities, the education process, and the consultation process (AOTA, 2002).

Therapeutic Use of Occupations and Activities

Therapeutic use of occupations and activities (play and leisure as means) can be used to facilitate clients' play and leisure as ends. As was described previously, they are means to address clients' impairments and limitations in body functions and structures, performance skills, and performance in the areas of occupation of play and leisure. A survey indicated that 35% of 77 occupational therapists reported using leisure activity as means in intervention to promote their clients' future participation in leisure as ends (Turner et al., 2000). Performance in other areas of occupation are also means to enhance play and leisure as ends. For example, practitioners may engage in their clients in activities of daily living, such as dressing or toileting, or in instrumental activities of daily living, such as driving or money management, to improve their ability to participate in play and leisure in home, school, work, and community settings. In fact, older people's ability to live active and healthy lives, including participation in the area of occupation of leisure, can be negatively affected by limitations in their community mobility (Iwarsson, Stahl, & Carlsson, 2003). Occupational therapy practitioners who work with their older clients to facilitate their community mobility can also enhance their ability to participate in leisure in community settings.

Education Process

The education process is a type of occupational therapy intervention (AOTA, 2002) that is used with clients, family members, friends, teachers, coworkers, or other people of significance to clients. Practitioners employ a variety of strategies to promote skill acquisition and structure the teaching-learning situation (Poole, 1995). They teach their clients skills that are required for play and leisure participation, such as how to throw and catch a ball or how to access leisure opportunities in the community. They teach other people (parents, other family members, teachers, and peers) how to facilitate clients' play and leisure participa-

children's participation in play as an outcome of intervention (Couch et al., 1998). Additionally, a search of two major North American occupational therapy journals from the 1980s and 1990s identified fewer than eight articles related to leisure (Suto, 1998). A similar search of these journals for the past eight years (1999–2006) revealed no new articles related to the use of leisure in occupational therapy. Literature outside occupational therapy, dating

tion by modeling playful interactions (CAOT, 1996). Practitioners also teach clients and others how to use adaptive equipment in play and leisure, such as computer games, toys with switches, and adaptive sports equipment (Deitz & Swinth, 1997). Leisure education programs educate clients about leisure, its potential benefits, and personal and community resources for and barriers to leisure and how to access or overcome them (Bundy, 2001a). These programs exemplify the occupational therapy intervention approach of *maintain* by supporting clients' continued participation in leisure in community settings.

Consultation Process

The consultation process is a type of occupational therapy intervention (AOTA, 2002) through which practitioners collaborate with clients and others in their home, school, work, and community settings to identify issues that affect their successful participation in play and leisure and then to plan solutions that address those issues (Barris, Kielhofner, & Watts, 1988). The focus is on clients' participation in play and leisure outside of therapy in the context of their daily lives (Kielhofner, 1997). Leisure counseling is a specific form of consultation that helps clients to identify and clarify leisure values, interests, and attitudes; determine their abilities and skills for leisure participation; improve or refine their skills as needed; and locate and access community resources for leisure (Barris et al., 1988; Caldwell & Smith, 1988).

Practitioners also use the consultation process to address contextual features that facilitate or hinder clients' successful participation in play and leisure in home, school, work, and community settings. As consultants and advocates for change (Law, Stewart, & Strong, 1995), practitioners advise, coordinate, educate, and collaborate with clients and others to remove barriers and shape supportive environments that facilitate clients' access to and inclusion in play and leisure opportunities (CAOT, 1996; Rigby & Huggins, 2003). For example, using the intervention approach of *create/promote,* practitioners advocate for accessible community playgrounds and collaborate with parents, teachers, and other adults to facilitate children's inclusion in play with peers and ensure protected play time (Blanche, 1997). Additionally, practitioners use the intervention approach of *prevent* to advise employers on the requirement of the Americans with Disabilities Act of 1990 to include clients with disabilities in all employment-related activities, including holiday parties, sports events, and business trips (Figure 52.4) (Crist & Stoffel, 1992).

Summary of Play and Leisure Intervention

Play and leisure in intervention may be lures or rewards, means, or ends. As lures, they motivate clients to engage in therapeutic activities; as rewards, they reinforce their participation in intervention. They are therapeutic means to achieve intervention goals related to clients' impairments

PRACTICE DILEMMA

LEISURE COUNSELING PROGRAM

You are an occupational therapy practitioner working on a mental health unit for adults with psychiatric disorders. You are asked to develop a leisure counseling program, focusing on leisure exploration and leisure participation (AOTA, 2002) for a group of adults with the following diagnoses:

◆ A 23-year-old woman with posttraumatic stress disorder
◆ A 35-year-old man with alcohol-related disorder
◆ A 28-year-old woman with major depression
◆ A 19-year-old woman with anorexia nervosa
◆ A 30-year-old man with panic disorder

Develop an intervention session plan for this group. Describe the activities that you would use and how you would present them to the group.

and limitations in body functions and structures, performance skills, and play and leisure performance. Play and leisure as ends are the goals or outcomes of intervention when practitioners promote clients' play and leisure participation for its own sake, not as means to some other end.

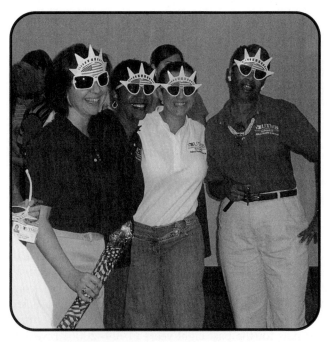

FIGURE 52.4 Play and leisure at work, such as participation in holiday parties and special events, is a significant feature of adults' participation in play and leisure.

CASE STUDY: *Putting it All Together: Evaluating and Designing Interventions for a Child's Participation in Play*

Alvin is a 4-year, 6-month-old boy with a diagnosis of autism. He has a fraternal twin brother who does not have autism. During the occupational therapy evaluation, the occupational therapist asks Alvin's parents about his play behaviors. They report that he essentially ignores other children and rarely engages in play with them. He prefers to play alone, choosing toys such as animal figurines or computer games. When he is around other children, he is likely to interact with those who are younger than he and is most comfortable interacting with others in structured play situations, such as preschool activities, and outdoor activities, such as tag, hide-and-seek, and jumping on the trampoline in their backyard. They also report that Alvin does not have any friends outside of structured play situations that occur in his preschool or that they set up for him at home. Although they state that he demonstrates playfulness, he rarely engages in the play behaviors that they observe in his twin brother's interactions with his peers. They report that

Alvin is unable to make or keep friends, yet that is their wish for him: to have friends outside of the structured activities in which they involve him.

Questions and Exercises

1. What do you know about Alvin's characteristics of play participation, his play contexts, and his play activity and experience? Organize this information according to the parameters for evaluation of play and leisure provided in this chapter.

2. What do you need to know to develop and implement an intervention plan to address Alvin's performance in play and how will you obtain this information? Refer to Table 52.1 for specific assessments that you could use.

3. How could you use play in your intervention with Alvin and what types of intervention would you use?

Therapeutic use of occupations and activities, the education process, and the consultation process are types of occupational therapy intervention that facilitate clients' play and leisure as ends. Practitioners choose among these purposes of play and leisure as lures or rewards, means, or ends to design interventions that lead to outcomes directly related to clients' participation and occupational engagement in home, school, work, and community settings.

ACKNOWLEDGMENT

I acknowledge Janice M. Ferguson, MS, OT(C), for her contributions to our previous conceptualization of occupation as ends that is the basis for this discussion of play and leisure as ends.

PROVOCATIVE QUESTION

1. Occupational therapy practitioners work in a variety of practice settings with different systems of payment for occupational therapy services (see Unit XVI and Chapter 69). How can practitioners address their clients' problems in play and leisure participation within the funding parameters of each setting? Describe how this might occur for the following settings and payment systems:
   a. Skilled nursing facility funded by Medicare
   b. Private, community-based center for children funded by individual health insurance plans
   c. Adult day care program funded by for-profit business

   d. Group homes for adults with developmental disabilities

REFERENCES

American Occupational Therapy Association. (2002). Occupational therapy practice framework: Domain and process. *American Journal of Occupational Therapy, 56,* 609–639.

Atwal, A., Owen, S., & Davies, R. (2003). Struggling for occupational satisfaction: Older people in care homes. *British Journal of Occupational Therapy, 66,* 118–124.

Barris, R., Kielhofner, G., & Watts, J. H. (1988). *Occupational therapy in psychosocial practice.* Thorofare, NJ: Slack.

Beard, J. G., & Ragheb, M. G. (1980). Measuring leisure satisfaction. *Journal of Leisure Research, 12,* 20–33.

Blanche, E. I. (1997). Doing with—not doing to: Play and the child with cerebral palsy. In L. D. Parham & L. S. Fazio (Eds.), *Play in occupational therapy for children* (pp. 202–218). St. Louis: Mosby-Year Book.

Brown, B. A., & Frankel, B. G. (1993). Activity through the years: Leisure, leisure satisfaction, and life satisfaction. *Sociology of Sport Journal, 10,* 1–17.

Bundy, A. C. (1993). Assessment of play and leisure: Delineation of the problem. *American Journal of Occupational Therapy, 47,* 217–222.

Bundy, A. C. (1997). Play and playfulness: What to look for. In L. D. Parham & L. S. Fazio (Eds.), *Play in occupational therapy for children* (pp. 52–66). St. Louis: Mosby-Year Book.

Bundy, A. C. (2001a). Leisure. In B. R. Bonder & M. B. Wagner (Eds.), *Functional performance in older adults* (2nd ed., pp. 196–217). Philadelphia: F. A. Davis.

Bundy, A. C. (2001b). Measuring play performance. In M. Law, C. Baum, & W. Dunn (Eds.), *Measuring occupational per-*

formance: Supporting best practice in occupational therapy* (pp. 89–102). Thorofare, NJ: Slack.

Burke, J. P., & Schaaf, R. C. (1997). Family narratives and play assessment. In L. D. Parham & L. S. Fazio (Eds.), *Play in occupational therapy for children* (pp. 67–84). St. Louis: Mosby-Year Book.

Caldwell, L. L., & Smith, E. A. (1988). Leisure: An overlooked component of health promotion. *Canadian Journal of Public Health, 79,* S44–S48.

Canadian Association of Occupational Therapists. (1996). Practice paper: Occupational therapy and children's play [Insert]. *Canadian Journal of Occupational Therapy, 63,* 1–20.

Coleman, D., & Iso-Ahola, S. E. (1993). Leisure and health: The role of social support and self-determination. *Journal of Leisure Research, 25,* 111–128.

Coster, W. (1998). Occupation-centred assessment of children. *American Journal of Occupational Therapy, 52,* 337–344.

Couch, K. J., Deitz, J. C., & Kanny, E. M. (1998). The role of play in pediatric occupational therapy. *American Journal of Occupational Therapy, 52,* 111–117.

Crist, P. A. H., & Stoffel, V. C. (1992). The Americans with Disabilities Act of 1990 and employees with mental impairments: Personal efficacy and the environment. *American Journal of Occupational Therapy, 46,* 434–443.

Csikszentmihalyi, M. (1975). *Beyond boredom and anxiety.* San Francisco: Jossey-Bass.

Csikszentmihalyi, M. (1988). The flow experience and its significance for human psychology. In M. Csikszentmihalyi & I. S. Csikszentmihalyi (Eds.), *Optimal experience: Psychological studies of flow in consciousness* (pp. 15–35). New York: Cambridge University Press.

Desha, L., Ziviani, J., & Rodger, S. (2003). Play preferences and behavior of preschool children with autistic spectrum disorder in the clinical environment. *Physical & Occupational Therapy in Pediatrics, 23*(1), 21–42.

Di Bona, L. (2000). What are the benefits of leisure? An exploration using the Leisure Satisfaction Scale. *British Journal of Occupational Therapy, 63,* 50–58.

Dietz, J. C., & Swinth, Y. (1997). Accessing play through assistive technology. In L. D. Parham & L. S. Fazio (Eds.), *Play in occupational therapy for children* (pp. 219–232). St. Louis: Mosby-Year Book.

Driver, B. L., Brown, P. J., & Peterson, G. L. (Eds.). (1991). *Benefits of leisure.* State College, PA: Venture.

Driver, B. L., Tinsley, H. E. A., & Manfredo, M. J. (1991). The Paragraphs about Leisure and Recreation Experience Preference Scales: Results from two inventories designed to assess the breadth of the perceived psychological benefits of leisure. In B. L. Driver,, P. J. Brown, & G. L. Peterson (Eds.), *Benefits of leisure* (pp. 263–286). State College, PA: Venture.

Dunn, W. (1998). Person-centered and contextually relevant evaluation. In J. Hinojosa & P. Kramer (Eds.), *Evaluation: Obtaining and interpreting data* (pp. 47–76). Bethesda, MD: American Occupational Therapy Association.

Fine, J. (2000). The effect of leisure activity on depression in the elderly: Implications for the field of occupational therapy. *Occupational Therapy in Health Care, 13*(1), 45–59.

Florey, L. L., & Greene, S. (1997). Play in middle childhood: A focus on children with behavior and emotional disorders. In L. D. Parham & L. S. Fazio (Eds.), *Play in occupational*

therapy for children (pp. 126–143). St. Louis: Mosby-Year Book.

Gooch, P., & Living, R. (2004). The therapeutic use of video-games within secure forensic settings: A review of the literature and application to practice. *British Journal of Occupational Therapy, 67,* 332–341.

Gray, J. M. (1998). Putting occupation into practice: Occupation as ends, occupation as means. *American Journal of Occupational Therapy, 52,* 354–364.

Griffin, J., & McKenna, K. (1998). Influences on leisure and life satisfaction of elderly people. *Physical & Occupational Therapy in Geriatrics, 15*(4), 1–16.

Gunter, B. G., & Stanley, J. (1985). Theoretical issues in leisure study. In B. G. Gunter, J. Stanley, & R. St. Clair (Eds.), *Transitions to leisure: Conceptual and human issues* (pp. 35–51). Lanham, MD: University Press of America.

Hackett, J. (2003). Perceptions of play and leisure in junior school aged children with juvenile idiopathic arthritis: What are the implications for occupational therapy? *British Journal of Occupational Therapy, 66,* 303–310.

Harris, K., & Reid, D. (2005). The influence of virtual reality play on children's motivation. *Canadian Journal of Occupational Therapy, 72,* 21–29.

Headey, B., Veenhoven, R., & Wearing, A. (1991). Top-down versus bottom-up theories of subjective well-being. *Social Indicators Research, 24,* 81–100.

Henderson, K. A., Bialeschki, M. D., Shaw, S. M., & Freysinger, V. J. (1996). *Both gains and gaps: Feminist perspectives on women's leisure.* State College, PA: Venture.

Hess, L. M., & Bundy, A. C. (2003). The association between playfulness and coping in adolescents. *Physical & Occupational Therapy in Pediatrics, 23*(2), 5–17.

Hodgson, S., Lloyd, C., & Schmid, T. (2001). The leisure participation of clients with a dual diagnosis. *British Journal of Occupational Therapy, 64,* 487–492.

Hoppes, S. (1997). Can play increase standing tolerance? A pilot study. *Physical & Occupational Therapy in Geriatrics, 15*(1), 65–73.

Iso-Ahola, S. E. (1979). Basic dimensions of definitions of leisure. *Journal of Leisure Research, 11,* 28–39.

Iso-Ahola, S. E., & Weissinger, E. (1990). Perceptions of boredom in leisure: Conceptualization, reliability, and validity of the Leisure Boredom Scale. *Journal of Leisure Research, 22,* 1–17.

Ivarsson, A., Carlsson, M., & Sidenvall, B. (2004). Performance of occupations in daily life among individuals with severe mental disorders. *Occupational Therapy in Mental Health, 20*(2), 33–50.

Iwarsson, S., Stahl, A., & Carlsson, G. (2003). Accessible transportation: Novel occupational therapy perspectives. In L. Letts, P. Rigby, & D. Stewart (Eds.), *Using environments to enable occupational performance* (pp. 235–251). Thorofare, NJ: Slack.

Kielhofner, G. (1997). *Conceptual foundations of occupational therapy* (2nd ed.). Philadelphia: F. A. Davis.

Kielhofner, G., Borell, L., Burke, J., Helfrich, C., & Nygard, L. (1995). Volition subsystem. In G. Kielhofner (Ed.), *A model of human occupation: Theory and application* (2nd ed., pp. 39–62). Baltimore: Williams & Wilkins.

Kielhofner, G., & Burke, J. P. (1983). The evolution of knowledge and practice in occupational therapy: Past, present, and future. In G. Kielhofner (Ed.), *Health through occupation: Theory and practice in occupational therapy* (pp. 3–54). Philadelphia: F. A. Davis.

Law, M., Baptiste, S., McColl, M., Opzoomer, A., Polatajko, H., & Pollock, N. (1990). The Canadian Occupational Performance Measure: An outcome measure for occupational therapy. *Canadian Journal of Occupational Therapy, 57*, 82–87.

Law, M., Stewart, D., & Strong, S. (1995). Achieving access to home, community, and workplace. In C. A. Trombly (Ed.), *Occupational therapy for physical dysfunction* (4th ed., pp. 361–375). Baltimore: Williams & Wilkins.

Leipold, E. E., & Bundy, A. C. (2000). Playfulness in children with attention deficit hyperactivity disorder. *Occupational Therapy Journal of Research, 20*, 61–82.

Lloyd, K. (1996). Planning for leisure: Issues of quality of life. *Social Alternatives, 15*, 19–22.

Marans, R. W., & Mohai, P. (1991). Leisure resources, recreation activity, and the quality of life. In B. L. Driver, P. J. Brown, & G. L. Peterson (Eds.), *Benefits of leisure* (pp. 351–363). State College, PA: Venture.

Matsutsuyu, J. S. (1969). The interest check list. *American Journal of Occupational Therapy, 23*, 323–328.

Morrison, C. D., & Metzger, P. (2001). Play. In J. Case-Smith (Ed.), *Occupational therapy for children* (4th ed., pp. 528–544). St. Louis: Mosby-Year Book.

O'Brien, J., Coker, P., Lynn, R., Suppinger, R., Pearigen, T., Rabon, S., et al. (2000). The impact of occupational therapy on a child's playfulness. *Occupational Therapy in Health Care, 12*(2/3), 39–51.

Okimoto, A. M., Bundy, A. C., & Hanzlik, J. (2000). Playfulness in children with and without disability: Measurement and intervention. *American Journal of Occupational Therapy, 54*, 73–82.

Parham, L. D. (1996). Perspectives on play. In R. Zemke, & F. Clark (Eds.), *Occupational science: The evolving discipline* (pp. 71–80). Philadelphia: F. A. Davis.

Parham, L. D., & Fazio, L. S. (Eds.). (1997). *Play in occupational therapy for children.* St. Louis: Mosby-Year Book.

Parham, L. D., & Primeau, L. A. (1997). Play and occupational therapy. In L. D. Parham & L. S. Fazio (Eds.), *Play in occupational therapy for children* (pp. 2–21). St. Louis: Mosby-Year Book.

Parker, C. J., Gladman, J. R. F., & Drummond, A. E. R. (1997). The role of leisure in stroke rehabilitation. *Disability and Rehabilitation, 19*, 1–5.

Passmore, A., & French, D. (2003). The nature of leisure in adolescence: A focus group study. *British Journal of Occupational Therapy, 66*, 419–426.

Pierce, D. (1997). The power of object play for infants and toddlers at risk for developmental delays. In L. D. Parham & L. S. Fazio (Eds.), *Play in occupational therapy for children* (pp. 86–111). St. Louis: Mosby-Year Book.

Pieris, Y., & Craik, C. (2004). Factors enabling and hindering participation in leisure for people with mental health problems. *British Journal of Occupational Therapy, 67*, 240–247.

Poole, J. L. (1995). Learning. In C. A. Trombly (Ed.), *Occupational therapy for physical dysfunction* (4th ed., pp. 265–276). Baltimore: Williams & Wilkins.

Primeau, L. A. (1989). *A description and comparison of game playing behavior of preadolescent boys 9 to 11 years of age with and without developmental dyspraxia.* Unpublished master's thesis, University of Southern California, Los Angeles.

Primeau, L. A. (1995). *Orchestration of work and play within families.* Unpublished doctoral dissertation, University of Southern California, Los Angeles.

Primeau, L. A. (1996). Work and leisure: Transcending the dichotomy. *American Journal of Occupational Therapy, 50*, 569–577.

Primeau, L. A., & Ferguson, J. M. (1999). Occupational frame of reference. In P. Kramer & J. Hinojosa (Eds.), *Frames of reference for pediatric occupational therapy* (2nd ed., pp. 469–516). Philadelphia: Lippincott Williams & Wilkins.

Read, D. L. (1996). Play as phenomenon in occupational therapy literature: A literature review. *New Zealand Journal of Occupational Therapy, 47*(1), 15–17.

Reilly, M. (1974). An explanation of play. In M. Reilly (Ed.), *Play as exploratory learning: Studies of curiosity behavior* (pp. 117–149). Beverly Hills, CA: Sage.

Rigby, P., & Huggins, L. (2003). Enabling young children to play be creating supportive play environments. In L. Letts, P. Rigby, & D. Stewart (Eds.), *Using environments to enable occupational performance* (pp. 154–176). Thorofare, NJ: Slack.

Rubin, K. H., Fein, G. G., & Vandenberg, B. (1983). Play. In P. H. Mussen (Series Ed.) & E. M. Hetherington (Vol. Ed.), *Handbook of child psychology: Vol. 4. Socialization, personality, and social development* (4th ed., pp. 693–774). New York: John Wiley.

Sakemiller, L. M., & Nelson, D. L. (1998). Eliciting functional extension in prone through the use of a game. *American Journal of Occupational Therapy, 52*, 150–157.

Samdahl, D. M. (1988). A symbolic interactionist model of leisure: Theory and empirical support. *Leisure Sciences, 10*, 27–39.

Sandqvist, G., Akesson, A., & Eklund, M. (2005). Daily occupations and well-being in women with limited cutaneous systemic sclerosis. *American Journal of Occupational Therapy, 59*, 390–397.

Saunders, E. B. (1922). Psychiatry and occupational therapy. *Archives of Occupational Therapy, 1*, 99–114.

Saunders, I., Sayer, M., & Goodale, A. (1999). The relationship between playfulness and coping in preschool children: A pilot study. *American Journal of Occupational Therapy, 53*, 221–226.

Segal, R., Mandich, A., Polatajko, H., & Cook, J. V. (2002). Play time. *Rehab Management: The Interdisciplinary Journal of Rehabilitation, 15*(8), 44–45, 65.

Shaw, S. M. (1985). The meaning of leisure in everyday life. *Leisure Sciences, 7*, 1–24.

Sietsema, J. M., Nelson, D. L., Mulder, R. M., Mervau-Scheidel, D., & White, B. E. (1993). The use of a game to promote arm reach in persons with traumatic brain injury. *American Journal of Occupational Therapy, 47*, 19–24.

Slagle, E. C. (1922). Training aides for mental patients. *Archives of Occupational Therapy, 1*, 11–17.

Specht, J., King, G., Brown, E., & Foris, C. (2002). The importance of leisure in the lives of persons with congenital physical disabilities. *American Journal of Occupational Therapy, 56*, 436–445.

Stagnitti, K. (2004). Understanding play: The implications for play assessment. *Australian Occupational Therapy Journal, 51,* 3–12.

Stagnitti, K., & Unsworth, C. (2000). The importance of pretend play in child development: An occupational therapy perspective. *British Journal of Occupational Therapy, 63,* 121–127.

Stagnitti, K., Unsworth, C., & Rodger, S. (2000). Development of an assessment to identify play behaviors that discriminate between the play of typical preschoolers and preschoolers with pre-academic problems. *Canadian Journal of Occupational Therapy, 67,* 291–303.

Sturgess, J. L. (1997). Current trends in assessing children's play. *British Journal of Occupational Therapy, 60,* 410–414.

Suto, M. (1998). Leisure in occupational therapy. *Canadian Journal of Occupational Therapy, 65,* 271–278.

Tinsley, H. E. A., & Tinsley, D. J. (1982). A holistic model of leisure counseling. *Journal of Leisure Research, 14,* 100–116.

Tinsley, H. E., Hinson, J. A., Tinsley, D. J., & Holt, M. S. (1993). Attributes of leisure and work experiences. *Journal of Counseling Psychology, 40,* 447–455.

Townsend, E. (1997). *Client-centred occupational assessment.* Unpublished manuscript, School of Occupational Therapy, Dalhousie University, Halifax, Nova Scotia, Canada.

Trombly, C. (1993). Anticipating the future: Assessment of occupational function. *American Journal of Occupational Therapy, 47,* 253–257.

Trombly, C. A. (1995). Occupation: Purposefulness and meaningfulness as therapeutic mechanisms. *American Journal of Occupational Therapy, 49,* 960–972.

Turner, H., Chapman, S., McSherry, A., Krishnagiri, S., & Watts, J. (2000). Leisure assessment in occupational therapy: An exploratory study. *Occupational Therapy in Health Care, 12*(2/3), 73–85.

World Health Organization. (2001). *ICF: International Classification of Functioning, Disability, and Health.* Geneva: Author. Retrieved April 23, 2007, from www.who.int/icidh

Ziegler, L. H. (1924). Some observations on recreations. *Archives of Occupational Therapy, 3,* 255–265.

Ziviani, J., Boyle, M., & Rodger, S. (2001). An introduction to play and the preschool child with autistic spectrum disorder. *British Journal of Occupational Therapy, 64,* 17–22.

Ziviani, J., Rodger, S., & Peters, S. (2005). The play behavior of children with and without autistic disorder in a clinical environment. *New Zealand Journal of Occupational Therapy, 52*(2), 22–30.

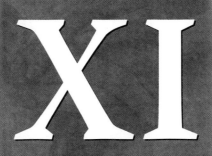

XI

OT Evaluation and Intervention: Personal Factors

" In order to understand anything well, you need at least three good theories. "

William Perry

" What we understand the world to be like is determined by many things: our sensory organs, our ability to move and to manipulate objects, the detailed structure of our brain, our culture, and our interactions with the environment. . . "

George Lakoff & Mark Johnson

Overview of Personal Factors Affecting Performance

53

BARBARA A. BOYT SCHELL,
ELLEN S. COHN, AND
ELIZABETH BLESEDELL CREPEAU

Learning Objectives

After reading this chapter, you will be able to:

1. Discuss how personal factors are related to occupations.
2. Discuss how knowledge and theories about personal factors are used in occupational therapy evaluation and intervention.
3. Identify examples of body functions and structures that are considered in the occupational therapy process.

INTRODUCTION

The chapters in this unit discuss various personal factors that affect occupational performance. The term **personal factors** is a broad term that we use here to encompass several aspects of the human condition. In part, personal factors include our **body structures**, which are the anatomical parts of our bodies, such as bones and organs (World Health Organization, 2001). In part, personal factors include our **body functions**, which are the physiological processes of the body (WHO, 2001). Chapters in this unit focus on body functions and structures and how those two sets of personal factors influence us as we engage in occupations. Our bodily structures and functions play an important role in how we conduct our daily lives. This becomes strikingly evident when our bodies and related abilities are different from those of our peers, become impaired, or otherwise change from what we have come to expect. It is important to understand body functions and structures in order to use occupation as therapy.

We also use the term *personal factors* to refer to the characteristics of the social and cultural context that each individual absorbs into his or her identity as a person. Because many of the chapters in Unit I addressed how social and cultural contexts affect individuals, these factors are only briefly summarized here as a reminder before we discuss body functions and structures.

THE WHOLE IS GREATER THAN THE SUM OF THE PARTS

Personal factors do not operate in isolation. People rarely take their arms and legs anywhere that their brains, eyes, and ears don't go as well! Anyone who has tried to maneuver in unfamiliar space in the dark (such as finding the bathroom in a dark hotel room in the middle of the night) can attest to the importance of vision to movement. All bodily factors work synergistically, which is why it is difficult to generate a definitive list of factors for practitioners to attend to. That is the case in this chapter as well, and the selected lists of factors and descriptions are presented to prompt your thinking. The categorizations that are presented here are not, nor can they be, a complete list of all the factors that affect human behavior. They are, at best, suggestions of factors to consider in analyzing occupational performance.

Practitioners can consider all of these factors from an **objective** standpoint or as **subjectively experienced** by the client. When considering personal factors objectively, practitioners observe or measure body functions and structures in ways that other observers can replicate. (Unit IX addresses the importance of using reliable and valid measures.) Although objective approaches are undeniably useful for informing professional reasoning, the client's subjective experience is also important. Skilled practitioners consider both. Box 53.1 provides some examples of objective and subjective reports related to body functions and structures.

Our job as occupational therapy practitioners is twofold. First, we must understand how bodily structures and functions support humans as they engage in occupations and, simultaneously, how occupational engagement can

---

BOX 53.1

OBJECTIVE AND SUBJECTIVE REPORTS OF BODY FUNCTIONS AND STRUCTURES

"I Didn't Have a Clue"

In a study seeking to understand the subjective experience of regaining self-care skills after a stroke or spinal cord injury, Guidetti, Asaba, and Tham (2007) reported numerous examples of what it felt like for the study participants to attempt familiar tasks with various impairments. For instance, one participant who was recovering from a stroke appears to have had what objectively might be documented as a sensory loss, along with neglect of the affected upper extremity (a perceptual impairment). She described her experience this way: "I didn't have a clue where it [her hand] was, it was behind my back and like this, so the first night it could have been anybody's hand" (Guidetti et al., 2007, p. 3).

"When You're Sitting There by Yourself, You're Just Eating"

In a study examining supported socialization for people with mental illness, Davidson and his colleagues (2004) argued that people with persistent mental illness are lonely and isolated, not by choice (or objective impairments) but because of lack of opportunity and encouragement. When viewed solely from an objective perspective, people with persistent mental illness have been described as having impairments in volition, self-awareness, or coping (affective and cognitive impairments) and are thought to no longer desire human connection, with a preference for being alone. In a randomized control trial of supported socialization intervention, Davidson and colleagues found that people with mental illness desire friendships. One participant in the study commented that eating with her friend was better than eating alone at Burger King: "I'm alone. I sit down at the table, I eat a hamburger. But when I go with somebody else, and I'm sitting there at the table and eating it, she'll say 'Oh, is your hamburger good?' Then it becomes, the hamburger becomes noticeable, and then your mind starts to think about the taste. But when you're sitting there by yourself, you're just eating" (Davidson et al., 2001, p. 380).

This woman's description of eating with a friend illustrates the importance of considering clients' subjective experience. Without consideration of the subjective experience, intervention could run the risk of negating what was meaningful to this woman.

be disrupted by impairments. Second, we must go beyond the generic labeling and understandings of diagnostic conditions to a deeper and more personal understanding of how clients feel in their specific situations. As an acquaintance once noted to the first author, when describing her experience with occupational therapy, "Occupational therapy is such an intimate profession. My OT really understood how this whole thing affected me."

REASONING ABOUT PERSONAL FACTORS: OCCUPATIONAL THERAPY AS A BRIDGE

Occupational therapy practitioners like to say that they treat the "whole person," While other professions (such as nursing) legitimately make a similar claim, occupational therapy is unique in its focus on how daily occupations are the synergistic product of personal factors within the individual and factors that are external to the person in the larger context.

Another way to think about occupational therapy and how we consider the factors under discussion is to contrast occupational therapy with other professions. Think of occupational therapy as a bridge between the medical world and the life world. In the medical world, there are many professions that focus on particular sets of body structures and functions. The field of medicine has obvious examples, with specialties in dermatology, endocrinology, gynecology, and the list goes on and on. But other professions can also be examples. For instance, ophthalmologists focus on the visual system, physical therapists focus on the neuromuscular and musculoskeletal systems, nutritionists focus on the digestive system, and speech-language pathologists focus primarily on the cognitive and oral-motor systems as they relate to communication. Although all of these professionals are interested in improving an individual's function, their contribution is very specific and their knowledge about body functions and structures within their specific scope is typically quite extensive. In general, people in the medical professions focus primarily on disease and reduction of impairment (Fleming, 1991) and secondarily on the use of devices or techniques to compensate for impairments related to their chosen scope of practice.

In contrast, other professions organize themselves around major roles or tasks of life. For instance, vocational evaluators and rehabilitation counselors focus on work-related concerns, educators focus on helping people learn to become productive citizens, recreation professionals focus on play and leisure, and social workers focus on family and community life. These professionals may attend to the impact of personal factors. Special educators, for example, are particularly aware of the impact of cognitive abilities and limitations for students in the classroom. However, for the most part, people in these professions are very different from those in the medically oriented fields in that they typically have little or no background related to anatomy, physiology, and the specific impact of different health conditions on performance. Rather, they have broad working knowledge about the skills and social demands that are required for their area of interest. So, for example, practitioners with a work focus know a great deal about job demands, employer requirements, and government standards related to work. Similarly, recreation therapists are quite knowledgeable about recreational spaces and places, the value of leisure in life, and the kinds of equipment that individuals might use to pursue leisure interests.

Complexity: An Asset and a Challenge

Occupational therapy is unique as a profession in its willingness to consider all personal factors along with all contextual factors as they shape engagement in the daily activities and routines of life. It is this appreciation of the transactional nature of occupational performance that makes occupational therapy so customized and effective for helping to solve complex problems of daily life. This uniqueness is a tremendous asset. However, for new practitioners and even some experienced ones, it can be challenging not to get absorbed in one aspect and thus lose sight of the larger picture. It is tempting, because there is so much to know. When this happens, you start to see practitioner refer to themselves by the particular aspect—for instance, hand therapy, cognitive therapy, or vision therapy. Recognizing that depth of knowledge about the personal factors is very important to expert practice; we maintain that our clients are best served when we view these factors in relation to the use of occupation as a means for intervention. Examples of such reasoning are provided through the practitioners' narratives in Unit XIII. All of these practitioners indicate a deep understanding of body functions and structures that are relevant to their clients, but they view these personal factors in relation to performance. Furthermore, occupational therapy practitioners grade their use of interventions in a way that is mindful of the person's development, impairments, potential for recovery, and/or need for adaptive approaches. Practitioners also are very in tune with how social and cultural contexts influence their clients' lives. Thus, occupational therapy practitioners specialize not in body parts or body functions, but in supporting health and participation in life through engagement in occupation.

Intertwining Knowledge and Theories

For occupational therapy practitioners to work effectively with people who have impairments or developmental conditions that affect their performance, practitioners must intertwine knowledge about occupation with knowledge about the client's particular health problems. Thus, the quotation from William Perry that opened the unit, stating that you "must have at least three good theories" to understand anything, seems written for occupational therapy practice. The therapists' narratives in Unit XIII provide examples of using different theories to guide practice. Readers might want to look at those chapters for examples of how to integrate theories about body functions and structures into an occupational therapy intervention. For instance, Mary Muhlenhaupt (Chapter 63) first obtained information about Davey, a third-grade student (occupation), from his teachers and parents and from her direct observation of him (occupational performance) in a variety of school settings (physical and social context). On the basis of his occupational abilities and performance problems, she suspected that a sensory processing problem (neurological system) was affecting his performance. Winifred Schultz-Krohn (Chapter 64) demonstrates an understanding of how many factors, both personal and contextual, contribute to stressful living for individuals in homeless shelters and uses her understanding as the basis for group programming. Karen Garren (Chapter 65) helped Dan to recover from a devastating hand injury (body

structure) in order to regain coordinated use (musculoskeletal function) of his hand so that he could return to being a master carpenter (occupation). Coralie Glantz (Chapter 66) received information from a family member (social context) who was worried about her mother's memory (cognitive function). As it turned out, the client had Alzheimer's disease (neurological impairment). Coralie's knowledge of the typical course of this disease helped her to anticipate and deal with the client's occupational performance problems. The professional reasoning processes that these four practitioners describe demonstrate the complexity and the richness of the occupational therapy process.

PERSONAL FACTORS THAT ARE COMMONLY CONSIDERED

In this section, we provide several tables that readers might find helpful to prompt consideration of one or more personal factors (see Tables 53.1, 53.2, and 53.3). Readers

TABLE 53.1. EXAMPLES OF PERSONAL FACTORS (EXCLUDING BODY FUNCTIONS AND STRUCTURES) THAT ARE CONSIDERED IN OCCUPATIONAL THERAPY

Factor	Common Categories or Descriptors
Age	Historical cohort (e.g., people who lived through the Depression and how that experience affects their worldview) Internalization of societal expectations regarding development and achieving a particular developmental milestone at a given time in the life course Personal expectations about age-related behavior
Gender	Personally adopted social/cultural norms regarding gender
Values	Meanings associated with physical and social spaces Importance of family Standards of conduct
Beliefs	Knowledge that is held to be truth Beliefs about causes and interventions related to illness Perceived locus of control
Spirituality	Beliefs about the meaning of life Religious and sacred beliefs
Family and significant others	Internalized family experiences that shape worldview Internalized expectations about relationships
Socioeconomic status	Financial status Work status Educational attainment
Ethnicity	Internal beliefs about membership in groups of common descent; can include race, culture, language, religion, and politics
Sexual orientation	An individuals sexuality, usually related to the sex or gender of the person the individual finds sexually attractive

TABLE 53.2.   EXAMPLES OF BODY STRUCTURES CONSIDERED IN OCCUPATIONAL THERAPY

Structure	Common Categories or Descriptors Addressed Within OT Process
Nervous system	Central (brain, spinal cord) Peripheral Autonomic (sympathetic, parasympathetic)
Eye, ear, nose, throat	Eye (retina, cornea, lens) Ear (inner, middle, outer) Mouth (lips, cheek,tongue, teeth) Nose Pharynx, esophagus Larynx
Cardiovascular, immunological, respiratory	Heart Veins Arteries Lungs Trachea Bronchial tubes Lymph system
Digestive, metabolic, endocrine	Esophagus Stomach Intestine Many glands
Genitourinary, reproductive	Bladder, ureters, urethra Reproductive structures, including glands
Movement-related structures	Bones Joints Muscles Tendons Ligaments Fascia
Skin and related structures	Skin layers Skin glands Hair Sensing organs in skin

Source: AOTA (in press), WHO (2001), Sloan, E. (1994)

will likely find the language useful in communicating about personal factors. As was discussed earlier, there is no practical way to make a comprehensive list, so we make no claim that the tables are all inclusive. Information for these tables was drawn primarily from the International Classification of Function (WHO 2001), the Occupational Therapy Practice Framework (American Occupational Therapy Association, in press), and topical areas that are addressed in this unit as well as chapters from Unit I. The factors that are listed in the tables provide a starting place. Occupational therapy practice, by nature, requires ongoing inquiry

to gain needed knowledge to respond to the challenges of practice.

Cues to personal factors that could be affecting performance are gained from at least three sources:

♦ **Reason for referral.** Referral information may contain a medical, psychological, or educational diagnosis and sometimes precautions to consider during intervention. Even when precautions, symptoms, or other descriptors are not included, knowledge about typical body structures and functions that are affected

TABLE 53.3.   EXAMPLES OF BODY FUNCTIONS ADDRESSED BY OCCUPATIONAL THERAPISTS

ICF Category		Examples
Mental (affective, cognitive, perceptual)	Consciousness	Arousal level
	Orientation	Person
		Place
		Time
		Self
		Others
		Past
		Present
	Excitation and inhibition	Balance between
	Centrifugal control	Suppression
		Divergence
		Convergence
	Attention	Alertness
		Selectivity
		Sustainability
		Shifting
		Tracking
	Memory	Short term
		Long term
		Working
	Perception	Discrimination
		Sensory memory
		Spatial relationships
		Temporal relationships
		Constancy
		Figure-ground
		Closure
	Sensory processing	Reception
		Organization
		Assimilation
		Integration
	Thought	Praxis (ideation and planning)
	Executive function/higher level	Volition
		Planning
		Purposeful action
		Self-awareness
		Self-monitoring
		Decision making
		Problem solving
	Emotional	Coping
		Behavioral regulation
Sensation and pain	Taste	Quality
		Intensity
	Smell	Quality
		Intensity

Continued

TABLE 53.3.   EXAMPLES OF BODY FUNCTIONS ADDRESSED BY OCCUPATIONAL THERAPISTS   *Continued*

ICF Category		Examples
Sensation and pain *(continued)*	Touch	Light Deep pressure
	Temperature	Hot Cold
	Pain	Sharp Stabbing Aching Burning
	Proprioception	Quick Sustained
	Vestibular	Linear Angular
	Visual	Acuity Intensity Contrast
	Auditory	Acuity Intensity Contrast Rhythm
Neuromuscular and movement	Joint mobility	Passive ROM Active ROM
	Muscle strength	Pinch Grip Force
	Muscle tone	Quality
	Voluntary motor control	Coordination (dexterity, gross motor, bilateral integration) Motor execution (mobility)
	Involuntary motor control	Reflexes Unconscious movement
	Posture	Alignment Orientation Stability Control Balance Adaptation
	Reaction time	
Cardiovascular, immunological, respiratory	Heart rate	
	Blood pressure	Tension
	Respiration	Rate Rhythm Depth

Source: Based on AOTA (in press), Dunn (2000), WHO (2001), chapters in this text (J. Poole, Chapter 54; C, Guiffrida & M. Rice, Chapter 55; B. White, Chapter 56; J. Toglia, K. Golisz, & Y. Goverover, Chapter 57; W. Dunn, Chapter 58; S. Smith Roley & E. Jacobs, Chapter 59.).

by the condition can guide practitioners about factors to consider.

♦ **Client self-report.** Clients themselves, their families, and other key people in their social environments (e.g., teachers, employers, caregivers) often give practitioners information about factors that they believe are affecting client performance.

♦ **Observation of client.** Observations of the client engaging in occupations often prompt practitioners to consider one or more factors that are affecting performance.

Skillful intervention requires that practitioners respond to these cues and then use credible resources to obtain needed objective information. This information, combined with the subjective data provided by the client, is then synthesized to develop interventions that enable clients' occupational performance

CONCLUSION

Occupational therapy practitioners routinely consider body functions, structures, and other personal factors during intervention. By integrating knowledge and theories about these factors with theories that relate to occupation and occupational contexts, practitioners provide a unique contribution to society and to the clients they serve.

REFERENCES

American Occupational Therapy Association. (in press). Occupational therapy practice framework: Domain and process (2nd ed.). *American Journal of Occupational Therapy.*

Davidson, L., Shahar, G., Stayner, D. A., Chiman, M. J., Rakfeldt, J., & Tebes, J. K. (2004). Supported socialization for people with psychiatric disabilities: Lessons from a randomized control trial. *Journal of Community Psychology, 31,* 453–477.

Davidson, L., Stayner, D. A., Nickou, C., Styron, T. H., Rowe, M., & Chinman, M. L. (2001). "Simply to be let in": Inclusion as a basis for recovery. *Psychiatric Rehabilitation Journal, 24,* 375–388.

Dunn, W. (2000). Best practice occupational therapy in community service with children and families. Thorofare, NJ: Slack.

Fleming, M. H. (1991). Clinical reasoning in medicine compared with clinical reasoning in occupational therapy. *American Journal of Occupational Therapy, 45,* 988–995.

Guidetti, S., Asaba, E., Tham, K. (2007). The lived experience of recapturing self-care. *American Journal of Occupational Therapy 61,* 303–310.

Sloan, E. (1994). *Anatomy and physiology: An easy learner.* Boston Jones & Bartlett Publishers [Electronic Version] Retrieved Oct 5, 2007 from http://library.brenau.edu/cgi-bin/Pwebrecon.cgi?v1=4&ti=1,4&Search%5FArg=Human%20Anatomy%20and%20Phys&SL=Submit%26LOCA%3D Electronic%20Resources%7C3&Search%5FCode=FT%2A&CNT=25&PID=2880&SEQ=20071005185045&SID=1

World Health Organization. (2001). *International classification of functioning, disability and health (ICF).* Geneva: Author.

Musculoskeletal Factors

JANET L. POOLE

54

Learning Objectives

After reading this chapter, you will be able to:

1. Identify assessments for individuals with musculoskeletal impairments.
2. Recommend intervention approaches for individuals with musculoskeletal impairments.
3. Evaluate the evidence for interventions for individuals with musculoskeletal impairments.

Musculoskeletal impairments can be present in individuals of all ages as a result of an injury or disease or during a recovery stage after surgery (e.g., hip precautions after a total hip replacement) or immobility (e.g., fracture). These impairments can include an injury or amputation of the upper extremity or extremities, amputation of the lower extremity or extremities, arthritis, fractures, joint surgery, or repetitive motion disorders. Regardless, musculoskeletal impairments can limit performance of basic activities of daily living, productivity, and/or leisure activities.

THEORIES

The traditional approaches to evaluation and treatment of individuals with musculoskeletal problems include the biomechanical and the rehabilitative frames of reference. The biomechanical frame of reference is used to assess and treat individuals who have activity limitations due to musculoskeletal impairments such as limited range of motion and strength and decreased dexterity and endurance (James, 2003). The main tenet of this frame of reference is that occupational performance can be regained through addressing the underlying impairments that limit performance of daily activities (Hagedorn, 1997; James, 2003; Trombly, 1995). Thus, assessment would focus on the impairments that appear to be the causes for the deficits in occupational performance and on intervention aimed at reducing these impairments. For example, if decreased upper extremity range of motion is noted and determined to be the reason why an individual with arthritis is having difficulty with bathing, then intervention would consist of a variety of stretching and range of motion exercises and exercises to increase joint motion. Other interventions that use a biomechanical frame of reference include **splints** and **orthotics**, range of motion exercises, strengthening and endurance exercises, stretching, **physical agent modalities**, and edema reduction techniques. However, what is not clear is whether a reduction in a biomechanical impairment corresponds to an improvement in occupational performance.

For individuals who have musculoskeletal impairments, the rehabilitative frame of reference aims to achieve maximum function in the performance of daily tasks. Through assessment, the client's goals are identified, and intervention focuses on compensatory methods, assistive devices, and environmental modifications (Seidel, 2003). Therefore, for the person with arthritis who is having difficulty bathing because of limitations in joint motion, the occupational therapist, using a rehabilitative frame of reference, might provide a long-handled sponge and a wash mitt to eliminate holding a washcloth and might suggest a hand-held shower. A rehabilitative frame of reference might be appropriate when an underlying impairment cannot be reduced. In addition, the introduction of potentially new strategies, techniques, and/or equipment involves the teaching-learning process. Box 54.1 lists strategies that therapists can use to facilitate learning of new skills (Poole, 1991, 1995).

BOX 54.1 STRATEGIES FOR TEACHING AN OCCUPATION BASED ON PRINCIPLES OF MOTOR LEARNING

1. Make sure the client understands the goal and critical aspects of the occupation.
2. Provide feedback.
3. Organize practice of an occupation, strategies, techniques, and/or equipment so that clients will retain and generalize the information to other occupations or new environments.
4. Assess whether material or techniques have been learned correctly.

These strategies may also be useful in teaching clients biomechanical inventions such as home exercise programs. Following are some examples of these strategies in use:

- **Make sure the client understands the goal and critical aspects of the occupation.** For example, in teaching a person with a total hip replacement to put on pants using a reacher, the critical aspects are adhering to the hip precautions and making sure the reacher has a good grip on the pants. In teaching a person to use an upper extremity **prosthesis** to use utensils for eating, the critical aspects of the occupation are to look for the flat surface of the utensil before deciding how to preposition the **terminal device**. In teaching a client techniques for behavioral changes, such as **joint pro-**

tection, **energy conservation**, total hip precautions, or body mechanics, make sure the client understand why these are important for him or her.

- **Provide feedback.** When a client is first learning a new technique or to use a piece of adapted equipment or a new exercise program, feedback should be given fairly frequently so that the learner understands the correct performance. However, wait a few minutes after the task is completed so that the person can process internal feedback. As the client becomes more proficient, feedback should be withdrawn so that the client does not become dependent on the feedback.

- **Organize practice of an occupation, strategies, techniques, and/or equipment use so that clients will retain the information and be able to generalize to other occupations or new environments.** For example, a client transfers to and from a toilet and a wheelchair several times. This is called **blocked practice**, in which the same occupation is practiced over and over again. Or a client transfers from the wheelchair to a toilet, tub bench, chair, and bed in succession. This type of practice, referred to as **random practice**, involves practicing variations of an occupation. Studies have shown that blocked practice can be helpful when someone is learning something new but that random practice results in better retention and generalization (Hanlon, 1996; Lee & Magill, 1983; Shea & Morgan, 1979).

When specific strategies for behavior change are taught, practice is also necessary. Sometimes clients are just given verbal or written instructions on body mechanics, joint protection, and energy conservation, for example. Clients need to pick up objects to use proper body mechanics and actually practice principles of joint protection. Hammond and Freeman (2001) have shown that supervised practice of joint protection principles in addition to verbal and visual instruction results in actual incorporation of these principles during daily tasks. Furthermore, principles of **motor learning** can be used in educating clients' families and/or caregivers. The therapist should direct families to practice the intervention they are being taught, such as a transfer, pushing a wheelchair up a curb, or putting on a splint with the therapist present and giving feedback.

- **Assess whether material or techniques have been learned correctly:** The therapist should ask the client, family, and/or caregiver to demonstrate what they have learned so that the therapist can determine whether they can apply this new technique to other situations.

Chapter 55 provides more information about motor control and motor learning theories.

ASSESSMENT

As is discussed in Units IX and X, the occupational therapy evaluation is guided by attention to those activities that the person wants or needs to perform. Additionally, in dealing with individuals with musculoskeletal impairments, it is critical that the occupational therapist follow appropriate precautions. For instance, individuals who recently had joint replacements might need to avoid resistive or weight-bearing activities for a period of time. Further, as part of the assessment, the therapist will likely need to determine whether and how musculoskeletal factors are inhibiting the performance. Important musculoskeletal factors to consider are joint motion, muscle strength, dexterity and endurance. Finally, in deciding what assessment to use to with people with musculoskeletal conditions, consider the ability of the assessment to detect change when it has occurred. Activity or occupation level outcome measures have been found to be more sensitive to short-term changes than are impairment (i.e., personal factor) level assessments such as range of motion and strength (Amadio, Silverstein, Ilstrup, Schleck, & Jensen, 1996).

Range of Motion

Range of motion for a joint is the arc of motion through which a joint moves. The motion at a joint is determined by the structure of the joint and the integrity of the surrounding capsule (Flinn, Trombly Latham, & Podolski, 2007; Killingsworth & Pedretti, 2006a;). There are two types of range of motion: **passive range of motion (PROM)** and **active range of motion (AROM)**. PROM is the motion available in a joint when it is moved by an outside force. PROM provides information about the extensibility of the joint capsule, associate ligaments, and muscles (Norkin & White, 1995). AROM is the range through which a client can move a joint using his or her muscle power; it provides additional information about muscle strength and functional ability. Range of motion is measured by a **goniometer**. Detailed instructions for placement of goniometers to measure each joint and norms for range of motion can be found in several sources (Flinn et al., 2007; Kohlmeyer, 2003; Norkin & White, 2005; Killingsworth & Pedretti, 2006a).

Range of motion is evaluated to determine limitations that affect function and whether additional motion is needed; to determine the need for splints, assistive devices, or both; to determine limitations that might produce deformity; and to document progress (Kohlmeyer, 2003). AROM can be observed during activities of daily living or performing a functional range of motion assessment in which a client moves through various positions (Killingsworth, 2006). All joints can be moved though their respective motion to briefly assess PROM.

Not every client needs a formal assessment of joint motion. However, certain diagnoses may result in deficits in range of motion such as arthritis, fractures, stroke, and spinal cord injury, and a formal assessment would be warranted. When range of motion measurements are below the norms and interfere with the performance of activities of daily living and other occupations, the therapist should determine the cause of the decreased range. Causes may include pain, edema, muscle weakness, skin adhesions, spasticity, bony obstruction or destruction, or soft tissue contractures (Kohlmeyer, 2003). If the cause is modifiable, therapy might be able to increase the active motion or prevent further loss of motion by stretching, strengthening, orthotics, casts, or physical agent modalities such as heat or neuromuscular electrical stimulation. If it is determined that it might not be possible to increase the joint motion, therapists might want to consider adaptive techniques or equipment to perform daily tasks (Flinn et al., 2007).

Muscle Strength

Muscle strength, or the power of a muscle to resist movement, is evaluated by manual resistance, **isokinetics exercises**, pinch meters, and **dynamometers**. Resistance can be provided by a therapist, who scores the strength of a muscle on the basis of the amount of resistance and whether the movement is against or with gravity (Daniels & Worthington, 1986; Flinn et al., 2007; Kendall, McCreary, & Provance, 1993; Killingsworth & Pedretti, 2006b). Hand strength can also be assessed by using an adjustable handle dynamometer, and pinch strength can be measured with a pinch meter. Generally, three types of pinch are tested: thumb to index finger (palmar pinch), thumb to lateral side of index finger (lateral pinch), and thumb to tips of index and middle fingers (three-point pinch). Standardized procedures for using a dynamometer and a pinch meter and normative data are provided in the occupational therapy literature (Flinn et al., 2007; Killingsworth & Pedretti, 2001b; Mathiowetz, Kashman, Volland, Weber, Dowe, & Rogers 1985).

Muscle strength is evaluated to do the following:

◆ Facilitate diagnosis in some neuromuscular conditions (e.g., spinal cord injury, peripheral nerve injury)
◆ Establish a baseline and assess intervention effectiveness
◆ Determine whether weakness is limiting performance
◆ Determine the need for compensatory measures or assistive devices on a temporary or long-term basis
◆ Identify muscle imbalances that might require strengthening, if possible
◆ Determine appropriate orthotic intervention to prevent deformity (Kohlmeyer, 2002).

Muscle weakness is often seen in people with lower motor neuron disorders, primary muscle diseases, neurological diseases, and conditions that result in muscle weakness through disuse or immobilization such as burns, arthritis and amputations (Flinn et al., 2007; Pedretti, 2001b).

Dexterity

Several tests are available to evaluate dexterity or fine motor coordination (Table 54.1). The majority of these tests are

TABLE 54.1   FINE MOTOR COORDINATION TESTS

Dexterity Assessment	Description and Features
Crawford Small Parts Dexterity Test	◆ Measures eye-hand coordination and manipulation of small hand tools ◆ Designed for teenagers and adults ◆ Uses pins, collars, screws, tweezers, screwdriver ◆ Client is timed on tasks such as inserting a pen in a hole in a metal plate with tweezers, covering with a collar, threading screws
Erhardt Developmental Prehension Assessment	◆ Measures components and skills of hand function development ◆ Designed for birth to 6 years ◆ Uses a variety of objects (e.g., small suitcase, plastic pail, toy hammer, key, beads, aluminum can, rubber ball, stacking rings) to measure grasp, reflex, and manipulation skills
Fine Dexterity Test	◆ Assesses fine finger movements of adults
Grooved Peg Board Test	◆ Measures eye-hand coordination and finger dexterity ◆ Client places grooved pegs in a 25-hole peg board in various random positions ◆ Measures speed of eye-hand coordination and color matching for all age groups
Purdue Peg Board Test	◆ Measures movements of arms, hands, fingers, and fingertip dexterity ◆ Norms for adults and children ages 5–15 years, 11 months ◆ Client places pins in a peg board; assembles pins, washers, and collars
Box and Block Test	◆ Tests manual dexterity ◆ Norms for children ages 7–9 years, adults, and adults with neuromuscular involvement ◆ Client picks up one block at a time and places it in an attached compartment
Nine Hole Peg Test of Fine Motor Coordination	◆ Measures fine dexterity ◆ Norms for adults older than 20 years ◆ Timed score to place nine 11/4-inch pegs in a 5 × 5-inch board and remove them
Jebsen-Taylor Hand Function Test	◆ Evaluates functional capabilities ◆ Subtests include writing, card turning, picking up small objects, simulated feeding, stacking checkers, and picking up light and heavy objects
Minnesota Rate of Manipulation Test	◆ Measures dexterity ◆ Assesses placing, turning, displacing, one-hand turning and placing, and two-hand turning and placing of round blocks
Arthritis Hand Function Test	◆ Functional capabilities plus grip and pinch strength ◆ Items: peg board dexterity, cut putty, lace and tie bow on shoe, use coins, pour water, lift tray of cans, open and close safety pins, unbutton and button buttons
TEMPA	◆ Evaluates routine daily tasks ◆ Tasks: pick up and move jar, open jar and spoon coffee, pour water from pitcher, open lock and take top off pill box, write and affix stamp, put scarf around neck, shuffle and deal cards, use coins, pick up and move small objects

Source: Reprinted and adapted from Kohlmeyer, K. (2003). Sensory and neuromuscular function. In E. B. Crepeau, E. S. Cohn, & B. A. B. Schell (Eds.), *Willard & Spackman's occupational therapy* (10th ed., pp. 365–426). Baltimore: Lippincott Williams & Wilkins. See appendix A for author, source, and descriptions of assessments.

timed and involve object manipulation, grasp and release, prehension patterns, and hand posture. Many are standardized and have norms. However, the majority of them do not assess fine motor function as occurs in daily tasks. The Arthritis Hand Function Test (Backman, Mackie, & Harris, 1991) and the Test d'Évaluation des Membres Supérieurs des Personnes Agées (TEMPA) (Desrosiers, Hébert, Dutil, & Bravo, 1993) are two more recently developed tests that do use tasks in daily living but are not commercially available and require assembly and fabrication to simulate daily tasks.

Endurance

Endurance is the ability to sustain a given activity over time. It can be compromised by inactivity, immobilization, cardiorespiratory deconditioning, muscular deconditioning, and diminished flexibility (Kohlmeyer, 2003). Table 54.2

TABLE 54.2 MET VALUES FOR SOME OCCUPATIONAL PERFORMANCE AREAS

METs	Oxygen Consumed (mL/kg/min)	Level of Activity	Self-Care Activities	Instrumental Activities of Daily Living and Work Activities	Play and Leisure Activities
1.5–2.0	4–7	Very light, minimal	Eating, shaving, grooming, getting in and out of bed, dressing, undressing, standing, walking 1 km/h or 1.6 mph	Working at desk, typing, writing	Playing cards, sewing, knitting
2–3	7–11	Light	Showering in warm water, level walking 2 km/h or 3.25 mph	Ironing, light woodworking, using riding lawnmower	Level bicycling 8 km/h or 5 mph, playing billiards, bowling, golfing with power cart
3–4	11–14	Moderate	Walking 5 km/h or 3.5 mph	Cleaning windows, making beds, mopping floors, vacuuming, bricklaying, doing machine assembly	Bicycling 10 km/h or 6 mph, fly fishing standing in waders, horseshoe pitching
4–5	14–18	Heavy	Showering in hot water, walking 5.5 km/h or 3.5 mph	Scrubbing floors, hoeing, raking leaves, doing light carpentry	Bicycling 13 km/h or 8 mph, table tennis, doubles tennis
5–6	18–21	Heavy	Walking 6.5 km/h or 4 mph	Digging in garden, shoveling light earth	Bicycling 16 km/h or 10 mph, canoeing 6.5 km/h or 4 mph, ice skating or roller skating 15 km/h or 9 mph
6–7	21–25	Very heavy	Walking 8 km/h or 5 mph	Shoveling snow, splitting wood	Bicycling 17.5 km/h or 11 mph, light downhill skiing, ski touring 4 km/h or 2.5 mph

mL/kg/min = milliliters per kilogram body weight per minute; km/h = kilometers per hour; mph = miles per hour.

Source: Data from Ainsworth et al., 1998; Wilmore & Costill, 1999. Reprinted from Kohlmeyer, K. (2003). Sensory and neuromuscular function. In E. B. Crepeau, E. S. Cohn, & B. A. B. Schell (Eds.). *Willard & Spackman's occupational therapy* (10th ed., p. 390). Baltimore: Lippincott Williams & Wilkins.

provides a summary of cardiorespiratory endurance, metabolic equivalent capacity values, and biomechanical and neuromuscular endurance (Kohlmeyer, 2003). For occupational therapists, observation of endurance, or how long clients can participate in daily activities, is probably the most pertinent clinical assessment (Kohlmeyer, 2003).

INTERVENTION

Much like assessment, the intervention process is one that blends attention to the client's occupational performance and to the underlying musculoskeletal factors affecting performance. The time and sequencing of these interventions are related to the acuity or chronicity of the impairment as well as to client priorities.

Splints and Orthotics

Splints and orthotics are external devices that are applied to the body to immobilize, restrain, or support injured tissues; align or correct deformities; and improve function (Anderson, Anderson, & Glanze, 1998; O'Toole, 1997). With regard to musculoskeletal conditions, splints and orthoses may be used to support healing. Basic anatomical and biomechanical considerations for fit and fabrication of splints are provided in Box 54.2.

In some musculoskeletal conditions, such as arthritis and cumulative trauma disorders, splints can be used to reduce stress on joints such as wrist support splints for

---

BOX 54.2 BASIC ANATOMICAL AND BIOMECHANICAL CONSIDERATIONS WHEN MAKING A SPLINT

- Preserve palmar arches.
- Use hand creases as landmarks for splint design and molding.
- Maintain antideformity position.
- Properly position and tighten straps to allow blood flow or venous return.
- Properly contour splints.
- Avoid or minimize pressure over bony prominence.
- Allow motion out of the splint when possible.

Reprinted from Emerson, S., & Shafer, A. (2003). Splinting and orthotics. In E. B. Crepeau, E. S. Cohn, & B. A. B. Schell (Eds). Willard & Spackman's Occupational Therapy (10th ed. pp. 677). Baltimore: Lippincott Williams & Wilkins.

---

carpel tunnel syndrome and arthritis pain. Thumb splints may be indicated for CMC arthritis or deQuervain's tendinitis. Splints can also be used to align or correct deformities; for example, ulnar deviation splints can be used for clients with rheumatoid arthritis (Figure 54.1).

Range of Motion and Strength Exercises

Although it is nice to think that performing everyday occupations maintains motions in the joints of the extremities, full range is usually not achieved during everyday tasks. Therefore, individuals who have deficits with joint motion might need passive, active assistive, or active range of motion exercises. To improve range of motion, activities must be graded by positioning materials and equipment to demand greater reach. However, compliance with exercise programs also needs to be considered. Self-efficacy, or the belief that one can perform the exercises, and the convenience of fitting an exercise program into one's daily routine are important factors to consider (Chen, Neufield, Feeley, & Skinner, 1999). For example, it might be easier for a mother with two young children to do her shoulder exercises in the morning during a shower where she can walk her fingertips up to a point on the shower wall, before her children wake up. On the other hand, a person who is retired might choose to do her exercises in the middle of the morning after a leisurely breakfast. Support from family and friends can also help with compliance. Therefore, therapists should make sure clients and families or caregivers understand the exercises and should provide them with written or picture instructions. Setting realistic weekly goals and reviewing them on a regular basis have been shown to be important factors in compliance with exercise programs (Chen et al., 1999).

For some clients, if the underlying reasons for the decreased motion are scar tissue or pain, physical agent modalities such as ultrasound or heat (e.g., a paraffin bath) may also be indicated (see Table 54.3). Physical modalities should be used as an adjunct to therapy, and therapists are encouraged to pursue professional education, including supervised use of modalities before using them (American Occupational Therapy Association, 2003).

A rehabilitation approach would be to provide an individual with long-handled assistive devices such as reachers or built-up handles on tools to compensate for range of motion deficits. Numerous assistive devices are available to compensate for decreased range of motion, such as long-handled utensils, shoehorns, combs and brushes, dressing sticks, reachers, sock aids, and long-handled sponges. The use of these items and other strategies are discussed in Chapter 49.

However, in determining which frame of reference to use, therapists must consider the reason for and duration of the joint limitation and the goals. It might not be possible to increase joint motion in a person who has had rheumatoid

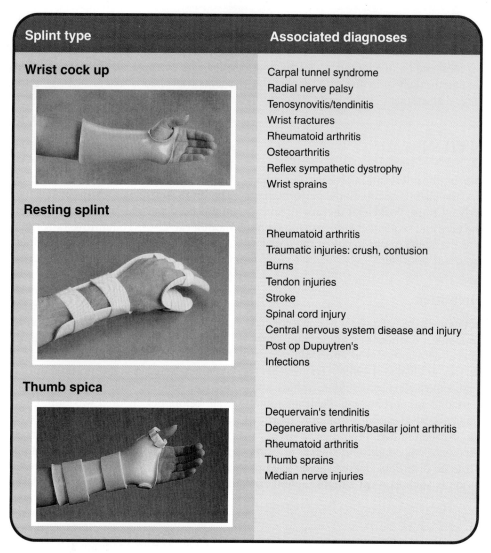

Splint type	Associated diagnoses
Wrist cock up	Carpal tunnel syndrome Radial nerve palsy Tenosynovitis/tendinitis Wrist fractures Rheumatoid arthritis Osteoarthritis Reflex sympathetic dystrophy Wrist sprains
Resting splint	Rheumatoid arthritis Traumatic injuries: crush, contusion Burns Tendon injuries Stroke Spinal cord injury Central nervous system disease and injury Post op Dupuytren's Infections
Thumb spica	Dequervain's tendinitis Degenerative arthritis/basilar joint arthritis Rheumatoid arthritis Thumb sprains Median nerve injuries

FIGURE 54.1 Common static splints associated with diagnostic conditions. (Photos courtesy of the Rehabilitation Division of Smith & Nephew, Germantown, WI.)

TABLE 54.3 PHYSICAL AGENT MODALITIES

Modality	Indications	Contraindications/ Precautions	Evidence for Effectiveness of the Modality
Superficial heat Hot packs, heating pads Paraffin wax Fluidotherapy Whirlpool	Prior to active exercise, passive stretching, and joint mobilization Before traction and soft tissue mobilization Reduce pain and muscle spasms After acute inflammation to increase tissue healing	Decreased circulation Decreased sensibility Altered cardiorespiratory status Open wounds or recently healed burns (paraffin) Significant areas of edema Over tissue during acute inflammation	Limited evidence for fluidotherapy Some evidence that superficial heat and paraffin wax reduce pain and increase motion in persons with arthritis (Minor & Sanford, 1993; Steultjens et al., 2002)

Continued

TABLE 54.3 PHYSICAL AGENT MODALITIES *Continued*

Modality	Indications	Contraindications/ Precautions	Evidence for Effectiveness of the Modality
Deep heat Ultrasound	Soft tissue tightness Subacute and chronic inflammation (e.g., tendinitis) Bone fracture Wound healing	Do not use over or near the eyes, ears, heart, pregnant uterus, testes, known or expected malignant tumor, pacemaker, joint replacements or metal implants, or insensate areas	Review by Robertson and Baker (2001) found eight articles that showed ultrasound to be no more effective than placebo in promoting tissue healing and decreasing pain, and two studies showed ultrasound to be beneficial. For people with rheumatoid arthritis, ultrasound to both surfaces of the hand increased grip strength (Casimiro et al., 2002).
Therapeutic cold Cold packs and cold baths Ice massage	Minimize acute inflammation associated with therapeutic intervention Reduce edema and bleeding Reduce spasticity	Temperature sensation deficits Circulation deficits Altered cardiorespiratory status Cold hypersensitivity such as Raynaud's phenomenon	Inconclusive evidence. Several systematic reviews (Bleakley, McDonough, & MacAuley, 2004; Hubbard, Aronson, & Denegar, 2004; Hubbard & Denegar, 2004) report some evidence for physiological responses to cold on blood flow, tissue temperature, and swelling, but few studies document a return to participation in valued occupations. Studies vary in duration, intensity, and mode, which limits conclusions that can be made.
Contrast baths	Promotes tissue healing	Cardiovascular problems as fluctuations in pulse and blood pressure may occur Peripheral vascular diseases Loss of sensation Pregnancy Cold hypersensitivity such as Raynaud's phenomenon	Inclusive evidence
Electrotherapy Iontophoresis	Modulate pain Decrease inflammation (e.g., bursitis, tendinitis) Reduce edema	Do not use over or near the eyes, ears, chest of person with cardiac disease, pregnant uterus, wounds or skin breaks, known or expected malignant tumor, pacemaker, blood vessels susceptible to hemorrhage, thrombosis or embolus, or insensate areas	Few studies available

ETHICAL DILEMMA

How Much Knowledge is Needed to Use Modalities?

You are an occupational therapy student at a hand rehabilitation center. Your supervisor is at a meeting at the moment, and you are to treat her client. The client has arrived, and the first intervention is ultrasound to the scar tissue on the client's hand. You had a brief lecture in school on ultrasound and tried it on one of your classmates. The technician in the room says that she has set the client up several times with ultrasound and can help you get started. What do you do?

---

arthritis for many years and has joint destruction; for this person, the goal might be to prevent further deformities and functional limitations and use compensatory methods. Similarly, for an adolescent who was recently diagnosed with rheumatoid arthritis, the goal would be to prevent joint limitations and destruction. On the other hand, for a person who has undergone recent surgery or has been in a cast because of a fracture, the decrease in joint motion is due to temporary immobilization and is probably amenable to change. For this person, more aggressive therapy using a physical agent modality (i.e., a hot pack) along with activities or exercise would be indicated to improve motion. Shiraishi, Fujii, and Kobayashi (2002) found that despite aggressive occupational therapy intervention to improve strength and motion after reconstructive surgery of the shoulder joint, a rehabilitative frame of reference was necessary to help clients maximize use of the contralateral intact upper extremity, as was education regarding use of assistive devices.

Strengthening and Endurance

In designing an intervention program for a person who needs strengthening, the occupational therapist must consider the role of resistance, the effect of gravity, and the type and speed of muscle contractions. Resistance is often used to stimulate muscle contractions and increase the firing of additional motor units to increase strength. In addition, muscles have to work harder to move a body part against gravity than to move in a gravity-eliminated or horizontal plane (O'Mahony, 2003). Most occupations require a combination of **isometric** (holding contractions) and **concentric** (shortening) contractions against a force. Thus, the occupational therapist must consider the strength of a muscle or muscles, precautions for movement, prognosis, and occupational demands (O'Mahony, 2003). See Table 54.4 for descriptions of

specific exercise programs including passive exercise, isotonic active assistive exercise, **isotonic** active exercise, isotonic resistive exercise, and isometric exercises. The occupational therapy practitioner can structure the exercise program using active motion by adding resistance as indicated. The resistance can be weights; Thera-Band, Thera-Tubing, or Theraputty; or springs. The therapist can also structure an occupation to grade the type of muscle contractions or amount of resistance, such as wiping off a table in a gravity-eliminated plane (isotonic active exercise), putting cans of food away on a cupboard shelf that is above shoulder height (isotonic resistive exercise), or cleaning a mirror above shoulder height (holding the shoulder in flexion and wiping from right to left would be isometric resistive exercise for the deltoid muscle). The resistance may be a weight, a spring, Thera-Tubing or Theraputty, or simply the weight of a limb. Therapists can also increase resistance by using tools of differing weights (e.g., a light versus a heavy hammer or sanding blocks of different weights or grade of sandpaper) or varying the resistance of a material (stiff versus soft cookie or bread dough or Theraputty).

In occupation-based approaches, relevant activities can be graded to increase strength, or assistive devices can be provided to compensate for the strength or endurance deficits. An individual might vacuum with a heavy or lightweight vacuum cleaner or use electric appliances to open cans and jars. However, the resistance offered by the occupation is often not great enough to increase strength in larger or stronger muscles. For example, a young man with a spinal cord injury at the C6 level needs to have enough strength in his shoulders, biceps, and wrist extensor muscles to be able to move and lift his body and legs for dressing and transferring his body to different surfaces. Although he can practice these occupations repetitively, which will lead to greater strength, actual strengthening exercises will

TABLE 54.4   EXERCISE PROGRAMS

Type	Definition	Resistance	Muscles Grades	Precautions
Passive exercise	Involves passive range of motion and passive stretch, usually done by a practitioner	None Stretch may be held 15–30 seconds	Zero Trace	Inflammation Limited sensation for pain Prolonged immobilization
Isotonic active assistive exercise	Client moves the joint as far as possible, then an outside force such as a practitioner or equipment assists with moving the joint through the rest of the range	None	Trace Poor minus Fair minus	None
Isotonic active exercise	Client moves the joint through available range of motion without any assistance. The muscle shortens and lengthens.	None	Poor Fair	Poor muscles: Move in gravity eliminated plane Fair muscles: Move in against gravity plane
Isometric without resistance	Client contracts the muscle, increasing the tension, and holds the position for 5 seconds. Used when motion of a joint is prohibited.	None	Trace Poor Fair Good	Clients with cardiac conditions and high blood pressure
Isotonic resistive exercise	An isotonic contraction against resistance	Resistance provided by wrist weights, dumbbells, Thera-Band, Theraputty, elastic bands, springs, weights	Fair plus Good	Inflammation Unstable joint Recent or unhealed fracture Use with caution with conditions that are exacerbated by fatigue
Isometric resistive exercise	An isometric contraction against a load	Resistance could be an immovable surface (e.g., pushing the palm against a wall).	Fair plus Good	Clients with cardiac conditions and high blood pressure
Isokinetic exercise	Exercise that uses a machine that controls the speed of contraction within the range of motion	Resistance controlled by machine and is variable in proportion to the change in muscle length throughout the range of motion	Fair plus Good	Inflammation Unstable joint Recent or unhealed fracture Use with caution with conditions that are exacerbated by fatigue

improve his strength faster and lead to faster achievement of independence and could preserve independence (Nyland et al., 2000). In these situations, optimum therapy thus involves both exercise and engagement in desired occupational activity.

Other compensatory approaches to treat strength and endurance impairments might consist of using lighter-weight tools; using electric appliances; and client education regarding joint protection, energy conservation, and work simplification (Tables 54.5 and 54.6).

TABLE 54.5 PRINCIPLES FOR JOINT PROTECTION

Principles	Examples
1. Respect pain.	If pain persists more than 2 hours after performing an activity, modify the activity by spending less time on it, using adaptive equipment, or resting during activity.
2. Use proper body mechanics and use joints in good alignment.	Lean forward to put weight over the feet, and use armrests on chairs to come to standing. Use the palms of the hands on the armrests to push up to standing. Push or pull objects, rather than lifting. Avoid bending, reaching, and twisting.
3. Avoid holding one position for a long time and prolonged repetitive motions.	Alternate sitting and standing during an activity, or shift around. Relax and stretch the hands every 5 minutes when doing an activity that requires holding objects or tools such as holding cards, pencils, telephone, knitting or crochet needles, garden, kitchen, or hand tools. Avoid kneeling to scrub the floor or to garden; instead, sit on a stool and use longer-handled tools
4. Avoid positions and stress that cause deformity.	Avoid pressures along the lateral (thumb) side of fingers that encourage ulnar deviation such as turning keys, doorknobs, and screwdrivers. Avoid pressure against the back of the fingers and wrist, such as propping the chin on the back of the hand. Avoid excessive and constant pressure against the pad of the thumb. Avoid positions of ulnar deviation of the wrist, such as cutting with scissors or cutting with knives.
5. Use the larger and strongest muscles and joints.	Carry a briefcase or purse over one or both shoulders instead of holding it with the fingers. Use the palm of the hands to lift pots and pans. Lift objects using leg muscles instead of back muscles.
6. Balance rest and activity.	Exercise and activity are important for joint mobility and strength, but leisure and work should be balanced with periods of rest.
7. Never begin an activity that cannot be stopped immediately if needed.	Preplan and pace activities. Try to slide, push, or pull objects rather than lifting. Also see energy conservation principles.

Dexterity

In designing an intervention program to improve dexterity, key factors are practice and repetition. In addition, during practice, the occupational therapist might want to consider changing the level of difficulty or complexity of the occupation or activity. Retraining a client's ability to keyboard might require practice using only a few fingers at a time to relearn finger placement. In the beginning, a client might type only individual letters or three- to four-letter words and then progress to longer words, sentences, and paragraphs. In this particular activity, speed might be an important factor to be considered, so another way to grade the activity would be to increase speed requirements of keyboarding. For other types of clients, the size or shape or even texture of the objects might also be altered. For example, in training a person to use a prosthesis, the therapist might start by having the client pick up one-inch cubes with flat sides and then progress to round objects such as pegs and then to flat objects such as checkers. The size of each of these objects could be decreased, and the texture could be changed by using a cube of cheese, a paper cup, or a flat cracker.

Compensatory approaches to dexterity impairments might consist of using adapted equipment such as button hooks, zipper pulls, and elastic laces to help manage fasteners during dressing. A therapist might also suggest that clients eliminate fasteners altogether by wearing pullover shirts, pants with an elastic waistband, and/or slip-on shoes. Other suggestions might include utensil holders or universal cuffs, weighted utensils if stability is needed, plate guards, stabilizers for plates and glasses, wash mitts,

TABLE 54.6   PRINCIPLES AND EXAMPLES OF ENERGY CONSERVATION

Principles	Examples
1. Plan ahead.	Gather all items needed before an activity. Spread heavy and light tasks throughout the day and week.
2. Pace yourself.	Perform energy-demanding tasks earlier in the day. Plan the day to balance rest and activity. Break activities into smaller units that can be done over a number of days. Pace yourself during activities, and do not rush. Take frequent rest breaks.
3. Prioritize.	Decide activities that are important to be completed and ones that can be completed later or eliminated. Delegate tasks to other family members.
4. Sit when possible.	Use a seat in the shower. Sit on the bed or a chair to get dressed. Consider using a high stool.
5. Use work simplification techniques.	Eliminate unnecessary tasks (e.g., buy permanent-press clothes, precut vegetables). Work in a well-lit and well-ventilated environment.
6. Maintain good posture.	Avoid a prolonged stooped posture. Avoid excessive reaching and bending by prearranging work centers to be at an appropriate height and keeping frequently used items at comfortable heights.

electric razors instead of safety razors, and voice-operated computer systems. See Chapter 48 for more ideas for compensation.

Activities of Daily Living

Assisting individuals to improve occupational performance or resume their occupations is the primary objective for occupational therapists working with individuals with musculoskeletal impairment (see Case Studies pp. 670–671). In conjunction with the suggestions provided in Chapter 48, the following should be considered in working with people who have musculoskeletal impairments:

- Application and removal of splints, orthoses, and/or prosthetics
- Use of long-term splints and prostheses
- Performing tasks with adaptive devices
- Developing adaptive techniques for temporary use following a recoverable injury
- Understanding precautions relevant to the impairment, such as encouraging a client to use total hip precautions
- Energy conservation and work simplification procedures, especially for people with arthritis or when endurance is an issue, such as with older adults

- Principles of motor learning, especially in training or retraining activities of daily living (see Box 54.1).

Table 54.7 lists musculoskeletal conditions of the lower extremities, back, and pelvis that are commonly treated by occupational therapists and describes intervention considerations and equipment. Dohli and colleagues (2003) stated that for these conditions, the areas of occupation that should be addressed include bed mobility, lower body bathing and dressing, transfers, home management, care of others or pets, childrearing, community mobility, meal preparation and cleanup, safety procedures and emergency responses, sexual activity, shopping, work or school, play, leisure, and social participation.

Table 54.8 shows musculoskeletal conditions of the upper extremities and intervention considerations and equipment. Since upper extremity and hand use is critical to the performance of occupations, limitations or loss of independence will be a primary concern. Individuals might experience a temporary or permanent change in hand dominance and need to compensate with the less involved extremity. Bilateral capabilities are compromised, and safety and speed of performance are therefore affected. Work and social participation can be disrupted, leading to anxiety and depression. Depending on the condition, deformities, amputations, or severe scarring can result in changes in appearance.

CASE STUDY: *Marita: A Client with a Total Hip Replacement*

Occupational therapy referral: The occupational therapy consult is "status post left total hip replacement as a result of degenerative joint disease."

Occupational profile: Marita is a divorced 63-year-old who resides alone in a two-story home. Premorbidly, she completed all housekeeping independently, including cooking, cleaning, and shopping. She attends weekly group activities at the senior citizens' center and engages in church activities.

Treatment setting: Inpatient rehabilitation hospital.

Disposition setting: Home.

Occupational therapy goals: While observing hip precautions and weight bearing as tolerated, Marita will, in 1 week, be able to:

◆ Prepare a frozen food entrée in the microwave with minimal assistance while ambulatory using a standard walker and walker basket.

◆ Independently don and doff shoes and socks using adaptive equipment while seated in an armchair.

◆ Develop a plan with minimal assistance for securing temporary help from others for obtaining groceries and mail.

Source: Reprinted from Dohli, C., Leibold, M. L., & Schreiber, J. (2003). Adult orthopedic dysfunction. In E. B. Crepeau, E. S. Cohn, & B. A. B. Schell (Eds.), Willard & Spackman's occupational therapy *(10th ed., p. 791). Baltimore: Lippincott Williams & Wilkins.*

CASE STUDY: *Joy: A Client with a Lower Extremity Amputation*

Occupational therapy referral: The occupational therapy consult is "status post left below the knee amputation because of diabetes." The client is in the prosthetic training phase.

Occupational profile: Joy is a widowed 78-year-old who lives alone in a third-floor apartment; she receives Meals-on-Wheels. She is a retired high school teacher who enjoys TV game shows and reading the Bible. Her two adult daughters reside out of state.

Treatment setting: Skilled nursing facility (while endurance is low).

Disposition setting: Inpatient rehabilitation center (when she is able to tolerate 3 hours of treatment per day).

Occupational therapy goals: Joy, in 1 week, wearing the prosthesis will be able to:

◆ Complete her morning grooming activities while standing at the bathroom sink with moderate assistance for maintaining standing balance.

◆ Complete lower body dressing while seated in an armchair at bedside with moderate assistance using adapted methods.

◆ Inspect her left lower extremity residual limb with a mirror and correctly identify areas of potential skin breakdown to the therapist with minimal assistance.

Source: Reprinted from Dohli, C., Leibold, M. L., & Schreiber, J. (2003). Adult orthopedic dysfunction. In E. B. Crepeau, E. S. Cohn, & B. A. B. Schell (Eds.), Willard & Spackman's occupational therapy *(10th ed., p. 792). Baltimore: Lippincott Williams & Wilkins.*

CASE STUDY: *Joe: A Client with a Hand Injury*

Occupational therapy referral: The occupational therapy consult is "for a right hand splint to increase flexion of fractured fourth and fifth metacarpals as a result of an injury at work." His cast for his right hand has been removed.

Occupational profile: Joe is a single 25-year-old who worked in construction. He lives alone and enjoys watching TV and playing games on the PlayStation.

Treatment setting: Outpatient clinic
Disposition setting: Home
Occupational therapy goals: Joe, in 1 week, will be able to:
- Independently don and doff hand splint.
- Complete morning grooming and hygiene activities independently using right hand to hold tools.
- Demonstrate an increase of 5 pounds of grip strength in order to hold a pair of pliers.

CASE STUDY: *Lee Ann: A Client with Arthritis*

Occupational therapy referral: The occupational therapy consult is "diagnosis of rheumatoid arthritis."

Occupational profile: Lee Ann is a 41-year-old who is married and has two children, aged 11 and 13 years. She lives in a one-story, three-bedroom home and works part time as an educational assistant at her daughters' school. She loves to bake. The pain in her hands makes it difficult for her to write and cut with scissors, tasks that she needs to do for her job. She fatigues easily.

Treatment setting: Inpatient rehabilitation setting

Disposition setting: Home
Occupational therapy goals: Lee Ann, in 1 week, will be able to:
- Utilize joint protection techniques 80% of the time while performing a baking task.
- Identify 2 styles of writing tools and adapted scissors in order to write and cut without pain.
- Utilize energy conservations techniques 80% of the time during daily living skills.

CASE STUDY: *Michelle: A Client with Tendinitis of the Abductor Pollicis Longus and Extensor Pollicis Brevis Tendons of the Thumb (DeQuervain's)*

Occupational therapy referral: The occupational therapy consult is "pain and swelling of the abductor pollicis longus and extensor pollicis brevis tendons."

Occupational profile: Michelle is a 37-year-old who is married. She works as a beautician 20–25 hours a week. In the last few weeks, she has scheduled all her appointments into three days because she started another part-time job in a store with home furnishings and accessories. The second job is "just for fun," as she really loves to work on hair. The pain in her thumbs is so bad that she can hardly cut hair.

Treatment setting: Outpatient setting

Disposition setting: Home
Occupational therapy goals: Michelle, in 1 week, will be able to:
- Wear her forearm-based thumb spica splint while performing her second job and in the evenings.
- Apply ice for 5–10 minutes between hair appointments if possible and rest her thumb.
- Identify two types of ergonomic scissors in order to cut hair without pain.
- Develop a schedule to spread out the time spent in both jobs more evenly throughout the week.

TABLE 54.7   OCCUPATIONAL THERAPY CONSIDERATIONS FOR CLIENTS WITH ORTHOPEDIC CONDITIONS OF THE BACK AND LOWER EXTREMITIES

Condition	Description	Precautions	Intervention Considerations and Equipment
Hip fracture with closed reduction	Break in any portion of femur that can be manipulated into its natural position without major surgery	Weight bearing established by physician; hip precautions	◆ Eating, grooming, and upper body dressing typically require assistance from another person for gathering, setting up, and putting away needed supplies; client can then complete tasks either long sitting in bed with an over-the-bed table or seated on the edge of the bed, seated in a wheelchair, or seated in an armchair at a table or sink.
Total hip replacement or total hip arthroplasty	Surgical removal of a diseased or injured hip joint, which is replaced with a prosthetic appliance		◆ Lower body dressing can be accomplished with equipment or adaptations as needed (e.g., reacher, dressing stick, sock aid, long shoehorn, elastic shoelaces, and/or hook-and-loop tape shoe closures); oversize clothing may ease dressing; standing should be encouraged during dressing (client can alternate sitting and standing during activities). ◆ Toileting equipment must enable client to maintain hip precautions; options include standard elevated toilet seat (or model designed for hip injuries) with bilateral arm supports or bedside commode with adjustable legs for use alone or positioned over toilet. ◆ Bathing may be completed by using a transfer tub bench, hand-held shower, nonskid mat, and long-handled sponge; client may choose to sponge-bathe at the sink or bedside instead. ◆ Abduction wedge pillow can be used to prevent internal rotation of the affected hip while in bed or seated. ◆ Walker bag or basket and/or wheeled cart can be used to retrieve and transport items safely.
Hip fracture with open reduction and internal fixation	Surgical procedure that uses wires, screws, or pins applied directly to fractured bone segments to keep them in place	Weight bearing established by physician	◆ Clients often do not require strict hip precautions; treatment considerations as described above may be implemented to enhance performance and minimize pain; this may be especially beneficial immediately post surgery, and equipment can be loaned to the client.

TABLE 54.7 OCCUPATIONAL THERAPY CONSIDERATIONS FOR CLIENTS WITH ORTHOPEDIC CONDITIONS OF THE BACK AND LOWER EXTREMITIES *Continued*

Condition	Description	Precautions	Intervention Considerations and Equipment
Knee replacement	Implantation of device to substitute for damaged joint surfaces	Weight bearing established by physician	◆ Typically, active movement of the knee is encouraged during *all* activities; the client's ability or willingness to flex knee may initially be limited because of fear or pain; twisting motions that put undue stress on the joint should be avoided. ◆ All activities of daily living (ADLs) and instrumental activities of daily living (IADLs) can be completed in a manner selected by the client once safety has been demonstrated and knee flexion has been promoted. Completion without the use of adaptive equipment is encouraged to promote normal movement; however, it may be used initially in some instances to enhance performance, encourage participation, and minimize pain. ◆ Walker bag or basket and/or wheeled cart may be used to retrieve and transport items safely while the client uses an ambulation device. ◆ If needed, equipment may be used on a long-term basis for independence.
Vertebral compression fracture (without CNS involvement)	Fracture of vertebral body, often associated with osteoporosis	Rolling in bed restricted to log-rolling technique; orthotic device may be used to restrict vertebral mobility (e.g., corset type or rigid body jacket); wearing schedule determined by physician	◆ Eating, grooming, and upper body dressing typically require assistance from another person for gathering, setting up, and putting away needed supplies; client can then complete tasks either long sitting in bed with an over-the-bed table or seated on the edge of the bed, in a wheelchair, or in an armchair at a table or sink. ◆ If an orthotic device is worn only when out of bed, the following sequence is recommended: Client lies in bed without the device; completes upper body bathing while semireclined; dons a thin T-shirt or undershirt; resumes a supine position, log–rolls, and dons the orthotic device; returns to supine and fastens the orthotic device; the client is now ready to assume a seated position on the edge of the bed.

Continued

TABLE 54.7 OCCUPATIONAL THERAPY CONSIDERATIONS FOR CLIENTS WITH ORTHOPEDIC CONDITIONS OF THE BACK AND LOWER EXTREMITIES *Continued*

Condition	Description	Precautions	Intervention Considerations and Equipment
			◆ Lower body dressing can be accomplished with equipment or adaptations as needed (e.g., a reacher, dressing stick, sock aid, long shoehorn, elastic shoelaces, and/or hook-and-loop tape shoe closures); oversize clothing may help to accommodate an orthotic device. ◆ Standing should be encouraged during dressing; the client can alternate sitting and standing during activities. ◆ Use of an elevated toilet seat and bilateral arm supports for toileting may enhance performance by increasing safety, decreasing anxiety, and increasing confidence. ◆ Bathing is restricted to long sitting in bed without the brace or sitting in a chair with the orthotic device in place. ◆ A walker bag or basket and/or wheeled cart may be used to retrieve and transport items safely.
Pelvic fracture	Break in any part of the pelvic ring or acetabulum	Hip flexion limited to 60 degrees; non-weight-bearing for both lower extremities	◆ Eating, grooming, and upper body dressing typically require assistance from another person for gathering, setting up, and putting away needed supplies; the client can then complete tasks long sitting in bed with the bed inclined to 60 degrees to adhere to precautions. ◆ Lower body dressing and bathing can be accomplished long sitting in bed with the bed inclined to 60 degrees and with equipment and adaptations as needed (e.g., reacher, dressing stick, sock aid, long shoehorn, elastic shoelaces, hook-and-loop tape shoe closures, and/or long-handled sponge); the client typically requires assistance with lower extremity dressing and bathing in conjunction with long-handled equipment. ◆ Toileting is managed either in bed with a bedpan or using a bedside commode with drop arms and a backrest that allows the client to maintain hip flexion at 60 degrees.

TABLE 54.7 OCCUPATIONAL THERAPY CONSIDERATIONS FOR CLIENTS WITH ORTHOPEDIC CONDITIONS OF THE BACK AND LOWER EXTREMITIES *Continued*

Condition	Description	Precautions	Intervention Considerations and Equipment
			◆ Bed mobility may be enhanced by use of a trapeze bar placed on a hospital bed. ◆ A reclining wheelchair is necessary for mobility to adhere to precautions; choice of proper wheelchair cushion is necessary to maintain skin integrity due to non-weight-bearing status. ◆ Completing functional transfers usually requires another person to assist with lower extremities during transfer; a sliding board may also be necessary to secure safe, confident transfers.
Lower extremity amputation: preprosthetic training phase	Loss of any part of the legs or feet (before artificial limb replacement)	Balance precautions owing to change in center of gravity; fall risk owing to phantom limb sensation and balance deficits	◆ Addition of antitipper bars and/or counterbalancing to the wheelchair to avoid tipping should be considered to accommodate for change in the center of gravity. ◆ All ADLs and IADLs can be completed in a manner selected by the client once safety has been demonstrated; the client completes tasks either from a wheelchair or ambulatory level, depending on a variety of factors (e.g., medical condition, balance, activity tolerance, cognition, and environmental accessibility). ◆ Use of an elevated toilet seat and bilateral arm supports for toileting may enhance performance by increasing safety, decreasing anxiety, and increasing confidence. ◆ Bathing may be completed with use of a tub transfer bench, tub seat, or sponge-bathing.
Lower extremity amputation: prosthetic training phase	Period in which client learns to use lower extremity prosthesis	Preprosthetic precautions as applicable; maintenance of skin integrity, especially during prosthetic use	◆ All ADLs and IADLs can be completed in a manner selected by the client once safety has been demonstrated; the client completes tasks either from a wheelchair or ambulatory level, depending on a variety of factors (e.g., medical condition, balance, activity tolerance, cognition, and environmental accessibility).

Continued

TABLE 54.7 OCCUPATIONAL THERAPY CONSIDERATIONS FOR CLIENTS WITH ORTHOPEDIC CONDITIONS OF THE BACK AND LOWER EXTREMITIES *Continued*

Condition	Description	Precautions	Intervention Considerations and Equipment
			◆ The following dressing procedures are recommended: Client with one prosthesis sits on the edge of the bed or in an armchair, dresses the prosthesis first, then dons the device and dresses the other leg; client with bilateral prostheses sits in an armchair or in bed, dresses both prosthetic devices, and then dons them; socks and shoes on a prosthesis should be inspected, cleaned, and changed as needed. ◆ Use of an elevated toilet seat and bilateral arm supports for toileting may enhance performance by increasing safety, decreasing anxiety, and increasing confidence. ◆ Bathing may be completed with the use of a tub transfer bench, tub seat, or sponge-bathing; cleaning of the prosthesis is done regularly as instructed by the prosthetist; the residual limb should be kept dry to maintain skin integrity and avoid skin breakdown; the client's bathing schedule should be arranged to allow a maximum amount of time so that the residual limb and prosthesis may dry thoroughly.

Source: Reprinted from Dohli, C., Leibold, M. L., & Schreiber, J. (2003). Adult orthopedic dysfunction. In E. B. Crepeau, E. S. Cohn, & B. A. B. Schell (Eds.), *Willard & Spackman's occupational therapy* (10th ed., pp. 793–795). Baltimore: Lippincott Williams & Wilkins.

TABLE 54.8 OCCUPATIONAL THERAPY CONSIDERATIONS FOR CLIENTS WITH SELECTED ORTHOPEDIC CONDITIONS OF THE UPPER EXTREMITIES

Condition	Description	Precautions	Intervention Considerations and Equipment
Shoulder: rotator cuff repair	Surgical repair of a tear in one of the rotator cuff muscles	Immobilized in sling PROM; progression to active-assist and isometric/isotonic	There might be a temporary change in hand dominance. Compensation with the less involved extremity. Bilateral capabilities affected. Sling and abduction pillow at night. Might need to wear front buttoning oversized shirts because they are easier to put on and can fit over the sling if necessary. Eliminating socks and wearing slip-on shoes will be easier initially; a long-handled shoes horn might help. Elastic waist pants might be easier to put on and remove, although usually the hand on the operated side is not enclosed by the sling. Bathing might require a long-handled sponge

TABLE 54.8 OCCUPATIONAL THERAPY CONSIDERATIONS FOR CLIENTS WITH SELECTED ORTHOPEDIC CONDITIONS OF THE UPPER EXTREMITIES *Continued*

Condition	Description	Precautions	Intervention Considerations and Equipment
Hand: laceration, penetration, compression	Direct trauma	Insensitivity Safety issue Pain Skin integrity Edema Immobility	There might be a temporary or permanent change in hand dominance. Compensation with the less involved extremity. Bilateral capabilities affected, so adapted equipment might be required to stabilize or compensate, such as elastic shoelaces, suction brush sponge, rocker knife, electric can opener, plastic disposable dental flossers. Client and/or family might have to be able to remove and apply a splint or orthotic device.
Repetitive use of upper extremity/ies	Inflammation of tendon cumulative effect of repeated stress on tissue	Inflammation Pain Swelling Sensory impairment Motor involvement	Ergonomic assessment modification of work station, job site, tools, and hand positions may be indicated. Splints may be needed in acute phase. An assessment should also be made of everyday activities to determine repetitive patterns.
Arthritis	Inflammation in joints	Sensory impairments Pain Swelling Deformities	Clients need to be instructed in and use principles of joint protection and energy conservation in all daily occupations. Adapted equipment should be used only to protect joints or improve function. A warm shower in the morning can help to loosen up joints, but client might need long-handled sponge. Dressing might be easier with pullover shirts, elastic waists on pants, slip-on shoes; however, assistive devices such as button hook, long shoehorns, dressing sticks may be used. Client and/or family might have to be able to remove and apply a splint or orthotic device. Involvement of the lower extremities might require a raised toilet seat and/or grab bars. Because of the chronic nature of the disease, psychological adjustment to the progressive disability and lifestyle changes may occur.
Upper extremity amputation	Loss of any part of the arm or hand	Insensitivity Pain Skin integrity Postural changes	Loss of any part of a limb can result in changes in body image. There might be a permanent change in hand dominance. Compensation with the unamputated limb. Bilateral capabilities are affected when the prosthesis is not worn, so adapted equipment might be required to stabilize or compensate, such as elastic shoelaces, suction brush sponge, rocker knife, electric can opener, plastic disposable dental flossers. Client and/or family might have to be able to remove and apply the prosthesis. Client must determine which occupations can be performed with and without the prosthesis.

COMMENTARY ON THE EVIDENCE

Interventions for Clients with Musculoskeletal Impairments

Although the effectiveness of interventions for musculoskeletal impairments is scarce in the occupational therapy literature, numerous studies do exist in the hand therapy and rheumatology literature that examine the effectiveness of range of motion and strengthening and endurance programs. Paraffin baths with and without a combined hand exercise program have been shown to be effective in increasing joint motion, strength, and hand function in people with rheumatoid arthritis (Buljina, Taljanovic, Avdic, & Hunter, 2001; Dellhag, Wollersjo, & Bjelle, 1992), osteoarthritis (Stamm, 2002), and scleroderma (Sandqvist, Akesson, & Eklund, 2004).

In a systematic review of hand exercises for people with rheumatoid arthritis, Wessel (2004) reported that of the nine studies that met her criteria for review, there were improvements in hand joint motion, strength, and dexterity. However, a number of different outcomes were studied, follow-up periods varied, therapist bias was present, power analyses were not done, and the impact on everyday activities was not studied. Michlovitz, Harris, and Watkins (2004) investigated the effectiveness of various interventions to increase joint range of motion in people with more varied types of diagnoses (fracture, fracture/dislocation, joint injury, or soft tissue injuries). The following interventions were reviewed for the above-mentioned diagnoses: splints and casts, joint mobilization, continuous passive motion, injection versus other therapist, and in-clinic versus home exercise. They reported moderate support for splints and casts and passive exercise and insufficient evidence to support continuous passive motion. They found no studies that assessed heat modalities such as hot packs, paraffin, fluidotherapy, ultrasound, or stretch for the diagnoses that were studied. Other studies have compared the effectiveness of exercise program versus activities or games and computer games in improving motion and strength (Jaris, Shavit, & Ratzon, 2000). Edema, motion, and grip strength improved after a five-week treatment for wrist movements regardless of which intervention was used.

The effectiveness of client-centered occupational therapy services for people with hand injuries showed improvements in functional measures after six to eight weeks of therapy (Case-Smith, 2003). The Canadian Occupational Performance Measure was used as an outcome measure and to identify individual functional goals. The interventions consisted of splints, therapeutic exercise and activities, manual therapy, activities of daily living, and physical agent modalities, primarily ultrasound. At the end of six to eight weeks, individuals made significant improvements in functional activities, and 80% of subjects returned to work (Case-Smith, 2003).

Steultjens, Dekker, Bouter, Van Schaardenburg, Van Kuyk, and Van Den Ende (2002) conducted a systematic review of controlled clinical and randomized control trials of occupational therapy intervention for people with rheumatoid arthritis. Studies were categorized into themes: comprehensive occupational therapy, training of motor function such as exercise, instruction in joint protection and energy conservation, assistive devices, and splints. They reported limited evidence for the effectiveness of comprehensive occupational therapy in functional ability, no evidence for the effects of exercises on pain and functional ability, limited evidence that joint protection leads to improvement in performing occupations, and insufficient data in the use of assistive devices. Evidence was found that splints reduce pain and increase grip strength but reduce dexterity. However, Steultjens and colleagues (2002) rated the overall methodological quality of studies as weak and without power.

CONCLUSION

Occupational therapists frequently encounter individuals who have musculoskeletal impairments that limit the performance of daily activities. An important factor to consider in working with individuals who have such impairments is to ensure that appropriate precautions are followed, especially after surgery. Regardless of what theoretical framework is used to evaluate and treat individuals with these impairments, the goal is to improve performance in desired occupations within the constraints of the precautions and musculoskeletal impairments themselves.

ACKNOWLEDGMENTS

The author appreciates the contributions of Cathy Dolhi, Karen Kolhmeyer, Mary Lou Leibold, and Jody Schreiber from their work in the Tenth Edition of *Willard and Spackman*. Aspects of their work have been embedded in this chapter.

PROVOCATIVE QUESTIONS

1. Compare and contrast frames of references for intervention for a person with rheumatoid arthritis who has had the disease for 15 years and has joint limitations and mild hand deformities versus a person who has had the disease for 1 year and has similar joint limitations and hand deformities.
2. Discuss how you might use principles of motor learning to teach transfers to a client who has had a recent hip replacement with a posterior approach.

REFERENCES

Ainsworth, B., Haskell, W., Leon, A., Jacobs, Jr., kd., Montoye, H., Sallis, J., & Paffenbarger, R. Jr. (1998). Compendium of physical activities: Classification of energy costs of human physical activities. In J. Roitman (Ed.), *ACSM' resource manual for exercise testing and prescription* (pp. 657–665). Baltimore: Williams & Wilkins.

Amadio, P. C., Silverstein, M. D., Ilstrup, D. M., Schleck, C. D., & Jensen, L. M. (1996). Outcome assessment for carpal tunnel surgery: The relative responsiveness of generic, arthritis-specific disease-specific and physical examination measures. *Journal of Hand Surgery, 21A*, 338–346.

American Occupational Therapy Association. (2003). Physical agent modalities: Position paper. *American Journal of Occupational Therapy, 57*, 650–651.

Anderson, K., Anderson, L., & Glanze, W. (Eds.). (1998). *Mosby's medical, nursing, and allied health dictionary* (5th ed.). St. Louis: Mosby.

Backman, C., Mackie, H., & Harris, J. (1991). Arthritis Hand Function Test: Development of a standardized assessment tool. *Occupational Therapy Journal of Research, 11*, 245–255.

Bleakley, C., McDonough, S., & MacAuley, D. (2004). The use of ice in the treatment of acute soft-tissue injury: A systematic review of randomized controlled trials. *The American Journal of Sports Medicine, 32*, 251–261.

Buljina, A. I., Taljanovic, M. S., Avdic, D. M., & Hunter, T. B. (2001). Physical and exercise therapy for treatment of the rheumatoid hand. *Arthritis Care and Research, 45*, 392–397.

Case-Smith, J. (2003). Outcomes in hand rehabilitation using occupational therapy services. *American Journal of Occupational Therapy, 57*, 499–506.

Casimiro, L., Brosseau, L., Robinson, V., Milne, S., Judd, M., Wells, G., et al. (2002). Therapeutic ultrasound for the treatment of rheumatoid arthritis. *Cochrane Database System Reviews, 3*, CD003787.

Chen, C. Y., Neufeld, P. S., Feely, C. A., & Skinner, C. S. (1999). Factors influencing compliance with home exercise program among patients with upper-extremity impairment. *American Journal of Occupational Therapy, 53*, 171–180.

Daniels, L., & Worthington, C. (1986). *Muscle testing: Techniques of manual examination* (5th ed.). Philadelphia: Saunders.

Dellhag, B., Wollersjo, I., & Bjelle, A. (1992). Effect of active hand exercise and wax bath treatment in rheumatoid arthritis. *Arthritis Care and Research, 2*, 87–91.

Desrosiers, J., Hébert, R., Dutil, E., & Bravo, G. (1993). Development and reliability of an upper extremity function test for the elderly: The TEMPA. *Canadian Journal of Occupational Therapy, 60*, 9–16.

Dohli, C., Leibold, M. L., & Schreiber, J. (2003). Adult orthopedic dysfunction. In E. B. Crepeau, E. S. Cohn, & B. A. B. Schell (Eds.), *Willard & Spackman's occupational therapy* (10th ed., pp. 789–796). Baltimore: Lippincott Williams & Wilkins.

Emerson, S., & Shafer, A. (2003). Splinting and orthotics. In E. B. Crepeau, E. S. Cohn, & B. A. B. Schell (Eds.), *Willard & Spackman's occupational therapy* (10th ed., pp. 676–687). Baltimore: Lippincott Williams & Wilkins.

Flinn, N. A., Trombly Latham, C. A., & Podolski, C. R. (2007). Assessing abilities and capacities: Range of motion, strength, and endurance. In M. V. Radomski & C. A. Trombly Latham (Eds.), *Occupational therapy for physical dysfunction* (6th ed., pp. 91–85). Philadelphia: Lippincott Williams & Wilkins.

Hagedorn, R. (1997). *Foundations for practice in occupational therapy* (2nd ed.). New York: Churchill Livingstone.

Hammond, A., & Freeman, K. (2001). One-year outcomes of a randomized controlled trial of an educational-behavioural joint protection programme for people with rheumatoid arthritis. *Rheumatology, 40*, 1044–1051.

Hanlon, R. E. (1996). Motor learning following unilateral stroke. *Archives of Physical Medicine and Rehabilitation, 77*, 811–815.

Hubbard, T. J., Aronson, S. L., & Denegar, C. R. (2004). Does cryotherapy hasten return to participation?: A systematic review. *Journal of Athletic Training, 39*, 88–94.

Hubbard, T. J., & Denegar, C. R. (2004). Does cryotherapy improve outcomes with soft tissue injury? *Journal of Athletic Training, 39*, 278–279.

James, A. B. (2003). Biomechanical frame of reference. In E. B. Crepeau, E. S. Cohn, & B. A. B. Schell (Eds.), *Willard & Spackman's occupational therapy* (10th ed., pp. 240–242). Baltimore: Lippincott Williams & Wilkins.

Jarus, T., Shavit, S., & Ratzon, N. (2000). From hand twister to mind twister: Computer-aided treatment in traumatic wrist fracture. *American Journal of Occupational Therapy, 54*, 176–182.

Kendall, F. P., McCreary, E. K., & Provance, P. G. (1993). *Muscles testing and function* (4th ed.). Baltimore: Williams & Wilkins.

Killingsworth, A. P. (2006). Occupation-based functional motion assessment. In H. M. Pendleton & W. Schultz-Krohn (Eds.), *Pedretti's Occupational therapy: Practice skills for physical dysfunction* (6th ed., pp. 429–436). St. Louis: Mosby.

Killingsworth, A. P. & Pedretti, L. W. (2006a). Joint range of motion. In H. M. Pendleton & W. Schultz-Krohn (Eds.). Pedretti's Occupational therapy: Practice skills for physical dysfunction (6th ed. pp. 437–468). St. Louis: Mosby.

Killingsworth, A. P., & Pedretti, L. W. (2006b). Evaluation of muscle strength. In H. M. Pendleton & W. Schultz-Krohn (Eds.). Pedretti's Occupational therapy: Practice skills for physical dysfunction (6th ed. pp. 469–512). St. Louis: Mosby.

Kohlmeyer, K. (2003). Sensory and neuromuscular function. In E. B. Crepeau, E. S. Cohn, & B. A. B. Schell (Eds.), Willard & Spackman's occupational therapy (10th ed., pp. 365–426). Baltimore: Lippincott Williams & Wilkins.

Lee, T. D., & Magill, R. A. (1983). The locus of contextual interference in motor-skill acquisition. Journal of Experimental Psychology, 9, 730–746.

Mathiowetz, V., Kashman, N., Volland, G., Weber, K., Dowe, M., & Rogers, S. (1985). Grip and pinch strength: Normative data for adults. Archives of Physical Medicine and Rehabilitation, 66, 69–74.

Michlovitz, S. L., Harris, B. A., & Watkins, M. P. (2004). Therapy interventions for improving joint range of motion: A systemic review. Journal of Hand Therapy, 17, 118–131.

Minor, M. A., & Sanford, M. K. (1993). Physical interventions in the management of pain in arthritis. Arthritis Care & Research, 6, 197–206.

Norkin, C. C., & White, D. J. (1995). Measurement of joint motion: A guide to goniometry (2nd ed.). Philadelphia: F. A. Davis.

Nyland, J., Quigley, P., Huang, C., Lloyd, J., Harrow, J., & Nelson, A. (2000). Preserving transfer independence among individuals with spinal cord injury. Spinal Cord, 38, 649–657.

O'Mahony, D. P. (2003) Strengthening. In E. B. Crepeau, E. S. Cohn, & B. A. B. Schell (Eds.), Willard & Spackman's occupational therapy (10th ed., pp. 581–586). Baltimore: Lippincott Williams & Wilkins.

O'Toole, M. (Ed.). (1997). Miller and Keane encyclopedia and dictionary of medical nursing and allied health (6th ed.). Philadelphia: Saunders.

Poole, J. L. (1991). Application of motor learning principles in occupational therapy. American Journal of Occupational Therapy, 45, 531–537.

Poole, J. L. (1995). Learning. In C. A. Trombly (Ed.), Occupational therapy for physical dysfunction (4th ed., pp. 265–276). Baltimore: Williams & Wilkins.

Robertson, V. J., & Baker, K. G. (2001). A review of therapeutic ultrasound: Effectiveness studies. Physical Therapy, 81, 1339–1350.

Sandqvist, G., Akesson, A., & Eklund, M. (2004). Evaluation of paraffin bath treatments in patients with systemic sclerosis. Disability and Rehabilitation, 26, 981–987.

Seidel, A. C. (2003). Rehabilitative frame of reference. In E. B. Crepeau, E. S. Cohn, & B. A. B. Schell (Eds.), Willard & Spackman's occupational therapy (10th ed., pp. 238–240). Baltimore: Lippincott Williams & Wilkins.

Shea, J. B., & Morgan, R. L. (1979). Contextual interference effects on the acquisition, retention, and transfer of motor skill. Journal of Experimental Psychology, 5, 179–187.

Shiraishi, H., Fujii, S., & Kobayashi, R. (2002). Function of the upper extremity and ability to perform housework following reconstructive surgery of the shoulder joint using a free vascularized fibula bone graft: A case report. Journal of Hand Therapy, 15, 274–281.

Stamm, T. A. (2002). Joint protection and home hand exercises improve hand function in patients with hand osteoarthritis: A randomized controlled trial. Arthritis Care and Research, 47, 44–49.

Steultjens, E. M. J., Dekker, J., Bouter, L. M., van Schaardenburg, D., van Kuyk, M. H., & van Den End, C. H. M. (2002). Occupational therapy for rheumatoid arthritis: A systemic review. Arthritis Care and Research, 47, 672–683.

Trombly, C. A. (1995). Theoretical foundations for practice. In C. A. Trombly (Ed.), Occupational therapy for physical dysfunction (4th ed., pp. 15–27). Baltimore: Williams & Wilkins.

Wessel, J. (2004). The effectiveness of hand exercises for persons with rheumatoid arthritis: a systemic review. Journal of Hand Therapy, 17, 174–180.

Wilmore, J. H., & Costill, D. L. (1999). Physiology of sports and exercise (2nd ed.). Champaign, IL: Human Kinetics.

Motor Skills and Occupational Performance: Assessments and Interventions

CLARE G. GIUFFRIDA
AND MARTIN S. RICE

Learning Objectives

After reading this chapter, you will be able to:

1. Discuss the emergence, control, and learning of motor skills from a systems perspective.
2. Identify the different terms that are used to describe movement organization and motor behaviors that contribute to skilled performance.
3. Identify the role of the occupational therapy practitioner in assessing and treating people with performance deficits in everyday skills and routines secondary to motor impairments.
4. Describe various types of motor dysfunction that are seen in people with central nervous system dysfunction and developmental disorders.
5. Identify the different strategies and measurement tools that are used to assess patients with deficits in skilled performance.
6. Discuss the influence of neuroscientific and movement scientific findings as well as evidence-based practices on occupational therapy assessment and interventions focused on everyday skill recovery and learning.
7. Discuss the strategies that are used by the neurophysiological and task-related systems approaches to intervention and the recovery of everyday skill.

Outline   *Continued*

Occupational therapy practitioners assess and treat patients with a variety of neuromotor impairments that interfere with movement control and organization. These deficits are displayed by both children and adults with specific difficulties such as tone irregularities, loss of postural and or limb control, motor planning problems, and motor coordination deficits as well as by children and adults with delayed sensory motor development. From an occupational therapy perspective, movement problems can interfere with the individual's performance of everyday tasks and the organization of purposeful and meaningful activities into daily occupations.

This chapter focuses on identifying common elements of movement control and organization that are essential to an individual's motor development and attainment of fundamental motor skills as well as life skills.

THE EMERGENCE OF MOTOR SKILLS

Conceptually, the development of motor skills, regardless of one's age, is essential for success in any type of occupation that requires a motor component. This statement hints at the foundation on which much occupational therapy treatment is based. Numerous factors contribute to success in motor skills, not the least of which is an intact central nervous system (CNS). As the CNS develops from infancy through early adulthood, there are associated increases in **motor skill** ability. Although motor skills per se are not automatically developed, their age-appropriate emergence is limited to the maturational level of the various systems of the body, including the CNS. The integrity of the CNS is the ultimate rate-limiting factor in determining any potential success in acquiring motor skills. It has been proposed that motor skills are not actually *developed* at all; rather, they are *acquired*. For example, a child who is beginning to learn how to walk will make many attempts at taking his or her first step before actually being successful. In the process of these attempts, the child is learning consciously and subconsciously about the limits of his or her **stability**, **postural control**, and **balance**. Once these (and several other factors) have been at least marginally accounted for, the

child will be successful in acquiring the ability to actually take that first step.

The development of motor abilities, however, is based on more than just CNS maturation. Many systems develop and change simultaneously along with the CNS, including, but not limited to, the muscular, skeletal, and endocrine systems. Each system within the body develops at its own rate and experiences periods of varying degrees of change across time. For any given motor skill, success with acquiring that skill rests on the critical maturation of any number of underlying systems (e.g., skeletal size, muscle strength, and postural stability). When each of the systems has reached a level of development that supports the acquisition of the new skill, the child then has the capability to acquire that new skill (Thelen, 1995). A large part of learning requires that the child learn what his or her body can and cannot do, given the constraints of the environment and the task at hand. Once the child's systems have the developmental maturity to allow the child to have the capability to learn a new skill and the child experiences the environmental constraints (physical constraints, social constraints, and task constraints), then all of the ingredients for successful learning are in place. Stated another way, once experimentation occurs, the child will learn how to succeed, given his or her developmental maturation and environmental constraints.

Reflexes, Myelination, and Maturational Processes in Motor Development

Interestingly, when a child is newly born, the number of neurons within the CNS is approximately 100 billion (Nolte, 2002). After birth, these neurons are believed to be unable to divide and reproduce themselves. Additionally, as a person traverses the decades of his or her life starting in the second decade, the CNS tends to lose neurons. This is considered to be a part of the normal aging process associated with the CNS. The point here, though, is that when a baby is born, it essentially has all of its neurons at the first day of its life. The question then becomes: If the infant has all of its neurons, then why does the child need to learn? Clearly, there are many processes involved in the development of the child. This is particularly true in the child's motor development.

Some of the earliest patterns of movement or positioning are in the form of **primary reflexes**. These primary reflexes are often conspicuous when one views the positioning of a child younger than six months of age. Two common primitive reflexes are known as the asymmetrical tonic neck reflex and the symmetrical tonic neck reflex. These two reflexes affect the position of the upper and lower extremities and are elicited or determined by the position of the head. Although these reflexes remain with us throughout life, their influence on the positioning of the body is not as apparent after the age of approximately six months. Sometimes these reflexes can emerge in older children or adults after an injury to the brain occurs.

There are several theories as to why these primitive reflexes become integrated. One of the most prevalent theories has to do with the rapid myelination of the brain within the first few years of life. The average mass of a human brain at birth is about 400 grams, and by the end of the third year, the mass has increased to approximately 1,200 grams (Nolte, 2002). Much of this increase is thought to come from the myelination of the CNS neurons. Myelination is thought to continue at least into the second decade of life. Further, it is believed that as the individual ages, the rapidity of myelination decreases.

Why is myelination so important? Once myelin is established, the ease of neuronal depolarization and the rate of the neuronal propagation increase dramatically. This results in the ability of the neurons to communicate with each other more efficiently. Simultaneously the establishment and proliferation of neuronal dendrites occur at a relatively intense rate during the early years of life. The more dendrites there are, the more connections there are to other neurons. Whereas the myelin facilitates the speed at which depolarization travels down the neuronal axon, the dendrites act as connections between other neurons. The increase in myelin and dendrites results in more efficient communication to many more neurons, which in turn means that the brain can process much more information much more efficiently. Pragmatically speaking, this results in being able to process more information, allows for greater coordination of movement, and facilitates the ability to learn new skills at a quicker rate.

As these neuronal changes are rapidly developing in typically developing children, growth charts provide some insight into the physical development in terms of height and weight. From birth to approximately age 20, there are two large growth spurts, which can be readily seen in Figure 55.1 and Figure 55.2. Specifically, the rate of

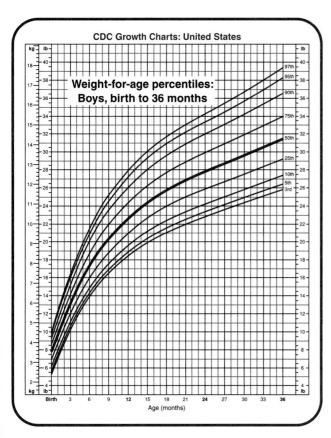

FIGURE 55.1 Centers for Disease Control weight-for-age percentile growth chart for boys from birth to 36 months.

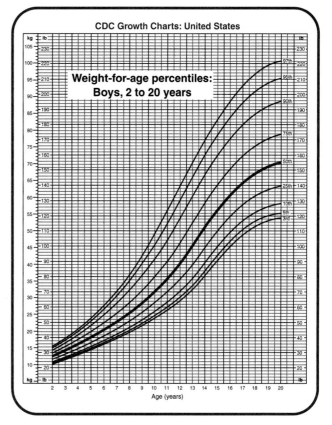

FIGURE 55.2 Centers for Disease Control weight-for-age percentile growth chart for boys from 2 to 20 years.

weight increase is greatest from birth to approximately 18 months, when it begins to plateau. Weight tends to stay relatively stable until approximately age 10 or 11 years; that is, the increase in weight is not as dramatic as it was in the earlier months of life (Figure 55.2). The child continues to develop between the ages of approximately 18 months and age 11, and then a second dramatic weight increase occurs throughout the years of puberty. Much of this weight gain is due to a rapid increase in muscle mass and skeletal growth. Accompanying this weight gain during these pubescent years are substantial maturational changes within the endocrine system.

How Body Systems Change with Motor Development

Once the person has successfully navigated puberty and enters the twenties, many of the body's systems (i.e., muscle mass, skeletal size, CNS myelination) remain relatively stable for the next several decades. However, detrimental changes in muscle mass can been seen as early as age thirty, when loss of muscle fibers begins, continuing to decrease at least through age 75 years (Abrams, Beers, Berkow, Fletcher, & Besdine, 1995). Bone mass is another area that changes, especially for menopausal women, but both sexes normally experience slow progressive loss of bone mass beginning at about age 50 years. Brain mass tends to decline by approximately 10% between the ages of 25 and 90 years (Abrams et al., 1995). This reduction in brain mass is not necessarily associated with decreased cognitive function, though some cognitive changes do occur with the normal aging process. As an example, people with large ventricles can still function normally, while those with "normal" sized ventricles have been known to have severe dementia. Therefore, normal age-related loss of brain mass does not necessarily mean loss of cognitive function.

Although we just touched on three systems that change across the life course (bone mass, muscle mass, and brain mass), changes occur in every organ and system throughout the life course, including, but not limited to, the cardiovascular system, the kidneys, the gastrointestinal system, the skin, and the immune system. Just as when the development of the child's subsystems provides the potential to acquire skills, the opposite can be true as the person traverses the fifth and sixth decades (and beyond). For instance, as the individual ages and experiences age-related organ and system changes, the potential for either learning new skills or maintaining the ability to perform skills learned earlier in life may decline. Having discussed some developmental, growth, and maturational issues that occur throughout life, we turn in the following section to motor control concepts that are specific to functional movement and skills.

THE INTERACTION OF MOTOR TASKS WITH THE ENVIRONMENT AND THE PERSON

Movement, with all its exquisite manifestations, is essential to the performance of everyday activity and skills. Occupational activities, such as writing and typing, require developing and organizing movements or actions that adapt to the task demands. For example, writing on a piece of paper requires organizing several actions: (1) reaching for a pen, (2) orienting, (3) grasping and (4) holding a pen to write on the surface of a piece of paper, (5) generating thoughts to write with the pen on the paper, (6) forming and initiating the plan to write, (7) executing the action plan for writing, (8) completing and stopping writing. In current scientific thought, movement emerges from the interaction of the individual with the task and the environment (Shumway-Cook & Woollacott, 1995). How we write will depend on the tool we grasp, the surface we write on, the message we want to convey, and what we know about the act of writing. The organization of each movement we make varies depending on the person and the task and reflects the multiple influences of the physical, social, and cultural environment on the person and the task. Movements are task specific, context dependent, and constrained by factors inherent to the situation. For example, the act of reaching depends on the posture, position, location, and size of the person reaching, as well as the size and placement of the object being reached for and its location relative to the person reaching. If a person has a disability that interferes with or disrupts the ability to move, then that person's initiation and/or task performance is affected. All individuals generate movements in line with task demands, and each person's ability to adapt to changing task demands on a daily basis reflects his or her functional capabilities and limitations. Current thinking highlights the expression of movement as a function of the integrity of the individual, the task, and the environment and not solely as the expression of neuromotor and musculoskeletal processes within the person. The scientific thinking that guided therapeutic practice from the 1950s through the 1980s relied heavily on the understanding of movement as both neuromotor and musculoskeletal derived. However, contemporary thinking highlights a multidimensional systems approach to motor development and motor control. Figure 55.3 illustrates this fundamental thought about a systems and multifactorial approach to the organization of movement and factors controlling movement.

Motor Control and Individual Constraints on Movement

Motor control involves both the study and understanding of the nature and regulation of movement. Motor

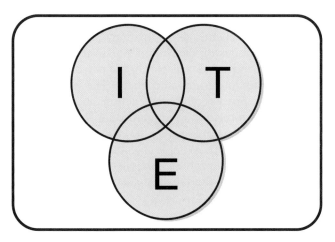

FIGURE 55.3 Interaction of the individual, the task, and the environment. (I = individual, T = task, E = environment).

control is seen as the end product of a dynamic interaction between the person's cognitive-perception-action systems, the task at hand, and the environment (Heriza, 1991; Shumway-Cook & Woollacott, 2001). An overview of the different body systems within the individual that contribute to movement follows.

Movement and Sensation/Perception

Most motor control theories propose several roles for sensory input and feedback in movement regulation. The sensory channels provide information from the environment and the body that is useful in initiating and maintaining movement. Sensory input not only has a role in initiating movement, but also has a role as sensory feedback in controlling the movement as the movement occurs.

Perception is the integration of sensory impressions from the different sensory sources into psychologically meaningful information. Both the perceptual and sensory systems provide information about the state of the body and features of the environment that influence movement control. Sensation and perceptual information are important to action just as action is essential to perceptual information (Rosenbaum, 1991). We act on what we perceive, and we perceive and act on our perceptions. Therefore, understanding movement requires an understanding of the systems that control sensation and perception and how these systems influence and form action.

Movement and Action

Movements are housed within actions, and for the occupational therapy practitioner, the focus on movement control is to understand how the individual organizes movements into meaningful and purposeful actions, activities, and routines within different occupations. Also, movements are described and best understood within the context of accomplishing goal-directed actions. Movement control is studied within the context of an action, such as reaching, with the

assumption that the control processes that are involved in this function will provide insight into principles related to how similar movements are controlled.

Understanding the control of action implies understanding how the motor output is based on musculoskeletal and neuromuscular components, including movement synergies and the motor programming systems. The musculoskeletal system includes joint and muscle properties, such as joint and muscle lengthening flexibility, contributing to the organization of the movement. There are numerous joints and muscles in the body, and these must be controlled during the execution of coordinated, functional movement. The problem of coordinating many muscles and joints into a **coordinative structure**, called the **degrees of freedom** problem, is a major research issue for motor control researchers.

Another movement structure that is relevant to action are **synergies**, which are categories of movement that require the action of more than one muscle. As defined by Shumway-Cook and Woollacott (2007), synergies are functional couplings of groups of muscles constrained to act as a unit and reflect preferred strategies for moving. Examples include grasping an object and throwing a ball. Synergies are characterized by spatial and temporal characteristics that allow for both stability and flexibility in movement. Flexibility in synergistic patterns allows the coordinated structure to adapt to the environmental demands, while stability is evidenced by the reliability of the spatial and temporal ordering of the specific movement. In the standing position, lower extremity stability is provided by the distal-to-proximal muscle sequence activation, while flexibility allows for walking on an uneven surface (Shumway-Cook & Woollacott, 2007). In occupational therapy literature, atypical synergies associated with impaired movement control have frequently been described, particularly in populations with stroke and cerebral palsy. These atypical flexion- and extension-dominated synergies are groups of muscles acting as mass movement patterns that reflect the individual's response to reorganization of movement control subsequent to brain injury. Such synergies are marked by lack of flexibility and stability and can result in muscle shortening and musculoskeletal deformity as set postures emerge and normal reciprocal movements and sequences do not occur as part of movement control.

Motor Program and Plans

Motor programs and plans are also part of the action system that is hypothesized to influence movement control. Several definitions of motor programs have been offered in the literature. According to Brooks (1986), **motor programs** have been defined as "communications within the central nervous system that are based on past experiences and can generate planned postural adjustments and movements" (p. 7). Alternatively, in motor control literature, motor programs are defined as abstract representations that when initiated result in the production of a coordinated movement sequence (Keele, Cohen, & Ivry, 1990; Schmidt & Lee, 2005). Much of motor control research has focused on examining the hypothesized invariant characteristics of motor programs and their role in movement planning and control. Invariant characteristics of motor programs include the relative timing, the order, and the relative force of an action. Such elements characterize categories of movements, such as throwing. Throwing is the motor programming action, and this action is generalized so that "throwing" can include throwing a football, throwing laundry into a hamper, or throwing a snowball at a friend. Several motor control theorists question the usefulness of the programming construct or the abstract representations of movements. However, the concept of a motor program or a stored representation of movement is central in cognitive approaches to movement planning and control. It is thought that the individual uses existing motor programs to organize motor behavior when faced with novel actions and tasks in the environment. Although there is neurobehavioral evidence to support the notion of motor programs in the individual, how motor programs develop and where they are stored in the individual remain controversial (Shea & Wulf, 2005). Along with movement plans and programs, an understanding of posture, stability, and postural control informs our understanding of movement.

Postural control involves controlling the body's position in space to maintain stability and orientation. Horak and Macpherson (1996) have defined *postural orientation* as the ability to maintain an appropriate relationship between body segments and between the body and the environment for a task. Postural stability or balance is the ability to maintain the body in equilibrium. Maintaining postural control requires two separate sensory motor processes: the sensory organization process and the motor adjustment process. The sensory organization process involves the interplay of one or more of the orientation senses (vision, somatosensory, and vestibular), their integration within the CNS, and their contributions to postural control. The motor adjustment process involves the ability to execute coordinated and properly scaled musculoskeletal responses. The motor responses are automatic processes that develop early in childhood, while the sensory processes develop over time in children and are not fully developed until a child is about 14 or 15 years of age. Both sensory and motor processes are essential to developing and maintaining postural control. Disruptions in these sensory or motor systems due to injury, disease or delay will result in inadequate postural control strategies.

The term *posture* is most often used to describe both the biomechanical alignment of the body and the orientation of the body to the environment. For example, the occupational therapy practitioner might describe the client's posture as sitting, standing, or lying down. When working with a client, the occupational therapy practitioner might focus on developing postural control and coordinative movements as part of the person's need to develop motor programs and plans. The practitioner considers the process of posture, action, and movement organization in relation to an individual's performance of a task and does not focus on the execution of a single movement or posture. What is essential is the therapist's supporting the organization of the client's movement relative to the task and the activity demands associated with different tasks.

Cognition and Action

Actions can occur as a result of external prompts, such as seeing a toothbrush and reaching for it, or reflexively in response to an external stimulus, or as a result of an internal intent or motivation, such as wanting to brush one's teeth in the morning and looking for and reaching for a toothbrush. Cognitive processes that are important to action include attention, memory, motivation, and the emotional aspects of motor control underlying the establishment of the person's intent or goals (Shumway-Cook & Woollacott, 2001). Also, the ability to attend to the relevant cues of a task and the performance environment and the ability to make task comparisons, to evaluate one's own performance, and to identify errors in movement planning are cognitive strategies that are useful in skill learning and relearning.

Reaction Time

One example of cognition and action that has been relatively well researched as a measure of cognitive processing is **reaction time**. Reaction time is considered to be a measure of how efficiently the CNS is working. Reaction time is defined as the time from when a stimulus is given to the time when a movement begins in reaction to the stimulus. There are different types of reaction time. For instance, *simple reaction time* is the reaction time when there is a single stimulus associated with a solitary specific response. For example, suppose that when a person sees a light turn on, he or she is required to reach forward; in this case, there is a one-to-one relationship between the stimulus and the response. *Choice reaction time* is somewhat more complex, occurring when a number of potential stimuli are present and the motor response is unique for each of the different stimuli. For example, there might be three potential stimuli involving a red light, a green light, and a blue light. The directions might be that when he or she sees the red light, the participant is required to lift his or her arm straight up; when he or she sees the green light, the participant is supposed to move his or her arm to the left; and when he or she sees the blue light, the participant is supposed to move his or her hand to the right. It has been shown that a person's choice reaction time performance is typically longer than his or her simple reaction time performance. It has also been shown that the best reaction times occur during the late teens and early twenties and that the reaction time increases each decade thereafter. Men tend to have faster reaction times than women. It also appears that the more education a person has, the better is his or her reaction time (Fozard, Vercryssen, Reynolds, Hancock, & Quilter, 1994; Houx & Jolles 1993) Within the individual movement is the product of many systems that need to be examined as they interact and contribute to movement organization and control. Deficits in one system affect the function of other systems. To understand motor control and organization, the perceptual, cognitive, and action components of motor control must be considered and synthesized as part of the full picture of motor control. In addition to individual body factors affecting control, different tasks as well as the environment impose constraints on motor control (see Figure 55.3).

Task and Environmental Constraints on Movement

Essential to movement control is the nature of the task and the task requirements. Within occupational therapy, the practitioner's role is to help the client be successful with tasks that are important to the client's occupations from basic activities of daily living to complex work or leisure routines. For instance, a therapist might have a child catch a ball while standing still or have the child catch a ball while he or she is running.

In motor behavior research, tasks are categorized according to task features and activity demands. These classifications are based on task attributes that affect postural and movement control and learning. Also, **motor learning** research has focused on examining optimal practice environments and feedback conditions for the learning of different tasks according to task attributes. This framework is helpful for understanding movement control; however, the research that has been done in this area with patient populations while performing activities of daily living and functional tasks is limited.

Discrete, Serial, and Continuous Movement Tasks

Discrete tasks are those with a recognizable beginning and end. For example, going from a sitting to a standing position, lying down in bed, and turning on the ignition of a car with a key are examples of discrete movements. A series of discrete movements performed together are referred to as **serial tasks**. An example is the sequence of inserting contact lenses; the steps involved might include removing the contact lens from the case, rinsing it with solution, orienting the contact lens on the finger, and finally applying the lens to the cornea of the eye. According to Schmidt and Lee (2005), serial tasks are composed of an ordered set of discrete movements. Most actions in basic and instrumental activities of daily living such as hygiene and dressing are serial in nature. Continuous tasks are those that have no

recognizable beginning or end; these include walking, running, biking, and, in the realm of hygiene, brushing or combing the hair. In these cases, the beginning and the end of the task are determined by the performer. In all tasks, the nature of the task defines the action needed and the organization of the action. How one learns or relearns tasks is also affected by the type of task.

Open Versus Closed Tasks or Skills

Another task classification system that is used in motor behavior research is based on the task environment interaction defined by Schmidt and Lee (2005) and later elaborated on by Gentile (1992). In this classification system, closed movement tasks are characterized by fixed habitual patterns of movement that are performed in relatively fixed environments. **Closed skills** are somewhat stereotypical, show little trial variability, have low information-processing demands, and require less cognitive attention than open skills. **Open skills** are those that are performed in a constantly changing environment, require the performer to adapt his or her behavior to a constantly changing environment, have high information-processing demands, and are attention demanding. Most basic activities of daily living, such as turning on faucets to wash one's face, are closed skills, while instrumental activities such as driving or maneuvering a grocery cart in a crowded store are open skills. To be successful with open skills, the client must develop a repertoire of movements that allow for adaptation to changing environmental conditions, such as hitting a ball with a bat (Figure 55.4).

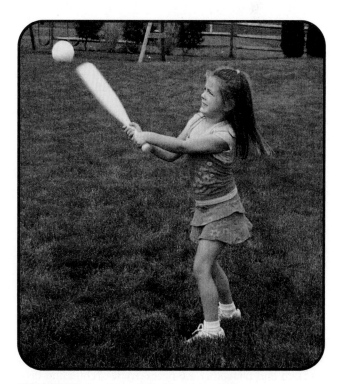

FIGURE 55.4   Open skill of batting a ball.

Stability Versus Mobility Tasks and Manipulation Demands

In classifying tasks and movement demands, Gentile (1992) also introduced a task dimension based on whether the person's base of support is still or in motion. Stability tasks such as sitting or standing are performed with a non-moving base of support. However, mobility tasks, such as walking or running, have a moving base of support. Also, Gentile (1992) took into account the amount of upper extremity manipulation involved in a task, as well as the degree of accuracy and speed necessary for functional performance of tasks. Manipulation tasks such as keyboarding that require speed and accuracy increase demands on the postural system, since body stabilization is critical to task performance.

Regulatory and Nonregulatory Environmental Constraints

As tasks are performed, environmental constraints can influence the person's performance in various ways. Some of these constraints directly regulate the movement, while others may affect performance more indirectly. For example, reaching is constrained by the size shape and weight of a glass that is to be used for drinking. The features of the glass regulate the movement. If the environment is noisy, however, reaching might not be directly affected; in this case, noise is a nonregulatory aspect of the environment. To plan effective interventions, it is necessary to understand the environment and its contribution to movement and to prepare patients to move in a variety of environments.

The Person, the Task, and the Environment

Skill acquisition is dependent on several factors. Practitioners help patients to learn skills, and these skills have multiple dimensions that influence reacquisition. Understanding the types and requirements of tasks as well as the regulatory features of the environment that affect task performance allows the practitioner to plan with the patient the optimal environment for skill learning. Also, understanding how movement control is affected in the client with a neurological disorder and what body systems have been affected helps the practitioner to plan effective multisystems interventions for skill learning.

Along with using task analysis, a task taxonomy can be useful for retraining functional movements in the patient with a neurological disorder. Using the three continuums of closed to open skills, stability to mobility, and no manipulation versus manipulation, the practitioner could assess a client's capability and skill level across many basic and instrumental activities of daily living. By systematically varying the regulatory features of the task and the environment, the practitioner, can help the patient to develop the motor program and plans that are necessary for rebuilding task routines. Now that we have reviewed some fundamental aspects of motor learning and control and its development

from a theoretical perspective, the next section focuses on defining and assessing motor skills and motor performance.

DEFINING AND ASSESSING MOTOR SKILLS AND MOTOR PERFORMANCE PROBLEMS

This section presents concepts from the **International Classification of Function (ICF)** to provide a framework for understanding motor skills and how neuromotor impairments that affect motor skills are defined and assessed. The ICF integrates medical and social models of disability by specifying the nature and parallels between functional ability and disability, as well as the impact of social and environmental factors on performance. According to the ICF, **function** reflects the composite of one's body functions, activity and participation, whereas **disability** reflects impairments, limitations of activity and function, and activity restrictions (Figure 55.5). Within the ICF classification, the person's achievement of a level of function that affords independence and quality of life is the determinant of a successful rehabilitation outcome. The ICF's focus on health and quality of life resonates with the focus of the occupational therapy profession on health and wellness, as well as its focus on the multifaceted aspects of function and occupational performance.

In assessing, treating, and determining client outcomes, the practitioner focuses on understanding the client factors, the client's occupational activity demands, the client's occupational performance contexts, the client's occupational performance patterns, the client's occupational performance skills, and the client's actual performance of and participation in personal tasks and meaningful occupations. Also, in assessing and treating the client, the practitioner observes what the client can and cannot do and what enables or interferes with the client's performances of his or her occupations. In understanding motor control and organization, this means that the practitioner integrates his or her understanding of the individual, the task, and the environment as it relates to movement control and motor skill to address the client's motor issues that interfere with the ability for participation in occupation. It is this integration that uniquely defines the art of occupational therapy as a profession.

This section lists the primary motor terms that are used to explain motor skills Additionally, client factors, including body structures, functions, and impairments that interfere with motor skill acquisition and performance, are defined. This is so that the reader has an understanding of both typical motor skill and the impairments that interfere with motor performance and result in inefficient movements.

From the practitioner's perspective, motor skills are clients' skills in moving and interacting with task, objects, and environment specific to their engagement in the occupations that are meaningful and necessary to their life roles and participation and satisfaction with their life. Also, clients' skilled performance in their occupations will

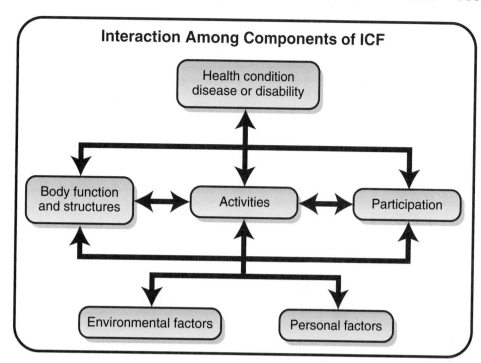

FIGURE 55.5 International Classification of Function.

depend on the integrity of their different body systems (client factors), the composite of activity demands of their occupations, and the influence of and the contexts in which they function.

Motor skill is defined as a goal-related volitional movement that requires both motor and sensory input for success. Motor skills are learned and can wax and wane depending on practice and experience. There can be multiple client factors that interfere with the performance of motor skills, as motor control and organization are integrally involved with the body systems and mental functions contributing to task performance. Not the least of these are neuromotor factors or impairments at the neuromuscular and postural levels that can interfere with motor skill. For instance, in addition to problems with motor planning (e.g., problems with praxis), the disruption of skilled performance can result from postural instability and malalignment, limited functional trunk and limb mobility, dyscoordination of the upper extremities, problems with in-hand manipulation, limb and body weakness, the inability to grade and sustain muscle coactivation and force, and the inability to sequence muscle activity. The following discussion defines terms and impairments that help the practitioner to understand the components of posture, movement, and skill, as well as what neuromuscular impairments can interfere with efficient and skilled movement. The typical components of postural control include posture, alignment, and adaptation.

Posture is a composite of the positions of all the joints of the body at any given time. It is the static position that is assumed by any body part at any time. Therapists must evaluate spinal alignment and curves, pelvis, trunk, head, neck, and upper extremity posture alone and in relation to each other in positions of standing, sitting, and lying down and in the context of occupational performance.

Good body and **postural alignment** occurs when the center of gravity of each body segment is over the supporting base of the body. In the case of a child with cerebral palsy, postural alignment can be limited by the presence of interfering reflexes, such as an asymmetrical tonic neck reflex, which results in the child's body being dominated by more extensor tone on the side of the body to which the head is turned and more flexion tone on the other side of the body (Preston, 2006). Similarly, in a person who has sustained a stroke, atypical muscle synergies can result in an atypical and sustained increase of flexion and or extension tone in different groupings of muscles, leading to postural asymmetries as the client is sitting or standing.

Postural adaptation refers to the ability of the body to maintain balance automatically and remain upright during alterations in positions and challenges to stability. Normal control and adaptation involve the ability to produce movements through adequate ranges and to control movements throughout the ranges. Also, they involve the ability to differentiate and selectively control different body parts; to initiate, stop, and hold a limb in action; and to have normal tone in the body to stabilize the body and support limb movements while the body is stationary or moving. As defined by Howle (2002), **postural control** consists of (1) proactive reactions or postural orientation, which helps to anticipate the appropriate relationship between body segments that is task specific; (2) postural stability, which is the ability to maintain the center of mass within the limits of the base of stability; and (3) reactive postural adjustments, which are flexible and varied responses to perturbations from the environment, self-initiated movements or a moving surface.

When evaluating a client, the practitioner needs to observe the client's posture in the context of his or her everyday actions, such as sitting at a computer, standing, pushing a grocery cart, or lying in bed. During these observations, the practitioner observes what is occurring in the client's body and whether the client is able to move efficiently and easily while also having a goal such as getting out of bed or typing while sitting. In this context, observations are made of the client's postural alignment, initiation of movement, selective and independent control of his or her limbs, and ability to terminate actions. Practitioners should look at the client's posture, alignment, and balance while the client is on stable, hard surfaces and when the client is on an unstable surface or a slippery surface. A difficulty in determining balance deficits is that balance has both sensory and motor components. Appropriate postural control depends on inputs from visual and somatosensory receptors and the vestibular system and

on the ability of the CNS to interpret the relative importance of each. To fully assess balance, the practitioner needs to evaluate all contributions to balance, including perturbations to balance and both sensory and motor influences on postural control. The client's ability to bend and tie shoes and to get into and out of the bathtub should also be assessed as part of the observation of the dynamic nature of postural control. Table 55.1 describes several clinical assessment tools that evaluate postural control.

Tone can be defined in several ways; varies from person to person; and can depend on age, gender, and occupation. Muscle tone is characterized by the stiffness or tension with which a muscle resists being lengthened. Both neural and nonneural mechanisms contribute to muscle tone (Lin, Brown, & Brotherstone, 1994). Normal tone

TABLE 55.1   POSTURAL CONTROL ASSESSMENTS

Assessment	Age Range	Description
Sensory Organization Test (SOT)	Adult	◆ Defines six different sensory conditions or environments to measure postural sway ◆ Assesses influence of vision and somatic and vestibular sensory information
Clinical Testing for Sensory Integration and Balance (CTSIB)	All	◆ A foam surface is used to disrupt somatic sensation ◆ A visual conflict done with dots or lines is used to disrupt vision ◆ Measures client's ability to maintain balance under six conditions
Functional Reach	Adults	◆ Measures the distance that can be reached in standing in a forward direction. It indicates the extent to which the center of the body mass can be moved in a forward direction toward the limit of stability
Timed "Up and Go" Test (TUG)	Adults	◆ Measures the time it takes to stand up from a seat, walk off, and sit down again. It indicates the ability to balance during body translation from one place to another, the ability to balance being interpreted as the time taken to perform the entire sequence
Tinetti's Balance and Gait Evaluation	Adult	◆ Client is asked to do a variety of tasks (e.g., move from sitting to standing and ambulate) ◆ Has high predictive validity for frail elderly at risk for falls
Berg Balance Scale	Adults	◆ Client is asked to complete 14 different tasks; each task is scored by using a four-point scale ◆ Client is asked to complete 14 different tasks; each task is scored using a four-point scale
Limits of Stability Test	Adult	◆ Client stands, and a computerized force plated center of gravity is calculated ◆ Client volitionally shifts weight toward a series of targets ◆ Monitors movement for smoothness and accuracy of postural movements
Fugl-Meyer Sensori-motor Assessment	Adults	◆ Balance subtest measures the amount of assistance and time tolerated using static standing balance and tilting reactions

is characterized by ability to move against gravity, shift between stability and mobility, use muscles in groups or selectively, and balance between agonist and antagonist tone (Preston, 2006). Tone in a muscle can be affected by damage to the nervous system and can increase and decrease as well as vary under different task and environmental conditions (Figure 55.6).

Hypotonia reflected in low-tone clients is a decrease in the sensation of a muscle's resistance to stretch as the joint is moved through the range of motion and the client's inability to recruit adequate force to move against gravity. Clinically, muscles appear soft, joints are lax as cocontraction around the joints is less than optimal because of inadequate force generation, and deep tendon reflexes are absent or diminished. Hypotonia is observed in lesions of the cerebellar pathways, primary muscle diseases, lower motor neuron disorders, and the acute phases of stroke and spinal cord injury. Hypotonia can also be observed as a transient phase in infants with cerebral palsy.

Hypertonia in contrast to hypotonia, is characterized by increased resistance to stretch, a feeling of stiffness, and limits to the range and variety of movements. **Spasticity** is a motor disorder that is characterized by a velocity dependent increase in tonic stretch reflexes with exaggerated tendon jerks resulting from a hyperexcitability of the stretch reflex. Clinically, spasticity is characterized by hypertonic muscles, hyperactive deep tendon reflexes, **clonus**, abnormal spinal reflexes, increased resistance to passive movement, and decreased coordination. Spasticity is influenced by the client's postural status and by extrinsic factors such as anxiety, pain, and temperature extremes. It can be mild, moderate, or severe.

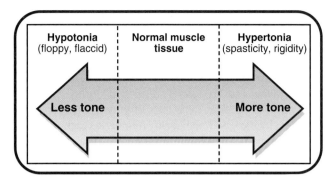

FIGURE 55.6 Tone continuum.

Rigidity is defined as the simultaneous increase of muscle tone in the agonist and antagonist muscles that results in increased resistance to passive motion in any direction. Rigidity occurs in extrapyramidal system lesions such as Parkinson's disease, encephalitis, and tumors. Rigidity that is characterized by a feeling of constant stiffness throughout the range is called *lead pipe rigidity,* whereas rigidity that is characterized by alternating contraction and relaxation is called *cogwheel rigidity.* There are many challenges to assessing muscle tone, as tone can vary and depends on intrinsic and extrinsic factors.

Observation of tone can be evaluated directly by using the Ashworth Scale of Spasticity (Ashworth, 1964) and the Modified Ashworth Scale of Spasticity (Bohannon & Smith, 1987). These scales provide a way to loosely quantify the level of spasticity in muscle. The Modified Ashworth Scale of Spasticity is fairly commonly cited in the literature and is fairly straightforward in its application and interpretation (Table 55.2).

TABLE 55.2 ASHWORTH SCALE OF SPASTICITY AND MODIFIED ASHWORTH SCALE OF SPASTICITY

Ashworth Scale of Spasticity (Ashworth, 1964)	Description	Modified Ashworth Scale of Spasticity (Bohannon & Smith, 1987)
1	"Slight increase in muscle tone with a 'catch' when the limb is moved"	0
	"Slight increase in muscle tone, manifested by minimal resistance at the end of the range of motion when the affected part(s) is moved in flexion or extension"	1
	"Light increase in muscle tone, manifested by a catch, followed by minimal resistance throughout the remainder (less than half) of the range of motion"	1+
2	"More marked increase in muscle tone, but the limb is easily flexed"	2
3	"Considerable increase in muscle tone"	3
4	"Rigid in flexion or extension"	4

Another scale for assessing spasticity is the Tardieu scale (Tardieu, Shentoub, & Delarue, 1954), later adapted by Held and Pierrot-Deseilligney (1969). This scale involves testing spasticity using three separate velocities (V1: as slow as possible, V2: velocity of limb as if it were falling under gravity, and V3: velocity of the limb as fast as possible, that is, faster than the effects of gravity). Under these various velocities, both the quality of muscle reaction ("X") and the angle of the muscle reaction ("Y") are recorded. The quality of muscle reaction uses a five-point scale from zero to four. Zero refers to "no resistance throughout the course of the passive movement." One refers to "slight resistance through the course of the passive movement, with no clear catch at a precise angle." Two refers to a "clear catch at a precise angle, interrupting the passive movement, followed by release." Three refers to "fatigable clonus (<10 seconds when maintaining pressure) occurring at a precise angle." Four refers to "infatigable clonuses (>10 seconds when maintaining pressure) occurring at a precise angle" (Gracies et al., 2000, p. 1555). The angle of muscle reaction is "measured relative to the position of minimal stretch of the muscle (corresponding to angle 0) for all joints except hip, where it is relative to the resting anatomic position" (Gracies et al., 2000, p. 1555.). **Gross coordination** is the combined activity of many muscles into smooth patterns and sequences of motion and is described as smooth, directed, and fluid actions supporting everyday activities. Also, coordinated movement is characterized by rhythm, appropriate muscle tension, appropriate postural tone, and refinement to the minimal number of muscle groups necessary to produce the desired movements and equilibrium. **Coordination** is an automatic response that is monitored primarily through proprioceptive sensory feedback. Visual and tactile sensory feedback, body scheme, and ability to judge and move the body through space also affect overall coordination. **Incoordination** is a broad term that is used for extraneous, uneven, or inaccurate movements. Neurological disorders and trauma such as muscle or peripheral nerve disease and lesions of the cerebellum, spinal cord, and frontal or postcentral cortex can cause unique disturbances in coordination. See Table 55.3 for examples of neurological disorders and their stereotypical coordination patterns.

TABLE 55.3   NEUROLOGICAL DISORDERS AND THEIR STEREOTYPICAL COORDINATION PATTERNS

Category	Description	Test
CEREBELLAR DYSFUNCTION		
Intention tremor	◆ Occurs during voluntary movement, is less apparent or absent during rest, and intensifies at the termination of the movement. ◆ Evident in multiple sclerosis.	◆ Finger-to-finger test, finger-to-nose test. ◆ May have trouble performing tasks that require accuracy and precision of limb placement (e.g., drinking from a cup or inserting a key in a lock).
Essential familial tremor	◆ Inherited as an autosomal-dominant trait, visible when client is carrying out a fine precision and accuracy task.	◆ Have the person reach for an item. Positive if tremors are present during the reach.
Adiadochokinesis	◆ Inability to perform rapid alternating movements, e.g. pronation/supination, elbow flexion/extension.	◆ Tests by counting how many cycles of alternating movements in 10-second time frame. Best to test unaffected/less affected side first, then compare performance to affected side.
Dysdiadochokinesia	◆ Decreased ability to perform rapid alternating movements smoothly.	◆ Supinate/pronate, flex/extend elbow, grasp/release hand, alternating bilateral tasks. Number of alternations within a time period and the differences between extremities are noted.
Dysmetria	◆ Inability to control muscle length results in overshooting when pointing to target objects. ◆ Inability to estimate range of motion necessary to reach a target. Two types include hypermetria (overshoot) and hypometria undershoot).	◆ Finger–to-finger or finger-to-nose tests.

TABLE 55.3   NEUROLOGICAL DISORDERS AND THEIR STEREOTYPICAL COORDINATION PATTERNS *Continued*

Category	Description	Test
Dyssynergia	◆ Movements are broken up into their component parts and appear jerky. Jerky movements are due to lack of synergy between agonist/antagonist. ◆ Can cause problems in articulation and phonation.	◆ Alternating movement, finger-to-nose, finger-to-finger tests.
Ataxia	◆ Delayed initiation of movement responses, errors in range and force of movement, errors in rate and regularity of movement. Poor agonist/antagonist coordination, results in jerky, poorly controlled movements, poor postural stability.	◆ When reaching for object, shortest distance between the client and object is not a straight line.
Ataxic gait	◆ Unsteady, wide-based gait, tendency to veer or fall toward side of lesion. ◆ Staggering, wide-based gait with reduced or no arm swing, uneven step length and tendency to fall.	◆ Observation of walking, turning quickly, walking toe to heel along straight line.
Rebound phenomenon of Holmes	◆ Lack of a check reflex. ◆ Inability to stop a motion quickly to avoid striking something.	◆ Therapist releases resistance to client's elbow flexion unexpectedly, client's hand hits his or her own chest if unable to check motion.
Hypotonia	◆ Decreased muscle tone, decreased resistance to passive movement	◆ Can observe clinically and perform a quick stretch.
Nystagmus	◆ Involuntary (oscillating) movement of eyes. Interferes with head control and balance. Can occur as result of vestibular system, brainstem, or cerebellar lesions.	◆ Can observe by having the person look at a fixed object. Is positive if the eyes make small rapid oscillations (tremorlike movements).
Dysarthria	◆ Explosive or slurred speech caused by incoordination of the speech mechanism. ◆ Speech may vary in pitch, seem nasal or tremulous.	◆ Can observe if ability to articulate words due to the oral-motor and/or larynx musculature. This is a motor problem, not due to aphasia.
POSTERIOR COLUMN DYSFUNCTION		
Ataxia	◆ Wide-based gait results from loss of proprioception, but client can self-correct using vision by watching their feet (compare with cerebellar dysfunction).	◆ Can observe in any part of the body. Is characterized by "large" tremors.
Romberg sign	◆ Inability to maintain standing balance with feet together and eyes closed.	◆ The test is the same as the definition.
BASAL GANGLIA DYSFUNCTION		
Athetoid movements	◆ Continuous, slow, wormlike, arrhythmic movements that primarily affect the distal portions of the extremities. Occur in the same patterns in the same subject, not present during sleep. Co-occurrence with athetosis = choreoathetosis.	◆ Therapist should note proximal or distal involvement extremities involved, pattern of motions, and which stimuli increase/decrease abnormal movements. Its occurrence can be documented through observation.

Continued

TABLE 55.3 NEUROLOGICAL DISORDERS AND THEIR STEREOTYPICAL COORDINATION PATTERNS *Continued*

Category	Description	Test
Dystonia	◆ A form of athetosis that causes twisting movements of the trunk and proximal muscles of the extremities, distorted postures and torsion spasms. ◆ Persistent posturing of the extremities (e.g., hyperextension of hyperflexion of the wrist and fingers) often with concurrent torsion of the spine and twisting of the trunk. Movements are often continuous and seen in conjunction with spasticity. Subtypes included segmental, generalized, focal, and multifocal.	◆ Its occurrence can be documented through observation.
Chorea	◆ Irregular, purposeless, involuntary, coarse, quick, jerky, and dysrhythmic movements of variable distribution. May occur in sleep.	◆ Its occurrence can be documented through observation.
Ballism	◆ A rare symptom produced by continuous, abrupt contraction of axial and proximal musculature of the extremity. Causes the limb to fly out suddenly. Occurs on one side (hemiballism) and is caused by lesions of the opposite subthalamic nucleus.	◆ Its occurrence can be documented through observation.
Resting tremors	◆ Stop at the initiation of voluntary movement, resume during holding phase of motor task (e.g., pill rolling tremor of Parkinsonism). ◆ Occurs at rest and subsides when voluntary movement is attempted. Seen in Parkinson's disease.	◆ Have the person reach for an item. Positive if tremors are present before initiation of the reach but stop when the reach begins.
Bradykinesia	◆ Movement is very slow or even nonexistent, with accompanying rigidity.	◆ Ask the person to move; on attempting to move, the person's motions are extremely slow, if at all. Tone appears to be high.

In addition to direct observation of the client's smooth and fluid movements during life activities and any notable deviations such as tremor at rest, lurching, and overshooting, there are several standardized tests that use speed and accuracy in functional tasks to determine performance, as shown in Table 55.4.

Fine coordination is defined as the smooth and harmonious action of groups of muscles working together to produce a desired motion, whereas **dexterity** is defined as a type of fine coordination that is mostly demonstrated in the use of the upper extremity. Coordination problems can be manifested in irregularity in rate of movement, excessive force, incorrect sequencing, and sudden corrective movements. Practitioners use several standardized tests to assess speed of object manipulation, grasp and release, accuracy of movement, prehension patterns, writing skills, and hand posture, as shown in Table 55.5.

Besides standardized tests that are performance based, it is important to observe the client using the upper extremities in self-help tasks such as buttoning, keyboarding, manipulating change, and writing. The Assessment of Motor and Process Skills, a standardized test based on the client's preferred task to perform, is a tool that was developed by an occupational therapist, Dr. Anne Fisher. The therapist grades the client's performance across tasks according to process, motor, and communication skills. This partitions task performance across the dimensions of posture, mobility coordination, strength, and energy. However, to administer this test, special training is required, which limits the applicability of this tool across populations.

TABLE 55.4 STANDARDIZED TESTS OF MOTOR CONTROL AND SKILL

Assessment	Age Range	Description
Bruininks-Oseretsky Test of Motor Proficiency	4.6–14.5 years	◆ Assesses gross and fine coordination, dexterity, upper limb speed, visual motor control, muscle strength running, balance.
BOT-2: Bruininks-Oseretsky Test of Motor Proficiency, Second Edition	4–21	◆ Covers a broad array of fine and gross motor skills, providing composite scores in four motor areas and one comprehensive measure of overall motor proficiency. These composites are Fine Manual Control, Manual Coordination, Body Coordination, Strength and Agility, and a Total Motor Composite.
Movement ABC	4–12	◆ Identifies and evaluates the movement problems that can determine a child's participation and social adjustment at school and to plan programs for remediation and management. It provides a comprehensive assessment for those who are identified as being at risk, yielding both normative and qualitative measures of movement competence, manual dexterity, ball skills, and static and dynamic balance.
Miller Assessment for Preschoolers	Preschool	◆ Assesses 27 items (e.g., walking a line, stepping, hand-to-nose test) and gross motor assessment.
Quick Neurological Screening Test	5 years–adult	◆ Screens neurological integration (attention, balance, spatial organization, rate and rhythm of movement, motor planning, coordination).
Assessment of Motor and Process Skills	Adults, adolescents, and older children; there is also a school version.	◆ Measures both process and motor skills as they relate to task performance, provides information on how the person is performing in a given context, and is used to predict performance in activities of daily living.
Test of Motor Impairment	5–14 years	◆ Assesses motor deficits (static and dynamic balance, manual dexterity, speed of movement, eye-hand coordination, problem solving ability).

TABLE 55.5 STANDARDIZED TESTS OF UPPER LIMB FUNCTION AND FINE MOTOR COORDINATION

Dexterity Assessment	Age Range	Description and Features
Crawford Small Parts Dexterity Test	Adults	◆ Measures eye-hand coordination and manipulation of small hand tools. ◆ Designed for teenagers and adults. ◆ Uses pins, collars, screws, tweezers, screwdriver. ◆ Client is timed on tasks such as inserting a pin in a hole in a metal plate with tweezers, covering with a collar, threading screws.
Erhardt Developmental Prehension Assessment	Birth–6 years	◆ Measures components and skills of hand function development. ◆ Used for birth–6 years. ◆ Uses a variety of objects (e.g., small suitcase, plastic pail, toy hammer, key, beads, tin can, rubber ball, stacking rings) to measure grasp, reflex, and manipulation skills.

Continued

TABLE 55.5   STANDARDIZED TESTS OF UPPER LIMB FUNCTION AND FINE MOTOR COORDINATION   *Continued*

Dexterity Assessment	Age Range	Description and Features
Melbourne Assessment of Unilateral Upper Limb Function	5–15 years	◆ Measures unilateral upper extremity quality of movement in children from 5 to 15 years of age. It is useful for children who are challenged by any neurological dysfunction.
Pediatric Evaluation of Disability Inventory (PEDI)		◆ Outcome measure that quantifies a child's level of ability and dependence in many functional activities of daily living. PEDI measures task performance in the areas of self-care, mobility, and social functioning.
Arm Motor Ability Test (AMAT)	Adult	◆ Measures ability to perform 13 activities of daily life composed of 1 to 3 component parts. The time taken to complete each task is measured using a stopwatch, and the actions are videotaped and rated on a scale of 1 to 6.
Actual Amount of Use Test (AAUT)	Adults	◆ Measures actual use of the limb on 21 items using a 3-point scale. Patients are videotaped.
Motor Activity Log: Amount of Use Scale (AOU)	Adult	◆ Provides information about actual use of the limb in everyday life situations. Patient reports in a semistructured interview about whether and how well, on a 6 point scale (0–5), 14 daily life activities were performed during a specified period.
Action Research Arm Test (ARA)	1	◆ Three subtests (grasp, grip, and pinch) measure the ability to grasp, move, and release objects of different size, weight, and shape. Scoring is on a 4-point scale (0–3).
Grooved Peg Board Test	5–adult	◆ Measures eye-hand coordination and finger dexterity. ◆ Client places grooved pegs in a 25-hole peg board in various random positions.
Purdue Peg Board Test	5 years +	◆ Measures movements of arms hands, fingers and fingertip dexterity. ◆ Normed for adults and children 5–15 years, 11 months. ◆ Client places pins in a peg board and assembles pins, washers, and collars.
Box and Block Test	7–9 years and adults	◆ Tests manual dexterity ◆ Normed for children 7–9 years, adults and adults with neuromuscular involvement. ◆ Client picks up one black at a time and places it in an attached compartment.
Nine Hole Peg Test of Fine Motor Coordination	Adult	◆ Measures fine dexterity. ◆ Normed for adults >20 years. ◆ Timed score to place nine 1-1/4 inch pegs in a 5 × 5 inch board and remove them.
Jebsen-Taylor Hand Function Test	5 years +	◆ Evaluates functional capabilities. ◆ Subtests include writing, card turning, picking up small objects, simulated feeding, stacking checkers, and picking up light and heavy objects.
Minnesota Rate of Manipulation Test	13 years +	◆ Measures dexterity. ◆ Assesses placing, turning, displacing, one-hand turning and placing, and two-hand turning and placing of round blocks.

Some assessments are more comprehensive that evaluate a number of the issues referred to above, whereas several assessments are easily categorized by problems specific to motor function, motor impairment, motor coordination, and motor control.

INTELLECTUAL HERITAGE AND OCCUPATIONAL THERAPY THEORETICAL FRAMES OF REFERENCE GUIDING NEUROMOTOR INTERVENTIONS

The field of motor control draws from a wide range of disciplines and reflects the scholarly and research activities of scientists who are interested in motor behavior. Research findings and theories about motor control and recovery of function have had an ongoing influence on the practice of occupational therapy focused on adults and children with motor control disorders. In the years following World War II, the dominant therapeutic approach that was used in the field of physical disabilities was muscle reeducation. This approach, although useful for polio, was not appropriate for treating people with disorders of the CNS with resultant paresis. Because of the inadequacies of applying muscle reeducation principles to CNS disorders, a few occupational and physical therapy practitioners (e.g., Ayers, 1972; Bobath, 1965; Brunnstrom, 1970; Knott, 1956; Rood, 1952; Voss, Ionata, & Myers, 1965) began to study and hypothesize about how the nervous system controls movement and applied these principles to clinical practice. As a result of their efforts, the development of organized approaches and techniques to restore CNS function emerged in the therapy fields. The period from the mid-1950s through the 1980s was marked by the development and teaching of specialized neurotherapeutic approaches such as proprioceptive neuromuscular facilitation, neurodevelopmental therapy, and Brunnstrom's movement therapy. These approaches were situated in the knowledge of the time focused on specific sensorimotor techniques and assumptions about the CNS and the organization of motor behavior. More recently, these approaches have been less favored, as there are more current theoretical approaches that have better research evidence supporting their use.

The field of motor control and learning tries to explain both the regulation and control of normal movements, as well as the factors and processes that are involved in normal motor learning. Motor learning is commonly defined as the processes associated with permanent changes in motor behavior resulting from practice and experience. The reader is referred to texts that provide in-depth explanations of the motor learning process and the research that supports learning using different practice conditions and the salient factors such as feedback that affects motor learning (e.g., Brooks, 1986; Schmidt & Lee, 2005).

The motor control approaches that are used in occupational therapy reflect an integration of ideas that explain the nature and regulation of movement. There is no one singular motor control theory of occupational therapy; rather, there are several applied motor learning and control approaches and models. These approaches are supported by motor learning and control research drawn from the movement and therapeutic sciences and provide evidence supporting different occupational therapy interventions.

Understanding motor control implies knowledge about what is controlled and how the controlling processes are organized (Horak, 1991). **Motor control** involves the ability to regulate or direct the mechanisms that are essential to movement. Rosenbaum (1991) has proposed that the central issues in motor control revolve around the multiple factors that determine movement selection, movement sequencing, and the coordination of perception and action in goal-directed activities. For instance, a fundamental question for motor control theorists is how stability is maintained and controlled while the individual acts in and on the environment. In the context of occupational performance, this question becomes "How are postural stability and movement regulated and controlled for in an individual engaged in an everyday daily life activity such as dressing while sitting on a stable or unstable surface such as a chair or soft mattress?"

Motor learning is directed more toward understanding how movements are acquired and modified with practice. Schmidt (1988) has defined motor learning as a set of processes associated with practice or experience leading to permanent changes in the capability for skilled acts. Shumway-Cook and Woollacott (2001) have proposed that motor learning develops from a complex set of perceptual, cognitive, and action that are processes developed in response to individual-task-environment interactions.

The field of motor control and learning continues to provide occupational therapy with new ideas for understanding the nature, cause, acquisition, and modification of movement supporting optimal occupational performance. The following section provides a synopsis of the prevailing motor learning and control theories and their implications for occupational therapy treatment. Theories are organized according to whether the control is centralized within the CNS or dispersed throughout the CNS and or other systems.

Motor development is the culmination of a number of underlying subsystems. These underlying subsystems all develop and mature at their own rates relative to other subsystems. Examples of these subsystems include, but are not limited to, the skeletal system, the muscular system, the central and peripheral nervous systems, the endocrine system, and the sensory systems (visual, auditory, gustatory, olfactory, haptic, proprioceptive, and vestibular systems).

Historically, motor development was thought to occur through specific and prescribed stages. Gessell (1928) and others (Gessell & Ames, 1947; McGraw, 1935) developed ontogenetic stages that depict developmental milestones for children from approximately 6 months to 6 years of age. These developmental milestones include postural and motor abilities that are believed to be stereotypical of various stages of development. The typical development follows certain directions, specifically cephalocaudal (head to tail) and proximodistal (axial to extremities). In other words, developmentally, a child gains control of the head before gaining control of the lower parts of the body (e.g., the ability to walk). In a similar vein, developmental milestones show that proximal stability is required before the affordance of distal mobility. If the trunk is not stable, the ability to successfully reach for an object will be diminished. These directionally dependent constructs require that the CNS organization is largely hierarchical in nature. That is, higher, more complex parts of the brain control or have some dominion over lower centers of the brain. Most primitive reflexes have their neuroanatomical origin in the midbrain, cerebellum, and medulla. As was stated earlier, if damage occurs to a higher area of the brain (e.g., the cerebral cortex), then the reemergence of primitive reflexes is not uncommon. This gave empirical evidence that reaching developmental milestones within the "normal" stereotypical time periods was a good indication of the child's overall development. Further, the evaluation and assessment of primitive reflexes and developmental milestones was believed to be a reliable method for evaluating the potential for success in age appropriate occupations (Capute et al., 1982).

Recently, however, there has been some question as to the veracity of this assumption (Bartlett, 1997). Bartlett evaluated 156 infants who were believed to be developing normally on the Primitive Reflex Profile and the Alberta Infant Motor Scale. Assessments were at 6 weeks and at 3 and 5 months. Bartlett found no statistical correlation between the developmental scale scores and the primitive reflex scores. Thus, Bartlett concluded that there was no relationship between motor development and the presence of primitive reflexes. Along the same lines, Thelen (1986) found that when a 6- to 7-month-old infant was supported over a treadmill, the infant demonstrated a relatively mature bipedal stepping motion. This is particularly interesting because the traditionally held ontogeny of developmental milestones asserted that the stepping motion normally appears as a newborn but then disappears at approximately 2 months only to reappear at approximately 12 months of age (Strauss, 1982). What Thelen has shown was that when the environment was manipulated (e.g., by supporting the child's body weight, thereby reducing the effects of gravity), the child spontaneously demonstrated a precocious bipedal stepping motion. Because it is illogical to think that the CNS matured only while the child was supported, it is clear that the assumed hierarchical organization of the CNS is not the exclusive factor or control mechanism in motor development.

Another line of evidence regarding grip configuration questions the traditionally held belief that there is a stereotypical sequence of hand grasp configurations (J. S. Connolly & Elliott, 1972; K. J. Connolly, 1973; Gessell, 1928). This sequence involves the initial use of a gross grasp/clawlike configuration and ending up with a mature finger-thumb opposition configuration. One group of researchers (Newell, Scully, Tenenbaum, & Hardiman, 1989) developed an interesting experiment in which the participants were asked to grasp blocks of varying sizes from 0.8 cm to 24.2 cm in width. Participants included 26 preschoolers aged 3 years 3 months to 5 years 4 months and 22 adults aged 18 to 46 years. These researchers found that when the ratio of the width of the block to the size of the hand was the same, similar types of grip configurations were elicited regardless of the age of the participant. These results demonstrated that if the child's environmental constraints are manipulated to match the constraints that an adult would face, the child will demonstrate grip configurations similar to those that the adult employed. Subsequent studies have shown similar results (Cesari & Newell, 2000; Newell, McDonald, & Baillargeon, 1993; Newell, Scully, McDonald, & Baillargeon, 1989).

Conceptually, these studies by Thelen, Newell, and others offer a departure from the belief that development is based on hierarchical organization of the CNS. On the basis of theoretical work by Bernstein (1967), these more contemporary theorists believe that the "system" (meaning the various organ, tissue, and bodily systems) is organized in a heterarchical fashion. This means that the method by which a person successfully plans and executes a motion requires the input of many subsystems (e.g., muscle groups, nervous systems), each of which contributes to the movement solution as the task requires. The subsystems are not necessarily under the direct control of the cerebral cortex; that is, the cerebral cortex or consciousness regarding the motor plan does not prescribe the specific details of what each subsystem must do for a successful motor action. Bernstein (1967) argued that although the "executive function" knows the general goal of the task at hand, it does not have the capability of knowing the precise myriad of details required by each of the subsystems. The executive function knows the goal of the task and can direct in a very general manner, but the subsystem is what handles the small details, such as how much range of motion is required at each joint, how much force is required with each muscle, and how many motor neurons to recruit, the sequential timing of the agonist and antagonist muscles.

Bernstein (1967) further argued that the subsystems tend to work together in synergistic patterns. For example, suppose that a person is sitting on a sofa and reaches for a television remote control that is two feet in front of the person on top of a coffee table. Certain muscle groups are recruited, such as the anterior deltoids and the triceps, as the primary muscles to fling the arm forward to the remote. Now suppose that the person is lying on his or her side on the sofa instead of sitting. The person reaches for the remote as in the previous example, but because the position of the arm in relation to the remote and to gravity is different, a different set of primary muscles is recruited (namely, the medial deltoid to counteract the direct pull of gravity, along with the anterior deltoid and the triceps) to move the arm in the direction of the remote. If one were to compare the electrical activity of the anterior deltoid and triceps between the two conditions, the electromyography would be completely different. An important thing to remember in this example is that although the goal was the same in both situations (i.e., grab the remote), different subsystems were recruited depending on what the situation required. The following section provides more information about some specific models of motor control that take these concepts into account.

DISTRIBUTED AND SYSTEM MODELS OF MOTOR CONTROL

General Description of Distributed Models of Motor Control

In this model, control of movement is not peripheral or central. As scientists examined different motor behaviors along with task and environmental constraints, a concept of distributed control of movement emerged; that is, the internal and external forces acting on this system were considered (Keshner, 1991). Distributed models of motor control are not unidirectional. Rather, they allow for communication within the nervous system to take place in ascending, descending, and lateral arrangements. The control hierarchy is perceived not as a descending chain of command but as an overlapping circular network in which each level influences those above and below it. Various sites within and throughout the system are part of the process underlying and controlling movement. Some models of distributed control, however, minimize the relevance of the nervous system. Others, such as neural network models, continue to rely heavily on processing units that consist of neurons and their extensive system of linked dendrites (Bate, 1997). Control of movement in these models is seen as being distributed throughout many working systems, which can include mechanical and environmental factors as well as nervous system factors. The following subsections contain a brief description of a few of many theories involving distributed control of movement.

General Description of Systems Theory

Bernstein, a Russian scientist, was among the first to look at internal and external forces acting on the body to understand the characteristics of the system being moved. The body was regarded as a mechanical system with mass and subject to external forces, such as gravity, as well as inertial and movement-dependent forces. Bernstein asked

questions related to (1) the function of the system in a continually changing environment, (2) the properties of the initial conditions affecting movement, and (3) the body as a mechanical system influencing the control process (Shumway-Cook & Woollacott, 2001).

Bernstein (1967) was also responsible for identifying what is known as the degrees of freedom problem. In describing the mechanics of the system, Bernstein noted that many degrees of freedom need to be controlled for coordinated movement to occur. For example, there are many joints that can flex, extend, and/or rotate, and these multiple options complicate the control of movement. Control therefore involves converting the body into a "controllable" system (Schmidt, 1988).

Bernstein's solution to this problem was proposing that hierarchical control exists to simplify the body's multiple degrees of freedom. He proposed that (1) groups of muscle are constrained to act together as a unit, and (2) these units are activated at lower levels in the system.

Description of Dynamic Pattern Theory

This is an operational approach to the study of coordinated movement (Keshner, 1991) as used in the movement sciences. The impact of this theory is seen in a variety of research areas, including development (Thelen & Smith, 1994), aging (L. S. Greene & Williams, 1996), rehabilitation (Scholz, 1990), and coordination research (Lee, 1998; Sternad, 1998; Walter, 1998). Dynamic pattern theory incorporates aspects of Bernstein's systems theory and the study of dynamics and synergistics. It is an attempt to define terms and provide behavioral and mathematical predictions for coordinated movement patterns. The following basic concepts are fundamental to many dynamical systems approaches and motor control research.

1. The human system exhibits self-organizing behavior.
2. The human system is a many element system that can be described by a few elements, which are referred to as *collective variables*. Collective variables are the fewest number of variables that completely describe the behavior. For example, Heriza (1991) proposes that for humans, walking is a highly complex behavior that is characterized by a specific movement pattern. The new walker compresses the many degrees of freedom available from the muscles, bones, joints, tendons, neurons, and motor units into a relatively few degrees of freedom that can be observed in walking. In this example, a complex behavior—walking— becomes characterized by a description of the behavior: the specific movement pattern.
3. Collective variables characterize movement patterns and capture the systems that cooperate to produce the movement, as movement is more than just muscles and motor neurons. For example, kicking, stepping, and throwing a ball are examples of coordinated movement patterns. Again, an example by Heriza (1991)

helps to clarify this. In intralimb coordination, as seen within one limb in kicking or stepping, the identified collective variables are the timing of the individual movement phases, such as flexion and extension; phase lags, defined as the time between the onset of movement of one joint and that of another joint; and the relationship of individual joints to each other.

4. The identification of phase transitions is basic to understanding behavior. Control parameters are variables that shift the movement from one form to another movement form. Control parameters act to reorganize the system. In the example of intralimb coordination as well as in interlimb coordination, behavioral states can drive the system. For instance, when an infant is asleep or drowsy, little kicking is noted. If the infant is aroused, the spatial and temporal pattern of kicking is observed. If the infant is in a crying state, a new pattern emerges that is described as a rigid coactivation of all the muscles into stiff mobility. Therefore, control parameters can be defined as components that are essential but nonspecific to the movement behavior. In this example, the control parameters can reside in the individual, such as behavioral state; in the environment, such as gravity; in the social environment, such as the caretaker; or in the goal or in the task. New coordinated patterns emerge because old patterns become unstable and the system is driven to a new state. Changes in the control parameters push the system to a new state. During these shifts in phase or phase transitions, the prevailing movement pattern becomes less stable and more easily perturbed by the control parameter (Heriza, 1991).

5. The study of the stability or instability of behavior during transition periods is essential to understanding pattern change in complex systems. In this approach, movement behavior and control can be aptly described by a set of collective variables and control variables associated with phase transition (Haugen & Mathiowetz, 1995).

IMPLICATIONS. Dynamical systems are systems in which behaviors evolve over time and are marked by their capacity to change states. Systems theories take into account factors other than the nervous system in regulating movement, for example, the physical characteristics such as the mass of the system being moved. These theories have enlarged the understanding of the multiple factors that are responsible for controlled movement. The individual is seen as active within the environment with movement an emergent product of many systems. These theories may be helpful in taking into account the passive components of a patient's biomechanics and factoring these components into explanations for movement stability and instability (Bate, 1997).

LIMITATIONS. The role of the nervous system is minimized in these theories. Transitions in movement patterns are explained in terms of physical causality, mathematical functions, and variables. These theories primarily seek physical explanations contributing to movement characteristics and thus seem more aligned with biomechanical interpretations of movement. However, several recent reviews of motor control theories suggest that dynamical motor control views and alternative information-processing views are not necessarily mutually exclusive (Walter, 1998). Furthermore, Walter contends that the relative role, as well as the strengths and weaknesses, of each theoretical account of motor control needs to be determined.

Parallel Distributed Processing Theory

Computer analysis and simulations are also providing models and theories for motor control. These have been recent efforts to develop models of higher-level processes that are based on an understanding of neural processing and patterns of neural activity provided by imaging studies. These attempts start by asking how the brain might achieve higher-level processing rather than by asking how the brain actually achieves such processing. Modeling starts from a basic understanding of how neurons work and asks: How could higher-level function be achieved by connecting basic elements like neurons together (Anderson, 1995)?

The parallel distributed processing (PDP) theory of motor control describes how the nervous system, as a network, processes information for action. It reflects current knowledge in neuroscience about the serial and parallel processing of the nervous system. Serial processing is the simultaneous processing of information through a single pathway while parallel processing is processing information through many pathways (Kandel, Schwartz, & Jessel, 2000). Parallel distributed processing is unique in its emphasis on explaining neural mechanisms associated with motor control. Neural modeling, that is, computer simulation of nervous system functioning, has correctly predicted aspects of processing in both the perception and action systems. As neural modeling develops, it could provide further knowledge as to how the nervous system solves particular problems.

Implications

Modeling of function and dysfunction can be integrated into clinical practice Shumway-Cook and Woollacott (1995) propose that a PDP model could be used to predict how changes within the nervous system affect function. As an example, the theory predicts that parallel redundant pathways exist in the system and that a loss of a few elements will not necessarily affect function. The loss of additional elements or loss once a certain threshold is attained, however, could affect the capacity of the system to function. This idea—threshold of dysfunction—is demonstrated in many pathological cases, such as in Parkinson's disease.

Limitations

PDP theory is a tool to think about the way in which the nervous system works. Some of the proposed functions are not replicated in nervous system processing, and modeling cannot fully account for what is known about nervous system processing.

Ecological Theory

Ecological theory, which was developed by James Gibson (1966), explores the interaction between the motor (action) system and goal-directed behavior. Gibson's research focused on how we detect environmental information and how we use that information to control our movements. Environmental information was seen as relevant to action in the environment. Perception rather than sensation is important to the individual acting on the environment. From this perspective, determining how the individual detects information in the environment, the form of this environmental information, and how this information is used to modify and control movement are important. In ecological theory, the organization of movement depends on the active exploration of tasks, the environment, and the individual's multiple ways to accomplish a task. Perception guides action and action guides perception. Therefore, movement disorders are not only the consequences of structural changes, but also can be understood as an atypical spatial temporal organization in the perception–action coupling and in movement coordination (Wagennar & van Emmerik, 1996). This approach has broadened our understanding of nervous system function from depending on sensory motor control to that of a more global perception action system that actively explores the environment to satisfy its goals. Likewise, disordered motor control is a disruption in the perception action system and not at the level of the CNS.

Implications

A major contribution of this perspective is seeing the individual as active in the environment and the environment as crucial in determining movements. Active exploration of the environment allows the individual to develop multiple ways to accomplish a task.

Limitations

This approach has enlarged the understanding of the interaction between the organism and environment. Research is at the level of the organism-environment interface. It has contributed less to the knowledge of the organization and function of the nervous system, which is a primary concern of therapists intervening in motor control problems, based on traditional neurotherapeutic approaches.

Task-Oriented Theory

In task-oriented theory, motor control is understood by identifying what problems the CNS has to solve in order to accomplish a motor task. By the term *task,* P. H. Greene (1972) was referring to the fundamental problems, such as the degrees of freedom problem described by Bernstein, that the CNS is required to solve in order to accomplish a motor task. Peter Greene (1972) proposed that this approach could provide the basis for a more coherent picture of the motor system.

Implications

This perspective suggests practicing functional tasks for retraining in therapy. It acknowledges the role of perceptual, cognitive, and action systems to accomplish tasks (P. H. Greene, 1972). It requires an understanding of motor strategies that are used to accomplish a task, as well as an understanding of the perceptual basis for action and the cognitive contributions to actions.

Limitations

There is a lack of agreement as to the fundamental tasks of the CNS. There is also lack of agreement as to the essential elements that are being controlled within a task. For example, in studying postural control, some scientists consider that the essential goal of the postural system is to control head position. Other scientists studying postural control think that controlling center of mass position to attain body stability is the essential goal of postural control (Shumway-Cook & Woollacott, 1995).

Perceptual Motor Workspace

How does the body know how to do something? In other words, how does the body know which subsystems need to be recruited in any given situation? A model proposed by Turvey, Kugler, McDonald, and Newell (Kugler & Turvey, 1987; Newell & McDonald, 1994; Turvey & Kugler, 1984) called the *perceptual motor workspace* has its basis in the dynamical systems theory (Gleick, 1987) as well as the ecological approach to perception and action (Gibson, 1979, 1982). In simple terms, the perceptual motor workspace model states that the motion solution that is employed for any given task is a direct result of how the person perceives (both consciously and unconsciously) the constraints of the task, the environment, and the constraints within himself or herself. Newell (1986) defined constraints as being information that provides boundaries. Further, Newell argues that constraints provide opportunity as well. Constraints give information that allow a person to size up the situation; that is, constraints yield an awareness regarding the unique characteristics of the object or situation. Once the person perceives these constraints, the person's nebulous "system" then calls into action specific subsystems (e.g., portions of the CNS and muscle groups) to interact with each other, a process that culminates in a solution that is uniquely attuned to the specific task and environment at hand.

Implications

Part of this model requires that the person accurately perceive the constraints in the environment. If the person misperceives a constraint, such as the location of the remote control, he or she will either overshoot, undershoot, or otherwise miss the remote control. In another common experience, if a person attempts to lift up a paint can, believing that it is full when in reality it is empty, the person will lift the can up with greater force than necessary, resulting in the can's accelerating in an unanticipated manner. Similarly, if a child does not have a good sense of where his or her body is in space, then he or she might be considered to be clumsy. It is quite possible that once the child is allowed to explore the limits of his or her body, the child will have a better sense of where his or her body is in relation to the surrounding environment. The resulting change will be fewer uncoordinated motions. The idea of misperceiving the environment is not uncommon. One of the authors of this chapter remembers an instance during a summer campout at a state park involving an accompanying niece, who was from a large metropolitan area and had little camping experience. When first arriving at the campsite, the niece saw the fire grate, but she did not recognize it as a fire grate. She perceived the fire grate's height to afford her a nice seat, on which she sat while wearing her white shorts (don't worry—there was no fire). The consequence was that she had a seat of appropriate height, but unfortunately for her, the back side of her shorts gave the illusion of a zebralike pattern. Here the environmental perception of the height of the fire grate was accurate, the task perception of sitting down was accurate (she successfully sat down), but she apparently had no previous experience with fire grates—hence, the "mistake" was made. The author has been informed that this error has not occurred a second time. This brings up an important point: that having memories on which to draw is an important constraint of the person when mapping perception to action.

Limitations

There is no evidence to support this model from a rehabilitation or clinical point of view. Therefore, this model currently has limited applicability to rehabilitation and other types of clinical settings.

MOTOR CONTROL APPROACHES PROPOSED FOR THERAPEUTIC INTERACTION

New approaches to intervening with motor performance deficits that affect occupational performances have evolved. These therapeutic approaches are based on both motor learning principles and on more contemporaneous models and research about the control of movements in both typical populations and populations with movement disorders.

Task-Oriented Model

The task-oriented model (Gordon, 1987; Horak, 1991; Shumway-Cook & Woollacott, 2001) targets both peripheral and central control systems. In line with system models of motor control, the task-oriented model assumes that control of movement is organized around goal-directed functional tasks. Clients are taught to accomplish goals for functional tasks. By practicing a wide variety of movements, the client solves different types of motor problems. The assumptions seen in Table 55.6 guide treatment.

Along with these assumptions and guidelines, Horak (1991) suggests organizing questions around several areas in treating clients with motor performance deficits. These areas are the client's behavioral goals, movement strategies, musculoskeletal constraints, compensatory strategies, and need for adaptations. Examples of questions about these areas are as follows:

1. **Behavioral goals:** Are the therapist's and client's goals the same? This might entail the practitioner incorporating the use of the Canadian Occupational Performance Measure (COPM) and the Assessment of Motor and Process Skills. Using both would allow the practitioner to determine what is important to the client and what are the strengths and weaknesses in the client's motor and process skills.
2. **Movement strategy:** What are the organizing principles of a normal movement strategy?
3. **Musculoskeletal constraints:** How much of the motor deficit in a patient with neurological deficits is due to a deficit in the musculoskeletal system rather the neural components?
4. **Compensatory strategies:** Has the patient found the most effective strategy?
5. **Adaptation:** How must a movement strategy be adapted to accomplish a task in a new environmental context?

Motor Re-Learning Program

The Motor Re-Learning Program (Carr & Shepherd, 1987) is a synthesis of the prevalent contemporary models of motor control and the motor learning process (Sabari, 1995). It is specific to the rehabilitation of patients following stroke. The program is based on four factors that are thought to be essential for the learning of motor skill and assumed to be essential for the relearning of motor control: (1) elimination of unnecessary muscle activity, (2) feedback, (3) practice, and (4) the interrelationship of postural adjustment and movement. In this program, treatment is directed toward relearning of control rather than to activities incorporating exercise or to facilitation or inhibition techniques.

Treatment is directed toward enhancing motor performance, and the emphasis is on the practice of specific

TABLE 55.6   ASSUMPTIONS GUIDING THE TASK-ORIENTED APPROACH

Assumptions	Treatment Principles
◆ Movement is controlled by the individual's goals. ◆ A wide variety of movement patterns can be accomplished with a task. ◆ Facilitation of normal movements is not necessary. ◆ The nervous system adapts continually to its environment and musculoskeletal constraints. ◆ The nervous system is not a passive recipient of sensory stimuli but actively seeks to control its own perception and actions. ◆ Voluntary and automatic control systems are interrelated. ◆ Multiple system involvement results in movement. ◆ The nervous system is exposed to its own specific environment. ◆ The nervous system seeks to accomplish goals with remaining systems after injury.	◆ The goal of therapy is to teach clients to accomplish goals for functional tasks. ◆ Therapists do not treat or limit therapy to one normal movement pattern. ◆ Therapists try to teach the nervous system how to solve different motor problems by practicing in a wide variety of situations. ◆ The therapist seeks to manipulate these environmental and musculoskeletal systems to allow for efficient, purposeful behavior. ◆ The client needs to practice motor behaviors motivated by the goal of task accomplishment. ◆ Clients are encouraged to assist voluntarily in accomplishing a motor behavior with therapist's encouragement. ◆ The therapist and the environment provide feedback. ◆ The therapist must design interventions in which practice of controlled movements is outside structured sessions. ◆ The therapist helps the patient to identify and use compensatory strategies.

Source: Horak, 1991, Gordon, 1987.

CASE STUDY: *Emily: A Toddler with Problems Walking*

Emily, a 2-year, 1-month-old girl with a recent diagnosis of athetoid cerebral palsy, was referred to a pediatric medical center for a diagnostic workup by an early intervention team that included an occupational therapist. The child's parents were concerned that Emily was not able to walk but that she seemed okay in other areas of development. She appeared playful and responsive and enjoyed playing and moving around the play area. Although she was not pulling to stand and was obviously delayed in her ability to walk, Emily's language, feeding ability, and play patterns seemed near age level.

Team Evaluation

The diagnostic team that gathered to assess Emily decided to use several tools that would provide an overview of her cognitive, sensorimotor, adaptive, and social-emotional developmental functioning and play behaviors. Because Emily appeared typical in her behavioral responses and play interests, the team did not have her parents complete a sensory profile on Emily, as she did not seem overly responsive or underresponsive to sensory stimuli and appeared not to have regulation problems. Mostly, she appeared to be a typical child who was significantly delayed in her ability to walk. However, she was able to come to a sitting position independently, and she negotiated the environment by either rolling or coming into an all-fours position and then collapsing but moving forward. She was able to bear weight on all four extremities when in quadriped, but she was unable to maintain that position for more than a few seconds or to crawl. The team decided to use the Bayley Scales of Infant Development to assess Emily's development in all areas and also decided to observe her in a natural play environment with both her parents present. The team administered the Bayley Scales with several of the team members present. Also, the speech therapist and occupational therapist observed Emily eating a snack to determine whether there were any problems with the task of eating. Emily's performance in all areas was remarkable in that she completed all tasks at her age level other than the movement tasks that seemed to precede walking or coming to a stand. Emily was able to finger-feed and sip from a cup. It was noted that weakness and athetoid movements were interfering more with her use of the lower limbs and only her ability to crawl, pull to stand, or walk.

Continued

CASE STUDY: *Emily: A Toddler with Problems Walking*   *Continued*

She was responsive to coming to all fours and to a stance when manually guided or directed through age-appropriate play activities, but she was limited in her ability to self-initiate or maintain these positions independently. However, when a large rectangular cushion was placed in front of her, Emily pulled up on her knees independently and played for several minutes with the Fisher-Price busy box that was on the cushion in front of her.

The Occupational Therapist's Reasoning

After assessing this child, the occupational therapist had several decisions to make:

1. Was Emily an appropriate candidate for services?
2. Would it be necessary for the occupational therapist to see Emily twice a week, once a week, or not at all?
3. Could the occupational therapist function more as a collaborator/consultant with the family and or other team members?

Even though the parents had expressed concerns only about Emily's walking, the occupational therapy practitioner wondered whether the family might have some other concerns and thought that administering the COPM to them could provide additional insight into their concerns about Emily's performance in different domains. Emily was limited in mobility but overall at age level in other areas, and the occupational therapist thought that she herself could collaborate most effectively with the team and the family on tasks and environmental challenges that might foster Emily's ability to pull up on all fours and to stand.

Occupational Therapy Intervention: Family Education

The occupational therapist decided to speak to the parents further. She emphasized that Emily had many strengths and that her movements appeared to be constrained by her weakness and instability in her lower extremities. How-ever, the occupational therapist also suggested that Emily's use of her lower extremities could be enhanced by using the natural home environment and play opportunities that challenged her use of her lower body. She reviewed with the parents how to structure the home environment so that Emily had to move in an environment that gave her the opportunities to come up on her knees, pull to stand, and cruise safely. Also, the occupational therapist emphasized that many factors contributed to Emily's difficulty with crawling and standing and that giving her opportunities to move and use her body while also being engaged in play would help Emily to grow and develop in her natural context. The therapist also spoke to the family about more recent research that suggests that motor learning occurs with practice and that having Emily "practice" and try out different movements while engaged in play would help her to develop.

The Six-Month Plan

The therapist with the team recommended that Emily be seen in six months to determine whether her play and development continued on course and whether she had achieved measurable goals in regards to being able to crawl and to stand independently. To monitor progress, the team decided that the physical therapist would see Emily in the home once a week and provide movement opportunities for Emily as well as modeling for her parents ways to challenge Emily so that she would learn to move in a goal-directed way. The occupational therapist planned to meet with the family when Emily was scheduled for follow-up and at that time administer the COPM to determine whether there were other performance concerns that the family has about Emily. Also, the occupational therapist would periodically speak with the treating physical therapist to discuss Emily's progress and provide suggestions in regard to play and challenges to be incorporated into the environment.

---

tasks, the training of controllable muscle action, and control over the movement components of these tasks. The major assumptions about motor control underlying this approach are listed in Box 55.1.

To provide this program, a four-step sequence is followed for skill acquisition. Step 1 is an analysis of the task, including observation. Step 2 is practice of missing components, including goal identification, instruction, practice, and feedback with some manual guidance. Step 3 is practice of the task with the addition of reevaluation and encouraging of task flexibility. Step 4 targets transfer of training (Carr & Shepherd, 1987).

Contemporary Task-Oriented Approach

Description

Haugen and Mathiowetz (1995) have proposed a task-oriented approach based on a systems model of motor control and influenced by contemporary developmental and motor learning theories. This model takes into account the interaction between the personal characteristics or systems of the person such as the sensorimotor system and the performance context. Occupational performance emerges from the interaction between personal characteristics and performance contexts as seen in Table 55.7.

BOX 55.1 ASSUMPTIONS UNDERLYING THE MOTOR RE-LEARNING APPROACH WITH GUIDELINES FOR EXERCISE AND TRAINING TO OPTIMIZE MOTOR SKILL

- In regaining motor control, learning is required. This learning follows the same principles and factors as those incurred in normal learning. Therefore, practice, receiving feedback, and understanding the goal are essential for treatment.
- Motor control is exercised in both anticipatory and ongoing modes.
- Sensory input is related to motor output and helps to modulate action.
- Control of a specific task can be effectively regained by practice of that specific motor task in various contexts.
- Conscious practice of tasks builds up awareness of the ability to elicit motor control activity.
- Progression of practice is from conscious awareness to practice at a more automatic level in order to ensure that a skill is learned.
- Cognitive function is emphasized. If the client is to learn, then the environment must encourage the learning process.

- When clients can perform a task effectively and efficiently without thinking about it in a variety of contexts, learning has occurred.
- Contemporary theories of motor control emphasize distributed control rather than a top-down or bottom-up approach. Therefore, in the Motor Re-Learning Program, recovery is directed to relearning control through many systems.
- The client is defined as an active participant in the treatment process. The major goal in rehabilitation is to relearn effective strategies for performing functional activities.
- The role of the therapist is to prevent the use of inefficient strategies by the client.
- The program addresses seven categories of functional daily activities: upper limb function, orofacial function, sitting up over the side of the bed, balanced sitting, standing up and sitting down, balanced standing, and walking.

Source: Carr & Shepherd (1987, 2003).

The Task-Oriented Approach (Mathiowetz, 2004) considers the person's role performance as well as the performance in areas of occupation. In addition, this model espouses that a task analysis be performed to determine the factors (from the person, the environmental context, and the task itself—the same three factors as in the perceptual motor workspace) that either facilitate or restrict performance. The treatment focus of this approach involves any individual or combination of the following:

- Environmental modification
- Manipulating or grading the task
- Remediating skills/abilities that are particularly limiting within the person

Implications

Specific strategies are espoused for the remediation of limiting factors within the person. Many of these strategies are founded in the motor learning body of knowledge. Some of these strategies involve how feedback is given. For instance, it has been shown (particularly with nondisabled populations) that reduced feedback actually results in better retention and transfer of the motor skill being learned (Rice, 2003; Rice & Hernandez, 2006; Winstein & Schmidt, 1990; Wulf, Schmidt, & Deubel, 1993). See Shea and Wulf (2005) for a review. Another motor learning strategy involves presenting tasks to be learned or practiced in a random fashion (e.g., moving from task to task without providing repeated trials on any given task) rather than giving multiple trials of the same task before moving on to another task.

Limitations

Much of the motor learning research has been performed on healthy college students, and the tasks have usually involved simple rote motor skills that do not represent normal occupationally oriented activities. Therefore, the generalization of these strategies to special populations should be done with caution until a greater body of evidence supports their use with special populations.

TABLE 55.7 ASSUMPTIONS GUIDING A CONTEMPORARY TASK-ORIENTED APPROACH

Assumptions	Treatment Principles
◆ Functional tasks help to organize behavior. Recent research suggests that parameters of motor behavior are not performance components but in fact functional goals (Burton & Davis, 1992; Gentile, 1992; Heriza, 1991; Thelen, 1989). ◆ Occupational performance emerges from the interaction of multiple systems that represent the unique characteristics of the person and the performance context. ◆ After CNS damage or other changes in personal or environmental systems, clients' behavioral changes reflect their attempts to compensate and achieve functional goals. ◆ Personal and environmental systems are hetarchically organized. There is no inherent ordering of the personal and environmental systems in terms of their influence on motor behavior. There is also no inherent ordering within the system, even within the CNS. ◆ A person must practice and experiment with varied strategies to find optimal solutions for motor problems and develop skill in performance.	◆ Because the primary purpose of motor behavior is to achieve functional goals, therapists begin and end therapy by focusing on occupational performance. The emphasis on task performance and evaluation is primarily at the disability level, using the World Health (1980) Organization Model of Disablement. ◆ The therapist assesses all systems that are contributing to problems in functional performance or supporting optimal performance, keeping in mind the tasks the person currently does or will be doing in the future. Because the client brings to the situation a unique constellation of characteristics, the therapist makes the client's perspective the focus of assessment. The client determines the important goals and roles necessary for occupational performance. ◆ Movement patterns that are used for compensation and achievement of functional goals must be understood fully. The evaluation of occupational performance must include an examination of the process (actual movement patterns), the outcome, and the stability or instability of observed motor behavior. ◆ Evaluation strategies consider all personal and environmental systems. The ones that interfere the most with performance are evaluated first. ◆ As part of treatment, clients practice, experiment, and problem-solve in order to achieve functional goals. Treatment planning is to develop and implement learning opportunities for clients with problem-solving abilities. When clients are unable to problem solve, the therapist might need to train them to use given routines.

Source: Haugen & Mathiowetz (1995).

Constraint-Induced Movement Therapy

Description

Constraint-induced movement therapy (CIMT) is a relatively new model of practice that focuses on restoration of the affected limb in individuals with unilateral stroke or brain injury. Many techniques have traditionally employed compensatory strategies for helping a person gain function, for example, teaching one-handed techniques with the unaffected limb to perform functional tasks. CIMT focuses on the function of the affected or paralyzed limb. The basic idea is to constrain (specifically, to splint, sling, or otherwise immobilize) the unaffected limb for a period of time while the affected limb is free to engage in activities, tasks, and occupations unilaterally. Although this idea is radically different from traditional neurorehabilitation approaches, its efficacy is beginning to be established in the literature (Broeks, Lankhorst, Rumping, & Prevo,1999; Taub, Crago, & Uswatte, 1998; Taub, Miller, et al., 1993; Taub & Morris, 2001; Taub, Uswatte, & Pidikiti, 1999; Taub & Wolf, 1997; Wolf, LeCraw, & Barton, 1989; Wolf, Thompson, et al., 2005). The general procedure involves a two-week period of constraining the unaffected limb during all waking hours. During this period, patients are engaged in what are termed *shaping techniques* with the affected limb for up to six hours per day for five days per week. Shaping involves the selection of tasks and motor skills in an area that a therapist deems to require functional and motor improvement for that individual. Common inclusion criteria for the above-mentioned studies

CASE STUDY: *Aetos: A Man with a Gunshot Wound to the Head*

Aetos is a 22-year-old man who immigrated to the United States from Cyprus. He worked in a convenience store, where he sustained a gunshot wound to his head when someone robbed the store during his shift. He was transported to a local trauma hospital and was stabilized. He was comatose for three weeks, after which he became cognitively responsive. Currently, he is the Ranchos–Los-Amigos cognitive scale level 6 (Confused-Appropriate). He presents with left-upper extremity hemiparesis. Although he has gross grasp abilities in his left hand, his fine motor control is limited. He requires minimum assistance for dressing and self-care. Before his injury, Ryan independently maintained his own apartment and enjoyed hosting parties for his friends. He particularly enjoyed planning and preparing the food for these parties.

Two possible approaches to addressing this case in occupational therapy are focusing on the impairment of the client or using a more client-centered and contextually sensitive approach.

Impairment-Focused Approach

The impairment-focused approach can involve evaluating and assessing the specific client and body factors, such as range of motion, strength, fine motor skill, sensation, visual perception, and cognitive function (specifically, memory, attention, and the ability to concentrate). On the basis of these evaluations, therapy is directed toward improving the patient's performance in these specific areas with the hope that these improvements will translate into functional improvements. The therapeutic milieu involves grading the tasks on the basis of the perceived "just right challenge" for the patient in these separate treatment areas. Throughout the session, the therapist provides feedback to encourage participation in these various domain-specific treatment areas. The majority of occupational

therapy treatment occurs in the rehabilitation gym using domain-specific rehabilitation equipment and supplies. Additionally, a SaeboFlex splint was ordered, and practice sessions occurred using the supplied balls and baskets. Discharge from occupational therapy will be based on accomplishment of measurable goals in these treatment areas (strength, coordination, memory, etc.) as well as predetermined functional independence measure goals.

Client-Centered Approach

The client-centered and contextually sensitive approach is more organized according to the client's stated goals. In this case, it might be a goal related to food preparation for a party. The therapist and the client plan several of the treatment sessions to be organized specifically around preparing vegetables to garnish hamburgers. The majority of the occupational therapy sessions will therefore occur in the rehabilitation clinic's therapeutic kitchen. One of the chosen occupationally embedded tasks is cutting tomato slices. The therapist grades the task by choosing a large enough tomato that the client can safely grasp it with the affected limb while slicing the tomato with the non-affected limb. Grading this task can be accomplished by using tomatoes of various sizes and degrees of ripeness. Additionally, the style and size of the knife can be manipulated to provide the "just right challenge." Safety and cognition can also be addressed, as well as task sequence. Repetition can be based on how many hamburgers have been planned, and variability can be manipulated through the use of multiple tomatoes as well as the inclusion of other vegetable garnishes. Discharge from occupational therapy will be based on the accomplishment of measurable goals regarding the successful and safe food preparation tasks as well as predetermined functional independence measure goals.

---

require that the person have at least 10 degrees of active metacarpal extension and at least 20 degrees of wrist extension. Participants in these studies have, for the most part, demonstrated remarkable improvement in their affected limb's motor function following the two-week period. Furthermore, some of these studies have shown the retainment of motor function at two years after the CIMT treatment (Taub, Miller, et al., 1993). There are several theories as to why success occurs in improving the function of the affected limb. These theories are based on the concepts of learned nonuse (Morris, Crago, DeLuca, Pidikiti, & Taub, 1997; Taub, 1994) and cortical reorganization (i.e., brain plasticity) (Liepert, 2006; Liepert, Bauder, et al., 2000; Liepert, Miltner, et al., 1998).

Implications

CIMT is an excellent example of an evidence-based model of practice. This approach has been exclusively driven by research findings from controlled research studies. For participants who meet the inclusion criteria, there is strong evidence that this treatment approach is effective in facilitating functional return to hemiparetic limbs.

Limitations

The inclusion criteria that are in the research studies mentioned above are relatively narrow. That is, this approach has been documented as effective only for participant who have a minimum of 10 to 20 degrees of extension at their metacarpals and wrist, respectively. Some critics would argue that individuals with this type of return already are experiencing spontaneous recovery anyway. Additionally, this treatment approach requires a high level of motivation on the part of the patient in order to tolerate what is undoubtedly a frustrating experience with constraining the unaffected limb during all waking hours.

Orthotic Approaches

Description

Some of the most recent approaches to upper limb control and skill learning are based on the use of repetition with functional practice and the principle of activity-dependent plasticity. Specific protocols such as the Functional Tone Management Arm (F.T.M.) Training Program incorporate use of a dynamic orthosis, the SaeboFlex, with specific repetitive practice (Hoffman & Farrell, 2005). The SaeboFlex is a custom dynamic resting hand orthosis that features a spring-loaded finger extension system (Figure 55.7). The extensor spring system assists in opening the fingers following functional grasp. When using the SaeboFlex, the client grasps an object using voluntary flexor control, places the object in a specified location, and then relaxes flexor tone enough to allow the extensor springs to assist in extending the fingers.

Like the CIMT protocol, the F.T.M. protocol was designed to decrease learned nonuse; increase learned use;

reduce spasticity; improve range of motion, strength, and control; improve functional arm use; and improve quality of life for individuals with some shoulder and elbow function but minimal hand movement. To qualify for this protocol, individuals must exhibit active shoulder elevation of 15 degrees, 10 degrees of active shoulder abduction, and active elbow flexion of 15 degrees with full passive range of motion into elbow flexion and be able to flex their digits at least a quarter of their range in a fist position (Hoffman & Farrell, 2005). Also, a minimum of 15 degrees of wrist extension with the fingers fully extended is required for F.T.M. training. The training protocol incorporates evaluating the patient's use of the hand without the orthosis, fitting the individual with the orthosis, and then having the client, with the orthosis, engage in one of four levels of crate activity that incorporates the client repetitively grasping and releasing specified objects. The program focuses on performing high-repetition strengthening exercises involving weak muscle groups. The gross motor items that are used with the protocol are assumed to effectively challenge the individual to achieve the motor function essential to complete the task. Completion of these tasks is assumed to translate into the individual's better functional use of the upper limb. Colorful study equipment used with the protocol includes the Height Adjustable Target (H.A.T.), the Multi-Purpose Exercise Device, the Four Tier Ball Activity, and the Five Ball Peg Activity (Figure 55.8).

Implications

The F.T.M. is an example of the use of an orthosis with a specific activity-oriented program that facilitates constant repetition and practice of grasp, placement, and release. It is proposed as a protocol to be used with clients who present with limited arm and hand function secondary to a stroke or traumatic brain injury. The approach, developed by two occupational therapists, is based on reasoning derived from research evidence about the efficacy of training techniques permitting repetitive selective muscular activation, recruitment of muscular activity versus inhibition and strengthening the arm (Fowler, Ho, Nwigwe, & Dorey, 2001). It may be of benefit to clients who have some use of their arm and are motivated to use their hand with an assisting orthosis both in the clinic setting and at home.

Limitations

Although this approach is based on evidence about the impact of repetition and strengthening on functional upper limb use, the evidence base for the specific protocol is limited. Research using this protocol has been primarily at the lower levels of research evidence using both case studies and single-subject design. However, this approach is one of the newer ways to treat and more than likely will undergo more rigorous research as

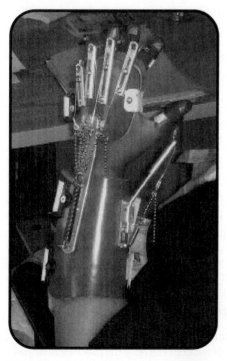

FIGURE 55.7   The SaeboFlex splint.

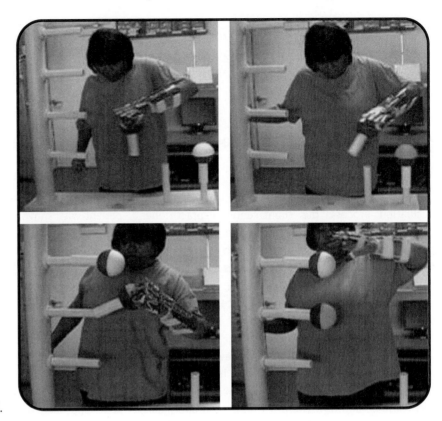

FIGURE 55.8 Saebo protocol.

it evolves and randomized controlled studies can be undertaken.

Robot-Aided Motor Training

Another recent addition to the techniques that are used to foster skill return is the use of robotic manipulators for providing training of arm movements. Robot manipulators have been used primarily in experimental paradigms that are attempting to examine the mechanisms underlying normal motor control and learning as well as attempting to examine the mechanisms underlying disorders of upper limb movements in patients with movement disorders. However, since the 1997 pioneering study of the MIT-Manus robotic manipulator at the Massachusetts Institute of Technology, the number of research groups engaged in this area with patient populations has substantively increased. Also, more devices have been developed for automated training for arm and wrist movements following stroke. The range of robotic possibilities is promising, as robots are precise and tireless and can easily simulate what a therapist can do in assisting movement (Patton, Kovic, & Mussa-Ivaldi, 2006). Also the research in this area has demonstrated that robot-assisted movement training improves movement ability following acute and chronic stroke (Kahn, Lum, Rymer, & Reinkensmeyer, 2006). Training is assumed to follow two interacting

processes: the patient trying to move and the robot applying forces. A fundamental motor learning principle involved in robot-assisted movement is that movement practice improves motor function. Evidence to date with this therapy suggests that active participation is required and that progressive training that is robot assisted and based on measures of movement coordination yields substantively improved outcomes. Recent research suggests that the most appropriate focus for robotic therapy might be movement coordination rather than muscle activation (Hogan et al., 2006).

Implications

There is limited evidence that robot-assisted movement affects change in both the acute and chronic stages of stroke recovery. Also, use of this technology has been helpful in examining the processes that are involved in learning and movement recovery.

Limitations

If movement practice is the primary stimulus for movement recovery, robotic devices that incorporate practice with the application of forces might be both unnecessary and expensive. Indeed, nonrobotic technology, including hand cycles, low-cost movement monitors, virtual reality systems, and passive antigravity devices such as the tradi-

Therapeutic Approaches to Improve Motor Control in Daily Life

Practitioners often apply scientific principles and thinking to practice. As part of the assessment and evaluation process, the client-centered practitioner frames the patient's occupational therapy performance problems with the patient and considers alternative intervention strategies that may be of help. Likewise, practitioners engage in hypothesizing how they can most effectively help the client learn or recover habits and skills that support their full participation in everyday life activities.

However, in the past 20 years, the evolving sciences of movement science and neuroscience have challenged the practitioner's understanding of movement control and learning, and how the practitioner can apply current scientific thinking to skill learning (Bate, 1997; Shumway-Cook & Woollacott, 2007). Our basic understanding of the principles guiding movement organization and recovery has shifted, and this shift has influenced the research as well as the more current approaches to intervention that are being proposed for occupation-based skill learning and recovery. Also, the evidence to support the influence of neuromotor techniques guiding occupation-based practice and recovery of function is limited, while evidence has accumulated supporting the importance of using context, repetition, and variability in the practice context to foster skill learning and control (Giuffrida, Shea & Fairbrother, 2002; Wolf et al., 2005). In this section, we highlight the surprising but ongoing influence of the neurofacilitation techniques on the practice of therapy and the increasing evidence for current strategies and approaches that promote skill learning and control.

Although occupational therapy was still a relatively young discipline during the early 1960s, the neurofacilitation and neurodevelopment therapeutic approaches based on the movement science of the time were developed (Mathiowetz, 1995; Woollacott & Shumway-Cook, 2007). These approaches resulted in a dramatic change in clinical interventions targeting those with neurological impairments. Prior to the development of the neurofacilitation approaches, therapy for those with neurological impairments was directed toward changing function at the level of the muscle. Current approaches were focused on muscle re-education, were more suited to the patient with movement disorders resulting from polio, and had less impact on altering movement patterns for those with upper motor neuron lesions such as stroke or cerebral palsy (Horak, 1991). The neurofacilitation techniques developed both in response to a clinician's dissatisfaction with seemingly non-impactful muscle re-education techniques and a desire to develop approaches that were more useful for those with movement problems secondary to a neurological dysfunction.

Neurofacilitation approaches include the Bobath approach developed by Karl and Berta Bobath (1965), the Road approach developed by Margaret Rood (Stockmeyer, 1967), Brunnstrom's approach developed by Signe Brunnstrom (1966), proprioceptive neuromuscular facilitation (PNF) developed by Voss (Voss et al., 1985), and the sensory integration theory developed by Jean Ayres (1972). These approaches were based largely on assumptions drawn from the then prevailing theories of motor control, the reflex and hierarchical models of motor control.

These approaches focused on retaining motor control and modifying the CNS through techniques designed to facilitate or inhibit movement patterns. As these approaches were associated with both the reflex and hierarchical theories of motor control, clinical practices were developed based on the importance of reflexes and hierarchical control in normal and abnormal motor control and the recovery of function (Mathiowetz, 1995; Montgomery, 1991). In these approaches, several key assumptions prevailed: (1) functional skills will return if abnormal movement patterns are inhibited and normal movement patterns are facilitated; (2) repetition of the normal movement pattern will result in the transfer to functional skills (Shumway-Cook & Woollacott 2007). Along with these assumptions, practice was guided by the prevailing thoughts about the importance of reflexes and hierarchical control in movement control (Bartlett, 1997; Easton, 1972; Gordon, 1987). Therefore, in these approaches, there is a focus on identifying the presence or absence of normal and abnormal reflexes controlling movements. Intervention is

COMMENTARY ON THE EVIDENCE   *Continued*

directed toward modifying the reflexes controlling movement and sensory input is used to direct and influence motor output. Use of a hierarchical theory suggests that a goal of therapy is to regain control of movement by higher centers of the CNS. Thus, the patient gains movement control and also recovers functionally, as patterns of movement are basic to function and development.

Although the evidence to support reflex and hierarchical motor control approaches to intervention is limited, these approaches still influence the way practitioners assess and intervene with patients with neuromotor problems (Shumway-Cook & Woollacott, 2007). However, many of the approaches have changed their approach to practice to incorporate more current scientific thinking about the nature and cause of movement. Within the neurofacilitation approaches today, there is more of an emphasis on training for functional recovery and less emphasis on inhibiting reflexes and facilitating normal patterns of movement (Howle, 2002). Also, there is more incorporation of motor learning principles into treatment interventions. Explanations and assumptions guiding the use of these neuromotor approaches have shifted to incorporate more of the current understanding of motor control, organization, and learning. However, rigorous scientific evidence supporting the use of these interventions is limited, while an increasing body of evidence supports CIMT interventions focused on the intensity and duration of functional treatments, repetition in practice as demonstrated in robotic training and the Sabo protocol, and the importance of the interaction of the person with the task and the environment, as evident in the task-oriented and systems approaches (Hoffman & Farrell, 2005; Morris et al., 1997; Sabari, 1995; Taub, Uswatte & Pidikiti, 1999). The more recent studies based on current motor control and learning science support more the tenets of occupation-based practice and the multiple, reciprocal, and distributed personal, task, and environmental influences that support the person's functional recovery, allowing fuller participation in all aspects of life. This evidence, as well as the paradigmatic shift in scientific thinking that has occurred regarding movement control and learning, highlights for the practitioner the importance of being current with the scientific thinking of the time if science and evidence is to continue to guide occupational therapy practice.

---

tional mobile arm supports and overhead slings, could provide the advantages of movement practice at a much lower cost than robotic technology.

CONCLUSION

To foster motor skills in clients, the practitioner must understand the interaction of motor development, control, and learning and the contextual factors that influence skill acquisition and reacquisition. The evolving science of movement science and research on neuroplasticity have dramatically altered our understanding of movement organization, control, and learning and how we as practitioners can foster skill recovery. Practitioners need to be aware that as scientific knowledge about movement evolves, new models of practice may emerge. Practitioners need to keep up to date on motor control and learning research so that they can provide clients with the most effective treatment possible for motor deficits. Likewise, practitioners need to keep current on the amount and quality of the levels of research evidence supporting all motor interventions. With the client's input, therapists can select among evidence-based approaches or combination of approaches that are best suited to assisting the client to maintain and or recover everyday routines and skills.

REFERENCES

Abrams, W. B., Beers, M. H., Berkow, R., Fletcher, A. J., & Besdine, R. W. (1995). *The Merck manual of geriatrics* (2nd ed.). Whitehouse Station, NJ: Merck Research Laboratories.

Anderson, J. R. (1995). *Cognitive psychology and its implications.* New York: W. H. Freeman.

Ashworth, B. (1964). Preliminary trial of carisoprodel in multiple sclerosis. *The Practitioner, 192,* 540–542.

Ayers, A. J. (1972). *Sensory integration and learning disorders.* Los Angeles: Western Psychological Services.

Bartlett, D. (1997). Primitive reflexes and early motor development. *Journal of Developmental and Behavioral Pediatrics: JDBP, 18*(3), 151–157.

Bate, P. (1997). Motor control theories: Insights for therapists. *Physiotherapy, 83,* 397–405.

Bernstein, N. A. (1967). *The coordination and regulation of movements.* London: Pergamon Press.

Bobath B. (1965). *Abnormal postural reflex activity caused by brain lesions.* London: Heinemann.

Bohannon, R. W., & Smith, M. B. (1987). Interrater reliability of a modified Ashworth scale of muscle spasticity. *Physical Therapy, 67*(2), 206–207.

Broeks, J. G., Lankhorst, G. J., Rumping, K., & Prevo, A. J. (1999). The long-term outcome function after stroke: Results of a follow-up study. *Disability and Rehabilitation, 21,* 357–364.

Brooks, V. B. (1986). *The neural basis of motor control.* New York: Oxford University Press.

Brunnstrom S. (1970) *Movement therapy in hemiplegia: A physiological approach.* New York: Harper & Row.

Burton, A. W., & Davis, W. E. (1992) Optimizing the involvement and performance of children with physical impairments in movement activities. *Pediatric Exercise Science, 4,* 236–248.

Capute, A. J., Shapiro, B. K., Accardo, P. J., Wachtel, R. C., Ross, A., & Palmer, F. B. (1982). Motor functions: Associated primitive reflex profiles. *Developmental Medicine and Child Neurology, 24*(5), 662–669.

Carr, J. H., & Shepherd, R. B. (1987). *A Motor re-learning program for stroke* (2nd ed.). Rockville, MD: Aspen.

Carr, J. H., & Shepherd, R. B. (2003). *Stroke rehabilitation: Guidelines for exercise and training to optimize motor skill* (1st ed.). New York: Butterworth-Heinemann.

Cesari, P., & Newell, K. M. (2000). Body scaling of grip configurations in children aged 6–12 years. *Developmental Psychobiology, 36*(4), 301–310.

Connolly, J. S., & Elliott, J. M. (Eds.). (1972). *Evolution and ontogeny of hand function.* London: Cambridge University Press.

Connolly, K. J. (Ed.). (1973). *Factors influencing the learning of manual skills by young children.* London: Cambridge University Press.

Fozard, J. L., Vercryssen, M., Reynolds, S. L., Hancock, P. A., & Quilter, R. E. (1994). Age differences and changes in reaction time: The Baltimore Longitudinal Study of Aging. *Journal of Gerontology, 49*(4), 179–189.

Fowler, E. G., Ho, T. W., Nwigwe, A. I., & Dorey, F. J. (2001). The effect of quadriceps femoris muscle strengthening exercises on spasticity in children with cerebral palsy. *Physical Therapy, 81,* 1215–1223.

Gentile, A. (1992). The nature of skill acquisition: Therapeutic implications for children with movement disorders. In H. Forssberg & H. Hirschfield (Eds.), *Movement disorders in children* (pp. 31–41). Basel: S. Karger.

Gessell, A. (1928). *Infancy and human growth.* New York: Macmillan.

Gessell, A., & Ames, L. B. (1947). The development of handedness. *Journal of Genetic Psychology, 70,* 155–175.

Gibson, J. J. (1966). *The senses considered as perceptual systems.* Boston: Houghton Mifflin.

Gibson, J. J. (Ed.). (1979). *The theory of affordances.* Hillsdale, NJ: Lawrence Erlbaum Associates.

Gibson, J. J. (1982). Notes on affordances. In E. Reed & R. Jones (Eds.), *Reasons for realism* (pp. 401–419). Hillsdale, NJ: Lawrence Erlbaum Associates.

Gleick, J. (1987). *Chaos: Making a new science.* New York: Penguin Books.

Gordon, J. (1987). Assumptions underlying physical therapy intervention: Theoretical and historical perspectives. In J. H. Carr, R. B. Shepherd, J. Gordon, A. M. Gentile, & J. M. Held (Eds.), *Movement science: Foundation for physical therapy in rehabilitation* (pp. 1–30). Rockville, MD: Aspen.

Gracies, J. M., Marosszeky, J. E., Renton, R., Sandanam, J., Gandevia, S. C., & Burke, D. (2000). Short-term effects of dynamic Lycra splints on upper limb in hemiplegic patients. *Archives of Physical Medicine and Rehabilitation, 81*(12), 1547–1555.

Greene, L. S., & Williams, H. G. (1996). Aging and coordination from the dynamical pattern perspective. In A. M. F. N. Teasdale (Ed.), *Changes in sensory motor behavior in aging* (pp. 89–131). Amsterdam: Elsevier.

Greene, P. H. (1972). Problems of organization of motor systems. In R. Rosen & F. M. Snell (Eds.), *Progress in theoretical biology* (pp. 304–338). San Diego: Academic Press.

Haugen, J. B., & Mathiowetz, V. (1995). Contemporary task-oriented approach. In C. Trombly (Ed.), *Occupational therapy for physical dysfunction* (pp. 510–529). Baltimore: Williams & Wilkins.

Held, J., & Pierrot-Deseilligny, E. (1969). *Reeducation motrice des affections neurologiques.* Paris: J. B. Baillere.

Heriza, C. (1991). Motor development: traditional and contemporary theories. In L. MJ Lister (Ed.), *Proceedings of the II STEP Conference: Contemporary Management of Motor Control Problems* (pp. 99–126). Alexandria, VA: Foundation for Physical Therapy.

Hoffman, H., & Farrell, J. (2005). *Improving upper extremity motor recovery following stroke: A novel approach to stroke treatment using the SaeboFlex arm training program.* Paper presented at the Functional Tone Management Arm Training Program, Chicago.

Hogan, N., Krebs, H. I., Rohrer, B., Palazzolo, J. J., Dipietro, L., Fasoli, S. E., et al. (2006). Motions or muscles?: Some behavioral factors underlying robotic assistance of motor recovery. *Journal of Rehabilitation Research and Development, 43*(5), 605–618.

Horak, F. (1991). Assumptions underlying motor control for neurological rehabilitation. In M. Lister (Ed.), *Contemporary management of motor control problems* (pp. 11–28). Alexandria, VA: American Physical Therapy Association.

Horak, H. B., & Macpherson, J. M. (1996). Postural orientation and equilibrium. In J. Shepard & L. Rowell (Eds.), *Handbook of physiology. Section 12. Exercise: Regulation and integration of multiple systems* (pp. 255–292). New York: Oxford University Press.

Houx, P. J., & Jolles, J. (1993). Age-related decline of psychomotor speed: effects of age, brain health, sex, and education. *Perceptual and Motor Skills, 76*(1), 195–211.

Howle, J. M. (2002). *Neuro-developmental treatment approach* (1st ed.). Laguna Beach, CA: NDTA.

Kahn, L. E., Lum, P. S., Rymer, W. Z., & Reinkensmeyer, D. J. (2006). Robot-assisted movement training for the stroke-impaired arm: Does it matter what the robot does? *Journal of Rehabilitation Research and Development, 43*(5), 619–630.

Kandel, E., Schwartz, J. H., & Jessel, T. M. (Eds.). (2000). *Principles of neuroscience* (4th ed.). New York: Elsevier.

Keele, S. W., Cohen, A., & Ivry, R. (1990). Motor programs: Concepts and issues. In *Attention and performance XIII: Motor representation and control* (pp. 77–110). Hillsdale, NJ: Lawrence Erlbaum Associates.

Keshner, E. (1991). How theoretical framework biases evaluation and treatment. In M. Lister (Ed.), *Contemporary management of motor control problems* (pp. 37–49). Alexandria, VA: American Physical Therapy Association.

Knott, M., & Voss, D. E. (1956). Proprioceptive neuromuscular facilitation: patterns and techniques. New York: Hoeber.

Kugler, P. N., & Turvey, M. T. (1987). *Information, natural law, and the self-assembly of rhythmic movement*. Hillsdale, NJ: Lawrence Erlbaum Associates.

Lee, T. D. (1998). On the dynamics of motor learning research. *Research Quarterly for Exercise and Sport, 69*(4), 334–337.

Liepert, J. (2006). Motor cortex excitability in stroke before and after constraint-induced movement therapy. *Cognitive and Behavioral Neurology: Official Journal of the Society for Behavioral and Cognitive Neurology, 19*(1), 41–47.

Liepert, J., Bauder, H., Wolfgang, H. R., Miltner, W. H., Taub, E., & Weiller, C. (2000). Treatment-induced cortical reorganization after stroke in humans. *Stroke, 31*(6), 1210–1216.

Liepert, J., Miltner, W. H., Bauder, H., Sommer, M., Dettmers, C., Taub, E., et al. (1998). Motor cortex plasticity during constraint-induced movement therapy in stroke patients. *Neuroscience Letters, 250*(1), 5–8.

Lin, J. P., Brown, J. K., & Brotherstone, R. (1994). Assessment of spasticity in hemiplegic cerebral palsy: I. Proximal lower-limb reflex excitability. *Developmental Medicine and Child Neurology, 36*(2), 116–129.

Mathiowetz, V. (2004). Task-oriented approach to stroke rehabilitation. In G. Gillen & A. Burkhardt (Eds.), *Stroke rehabilitation: A function-based approach* (2nd ed.). St. Louis: Mosby.

McGraw, M. (1935). *Growth: A study of Johnny and Jimmy*. New York: Appleton-Century-Crofts.

Montgomery, P. (1991). Neurodevelopmental treatment and sensory integrative theory. In M. Lister (Ed.), *Contemporary management of motor control problems* (pp. 135–137). Alexandria, VA: American Physical Therapy Association.

Morris, D. M., Crago, J. E., DeLuca, S. C., Pidikiti, R. D., & Taub, E. (1997). Constraint-induced movement therapy for motor recovery after stroke. *Neurorehabilitation, 9,* 29–43.

Newell, K. M. (1986). Constraints on the development of coordination. In M. G. Wade & H. T. A. Whiting (Eds.) *Motor development in children: Aspects of coordination and control*. (pp. 341–360). Boston: Nijhoff.

Newell, K. M., & McDonald, P. V. (1994). Learning to coordinate redundant biomechanical degrees of freedom. In S. P. Swinnen & P. Casaer (Eds.) *Interlimb coordination: neural, dynamic and cognitive constraints*. (pp. 515–535). San Diego: Academic Press.

Newell, K. M., McDonald, P. V., & Baillargeon, R. (1993). Body scale and infant grip configurations. *Developmental Psychobiology, 26*(4), 195–205.

Newell, K. M., Scully, D. M., McDonald, P. V., & Baillargeon, R. (1989). Task constraints and infant grip configurations. *Developmental Psychobiology, 22*(8), 817–831.

Newell, K. M., Scully, D. M., Tenenbaum, F., & Hardiman, S. (1989). Body scale and the development of prehension. *Developmental Psychobiology, 22*(1), 1–13.

Nolte, J. (2002). *The human brain: An introduction to its functional anatomy* (5th ed.). St. Louis: Mosby.

Patton, J. L., Kovic, M., & Mussa-Ivaldi, F. A. (2006). Custom-designed haptic training for restoring reaching ability to individuals with poststroke hemiparesis. *Journal of Rehabilitation Research and Development, 43*(5), 643–656.

Preston, L. A. (2006). Evaluation of Motor Control. In H. M. Pendleton & W. Schultz-Krohn (Eds.), *Pedretti's Occupational Therapy: Practice skills for physical dysfunction* (6th ed., pp. 403–428.) St. Louis: Mosby Elsevier.

Rice, M. S. (2003). Motor learning strategies for well elderly: A pilot study. *Physical & Occupational Therapy in Geriatrics, 21*(3), 59–74.

Rice, M. S., & Hernandez, H. G. (2006). Frequency of knowledge of results and motor learning in persons with developmental delay. *Occupational Therapy International, 13*(1), 35–48.

Rood, M. (1952). Occupational therapy in the treatment of the cerebral palsied. *The Physical therapy review vol. 32,* 76–82.

Rosenbaum, D. A. (1991). *Human motor control.* San Diego: Academic Press.

Sabari, J. (1995). Carr and Shepherd's motor relearning programme for individuals with stroke. In C. Trombly (Ed.), *Occupational therapy for physical dysfunction* (pp. 501–510). Baltimore: Williams & Wilkins.

Schmidt, R. A. (1988). *Motor control and learning: A behavioral emphasis.* Champaign, IL: Human Kinetics.

Schmidt, R. A., & Lee, T. D. (2005). *Motor control and learning: A behavioral emphasis* (4th ed.). Champaign, IL: Human Kinetics.

Scholz, J. P. (1990). Dynamic pattern theory: Some implications for therapeutics. *Physical Therapy, 70*(12), 827–843.

Shea, C. H., & Wulf, G. (2005). Schema theory: A critical appraisal and reevaluation. *Journal of Motor Behavior, 37*(2), 85–101.

Shumway-Cook, A., & Woollacott, M. (1995). *Motor control: Theory and practical application.* Baltimore: Williams & Wilkins.

Shumway-Cook, A., & Woollacott, M. H. (2001). Motor learning and recovery of function. In A. Shumway-Cook & M. H. Woolacott (Eds.) *Motor control: Theory and practical applications* (pp. 23–43). Baltimore, MD: Williams & Wilkins.

Shumway-Cook, A., & Woollacott, M. (2007). *Motor control: Translating research into clinical practice* (3rd ed.). Baltimore: Lippincott Williams & Wilkins.

Sternad, D. (1998). A dynamic systems perspective to perception and action. *Research Quarterly for Exercise and Sport, 69*(4), 319–325.

Strauss, S. (1982). *U-Shaped behavioral growth.* New York: Academic Press.

Tardieu, G., Shentoub, S., & Delarue, R. (1954). A la recherche d'une technique de mesure de la spasticite. *Revista de Neurologia, 91,* 143–144.

Taub, E. (1994). Overcoming learned nonuse: A new approach to treatment in physical medicine. In J. G. Carlson, A. R.

Seifert, & N. Birbaumer (Eds.), *Clinical applied psychophysiology* (pp. 185–219). New York: Plenum Press.

Taub, E., Crago, J. E., & Uswatte, G. (1998). Constraint-induced movement therapy: A new approach to treatment in physical rehabilitation. *Rehabilitation Psychology, 43*(2), 152–170.

Taub, E., Miller, N. E., Novack, T. A., Cook, E. W., Fleming, W. C., Nepomuceno, C. S., et al. (1993). Technique to improve chronic motor deficit after stroke. *Archives of Physical Medicine and Rehabilitation, 74*(4), 347–354.

Taub, E., & Morris, D. M. (2001). Constraint-induced movement therapy to enhance recovery after stroke. *Current Atherosclerosis Reports, 3*(4), 279–86.

Taub, E., Uswatte, G., & Pidikiti, R. (1999). Constraint-induced movement therapy: A new family of techniques with broad application to physical rehabilitation—A clinical review. *Journal of Rehabilitation Research and Development, 36*(3), 237–251.

Taub, E., & Wolf, S. L. (1997). Constraint induced movement techniques to facilitate upper extremity use in stroke patients. *Topics in Stroke Rehabilitation, 3*(4), 38–61.

Thelen, E. (1986). Treadmill-elicited stepping in seven-month-old infants. *Child Development, 57*(6), 1498–1506.

Thelen, E. (1989). Self-organization in developmental processes: Can systems approaches work? In M. R. Gunnar & E. Thelen (Eds.), Systems and development (pp.77–117). Hillsdale, NJ: Lawrence Erlbaum.

Thelen, E. (1995). Motor development: A new synthesis. *The American Psychologist, 50*(2), 79–95.

Thelen, E., Kelso, J., & Fogel, A. (1987). Self-organizing systems and infant motor development. *Developmental Review, 7,* 39–65.

Thelen, E., & Smith, L. B. (1994). *A dynamic system approach to the development of cognition and action.* Cambridge, UK: Bradford.

Turvey, M. T., & Kugler, P. N. (1984). An ecological approach to perception and action. In H. T. A. Whiting (Ed.), *Human motor actions* (pp. 373–407). New York:

Voss, D., Ionata, M., & Myers, B., (1985) *Proprioceptive neuromuscular facilitation: Patterns and techniques* (3rd ed.). Philadelphia: Harper & Row.

Wagennar, R. C., & van Emmerik, R. E. A. (1996). Dynamics of movement disorders. *Human Movement Science, 15,* 161–175.

Walter, C. (1998). An alternative view of dynamical systems concepts in motor control and learning. *Research Quarterly for Exercise and Sport, 69,* 326–333.

Winstein, C. J., & Schmidt, R. A. (1990). Reduced frequency of knowledge of results enhances motor skill learning. *Journal of Experimental Psychology, 16*(4), 677–691.

Wolf, S. L., LeCraw, D. E., & Barton, L. A. (1989). Comparison of motor copy and targeted biofeedback training techniques for restitution of upper extremity function among patients with neurologic disorders. *Physical Therapy, 69*(9), 719–735.

Wolf, S. L., Thompson, P. A., Morris, D. M., Rose, D. K., Winstein, C. J., Taub, E., et al. (2005). The EXCITE trial: Attributes of the Wolf Motor Function Test in patients with subacute stroke. *Neurorehabilitation and Neural Repair, 19*(3), 194–205.

World Health Organization. (1980). *International Classification of Impairments, Disabilities, and Handicaps: A Manual of Classification Relating to the Consequences of Disease.* Geneva: World Health Organization.

Wulf, G., Schmidt, R. A., & Deubel, H. (1993). Reduced feedback frequency enhances generalized motor program learning but not parameterization learning. *Journal of Experimental Psychology: Learning Memory, and Cognition, 19*(5), 1134–1150.

Psychobiological Factors

56

BARBARA PRUDHOMME WHITE

Learning Objectives

After reading this chapter, you will be able to:

1. Describe a number of psychobiological factors that arise from the autonomic nervous system (ANS), including prominent signs of stress.
2. Describe some of the relationships between ANS and central nervous system (CNS) processes.
3. Describe some of the physical and psychological reasons for ANS disturbance.
4. Describe strategies that therapists can employ to support ANS stability during intervention.
5. Define and describe several examples of human biomarkers that are of interest to occupational science and therapy research.

INTRODUCTION

Imagine your typical day. Did you have to hurry to get to a class on time? Did you get enough sleep that you felt rested? Did you have a paper due or an exam to take? Are you worried about someone? Did you think about someone special? Are you angry with a friend? Are you excited about going on a vacation? Each of these questions should evoke some sort of response from you—either a neutral "No, that's not me" or a quickening heart rate, increased breathing, and tension as you recognized something relevant about which you are concerned. Possibly, one of these questions made you feel a sensation of love, all warm and fuzzy inside with an increased heart rate. This chapter addresses the internal responses that humans have in relation to real-world events, memories, or imagined possibilities. The human body is in continual dialogue with both the outside and inside environments. How we respond is shaped by both how we are constructed in our mother's womb, including our genetic potentials from our parents and our fetal experiences and nutrition, and how we are, moment by moment, influenced by our experiences from our birth forward. The dynamics of what is happening to our bodies in transactions with the environment are intimately linked with each other and not easily teased apart. However, as occupational therapists, we have an interest in this dialogue between the body and the internal and external environments because it influences why people do what they do (engage in activities and occupations) and how successfully they do them.

Psychobiological factors refer to the body function level in the OT Practice Framework (American Occupational Therapy Association, 2007) and pertain to the anatomical and physiological interconnections among brain and body structures as they transact with the environment. Environments are defined as both external (the world) and internal (what we perceive, think, or feel). Psychobiological factors in an individual describe physical responses as our bodies interact with both our internal and external environments and can be broken down into biological and psychological components. *Body functions* in the OT Practice Framework include sensory, cardiovascular, respiratory, pain, visual, auditory, vestibular, olfactory, oral, cognitive, and endocrine (e.g., hormone) functions.

Biological responses (e.g., our internal biophysiology) arise from the body's interaction with the external environment moment by moment in terms of nervous system arousal, engagement, brain response, neurotransmitters and hormone response, and so on. For example, a person who exercises regularly increases demands to the heart muscle and vascular system, and the body becomes stronger and accustomed to this demand. These changes are both immediate (an increase in heart rate to deal with the exercise) and long-term (repeated exercise influences the cardiovascular system's response over time by increasing the size and amount of heart and leg muscle cells as well as blood-pumping efficiency). However, the system remains adaptive; for instance, if the person goes to a higher altitude, the cardiovascular system has to adapt again; less oxygen in higher altitudes means that the heart has to pump faster. In addition, the person experiences accommodations in blood chemistry so that more oxygen-carrying hemoglobin is available. Thus, contextual demands induce physical adaptation in heart rate and internal blood chemistry so that the individual can function effectively in different environments.

Psychological influences to biological responses are those linked with cognition, perception, and emotion instead of, or in addition to, environmental demands. The term implies a certain degree of higher-order "thinking" and its subsequent reaction throughout the body, but this is not necessarily so. For example, we sometimes have emotional reactions to smells and touch sensations for which we are not always aware of the reason. Indeed, neuroanatomical connections exist among structures in the brain that process emotion, which suggests that being aware of the environment is not always necessary to establish an emotional response. Furthermore, relationships with other beings often trigger emotional responses that influence our bodies. Love or feelings of affiliation are associated with high amounts of the hormone oxytocin in the limbic portion of the brain, which cause physical reactions in our body, including increased heart rate and

facial flushing. Sometimes, our perceptions influence our responses. For example, when you see a cat, your physical responses (e.g., heart rate, epinephrine release) are mediated by whether you learned to be fearful of cats or are fond of them. Sometimes we can increase our physical reactions by merely thinking about a task (a midterm exam!) that we have to do, often in the middle of the night when there is no external environmental reason to have a racing heart rate.

REGULATION OF BODY SYSTEMS AND BEHAVIOR

Simply put, *regulation* refers to a dynamic balance between systems that are on "go" and those that are on "rest" (Figure 56.1). For example, when a person is exposed to bacteria, the immune system needs to be on "go" to capture and destroy the invading cells. Once the threat is over, the immune system needs to replenish itself and "rest" in wait for the next attack. These states are defined medically as *allostasis* ("go") and *homeostasis* ("rest"), the balance of which is generally managed unconsciously through the autonomic nervous system (ANS). This is a good thing; otherwise, in addition to remembering to do your laundry and study for an upcoming exam, you would have to add, among a thousand other tasks, "monitor body temperature," "mend radial bone crack," "make more white blood cells, killer-T variety," and "check those cortisol levels in the bloodstream" to your already busy day.

The ANS has two major branches that coregulate each other through homeostatic and allostatic processes: the sympathetic branch (SNS) (also referred to as the sympathetic-adrenomedullary system [SAM]) and the parasympathetic branch (PNS) (Kandel, Schwartz, & Jessell, 2000). Each system serves purposes that are antagonistic to or the opposite of each other; therefore, at any time, one system takes precedence over the other. However, at the same time, the SNS and PNS branches work together to support physiological, emotional, and

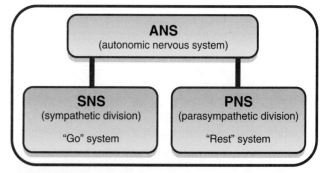

FIGURE 56.1 Autonomic nervous system with sympathetic ("go") and parasympathetic divisions ("rest/chill").

behavioral functioning. In synergistic fashion, both systems adjust and fine-tune what happens in our bodies while we are awake and when sleeping to ensure our capacity to adapt and survive in our environment (Figure 56.2). The SNS drives the fear, flight, or fight responses with increased respiration, cardiac activity, and metabolic activity, among others. Connections between the SNS and the adrenal glands produce the primary stress hormones, epinephrine (also known as adrenalin) and norepinephrine (also known as noradrenalin). Conversely, the PNS branch is concerned

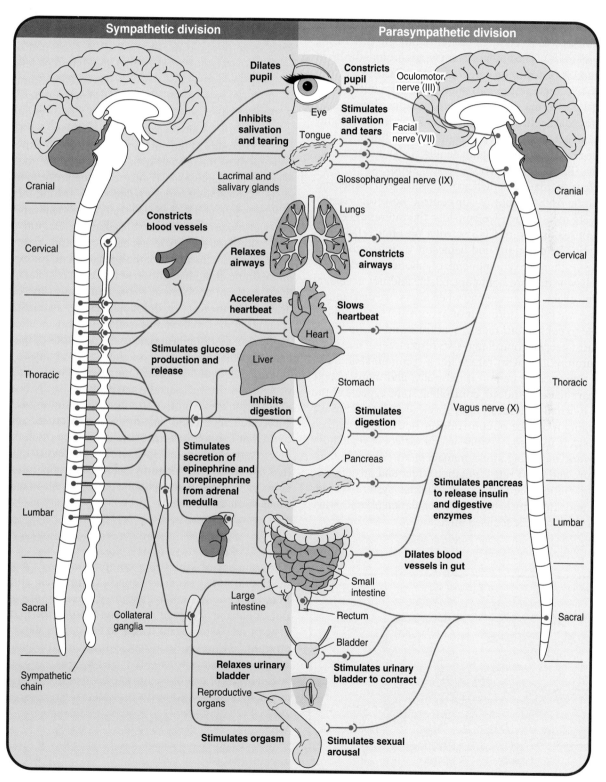

FIGURE 56.2 The autonomic nervous system and its primary functions.

with generalized *homeostasis,* or the state in which primary goals are the conservation and restoration of energy, the digestion and absorption of nutrients, body repair and healing, sexual reproduction, and excretion of waste. Often, the limbic system is included in the structural description of what supports stress responses (see Figure 56.3). The limbic system comprises a number of brain structures that are responsible for emotion formation and emotional behavior as well as complex cognitive thought processing (e.g., memory). The limbic system wraps around the brain stem and is beneath the cerebral cortex. Parts of the limbic system include the cingulate gyrus, the parahippocampal gyrus, the dentate gyrus, the hippocampus, and the amygdala. The parts of the limbic system are highly interconnected with other structures in the brain, including the cerebral cortex, hypothalamus, thalamus, and basal ganglia (Kandel, Schwartz, & Jessell, 2000).

Most regulatory activities of allostasis and homeostasis via the ANS are out of our control; however, regulation gets messy when we consider the interconnections with consciousness, or CNS activity. We often refer to the regulation of emotions and behaviors as *self-regulation.* However, there are components of emotional and physical behavior that are both controllable and not necessarily controllable. For example, when angry, we can control whether we yell or storm out of a room, but we might not be able to control our racing heart rate and flushed face. For most people, controlling ANS responses such as body temperature and heart rate is not a common skill; however, some people can do it naturally, and many people can learn to do it. Indeed, controlling some aspects of the ANS is what underlies biofeedback as a technique for managing a degree of control over body systems. Biofeedback is used successfully with a variety of regulatory behaviors, including stress management (via body temperature and heart rate regulation), fear and anxiety (via cognitive appraisal and stress response system regulation), and attending behavior (via regulation of brain wave states that promote focused attention).

Self-Regulation and Psychobiological Systems

Most psychobiological factors tap into systems that support self-regulation in each environmental context in which an individual finds himself or herself. Self-regulation is critical in supporting functional, adaptive behaviors in occupations and occupational tasks. Thus, understanding more about the body structures and physiology that support self-regulation is in the interest of occupational science and occupational therapists. Self-regulation is defined in this chapter within three primary domains, although in reality, these domains function in tandem (Barkley, 1998; Rothbart, 1981; Rubia et al., 2001). Self-regulation of behavior is the ability to adjust one's activity level to contextual demands of the environment. Sitting relatively still and quietly as the teacher speaks in front of the class is an example of adaptive self-regulation of behavior in a classroom. The child who gets up and walks around the room or fidgets so much that she falls out of her chair represents less well-adapted behavioral regulation. Cognitive self-regulation is the ability to generate or maintain attention skills that meet the needs of the environment, for example, maintaining enough attention to the teacher in the front of the classroom so that one hears and retains the content delivered by the teacher. Emotional self-regulation involves generating and maintaining suitable affect or emotional expression that is appropriate to the demands of the social environment. An example of this is the ability to know when, where, and at what intensity to show happiness or sadness. In a classroom environment, it is not suitable or socially adaptive to burst out laughing because someone tripped and hurt himself. Structures and systems that support self-regulation skills are often the target of psychobiological measures. Self-regulation skills that blend physical, cognitive, and emotional influences support successful occupational engagement in environmental contexts (see Box 56.1).

Stress

The concept of stress is a complicated one. A simple description of stress is as a condition in which either regulatory systems, self-regulatory capacities, or both are out of balance. Most of us use the word *stress* to denote a negative state, as in "I am so stressed I can't think straight." However, in its true definition, stress comes in all forms, many of which are positive. When you are falling in love, for example, you experience a form of stress. Exercise is also a good form of stress; exercise initially takes a toll on the body, but after exercise, we experience a rebound effect in the PNS that is responsible for homeostasis. In other words, after working out, our bodies are replenished with all sorts of hormonal benefits that make us feel good (e.g., endorphins) as well as strengthening and repairing body structures and restoring needed glu-

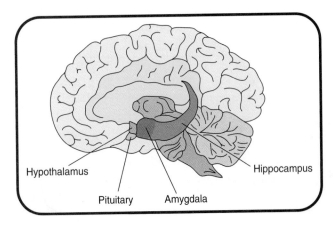

FIGURE 56.3 The limbic system.

SELF-REGULATION

Many children have difficulty regulating their behavior, emotions, and cognitive state in varying contexts. Self-regulation emerges over time, drawing on the development of frontal areas in the brain; young children are not yet very good at it, while older children and adults are expected to have quite a bit of skill in self-regulation. Sometimes, otherwise typically developing children have trouble regulating emotions, attention, and behavior, leading many parents and professionals to describe them as having an attention disorder. In reality, an attention disorder reflects problems regulating more than just attention; behavior, emotions, and cognitive arousal states are frequently clustered together and observed as impaired self-regulation skills. Self-regulation skills can be developed and/or improved through intervention; indeed, the ability to adapt self-regulation skills provides the rationale for an intervention strategy developed by occupational therapists called "How Does Your Engine Run?" This intervention approach, developed for children, provides an understandable structure to help clients recognize their internal arousal states and learn to manage them more effectively in specific environments. (Shellenberger & Williams, 2007).

cose and other nutrients in our blood and cells. Moreover, exercise has the added benefit of helping us to use up unnecessary fat stores. Stress responses support action and, in just the right amount, make us effectively productive. Too much stress, however, takes its toll on functional performance and can degrade the body through excessive wear and tear. There are two stress response systems that are engaged when we encounter a stressor. A primary one is the sympathetic-adrenomedullary branch of the ANS (SAM axis), described previously, which produces epinephrine and norepinephrine. This response is designed to be a fast (within milliseconds) mobilizer of the body for fight, fright, flight, and sex—known with affection as the 4-Fs of the stress system. The SAM axis is designed to be short-lived and highly responsive. Another system, the hypothalamic-pituitary-adrenal (HPA) axis (Figure 56.4), is designed for more sustained body mobilization and is engaged minutes or more after a stressor is encountered or imagined, primarily by releasing cortisol, the major corticosteroid in the human body. Cortisol raises blood sugar by triggering the release of stored fats, as well as by breaking down stored body tissue proteins and triggering the liver to covert them into blood glucose. Cortisol also suppresses the immune system and places most homeostatic functions on hold, including digestion and cell replenishment and repair. The effects of cortisol on the body and brain are extensive and, when long lasting, eventually cause excessive wear and tear on most body structures and systems.

Imagine chronic stress, or allostatic load, as an extended activation of the longer-lasting stress response system, a "go" state in which little if any time is spent on replenishment, growth, and repair. Because of its many functions, it is easy to appreciate why chronic stress has a systemic effect on the body. However, as was previously noted, certain amounts of stress are positive and normal. Optimal stress has been described by a U-shaped curve, borrowed from a description of how much optimal strength of a stimulus is necessary for learning to occur. Referred to as the Yerkes-Dodson principle (Figure 56.5), it also applies nicely to the characteristic of stress, such that increasing amounts of it support and enhance functional behavior until it reaches a peak. After the peak, increased amounts of stress and stress hormones begin to degrade performance and function, leading to imbalances in physiology that also affect health. Chronic increases in stress and cortisol, for example, are linked with immune system dysfunction, cardiac disease, metabolic syndromes including diabetes, and cancer and autoimmune disorders (McEwen, 2002; Sapolsky, 2004).

Stress is also a function of the balance between the type of stressor and the environment paired with the individual's coping resources, attitude, and mood (Figure 56.6). Thus, when faced with a situation, a person weighs environmental information, the nature of the stressor, and his or her own capacities in order to behave adaptively. Often, this appraisal process occurs on an unconscious level. As you can imagine when you think of individuals who thrive in high-stress jobs, one person's stress is another person's delight. Conversely, what may overwhelm one individual might seem like a mere irritant or not even be noticeable to another. A large part of this complexity comes from the capacities and attitudes with which we engage the world around us.

Imagine this scenario: You are taking a course in neurology; you feel fully skilled in your study habits, have put in the time necessary to do all of the readings, and have attended all of the lectures; you feel respected by the instructor; you eat well and get enough sleep; and you

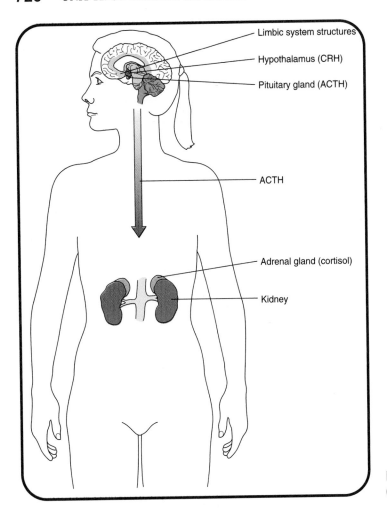

FIGURE 56.4   The hypothalamus-pituitary-adrenal (HPA) axis.

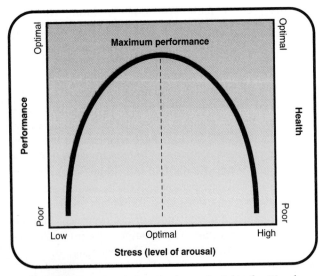

FIGURE 56.5   The Yerkes-Dodson principle of optimal arousal is linked to performance and health. (Source: Adapted from Yerkes, R. M., & Dodson, J. D. (1908). The relation of strength of stimulus to rapidity of habit-formation. *Journal of Comparative Neurology and Psychology, 18,* 459–482.)

have a good idea of what will be expected of you on an upcoming exam. You appear to have the "just right" resources in place to do well, and in this situation, you probably feel energized by taking an exam in the course. However, any variations of this scenario might place you in a less-prepared situation, and as a result, you might feel heightened stress at the prospect of taking an exam.

Personal capacities and resources vary from intellect and social skills to environmental characteristics. Essentially, anything that contributes in a positive way to an individual's ability to adapt to environmental demands can be thought of as a resource and can lead to resilience in the face of threats or challenges. Conversely, characteristics of a person or environment that overwhelm the person may be risks or liabilities. Balancing personal resources with "just right" challenges leads to effective and meaningful engagement in activities and occupations. Being aware of weaker capacities can lead to targeted skill development, improved self-regulation, and accommodations that may lessen the possibility of chronic stress experiences.

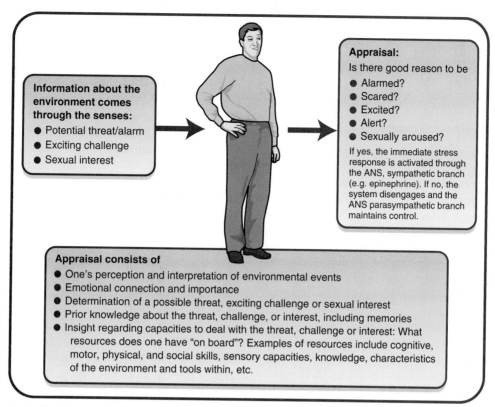

FIGURE 56.6   The physical, emotional, and cognitive factors that are related to stress.

Occupational therapy practitioners are most concerned with *occupational engagement,* or the "doing" of occupations in real contexts. We are most interested in the dynamics between the person; motivation to participate; functional, adaptive behavior; and the environment. Thus, the technologies that allow us to evaluate questions that address real-time participation and engagement in relevant occupations are ones that are likely to be most attractive for us in clinical practice and research. In practical terms, occupational therapy practitioners, as well as occupational scientists, are keen observers of purposeful human behavior. However, this chapter presents information about "internal" and sometimes "hidden" processes that also support functional behavior. These internal states of operation are managed by either the ANS or the CNS and ANS together and are important clues to how well a person's body, emotions, and behavior are both regulated and self-regulated to the context and task demands at hand. The extent to which an occupational therapy practitioner is aware of and can adapt for these internal working states can determine how successfully an individual client will engage in activities and occupations. The next section presents common signs and symptoms of ANS and CNS dysregulation in the clinic or home setting and offers a variety of appropriate response options that can support an individual's engagement in intervention.

POSSIBLE PSYCHOBIOLOGICAL FACTORS THAT ADDRESS THE CONCERNS OF OCCUPATIONAL THERAPISTS

This section describes two sets of psychobiological factors that influence occupational behavior. While these are not intended to be exhaustive lists, the factors that are described are ones that are most commonly identified by clinicians and researchers. OT practitioners should note that any psychobiological factor might be influenced by medication. Therefore, an assessment of medications and their possible influences on heart rate, respiration, temperature, sweating, and emotional expression, among others, is a critical part of understanding psychobiological factors. *Clinically relevant psychobiological factors* are the factors that can be observed in the clinic or community setting without special equipment; these are critical for practitioners to be aware of when working with clients. A second set of *research relevant psychobiological factors,* also referred to as *biomarkers,* are ones that are often used in medical and psychological research, including occupational science and therapy research, to learn how body systems work and adapt meaningfully in response to contextual demands. These biomarkers can also be used in shaping intervention practices by conducting research that suggests to us how and why different intervention strategies are effective in producing meaningful and functional behavior.

Clinically Relevant Psychobiological Factors

Heart Rate and Blood Pressure

Most of us are aware of our resting heart rates and can detect changes as we move around, exert ourselves, or are suddenly emotionally aroused by someone we care about or with whom we have had an argument. Heart rate is adaptive and changes continuously in response to internal or environmental demands. A cardiologist is interested in heart rate and blood pressure as a person increases his or her demand on the cardiovascular system. For example, how hard does the heart have to pump when this person climbs a set of stairs? This is a basic example of the external environment (stairs) influencing the body (increased heart rate). The technology that is available to measure what is happening in the heart includes electrocardiography (abbreviated ECG or EKG), blood pressure measurement, and ultrasound. However, we might also think about another way in which the heart is influenced: by whether the person is angry or frightened—a psychological influence. Thus, changes in heart rate can be triggered by an external event (climbing stairs), by an internal event (having a fear of spiders and thinking of them or seeing them), or both (climbing the stairs to escape the spiders). ECG, blood pressure, or ultrasound does not easily measure only psychological influences; rather, as described above, these measures are based on detecting functional changes because of psychological influences or environmental demands. How might we measure the psychological influences on the heart and tap into an individual's perception of meaning and context? Later in the chapter, a sophisticated method (i.e., vagal tone or respiratory sinus arrhythmia [RSA]) is described that measures the relative contribution of psychological processes to heart rate variability. How might this knowledge inform what a clinician observes in clients within a community or therapeutic context? For one thing, therapists can appreciate that heart rate changes have psychological influences as well as physical ones. For example, if a person who is in cardiac rehabilitation following bypass surgery begins to have racing heart symptoms, it might be caused by the person being nervous or frightened to challenge his or her fragile heart as well as by the physical condition of the heart. A great example of this phenomenon is portrayed in the movie *Something's Got to Give,* in which Jack Nicholson plays an older man recovering from a heart attack who falls in love for the first time with a woman his own age, played by Diane Keaton. During the period in which they are broken up, he has multiple heart "events" that he perceives to be other heart attacks, which in reality they are not. In fact, he is in love and reacts to his emotions with a racing heart and sweaty palms when he sees the woman.

However, increases or decreases in heart rate can be signs of ANS dysregulation and physical stress. For example, in individuals with spinal cord injury, a decreased heart rate may be a sign of autonomic dysreflexia (AD), also known as hyperreflexia, a condition that is unique to individuals with spinal cord injury at C5–C6 or above. AD is a life-threatening condition in which the ANS responds to a physical stressor, often a blocked urinary catheter, a skin lesion, or extremely cold or hot ambient temperatures. Other symptoms of AD include pale skin color below the level of spinal cord injury and flushed skin above, disorientation and/or fainting, headache, increased blood pressure, and sweating above the injury level. This physical stress condition is serious and requires immediate medical assistance.

An increase in heart rate or blood pressure is observed by an accompanied increased breathing rate, reddened skin color changes, nonverbal grimacing or grunting, skin temperature changes, sweating, and complaints of a racing heart and/or a pounding headache. Therapists should quickly determine whether the person's life is threatened by accessing appropriate medical personnel and emergency services. Once an individual has been cleared medically, meaning that the symptoms are not the result of a physical life-threatening cause (e.g., heart attack, extreme high blood pressure), then careful assessment should be used to gather information about any possible psychological influences. In collaboration with the client and other clinicians, the occupational therapist should attend to the clinical symptom through close communication, paving the way for therapeutic intervention to proceed effectively. See Tables 56.1 and 56.2 for information on how to monitor cardiac function.

Sweating

Only the sympathetic branch of the ANS innervates human sweat glands in the skin. This means that only under "stress" do we sweat. However, stress to the body takes many different forms, not all of which are psychological. Body temperature outside of the optimal range (e.g., 98.6°F core temperature) is a form of stress. Therefore, in overheated environments, the body sweats to regulate body temperature by causing sweat on the skin to evaporate, thus cooling the skin and body in the process. Illness is a state of physical stress to the body, as is also the immune system's response to any pathogen that makes us ill. As the immune system triggers a fever to kill off invading pathogens, the body responds by sweating to reduce the increased body temperature. The same mechanism is triggered when the body is heated from exercise. Exercise is also a form of physical stress, albeit a good one. Research shows that individuals who are in good physical condition typically have highly responsive sweating capacity,

TABLE 56.1   CARDIAC INDICATORS

How to Measure Heart Rate via Pulse	Normal Heart Rate by Age	Maximum Heart Rate	Target Heart Rate	Normal Blood Pressure (18 years of age and older)
Carotid pulse (neck): Place your first two fingers horizontally beneath the chin, near the ear. Radial pulse (wrist): Place your first two fingers across the wrist, with finger pads under the thumb. Measure for 10 seconds and multiply by 6 for beats per minute.	Newborn: 120–160 0–5 months: 90–140 6–12 months: 80–140 1–3 years: 80–130 3–5 years: 80–120 6–10 years: 70–110 11–14 years: 60–105 14+ years: 60–100	Maximum heart rate (MHR) is the highest rate that a person should achieve during physical exertion. It is linked to both age and physical fitness. A rough estimate of maximum heart rate is to subtract one's age from 220. However, other factors, including weight and fitness, also need to be considered. 220 – age = MHR Refer to Table 56-2 for maximum heart rate per age.	Target heart rate (THR) is a percentage of an individual's maximum heart rate. It is used for fitness training purposes. Depending on a person's age and overall baseline fitness level, THR will fall somewhere within 50–85% of maximum heart rate. Refer to Table 56-2 for target heart rate per age.	Systolic pressure < 120 Diastolic pressure < 80

TABLE 56.2   TARGET HEART RATE AND AVERAGE MAXIMUM HEART RATE PER AGE GROUP

Age	Average Maximum Heart Rate (100%)	Approximate Target Heart Rate Zone (50–85%)
20 years	200 beats per minute	100–170 beats per minute
25 years	195 beats per minute	98–166 beats per minute
30 years	190 beats per minute	95–162 beats per minute
35 years	185 beats per minute	93–157 beats per minute
40 years	180 beats per minute	90–153 beats per minute
45 years	175 beats per minute	88–149 beats per minute
50 years	170 beats per minute	85–145 beats per minute
55 years	165 beats per minute	83–140 beats per minute
60 years	160 beats per minute	80–136 beats per minute
65 years	155 beats per minute	78–132 beats per minute
70 years	150 beats per minute	75–128 beats per minute

Source: Adapted from the American Heart Association. Retrieved 8/10/2007 from http://www.americanheart.org/presenter.jhtml?identifier=4736

CASE STUDY: *Callie: Exercise and Activity After a Bilateral Knee Replacement*

Callie, age 62, was diagnosed with severe osteoarthritis in both knees. Because she was in so much pain and her mobility was significantly compromised, Callie was referred for bilateral knee replacements. She had both knees replaced without complications and recovered quickly, moving into outpatient rehabilitation about a week after surgery. There, Callie received both physical and occupational therapy, with a focus on personal activities of daily living (ADLs) and functional mobility around her home. Callie's physician determined that Callie was stable enough to participate four times per week in rigorous exercise and occupational engagement. Callie attended a local rehab clinic and participated in 30 minutes of cycling and upper extremity weight lifting as well as walking with supervision for 30 minutes followed by a gardening activity in which she weeded the clinic's vegetable and flower garden. During gardening, her occupational therapist noted that Callie began to sweat visibly, become flushed, and increase her breathing rate. Even though Callie said that she felt "just fine, thank you" when asked, her occupational therapist was concerned, observing Callie carefully. What might be a possible reason(s) for Callie's apparent discomfort? Is it possible that Callie's activity level is too much for her at this time? What are possible steps you would take next, assuming that Callie's color was not typical and her breathing rate continued to be too fast?

making them more likely to sweat a lot during exercise. However, it is also true that there is a lot of variability in the amount that individuals sweat during exercise.

People sweat during psychological stress as well. Think about what happens to most of us when we have to stand in front of a group of people and speak. Individuals might also sweat when anxious about their performance in activities or occupations, especially during assessments. For reasons that are not fully understood, women going through menopause also tend to become overheated periodically and may increase the amount that they sweat during hot flashes.

Sweat happens, and in most instances, it is the natural response to a warm environment, physical exercise, illness, or some degree of typical psychological stress. However, is important to recognize that sweat is also an easily observed sign of stress and anxiety due to extraordinary psychological disturbance. If an individual sweats in the presence of an occupational therapy practitioner, the practitioner should determine the reasons for sweating. If the sweating does not appear to be due to warmth, exertion, menopause, or any other identified cause, then the therapist might consider it to be possibly due to psychological stress. Observed examples of sweating and generalized anxiety due to nervousness from being in a hospital or clinical setting are fairly common among the elderly, people who come from rural areas, and those who come from impoverished backgrounds. Even for people who are familiar with modern health care facilities and personnel, there may be personal reasons for anxiety in these places. It is easy to become comfortable in health care settings when you work there and you understand the people and the culture. However, for many people, hospitals, rehabilitations centers, and outpatient clinics are sources of unknown expectations and loss of control. An astute practitioner never loses his or her perspective that clients and patients may be highly stressed and anx-

ious about being in a health care facility and will consider this in his or her assessment and intervention approaches with the client and the client's family.

Skin Color: Pale or Flushed

Skin color is largely due to how much pigment is present in the dermis, or uppermost layer of the skin. However, baseline skin color can redden or pale perceptively by alterations in blood flow within the skin in response to physical stress or emotions. Although changes may be easier to detect in individuals with lighter pigmentation (e.g., Asian or Caucasian), all people have subtle skin color changes, especially in the face, which are possible to see with careful observation. Some diagnoses—Raynaud's syndrome, for example—can cause skin color changes that are seen typically as blanching in the hands and feet, especially in colder environments. Individuals with Raynaud's syndrome sometimes respond to biofeedback intervention in which they learn to exert some degree of control over their ANS by engaging PNS influences to relax capillaries in their extremities. Skin color and texture changes are also common in individuals with complex regional pain syndrome, a poorly understood condition that affects mostly women in their middle to senior years. In the absence of a known medical condition for atypical skin color changes, most changes can be assumed to be the result of ANS stimulation. Blood vessels in the skin generally constrict when the SNS is engaged, for shunting blood to larger muscles and organs in the body. This effectively supplies blood where it is most needed for physical action. Conversely, blood vessels relax and open under parasympathetic control, allowing for nourishment of all body cells and structures. However, physical stressors such as exercise or fever can cause facial reddening, as can disturbances in cardiac or respiratory activity. Sudden paling may also be a sign of internal physical stress, such as acute

---

CASE STUDY: *ANS Stability in a Premature Infant*

Sam is a male infant who was born prematurely at 28 weeks gestational age. Now, two weeks after delivery, Sam is able to be taken out of his isolette for cuddling by his parents. Sam is beginning to show signs of rooting and sucking on his pacifier, and his mother has expressed a desire to begin feeding him as soon as possible. The occupational therapist and Sam's primary nurse have been observing his reaction to environmental and social stimuli to see whether he is able to regulate body functions such as breathing, color maintenance, and muscle tone as well as to sustain an awake, alert state for short periods. So far, Sam has been doing well at maintaining stability in his ANS while in his isolette, and he is showing signs of purposeful interaction with his caregivers (e.g., visual regard, rooting toward the nipple). However, during one recent snuggle session with his parents outside of his isolette, Sam's heart rate dropped significantly, and his color paled. Why is it important to pay attention to Sam's ANS stability before proceeding to more demanding interactions? What methods might you employ to ensure that Sam is introduced to social interactions successfully?

---

or severe pain. Certain emotions, such as love and anger, can cause sudden reddening of the skin or blushing. At the same time, other emotions, such as fear or anxiety, can pale the skin. It is important that occupational therapy clinicians attend to skin color changes and determine reasons for the changes. Color change may be the first indicator, for example, that an individual client is experiencing pain during movement or activity. In addition, it can be possible that an individual is angry or embarrassed and will not otherwise express the emotion. Furthermore, some individuals might ignore physical symptoms of cardiac or respiratory distress and attempt to push through the warning signals. A clinician who pays close attention to skin color, as well as other psychobiological factors discussed in this chapter, can be instrumental in identifying underlying barriers to successful occupational performance.

Breathing

Respiratory rate is linked with environmental conditions and oxygen levels, physical fitness, cardiac strength and condition, health state of the lungs, and amount of red blood cells and iron available, as well as other health and environmental factors. For example, problems with respiration may be indicative of chronic obstructive pulmonary disease (COPD), which is a term that refers to both chronic bronchitis and chronic emphysema. COPD is caused by obstruction to airflow that interferes with normal breathing. Asthma, another airflow obstructive disease, can also affect respiration rate and is common in children and many adults.

The respiratory rate can also be affected by stress and anxiety; links with cardiac changes make this inevitable. However, respiration is also affected by direct connections from both sympathetic and parasympathetic branches of the ANS. The SNS innervates the lung to open up airways for deep breathing, anticipating hard work in the form of exercise, and either escaping or fighting the threat at hand. In contrast, the PNS constricts airways for more energy-efficient breathing associated with calmer states.

Individuals experiencing psychological stress and anxiety have a similar stress response, just as if they were exercising; they experience faster, deeper breathing to accompany their increased heart rate and in response to sympathetic inputs. Occupational therapy practitioners should ascertain the nature of increased breathing and follow the same clinical reasoning as described for cardiac signs and symptoms. Once physical threats to respiratory stability have been ruled out, the symptom may be determined psychological in nature and indicative of an emotional response (e.g., anger, fear, stress, or anxiety). Respiratory rate is also used in research along with skin conductance and heart rate, as part of what is commonly known as a lie detector test. Respiratory rate is rarely used alone; its meaning is more thoroughly understood in the context of cardiac, skin color, and skin resistance changes.

Skin Temperature: Hot or Cold, Wet/Clammy or Dry

Body and skin temperature is regulated by neurons in the brain stem and the hypothalamus, with connections to other structures within the ANS. Temperature regulation happens in concert with autonomic, endocrine, and motor systems. Temperature feedback sensors are located throughout the body, many of them in the skin as well as in the hypothalamus. Thus, there is constant feedback from the body to the brain regarding temperature, and adjustments are made accordingly. This feedback happens neurochemically, as well as through direct nervous connections. For example, cold temperatures cause the hypothalamus to make thyroxin, a thyroid hormone that increases metabolic rates. Other hormones also affect body and skin temperature; as a result, body temperatures, including subsequent sweating, can vary in women during their menstrual cycles as well as during perimenopause. Shivering is an involuntary response that is driven by the ANS to muscles to increase body temperature, although shivering can also be caused by generalized body temperature disturbance, as in the case

CASE STUDY: *Anxiety in a Woman with an Eating Disorder*

Maggie is a 20-year-old woman with an anorexia-type eating disorder. She was hospitalized recently for severe weight loss and has been silent regarding her feelings about her eating disorder. At the hospital, Maggie attends occupational therapy regularly. One of her goals is to develop her skills in painting, and she and her therapist, Janna, recently went shopping for art materials and had lunch at a local art gallery. Another occupational therapist, Michael, also began working with Maggie. At first, Maggie seemed enthusiastic working with Michael. However, Michael noticed that each time he entered a room where Maggie was, her behavior changed. He observed that Maggie appeared agitated and that her color flushed when he was close by. When asked about it, Maggie admitted that she felt funny, had racing heartbeats, could not breathe well, and became cold and sweaty when Michael came nearby. He encouraged Maggie to discuss her reactions with her counselor, and as a result, Maggie was able to recount a history of sexual abuse by a male family member that she had not previously acknowledged to her caregivers. Maggie said that she felt embarrassed talking about it and thought initially that it had nothing to do with her eating disorder.

Even though Maggie had insisted at first that nothing was wrong when Michael was present, careful attention to her stress signals revealed that she was more upset than she revealed; her body was unable to hide her feelings, and an observant occupational therapist was able to uncover key information that was critical to Maggie's recovery. Can you think of other situations in which subtle signals of distress in another person betrayed feelings and emotions that were otherwise not acknowledged? What are some of the typical signals you might look for in someone who is angry or scared?

An intervention approach that Michael suggested to Maggie was biofeedback training. Michael instructed Maggie in deep breathing exercises and meditation to help manage her racing heart and her shallow breathing. He attached a biofeedback thermometer to her index finger and asked her to mindfully increase the temperature of her fingers. Since warm hands are associated with high PNS influence and increased blood flow, an increase in her distal finger temperature would be a good indicator that Maggie was able to influence her body into a relaxation response. The use of a biofeedback thermometer allowed Maggie to see her success at raising her own finger temperature through purposeful thinking. Once she mastered the technique, Maggie was able to use the technique in other situations in which she felt anxious, allowing her a degree of control over her emotional reaction.

---

of fever-induced shivering. The immune system also influences body and skin temperature by producing substances that cause fever. Fever is indicated by hot, dry skin and feelings of malaise as the body attempts to kill off invading pathogens by increasing body temperature. The typical baseline temperature for humans is 98.6°F, although body temperature drops lower naturally during nighttime sleep.

Cold hands and feet can happen for a variety of reasons, including personal baseline temperature variation and conditions such as Raynaud's syndrome. Other medical conditions that affect blood perfusion in the extremities, including diabetes, can also affect skin temperature in the extremities. However, SNS engagement during stress or anxiety can also cause cold hands and feet. Indeed, acute stress can be accompanied by feeling cold all over. The SNS constricts blood vessels, especially in the extremities, in response to stress. If a client complains of being cold, especially in the hands and feet, or if shivering is observed, the occupational therapy practitioner needs to determine what could be a physical cause. For instance, is the person thin and susceptible to cold? Is the person ill and feverish? Once physical causes have been eliminated, the clinician may reason that cold extremities could be indicative of a stress reaction.

Tears, Salivation, and Digestion

Only the parasympathetic branch of ANS produces tears and saliva. As you recall, the PNS and SNS override each other such that only one system can be "in control" at any one time. Thus, crying with tears does not happen during acute stress. The same is true for salivation and digestion; in fact, the SNS inhibits salivation in the mouth, blood flow to the stomach, and stomach acid production, thus inhibiting digestion during acute stress. This explains why we often experience a dry mouth and indigestion when we feel highly stressed. Only after acute stress, when parasympathetic input is restored, do we experience normal digestion, elimination, and crying with tears. The astute reader might be thinking that people cry during chronic stress and depression, however. This is true, and it brings up a good point about differences between chronic and acute stress. The acute stress response system through the SNS is designed for short-term engagement only. The longer-lasting stress response that is mediated through the HPA system (see Figure 56.4) is designed for more sustained arousal. However, it cannot possibly be on "go" the entire time a person perceives stress. Humans would literally burn themselves out by depleting all nutrients and running internal body systems in high gear. Therefore, chronic stress is riddled periodically by parasympathetic

CASE STUDY: *A Healthy Stress Response*

Torrance is a 35-year-old Iraq war veteran who is currently in outpatient rehab to learn how to use his new upper extremity prostheses. One of Torrance's goals in therapy is to reestablish a busy lifestyle with his children, including his favorite leisure occupation, skiing. His occupational therapist, Selena, along with Torrance's family, planned a ski trip to a local mountain ski resort that specializes in adaptive sports. At the top of the mountain, before his first run, Torrance began unexplainably to cry, sweat, and complain that his heart was racing. Selena noted that this was an expected reaction and began to talk Torrance through the challenge at hand. In addition, she gave him a deep breathing exercise and asked him to focus on his prior skills in skiing. Once Torrance seemed relatively in control, Selena asked him to head down the fall line of the mountain. Was Torrance's life at risk in any way, or was he having a healthy stress response? In pointing out Torrance's capacities, which included an expert level of skiing prior to his injury, what was Selena trying to do? Why did she explain to Torrance that his reactions were normal and expected? How can you prepare for situations like this?

rebounds that allow some degree of restoration to support survival. It is during these intermittent periods that the chronically stressed person is likely to cry tears. Indeed, some researchers suggest that crying is one way in which the PNS mobilizes a return to homeostasis; in other words, crying is a self-regulatory action that produces hormones to make us feel less upset after a stressful situation. This makes sense in light of the old saying "You'll feel better after a good cry." Indeed, most of the time, we do.

Humans are the only animals that cry with tears. Obviously, crying has strong links with emotional experiences. Sometimes we cry when we are happy, and often we cry when we are sad, but there is always a strong emotional experience. Researchers have noted that the chemical constitution of tears changes depending on the reasons for crying, such that happy tears are different from sad ones, which are also different from the tears we produce when cutting an onion. Though the reason for tears has perplexed researchers, and a number of theories have been produced, most researchers agree that tears serve as a communication signal to others. Researchers who are interested in why behaviors develop from an evolutionary perspective believe that tears are a social signal to others that sends a message about true emotional expression. Indeed, crying is hard, if not impossible, to fake unless you "call up" emotional memories to make yourself sad. Therefore, we assume that people who cry tears are expressing their emotions in an honest manner, and we are compelled to act supportively.

Knowing this information about tears, salivation, and digestion should make the occupational therapy practitioner more aware of what subtle behaviors can be observed clinically or in community settings. For example, a dry mouth accompanied by indigestion could be a number of things; for example, medications often have these symptoms as side effects. However, it might also be a signal that an individual is experiencing high amounts of stress and is not expressing this verbally or through other behavioral means. In a similar fashion, crying with tears can be a sign of emotional distress, or it may be the result of emotional lability resulting from neurological damage to limbic system structures and/or the right hemisphere in the brain (i.e., primary locations for emotional regulation). Occupational therapy practitioners need to be aware of the reasons for the emotional expression and address intervention accordingly.

Vision

Any number of things, including age, medications, and disease, can cause changes in visual acuity. However, there are also visual implications related to mood and stress. The SNS dilates the pupil in the eye to support long-distance vision and vigilant behavior. This makes sense because in challenging or stressful situations, an individual needs to be "on guard" for what is happening in the environment. In addition to vision, all senses are heightened so that the person is ready to react. As a result, a highly stressed individual might be less able to focus visually on nearby items and might be unable to attend well or concentrate adaptively to various task demands. In fact, the person might seem agitated and flighty. Conversely, the PNS constricts the pupil and allows for more focused vision, supporting close-up work and social interaction. A calm person is also one who can visually attend for longer periods.

Pain: Grimace and Other Nonverbal (or Verbal) Expressions of Pain

The 2001 Joint Commission on Accreditation of Health Care Organizations report recommended that pain be considered a fifth vital sign, along with pulse, respiration, blood pressure, and temperature, in the physical assessment of patients. Pain is commonly defined as an unpleasant sensory and/or emotional experience that is often associated with damage to body tissues (Figure 56.7). However, many definitions separate pain *sensation* from pain *perception*

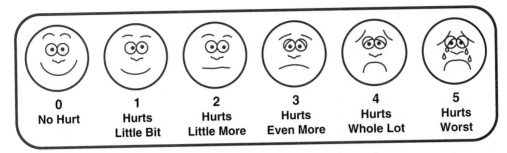

FIGURE 56.7 Wong-Baker FACES Pain Rating Scale. Many health care providers assess pain through scales, especially because pain is difficult to describe and explain in terms of magnitude. Some scales use a numbering system (0 = no pain to 10 = intolerable pain); others use words (low to excruciating). This example provides a visual scale for pain assessment that is used effectively with clients from age 3 years through adulthood. (Source: Hockenberry, M. J., Wilson, D. & Winkelstein, M. L. (2005). *Wong's Essentials of Pediatric Nursing*, ed. 7, p. 1259. Copyright, Mosby: St. Louis. Used with permission.) Done

because pain is an experience that is open to interpretation by other sensations, feelings, and thoughts that coincide with the pain. In other words, the perception of pain changes with environmental context, mood, and stress levels, among other things.

For example, imagine this scenario: You stub your big toe on the way to class and experience sudden, intense pain. However, you are late and shrug off the pain sensation in order to run to class on time. In fact, you hardly feel your bruised big toe at all over the next 30 minutes as you hurry to class. Once you settle in your seat, greet your friends, gather your materials, and begin listening to your professor, your body quiets. Slowly, or perhaps abruptly, you become aware of a throbbing pain in your big toe. What changed? The nerve impulses carrying pain sensations from your big toe did not change since you stubbed it; the nerves continued to respond to the slight swelling and development of a bruise indicating mild damage to the tissues of the big toe. What changed was your perception of the pain in the quieter classroom context with fewer competing sensory perceptions, along with a quieter state of mind and body in which you were more receptive to the pain sensations. Indeed, we are often unaware of slight bumps, bruises, and cuts until we go to bed, where the quiet environment and stillness of our bodies allow pain sensations to jump to the forefront of our awareness. The characteristics of pain that make it adaptable to mood and context along with individual interpretations of perception make pain, especially chronic pain, difficult to assess, understand and manage.

Acute pain is short-term (e.g., minutes, hours, days) and is typically related to injury, disease, or surgery. Acute pain functions as a signal to stop whatever you are doing and rest the damaged body area so that it may heal (Britt, 2006). In this way, pain is a useful messenger. However, chronic pain provides more of a challenge. By definition, chronic pain lasts beyond body damage and repair; furthermore, it is often associated with psychosocial disorders and

might not always connect to an actual physiological event (Britt, 2006). Phantom limb pain, for example, exists long after the wound from an amputation has healed. Identifying the source or reason for back pain is often a mystery for health practitioners. It is clear, however, that psychological stress, depression, anxiety, and negative mood affect pain perception. Occupational therapy practitioners need to pay attention to a person's overall mood and perceived stress level in order to understand the nature and magnitude of the person's pain. To help individuals manage pain, especially during ADLs and other daily occupations, clinicians should be mindful of addressing the individual's stress and anxiety level, mood orientation, and social network (including supports and nonsupports) in addition to the physical aspects of pain management.

Short-term physical stress, including exercise, blunts pain perception through the release of beta-endorphins. These substances, released by the pituitary gland and throughout the body, are internally produced pain relievers, also known as endogenous opiates. Thus, during periods of acute stress, beta-endorphins provide a degree of short-lasting pain relief. Chronic stress, on the other hand, is associated with increased cortisol levels in the body, which appear to make many people hypersensitive to pain perception. As a result, pain thresholds, or the amount of tolerable pain an individual can handle without functional impairment, are lower in the presence of chronic stress.

Intervention Responses to Psychobiological Factors

Stress management, relaxation, and self-regulatory interventions should always be guided by client choice.

Psychobiological Changes Related to Physical Stress

Examples of psychological changes related to physical stress include changes in breathing (too fast or too slow),

CASE STUDY: *Pain in a Woman with Carpal Tunnel Syndrome*

Truth was referred to your clinic for evaluation and possible therapy for bilateral carpal tunnel syndrome. Truth is a 40-year-old woman who works as an administrative assistant to several attorneys in a busy law firm. She has held this position for 12 years and stated that she loves her job; however, she was worried that she would not be able to continue in her position if her condition progressed. She confessed that she was highly anxious about her future job security. Truth had also recently divorced and was sharing custody of two young children with her husband. She was the provider of health benefits for her children. Truth was compliant with her exercises and splinting routine and, as a result, began to show modest improvements in her wrist pain. However, she reported that she did nothing but work, giving up her normal exercise routine as well as cooking for her family

because she was fearful that if she used her wrists and hands too much, the pain would increase and she would be unable to work. As a result, Truth appeared worried most of the time. During therapy, her occupational therapist noticed that Truth became dry-mouthed, unable to pronounce words clearly, and asked for water. Truth also was unable to sit still, seemed distracted in therapy, and appeared on edge. At one point during a therapy session, Truth stated that she felt faint and that her heart was racing.

What might be happening? How might Truth's psychological state be affecting her recovery? What are some strategies that her occupational therapist could use with Truth to address her anxiety? What are the possible physical implications for healing if Truth remains anxious and possibly depressed?

cardiac changes (heart rate too fast or slow, blood pressure too low or high), temperature, sweating, skin color changes, vision changes, emotional lability, indigestion, and complaints of pain.

Intervention Suggestions

- Ascertain whether the client is in any immediate life-threatening danger. If so, access medical help.
- Instruct the individual on how to self-monitor his or her activity level within the range specified by his or her care providers (e.g., know and measure target heart rate).
- Instruct the client on energy conservation techniques for basic and instrumental ADLs.
- Instruct the client in various techniques for stress management, including breathing exercises, relaxation response training, and biofeedback training as appropriate.
- Instruct the client in time management to ensure adequate time spent in leisure occupations and social activities.
- Suggest a pet or other social companion.
- Instruct the client in cognitive-behavioral techniques to promote optimistic mood orientations and prosocial attitudes.
- Instruct the client in reframing techniques to develop better self-control.
- Instruct the client on the importance of sleep, nutrition, and exercise.
- Assist the client in incorporating the suggestions of other professionals (e.g., dietician, nursing, physician, social worker, physical therapist, psychologist) into daily routines, activities and occupations.
- Explore the possible use of complementary alternative medicine approaches such as acupuncture and massage.

Psychobiological Changes Related to Psychological Stress or Problems in Self-Regulation

Examples of psychobiological changes related to psychological stress or problems in self-regulation include changes in breathing (too fast or too slow), cardiac changes (heart rate too fast or slow, blood pressure too low or high), temperature, sweating, skin color changes, vision changes, complaints of pain, mood changes, emotional lability, crying, distractibility, and hyperactivity.

Intervention Suggestions

- Instruct the client to self-monitor internal physical and psychological states.
- Teach the client techniques to modify internal states as appropriate to environmental contexts.
- Instruct the client in various techniques for stress management, including breathing exercises, relaxation response training, and biofeedback training as appropriate.
- Instruct the client in time management to ensure adequate time spent in leisure occupations and social activities.
- Instruct the client on the importance of sleep, nutrition, and exercise.
- Assist the client in incorporating the suggestions of other professionals (e.g., dietician, nursing, physician, social worker, physical therapist, psychologist) into daily routines, activities, and occupations.
- Suggest a pet or other social companion.
- Explore the possible use of complementary alternative medicine approaches such as acupuncture and massage.
- Instruct the client in cognitive-behavioral techniques to promote optimistic mood orientations and prosocial attitudes.
- Instruct the client in reframing techniques to develop better self-control.

♦ Assist the client in broadening his or her activity and occupational repertoire.

♦ Assist the client in managing drug and alcohol abuse by helping him or her to incorporate necessary life changes into daily routines and healthy habits.

RESEARCH RELEVANT PSYCHOBIOLOGICAL FACTORS: BIOMARKERS

Occupational science and occupational therapy research, from a psychobiological perspective, concerns itself primarily with structures and processes that support occupational behavior. Essentially, the questions that drive research are ones about what is going on inside a person's body or brain that supports or drives the behaviors we see. Technological advances give us tremendous insight into body structures, but we are still limited in measuring internal processes as people *do* something. As a result, some psychobiological-based measures lend themselves more easily to addressing this interest in *understanding the doing* than perhaps do others. Some measures are technically difficult to obtain or measure things that might not be relevant specifically to occupational therapy. For example, a computed tomography (CT) scan gives a detailed picture of body structures that are essential in identifying normal versus atypical growth and development. However, a CT scan does not give information regarding how they the body structures work in context (a question that is relevant to occupational therapy). Similarly, a functional magnetic resonance image (fMRI) assesses body structure and function, but does not address contextual functional performance in the way occupational therapists define *function*. Though a great tool for investigating functional skills that can be performed in an MRI bed and tube, with only finger movement for pointing, the fMRI limits the sort of questions that might be asked of people who are performing meaningful tasks within typical environments. Can you imagine trying to measure a person's brain function with an fMRI scanner under the task demand of making a peanut butter sandwich?

Some measures are too intrusive for occupational therapists to obtain regularly. For example, unless an occupational therapy practitioner or researcher works in an acute care setting and has direct access to blood and urine samples, these measures would not be feasible to collect. Saliva samples, on the other hand, as well as cardiac measures, lend themselves to greater possibilities for use as measures in occupational therapy research. Thus, the extent to which occupational scientists and occupational therapy practitioners can measure psychobiological factors is influenced by available technology, as well as by our interest in certain behaviors. This next section describes a selection of psychobiological measures that can give us a window into internal processes. When measures are based on psychobiological processes, we label them *biomarkers*. Some biomarkers are direct and "up close" to what is the target for measurement. For example, a test of the number and type of blood cells in the body (or complete blood count, or CBC) measures red and white blood cells in a sample of blood; this is pretty straightforward as biomarkers go. On the other hand, some biomarkers are more "distal" in nature, meaning that they measure something that is one or more steps removed (distal) from the actual process of interest. Cortisol is an example of a distal biomarker. Often measured in saliva as an unobtrusive biomarker, salivary cortisol is an estimate of the cortisol in blood that is related to the amount of the precursor hormone adrenocorticotropin hormone (ACTH) in the body. ACTH is sent to the adrenals from the pituitary gland because of how much of the precursor corticotropin-releasing hormone (CRH) is sent from the hypothalamus. CRH was released because of messages sent to the hypothalamus from the ANS to sustain a heightened stress state. This might seem complicated, but you get the point. In a perfect situation, we would rather assess the amount of CRH that is sent from the hypothalamus to the pituitary in response to a stressor, because this would be a more direct measure of a stress response. However, we cannot ethically tap into people's brains to measure these processes in healthy adults. Therefore, we need to rely on biomarkers that are more distal. Distal biomarkers are still relevant, but they can be tricky to understand because they are not the immediate measure of a response but rather are a measure of something that happened a few steps back. However, research ethics preclude the type of research that measure biomarkers within brain structures and other organs; this is one of the reasons why animal research can be so valuable.

The following sections discuss selected examples of psychobiological measures that are used in research.

Electrodermal Response

Because sweat glands are innervated by the SNS (the "go" system) and thus affect the tension of the skin, many researchers have been interested in using skin resistance via sweat glands as a stress response biomarker. Electrodermal response (EDR), also known as galvanic skin response (GSR), refers to a measurement of the electrical conductance of skin, specifically related to the sweat glands. The preferred term is *EDR* or *electrodermal activity*. Sweat glands respond to ANS activity by fluctuations in salt and water concentrations that lead to either sweaty or dry skin. The concept that supports EDR is that emotional arousal and subsequent ANS activity from the SNS causes changes in skin conductance. Some evidence suggests that brain circuitry originating in the prefrontal cortex and limbic structures mediates the electrodermal response through the SNS (Critchley, 2002). Higher SNS stimula-

CASE STUDY: *Depression in Individuals with Acquired Brain Injury*

Liz works as an occupational therapist in a rehabilitation facility. Her primary caseload is with individuals who have acquired brain injury, either from trauma or from a stroke. Within this setting, her team is noticing that a large number of individuals are depressed following the injury, and they suspect that it is more than just depression due to ability and lifestyle changes. The rehabilitation team has followed recent research regarding depression and links to dysregulation in the stress response system. They would like to include a psychobiological measure, or biomarker, in a research study, and the local university is willing to assist them. What are possible psychobiological measures that would address stress physiology and possibly depression? What ones are more feasible for use, on the basis of Liz's need to be as nonintrusive as possible? What other measures would be appropriate to include?

tion (e.g., arousal or stress) is associated with skin sweating, a lowered skin electrical resistance, and therefore increased electrical conductance. A relaxation state or higher PNS is associated with drier skin and higher electrical skin resistance, resulting in decreased electrical skin conductance. Unfortunately, a number of emotions (e.g., sexual desire, anger, fear) produce the same response (e.g., SNS arousal), making an interpretation of the results difficult. For example, an individual's response could be based on fear, happiness, or the need to go to the bathroom, which are all SNS-arousing events but for very different reasons. The most common application of EDR is as part of a polygraph assessment, or lie detector test. The polygraph uses cardiac and respiratory information as well as EDR. However, the polygraph is considered a controversial assessment for legal use because of its unreliability in discerning the source of an individual's response. In a novel application of this biomarker, a recent study (Marci & Riess, 2005) used EDR to objectively measure the degree of connectedness in developing therapeutic rapport between a therapist and a client.

EKG/ECG and Vagal Tone

Previously, we asked, "How might therapists measure the psychological influences on the heart that tap into an individual's perception of meaning and context?" This question has driven a number of researchers, including some occupational therapists, to learn measurement strategies that assess the unique contribution of cognitive and emotional appraisal to heart rate variation. This psychobiological measure, called *vagal tone,* is a derived estimate of heart rate variability that is due not to physical reasons, but rather to psychological ones. Thus, vagal tone is an example of a biomarker that estimates psychological influences (e.g., cognition and emotions) on a body system (e.g., heart rate).

EKG/ECG does not easily measure psychological influences on heart rate; rather, as was described previously, it is based primarily on measuring functional changes in heart rate in response to immediate environmental demands (e.g., blood oxygen levels, climbing stairs). The vagus nerve (tenth cranial) provides a direct nervous system connection to the heart, and is primarily influenced by the PNS. While both branches of the ANS influence the heart, the SNS contributions increase heart rate and blood pressure, while the PNS slows down the heart and thus influences the resting heart rate. Heart rate variability is measured in periods, also referred to as R-R intervals or interbeat intervals. In a simple example, if a person experiences an environmental threat, the SNS takes precedent and increases heart rate; in contrast, when a person is relaxed, the PNS is predominant and slows the heart rate.

Porges (1992) as well as other researchers have developed algorithms that calculate a measure of RSA or vagal tone. These require EKG/ECG readings that are then further analyzed to factor out heart rate variability contributions that can be attributed to vagal nerve inputs. An overall measure of RSA is then computed. In general, lower measures of heart rate variability are associated with less adaptable behaviors and poorer developmental capacities. Highly competent parasympathetic reactions appear to be faster and more flexible and are thus reflected in higher values of heart rate variability. Another technique for quantifying heart rate variability uses spectral analysis of cardiac electrical frequencies (Zhuravlev, Rassi, Mishin, & Emery, 2002). The parasympathetic and sympathetic branches of the ANS oscillate at different frequencies and can be captured by using EKG/ECG heart rate monitors and computerized analysis. The results are displayed as power spectrums of low- and high-frequency bandwidths that disentangle the sympathetic and parasympathetic components. While this biomarker is useful for research purposes, it cannot be used clinically because it requires specialized computers, ECG/EKG connections, and technical expertise.

Cortisol

Cortisol is a glucocorticoid hormone (i.e., steroid) that is released by the adrenal glands that sit on top of each kidney. The hormone is released as part of a complex system called the hypothalamic-pituitary-adrenal axis (see Figure 56.4). The purpose of this hormone is to sustain metabolic activity, increased vigilance, and increased blood pressure, among other things, such that the individual can

COMMENTARY ON THE EVIDENCE

Examples of Relevant Research Using RSA (Vagal Tone)

Schuetze (2006) examined RSA in young infants (4–8 weeks) with and without prenatal cocaine exposure and found that differences existed in RSA between both groups, depending on the extent of cocaine exposure. In general, infants with greater cocaine exposure displayed lower RSA variability when compared to typical children and to those with lower amounts of cocaine exposure (Schuetze & Eiden, 2006). The same researchers also found that 2- to 4-week-old infants who were exposed to prenatal maternal smoking as well as environmental smoke after birth had lower RSA values when compared to nonexposed infants. In addition, although both boys and girls appeared affected by smoke exposure, they found a greater effect for boys, suggesting greater vulnerability. Smith (2003) found that very low-birth-weight premature infants also had lower vagal tone, suggesting potential risks for developmental outcomes.

In one study of typical 2-year-old children, researchers found that vagal tone differed as a result of maternal interaction style (Calkins, Smith, Gill, & Johnson, 1998). Children's behavioral and emotional regulation was linked to lower vagal tone in children whose mothers were more negative in their interactions. This study highlights a potentially important variable of parenting style in the development of self-regulation skills and opens discussion for abilities such as self-regulation to be adaptive to environmental influences. Other researchers have noted the influence of parents and social environments in the development of self-regulation abilities, especially in relation to attention and behavioral regulation (Quas, Bauer, & Boyce, 2004).

DeGangi, Porges, Sickel, and Greenspan (1993) used a measure of vagal tone with infants who had been determined to have some degree of regulation disorder at 8–11 months. Regulation problems included disturbances in sleeping, self-calming, and state-transition control, as well as early signs of sensory processing problems. The infants were untreated and were assessed again at 4 years of age and compared to typical peers. Their results suggested that low vagal tone assessed earlier in infancy was associated with poorer developmental outcomes and behavior regulation skills at 4 years of age in comparison to typical children. These data, though based on a small sample, suggest that vagal tone might be a reasonable biomarker for potential developmental difficulties, as related to behavior regulation. Schaaf, Miller, Seawell, and O'Keefe (2003) used vagal tone measures in children with problems in sensory processing. Although it was a small pilot study, they also found lower vagal tone in children with sensory processing problems when compared to children without problems, and documented the need for further research in this area.

---

deal with environmental challenges. Cortisol is released in pulses or surges throughout the day and night as part of a circadian cycle as well as in response to both internal and external events, such as feelings of excitement or worry or a police siren and lights pulling up behind you on the freeway.

Salivary α-Amylase

Salivary α-amylase has recently been studied as a marker of SNS activation or stress system responding. Generally, catecholamines provide a reliable marker for SNS activity in research by measuring epinephrine and norepinephrine in urine or blood. However, collection of blood and urine is either too invasive and/or impractical for many human research endeavors. α-Amylase is a protein-based digestive enzyme that is produced by the salivary glands (e.g., the parotid glands) in response to SNS activity, thereby increasing the amounts of α-amylase in saliva for the purpose of breaking down sugars in the digestive tract so that energy is released to support "fight-or-flight" behavior. In contrast, parasympathetic activation of the salivary glands increases the saliva flow rate and thus reduces the amount of α-amylase in saliva (Rohleder, Nader, Wolf, Ehlert, & Kirschbaum, 2004). Salivary α-amylase appears sensitive to both physical (e.g., exercise) and social stressors in studies of typical individuals (Granger et al., 2006; Rohleder et al., 2004; Wetherell et al., 2006). Normal secretions of α-amylase appear to follow a reliable daily release pattern in typical adult individuals (Granger et al.,

COMMENTARY ON THE EVIDENCE

Relevant Research Using Salivary Cortisol

There is converging evidence from multiple well-conducted research efforts that suggest that HPA dysregulation is real in people with stress-related and other health conditions and that it links well with what is known from animal studies (Gunnar & Vazquez, 2006; Schneider, Moore, Kraemer, Roberts, & DeJesus, 2002). Furthermore, we can use this research to help shape interventions. For example, in individuals who are recovering from cancer, depression is linked with rates of recovery and survival (Jehn et al., 2006). One of the emerging biomarkers for depression in cancer patients is cortisol along with an immune system biomarker, interleukin-6 (Jehn et al., 2006). Researchers have proposed that these biomarkers can be used to identify people with cancer who are at risk for depression and then intervene proactively. Although further research is needed to better understand whether HPA dysregulation is the cause or a symptom of health disorders, researchers seem to agree that it is a mixture of both.

Another relevant use of cortisol in research might be as a psychobiological measure to mark, among many occupational therapy interventions, the potential effects of social participation and occupational engagement. HPA reactivity appears to be sensitive to environmental influence and interventions. Gitau, Modi, Gianakoulopoulos, Bond, and Glover (2002) demonstrated that cortisol levels were modifiable in preterm infants through skin-to-skin contact with mothers. In children, the social environment appears to influence responses to stress (Braarud & Stormark, 2006; Nachmias, Gunnar, Mangelsdorf, Parritz, & Buss, 1996; Young, Vazquez, Jiang, & Pfeiffer, 2006) through both supportive (e.g., sensitive) and nonsupportive (e.g., parental depression) caregiving patterns. In adults, the HPA appears to be sensitive to social mediators as well, in the form of supportive friendships (Heinrichs, Baumgartner, Kirschbaum, & Ehlert, 2003). In other words, in the presence of supportive relationships, people appear to be able to lower their overall stress state, at least as measured by their stress-related hormones.

CASE STUDY: *Sensory Modulation Disorder in a 5-Year-Old Girl*

Gillian is a 5-year-old girl with some peculiar behaviors. Her parents are not quite sure how to understand her and think that at times she acts strangely for attention. However, they recently inquired about the possibility that Gillian has a sensory modulation disorder. As they describe her behavior to her pediatrician, it becomes clear that Gillian's behavior crosses a line into a functional impairment. For example, Gillian refuses to wear any clothes but two outfits, and she prefers that they be unwashed. She refuses all socks on her feet, stating that they "hurt." She protests if her mother attempts to wash her bedsheets, and she cannot tolerate having any windows open in the house. In addition, certain lights "hurt her ears," especially in grocery stores, and she is fearful of public places and anywhere there is the possibility of loud noises. To her parents' dismay, she does not like to be hugged or cuddled, and her diet is restricted to solid, firm foods such as apples, bread, and cheese. Her parents have also noticed that she seems to be developing anxiety around leaving the house. For example, she is now complaining about headaches and stomachaches, and she seems to become anxious and jittery for no apparent reason.

What are some psychobiological indicators that are possibly associated with Gillian's behavior? How would you determine whether she is experiencing stress responses related to otherwise non-threatening things in her environment? How might you incorporate stress management interventions to help Gillian with her sensory disturbances? Can you think of ways to use any psychobiological factor as an indicator of possible effectiveness of sensory integration intervention?

CASE STUDY: *Weight Loss and Obesity Prevention*

Jay is an occupational therapist working in a community-based outreach program for individuals with low incomes. Jay is interested in using a number of outcome measures that would demonstrate the effectiveness of an intervention program that he directs along with a dietitian, a nurse, and a social worker. The program's key purposes are to promote weight loss in low-income single mothers, to prevent obesity in children through participation in exercise that is embedded in daily routines, and to teach healthier eating habits. For example, participants learn to take the stairs when possible and to avoid elevators unless they need to go above five floors in a building. In addition, Jay teaches participants how to shop for healthy foods on a budget as well as low-fat meal preparation. The intervention group also works with the mothers on time management skills and on other forms of exercise. Many of the women and children in the program report high stress and anxiety levels that affect them daily. The team, in consultation with community physicians and university researchers, would like to include psychobiological measures as a part of their research approach, in addition to a number of other measures, including weight loss. Many of the mothers have elevated blood fats and are showing signs of developing type 2 diabetes.

◆ What questions could you ask about psychobiological factors in these women and children that are related in some way to their occupations and activities?

◆ What would you hope to see change if this program is effective?

◆ Are any psychobiological measures presented here that could address your questions?

◆ Where might you look for further information on psychobiological factors and obesity?

◆ How could occupational therapy practitioners complement research that is being done in other science areas?

2006). This pattern appears to run opposite to that of salivary cortisol; whereas cortisol peaks in the morning and gradually declines throughout the day, typical α-amylase patterns appear to demonstrate lower levels in the morning and higher levels in the afternoon and evening (Rohleder et al., 2004). To date, studies using α-amylase levels in typical children are just emerging (Granger et al., 2006), and nothing has been published regarding atypically developing children. There is also preliminary research using salivary α-amylase in pregnant women. The use of α-amylase as a biomarker appears promising, but there are obvious needs for future research in multiple samples across the life course.

Functional MRI

Functional MRI (fMRI) measures increased blood flow and oxygen use in different parts of the brain under stimulus-response conditions. This increased blood flow that supports the neural activity is accompanied by a characteristic decrease in a substance called deoxyhemoglobin, a normal by-product that is produced when cells extract oxygen from hemoglobin in the blood. Deoxyhemoglobin has weak magnetic properties that provide the source of the signal for the fMRI. The process is different from regular MRI in that no radioisotopes are injected into blood circulation. To collect fMRI data, an individual lies flat in an MRI scanner (Figure 56.8). A variety of auditory, visual, and touch stimuli (depending on the purpose of the fMRI) are introduced to the individual while he or she lies still in the apparatus. The individual then generates a response either by moving fingers (e.g., touching a clicker to respond "yes" to a question) or by saying something aloud (Figure 56.9).

Electroencephalography, Magnetoencephalography, and Event-Related Potential

An electroencephalograph (EEG) provides a noninvasive method of looking at brain activity. The EEG records the brain's natural electrical activity through electrodes that are strategically placed on an individual's scalp. EEG research has documented characteristic electrical signals or patterns for various states such as awake and sleep such that individual EEG signals can be compared to typical expectations. EEG is useful in displaying how long it takes and, broadly, what regions are important in processing various kinds of information in the brain. However, EEG does not show specific structures or which specific regions of the brain do specific tasks.

Magnetoencephalography (MEG) is a new technology that measures natural magnetic signals that are emit-

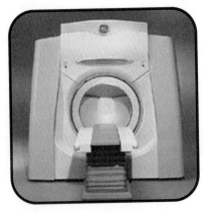

FIGURE 56.8 Magnetic resonance imaging (MRI) scanner.

COMMENTARY ON THE EVIDENCE

Relevant Research Using MRI or fMRI

Functional MRI (fMRI) is being used in a number of research studies related to human behavior. Recently, Aron, Gluck, and Poldrack (2005) noted that fMRI can be a stable measure over time in individuals, suggesting that it can be a reliable marker of brain development as well as neurodegeneration over time. Thus, fMRI might be a suitable biomarker for outcome-based research on the efficacy of occupational therapy interventions. For example, Talati, Valero-Cuevas, and Hirsch (2005) investigated brain function in normal individuals performing an in-hand manipulation of a spring that required calibration of force and fine motor accuracy. The researchers altered trials such that the participants performed the tasks sometimes under visual guidance and sometimes under tactile-only conditions. The findings noted that the neural networks to produce accurate fine motor performance required a highly distributed and integrated neural complex that included multiple structures in the brain, which sometimes differed depending on whether the participants used vision to guide their motor actions. This suggests that fine motor dexterity is interdependent on sensory input and that the processing of sensory input takes place in multiple areas. From a therapeutic standpoint, we might use this information to support using rich sensory experiences when helping others acquire or relearn fine motor skills. Erickson

and colleagues demonstrated, using fMRI as a psychobiological measure, that skills training in older individuals lessened cognitive decline, which is often associated with aging (Erickson, Colcombe, Elavsky, et al., 2007; Kramer, Colcombe, McAuley, Scalf, & Erickson, 2005). The results suggested that fMRI could detect beneficial changes in prefrontal areas in the brain as a result of training, as well as demonstrating that the aging brain was still capable of plasticity, or adaptive changes in response to the environment (Erickson, Colcombe, Wadhwa, et al., 2007).

Researchers who investigated specific brain regions associated with social interactions (Walter et al., 2004) provided another interesting example of fMRI use in behavioral studies. Their findings suggested that social interaction appraisal (e.g., understanding other people's intentions in social interactions) is supported by specific brain regions in the prefrontal cortex (e.g., the paracingulate gyrus area in the brain). Social intention understanding is important for a theory of mind (e.g., understanding that what others might be thinking may be different from your own thoughts) and is one of the significant deficits identified in individuals with autism spectrum disorders. A clearer understanding of the brain areas that may be impaired in diagnoses such as autism will help with diagnosis as well as contributing to new treatments and interventions.

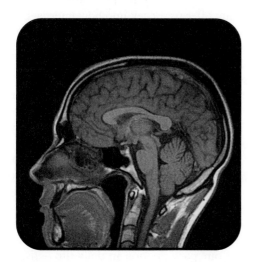

FIGURE 56.9   MRI image of an individual's brain.

ted from brain activity. Although MEG produces a highly accurate record of brain cell activity, only a few machines are currently available worldwide because of cost (millions of dollars), size (eight tons or more), and advanced technology (a specialized quantum physics apparatus is needed). As with other machines that measure brain activity, MEG is impractical for investigating brain function under contextual demands such as meal preparation, self-care activities, and other occupations. However, it might prove useful for limited questions of functional performance similar to those posed in fMRIs.

The event-related potential (ERP) is similar to EEG in that it is a measure of electrical activity in the brain. However, the ERP is a neural signal that reflects the coordinated pattern of activity in groups of neurons as they respond to a meaningful event. Meaningful events for ERP analyses are usually noises or visual stimuli, but they can

---

CASE STUDY: *Constraint-Induced Techniques*

Tim works with adult stroke patients in an outpatient rehabilitation facility. He has recently learned how to use constraint-induced techniques with his patients and believes that he is seeing improvement of function. However, there is little information in the research literature that links this intervention approach to behavioral changes as well as the possible neural plastic changes that would support improved motor behavior. Tim contacts Rowan, a researcher in the area who is interested in the similar issues, and they decide to work as a team. Rowan and Tim decide to write a grant together and develop a research plan. What specific questions can you develop for their research topic that might use a psychobiological measure? How would you use this measure(s)? What are some of the behavioral measures that you would use in addition to your biomarkers?

---

also reflect emotional states or other internally generated "events." A type of ERP is the auditory evoked potential, which measures specifically brain activity to sounds. This is a powerful tool in determining the potential for hearing in people who otherwise cannot state whether they can hear (e.g., infants, nonverbal adults). One strength of ERP is the ability to see cortical networks as they engage and disengage depending on the events or the tasks that the person is doing. However, during assessment, an individual is connected with an elaborate head covering in which the electrodes are strategically placed, limiting the questions that can be posed of brain function while the person is engaged in occupational "doing."

Oxytocin

Oxytocin is a mammalian peptide composed of amino acids that is produced by the pituitary gland. It is a potent hormone in the body and neurohormone in the brain, responsible for sexual reproduction and supporting caregiving behavior, including stimulating milk production for breastfeeding. In both males and females, orgasm releases large of amounts of oxytocin. Moreover, if you have ever experienced the feeling of "love," you have experienced a rush of oxytocin in the emotional centers of your brain. Oxytocin is similar to vasopressin, another pituitary hormone/neurohormone that is responsible for salt and fluid regulation in the body as well as blood pressure. One of the effects of oxytocin in the brain is to suppress the HPA axis, thereby reducing levels of cortisol (Detillion, Craft, Glasper, Prendergast, & De Vries, 2004; Heinrichs et al., 2003) as well as blood pressure. Because oxytocin is associated with social behavior, it is an attractive psychobiological measure for studying human behavior in social contexts. The research is somewhat limited at the current time only because it is not an easy measure to collect. However, in concept, oxytocin would be an excellent biomarker for studies investigating the effects of social participation and occupational engagement in individuals with a variety of disorders that especially influence social abilities, including autism spectrum disorder, obsessive-compulsive disorder, and schizophrenia. More-

over, it would be an effective biomarker for documenting the effects of stress management interventions, since studies document that oxytocin acts as a buffer for the stress hormone cortisol (Heinrichs et al., 2003; Kiecolt-Glaser et al., 2005), especially when individuals have companionship.

Oxytocin can only be measured in blood or cerebral spinal fluid at this time, and levels of oxytocin appear to change within seconds and/or within a few minutes in response to an environmental stimulus, making its use as a psychobiological measure somewhat limited in human studies.

SUMMARY

Sophisticated and adaptive mind-body connections in humans allow for the richest and most complex behaviors on the planet. Indeed, we are such elaborate thinkers and doers that we risk underappreciating and perhaps even missing the more subtle aspects of our behavior. Moreover, we can sometimes use our language skills to either dismiss or cover up our "true" feelings in certain situations. This chapter presented information about the subtle signs and "hidden" indicators linked with human behavior that offer us a peek into how internal body processes support interest, motivation, and engagement in activities and occupations. Sometimes individuals are not aware of the influences that, for example, a health condition might be having on their performance. Some people might not be aware of psychological reasons that can influence participation and fulfillment. Others might mask their true feelings for a variety of reasons, and unless voiced, these feelings can impede daily functioning. Moreover, some individuals certainly attempt to dull or bury unmanaged stress, anxiety, worry, or pain by abusing alcohol or drugs, by overeating or undereating, or by participating in other risky activities that can impair their health and well-being. We might not care so much about these subtle psychobiological factors if they did not have so much influence on our participation in daily life activities and occupations and on our overall health. Indeed, many of these psychobiological factors, as we discussed in this chapter, are related to either physical or psychological stress that can greatly affect our health and well-being. The extent to which occupational therapy practitioners are aware of subtle psychobiological factors will influence and shape their practice. It is important that practitioners appreciate the ways in which psychobiological factors may be observed and understand the potential messages that they can impart about their clients' wellness, health, and participation in life activities and occupations. Furthermore, practitioners should know a wide variety of stress management techniques and be prepared to use them along with other practice skills in any area of occupational therapy practice. Finally, an enhanced appreciation of psychobiological factors and their potential in research will help to define the next generation of occupational science scholars and therapy practitioners by giving us a better understanding of mind-body relations in human functional performance as well as by adding to objective documentation of the effectiveness of therapy intervention.

REFERENCES

American Occupational Therapy Association. (2007). *Occupational Therapy Practice Framework: Domain and Process.* Bethesda, MD: Author.

Aron, A. R., Gluck, M. & Poldrack, R. A. (2005). Long-term test-retest reliability of functional MRI in a classification learning task. Neuroimage, 29, 1000–1006.

Barkley, R. A. (1998). *Attention deficit/hyperactivity disorder: A handbook for diagnosis and treatment.* New York: Guilford Press.

Braarud, H. C., & Stormark, K. M. (2006). Maternal soothing and infant stress responses: Soothing, crying and adrenocortical activity during inoculation. *Infant Behavior and Development, 29*(1), 70–79.

Britt, R. R. (2006). *The pain truth: How and why we hurt.* Accessed July 30, 2007, from http://www.livescience.com/health/060131_pain_truths.html

Calkins, S. D., Smith, C. L., Gill, K. L., & Johnson, M. C. (1998). Maternal interactive style across contexts: Relations to emotional, behavioral and physiological regulation during toddlerhood. *Social Development, 7*(3), 350–369.

Critchley, H. D. (2002). Electrodermal responses: What happens in the brain. *The Neuroscientist, 8*(2), 132–142.

DeGangi, G. A., Porges, S. W., Sickel, R. Z., & Greenspan, S. I. (1993). Four-year follow-up of a sample of regulatory disordered infants. *Infant Mental Health Journal, 14*(4), 330–343.

Detillion, C. E., Craft, T. K., Glasper, E. R., Prendergast, B. J., & De Vries, A. C. (2004). Social facilitation of wound healing. *Psychoneuroendocrinology, 29,* 1004–1011.

Erickson, K. I., Colcombe, S. J., Elavsky, S., McAuley, E., Korol, D. L., Scalf, P. E., et al. (2007). Interactive effects of fitness and hormone treatment on brain health in postmenopausal women. *Neurobiology of Aging, 28*(2), 179–185.

Erickson, K. I., Colcombe, S. J., Wadhwa, P. D., Bherer, L., Peterson, M. S., Scalf, P. E., et al. (2007). Training-induced plasticity in older adults: Effects of training on hemispheric asymmetry. *Neurobiology of Aging, 28*(2), 272–283.

Gitau, R., Modi, N., Gianakoulopoulos, X., Bond, C., & Glover, V. (2002). Acute effects of maternal skin-to-skin contact and massage on saliva cortisol in preterm babies. *Journal of Reproductive and Infant Psychology, 20*(2), 83–88.

Granger, D. A., Kivlighan, K. T., Blair, C., El-Sheikh, M., Mize, J., Lisonbee, J. A., et al. (2006). Integrating the measurement of salivary alpha-amylase into studies of child health, development, and social relationships. *Journal of Personal and Social Relationships, 23,* 267–290.

Gunnar, M. R., & Vazquez, D. M. (2006). Stress neurobiology and developmental psychopathology. In D. Cicchetti & D. Cohen (Eds.), *Developmental psychopathology: Developmental neuroscience* (pp. 533–577). New York: Wiley.

Heinrichs, M., Baumgartner, T., Kirschbaum, C., & Ehlert, U. (2003). Social support and oxytocin interact to suppress cortisol and subjective responses to psychosocial stress. *Biological Psychiatry, 54,* 1389–1398.

Jehn, C. F., Kuehnhardt, D., Bartholomae, A., Pfeiffer, S., Krebs, M., Regierer, A. C., et al. (2006). Biomarkers of depression in cancer patients. *Cancer, 107*(11), 2723–2729.

Kandel, E. R., Schwartz, J. H., & Jessell, T. M. (2000). *Principles of neural science* (4th ed.). New York: McGraw-Hill. Done

Kiecolt-Glaser, J. K., Loving, T. J., Stowell, J. R., Malarkey, W. B., Lemeshow, S., Dickinson, S. L., et al. (2005). Hostile marital interactions, proinflammatory cytokine production, and wound healing. *Archives of General Psychiatry, 62*(12), 1377–1384.

Kramer, A. F., Colcombe, S. J., McAuley, E., Scalf, P. E., & Erickson, K. I. (2005). Fitness, aging and neurocognitive function. *Neurobiology of Aging, 26,* 124–127.

Marci, C., & Riess, H. (2005). The clinical relevance of psychophysiology: Support for the psychobiology of empathy and the psychodynamic process. *American Journal of Psychotherapy, 59*(3), 53–60.

McEwen, B. (2002). *The end of stress as we know it* (1st ed.). Washington, DC: Joseph Henry Press.

Nachmias, M., Gunnar, M. R., Mangelsdorf, S., Parritz, R., & Buss, K. A. (1996). Behavioral inhibition and stress reactivity: Moderating role of attachment security. *Child Development, 67,* 508–522.

Porges, S. W. (1992). Vagal tone: A physiological marker of stress vulnerability. *Pediatrics, 90,* 498–504.

Quas, J. A., Bauer, A., & Boyce, W. T. (2004). Physical reactivity, social support and memory in early childhood. *Child Development, 75*(3), 797–814.

Rohleder, N., Nader, U. M., Wolf, J. M., Ehlert, U., & Kirschbaum, C. (2004). Psycho-social stressed-induced activation of salivary alpha-amylase: An indicator of sympathetic activity? *Annals of the New York Academy of Sciences, 1032,* 258–263.

Rothbart, M. K. (1981). Measurement of temperament in infancy. *Child Development, 52,* 569–578.

Rubia, K., Taylor, E., Smith, A. B., Oksannen, H., Overmeyer, S., & Newman, S. (2001). Neuropsychological analyses of impulsiveness in childhood hyperactivity. *British Journal of Psychiatry, 179,* 138–143.

Sapolsky, R. M. (2004). *Why zebras don't get ulcers* (3rd ed.). New York: Henry Holt.

Scaaf, R. C., Miller, L. J., Seawell, D., & O'Keefe, S. (2003). Children with disturbances in sensory processing: A pilot study examining the role of the parasympathetic nervous system. *American Journal of Occupational Therapy, 57,* 442–449.

Schneider, M. L., Moore, C. F., Kraemer, G. W., Roberts, A. D., & DeJesus, O. T. (2002). The impact of prenatal stress, fetal alcohol exposure, or both on development: Perspectives from a primate model. *Psychoneuroendocrinology, 27*(1–2), 285–298.

Schuetze, P., & Eiden, R. D. (2006). The association between maternal cocaine use during pregnancy and physiological regulation in 4- to 8-week old infants: An examination of possible mediators and moderators. *Journal of Pediatric Psychology, 31*(1), 15–26.

Shellenberger, S., & Williams, M. S. (2007). *How does your engine run?* Albuquerque, NM: Therapyworks.

Smith, S. L. (2003). Heart period variability of intubated very-low-birth-weight infants during incubator care and maternal holding. *American Journal of Critical Care, 12,* 54–64.

Talati, A., Valero-Cuevas, F. J., & Hirsch, J. (2005). Visual and tactile guidance of dexterous manipulation tasks: an fMRI study. *Perceptual and Motor Skills, 101,* 317–334. Walter, H., Adenzato, M., Ciaramidaro, A., Enrici, I., Pia, L., & Bara, B. G. (2004). *Understanding intentions in social interactions: The role of the anterior paracingulate cortex. Journal of Cognitive Neuroscience, 16* (10), 1854–1863.

Wetherell, M. A., Crown, A. L., Lightman, S. L., Miles, J. N. V., Kaye, J., & Vedhara, K. (2006). The four-dimensional stress test: Psychological, sympathetic-adrenal-medullary, parasympathetic and hypothalamic-pituitary-adrenal responses following inhalation of 35% CO_2. *Psychoneuroendocrinology, 31,* 736–747.

Young, E. A., Vazquez, D. M., Jiang, H., & Pfeiffer, C. R. (2006). Saliva cortisol and response to dexamethasone in children of depressed patients. *Biological Psychiatry, 60*(8), 831–836.

Zhuravlev, Y. E., Rassi, D., Mishin, A. A., & Emery, S. J. (2002). Dynamic analysis of beat-to-beat fetal heart rate variability recorded by a squid magnetometer: Quantification of sympatho-vagal balance. *Early Human Development, 66,* 1–10.

Evaluation and Intervention for Cognitive Perceptual Impairments

57

JOAN PASCALE TOGLIA,
KATHLEEN M. GOLISZ, AND
YAEL GOVEROVER

Learning Objectives

After reading this chapter, you will be able to:

1. Define cognition and describe its association with activity limitation and participation.
2. Discuss the role of occupational therapy practitioners in cognitive rehabilitation.
3. Describe the key characteristics of three evaluation approaches that can be used in cognitive rehabilitation.
4. Discuss the difference among the main three intervention approaches: remedial, functional, and multicontext.
5. Discuss the factors that need to be considered when choosing evaluation and intervention approaches.
6. Define specific cognitive and perceptual skills, identify possible assessments to evaluate these skills, and discuss the different approaches for therapy that are described for each cognitive and perceptual skill.

"Thinking, remembering, reasoning, and making sense of the world around us are fundamental to carrying out everyday living activities" (Unsworth, 1999, p. 3). **Cognition** consists of interrelated processes including the ability to perceive, organize, assimilate, and manipulate information to enable the person to process information, learn, and **generalize** (Abreu & Toglia, 1987). Because so much of rehabilitation in general requires learning and generalization, the principles of intervention that are discussed in this chapter are important to consider with a wide spectrum of clients and are not limited to those who are typically identified with cognitive impairments. Cognitive impairments may be seen as a result of developmental or learning problems, brain injury or disease, psychiatric dysfunction, or sociocultural conditions (American Occupational Therapy Association, 1999). Cognitive impairments can result in significant activity limitations and participation restrictions in all aspects of the client's life, potentially compromising safety, health, and well-being. For example, decreased abilities to recognize potential hazards, anticipate consequences of actions and behaviors, follow safety precautions, and respond to emergencies are often major factors that interfere with independence. Cognitive limitations can also diminish one's sense of competence, self-efficacy, and self–esteem, further compounding difficulties in adapting to the demands of everyday living. The influence of cognitive symptoms can be observed across all aspects of the domain of occupational therapy practice. The aim of occupational therapy intervention for people with cognitive-perceptual impairments is to decrease activity limitations, enhance participation in everyday activities, and assist individuals to gain the abilities they need to take control over their lives and develop healthy and satisfying ways of living. Although the ultimate goal of intervention with this population is clear, there are different perspectives and rehabilitation approaches to accomplish the goal. These approaches are discussed in detail in this chapter.

OCCUPATIONAL THERAPY ROLE WITHIN A MULTIDISCIPLINARY TEAM

Currently, there is no single discipline that is responsible for the evaluation and intervention of cognitive-perceptual impairments. Multiple team members have the potential to make valuable contributions to understanding the client who has a cognitive-perceptual impairment. A strong interdisciplinary approach is needed to address the complex of issues that arise from cognitive-perceptual problems. Team goals should be identified, as well as specific discipline goals. The family and client are also members of the team and should be involved in team discussions and provide input into the overall intervention plan.

Occupational therapists provide a unique contribution to the evaluation and rehabilitation of cognitive perceptual process skills because of their educational background, knowledge of occupation, training in activity analysis, and ability to analyze how cognitive-perceptual symptoms are affected by changes in activity demands and context. The role of the occupational therapist in evaluating cognition and perception is to provide clear, comprehensive information on the effect of cognitive-perceptual impairments on activities of daily living (ADLs), instrumental activities of daily living (IADLs), education, work, play and leisure, and social participation. The work environment in which the therapist practices may determine the depth of the occupational therapist's involvement because of the nature of the practice setting and the client's length of stay.

An interdisciplinary intervention program should emphasize the same major goals during intervention rather than working on separate skills. For example, the speech-language pathologist might address **attention** problems within the context of language material, such as listening to tapes or conversations; the neuropsychologist might use remedial attentional exercises; the physical therapist might reinforce attention through motor tasks; and the occupational therapy practitioner might address attentional strategies within the context of self-care, leisure, community, or work activities. An integrated approach that assists the person in seeing patterns of behaviors across different activities is strongly advocated, rather than one that reinforces the fragmentation that the client already perceives.

The occupational therapy assistant works in cooperation with the occupational therapist to contribute to the evaluation process and implement aspects of the occupational therapy intervention plan (AOTA, 1999). If state licensure permits and service competency has been demonstrated, an occupational therapy assistant can administer selected portions of cognitive assessments as directed by the occupational therapist, provide clinical observations, and complete behavioral checklists. Once the targeted behaviors for intervention have been clearly identified, the occupational therapy assistant and occupational therapist collaborate to choose a variety of different activities that can be used to reinforce the desired behaviors.

THE PROCESS OF COGNITIVE REHABILITATION

Evaluation

This section provides detailed information about cognitive evaluation issues that are necessary for practitioners to understand before choosing and performing appropriate evaluations and assessments. We present the importance of the evaluation process, its goals, and important considerations in choosing an assessment.

The evaluation process begins with an occupational profile that considers the client's typical routines and occupations (AOTA, 2002). The client is usually asked to identify everyday activities that he or she is most concerned about or would like to be able to do with greater ease. However, people with cognitive impairments often have limited awareness of their impairments and limited understanding of the implications of these impairments (Goverover, Chiaravalloti, & DeLuca, 2005); therefore, a close relative or friend should participate in identifying concerns and priorities for intervention. It should be kept in mind that in inpatient settings, clients and their relatives might be unaware of the presence of mild cognitive impairments. Subtle cognitive symptoms tend to be apparent only in higher-level activities such as driving, social participation, shopping, or using public transportation. A client in an acute or rehabilitation inpatient setting has not yet had the opportunity to resume these higher-level activities.

Comprehensive cognitive evaluations are needed for two primary reasons. First, evaluations provide evidence and information about the presence of impairments and competencies. Such information can be used to establish baselines, to plan discharge, and to measure intervention effectiveness (e.g., rehabilitation outcomes). Second, evaluations are needed to gather information for intervention planning. Models for cognitive intervention in occupational therapy often guide the focus of evaluation. For example, the cognitive disability model (Allen, 1985) and the neurofunctional model (Giles, 2005) focus on occupational performance and are not concerned with identifying specific cognitive impairments. The cognitive disability approach (Allen, 1985) describes hierarchical levels of cognitive function. Evaluation focuses on identifying the cognitive level at which the person is functioning. The neurofunctional approach (Giles, 2005) emphasizes training functional skills and habits within naturalistic settings; therefore, evaluation emphasizes observation of real-life functioning. The quadrophonic approach (Abreu & Peloquin, 2005) and the cognitive retraining model (Averbuch & Katz, 2005) are concerned with identifying and understanding the cognitive impairments that are influencing occupational performance. Measures of cognitive impairment are examined in combination with broader measures of occupation to guide intervention. The multicontext approach (Toglia, 2005) is concerned with facilitating transfer of learning, so evaluation emphasizes evaluation of learning potential or dynamic assessment. Each of these perspectives is described in greater detail later in the chapter.

Approaches to Evaluation of Cognitive Impairments

Traditional Approaches to the Evaluation Process

Standardized cognitive assessments have specific administration guidelines and compare the client's performance to normative data. They are static in nature, evaluating "here and now" performance. Standardized assessments can help the occupational therapist to determine whether a cognitive impairment exists and to quantify the severity of such impairments. These types of assessments are also useful as baselines against which changes in condition or ability can be measured over time. Examples of standardized assessments are summarized in Table 57.1.

Cognitive-screening assessments are a type of standardized assessment designed to identify problems that need special or further attention. They typically comprise subtests that are divided into specific cognitive subskills such as attention, visual processing, **memory**, and **executive functions**. These assessments are either general in nature, addressing all cognitive subskills, such as the Lowenstein Occupational Therapy Cognitive Assessment,

(Katz, Itzkovich, Averbuch, & Elazar, 1990), or more focused evaluations of a particular subskill, such as the Motor Free Visual Perception Test (Colarusso & Hammill, 2002). Impaired performance on a specific task or subtest is typically used to define the impairment. For example, difficulty differentiating foreground objects or figures from background objects (e.g., picking up a white sock off a white sheet) would be identified as a figure-ground impairment (Zoltan, 1996).

Many cognitive-screening assessments were designed to be used with specific populations, such as clients with strokes (Hajek, Rutman, & Scher, 1989), multiple sclerosis (Rao, Leo, Bernardin, & Unverzagt, 1991), dementia (Mattis, 1976), or traumatic brain injury (Ansell & Keenan, 1989) or elderly clients (Golding, 1989). These assessments have subtests that focus on areas of impairment that are typically seen within the diagnostic population.

Mental status exams, such as the popular Mini-Mental State Exam (Folstein, Folstein, & McHugh, 1975) and cognitive screening assessments have some disadvantages, as they rely heavily on verbal skills, can be culturally biased (owing to comparison to normative populations), and have substantial false-negative rates (i.e., missing possible cognitive impairments). The deficits of clients with focal lesions, particularly right-hemisphere lesions, or mild diffuse cognitive disorders are often missed (Nelson, Fogel, & Faust, 1986). Cognitive-screening assessments usually miss more subtle impairments that are displayed by higher-level, clients as the breadth and depth of item content are limited (Doninger, Bode, Heinemann, & Ambrose, 2000).

Direct Observation of Function

Direct observation of function is an alternative method that is used to identify cognitive-perceptual impairments. A variety of standardized functional assessments (presented in Table 57.1) use a numerical or descriptive scale to rate performance and the amount of cognitive cueing and/or physical assistance required to complete a particular task. Some functional assessments are designed to identify the cognitive and perceptual impairments that interfere with successful performance on such tasks. For example, in the OT-ADL Neurobehavioral Evaluation (A-ONE) (Arnadottir, 1990), a client is observed performing a basic ADL activity (e.g., putting on a shirt) for possible cognitive impairments such as spatial relation difficulties, unilateral spatial or body neglect, and the like. The Executive Function Performance Test (Baum, Edwards, Morrison, & Hahn, 2003; Goverover et al., 2005) is another functional performance test that analyzes cognitive impairments such as initiation, organization, and safety by observing client performance on IADL activities such as making a phone call.

Functional tasks require the integration of a variety of skills, so it can be difficult to isolate the specific cognitive problems interfering with performance. Some functional assessments try to identify broad areas of cognitive and

TABLE 57.1   COGNITIVE PERCEPTUAL ASSESSMENTS

STANDARDIZED COGNITIVE SCREENING INSTRUMENTS

Blessed Dementia Rating Scale (Blessed, Tomlinson, & Roth, 1968)
Brief Test of Head Injury (BTHI) (Helm-Estabrooks & Hotz, 1991)
Cognitive Assessment of Minnesota [CAM] (Rustad et al., 1993)
Cognitive Competency Test [CCT] (Wang, Ennis, & Copland, 1992)
Galveston Orientation and Amnesia Test [GOAT] (Levin, O'Donnell, & Grossman, 1979)
Lowenstein Occupational Therapy Cognitive Assessment [LOTCA] (Katz et al., 1990)
Middlesex Elderly Assessment of Mental State [MEAMS] (Golding, 1989)
Mini Mental State Exam [MMSE] (Folstein, Folstein, & McHugh, 1975)
Modified Mini-Mental Examination [3MS] (Teng & Chui, 1987)
COGNISTAT [Neurobehavioral Cognitive Status Screening Examination] (Kiernan, Mueller, & Langston, 1983)
Repeatable Battery for the Assessment of Neuropsychological Status [RBANS™] (Randolph, 1998)

STANDARDIZED FUNCTION-BASED COGNITIVE SCREENING INSTRUMENTS

Allen Cognitive Level Test [ACL] (Allen, Earhart, & Blue, 1992)
Assessment of Motor and Process Skills [AMPS] (Fisher, 1993a, 1993b)
Cognitive Performance Test [CPT] (Allen, Earhart, & Blue, 1992)
Executive Function Performance Test [EFPT] (Baum, Edwards, Morrison, & Hahn, 2003)
Independent Living Scales (ILS) (Loeb, 1996)
Kitchen Task Assessment [KTA] (Baum & Edwards, 1993)
OT-ADL Neurobehavioral Evaluation [A-ONE] (Arnadottir, 1990)
Rabideau Kitchen Evaluation [RKE-R] (Neistadt, 1992b)

STANDARDIZED ASSESSMENTS FOR SPECIFIC COGNITIVE IMPAIRMENTS

Orientation Assessments

Orientation Log [O-Log] (Jackson, Novack, & Dowler, 1998)
Test of Orientation for Rehabilitation Patients [TORP] (Deitz, Beeman, & Thorn, 1993)

Attention Assessments

Comprehensive Trail-Making Test [CTMT] (Reynolds, 2002)
Paced Auditory Serial Addition Test [PASAT] (Gronwall, 1977)
Test of Everyday Attention [TEA] (Robertson, Ward, Ridgeway, & Nimmo-Smith, 1994)

Unilateral Neglect Assessments

The Baking Tray Test (Tham & Tegner, 1996)
The Balloons Test (Edgeworth, Robertson, & McMillan, 1998)
Behavioral Inattention Test [BIT] (Wilson, Cockburn, & Baddley, 1987)
The Bells Test (Gauthier, Dehaut, & Joanette, 1989)
Indented Paragraph Test (Caplan, 1987)
Line Cancellation (Albert, 1973)
Verbal and Nonverbal Cancellation Tasks (Mesulam, 2000)

Memory Assessments

Contextual Memory Test [CMT] (Toglia, 1993b)
Hopkins Verbal Learning Test–Revised [HVLT-R] (Brandt & Benedict, 2001).
Prospective Memory Screening [PROMS] (Sohlberg & Mateer, 1989b).
Rivermead Behavioral Memory Test–Extended Version (RBMT-E) (Wilson, Clare, Baddeley, Watson, & Tate, 1998)

TABLE 57.1   COGNITIVE PERCEPTUAL ASSESSMENTS   *Continued*

Visual Perception Assessments

Brain Injury Visual Assessment Battery for Adults [biVABA] (Warren, 1998)
Motor Free Visual Perception Test [MVPT-3] (Colarusso & Hammill, 2002).

Executive Function Assessments

Behavioral Assessment of Dysexecutive Syndrome [BADS] (Wilson et al., 1996)
Behavior Rating Inventory of Executive Function–Adult Version [Brief-A] (Roth, Isquith, & Gioia, 2005)
Executive Function Route Finding Task [EFRT] (Boyd & Sautter, 1993)
Multiple Errands Test [MET] (Shallice & Burgess, 1991)
Profile of Executive Control System [PRO-EX] (Branswell et al., 1992)
Revised Observed Tasks of Daily Living [OTDL-R] (Diehl, Willis, & Schaie, 1995)
Toglia Category Assessment [TCA] (Toglia, 1994)

Awareness Assessments

Assessment of Awareness of Disability (ADD) (Tham, Bernspang, & Fisher, 1999)
Awareness Questionnaire [AQ] (Sherer, Bergloff, Boake, High, & Levin, 1998)
Patient Competency Rating Scale [PCRS] (Prigatano, 1986)
Self-Awareness of Deficits Interview [SADI] (Fleming, Strong, & Ashton, 1996)

Motor Planning Assessments

Benton Constructional Praxis Test (Benton, Hamsher, Varney, & Spreen, 1983)
Test of Oral and Limb Apraxia [TOLA] (Helm-Estabrooks, 1992)

---

perceptual strengths and weaknesses by identifying the underlying processes that contribute to difficulty in performing functional tasks. Therefore, subtle cognitive impairments might not be readily apparent in familiar activities. Functional assessments that simulate performance in a treatment setting might not be predictive of performance in natural **contexts** in which the person has to set goals, plan, initiate, problem-solve, and deal with subtle and complex environmental cues.

Situations that require higher-level cognitive-perceptual skills are difficult to capture in structured treatment environments. In addition, contextual factors can increase or decrease cognitive demands of performance, so it important to consider the context in which an activity is performed. Hamera and Brown (2000) developed the Test of Grocery Shopping Skills as a real-world measure of community function for people with chronic schizophrenia. Clients are asked to shop for a list of 10 grocery items in a natural context. In hospital-based treatment settings, the occupational therapist might not be able to create a close enough approximation of a real-world environment. The contextual influence on performance needs to be kept in mind, and if feasible, performance should be observed across real-world contexts.

Other tools that involve direct observation of performance have been developed to measure the cognitive levels associated with the cognitive disability model. For example, the Allen Cognitive Level Screen (ACLS) (Allen, 1985) uses a leather-lacing task to provide a quick measure of learning and an initial estimate of cognitive function. The ACLS screen is then validated by further observations of performance in craft activities or ADL/IADL activities using additional tools such as the Routine Task Inventory (RTI), Allen Diagnostic Module craft projects, or the Cognitive Performance Test (Allen, 1993; Allen, Earhart, & Blue, 1992).

These tools are interpreted within Allen's conceptual framework and focus on broadly identifying the person's cognitive level or general information-processing capacities. In contrast to functional assessments that are concerned with rating specific cognitive skills or the degree of assistance that is required on specific functional tasks, assessment of the person's cognitive level involves global functional abilities and is meant to explain and predict ability to function in various activities and contexts (Levy & Burns, 2005).

See Table 57.1 for detailed information about performance-based ADL evaluations.

Dynamic Assessment

Dynamic assessment is a nontraditional approach to evaluation that uses cues, mediation, feedback, or alterations of activity demands during assessment to examine changes in performance. Unlike standardized assessments, the focus is not on the outcome of performance but on the processes of learning and change. Dynamic assessment has also been referred to as assessment of learning potential or cerebral plasticity.

Dynamic assessment investigates a person's ability to learn certain tasks and identifies the conditions that facilitate such learning. The objective is to discover what the person is capable of doing with assistance, or under favorable conditions to determine the full range of performance potential. Because dynamic assessment is interested in *how* performance can be facilitated, it is naturally linked to intervention. During an evaluation, the therapist intervenes to change, guide, or improve the person's performance by demonstrating strategies, providing cues, or modifying the activity (Tzuriel, 2000). This information directly relates to intervention planning. For example, if performance cannot be modified through dynamic procedures, then an intervention approach that seeks to change the environment or train caregivers might be more appropriate than an approach that focuses on changing a person's abilities or behaviors. Dynamic assessment methods have been applied to a wide range of ages and people with cognitive disabilities, including those with developmental disabilities (Hessels-Schlatter, 2002), schizophrenia (Rempfer, Hamera, Brown, & Bothwell, 2006; Wiedl, 2003), stroke, brain injury (Haywood & Miller 2003; Toglia, 2005), and Alzheimer's disease (Fernandez-Ballesteros, Zamarron, & Tarraga, 2005). However, research applications and specific tools are limited. Toglia (2005) describes the use of a dynamic assessment approach for people with brain injury within the framework of a dynamic model of cognition. Dynamic assessment and intervention within this model involve investigating self-perceptions of abilities before and after activity experiences, facilitating change in performance if a person has difficulty, and investigation and analysis of strategy use. The Contextual Memory Test (Toglia, 1993b) and Toglia Category Assessment (Toglia, 1994) are two examples of dynamic assessments (Table 57.1). Other resources by Toglia (2005) provide information on how to apply the dynamic assessment process in practice.

Proponents of dynamic assessment claim that conventional static assessments are incomplete in describing the range of performance potential. There is a considerable difference between identifying and quantifying deficits and making specific recommendations for intervention. A more comprehensive picture of the person's ability, including responsiveness to learning situations, is needed to provide guidance for intervention (Kolakowsky, 1998; Lidz, 1991; Tzuriel, 2001). Dynamic assessments therefore do not replace standardized tests but supplement the information that is obtained and provide direct guidance for intervention planning.

Choosing the Most Appropriate Type of Assessment

In selecting the most appropriate type of assessment, an occupational therapist must first decide what questions

need to be answered. The therapist can then select the assessment that will most effectively address such questions. Some factors to consider before choosing an assessment include questions such as the following:

1. *Does the therapist need to clarify the presence of cognitive impairments?* To answer this type of question, a traditional evaluation approach can provide the therapist with a normative comparison. The extent to which the person's scores deviates from expected performance within the person's age group identifies the presence and severity of cognitive impairments.

2. *Does the therapist need to understand the effect of cognitive-perceptual impairments on occupational performance (i.e., the activity limitation and participation restrictions from the International Classification of Function (ICF) (World Health Organization, 2001)?* This question could be answered by through direct observation of function. This top-down approach to evaluation permits the evaluator to determine how cognitive impairment affects functional performance or activity participation (Goverover, 2004; Goverover et al., 2005).

3. *Does the therapist need information to guide intervention?* The model of cognitive intervention that the therapist is using, often guides the selection of evaluation tools. Dynamic assessments emphasize the processes that are involved in learning and change (Grigorenko & Sternberg, 1998) and may provide information that is needed to plan and guide intervention that focuses on changing skills or behaviors.

4. *Does the therapist need to establish a baseline as a measurement of change or outcome of intervention?* To answer this question, the therapist needs to take into consideration short-term and long-term intervention goals. In documenting outcomes, it is important to take into consideration the three levels of disability described by the ICF: impairment, activity limitation, and participation restriction. Therefore, a cognitive perceptual evaluation that includes these three components will provide a more comprehensive view of the person's functioning.

OVERVIEW OF INTERVENTION APPROACHES

Interventions for people with cognitive dysfunction differ in the areas that are targeted for intervention and in the underlying assumptions about individuals' abilities to learn and generalize information. The characteristics and underlying assumptions of the different intervention approaches are explored in this section. Factors that are critical in the selection of these intervention approaches as well as methods for systematically integrating them are also discussed. As you read this section, review the case study on cognition and performance context.

CASE STUDY: *Cognition and Performance Contexts*

Scenario 1

Mr. James is a 24-year-old man with a 10-year history of attention and memory problems related to a head trauma that he sustained at age 14. He has difficulty recalling conversations and events that occurred just hours before. During performance of a task, he easily loses track of the steps and repeats some steps twice while omitting other steps altogether. Mr. James denies any difficulty with his concentration or memory and would like to return to school. He currently lives with his parents, who care for him.

Scenario 2

Mr. Cornwall is a 64-year-old man with attention and memory problems related to a head trauma that he sustained three weeks ago. He has difficulty recalling conversations and events that occurred just hours before. During performance of a task, he easily loses track of the steps and repeats some steps twice while omitting other steps altogether. Mr. Cornwall is well aware of his difficulties and is depressed by them. For example, he states, "I can't even remember what I ate for breakfast. What good am I? If I have to give up my business, my life is over." Mr. Cornwall was recently widowed and lived alone before his accident.

Questions

The two scenarios describe the same clinical symptoms, but the performance contexts are different.
1. How do the differences in context influence the emphasis in intervention that you would use?
2. What influenced your selection?

Discussion

There are no absolute right or wrong answers to these questions. In scenario 1, Mr. James is 10 years postinjury, so the potential for change in the underlying cognitive skills is assumed to be minimal. A remedial approach that focuses on improving memory and attention skills would not be warranted unless there was some evidence of potential for

further improvement. Compensatory strategies, such as use of a memory notebook or a checklist, could be considered. However, Mr. James denies any difficulty in memory or attention. This lack of self-awareness will present a major obstacle to independent initiation and use of compensatory strategies.

Caregiver training, task and environmental adaptation, and the possibility of functional skill training to increase performance on a specified task appear to be the most appropriate areas for intervention. Techniques to increase awareness may be attempted as a prerequisite for using compensatory aids. External memory aids, such as memory notebook training, may be introduced by using task-specific training methods in combination with maximum prompts and external cues for their use; however, success likely depends on Mr. James's ability to gain some awareness and acceptance of his disability.

In scenario 2, Mr. Cornwall is only three weeks post-injury, so that the potential for change in the underlying skills is presumably present. In addition, Mr. Cornwall is well aware of his problems. This would appear to make him a prime candidate for remedial techniques. However, he is also depressed by his difficulties. He might not be able to cope emotionally with an approach that focuses on the underlying client factors.

An approach that will provide greater opportunities for success and control over his environment could be the initial intervention emphasis. For example, adaptive techniques in which the caregiver or practitioner presents directions one step at a time might make it easier for Mr. Cornwall to follow task instructions. Training in the use of compensatory strategies, such as use of a memory notebook to keep track of daily events and conversations and in use of a checklist to assist in keeping track of task steps that have already been completed, might enhance task performance. As Mr. Cornwall gains self-confidence and control, remedial tasks that focus on improving attention may be gradually introduced if he is able to tolerate them.

Capitalizing on the Assets: The Functional Approach

The functional approach capitalizes on the person's assets to improve occupational performance. The emphasis is on reducing activity limitations and participation restrictions rather than on remediating or restoring impaired skills (Figure 57.1). The functional approach can be subdivided into three intervention techniques: adaptation of the activity or context, functional task training, and compensation. The Cognitive Disability Model (Allen, 1985) emphasizes use of adaptation, while the Neuro-

functional Approach (Giles, 2005) focuses on functional task training.

Adaptation of the Activity or Context

Adaptation involves changing, altering, or structuring the activity demands or context to prevent disruptive behaviors or accidents, minimize cognitive or perceptual demands of a task, minimize caregiver burden, and maintain the client's level of functioning (Erikson, Karlsson, Soderstrom, Tham, 2004; Radomski, Dougherty, Fine, & Baum, 1993). Rather than providing direct intervention to the client, the focus

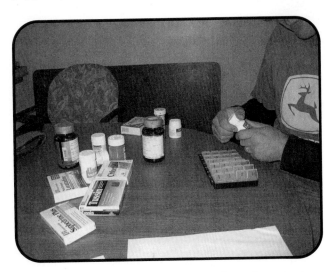

FIGURE 57.1 A pill box organizer can be an important contextual cue to help those with memory impairments safely self-administer medications.

is on providing support, education, and training to the caregiver, family, or employer (Sohlberg, Glang, & Todis, 1998). Adaptations should directly address the problems and needs that have been identified by the client or significant other and be designed in collaboration with them (Campbell, Duffy, & Salloway, 1994) Adaptations might be fixed (e.g., installing an alarm on a door to prevent wandering), or they might require ongoing implementation and monitoring (e.g., preselecting clothes from the closet on a daily basis). In the latter case, implementation depends on the ability, consistency, and reliability of another person.

In some cases, a significant other can be trained to alter or structure the activity demands or context to maintain the person's performance capabilities. For instance, the person might not be able to attend to the task of preparing a meal but might be able to perform individual components, such as mixing the salad or folding napkins in half for the table setting. Engagement in such meaningful activity components can help to maintain the client's performance capabilities and prevent disruptive behaviors (Levy & Burns, 2005). Although adaptations can produce rapid changes in function, the effects are limited to the activity or environment that is adapted, and success often depends on the extent to which other people are able to consistently follow through with the adaptations.

Adaptation: The Cognitive Disability Approach

Allen (1985, 1993) designed a cognitive disability approach that provides guidelines for matching and adapting the individual's cognitive level with activity demands. This approach for evaluation and intervention was designed initially for people with psychiatric disorders and chronic cognitive disabilities (e.g., dementia) and later was expanded

for individuals with different central nervous system problems resulting in cognitive impairments (e.g., stroke).

In this model, function is organized into six ordinal levels of global function ranging from normal (level 6) to profoundly disabled (level 1). Modes of performance within each level further qualify behavior variations and allow for more sensitive measurement of the person's capacity. To get an elaborated description of the Allen Cognitive Level, refer to Allen (1985) and Levy and Burns (2005). Each of Allen's cognitive levels has three components: attention, motor control, and verbal performance. The person's cognitive progress can be seen as a continuum along two dimensions, motor and verbal performance, which are linked by attention.

The six cognitive levels are used to describe functional profiles of capacities and limitations that help to clarify and direct interventions and care. Allen's model provides clinicians with intervention guidelines for different levels of cognitive function. For example, the cognitive levels identify the required assistance needed, as well as what the person is still able to do safely. This information is used to educate and train caregivers and to make recommendations for assistance and environmental adaptations to optimize function and safety. It is also used to select activities that match the person's cognitive level and maximize participation in meaningful occupations (Allen, 1985; Allen et al., 1992; Levy & Burns, 2005).

Functional Task Training: The Neurofunctional Approach

Giles (2005) describes a neurofunctional approach that emphasizes the use of task-specific training or rote repetition of a specific task or routine within natural contexts to develop habits or functional behavioral routines. Emphasis is on the mastery of functional task performance through practice rather than on the underlying skills that are needed to perform the task. Giles (2006) states that development of new functional habits and routines can occur in clients who have decision-making deficits and only minimal awareness of their impairments. Behavioral techniques, including reinforcement and chaining, are incorporated into practice sessions. Intervention involves breaking down a functional task into small subcomponents (Giles, 2005; Glisky, Schacter, & Butters, 1994). Techniques such as errorless learning or the method of vanishing cues may be used. In errorless learning, the person is prevented from making incorrect or inappropriate responses during the learning process. The vanishing cue method involves systematically reducing or fading the cues that are required to perform a task. There is evidence that errorless learning techniques are more effective than the vanishing cue method in people with severe memory impairment (Evans, Levine, & Bateman, 2004; Kessels & de Haan, 2003; Page, Wilson, Sheil, Carter, & Norris, 2006).

Functional task training capitalizes on procedural or implicit memory. Case studies have demonstrated that functional task training can produce significant changes in activities of daily living and work tasks in people with severe impairments (Giles, 2005; Giles, Rideley, Dill, & Frye, 1997; Giles & Shore, 1989; Glisky et al., 1994; Hallgren & Kottorp, 2005; Kottorp, Hallgren, Bernspang, & Fisher, 2003). However, intervention addresses only one task or routine at a time, and extensive training, time, and effort may be required to achieve success within one task sequence and environment. The person might have difficulty in dealing with minor changes in the task stimuli or the environment. Proponents of this method argue that people with cognitive impairment should be treated in the natural context in which they will function, because people with brain injury have difficulty generalizing learning (Giles, 2005; Glisky et al., 1994).

Compensation

Compensation teaches the person to bypass or minimize the effects of the impairment by modifying the method that is used to perform an activity. The client is expected to initiate and implement the use of an external aid or strategy to enhance occupational performance in a variety of different situations (AOTA, 1999). The complexity of the task and the compensatory strategy may require awareness and acceptance to be generalized and independently applied to a variety of situations (Birnboim & Miller, 2004; Toglia, 1993a). For example, a memory notebook could be used to compensate for memory loss. Independent use requires that the person recognize that he or she is having difficulty with memory and perceive the need to write things down to aid in remembering. It also requires initiation of use of the book in multiple situations. Clients with more severe cognitive impairments can be trained, through rote repetition and errorless learning, to use simplistic compensatory strategies and modifications with minimal awareness of why the strategy is needed (Giles, 2006; Hallgren & Kottorp, 2005; Kottorp et al., 2003). In these clients, the compensatory strategy becomes automatic and integrated into the person's habits or functional routines.

Addressing the Cognitive Perceptual Impairment

The Remedial Approach

Remedial approaches place an emphasis on restoring impaired cognitive-perceptual skills (Unsworth, 2007). The emphasis is on changing the person's underlying skills rather than on manipulating the activity demands or context (Neistadt, 1990; Zoltan, 1996).

In traditional cognitive-perceptual remedial approaches, cognitive skills are conceptualized in terms of higher cortical skills, which are divided into a hierarchy of discrete subskills such as attention, discrimination, memory, sequencing, categorization, concept formation, and problem solving. The lower-level skills provide the foundation for more complex skills and behaviors (Toglia, 1998). For example, attention skills are addressed before higher-level cognitive skills such as problem solving. Intervention emphasizes practice of the specific cognitive or perceptual skills that are deficient, using worksheets, computerized exercises, and electronic scanning devices. One example of a remedial training program is the Attention Process Training Program (Sohlberg & Mateer, 1989a, 2001). This program includes graded worksheets and audiotapes that are systematically graded to place increasing demands on different aspects of attention.

It is assumed that improvement in underlying cognitive perceptual skills will have a greater influence on behavior than will direct training of functional task training because learning will spontaneously generalize to a wider range of activities. For example, if block design construction improves during remedial treatment, it is assumed that there will also be improvement on a wide range of other tasks involving constructional skills, such as dressing or making a sandwich. Remedial training has also been referred to as the transfer training approach (Toglia, 1998).

Improving underlying cognitive or perceptual deficits is thought to promote recovery or reorganization of the impaired skill. Information on functional reorganization and adult brain plasticity supports this view. For example, it has been postulated that some parts of the brain may assume new functions or work together in different ways as a result of environmental experiences (Luria, 1973). Functional magnetic resonance imaging that show changes after cognitive rehabilitation provides preliminary support for this premise (Laatsch, Little, & Thulborn, 2004; Laatsch, Thulborn, Krisky, Shobat, & Sweeney, 2004; Wykes et al., 2002). However, Neisdadt (1994) observed that "because both remedial and adaptive intervention approaches stimulate clients to learn new behaviors, neither approach can claim to take advantage of adult brain plasticity more than the other" (p. 426). Dirette, Hinojosa, and Carnevale (1999) compared remedial and compensatory training and found no significant difference between the two approaches. It was observed that participants in the remedial group began to use compensatory strategies, thus confounding results. Remedial activities focus on the area of impairment and provide structured tasks that accentuate the problem areas; therefore, awareness and insight into one's impairments may improve as a secondary effect. The emergence of awareness could allow some individuals to initiate use of compensatory strategies.

There is some evidence that supports the effectiveness of remedial intervention for specific cognitive skills, such as attention and visual scanning. However, intervention has been found to be more effective when it incorporates use of self-monitoring techniques and strategy training across a variety of activities (Cicerone et al., 2005). Studies have not supported the isolated use of repetitive graded memory drills, computerized memory games, logic games, or other cognitive remedial activities.

Recently, occupational therapists have described several models that utilize a combination of approaches. These include the cognitive retraining model, the quadraphonic approach, and the multicontext approach.

The Cognitive Retraining Model

Averbuch and Katz (2005) describe a comprehensive occupational therapy cognitive retraining model for adolescents and adults with neurological disabilities that integrates cognitive remedial training with strategy use and awareness of abilities to broaden the capacity for learning. The model draws on neurophysiological, neurobiological, and neuropsychological theories to provide a framework for cognitive learning. Training is directed at initially improving impaired cognitive functioning and may involve systematic and structured training in visual scanning, categorization or classification, sequencing, planning or thinking operations. Cognitive training gradually increases the amount and complexity of information presented but, at the same time, teaches new strategies to improve impaired functioning. Once clients learn to use strategies within a variety of activities within the clinic, they practice these strategies in real-life situations. The authors use a combination of paper-and-pencil exercises, tabletop and computer activities, and functional activities. If the client is incapable of using specific remedial-based strategies, procedural strategies that focus on training the components parts of a task are used to promote the ability to perform activities of daily living (Katz & Hartman-Maeir, 2005).

The Quadraphonic Approach

The quadraphonic approach incorporates a micro perspective that provides guidelines for addressing cognitive impairments as well as a macro perspective that provides a holistic perspective. The micro perspective integrates information from information-processing, teaching-learning, neurodevelopmental, and biomechanical theories to provide guidelines for evaluation and treatment of cognitive perceptual skills (e.g., attention, memory, problem solving, and motor planning) and postural control dysfunction. The macro perspective embraces an individualized, client/learner-centered model of therapy within a holistic occupational framework. There is a focus on the client-therapist relationship, occupational engagement, and health adaptation or wellness. The macro perspective examines the person's satisfaction, subjective well-being, meaningful occupations, and lifestyle through the use of interviews, storytelling, storymaking, and narrative analysis. The model conceptualizes a fluid, dynamic movement back and forth between the micro and macro perspectives and argues that performance skills and whole-person engagement in occupation need to be considered together (Abreu & Peloquin, 2005).

The Multicontext Approach

The multicontext approach is based on the dynamic interactional model of cognition (Toglia, 2005). This model draws heavily from cognitive and educational psychology. It emphasizes the dynamic nature of cognition and explains how cognitive symptoms and occupational performance change depending on a combination of person factors (unique characteristics of the person such as lifestyle, personality, beliefs, and values; information-processing capacity, self-awareness, and strategy use) as well as activity demands and environmental factors. Intervention based on this model may emphasize the person, task, or environment or a combination of all three. The multicontext approach is based on this model but is narrower in focus and provides specific guidelines for facilitating awareness and strategy use within activities or environments that might need to be modified so that they are at a "just right" challenge level (i.e., activities that are not too difficult but also not too easy) for the client. This approach emphasizes facilitating transfer of learning.

For example, in the multicontext approach, the person practices application of a targeted strategy such as use of a checklist, mental rehearsal, or self cues across purposeful and occupation-based activities that systematically differ in appearance yet remain at a similar level of difficulty. This places gradual demands on the ability to transfer learning because the more two situations or activities are physically similar, the easier it is to transfer strategies learned in one situation to another (Davidson & Sternberg, 1998; Toglia, 1991b). Table 57.2 shows an example of intervention activities presented along the transfer continuum. Activity demands are not graded in difficulty until evidence of spontaneous strategy use along the entire transfer continuum is observed. The use of awareness training techniques to facilitate self-monitoring skills and self-evaluation is deeply embedded throughout intervention.

The multicontext approach has been used with adults with brain injury (Toglia, 2005) and schizophrenia (Josman, 2005) as well as with children and adolescents (Cermak, 2005; Josman, 2005). It has also been utilized to guide individual as well as group treatment programs (Harrison et al., 2005; Landa-Gonzalez, 2001; Toglia, 2005).

SELECTING INTERVENTION APPROACHES

In planning intervention, the clinician considers the following questions: How much change is expected from the person? How much learning and generalization are expected? How much do the activity demands or context need to be changed or altered to meet the person's capabilities? Is the person responsive to cues? Is the person

TABLE 57.2   THE TRANSFER CONTINUUM

Strategy emphasized in all activities: Use a checklist to gather and keep track of items to:

Very Similar		Somewhat Similar		Different		Very Different	
Make vegetable salad (6–8 items)	Make fruit salad (6–8 items)	Set a table for dinner (For 6–8)	Pack 6–8 items in a lunch-box	Pack 6–8 items in a bag for an over-night stay	Put a list of 6–8 appoint-ments in a calendar	Use a list to complete 6–8 party invitations	Use a list to complete 6–8 errands

aware of his or her difficulties? If the person is completely unaware of his or her difficulties, is unresponsive to cues, or does not show potential for change within the intervention time frame, a treatment approach that targets change in strategy use such as the multicontext approach or cognitive retraining approach might not be appropriate. It might be more appropriate to use the cognitive disability model or an approach that changes the environment or activity rather than the person. The neurofunctional approach, which uses repetitive practice to change performance on a specific task, might also be indicated. Assumptions regarding awareness and learning within intervention models need to be carefully considered in planning intervention (Toglia, 2005). This is reflected in Case Study 57-1.

COGNITIVE IMPAIRMENTS: DEFINITIONS, EVALUATIONS, AND INTERVENTIONS

In this section, the main constructs involved in cognition will be discussed in terms of their definitions, evaluation, and treatment. Self-awareness will be discussed first because lack of awareness can affect the motivation, effort, and sustained participation that are needed for intervention.

Following discussion of self-awareness, the areas of **orientation**, attention, memory, executive functions, **motor planning**, **unilateral neglect**, and visual processing will be reviewed. Some of these concepts are also described and summarized in Table 57.3. Although these areas are discussed separately for the purposes of description, it should be kept in mind that cognitive problems are interrelated and rarely occur in isolation.

Evidence-based reviews in cognitive rehabilitation have found that training in strategies, and self-monitoring or self-regulatory skills are key characteristics of studies demonstrating the effectiveness of cognitive rehabilitation (Cicerone et al., 2000, 2005). These interventions will therefore be emphasized. It should be kept in mind that the context of the person's life needs to be considered in plan-

ning and choosing intervention activities (Johnston, Goverover, & Dijkers, 2005). This includes the person's occupations, personality, interests, premorbid level of functioning, culture, values, external supports, and resources. Interventions that address cognitive impairments need to be blended with those that address interpersonal skills, social participation, and everyday activities, routines, and roles (Abreu & Peloquin, 2005).

Self-Awareness

Impaired self-awareness associated with neurological dysfunction includes lack of knowledge about one own physical or cognitive-perceptual impairments and/or their functional implications as well as inability to anticipate difficulties, recognize errors, or monitor performance within the context of an activity (Toglia & Kirk, 2000). Impaired self-awareness presents obstacles to adjustment, collaborative goal setting, and active participation in intervention. Decreased awareness results in poor motivation and compliance, lack of sustained effort, unrealistic expectations, incongruence between goals of the client and family, impaired judgment and safety, and inability to adopt use of compensatory strategies (Hartman-Maeir, Soroker, Oman, & Katz, 2003; Sherer, Oden, Bergloff, Levin, & High, 1998; Toglia & Kirk, 2000). A number of studies support the association between awareness and functional outcome (Fischer, Gauggel, & Trexler, 2004; Goverover, 2004; Hoofien, Gilboa, Vakil, & Barak, 2004; Noe et al., 2005; Tham, Ginsberg, Fisher, & Tegner, 2001). Unawareness may be related to psychological or neurological sources. Denial is a psychological defense mechanism that is related to premorbid personality traits and is characterized by overrationalization, hostility, resistance to feedback, and an unwillingness to confront problems (Prigatano, 1999). A person who has a history of denying inadequacies and resisting help from others and a strong desire to be "in control" is more likely to use denial as a coping strategy. Impaired self-awareness resulting from neurological lesions, represents a lack of access to information

TABLE 57.3 COGNITION: CLINICAL SIGNS AND FUNCTIONAL OBSERVATIONS

Area of Cognitive Impairment	Clinical Signs/Observations	Sample Strategies	Sample Adaptations
Orientation: the ability to understand the self and the relationship between the self and the past and present environment.	Client might think he/she is home in own house rather than a hospital. May confuse the hospital staff with relatives and may believe each time he/she wakes up from a short nap that it is a new day. Client might not initiate basic ADLs because of confusion about time.	Teaching person to look for key cues in the environment when he/she feels confused or has difficulty recalling information.	A talking watch or alarm clock that automatically announces the date and time on an hourly basis; a large, brightly colored sign with the day and date can be placed in a key location; large clock. Orientation poster with key personal data listed (e.g., photos of family members, friends).
Attention: multidimensional capacity that involves several components: alertness (detection and reaction), sustained attention, shifting of attention, selective attention, and mental tracking.	Perseveration or difficulty switching between tasks during grooming activities such as shifting from brushing teeth to washing one's face. Difficulty selectively attending and sustaining attention to a task such as a work activity while ignoring music playing or people talking. Simultaneously performing two tasks and mentally tracking one's performance in both (e.g., holding a conversation while driving and looking for a street sign).	Taking time-outs from a task when concentration begins to fade. Remembering to get a sense of the whole situation before attending to the parts. Saying each step of a task aloud to focus attention on the task and inhibit distractions.	Reducing the number of items or choices presented to the client at any one time. Preselecting relevant objects needed for tasks, and task segmentation or presenting only one component or step of a task at a time.
Neglect: failure to orient to, respond to, or report stimuli presented on the side contralateral to the cerebral lesion in clients who do not have primary sensory or motor impairments.	Clients may display asymmetry in functional activities, such as difficulty locating items on the left side of the food tray; shaving only the right side of the face and combing only the right side of the head. May display difficulty scanning left to right while going down grocery store isle; must turn at end of isle and scan for items previously on left (now on right).	Teaching client to find the edges of a page or periphery of stimuli before beginning a task; marking it with an anchor such as colored tape, a colored highlighter, a bright object, or placement of his or her arm.	Placing a vibrating or auditory beeper on the left side (Seron, Deloche, & Coyette, 1989). Using a large colored tape on the edges of tables, corners Lennon (1994).

Function	Difficulty	Intervention
Memory: gives us the ability to draw upon past experiences and learn new information.	Client may display rapid forgetting of conversations, information read, TV shows watched, or recently met people. May confabulate information. May have difficulty learning new information and remembering to take medications, show up for scheduled appointments, where items are placed, or how to get to particular locations.	Chunking or grouping similar items together; the story method or linking a series of facts or events into a story; rehearsal or repeating information over and over to oneself; rhymes or recalling a fact by changing the fact into a rhyme; and visual imagery.	Cue cards or signs in key places, devices with preprogrammed alarms or alarm messages, electronic devices such as pagers, mobile phones, PDAs, computers, pill box organizers, lists, daily planners, and notebooks.
Visual processing: involves the reception, organization, and assimilation of visual information.	Difficulty locating objects on bathroom sink despite being able to name the item being sought. Difficulty detecting gross differences in size, position, direction, angles, and rotations. Difficulty finding items on a crowded refrigerator shelf, closet, or supermarket shelf. Difficulty identifying objects partially hidden or overlapping on a counter or in a drawer.	Getting a sense of the whole before looking at the parts, teaching the person to partition space before localizing details; using one's finger to trace visual stimuli; covering or blocking out visual stimuli when too much information is presented at once; verbalizing salient visual features or subtle differences and mentally visualizing a particular item prior to looking for it.	Colored tape on buttons to operate appliances; salient color cues on objects to make them easier to locate and discriminate (e.g., bright pink tape on a medication bottle); increased spaces between lines; using a felt-tip pen instead of a pencil to provide greater contrast. Visual stimuli, arranged in an organized manner, with large spaces between items, are easier to perceive.
Executive function: broad band of performance skills that allow a person to engage in independent, purposeful, self-directed behavior (i.e., volition, planning, purposeful action, and self-awareness and self-monitoring).	Difficulty planning and initiating activities that the client needs or wants to complete. Difficulty anticipating consequences, weighing and making choices, conceiving of alternatives, sustaining attention, and sequencing the activity. May appear very passive, may rarely initiate conversation, may appear to have lost his/her sense of humor, is disorganized and unable to get things done once cued to start tasks.	Verbal mediation, self-instruction.	Preorganize an activity or activity materials; audiotape instructions that cue the person to initiate an activity and perform each step at a time in its proper sequence; predictable and structured daily routine.

Continued

TABLE 57.3   COGNITION: CLINICAL SIGNS AND FUNCTIONAL OBSERVATIONS   *Continued*

Area of Cognitive Impairment	Clinical Signs/Observations	Sample Strategies	Sample Adaptations
Motor planning: ability to figure out how to get one's body to do what one wants it to do.	May position limb awkwardly in relation to object (e.g., reach with right hand to the left side of the glass) or perseverate on a movement (production errors). May use a body part for the object (e.g., use finger as a toothbrush) when asked to pantomime. Shows spatiotemporal errors during sequencing of a series of actions (e.g., pouring coffee into a cup, adding sugar and milk, stirring, and drinking it). May display conceptual errors when using objects (using a knife as a spoon), have difficulty matching demonstrated gesture to picture or object, or missequence functional tasks such as brushing one's teeth, donning clothes, shaving face, or applying makeup.	Mental practice strategy: before performing an activity, the client imagines him or herself performing the activity in a smooth, accurate, and coordinated manner or imagines how his/her hand will grasp an object. Associate the movement pattern with a rhyme, rhythm, musical tune, visual image, or word. Guide the movement with self-verbalizations.	Colored tape on the handle of a drawer, utensil, or faucet or other salient feature of an object. Adaptations such as elastic-waist trousers, elastic buttons, Velcro fasteners, wash mitts, slip-on shoes, or elastic shoelaces that simplify the task.
Awareness: the degree of understanding one has regarding one's own physical or cognitive-perceptual impairments.	Clients with poor awareness might independently attempt to transfer themselves to the toilet despite dense hemiplegia and the need for physical assistance from a health care worker. Clients might not initiate use of compensatory strategies during home and community activities, thus causing safety risks.	Self-prediction of performance before and after specific tasks. Self-rating of performance for specific tasks. Self-reflection of videotaped performance.	A posted list of self-evaluation questions (e.g., Have I attended to all the necessary information?; Did I check over my work?)

regarding one's cognitive state, and is characterized by surprise, indifference, or perplexity in response to feedback (Prigatano, 1999). In many cases, the neurological and psychological sources of unawareness coexist and cannot be easily differentiated. If denial is the predominant source of unawareness, methods of awareness training might not be effective (Lucas & Fleming, 2005).

Crosson and coauthors (1989) described a hierarchical pyramid model of awareness that distinguishes between three aspects of awareness that are important to consider in evaluation and intervention: intellectual awareness, emergent awareness, and anticipatory awareness. *Intellectual awareness* is knowledge that a particular function is impaired. It is reflected in the ability to verbally describe limitations in functioning. Intellectual awareness is a foundation for emergent and anticipatory awareness. *Emergent awareness* is the ability to recognize a problem only when it is actually happening. It is thought that a minimum level of emergent awareness must be present to be able to recognize the need for compensatory strategies (Bruce, 1993). *Anticipatory awareness* is the ability to anticipate that a problem will likely occur as the result of an impairment before performing a given activity (Crosson et al., 1989). This involves the ability to judge task difficulty in relationship to one's abilities. The hierarchical nature of this model has not been empirically demonstrated, and there is some indication that the interrelationship between these concepts is complex and nonhierarchical (Abreu et al., 2001).

Toglia and Kirk (2000) proposed a dynamic model of awareness that includes self-knowledge or beliefs about knowledge and abilities that exists prior to an activity (i.e., intellectual awareness) and "online" awareness that includes self-monitoring and self-regulatory processes that are activated within the context of an activity. This view of awareness is nonhierarchical and proposes that levels of awareness vary across different tasks and contexts within the same domain. It implies that awareness needs to be assessed both outside and inside the context of an activity (Toglia & Kirk, 2000).

Interview and rating scales for awareness (see Table 57.1) generally evaluate awareness of limitations and strengths, the ability to generalize the impact of limitations on functional tasks, and concerns regarding disability judgment (intellectual awareness). Typically, the person's self ratings are compared to those of a relative or clinician (Bogod, Mateer, & MacDonald, 2003). For example, a client might be asked to rate how much of a problem he or she has in preparing meals, doing laundry, or remembering names. Discrepancy between the client's self ratings and the ratings of others is considered to be an indicator of an awareness deficit, greater discrepancies indicating more severe deficits in awareness. Alternatively, some scales, such as the Self Awareness Deficits Interview (Fleming, Strong, & Ashton, 1996), use a semistructured interview in which the clinician directly rates

the person's level of awareness, depending on the response to questions. Both of these methods of assessing awareness examine intellectual awareness outside the context of an activity.

Although interviews and rating scales are the most common method of assessing awareness, it can also be assessed within the context of an activity by asking the client to estimate his or her performance before (i.e., anticipatory awareness) and immediately after (i.e., emergent awareness) performing a task. Differences between estimated performance and actual performance are compared. Task estimation, including normative comparison, is used within the Contextual Memory Test (Toglia, 1993b) and the Assessment of Awareness of Disability (Tham, Bernspang, & Fisher, 1999). Changes in awareness that may occur during the experience of an activity can be examined by comparing responses to awareness questions before, during, and immediately after performance.

A comprehensive evaluation of awareness plays a key role in guiding and selecting methods of intervention. In some cases, potential for changes in awareness may be limited, particularly within the intervention time frame. In these situations, intervention methods that do not require awareness, such as functional skill training, errorless learning, or adaptation of the environment, might be most appropriate in facilitating occupational performance. If a lack of understanding of his or her own strengths and limitations prevents a person from choosing goals that are realistic and attainable, the therapist should assist the client in focusing on skills or tasks that are needed for the "here and now."

Awareness training involves helping a person with neurological impairment to learn about the changes that have occurred. It involves helping clients to get to know themselves again. Intervention should be directed toward helping people with cognitive-perceptual deficits to discover their own errors. This is most likely to occur in tasks that are familiar so that the person has a basis for comparison of performance (Tham et al., 2001; Toglia & Kirk, 2000). In addition, the therapist should select activities at a "just right challenge" level so that the person is able to integrate and assimilate the experience. As awareness emerges, the client gradually assumes greater responsibility in the goal-setting and intervention-planning process.

Directly pointing out errors or telling clients that they have problems is least effective in increasing awareness. Direct confrontation tends to elicit defensive reactions (Toglia & Kirk, 2000). There might be times when a person rationalizes his or her mistakes and is difficult to engage in treatment. Impairments should be introduced slowly and indirectly within structured experiences while simultaneously emphasizing strategies to control and monitor the emergence of cognitive symptoms.

Systematic investigation of the effectiveness of awareness training is limited. Initial studies indicate that direct intervention for awareness can be effective in some groups of clients (Cicerone & Giacino, 1992; Fleming, Lucas, & Lightbody, 2006; Fleming, Shum, Strong, & Lightbody, 2005; Schlund, 1999; Tham & Tegner, 1997; Tham et al., 2001). Following are descriptions of some of the techniques that can be used in a wide range of activities to enhance awareness. These techniques are often used in combination with one other.

Self-Prediction

Self-prediction involves asking the person to anticipate difficulties or predict his or her performance on a task. The client might be asked to indicate on a rating scale whether the activity will be easy or hard or to predict specific parameters of performance. For example, the accuracy of performance, the time required to complete the task, the number of verbal cues required, or the type of difficulties that one might encounter can be estimated and discussed before actually performance of an activity.

Immediately following performance, the actual results are compared with predicted results, and any discrepancies are discussed (Toglia, 1991a, Toglia, 2005). Case studies using self-prediction have been reported in people with executive dysfunction, memory deficits, and unilateral neglect (Cicerone & Giacino, 1992; Rebmann & Hannon, 1995; Schlund, 1999; Sohlberg & Mateer, 2001; Tham et al., 2001).

Specific Goal Ratings

Daily or weekly self-ratings of clearly defined behaviors or targeted strategies can be used to help a person focus on what he or she can do in the present. Goal attainment scales offer a concrete, individualized focus that can increase self-awareness and realistic goal orientation (Malec, Smigielski, DePompoplo, 1991; Rockwood, Joyce, & Stolee, 1997). Client self-ratings of goal attainment can be compared to the ratings of the therapist or of a significant other, and any discrepancies can be discussed. For example, suppose a client with moderate memory deficits continually relies on others to remember events and does not use a memory notebook. If the targeted behavior is to rely less on others for information, the client might be asked to rate himself or herself weekly on a scale of 1 (relies on others all the time or does not use the book) to 5 (does not rely on others for information or consistently uses the book). The client's rating can be compared to the rating of a significant other, and any discrepancies can be discussed. Self-ratings can be charted or graphed over time and tracked to improve awareness (Sohlberg & Mateer, 2001).

Videotape Feedback

A videotape of a client that illustrates problems in performing and activity may be used to enhance awareness. Videotape feedback is concrete, and it allows clients to reexperience their performance and evaluate their diffi-

culties as they are occurring rather then simply discussing them after the fact. Videotape feedback has been used successfully in treating people with stroke and brain injury (Liu, Chan, Lee, Li, & Hui-Chan, 2002; Tham & Tegner, 1997).

Self-Evaluation

The practitioner provides a structured system such as a set of questions, a checklist, or a rating system that the client uses as a guide to evaluate his or her own performance (Toglia, 1991a, 1998). Sample self-evaluation questions might include "Have I attended to all the necessary information?" and "Did I check over my work?"

Self-Questioning

Questions that are designed to cue the client to monitor his or her behavior may be written on an index card or memorized. At specific time intervals during the task, the client is expected to stop and answer the same two or three questions, such as "Am I sure that I am looking all the way to the left?," "Am I paying attention to the details?," and "Am I going too quickly?" (Fertherlin & Kurland, 1989).

Journaling

The client keeps a journal in which he or she records activity experiences and performance results. The client is encouraged to reflect on and interpret activity experiences, think about what he or she has learned about himself or herself, and summarize strengths and weaknesses (Tham et al., 2001; Ylvisaker & Feeney, 1998).

Awareness training techniques can be blended with strategy training and incorporated into all treatment sessions. The multicontext approach provides additional guidelines for simultaneously addressing awareness and strategy use (Toglia, 2005).

Orientation

Orientation is the ability to understand the self and the relationship between the self and the past and present environment. Orientation depends on the integration of several mental activities that are represented in different areas of the brain. Disorientation is indicative of significant impairments in attention and memory (Lezak, Howieson, & Loring, 2004). For example, disoriented clients might think they are home rather than in a hospital, might confuse the hospital staff with relatives, or might believe it that is a new day each time they wake up from a short nap.

Evaluation

Evaluation of orientation traditionally includes the client's orientation to person, place, and time. Orientation to person involves both the self and others. Is the client able to report personal facts and events and describe his or her previous lifestyle? Does the client recognize people and associate them with their role and name? Orientation to place is demonstrated by the client's ability to understand the type of place he or she is in (e.g., a hospital), to report the name and location of the place, and to appreciate distance and direction. Orientation to time requires an ability to report the current point in time (e.g., day, month, and year), to show understanding of the continuity and sequence of time (i.e., estimation), and to associate events with time.

Topographical orientation, often considered a component of orientation to place, is the ability to follow a familiar route or a new route once given an opportunity to become familiar with it. Functionally, the person might not be able to find his or her way from the therapy area to his or her room or describe and draw the layout of a familiar room or route (Unsworth, 2007). Difficulties with the visual-spatial and memory aspects of topographical orientation need to be distinguished during evaluation (Brunsdon, Nickels, & Coltheart, 2007; Unsworth, 2007).

Orientation assessments are traditionally covered in **mental status examinations**. Table 57.1 provides a list of standardized screening tools for orientation. However, occupational therapists frequently use nonstandardized measures of orientation, such as interviews with open-ended questions asked in a conversational or informal manner. Most practitioners use cues to determine the severity of the disorientation. If the client is unable to answer the questions independently, the practitioner might offer a multiple-choice array or verbal cues. Cues usually move from general or abstract to more concrete, as determined by the severity of disorientation (e.g., "Today is the beginning of the work week" versus "Today is the day after Sunday"). The number and type of cues offer a method for scoring and monitoring progress. Fluctuations in orientation during the day should be noted, as clients might experience **sundowning**, in which they become confused in the evening because of fatigue.

Intervention

STRATEGY TRAINING AND/OR ADAPTATIONS OF TASK OR ENVIRONMENT. Strategy training for disorientation involves teaching the person to look for external cues when he or she is feeling confused or is having difficulty recalling orientation information. For example, an information poster that contains orientation facts can be placed on a wall, in a closet, or eventually inside a notebook. When the client is asked orientation information, he or she is expected to locate the information poster to verify responses or to find the correct answers. A memory book, containing pictures and names of familiar people or important life events, can also be placed in a key location within the room. As an alternative, an audiotape or videotape can be created by a family member to review orientation information at set times during the day or used whenever the person feels confused. An alarm that is pre-

programmed to ring several times a day can be used to cue the person to read his or her orientation fact book or listen to the audiotape. Orientation questions with use of cueing strategies can also be incorporated into a bean bag toss game, a board game, or a "Family Feud" style game within a group format (Toglia & Golisz, 1990).

A calendar posted on the wall or closet may be helpful in orienting the person to time. If the client has poor selective attention, a single piece of paper with the day and date written daily, rather than a monthly calendar, might be needed.

To assist the client in finding his or her room, directional arrows can be placed in the hallway, and tape indicating the route to his or her room can be placed on the floor. Key landmarks can be pointed out and made more salient with arrows or colored tape.

The therapist needs to immediately reinforce initiation or use of any of these external cues by praising the client (or rewarding points), and each time the client initiates the use of an external cue, the therapist should keep track of it by recording it on a chart or visual graph. The use of external cues should be gradually faded until the orientation information is internalized. In addition, the person should be trained to look for orientation cues (e.g., clocks, calendars) in different environments. Spaced retrieval techniques can be used to train use of strategies and external aids, such as using a daily calendar. Spaced retrieval involves systematically lengthening the period of retention and recall. There is evidence that this technique is more effective than cueing hierarchies in treating people with dementia (Bourgeois et al., 2003).

Attention

Attention is a multidimensional capacity that involves several components:

1. *Detect/react:* the ability to detect and react to gross changes in the environment, such as a telephone ringing, a name being called, or a ball that is thrown.
2. *Sustained attention:* the ability to consistently engage in an activity over time, such as reading for 15 minutes without losing concentration. Repetitive and predictable activities, such as stuffing envelopes or folding letters, place less demands on sustained attention.
3. *Selective attention:* the ability to attend to relevant stimuli while inhibiting distractions or irrelevant information. Examples include selecting specific locations on a map, finding items within a certain price range on a menu, choosing all the red or even playing cards, and finding specific ingredients in a closet. Selective attention demands are increased as the number of items presented simultaneously is increased and as the saliency of the target stimuli is decreased.
4. *Shifting of attention:* the ability to shift or alternate attention between tasks with different cognitive and/or

motor requirements. Examples include the ability to shift between adding and subtracting when balancing a checkbook, answering the telephone and typing, and making a salad while cooking something on the stove.

5. *Mental tracking:* the ability to simultaneously keep track of two or more stimuli during ongoing activity. Examples include keeping track of what has already been done in a multistep cooking task and listening to the radio while cooking a meal.

During evaluation (see Table 57.1) and intervention, it is important to keep these different aspects of attention in mind.

Attentional symptoms vary with anxiety and fatigue as well as with the task and context. Symptoms that reflect impairments in attention include distractibility; impulsivity; attentional lapses; and a tendency to become sidetracked, wander off task, overfocus on parts of a task, omit details, and lose track of something that was just done. In general, routine and repetitive activities place fewer demands on attentional capacity than do activities that are unfamiliar or unpredictable. For example, attentional symptoms might not be observed in basic self-care activities, but the same client might show attentional symptoms during a higher-level activity such as searching on the Internet for information.

Evaluation

Because attention is a multidimensional skill, therapists should ensure that they evaluate all components for potential impairments. More severe impairments in components such as sustaining attention may be easily observable in functional performance; however, more subtle impairments might be missed. Assessments such as the Test of Everyday Attention (Robertson, Ward, Ridgeway, & Nimmo-Smith, 1994) evaluate multiple components of attention.

Intervention

Strategy Training for Attention.   Attention strategy training involves helping a person learn to control, monitor, or prevent the emergence of attentional symptoms. For example, awareness training techniques described earlier, including self-prediction, self-questioning, specific goal setting and self-evaluation, can be embedded within strategy training to help a client monitor and regulate attentional lapses. Strategy training can be integrated into a wide range of simulated or occupation-based activities, during which the practitioner assists the client in monitoring and recording the frequency with which the targeted strategy or behavior is initiated and used. Examples of simulated functional activities include looking though a random stack of greeting cards for a particular holiday card; looking through a stack of recipe cards for recipes that match ingredients on a list; and looking up information in a telephone directory, calendar, or TV guide while simultaneously keeping track of the items found or while listening to the radio.

Strategies that may be emphasized include the following:

◆ Taking a time-out from a task when concentration begins to fade
◆ Remembering to get a sense of the whole situation before attending to the parts
◆ Monitoring a tendency to become distracted by internal thoughts or external stimuli
◆ Monitoring the ability to stay on task
◆ Remembering to look all over and actively search for additional information before responding
◆ Self-instruction or saying self-cues or each step of a task (aloud and then to self)
◆ Time pressure management techniques (Fasotti, Kovacs, Eling, & Brouwer, 2000)

Evidence supports the effectiveness of attention training for people with traumatic brain injury, in the postacute phase of rehabilitation. Successful interventions included strategy training, self-awareness techniques such as training participants to recognize when they are experiencing information overload or when they are off task (Cicerone et al., 2005). Similarly, Silverstein and colleagues (2005) demonstrated that attention training for people with schizophrenia combined with shaping techniques, including specific goal setting and feedback regarding on task behaviors, was more effective than attentional exercises alone.

Adaptations of Task or Environment.   Adaptations can be used to minimize attention demands within everyday activities. Techniques that include increasing saliency of items that require attention and reducing or limiting the amount of information presented to the client at one time can be used. Examples include the following (Toglia, 1993a):

◆ Modifying the environment to reduce visual clutter, interruptions, and auditory distractions
◆ Simplifying task instructions so that only one step is presented at a time
◆ Reducing the number of items or choices presented to the client at one time
◆ Preselecting relevant objects needed for tasks
◆ Task segmentation (e.g., presenting only one component of a task at a time) (Moulton, Taira, & Grover, 1995; Toglia, 1993a)
◆ Placing colored tape on house keys or on operating buttons of appliances

The enhancement of salient cues in the environment can be used to promote desired behaviors. In the task of brushing teeth, for example, unnecessary items should be removed from the sink, and the items that are required for use should be made salient with contrasting colors. The contrasting colors of the toothbrush, toothpaste, and cup

ETHICAL DILEMMA

How Can a Practitioner Balance Conflicting Ethical Obligations?

Mr. Grahm, who sustained a stroke and has resulting left hemiparesis and unilateral left neglect, is receiving outpatient occupational therapy services. He is driven to therapy by a daughter who lives nearby, but Mr. Grahm is living alone. Mr. Grahm tells you that although his daughter took his car keys, he has another set that she doesn't know about and he plans on driving to visit a friend this weekend. The occupational therapist knows that the driving assessment, completed when Mr. Grahm was an inpatient, advised him not to drive owing to his left neglect.

Questions

1. The occupational therapy practitioner has obligations and duties to several individuals and groups. Identify them. Which group or individual should receive the highest priority? Why?

2. What are the ethical principles that are in conflict in this situation?

3. What legal obligations might the therapist have in addition to ethical obligations?

provide a cue to assist the client in attending to the different items.

Unilateral Neglect

Unilateral neglect is a failure to orient to, respond to, or report stimuli that are presented on the side contralateral to the cerebral lesion in clients who do not have primary sensory or motor impairments (Heilman, Watson, & Valenstein, 2003). The term *neglect* connotes a volitional component to the disorder, but this is a misnomer. The client with unilateral neglect is unaware of the incompleteness of his or her perception of, and responses to, the environment. He or she often behaves as though one half of the world does not exist (Corben & Unsworth, 1999). For example, following right-hemisphere strokes, clients often begin scanning on the right side and miss or fail to explore most of the stimuli on the left. Asymmetry may be observed in functional activities, drawing tasks, reading, or writing. In severe cases, clients may eat food on one side of their plate, shave half their face, or dress half of their body without recognizing that anything is wrong. In milder cases, they may misread the first letter of a particular word or fail to attend to information while crossing a street, shopping, or driving (see the Ethical Dilemma). Many clients with unilateral neglect also exhibit anxiety or flattened affect.

Unilateral neglect has been identified as a major factor impeding functional recovery in clients who have sustained strokes (Chen Sea, Henderson, & Cermack, 1993; Cherney, Halper, Kwasnica, Harvey, & Zhang, 2001). Those with unilateral neglect have more difficulty resuming activities of daily living, have longer hospital stays

(Gillen, Tennen, & McGee, 2005; Katz et al., 1999), and are at increased risk for accidents (Webster et al., 1995).

Unilateral neglect has been described as a heterogeneous disorder that includes different clinical subtypes and behavioral components (Mesulam, 1994; Pierce & Buxbaum, 2002; Stone, Halligan, Marshall, & Greenwood, 1998). Unilateral neglect can involve one or more modalities, may vary with the nature of the stimuli (e.g., verbal versus nonverbal), and can encompass single objects or different spatial frames of space: extrapersonal or large space, peripersonal or space within reach, and personal or body space (Mesulam, 2000; Plummer, Morris, & Dunai, 2003). For example, some clients demonstrate neglect symptoms in large spaces, such as a room (extrapersonal neglect), but do not have reduced awareness of their body (personal neglect) or difficulty on paper-and-pencil tasks (peripersonal neglect). Neglect subtypes have also been proposed that involve internal mental images (representational neglect), decreased movement into or toward the contralesional space (motor neglect), or decreased ability to perceive sensory stimuli in contralesional space (sensory neglect) (Mesulam, 1994).

Evaluation

Occupational therapists evaluating clients with unilateral neglect must first distinguish between hemianopsia and unilateral neglect. Visual field cuts (hemianopsia) are hemiretinal, while neglect is hemispatial. Clients with visual field cuts typically have awareness of their visual field loss and make compensatory head movements and turns. Unilateral neglect may exist with or without hemianopsia, and one syndrome does not cause the other. Assessment of unilateral neglect typically involves cancellation tasks that require detection of target stimuli, distributed on both sides of space (see Table 57.1). Typically, the majority of targets on the contralesional side of space are missed. The complexity of unilateral neglect symptoms is not fully captured by traditional tests of neglect. Therefore, it is important not to rely completely on test instruments in identifying unilateral neglect. The different behavioral manifestations and subtypes of neglect need to be kept in mind during observation of performance (Appelros, Nydevik, Karlsson, Thorwalls, & Seiger, 2003; Plummer et al., 2003).

Dynamic assessment of unilateral neglect provides information about task conditions that increase or decrease the symptoms of unilateral neglect as well as the person's ability to respond to different types of cues or implement and carryover learned strategies to different situations. Toglia (2005) has described a dynamic object search task that analyzes the ability to learn and apply a strategy across a series of search tasks in people with unilateral neglect.

Intervention

Specific skill training is emphasized in this section because evidence exists to support the use of visual scanning training to remediate disorders of unilateral neglect.

In unilateral neglect, clients demonstrate decreased eye movements to the affected side. This decrease in eye movements reflects a decrease in attention to one side of the environment (Antonucci et al., 1995; Toglia, 1991b). A scientific literature review by Cicerone and colleagues (2000, 2005) concluded that there is level 1 evidence to support use of visuospatial interventions that include practice in visual scanning because it improves compensation for unilateral neglect and generalizes to everyday activities. Therefore, they recommended visuospatial rehabilitation with visual scanning as a practice standard for clients with visual neglect after right-hemisphere stroke. The combination of forced limb activation or movements of the left arm or hand on the left side of space in conjunction with visual scanning also shows positive results (Cicerone et al., 2005; Robertson, Hogg, & McMillan, 1998). Intervention appears to be most effective when a wide combination of intervention activities, including everyday tasks, is used (Antonucci et al., 1995; Pizzamiglio et al., 1992). Programs with greater levels of intensity have generally produced more positive outcomes. However, even with intensive training, it has been demonstrated that people with unilateral neglect have poorer functional outcome than do other people with stroke (Paolucci, Antonucci, Grasso, & Pizzamiglio, 2001).

Weinberg and colleagues (1977) designed systematic training techniques that incorporated a combination of remedial worksheets and strategy training techniques during reading and scanning tasks. For example, they used graded anchoring, pacing the speed of scanning, feedback, and decreasing the density of the stimulus. Anchoring, or teaching the person to use a spatial reference point, such as a colored line on the left side, is a common strategy in visual scanning training.

Gross motor activities involving vestibular input and whole-body movement in space increase general arousal and alertness and have been used in combination with visual scanning activities to increase gaze and attention to the affected side (Cappa, Sterzi, Vallar, & Bisiach, 1987). Activities such as balloon volleyball, with the client hitting the balloon with his or her hands clasped together, is an example of such an activity.

Other intervention techniques that have been recommended for clients with unilateral neglect include use of prisms and visual occlusion techniques (Pierce & Buxbaum, 2002). Prisms cause an optical deviation of the visual field to the right so that objects appear to be moved farther to the right than they actually are (Redding & Wallace, 2006). Partial visual occlusion methods attempt to force the person to use the neglected visual field by patching the eye ipsilateral to the lesion, patching the nonneglected half field of eyeglasses (Beis, Andre, Baumgarten, & Challier, 1999), or darkening the nonneglected half field of eyeglasses (hemispatial sunglasses) (Arai, Ohi, Sasaki, Nobuto, & Tanaka, 1997).

Recently, computer-assisted training programs for street crossing and wheelchair navigation have been described. Trained subjects with unilateral neglect performed better on real-life tasks after virtual reality training than control subjects did. The use of virtual reality–based technology appears to show potential for clients with unilateral neglect (Katz et al., 2005; Webster et al., 2001).

STRATEGY TRAINING.   Strategies for unilateral neglect can be practiced within everyday tasks such as setting a table for several people, dealing a deck of cards to six people, identifying appointments on a wall calendar, reading a newspaper, addressing envelopes of different sizes, or identifying all the pictures or chairs in the room. Because unilateral neglect symptoms vary with the size of space, arrangement of space, and amount and density of information presented, these activity parameters need to be matched with the neglect symptoms and systematically varied and graded in treatment. In some cases, treatment activities should emphasize large-space activities; in other situations, activities should focus on tabletop tasks that involve visual detail. In general, activities that are unpredictable or involve stimuli randomly scattered on a table or page are more sensitive to the symptoms of unilateral neglect than are activities that are arranged in a predictable, structured, or horizontal array (Ferber & Karnath, 2001). Intervention should include practice in identifying situations in which neglect symptoms are most likely to occur, such as filling multiple bowls with salad, placing cookie dough on a baking sheet, or arranging photographs in a picture album.

Individuals with unilateral neglect do not always know when they are attending to the left side. Intervention needs to assist clients in finding external cues that will provide feedback about when they are indeed attending to the left. An emphasis in intervention should be teaching the client to find the edges of a page or a table or the periphery of stimuli before beginning a task and to mark it with spatial point of reference, such as colored tape, a colored highlighter, a bright object, or placement of his or her arm on the left border. Auditory cueing, utilizing a beeper or alarm device, can be combined with strategy training to remind the person to use a strategy or visual cue. The alarm device can require the client to scan space and attend to the left to turn off the sound (Seron, Deloche, & Coyette 1989).

Other intervention strategies for unilateral neglect include tactile search, use of mental imagery, and general alerting techniques. Tactile search includes teaching the client to feel the left side of space with eyes closed or to feel the left edges of objects before visual search. Visual imagery teaches imagining and describing familiar scenes or routes and using mental images during movement of limbs or visual scanning (Niemeier, 1998; Smania, Bazoli, Piva, & Guidetti, 1997). For example, reduction in neglect symptoms and increased performance on functional tasks were reported after a mental imagery program that involved teaching people with neglect to imagine their eyes as sweeping beams of a lighthouse from left to right across the visual field. Clients were cued to use this mental image during functional and therapy training tasks (Niemeier, 1998; Niemeier, Cifu, & Kishore, 2001). In addition to strategies specifically aimed at facilitating attention to the left side, strategies that focus on the general ability to sustain attention have also been found to reduce unilateral neglect. For example, Robertson, Tegner, Tham, Lo, and Smith (1995) taught clients with chronic unilateral neglect to mentally tell themselves to "pay attention" and to tap loudly on a table.

It has been observed that response to strategy training depends on whether people with unilateral neglect show improvements in their awareness (Tham et al., 2001; Robertson & Halligan, 1999). This underscores the importance of deeply embedding awareness training techniques, such as those described earlier, into all intervention activities.

ADAPTATIONS OF TASK OR ENVIRONMENT. To minimize the need to attend to the left, it has been suggested that the environment be rearranged so that key items (e.g., the telephone, the nurse call button) are on the unaffected side. However, a study by Kelly and Ostreicher (1985) found no significant difference in functional outcome in clients whose hospital rooms were rearranged in this way. Lennon (1994) described the successful use of large colored paper markings on the edges of tables, corners, and elsewhere to prevent collision for clients with unilateral neglect. The client was trained to look for these markers. Markers were gradually faded. Performance improved and was maintained with removal of markers; however,

effects did not generalize to other environments. Calvanio, Levine, and Petrone (1993) described the use of an adapted plate to increase feeding skills in a client with a severe case of left inattention and a dense left hemianopsia. The plate was mounted on a lazy Susan so that it could be rotated. As the client pushed at the food with a fork, the plate rotated so that all the food eventually came into view, thus eliminating the need for scanning to the left. Other environmental adaptations include placing red tape on the client's wheelchair brakes or placing brightly colored objects such as a napkin or cup on the left side (Golisz, 1998).

Visual Processing

Visual perception is viewed on an information-processing continuum involving the reception, organization, and assimilation of visual information. On one end of the continuum, simple visual-processing tasks such as matching shapes or objects occurs quickly and automatically, with minimal effort. On the opposite end of the continuum, complex visual tasks that include unfamiliar stimuli or subtle discriminations within visually crowded arrays require slower and effortful processing. In this conceptualization, visual-processing dysfunction is defined as a decrease in the amount that the visual system is able to assimilate at any one time (Toglia, 1989). To understand the client's **visual perceptual** skills and the effects of impairments on functioning, we need to analyze the activity conditions (complexity, amount, familiarity, and predictability) rather than the type of activity (visual spatial, visual discrimination, visual motor, or visual gestalt).

Problems in simple visual processing include difficulty in discriminating between objects, pictures of objects, and basic shapes; difficulty in detecting gross differences in size, position, direction, angles, and rotations; decreased ability to visually locate single visual targets in space or judge gross distance between two objects; and decreased ability to detect simple part-whole relationships in objects or basic shapes. The person may have difficulty in familiar and routine activities and may easily misinterpret or misidentify objects. Failure to recognize an object is labeled visual **agnosia**. Toglia (1989) proposes that labels such as visual agnosia are too broad for the purposes of intervention because there are many different underlying reasons for object recognition difficulties. For example, a person might fail to attend to the critical feature of an object or the part of the object that tells what it is (e.g., prongs of a fork). Attention might be captured by salient but irrelevant aspects of the object (e.g., the utensil's decorative handle). There might be an inability to process the overall shape and the details simultaneously, so the person might miss important details.

Complex visual processing skills are required in visually confusing environments; when there is abstract, unfamiliar, or detailed visual information; or in conditions under which the distinctive visual features are partially obscured (e.g., the object is rotated and partially hidden on a crowded desk). Dysfunction of complex visual perceptual skills may include decreased ability to detect subtle differences in abstract shapes and objects or angles, size, distance, and position. A client might have difficulty making sense out of ambiguous, incomplete, fragmented, or distorted visual stimuli. The client might misinterpret an object when it is in an unusual position or partially hidden. The person might experience increased difficulty in visually confusing or crowded environments. Functional tasks such as finding items in a crowded closet, drawer, desk, or supermarket shelf and locating key information on a bill, map, or schedule might present difficulty. On these tasks, the person might misinterpret information, miss key visual details, or become sidetracked by irrelevant visual stimuli.

Visual Motor

Visual motor skills include drawing tasks (e.g., drawing a map, copying a design) or construction of three-dimensional figures (e.g., assembling a coffeepot). Clients may demonstrate difficulty on visual motor tasks for many reasons. For example, a client might have difficulty constructing a block design because of a poor ability to scan the complete design, decreased planning and organization, unilateral neglect, or impaired discrimination of size, angles, and rotations. The term *constructional apraxia* is used to refer to difficulty with drawing or assembly tasks that cannot be attributed to primary motor or sensory impairment, ideomotor apraxia, or general cognitive impairments (Farah, 2003). Constructional abilities are closely related to ADL performance (Neistadt, 1992a; Warren, 1981). Clients may have difficulty dressing (dressing apraxia), orienting clothes correctly on a hanger, or assembling a sandwich or coffeepot. People with left-hemisphere parietal lesions tend to omit individual pieces or details in constructional tasks, whereas those with right-hemisphere lesions demonstrate spatial disorganization of the pieces and lose the overall gestalt (Kramer, Kaplan, & Blusewicz, 1991). Constructional apraxia is not a unitary syndrome. Impairments in different types of perceptual processing or spatial relations are thought to underlie constructional apraxia in both right- and left-hemisphere lesions (Laeng, 2006).

Evaluation

Evaluation for people with visual perceptual impairments should examine visual foundations skills, visual abilities without a motor response, and visual motor skills. Visual foundation skills, including visual acuity, oculomotor skills, and visual fields, should be evaluated prior to a visual-processing evaluation to screen out visual problems that will interfere with the accuracy of perceptual testing (Cate & Richards, 2000). Several clinical observations during functional tasks can alert occupational therapists to the need for a formal visual assessment: compensatory head

movements and tilting, squinting, shutting of one eye, or a tendency to lose one's place while reading. A basic screening can be performed by the occupational therapist (i.e., visual acuity, range of motion of the eyes, ocular alignment, visual pursuits or smooth tracking of moving objects, saccades or quick eye movements to place an object of interest in view, and visual-scanning functions). Any disruptions of these foundational skills will affect interpretations of higher level visual-processing assessments (Warren, 1993).

Standardized nonmotor assessments of visual perception (see Table 57.1) categorize visual perception into specific skills such as figure-ground, position in space, form constancy, spatial relations, and visual recognition. Adults with neurological lesions may have difficulty performing various types of visual processing tasks for similar reasons (e.g., a tendency to overfocus on parts, a tendency to miss visual details, failure to simultaneously attend to the details as well as the whole). Therefore, Toglia (1989) recommends an approach that conceptualizes visual processing on a continuum and evaluates both conventional and unconventional objects under a variety of different activity conditions. In a dynamic approach to visual perception, the therapist systematically manipulates activity parameters and analyzes responses to cues to understand why a client is having difficulty accurately discriminating objects or visual stimuli (Kline, 2000; Toglia, 1989; Toglia & Finkelstein, 1991). Visual perceptual assessment should examine responses to activities with and without a motor response to examine differences in performance. Visual motor skills are typically evaluated with block designs, puzzles, or copying designs. The therapist needs to observe how the person begins and how he or she proceeds. For example, does the client begin by drawing the details rather than attending to the overall shape of the figure? Informal observations in tasks such as copying a map route, assembling a coffeepot or woodworking project, wrapping a package, packing a lunchbox, or folding clothes can provide additional information on visual motor abilities (Figure 57.2). Symptoms may include angular deviations; improper position, location, spacing, or alignment of parts; and spatial distortions. The client's ability to recognize and correct errors in alignment or position should be investigated. For example, some clients do not recognize visual spatial errors even when attention is directed to the problem area, whereas other clients recognize errors but are unable to correct them.

Intervention

Interventions may address visual foundations skills or visual processing skills with or without a motor response.

VISUAL FOUNDATION SKILLS.   Treatment of visual foundation skills such as visual acuity and contrast sensitivity, oculomotor skills, and visual fields generally involves adaptations a such as large-print reading materials; mag-

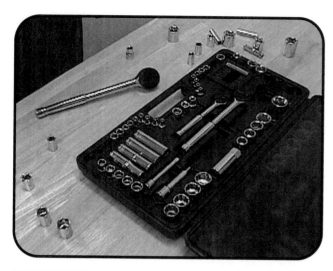

FIGURE 57.2 Organizing the components of a ratchet tool kit requires perception of size and shape as well as organizational skills.

nifiers; talking devices; increasing contrast of edges, borders, or backgrounds; and changes in lighting. However, remedial exercises may be recommended for individuals with oculomotor or visual field deficits. For example, range-of-motion eye exercises to the involved muscle have been advocated for individuals with eye muscle paresis. Occlusion of the intact visual field with eye patching has been used to force use of the impaired visual field (Warren, 1993).

STRATEGY TRAINING. Strategies that maximize the client's ability to process visual information can be trained within everyday activities that involve choosing among objects that are similar in shape and size (e.g., matching socks, sorting teaspoons and soupspoons); locating information within supermarket circulars, calendars, maps, or schedules; arranging information within grids or spreadsheets; copying patterns in arts and craft activities; or finding information in crowded draws, shelves, tables, or bulletin boards.

Strategies can include getting a sense of the whole before looking at the parts; teaching the person to partition space before localizing details; using one's finger to scan, trace visual stimuli, or focus on details; covering or blocking visual stimuli when too much information is presented at once; verbalizing salient visual features or subtle differences; and mentally visualizing a particular item before looking for it (Toglia, 1989, 1998). Intervention involves careful manipulation of activity parameters. Activities that involve familiar items or contexts, high contrast (e.g., red socks and white socks), distinctive features, little detail, and solid colors or backgrounds require less attention, effort, and visual analysis than do activities that involve choosing among items that have low contrast (e.g., light beige and white socks), are in unusual posi-

tions, are embedded within crowded or distracting visual backgrounds, or are partially obscured. Changes in the familiarity, number of items, and degree of detail can place greater demands on visual processing. In addition, verbal mediation, including repeating a list of step-by-step instructions during a functional activity such as dressing, capitalizes on strengths in verbal abilities and can be effective in facilitating functional performance (Sunderland, Walker, & Walker, 2006).

ADAPTATION OF TASK OR ENVIRONMENT. The key guideline in minimizing the effects of visual perceptual difficulties is to make the distinctive features of objects more salient with color cues. An example is placing colored tape on buttons to operate appliances or using salient color cues on objects to make them easier to locate and discriminate (e.g., bright pink tape on a medication bottle). Cues such as colored marks or tape at spatial landmarks (e.g., tape recorder, wheelchair footrests, or label of a shirt) reduce spatial demands and make it easier to orient and align parts of an item. Visual stimuli such as items on a shelf or sentences on a page that are large and arranged in an organized manner with large spaces between items are easier to perceive. Consistent locations for objects in the refrigerator, closet, or drawer or a countertop increase predictability and provide contextual cues for recognition. Significant others should be instructed to decrease visual distractions in the room or within a task by limiting designs and patterns and by using solid colors with high contrast. Patterns, designs, and decorations make it harder to select and recognize critical features of an object. Significant others should also be trained to introduce only a small amount of visual information at one time.

Motor Planning

Motor planning, or praxis, is the ability to execute learned and purposeful activities. **Apraxia** is defined as a disorder of skilled movement that cannot be adequately explained by primary motor or sensory impairments, visual spatial problems, language comprehension difficulties, or cognitive problems alone (Heilman & Rothi, 2003). Damage to the association areas of the brain (affecting the cognitive aspects of motor control) is thought to cause apraxia (Kertesz, 1982). Apraxia may be seen after strokes in either hemisphere, although it is more commonly seen in clients who have sustained a left-hemisphere lesion. Aphasia is often associated with apraxia, since the left hemisphere is also dominant for language (Heilman & Rothi, 2003). People with apraxia can improve performance of skilled movement over time (Basso, Burgio, Paulin, & Prandoni, 2000); however, they frequently continue to have significant functional limitations in both the learning of new motor tasks, such as one-handed shoe tying (Poole, 1998), and in the performance of motor acts to verbal command or demonstration (Poole, 2000).

Roy (1978) identifies two major subsystems in apraxia: the conceptual and the production subsystems. The symptoms of apraxia may reflect disorders in one or both of these subsystems. The production aspect of motor planning, traditionally called *ideomotor apraxia,* involves generating the action plan, sequencing and organizing the appropriate elements, and carrying out the plan (e.g., reaching for a glass of water to take a drink). The greatest difficulty is observed when the client is asked to pretend use of a tool or object or to perform limb gestures. Some improvement may be seen when the client is asked to imitate the motion or perform the motion with the actual object, but the movement is still imprecise. These clients know what they want to do, but actions are carried out in an awkward, inefficient, or clumsy manner. Errors of preservation, sequencing, or omissions may be observed.

The conceptual aspect of motor planning (Roy, 1978) includes knowledge about the functional properties of an object, the object action, and the sequence of action. Conceptual errors, traditionally called *ideational apraxia,* involve object function, action knowledge, and knowledge of sequence. Clients might be able to accurately identify and match objects, but inappropriate use of objects is frequently observed. For example, the client might try to brush his or her hair with a toothbrush. Although object recognition may be intact, the person might be unable to associate the object with its correct action plan.

Dressing apraxia and constructional apraxia are additional subtypes of apraxia, previously described in the section on visual processing. Traditional labels of apraxia are narrow in scope and do not account for the wide range of skills that underlie motor planning and constructional abilities.

Evaluation

The classic definition of apraxia includes motor-planning problems that cannot be accounted for by weakness, increased tone, incoordination, sensory loss, or other cognitive-perceptual impairments. The clinician is urged to analyze underlying reasons for difficulties in performance rather than attempting to classify clients within traditional categories. In clinical practice, most clients have associated difficulties that contribute to difficulty in motor planning. Information on the client's language skills should be obtained from the speech-language pathologist or be screened for by testing for "yes" or "no" comprehension and ability to follow one-step commands, since apraxia and aphasia often coexist.

In evaluating apraxia, the clinician typically observes the client's performance of different types of movements, noting the method of evocation (e.g., command, imitation, or object use) and type of errors made (Haaland, 1993). Assessments for apraxia are listed in Table 57.1. An observational method for assessing apraxia in ADL activities, adapted from the Arnadottir OT Neurobehav-ioral Evaluation (A-ONE), has been validated for people with stroke (van Heugten et al., 2000).

A dynamic assessment approach attempts to identify the activity conditions under which the limb apraxia symptoms emerge, the client's response to cueing, and the client's awareness of his or her activity performance (Toglia, 1998).

Intervention

Interventions to overcome motor-planning deficits may emphasize either the production aspect or the conceptual aspect of motor planning (Roy, 1985). Techniques that address the orientation of an object or limb in space or the timing, sequence, and organization of the motor elements aim to enhance the production aspect of motor planning. For example, the practitioner might provide physical contact (i.e., hand-over-hand assistance or light touch) to limit inappropriate or extraneous movements while simultaneously using guiding methods to facilitate a smooth motor pattern or to guide the manipulation of objects. Through repeated practice in different tasks, the client begins to learn the movement patterns that feel "right," and the practitioner gradually withdraws assistance. Deep proprioceptive input and contact have an inhibitory effect on normal people, whereas light touch tends to have a more facilitatory effect (Farber, 1993).

Familiar tasks that are performed in context are easier for people with motor-planning disorders because the context provide cues that facilitate the desired action (Ferguson & Trombly, 1997). Interventions can be graded by gradually introducing activities and environments that have less stability and predictability, such as negotiating around obstacles in a crowded store.

Intervention addressing the conceptual aspect of motor planning focuses on facilitating the client's understanding of how an object is used or how a gesture is performed (Helm-Estabrooks, 1982; Pilgrim & Humphreys, 1994; Smania, Girardi, Domenicali, Lora, & Aglioti, 2000).

STRATEGY TRAINING.   Clients may be taught to use verbal, visual, or tactile cues to enhance movement. For example, before performing an activity, the client might mentally practice or imagine the task performance; or the client might imagine how an object should look in his or her hand before picking it up. Incorrect patterns of movement, such as holding an object the wrong way, can also be visualized, with an emphasis on having the client mentally practice correcting the movement. Talking a client through action sequences or use of step-by-step written lists or illustrations can be useful in facilitating functional performance in tasks such as drinking from a cup (Butler, 1999). The person can be taught to verbally rehearse an action sequence or associate the movement with a rhyme, rhythm, or musical tune with a gradual fading of the verbalization. Self-monitoring strategies can be used to teach a client to monitor unnecessary cocontraction, incomplete actions, or difficulty in switching direction of movements. Preliminary studies indicate that strategy training is effective in improving everyday function (Donkervoort, Dekker, Stehmann-Saris, & Deelman, 2001; Geusgens et al., 2006). For example, in a randomized study design, changes on nontrained ADL activities were greater in a group of people with stroke who had received strategy training as compared with those receiving usual occupational therapy. This suggests that the strategies generalized to everyday activities (Geusgens et al., 2006).

ADAPTATION OF TASK OR ENVIRONMENT.   Simple adaptations to objects that draw attention to the critical features of the object or activity can facilitate action and motor planning (e.g., colored tape on the knife handle or toothbrush handle). Patterns and designs on utensils or clothing might draw attention to the wrong detail and result in an inappropriate motor response.

Tool use should be minimized (Poole, 2000), and adaptive equipment should be selected with caution for the apraxic client. For example, some adaptations, such as a button hook, one-handed shoe tying, or a one-arm-drive wheelchair, might be confusing for clients with apraxia and place greater demands on motor-planning abilities. Other adaptations, such as adaptive clothing closures, may simplify the task or motor pattern required to manipulate or hold objects, reduce the number of steps, and facilitate function in the client with apraxia.

Other adaptations include training the caregiver to modify instructions so that the activity is broken into one command at a time (Unsworth, 2007). Simple whole commands (e.g., "Get up") can put the activity on an automatic level and effectively enhance motor planning (Zoltan, 1996).

Memory

Memory gives us the ability to draw on past experiences and learn new information (Toglia, 1993a). This provides us with a sense of continuity in the environment and frees us from dependency in here-and-now situations. Memory is conceptualized as a multistep process involving encoding (i.e., input of information), storage (i.e., holding information), and retrieval (i.e., getting information) (Levy, 2005b). There are different types of memory. Working memory is the temporary storage of information while one is working with it or attending to it. It includes the ability to recall information immediately after exposure. It allows one to focus conscious attention and keep track of information as one is performing an activity. Declarative memory is one aspect of long-term memory and includes conscious memory for events, knowledge, or facts. Procedural (nondeclarative) memory involves the ability to remember how to perform an activity or procedure without conscious awareness. Prospective memory

involves the ability to remember intentions or activities that will be required in the future (Levy, 2005b).

Evaluation

It is important to distinguish whether everyday memory problems are due to failures to recall past events or conversations or failures in carrying out future activities (e.g., prospective memory). A comprehensive evaluation of memory, whether static or dynamic, must address the different types of memory and methods of retrieval (Table 57.1). Assessments must consider factors such as the modality in which the information is presented (auditory or visual), the type of instructions (general or specific), the amount of stimuli presented, the familiarity and meaningfulness of the information, the presence of contextual cues during recall phases, the type of information to be remembered (factual or skill related), and the length of retention. Dynamic assessment of memory, such as Toglia's (1993b) Contextual Memory Test, evaluates awareness of memory capabilities and use of strategies.

Intervention

Memory impairments can be closely related to other cognitive impairments, particularly attention. Some investigators have suggested that an indirect approach that addresses other cognitive skills, such as attention or organization, rather than memory, may be effective. For example, Sohlberg and Mateer (1989a) reported improvement in memory function after attentional training. Interventions for memory impairments include memory strategy training, external aids and devices, and adaptations, as well as techniques of errorless learning, vanishing cues, and spaced retrieval that were discussed earlier in this chapter.

STRATEGY TRAINING.   Training of internal memory strategies is most appropriate for people with mild memory deficits or those in whom other areas of cognition are intact (Cicerone et al., 2000, 2005). The client practices one or two targeted memory strategies in a variety of different tasks, such as remembering telephone numbers, news headlines, a sequence of errands, items that need to be bought in a store, or instructions to an activity. During practice on different memory tasks, a variety of awareness training techniques may also be used. Memory strategies may be directed primarily at encoding operations (i.e., getting information in) or the retrieval phase of memory (i.e., getting information out). Encoding strategies include the following:

◆ Chunking or grouping similar items
◆ The story method, or linking a series of facts or events into a story
◆ Rehearsal, or repeating information over and over silently

- Rhymes, or recalling a fact by changing the fact into a rhyme
- Visual imagery

Retrieval strategies include the following:

- Alphabetical searching, or going through the alphabet to find the first letter of a forgotten item
- Retracing one's steps to find a missing object or to recall an event
- Thinking of associated information to cue the recall of a new fact or event
- Self-generating words, concepts, or items to improve learning and memory (Chiaravalloti & DeLuca., 2002)

MEMORY EXTERNAL STRATEGIES AND AIDS.   External aids such as notebooks, tape recorders and computers store information that the person might have difficulty remembering. Other aids such as pagers or alarm signals serve to remind a person to perform an action (prospective memory) (Toglia, 1993a). The success of an intervention program that utilized a combination of external aids and strategies with awareness training to improve prospective memory was recently described by Fleming, Shum, Strong, and Lightbody (2005). External memory aids include the following: timers, tape recorders, devices with preprogrammed alarms or alarm messages, electronic devices such as pagers, mobile phones, palm pilots, and cell phones, computers, pill box organizers, lists, daily planners, and notebooks (Figure 57.3). Case studies have documented the effectiveness of external aids (McKerracher, Powell, & Oyebode, 2005; Wade & Troy, 2001; Wilson, Emslie, Quirk, & Evans, 2001). Intervention is most effective when the client is motivated, involved in identifying the memory problem, and fairly independent in daily function (Cicerone et al., 2000, 2005).

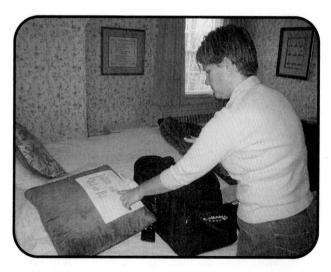

FIGURE 57.3   Use of a list of clothing and other items to pack assists this client with memory and executive function impairments.

Evidence obtained from case studies supports the use of memory notebooks and other external aids in reducing everyday memory failures for people with moderate to severe memory impairments (Cicerone et al., 2000, 2005, McKerracher et al., 2005; Wade & Troy, 2001; Wilson et al., 2001). However, the successful use of an external memory aid may require extensive training. The client may need to practice initiating and using the aid in a variety of different situations.

The use of external aids might need to be graded. In the initial stages, the client might be expected to use the aid only when it is initiated by another person. Gradually, the client might be trained to initiate the use of the aid independently. Errorless learning, spaced retrieval, and other task-specific training methods that capitalize on procedural memory, may be used in training clients with moderate or severe memory impairments to use an external aid.

The most commonly used external memory strategy is the memory notebook. The memory notebook needs to be designed with the person's needs and lifestyle in mind (McKerracher et al., 2005). Sample sections in a memory notebook are as follows: personal facts, names of people to remember, calendar and schedule, things to do/important events (daily, within the next week), daily log of important events, conversations, summary of readings (articles, newspaper), medication schedule, and directions to frequently traveled places. Initially, the notebook should begin with one or two sections and gradually increase.

Memory notebook training needs to take place in the context of a variety of everyday activities. Therapy sessions should include role-playing and practice in use of the notebook. In addition, the client may be asked questions that involve reviewing and rereading the memory notebook. Specific memory notebook training protocols have been described in the literature (Donaghy & Williams 1998; Sohlberg & Mateer, 2001).

ADAPTATIONS OF TASK OR ENVIRONMENT.   Tasks and environments can be rearranged so that they place fewer demands on memory:

- Cue cards or signs in key places (e.g., a sign on door where it will be seen before leaving: "Take keys and . . .")
- Labeling the outside of drawers or closets to minimize the need to recall the location of items
- Providing step-by-step directions to reduce memory demands
- Providing checklists to assist in keeping track of task steps

Significant others can be trained to use methods that increase the likelihood that the client will remember material, such as asking the client to repeat any instructions or important information in his or her own words; encouraging the client to ask questions; and presenting material in small groups, clusters, or categories (Levy, 2005a).

Executive Functions, Organization, and Problem Solving

Executive functions are a broad band of performance skills that allow a person to engage in independent, purposeful, and self-directed behavior. Higher-level cognitive skills, including planning, cognitive flexibility, organization, problem-solving, and self–regulation, are fundamental components of executive function (Katz & Hartman-Maeir, 2005). Lezak and colleagues (2004) identifies four primary components of executive functions: volition, planning, purposeful action, and self-awareness and self-monitoring. Impairments are associated with prefrontal lesions and may be seen in all of these components, with one or two areas of impairment especially prominent (Lezak et al., 2004). Volition is the capacity to formulate an intention or goal and to initiate action. Planning involves the ability to efficiently organize the steps or elements of a behavior or activity and includes the ability to look ahead, anticipate consequences, weigh and make choices, conceive of alternatives, sustain attention, and sequence the activity. Purposeful action is the translation of an intention into an activity, requiring the ability to initiate, switch, and stop sequences (flexibility), as well as self-regulation. Self-regulation involves the ability to monitor, self-correct, and evaluate performance.

Executive function impairments significantly influence social participation, daily activity, and functional outcome (Goverover, 2002, 2004; Reeder, Newton, Frangou, & Wykes, 2004). Clients who display executive dysfunction may be able to verbalize plans but have difficulty carrying them out. There is often a disassociation between stated intentions and actions. This creates gaps between what a person needs to do or wants to do and what the person actually does (Eriksson, Tham, & Borg, 2006). Decreased initiation, flexibility, impulsivity, or **perseveration** may be observed during performance. Often, the client's approach is haphazard or consists of trial and error, and there is decreased ability to maintain goal-directed actions and to monitor or modify behaviors. For example, when grocery shopping, the client might proceed in an unorganized manner, not using a list or the aisle headings and reentering the same aisle multiple times. The client might have difficulty deciding on appropriate substitute items, buy items that are not needed, and forget items that were needed (Sohlberg & Mateer, 2001). Rempfer, Hamera, Brown, and Cromwell (2003) found that grocery shopping accuracy and efficiency were significantly associated with measures of executive functions in people with chronic schizophrenia. In addition, limitations in the ability to view information from different perspectives, generate alternative solutions, and respond flexibly can reduce the ability to cope, adapt to everyday demands, and relate to others.

Executive functions impairments represent a distinct challenge because they can be masked within familiar ADLs or routines but are most apparent when the client is required to function in situations that are less structured, require multitasking, or require dealing with novelty and unexpected situations (Burgess et al., 2006; Katz & Hartman-Maeir, 2005). Examples of activities that might present difficulty include following directions to a new location; selecting and ordering a gift from a catalogue; organizing a day's activities; planning a menu, lunch, picnic, vacation, or social gathering; investigating and comparing prices for delivery of flowers; mailing a package; or purchasing an electronic device.

Evaluation

Most standardized cognitive assessments are structured and do not adequately examine the area of executive functions (Sohlberg & Mateer, 2001) (see Table 57.1). Several assessments for executive functions have recently been developed (Bamdad, Ryan, & Warden, 2003; Birnboim & Miller, 2004; Wilson, Alderman, Burgess, Emslie, & Evans, 1996). Although these assessments appear more "ecologically valid" (i.e., able to predict behavior in everyday situations) than previous assessments were, further research data on the reliability and validity of these assessment tools are needed.

Intervention

STRATEGY TRAINING. Strategies that maximize executive functioning can be practiced in a variety of unstructured tasks that require initiation, planning, organization, and decision making, such as organizing medications according to a schedule, planning an overnight trip and packing a suitcase, obtaining and organizing a list of local business phone numbers, and organizing tools (Figure 57.4).

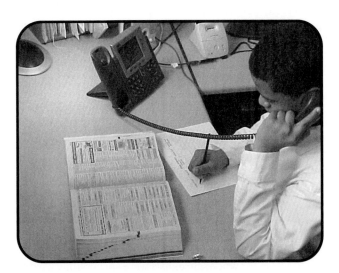

FIGURE 57.4 A checklist helps this young client to ensure that he obtains all the required information as he makes phone calls.

Verbal mediation has been reported to be an effective strategy in improving executive function and self-regulation deficits. For example, Cicerone and Wood (1987) reported the successful use of a self-instructional procedure in a client with impaired planning ability and poor self-control secondary to brain injury. Intervention involved requiring the client to verbalize a plan of action before and during execution of a task. Gradually, the client was instructed to whisper rather than talk aloud. Generalization to real-life situations was observed after an extended period of time that included training in self-monitoring.

Training in problem-solving strategies involves teaching the person to break down complex activities into smaller, more manageable steps. Strategies may also aim to help the person to maintain the focus of goals and intentions (Katz & Hartman-Maeir, 2005). An evidenced-based review (Cicerone et al., 2000, 2005) concluded that there is evidence to support the use of formal problem-solving training with application to everyday activities. The authors recommended such training as a practice guideline for people with stroke or brain injury during postacute rehabilitation. The intervention goal is to replace an impulsive, disorganized approach with a systematic and controlled approach to planning activities, maintaining goal intentions, and solving problems. The steps of the problem-solving process are reinforced with use of self-questioning techniques. For example, self-questioning cue cards with the following types of questions can be used during problem-solving tasks: What do I need to do? Do I need more information? What do I have to do next? Have I identified all the critical information? Do I understand the problem? What are all the possible solutions? Did I choose the best one?

Broad checklists or task guidance systems are commonly used to assist the client in initiating, planning, and carrying out an activity systematically. Checklists may be specific to a particular activity (e.g., following steps to operate a computer program), or they may be designed broadly so that they can be used in a variety of similar activities (e.g., a checklist for food preparation or cooking activities).

Interventions should incorporate practice in identifying the situations or activities in which use of a checklist could be helpful. The client may be given the opportunity to practice the same activity with and without the use of a checklist to enhance awareness. Initially, the goal might be to have a client follow a checklist established by the practitioner or significant other. Eventually, the client might be given checklists with missing steps and be asked to review the lists to identify the missing components. Finally, the client might be required to create a checklist independently. Burke, Zencius, Wesolowskis, and Doubleday (1991) describe four cases of individuals with executive dysfunction for whom checklists were successfully used to improve the ability to carry out routine vocational tasks.

Decreased initiation, one of the hallmark features of executive dysfunction, can significantly interfere with the ability to use and apply a learned strategy. For example, a person with deficits in executive functions might use a strategy effectively when cued but not use the strategy spontaneously because of a failure to initiate its use. External cues such as alarm signals can be used to prompt the client to initiate a task, switch to a different task component, or use a particular strategy within an activity (Evans, Emslie, & Wilson, 1998; Manly, Hawkins, Evans, Wodlt, & Robertson, 2002).

ADAPTATIONS OF TASK OR ENVIRONMENT. Adaptations that minimize demands on executive functions include training a significant other to preorganize an activity or activity materials. For example, all the items needed for grooming can be prearranged on the sink in the sequence in which they are used. As an alternative, one task step can be introduced at a time. These adaptations limit the need for planning and organization (Sohlberg & Mateer, 2001).

People who have difficulty with initiation, organization, and decision making require structure. Open-ended questions such as "What do you want to eat" should be avoided. Clients who have difficulty in initiation will have a great deal of difficulty in answering open-ended questions. Questions should provide a limited number of choices whenever feasible.

A predictable and structured daily routine enhances the client's ability to initiate tasks and should be established and monitored by a significant other. Audiotape instructions that cue the client to initiate an activity and perform each step at a time in its proper sequence have been reported to be successful within the context of daily routines (Schwartz, 1995).

GROUP INTERVENTIONS

Cognitive rehabilitation principles and strategies can be incorporated within group programs and combined with psychosocial or psychoeducational interventions. The group format can be used to target specific cognitive skills, or it can be used to teach compensatory strategies (Revheim & Marcopulos, 2006; Schwarztberg, 1999; Stuss et al., 2007). Group activities can emphasize interpersonal skills within cooperative tasks, such as planning a bake sale or publishing a newsletter, or role-playing scenarios involving interviews, conflicts, or on-the-spot problem solving. Strategies that include monitoring the tendency to respond impulsively, become stuck in one viewpoint, or wander off task can be practiced within social contexts (Toglia, 2005). Group programs that center on teaching self-monitoring techniques and strategies for paying attention, remembering, organization, or problem solving can be applied to a wide spectrum of clients. Activities such as remembering names and facts about group members, recalling directions for operating a new electronic device, or creating a checklist for a complex task can provide opportunity to practice

Evidence and Expanding Literature on Executive Function, Awareness, and Subtle Cognitive Impairments

Throughout this chapter, we cited evidence-based reviews (Cappa et al., 1987, 2005; Cicerone et al., 2000, 2005) and studies that support the effectiveness of interventions designed to address different cognitive perceptual symptoms. In this section, we highlight the evidence regarding executive functions and awareness. We also discuss the expanding literature on cognitive impairments across different populations and its implications.

Executive impairments have been found to consistently predict function (Boyle, Paul, Moser, & Cohen, 2004; Goverover, 2004; Laes & Sponheim, 2006; Royall, Palmer, Chiodo, & Polk, 2004). Significant relationships between executive function and social participation (Laes & Sponheim, 2006; Ucok et al., 2006; Yeates et al., 2004), academics (Biederman et al., 2004), IADLs (Jefferson, Paul, Ozonoff, & Cohen, 2006; Rempfer et al., 2003), employment (DeBattista, 2005; Eriksson et al., 2006), and quality of life (Sherman, Slick, & Eyrl, 2006) have been documented. The strong association between executive impairments and function that has been documented across different ages and populations highlights the critical need for occupational therapists to include executive function in evaluation and intervention planning.

Most standardized ADL assessments are structured and are not sensitive to the effects of executive function problems. Occupational therapists are encouraged to embrace the challenge of investigating tasks that adequately capture the cognitive demands of higher-level real-life activities. The use of ecologically relevant problem and situational simulations to examine the demands of higher-level everyday functioning is an important and promising direction for future research.

Self-awareness has been linked to daily functioning, involvement in productive activities, and outcome (Hoofien et al., 2004; Petrella, McColl, Krupa, & Johnston, 2005). Recently several pilot studies (Fleming et al., 2006; Goverover, Johnston, Toglia, & DeLuca, 2007; Ownsworth, Fleming, Desbois, Strong, & Kuipers, 2006; Tham et al., 2001) have investigated the use of occupation-based intervention to enhance self-awareness and occupational performance.

Occupation-based self-awareness studies support the premise that awareness gradually emerges within activities that are familiar because clients have a benchmark of comparison for self-evaluation (Ownsworth et al., 2006; Tham et al., 2001). This is important for occupational therapists because occupation-based self-awareness intervention appears to have potential for enhancing functional outcome. However, it is important to note that more research is needed to increase sample size and employ a more rigorous methodology to enhance the level of the evidence.

Although initial research in cognitive rehabilitation has been in the area of traumatic brain injury and stroke, cognitive rehabilitation principles are now being applied to other populations, such as those with schizophrenia (Penades et al., 2006), multiple sclerosis (Chiaravalloti, DeLuca, Moore, & Ricker, 2005), Parkinson's disease (Sinforiani, Banchieri, Zucchella, Pacchetti, & Sandrini, 2004), lupus (Harrison et al., 2005), learning disabilities (Cermak, 2005), mild cognitive impairment, and Alzheimer's disease (Bier, Desrosiers, & Gagnon 2006) and the well elderly population (Willis et al., 2006; Winocur et al., 2007).

Recently, subtle cognitive impairments that affect the ability to learn and integrate new information have been identified in people without brain injury, including conditions such as rheumatoid arthritis (Appenzeller, Bertolo, & Costallat, 2004), chronic fatigue syndrome (Capuron et al., 2006), Lyme disease (Fallon, Keilp, Prohovnik, Heertum, & Mann, 2003), cardiac failure (Vogels, Scheltens, Schroeder-Tanka, & Weinstein, 2006), muscular dystrophy (D'Angelo, & Bresolin, 2006), amyotrophic lateral sclerosis (Ringholz et al., 2005), diabetes (Munshi et al., 2005), critical illness (Hopkins & Brett, 2005), chronic obstructive pulmonary disease (Orth et al., 2006), and fibromyalgia (Katz, Heard, Mills, & Leavitt, 2004). In addition, subtle cognitive changes have been associated with chemotherapy treatments (Bender et al., 2006; Jansen, Miaskowski, Dodd, Dowling, & Kramer, 2005), radiation (Spiegler, Bouffet, Greenberg, Rutka, & Mabbott, 2004), and hemodialysis (Murray et al., 2006). Although cognitive impairments have been recognized as a core feature of schizophrenia, cognitive impairments are also now identified in across a wider range of mental health conditions, including depression (Kiosses, Klimstra, Murphy, & Alexopoulos, 2001), bipolar disease (Martinez-Aran et al., 2004), and obsessive-compulsive disorder (Boldrini et al., 2005), as well as in people with past histories of substance abuse (Davies et al., 2005).

different strategies and share experiences within a group context. Group members can be encouraged to reflect on performance and identify strategies that would be useful in their everyday activities. Group interventions that simultaneously address subtle cognitive difficulties and emotional issues have demonstrated value in improving self-awareness, self-efficacy, coping skills, psychosocial skills, and perceived daily functioning (Harrison et al., 2005; Rath, Smon, Langenbahn, Sherr, & Diller, 2003; Toglia, 2005).

SUMMARY

Recently, there has been a move away from intervention programs that focus exclusively on remediation of cognitive impairments. There is increasing evidence that supports the use of comprehensive and holistic cognitive rehabilitation programs that address a combination of cognitive, emotional, functional, and social participation skills in people with brain injury (Cappa et al., 2005; Cicerone et al., 2005, Cicerone, Mott, Azulay, & Friel, 2004; Sarajuuri et al., 2005; Tiersky et al., 2005). The need to blend cognitive interventions with those that address interpersonal and real-world functioning has been emphasized in recent literature; however, the outcome of cognitive rehabilitation is most commonly measured at the impairment level. As occupational therapists return to more community-focused intervention, we need to widen our perspective on the influence that cognitive perceptual impairments have on our clients' ability to engage in the occupations they need or want to do within the contexts of their lives. We need to explore the effect of cognitive rehabilitation on occupational engagement and social participation, for even subtle cognitive impairments can decrease satisfaction, participation, and quality of life, preventing our clients from leading enriching lives (McDowd, Filion, Pohl, Richards, & Stiers, 2003).

The outcome or benefit of cognitive rehabilitation needs to be examined broadly across different populations, including effects on changing existing habits; routines or increasing productive activity patterns; increasing the frequency and quality of social participation; decreasing caregiver assistance, stress, or burden; improving subjective well-being, including self-efficacy, self-esteem, satisfaction and quality of life; and preventing functional decline.

PROVOCATIVE QUESTIONS

1. The neuropsychologist reports that the client performed within normal ranges on a standardized test of executive function. Your occupational therapy evaluation included observation of real-life activities, during which the client showed difficulties in initiating, planning, and organization. How would you explain this discrepancy to team members? Explain how executive skills are linked to performance areas, providing examples. Describe how these skills can be evaluated and addressed in a client-centered intervention program within an inpatient or outpatient setting.

2. Your client who sustained a traumatic brain injury and has both hemiplegia and cognitive limitations tells you that he wants to work only on improving his arm movement. He appears unaware of his cognitive limitations and refuses to work on any activities that involve memory or problem solving because it is "not necessary." The client's family is concerned about his cognitive limitations and ability to return to his previous job, drive in his community, and be left alone at home. How would you respect your client's right to autonomy while addressing his impairments? What would be the goals of intervention? What might your intervention plan look like for this client?

REFERENCES

Abreu, B. C., & Peloquin, S. M. (2005). The Quadraphonic Approach: A holistic rehabilitation model for brain injury. In N. Katz (Ed.), *Cognition and occupation across the life span* (2nd ed., pp. 73–112). Bethesda, MD: AOTA.

Abreu, B. C., Seale, G., Scheibel, R. S., Huddleston, N., Zhang, L., & Ottenbacher, K. (2001). Levels of self-awareness after acute brain injury: How patients' and rehabilitation specialists' perceptions compare. *Archives of Physical Medicine and Rehabilitation, 82,* 49–56.

Abreu, B., & Toglia, J. P. (1987). Cognitive rehabilitation: A model for occupational therapy. *American Journal of Occupational Therapy, 41,* 439–448.

Albert, M. L. (1973). A simple test of visual neglect. *Neurology, 23,* 658–665.

Allen, C. K. (1985). *Occupational therapy for psychiatric diseases: Measurement and management of cognitive disabilities.* Boston: Little Brown.

Allen, C. K. (1993). Creating a need-satisfying, safe environment management and maintenance approaches. In C. B. Royeen (Ed.), *AOTA self-study series: Cognitive rehabilitation* (Lesson 11). Rockville, MD: AOTA.

Allen, C. K., Earhart, C. A., & Blue, T. (1992). *Occupational therapy treatment goals for the physically and cognitively disabled.* Rockville, MD: AOTA.

American Occupational Therapy Association. (1999). Management of occupational therapy services for persons with cognitive impairments (statement). *American Journal of Occupational Therapy, 53,* 601–607.

American Occupational Therapy Association. (2002). Occupational therapy practice framework: Domain and process. *American Journal of Occupational Therapy, 56,* 609–639.

Ansell, B. J., & Keenan, J. E. (1989). The Western Neuro Sensory Stimulation Profile: A tool for assessing slow-to-recover head injured patients. *Archives of Physical Medicine and Rehabilitation, 70,* 104–108.

Antonucci, G., Guariglia, A., Magnotti, L., Paolucci, S., Pizzamiglio, L., & Zoccolotti, P. (1995). Effectiveness of neglect rehabilitation in a randomized group study. *Journal of Clinical and Experimental Neuropsychology, 17,* 383–389.

Appelros, P., Nydevik, I., Karlsson, G. M., Thorwalls, A., & Seiger, A. (2003). Assessing unilateral neglect: shortcomings of standard test methods. *Disability and Rehabilitation, 25,* 473–479.

Appenzeller, S., Bertolo, M. B., & Costallat, L. T. (2004). Cognitive impairment in rheumatoid arthritis. *Methods and Findings in Experimental and Clinical Pharmacology, 26,* 339–343.

Arai, T., Ohi, H., Sasaki, H., Nobuto, H., & Tanaka, K. (1997). Hemispatial sunglasses: Effect on unilateral spatial neglect. *Archives of Physical Medicine and Rehabilitation, 78,* 230–232.

Arnadottir, G. (1990). *The brain and behavior: Assessing cortical dysfunction through activities of daily living.* St. Louis: Mosby.

Averbuch, S., & Katz, N. (2005). Cognitive Rehabilitation: A retraining model for clients with neurological disabilities. *Cognitive and occupation across the life span: Models for intervention in occupational therapy* (pp. 113–138). Bethesda, MD: AOTA.

Bamdad, M. J., Ryan, L. M., & Warden, D. L. (2003). Functional assessment of executive abilities following traumatic brain injury. *Brain Injury, 17,* 1011–1020.

Basso, A., Burgio, F., Paulin, M., & Prandoni, P. (2000). Long-term follow-up of ideomotor apraxia. *Neuropsychological Rehabilitation, 10,* 1–13.

Baum, C., & Edwards, D. F. (1993). Cognitive performance in senile dementia of the Alzheimer's type: The Kitchen Task Assessment. *American Journal of Occupational Therapy, 47,* 431–436.

Baum, C., Edwards, D., Morrison, T., & Hahn, M. (2003). *Executive Function Performance Test.* St. Louis: Washington University School of Medicine.

Beis, J., Andre, J., Baumgarten, A., & Challier, B. (1999). Eye patching in unilateral spatial neglect: Efficacy of two methods. *Archives of Physical Medicine and Rehabilitation, 80,* 71–76.

Bender, C. M., Sereika, S. M., Berga, S. L., Vogel, V. G., Brufsky, A. M., Paraska, K. K., et al. (2006). Cognitive impairment associated with adjuvant therapy in breast cancer. *Psychooncology, 15,* 422–430.

Benton, A. L., Hamsher, K. deS., Varney, N. R., & Spreen, O. (1983). *Contributions to neuropsychological assessment: Clinical manual.* New York: Oxford University Press.

Biederman, J., Monuteaux, M. C., Doyle, A. E., Seidman, L. J., Wilens, T. E., Ferrero, F., et al. (2004). Impact of executive function deficits and attention-deficit/hyperactivity disorder (ADHD) on academic outcomes in children. *Journal of Consulting and Clinical Psychology, 72,* 757–766.

Bier, N., Desrosiers, J., & Gagnon, L. (2006). Cognitive training interventions for normal aging, mild cognitive impairment and Alzheimer's. *Canadian Journal of Occupational Therapy, 73,* 26–35.

Birnboim, S., & Miller, A. (2004). Cognitive strategies application of multiple sclerosis patients. *Multiple Sclerosis, 10,* 67–73.

Blessed, G., Tomlinson, B. E., & Roth, M. (1968). The association between quantitative measures of dementia and of senile change in the cerebral gray matter of elderly subjects. *British Journal of Psychiatry, 114,* 797–811.

Bogod, N. M., Mateer, C. A., & Macdonald, S. W. S. (2003). Self-awareness after traumatic brain injury: A comparison of measures and their relationship to executive functions. *Journal of the International Neuropsychological Society, 9,* 450–458.

Boldrini, M., Del Pace, L., Placidi, G. P., Keilp, J., Ellis, S. P., Signori, S., et al. (2005). Selective cognitive deficits in obsessive-compulsive disorder compared to panic disorder with agoraphobia. *Acta Psychiatrica Scandinavica, 111,* 150–158.

Bourgeois, M. S., Camp, C., Rose, M., White, B., Malone, M., Carr, J., et al. (2003). A comparison of training strategies to enhance use of external aids by persons with dementia. *Journal of Communication Disorders, 36,* 361–378.

Boyd, T. M., & Sautter, S. W. (1993). Route-finding: A measure of everyday executive functioning in the head-injured adult. *Applied Cognitive Psychology, 7,* 171–181.

Boyle, P. A., Paul, R. H., Moser, D. J., & Cohen, R. A. (2004). Executive impairments predict functional declines in vascular dementia. *Clinical Neuropsychology, 18,* 75–82.

Brandt, J., & Benedict, R., H., B. (2001). *The Hopkins Verbal Learning Test–Revised (HVLT-R).* Lutz, FL: Psychological Assessment Resources.

Branswell, D., Hartry, A., Hoornbeek, S., Johansen, A., Johnson, L., Schultz, J., et al. (1992). *The profile of executive control system.* Puyallup, WA: Association for Neuropsychological Research and Development.

Bruce, M. G. (1993). Cognitive rehabilitation: Intelligence, insight, and knowledge. In C. B. Royeen (Ed.), *AOTA self-study series: Cognitive rehabilitation* (Lesson 5). Rockville, MD: AOTA.

Brunsdon, R., Nickels, L., & Coltheart, M. (2007). Topographical disorientation: Towards an integrated framework for assessment. *Neuropsychological Rehabilitation, 17,* 34–52.

Burgess, P. W., Alderman, N., Forbes, C., Costello, A., Coates, L. M., Dawson, D. R., et al. (2006). The case for the development and use of "ecologically valid" measures of executive function in experimental and clinical neuropsychology. *Journal of the International Neuropsychological Society, 12,* 194–209.

Burke, W. H., Zencius, A. H., Wesolowskis, M. D., & Doubleday, F. (1991). Improving executive function disorders in brain injured clients. *Brain Injury, 5,* 241–252.

Butler, J. A. (1999). Evaluation and intervention with apraxia. In C. Unsworth (Ed.), *Cognitive and perceptual dysfunction* (pp. 257–298). Philadelphia: F. A. Davis.

Calvanio, R., Levine, D., & Petrone, P. (1993). Elements of cognitive rehabilitation after right hemisphere stroke. *Neurologic Clinics, 11,* 25–57.

Campbell, J. J., Duffy, J. D., & Salloway, S. P. (1994). Treatment strategies for patients with dysexecutive syndromes. *Journal of Neuropsychiatry and Clinical Neurosciences, 6,* 411–418.

Caplan, B. (1987). Assessment of unilateral neglect: A new reading test. *Journal of Clinical and Experimental Neuropsychology, 9,* 359–364.

Cappa, S. F., Benke, T., Clarke, S., Rossi, B., Stemmer, B., & van Heugten, C. M. (2005). EFNS guidelines on cognitive rehabilitation: Report of an EFNS task force. *European Journal of Neurology, 12,* 665–680.

Cappa, S., Sterzi, R., Vallar, G., & Bisiach, E. (1987). Remission of hemineglect and anosognosia during vestibular stimulation. *Neuropsychologia, 25,* 775–782.

Capuron, L., Welberg, L., Heim, C., Wagner, D., Solomon, L., Papanicolaou, D. A., et al. (2006). Cognitive dysfunction relates to subjective report of mental fatigue in patients with chronic fatigue syndrome. *Neuropsychopharmacology, 31,* 1777–1784.

Cate, Y., & Richards, L. (2000). Relationship between performance on tests of basic visual functions and visual-perceptual processing in persons after brain injury. *American Journal of Occupational Therapy, 54,* 326–334.

Cermak, S. A. (2005). Cognitive rehabilitation of children with attention-deficit/hyperactivity disorder. In N. Katz (Ed.), *Cognition and occupation across the lifespan: Models for intervention in occupational therapy* (2nd ed., pp. 277–302). Bethesda, MD: AOTA.

Chen Sea, M. J., Henderson, A., & Cermack, S. A. (1993). Patterns of visual spatial inattention and their functional significance in stroke patients. *Archives of Physical Medicine and Rehabilitation, 74,* 355–360.

Cherney, L. R., Halper, A. S., Kwasnica, C. M., Harvey, R. L., & Zhang, M. (2001). Recovery of functional status after right hemisphere stroke: Relationship with unilateral neglect. *Archives of Physical Medicine and Rehabilitation, 82,* 322–328.

Chiaravalloti N., & DeLuca, J. (2002) Self-generation as a means of maximizing learning in multiple sclerosis: An application of the generation effect. *Archives of Physical Medicine and Rehabilitation, 83,* 1070–1079.

Chiaravalloti, N. D., DeLuca, J., Moore, N. B., & Ricker, J. H. (2005). Treating learning impairments improves memory performance in multiple sclerosis: A randomized clinical trial. *Multiple Sclerosis, 11,* 58–68.

Cicerone, K. D., Dahlberg, C., Kalmar, K., Langenbahn, D. M., Malec, J. F., Bergquist, T. F., et al. (2000). Evidence-based cognitive rehabilitation: Recommendations for clinical practice. *Archives of Physical Medicine and Rehabilitation, 81,* 1596–1615.

Cicerone, K. D., Dahlberg, C., Malec, J. F., Langenbahn, D. M., Felicetti, T., Kneipp, S., et al. (2005). Evidence-based cognitive rehabilitation: Updated review of the literature from 1998 through 2002. *Archives Physical Medicine & Rehabilitation, 86,* 1681–1692

Cicerone, K. D., & Giacino, T. J. (1992). Remediation of executive function deficits after traumatic brain injury. *Neuro-Rehabilitation, 2,* 12–22.

Cicerone, K. D., Mott, T., Azulay, J. & Friel, J. C. (2004). Community integration and satisfaction with functioning after intensive cognitive rehabilitation for traumatic brain injury. *Archives of Physical Medicine and Rehabilitation, 85,* 943–950.

Cicerone, K. D., & Wood, J. C. (1987). Planning disorder after closed head injury: A case study. *Archives of Physical Medicine and Rehabilitation, 68,* 111–115.

Corben, L., & Unsworth, C. (1999). Evaluation and intervention with unilateral neglect. In C. Unsworth (Ed.), *Cognitive and perceptual dysfunction* (pp. 357–392). Philadelphia: F. A. Davis.

Colarusso, R. P., & Hammill, D. D. (2002). *Motor-Free Visual Perception Test (MVPT-3).* Austin, TX: PRO-ED

Crosson, C., Barco, P. P., Velozo, C., Bolesta, M. M., Cooper, P. V., Werts, D., et al. (1989). Awareness and compensation in postacute head injury rehabilitation. *Journal of Clinical and Experimental Neuropsychology, 2,* 355–363.

D'Angelo, M. G., & Bresolin, N. (2006). Cognitive impairment in neuromuscular disorders. *Muscle Nerve, 34,* 16–33.

Davidson, J. E., & Sternberg, R. J. (1998). Smart problem solving: How metacognition helps. In D. J. Hacker, J. Dunlosky, & A. G. Graesser (Eds.), *Metacognition in educational theory and practice* (pp. 47–68). Mahwah, NJ: Lawrence Erlbaum Associates.

Davies, S. J., Pandit, S. A., Feeney, A., Stevenson, B. J., Kerwin, R. W., Nutt, D. J., et al. (2005). Is there cognitive impairment in clinically 'healthy' abstinent alcohol dependence? *Alcohol & Alcoholism, 40,* 498–503.

DeBattista, C. (2005). Executive dysfunction in major depressive disorder. *Expert Review of Neurotherapeutics, 5,* 79–83.

Deitz, T., Beeman, C., & Thorn, D. (1993). *Test of Orientation for Rehabilitation Patients.* Tucson, AZ: Therapy Skill Builders.

Diehl, M., Willis, S. L., & Schaie, W. (1995). Everyday problem solving in older adults: Observational assessments and cognitive correlates. *Psychology and Aging, 10,* 478–491.

Dirette, D. K., Hinojosa, J., & Carnevale, G. J. (1999). Comparison of remedial and compensatory interventions for adults with acquired brain injuries. *Journal of Head Trauma Rehabilitation, 14,* 595–601.

Donaghy, S., & Williams, W. (1998). New methodology: A new protocol for training severely impaired patients in the usage of memory journals. *Brain Injury, 12,* 1061–1076.

Doninger, N. A., Bode, R. K., Heinemann, A. W., & Ambrose, C. (2000). Rating scale analysis of the Neurobehavioral Cognitive Status Examination. *Journal of Head Trauma Rehabilitation, 15,* 683–695.

Donkervoort, M., Dekker, J. Stehmann-Saris, F. C., & Deelman, B. G. (2001). Efficacy of strategy training in left hemisphere stroke patients with apraxia: A randomised clinical trial. *Neuropsychological Rehabilitation, 11,* 549–566.

Edgeworth, J. A., Robertson, I., H., & McMillan, T. M. (1998). *The Balloons Test.* Bury St. Edmunds, UK: Thames Valley Test Company.

Erikson, A., Karlsson, G., Soderstrom, M., & Tham, K. (2004). A training apartment with electronic aids to daily living: Lived experiences of persons with brain damage. *American Journal of Occupational Therapy, 58,* 261–271.

Eriksson, G., Tham, K., & Borg, J. (2006). Occupational gaps in everyday life 1–4 years after acquired brain injury. *Journal of Rehabilitation Medicine, 38,* 159–165.

Evans, J. J., Emslie, H., & Wilson, B. A. (1998). Case study: External cueing systems in the rehabilitation of executive impairments of action. *Journal of the International Neuropsychological Society, 4,* 399–408.

Evans, J., Levine, B., & Bateman, A. (2004). Research digest: Errorless learning. *Neuropsychological Rehabilitation, 14,* 467–476.

Fallon, B. A., Keilp, J., Prohovnik, I., Heertum, R. V., & Mann, J. J. (2003). Regional cerebral blood flow and cognitive deficits in chronic Lyme disease. *Journal of Neuropsychiatry and Clinical Neurosciences, 15,* 326–332.

Farah, M. J. (2003). Disorders of visual-spatial perception and cognition: Visuoperceptual, visuospatial, and visuoconstructive disorders. In K. M. Heilman and E. Valenstein (Eds.), *Clinical neuropsychology* (4th ed., pp. 146–160). New York: Oxford University Press.

Farber, S. (1993). *Occupational therapy intervention for individuals with limb apraxia*. Paper presented at the AOTA Neuroscience Institute: Treating Adults with Apraxia, March 20, Baltimore, MD.

Fasotti, L., Kovacs, F., Eling, P., & Brouwer, W. H. (2000). Time pressure management as a compensatory strategy training after closed head injury. *Neuropsychological Rehabilitation, 10*, 47–65.

Fernandez-Ballesteros, R., Zamarron, M. D., & Tarraga, L. (2005). Learning potential: A new method for assessing cognitive impairment. *International Psychogeriatrics, 17*, 119–128.

Ferber, S., & Karnath, H. (2001). How to assess spatial neglect: Line bisection or cancellation tasks? *Journal of Clinical and Experimental Neuropsychology, 23*, 599–607.

Ferguson, J. M., & Trombly C. A. (1997). The effect of added purpose and meaningful occupation on motor learning. *American Journal of Occupational Therapy, 51*, 508–515.

Fertherlin, J. M., & Kurland, L. (1989). Self-instruction: A compensatory strategy to increase functional independence with brain injured adults. *Occupational Therapy Practice, 1*, 75–78.

Fischer, S., Gauggel, S., & Trexler, L. E. (2004). Awareness of activity limitations, goal setting and rehabilitation outcome in patients with brain injuries. *Brain Injury, 18*, 547–562.

Fisher, A. G. (1993a). Functional measures: Part 1. What is function, what should we measure and how should we measure it? *American Journal of Occupational Therapy, 46*, 183–185.

Fisher, A. G. (1993b). Functional measures: Part 2. Selecting the right test, minimizing the limitations. *American Journal of Occupational Therapy, 46*, 278–281.

Fleming, J. M., Lucas, S. E., & Lightbody, S. (2006). Using occupation to facilitate self-awareness in people who have acquired brain injury: A pilot study. *Canadian Journal of Occupational Therapy, 73*, 44–55.

Fleming, J. M., Shum, D., Strong, J., & Lightbody, S. (2005). Prospective memory rehabilitation for adults with traumatic brain injury: A compensatory training programme. *Brain Injury. 19*, 1–13.

Fleming, J. M., Strong, J., & Ashton, R. (1996). Self-awareness of deficits in adults with traumatic brain injury: How best to measure? *Brain Injury, 10*, 1–15.

Folstein, M. F., Folstein, S. E., & McHugh, P. R. (1975). Mini-mental state: A practical method for grading the cognitive state of patients for the clinician. *Journal of Psychiatric Research, 12*, 189–198.

Gauthier, L., Dehaut, F., & Joanette, Y. (1989). The Bells Test: A quantitative and qualitative test for visual neglect. *International Journal of Clinical Neuropsychology, 11*, 49–54.

Geusgens, C., van Heugten, C., Donkervoort, M., van den Ende, E., Jolles, J., & van den Heuvel, W. (2006). Transfer of training effects in stroke patients with apraxia: an exploratory study. *Neuropsychological Rehabilitation, 16*, 213–229.

Giles, G. M. (2005). A neurofunctional approach to rehabilitation following severe brain injury. In N. Katz (Ed.), *Cognitive and occupation across the life span: Models for intervention in occupational therapy* (pp. 139–165). Bethesda, MD: AOTA.

Giles, G. M. (2006). Habit, routine, and context in neurorehabilitation. In G. M. Giles (Ed.), *Neurorehabilitation self-paced clinical course*. Bethesda, MD: AOTA.

Giles, G. M., Ridley, J. E., Dill, A., & Frye, S. (1997). A consecutive series of adults with brain injury treated with a washing and dressing retraining program. *American Journal of Occupational Therapy, 51*, 256–266.

Giles, G. M., & Shore, M. (1989). A rapid method for teaching severely brain injured adults how to wash and dress. *Archives of Physical Medicine and Rehabilitation, 70*, 156–158.

Gillen, R., Tennen, H., & McKee, T. (2005). Unilateral spatial neglect: Relation to rehabilitation outcomes in patients with right hemisphere stroke. *Archives of Physical Medicine & Rehabilitation, 86*, 763–767.

Glisky, E. L., Schacter, L. D., & Butters, A. M. (1994). Domain-specific learning and remediation of memory disorders. In M. J. Riddoch & G. W. Humphreys (Eds.), *Cognitive neuropsychology and cognitive rehabilitation* (pp. 527–548). East Sussex, UK: Lawrence Erlbaum Associates.

Golding, E. (1989). *The Middlesex Elderly Assessment of Mental State*. Bury St. Edmunds, UK: Thames Valley Test Company.

Golisz, K. M. (1998). Dynamic assessment and multicontext treatment of unilateral neglect. *Topics in Stroke Rehabilitation, 5*, 11–28.

Goverover, Y. (2004). Categorization, deductive reasoning and self-awareness: Association to everyday competence in persons with acute brain injury. *Journal of Clinical and Experimental Neuropsychology, 26*, 737–749.

Goverover Y., Chiaravalloti, N., & DeLuca, J. (2005). The relationship between self-awareness of neurobehavioral symptoms, cognitive functions and emotional symptoms in multiple sclerosis. *Multiple Sclerosis, 11*, 203–212.

Goverover, Y., & Hinojosa, J. (2002). Categorization and deductive reasoning: Can they serve as predictors of Instrumental Activities of Daily Living performance in adults with brain injury? *American Journal of Occupational Therapy, 56*, 509–516.

Goverover, Y., Johnston, M. V., Toglia, J., & DeLuca, J. (2007). *Treatment to improve self-awareness and functional independence for persons with TBI: A pilot randomized trial*. Paper presented at the Neuropsychological Society 35th Annual Meeting, Portland OR, Feb. 7–10.

Grigorenko, E. L., & Sternberg, R. J. (1998). Dynamic testing. *Psychological Bulletin, 124*, 75–111.

Gronwall, D. M. A. (1977). Paced Auditory Serial Addition Task: A measure of recovery from concussion. *Perceptual and Motor Skills, 44*, 367–373.

Haaland, K. Y. (1993). *Assessment of limb apraxia*. Presentation at the AOTA Neuroscience Institute Treating Adults with Apraxia, March 20, Baltimore, MD.

Hajek, V. E., Rutman, D. L., & Scher, H. (1989). Brief assessment of cognitive impairment in patients with stroke. *Archives of Physical Medicine and Rehabilitation, 70*, 114–117.

Hallgren, M., & Kottorp, A. (2005). Effects of occupational therapy intervention on activities of daily living and awareness of disability in persons with intellectual disabilities. *Australian Occupational Therapy Journal, 52*, 350–359.

Hamera, E., & Brown, C. E. (2000). Developing a context-based performance measure for persons with schizophrenia: the test of grocery shopping skills. *American Journal of Occupational Therapy, 54*, 20–25.

Harrison, M. J., Morris, K. A., Horton, R., Toglia, J., Barsky, J., Chait, S., et al. (2005). Results of an intervention for lupus patients with self-perceived cognitive difficulties. *Neurology, 65,* 1325–1327.

Hartman-Maeir, A., Soroker, N., Oman, S. D., & Katz, N. (2003). Awareness of disabilities in stroke rehabilitation: A clinical trial. *Disability and Rehabilitation, 25,* 35–44.

Haywood, H. C., & Miller, M. B. (2003). Dynamic assessment of adults with traumatic brain injuries. *Journal of Cognitive Education and Psychology Online, 3,* 137–158.

Heilman, K. M., & Rothi, L. J. (2003). Apraxia. In K. M. Heilman & E. Valenstein (Eds.), *Clinical neuropsychology* (4th ed., pp. 215–245). New York: Oxford University Press.

Heilman, K. M., Watson, R. T., & Valenstein, E. (2003). Neglect and related disorders. In K. M. Heilman & E. Valenstein (Eds.), *Clinical neuropsychology* (4th ed., pp. 296–346). New York: Oxford University Press.

Helm-Estabrooks, N. (1982). Visual action therapy for global aphasics. *Journal of Speech and Hearing Disorders, 47,* 385–389.

Helm-Estabrooks, N. (1992). *Test of Oral and Limb Apraxia (TOLA).* Chicago: Riverside.

Helm-Estabrooks, N., & Hotz, G. (1991). *Brief Test of Head Injury (BTHI).* Chicago: Riverside.

Hessels-Schlatter, C. (2002). A dynamic test to assess learning capacity in people with severe impairments. *American Journal on Mental Retardation, 107,* 340–351.

Hoofien, D., Gilboa, A., Vakil, E., & Barak, O. (2004). Unawareness of cognitive deficits and daily functioning among persons with traumatic brain injuries, *Journal of Clinical and Experimental Neuropsychology, 26,* 278–290.

Hopkins, R. O., & Brett, S. (2005). Chronic neurocognitive effects of critical illness. *Current Opinion in Critical Care, 11,* 369–375.

Jackson, W. T., Novack, T. A., & Dowler, R. N. (1998). Effective serial measurement of cognitive orientation in rehabilitation: The Orientation Log. *Archives of Physical Medicine and Rehabilitation, 79,* 718–720.

Jansen, C. E., Miaskowski, C., Dodd, M., Dowling, G., & Kramer, J. (2005). A meta-analysis of studies of the effects of cancer chemotherapy on various domains of cognitive function. *Cancer, 104,* 2222–2233.

Jefferson, A. L., Paul, R. H., Ozonoff, A., & Cohen, R. A. (2006). Evaluating elements of executive functioning as predictors of instrumental activities of daily living (IADLs). *Archives of Clinical Neuropsychology, 21,* 311–320.

Johnston, M. V., Goverover, Y., & Dijkers, M. (2005). Community activities and individuals' satisfaction about them: Quality of life in the first year after traumatic brain injury. *Archives of Physical Medicine & Rehabilitation, 86,* 735–745.

Josman, N. (2005). The dynamic interactional model for children and adolescents. In N. Katz (Ed.), *Cognition and occupation across the lifespan: Models for intervention in Occupational Therapy* (2nd ed., pp. 261–276). Bethesda, MD: AOTA.

Katz, N., & Hartman-Maeir, A. (2005). Higher-level cognitive functions: Awareness and executive functions enabling engagement in occupation. In N. Katz (Ed.), *Cognition and occupation across the life span* (2nd ed., pp. 3–25). Bethesda, MD: AOTA.

Katz, N., Hartman-Maeir, A., Ring, H., & Soroker, N. (1999). Functional disability and rehabilitation outcome in right hemisphere damaged patients with and without unilateral spatial neglect. *Archives of Physical Medicine & Rehabilitation, 80,* 379–384.

Katz, R. S., Heard, A. R., Mills, M., & Leavitt, F. (2004). The prevalence and clinical impact of reported cognitive difficulties (Fibrofog) in patients with rheumatic disease with and without fibromyalgia. *Journal of Clinical Rheumatology, 10,* 53–58.

Katz, N., Itzkovich, M., Averbuch, S., & Elazar, B. (1990). *Lowenstein Occupational Therapy Cognitive Assessment (LOTCA) manual.* Pequannock, NJ: Maddak.

Katz, N., Ring, H., Naveh, Y., Kizony, R., Feintuch, U., & Weiss, P. L. (2005). Interactive virtual environment training for safe street crossing of right hemisphere stroke patients with unilateral spatial neglect. *Disability and Rehabilitation, 27,* 1235–1243.

Kelly, M., & Ostreicher, H. (1985). Environmental factors and outcomes in hemineglect syndromes. *Rehabilitation Psychology, 30,* 35–37.

Kertesz, A. (1982). *Western Aphasia Battery.* San Antonio, TX: Psychological Corporation.

Kessels, R., & de Haan, E. (2003). Implicit learning in memory rehabilitation: A meta-analysis on errorless learning and vanishing cues methods. *Journal of Clinical & Experimental Neuropsychology, 25,* 805–814.

Kiernan, R. J., Mueller, J., & Langston, J. W. (1983). *The Neurobehavioral Cognitive Status Examination.* San Francisco: Northern California Neurobehavioral Group.

Kiosses, D. N., Klimstra, S., Murphy, C., & Alexopoulos, G. S. (2001). Executive dysfunction and disability in elderly patients with major depression. *American Journal of Geriatric Psychiatry, 9,* 269–274.

Kline, N. K. (2000). Validity of the Modified Dynamic Visual Processing Assessment. *The Israel Journal of Occupational Therapy, 9,* 69–88.

Kolakowsky, S. A. (1998). Assessing learning potential in patients with brain injury: Dynamic assessment, *Neurorehabilitation, 11,* 227–238

Kottorp, A., Hallgren, M., Bernspang, B., & Fisher, A. G. (2003). Client-centered occupational therapy for persons with mental retardation: Implementation of an intervention programme in activities of daily living tasks. *Scandinavian Journal of Occupational Therapy, 10,* 51–60.

Kramer, J. H., Kaplan, E., & Blusewicz, M. J. (1991). Visual hierarchical analysis of block design configural errors. *Journal of Clinical and Experimental Neuropsychology, 13,* 455–465.

Laatsch, L, Little, D., & Thulborn, K. (2004). Changes in fMRI following cognitive rehabilitation in severe traumatic brain injury: A case study. *Rehabilitation Psychology, 49,* 262–267.

Laatsch, L, Thulborn, K. R., Krisky, C. M., Shobat, D. M., & Sweeney, J. A. (2004). Investigating the neurobiological basis of cognitive rehabilitation therapy with fMRI. *Brain Injury, 18,* 957–974.

Laeng, B. (2006). Constructional apraxia after left or right unilateral stroke. *Neuropsychologia, 44,* 1595–1606.

Laes, J., & Sponheim, S. (2006). Does cognition predict community function only in schizophrenia?: A study of schizophrenia patients, bipolar affective disorder patients, and community control subjects. *Schizophrenia Research, 84,* 121–131.

Landa-Gonzalez, B. (2001). Multicontextual occupational therapy intervention: A case study of traumatic brain injury. *Occupational Therapy International, 8,* 49–62.

Lennon, S. (1994). Task specific effects in the rehabilitation of unilateral neglect. In M. J. Riddoch & G. W. Humphreys (Eds.), *Cognitive neuropsychology and cognitive rehabilitation* (pp. 187–203). East Sussex, UK: Lawrence Erlbaum Associates.

Levin, H. S., O'Donnell, V. M., & Grossman, R. G. (1979). The Galveston Orientation and Amnesia Test: A practical scale to assess cognition after head injury. *Journal of Nervous and Mental Diseases, 167,* 675–684.

Levy, L. L. (2005a). Cognitive aging in perspective: Implications for occupational therapy practitioners. In N. Katz (Ed.), *Cognition and occupation across the life span* (2nd ed., pp. 327–346). Bethesda, MD: AOTA.

Levy, L. L. (2005b). Cognitive aging in perspective: Information processing, cognition and memory. In N. Katz (Ed.), *Cognition and occupation across the life span* (2nd ed., pp. 305–325). Bethesda, MD: AOTA.

Levy, L. L., & Burns, T. (2005). Cognitive disabilities reconsidered. In N. Katz (Ed.), *Cognition and occupation across the life span* (2nd ed., pp. 347–385). Bethesda, MD: AOTA.

Lezak, M. D., Howieson, D. B., & Loring, D. W. (2004). *Neuropsychological assessment* (4th ed.). New York: Oxford University Press.

Lidz, C. (1991). *Practitioner's guide to dynamic assessment.* New York: Guilford Press

Liu, K. P. Y., Chan, C. C. H., Lee, T. M. C., Li, L. S. W., & Hui-Chan, C. W. Y. (2002). Self-regulatory learning and generalization for people with brain injury. *Brain Injury, 16,* 817–824.

Loeb, P. A. (1996). *Independent Living Scales.* San Antonio, TX: Psychological Corporation.

Lucas, S. E., & Fleming, J. M. (2005). Interventions for improving self-awareness following acquired brain injury. *Australian Occupational Therapy Journal, 52,* 160–170.

Luria, A. R. (1973). *The working brain* (Basil Haigh, Trans.). New York: Basic Books.

Malec, J. F., Smigielski, J. S., & DePompolo, R. W. (1991). Goal attainment scaling and outcome measurement in postacute brain injury rehabilitation. *Archives of Physical Medicine and Rehabilitation, 72,* 138–143.

Manly, T., Hawkins, K., Evans, J., Wodlt, K., & Robertson, I. H. (2002). Rehabilitation of executive function: Facilitation of effective goal management on complex tasks using periodic auditory alerts. *Neuropsychologia, 40,* 271–281.

Martinez-Aran, A., Vieta, E., Colom, F., Torrent, C., Sanchez-Moreno, J., Reinares, M., et al. (2004). Cognitive impairment in euthymic bipolar patients: Implications for clinical and functional outcome. *Bipolar Disorders, 6,* 224–232.

Mattis, S. (1976). Mental status examination for organic mental syndromes in the elderly patient. In L. Bellak & T. E. Karasu (Eds.), *Geriatric psychiatry* (pp. 77–121). New York: Grune & Stratton.

McDowd, J. M., Filion, D. L., Pohl, P. S., Richards, L. G., & Stiers, W. (2003). Attentional abilities and functional outcomes following stroke. *Journal of Gerontology, Series B, Psychological Sciences and Social Sciences, 58,* 45–53.

McKerracher, G., Powell, T., & Oyebode, J. (2005). A single case experimental design comparing two memory notebook formats for a man with memory problems caused by traumatic brain injury. *Neuropsychological Rehabilitation, 15,* 115–128.

Mesulam, M. M. (1994). The multiplicity of neglect phenomena. *Neuropsychological Rehabilitation, 4,* 173–176.

Mesulam, M. M. (2000). Attentional networks, confusional states and neglect syndromes. In: M. Mesulam (Ed.), *Principles of behavioral neurology* (2nd ed., pp. 174–256). New York: Oxford University Press.

Moulton, H. J., Taira, E. D., & Grover, R. (1995). *Utilizing occupational therapy and families at mealtimes with nursing home residents with dementia.* Presentation at Gerontological Society on Aging, Annual Conference, November, Los Angles, CA.

Munshi, M., Grande, L., Hayes, M., Ayres, D., Suhl, E., Capelson, R., et al. (2006). Cognitive dysfunction is associated with poor diabetes control in older adults. *Diabetes Care, 29,* 1794–1799.

Murray, A. M., Tupper, D. E., Knopman, D. S., Gilbertson, D. T., Pederson, S. L., Li, S., et al. (2006). Cognitive impairment in hemodialysis patients is common. *Neurology, 67,* 216–223.

Neistadt, M. E. (1990). A critical analysis of occupational therapy approaches for perceptual deficits in adults with brain injury. *American Journal of Occupational Therapy, 44,* 299–304.

Neistadt, M. (1992a). Occupational therapy treatments for constructional deficits. *American Journal of Occupational Therapy, 46,* 141–148.

Neistadt, M. E. (1992b). The Rabideau Kitchen Evaluation–Revised: An assessment of meal preparation skill. *The Occupational Therapy Journal of Research, 12,* 242–255.

Neistadt, M. (1994). Perceptual retaining for adults with diffuse brain injury. *American Journal of Occupational Therapy, 48,* 225–233.

Nelson, A., Fogel, B. S., & Faust, D. (1986). Bedside cognitive screening instruments: A critical assessment. *Journal of Nervous and Mental Disease, 174,* 73–83.

Niemeier, J. P. (1998). The lighthouse strategy: Use of a visual imagery technique to treat visual inattention in stroke patients. *Brain Injury, 12,* 399–406.

Niemeier, J. P., Cifu, D. X., & Kishore, R. (2001). The lighthouse strategy: Improving the functional status of patients with unilateral neglect after stroke and brain injury using a visual imagery intervention. *Topics in Stroke Rehabilitation, 8*(2), 10–18.

Noe, E., Ferri, J., Caballero, M. C., Villodre, R., Sanchez, A., & Chirivella, J. (2005). Self awareness after acquired brain injury: Predictors and rehabilitation. *Journal of Neurology, 252,* 168–175.

Orth, M., Kotterba, S., Duchna, K., Widdig, W., Rasche, K., Schultze-Werninghaus, G., et al. (2006). Cognitive deficits in patients with chronic obstructive pulmonary disease (COPD). *Pneumologie, 60,* 593–599.

Ownsworth, T., Fleming, J., Desbois, J., Strong, J., & Kuipers, P. (2006). A metacognitive contextual intervention to enhance error awareness and functional outcome following traumatic brain injury: A single-case experimental design. *Journal of the International Neuropsychological Society, 12,* 54–63.

Page, M., Wilson, B. A., Sheil, A. Carter, G., & Norris, D. (2006). What is the locus of the errorless learning advantage? *Neuropsychologia, 44,* 90–100.

Paolucci, S., Antonucci, G., Grasso, M. G., & Pizzamiglio, L. (2001). The role of unilateral spatial neglect in rehabilitation of right brain-damaged ischemic stroke patients: A matched comparison. *Archives of Physical Medicine and Rehabilitation, 82,* 743–749.

Penades, R., Catalan, R., Salamero, M., Boget, T., Puig, O., Guarch, J., et al. (2006). Cognitive remediation therapy for outpatients with chronic schizophrenia: A controlled and randomized study. *Schizophrenia Research, 87,* 323–331.

Petrella, L., McColl, M. A., Krupa, T., & Johnston, J. (2005). Returning to productive activities: Perspectives of individuals with long-standing acquired brain injuries. *Brain Injury, 19,* 643–655.

Pierce, S. R., & Buxbaum, L. J. (2002). Treatments of unilateral neglect: A review. *Archives of Physical Medicine and Rehabilitation, 83,* 256–268.

Pilgrim, E., & Humphrey's, G. W. (1994). Rehabilitation of a case of ideomotor apraxia. In M. J. Riddoch & G. W. Humphreys (Eds.), *Cognitive neuropsychology and cognitive rehabilitation* (pp. 271–315). East Sussex, UK: Lawrence Erlbaum Associates.

Pizzamiglio, L., Antonucci, G., Judica, A., Montenero, P., Razzano, C., & Zoccolotti, P. (1992). Cognitive rehabilitation of the hemineglect disorder in chronic patients with unilateral right brain damage. *Journal of Clinical Experimental Neuropsychology, 14,* 901–923.

Plummer, P., Morris, M., & Dunai, J. (2003). Assessment of unilateral neglect. *Physical Therapy, 83,* 732–740.

Poole, J. L. (1998). Effect of apraxia on the ability to learn on-handed shoe tying. *Occupational Therapy Journal of Research, 18,* 99–104.

Poole, J. L. (2000). A comparison of limb praxis abilities of persons with developmental dyspraxia and adult onset apraxia. *Occupational Therapy Journal of Research, 20,* 106–120.

Prigatano, G. P. (1986). *Neuropsychological rehabilitation after brain injury.* Baltimore: Johns Hopkins University Press.

Prigatano, G. P. (1999). *Principles of neuropsychological rehabilitation.* New York: Oxford University Press.

Radomski, V. M., Dougherty, M. P., Fine, B. S., & Baum, C. (1993). Case studies in cognitive rehabilitation. In C. B. Royeen (Ed.), *AOTA self-study series: Cognitive rehabilitation* (Lesson 10, pp. 4–68). Rockville, MD: AOTA.

Randolph, C. (1998). Repeatable Battery for the Assessment of Neuropsychological Status [RBANS™]. San Antonio, TX: Psychological Corporation.

Rao, S. M., Leo, G. J., Bernardin, L., & Unverzagt, F. (1991). Cognitive dysfunction in multiple sclerosis. *Neurology, 41,* 684–691.

Rath, J. F., Simon, D., Langenbahn, D. M., Sherr, R. L., & Diller, L. (2003). Group treatment of problem solving deficits in outpatients with traumatic brain injury: A randomized outcome study. *Neuropsychological Rehabilitation, 13,* 461–488.

Rebmann, M. J., & Hannon, R. (1995). Treatment of unawareness of memory deficits in adults with brain injury: Three case studies. *Rehabilitation Psychology, 40,* 279–287.

Redding, G. M., & Wallace, B. (2006). Prism adaptation and unilateral neglect: Review and analysis. *Neuropsychologia, 44,* 1–20.

Reeder, C., Newton, E., Frangou, S., & Wykes, T. (2004). Which executive skills should we target to affect social functioning and symptom change?: A study of cognitive remediation therapy program. *Schizophrenia Bulletin, 30,* 87–100.

Rempfer, M., Hamera, E., Brown, C., & Bothwell, R. J. (2006). Learning proficiency on the Wisconsin Card Sorting Test in people with serious mental illness: What are the cognitive characteristics of good learners? *Schizophrenia Research, 87,* 316–322.

Rempfer, M. V., Hamera, E. K., Brown, C. E., & Cromwell, R. L. (2003). The relations between cognition and the independent living skill of shopping in people with schizophrenia. *Psychiatry Research, 117,* 103–112.

Revheim, N., & Marcopulos, B. A. (2006). Group treatment approaches to address cognitive deficits. *Psychiatric Rehabilitation Journal, 30,* 38–45.

Reynolds, C. R. (2002) *Comprehensive Trail-Making Test (CTMT).* Austin, TX: PRO-ED.

Ringholz, G. M., Appel, S. H., Bradshaw, M., Cooke, N. A., Mosnik, D. M., & Schulz, P. E. (2005). Prevalence and patterns of cognitive impairment in sporadic ALS. *Neurology, 65,* 586–590.

Robertson, I. H., & Halligan, P. W. (1999). *Spatial neglect: A clinical handbook for diagnosis and treatment.* East Sussex, UK: Psychology Press

Robertson, I. H., Hogg, K., & McMillan, T. M. (1998). Rehabilitation of unilateral neglect: Improving function by contralesional limb activation. *Neuropsychological Rehabilitation, 8,* 19–29.

Robertson, I. H., Tegner, R., Tham, K., Lo, A., & Smith, N. I. (1995). Sustained attention training for unilateral neglect: Theoretical and rehabilitation implications. *Journal of Clinical Neuropsychology, 17,* 416–430.

Robertson, I. H., Ward, T., Ridgeway, V., & Nimmo-Smith, I. (1994). *The Test of Everyday Attention (TEA).* Bury St. Edmunds, UK: Thames Valley Test Company.

Rockwood, K., Joyce, B., & Stolee, P. (1997). Use of goal attainment scaling in measuring clinically important change in cognitive rehabilitation patients. *Journal of Clinical Epidemiology, 50,* 581–588.

Roth, R. M., Isquith, P. K., & Gioia, G. A. (2005). *Behavior Rating Inventory of Executive Function–Adult Version.* Lutz, FL: Psychological Assessment Resources.

Roy, E. A. (1978). Apraxia: A new look at an old syndrome. *Journal of Human Movement Studies, 4,* 191–210.

Roy, E. A. (1985). *Neuropsychological studies of apraxia and related disorders.* Amsterdam: Elsevier Science Publishers.

Royall, D. R., Palmer, R., Chiodo, L. K., & Polk, M. J. (2004). Declining executive control in normal aging predicts change in functional status: The Freedom House Study. *Journal of the American Geriatric Society, 52,* 346–352.

Rustad, R. A., DeGroot, T. L., Jungkunz, M. L., Freeberg, K. S., Borowick, L. G., & Wanttie, A. M. (1993). *The Cognitive Assessment of Minnesota.* Tucson, AZ: Therapy Skill Builders.

Sarajuuri, J. M., Kaipio, M. L., Koskinen, S. K., Neimela, M. R., Servo, A. R., & Vilkki, J. (2005). Outcome of a comprehensive neurorehabilitation program for persons with traumatic brain injury. *Archives of Physical Medicine and Rehabilitation, 86,* 2296–2302.

Schlund, M. W. (1999). Self awareness: Effects of feedback and review on verbal self reports and remembering following brain injury. *Brain Injury, 13,* 375–380.

Schwartz, M. S. (1995). Adults with traumatic brain injury: Three case studies of cognitive rehabilitation in the home setting. *American Journal of Occupational Therapy, 49,* 655–668.

Schwartzberg, S. (1999). Use of groups in rehabilitation of persons with head injury: Reasoning skills used by the group facilitator. In C. Unsworth (Ed.), *Cognitive and perceptual dysfunction* (pp. 455–471). Philadelphia: F. A. Davis.

Seron, X., Deloche, G., & Coyette, F. (1989). A retrospective analysis of a single case of neglect therapy: A point of theory. In X. Seron & G. Deloche (Eds.), *Cognitive approaches in neuropsychological rehabilitation.* Hillsdale, NJ: Lawrence Erlbaum Associates.

Shallice, T., & Burgess, P. (1991). Deficits in strategy application following frontal lobe damage in man. *Brain, 114,* 727–741.

Sherer, M., Bergloff, P., Boake, C., High, W., & Levin, E. (1998). The Awareness Questionnaire: Factor structure and internal consistency. *Brain Injury, 12,* 63–68.

Sherer, M., Oden, K., Bergloff, P., Levin, E., & High, W. M. (1998). Assessment and treatment of impaired awareness after brain injury: Implications for community re-integration. *NeuroRehabilitation, 10,* 25–37.

Sherman, E. M., Slick, D. J., & Eyrl, K. L. (2006). Executive dysfunction is a significant predictor of poor quality of life in children with epilepsy. *Epilepsia, 47,* 1936–1942.

Silverstein, S. M., Hatashita-Wong, M., Solak, B. A., Uhlhaas, P., Landa, Y., Wilkniss, S. M., et al. (2005). Effectiveness of a two-phase cognitive rehabilitation intervention for severely impaired schizophrenia patients. *Psychological Medicine, 35,* 829–837.

Sinforiani, E., Banchieri, L., Zucchella, C., Pacchetti, C., & Sandrini, G. (2004). Cognitive rehabilitation in Parkinson's disease. *Archives of Gerontology and Geriatrics, Supplement 9,* 387–391.

Smania, N., Bazoli, F., Piva, D., & Guidetti, G. (1997). Visuomotor imagery and rehabilitation of neglect. *Archives of Physical Medicine and Rehabilitation, 78,* 430–436.

Smania, N., Girardi, F., Domenicali, C., Lora, E., & Aglioti, S. (2000). The rehabilitation of limb apraxia: A study in left-brain-damaged patients. *Archives of Physical Medicine and Rehabilitation, 81,* 379–388.

Sohlberg, M. M., Glang, A., & Todis, B. (1998). Improvement during baseline: Three case studies encouraging collaborative research when evaluating caregiver training. *Brain Injury, 12,* 333–346.

Sohlberg, M. M., & Mateer, C. A. (1989a). *Attention process training.* San Antonio, TX: Psychological Corporation.

Sohlberg, M. M., and Mateer, C. (1989b). *Introduction to cognitive rehabilitation: Theory and practice.* New York: Guilford Press.

Sohlberg, M. M., & Mateer, C. A. (2001). *Cognitive rehabilitation: An integrative neuropsychological approach.* New York: Guilford Press.

Spiegler, B. J., Bouffet, E., Greenberg, M. L., Rutka, J. T., & Mabbott, D. J. (2004). Change in neurocognitive functioning after treatment with cranial radiation in childhood. *Journal of Clinical Oncology, 22,* 706–713.

Stone, S. P., Halligan, P. W., Marshall, J. C., & Greenwood, R. J. (1998). Unilateral neglect: A common but heterogeneous syndrome. *Neurology, 50,* 1902–1905.

Stuss, D. T., Robertson, I. H., Craik, F. I., Levine, B., Alexander, M. P., Black, S., et al. (2007). Cognitive rehabilitation in the elderly: A randomized trial to evaluate a new protocol. *Journal of International Neuropsychological Society, 13,* 120–131.

Sunderland, A., Walker, C. M., & Walker, M. F. (2006). Action errors and dressing disability after stroke: an ecological approach to neuropsychological assessment and intervention. *Neuropsychological Rehabilitation, 16,* 666–683.

Teng, E., & Chui, H. (1987). The Modified Mini-Mental State (3MS) Examination. *Journal of Clinical Psychiatry, 48,* 314–318.

Tham, K., Bernspang, B., & Fisher, A. G. (1999). Development of the assessment of awareness of disability. *Scandinavian Journal of Occupational Therapy, 6,* 184–190.

Tham, K., Ginsburg, E., Fisher, A., & Tegner, R. (2001). Training to improve awareness of disabilities in clients with unilateral neglect. *American Journal of Occupational Therapy, 55,* 46–54.

Tham, K., & Tegner, R. (1996). The baking tray task: A test of spatial neglect. *Neuropsychological Rehabilitation, 6,* 19–25.

Tham, K., & Tegner, R. (1997). Video feedback in the rehabilitation of patients with unilateral neglect. *Archives of Physical Medicine and Rehabilitation, 78,* 410–413.

Tiersky, L. A., Anselmi, V., Johnston, M. V., Kurtyka, J., Roosen, E., Schwartz, T., et al. (2005). A trial of neuropsychologic rehabilitation in mild spectrum traumatic brain injury. *Archives of Physical Medicine and Rehabilitation, 86,* 1565–1574.

Toglia, J. P. (1989). Visual perception of objects: An approach to assessment and intervention. *American Journal of Occupational Therapy, 43,* 587–595.

Toglia, J. P. (1991a). Generalization of treatment: A multicontextual approach to cognitive perceptual impairment in the brain injured adult. *American Journal of Occupational Therapy, 45,* 505–516.

Toglia, J. P. (1991b). Unilateral visual inattention: Multidimensional components. *Occupational Therapy Practice, 3,* 18–34.

Toglia, J. P. (1993a). Attention and memory. In C. B. Royeen (Ed.), *AOTA self-study series: Cognitive rehabilitation* (Lesson 4, pp. 4–72). Rockville, MD: AOTA.

Toglia, J. P. (1993b). *The Contextual Memory Test.* Tucson, AZ: Therapy Skill Builders.

Toglia, J. P. (1994). *Toglia Category Assessment (TCA).* Pequannock, NJ: Maddak.

Toglia, J. P. (1998). A dynamic interactional model to cognitive rehabilitation. In N. Katz (Ed.), *Cognition and occupation in rehabilitation: Cognitive models for intervention in occupational therapy* (pp. 5–50). Bethesda, MD: AOTA.

Toglia, J. P. (2005). A dynamic interactional model to cognitive rehabilitation. In N. Katz (Ed.), *Cognition and occupation across the life span* (2nd ed., pp. 29–72). Bethesda, MD: AOTA.

Toglia, J. P., & Finkelstein, N. (1991). *Manual for the dynamic visual processing assessment.* Unpublished manuscript.

Toglia, J. P., & Golisz, K. M. (1990). *Cognitive rehabilitation: Group games and activities.* Tucson, AZ: Therapy Skill Builders.

Toglia, J., & Kirk, U. (2000). Understanding awareness deficits following brain injury. *NeuroRehabilitation, 15,* 57–70.

Tzuriel, D. (2000). Dynamic assessment of young children: Educational and intervention perspectives. *Educational Psychology Review, 12,* 385–435.

Tzuriel, D. (2001). Dynamic assessment is not dynamic testing. *Issues in Education, 7,* 237–250.

Ucok, A., Cakir, S., Duman, Z. C., Discigil, A., Kandemir, P., & Atli, H. (2006). Cognitive predictors of skill acquisition on social problem solving in patients with schizophrenia. *European Archives of Psychiatry and Clinical Neuroscience, 256,* 388–394.

Unsworth, C. (1999). Introduction to cognitive and perceptual dysfunction: Theoretical approaches to therapy. In C. Unsworth (Ed.), *Cognitive and perceptual dysfunction* (pp. 1–41). Philadelphia: F. A. Davis.

Unsworth, C. (2007). Cognitive and perceptual dysfunction. In S. B. O'Sullivan & T. J. Schmitz (Eds.), *Physical rehabilitation* (5th ed., pp. 1151–1188). Philadelphia: F. A. Davis.

van Heugten, C., Dekker, J., Deelman, B. G., van Dijk, A. J., Stehmann-Saris, J. C., & Kinebanian, A. (2000). Measuring disabilities in stroke patients with apraxia: A validation study of an observational method. *Neuropsychological Rehabilitation, 10,* 401–414.

Vogels, R. L., Scheltens, P., Schroeder-Tanka, J. M., & Weinstein, H. C. (2006). Cognitive impairment in heart failure: A systematic review of the literature. *European Journal of Heart Failure.* Retrieved January 29, 2007, from doi:10.1016/j.ejheart.2006.11.001

Wade, T. K., & Troy, J. C. (2001). Mobile phones as a new memory aid: A preliminary investigation using case studies. *Brain Injury, 15,* 305–320.

Wang, P. L., Ennis, K. E., & Copland, S. L. (1992). *Cognitive Competency Test [CCT].* North York, Ontario: Paul Wang.

Warren, M. (1981). Relationship of constructional apraxia and body scheme disorders to dressing performance in CVA. *American Journal of Occupational Therapy, 35,* 431–442.

Warren, M. (1993). Visuospatial skills: Assessment and intervention strategies. In C. B. Royeen (Ed.), *AOTA self-study series: Cognitive rehabilitation* (Lesson 7, pp. 6–76). Rockville, MD: AOTA.

Warren, M. (1998). *The Brain Injury Visual Assessment Battery for Adults.* Lenexa, KS: visABILITIES Rehab Services.

Webster, J. S., Roades, L. A., Morrill, B., Rapport, L. J., Abadee, P. S., Sowa, M. V., et al. (1995). Rightward orienting bias, wheelchair maneuvering, and fall risk. Archives of Physical Medicine and Rehabilitation, 76, 924–928.

Webster, J. S., McFarland, P. T., Rapport, L. J., Morrill, B., Roades, L. A., & Abadee, P. S. (2001). Computer-assisted training for improving wheelchair mobility in unilateral neglect patients. *Archives of Physical Medicine and Rehabilitation, 82,* 769–775.

Weinberg, J., Diller, L., Gordon, W. A., Gerstman, L. J., Lieberman, A., Lakin, P., et al. (1977). Visual scanning training effect on reading related tasks in acquired right brain damage. *Archives of Physical Medicine and Rehabilitation, 58,* 479–486.

Wiedl, K. H. (2003). Dynamic testing: A comprehensive model and current fields of application. *Journal of Cognitive Education and Psychology Online, 3,* 93–119.

Williams, T. A. (1995). Low vision rehabilitation for a patient with a traumatic brain injury. *American Journal of Occupational Therapy, 49,* 923–926.

Willis, S. L., Tennstedt, S. L., Marsiske, M., Ball, K., Elias, J., Koepke, K. M., et al. (2006). Long-term effects of cognitive training on everyday functional outcomes in older adults. *Journal of the American Medical Association, 296,* 2805–2814.

Wilson, B. A., Alderman, N., Burgess, P., Emslie, H., & Evans, J. (1996). *Behavioural Assessment of the Dysexecutive Syndrome.* Bury St. Edmunds, UK: Thames Valley Test Company.

Wilson, B. A., Clare, L., Baddeley, A. Watson, P., & Tate, R. (1998) *The Rivermead Behavioral Memory Test–Extended Version (RBMT-E).* Bury St. Edmunds, UK: Thames Valley Test Company.

Wilson, B., Cockburn, J., & Baddeley, A. (1987). *Behavioral Inattention Test (BIT).* Bury St. Edmunds, UK: Thames Valley Test Company.

Wilson, B. A., Emslie, H. C., Quirk, K., & Evans, J. J. (2001). Reducing everyday memory and planning problems by means of a paging system: A randomised control crossover study. *Journal of Neurology, Neurosurgery & Psychiatry, 70,* 477–482.

Winocur, G., Craik, F. I., Levine, B., Robertson, I. H., Binns, M. A., Alexander, M., et al. (2007). Cognitive rehabilitation in the elderly: Overview and future directions. *Journal of the International Neuropsychology Society, 13,* 166–171.

World Health Organization. (2001). *ICIDH-2: International classification of functioning, disability and health.* Geneva, Switzerland: Author.

Wykes, T., Brammer, M., Mellers, J., Bray, P., Reeder, C., Williams, C., et al. (2002). Effects of the brain of a psychological treatment: Cognitive remediation therapy: functional magnetic resonance imaging in schizophrenia. *British Journal of Psychiatry, 181,* 144–152.

Yeates, K. O., Swift, E., Taylor, H. G., Wade, S. L., Drotar, D., Stancin, T., et al. (2004). Short- and long-term social outcomes following pediatric traumatic brain injury. *Journal of the International Neuropsychological Society, 10,* 412–426.

Ylvisaker, M., & Feeney, T. J. (1998). *Collaborative brain injury intervention.* San Diego: Singular.

Zoltan, B. (1996). *Vision, perception and cognition: A manual for the evaluation and treatment of the neurologically impaired adult* (3rd ed.). Thorofare, NJ: Slack.

Sensation and Sensory Processing

WINNIE DUNN

Learning Objectives

After reading this chapter, you will be able to:

1. Identify the major features of sensory systems.
2. Explain the alerting and discriminating aspects of each sensory system.
3. Describe the mechanisms of receiving, organizing, and using sensory input.
4. Categorize patterns of sensory processing based on evidence.
5. Link sensory-processing patterns to behaviors in everyday life.
6. Appreciate the significant contribution of sensation and sensory processing to one's ability to function during occupational performance.

SENSATION AND SENSORY PROCESSING ARE CRITICAL ASPECTS OF PERFORMANCE

There are many ways to characterize the human experience. We can consider the psychological, physical, and cognitive aspects of being human. Regardless of which perspective we take, sensation is the fuel that feeds all of these experiences. The way we have information about our psychological, physical, and cognitive experiences is from our senses. This is why occupational therapists must understand how the sensory systems work. We cannot understand people's experiences in their lives without understanding how their nervous systems are receiving, processing, and making meaning out of the sensory information that is available to them. Sensation and sensory processing provide the infrastructure for our experiences and therefore also provide critical tools for occupational therapy practice.

BASIC PRINCIPLES UNDERLYING THE FUNCTIONS OF THE SENSORY SYSTEMS

The sensory systems are the input mechanisms for the nervous system. The nervous system has several functions that direct how the sensory systems operate, including **centrifugal control** and balancing **excitation** and

inhibition. When we understand these neurological actions, we can also understand how to design activities that will take advantage of how the brain operates, thus creating an internal mechanism for supporting the person's performance.

Centrifugal Control

Centrifugal control is the most basic operation of the central nervous system (CNS) and is the brain's ability to regulate its own input. The brain accomplishes centrifugal control with suppression, divergence, and convergence (Noback & Demarest, 1981).

Suppression is the ability of the CNS to dampen some stimuli so that others are easier to detect. People receive continuous and variable sensory input; with suppression, we can filter through all the input to the brain, which determines which stimuli warrant attention and which can be ignored safely. Distractibility is related to poor suppression. Difficulty staying on a task occurs because attention is distributed to all the stimuli that are available in the environment.

Divergence is the brain's ability to transmit sensory input to many parts of the brain so that the input can affect multiple places at once. When a person is in danger, a small stimulus (e.g., the faint smell of smoke) needs to recruit lots of activity; we refer to these high activity levels as a *fight-or-flight response*. Divergence also allows an entire muscle works rather than one muscle fiber.

Convergence is the phenomenon of bringing input together from many sources. It is as if the brain is seeking confirmation by getting information from several sensory systems and is being careful to act only when there is enough input to tell a clear story. Convergence prevents us from reacting inappropriately when only partial stimuli are available and keeps us from reacting to every stimulus that comes along. In the sensory systems, inputs from multiple sensory inputs converge so that the brain can create a more organized response.

Balance of Excitation and Inhibition

The brain depends on a balance of excitation and inhibition to mediate input and output. With too much excitation, we overreact; and with too much inhibition, we will fail to notice and respond to the world around us. At each synapse and within neuron systems, there is a continuous negotiation between the excitation and inhibition messages that are available. There has to be enough excitation to override the inhibition in order to get an action.

When we consider this balancing at a systems level, we also see a balance of power in the complementary functions of the brain as a whole. Some parts of the brain are responsible for increasing our attention, while others are responsible for scanning the environment. These systems remain balanced because of the excitation and inhibition patterns between these parts of the brain. When brain injury disrupts typical function, people experience a release phenomenon. This means that one function is set free from the excitatory and inhibitory controls of its complementary parts of the brain. Heightened or dampened reactions occur when there is a release phenomenon.

Another way to balance excitation and inhibition is through feed forward and feedback mechanisms. The brain has connections that enable it to "listen in" to input and reactions. This allows the brain to monitor itself and make adjustments in plans for acting. Feed forward circuits send a message ahead of the primary sensory message either to alert higher centers about incoming input (i.e., "pay attention") or to create an inhibitory path so that the sensory message gets stronger (i.e., "notice only THIS"). Feedback circuits send a message back to modulate the strength of a response (Dunn, 2000). For example, feedback occurs after you have completed a movement and allows the brain to evaluate how effective that movement was to reaching your goal. On the basis of feedback, the system will make adjustments in how the message gets sent the next time (e.g., "a little more of those muscles, a little less of these muscles").

BASIC FEATURES OF SENSORY SYSTEMS IN THE NERVOUS SYSTEM

Even though each sensory system has unique functions, they have basic functions that they share. They all have an input structure that transmits information into the nervous system, and each sensory system has multiple types of input to transmit. They all have several levels in the brain for processing the input. Every sensory system operates to make the brain aware of stimuli that are available in the environment (i.e., the arousal/alerting function), and to construct maps of the body and the environment (i.e., the discriminating and mapping function). With this information and the maps that are created, a person can design effective responses to the demands of life.

Under typical circumstances, the arousal/alerting and discriminating/mapping functions complement each other, forming a balance of power. People use their sensory maps to figure out what is happening and how to react appropriately. The discriminating/mapping function guides behavior during everyday activities. The arousal/alerting function enables people to become aware of a new, unfamiliar, or potentially harmful stimulus so that they can be more aware and possibly create alternative responses (e.g., fight-or-flight responses). Arousal/alerting stimuli generate "noticing" behaviors, that is, attention is drawn toward the stimulus, which can disrupt ongoing behavior. Arousal/alerting stimuli make it possible for the brain to orient to stimuli in case a protective response will be needed.

Discriminatory/mapping stimuli make it possible to gather data that will support and design functional behaviors. The information combines to create maps of body and environment, which can be used to create purposeful movement. Discriminating and mapping stimuli are more organizing for the brain.

Table 58.1 provides a summary of the arousal/alerting and discriminating/mapping components of each sensory system, with a simple definition and example of each. Table 58.2 is in the same format and provides information about when to use each sensory component in a therapeutic way. Remember that every sensory input can be useful or harmful. When we understand the characteristics of each sensory input, we can harness that input positively for a therapeutic purpose, that is, to support occupational performance.

SPECIFIC FEATURES OF SPECIFIC SENSORY SYSTEMS

Each sensory system has specific functions. The sensory neurons transmit information into the nervous system, and this information reaches higher brain centers. However, we must remember that **sensory processing** is different from sensory input itself. Sensation involves transmitting physical properties of a stimulus to the brain. Once in the brain, stimuli are changed (through excitation and inhibition),

TABLE 58.1 AROUSAL/ALERTING AND DISCRIMINATION/MAPPING DESCRIPTORS OF THE SENSORY SYSTEMS

Sensory System	Arousal/Alerting Descriptors*	Discrimination/Mapping Descriptors†
For all systems	*Unpredictable:* The task is unfamiliar; the child cannot anticipate the sensory experiences that will occur in the task.	*Predictable:* Sensory pattern in the task is routine for the child, such as diaper changing—the child knows what is occurring and what will come next.
Somatosensory	*Light touch:* gentle tapping on skin; tickling (e.g., loose clothing making contact with skin) *Pain:* brisk pinching; contact with sharp objects; skin pressed in small surface (e.g., when skin is caught in between chair arm and seat). *Temperature:* Hot or cold stimuli (e.g., iced drinks, hot foods, cold hands, cold metal chairs). *Variable:* Changing characteristics during the task (e.g., putting clothing on requires a combination of tactile experiences). *Short duration stimuli:* Tapping, touching briefly (e.g., splashing water). *Small body surface contact:* Small body surfaces, as when using only fingertips to touch something.	*Touch pressure:* Firm contact on skin (e.g., hugging, patting, grasping). Occurs both when touching objects or persons, or when they touch you. *Long duration stimuli:* Holding, grasping (e.g., carrying a child in your arms. *Large body surface contact:* Large body surfaces include holding, hugging; also includes holding a cup with the entire palmar surface of hand.
Vestibular	*Head position change:* The child's head orientation is altered (e.g., pulling the child up from lying on the back to sitting). *Speed change:* Movements change velocity (e.g., the teacher stops to talk to another teacher when pushing the child to the bathroom in his wheelchair). *Direction change:* Movements change planes, such as bending down to pick something up while carrying the child down the hall. *Rotary head movement:* head moving in an arc (e.g., spinning, turning head side to side).	*Linear head movement:* Head moving in a straight line (e.g., bouncing up and down, going down the hall in a wheelchair). *Repetitive head movements:* Movements that repeat in a simple sequence (e.g., rocking in a rocker).

Continued

TABLE 58.1   AROUSAL/ALERTING AND DISCRIMINATION/MAPPING DESCRIPTORS OF THE SENSORY SYSTEMS   *Continued*

Sensory System	Arousal/Alerting Descriptors*	Discrimination/Mapping Descriptors†
Proprioception	*Quick stretch:* Movements that pull on the muscles (e.g., briskly tapping on a muscle belly).	*Sustained tension:* Steady, constant action on the muscles pressing or holding on the muscle (e.g., using heavy objects during play). *Shifting muscle tension:* Activities that demand constant change in the muscles (e.g., walking, lifting, moving objects).
Visual	*High intensity:* Visual stimulus is bright (e.g., looking out a window on a bright day). *High contrast:* A difference between the visual stimulus and surrounding environment (e.g., cranberry juice in a white cup). *Variable:* Changing characteristics during a task (e.g., a TV program is a variable visual stimulus).	*Low intensity:* Visual stimulus is subdued (e.g., finding objects in the dark closet). *High similarity:* Small differences between visual stimulus and its surrounding environment (e.g., oatmeal in a beige bowl). *Competitive:* The background is interesting or busy (e.g., the junk drawer, a bulletin board).
Auditory	*Variable:* Changing characteristics during a task (e.g., a person's voice with intonation). *High intensity:* The auditory stimulus is loud (e.g., siren, high volume radio). *Competitive:* The environment has a variety of recurring sounds (e.g., the classroom, a party)	*Rhythmic:* Sounds repeat in a simple sequence/beat (e.g., humming; singing nursery songs). *Constant:* The stimulus is always present (e.g., a fan noise). . *Noncompetitive:* The environment is quiet (e.g., the bedroom when all is ready for bedtime). *Low intensity:* The auditory stimulus is subdued (e.g., whispering).
Olfactory/gustatory	*Strong intensity:* The taste/small has distinct qualities (e.g., spinach).	*Mild intensity:* The taste/smell has nondistinct or familiar qualities (e.g., cream of wheat).

Note: *Arousal/alerting stimuli tend to generate "noticing" behaviors. The individual's attention is at least momentarily drawn toward the stimulus (commonly disrupting ongoing behavior). These stimuli enable the nervous system to orient to stimuli that may require a protective response. In some situations, an arousing stimulus can become part of a functional behavior (e.g., when the arousing somatosensory input from putting on shirt becomes predictable, a discriminating/mapping characteristic).

†Discriminatory/mapping stimuli are those that enable the individual to gather information that can be used to support and generate functional behaviors. The information yields spatial and temporal qualities of body and environment (the content of the maps), which can be used to create purposeful movement. These stimuli are more organizing for the nervous system.

Source: Dunn, W. (1991). The sensorimotor systems: A framework for assessment and intervention. In F. P. Orelove & D. Sobsey (Eds.), *Educating children with multiple disabilities: A transdisciplinary approach* (2nd ed.). Baltimore: Paul H. Brookes. Reprinted with permission.

organized, and compared to past experiences to determine the meaning of the sensory input. This is the sensory-processing part of the actions and is the aspect that we consider when observing behavior.

SENSORY INPUT MECHANISMS

The sensory systems are designed to transmit an exact kind of information. The chemical senses transmit information about tastes and smells. The body senses inform the brain about the skin, muscles, and body placement. The environmental senses provide information about the surround.

The Chemical Senses

The chemical senses separated into taste (gustatory) and smell (olfactory) when organisms moved from the sea to land during evolution. The taste system was the final check point for foods entering the body, while the smell system served to identify the location and direction of food or predators (Coren, Porac, & Ward, 1984).

TABLE 58.2   REASONS FOR INCORPORATING VARIOUS SENSORY QUALITIES INTO INTEGRATED INTERVENTION PROGRAMS*

Sensory System	Arousal/Alerting Descriptors	Discrimination/Mapping Descriptors
For all systems	*Unpredictable:* To develop an increasing level of attention to keep the child interested in the task/activity (e.g., change the position of the objects on the child's lap tray during the task).	*Predictable:* To establish the child's ability to anticipate a programming sequence or a salient cue; to decrease possibility to be distracted from a functional task sequence (e.g., use the same routine for diaper changing every time).
Somatosensory	*Light Touch:* To increase alertness in a child who is lethargic (e.g., pull cloth from child's face during peek-a-boo). *Pain:* To raise from unconsciousness; to determine ability to respond to noxious stimuli when unconscious (e.g., flick palm of hand or sole of foot briskly). *Temperature:* To establish awareness of stimuli; to maintain attentiveness to task (e.g., use hot foods for spoon eating and cold drink for sucking through a straw). *Variable:* To maintain attention to or interest in the task (e.g., place new texture on cup surface each day so child notices the cup). *Short duration:* To increase arousal for task performance (e.g., tap child on chest before giving direction). *Small body surface contact:* To generate and focus attention on a particular body part (e.g., tap around lips with fingertips before eating task).	*Touch pressure:* To establish and maintain awareness of body parts and body position; to calm a child who has been overstimulated (e.g., provide a firm bear hug). *Long duration:* To enable the child to become familiar, comfortable with the stimulus; to incorporate stimulus into functional skill (e.g., grasping the container to pick it up and pour out contents). *Large body surface contact:* To establish and maintain awareness of body parts and body position; to calm a child who has been overstimulated (e.g., wrap child tightly in a blanket).
Vestibular	*Head position change:* To increase arousal for an activity (e.g., position child prone over a wedge). *Speed change:* To keep adequate alertness for functional task (e.g., vary pace while carrying the child to new task). *Direction change:* To elevate level of alertness for a functional task (e.g., swing child back and forth in arms prior to positioning him or her at the table for a task).	*Linear head movement:* To support establishment of body awareness in space (e.g., carry child around the room in fixed position to explore its features). *Repetitive head movement:* To provide predictable and organizing information; to calm a child who has been overstimulated (e.g., rock the child).
Proprioception	*Quick stretch:* To generate additional muscle tension to support functional tasks (e.g., tap muscle bell of hypotonic muscle while providing physical guidance to grasp).	*Sustained tension:* To enable the muscle to relax, elongate, so body part can be in more optimal position for function (e.g., press firmly across muscle belly while to objects being manipulated). *Shift muscle tension:* To establish functional movements that contain stability and mobility (e.g., prop and reach for a top; reach, fill, and lift spoon to mouth).

Continued

TABLE 58.2 REASONS FOR INCORPORATING VARIOUS SENSORY QUALITIES INTO INTEGRATED INTERVENTION PROGRAMS* *Continued*

Sensory System	Arousal/Alerting Descriptors*	Discrimination/Mapping Descriptors[†]
Visual	*High intensity:* To increase opportunity to notice object; to generate arousal for task (e.g., cover blocks with foil for manipulation task). *High contrast:* To enhance possibility of location object and maintaining attention to it (e.g., place raisins on a piece of typing paper for prehension activity). *Variable:* To maintain attention to or interest in the task (e.g., play rolling catch with a clear ball that has moveable pieces inside).	*Low intensity:* To allow visual stimulus to blend with other salient features; to generate searching behaviors, since characteristics are less obvious (e.g., find own cubby hole in back of room). *High similarity:* To establish more discerning abilities; to develop skills for naturally occurring tasks (e.g., scoop applesauce from beige plate). *Competitive:* To facilitate searching; to increase tolerance for natural life circumstances (e.g., obtain correct tools from equipment bin).
Auditory	*Variable:* To maintain attention to or interest in the task (e.g., play radio station after activating a switch). *High intensity:* To stimulate noticing the person or object, to create proper alerting for task performance (e.g., ring a bell to encourage the child to locate the stimulus).	*Rhythmic:* To provide predictable/organizing information for environmental orientation (e.g., sing a nursery rhyme while physically guiding motions). *Constant:* To provide a foundational stimulus for environmental orientation, especially important when other sensory systems (e.g., vision, vestibular) do not provide orientation (e.g., child recognizes own classroom by fan noise and calms down). *Competitive:* To facilitate differentiation of salient stimuli; to increase tolerance for natural life circumstances (e.g., after child learns to look when his or her name is called, conduct activity within busy classroom).
Olfactory/gustatory	*Strong intensity:* To stimulate arousal for task (e.g., child smells spaghetti sauce at lunch).	*Noncompetitive:* To facilitate focused attention for acquiring a new and difficult skill; to calm a child who has been overstimulated (e.g., move child to quiet room to establish vocalizations). *Low intensity:* To allow the auditory stimulus to blend with other salient features; to generate searching behaviors since stimulus is less obvious (e.g., give child a direction in a normal volume). *Mild intensity:* To facilitate exploratory behaviors; to stimulate naturally occurring activities (e.g., smell of lunch food is less distinct, so child is encouraged to notice texture, color).

Source: Adapted from Dunn, W. (1991). The sensorimotor systems: A framework for assessment and intervention. In F. P. Orelove & D. Sobsey (Eds.), *Educating children with multiple disabilities: A transdisciplinary approach* (2nd ed.) Baltimore. Paul H. Brookes. Reprinted with permission.

The Gustatory System

We identify tastes by how the chemicals break down within our systems in the categories of sweet, salty, sour, and bitter (Coren et al., 1984). Taste buds receive the chemicals; 10,000 taste buds are available to young people, and the number diminishes with age. Taste goes from the taste buds to the brain stem, then to the thalamus, and on to the sensory homunculus in the parietal lobe (Heimer, 1983). Taste is compromised when there is brain stem trauma and with degenerative diseases that affect the thalamic and cortical regions that serve taste.

Taste on the tongue has been mapped many times, but functionally, food appeals to us because of the overall experience we have with the food, including not only the taste, but also the texture, temperature, and smell (i.e., intersensory integration of other senses with taste). People do not have universal reactions to tastes; for example, researchers have reported that some people taste caffeine and others do not (Blakeslee & Salmon, 1935; Coren et al., 1984; Hall, Bartoshuk, Cain, & Stevens, 1975). Older adults often complain about foods being bland; this is because the reduction of taste receptor viability. Because the taste receptors recover in about 10 seconds, changing the flavors in the mouth during the meal (e.g., salty, then sweet) can keep food interesting.

Olfactory Sense

We identify smells from the environment through a chemical reaction with the cells at the top of the nose. These cells project directly to higher brain centers, bypassing the thalamus; this is the only sensory system that does not relay through the thalamus en route to the cortex (Coren et al., 1984). Olfaction is the most sensitive system, but researchers have yet to be able to categorize the way in which people smell. We have a tendency to take our smell sensations for granted, but smell is critical to many human functions. With the connection of the olfactory system to the limbic system, smells associate with our emotions and with our memories. An odor can bring back very vivid images of past events. The olfactory system is also directly linked to arousal mechanisms, which is why it can be so helpful in getting a response out of people who are comatose.

It is this powerful influence on our emotions and memories that we must keep in mind in practice. Clients might react strongly to smells that we are not even aware of, including personal hygiene products that we use. An acutely ill person or a person with severe disabilities might recognize people by their smells as well, providing grounding and comfort in a confusing world. We must also be aware of the unfamiliar odors of a sterile environment and the comfort of familiar odors, even if those odors are unpleasant to us. Entering a family's home can expose the therapist to many unfamiliar odors; we might need to set our discomfort aside to consider how this olfactory environment is affecting the family members.

The Body Senses

The body senses tell the brain about where your body parts are and what they are doing. The somatosensory, or touch, system tells where you end and where the world begins because the receptors are within your skin. The proprioceptive system tells where your muscles and joints are, thus contributing additional information about the body's positions in space. The vestibular system tells where you are in relation to gravity; this adds a dynamic dimension to the body map.

The Somatosensory System

There are many types of touch receptors, and this variety allows the brain to know exactly what is happening to the skin. There is an elaborate system of receptive fields on the skin whose job it is to locate the touch experiences. A receptive field is the area on the surface of the skin served by one sensory neuron. In some places on your skin, the receptive fields overlap a lot (i.e., the mouth, face, hands, genitals); in other places, they barely overlap (e.g., the back). The brain compares the receptive fields of all the active neurons to detect the location of the touch; so when they overlap a lot, we know exactly where touch occurs, and when they overlap little, we can tell only the general area of touch. When we have an itch on a high-density area, we can get right to the spot to scratch, but when we have an itch on our back, we have to feel around a little to find the right spot. This is because of the receptive fields.

Since the touch receptors are all over the body surface, these sensory neurons transmit information into and up the spinal cord. Information travels to the brain stem, the thalamus, and then the sensorimotor cortex, specifically the parietal lobe. Traditionally, neuroscientists divided this system into the posterior and anterolateral systems, the posterior portion being responsible for touch pressure and proprioception (see the next section) and the anterolateral portion being responsible for light touch, pain, and temperature reception. We now understand that those divisions provide general guidance and recognize that individual experiences are unique.

Generally, the dorsal column system provides specific information about the surface of the skin and about the muscles and joints (see the section on proprioception). In reference to Tables 58-1 and 58-2, this system transmits the discriminating and mapping information. The input that travels through the dorsal columns goes directly to the thalamus and on to the parietal lobe in a very specific pattern, creating the sensory homunculus (a map of the body from a sensory point of view).

The anterolateral system transmits information for arousal and alerting the brain (see Tables 58.1 and 58.2 for examples). This input travels into the spinal cord and from there to the reticular formation of the brain stem. The reticular formation is responsible for generalized arousal of the brain, so these connections are less specific and more diffuse. The anterolateral input is important when people need more arousal to participate, and it is input to be avoided when people are already agitated or have heightened responsiveness.

The Proprioceptive System

Inside the muscles, tendons, and joints are sensory receptors that keep track of what is going on with your body parts. They detect how long a muscle is, how fast it is moving, and the direction in which the limb is moving, which creates knowledge about where the body parts (particularly the limbs) are in space. We always think about the muscles and joints as part of the musculoskeletal system, but the sensory part of this system enables us to know where and how our bodies are moving. We do not just move; we have awareness of our own movements from the proprioceptive sensory receptors.

The muscle spindles detect length changes in the muscle. The muscle spindles are the sensory component of the reflex arc that supports muscle tone. The motor centers of the brain control the actions of the muscles by dampening the activity of the reflex arcs. When the motor centers of the brain are damaged, the reflex arc continues to activate without inhibitory control; this mechanism creates spasticity (Crutchfield & Barnes, 1984).

The Golgi tendon organs (GTO) are the sensory receptors in the tendons around the joints. The GTO detects changes in tension of the muscle pulling on the tendons. This action is important in cramp relief. During cramping, the muscle contains a high degree of tension. When you slowly and consistently stretch a cramped muscle, you pull on the tendon, which activates the GTO. This sensory message creates increased inhibition to the muscle, enabling the muscle to relax. This is the mechanism that we are harnessing when we use sustained stretch with people who have spasticity (Crutchfield & Barnes, 1984).

The cerebellum plays an important role in processing proprioceptive information. The cerebellum receives sensory input before the input is processed in the higher brain centers. This raw sensory input enables the cerebellum to be very precise in how it organizes motor actions. The cerebellum makes adjustments on the basis of what is actually happening (as told by the sensory input), which is why our motor planning can be so accurate. The cerebellum also gets information from the brain about the proposed movement plans and compares the plan and the sensation to determine whether an alteration must occur (Dunn, 2000). We can make just the right step because the cerebellum is fine-tuning the plan just before we need to act.

The Vestibular System

The vestibular system is responsible for our orientation in space. By detecting our relationship to gravity, the vestibular system keeps track of the body's movements. The vestibular organ, which is housed in the inner ear,

contains one structure (the semicircular canals) that responds to angular movement such as swinging, spinning, and rolling and another structure (the chambers) that responds to linear movement such as jumping and running. Together, they record direction, angle, and speed of movement, with particular attention to the position of the head (Goldberg & Fernandez, 1984; Heimer, 1983; Kornhuber, 1974).

Like the proprioceptive system, the vestibular organ sends sensory input to the brain stem and cortex as well as the cerebellum. The connections with the cerebellum contribute to postural control through a continuous processing of sensory input (i.e., where the muscles and joints are, where the head is). Postural control is a basic building block for human behavior; although we tend to think of postural control as a motor operation, it is important to remember that postural control is built on accurate sensory input. Sometimes poor postural stability is due to weakness of muscles or poor biomechanical positioning, but equally likely is the possibility that inaccurate or unreliable sensory input makes it impossible to create postural control. When sensory processing is the source of the problem, our interventions must involve sensory-based strategies in order for postural control to improve. Without postural control, all other actions will be poorly orchestrated because there will be no stability on which to build movements. The sensory systems are the silent partners during occupational performance, creating a background on which to build purposeful movement (Kornhuber, 1974).

Another important function of the vestibular system is to coordinate with the visual system. Head position and eye position have to be in concert with each other to stay oriented in space. In addition to connecting with the cerebellum, vestibular input connects with the cranial nerves that serve the eye muscles (specifically cranial nerves III, IV, and VI). These connections enable us to determine whether our eyes are moving, our head is moving, or the world is moving. People who have motion sickness have more difficulty resolving this potential conflict.

The Environmental Senses

The environmental senses are responsible for providing information about the world around us. Technically, we could say that all sensation comes from the environment, but the function of the chemical and body senses is ultimately related to the body (e.g., determining how to get food for fuel, whether something is edible, where one's body is). The environmental senses map the world for us. The visual system informs us about the objects and people around us in a spatial context, and the auditory system informs us about the world in a temporal way. The visual system is concerned with size, shape, color, and placement. The auditory system is concerned with distance, intensity, and range. These senses work in concert with the chemical and body senses by providing the maps about where we are so that we can understand what our bodies might need to do in response to environmental demands.

The Visual System

The visual system is responsible for mapping the spatial relationships in the world for us. The visual system has three characteristics that make it unique among the sensory systems. First, with more sensory nerves than all the other sensory systems, the visual system is very prominent and important to human function. Second, the visual pathways move from front to back in the brain, making it an excellent marker for site of lesions in the brain (Kandel, Schwartz, & Jessell, 2000). Third, the retinal cells, which are the input receptors for the visual system, can be seen by looking into the eyeball, making this the only place that we can view the central nervous system directly. Because of this accessibility, physicians use the retina to determine what might be going on systemically in the brain.

The visual pathways include the optic nerve, which carries information from each eyeball separately; the optic chiasm, which contains the combined fibers from both eyeballs as the pathways converge together; and the optic tract, which contains a new configuration of fibers from each eyeball. The optic tracts contain fibers from both eyes; the fibers in the left optic tract transmit information from the right visual world, and the fibers in the right optic tract transmit information from the left visual world. This pattern of fibers converging and reorganizing leads to specific visual losses with brain damage; occupational therapists must understand these patterns so that they can hypothesize about what functional challenges an individual might face with particular losses. For example, without use of the left eye (close your left eye to see what it is like), the person cannot see to the left side. The right eye's visual span covers part of the space in front of the left eye, so the person does not lose all vision to the left. Neuroscience textbooks have diagrams that break down the visual pathway losses and corresponding visual losses (e.g., Kandel et al., 2000). Figure 58.1 illustrates the classic lesions and visual deficits patterns.

The visual system is designed to recognize contrasts (Dunn, 1997; Kandel et al., 2000). The cells search diligently for the most contrasting areas, just as a digital camera searches for contrast to focus itself. The eyeball is moving continuously so that new retinal cells can be activated, keeping a steady flow of input to the brain about the visual world. The visual system is most challenged by lack of contrast (e.g., misty, homogeneous environments) and also by overly busy environments (e.g., the contents of the junk drawer). Knowing this, therapists can be attentive to the contrasts in the visual environment to increase the chances that the person can detect important cues. For example, we can place a dark cloth on the work table to highlight white paper and writing utensils. We can also offer organizing strategies (e.g., sectioning off draw-

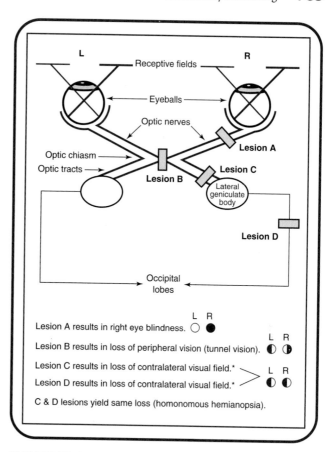

FIGURE 58.1   Neural lesions of visual field deficits. Source: Reprinted with permission from Dunn W. Implementing neuroscience principles to support habilitation and recovery. In: Christiansen C, Baum C, eds. *Occupational Therapy: Enabling Function and Well-Being.* 2nd ed. Thorofare, NJ: Slack, 1997.

ers) to increase the chances of finding things when they are needed.

The Auditory System

The auditory system processes sounds by detecting distance, direction, and sound quality; this enables us to orient within the environment (Kiang, 1984). The auditory system transmits air waves into pressure waves within the auditory receptors in the inner ear. The cochlea is shaped like a snail, and the different parts are situated so that we can detect all different tones.

The unique characteristic of the auditory system is the bilateral connections within the nervous system. Other sensory system input crosses to the opposite side of the brain when traveling to the cortex. When auditory input reaches the brain stem, information travels bilaterally to the cortex. This is important because bilateral connections create a safeguard for auditory input; both sides of the brain receive sounds from both sides of the world. When some auditory input is lost, we lose the ability to localize sounds, but the brain continues to receive input bilaterally. The auditory system also has a feedback loop that sends information back to the cochlea; this feedback loop dampens the actions of some noises so that other sounds can be processed more clearly. This process, called *auditory figure-ground perception*, enables people to focus on the important sounds (e.g., the musician) and dampen the potentially interfering sounds (e.g., the person whispering next to you).

Other professionals serve as experts about how the auditory system works. Occupational therapists consider the functional use of auditory input. We might choose a quieter auditory environment if someone is more distractible to sounds. We might also work in a natural environment with random background noise to increase a person's ability to manage in a classroom, worksite, or social situation. By considering the contribution or interference of the auditory input, we increase the capacity of our interventions to be successful. For example, we might suggest that a worker use earphones with music during work hours to increase focus on work and decrease distraction from other environmental sounds (because the music will be louder in the ears). We might suggest that a teacher give a student easier seatwork when working in the classroom and send the student to do more challenging work in the library. Thus, we can manipulate the auditory environment in many ways to support performance.

Summary of Sensory Input Mechanisms

Each sensory system processes a certain type of input to inform the brain about our bodies and the world around us. Occupational therapists need to understand these input mechanisms because they provide the brain with all the material that is needed to design adaptive responses that enable us to participate successfully in our lives. When sensory input is impaired, the brain has inaccurate or unreliable input, and this can lead to maladaptive behaviors. When occupational therapists understand the sensory systems, they can design and adapt activities and environments to support more successful participation.

A MODEL FOR SENSORY PROCESSING

Once we understand the sensory input mechanisms, the next step is to understand how the brain manages this information. Sensory processing is the mechanism of organizing, making meaning, and responding to sensory experiences. The sensory systems themselves are important because people have specific reactions to touch, sounds, and other input. However, we also have learned that the brain has ways of responding that are separate from the sensory systems; these ways of responding reflect how the brain detects input and how the brain regulates the input for responding.

In studies with infants, toddlers, children, and adults, Dunn and colleagues (Brown, et al. 2001; Dunn 1997; Dunn 1999; Dunn 2001; Dunn 2002; Dunn & Bennett 2002; Dunn & Brown 1997; Dunn, Myles, et al. 2002; Dunn, Saiter, et al. 2002; Ermer & Dunn 1998; Kientz & Dunn 1997; McIntosh, et al. 1999; Myles, Hagiwara et al. 2004; Pohl, Dunn et al. 2001) identified four ways in which people process sensory information. The four patterns reflect a combination of nervous system thresholds and self-regulation strategies.

Underlying Concepts for Sensory-Processing Patterns

The sensory processing patterns are based on how the nervous system reacts to input (i.e., the neurological thresholds) and how the person responds to input (i.e., the self-regulation strategies).

Nervous System Thresholds

Individual neurons, neuron groups, and systems within the brain all have thresholds for responding. This means that it takes a certain amount of excitatory input to activate the neurons. For some people, it takes very little input to activate neurons, so we say that they have low thresholds. For other people, it takes a lot of input to activate the neurons, so we say that they have high thresholds. Thresholds for responding occur along a continuum rather than at extremes, and a person may have lower thresholds for some inputs and higher thresholds for other inputs. For example, one might be more sensitive to touch input yet might not notice sounds as easily.

Self-Regulation Strategies

In addition to thresholds, we act on the basis of self-regulation strategies. Some people actively control the amount of sensory input they receive; other people are passive, letting things happen and then responding. Self-regulation also occurs along a continuum rather than as only active or passive responding. For example, one person might leave the room to actively limit the amount of auditory input he or she is receiving, while another person might become irritable because of too much sound.

Patterns of Sensory Processing from Dunn's Model

Where the neurological thresholds continuum and the self-regulation continuum intersect, there are four basic patterns of sensory processing. **Sensation seeking** represents high thresholds and an active self-regulation strategy. **Sensation avoiding** represents low thresholds and an active self-regulation strategy. **Sensory sensitivity** represents low thresholds and a passive self-regulation strategy. **Low registration** represents high thresholds and a passive self-

COMMENTARY ON THE EVIDENCE

Linking Neuroscience to Everyday Life with Sensory Processing Knowledge

The neuroscience literature provides a wealth of knowledge about how the brain and nervous system work to support the human experience. One of the definitive texts to have as a reference is *Principles of Neural Science* by Kandel, Schwartz, and Jessell (2000); this text provides clear explanations of brain anatomy and function and summarizes the studies that have demonstrated the phenomena that are under discussion. As occupational therapists, we rely on the evidence provided by neuroscientists about how the nervous system operates.

When we take the neuroscience knowledge and begin to apply it to the human condition, this is where we create and test our hypotheses. The studies that have used the Sensory Profile measures have provided evidence that there seem to be specific patterns of sensory processing and that these patterns are present in people of all ages, from infants to older adults, who do not have disabilities (Dunn & Brown 1997; Dunn 1999; McIntosh, Miller et al. 1999; Dunn 2001; Dunn & Daniels 2001; Pohl, Dunn et al. 2001; Brown & Dunn 2002; Dunn 2002). Studies have also shown that people with specific disabilities demonstrate some of the same patterns of sensory processing but are more likely to experience extreme versions of the same patterns (Kientz & Dunn 1997; Ermer & Dunn 1998; Brown, Tollefson et al. 2001; Dunn, Myles et al. 2002; Myles, Hagiwara et al. 2004). Some authors have tested the validity of the sensory-processing patterns in Dunn's model of sensory processing and have found relationships between particular patterns of brain activity (using skin conductance measures) and Sensory Profile scores (Brett-Green, Schoen et al. 2004; Brown, Tollefson et al. 2001; McIntosh, Miller et al. 1999; Schaaf, Miller et al. 2003). These findings suggest that the Sensory Profile questionnaires are capturing behavioral responses that are consistent with differential brain activity. Further studies with more advanced technology will provide additional evidence of this validity.

We can also apply neuroscience knowledge within practice. Several recent studies have demonstrated preliminary support for applying our knowledge about sensory processing within natural environments. In two studies, researchers showed that using weighted vests in school contexts contributed to increased attention on task behavior and decreased self-stimulation (Fertel Daly, Bedell et al. 2001; VandenBerg, 2001). Both of these studies also present a rationale for linking the sensations from the vest to organizing nervous system responses. In a related preliminary study with adults who have sensory sensitivities, researchers report that providing deep pressure in the form of a weighted blanket mediates skin conductance responses to normal levels (Smith, 2005). Researchers have also demonstrated that using ball chairs for seating improved students' on-task behaviors in children both with and without disabilities (Schilling, Washington, et al. 2003). These authors hypothesized about the relationship between the sensory activation and the children's behaviors. Taken together, these studies provide some evidence that applying neuroscience knowledge within the natural context can be an effective way to support participation.

regulation strategy. These four patterns exist in people without disabilities across the life course, so we cannot think of them as a dysfunction or characteristic of disability. Although it is true that people with particular disabilities (e.g., autism, Asperger syndrome, schizophrenia) exhibit more intense sensory-processing patterns in general, we must remember that the patterns themselves reflect the general human experience. Our personal sensory-processing patterns can contribute to or interfere with our ability to participate in our daily lives. Let's discuss each pattern in turn. Figure 58.2 illustrates Dunn's model of sensory processing.

Sensation Seeking

People with a sensation-seeking pattern of sensory processing select behavior to increase the amount and intensity of the sensory experiences in their daily routines. They might add movement, sound, tactile input, or visual input to an experience, such as humming and rubbing the wall while skipping down the hall or chewing on a pencil or fiddling with objects during work. They engage in these behaviors to increase their sensory experiences during life routines and derive pleasure from the additional sensory input.

PRACTICE DILEMMA

MOVING EVIDENCE INTO EVERYDAY PRACTICE

A family has been reading on the Internet and tells you that they want you to provide a sensory technique that you know has no evidence to support it. Discuss how you will handle this situation. Include how you will talk about the technique to the family, what other information you might provide for them, and alternatives that you might offer.

Because they have high sensory thresholds, more sensory input enables people with sensation-seeking patterns to reach their high thresholds and therefore be more responsive within their daily activities. For sensation seekers, it is more comfortable to have more sensory input. People with sensation-seeking patterns might play music while cooking or layer their clothing to provide more input to the skin throughout the day.

Sometimes people lack insight about their need for sensation seeking. They might get distracted from their daily life activities as they seek sensory input. For example, a person who seeks movement and body position input might be distracted from his desk job tasks because sitting at the computer does not provide enough input. This person might get up many times during the day to get more vestibular and proprioceptive input; if the person has a desk job, these frequent breaks could affect productivity. An occupational therapist might suggest that this person sit on a flexible cushion or a rocking chair at the desk to provide needed sensory input while working. We might also suggest that the person work at a standing desk to increase body input while working. We support participation when we find ways to provide needed sensory input within daily activities so that sensation seekers can continue to participate while getting the sensory experiences they need.

Low Registration

People with a low registration pattern of sensory processing fail to detect sensory experiences around them, so their behaviors might seem mismatched to situations. They will be calm in situations that would be disconcerting to others. It might also seem that people with low registration are uninterested, when in fact they are not noticing things that others notice quickly. For example, a person with low registration would be slower to intervene with children who are bickering, which could have the effect of providing time for the children to work things out for themselves.

People with low registration will be comfortable in more situations than others will. Because it takes a lot of sensory input for them to notice, they have a much wider range of tolerance. Behaviors that might be noticeable or irritating to others will go unnoticed, so some situations will not become charged for a person who has low registration. One family member could be watching TV while another is listening to the radio in an adjoining room; for a family member with low registration for sounds, this situation would be fine for continuing to pay bills or write a letter.

People with low registration are not getting enough activation to meet their sensory thresholds; and with a passive self-regulation strategy, they are less likely to pursue additional sensory input. Missing cues around them could interfere with their daily routines. For example, a person might burn parts of the dinner, missing the fact that what is in the pot is getting dry or the oven timer has been beeping. When low registration interferes with a person's daily life participation, occupational therapists can provide sup-

Neurological thresholds	Self Regulation Strategies	
	PASSIVE	**ACTIVE**
HIGH	Low registration	Sensation seeking
LOW	Sensory sensitivity	Sensation avoiding

FIGURE 58.2 Dunn's model of sensory processing. Source: Reprinted with permission: Dunn, W. (1997). The impact of sensory processing abilities on the daily lives of young children and families: A conceptual model. *Infants and Young Children, 9*(4), 23–35.

port by creating ways to intensify the sensory environment to make it easier to notice what is happening. In the kitchen example, we could change to a cooking timer that has an irregular sound (rather than even beeping sounds) and make it louder. We could also add a programmable timer that talks to indicate when it is time to check on the food. Adding music could also increase sensory intensity, making it easier for the person to notice what is going on in the kitchen. As with sensation seekers, we want to make it possible for the person with low registration to continue participating while getting the increased intensity they need.

Sensation Avoiding

People with a sensation-avoiding pattern of sensory processing select behavior to minimize the chances for new or unexpected sensory experiences. Sensation-avoiding people will withdraw from situations to reduce sensory input. When withdrawing is not possible, they might become aggressive to get others' help to remove them from the overwhelming situation. Having only predictable and familiar sensory input is the most comfortable situation for a person with sensation-avoiding patterns.

Because they have low sensory thresholds, less sensory input enables people with sensation-avoiding patterns to be more responsive within their daily activities. For avoiders, doing things the exact same way every time is comforting; the sensory experiences of getting dressed in the same clothing would be desirable. New clothing would represent new and unfamiliar tactile input.

Sensation avoiding can interfere with daily routines because it is hard to have everything be the same from day to day. If the person feels the need to withdraw at the first sign of unfamiliar sensory input, it can be hard to get any tasks completed. Occupational therapists can provide support for participation in several ways. First, we can help the person to identify ways to get respite from intense sensory environments during the day (e.g., a getaway space at home, a place to take a walk). Second, we can learn what sensations are acceptable for the person and work together to find ways to increase these sensations during daily routines. For example, if a person is overwhelmed by light touch on the skin, we can work on developing a wardrobe that provides even, firm touch pressure input to the skin. (Remember that light touch activates the arousal mechanisms and therefore can become overwhelming very quickly, while touch pressure provides more organized body scheme input without providing additional arousal.) We can suggest Lycra undergarments and stretchy, form-fitting shirts and tights; the additional benefit of these suggestions is that touch pressure input makes it harder to receive the arousing input that is bothersome. So we support participation for sensation avoiders when we find ways to provide acceptable sensory input while reducing the chances for difficult sensory input during daily routines.

Sensory Sensitivity

People with a sensory sensitivity pattern of sensory processing react to the sensory experiences around them. They notice sensations quite readily, so they can seem distractible or bothered a lot of the time. People with sensitivity will comment on the things that are going on around them because they are so aware of sensations. For example, at a concert, the person will notice others pulling out a tissue, shuffling their feet, flipping through the program, and adjusting in their seats. Sometimes the sensation from all these associated actions can keep the person from being able to hear and enjoy the concert.

People with sensory sensitivity do best with precise circumstances. They are less likely to withdraw like avoiders yet still want to keep their sensory experiences within ranges they can handle. For people with sensory sensitivity, it is more comfortable when they know their own limits and can manage the amount of sensory input that is comfortable in each life circumstance. For example, they will plan a family outing in great detail to make sure everything is just right for them. (An avoider will get out of going altogether.)

When a person has sensitivity, precision in everyday life becomes important. A person might go through several showerheads, towels, soaps, and other hygiene products before finding the ones that are "just right." These individuals may also be unhappy when companies change their product lines because it means finding another acceptable product. Occupational therapists can support people with sensitivity by helping them to characterize the details of their sensory needs and to find additional products, furniture, supplies, and situations that contain what sensory input they need without containing too much sensory input or undesirable sensory input. For example, we could look at all the person's personal hygiene products to identify similarities among them and then collaborate to identify other products, foods, and supplies that have these characteristics. If all the items are unscented and creamy, we can use this information in other situations. Knowing the sensory characteristics is a powerful tool for people with sensitivity.

PROVOCATIVE QUESTIONS

1. Think about your daily routines as a continuous sensory-processing experience. What do you gravitate toward? What do you shy away from? What sensory-processing strategies are embedded in your daily routines? What sensory experiences seem to interrupt your flow?
2. Think about a situation that you find very difficult to deal with. Using a sensory-processing point of view, how could you change that situation to make it more manageable for you?

CASE STUDY: *Danielle, Please Join Us for Dinner*

Danielle is a 5-year-old girl who lives with her older sister and her parents. Her mother, Sandy, wants some help in figuring out how to get Danielle to be engaged with the family during the evening meal. This is the only time when all the family members are together and can check in with each other about their days.

In an initial phone conversation, Sandy tells Mona, the occupational therapist, about what happens when they get home. Typically, the older sister is in her room on her computer, listening to music and talking on the phone. Danielle comes home with Sandy, and although they talk in the car, Danielle becomes less interactive once they get home. Sandy gets busy working on dinner, and Danielle watches TV. Dad is not home from work yet.

They sit down to dinner, and Danielle has to be called several times to get her to the table. Once Danielle gets to the table, she hangs on the chair and lays her head on the table, and her parents continue to have a hard time getting her attention.

Mona comes to the house for a dinnertime visit so that she can observe the family routines and gather more information. She also sends the parents a Sensory Profile to complete about Danielle, because she wonders whether low registration might be making it hard for Danielle to stay engaged within her contexts. Mona notices that Danielle is talking to Sandy when they come in the door, but then Danielle gets more placid as she lies in front of the TV. When Mona asks Danielle to sit up on a pillow, this seems to help a bit, and when they both start talking back to the TV show to answer the questions the program asks of its audience, Danielle becomes a little more animated. Mona knows that her being new in the home is also contributing to Danielle's higher engagement.

Mona's hypothesis about low registration turns out to be correct; the Sensory Profile scores, the parents' descriptions, and Mona's observations all converge to paint a consistent picture of a child who needs more intense sensory input to stay engaged. Because Danielle responds to prompting by others (e.g., to sit up, to talk back) and becomes more engaged, this gives Mona some ideas about how to help this family.

When Mona and Sandy meet, they discuss Danielle's need to have more sensory input. Mona explains that when they are in the car, Sandy is talking, pointing out things to look at, and playing the radio, and all these things help to keep Danielle active and engaging. When they get home and Danielle is left on her own, she does not seek extra input for herself, so she becomes less engaged and misses things going on around her. This is not a good situation leading up to dinner, because Danielle cannot get enough sensory input from just walking into the dining room.

Mona makes several suggestions for increasing the sensory experiences Danielle has leading up to dinner that could make it easier for her to interact during the meal. They talk about ways in which Danielle can help with dinner, such as stirring pots, getting out utensils, and carrying plates to the table, so that Danielle's system can have continuous sensory input from walking, carrying, talking, and feeling the objects as she works. Mona also explains that using contrasting placemats and plates with the food will make the table more visually interesting. Sandy really responds to the plan and even starts to add her own ideas. She puts food coloring into Danielle's milk to surprise her at the table, and the family starts a guessing game about what foods are in the dishes. All these things keep Danielle engaged because she is getting a continuous and intense amount of sensory input while they are preparing and eating the meal. This enables Danielle to stay alert at dinner and talk with her family more actively.

Questions

1. Do you have other ideas that Danielle's parents could try to increase Danielle's sensory input before or during dinner?
2. Mona would need to help the parents know how to detect overstimulation as well. What would be some behaviors that might be warning signs to the parents that Danielle is getting overstimulated?

---

3. What evidence in the literature supports the changes you might make in your life to make a situation more manageable for you?

REFERENCES

Blakeslee, A. F., & Salmon, T. H. (1935). Genetics of sensory thresholds: Individual taste reactions for different substances. *Proceedings of the National Academy of Sciences of the U.S.A., 21,* 84–90.

Brett-Green, B., Schoen, S., et al. (2004). Psycho-physiological variability in children with Asperger's syndrome. *Psychophysiology* 41(abstract).

Brown, C. & Dunn, W. (2002). *The Adult Sensory Profile.* San Antonio, TX: Psychological Corporation.

Brown, C., Tollefson, N., et al. (2001). The Adult Sensory Profile: Measuring patterns of sensory processing. *American Journal of Occupational Therapy* 55(1): 75–82.

Dunn, W. (1997). The impact of sensory processing abilities on the daily lives of young children and families: A conceptual model. *Infants and Young Children* 9(4): 23–35.

Dunn, W. (1999). *The Sensory Profile Manual.* San Antonio, TX: Psychological Corporation.

Dunn, W. (2001). The sensations of everyday life: theoretical, conceptual and pragmatic considerations. *American Journal of Occupational Therapy* 55(6): 608–620.

Dunn, W. (2002). *The Infant Toddler Sensory Profile.* San Antonio, TX: Psychological Corporation.

Dunn, W., & Bennett, D. (2002). Patterns of sensory processing in children with attention deficit hyperactivity disorder. *Occupational Therapy Journal of Research 22*(1): 4–15.

Dunn, W., & Brown, C. (1997). Factor analysis on the Sensory Profile from a national sample of children without disabilities. *American Journal of Occupational Therapy 51*(7): 490–495.

Dunn, W., & Daniels, D. (2001). Initial development of the Infant Toddler Sensory Profile. *Journal of Early Intervention 25*(1): 27–41.

Dunn, W., Myles, B., et al. (2002). Sensory processing issues associated with Asperger Syndrome: A preliminary investigation. *American Journal of Occupational Therapy 56*(1): 97–102.

Dunn, W., Saiter, J., et al. (2002). Asperger syndrome and sensory processing: A conceptual model and guidance for intervention planning. *Focus on Autism and other Developmental Disabilities 17*(3): 172–185.

Ermer, J., & Dunn, W. (1998). The Sensory Profile: A discriminant analysis of children with and without disabilities. *American Journal of Occupational Therapy 52*(4): 283–290.

Fertel Daly, D., Bedell, G., et al. (2001). Effects of a weighted vest on attention to task and self stimulatory behaviors in preschoolers with pervasive developmental disorders. *American Journal of Occupational Therapy 55*(6): 629–640.

Kientz, M. A., & Dunn, W. (1997). Comparison of the performance of children with and without autism on the Sensory Profile. *American Journal of Occupational Therapy 51*(7): 530–537.

McIntosh, D. N., Miller, L. J., et al. (1999). Overview of the Short Sensory Profile (SSP). In *The Sensory Profile.* W. Dunn (ed.). San Antonio, TX: Psychological Corporation: 59–74.

Myles, B. S., Hagiwara, T., et al. (2004). Sensory Issues in children with Asperger syndrome and autism. *Education and Training in Developmental Disabilities 3*(4): 283–290.

Noback, C., & Demarest, R. (1981). *The Human Nervous System: Basic Principles of Neurobiology.* New York: McGraw-Hill.

Pohl, P., Dunn, W., et al. (2001). The role of sensory processing in the everyday lives of older adults. *Occupational Therapy Journal of Research 23*(3): 99–106.

Schaaf, R. C., Miller, L. J., et al. (2003). Preliminary study of parasympathetic functioning in children with sensory modulation dysfunction and its relation to occupation. *American Journal of Occupational Therapy 57*: 442–449.

Schilling, D., Washington, K., et al. (2003). Classroom seating for children with attention deficit hyperactivity disorder: Therapy balls versus chairs. *American Journal of Occupational Therapy 57*(5): 534–541.

Smith, S. (2005). *Psychophysiological Evidence about Sensory Sensitivities in Adults.* Supply city name, California: American Occupational Therapy Association.

VandenBerg, N. (2001). The use of a weighted vest to increase on-task behavior in children with attention difficulties. *American Journal of Occupational Therapy 55*(6): 621–628.

Sensory Integration

SUSANNE SMITH ROLEY AND S. ESSIE JACOBS

Learning Objectives

After reading this chapter, you will be able to:

1. Describe the significance of sensory processing to learning and behavior.
2. Identify concepts that are central to sensory integration theory.
3. List ways to assess sensory integrative dysfunction.
4. Distinguish intervention using sensory integration principles from those using other frames of reference.
5. Recognize the evidence that supports and guides the use of sensory integration theory and principles in occupational therapy practice.

INTRODUCTION

Sensory integration (SI) theory is a dynamic and ecological theory that specifies the critical influence of **sensory processing** on human development and function. This theory emphasizes a person's ability to appropriately process sensory information from the body and integrate it with information about what is going on around the person so that he or she can effectively act on the environment. It contributes to our understanding of how sensation affects learning, social-emotional development, and neurophysiological processes such as motor performance, attention, and **arousal**. Occupational therapists commonly use sensory integration theory in practice as a frame of reference that can be used to both assess and intervene with people who have sensory integrative or sensory processing dysfunction that adversely affects function (Parham & Mailloux, 2005). It is important to be clear what one is referring to when using the term *sensory integration,* as this singular term has been used to refer to a theory, a neurological process, a disorder, and an intervention approach (Bundy, 2002; Mulligan, 2003).

The theoretical principles that support the use of this frame of reference draw on evidence from neuroscience as Dr. Ayres recognized that behavior and emotions are regulated by brain mechanisms. Advances in neuroscience continue to expand and support Dr. Ayres' original hypotheses, contributing to evidence-based practice (Bauman, 2005; Schneider, 2005). Dynamic systems theories have emerged that provide an understanding of the complexity of development (Thelen & Smith, 1994) and help to explain the complexity of the way in which this intervention effects change in children (Spitzer, 1999). SI is now commonly applied in educational settings with children who have learning and behavior disorders (American Occupational Therapy Association, 2003), as well as in private settings.

While education in sensory integration theory and intervention principles is part of the entry-level curricula for occupational therapists and occupational therapy assistants, postgraduate training is recommended for those specializing in the use of SI intervention in clinical practice. Occupational therapists with sensory integration certification and mentorship with a master clinician are best prepared to evaluate and provide SI intervention. Occupational therapy assistants may provide intervention using SI principles with appropriate supervision by an occupational therapist (Miller-Kuhaneck & Smith Roley, 2005).

A. JEAN AYRES

In the 1960s, Dr. A. Jean Ayres (1920–1988), an occupational therapist and educational psychologist, recognized and described hidden disabilities, referring to them as *dysfunction in sensory integrative processes* (Ayres, 1963, 1968) and later as *sensory integrative dysfunction* (Ayres, 2005). Her insights and subsequent theory development were made through keen observation of behavior; review of the neurophysiological underpinnings of behavior; synthesis of literature from neurology, psychology, neurophysiology and education; ongoing research on assessment; and statistical analysis of patterns of dysfunction (Ayres, 1972, 1974) (Figure 59.1).

In 1979, Dr. Ayres published *Sensory Integration and the Child,* a book "to help parents recognize sensory integrative problems in their child, understand what is going on, and do something to help their child" (2005, p. 12). Dr. Ayres anticipated that as our understanding of the central nervous system advanced, our understanding of the neurological basis of sensory integration theory, assessment, and intervention would become more refined. The basic premises of her work stand today. In the 25th Anniversary Edition of *Sensory Integration and the Child: Understanding Hidden Sensory Challenges* (2005), Dr. Ayres is described as a "developmental theorist" (Knox, 2005), a "pioneer in affective neuroscience" (Schneider, 2005), a "pioneer in our understanding of developmental **dyspraxia**" (Cermak, 2005), "one of the original perceptual-motor theorists" (Smith Roley, 2005), and "an astute observer of human behavior and neurological development" (Bauman, 2005). Her work made major inroads into our understanding of clinical neuroscience, the importance of experience in brain development, the role of **tactile defensiveness** and **sensory modulation** disorders as contributors to behavioral disorders, and the impact of **sensory registration** in autism, among others.

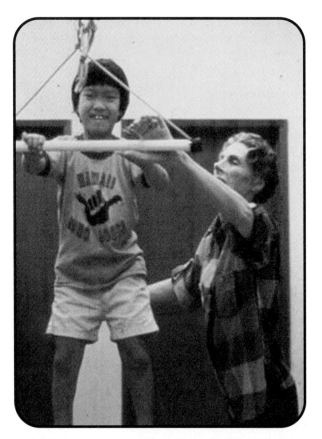

FIGURE 59.1 Dr. Ayres applied her theories through precise evaluation that guided the intervention that is characterized by playful self-motivated motor engagement in sensory activities.

SENSORY INTEGRATION THEORY

Dr. Ayres developed a theory of sensory integration to explain the link between the nervous system and behavior. Five basic assumptions formed the theoretical basis for Dr. Ayres' thinking:

1. The remarkable potential for change of the developing brain, or **neuroplasticity**, which has recently been found to be true of the adult brain as well (for reviews, see Buonomano & Merzenich, 1998; Cruikshank & Weinberger, 1996; Gross, 2000)

2. Interactions between the "higher-order" (cortical) areas of the brain and those in the "lower" subcortical areas as fundamental to adequate sensory integration

3. Neurophysiological development of sensory integrative functions that occur in a natural order and follow a basic sequence

4. An **adaptive response**, which is "the ability to adjust one's action upon environmental demand" (Ayres, 1972, p. 8) and promotes a higher level of integration as a consequence of the **feedback** to the central nervous system

5. Presence of an **inner drive** to meet and master a challenge, which fosters the development of sensory integration

Neuroplasticity

Dr. Ayres' appreciation of the importance of experience as a major determinant of cortical organization and resulting function remains a bedrock principle in the field of neuroscience today. This "experience-dependent plasticity in the cerebral cortex reflects the importance of learning in our mental life and behaviors" (E. K. Miller, 2000, p. 1067). During the period when Dr. Ayres studied neuroplasticity, researchers thought that the brain's ability to be modified was robust during childhood but, after a critical period of development, became quite limited. It is now known that the brain has the capacity to be modified throughout the life course (Bear, Connors, & Paradiso, 2006; Gilbert & Wiesel, 1992).

Organization of the Brain

Although our nervous systems are almost constantly being bombarded by sensation, not all of this sensation reaches the cortex. If the cortex had to process every sensation a person experienced, it would not be able to perform higher-level tasks, such as thought and action. Neuroscientists have long explored the hierarchical organization of the brain. Dr. Ayres understood that higher brain levels, as they develop, remain dependent on lower brain levels (Ayres, 1972, 2004, 2005). Before many of the incoming sensory messages ascend or somewhere along their ascent toward the thalamus and then the cortex, other neurons are acting on them to either dampen their activity (**inhibition**) or, in some cases, enhance their activity (**facilitation**). Dr. Ayres described this process of inhibition and facilitation as a central nervous system process of self-organization (2005). In this way, the subcortical structures are important drivers of the information that higher cortical levels might have to act on.

On the basis of her understanding that perception of any sensory input requires facilitation of some input and inhibition of other input, Dr. Ayres designed intervention that would incorporate these mechanisms and would therefore promote more integrated functioning of the brain as a whole. Using stimuli that have an inhibitory effect and using a task on which the child can focus that elicits an **adaptive response** were proposed by Dr. Ayres as early therapeutic principles to advance central nervous system organization. These principles remain today as core elements of occupational therapy using a sensory integration approach.

To date, there has been no change in our appreciation of the role of the subcortical structures to provide the foundation for efficient functioning. However, there is currently a greater focus on the reciprocal interdependence between higher and lower brain levels (Middleton & Strick, 2000; Wall, Xu, & Wang, 2002). This interplay of activity between the higher-level cortex and subcortical structures (in particular, the thalamus) further contributes to the self-organizing processes of the brain. In this way, the brain is able to develop representations that impart deeper meaning than is provided by the multisensory information alone. For example, suppose we have an object that is orange and round (vision), has a citrus scent (olfaction), and has a slight bumpiness along its surface (tactile); the interplay in the brain contributes to our associating these qualities with an orange.

Dr. Ayres believed that the therapeutic use of appropriate multisensory activities might be the most effective way to promote sensory integration. The research that guided her thinking suggested that there were common integrating sites within the central nervous system where information from separate sensory sources converged onto neurons that had the potential to respond to inputs from multiple sensory sources. These were referred to as "convergent" or "polysensory" neurons and were considered important sites for the coordination of several different types of information (Ayres, 1972). Over the past 25 years, there has been extensive research into cross-modality or multisensory convergence, and findings demonstrate that this process takes place at sites in the midbrain, thalamus, and cortex (for a review, see Stein and Meredith, 1993). At every such site, there is the opportunity for cross-modality or multisensory integration.

One of the best-studied groups of multisensory neurons is in the superior colliculus (SC) (Sparks & Groh, 1995; Stein, 1984; Wallace, Meredith, & Stein, 1993). This midbrain structure is classically divided into superficial layers predominantly containing visual neurons and deep layers containing multisensory (visual, somatosensory, and/or auditory) and premotor neurons. Investigation into the SC has demonstrated how signals from the different senses are combined and used to guide adaptive motor responses, such as hearing a sound and turning to visually locate the source (King & Palmer, 1985; Meredith & Stein, 1986; Stein, Meredith, Huneycutt, & McDade, 1989; Stein, Huneycutt, & Meredith, 1988; Wallace et al., 1993). In this example of the orienting response, when the auditory and visual stimuli occur close together in space and time, their combination enhances the ability to detect and identify the external stimuli. Conversely, cross-modality cues that are significantly discordant (e.g., spatially disparate) can have the opposite effect and depress responses (Stein et al., 1989). Whether the response is enhanced or depressed, an important behavioral consequence of the synthesis (or discordance) of the sensory information is closely related to changes in attention (Stein et al., 1989).

Recent studies by Stein (2005) exploring multisensory integration demonstrate that the cortex plays an important role in mediating convergence of sensory inputs at the level of the superior colliculus. By temporarily deactivating the information flow from the cortex to SC neurons, response enhancement is compromised. As a consequence, the ability to use cross-modal stimuli to enhance SC-mediated behavioral performance is also compromised. As Dr. Ayres suspected and the ongoing research has confirmed, the process of multisensory integration is highly adaptive, "knitting together information from different sensory channels to better detect, identify and react to environmental events. . . . Sensory integration is critical to perception and behavior" (Stein et al., 1989, p. 12).

We have come to recognize that primary sensory pathways, rather than merely transmitting sensation in an inflexible manner, are sending impulses that are constantly being adjusted in relation to attention, arousal, and anticipation as well as thought and planning. Eide notes that "when the sensory system is working effectively, crossmodality improves our responsiveness and interaction with our environment. However, when sensory systems are underactive or overactive (**sensory defensiveness**), attention becomes inappropriately directed or diverted" (2003, pp. 1–2). Eide proposes that therapeutic interventions focused on environmental adaptations and appropriate sensory strategies "are often children's best hope of reducing bodily 'distractions' so that they can focus on learning and socialization" (2003, p. 2).

Over the past two decades, findings from neuroscience research indicate that sensory information (such as that which allows us to perceive an object as an orange) is distributed as serial and parallel streams of information (Felleman & Van Essen, 1991; Pons et al., 1987; for a review, see Mesulam, 1998). Even though this distributed processing model of brain structure and function was not specified at the time, in 1972, Dr. Ayres wrote, "Organization must and does occur vertically among the levels of the brain as well as horizontally between two structures at the same level" (p. 27), demonstrating an understanding of the integrative and reciprocal complexity of the brain. Bundy and Murray (2002) comment that a systems approach to nervous system organization, in which "systems interact, and both cortical and subcortical structures contribute to sensory integration" (p.11), is consistent with Dr. Ayres' theory.

Developmental Progression

Viewing development as a process that the brain undergoes, Dr. Ayres noted that "each child's brain is designed to follow an orderly, predictable, interrelated sequence of development that results in the capacity for learning" (1972, p. 4). Given an enriched, supportive environment, children will grow and develop sensory and motor memories that help the children adapt to their own growth and interests in the context of an ever-changing environment. Whereas Dr. Ayres focused on the first seven years of life as the time frame in which this occurred, we now know that the brain continues to develop throughout the life

course (Bear et al., 2006; Gilbert & Wiesel, 1992). A critical aspect of this process is that the child experience sensations, which places a demand on the brain to organize the incoming stimuli into **percepts**. Depending on the context in which the stimuli are experienced, the child might focus on and attend to the input (**sensory detection** as a central nervous system process; sensory registration as inferred from the child's behavior), or if they are not relevant, the stimuli might be ignored (inhibition centrally, sensory modulation behaviorally) (Lane, Miller, & Hanft, 2000; Miller & Lane, 2000). For example, a child who is riding a bicycle typically attends to visual and auditory inputs along the ride (sensory registration) while ignoring the feel of the shirt as it is blown by the wind (inhibition). If the child's brain is unable to organize incoming sensation efficiently, these "filtering out" and "attending to" processes might be inadequate. In this example, the child who is unable to tolerate the tactile input from the shirt's movement against the body will have difficulty attending to the important visual and auditory information in the environment that are necessary for both safety and skill. Until the tactile sensation is discriminated as "safe," the child is considered to remain in a more primitive "fight-or-flight" mode. In general, this primitive state undermines both the development of skills and emotions as it is through the ability of the brain to organize sensations that "the child gains control over his emotions" (Ayres, 2005, p. 14).

Adaptive Response

Our ability to make adaptive responses to ever-changing environmental demands and challenges allows us to learn something new and, in turn, change the environment (Ayres, 1972, 1979, 2005). Spitzer (1999) discusses the congruence between the concept of self-organization in dynamic systems theory with Dr. Ayres' concept of the adaptive response in sensory integration theory. In both theories, feedback from the individual's spontaneous, active adjustments contributes to self-organization of the brain (Smith & Thelen, 1993; Ayres, 1979, 2005). Dr. Ayres stressed the importance of "organizing adaptive responses to increasing complexity" (1972, p. 128) as a key component of intervention. She was guided by neuroscience research suggesting that inefficiency in **synaptic activity** along anatomical pathways might be contributing to poor integration of sensory information and proposed that focusing on eliciting a response that was not yet well developed might enhance **synaptic function** (Ayres, 1972; Katz & Shatz, 1996; Schlaug, 2001). While an adaptive response occurs most typically during a motor task, it is also apparent with demands arising in other domains (e.g., emotional regulation, cognitive, and social interaction).

"Therapy using a sensory integration approach is a natural process" (Ayres, 2005, p. 140). Dr. Ayres stated that if the child is not able to integrate his or her nervous system successfully in typical environments, "[h]e needs a highly specialized environment, tailor-made for his nervous system" (Ayres, 2005, p. 141). This style of therapy requires that the occupational therapist or occupational therapy assistant design a rich set of sensory-based activities and facilitate the child's self-organization and physical engagement with the environment. While classic intervention using sensory integration is provided in a carefully designed clinic setting (Parham & Mailloux, 2005), sensory integration principles and activities can be adapted to be used in a variety of sensory-based activities in natural settings such as at home or at school (Pediatric Therapy Network, 2004). It is difficult to use SI interventions, however, if the child does not have room to safely move, jump, and crash or cannot rearrange the objects to interact in novel ways.

Inner Drive

A child cannot be forced to self-organize or to generate an adaptive response. Rather, it is the drive for mastery or the motivation to explore that elicits in the individual the willingness to participate. "Organizing and evincing an adaptive response which is more mature and complex than any emitted before requires effort—the kind of effort that a child gladly summons when he is emotionally involved in the task and believes he can cope with it" (Ayres, 1972, p. 127). Embedded in this statement are two important concepts of intervention. One is the concept of the "**just-right challenge**," whereby the task is beyond what the child is already capable of achieving yet is maximally demanding to promote central nervous system integration. The other concept is the child-led nature of SI-based intervention, during which the therapist allows the child the freedom to choose and engage in activities as long as they are appropriately challenging, foster increasingly complex adaptive behaviors, and generally further the development of sensory integration (Stein & Meredith, 1993; Stein, 1998).

SENSORY INTEGRATION AND OCCUPATION

Sensory integration is fundamental to interpreting information from the environment and for learning. Dr. Ayres defined sensory integration as "the neurological process that organizes sensations from one's body and from the environment and makes it possible to use the body effectively in the environment" (2004, p. 9). Sensation is used to guide an individual's engagement with people and objects in the environment, in other words, to engage in needed and desired occupations (Figures 59.2 and 59.3). Table 59.1 lists the functions of the different sensory systems.

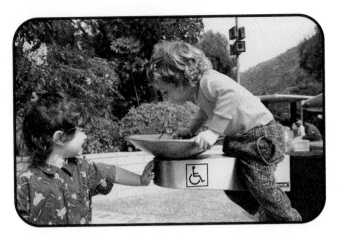

FIGURE 59.2 Children need a variety of experiences to learn how to use their bodies in novel ways; balance, adjust, and coordinate their actions with the way things feel; and come up with new ways to interact with the environment. Interacting cooperatively with other people might require the most adaptive responses of all these skills.

OCCUPATIONAL THERAPY USING SENSORY INTEGRATION PRINCIPLES

The sensory integration frame of reference consists of three interrelated components of occupational therapy practice:

1. Application of theoretical concepts supporting evidence-based practice
2. Assessment tools to assess the sensory integrative functions in individuals, such as:
   - **The Sensory Integration and Praxis Tests** (SIPT) (Ayres, 1989), a series of 17 standardized tests designed to assess sensory discrimination and praxis including visual perception, visual motor skills, **vestibular** functions, **proprioception**, tactile discrimination, fine and gross motor skills, and praxis
   - Measures of sensory processing, particularly modulation, such as the Sensory Profile (Brown & Dunn, 2002; Dunn, 1999, 2002a, 2002b), Sensory Processing Measure (SPM)—Home (Parham & Johnson-Ecker, 2007), SPM School Editions (Miller-Kuhaneck, Henry, & Glennon, 2007) [portions previously published as the Evaluation of Sensory Processing (Johnson-Ecker & Parham, 2000)], and questionnaires completed by the caregivers that indicate a child's sensitivity and responsiveness to various sensations and sensory situations
   - Clinical observations of neuromotor functions, praxis, and play (Blanche, 2002; Windsor, Smith Roley, & Szklut, 2001), a series of structured and unstructured observations that include classic neuromotor abilities, sensory responsiveness, and **motor planning** abilities

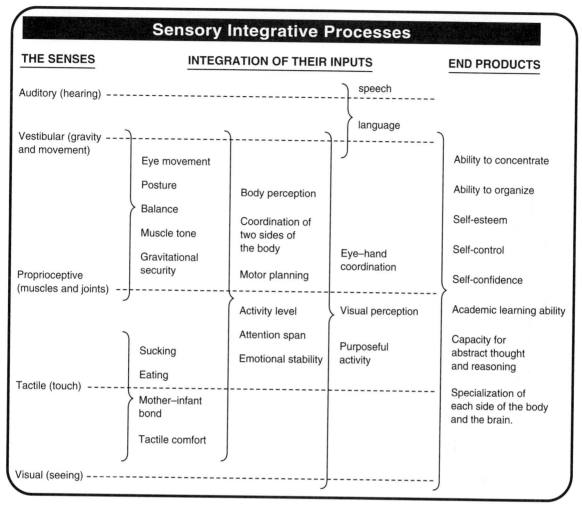

FIGURE 59.3   Ayres' flowchart. *The Senses, Integration of Their Inputs, End Products* copyright (c) 1979 by Western Psychological Services. Reprinted by permission of the publisher, WPS, 12031 Wilshire Boulevard, Los Angeles, CA 90025, www.wpspublish.com No additional reprinting without WPS's prior, written authorization. All rights reserved.

3. Intervention strategies (Bundy, Lane, & Murray, 2002; Koomar & Bundy, 2002; Smith Roley, Blanche, & Schaaf, 2001)

IDENTIFYING SENSORY INTEGRATION DYSFUNCTION

Dr. Ayres analyzed test scores and clinical observations of children with learning disabilities to empirically identify patterns of dysfunction (Ayres, 1974, 1989). Later, Mulligan (1998a, 1998b, 2000) conducted confirmatory factor and cluster analyses that supported Dr. Ayres' original patterns of dysfunction. Consequently, the strongest research in sensory integration is in the identification of the types and patterns of sensory integration dysfunction using the Sensory Integration and Praxis Tests (Ayres, 1989; Mulligan, 1998a, 1998b, 2000). Various types and patterns of sensory processing dysfunction continue to be

examined (Ayres & Tickle, 1980; Brown & Dunn, 2002; Dunn, 1999, 2002a, 2002b; Miller, McIntosh, McGrath, Shyu, Lampe, & Taylor, 1999; Miller & Summers, 2001). These studies suggest that sensory integrative dysfunction is not a single disorder but a spectrum of disorders (Parham & Mailloux, 2005) related to the following processes.

Sensory Modulation

Dr. Ayres (1979, 2005) proposed that the "combination of facilitatory and inhibitory messages produces modulation, which is the nervous system's process of self-organization" (2005, p. 36). Sensory modulation disorder is one type of SI dysfunction characterized by fluctuating or extremes in the responsiveness to the intensity of one or more sensations. Difficulties with sensory modulation are often observed during everyday activities such as grooming, social events, or transitions. Specific behaviors may include **auditory hypersensitivity or tactile defensiveness, gravita-**

TABLE 59.1   FUNCTIONS OF SPECIFIC SENSORY SYSTEMS

FUNCTIONS OF THE:

Vestibular System	Proprioceptive System	Tactile System	Visual System	Auditory System	Olfactory and Gustatory Systems
Detects gravity Detects head position and movement Modulates postural tone Head/neck/ eye control Righting and equilibrium reactions Auditory connections for spatial orientation Arousal regulation	Provides sensations for **body scheme,** body concept Essential for precisely graded movement Interacts with vestibular system for postural control Interacts with the tactile system for finely graded movements	Emotional development Body scheme Skills associated with: Tactile perception Motor planning Sequencing Organization Visual perception	Bonding Spatial orientation Movement through space Social skills Communication	Language development Sound modulation Spatial orientation	Caregiver-infant bonding Protection from noxious substances Attraction to potentially nurturing substances

tional insecurity, aversion to movement, or feeling overwhelmed in high-stimulus environments such as shopping malls (Koomar, 1995; Weisberg, 1984). Sensory modulation disorders are seen in conjunction with arousal, external regulation, or **self-regulation** issues, including colic and poor rhythmic respiration, digestion, and elimination; arousal and attention deficits; hyperactivity; anxiety and other signs of emotional instability; and social problems (DeGangi, 2000; DeGangi & Greenspan, 1988; Schaaf & Anzalone, 2001; Schaaf, Miller, Seewal, & O'Keefe, 2003; Williamson & Anzalone, 2001; see also Chapter 59).

Sensory Discrimination

Sensory discrimination is the interpretation of sensory information that allows you to know efficiently and accurately where your body is, where other people are, and details about the environment from multiple sensory channels. Sensory discrimination disorders are a result of slow and inaccurate processing of one or more types of sensory information, **underresponsiveness** to sensation, inadequate perception formation, and poor sensory associations. Patterns of dysfunction that have been identified through factor and cluster analyses indicate that poor vestibular proprioceptive processing is often associated with poor anticipatory and reactive **postural control** and inadequate

bilateral integration and sequencing. Tactile discrimination deficits are often associated with poor fine motor skills and praxis. It is as if the child is trying to do precise work with his or her hands while wearing winter gloves. Visual perceptual deficits are associated with poor visual **construction ability** and visual motor skills. Auditory perceptual deficits often contribute to poor auditory language skills.

Praxis

Praxis is the ability to conceptualize, plan, and execute skilled tasks. It underlies engagement in purposeful activity. Any nonhabitual motor task that the child needs to think through requires praxis. The child who is learning how to dive needs to stand at the water's edge, get the arms in position over the head, shift the weight forward, tuck the chin against the chest, and then maintain this position as he or she falls head first into the water. All of this requires cognitive effort as well as physical coordination. Dr. Ayres (1972) hypothesized that sensory discrimination, particularly of tactile, vestibular, and proprioceptive sensations along with visual input, was the foundation for praxis. The resulting sensation from the activity is processed by the brain, and this further informs individuals about their body in relation to itself as well as to other people and objects in the environment (Ayres, 1989, 2004). Through her factor analyses, she later found a consistent relationship, particularly between the tactile system and praxis.

There are a variety of different types of praxis disorders, including poor ideation of creative or novel activities (e.g., the child in the sandbox who shovels sand into the pail and then pours it out and repeats the process but does not come up with the idea that she can "make a cake" by filling the pail with sand and then turning the pail over to form a mound that she can then decorate); **somatodyspraxia**, or poor use of the body to motor plan action sequences; poor use of language for sequencing and planning; poor ability to modify an action while in motion to enhance skill and precision; poor visual construction (e.g., difficulty replicating a block design); and poor ability to organize behavior in future time and space. Conceptualizing an action, or forming the idea about *what* one wants to do, is a critical aspect of praxis. This is **ideation**, and it is a cognitive function (May-Benson, 2001). Planning *how* one intends to engage in the task is also cognitive. A child observing a newly constructed playground with swings, slides, tree house, poles, and sand will have 101 ideas about what to do and will want to do them all. The actual execution of the activity is the part of praxis that we can observe, and this is the part that is assessed to determine a child's skill for motor tasks. The child then sequences these ideas into swinging, sliding, and digging activities and modifies the sequence or the challenge so that it is more fun and successful.

ASSESSMENT

The process of sensory integration cannot be observed directly, which is why Dr. Ayres used the term "hidden disabilities" when referring to SI dysfunction (Ayres, 2005).

CASE STUDY: *Larissa: A 3-Year-Old Girl Not Interested in Play with Others*

Referral

Larissa is an energetic 3-year-old girl who loves to play but does not seek out play with other children. She does not seem to mind them, but she is happy playing alone or alongside others. She has good attachment to her mother and relies on her for guidance and nurturing, which her mother readily and effectively provides. Larissa is happiest if she is close to her mother day and night. Household routines are difficult for the family. Larissa loves to take a bath and often does not want to get out. Larissa does not want to stop playing to do general hygiene tasks, making routine activities such as tooth brushing difficult. Errands, shopping, or spontaneous outings are problematic, as Larissa is overly active and tires easily when she has to stand in line or wait. Larissa's mother has learned to give her three children time to prepare for transitions; otherwise, Larissa or one of her older brothers, ages five and eight, might have a tantrum.

Larissa's mother requested an occupational therapy evaluation to determine whether services were available that provided assistance with parenting and to support her child's development. She reported that her life was very difficult. She had always had difficulty organizing herself, but now with three children and a husband, she sometimes felt that her life was unmanageable. She decided to focus on services for the youngest child first but felt that all of her children and herself needed assistance to varying degrees.

Occupational Profile:

When asked what Larissa likes to do during the day, her mother replied:

"If I'm not in the room when she wakes up, she will cry or whine "Mommy" until I come in. She then wants to nurse until she is completely awake. I usually carry her downstairs, and she starts playing with little toys. It's a little hard to stop playing, but she usually climbs into her chair for breakfast and eats neatly. When she's done, she sometimes puts her hands in her warm cereal and smears it on herself, the table, her head . . . and has a good time with it. She likes to touch everything wherever we go. She *loves* to play out back with water, dirt, and mud. She usually gets herself all wet with the hose and has several changes of clothes a day. She likes to play in the sand, lie in the sand with her face in the sand, and eat the sand. She loves the bath, but I usually have to take her out early for hitting her brothers or pouring water out of the tub. Then she screams, cries, and tries to get back in the bath. Eventually, she calms down and lies down or jumps on the bed. She never wants to put her clothes on, but when she is very tired, she will."

The therapist determined that Larissa's high activity level, anxiety, and sensory-seeking behaviors were interfering with her ability to cope with and engage in typical daily occupations. Additionally, her behaviors created situations in which her mother was unable to carry out her own daily activities without upset, contributing to family stress. The therapist recommended intervention and requested that a standardized evaluation using the Sensory Integration and Praxis Tests be completed in approximately one year when Larissa was old enough, in order to have standardized measures of her abilities. Her scores indicate a subtle but significant problem in sensory integration (Figure 59.4).

Analysis of Occupational Performance:

Larissa is an intelligent child who has subtle difficulties with vestibular-proprioceptive processing that affect fine motor skill development and **bilateral motor coordination**, age-appropriate social play, self-organization, and self-regulation. This may become more pronounced when she is expected to function independently and pay attention and engage in skilled tasks in high-stimulus social environments.

CASE INFORMATION

Child's first name: __Larissa__

Child's age: __3 years 2 months__

Child's year in school: __pre-K__

Parent/guardian(s) name: _____

EVALUATION

Reasons for referral (include the occupational concerns/desires for the child and family):
Clingy, tantrums easily, fights with siblings, difficulty taking her to grocery store, not interested in playing with other children.

Background Information

Medical history: OK

Developmental history: Normal milestones. Concerns regarding balance, activity level, self-regulation, and social skills

Educational history: N/A

Occupational history/profile: see above narrative

Evaluation of Occupational Performance

Interview Data

- ◆ Teacher report:
- ◆ Guardian Report:
  See above
- ◆ Others:

Observation Data

Strengths:
Bright
Affectionate
Good attachment with parents
Good fine motor
Enjoys tactile play

Challenges:
Does not seek interactions with other
  children
Sensitivity to sounds
Excessively seeks tactile play
Poor interactions with other children
Inattention to task
Poor sustained sitting
Difficulty adapting to transitions and
  high stimulus environments

Test Data

Structured assessments:
See SIPT scores

Unstructured assessment:
Mildly low muscle tone
Difficulty imitating movement
  sequences

Interpretation:
Vestibular and bilateral integration
  and sequencing issues

INTERVENTION

Goals and Objectives

By (date): To demonstrate improved fine motor and self-care skills, Larissa will use two hands to independently don and doff socks and shoes when given minimal physical assistance, 4/5 opportunities.

OT Intervention Plan

Includes the following:

Setting:
Specialized clinic 2x/wk

Duration:
6 months with reevaluation at that
  time to determine the need for
  further therapy

*OT Intervention Process
and Strategies*

Therapeutic Activities:
In the process of play include:
Vigorous swinging using flexion
  swing, platform swing.

Continued

INTERVENTION

Goals and Objectives

By (date): To demonstrate improved organization of behavior during social interactions, Larissa will engage in play with another child, for 10 minutes of turn-taking interaction when given no more than 3 prompts, 4/5 opportunities.

By (date): To demonstrate improved balance and postural/protective reactions for increased preschool participation, Larissa will execute smooth and efficient movement patterns with her trunk and upper extremities (imitating motions to songs, etc.) while maintaining a cross-legged sitting posture on the floor for 5 minutes with minimal verbal and/or visual prompting, 4/5 opportunities.

OT Intervention Plan

Discharge plan:

Create an enriched sensory environment in the home and at school with a sensory diet in place that is adjusted as needed or at least every 6 months.

Referrals:

Psychoeducational testing

OT Intervention Process and Strategies

Therapeutic activities:

A variety of textures along with vibration toys and messy materials

Stereognosis games

Static and dynamic balance activities

Obstacle courses that include gross motor sequences

Environmental Modifications:

Provide picture/word schedule of daily routines

Provide swinging equipment in the home

Enrich the tactile play by including interactive and shape or object-identifying games

Mobile seating devices such as a peanut ball during mealtimes

OUTCOMES

Expected or Reported Outcomes

◆ Occupational Performance: Improve social skills, dressing skills, grooming activities, and participation in daily events without emotional outbursts

◆ Client Satisfaction: Mother report on usefulness of the information and strategies provided by the OT/OTA

◆ Adaptability/Generalized Skills: Improve tolerance to outings that include shopping, increased harmony in home due to acceptance of routine and changes in routine

◆ Impact on Family Life (including the occupations of other family members): Mother report of improved life satisfaction, stress reduction, improved coping, and improved organization

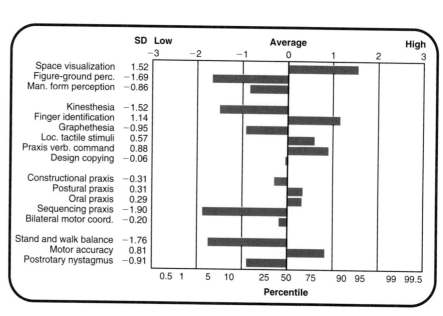

FIGURE 59.4 Larissa's SIPT scores at age five.

The therapist must rely on information from interviews, direct observations and structured and unstructured assessments of skills and abilities related to occupational performance in order to understand the way in which the individual is processing information (Windsor et al., 2001).

INTERVENTION PLANNING

Occupational therapy using a sensory integrative approach is guided by the evaluation data. On the basis of the information from the occupational profile, the therapist considers the identified occupationally related outcomes that are important to the client, the family, and the reimbursement agency. The analysis of performance provides detailed information on client factors, performance skills, and patterns that contribute to the development of client-directed interventions, therapeutic activities, and environmental modifications. Additionally, education and consultation are required so that the team understands the relationship of the child's sensory integrative functions to participation in daily life activities.

Therapeutic activities to address the identified deficits are designed with specific attention to the contribution of the tactile, proprioceptive, and vestibular sensations to function (Figures 59.5, 59.6, and 59.7).

- ◆ Special consideration is given to including proprioception in the form of active movement and heavy work activities. Proprioception exerts a regulatory influence on other sensations (Blanche & Schaaf, 2001).
- ◆ Vestibular activities are especially important so that the child can develop the capacity to hold the body upright against gravity while holding still and while moving (Ayres, 1972). Processing vestibular information is important for the development of the sense of space and navigation (Berthoz, 2000).
- ◆ Tactile information is essential for refined interactions with the external social and physical environment (Ayres, 1972, 2005; Montegue, 1986).

Tables 59.2, 59.3, and 59.4 provide information on the various considerations that should be used in grading sensory-based activities.

INTERVENTION

Central to intervention using sensory integration principles is a unique philosophy that reflects Dr. Ayres' sense of trust, compassion, and respect for children (Spitzer & Smith Roley, 2001). She proposed that intervention delivered in a playful style at the child's level could elicit the child's "inner drive" to learn and develop. In this way,

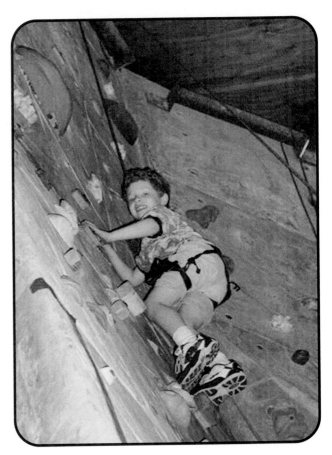

FIGURE 59.5   Rock climbing is a proprioceptive activity that requires muscular exertion, body awareness, and resisting the pull of gravity to help the climber stay organized and alert while concentrating on foot and hand placement.

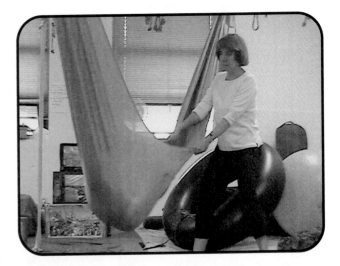

FIGURE 59.6   Swings provide multisensory play opportunities that are both calming and alerting by providing deep pressure, vestibular sensations, and the opportunity for increased proprioceptive awareness.

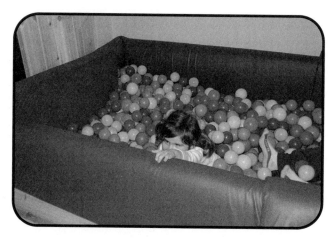

FIGURE 59.7   Playing in a ball pit provides transient deep pressure tactile sensations and resistance to movement, increasing the child's body awareness.

we facilitate enhanced neuronal growth and development that lead to increased skill and independence in daily life activities (Ayres, 1972). The therapeutic environment designed by Dr. Ayres was unique in its ability to safely provide opportunities for vestibular, proprioceptive, and tactile sensations and adaptive motor responses. She used simple and readily available objects such as tires, ropes, wood, hula hoops, and rocker boards and created unusual obstacle courses and games with them. She used ceiling beams and devices so that she could suspend equipment that allowed the child to swing safely through space. She invented this equipment as the need arose for individual clients.

Although a clinic filled with ceiling hooks, swings, mats, carpeted barrels, scooter boards, ramps, and pillows is commonly associated with pediatric occupational therapy using "classic" SI intervention methods, the environment alone is not sufficient to define intervention using sensory integration theory. Dr. Ayres described not only the environment, but also what might be considered the therapeutic alliance. Parham and her colleagues (2007) report that intervention using sensory integration principles should be faithful to the methods and principles that are considered essential and distinctive to this particular therapeutic method. The authors examined the literature and gathered expert opinion to specify the essential and distinctive sensory integration methods and principles. By using these principles, a therapist is demonstrating **fidelity** to the intervention. Classic SI intervention comprises both structural processes (e.g., length of the session, therapist's training, equipment used) and therapeutic processes (e.g., therapist creates an environment that invites play and ensures safety, fosters a therapeutic alliance). Establishing fidelity helps to clearly delineate the qualities that must be present to define the intervention as sensory integration, and for the practitioner, it clearly articulates the specific strategies and process that are linked to an underlying theoretical base and supporting evidence.

TABLE 59.2   VARIABLES RELATED TO VESTIBULAR SENSATIONS

Client Factors	Types of Vestibular Sensations	Environmental Condition
Head Position Prone Supine Upright Standing Quadruped Head tilted Side lying Inverted	Linear (vertical and horizontal) Rotary (around in circles) Axial (around the body) Orbital (in an axis outside of the body) Arc Coreolis (three types at once)	**Visual Field** Stable Moving
Head Movement Static Transient In motion		
Body Status Static Moving Passive Active	Speed, intensity Duration, rhythmicity Stop and start Changes in direction	**Physical Environment** Stable Moving

TABLE 59.3   VARIABLES RELATED TO PROPRIOCEPTIVE SENSATIONS

Client Factors	Types of Proprioceptive Sensations	Environmental Condition
Muscles	Stretch	Distance/size/dimension
Tendons	Traction—pull	With or against gravity
Joints	Compression—push	Time
At rest	Coactivation—cocontraction	Physical environment
Transient	Isometric/isotonic	Stable
In motion	Speed, intensity	Moving
Static/dynamic	Duration/rate/rhythm	
Active/passive	Direction	
Effort exerted	Resistance	
Motivation or purpose	Tension/weight-bearing load	

Hallmark Features of Intervention Using Sensory Integration

Intervention using SI should include the following:

◆ A qualified therapist with an understanding of the neurobiological principles of sensory integration theory and its methods. Postgraduate certification in sensory integration is available for occupational therapists, speech and language therapists, and physical therapists only.

◆ The use of sensory opportunities that feature varied and appropriate vestibular, tactile, and proprioceptive sensations, including thick mats, large overstuffed pillows, swings, ramps, ladders, ropes, targets, manipulatives, balls, vibrating toys, various textures such as stretchy soft or furry fabrics, brushes, props, and materials that are used during daily routines.

◆ Opportunities to move through space so that the child can achieve increasingly complex somatomotor adaptive responses.

◆ The therapist's scaffolding of success emotionally, physically, cognitively, and socially.

◆ Facilitating the just-right challenge: The therapist collaborates with the child on choice and sequence of activities and equipment and adjusts the intervention accordingly to ensure success.

◆ Providing **environmental affordances** (the opportunities that the environment affords children to do things)

TABLE 59.4   VARIABLES RELATED TO TACTILE SENSATIONS

Client Factors	Types of Tactile Sensations	Environmental Condition
Head	Light touch	Familiar versus unfamiliar object
Face including cheeks, mouth, tongue, and ears	Deep pressure	Familiar versus unfamiliar person
Hands	Texture	Intensity of other stimuli in the environment
Feet	Temperature	Task demands
Limbs	Sharp/dull/pain/numbness	Intention of person touching
Front	One- and two-point	Time of day
Back		Cultural norms
*Avoid ventral midline		
While stressed or relaxed (existing arousal level and arousability)	Transient	
Amount of surface area	Sustained	
Anticipated versus expected	Intermittent	
Unanticipated versus unexpected	Duration	
Self versus other initiated	Rhythm	
Prior experiences	Frequency	

that invite interactions with the environment, including space to move, jump, and crash and items that stimulate creativity and engagement.

♦ Assisting in organization of behavior relative to physically interacting with objects and people in time and space, including the opportunity to rearrange the environment and the way in which it is used (Parham et al., 2007).

Guiding Principles of the Actual Intervention

Intervention based on sensory integration theory is *child-directed*. This concept has often been misunderstood. It does not mean that there is no structure. Rather, it means that the therapist vigilantly observes the child to understand the child's current capabilities, structures the activities around the child's interests and abilities, and engages the child by eliciting his or her *intrinsic motivation* to play. Sensory integration methods are provided in the *context of play,* and the therapist, who is inviting the child's *active participation,* is focused on the desired outcome of an *adaptive response.* "When the therapist is doing her job effectively and the child is organizing his nervous system, it looks as if the child is merely playing" (Ayres, 2005, p. 142).

Basic Tenets of Sensory Integration

Following are the classic principles of intervention using a sensory integration approach:

♦ *Integrated sensation* is "nourishment for the brain" (Ayres, 1979).
♦ *Adaptive responses* are required to successfully meet challenges essential for growth and development (Ayres, 1972). The adaptive response is essential to increased sensory integration.
♦ The *inner drive* of the human being invites the experience of life. It is this motivation to enjoy life that Dr. Ayres wished to engage during intervention.
♦ *Active participation* promotes organization.
♦ *Artful vigilance* is essential on the part of the therapist to facilitate the just-right challenge.

When using sensory integration intervention strategies, the practitioner will provide a balance of structure and freedom so that the child has opportunities to problem-solve and make some of his or her own choices. Some essential characteristics that differentiate sensory integration methods from other frames of reference are freedom within the structure of a sensory-rich environment, the ability to physically move through space and move objects in space, and the assistance of the practitioner so that the child can learn to use his or her body in new and novel ways so that increasingly complex possibilities for physical engagement emerge. Sensory integration is not sensory stimulation, due to the imperative of the adaptive response

and modification of the activity based on the child's reaction (Anzalone & Murray, 2002). It is not adult planned and designed; rather, the adult sets up the structure and possibilities in which the child's interests and ability to cope with the sensory, motor, and organization demands dictate the level of challenge and intensity of the activities. Therefore, the equipment does not stay in the same place each time, and the therapy does not follow an orderly and predictable sequence, so each session is somewhat novel. The intervention is not provided with the expectation of a subsequent reward. The activities are intended to be fun and inviting and therefore are rewarding in and of themselves. Play is one of the most important and powerful parts of the process of intervention using sensory integration strategies and one that facilitates the intrinsic reward of this kind of occupational engagement (Bundy, 2002).

Sensory integrative dysfunction commonly occurs in children with diagnoses such as autism, fragile X syndrome, and cerebral palsy. These children will benefit from a variety of approaches in addition to sensory integration methods (Mailloux, 2001; Mailloux & Smith Roley, 2004; Schaaf & Smith Roley, 2006; Smith Roley et al., 2001). During a typical occupational therapy session, sensory integration methods are often used in conjunction with complementary methods such as neurodevelopmental treatment (Blanche, Botticelli, & Hallway, 1995), play-based approaches (Burke & Mailloux, 1997; Knox & Mailloux, 1997), developmental and behavioral approaches (Anzalone & Murray, 2002), and cognitive approaches such as the Alert Program for Self-Regulation (Williams & Shellenberger, 1996). This is especially true for children with multiple impairments.

GOALS OF OCCUPATIONAL THERAPY USING SENSORY INTEGRATION STRATEGIES

Sensory integration principles applied within occupational therapy practice results in improved occupational engagement and social participation (Figure 59.8).

To accomplish the overarching goals of occupational therapy, sensory integration strategies are used to facilitate adaptive responses in various domains. In addition to the somatomotor adaptive response described by Ayres (1972), Parham & Mailloux (2005, p. 393) identified the following expected goals as a result of intervention using SI that could be used as outcome measures:

♦ Increase in the frequency or duration of adaptive responses
♦ Cognitive, language, and academic skills
♦ Gross and fine motor skills
♦ Self confidence and self-esteem
♦ Enhanced occupational performance and social participation
♦ Enhanced family life

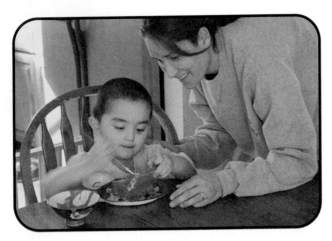

FIGURE 59.8 Following vigorous play, this child more easily engages in this activity with his mother that involves tactile media, spatial organization, and visual motor control.

The diverse array of possibilities makes it difficult to predict exactly the areas of life that may change as a result of intervention using sensory integration strategies (Mailloux et al., 2007). Traditionally, evaluations of the effectiveness of pediatric occupational therapy intervention have focused on performance skills such as improved handwriting or improved balance or ball skills. These measures are not sufficient to capture the potential change in an individual's quality of life. Reports from parents include comments such as the following:

"My life is easier."
"My child now has friends."
"I can actually cook dinner without disruption."
"My kids play together longer without needing me to intervene."
"I feel like I am brave enough to try a family vacation."

" Occupational therapy is the first place I've been where I feel like they understood what I'm going through."
"It is nice to see someone playing with my child, and it showed me another way to view my child in a more positive light."

Cohn, Miller, & Tickle-Degnen (2000) found that the outcomes identified by parents of children receiving services included those that support the child's participation in typical contexts and the way in which the child affects parenting and family life. In this study, the parents reported that they wanted strategies that supported and validated their parenting skills in addition to helping their child achieve increased social participation, self-regulation, and competence. In a subsequent study, Cohn (2001a, 2001b) found that parents valued an improved understanding of their child's behavior as well as the validation of their parenting efforts and being able to advocate for services for their children. She identified that the ritual of waiting for their children in the waiting room at the clinic site afforded the parents the opportunity to share resources, validate their experiences, and engage in social dialogue with others. In fact, this experience helped to reframe their views of their children. This work broadens the potential outcomes related to occupational therapy using a sensory integrative approach.

While structured and unstructured observations of occupational performance continue to be valid ways to measure progress, for certain children such as those with autism the progress will never approach normal development. Mailloux and colleagues (2007) propose that the method of Goal Attainment Scaling (GAS) might serve as a useful method to measure achievement. GAS is a method of setting achievable goals in conjunction with the family that may prove to be useful in capturing significant changes as the result of intervention.

CASE STUDY: *Todd: A 6-Year-Old-Boy Referred for a Developmental Evaluation*

Referral

Todd is a 6-year-old boy who was referred for a developmental evaluation because of difficulties with behavior and attention at school.

Occupational Profile

Todd's mother reported that as an infant, Todd liked being held. When he woke up at night, he had to be walked around because he did not calm easily just by having someone lie down with him. His motor skills were typical, although he used to bump into things and get hurt a lot, especially when his head was at the same height as the doorknob. She describes him as a quiet, happy child who is

easily frustrated and resistant to change. He likes to do things slowly and carefully. He likes to play with others once he knows them. When he is in a bad mood, it is hard to get him to recover. When he is frustrated, he loses his temper and sometimes hits or digs his nails into someone.

When asked about a typical day, Todd's mother provided the following narrative:

"He wakes up between 6 and 7 A.M. and starts playing with his older brother. Sometimes he wets the bed; otherwise, he wets the bed while playing. I try to prevent that by taking him to the bathroom, but he talks nonstop, and I have to yell to get him to hear me. He gets a reward for going to the bathroom. I get his sandals before he comes down, but he's too busy playing to remember or listen to me. I usually pull him downstairs and try

CASE STUDY: *Todd: A 6-Year-Old-Boy Referred for a Developmental Evaluation* *Continued*

to get him to sit in the chair. He wants macaroni and cheese every morning for breakfast. He uses his fingers instead of his fork to eat, but when I remind him, he uses it a little. He spills a lot of food on the table and keeps moving around and falling out of his chair. I open a book in front of him on the table, and he starts reading and stops moving around so much. He's still a messy eater. He is happy playing by himself. The kids put their clothes on the night before so they don't have to get dressed in the morning. After playing outside and pulling on the plants, I finally get him into the car and drive 5 minutes to school. He says he is tired, cold, and bored and won't leave my side. He wanders around a little watching the other kids but not joining in or talking to anyone except maybe adults or little kids. He doesn't seem to hear when anyone calls his name. He is usually the last child to leave class when school is over. I often get calls that his stomach hurts, and after school, he is so sad he only wants to go home. He usually doesn't eat lunch but will eat dinner. After we go upstairs to get ready for bed, he sometimes gets very wild. I lie down with him, but he starts fidgeting, and eventually I leave and he gets back up out of bed."

Todd was referred for an occupational therapy evaluation to assess his development and determine the need for occupational therapy services. His mother described him as a loving child who just seems not to know what to do with himself. He constantly asks how to do something and wants his mother to show him. He will follow others and tends to play best with younger children (Figure 59.9).

Analysis of Occupational Performance

Todd is a bright, active, engaging little boy who has strengths in visual perception, fundamental motor skills, language, and cognition. He specifically demonstrated difficulty in discrim-

inating vestibular-proprioceptive information and using that information rapidly, efficiently, and accurately; this impairs his ability to sort out everything that is going around him and figure out how to respond quickly. Todd's difficulties with vestibular-proprioceptive processing are interfering with ocular motor skills, focus (especially in busy environments), balance when an activity requires anticipating a postural adjustment to maintain balance or reacting to an unexpected postural change, and organization of actions, especially during transitions and social situations. He has difficulty in motor planning and organizing his materials. Although his sensory integrative problems significantly affect his development, they are not sufficient to explain all of his difficulties with social interactions and self-regulation.

Intervention Planning

Occupational therapy using sensory integration was recommended for two 60-minute sessions per week in the home and community settings. Specific activities were designed for Todd to engage in throughout his daily routine that included tactile activities combined with vestibular and proprioceptive activities to improve praxis and spatial awareness. Additional methods were incorporated to enhance his ability to participate more easily in daily routines without feeling sad or being disruptive.

Intervention

The occupational therapist scheduled consultations with the parents and the educational staff. In response to the evaluation results and the consultation, two separate

Continued

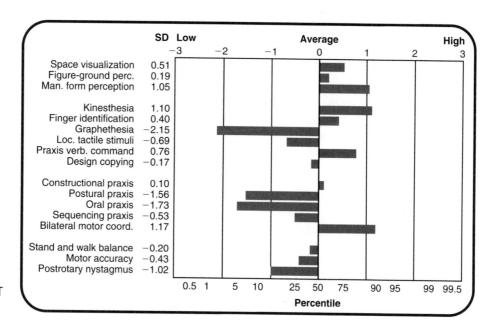

FIGURE 59.9 Todd's SIPT scores at age six.

programs were developed: sensory-based modifications for the home and a sensory diet for the classroom. The therapist monitored Todd's reactions to the program to ensure that he was more organized and performed better. The occupational therapist provided direct service with consultation on a regular basis. The occupational therapist scheduled a reevaluation at the end of 6 months to ensure that Todd was making progress and to determine the need for continued intervention services.

For the home, the therapist worked with Todd to develop picture and word schedules of daily routines that included dressing, meal preparation, and clean-up and bedtime rituals. Todd posted them in the appropriate room and negotiated with his parents the times when they were to be done. He made a book with pictures of self-regulatory strategies that included high-intensity physical activities; tactile play; swinging; jumping; and building with pillows, blankets, and cushions. He also included activities such as drinking a warm glass of milk, taking a walk, reading a book, and asking his father for a wrestling match, a piggyback ride, or a foot massage. His parents broke down activities that required sequencing, such as shoe tying, so that he could learn the steps; they then provided other opportunities with tying ribbons and laces so that he could generalize the skill. Resources for additional information were provided (Ayres, 2005; Ayres, Erwin, & Mailloux, 2004; Coleman, Mailloux, & Smith Roley, 2005; Williams & Shellenberger, 2001).

The home environment was modified in the following ways: Todd's mother created a Lycra™ hammock that he could sleep in at night. She also provided flannel sheets and a heavy comforter with big pillows for his bed. She put an old mattress on the floor of his bedroom so that he could jump. A swing was attached to a beam on the back porch so that he could swing before school, before meals, and an hour before bedtime. His mother set aside soap foam and various brushes and textured toys to play with in the bath, including cups and soap crayons. He was given a battery-operated toothbrush. His parents were taught strategies for calming and for alerting and determined the times in his day when he would get more physical activity and active play and how much time was needed afterward with inhibitory activities for him to calm down and pay attention or sleep. To help him discriminate better tactually, a variety of tactile games were created, such as a memory box that he had to reach into and, without looking, find familiar objects that were buried in dried rice and beans.

For the classroom, the teacher, parents of other children in the class, and the teaching assistant were provided a short in-service focusing on appropriate expectations in planning and organization for first graders. Included was information on how to determine whether there were sensory integration problems such as developmental dyspraxia. Strategies to help children develop and follow through on typical daily routines were included that could be applied to all the children in the class, including beginning time management strategies. Also included were the concepts related to **information processing** and sensory motor development that contribute to the development of praxis skills. An emphasis was placed on the need for a balance between sedentary and active tasks. Discussion of research on the benefits of recess was included (Jarrett, 2002; Pellegrini, 1993).

The classroom was a creative kindergarten with several simultaneous activities and children moving about the class throughout the day. Todd's teacher created a picture schedule and allowed him a quiet area with pillows to which he could retreat when overwhelmed or if he needed to complete his work. He was provided a peanut ball and an inflated cushion that he could use to sit on if he chose. He had a sensory box that included a variety of tactile and proprioceptive activities that he could use as long as he was not disruptive. He was allowed to take movement breaks outside in which he could run to the water fountain and back, do 25 jumping jacks, or ride on a Playskool Sit 'N Spin located directly outside the classroom as long as he returned within five minutes to do his class work.

The teacher soon found that these strategies were beneficial to many children in her classroom and that some children needed them more than others. Along with other valuable information on sensory integration, the therapist gave the teacher the article on the use of mobile seating devices with children with attention problems (Schilling, Washington, Billingsley, & Deitz, 2003). The teacher adapted her room so that children could have these choices and reported to the occupational therapist that this had dramatically reduced the time she spent correcting behavior (Bissell, Fisher, Owens, & Polcyn, 1998; Coleman, Mailloux, & Smith Roley, 2006; Pediatric Therapy Network, 2004; Williams & Shellenberger, 1996).

Direct intervention consisted predominantly of engagement in a variety of somatosensory and vestibular activities that gave Todd the sensory feedback he needed about his body and the environment. During these activities, Todd often lined and stacked large equipment and would crawl, climb, and swing his way through the obstacle course sequentially in three-dimensional space. For example, incorporating the concept of "1-2-3-go!," the therapist helped Todd to plan ahead and then time his actions. Once he had gone through it, Todd and the occupational therapy assistant (OTA) discussed what had gone well and what had not, made the necessary modifications, and then went back to do it again. At the end of the session, Todd and the OTA put together a picture sequence of the activities and planned what they might be able to do in the following session. She also helped him to think of ways in which he could use his new skills at home, asking him, "What do you have at home that you can use to do this amazing activity that you just finished? Let me know how it goes."

For the first three months, Todd spent the majority of his time in clinic-based services going from tactile activities to vestibular activities without accepting motor or motor-planning challenges. He was easily frustrated and acutely aware of his limitations. If the therapist encouraged him to do too much in these areas, he quit and wanted to go home. He preferred to sit and watch the therapist set up the activity and then passively enjoy the sensory play. He showed great imagination, and the therapist discovered that he had a lot of knowledge about a specific superhero. She asked him to teach her and show her what this superhero did. In this way, they together began to construct more complicated activities that included swinging from the trapeze into the ball pit but in which Todd had to move between pieces of equipment and figure out how to put things together in a way that was worthy of the special talents of the superhero. When something went wrong, it became the fault of those who wanted to thwart his powers. He eventually was so excited about his buildings that he began to draw them at home in preparation for the next therapy session. He wanted his mother and brother to come see one of the buildings once he had it working toward the end of the session. His self-esteem greatly improved, as did his muscle tone, balance, bilateral coordination, construction, and imitation skills. He began to think of ways in

which he could use objects as tools to accomplish more than he could with just his hands.

Outcomes

Todd's mother reported that after three months of occupational therapy, Todd sleeps better; stays dry, sits still and listens, transitions better, is more organized, is more secure, is less clingy, has improved play skills, has increased family engagement in active physical play activities, has increased tolerance of calming physical contact, has increased awareness of sensory conditions and their effect on behavior, and has increased adaptation of the sensory environment for more optimal learning and engagement. Additionally, his mother reported less yelling in the household because Todd listens better and more time to play due to smoother transitions. The household is more organized because Todd's progress has freed up time for his parents, and they feel more secure about their child, who is less clingy. His improved play skills offer hope that he will be able to make and keep friends, including family friends.

Todd's teacher reported that within two weeks of his beginning occupational therapy, she saw a happier child. He continued to show a low tolerance for frustration, but he recovered more rapidly and actually seemed to enjoy school. He continued to need adult guidance to begin and complete his work, but he did so in less time. He watched other children on the playground and expressed his desire to play some playground games, such as handball. Because the children knew that Todd was the reason they had new things in the class, such as the therapy balls, they showed him a bit more admiration. His teacher gave him the responsibility of checking out this equipment. She even noticed that at times, he suggested to another child that they might be able to listen better if they had a fidget or put the cushion on their chair to sit on.

CASE INFORMATION

Child's first name: __Todd__

Child's age: __6 years 10 months__

Child's year in school: __1st__

Parent/guardian(s) name:_____

EVALUATION

Reasons for referral: Todd was referred for an occupational therapy evaluation to assess his development and to determine the need for occupational therapy services. His mother described him as a loving child who seems like he just does not know what to do with himself. He is inattentive and disorganized. He will follow others and tends to play best with younger children.

Background Information

Medical history: Todd was born full term, the product of a normal delivery. He had difficulty breathing and required resuscitation but recovered quickly and did not require any hospital stay.

Developmental history: Todd was a clumsy baby who fell a lot. He cried often and was sensitive to many foods. He sat at 6 months and walked at 12 months. His fine motor skills emerged slowly, and he continues to prefer finger feeding to using utensils. He is slow to acquire gross motor skills, such as bike riding without training wheels or ball skills. He does not like organized sports activities. His language emerged typically. He is socially and emotionally immature.

Educational and intervention history: Todd is in a typical classroom. He is currently in the process of evaluations with a suspicion of ADHD. He has received no prior therapy services.

Occupational history/profile: (see above narrative)

Evaluation of Occupational Performance

Interview Data

◆ Teacher Report:
Main concern was that she thought he might be depressed. He often seemed sad and pretended to be sick so that he could go home and be with his mother. His stomachaches were worse when he had to do something that he hadn't done before or if there was an unfamiliar teacher leading the activity. He is a bright child but messy and often needed assistance to get his materials organized and an adult to help him get started on a project. Once started, he did well, and if he could sustain his attention, he completed the activity fairly well. His general knowledge is good.

◆ Guardian Report:
(see narrative above)

◆ Others:

Observation Data

Strengths:
Bright
Active
Plays well alone
Loving toward his family unless upset
Wants to please adults
Tries hard to do well
Likes routine and structure

Challenges:
Developmental dyspraxia
Motor planning
Time management
Sequencing
Imitation
Attention
Self-regulation
Often anxious and sad
Social skills
Poor use of tools such as utensils and
    writing implements
Slow performance

Test Data

Structured assessments:
SIPT (see scores)
ESP results indicated sensitivity to auditory and visual stimuli; seeks vestibular and proprioceptive activities and is sensitive to touch required in grooming activities but also seeks out touch by touching everything.

Unstructured assessment:
Immature play patterns. He waits to see what others are doing and then tries to imitate them. When he doesn't do it correctly, he gets mad, withdraws, whines, or yells. His neuromotor skills are age appropriate. He has slightly low tone, more so in flexor muscles. He has difficulty with ocular convergence.

Other:

CASE INFORMATION *Continued*

Intervention

Goals and Objectives

By (date): To demonstrate improved sequencing and motor-planning for increased school performance, Todd will independently begin an activity requiring 3 materials, such as pencil, paper, and scissors, and start the activity without adult assistance, 4/5 opportunities.

By (date): To demonstrate improved organization of behavior and attention for structured tasks, Todd will engage in games/activities/tasks with a peer, for 10 minutes of turn-taking interaction, when given no more than 3 prompts from the caregiver, 4/5 opportunities.

Given vestibular input, Todd will demonstrate a calm and alert state by following through on a 5-step familiar sequence without adult prompts during a necessary activity, 4/5 trials.

Todd will follow 3-step directions during selected activities with 1 or fewer verbal cues/rehearsals to remain on-task, 4/5 opportunities.

Given minimal cues (3 or fewer), Todd will engage for up to 10 minutes or until the activity is completed in tabletop activities without verbal complaint and/or leaving the activity, 4/5 opportunities.

OT Intervention Plan includes the following

Setting:

Duration:

Discharge plan:

Todd will engage in community-based activities that support his ability to adapt to novel environments and participate with peers in activities that are healthy, fun, and cooperative. It is estimated that occupational therapy will be discontinued within one year with systems in place at home, in the school, and in the community that will support his ongoing development. If concerns arise, occupational therapy services can be reinstated as needed.

Referrals:

Social skills training
Biomedical evaluation

OT Intervention Process and Strategies

Therapeutic activities:

Environmental modifications:

OUTCOMES

Expected or Reported Outcomes

◆ Occupational Performance: Ability to perform daily routines with minimal adult assistance.
◆ Client Satisfaction: Report
◆ Adaptability/Generalized Skills: Todd is able to adjust to routines in his new classroom and to extracurricular adult-led activities.
◆ Impact on Family Life (including the occupations of other family members): His mother is able to reduce the time getting ready to go to school by 30 minutes, and they arrive on time 100 percent of the time for the remainder of the school year.

See another case study of an eight-year-old boy with a diagnosis of autism on the Willard & Spackman Website.

REPORT PREPARATION

The following form will assist the reader in organizing information to prepare the report.

CASE INFORMATION

Child's first name: _____   Child's age: _____

Child's year in school: _____   Parent/guardian(s) name: _____

EVALUATION

Reasons for referral (include the occupational concerns/desires for the child and family):

Background Information

Medical history:

Developmental history:

Educational history:

Intervention history:

Occupational history/profile:

Evaluation of Occupational Performance

Interview Data
- Teacher Report:
- Guardian Report:
- Others:

Observation Data
Strengths:

Challenges:

Test Data
Structured assessments:

Unstructured assessment:

Other:

Intervention

Goals and Objectives

OT Intervention Plan includes the following
Setting:

Duration:

Discharge plan:

Referrals:

OT Intervention Process and Strategies
Therapeutic activities:

Environmental modifications:

OUTCOMES

Expected or Reported Outcomes

- Occupational Performance:
- Client Satisfaction:
- Adaptability/Generalized Skills:
- Impact on Family Life (including the occupations of other family members):

Sensory Integration

Dr. Ayres provided a model of evidence-based practice as she grounded her work in both basic and applied science and investigated her theory through rigorous methods of assessment and intervention (Henderson, Llorens, Gilfoyle, Myers, & Prevel, 1974). Consequently, sensory integration theory is the most widely researched area of occupational therapy (Mulligan, 2002, 2003; Parham & Mailloux, 2005).

Despite the volume of research in sensory integration (Mulligan, 2002, 2003; Parham & Mailloux, 2005), "evidence of the effectiveness of this intervention remains inconclusive" (Parham et al., 2007). Miller (2003) reported that over 80 studies addressed the effectiveness of sensory integration intervention methods. Most of these had one or more of the following deficiencies: (1) no homogeneous sample, (2) lack of replicable method of treatment that adheres to sensory integration principles, (3) inadequate outcome measures, and (4) methodological limitations (e.g. low power, lack of randomization, lack of control groups). Mulligan (2003) analyzed effectiveness studies or reviews of studies and found that these studies had mixed results.

A review of evidence on intervention using sensory integrative methods indicates that children with *autism* show less nonengaged behavior and more language and parallel play behavior with decreased self-stimulation after intervention (Ayres & Tickle, 1980; Case-Smith & Bryan, 1999); children with *mental retardation* showed gains in gross and fine motor skills as well as in postural control and stability (combined with neurodevelopmental treatment); and adults with *mental retardation* showed improved eye contact, vocalization, and postural control (Clark, Miller, Thomas, Kucherawy, & Azen, 1978; Montgomery & Richter, 1977; Norton, 1975). Schaaf, Merrill, and Kinsella (1987) presented a single case study of a child with a *learning disorder* that suggests that sensory integration approaches improved play, interactions with others and with toys and other objects, and tolerance for vestibular and proprioceptive sensations and led to greater sensory exploration of the environment.

By contrast, Polatajko, Law, Miller, Schaffer, and Macnab (1991) showed no difference in gains in academic or motor skills between children receiving the sensory integration versus perceptual-motor intervention, and Wilson, Kaplan, Fellowes, Gruchy, and Faris (1992) found no difference in academic or motor skills between sensory integration and tutoring in a randomized study. Although the sensory integration group did not make greater gains in the initial study, at follow-up two years later, Wilson and colleagues (1992) found that only the sensory integration group maintained their gross motor skills. Although an early meta-analysis of research on sensory integration treatment showed positive results (Ottenbacher, 1982), a later meta-analysis that included studies such as those mentioned above showed little or no effect (Vargas & Camilli 1999).

Recent studies have documented improved adaptive behavior and occupational performance (Roberts, King-Thomas, & Boccia, 2007) and improvement on cognitive, behavioral, and physiological measures (Miller, Coll, & Schoen, 2007) following occupational therapy using a sensory integration approach. Schilling and colleagues (2003) documented improved sustained sitting and improved writing legibility for the students with ADHD when they were seated on therapy balls that offer enhanced proprioceptive stimulation. Similar benefits in attention and engagement were found with children with autism spectrum disorder (Schilling & Schwartz, 2004). Smith, Press, Koenig, & Kinnealey (2005) demonstrated significantly reduced self-stimulating behaviors in children and youths with pervasive developmental delay when occupational therapy with a sensory integration approach was used compared to a control intervention of tabletop activities. The authors suggest that the sensory integration approach is effective in reducing self-stimulating behaviors, which interfere with the ability to participate in more functional activities.

Consistent with all areas of occupational therapy practice, sensory integration intervention requires further examination. For the field to move forward, collaborative research models that capitalize on researchers' strengths should be developed (Smith Roley et al., 2005). Parham and Mailloux (2005) suggest that further research is needed that predicts those who will respond best to sensory integration methods, determines more refined outcomes that can be expected, and elucidates potential types of long-term gains, especially those that are meaningful to families.

PROVOCATIVE QUESTIONS

1. How would you communicate your understanding of the evidence to parents who are seeking occupational therapy intervention that uses a sensory integration approach?
2. A characteristic behavior that is seen in children with autism is self-stimulatory behavior, such as hand flapping or repetitive rocking. How might you make the case that this is the result of inadequate neural inhibition? Can you make the converse case: that it is the result of inadequate neural facilitation?
3. What are the benefits to allowing a child to choose an activity versus guiding the child to an appropriate activity?

ACKNOWLEDGMENTS

We wish to acknowledge our mentors, Dr. A. Jean Ayres and Ginny Scardina, along with the many outstanding colleagues with whom we have collaborated.

ON THE WEB

◆ Case study of an eight-year-old boy with a diagnosis of autism

REFERENCES

American Occupational Therapy Association. (2003). Applying sensory integration framework in educationally related occupational therapy practice. *American Journal of Occupational Therapy, 57,* 652–659.

Anzalone, M. E., & Murray, E. A. (2002). In A. C. Bundy, S. J. Lane, & E. A. Murray (Eds.), *Sensory integration: Theory and practice* (pp. 371–394). Philadelphia: F. A. Davis.

Ayres, A. J. (1963). The Eleanor Clark Slagle Lecture. The development of perceptual-motor abilities: A theoretical basis for treatment of dysfunction. *American Journal of Occupational Therapy, 17,* 221–225.

Ayres, A. J. (1968). Sensory integrative processes and neuropsychological learning disability. *Learning Disorders, 3,* 41–58.

Ayres, A. J. (1972). *Sensory integration and learning disorders.* Los Angeles: Western Psychological Services.

Ayres, A. J. (1974). *The development of sensory integrative theory and practice: A collection of the works of A. Jean Ayres.* Dubuque, IA: Kendall/Hunt.

Ayres, A. J. (1979). *Sensory integration and the child.* Los Angeles: Western Psychological Services.

Ayres, A. J. (1989). *Sensory integration and praxis tests manual.* Los Angeles: Western Psychological Services.

Ayres, A. J. (2004). *Sensory integration and praxis tests manual: Updated edition.* Western Psychological Services: Los Angeles.

Ayres, A. J. (2005). *Sensory integration and the child: Understanding hidden sensory challenges* (rev. ed.). Los Angeles: Western Psychological Services.

Ayres, A. J., Erwin, P. R., & Mailloux, Z. (2004). *Love, Jean: Inspiration for families living with dysfunction of sensory integration.* Santa Rosa, CA: Crestport Press.

Ayres, A. J., & Tickle, L. S. (1980). Hyper-responsivity to touch and vestibular stimuli as a predictor of positive response to sensory integration procedures by autistic children. *American Journal of Occupational Therapy, 34,* 375–381.

Bauman, M. L. (2005). Commentary, Chapter 9: The child with autism. In A. J. Ayres (Ed.), *Sensory Integration and the child: Understanding hidden sensory challenges.* (p. 180). Los Angeles: Western Psychological Services.

Bear, M. F., Connors, B. W., & Paradiso, M. A. (2006). *Neuroscience: Exploring the brain* (3rd ed.). Baltimore: Williams & Wilkins.

Berthoz, A. (2000). *The brain's sense of movement.* Cambridge, MA: Harvard University Press.

Bissell, J., Fisher, J., Owens, C., & Polcyn, P. (1998) *Sensory motor handbook: A guide for implementing and modifying activities in the classroom* (2nd ed.). San Antonio, TX: Harcourt Assessment.

Blanche, E. I. (2002). *Observations based on sensory integration theory.* Torrance, CA: Pediatric Therapy Network.

Blanche, E. I., & Schaaf, R. C. (2001). Proprioception: A cornerstone of sensory integrative intervention. In S. Roley, E. I. Blanche, & R. C. Schaaf (Eds.), *Understanding the nature of sensory integration with diverse populations* (pp. 109–122). San Antonio, TX: Therapy Skill Builders.

Blanche, E. I., Botticelli, T. M., & Hallway, M. K. (1995). *Combining neuro-developmental treatment and sensory integration principles: An approach to pediatric therapy.* San Antonio, TX: Therapy Skill Builders.

Bronson, M. B. (2000). *Self-regulation in early childhood: Nature and nurture.* New York: Guilford.

Brown, C., & Dunn, W. (2002). *Adolescent/Adult Sensory Profile.* San Antonio, TX: The Psychological Corporation.

Bundy, A. C. (2002). Play theory and sensory integration. In A. C. Bundy, S. J. Lane, & E. A Murray (Eds.), *Sensory integration: Theory and practice* (pp. 227–240). Philadelphia: F. A. Davis.

Bundy, A. C., & Murray, E. A. (2002) Sensory integration: A. Jean Ayres' Theory Revisited. In A. C. Bundy, S. J., Lane, & E. A. Murray (Eds.), *Sensory integration: Theory and practice.* Philadelphia: F. A. Davis, pp. 3–29.

Bundy, A. C., Lane, S. J., & Murray E. A. (Eds.) (2002). *Sensory integration: Theory and practice.* Philadelphia: F. A. Davis.

Buonomano, D. V., & Merzenich, M. M. (1998). Cortical plasticity: From synapses to maps. *Annual Review of Neuroscience, 21,* 149–186,

Burke, J. P., & Mailloux, Z. (1997). Play and the sensory integrative approach. In L. D. Parham & F. S. Fazio (Eds.), *Play in occupational therapy for children.* pp. 112–125. St. Louis: Mosby-Year Book.

Calvert, G., Spence, C., & Stein, B. E. (Eds.). (2004). *The handbook of multisensory processes.* Cambridge, MA: MIT Press.

Case-Smith, J., & Bryan, T. (1999). The effects of occupational therapy with sensory integration emphasis on preschool-age children with autism. *American Journal of Occupational Therapy, 53,* 489–497.

Cermak, S. (2005). Chapter 6 Commentary in A. J. Ayres (Ed.). *Sensory integration and the child: Understanding hidden sensory challenges* (rev. ed.). p. 175 Los Angeles: Western Psychological Services.

Clark, F., Miller, L. R., Thomas, J. A., Kucherawy, D. A., & Azen, S. P. (1978). A comparison of operant and sensory integrative methods on developmental parameters in profoundly retarded adults. *American Journal of Occupational Therapy, 32,* 86–92.

Cohn, E. S. (2001a). From waiting to relating: Parents' experiences in the waiting room of an occupational therapy clinic. *American Journal of Occupational Therapy, 55,* 167–174.

Cohn, E. S. (2001b). Parent perspectives of occupational therapy using a sensory integration approach. *American Journal of Occupational Therapy, 55,* 285–294.

Cohn E. S., Miller, L. J., & Tickle-Degnen, L. (2000). Parental hopes for therapy outcomes: Children with sensory modulation disorders. *American Journal of Occupational Therapy, 54,* 36–43.

Coleman, G., Mailloux, Z., & Smith Roley, S. (2005). *Sensory integration: Answers for parents.* Santa Clara, CA: Crestport Press.

Coleman, G., Mailloux, Z., & Smith Roley, S. (2006). *Sensory integration: Answers for teachers.* Santa Clara, CA: Crestport Press.

Cruikshank, S. J., & Weinberger, N. M. (1996). Evidence for the Hebbian hypothesis in experience-dependent physiological plasticity of neocortex: A critical review. *Brain Research Reviews, 22,* 191–228.

DeGangi, G. (2000). *Pediatric disorders of regulation in affect and behavior: A therapist's guide to assessment and treatment.* San Diego: Academic Press.

DeGangi, G., & Greenspan, S. (1988). The development of sensory functioning in infants. *Physical & Occupational Therapy in Pediatrics, 8*(3), 21–33.

Dunn, W. (1999). *Sensory Profile.* San Antonio, TX: Therapy Skill Builders.

Dunn, W. (2002a). *Infant/Toddler Sensory Profile.* San Antonio, TX: Therapy Skill Builders.

Dunn, W. (2002b). *The Adolescent/Adult Sensory Profile.* San Antonio: TX: Therapy Skill Builders.

Eide, F. F. (2003). Sensory integration: Current concepts and practical implications. *Sensory Integration Special Interest Section Quarterly, 26,* 3, 1–3.

Felleman, D. J., & Van Essen, D. C. (1991). Distributed hierarchical processing in the primate cerebral cortex. *Cerebral Cortex, 1*(1), 1–47.

Gibson J. J. (1977). The theory of affordances. In R. Shaw & J. Bransford (Eds.), Perceiving, acting, and knowing (p. 67–82). Hillsdale, NJ: Erlbaum.

Gilbert, C. D., & Wiesel, T. N. (1992). Receptive field dynamics in adult primary visual cortex. *Nature, 356*(6365), 150–152.

Giuffrida, C. (2001). In S. Roley, E. I. Blanche, & R. C. Schaaf (Eds.), *Understanding the nature of sensory integration with diverse populations* (pp. 133–161). San Antonio, TX: Therapy Skill Builders.

Gross, C. G. (2000). Neurogenesis in the adult brain: Death of a dogma. *National Review of Neuroscience, 1,* 67–73.

Henderson, A., Llorens, L., Gilfoyle, E., Myers, C., & Prevel, S. (Eds.). (1974). *The development of sensory integrative theory and practice: A collection of the works of A. Jean Ayres.* Dubuque, IA: Kendall/Hunt.

Jarrett, O. S. (2002). *Recess in elementary school: What does the research say?* (EDO-PS-02-5). Washington, DC: ERIC/EECE Publications.

Johnson-Ecker, C. L., & Parham, L. D. (2000). The evaluation of sensory processing: A validity study using contrasting groups. *American Journal of Occupational Therapy, 54,* 494–503.

Katz, L. C., & Shatz, C. J. (1996). Synaptic activity and the construction of cortical circuits. *Science, 274*(5290), 1133–1138.

King A. J. & Palmer, A. R. (1985) Integration of visual and auditory information in bimodal neurones in the guinea-pig superior colliculus. *Experimental Brain Research Journal. Springer Berlin 60*(3), 492–500.

Knox, S., & Mailloux, Z. (1997). Play as treatment and treatment through play. In B. E. Chandler (Ed.), *The essence of play: A child's occupation* (pp. 175–204). Bethesda, MD: American Occupational Therapy Association.

Knox, S. H. (2005). Chapter 2 Commentary in A. J. Ayres, (Ed.). *Sensory integration and the child: Understanding hidden sensory challenges* (rev. ed.). p. 171 Los Angeles: Western Psychological Services.

Koomar, J. (1995). *Vestibular dysfunction is associated with anxiety rather than behavior inhibition or shyness.* Unpublished doctoral dissertation, Boston University, Boston, Massachusetts.

Koomar, J. A., & Bundy, A. C. (2002). Creating direct intervention from theory. In A. C. Bundy, S. J. Lane, & E. A. Murray (Eds.), *Sensory integration theory and practice* (2nd ed., pp. 261–306). Philadelphia: F. A. Davis.

Kopp C. (1982). Antecedents of self-regulation: A developmental perspective. *Developmental Psychology, 18,* 199–214.

Lane, S. J., Miller L. J., & Hanft B. E. (2000). Toward a consensus in terminology in sensory integration theory and practice: Part 2. Sensory integration patterns of function and dysfunction. *Sensory Integration Special Interest Section Quarterly, 23*(2), 1–3.

Mailloux, Z. (2001). Sensory integrative principles in intervention with children with autistic disorder. In S. Roley, E. I. Blanche, & R. C. Schaaf (Eds.), *Understanding the nature of sensory integration with diverse populations* (pp. 365–384). San Antonio, TX: Therapy Skill Builders.

Mailloux, Z. K., May-Benson, T. A., Summers, C. A., Miller, L J., Burke, J. P., Brett-Green, B., et al. (2007). Goal attainment scaling as a measure of meaningful outcomes for children with sensory integration disorders. *American Journal of Occupational Therapy 61* 254–259.

Mailloux, Z., & Smith Roley (2004). Sensory integration. In H. Miller-Kuhaneck (Ed.), *Autism: A Comprehensive Occupational Therapy Approach* (2nd ed.). Bethesda, MD: American Occupational Therapy Association.

Meredith M. A. & Stein, B. E. (1986). Visual, auditory, and somatosensory convergence on cells in superior colliculus results in multisensory integration. *Journal of Neurophysiology, 56*(3), 640–662.

May-Benson, T. A. (2001). A theoretical model of ideation in praxis. In S. Smith Roley, E. I. Blanche, and R. C. Schaaf (Eds.), *Understanding the nature of sensory integration with diverse populations* (pp. 163–181). San Antonio, TX: Therapy Skill Builders.

Mesulam, M. M. (1998). From sensation to cognition. *Brain, 121*(6), 1013–1052.

Middleton, F. A., & Strick, P. L. (2000). Basal ganglia and cerebellar loops: Motor and cognitive circuits. *Brain Research Reviews, 31*, 236–250.

Miller, E. K. (2000). Organization through experience. *Nature Neuroscience, 3*, 1066–1068.

Miller, L. J. (2003). Empirical evidence related to therapies for sensory processing impairments. *National Association of School Psychologists Communique, 31*(5), 34–36.

Miller, L. J., Coll, J. R., & Schoen, S. A. (2007). A randomized controlled pilot study of the effectiveness of occupational therapy for children with sensory modulation disorder. *American Journal of Occupational Therapy, 61*, 228–238.

Miller L. J., & Lane S. J. (2000). Toward a concensus [*sic*] in terminology in sensory integration theory and practice: Part 1. Taxonomy of neurophysiological processes. *Sensory Integration Special Interest Section Quarterly, 23*(1), 1–4.

Miller, L. J., McIntosh, D. N., McGrath, J., Shyu, V., Lampe, M., Taylor, A. K., et al. (1999). Electrodermal responses to sensory stimuli in individuals with fragile X syndrome: A preliminary report. *American Journal of Medical Genetics, 83*, 268–279.

Miller-Kuhaneck, H., Henry, D., & Glennon, T. (2007). *Sensory Processing Measure (SPM) School Form*. Los Angeles: Western Psychological Services.

Miller-Kuhaneck, H., & Smith Roley, S. (2005). A kindergartner with sensory integration dysfunction. In K. Sladyk & S. Ryan (Eds.), *Ryan's occupational therapy assistant: Principles, practice issues, and techniques* (4th ed.). Thorofare, NJ: Slack.

Montegue, A. (1986). *Touching: The human significance of the skin*. New York: Harper and Row.

Montgomery, R., & Richter, E. (1977). Effect of sensory integrative therapy on the neuromotor development of retarded children. *Physical Therapy, 57*, 799–806.

Mulligan, S. (1998a). Patterns of sensory integration dysfunction: A confirmatory factor analysis. *American Journal of Occupational Therapy, 52*, 819–828.

Mulligan, S. (1998b). Application of structural equation modeling in occupational therapy research. *American Journal of Occupational Therapy, 52*, 829–834.

Mulligan, S. (2000). Cluster analysis of scores of children on the Sensory Integration and Praxis Tests. *Occupational Therapy Journal of Research, 20*, 256–262.

Mulligan, S. (2002). Advances in sensory integration research. In A. C. Bundy, S. L. Lane, & E. A. Murray (Eds.), *Sensory integration: Theory and practice* (2nd ed., pp. 397–411). Philadelphia: F. A. Davis.

Mulligan, S. (2003a). Examination of the evidence for occupational therapy using a sensory integration framework with children: part one. *Sensory Integration Special Interest Section Quarterly, 26*(1). 1–4.

Mulligan, S. (2003b). Examination of the evidence for occupational therapy using a sensory integration framework with children: part two. *Sensory Integration Special Interest Section Quarterly, 26*(2), 1–5.

Norton, Y. (1975). Neurodevelopment and sensory integration for the profoundly retarded multiply handicapped child. *American Journal of Occupational Therapy, 29*, 93–100.

Ottenbacher, K. (1982). Sensory integration therapy: Affect or effect? *American Journal of Occupational Therapy, 36*, 571–578.

Parham, L. D., & Mailloux, Z. (2005). Sensory integration. In J. Case-Smith (Ed.), *Occupational therapy for children* (5th ed., pp. 356–411). St. Louis: Mosby.

Parham L. D., & Johnson-Ecker, C. L. (2007). *Sensory Processing Measure (SPM) Home Form*. Los Angeles: Western Psychological Services.

Parham, L. D., Cohn, E. S., Spitzer, S., Koomar, J., Miller, L. J., Burke, J. P., et al. (2007). Fidelity in sensory integration intervention research. *American Journal of Occupational Therapy, 61*, 206–227.

Pediatric Therapy Network. (2004). *Applying sensory integration principles where children live, learn and play* [DVD/video]. Torrance, CA: Author.

Pellegrini, A. D. (1993). School recess: Implications for education and development. *Review of Educational Research, 63*, 51–67.

Polatajko, H. J., Law, M., Miller, J., Schaffer, R., & Macnab, J. (1991). The effect of a sensory integration program on academic achievement, motor performance, and self-esteem in children identified as learning disabled: Results of a clinical trial. *Occupational Therapy Journal of Research, 11*, 155–176.

Pons, T. P., Garraghty, P. E., Friedman, D. P., & Mishkin, M. (1987). Physiological evidence for serial processing in somatosensory cortex. *Science, 237*, 417–420.

Roberts, J. E., King-Thomas, L., Boccia, M. L. (2007). Behavioral indexes of the efficacy of sensory integration. *American Journal of Occupational Therapy, 61*, 555–563.

Schaaf, R. C., & Anzalone M. (2001). Sensory integration with high-risk infants and young children. In (Eds.) S. Smith Roley, E. I. Blanche, & R. A. Schaaf, (Eds.). (2001). *Understanding the nature of sensory integration with diverse populations*. San Antonio, TX: Therapy Skill Builders p. 275–311.

Schaaf, R. C., Merrill, S., & Kinsella, N. (1987). Sensory integration and play behavior: A case study of effectiveness of occupational therapy using sensory integrative techniques. *Occupational Therapy in Health Care, 4*, 61–75.

Schaaf, R. C., Miller, L. J., Seewal, D., & O'Keefe, S. (2003). Children with disturbances in sensory processing: A pilot study examining the role of the parasympathetic nervous system. *American Journal of Occupational Therapy, 57*, 442–449.

Schaaf, R. C., & Nightlinger, K. M. (2007). Occupational therapy using a sensory integrative approach: A case study of effectiveness. *American Journal of Occupational Therapy, 61*, 239–246.

Schaaf, R. C., & Smith Roley, S. (2006). *Clinical reasoning: Applying sensory integration principles to practice with diverse populations*. San Antonio: TX: Psychological Corporation.

Schilling, D. L., & Schwartz, I. S. (2004). Alternative seating for young children with autism spectrum disorder. *Journal of Autism and Developmental Disorder, 34*, 423–432.

Schilling, D. L., Washington, K., Billingsley, F. F, & Deitz, J. (2003). Classroom seating for children with attention deficit hyperactivity disorder: Therapy balls versus chairs. *American Journal of Occupational Therapy, 57*, 534–541.

Schlaug, G. (2001). The brain of musicians: A model for functional and structural adaptation. *New York Academy of Sciences, 930*, 281–299.

Schneider, M. (2005). Commentary, Chapter 1: What is sensory integration? In A. J. Ayres (2005), *Sensory integration and the child: Understanding hidden sensory challenges.* Pp. 169–170. Los Angeles: Western Psychological Services.

Shumway-Cook, A., & Woollacott M. H. (2001). *Motor control: Theory and practical applications* (2nd ed.). Baltimore: Williams & Wilkins.

Smith, L. B., & Thelen, E. (Eds.). (1993). *A dynamic systems approach to development.* Cambridge, MA: MIT Press.

Smith S. A., Press, B., Koenig K., & Kinnealey, M. (2005). Effects of sensory integration intervention on self-stimulating and self-injurious behaviors. *American Journal of Occupational Therapy, 59,* 418–425.

Smith Roley, S. (2005). Chapter 8 Commentary in A. J. Ayres, (Ed.). *Sensory integration and the child: Understanding hidden sensory challenges* (rev. ed.). p. 179, Los Angeles: Western Psychological Services.

Smith Roley, S., Blanche, E. I., & Schaaf, R. C. (Eds.). (2001). *Understanding the nature of sensory integration with diverse populations.* San Antonio, TX: Therapy Skill Builders.

Smith Roley, S., Burke, J. P., Cohn, E. S., Koomar, J. A., Miller, L. J., Schaaf, R. C., et al. (2005). A strategic plan for research in a human service profession. *Sensory Integration Special Interest Section Newsletter, 28,* 1–3.

Sparks, D. L, & Groh, J. M. (1995). The superior colliculus: A window to problems in integrative neuroscience. In M. S. Gazzaniga (Ed.), *The Cognitive Neurosciences* (pp. 565–584) Cambridge, MA: MIT Press.

Spitzer S. L. (June 1999). Dynamic systems theory: Relevance to the theory of sensory integration and the study of occupation. *Sensory Integration Special Interest Section Quarterly, 22*(2) 1–4.

Spitzer, S., & Smith Roley, S. (2001). Sensory integration revisited: A philosophy of practice. In S. Smith Roley, E. I. Blanche, & R. C. Schaaf (Eds.), *Understanding the nature of sensory integration with diverse populations* (pp. 3–23). San Antonio, TX: Therapy Skill Builders.

Stein, B. E. (1998). Neural mechanisms for synthesizing sensory information and producing adaptive behaviors. *Experimental Brain Research, 123,* 124–135.

Stein, B. E., & Meredith, M. A. (1993). *The merging of the senses.* Cambridge, MA: MIT Press.

Stein, B. E. (1984). Development of the superior colliculus. *Annual Review of Neuroscience. 7,* 95–125.

Stein, B. E., Huneycutt, W. S. & Meredith, M. T. (1988). Neurons and behavior: The same rules of multisensory integration apply. *Brain Research, 448,* 355–358.

Stein, B. E. Meredith, M. A., Huneycutt, W. S. & McDade, L. (1989). Behavioral indices of multisensory integration: Orientation to visual cues is affected by auditory stimuli. *Journal of Cognitive Neuroscience. 1,* 12–24.

Thelen, E., & Smith, L. B. (1994). *A dynamic systems approach to the development of cognition and action.* Cambridge, MA: MIT Press.

Vargas, S., & Camilli, G. (1999). A meta-analysis of research on sensory integration treatment. *American Journal of Occupational Therapy, 53,* 189–198.

Wall, J. T., Xu, J., & Wang, X. (2002). Human brain plasticity: An emerging view of the multiple substrates and mechanisms that cause cortical changes and related sensory dysfunctions after injuries of sensory inputs from the body. *Brain Research Reviews, 39*(2–3), 181–215.

Wallace, M. T., Meredith, M. A., & Stein, B. E. (1993). Converging influences from visual, auditory, and somatosensory cortices onto output neurons of the superior colliculus. *Journal of Neurophysiology, 69*(6):1797–1809.

Weisberg, A. (1984). The role of psychophysiology in defining gravitational insecurity: A pilot study. *Sensory Integration Special Interest Section Newsletter, 7*(4), 1–4.

Williams, M. S., & Shellenberger, S. (1996). *"How does your engine run?": A leader's guide to the Alert Program for Self-Regulation.* Albuquerque, NM: TherapyWorks.

Williams, M. S., & Shellenberger, S. (2001). *Take five!: Staying alert at home and school.* Albuquerque, NM: TherapyWorks.

Williamson, G. G. & Anzalone, M. E. (2001). *Sensory integration and self regulation in infants and toddlers: Helping very young children interact with their environment.* Washington DC: Zero to Three.

Wilson, B. N., Kaplan, B. J., Fellowes, S., Gruchy, C., & Faris, P. (1992). The efficacy of sensory integration treatment compared to tutoring. *Physical and Occupational Therapy in Pediatrics, 12,* 1–36.

Windsor, M., Smith Roley S., & Szklut, S. (2001). Assessment of sensory integration and praxis. In S. Roley, E. I. Blanche, & R. C. Schaaf (Eds.), *Understanding the nature of sensory integration with diverse populations* (pp. 215–245). San Antonio, TX: Therapy Skill Builders.

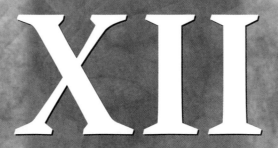

OT EVALUATION AND INTERVENTION: ENVIRONMENTS

> "Human occupation arises out of an innate, spontaneous tendency of the human system—
> the urge to explore and master the environment."
>
> *Gary Kielhofner & Janice P. Burke, 1980*

Physical Environments

PATTY RIGBY, SUSAN STARK, LORI LETTS, AND LAURIE RINGAERT

Learning Objectives

After reading this chapter, you will be able to:

1. Describe why the environment is critical to occupational performance.
2. Identify useful measures to assess the physical environment in the contexts of home, school, community, and workplace.
3. Describe the process for addressing the physical environment while planning for and implementing interventions.
4. Describe interventions that can be applied in various contexts across the life course (home, work, school, community).
5. Describe the evidence supporting specific intervention approaches.

INTRODUCTION: THE ROLE OF THE PHYSICAL ENVIRONMENT IN OCCUPATIONAL PERFORMANCE

Occupational therapists recognize that occupational performance is a function of the individual's abilities, the activities being performed, and the environment in which the performance occurs (American Occupational Therapy Association, 2002; Canadian Association of Occupational Therapists, 1997; Law et al., 1996). The environment is complex and multifaceted and can either challenge or support a person's competencies and performance in daily life. For example, flat surfaces such as a level, accessible entry to a building can support the performance of someone using a mobility aid such as a wheelchair. By contrast, the environment can create barriers to performance, as when older adults with low vision have trouble finding their way and ordering food in a dimly lit restaurant. **Environments**, as described in the International Classification System for Functioning, Disability and Health (ICF) (World Health Organization, 2001), can include physical elements (human-made environments, natural environments, equipment, and technology), social elements (social support and societal attitudes), and cultural, institutional, and economic elements.

Although in practice, the environment must be considered in its entirety, the focus of this chapter is on the **physical environment**. For discussions of social and political environments, refer to Chapter 63. Assistive technology, though part of the physical environment, is addressed in Chapter 62. We describe the assessment process as well as the role of occupational therapists in making **environmental modifications** to maintain and/or improve the occupational performance of their clients.

Not all health practitioners acknowledge the influence of the environment on performance. Medical models of health attribute disability (or the inability of individuals to perform daily activities) to the functional limitations caused by impairments. For example, a person who is blind is "disabled" merely due to loss of vision. In contrast, social models of disability suggest that disability is a construct imposed by circumstances, and consequently, the environment plays a role in performance (Stewart, 2003). In a social model, the disability occurs when the attributes of the person interact with an environment that is not compatible with the person's functional limitation(s). For an individual who is blind, a lack of Braille signage or audible cues in an elevator results in disability. With adequate environmental support, this person is just as "able" as his or her nonblind counterparts. In other words, people who use wheelchairs are not "disabled" on smooth, flat pathways. They become disabled when they encounter a flight of stairs.

Conceptually, disability can be viewed as a lack of fit between the person (P), the environment (E), and the person's daily occupations (O). In this approach, modifying the environment becomes an important intervention strategy to help manage chronic health conditions, maintain or improve functioning in daily life, and increase independence. Optimal **person-environment-occupation (PEO) fit** occurs when an individual's capacities are consistent with the demands and the opportunities of the occupation of interest and the environment (Law, et al., 1996). Conversely, when the demands of the environment exceed an individual's abilities, there is a lack of congruence, or lack of PEO fit.

How the environment influences an individual's ability to perform an activity was initially defined by psychologists as **environmental press** (Lawton & Nahemow, 1973). The environmental press model defines behavior and performance as functions of an individual's competence and environmental press. Thus, to optimize performance, environmental demands must match the individual's abilities. When demands are greater or less than an individual's skill level, negative outcomes or maladaptive behavior occurs, resulting in environmental interactions that minimize performance. For example, when a grab bar in a public washroom is located too far away (environmental demand) for a frail older person to reach (personal competency), the individual might lose his or her balance and fall or experience fear of falling. Consequently, the individual might require assistance in toileting or might avoid the toilet or that public location altogether (maladaptive behavior) (Lawton & Nahemow, 1973).

LEGAL RIGHTS TO AN ACCESSIBLE ENVIRONMENT

The rights of people with disabilities are typically protected in developed countries through human or civil rights laws. For example, the Americans with Disabilities Act (ADA, 1990) was designed to create equal opportunity and equal access to public environments, services, employment, accommodations, telecommunications, and transportation across the United States. The focus of this law, and of similar legislation in many countries, is to enable people with disabilities to achieve integration and independent living.

Titles II and III of the ADA outline how both public- and private-sector services, programs, and facilities must comply with and implement the ADA. The ADA/ABA (Architectural Board Act) Accessibility Guidelines provide the accessibility requirements for public and private facilities covered by Titles II and III (U.S. Access Board, 2004). Accessibility guidelines have also been developed for play areas, public rights of way, and outdoor recreation areas (U.S. Architectural and Transportation Barriers and Compliance Board, 2000).

In Canada, the National Building Code provides accessibility requirements, and all federally operated organizations and their owned and leased entities must comply with the Canadian standard of accessibility, "Accessible Design for the Built Environment" (Canadian Standards Association, (2004). In many Canadian provinces and cities, the accessibility requirements go beyond the federal requirements.

Building codes, guidelines, and standards all provide minimum levels of accessibility. However, they do not make accommodations for everyone. For example, most of the accessibility requirements for people with mobility impairments are based on the needs of young males with paraplegia. That is why we see one grab bar in the toilet stall of a public building rather than two pull-down bars, which would be better for many older adults who have to push themselves up off a toilet. Similarly, the space requirements in building standards and codes are based on the needs of a manual wheelchair user and not a power chair or scooter user (Ringaert, Rapson, Qiu, Cooper, & Shwedyk, 2001). These issues are important for the occupational therapist who is trying to understand accessibility in the built environment. Occupational therapists should become familiar with local legislation that promotes and supports accessibility and the inclusion of people with disabilities into all aspects of society, as these laws affect client expectations for occupational therapy services, and upon how we practice.

UNIVERSAL DESIGN

Universal design is a way to create products and environments that are more usable by everyone, regardless of age or ability (Mace, 1985). Universal design involves thinking about a range of human abilities before the environment is built. Today, universal design is considered across most environments, including housing, office buildings, airports, restaurants, parks, streetscapes, urban planning, and museums. It recognizes human differences in shapes, sizes, ages, abilities, and cultures and promotes inclusion and ergonomic design for all people.

Seven principles of universal design (Center for Universal Design, 1997) assist in designing new products and environments to be accessible for all (Figure 60.1). These principles offer occupational therapists useful guidelines to use in developing interventions for clients or organizations seeking to improve the receptivity of the environment.

Terms such as *accessible design, adaptable design,* and *barrier-free design* tend to refer to specialized populations and in some cases are used to add features to a building (e.g., a ramp added after the building was built). However, universal design represents designs that provide inclusion of all people during the design process. For example, the level entrance and power sliding doors at the entrance to

---

The design of products and environments should be usable by all people, to the greatest extent possible, without the need for adaption or specialized design.

PRINCIPLE 1: Equitable Use
The design is useful and marketable to people with diverse abilities.

Guidelines:
1a. Provide the same means of use for all users: identical whenever possible; equivalent when not.
1b. Avoid segregating or stigmatizing any users.
1c. Provisions for privacy, security, and safety should be equally available to all users.
1d. Make the design appealing to all users.

PRINCIPLE 2: Flexibility in Use
The design accommodates a wide range of individual preferences and abilities.

Guidelines:
2a. Provide choice in methods of use.
2b. Accommodate right- or left-handed access and use.
2c. Facilitate the user's accuracy and precision.
2d. Provide adaptability to the user's pace.

PRINCIPLE 3: Simple and Intuitive Use
Use of the design is easy to understand, regardless of the user's experience, knowledge, language skills, or current concentration level.

Guidelines:
3a. Eliminate unnecessary complexity.
3b. Be consistent with user expectations and intuition.
3c. Accommodate a wide range of literacy and language skills.
3d. Arrange information consistent with its importance.
3e. Provide effective prompting and feedback during and after task completion.

PRINCIPLE 4: Perceptible Information
The design communicates necessary information effectively to the user, regardless of ambient conditions or the user's sensory abilities.

Guidelines:
4a. Use different modes (pictorial, verbal, tactile) for redundant presentation of essential information.
4b. Provide adequate contrast between essential information and its surroundings.
4c. Maximize "legibility" of essential information.
4d. Differentiate elements in ways that can be described (i.e., make it easy to give instructions or directions).
4e. Provide compatibility with a variety of techniques or devices used by people with sensory limitations.

PRINCIPLE 5: Tolerance for Error
The design minimizes hazards and the adverse consequences of accidental or unintended actions.

Guidelines:
5a. Arrange elements to minimize hazards and errors: most used elements, most accessible; hazardous elements eliminated, isolated, or shielded.
5b. Provide warnings of hazards and errors.
5c. Provide fail safe features.
5d. Discourage unconscious action in tasks that require vigilance.

PRINCIPLE 6: Low Physical Effort
The design can be used efficiently and comfortably and with a minimum of fatigue.

Guidelines:
6a. Allow user to maintain a neutral body position.
6b. Use reasonable operating forces.
6c. Minimize repetitive actions.
6d. Minimize sustained physical effort.

PRINCIPLE 7: Size and Space for Approach and Use
Appropriate size and space is provided for approach, reach, manipulation, and use regardless of user's body size, posture, or mobility.

Guidelines:
7a. Provide a clear line of sight to important elements for any seated or standing user.
7b. Make reach to all components comfortable for any seated or standing user.
7c. Accommodate variations in hand and grip size.
7d. Provide adequate space for the use of assistive devices or personal assistance.

FIGURE 60.1   The Principles of Universal Design: Version 2.0. [Source: Center for Universal Design (1997).]

a grocery store makes the store accessible to everyone. In this case, the entrance design accomodates people who are pushing the grocery carts, those pushing baby carriages, or those moving large objects on a cart as well as those using wheelchairs or mobility devices. Having good way-finding features, such as clear paths of travel, color cues, and clear signage, is useful for anyone, especially for visitors to a new location who cannot read the local language.

Occupational therapists have the skills to assist in design and postoccupancy evaluations of public places as well as home environments (Ringaert, 2003). Occupational therapists must think at a societal level, not only at the level of the individual, to ensure that all of their clients are able to participate fully in society.

PROCESS FOR ASSESSMENT AND INTERVENTIONS DIRECTED AT THE PHYSICAL ENVIRONMENT

Understanding and describing the range of environmental factors that affect the performance of individuals is difficult, given the immeasurable potential combinations of environments in which clients will perform. Occupations occur within a context that is unique to each individual's circumstance(s). Each human lives in a life space that is built on a system of environments. The environments include a mix of physical and social elements. Physical elements can include the built environment, objects within the environment, and the geographical and climatic features of the natural environment. Social elements consist of people, including their attitudes and cultural values as well as social support offered by these people. Policies and services are also social and political elements of the environment.

Occupational therapists can intervene in the environment at several different levels. How do we organize and think about the factors that determine how the changes will be made? One strategy to use in considering environmental issues is to use an environmental hierarchical continuum (Stark, 2004). This organizing scheme, based on the work of occupational therapists (Hagedorn, 2000; McColl, 1997) and environmental psychologists (Bronfenbrenner, 1977; Lawton, 1980) organizes the environment from proximal to distal, the most proximal environments consisting of personal places that are used frequently and distal being the wider more expanded layer of the environment that includes community.

While each of these layers of the environment contains physical and social attributes, the physical environmental attributes are the focus of this chapter. The most proximal layer includes personal spaces such as an individual bedroom or bathroom in a home or a personal car. These spaces are likely to have the greatest influence on the performance of an individual and are most likely to be influenced by an individual. The personal environment is easily managed and manipulated by an individual and can be customized to an individual's needs. The second layer of the environment includes the semipersonal contexts. Semipersonal environments are the places through which individuals often move during their daily routines. These spaces can include workplaces, local stores that are visited often, or a religious institution. These places might be customized to suit an individual's needs. Individuals are likely known in these environments. These contexts naturally surround personal environments. Generally, these spaces provide less accommodation than personal spaces do but are often critical for the successful execution of occupational goals.

The third layer, the public sphere of performance, contains spaces an individual visits less frequently than those in the second layer. These are community spaces that are typically used by many individuals in a community, such as government facilities, arenas, or other areas of public accommodation. These are the places that are least likely to be customized to meet an individual's needs and more likely to meet general anthropometric guidelines.

To understand how the physical environment can affect the occupational performance of each individual, it is important to consider each element of the environment in the context that is relevant to that person. Although each of the elements can be assessed and modified, they continuously change and influence each other. Both people and environments are constantly changing. In part, the change is a result of the layers of the environment influencing each other.

ASSESSMENT OF PHYSICAL ENVIRONMENTS

Occupational therapy assessment follows a systematic process, starting with the identification of the client's occupational performance in valued activities (AOTA, 2002; Fearing & Clark, 2000). The next step involves analysis of the client's occupational performance, in which the goodness of PEO fit is examined. The assessment of the environment typically starts here. We have organized assessments of physical environments across home, school, workplace, and community settings and across the layers of proximity from personal spaces through to public spaces.

Table 60.1 lists standardized tools that have been designed to assess physical characteristics and features of the environment in the home, school, workplace, and community and indicates the purpose or focus of each tool, the targeted population and age group, and the methods for administration. Some tools focus on measuring discrete elements of the physical environment, such as those that affect accessibility or safety, while others assess the client's functional needs and abilities in relation to environmental factors for an examination of PEO fit. Assessment of the physical environment can utilize several approaches,

TABLE 60.1 ENVIRONMENTAL ASSESSMENTS

HOME

Assessment	Source	Purpose/Focus: P:E fit	Accessibility	Home Hazards/Client Safety	Solutions/Interventions/Recommendations	Population: All—non-specific	Multi-diagnosis	Mobility Impairment	Age	Administration: Interview	Self-report	On-site Observation	Performance	Caregiver or Proxy	Time to Administer
Ease 3.2 Basic/Deluxe	Christenson, 2005; http://www.lifease.com/lifease-home.html	✓			✓	✓			OA	✓		✓		✓	
Home-Fast	Mackenzie, Byles, Higginbotham, 2000 & Mackenzie, Byles, Higginbotham, 2002.			✓		✓			OA			✓			20m
Home Observation for Measurement of the Environment (HOME)	Caldwell & Bradley, 1984; http://www.ualr.edu/~crtldept/home4.htm	✓				✓			C	✓		✓			90–120m
Housing Enabler	Slaug & Iwarsson, 2001; http://www.enabler.nu/index.html	✓						✓	OA	✓		✓			1–2 hrs
The Multiphasic Environmental Assessment Procedure—Architectural Features Checklist	Moos & Lemke, 1996		✓	✓	✓	✓			OA			✓			
Maintaining Seniors' Independence Through Home Adaptation: A self-assessment guide	Canadian Mortgage and Housing Corporation, 2003; http://www.cmhc.ca	✓				✓			OA		✓	✓			

Instrument	Reference	Age	Time
Safety Assessment of Function and the Environment for Rehabilitation (SAFER Tool) and SAFER-HOME	Chui, Oliver, Marshall & Letts, 2001; http://www.cotahealth.ca	A – OA	45–90m
Westmead Home Safety Assessment	Clemson et al., 1999; http://www.therapybookshop.com/coordinates.html	OA	1 hr
COMMUNITY			
ADA Checklist for Existing Facilities, version 2.1	Adaptive Environments, 1995; http://www.usdoj.gov/crt/ada/checkweb.htm	All	Variable
Craig Hospital Inventory of Environmental Factors (CHIEF and CHIEF Short Form)	Craig Hospital Research Department, 2005; http://www.craighospital.org/Research/Disability/CHIEF%20Manual.pdf	A – OA	10–15m
Measure of Quality of the Environment (MQE)	Fougeyrollas, Noreau, St. Michel & Boschen, 1999	A – OA	<30m
Home and Community Environment Instrument (HACE)	Keysor, Jette & Haley, 2005	A – OA	
SCHOOL			
School Setting Interview (SSI), Version 3.0	Hemmingsson, Egilson, Hoffman,& Kielhofner, 2005. Available from the MOHO Clearinghouse	C	40 m

Continued

TABLE 60.1 ENVIRONMENTAL ASSESSMENTS *Continued*

WORKPLACE

Assessment	Source	P:E fit	Accessibility	Home Hazards/ Client Safety	Solutions/Interventions/ Recommendations	All—non-specific	Multi-diagnosis	Mobility Impairment	Age	Interview	Self-report	On-site Observation	Performance	Caregiver or Proxy	Time to Administer
						Population				Administration					
ADA Worksite Assessment	Jacobs, 1999	✓	✓		✓	✓			A			✓			
Work Experience Survey	Roessler & Gottcent 1994; Roessler, 1996. Available from The National Clearinghouse of Rehabilitation Training Materials http://shopping.netsuite.com/s.nl/c.392723/sc.1/.f	✓					✓		A	✓					30–60m
Work Environment Impact Scale (WEIS)	Kielhofner et al., 1998; MOHO Clearinghouse, UIC. http://www.moho.uic.edu/assess/weis.html	✓					✓		A	✓					30m

Legend:
C = child
A = adult
OA = older adult

sometimes in combination. These include interviews with the client and/or designated people who know the client and/or the environmental setting well; observation of the client engaged in occupational performance within that setting, noting the environmental influences; and evaluation of specific aspects of the setting based on a set or list of criteria (e.g., standards). While most of these assessments have been developed for occupational therapy practice, some tools have broader applications (e.g., the Multiphasic Environmental Assessment Procedure is typically used by a multidisciplinary team to assess a congregate residential setting, and the ADA checklist is widely used by various groups to assess public access to buildings in the community). The clinical utility of these assessments is discussed in the following sections. For a detailed critique of these and other environmental assessments, see Cooper, Letts, Rigby, Stewart, and Strong (2005).

In most circumstances, occupational therapists should use standardized tools to assess the physical environment to ensure that the assessment has been comprehensive, valid, and reliable. However, suitable, well-designed tools might not always be available, and time constraints can limit what the therapist is able to achieve during assessment. A systematic approach to occupational performance analysis helps to ensure that the environmental factors that are influencing a client's performance are carefully examined.

Assessing the Home Environment

Occupational therapists assess clients' home environments to ensure that the home environment is safe and ready for the client on discharge from an institutional setting, to assess for and recommend home modifications, and to assess the home environment in terms of the client's ability to remain in the home. In the case of discharge planning, the purpose of the assessment is to determine whether the client will be able to manage functional activities while living in the home environment and/or to determine whether the home environment is suitable as a discharge location for the client. This could include assessment of a client's home prior to admission or assessment of a congregate living facility that the client and family are considering as a home after discharge. Further, it might be to determine whether modifications (major or minor) are required in the home to ensure that the client is going to be able to manage after discharge.

Another common home assessment occurs when clients are living in their own home but there is some question about whether or not safety or accessibility problems can be addressed. In many situations, home safety and falls prevention are key considerations of the occupational therapist.

In many home assessments, there is often overlap between assessments of activities of daily living (ADLs) and instrumental activities of daily living (IADLs) and the home environmental assessment. This overlap exists because

occupational therapists focus their home assessments on the functional abilities of the client in the home environment. ADL, IADL, and home-based leisure or productivity activities become a focus to help the therapist understand how the physical environment in the home is used, what the requirements of the environment are depending on the client's activities and preferences, and the meaning of home and its components to the client. This exploration of the occupational profile and analysis of occupational performance of the client provides information for the occupational therapist to then use in considering the need for home modifications (Siebert, 2005).

Home assessments often begin with a focus on the home's location within its community context. For example, is the home located in an urban, suburban, or rural setting? Is the client able to access the community resources he or she requires? How close are the local shopping district and medical offices? Specific to the home itself, there are some commonly assessed components of the home environment. These include entry to and exit from the home, including considerations of emergency exits, circulation within the home, and access within specific areas of the home, including the bathroom, kitchen, bedrooms, laundry, and living spaces. Although clinicians vary in the order in which they conduct assessments, an assessment typically moves from more public areas (entrances, living room, kitchen) to more intimate spaces (bathroom and bedroom).

A number of standardized instruments are available to guide home assessments (see Table 60.1). For example, if home safety is the focus of the assessment, an instrument such as the SAFER (Chui, Oliver, Marshall, & Letts, 2001), HOME-FAST (Mackenzie, Byles, & Higginbotham, 2000), or Westmead (Clemson, Fitzgerald, & Heard, 1999) might be selected. The Housing Enabler (Iwarsson & Slaug, 2001) or Ease 3.2 (Christenson, 2005) might be preferred if accessibility is the issue. If a congregate living facility is being assessed, the Physical and Architectural Features Checklist of the MEAP (Moos & Lemke, 1996) could provide useful information. Standardized home assessments can be used in conjunction with photographs of the home environment to document the current situation in the home. Photographs can be particularly useful when home modifications or renovations are being considered as part of the intervention. The therapist can use them as a means to recall the exact layout of a space and to provide justification for recommendations to the client, funders, and contractors with specific information about what needs to be modified.

Although standardized home assessments are not always used in clinical practice, they provide a significant advantage by ensuring that a comprehensive home assessment has been conducted, providing documentation of the assessment, providing useful information to justify the need for home modifications, and creating opportunities for evaluation of outcomes.

Assessing the School Environment

Occupational therapists play a critical role in enabling students with disabilities to succeed in the school environment and to participate in classroom, playground, and extracurricular activities (Mu & Royeen, 2004). The school team typically establishes the student's educational needs and goals, and the occupational therapist contributes to the analysis of the student's needs and school performance by examining the environmental influences on the student's school experiences.

In many jurisdictions, legislation requires that schools must be accessible to and usable by people with disabilities. The Americans with Disabilities Act Checklist for Readily Achievable Barrier Removal (Adaptive Environments Center, 1995) is a useful tool for assessing the accessibility of public buildings, such as schools, and provides a list of possible solutions for increasing a building's accessibility.

Few tools are available to the occupational therapist who needs to assess the environment for an individual student. The School Setting Interview was developed to explore school environment–student fit for students with physical disabilities ranging in age from 10 to 18 years (Hemmingsson, Kottorp, & Bernspang, 2004). It uses a semistructured interview covering the accommodation needs of students in 11 areas of school performance (e.g., writing, reading, examinations, and doing homework). The psychometric properties, in terms of interrater reliability and content validity, are good. The School Function Assessment (Coster, Deeney, Haltiwanger, & Haley, 1998) focuses on functional behaviors in elementary school environments, including the classroom, bathroom, and playground. Although this is not an assessment of the school environment, the scores reflect a child's participation in school activities and the need for adaptations to the school environment.

Assessing the Work Environment

An occupational therapist might be asked to assess the physical characteristics of the workplace environment for a client who plans to work or return to work in that setting or for the purposes of examining accessibility, safety, and ergonomic factors in a broader sense for a workplace injury prevention program. At the individual client level, the occupational therapist conducts a worksite analysis of the physical environmental factors that help or hinder that individual's work performance. The Work Experience Survey (Roessler, 1996; Roessler & Gottcent, 1994) can be used to assess worksite accessibility and job accommodation needs. The Workplace Environment Impact Scale (Kielhofner et al., 1998) facilitates dialogue about the individual's experiences and perceptions of the work environment, which is particularly useful in examining issues related to return to work. The Americans with Disabilities Act Checklist for Readily Achievable Barrier Removal (Adaptive Environments Center, 1995) and the ADA Work-Site Assessment (Jacobs, 1999) are also recommended for examining accessibility of the worksite.

At the broader level, occupational therapists are consulted by industry to assess the physical environment of the worksite for the purposes of injury prevention. The occupational therapist might be invited to do a job site analysis to identify workplace accessibility, physical hazards, and workstation design, among other factors such as ergonomics and the psychological demands of the work environment. Therapists who assume this role should familiarize themselves with standards and guidelines developed to prevent workplace injury in their community, such as those published by the National Institute of Occupational Safety and Health, which are available from the organization's Website: http://www.cdc.gov/niosh/homepage.html. For more detail about the role of the occupational therapist in the workplace, please refer to Chapter 52.

Assessing Community

There are a variety of reasons why occupational therapists assess community environments. Some of the variation relates to whether or not the therapist is working with a specific individual client or the community site is the "client." In community-based practice with a single client, a community assessment might be required as part of the process of understanding an individual client's abilities and limitations in different contexts. For example, it can be useful to observe a client while grocery shopping to better understand the environmental constraints and facilitators that the client experiences in the grocery store that the client most commonly uses. The occupational therapist can then make recommendations to modify the client's approach to the task, the client's abilities, or the environment itself.

Community assessments can also be focused on the experiences of the individual client within the home and community. Assessments such as the Craig Hospital Inventory of Environmental Factors (Craig Hospital Research Department, 2001; Whiteneck, Harrison-Felix et al., 2004) and the Home and Community Environment Assessment (Keysor, Jette, & Haley, 2005) provide means for clients to report on their experiences in these environments. These types of assessment results can help occupational therapists to better understand the experiences of the client and to set priorities with the client to enhance participation in occupational performance across a number of settings.

Alternatively, the community site or setting may be the client, in which case the needs of many people with different types and degrees of disability may be considered. Although this type of assessment can be more complicated because there is no single client whose individual needs are being considered, it offers an opportunity to suggest environmental modifications that might meet the needs of a larger group of users of the environment.

A number of assessments are available that focus on the accessibility of community settings. For example, AIMFREE (Rimmer et al., 2004) was developed to measure the accessibility of fitness and recreation facilities and has been standardized with initial testing of its psychometric properties. The ADAAG Checklist provides the assessor with the technical requirements from the ADA-ABA Accessibility Guidelines to conduct the evaluation (U.S. Access Board, 2004). Access Guide Canada provides a number of forms to evaluate community settings such as restaurants, financial institutions, entertainment venues, parks, and places of worship. These forms can be obtained from http://enablelink.org/agc/index.php. The Access Guide Canada Website and project are a valuable resource and a model of how information about accessibility can be readily shared with others using the internet. Users can search by province and community and can review information submitted by volunteers on the basic accessibility of sites within the community. The project provides people with disabilities the opportunity to promote the accessible spaces in their community and to participate more fully in the communities in which they live and visit.

Community settings also include playgrounds. An accessible playground provides play opportunities for children of varying abilities and can facilitate social integration (see Figure 60.2). Occupational therapists who work with children with disabilities will find the Guide to ADA Accessibility Guidelines for Play Areas (U.S. Architectural and Transportation Barriers and Compliance Board, 2001) an excellent resource when working within a community setting toward creating accessible play areas. Accessible playground components include accessible routes throughout the play area to both ground-level and elevated play structures and using accessible surfaces such as wooden ramps and rubber tiles. Play tables for sand and water play and vertically mounted panels with activities that are easy to reach and manipulate provide access for children using wheelchairs and walkers. The playground should also be accessible for adults with disabilities. At times, there may be teachers, parents, or other caregivers at the play area who have disabilities and need to access different elements of the play area when children using the equipment need support, supervision, or help.

INTERVENTIONS

When the assessment process is complete, interventions focusing on the client's identified targeted occupational performance outcomes should be developed using a systematic approach such as the Occupational Therapy Practice Framework (AOTA, 2002) or the Occupational Performance Process Model (Fearing & Clark, 2000). The goal of improving PEO fit as it relates to occupational engagement guides the development of the intervention plan. Goals should be written to reflect the targeted occupational performance outcome (e.g., the client will be able to transfer using grab bars), not the intervention (e.g., install grab bars).

The client or person representing the end-user group plays an integral role in intervention planning and decision making (Ringaert, 2003). When addressing macro settings in the public sphere, the occupational therapist and other planners and designers consult with all end-user groups to help design an environment that is accessible and available to all.

In this section, we present various intervention strategies for the home, school, and workplace and for community settings. Although occupational therapists recommend interventions related to the context of an individual's home, there are several other important settings for environmental interventions. Some interventions can be applied at the personal or semipersonal level with individual clients, and others can be applied at the broader public level with communities or at a societal level.

Interventions in the Personal Environment: The Importance of Home

Home is the context for a broad range of occupations. These occupations can be basic and common, such as dressing and grooming, or complex, such as planning and executing family gatherings and celebrations, maintaining finances, and participating in sexual relations. Home is where we store and display treasured possessions and seek shelter from community stressors (Rowles, 2003). Home is frequently one of the most cherished environments in people's lives and has been associated with personal identity and values (Dovey, 1985). Often, the primary goal of most individuals in an inpatient setting is to go home; the goal of older adults with chronic conditions is to be able to stay home (American Association of Retired Persons, 2000). However, because of the cost of home visits by a

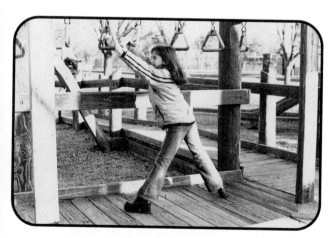

FIGURE 60.2 In an adapted playground, the ramps and boardwalk provide access for all children.

therapist, the home is often overlooked as a focus for intervention. Despite clinical reports of the value of home modifications (Siebert, 2005) and the evidence of the positive influence on occupational performance following intervention programs that occur in the home (e.g., Gitlin, Corcoran, Winter, Boyce, & Hauck, 2001; Mann, Ottenbacher, Fraas, Tomita, & Granger, 1999), therapists often rely on verbal reports from caregivers or clients to understand the complicated environmental influences facing a client who will be returning home. Ordering equipment or making recommendations for architectural modification without observing clients in context is not recommended, as this practice often results in poor outcomes for clients. Most individuals with new disabilities are not able to consider the range of possible barriers they will face in their home. As a result, many opportunities for useful modifications are missed.

Types of Homes

The range of housing options is considerable. Individuals can live in free-standing houses, mobile homes, townhouses, apartments, and condominiums. Homes can be designed for single or multiple families; can include retrofitted loft spaces in large cities or large single-family houses in rural farming communities. Homes can also be congregate living facilities such as assisted living facilities, homeless shelters, dormitories, and group homes. Unfortunately, most housing lacks features that support the performance of individuals with disabilities. Fewer than 10% of the 100 million existing private homes in the United States contain such modifications (Center for Universal Design, 1997), making home modification a priority for intervention for any client who will live with functional limitations as a result of a disability.

It is critical that the occupational therapist understands the policy and legal ramifications of making home modifications in various housing situations. For example, in a walk-up apartment, a person with a new spinal cord injury has the right under the Fair Housing Laws (U.S. Department of Housing and Urban Development, 2001) to add a ramp to reach the apartment building's front door at his or her own expense. Under the same law, an individual with multiple sclerosis who uses a support dog cannot be denied housing even if there is a "no pet" policy in a large apartment complex. The laws can vary depending on the housing situation. For example, dormitories and homeless shelters may be subject to the ADA (1990). Private housing may be subject to local building codes. It is important to understand individual rights with regard to accessible housing. If a law requires that accessible housing features be present but they are not, the therapist might have the role of assisting the client in advocating for accessible features.

Occupational therapists must also consider other residents in the dwelling who could be influenced by or will influence environmental modifications. People who live in single-family homes will likely have family members who cohabitate with them or visit on a frequent basis, apartment dwellers will share common space with other residents, and students might share bathroom facilities.

Person-Environment-Occupation Misfit in the Home

The goal of enabling clients with disabilities to live at home is threatened when the client's functional capacity does not match the demands of the environment. Often, the threat of occupational dysfunction can be attributed to a lack of environmental support (Connell, Sanford, Long, Archea, & Turner, 1993; Mann, Hurren, Tomita, Bengali, & Steinfeld, 1994). In some cases, valued occupations are relinquished because of environmental barriers. For example, a woman who is experiencing the complications of Parkinson's disease might no longer be able to wash her clothing independently because her laundry facilities are located in her basement. In other instances, clients might go to great lengths to continue doing vital activities of daily living, as in the example of an older woman who could no longer step safely into her large bathtub and would take trips to a fitness facility to safely use a walk-in shower. These are examples of poor PEO fit. The desired occupation is difficult or impossible, given the functional limitations of the client and the demands made by the environment. Many common environmental features, as shown in Table 60.2, become barriers when encountered by people with functional limitations.

How to Modify the Home

Home modifications can include changes to the physical environment (both spaces and objects within the environment), education about the physical environment and how to use it in a more efficient or safe way, or changing the social support in the environment to compensate for physical environmental barriers. Often, a blend of all three approaches is used in successful interventions. Interventions should be planned with consideration of the cultural, economic, institutional, political, and social context of the client and the family in relation to impairment and functional limitations associated with the client's acute or chronic condition.

Occupational therapists can use several approaches to change the physical environment in order to reduce demand. They can add features to an environment (e.g., add a bath bench), remove features of an environment (e.g., remove scatter rugs from a hallway), or modify existing features (e.g., paint the door frame a contrasting color). Features of the environment that are barriers to one individual might serve as supports to another. For example, an individual with back pain might benefit from the support that a 19-inch-high toilet (taller than a standard

TABLE 60.2 EXAMPLES OF BARRIERS IN THE HOME

ENTRANCES AND DOORWAYS IN THE HOME

Steps at entrances

Stairs with no railings or with inadequate railings

Narrow doorways

Heavy doors

Door hardware and locks that are difficult to manipulate

Thresholds over ½-inch high

GENERAL CIRCULATION THROUGHOUT THE HOME

Slippery floors

Uneven floor surfaces, multiple levels

Loose carpeting

Throw rugs

Poorly lit areas (e.g., hallway/stairway)

Lack of color contrast on edges of counters, doorways, etc.

Clutter on floors or stairs

BATHROOMS

Height of bathtub

Lack of grab bars by tub and toilet

Height of toilet

Lack of space in bathroom for wheelchair, walkers, assistant

Nonslip resistant flooring in bathtub/shower

KITCHENS

Counter heights either too low or too high

Lack of space for wheelchair, walkers

Height and depth of cupboards, shelves

Appliances that are difficult to use (e.g., handles/controls)

GENERAL

Loose cords (e.g., extension cords, cables)

Low-volume telephone/doorbell

Small-button telephone

Heights of seats including chairs, sofas

Small print on items (e.g., cleaning products/medications)

Sharp corners on furniture and fixtures

---

toilet) offers. The same 19-inch-high toilet might serve as a barrier to an individual who is short in stature and would need a step stool to achieve a sitting position. The goal of the intervention process is to determine the optimal environmental modifications that will support individuals with disabilities in achieving their occupational goals.

Adaptive equipment, such as a bath bench and hand-held shower for someone who is unable to enter and stand for a shower, is a common modification that occupational therapists provide. Adaptive equipment can include specialized medical equipment such as a raised toilet seat, specially designed equipment such as a reacher for someone who cannot bend or reach the floor, or off-the-shelf products that support performance such as an ultra-light vacuum cleaner for a person with arthritis. Architectural modifications range from simple modifications, such as adding stair handrails, to complicated modifications, such as the provision of ramps to enter the home, or the major remodeling of a home. Home renovations can include replacing a bathtub with a roll-in shower, adding an elevator, or building an accessible addition that includes a bedroom and bathroom for a family member who has a disability.

Occupational therapists can also modify how people use the physical environment by providing education about safety in the home. For example, they can teach individuals to make use of features of their existing environment in ways that make it safer or easier to perform daily activities. The conceptual framework for developing home modification developed by Sanford and Jones (2001) provides an organizing scheme to systematically analyze environmental features. The framework, as shown in Table 60.3, hierarchically organizes the architectural features of a room into the categories of spaces, products, controls, and hardware.

How to Decide Which Intervention Is Best

Once the therapist has identified potential intervention options that are most likely to support performance, the therapist reviews these with the client and presents the preferred interventions to potential funders. Often, there are multiple solutions to the occupational performance problems faced by the client. Consider this scenario: A young woman with multiple sclerosis has two primary occupational performance problems. She is unable to bathe independently and struggles to prepare simple meals. She has difficulty walking and uses a wheelchair for mobility. With the first problem, she is unable to transfer into her traditional-style bathtub and currently relies on an attendant to lift her into the tub and to bathe her. She finds the situation frightening and embarrassing and would like to be able to bathe independently. The occupational therapist met with this young woman and identified two environmental modifications that might support her occupational performance goal. The first option was a major

TABLE 60.3   ARCHITECTURAL FEATURES OF A ROOM

Spaces	**Described in terms of:** -Layout -Dimensions -Lighting -Ambient conditions (e.g., heat, light) -Finishes (carpet/wall covering) -Entry dimensions of a room or area **Examples:** -Rooms -Playground -Garage
Products	**Contained in the spaces and include:** -Fixtures -Appliances -Off-the-shelf items **Described in terms of:** -Type -Size -Force required to operate -Auditory or visual signals -Texture **Examples:** -Toilet -Refrigerator
Controls and hardware	Aspects of the environment where the human interfaces with the physical environment **Analyzed in terms of:** -Type -Fine motor skills (one versus two hands, pinch, grip strength) -Access to the item (height of dispenser) -Location of controls -Size -Force to operate -Operational characteristics (calibration/type of sensory feedback) **Examples:** -Doorknobs -Light switches

architectural renovation that involved removing her existing tub and building a roll-in shower with an integrated bench and adjustable hand-held shower. Her second choice was a transfer bench with a hand-held shower (Figure 60.3). Both options would help her to bathe independently. This scenario identifies numerous possibilities, but environmental constraints, such as economic, architectural, and social barriers, might influence the choices.

Funding is often the most challenging obstacle for individuals with disabilities who are attempting to make home modifications. Building renovations are expensive, and funding currently is not available through most insurance companies for modifications to the home. People often rely on personal resources or social service agencies to fund the modifications. Occupational therapists should be familiar with their local social service agencies that provide for such modifications.

The decision to make architectural modifications in the home is generally expensive. Therefore, it is important to plan for modifications that will continue to meet the needs of the client (and their family members) over time. Therapists should consider the possible course of a chronic dis-

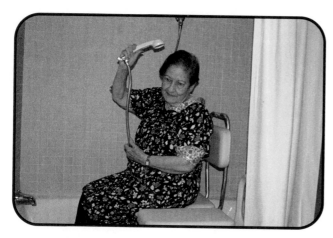

FIGURE 60.3 Bathroom aids: transfer bench and hand-held shower.

ease or how an individual with a disability might age and should recommend modifications accordingly.

The vast differences in housing construction methods can also pose challenges. Although therapists do not often oversee major modifications, they can advise their clients to consult building professionals to determine whether the home can accommodate the changes required before the clients proceed with implementing the recommendations. Questions of how to move plumbing or whether a structure will support a grab bar are important safety concerns and should be made in consultation with professionals.

The decision to make modifications to one's home can sometimes be difficult for homeowners who do not want their home to appear unattractive. Home is often an expression of self; displaying medical equipment or institutional-looking steel grab bars can be undesirable. When therapists offer choices for modifications, aesthetics are an important consideration. Presenting clients with a range of options allows them to weigh the costs in relation to their needs, priorities, aesthetic tastes, family goals, and values. Clients should have all of the information possible to assist them in their decision about modifying their home environment.

Visitability as a Universal Design Concept

Most homes have steps at every entrance, interior doorways that are too narrow for passage by someone using a wheelchair, and lack a bathroom on the main floor. These three barriers are the primary design habits that cause people who are disabled to become isolated from their neighbors and extended families and cause people who develop mobility impairments to become unable to reside safely in their own homes. Without intending to do so, the design of homes often forces people with disabilities and older people to be isolated rather than being integral parts of their communities. Fiscally, it costs much more to do home modifications and remove architectural barriers in inaccessible homes than to incorporate basic access features into new construction.

Visitability is an affordable and sustainable design strategy aimed at increasing the number of minimally accessible single-family homes and neighborhoods. The dual goals of visitability are to ensure access by people with mobility impairments to neighbors and family homes and to provide a basic "shell" of access to allow people to remain in their own homes if they develop a disability. Visitability does not offer total access but does allow people with disabilities to enter the first floor of a home without being lifted up and provides access to the rooms and bathrooms on the first floor (Smith, 2003).

Many communities around the globe have incorporated visitability standards that have resulted in a significant number of new homes designed with accessibility features (http://www.concretechange.org). Typically, visitability includes at least one accessible (or "zero-step") entrance into the home (as shown in Figure 60.4), 32-inch clearance doorways on the main level, and at least one half-bathroom on the main floor (Claar & Boan, 2005). Occupational therapists have many exciting opportunities to assist in community development, education and advocacy using the principles of universal design, and specifically visitability (Ringaert, 2003).

How to Make Going to School Achievable

In many Western societies, students with disabilities are entitled to public education in the least restrictive environment (e.g., Individuals with Disabilities Education Act [IDEA] of 1990 and the IDEA amendments of 1997 [P.L. 105-17], Section 504 of the Rehabilitation Act of 1973 [P.L. 93-112], and Ontarians with Disabilities Act [ODA; Government of Ontario, 2001]). The physical accessibility of schools and school playgrounds and access to barrier-free transportation to and from school are important steps toward achieving the integration of students with disabilities. In addition, the ADA requires school districts to provide programs and services that are readily accessible and usable by individuals with disabilities (Abend, 2001), thus enabling students, parents, teachers, and others with disabilities to access schools. The ADA-ABA Accessibility Guidelines (U.S. Access Board, 2004) are based on both adult and child dimensions and anthropometrics and should be applied in renovating or constructing new schools. Occupational therapists can consult about and advocate for architectural accessibility and the use of universal design principles within schools. For example, in Ontario, Canada, occupational therapists can consult with school boards to prepare annual accessibility plans, mandated by the ODA (Government of Ontario, 2001), or to assist in the design and planning of new schools and planning for major renovations to make schools more accessible.

ETHICAL DILEMMA

Should an Occupational Therapist Recommend Expensive Environmental Modifications?

Darrell is a 72-year-old man with post-polio syndrome. He lives with his wife, Edith. They have been married for 50 years. He uses a scooter for mobility. He has weakness and limited range of motion in his upper extremities, likely resulting from obesity and inactivity as well as the late effects of polio. Darrell has demonstrated a change in his cognitive status and has exhibited new behaviors that are not typical of his abilities (losing keys, unable to use the TV remote control). Edith has been Darrell's primary caregiver over the past 20 years. She lifts him, bathes him, helps him dress, prepares meals, and cares for laundry, their pets, and their home. Edith has begun to experience significant pain and dysfunction as a result of her rheumatoid arthritis. She has joint pain, swelling, and stiffness. She recently injured her back transferring Darrell from the bathtub.

Arven, an occupational therapist, received a referral from Darrell's doctor to evaluate Darrell's functional status. Darrell's doctor would like to consider nursing home placement to relieve the stress that Edith is feeling. The doctor also worries about Darrell wandering away, after Edith recently found him scooting along in a nearby park looking at the ducks in a pond.

On evaluation of Darrell, Edith, and their home, Arven discovers that there are many changes that could be made to the home that would relieve the physical strain on Edith. Arven discusses a plan for a bathroom modification that is fairly extensive, with an overhead lift system that will transfer Darrell safely to the toilet and tub. Arven also describes a new alarm system that will alert Edith if Darrell leaves the premises. They discuss the possibility of a new bed, some modifications in the kitchen that will give Darrell greater independence in preparing meals, and a new laundry machine that Darrell can operate from a seated position. All of these changes will relieve Edith of duties and keep Darrell engaged in his daily life. Edith tells Arven that she finally sees a ray of hope in their lives and is thrilled with the possibility of some quality time with her husband. The plan is reviewed, and both Darrell and Edith agree that the modifications will make important and meaningful changes in their lives. Arven sends a report to the physician indicating that the nursing home is not a necessary option and presents his environmental modification plan. Arven is shocked when he receives a call from his supervisor demanding a meeting with Arven to discuss his unethical behavior.

Arven meets with his supervisor and is told that the referring physician will no longer send referrals to the agency. The physician is angry that Arven gave the family hope to stay home and demands to know how Arven can guarantee Darrell's safety, given his functional limitations and likely cognitive changes. The physician is also furious because his patient has called him asking whether there are funds available to make these changes, since the family is on a fixed income and can barely afford the expensive medications that might make a slight change in Darrell's dementia course. The family has asked the doctor which they should spend their limited funds on: the medication or the modifications. Arven's supervisor has also given Arven a message from Edith asking whether he is aware of any available funds to help pay for the modifications. Arven explains to his supervisor that he has some ideas about funding for the project. He admits that he committed to calling the Alzheimer's Association, Darrell's church, and a few other local charitable organizations on Edith's behalf. Arven's supervisor advises him that he has already spent too much time on the case and informs him that looking for funding is not a reimbursable activity. Arven is told that he will not be permitted to look for funding for these clients.

Questions

1. Should Arven have discussed the possibility of expensive modifications when the family could not afford the changes?
2. Should Arven have followed the referral from the physician and focused his attention on how to make the transition to a nursing home as smooth as possible, even though his professional opinion is that Darrell does not need to be there?
3. Does Arven (and his therapy service) have an obligation to find funding for these modifications?
4. How can Arven defend the course of action he has taken with this client?

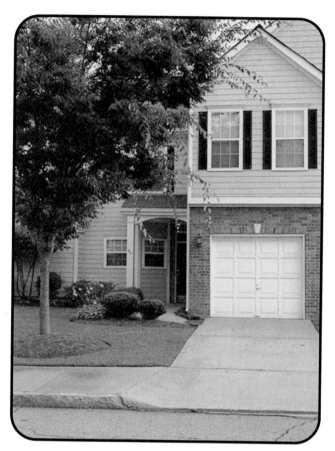

FIGURE 60.4 Visitability standard: "zero-step" entrance to new home.

Abend's (2001) guide, *Planning and Designing for Students with Disabilities,* provides useful design principles that are applicable to students with various disabling conditions, including physical, sensory, attention and/or learning impairments, and universal design principles. For example, Abend suggests that versatile classroom spaces with a small alcove off a large common classroom area can help to control noise and visual distractions for students with attention deficits. Modular furniture can be combined or separated to support a variety of activities, such as individual and group work, and can include accessible desks and computer workstations to accommodate students who use wheelchairs or who need writing aids such as laptop computers.

Several physical barriers that have been consistently identified by students with disabilities are steep ramps, heavy doors and raised door thresholds at school entrances, a lack of elevators to a second level, and inadequate accessibility on school playgrounds (Hemmingsson & Borell, 2000; Pivik, McComas, & LaFamme, 2002). School cafeterias should have wheelchair-accessible food aisles, food placed within reach of people who use a wheelchair, and accessible seating arrangements. Way-finding within a school can pose problems for many students, including those with visual, cognitive, and perceptual impairments. Clear signage in corridors that provides directions around the school and distinctive color-coding in sections of buildings can assist students and others to find their way around the school.

Occupational Therapy in the Schools with Individual Students

Occupational therapists play a critical role in enabling students with disabilities to succeed in the school environment and to participate in classroom, playground, and extracurricular activities (Mu & Royeen, 2004). A few examples provided below demonstrate how goodness of fit can be achieved by modifying the environment. Further information about school-based practice is provided in Chapters 51 and 64.

For students who use wheelchairs, school accessibility is critical. To facilitate bathroom accessibility, modifications such as installing an electronic door opener, installing grab bars and a raised toilet seat in the toilet stall, and lowering the sink and installing lever-style taps might be necessary. To facilitate group work with peers, the therapist might recommend a round or rectangular table to bring the group together at a level work surface. Classroom materials should be placed within reach of students.

Classroom environments can have high levels of sensory stimuli in terms of noise, visual clutter, and the physical activity of a classroom full of students, which can have a disorganizing effect for children with sensory-processing problems. Occupational therapists assess the classroom environment to identify the sensory features that either facilitate or hinder students' ability to complete schoolwork and recommend rearranging the physical environment to better fit students' sensory-processing needs. For example, sound-absorbing partitions and low lighting can enable some students to focus their attention while working on individual assignments. The therapist might recommend setting up a quiet space in the classroom where a student with autism can use a rocking chair to seek calming sensory input and put on a headset to listen to music or a taped story.

The occupational therapist should become familiar with the conditions and terms for funding environmental modifications and special or adapted furniture or equipment for schools. Some environmental modifications can be made at little cost, while others will involve applying to the school board or a government agency for special funding.

Accessibility at Colleges and Universities

Many colleges and universities have accessibility plans and special services for students, faculty, and staff with disabilities. For example, a college might have accessible student housing options and special services within the libraries to help with accessing books and other educational materials. Typically, occupational therapists work for the college or university with the role of providing specific services to students and employees or work for a health provider and have a student or college employee as a client. Occupational therapists can also provide consultation regarding the development of accessibility plans and special services, particularly for communal spaces such as libraries, cafeterias, bookstores, and student lounges. For example, the therapist might not only advise about creating accessible spaces, but might also recommend assistive technologies, such as closed-circuit televisions or screen readers for school libraries to support students and faculty with low vision.

When working with students or college employees, occupational therapists can examine their clients' occupational performance challenges in relation to their roles on campus and help clients to access special services. Therapists can use many of the strategies described in this chapter to address access to the home (which would apply to student dormitories and other student housing), access to classrooms and libraries, and participation in campus life in general. Colleges and universities, like other public spaces, are typically subject to the accessibility guidelines that are mandated in their jurisdiction, such as the ADA-ABA Accessibility Guidelines (U.S. Access Board, 2004).

Transportation to campus and around campus can pose challenges for people with physical disabilities. Occupational therapists can assist their clients to develop a transportation plan that might involve such strategies as arranging for accessible transportation to campus or obtaining a parking permit that allows a student to park next to an accessible entrance to a building in which the student has classes.

Interventions in the Workplace

For many people with disabilities, the ability to work is a primary occupational performance goal. However, the opportunity to work is denied to many individuals with disabilities; the rate of unemployment is significantly higher among people with disabilities than among their counterparts who do not have disabilities (U.S. Department of Labor, 2001). The presence of environmental barriers in the workplace influences a person's ability to perform the essential functions of his or her job. For example, steps at the entry to an office building act as a barrier to a person who uses a manual wheelchair for mobility. A person with low vision might have difficulty reading the small print of office signs. With environmental modification, these barriers can be removed, resulting in people with disabilities being able to successfully perform their jobs. Removing barriers by providing adaptive equipment or modification of the physical environment is typically easy and not expensive (Gray, Hollingsworth, & Morgan, 2001). Table 60.4 provides some typical examples of workplace modifications.

TABLE 60.4   EXAMPLES OF ENVIRONMENTAL MODIFICATIONS IN THE WORKPLACE FOR FUNCTIONAL IMPAIRMENTS

Impairment	Environmental Modifications in the Workplace
Cognitive impairment:	◆ Minimize distractions in a quiet, private space. ◆ Use the layout of the space to provide structure to the work day. ◆ Provide photographs in addition to words on signs or office name plates.
Fatigue/weakness:	◆ Use the layout of the space to efficiently complete tasks. ◆ Provide parking close to the worksite.
Fine motor impairment:	◆ Implement ergonomic workstation design. ◆ Provide large buttons or controls with lever-type handles and low force requirements to operate.
Gross motor impairment:	◆ Provide an accessible entrance (e.g., add ramp). ◆ Provide accessible parking on an accessible route of travel. ◆ Provide power-assist door openers. ◆ Provide an accessible restroom and break room.
Auditory impairment:	◆ Provide teletypewriter (TTY) with a visual alert system. ◆ Install an emergency alert system with visual or tactile signal. ◆ Encourage full use of visual aids, including films, overhead projectors, diagrams, and chalkboards.
Vision impairment:	◆ Install proper office lighting. ◆ Use high-contrast color on door frames. ◆ Provide large signs with high color contrast.

The ADA and similar human rights legislation in many countries support the individual's right to work by prohibiting discrimination against people with disabilities. In the United States, when people with disabilities can perform the essential functions of a job with accommodations, they are allowed to apply for and maintain a job. Under the ADA, an employer is responsible for providing the reasonable accommodations necessary for a qualified individual to perform the job.

When job accommodations are necessary, the occupational therapist can be invited to lead a team to identify the environmental barriers that influence an employee's ability to work and help to remove these barriers. The team members can include the occupational therapist, the employer, key employees, and the group that is responsible for implementing the environmental changes. The process of making workplace accommodations is similar to that of making home modifications. An occupational performance analysis is conducted, barriers are identified, and solutions are proposed.

Several strategies are useful for workplace modifications. It is possible to consider the use of adaptive equipment such as a telephone headset for a person with limited upper-extremity function (see also Chapter 62) or to modify the functions of the job by eliminating ancillary tasks that are impossible for the individual to perform. The existing job can also be restructured, as in the case of a person with cognitive impairment who had his workstation moved to an enclosed cubicle to minimize disruptions. The physical environment can also be modified to match the functional limitations experienced by an employee, such as installing power-assist doors for an employee who uses a power wheelchair. The Job Accommodation Network website (see http://www.jan.wvu.edu) provides an excellent resource for therapists, employers, and employees with disabilities.

The occupational therapist should consider all aspects of the work experience when making a plan for accommodations. The therapist must consider not only the employee's daily job duties, but also the administrative and practical functions. The therapist must evaluate the employee's ability to park or get from public transportation to the job site, eat lunch, take breaks, visit the human resources office, and receive communication about relevant work issues. The workstation and the worksite must be evaluated. The emergency evacuation plan must be reviewed to ensure that the worker is able to safely evacuate from the worksite in case of emergency.

Changing the physical environment is an expensive prospect, and the plan that the occupational therapist develops should take into account whether the employee's condition is progressive or stable. When a health condition is stable, the modifications that are made should serve the person's needs. In the case of progressive conditions, it is often important to consider a flexible accommodation that can change with time as a condition progresses.

Before starting the job accommodation process, the occupational therapist should have a clear understanding of pertinent legislation, how to apply it, and the limitations of the legislation. For example, under the ADA, workers are permitted "reasonable accommodations" as long as these do not cause "undue hardship" to the employer. A small employer that has a very small profit margin might not be required to pay for an elevator if it would cause the company bankruptcy, but the employer might be required to move the office of an employee with a mobility impairment to the first floor if space was available. Excellent resources are available from the Equal Employment Opportunity Commission (2005) about the ADA in the United States and from the Canadian Employment Programming for Persons with Disabilities (Human Resources and Skills Development Canada, 2005).

It is also important that the job accommodations leave the facility in compliance with regulations regarding accessibility and safety. A modification plan should be reviewed and approved by an individual who is knowledgeable about the regulations to which the facility must adhere. The outcome of the job accommodation should be evaluated, and the continued success of the accommodations should be monitored over time to ensure the best worker-job fit.

The Public Sphere of Occupational Performance: Community-Based Interventions

The public sphere of performance contains spaces in which people visit on a less frequent basis than the work or home environment. Examples of places included in this sphere of performance include government agencies, cultural venues, shopping complexes, and stores. Although people often spend less time in community spaces, they are important environments that serve as links between more private spaces such as work and home, and they also contain critical goods and services necessary for successful participation in community life. Community spheres are important for socialization, recreation, and civic and social engagement. Environments with poor accessibility can negatively affect the community participation of people with disabilities.

Public places are not customized to meet individual needs. Rather, public spaces are typically designed to meet the needs of average individuals and are based on general guidelines such as the ADA-ABA Accessibility Guidelines (U.S. Access Board, 2004) and building codes in Canada. Yet there are still many challenges in achieving accessible communities, as demonstrated in several articles that describe architectural barriers in food stores (McClain & Todd, 1990), restaurants (McClain, Cram, Wood, & Taylor, 1993), physicians' offices (Grabois, Nosek, & Rossi, 1999), and religious institutions (Harris Interactive, Inc.,

2004). We can achieve greater accessibility by working directly with clients, by working with community property owners or consultants, and by working as advocates in the community.

Transportation is a form of functional mobility and represents an important area of occupational performance. People with functional impairments may face challenges when navigating public transportation systems. Iwarsson, Ståhl, & Carlsson (2003) described collaborative work between occupational therapy, traffic planning, and engineering in an initiative to understand the accessibility of transportation systems. They used a travel chain perspective, which involves considering all steps in the process of traveling from the point of origin to the destination. Occupational therapists can also use occupational analyses to examine the steps involved in using public transportation in relation to the functional limitations experienced by people with disabilities with the goal of optimizing the accessibility and usability of these systems.

Another community setting in which occupational therapists can provide input is in sheltered living or long-term care facilities for older adults. Cooper and Day (2003) described a postoccupancy evaluation process involving assessment and recommendations to meet the needs of people with dementia and their caregivers for short-term respite. Their recommendations focused on promoting safety, self-care, way-finding, and quality of life through such strategies as clear signage, temperature control of water to prevent burns, specific products and devices in the bathroom to optimize independence, and the provision of a wandering path and therapeutic garden.

Occupational therapists who recognize the importance the community sphere plays in the participation of their clients with disabilities can also serve as advocates who promote accessible, livable communities. Occupational therapists can bring their knowledge of accessibility standards and theory to community agencies or organizations. Examples of advocacy include ensuring that polling stations are accessible for people with disabilities and preparing an accessibility guide for community restaurants. Although the advocacy role is often voluntary, it is an important service to the community and citizens with disabilities and is often an extension of direct service roles.

In working directly with clients, barrier removal might not always be possible. In some cases, if the environmental support is not part of a mandatory accessibility guideline, it might not be possible to make changes. For example, the elevator exemption in the ADA permits owners of some small businesses to operate on the second floor with no elevator access, making participation for a person with a mobility impairment impossible. It is the occupational therapist's role to understand current legislation and minimum standards and to help the client advocate for change. It is also possible to identify barriers through the assessment process to help clients make decisions about how they could access and use spaces. In this case, understanding the environment is the goal, even though modification might not be possible.

CASE STUDY: *Occupational Therapist Working with a Client Returning Home*

Gary Lau is a 30-year-old man who sustained a closed head injury with diffuse axonal injury as the result of a motor vehicle accident. Before his brain injury, Gary worked full-time as a mechanical engineer. He is married and lives with his wife; they have no children. In the past, he enjoyed participating in social activities with family and friends, playing sports, woodworking, and many outdoor activities. Gary perceives himself to be very independent, a risk taker, and stubborn at times.

The brain injury resulted in both cognitive and physical impairments. Following five months of intensive therapy, Gary was discharged home. Gary is left with some impairments that negatively affect his ability to be independent with his ADLs. The most limiting is Gary's left hemiplegia. He has decreased balance and an unsteady gait, and he uses a quad cane (a cane with four prongs) for walking. He has no voluntary spontaneous movement in his left hand, and he cannot grasp things with that hand. In addition to poor short-term memory, he has limitations in his executive function, including difficulty initiating tasks, poor organization, difficulty sequencing, and poor judgment and safety. He currently has decreased insight; he is aware of his deficits but has poor appreciation of how his deficits affect his occupational performance.

Currently, Gary requires assistance with his ADLs and IADLs. He is independent with most self-care tasks, including dressing, toileting, and grooming (in a seated position). However, he has difficulty with bathtub transfers, and he needs help to wash his legs, feet, and back. He requires assistance with all IADLs, including, laundry, meal preparation, and housekeeping chores.

Katya, who works as a home-care occupational therapist, met Gary and his wife in their 1-½ story bungalow home to assess the home environment and to provide recommendations to maximize Gary's functional independence at home. Katya interviewed the Laus using the

CASE STUDY: *Occupational Therapist Working with a Client Returning Home*   *Continued*

Canadian Occupational Performance Measure (Law et al., 1996), and from those results, the Laus identified the following occupational performance goals for Gary: (1) to become independent with bathing and (2) to be able to prepare a simple lunch for himself during the week when his wife returns to work.

Katya chose the Housing Enabler 1.0, a 188 item checklist that provides a reliable, and valid assessment of accessibility (Iwarsson, 2005; Iwarsson & Slaug, 2001), to assess Gary's functional abilities in relation to the physical aspects of the Laus' home environment. Katya first completed the form "Analysis of Personal Component of Accessibility" to identify Gary's impairments before examining these in relation to environmental barriers in his home and its close surroundings (see Figure 60.5). Katya went on to complete the form, "Environmental Component of Accessibility" (http://www.enabler.nu/; selected items are shown in the figure on the W&S Website). She analyzed the assessment findings by looking at Gary's profile of functional limitations in relation to the environmental barriers in the home; an assessment of person-environment fit. This allowed her to generate a list of the greatest accessibility problems for Gary. For example, the carpeted floor throughout the house and the very narrow hallways and door openings made it difficult

for Gary to maneuver with his cane throughout the home. In addition, the lighting on the stairway was poor, and the home was cluttered with a lot of furniture, loose scatter rugs on the carpeting, and electrical cords. Katya recommended increasing lighting on the stairway, moving furniture that was creating obstacles, removing the loose rugs, and taping electrical cords to the floor or walls to create a safer, more accessible environment.

The assessment of the bathroom and the kitchen revealed several barriers. In the bathroom the toilet was a standard height; there was no place to sit in the shower/bath; there were no grab bars located in the shower/bath or by the toilet; the handles to control the water temperature in the bathtub required high force and were extremely difficult to grasp; there was no nonslip bath mat in the bathtub; a very thick carpeted bath mat lay on the floor outside of the bathtub; the bathroom had a very low, small rounded sink with no counter space; and the mirror was located at a height that was useful only for someone in a standing position. Katya then analysed the accessibility of the bathroom in relation to Gary's occupational performance needs, which are described below. This analysis led her to identify a number of intervention strategies.

Occupational Performance	Recommendations/ Intervention to Enable Safety and Independence	Rationale for Intervention
Bathing ♦ Difficulty transferring into and out of bathtub. Gary was using a very unstable towel rack to help him transfer into and out of the bathtub.	♦ Install a bath transfer bench with back. ♦ Install a clamp-on bar on side of the tub and a vertical grab bar on the wall beside the tub. ♦ Put a nonslip bath mat or a rubber mat with suction cups in the bottom of the bathtub. ♦ Add a hand-held shower.	♦ Bench legs go over the side of the bathtub, which allows Gary to slide his legs over and into the bathtub while sitting without having to step in and out. ♦ Allows Gary to sit and shower, this helps to compensate for his impaired balance. Sitting on a shower bench is much safer than standing, and it helps to conserve energy and increases Gary's independence. ♦ Easy to use, portable, and makes transferring into and out of bathtub easier and safer ♦ Much safer and reduces Gary's chance of slipping and falling in a wet bathtub. ♦ Allows Gary to have control over where the water sprays, works well when using a bath bench because it allows him to wash and rinse himself independently.

Continued

Kitchen, laundry room, utility kitchen (pp. 131–35, 148)

	A	B1	B2	C	D	E	F	G	H	I	J	K	L	M	N	Notes
Insufficient manoeuvring areas around white goods/storage units (service area less than 1.2 m in front). Insufficient area because of furnishings is rated under C9.		3	3	3	3	3	1		3				3	4	1	
Wall-mounted cupboards and shelves placed extremely high (lowest shelf more than 0.5 m above the working surface).		3	3	4	4	3	3	2	4	3	4	3	3	4	3	◆ *The kitchen cupboards were installed very high and required standing on a stool to reach items on the top shelf.* ◆ *When working at the counter, reaching above shoulder height was required to reach greater than 50% of the items.* ◆ *There were no adjustable shelves within cupboards.* ◆ *Cupboards were very deep and required extensive reaching and twisting of body to retrieve items in back of cupboard.*
No surface at a height suitable for sitting work (0.85 m or higher is only suitable for standing; lower working height is required for sitting). Leg clearance is rated at C29.					1		1						3	3	1	◆ *The counters were all greater than 0.85 m in height.* ◆ *The counters were too high to sit and work.*
Low working surfaces (i.e. 0.84 m or lower).								3				3			1	◆ *Only low working surface available was kitchen table*
No working surfaces with leg room (clearance less than 0.65 m height, depth 0.6 m, width 0.8 m, p. 134).					2		2						2	3	2	◆ *Only working surface that had leg clearance and was at an appropriate height to sit and work was the kitchen table*
Working surfaces too deep (more than 0.6 m).									3	1	4		3	3		
Shelves too deep (i.e. more than 0.3 m). Deeper shelves require pullout shelves/turntable units.									4		4	3	3	3	1	
More than half of apparatus/controls in very high/inaccessible position (>1.2 m above the floor).								2	3	1			2	4	1	◆ *Inaccessible and unsafe access to electric outlets for use of small kitchen appliances* ◆ *Required stretching and twisting of body to access outlets located on back wall of the counter, and behind microwave stand*

FIGURE 60.5 Housing enabler: Analysis of personal component of accessibility (or person–environment fit) (from Iwarsson & Slaug, 2001. Printed with permission).

Hygiene area (pp. 64–70)

Item	Scores	Comments
No place to sit in shower/bath.	2	3	3	1	◆ *Bathtub with shower (no shower chair and no hand held shower)* ◆ *No place to sit in shower* ◆ *No grab Bars Installed in bathroom*
No grab bars at shower/bath and/or toilet.	1	1	4	4	4	4	1	
Controls/operable hardware in hygiene areas refers to permanent functions, e.g. taps, handles of bathroom cupboards etc. (pp. 111–15, 178).	2	3	
Illogical controls.	4	3	
High force required to activate controls (p. 113)	3	3	1	3	3	1	◆ *Handles to control the water temperature in the bathtub required high force to turn on and off, very short-lever arms*
Use requires intact fine motor control (pp. 112–13).	1	3	1	1	◆ *Pulling the drain plug out from the bottom of the bathtub and sink*
Complex manouvres (more than one operation/movement) and good precision required (p. 113).	2	1	2	1	1	1	◆ *Turning on and off bathtub and sink water faucets* ◆ *Pulling down handle to flush toilet* ◆ *Turning on/off light switch* ◆ *Opening cupboard door below the bathroom sink*
Use requires hands.	3	4	3	3	
Wash-basin placed at a height for use only when standing (top edge 0.81 m above the floor or higher).	3	3	◆ *Wash basin was at height for use only when standing. Also, it had no leg clearance space thus making it very difficult and uncomfortable to sit and complete grooming activities*
Toilet with standard height (0.41 m incl. seat) or lower.	3	3	1	◆ *Toilet was mounted onto wall at the standard height*
Mirror placed at a height for use only when standing (lower edge more than 0.9 m above the floor, p. 69).	2	2	3	
Toilet roll holder in inaccessible position (more than 0.4 m from toilet, other height than approx. 0.8 m above the floor, placed on the wall behind toilet, etc., p. 70).	1	1	1	2	1	1	2	
Storage cupboards, towel hooks, etc. inaccessibly placed (recommended height 0.9–1.2 m above the floor, p. 70).	1	1	3	◆ *Personal care items for completion of grooming tasks were not easily accessible (located below sink in the cupboard) and thus required reaching very low to retrieve*
Slippery floor surface (pp. 70, 96–97).	3	3	3	1	1	3	3	1	◆ *Thick carpeted rug lying on floor outside of bathtub— this will increase risk of tripping and falling*

FIGURE 60.5 *Continued*

CASE STUDY: *Occupational Therapist Working with a Client Returning Home*   *Continued*

Gary presents with decreased safety and independence with meal preparation secondary to both cognitive and physical deficits. On assessing the kitchen environment, Katya could see that some physical features were not a good fit for Gary with his current functional limitations. The kitchen in Gary's home is very small and cluttered, and it has very limited counter space.

Occupational Performance	Recommendations/Intervention to Enable Safety and Independence	Rationale for Intervention
Meal Preparation ◆ Mobility: Gary is ambulating around the kitchen with a quad cane, and he has impaired left hand function; therefore, he finds it difficult to transfer heavier items such as foods and plates.	◆ Recommend that Gary use a four-wheeled walker (rollator) with a tray/basket or a tea trolley. ◆ Consider purchasing lightweight pots, pans, and plates.	◆ Enable him to independently and safely transfer items to and from counter, stove, and refrigerator to the table. ◆ Enable him to safely lift and use while conserving energy.
◆ Cupboards' height of installation is very high, dishes (plates, glasses) are stored on the top shelves. Gary's ability to engage in overhead reaching is limited by decrease balance, unsteady gait, and decreased upper extremity fine and gross motor skills.	◆ Lower the height of the cupboards. ◆ Relocate items in the cupboards so the items that are most frequently used are in easy-to-reach places. ◆ A long-handled reacher can be used for overhead reaching of light items.	◆ Allow Gary to have easy access and promote safe reaching. ◆ Avoid unnecessary bending and reaching. ◆ Reduce risk of falls due to overreaching (loss of balance).
◆ Short-term memory deficits and executive function ◆ Gary sometimes forgets and needs to be reminded to turn off the stove.	◆ Place written sign above stove that reads "TURN OFF STOVE." ◆ Use a timer for reminder; when the timer sounds, that acts as a cue to turn off the stove. ◆ When preparing a meal while home alone, try to prepare something light that does not require use of the stove (e.g., a sandwich).	◆ Utilize compensatory strategies to enhance independence and safety.
◆ Executive function deficits	◆ Arrange the ingredients and place the objects and items that Gary uses most frequently in one area (in cupboard, in the refrigerator). ◆ Label drawers and cupboards so that Gary knows exactly where to look to retrieve the cooking utensils and ingredients that he needs. ◆ Gary and his wife could generate step-by-step instructions for commonly prepared items and place these in clear plastic jackets so that Gary can use an erasable marker to tick off steps as they are completed.	◆ Compensates for short-term memory deficits and increases independence. Katya discussed her recom-

CASE STUDY: *Occupational Therapist Working with a Client Returning Home*   *Continued*

mendations for environmental modifications with Gary and his wife. Although Gary's condition might improve, some of the modifications were considered essential for safety. Gary and his wife followed through with the recommended environmental modifications. Katya met with Gary and his wife and trained them both in the safe use of all the modifications in the home. As a result of this environmentally based intervention, Gary has made several advancements in his occupational performance. Gary has increased independence and improved safety with bathing activities and can

independently prepare a simple meal. He is less reliant on his wife to help him with these activities. Gary reports improved satisfaction and performance scores on the Canadian Occupational Performance Measure, although his personal abilities (cognition, strength, and range of motion) have not changed during this intervention. Gary and his wife are pleased with his increased independence and have expressed their appreciation for the extra time they now have to spend on family activities instead of on self-care.

CASE STUDY: *Occupational Therapy Consultation to a Community Group*

A community center in a small urban community has asked for an occupational therapist to join the design team for the redevelopment that is to occur at the center. The center serves as a focal point for seniors, people with disabilities, single parents, low-income families, new immigrants, and the general public. Programs and activities include a shared meal program, employment preparation classes, arts and crafts programs, evening movies and dance programs, exercise classes, healthy living classes, and counseling.

The present facility is in an old two-story building that has a very steep add-on ramp to the building, one "accessible" toilet stall that is not fully accessible, narrow 32-inch corridors, a lack of windows, and many other issues. The center has obtained a very large foundation grant to build a new facility. The design team will have the opportunity to decide the best location for the new facility and the best design features. Funding has been conditionally provided, given that this facility will be a showcase for universal design.

The design team provides expertise in design, while users of the facility provide firsthand knowledge of their needs and desires for the best functional design. Many designers do not fully understand the functional needs of people with disabilities and value the occupational therapist's knowledge and skills in this area.

Because this is a public building, the occupational therapist will first develop a conceptual analysis of the clients who will use the building, including their age range, their general abilities and functional challenges, and how they use the building. The occupational therapist will use her expertise in interviewing and in research to run focus groups with clientele from the existing facility (the user-experts) to determine their needs and wishes for the new facility. Design team members will attend the focus groups to hear from the user-experts directly. The occupational therapist will combine the information from the user-experts with her knowledge of disability and abilities and access issues and will share the synthesis with the design team. The occupational therapist will work with the design team throughout the design process and assist in site selection, building layout, space requirements, materials, and color selections. For example, site selection should consider where transportation can be most easily accessed. The occupational therapist can help to identify the best dimensional requirements for user groups and assist with specific selection of assistive technologies.

Questions

1. Describe more specific occupational therapy roles and areas of expertise for this case study.
2. What are the specific issues that the occupational therapist will want to ensure are addressed?

COMMENTARY ON THE EVIDENCE

The Effectiveness of Physical Environmental Modifications

Despite the widespread calls from occupational therapists and others for environmental modifications to promote independence and occupational performance in homes, schools, workplaces, and the community at large, evidence demonstrating the effectiveness of environmental modifications is still evolving. Available evidence tends to focus on home modifications related to outcomes of falls prevention, reducing caregiver burden, and optimizing productivity and participation primarily in the home environment.

Falls and Injury Prevention

Two reviews focus on falls prevention interventions for older adults (Gillespie et al., 2003; McClure et al., 2003), and one review addresses home modifications to prevent injuries in children, the general population, and older adults (Lyons et al., 2003). Together, these systematic reviews suggest that home hazard reductions may be most effective with older adults who have a history of falling. There is not yet sufficient evidence to support the reduction of home hazards to prevent injuries. Home hazards can be the single focus of the falls prevention intervention or more commonly as part of a larger, multifactorial intervention.

Reducing Caregiver Burden

Much of the literature about the effectiveness of environmental modifications to reduce caregiver burden focuses on caregivers of people with dementia. The Environmental Skill-Building Program (ESP), described by Gitlin and Corcoran (2005), is a structured intervention that involves working collaboratively with caregivers of people with dementia living in their own homes. The intervention includes education, environmental modifications, and skill training of the caregiver. The environmental focus includes a home hazards assessment and recommendations for equipment such as bathroom devices, lighting modifications, ramps, and intercom and communication systems. Overall, the ESP resulted in improvements for both care recipients and caregivers. For example, the three-month intervention resulted in reduced declines in IADL in the care recipients, while caregivers experienced reduced upset,

and female caregivers reported higher levels of self-efficacy (Gitlin et al., 2001). The six-month study noted reduced caregiver stress and subjective burden and reduced upset behaviors (Gitlin et al., 2003). A twelve-month follow-up demonstrated improved caregiver affect, trends towards maintained skills, and fewer behavioral problems for participants in the intervention group (Gitlin, Hauck, Dennis, & Winter, 2005).

Optimizing Participation and Productivity

There is growing evidence to support the relationship between physical environments and participation in home, community, and work environments in people who have had spinal cord injuries and traumatic brain injuries (Richards et al., 1999; Whiteneck, Gerhardt, et al., 2004; Whiteneck, Meade et al., 2004). Although physical environments are not the only environmental factors that influence participation, such factors as transportation and access to public buildings clearly influence participation and productivity.

There is growing evidence about the effectiveness of home modifications to promote occupational performance. For example, Gitlin, Miller, and Boyce (1999) found that bathroom renovations resulted in significant improvements in bathing, ADL performance, and transfers. Stark (2004) found that self-reported occupational performance scores improved after an intervention that involved home modifications to address environmental barriers in the homes of older adults. Fänge and Iwarsson (2005) found that while overall ADL dependence did not change as a result of home modifications, bathing dependence did improve, as did participants' perceptions of the usability of the home environment.

Barriers to the implementation of home modifications have also been identified. In particular, costs associated with home modifications can be prohibitive for some participants (Pynoos & Nishita, 2003). Lysack and Neufeld (2003) identified that people receiving publicly funded insurance were provided with fewer recommendations for home modifications and assistive devices than were people receiving private insurance. Therapists need to be alert

COMMENTARY ON THE EVIDENCE *Continued*

to these barriers and strategies that might be used to address them. For example, Stearns and colleagues (2000) suggest that home modifications resulted in reduced Medicare expenditures.

Despite some efforts to evaluate the implementation of recommendations for workstation modifications (e.g., Goodman et al., 2005), limited evidence is available that demonstrates the effectiveness of workstation modifications in improving productivity or work performance.

The least amount of evidence seems to be available to demonstrate the effectiveness of making community sites more accessible to people with differing abilities. For example, although principles of universal design have been described, there is less literature that demonstrates the effectiveness of universal design in outcomes such as social, leisure, or community participation. Some evidence is now accumulating about the accessibility of public spaces and strategies are emerging on how best to evaluate accessibility (Meyers et al., 2002; Thapar et al., 2004). The perspective of the users (client centeredness) and the use of theoretical models that include participa-

tion factors (such as the ICF) rather than audits of environmental features provide more meaningful information and are recommended. Because universal design and the ADA are relatively new initiatives, research should be conducted to evaluate the value of improving access for all in homes, workplaces, and the community at large.

Future Research Directions

For occupational therapists who are interested in generating new evidence related to the effectiveness of physical environmental modifications, many areas warrant further research. First, we need to know whether environmental modifications make a difference in areas of performance that are important to our clients. Further, while evidence is accumulating related to home modifications, less evidence is available to support environmental modifications in workplace, school, and community environments. As universal design principles are implemented, there will be opportunities to explore the effects of design on occupational performance and participation.

CONCLUSIONS AND FUTURE CONSIDERATIONS

Physical environments can create barriers or provide the necessary supports toward enabling optimal occupational performance. Occupational therapists have considerable experience and success with interventions to make homes more accessible and supportive of clients' occupational performance. As a profession, we are demonstrating leadership in addressing environmental factors that influence the participation of people with disabilities in their daily pursuits through the services that we provide in schools, communities, and workplace environments. Today, more people with disabilities are able to go to school, return to work, and participate in their communities through efforts made by occupational therapists to reduce environmental barriers and harness environmental resources. To provide this leadership, it is critical that occupational therapists maintain a strong working knowledge about key disability rights legislation, building codes, universal design initiatives, and accessibility guidelines that can

improve the overall participation and empowerment of persons with disabilities.

PROVOCATIVE QUESTIONS

1. Many occupational therapists spend a great deal of time involved in home modifications and the many frustrations that go with them, including lack of funding. Perhaps the occupational therapist could also advocate for visitable housing in the region so that there would be less need for as many home modifications. Is this an occupational therapist's role?

2. Although occupational therapists may be readily able to identify home modifications that promote occupational performance with a client, funding limitations might present significant barriers. How can occupational therapists ensure that they are not impeded in providing the best recommendations for clients because of perceived or real limitations in funding?

3. Universal design principles have been described in the literature, and occupational therapists can provide

insights into their implementation in public buildings and spaces. How can we evaluate the effectiveness of this type of service to justify our involvement?

4. Think about your own personal environmental hierarchical continuum. What are some of your proximal and distal environments? If you were suddenly unable to access these environments independently, how would this affect your life?

5. Think about your current home environment. If you used a manual wheelchair, would you still be able to live in your current home? What new limitations would you face? What if you were using a power wheelchair or a scooter? What adaptations would have to be made? Would you be able to continue independently engaging in your meaningful occupations?

REFERENCES

Abend, A. (2001). *Planning and designing for students with disabilities.* Washington, DC: National Clearinghouse for Educational Facilities. Retrieved August 17, 2005, from www.edfacilities.org

Adaptive Environments Center. (1995). *Americans with Disabilities Act checklist for readily achievable barrier removal.* Boston: Author. Retrieved May 2, 2005, from http://www.usdoj.gov/crt/ada/checkweb.htm or from http://www.adaptenv.org/index.php?option=Resource&articleid=226&topicid=30

American Association of Retired Persons. (2000). *Fixing to stay: A national survey on housing and home modification issues—Executive summary.* Washington, DC: Author.

American Occupational Therapy Association (AOTA). (2002). Occupational therapy practice framework: Domain and process. *American Journal of Occupational Therapy, 56,* 609–639.

Americans with Disabilities Act. (1990). P.L. 101-336, 42, U.S.C. 12101. Retrieved March 11, 2005, from http://www.usdoj.gov/crt/ada/adahom1.htm

Bronfenbrenner, U. (1977). Toward an experimental ecology of human development. *American Psychologist, 32,* 513–531.

Caldwell, B. M., & Bradley, R. H. (1984). *Administration manual (Rev. ed.): Home Observation for Measurement of the Environment.* Little Rock, AR: University of Arkansas.

Canadian Association of Occupational Therapists (CAOT). (1997). *Enabling occupation: An occupational therapy perspective.* Ottawa, ON: CAOT Publications ACE.

Canadian Mortgage and Housing Corporation. (2003). *Maintaining seniors' independence through home adaptations: A self-assessment guide.* Ottawa, ON: Author. Retrieved June 14, 2005, from http://www.cmhc.ca. The guide is available for free in pdf format.

Canadian Standards Association. (2004). *Accessible design for the built environment.* (CAN/CSA B651-04). Ottawa, ON: Author. Retrieved October 12, 2006, from http://www.csa-intl.org/onlinestore/GetCatalogItemDetails.asp?mat=2417157&Parent=1070

Center for Universal Design. (1997). *A blueprint for action: A resource for promoting home modifications.* Raleigh, NC: North Carolina State University.

Christenson, M. (2005). *EASE3.2.* Retrieved March 3, 2005, from http://www.lifease.com/lifease-home.html

Chui, T., Oliver, R., Marshall, L., & Letts, L. (2001). *Safety assessment of function and the environment for rehabilitation tool manual.* Toronto, ON: COTA Comprehensive Rehabilitation and Mental Health Services.

Claar, R. C., & Boan, J. S. (2005). *Visitability: The way of the future in home building: Village of Bolingbrook.* Retrieved January 17, 2005, from http://www.concretechange.org/Visitability1.pdf

Clemson, L., Fitzgerald, M. H., & Heard, R. (1999). Content validity of an assessment tool to identify home fall hazards: The Westmead Home Safety Assessment. *British Journal of Occupational Therapy, 62,* 171–179.

Connell, B. R., Sanford, J. A., Long, R. L., Archea, C. K., & Turner, C. (1993). Home modifications and performance of routine household activities by individuals with varying levels of mobility impairments. *Technology and Disability, 2*(4), 9–18.

Cooper, B. A., & Day, K. (2003). Therapeutic design of environments for people with dementia. In L. Letts, P. Rigby, & D. Stewart (Eds.), *Using environments to enable occupational performance* (pp. 253–268). Thorofare, NJ: Slack.

Cooper, B., Letts, L., Rigby, P., Stewart, D., & Strong, S. (2005). Measuring environmental factors. In M. Law, W. Dunn, & C. Baum (Eds.), *Measuring occupational performance: Supporting best practice in occupational therapy* (pp. 315–344). Thorofare, NJ: Slack.

Coster, W., Deeney, T., Haltiwanger, J., & Haley, S. (1998). *School Function Assessment.* San Antonio, TX: Psychological Corporation.

Craig Hospital Research Department. (2001). *Craig Hospital Inventory of Environmental Factors (CHIEF) Manual: Version 3.0.* Englewood, CO: Craig Hospital. Retrieved May 2, 2005, from www.tbims.org/combi/chief/

Dovey, K. (1985). Home and homelessness. In I. Altman. & C. M. Werner (Eds.), *Home environments, human behavior and environment: Advances in theory and research* (pp. 33–63). New York: Plenum.

Fänge, A., & Iwarsson, S. (2005). Changes in ADL dependence and aspects of usability following housing adaptation: A longitudinal perspective. *American Journal of Occupational Therapy, 59,* 296–304.

Fearing, V., & Clark, J. (Ed.) (2000). *Individuals in context: A practical guide to client-centered practice.* Thorofare, NJ: Slack.

Fougeyrollas, P., Noreau, L., St. Michel, G., & Boschen, K. (1999). *Measure of the quality of the environment: Version 2.* Unpublished tool. Available from author.

Gillespie, L. D., Gillespie, W. J., Robertson, M. C., Lamb, S. E., Cumming, R. G., & Rowe, B. H. (2003). Interventions for preventing falls in elderly people. *The Cochrane Database of Systematic Reviews 2003,* Issue 4, Art. No. CD000340. (DOI: 10.1002/14651858.CD000340).

Gitlin, L. N., & Corcoran, M. A. (2005). *Occupational therapy and dementia care: The home environmental skill-building program for individuals and families.* Bethesda, MD: AOTA Press.

Gitlin, L. N., Corcoran, M. A., Winter, L., Boyce, A., & Hauck, W. W. (2001). A randomized, controlled trial of a home environmental intervention to enhance self-efficacy and reduce upset in family caregivers of persons with dementia. *Gerontologist, 41,* 4–14.

Gitlin, L. N., Hauck, W. W., Dennis, M. P., & Winter, L. (2005). Maintenance of effects of the home environmental skill-building program for family caregivers and individuals with Alzheimer's disease and related disorders. *Journal of Gerontology: Medical Sciences, 60A,* 368–374.

Gitlin, L. N., Liebman, J. & Winter, L. (2003). Are environmental interventions effective in the management of Alzheimer's disease and related disorders? A synthesis of the evidence. *Alzheimer's Care Quarterly, 4,* 85–107.

Gitlin, L. N., Miller, K. S., & Boyce, A. (1999). Bathroom modifications for frail elderly renters: Outcomes of a community-based program. *Technology and Disability, 10,* 141–149.

Goodman, G., Landis, J., George, C., McGuire, S., Shorter, C., Sieminski, M., et al. (2005). Effectiveness of computer ergonomics interventions for an engineering company: A program evaluation. *WORK: A Journal of Prevention, Assessment & Rehabilitation, 24,* 53–62.

Government of Ontario (2001). *Ontarians with Disabilities Act.* Retrieved January 10, 2005, from http://www.e-laws.gov.on.ca/DBLaws/Statutes/English/01o32_e.htm

Grabois, E. W., Nosek, M., & Rossi, C. D. (1999). Accessibility of primary care physicians' offices for people with disabilities: An analysis of compliance with the Americans with Disabilities Act. *Archives of Family Medicine, 8,* 44–51.

Gray, D. B., Hollingsworth H. H., & Morgan, K. A. (2001). Independent living and assistive technology: Work context. *Rehabilitation Education; 15*(4), 1–19.

Hagedorn, R. (2000). *Tools for practice in occupational therapy: A structured approach to core skills and processes.* Edinburgh: Churchill Livingstone.

Harris Interactive, Inc. (2004). Access to religious services. In *N.O.D./Harris 2004 Survey of Americans with Disabilities.* Rochester, NY: Author.

Hemmingsson, H., & Borell, L. (2000). Accommodation needs and student-environment fit in upper secondary schools for students with severe physical disabilities. *Canadian Journal of Occupational Therapy, 67,* 162–172.

Hemmingsson, H., Egilson, S., Hoffman, O., & Kielhofner, G. (2005). *The School Setting Interview (SSI): Version 3.0.* Chicago IL: MOHO Clearinghouse. Retrieved August 24, 2005, from http://www.moho.uic.edu/assess/ssi.html

Hemmingsson, H., Kottorp, A., & Bernspang, B. (2004). Validity of the school setting interview: An assessment of the student-environment fit. *Scandinavian Journal of Occupational Therapy, 11*(4), 171–178.

Human Resources and Skills Development Canada. (2005). *Employment programming for persons with disabilities.* Retrieved November 1, 2005, from http://www.hrsdc.gc.ca/asp/gateway.asp?hr=en/on/epb/disabilities/programs.shtml&hs=hze

Iwarsson, S. (2005). A long-term perspective on person-environment fit and ADL dependence among older Swedish adults. *Gerontologist, 45 (3),* 327–36

Iwarsson, S. & Slaugh, B. (2001). *The Housing Enabler: An instrument for assessing and analyzing accessibility problems in housing.* Navlinge och Staffanstorp, Sweden: Veten & Skapen HB & Slaug Data Management.

Iwarsson, S., Ståhl, A., & Carlsson, G. (2003). Accessible transportation: Novel occupational therapy perspectives.

In L. Letts, P. Rigby, & D. Stewart (Eds.), *Using environments to enable occupational performance* (pp. 235–251). Thorofare, NJ: Slack.

Jacobs, K. (1999). Americans with Disabilities Act Work-Site Assessment. In K. Jacobs (Ed.), *Ergonomics for therapists* (2nd ed., pp. 345–354). Boston: Butterworth-Heinemann.

Keysor, J. J., Jette, A. M., & Haley, S. M. (2005). Development of the home and community environment (HACE) instrument. *Journal of Rehabilitation Medicine, 37,* 37–44.

Kielhofner, G., Lai, J., Olson, L., Haglund, L., Ekbadh, E., & Hedlund, M. (1998). Psychometric properties of the work environment impact scale: A cross-cultural study. *Work: A Journal of Prevention, Assessment, and Rehabilitation, 12,* 71–77.

Law, M., Cooper, B., Strong, S., Stewart, D., Rigby, P., & Letts, L. (1996). The Person-Environment-Occupation model: A transactive approach to occupational performance. *Canadian Journal of Occupational Therapy, 63*(1), 9–23.

Lawton, M. P. (1980). *Environment and aging.* Monterey, CA: Brooks-Cole.

Lawton, M. P., & Nahemow, L. (1973). Ecology and the aging process. In C. L. Eisdorfer & M. P. Lawton (Eds.), *Psychology of adult development and aging* (pp. 619–674). Washington, DC: American Psychological Association.

Lyons, R. A., Sander, L. V., Weightman, A. L., Patterson, J., Jones, S. A., Lannon, S., et al. (2003). Modification of the home environment for the reduction of injuries. *The Cochrane Database of Systematic Reviews* 2003, Issue 4. Art. No.: CD003600. (DOI: 10.1002/14651858.CD003600).

Lysack, C. L. & Neufeld, S. (2003). Occupational therapist home evaluations: Inequalities, but doing the best we can? *American Journal of Occupational Therapy, 57,* 369–379.

Mace, R. (1985) Universal design: Barrier-free environments for everyone. *Designer West, 3,* 147–152.

Mackenzie, L., Byles, J., & Higginbotham, N. (2000). Designing the Home Falls and Accidents Screening Tool (HOME FAST): Selecting the items. *British Journal of Occupational Therapy, 63,* 260–269.

Mackenzie, L., Byles, J., & Higginbotham, N. (2002). Professional perceptions about home safety: Cross-national validation of the Home Falls and Accidents Screening Tool (HOME FAST). *Journal of Allied Health, 31*(1), 22–28.

Mann, W. C., Hurren, D., Tomita, M., Bengali, M., & Steinfeld, E. (1994). Environmental problems in homes of elders with disabilities. *The Occupational Therapy Journal of Research, 14*(3), 191–211.

Mann, W. C., Ottenbacher, K. J., Fraas, L., Tomita, M., & Granger, C. V. (1999). Effectiveness of assistive technology and environmental interventions in maintaining independence and reducing home care costs for the frail elderly. *Archives of Family Medicine, 8,* 210–217.

McClain, L., Cram, A., Wood, J., & Taylor, M. (1993). Restaurant wheelchair accessibility. *American Journal of Occupational Therapy, 47,* 619–623.

McClain, L., & Todd, C. (1990). Food store accessibility. *American Journal of Occupational Therapy, 44,* 487–491.

McClure, R., Turner, C., Peel, N., Spinks, A., Eakin, E., & Hughes, K. (2003). Population-based interventions for the prevention of fall-related injuries in older people. *The Cochrane Database of Systematic Reviews 2003,* Issue 1,

Art. No.CD004441.pub2. (DOI: 10.1002/14651858. CD004441.pub2).

McColl, M. A. (1997). Social support and occupational therapy. In C. H. Christiansen & C. M. Baum (Eds.), *Occupational therapy: Enabling function and well-being* (2nd ed., pp. 508–528). Thorofare, NJ: Slack.

Meyers, A. R., Anderson, J. J., Miller, D. R., Shipp, K., Hoenig, H., Meyers, A. R., et al. (2002). Barriers, facilitators, and access for wheelchair users: Substantive and methodologic lessons from a pilot study of environmental effects. *Social Science & Medicine, 55,* 1435–1446.

Moos, R. H., & Lemke, S. (1996). *Evaluating residential facilities: The Multiphasic Environmental Assessment Procedure.* Thousand Oaks CA: Sage.

Mu, K., & Royeen, C. (2004). Facilitating participation of students with severe disabilities: Aligning school-based occupational therapy practice with best practices in severe disabilities. *Physical and Occupational Therapy in Pediatrics, 24,* 5–21.

Pivik, J., McComas, J., & LaFlamme, M. (2002). Barriers and facilitators to inclusive education. *Exceptional Children, 69,* 97–107.

Pynoos, J., & Nishita, C. M. (2003). The cost and financing of home modifications in the United States. *Journal of Disability Policy Studies, 14,* 68–73.

Rehabilitation Act of 1973, 29 U.S.C. §504 (1973).

Richards, J. S., Bombardier, C. H., Tate, D., Dijkers, M., Gordon, W., Shewchuk, R., et al. (1999). Access to the environment and life satisfaction after spinal cord injury. *Archives of Physical Medicine & Rehabilitation, 80,* 1501–1506.

Rimmer, J. H., Riley, B., Want, E., & Rauworth, A. (2004). Development and validation of AIMFREE: Accessibility instruments measuring fitness and recreation environments. *Disability and Rehabilitation, 26,* 1087–1095.

Ringaert, L. (2003). Universal design of the built environment to enable occupational performance. In L. Letts, P. Rigby, & D. Stewart (Eds.), *Using environments to enable occupational performance* (pp. 97–115). Thorofare, NJ: Slack.

Ringaert, L., Rapson, D., Qiu, J., Cooper, J., & Shwedyk, E. (2001) *Determination of new dimensions for universal design codes and standards with consideration of powered wheelchair and scooter users.* Winnipeg, MB: Universal Design Institute, University of Manitoba, Faculty of Architecture.

Roessler, R. T. (1996). The role of assessment in enhancing vocational success of people with multiple sclerosis. *Work, 6,* 191–201.

Roessler, R. T., & Gottcent, J. (1994). The Work Experience Survey: A reasonable accommodation/career development strategy. *Journal of Applied Rehabilitation Counseling, 25*(3), 16–21.

Rowles, G. D. (2003). The meaning of place as a component of self. In E. B. Crepeau, E. S. Cohn, & B. A. B. Schell (Eds.), *Willard and Spackman's occupational therapy* (10th ed., pp. 111–119). Philadelphia: Lippincott, Williams & Wilkins.

Sanford, J. A., & Jones, M. L. (2001). Home modifications and environmental controls. In D. A. Olson & F. DeRuyter (Eds.), *Clinician's guide to assistive technology* (pp. 405–423). Chicago: Mosby.

Siebert, C. (2005). *Occupational therapy practice guidelines for home modifications (Practice Guidelines Series).* Bethesda, MD: AOTA Press.

Smith, E. (2003). *Visitability defined: 2003.* Retrieved September 22, 2005, from http://www.concretechange.org/

Stark, S. (2004). Removing environmental barriers in the homes of older adults with disabilities improves occupational performance. *Occupational Therapy Journal of Research, 24*(1), 32–39.

Stearns, S. C., Bernard, S. L., Fasick, S. B., Schwartz, R., Konrad, R. T., Ory, M. G., et al. (2000). The economic implications of self-care: The effect of lifestyle, functional adaptations, and medical self-care among a national sample of Medicare beneficiaries. *American Journal of Public Health, 90,* 1608–1612.

Stewart, D. (2003). The environment: Paradigms and practice in health, occupational therapy, and inquiry. In L. Letts, P. Rigby, & D. Stewart (Eds.), *Using environments to enable occupational performance.* (pp. 3–15). Thorofare, NJ: Slack.

Thapar, N., Warner, G., Drainoni, M., Williams, S. R., Ditchfield, H., Wierbick, Y., et al. (2004). A pilot study of functional access to public buildings and facilities for persons with impairments. *Disability and Rehabilitation, 26,* 280–289.

U.S. Access Board. (2004). *ADA-ABA accessibility guidelines.* Retrieved March 5, 2005, from http://www.access-board. gov/ada-aba/final.pdf

U.S. Architectural and Transportation Barriers and Compliance Board. (2000). *Americans with Disabilities Act (ADA) Accessibility Guidelines for Buildings and Facilities: Play areas, final rule.* Retrieved August 17, 2005, from http:// www.access-board.gov/play/finalrule.pdf

U.S. Architectural and Transportation Barriers and Compliance Board. (2001). *Guide to ADA Accessibility Guidelines for Play Areas.* Retrieved August 17, 2005, from http://www. access-board.gov/play/guide/guide.pdf

U.S. Department of Labor. (2001). *Statistics about people with disabilities and employment.* Retrieved September 8, 2005, from http://www.dol.gov/odep/pubs/ek01/stats.htm

U.S. Department of Housing and Urban Development. (2001). *Fair housing and equal opportunity: People with disabilities.* Retrieved June 8, 2005, from http://www.hud.gov/offices/ fheo/disabilities/sect504.cfm

U.S. Equal Employment Opportunity Commission (2005). *The Americans with Disabilities Act, Titles I and V.* Retrieved November 12, 2005, from http://www.eeoc.gov/policy/ ada.html

Whiteneck, G. G., Gerhardt, K. A., Cusick, C. P. (2004). Identifying environmental factors that influence the outcomes of people with traumatic brain injury. *Journal of Head Trauma Rehabilitation, 19,* 191–204.

Whiteneck, G. G., Harrison-Felix, C. L., Mellick, D. S., Brooks, C. A., Charlifue, S. B., & Gerhart, K. A. (2004). Quantifying environmental factors: A measure of physical, attitudinal, service, productivity and policy barriers. *Archives of Physical Medicine & Rehabilitation, 85,* 1324–1335.

Whiteneck, G., Meade, M. A., Dijkers, M., Tate, D. G., Bushnik, T., Forchheimer, M. B. et al. (2004). Environmental factors and their role in participation and life satisfaction after spinal cord injury. *Archives of Physical Medicine & Rehabilitation, 85,* 1793–1803.

World Health Organization. (2001). *International classification of functioning, disability and health.* Geneva: Author. Retrieved January 30, 2005, from http://www.who.int/classification/icf/

RESOURCES

Adaptive Environments Center: http://www.adaptenv.org

American Printing House for the Blind (provides materials, alternative media, tools, and resources for individuals who are blind or visually impaired): http://www.aph.org/

Americans with Disabilities Act: http://www.usdoj.gov/crt/ada/adahom1.htm

Americans with Disabilities Act Document Center: http://janweb.icdi.wvu.edu/kinder/

Centre for Accessible Environments, UK: http://www.cae.org.uk/

Center for Universal Design at North Carolina State University: http://www.design.ncsu.edu:8120/cud/

Enforcement Guidance: Reasonable Accommodation and Undue Hardship Under the ADA: http://www.eeoc.gov/policy/docs/accommodation.html

Home Modification and Maintenance Information Clearing House in Australia: http://www.homemods.info/

Job Accommodation Network (JAN): www.jan.wvu.edu

IDEA Center at State University of New York: http://www.ap.buffalo.edu/idea/Home/index.asp

National Centre on Accessibility (promotes access for people with disabilities in recreation): http://www.ncaonline.org

Paths to Equal Opportunity, Government of Ontario: http://www.equalopportunity.on.ca/eng_g/index.asp

U.S. Architectural and Transportation Barriers Compliance Board (a federal agency committed to accessible design): www.access-board.gov/

Assistive Technology and Wheeled Mobility

MARY ELLEN BUNING

Learning Objectives

After reading this chapter, you will be able to:

1. Explain how the client's goals drive the selection of assistive technology and its use as an enabler of occupation and participation.
2. Describe assistive technology devices on the basis of their ability to help people compensate for challenges to occupational performance.
3. Describe how knowledge of occupational performance helps to identify and optimize the human-technology interface.

ASSISTIVE TECHNOLOGY: TECHNOLOGY TO ENABLE ACTIVITY AND PARTICIPATION

Assistive technology (AT) is a multidisciplinary intervention that helps people develop compensatory techniques to engage in activities that are important to them. Occupational therapists specializing in assistive technology use knowledge from human occupation, kinesiology and biomechanics, perception and learning theory, and skills in activity analysis and energy conservation to help people do the things they want to do. Occupational therapists guide clients in selecting AT solutions and integrating them into daily life. They emphasize activity and participation, not just the technology. Broad knowledge of human occupation is a valuable asset on an AT team.

Although AT is a relatively new area of occupational therapy practice, microprocessor-based technologies are now familiar and useful parts of daily routines and personal productivity. Concepts such as storing and sending data via the Internet, signaling garage doors with radio frequency, and beaming data between infrared ports on a personal digital assistant (PDA) are commonplace today. Technologies are an essential part of daily life and can be used to aid persons with impairments. Even when occupational therapists do not possess AT skills themselves, they should recognize when a client might benefit from AT and make an appropriate referral.

The HAAT Model

An engineer and an occupational therapist created the Human, Activity and Assistive Technology (HAAT) Model to explain and guide evaluation and delivery of AT services (Cook & Polgar, 2008) (Figure 61.1). The HAAT model, based on general systems theory in which change in one element creates a consequence in another, represents performance as an interaction between the person, the person's activities, the AT, and the environment (American Occupational Therapy Association, 2002; Cook & Polgar, 2008).

The client's desire to engage in occupations is often the starting point for an AT evaluation. Context includes the physical attributes of environment, such as temperature and moisture (affecting technology performance), and the social and cultural attributes, which are both external and within the individual (affecting expectations and tolerance for technology). For example, in the school setting, students need to answer questions and work with others in the classroom and want to talk with friends in the cafeteria and after school. Different settings require different types of communication and may require particular product features to meet the client's desire for participation and acceptance. To identify the features that are needed in an

AT device, it is important to understand the settings, the occupations, and the person's strengths (intrinsic enablers) and gaps in performance. When the AT device supports performance, it serves as an "extrinsic enabler." For example, a text-to-speech synthesizer added to a computer enables use of the computer by a client with a visual impairment or learning disability. Unimpaired performance skills and capacities (listening and remembering) are enlisted and used in combination with the adapted computer.

The HAAT Model describes the interaction between the four components of an AT device. The *human-technology interface* is the means by which the client interacts with the device—to either input or receive information or both. A computer keyboard and display are examples of common human-technology interfaces. The *processor* acts on the user input (e.g., pushing a joystick) and follows instructions or a program (e.g., the wheelchair's computer) to produce an activity output (e.g., motor-powered movement in the direction the joystick is pushed). The *activity output* of AT devices ranges from speaking selected words via digitized speech to launching a music CD in response to activation of a switch on a remote controller. Some AT devices have an *environmental interface*. This factor detects external information, interprets it, and delivers it back to the human through the human-technology interface. A page scanner that converts print into computer text for listening via speech synthesizer and an ultrasonic cane that detects obstacles for an individual without vision are examples of environmental interfaces.

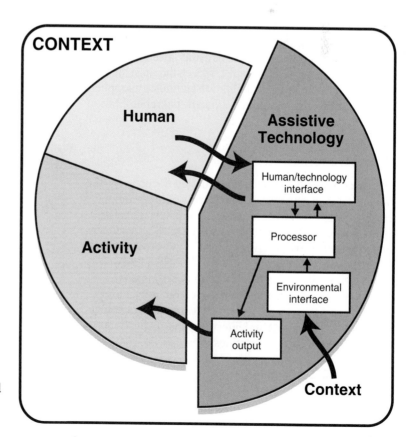

FIGURE 61.1 The HAAT model represents all the system factors that must be considered for successful assistive technology intervention.

Client-Centered Intervention

The desire for meaningful occupation facilitates motivation and the potential for successful use of an AT device. The positive experience of using AT to engage in valued occupations often opens the door to considering other forms of AT. For example, the stimulation of attending a baseball game in a new powered wheelchair might naturally lead to the desire to talk about teams or game statistics. This experience could lead a nonspeaking individual to consider using an augmentative or alternative communication (AAC) device to enhance the capacity for participation. The investment of time and effort in learning to use an AT device is returned when the client becomes even more motivated for activity and participation.

Multidisciplinary Teams

Because occupational therapists have broad expertise in human performance and activity analysis, they are involved in many aspects of AT practice. However, occupational therapists are not experts in the areas of hearing, speech and language, special education, or engineering. Multidisciplinary teams with broad expertise lead to client success. For example, a speech therapist will be better prepared to support a person who is learning to communicate with an AAC device when the speech therapist works with an occupational therapist who helps to identify the best selection method and the optimal device placement. The technical skills of engineers are useful in customizing or integrating two or more technical solutions. An interactive multidisciplinary team has greater problem-solving skills for meeting the client's needs. Depending on the client's age and activity and participation needs, the team might include a physical therapist, speech therapist, audiologist, special educator, rehabilitation technology supplier, rehabilitation engineer, and/or vocational rehabilitation counselor.

The AT Evaluation

The occupational therapist's evaluation focuses on the human-technology interface and activity output to support engagement in desired occupations. The occupational therapy evaluation identifies the performance skills and patterns that are needed to efficiently control an AT device and/or to individualize its activity output.

Because clients use AT in various settings, such as school, work environments, home, or community, the evaluation processes vary. Usually, one team member orients the client to the process and interviews the client about his or her activity goals; the settings in which the client will function; and his or her physical, sensory, or learning challenges. This lead role in the evaluation process is ideal for an occupational therapist. In the case of a child or a nonspeaking adult, family members or advocates actively participate in the evaluation. The lead therapist reviews reports from referring specialists, if they are available, looking for history and diagnostic data for prognosis or precautions or summaries of the client's strengths and abilities and then determines whether additional information is needed. The lead therapist identifies the other team members the client should meet. In collaboration with the client, the therapist summarizes the identified needs and outlines a plan for using AT to address them.

The therapist then develops a process for further assessing the client's needs and begins to identify categories of AT solutions. For example, if the client is a fifth grader with dysgraphia who is struggling to develop written language skills, the therapist might think about keyboarding, knowing that this will be an important lifelong strategy for written communication. The options to be considered might range from a desktop computer to an inexpensive portable word processor (Figure 61.2). A client with amyotrophic lateral sclerosis might also be struggling with writing. In this case, the therapist's knowledge of this disease and its rapid progression leads the therapist to consider a device with more features. The client with amyotrophic lateral sclerosis might initially use a keyboard but will soon need another technology interface, such as a single-switch scan to generate text, and eventually a way to convert that text into speech output.

In considering a range of AT options, it is helpful to use a principle called the *hierarchy of access,* which advises using the least technology required to do the job (Schmitt, 1992). Simpler solutions are easier to learn, cost less, and have fewer elements to malfunction, yet create the desired activity output for the client.

The Human-Technology Interface

As adults in a technologically sophisticated world, we are aware of the many means by which humans control devices:

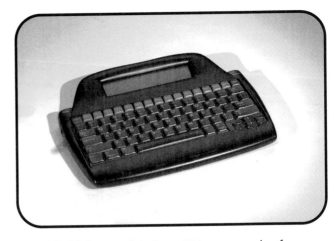

FIGURE 61.2   An AlphaSmart™ is an example of an inexpensive, portable word processor with adaptive features. It beams text to a computer, where it can be printed and saved.

keyboards, dials, two- or three-button mice, slider bars, push buttons, toggle switches, voice menus, touch screens, and more. When these controls are well designed, they fit the hand or finger, provide enough resistance to increase control, and provide feedback that gives knowledge of results to the user. We recognize a well-designed product because it requires minimal effort for successful use. Designing products for easy and effective use by the largest segment of the population is called **universal design** (Center for Universal Design, 1997). For example, a universally designed cell phone would have larger keys and a larger display, making it usable by elderly people and those with some impairment in vision or motor control as well as the typical user.

The human-technology interface, often called the *user interface* (UI), is central to the AT process and serves as a valuable way to categorize AT solutions (Cook & Hussey, 2002). The UI includes the means of input as well as the type of feedback or output to the user.

MODIFICATIONS TO SYSTEM INPUT: DIRECT AND INDIRECT SELECTION. A user who has good motor control can choose from among all options, and no modification is needed. This is called **direct selection**. When the requirements for direct selection are impaired, every effort is made to enable direct selection through the use of performance or **control enhancers** (Cook & Hussey, 2002). These are low-tech or positioning aids that augment or extend motor control. **Indirect selection** is used only as a last resort because of the inefficiency of waiting for the scan and the high cognitive load. Table 61.1 provides more information on these three types of user interfaces.

Selecting from a scanning array requires less motor control, but it is much more cognitively demanding. Scanning involves anticipating the presentation of an option and activating the switch at precisely the right time to select it, along with the intellectual ability to systematically build a word or sentence or select a path of travel. When scanning is required, occupational therapists should explore methods for increasing efficiency, such as presenting options in order of frequency of use or using word prediction to save keystrokes (Angelo, 1996, 2000). A single switch is placed where the client can activate it with a hand or upper extremity, chin, foot, knee, or eye blink. The occupational therapist identifies the ideal control site on the body, selects a switch type that complements it, and mounts the switch to optimize activation. Switches vary on many parameters. For example, a small, sensitive switch is selected for finger activation by a person with late-stage multiple sclerosis, and a bright, tough switch is selected for hand or foot activation by a preschooler with powerful athetoid movements.

MODIFICATIONS TO SYSTEM INPUT: PROPORTIONAL AND DIGITAL. Another characteristic on which human-technology interfaces vary is the signaling or control

TABLE 61.1 METHODS TO CONTROL ASSISTIVE TECHNOLOGY DEVICES

User Interface	Description	Examples	Requires
Direct selection	The user picks the desired options from a display of all options (the selection set) possible.	◆ Computer keyboard ◆ Phone number pad ◆ Pressing the TV channel number	Stability, reach, control, strength, control of a finger or body segment to accurately select
Control enhancers	An item that facilitates using a part of the body that could make a direct selection if enabled.	◆ Positioning a keyboard on an easel or platform ◆ Forearm or mobile arm supports ◆ Mouth/typing stick	Observing that a body segment has some but not all of the skills needed for direct selection
Indirect selection	The user is given subsets of the entire selection set. The subsets are presented in sequence. The user waits until the desired option is presented and then picks it by activating a switch; also called scanning.	◆ Repeat presses of "channel up" until reaching the desired channel ◆ Alphabet offered in subsets of five letters with branches to numbers and punctuation	◆ A body part with reliable and repeatable movement ◆ An appropriate single switch placed to facilitate accuracy ◆ The cognitive ability to anticipate and activate a switch and plan a sequence of steps

technology that the interface uses. Individuals with good motor control succeed with **proportional controls**. The typical wheelchair joystick is proportional, with speed and direction linked so that the farther the joystick is pushed, the faster the wheelchair moves. Easing up slows the movement. For people without precise motor control, a digital or microprocessor-based controller is used. Speed is preset, and the user chooses only direction.

MODIFICATIONS TO SYSTEM OUTPUT: USING ALTERNATE SENSORS.   When clients have sensory limitations, it is necessary to modify the system *output*. Just as vibration or flashing strobes can replace the sound of doorbells, clock alarms, and fire signals, so text-to-speech or refreshable Braille displays can substitute for reading text on a computer display. AT is a powerful tool for inclusion, employment, and education for people with sensory impairment, such as when text telephones in combination with relay operators enable clients without hearing to telephone anyone.

The Activity Output

Occupational therapists have affinity with AT because the device's activity output enables individuals to engage in occupations. To illustrate, consider the value of alternative computer access that bypasses the keyboard and mouse for an individual with C-4 quadriplegia. The AT solution could be speech recognition or Morse code sent via a sip-and-puff switch or a head-directed mouse paired with an on-screen keyboard. Regardless of the solution that is chosen, AT restores written communication for any purpose across occupational settings. Computer use enables e-mailing friends and family, writing about life in a journal, or writing advertising copy and participating via the office intranet in work projects. Restoration of written communication supports the client in the roles of friend, family member, and employee.

ASSISTIVE TECHNOLOGY SOLUTIONS

There are many AT solutions, and new or updated products arrive continuously. Because AT solutions change frequently, they are discussed here in categories, along with general guidelines for their use.

Posture

The body continuously cocontracts groups of muscles to maintain posture and enable occupational performance. In addition, an individual automatically shifts body position to relieve pressure, rebalance and stabilize, regain comfort, and improve function. Many occupations occur while seated, and sitting is the only option for clients who use wheelchairs.

Assessing Seating Needs

Many practitioners falsely believe that a client with good sitting posture sits with a vertical trunk and 90 degrees of flexion at the hips, knees, and ankles. This is a posture that many people do not tolerate—or not for very long. A client who is forced by the design of a wheelchair or seating system to sit continuously in one position will be uncomfortable and unable to reposition for tasks.

A physical motor assessment allows observing or checking for the following:

- Ability to transfer and sitting balance
- Bilateral symmetry and range of motion through the spine and pelvis:
  - A fixed asymmetry or deformity must be accommodated, whereas a flexible asymmetry should be corrected to prevent worsening.
- Signs of pressure or shear over bony areas of the pelvis
- Muscle tone, the presence of primitive reflexes, and other factors that affect sitting:
  - Decreased range of motion in the hips affects the seat-to-back angle.
  - Shortened hamstrings directly affect the angle of the footrest hanger.

Table 61.2 provides some examples of seating goals.

Seating for Soft Tissue Management

Individuals without sensation or the ability to reposition themselves are at high risk for pressure ulcers. In addition to ischemia, causes of pressure ulcers include **shear** created by sliding, heat and moisture, poor nutrition, and age-related soft tissue changes. Preventing pressure ulcers is much less expensive than treatment; time lost to healing is also a consideration (Allman, Goode, Burst, Bartolucci, & Thomas, 1999). Properly selected pressure-reducing cushions (rather than low-cost foam) reduce the incidence of pressure sores. (Brienza, Karg, Geyer, Kelsey, & Trefler, 2001; Conine, Herschler, Daechsel, Peel, & Pearson, 1994). Cushion features should be matched to a client's risk factors. Adjusting footrests, armrests, and seat angle also redistribute pressures.

Pressure mapping is a technology that is designed to estimate interface pressure created by gravity. A thin mat of pressure sensors connected to a computer is placed between the client and the seating surface. The computer displays pressure data, and a clinician uses these data to estimate pressure ulcers risk (Brienza et al., 2001; Conine et al., 1994). Mapping of data allows comparison among cushions for a particular client. A pressure map does not measure shear, heat, moisture, or postural stability, and these factors must also be considered.

TABLE 61.2 EXAMPLES OF SEATING GOALS

Structure	Function	Activity and Participation
Reduce potential for deformity or slow its progression	Increase sitting tolerance for activities	Enable greater participation in the community
Prevent pressure ulcers by dispersing peak pressures over larger areas of soft tissue	Decrease pain, enable use of seated posture, increase comfort and well-being	Support personal productivity in education or employment
Maintain vital organ function	Orient the head for visual input	Maximize independence in transfers and self-care activities

Seating for Pelvic Support

For some clients, stabilizing the pelvis in an optimal alignment is essential for functioning. Cushions provide external support to compensate for weakness or help to offset the force of spasticity or fluctuating tone. A neutral pelvis supports the natural curves in the spine and contributes to upper extremity function. Positioning belts can help to maintain pelvic position. Tilting the seat pan toward the rear also increases pelvic control and diminishes extensor tone. The only option for fixed pelvic and spinal deformities might be a custom-molded system that accommodates the shape of the trunk, distributes pressures, and optimizes orientation in space.

Matching Seating to Client Needs

Seating goals plus the material properties and shape of cushions underlie the selection of wheelchair cushions and seat backs. Sling upholstery, the most common seating, is popular because it collapses. In fact, sling upholstery is such a poor foundation for the pelvis that over time, it leads to postural deformity (Trefler, Hobson, Taylor, Monahan, & Shaw, 1993).

Today, a seat pan and cushion are used. Cushions include flat or contoured foams, air-filled bladders, viscous fluids, contoured plastic honeycombs, custom-contoured foam, and alternating pressure systems. They vary in their ability to distribute pressure, stabilize posture, insulate or conduct heat, and perform over time. Seat backs vary in height, lateral support, accommodation for spinal curves, and orientation to the seat pan. The certified rehabilitation technology supplier (CRTS) is an essential partner for the occupational therapist. The CRTS specializes in knowing available products and their features. When the occupational therapist works in partnership with a CRTS, this enables matching an active client with paraplegia with a very low wheelchair back that permits full arm mobility, torso rotation, and leaning with the upper body and a pressure relieving cushion. Alternatively, a client with significant trunk weakness is matched with the support of a taller, deeply contoured back.

Recline and Tilt-in-Space

Seating can also be modified with a wheelchair frame that enables recline or tilt-in-space, relieve pressure, manages posture, increases comfort, and helps with personal care activities. *Recline* changes the seat-to-back angle and, in powered wheelchairs, is user controlled. Reclining the seat back creates shear, so antishear mechanisms should be used. Recline helps to stretch hip flexors and enables attending to catheters and dressing. *Tilt-in-space* keeps the hip and knee angles constant while tilting the whole body. Reduced gravity makes it easier to reposition. A tilt of 35 degrees or more unweights the ischial tuberosities and facilitates extension in the spine, neck, and shoulders (Sprigle & Sposato, 1997). Individuals with sensation who are unable to shift their weight or change position require tilt-in-space for day-long comfort. Individuals with high-level spinal cord injury, amyotrophic lateral sclerosis, or advanced multiple sclerosis use tilt to manage dependent edema. In addition to a head rest, a tilt-in-space wheelchair usually creates the need for greater support for arms and legs.

Mobility

Many clients need support to accept and integrate wheeled mobility into daily life when ambulation is no longer safe and efficient. Wheelchairs enable many people to achieve occupational competence despite the loss of ambulation (Iezzoni, 1996). There are many factors to consider in choosing between manual and powered mobility, and it is sometimes a difficult decision (Buning, Angelo, & Schmeler, 2001). Skilled users of manual wheelchairs can maneuver in tight spaces and pull their chair into a car. Heavy powered wheelchairs require accessible environments but traverse hills and distances with ease (Figure 61.3). The user can focus on activities and interactions rather than propelling.

Therapists should not insist on manual propulsion just because a client has the ability to push. Long-term manual propulsion appears to be linked to repetitive strain

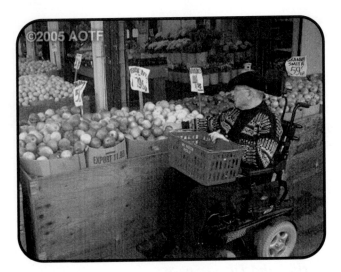

FIGURE 61.3 A powered wheelchair enables assuming many valued occupations and supports self-reliance but requires a supportive environment with ramps, elevators, and wider doors.

injuries (RSIs) and rotator cuff tears. These injuries abruptly end self-propulsion as well as transfers, lifting, and reaching (Boninger, Baldwin, Cooper, Koontz, & Chan, 2000).

The Human-Technology Interface: Controls

A primary difference in wheelchairs is the means of control. For manual wheelchairs, it is either a passive system in which someone else pushes or an active one in which the individual uses hands or a combination of hands and feet to self-propel. In a powered wheelchair, the motors are directed by a controller, which receives and translates input from the user. The typical controller is a joystick, but alternatives such as head movement or a sip-and-puff switch are available.

Table 61.3 categorizes wheelchair types, features, usability, and environmental requirements.

MANUAL WHEELCHAIRS. The Centers for Medicare and Medicaid Services (CMS) assigns product codes to all wheelchairs based on their features (Health Care Finance Administration & United Healthcare, 1998). All insurers now use these codes to categorize wheelchair features. Coding decisions are often controversial because they rigidly limit access to wheelchair types on the basis of the ability to transfer or other functional skills, which can impede independent mobility. For example, a standard wheelchair with large rear wheels appears suitable for self-propulsion. However, its weight, limited size options, sling upholstery, and nonadjustable axle position make it a poor choice for self-propulsion.

Axle adjustability is a valuable feature. Alignment of the rear axle directly below the shoulder improves access

to the pushrims throughout the push stroke and balances the muscle groups that are used in propulsion (Boninger et al., 2000). This increased efficiency results in fewer strokes for the distance traveled, which reduces the likelihood of RSI. When the axle is in this position, turns are easier, but so is tipping backward. The therapist must offer skills training and provide rear antitippers until the client is skilled. Axle adjustability is essential for long-term users, but few clients currently qualify because of CMS coding restrictions.

The body of scientific evidence favoring light, adjustable-axle manual wheelchairs is growing. Manual wheelchair users experience a 49–73% incidence of carpal tunnel syndrome (Boninger et al., 2000; Boninger, Cooper, Baldwin, Shimada, & Koontz, 1999). These individuals depend on their upper extremities for propulsion, transfers, and ADL. Carpal tunnel syndrome in wheelchair users leads to costly surgery, loss of productivity, and usually to powered mobility and the consequent changes in daily environments and lifestyle (Buning et al., 2001).

Boninger and colleagues (2000) found that rear axle placement relative to shoulder position is correlated with median nerve injury. The study also showed that proper rear axle position improved propulsion biomechanics. On a driving course, users of ultralight wheelchairs reported a significant positive difference in perceived comfort compared to users of standard wheelchairs (DiGiovine et al., 2000). When both types of wheelchairs were stressed to simulate 5 years of typical use, ultralightweight chairs proved to be far more durable and economical (Cooper et al., 1997).

POWERED WHEELCHAIRS. Motors were first added to wheelchairs in the 1950s and have continuously improved in performance and features since then (Cooper, 1998). People who use powered mobility have moderate to severe upper extremity limitations. Even when clients have some ability to propel short indoor distances, they rarely have sufficient strength and coordination to offset the risk for RSI or to maintain independent mobility over time.

The CMS recently released new codes for powered wheelchairs for Medicare beneficiaries with specific requirements for client functioning, such as ability to transfer, need for postural support, or powered seat functions (Centers for Medicare and Medicaid Services, 2006). Medicare reimbursement is tied to enabling mobility-related activities of daily living (MRADL) and is restricted to in-home use. The codes now require a face-to-face visit with a physician (who may refer the patient out to an occupational therapist) and home visits to determine home accessibility. Table 61.4 summarizes information on scooters and powered wheelchairs at present, though further changes may occur.

TABLE 61.3   TYPES OF WHEELCHAIRS: FEATURES, SUITABLE USES, AND ENVIRONMENTS

WC Type and Examples	Features	Suitable Uses	Suitable Environments
Dependent Mobility ◆ Transport wheelchair ◆ Adaptive stroller	◆ 6–8" wheels ◆ Sling seat ◆ Lighter than standard wheelchair ◆ Foldable ◆ May or may not have postural supports	◆ Temporary transport ◆ Sick or physically unable to propel ◆ Young children ◆ Cognitively impaired	◆ Hospital corridors ◆ Physician's office ◆ Airport ◆ Traveling ◆ Shopping malls ◆ Not for use as a vehicle seat unless crash tested
Dependent Mobility ◆ Standard wheelchair ◆ Depot chair ◆ Hemi-height wheelchair	◆ 24–26" rear wheel ◆ Heavy (>36 lb) ◆ Few sizes ◆ No or minimal adjustment ◆ Lower seat option for foot propulsion ◆ Foldable ◆ Sling seat	◆ Short-term use ◆ Able to transfer ◆ Able to reposition self ◆ For hemi-height, use of same side arm and leg	◆ Hospital corridors ◆ Physician's office ◆ Airport ◆ Home ◆ Community outings with pusher ◆ Not for use as a vehicle seat unless crash tested
Dependent Mobility ◆ Tilt-in-space (55-degree tilt) ◆ Recliner (seat back to 180 degrees)	◆ 24–26" or 10–12" rear wheel ◆ Long wheel base ◆ Heavy (40–60 lb) ◆ Few sizes ◆ Specialized seating ◆ Not foldable	◆ Long-term use ◆ High postural support needs ◆ Dependent with pressure management ◆ Unable to transfer or reposition self	◆ Home ◆ School ◆ Community outings with pusher ◆ Not for use as a transit seat unless crash tested
Dependent Mobility ◆ Heavy duty (for clients who weigh 250–650 lb)	◆ 24–26" rear wheel ◆ Heavy (>50 lb) ◆ Width: 24–30" ◆ Depth: 18–22" ◆ Double crossbars ◆ Stabilizer bar between seat canes ◆ Heavy tubing	◆ Long-term use ◆ Difficult to propel with arms so often used with foot propulsion ◆ Variable ability to transfer	◆ Inside the home ◆ Inside the office ◆ Hard, smooth surfaces ◆ Becomes dependent mobility in most community travel. ◆ Not for use as a transit seat unless crash tested
Independent Mobility ◆ Lightweight wheelchair	◆ 24–26" rear wheel ◆ Heavy (26–40 lb) ◆ Two height options: regular and hemi ◆ Two seat depth options. ◆ No axle adjustment ◆ Accepts removable seating/backrest	◆ Long-term use in limited environments ◆ Able to transfer ◆ Able to reposition self	◆ Inside the home ◆ Inside the office ◆ On hard or smooth surfaces. ◆ Reverts to dependent mobility in most community travel. ◆ Not for use as a transit seat unless crash tested
Independent Mobility ◆ Ultralightweight folding frame ◆ Ultralightweight rigid frame	◆ 24–26" rear wheel; may have quick release hubs ◆ Light (<30 lb, some <20 lb) ◆ Custom sizes for depth and width ◆ Axle position can adjust to shoulder position. ◆ Accepts removable seating/backrest	◆ With appropriate adjustment of axle, appropriate for long-term use in all community environments	◆ With ability to do a "wheelie," all indoor and most community ◆ With knobby tires, usable on packed trails and in snow ◆ Not for use as a transit seat; should transfer to vehicle seat

TABLE 61.4 SCOOTERS AND POWERED WHEELCHAIRS: FEATURES, SUITABLE USES, AND ENVIRONMENTS

Wheelchair Category and Examples	Features	Suitable Use	Suitable Environments
Scooters or Power-Operated Vehicles ◆ Three-wheeled scooters ◆ Four-wheeled scooters	◆ Front- or rear-wheel drive ◆ Steers with a tiller ◆ Large turning radius or three-point turns due to long wheelbase ◆ Disassembles for transport ◆ No options for postural support	◆ Required for MRADL "in the home" ◆ Unable to walk long distances because of pain, low endurance, etc. ◆ Able to transfer safely ◆ Able to maintain postural stability ◆ Home needs open floor plan	◆ Ramped, accessible environments only ◆ Three wheels: for smooth, flat surfaces ◆ Four wheels: for uneven or unpaved surfaces; not indoors ◆ Outdoors: shopping malls, sidewalks, etc. ◆ Not for use as a transit seat; client should transfer ◆ Medicare does not reimburse for four-wheeled scooters
Group I: Limited-Duty or Portable Powered Mobility	◆ Wheelchair size: <24" × 40" ◆ May fold or disassemble ◆ No part >55 lb ◆ Joystick only ◆ Electronics not upgradable ◆ Only "off-the-shelf" seating ◆ Obstacle climb: 20 mm ◆ Min. top speed 3mph	◆ Required for MRADL "in the home" ◆ Unable to propel manual wheelchair ◆ Is required for very light use ◆ Minimum range: 5 miles on a charge ◆ Ramps: 6 degrees	◆ Ramped accessible environments only ◆ Hard, smooth surfaces; climbs only a threshold ◆ Not for use as a seat in transit unless crash tested
Group II: Limited-Duty or Portable Powered Mobility ◆ Front-wheel drive ◆ Mid-wheel drive ◆ Rear-wheel drive	◆ Wheelchair size <34" × 48" ◆ May fold or disassemble ◆ No part >55 lb ◆ Joystick only ◆ Nonupgradable electronics ◆ Expandable electronics only at initial issue ◆ Skin protection and positioning cushions on sling or solid seats ◆ Obstacle climb: 40 mm ◆ Min top speed: 3mph	◆ Required for MRADL "in the home" ◆ Light use but with special seating ◆ Minimum range: 7 miles on a charge ◆ Ramps: 6 degrees	◆ Ramped accessible environments only ◆ Hard, smooth surfaces ◆ Inside the home ◆ Not for use as a seat in transit unless crash tested

TABLE 61.4 SCOOTERS AND POWERED WHEELCHAIRS: FEATURES, SUITABLE USES, AND ENVIRONMENTS *Continued*

Wheelchair Category and Examples	Features	Suitable Use	Suitable Environments
Group III: Medium-Duty Powered Mobility ◆ Front-wheel drive ◆ Mid-wheel drive ◆ Rear-wheel	◆ WC size <34" × 48" ◆ Suspension to dampen vibration ◆ Proportional joystick or alternate input ◆ May upgrade to expandable electronics ◆ Expandable controller at initial issue ◆ Customized seating possible ◆ May include powered seat functions: tilt and recline ◆ Obstacle climb: 60mm ◆ Min top speed: 4.5 mph ◆ Home visit and evaluation by OT/PT/MD/DO	◆ Required for MRADL "in the home" ◆ Neurological or myopathic diagnosis and inability to stand/pivot transfer ◆ Needs postural support and/or pressure relief. ◆ Minimum range: 12 miles ◆ Accommodates a ventilator ◆ Min range: 16 mi. on a charge ◆ Ramps <7.5 degrees	◆ Ramped accessible environments only ◆ Indoor and limited community use on hard surfaces with some uneven surfaces ◆ Not for use as a seat in transit unless crash tested
Group IV: Heavy-Duty Powered Mobility ◆ Front-wheel drive ◆ Mid-wheel drive ◆ Rear-wheel Also includes pushrim-activated power-assist wheels	◆ Need for drive wheel suspension ◆ Proportional joystick or alternative input ◆ May upgrade electronics ◆ Customized seating and powered seat functions ◆ Obstacle climb: 75 mm ◆ Min top speed: 6 mph ◆ Home visit evaluation by OT/PT/MD/DO	◆ Required for MRADL "in the home" and for community use ◆ Need for wheel suspension ◆ Unable to transfer ◆ Need for postural support and/or pressure relief ◆ Accommodates a ventilator ◆ Minimum range: 16 miles ◆ Ramps ≥9 degrees	◆ Ramps and accessible environments only ◆ Indoor and community use on most surfaces ◆ Available for use as a transit seat as this category must pass crash test ◆ Medicare does not reimburse for this category of wheelchair.

A powered base with mid-wheel drive is highly maneuverable and turns within its own footprint, making it ideal for small spaces. This is important because payment for a powered wheelchair is based on its necessity for MRADL. If the person is also using a powered chair in the community, the advantages of front- or rear-wheel drive should be considered. Wheelchair users will make significantly different demands on the batteries, motors, and torque offered by a powerbase, so knowledge of contexts and occupations is important.

An individual's need for postural support, pressure management, and comfort will also determine the category of wheelchair that is needed. A range of aftermarket products can customize pelvic position; head, back, and arm support; thigh placement; and foot support. Powered options for tilt-in-space, leg elevation, recline, seat elevation, and sit-to-stand should also be considered. The most commonly used powered wheelchair option is tilt-in-space as it redistributes pressure for individuals unable to transfer or shift weight.

A joystick is the typical control interface for a powered wheelchair and uses proportional control. When a client cannot use a joystick, the therapist, using the concepts presented previously, collaborates with the client and the CRTS to determine alternative control options. Interfaces such as a sip-and-puff straw or directional switches embedded in a head support allow the client to control direction and move at preset speeds. Powered wheelchair users can also use scanning interfaces in which they choose from the four directions as they are offered sequentially.

The Human Interface for Mobility

A client will not be fully successful with manual or powered mobility unless the client is confident that he or she can control its activity output. The therapist needs to teach mobility skills. Active manual wheelchair users need to learn to do a wheelie so that they can feel comfortable going down ramps, bouncing off a curb, or traveling over soft earth (Kirby, 2005). In dependent mobility systems, the therapist teaches the pusher, who must deal with these same barriers.

The equivalent with a powered wheelchair is programming the controller for the user's ability and environ- ments. Novice users should have driving parameters set conservatively and readjusted when skills improve. Clients who drive in hilly areas should have torque settings adjusted for better climbing performance. Those with progressive impairment should have settings adjusted periodically to compensate for weakness, lost range of motion, or tremors. These modifications show the benefit of having a smart processor as part of an AT solution. The processor modifies input or output as needed in response to changes in skills or the environment.

With powered wheelchairs that have more complex control interfaces, a partnership between the therapist and the CRTS is critical. The therapist conveys the client's needs and output requirements to the CRTS, who is able to recommend products with the needed features and performance attributes. The knowledge and ethics of a CRTS are valuable in ordering the wheelchair, negotiating payment, and later handling product warranty and repairs.

PRACTICE DILEMMA

WHEN *NO* DOESN'T MEAN *NO!*

Debra, a 58-year-old woman, has symptoms with no clear diagnosis. Her neurologist continues to do tests to rule out one diagnosis after another and meanwhile refers Debra to a seating and mobility clinic. Debra comes in using an ill-fitting borrowed manual wheelchair. She has tremors in her upper extremities, significant weakness in her legs, and paresthesias in her feet, and she can walk only a few feet. Tremors make it difficult for her hands to connect with the pushrims on the manual chair and coordinate self-propelling movements.

The occupational therapist interviews Debra and notes her occupations as homemaker, wife, and grandparent. Following a complete assessment, Debra, the occupational therapist, and the CRTS discuss several wheelchair options. After a driving trial, they agree that a small, mid-wheel drive powered wheelchair would maneuver within the dimensions of Debra's home yet have the power to get her out onto the rear deck, where she could watch her grandchildren play. The occupational therapist writes up the evaluation results and includes the CRTS's report from the home visit with a demo chair, the letter of justification, and the specifications for the wheelchair that meet Debra's needs.

Four weeks later, Debra calls saying she that has received a letter of denial from her health plan. The occupational therapist is stunned. Surely, a follow-up phone call will clarify Debra's need for a powered wheelchair. The health plan representative cites Debra's lack of diagnosis and her ability to walk short distances as reasons for denying the powered chair. The representative outlines the appeal process, and the occupational therapist immediately writes a letter of appeal to the health plan with a copy to Debra's neurologist.

Five days later, Debra calls again with more bad news. She has fallen while attempting to get clothes out of her dresser. She lay on the floor for several hours and was discovered only when her daughter stopped at the house. Debra bruised her right arm, fractured a rib, and blackened her right eye. She spent a night in the hospital and is quite distraught.

Questions

1. What ethics should guide this occupational therapist's behavior in this situation?
2. How can clinical findings be used to get the health plan to recognize its responsibility?
3. How will the occupational therapist be reimbursed for the time required for this appeal?

An important context for wheelchairs is transportation. Personal vans with lifts are ideal but are expensive. Other types of transportation include public buses, paratransit, and school buses. At a minimum, the therapist should be aware that wheelchairs to be used as seats in motor vehicles should meet transportation safety standards with crash-tested frames and securement points (RERC on Wheelchair Transportation Safety, 2000) (Figure 61.4).

Communication

Communication is essential for expressing needs; making choices; forming and maintaining relationships; and participating in education, employment, and community life. Communication happens through facial expression and gestures as well as through speech and writing (Beukelman & Mirenda, 1998). Speech-language pathologists who have specialized in AAC are the leaders of an AAC intervention team. They evaluate a client's potential to use an AAC device, which range from line drawings representing basic human needs to computer-based devices that can store and retrieve language (U.S. Society for Augmentative and Alternative Communication, 2005).

The Human-Technology Interface: Selection Methods

The ideal human-technology interface for an AAC device is direct selection. Clients with poor pointing accuracy or limited hand range of motion will need keys that are sized and located to match their capacity. Performance enhancers such as mouth sticks, head pointers, or mobile arm supports may augment residual abilities (Figure 61.5). Some high-end devices allow the use of electronic head pointing, in which sensors within the AAC device detect light from a reflective dot worn on the forehead. This input is equivalent to a key press. Touch screens allow customization of key size and location so that frequently used keys are placed where accuracy and range are better.

When a client cannot use direct selection methods, indirect selection or scanning methods are used. Users of AAC devices already speak very slowly, and scanning slows the process further. Scanning strategies such as row/column allow the user to first select the row with the desired icon and then move through columns until the icon is reached. Row/column is just one style of scanning array, and users with more skill can use other styles to increase their efficiency. AAC users who rely on scanning use word and icon prediction to decrease switch activations. A client with visual impairment uses a method called **auditory scanning**. The name of the icon or message is quietly announced to the device user, who then activates a switch to select it, which makes the AAC device speak aloud.

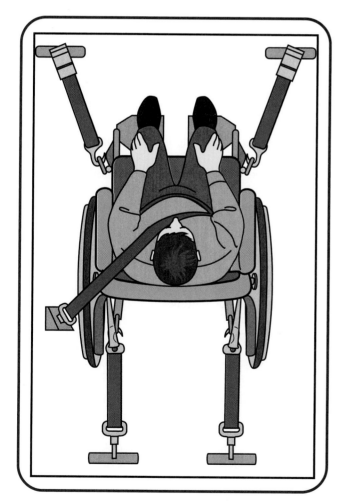

FIGURE 61.4 Using best practices in wheelchair securement and occupant restraint creates equivalent safety for individuals who cannot transfer to the motor vehicle seat. Wheelchairs are now available with the transit option.

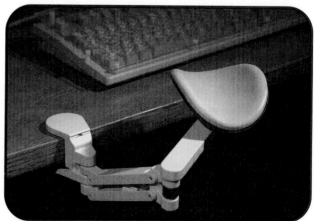

FIGURE 61.5 A forearm support paired with a polycarbonate keyguard on the keyboard functions as a performance enhancer to reduce effort and increase accuracy.

Visual perceptual skills should be considered in setting up communication boards or choosing the symbol set to represent stored sentences or words. Clients with good tactile and spatial awareness may soon memorize icon location on AAC devices with fixed displays.

The Human-Technology Interface: Mounting for Access and Function

Most AAC users use wheelchairs, so devices are mounted to its frame. Therapists recommend where to mount AAC devices so that they are positioned for optimal visual and motor access. AAC mounts should not obstruct driving, passing through doorways, completing transfers, or functions of the wheelchair, such as tilting. Mealtime is a natural context for communication, so the mounting system should make it possible to both eat and talk.

The Processor and Activity Outputs

It is important to remember that expensive AAC devices are wasted if clients are not expected or allowed to communicate. The people who are the communication partners of AAC users must learn to respect their speaking pace and avoid interrupting, guessing, ignoring, or peering at the display on a user's device. Helping family members, teachers, and personal care attendants to embed communication within occupations is another important role for occupational therapists. Everyone needs to reinforce the effort of learning to use an AAC device.

Manipulation

Another major area of AT intervention is helping people to compensate for hand skill limitations, such as paralysis, weakness, tremor, incoordination, and limited range of motion. These limitations make writing a message, reading a textbook, balancing a checkbook, or turning on the TV difficult or impossible. AT devices called *electronic aids to daily living* (EADLs) and alternative methods for accessing computers assist people with limited hand skills.

The Human-Technology Interface: Selection Methods

The selection methods for EADLs are similar to those that have already been discussed: a variety of direct selection methods and, if these are not possible, indirect selection. Speech recognition is sometimes used when physical limitations prevent controlling items in the environment. After configuring the interface, learning commands, and training the device, the user speaks commands such as "Dial Jack" or "TV on" to get results. Users without speech are often limited to indirect selection methods. Scanning arrays might need to offer pictures to clients who do not read.

Electronic Aids to Daily Living

Managing the telephone, controlling TV and music, exiting the house, and regulating lights and temperature create safety and comfort at home. Because home automation systems enable remote control of these electronic devices, therapists simply adapt the user interface to enable control for people with physical limitations. Previously, EADL devices were called *environmental control units.* The name change spotlights their function: using electronics to perform instrumental ADLs.

Evaluation for EADLs begins with a review of a person's daily environments and the activities and routines that occur in each setting. This information helps to identify the types of devices to be controlled and whether a stationary or portable system is needed. Assessing the person's motor and cognitive abilities helps to identify the requirements of the user interface. Because individuals who use EADLs often have significant physical limitations, it might be important to integrate the EADL with other equipment to make use of limited movement. Flexibility and expandability are important considerations in an EADL system. High-end devices are expensive, so thinking ahead is important when someone is learning how to use one or is faced with a progressive diagnosis (Bain & Leger, 1997; Cook & Hussey, 2002).

As is seen in Table 61.5, EADLs use several means to transmit a signal.

Figure 61.6 shows the two categories of EADLs. Simple EADLs use one signaling technology to control one type of device—the TV, a light, a toy, or a telephone. They succeed when needs are limited or when clients are young and learning. One example is a scanning telephone that enables using a switch to answer the phone or scan through prestored numbers to dial and make calls via speakerphone.

Complex EADLs control multiple devices using two or more signaling technologies. They use one control center to manage several systems: send electrical current to X-10 modules or send infrared (IR) signals to home entertainment appliances or an IR telephone. Wheelchair-mounted complex EADLs often incorporate radio frequency so that users can independently unlock and open doors. EADLs reduce attendant care and enable the satisfaction of safely spending time alone. Using EADLs, clients can call for help or exit the house in an emergency as well as independently manage daily activities.

EADLs can also be controlled through AAC devices, computers, and wheelchairs. High-end AAC devices have IR sending capacity and can be used to directly control any appliance with an IR receiver. The user interface on an AAC device is ideal, since picture symbols are used to represent the output (e.g., lights on, music on). In a similar way, computer software with a graphical user interface can drive hardware that sends several signal transmission technologies. Several manufacturers of high

TABLE 61.5 ELECTRONIC AIDS TO DAILY LIVING: SIGNAL TYPES

Signal Type	Description	Typically Used to Control	Requirements
Infrared (IR)	A light beam from an invisible part of the spectrum	TV, stereo, CD or DVD player	Clear line of sight Unique coded light bursts that are paired with a device function
Radio frequency (RF)	An electromagnetic signal sent from an antenna to a receiver using a very high-frequency radio wave	Garage and entry door openers, alarm systems, remote car entry, etc.	Transmits through solid materials Signal travels distance based on strength of transmitter
X-10	A short RF burst of digital information travels via the house wiring until it meets the coded module or receiver matched to the signal	Devices that plug into wall sockets such as a fan, table radio, or lamp. Also, X-10 units like an alert chime.	Lamps, etc. plug into coded modules that are plugged into electrical outlets. Used to control on/off devices; special modules dim lights and adjust thermostat.

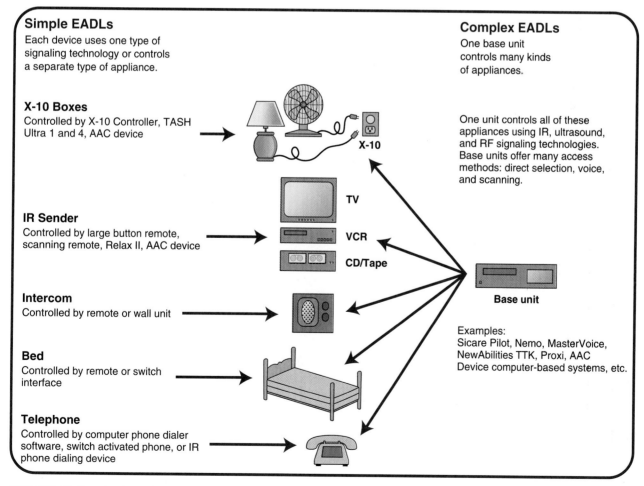

Simple EADLs

Each device uses one type of signaling technology or controls a separate type of appliance.

X-10 Boxes
Controlled by X-10 Controller, TASH Ultra 1 and 4, AAC device

IR Sender
Controlled by large button remote, scanning remote, Relax II, AAC device

Intercom
Controlled by remote or wall unit

Bed
Controlled by remote or switch interface

Telephone
Controlled by computer phone dialer software, switch activated phone, or IR phone dialing device

X-10

TV

VCR

CD/Tape

Complex EADLs

One base unit controls many kinds of appliances.

One unit controls all of these appliances using IR, ultrasound, and RF signaling technologies. Base units offer many access methods: direct selection, voice, and scanning.

Base unit

Examples:
Sicare Pilot, Nemo, MasterVoice, NewAbilities TTK, Proxi, AAC Device computer-based systems, etc.

FIGURE 61.6 Simple and complex EADLs.

end power wheelchairs have just started including this technology within the wheelchair controller.

Computers for Occupation

For people with disabilities, computer input or output can be adapted to accomplish tasks while increasing their access to the broader community and its resources. Computers can significantly enhance self-reliance and quality of life for people with disabilities.

Because clients who could benefit from alternative computer access may have varying abilities and interests, the first step is evaluation to identify goals and begin to narrow the options. A young child with cognitive limitations might need to learn cause and effect with the help of software or develop number concepts through early learning software. A middle-schooler with hemiplegia might need only a one-handed keyboarding application. An adult with spinal cord injury who is preparing for self-employment might want to use desktop publishing software, a spreadsheet to manage accounts, and computer-enabled phone dialing. Each of these activity goals and many more can be reached with knowledge of alternative computer access methods. The next step is to assess a client's performance skills to determine what types of adaptations might be needed.

INPUT MODIFICATIONS.   Computer input modifications can be categorized as a substitute for either the keyboard or the mouse. With the hierarchy of access in mind, it is important to start simple. The computer operating system (OS) control panels offer options that can compensate for mild limitations. For example, the sticky keys option helps a computer user who is typing with one hand or a mouthstick. The sticky keys option enables a user to replace simultaneous keystrokes (e.g., command+alt+delete) with the same keystrokes entered in sequence. All of the accessibility options are fully described on company Websites (Apple Computer Inc., 2005; Microsoft Corporation, 2005). Using a control enhancer such as an easel to reposition the keyboard and using a trackball to increase mouse control are other simple solutions.

Alternatives to the standard keyboard include miniature keyboards that require less range or reach, large keyboards that increase key size and adjust sensitivity to improve accuracy, and keyboards that make one-handed typing more efficient. When keyboard use is not successful, other methods of text entry, such as speech recognition, sending Morse code, pointing a cursor at the keys on an on-screen keyboard, and eye pointing, are considered.

The ability to control cursor movement is important in graphics and design applications, or it may be preferred for moving around a computer desktop. Alternative cursor or mouse control methods include mouse keys (a control panel option), joysticks, and several head-controlled technologies that use either reflected light or ultrasound.

Usually, these head-controlled mice are paired with an on-screen keyboard to allow writing text as well as fluid mouse movement. Keyboard shortcuts by-pass the need for a mouse for many common tasks.

These options are examples of direct selection. Users who do not have the ability to use these methods must revert to indirect selection. It is possible for a client using scanning software that interprets the switch activation to control every aspect of computer use or, with more limited goals, to work within just one application or perform one meaningful task.

THE PROCESSOR: THE COMPUTER'S CENTRAL PROCESSING UNIT.   The power and speed of microprocessors continue to increase, and devices such as modems, CD players, and wireless cards are now standard equipment on computers and give users many options. Many keyboard or mouse alternatives are hardware solutions paired with software for modifying settings or options. Other alternatives, such as the on-screen keyboard, rely only on software. Either way, alternatives must be compatible with the computer's OS and hardware.

THE ACTIVITY OUTPUT: INTEGRATING COMPUTERS INTO DAILY LIVES.   Occupational therapists help clients use computers to engage in activities. To illustrate, a student with significant motor impairment might use a scanning method with a computer at school. This student will need support to master an alphabet scan and then to move beyond just writing. Learning a scan that manages the computer environment will allow shifting between applications and functions, such as searching the Web for a geography assignment in one period and then taking and printing a spelling test in the next. This teaching role is well suited to an occupational therapist focused on integrating AT into school occupations and enabling the student's academic success.

Sensory

People with visual and auditory impairment need modifications to the computer output. AT developers have created excellent solutions in this area. The problem has been getting information and funding to clients who could benefit from using them.

The Human-Technology Interface: System Outputs

When using computers, individuals with low vision need enlarged print on the display or hard copy. Enlargement gives access to any information that can be acquired through a computer. The accessibility options within the OS control panel permit basic screen enlargement for someone who is an occasional user or one with minimal vision loss. Screen enlargement applications add many features that increase usability for individuals with greater needs.

Individuals without vision need substitutes for moving around desktops, icons, and menus. When you cannot see, pointing with a mouse is irrelevant. Impressive software enables navigating within and between documents and controlling functions such as saving or printing by using keys on the number pad. This software offers access to the text within word-processed documents or e-mails by either a speech synthesizer or a refreshable Braille display. Text can be sent to a Braille printer if hard copy is needed. Technology is also capable of scanning a page of text printed on paper, recognizing the image as letters and numbers, and converting the image into digital text using a process called optical character recognition (OCR). Once in digital format, text can be saved in large print, listened to via computer speech synthesizer, or converted to Braille. OCR creates access to printed materials any time the individual wants it, not just when a sighted reader is available.

Computer users with hearing impairment need captioning on multimedia software and visual alerts such as a blinking title bar rather than auditory signals such as a beep. The ability to communicate with hearing friends and colleagues via e-mail or cell phones with text messaging or short messaging service opens new possibilities for interaction. Video phones that enable direct communication in American Sign Language with other signers or relay operators are quickly changing telecommunication modes for individuals who are deaf.

The Human-Technology Interface: Activity Outputs

Closed-circuit television technology enlarges any item for individuals with low vision. Systems use a camera and flat-panel display to magnify whatever is under the camera—a greeting card, a household bill, or a crochet hook. Full-sized systems can be used only on a desktop, but small handheld models are easy to carry into the community for shopping.

Many commercially available products support independent living. These range from kitchen timers, alarm clocks, and telephones with large numbers for people with low vision to vibrating or flashing alerts for alarm clocks, doorbells, and fire alarms for people with hearing impairment. It is easy to get information about and purchase these items from the Internet.

Cognition

AT can be very useful for clients with cognitive impairments because the AT processor performs the missing skill. Many of the issues that affect the user interface are relevant to this area of AT. For example, when the human-technology interface is modified with icons and spoken

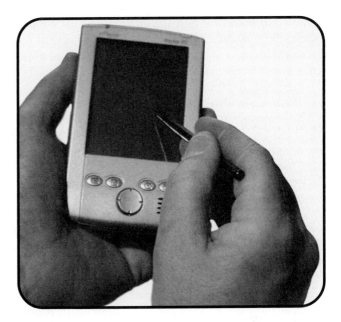

FIGURE 61.7 The PocketCompass™ offers pictures and stored speech as cognitive supports for sequencing activities. PDAs can also remind, report location, and support decisions.

menus, the same process that enables an individual with blindness to hear text also assists a person with a severe learning disability.

Mainstream technologies such as the PDA, pager, global positioning system, cellular telephone, and digital voice recorder are being modified and incorporated into AT devices for use by individuals with cognitive impairment (RERC on Cognitive Assistive Technology, 2006). For example, software written for a PDA allows customization of photos and digitized speech to depict the steps of a morning grooming routine or catching a bus (Figure 61.7). Repeating reminders can alert a person that it is time to take medications. Cellular phone with voice commands such as "call home" make it simpler to use the phone and have two-way communication with family or job coaches. Cell phone cameras can help with recall, and digital voice recorders can substitute for writing memos. Using mainstream technologies in this way can provide new options for safety, discrete assistance for remembering, and a means of remote supervision.

CUSTOMIZING AND INTEGRATING AT SOLUTIONS

Occupational therapy practice uses teaching and an understanding of the learning process to help clients make changes. This knowledge helps therapists in following up with clients as the clients learn to use an AT device and integrate it into meaningful routines and activities. Awareness of the interaction between individual and device and between an individual and the environment or context enables occupational therapists to modify aspects of AT devices. This ability to notice changes in social and physical settings where AT devices are used helps to solidify their use and usefulness.

When clients have significant levels of impairment, it is often necessary to combine AT solutions, as in a person with both low vision and motor impairment who wants to use a computer. It is very common for the same person who uses a powered wheelchair to also need an AAC device and want to control entertainment devices or doorways in his or her environment.

It is increasingly common for AT devices to work well with each other because of improved standards in OS design and control electronics. Technical support from manufacturers or rehabilitation technology suppliers is often helpful if conflicts do arise. The iterative process of product design with feedback from informed users and therapists has helped to improve AT devices. In reality, AT devices have very small markets, and the economies associated with mass-market products do not apply here. Therefore, this cycle of improvement is often slower than is desired.

PAYING FOR AT SOLUTIONS

Third-party payment for AT is essential, since the majority of individuals with disability survive on small incomes and AT devices tend to be proportionately expensive. Although funding systems have become more responsive, there is continued resistance to paying for AT devices. More studies are needed to demonstrate the outcomes or the long-term economic benefits to society that accrue when AT devices enable better education, improve or create skills for employment, and reduce the costs of dependent care. There are also the individual benefits of participation, expanded social networks, and improved emotional and mental health.

Occupational therapists will always have an important role in documenting the need for AT devices. Their skill set enables them to make a correlation between deficits in occupational performance and the features of AT devices that enable occupation and participation. The ability to use this logic in written letters of justification is effective in getting funding for AT devices. Photos and videos of clients accomplishing their goals during trial use have often strengthened these letters.

When attempting to identify a source of funding for AT devices and services, think about a client's age or occupations and the associated programs and resources. For example, a toddler might expect funding assistance as part of an early intervention program, whereas an adult seeking employment should look to vocational rehabilitation. It is important to remember the goals of the potential payment source in writing letters of justification. Schools want to know about the educational benefit of an AT device, and Medicaid wants to know about its medical necessity. Remember that a funding denial does not mean *no;* rather, it means that you must strengthen the case or ask for a higher level of review.

CONCLUSION

This chapter provides an introduction to the use of assistive technology. Even experts must constantly update their skills through continuing education, AT-oriented conferences, and advanced education. Often, a powerful motivator for learning more about AT is meeting a client who could really benefit from AT intervention. Either refer your client to an AT expert or work collaboratively with your client to gather information and learn more. With the use of OT concepts, the foundation that you have gained in this chapter, persistence, and your own experience with twenty-first century technologies will help you to incorporate AT in your practice.

CASE STUDY: *Making a Computer Work for Ted*

Ted, a 25-year-old man, uses a computer to e-mail and browse the Web. Significant health problems (rheumatoid arthritis, liver disease, and glaucoma) kept him at home when his high school peers left for college. His health is stable, and he wants to pursue his interest in art through an online course in art theory. His visual acuity is poor, and he leans in close to the display to see. His vocational rehabilitation counselor has referred him for assessment.

Following an intake interview, the occupational therapist shows Ted how to reduce the resolution on the display, which has the effect of magnifying everything on the display. She also shows him the magnifier option among the OS accessibility options. Using these together, Ted can see more detail at the location of the mouse or text cursor. There are screen enlargement applications that provide features such as text tracking and text-to-speech, but Ted says that he is not interested. He says that he will return for more powerful solutions if his vision worsens.

1. How does the therapist's approach demonstrate hierarchy of access?
2. Do you agree with the therapist's approach?

REFERENCES

Allman, R. M., Goode, P. S., Burst, N., Bartolucci, A. A., & Thomas, D. R. (1999). Pressure ulcers, hospital complications, and disease severity: Impact on hospital costs and length of stay. *Advances in Wound Care, 12*(1), 22–30.

American Occupational Therapy Association. (2002). Occupational therapy practice framework: Domain and process. *American Journal of Occupational Therapy, 56,* 609–639.

Angelo, J. (1996). *Assistive technology for rehabilitation therapists.* Philadelphia: F. A. Davis.

Angelo, J. (2000). Factors affecting the use of a single switch with assistive technology devices. *Journal of Rehabilitation Research and Development, 37*(5), 591–598.

Apple Computer Inc. (2005). *Apple Mac OS X universal access.* Retrieved October 19, 2005, 2005, from http://www.apple.com/macosx/features/universalaccess/

Bain, B., & Leger, D. (1997). *Assistive technology: An interdisciplinary approach.* Philadelphia: Churchill Livingstone.

Beukelman, D. R., & Mirenda, P. (2005). *Augmentative and alternative communication: Supporting children and adults with complex communication needs* (3rd ed.). Baltimore: Paul H. Brookes.

Boninger, M. L., Baldwin, M., Cooper, R. A., Koontz, A., & Chan, L. (2000). Manual wheelchair pushrim biomechanics and axle position. *Archives of Physical Medicine & Rehabilitation, 81*(5), 608–613.

Boninger, M. L., Cooper, R. A., Baldwin, M. A., Shimada, S. D., & Koontz, A. (1999). Wheelchair pushrim kinetics: Body weight and median nerve function. *Archives of Physical Medicine & Rehabilitation, 80*(8), 910–915.

Brienza, D. M., Karg, P. E., Geyer, M. J., Kelsey, S., & Trefler, E. (2001). Relationship between pressure ulcer incidents and buttock seat cushion interface pressure in at-risk elderly wheelchair users. *Archives of Physical Medicine & Rehabilitation, 82*(4), 529–533.

Buning, M. E., Angelo, J. A., & Schmeler, M. R. (2001). Occupational performance and the transition to powered mobility: A pilot study. *American Journal of Occupational Therapy, 55*(4), 339–344.

Center for Universal Design. (1997). *What is universal design?: The principles of universal design.* Retrieved October 3, 2005, from http://www.ncsu.edu/www/ncsu/design/sod5/cud/

Centers for Medicare and Medicaid Services. (2006). *New codes, fee schedule amounts and local coverage determinations (lcds) for power mobility devices.* Washington, DC: U.S. Department of Health and Human Services.

Conine, T. A., Herschler, C., Daechsel, D., Peel, C., & Pearson, A. (1994). Pressure ulcer prophylaxis in elderly patients using polyurethane foam or jay wheelchair cushions. *International Journal of Rehabilitation Research, 17*(2), 123–137.

Cook, A. M., & Polgar, J. M. (2008). *Assistive technology: Principles and practice* (2nd ed.). St. Louis: Mosby.

Cooper, R. A. (1998). Wheelchair research and development for people with spinal cord injury [editorial]. *Journal of Rehabilitation Research & Development, 35*(1), xi.

Cooper, R. A., Gonzalez, J., Lawrence, B., Rentschler, A., Boninger, M. L., & VanSickle, D. P. (1997). Performance of selected lightweight wheelchairs on ANSI/RESNA tests. *Archives of Physical Medicine and Rehabilitation, 78,* 1138–1144.

DiGiovine, M. M., Cooper, R. A., Boninger, M. L., Lawrence, B. M., VanSickle, D. P., & Rentschler, A. J. (2000). User assessment of manual wheelchair ride comfort and ergonomics. *Archives of Physical Medicine & Rehabilitation, 81*(4), 490–494.

Health Care Finance Administration & United Healthcare. (1998). *Medicare supplier manual: Region A DMERC* (rev. 008). Wilkes-Barre, PA: United HealthCare Insurance Company.

Iezzoni, L. I. (1996). When walking fails. *Journal of the American Medical Association, 276*(19), 1609–1613.

Kirby, L. (2005). *Wheelchair skills program* (ver. 3.2). Halifax, Nova Scotia: Queen Elizabeth II Health Sciences Center.

Microsoft Corporation. (2005). *Accessibility at Microsoft.* Retrieved October 23, 2005, from http://www.microsoft.com/enable/

RERC on Cognitive Assistive Technology. (2006). *Advancing cognitive assistive technologies.* Retrieved April 4, 2006, from http://www.uchsc.edu/atp/RERC-ACT/

RERC on Wheelchair Transportation Safety. (2000). *New transit wheelchair standard: ANSI/RESNA WC-19.* Retrieved October 18, 2005, from http://www.rercwts.org/RERC_WTS2_KT/RERC_WTS2_KT_Stand/WC19_Docs/WC19_PressRel.html

Schmitt, D. (1992, October). *Hierarchy of access.* Paper presented at Closing the Gap, Minneapolis, MN.

Sprigle, S., & Sposato, B. (1997). Physiologic effects and design considerations of tilt and recline wheelchairs. *Orthopedic Physical Therapy Clinics of North America, 6*(1), 99–122.

Trefler, E., Hobson, D. A., Taylor, S. J., Monahan, L. C., & Shaw, C. G. (1993). *Seating and mobility for persons with physical disabilities.* Tucson, AZ: Therapy Skill Builders.

U.S. Society for Augmentative and Alternative Communication. (2005). *What is AAC intervention and what should it include?* Retrieved August 1, 2005, from http://www.ussaac.org/

From Disability Rights to Empowered Consciousness

JOY HAMMEL, JIM CHARLTON,
ROBIN JONES, JESSICA M. KRAMER,
AND TOM WILSON

Learning Objectives

After reading this chapter, you will be able to:

1. Compare and contrast different models of framing disability, key terms within each model, and implications of each model for occupational therapy practitioners and for disabled people.
2. Describe the disability rights movement in the United States and its history as an example of a social movement's framing of the disability experience from within.
3. Describe the sociopolitical and social justice issues that disabled people as a minority group face in the effort to realize rights and improve participation opportunities and access in society.
4. Critically reflect on your practice as an occupational therapist, how you "treat" disability, and key points in the process of reflecting and incorporating sociopolitical, economic, and cultural perspectives into your practice.
5. Develop innovative strategies to collaborate with disability communities on systems change and community and empowered consciousness building.

INTRODUCTION

How you think about and construct disability significantly influences how you experience disability in your own life as well as how you "treat" disability and disabled people as an occupational therapy practitioner and as a member of society. Notice that we put the term *treat* in quotation marks.

INITIAL LEARNING ACTIVITY

Take out a piece of paper, and jot down what you think about when you hear the words *disability* and *independence*. What do these words mean to you? How are they defined and constructed in society (e.g., by the public or in the media)? How does the profession of occupational therapy view disability and independence?

Practitioners frequently use the term *treatment* to designate what therapists do to, or do in collaboration with, clients during therapeutic sessions. However, the term *treat* can also refer to how people are viewed and treated as a social group in society.

This chapter focuses on this sociological framing of treatment by exposing you to different models and framings of disability and the disability experience using a critical theory stance. Critical theory involves stepping back to critically reflect on how disability is constructed in society and your role as a professional in that construction. The chapter also introduces you to a sociological framing of the political, economic, social, and cultural issues that influence the disability experience of individuals and that of disabled people[1] as a collective minority group. Specifically, a critical theory framework will challenge you to reflect on every aspect of your evaluation and intervention as an occupational therapist to determine whether they authentically reflect the insider experiences, needs, priorities, issues, and goals of people with disabilities and what is most meaningful and relevant to them and to people with disabilities as a minority group.

COMPARING AND CONTRASTING MODELS OF DISABILITY

Individuals do not exist or operate in isolation from their social worlds, their communities, and the broader society with its expectations, norms, cultural beliefs, and socio-

political and economic realities. Nor do occupational therapists operate in isolation from their own beliefs or from the values and economic interests of the systems within which they work and the broader society in which they live. Yet we often try to achieve this isolation within the therapeutic context; that is, we try to focus in on individual rehabilitation goals, impairment remediation, or functional return without fully considering the holistic needs and desires of the individual as influenced by society.

We can look to different models and conceptual framings of disability to better understand this social phenomena and to critically examine how rehabilitation professionals such as occupational therapists have situated themselves in relation to disability and to disabled people.

From a historical perspective, some of the earliest documented societal framings of disability are situated within religious and cultural constructions (for detailed history accounts, see Longmore & Umansky, 2001; Oliver, 1990, 1996). Although different religious sects and cultures treat disability differently, one of the most important influences in defining disability has been that of Western Christianity and the *moral model* of disability. In the moral model, disability is seen as a moral marking. In most cases, the mark is seen as a negative one—one that designates a sinner or an evil or unclean presence within the person. Historically, the mark was used to validate the separation of that person from the rest of society lest the evil spread or to justify the need to cleanse the person from the evil spirit, a type of early cure. At the same time, however, the moral model asserted the responsibility of the religious community to have pity on the less fortunate and to take care of them, thus extending into the *charity model.* Together, these beliefs led to the formation of institutions, asylums, sanitariums, and segregated communities to isolate yet take care of people with disabilities.

The charity model was also reified by Western-influenced societies, such as the United States and United Kingdom, and in turn extended beyond religion into a societal practice within the *welfare model.* In this model, society assumes responsibility over the welfare of the less fortunate, who are otherwise deemed not to be capable of supporting themselves (Oliver, 1990, 1996). Using a welfare model, groups of people, including people with diverse disabilities and those labeled as *sick, feeble, poor, criminals,* and *the underclass* were often grouped, housed, and "treated" together, separate from the rest of society.

Although they were framed within a charity model, conditions in these institutions were often less than charitable, and since these individuals were not deemed to be a valid part of the productive workforce, financial supports were often limited and were cut back even more during times of societal depression. This trend toward a *political economic and materialist framing* of disability focuses on labor economics and on surplus or deficit in the labor market to define and "treat" disability (Hahn,

---

[1]Although the term *people with disabilities* often appears in the literature as recommended people-first language, *disabled people* and other "disability-centered" terms are increasingly preferred and used by many activists and scholars who promote positive disability identity as an act of resistance against disability oppression (e.g., the focus is not on the deficit in the individual but on the society that imposes disability on disabled people as a collective minority group).

1985; Oliver, 1990, 1996). In our capitalist society in the United States, the ability to work or not and the simultaneous value of independence have been central forces in defining and socially constructing disability and the treatment of disabled people.

Historically, as science and technology came to the fore and continued to progress within industrialized societies, we began to see the formulations of a more scientific approach to disability in the field of professionalized medicine (Foucault, 1973; Mechanic, 1974; Oliver, 1996). The scientific focus was based on a positivist framing that there are certain universal truths or facts that can be identified and proven. In this case, those truths relate to disability in the tenet that one can identify what is wrong, how it came to be wrong, and therefore how to treat and/or cure that wrong. In some branches of medicine, these tenets applied to treating physical ailments, conditions, and impairments. In psychology, similar tenets were applied to diagnosing and treating illnesses of the mind, such as psychiatric and cognitive conditions.

However, given the difficulties involved in trying to objectively explain social and psychological behaviors, other psychologists began to qualitatively examine how people interacted in the moment and how actions were shaped by and given meaning via social interactions with other people in everyday contexts (Blumer, 1969; Goffman, 1963). Concepts such as stigma, learned helplessness, self-efficacy, and social learning emerged, tying together the individual with the immediate social environment in an *ecological framing* (Bronfenbrenner, 1979). Sociologists and anthropologists challenged the focus on the individual, however, and began to focus on cultural and societal constructions of disability, pointing to the political, economic, and cultural influences of the society on individuals and groups of people in society. Concepts such as oppression, marginalization, and alienation were used to describe disabled people as a minority group. The *social model of disability* (Oliver, 1990, 1996) asserts that oppression occurs because of the political economy of societies that exclude disabled people and prevent them from moving out of welfare systems to the productive workforce, thus invalidating them as full citizens. The *minority group model of disability* (Hahn, 1985; Longmore, 1995) acknowledges the societal oppression of disabled people but, like other minority group social movements (e.g., by race, ethnicity, gender, or sexual identity), equally emphasizes the strengths, power, and pride of the group. Thus, the minority group model introduces concepts such as disability identity, culture, community, and pride as ways to reframe and own disability "from within." Feminist scholars further tie the individual and the society together via the slogan "The personal is political and the political is personal," pointing to the need to recognize how the personal experience of disability and gender intersect and, in turn, are heavily influenced by and constructed by societal beliefs, norms, and ideologies (Morris, 1992; Thomas, 1999). It is within these soci-

ological and cultural framings that disabled people as a social group and as insiders to the disability experience continue to assume control and power over reframing disability from an insider perspective according to a critical theory stance.

Although it is beyond the scope of this chapter to comprehensively review the history of medicine, rehabilitation, disability, and sociology, this brief history leads us to a contemporary critical analysis of disability models as shown in Table 62.1 that you can use to inform your everyday practice. The table presents three key models of disability: the medical model, the rehabilitation model, and the closely related social and minority group models, which are ascribed to and framed from within disability-led groups and social movements.

What is important to note is the location and construction of disability, moving from:

- A deficit or dysfunction within the individual to treat or cure within the medical model
- To a negative interaction of the person with his or her immediate environment within a rehabilitation model, pointing to the need to remediate, compensate, or normalize the individual
- To a societally constructed and imposed phenomena that can be addressed only through social and societal change within the social model
- To a collective social movement of empowered consciousness from within (e.g., disability culture and art, community building, identity, and pride) within a minority group cultural model.

Also note the shifts in power across the models, from the expert, professionally driven medical model to the professional-client relationship of the rehabilitation model (which can vary from professional-led to client-centered) to the disability constituency–led movements of social change and critical consciousness within the social and minority group models. Depending on which model you situate yourself within, terms such as *independence, participation,* and *empowerment* can take on different meanings as well. For example, *independence* can be defined as the individual ability to safely perform activities by oneself (as we frequently ascribe to in rehabilitation) or as a rights-based framing of freedom of choice, access, and opportunity in society, and autonomy in managing one's life decisions (as framed in a minority group model). It is important for occupational therapists to be aware of and responsive to the disability rights movement's conceptualizations and underlying philosophy of independent living as something that is not about the individual's impairment so much as about the individual's right to societal opportunities and the need to create environments and to change systems, rather than individuals, to support those rights. For example, an occupational therapist might focus exclusively on increasing a client's functional independence, that is, the client's ability to perform activities independently.

TABLE 62.1 COMPARISON OF DISABILITY AND INDEPENDENCE CONSTRUCTIONS

	Medical Model	Rehabilitation Model	Minority Group/Social Model
What is disability?	Disability is deficiency or abnormality.	Disability is loss or inability to functionally perform everyday activities independently or in a socially expected way (e.g., timely, safely, efficiently).	Disability is difference. (Some would argue for saying that *impairment* is difference, while *disability* occurs only when societally imposed barriers limit people.)
How is disability constructed?	Being disabled is negative.	Being disabled is negative and something to be overcome or to accept/adjust or adapt to its negative consequences within one's life.	Being disabled is neutral; negative constructions occur when society imposes barriers and oppresses participation; positive constructions occur when the personal and social world own difference and support and validate people.
Where is disability located?	Disability is in the individual body.	Disability is in the individual or in the interaction between the individual and the immediate environment.	Disability derives from the interaction between the individual and society. Disability is located in societal structures and practices that oppress.
What is the mechanism for change?	The remedy for disability-related problems is cure or normalization.	The mechanism for change for disability-related problems is to rehabilitate or remediate to normal and/or to become as physically/cognitively independent in everyday activities as possible.	The mechanism for change is changing the interaction between the individual and society.
Examples of change strategies	Surgery, medication, medical technology and intervention	Individual remediation and person/environment compensation or adaptation	Systems and social action change; collective activism; disability identity, pride and culture
Who/what are the agents of change?	The agent of remedy is the professional.	The agent of change is the professional in collaboration with the individual client and/or people in client's immediate social world (e.g., client-centered approach).	The agent of change can be the individual; an advocate or ally; any person or group of people that changes the interaction; the community; the society's sociopolitical structure and systems; and art, culture, and media.
What is independence?	Individual physical, cognitive, and mental ability to perform and capacity to make decisions	Individual physical and cognitive ability to perform everyday activities safely and in a reasonable amount of time	Freedom to do what you want to do, when, where, and with whom you want; choice; power over life decisions; control over everyday life and resources to support it

Source: Adapted by Joy Hammel & Access Living based on Gill (1999); Linton (1998); Longmore (1995); Oliver (1996); Rioux (1997).

If you assume a social or minority group model instead, disabled people would argue that *independence* to them means the freedom to make choices and to be in control of decisions, regardless of whether they can perform an activity by themselves. So as an occupational therapist, you might consider spending equal time collaborating with the consumer on whether he or she might want to use a personal attendant and how to access and get funding for this supportive resource to remain "independent."

THE DISABILITY RIGHTS HISTORY AND MOVEMENT: FROM RIGHTS TO EMPOWERED CONSCIOUSNESS

To better understand and apply these models, it is important to situate them within the history of the disability rights movement internationally. The history that follows represents a synthesis of accounts documented by disabled people with and about disabled people who were a part of this history (for detailed histories, see Charlton, 1998; Longmore, 1995; Longmore & Umansky, 2001).

The Organization of Empowerment

Out of the different and often hard realities of everyday life, organizations of people with disabilities have appeared in virtually every country in the world. Most of these organizations embrace the principles of empowerment and human rights, independence and integration, and self-help and self-determination, and these organizations form the core of the international disability rights movement. In a few places, people with disabilities have been politically active for many decades, but in most places, the disability rights movement is a recent phenomenon. Today, most activists locate the beginning of what constitutes the contemporary disability rights movement in the early 1970s.

Trying to pin any social movement down to a given period is complicated, but two periods stand out. It was during the early 1970s that people with disabilities in the United States and Europe, influenced by and directly involved in the civil rights, antiwar, and student movements, began to organize on disability-related issues. The year 1972 is associated with the founding of the Berkeley Center for Independent Living (CIL). It was also about then that the Boston Self-Help Center became interested in independent living as an alternative kind of organization. The independent living movement has been the linchpin of the disability rights movement (DRM) in the United States, and its leaders have had an influence on activists and leaders elsewhere. For example, the first disability rights–oriented group in Europe was established in England when Vic Finkelstein, Paul Hunt, and others initiated the Union of Physically Impaired Against Segregation in 1975. As activists in the United States and Europe began to take up major disability-related issues, the DRM began to develop and grow. Early on, these issues included the inaccessibility of public transportation; the lack of accessible, affordable housing; the institutionalizing of poor, young people with severe disabilities in nursing homes because of the prohibitive cost of personal assistance; the struggle for inclusion of students with disabilities in regular classrooms; and efforts to change the way in which the public relates to, perceives, and understands disability. The first center, Berkeley CIL, began in 1973, but most CILs in the United States were set up in the early 1980s. There are now more than 350 in the United States. CILs are the most important organizations within the U.S. DRM for two reasons. First, most of the early disability rights leaders were identified with CILs, and the philosophy of independent living formed much of the basic philosophical underpinning of the larger DRM. Second, CILs were and still are cornerstones of the DRM because of the sheer numbers of paid staff. These centers have extensive resources. Out of the work of early activists, legislation and legal mandates concerning the "handicapped" appeared. This happened in North America and northern Europe and to a lesser extent in the Third World. The most important legislation in North America was the Rehabilitation Act of 1973.[2]

The first half of the 1980s were also crucial. The year 1981 was designated the International Year of Disabled Persons (IYDP) by the United Nations. The significance of this was not lost on most disability rights activists in the United States. The year 1981 was very important to the DRM on the international front. In many cases, it was the first time efforts had been made to involve people with disabilities in disability-related projects and programs. Indeed, a crucial event had taken place earlier than the IYDP, in late June 1980, when there was a split in Rehabilitation International (RI), the most significant disability-related international body. RI was a large membership organization composed primarily of rehabilitation professionals. Through efforts of people from Sweden and Canada, RI for the first time made an attempt to bring people with disabilities to its conference in Singapore.

---

[2]It took a month-long sit-in and office takeover at the San Francisco office of the U.S. Department of Health, Education, and Welfare to force Secretary Joseph Califano to mandate enforcement of the act. There are a number of interesting accounts of this action. "More than 150 people took over the federal building and remained for twenty-eight days. Ed Roberts left his new office as Director of the California Department of Rehabilitation to join the protest. Judy Heumann crossed the Bay from Berkeley to become one of the leaders of the takeover. Early in action, Heumann, in a statement reminiscent of freedom fighters of all ages, declared that 'we will no longer allow the government to oppress disabled individuals. . . . We will accept no more discussion of segregation.' . . . The Black Panthers and the Gray Panthers brought in food donated by Safeway and assisted with personal care needs. The siege remains the longest takeover of a federal building by any group in American history" (Brown, 1992, pp. 57–58).

The largely token effort backfired. The few hundred participants who had disabilities demanded that RI mandate that 50% of its delegate assembly be composed of people with disabilities. This motion was overwhelmingly defeated by a vote of 61 to 37, a vote that probably represented the sentiments of the 3,000 other delegates at the convention. Those with disabilities and a few supporters led a split in RI, the outcome of which was the formation of Disabled Peoples' International (DPI).[3] DPI has seen impressive growth in the last 25 years. There are affiliated groups in dozens of countries and an international headquarters in Winnipeg, Canada.[4]

The early 1980s was also a time when many of the leading disability rights organizations were founded, such as the National Council of Disabled Persons Zimbabwe, the Organization of the Revolutionary Disabled in Nicaragua, the Self Help Association of Paraplegics (Soweto) (SHAP), the Program of Rehabilitation Organized by Disabled Youth of Western Mexico (PROJIMO), DPI-Thailand, the Southern Africa Federation of the Disabled (SAFOD), and the American Disabled for Accessible Public Transportation (now known as ADAPT). At the same time, different disability constituency groups began to form and further assert their voice and their rights, including groups such as People First and Self Advocates Becoming Empowered (SABE), representing people with intellectual disabilities, and groups such as MindFreedom and Mad-Nation, representing people with psychiatric disabilities. From many disparate beginnings and places, networks began to form, and the disability movement, as owned and framed from within, began to go public.

Many of these organizations started as a response to the simple need for survival, and their goals were limited to economic self-help and self-sufficiency. Others started as political groups that wanted to mobilize people with disabilities in their communities, cities, countries, or regions. These groups and purposes have gradually merged. All seek to link their work with the struggle for self-determination and human rights. With few exceptions, this is their common denominator. All the organizations within the DRM have a few basic things in common. Most important, they are organizations that are controlled by people with disabilities. Each, in its own way and in its own circumstances, confronts the everyday realities of disability oppression. Another crucial similarity is that each embraces the general philosophical principle that people with disabilities must have their own voice and have control in their lives.

Empowered Consciousness

The emergence of disabled people's organizations, the concomitant promotion of independence and empowerment, and the recognition of the centrality and imperative of speaking for themselves spawned a whole new generation of disabled people who rejected the paternalistic, medical model notions regarding disability. As hundreds of thousands or even millions of disabled people worldwide have come to understand that the "problems" of disability have little to do with them and much to do with how society is organized, large numbers of political activists with disabilities have come forward.

Out of similar and divergent experiences, people with disabilities have acquired a consciousness about themselves and the world around them. This new understanding has affected their aspirations and responsibilities. They have come to a raised consciousness of themselves not only as people with disabilities, but also as oppressed people. Moreover, they have become political activists because their raised consciousness has become empowered. (See Figure 62.1 for images of collective activism and empowered consciousness.) They no longer think of disability as a medical condition; instead, they see it as a human condition. They are no longer interested in the "welfare of the handicapped"; they are interested in the human rights of disabled people. They have joined a social movement to free people with disabilities from political, economic, and cultural oppression (Charlton, 1998).

For political activists, consciousness that resists the emasculation of the self by the dominant ideology, that is, raised consciousness, has been transformed into a consciousness of active opposition: empowered consciousness.[5] Empowered consciousness means acting collectively to empower an entire social group. This can mean educating people, creating disturbances, confronting institutions, and seeking group power in churches, schools, communities, and institutions. Empowered consciousness insists on the active, collective contestation for control over the necessities of life: housing, school, personal and family relationships, respect, independence, and more. People with empowered consciousness might still see only part of the larger world, but they understand that they can and should influence it. This does not mean that they insist on being leaders. It does mean that they want to empower others, especially other people who are experiencing disability. These people see the connections between themselves and others and begin to recognize a level of universality that was obscured in their consciousness. They begin to speak of "we" instead of "I" or "they." Some of these activists

---

[3]Diane Driedger's book *The Last Civil Rights Movement: Disabled Peoples' International* (1989, especially pp. 28–57) is a good history of the split and the subsequent formation of DPI.
[4]RI remains much larger and more influential than DPI. In recent years, RI has added people with disabilities to its executive committee, but it is still dominated by rehabilitation "professionals" (doctors, therapists, social workers, psychologists, etc.). Since the split, a number of disability rights activists have worked with both RI and DPI. RI is headquartered in New York City.

---

[5]Whenever and wherever this transformation occurs, it produces recognition of the self on both the personal and political levels. This transformation has been particularly important to feminist and multicultural studies. See Charles Taylor's "The Politics of Recognition" (Goldberg, 1994, 81–85).

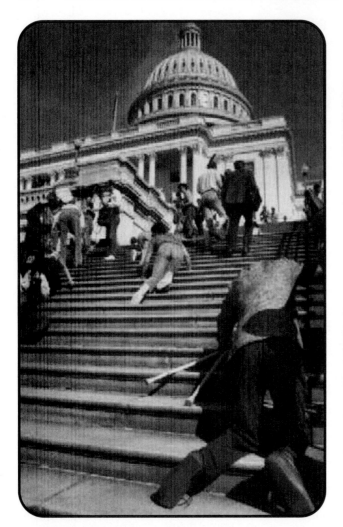
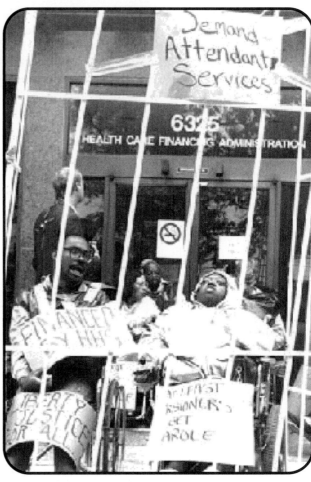

FIGURE 62.1 Collective disability activism took disability public during the fight to pass the Americans with Disabilities Act (left) and continues to do so in the ongoing movement to mandate and fund community-based living options with supports (right). (Copyright Tom Olin, Photographer.)

are motivated by personal experience (poverty, harassment, institutionalization, a personal loss, rape, indignity, etc.). Others are motivated by something they have learned by being exposed to injustice and oppression in school or out of an outraged sense of social injustice. Most people are politically active for a combination of these and other reasons. A consciousness of empowerment is growing among people with disabilities. (See Figure 62.2 for symbols of this empowered consciousness created from within.)

Empowered consciousness is, in Cheryl Marie Wade's words, being passed around on notes, and it has to do with being proud of self and having a culture that fortifies and spreads that feeling:

> Disability culture. Say, what? Aren't disabled people just isolated victims of nature or circumstance? Yes and no. True, we are far too often isolated. Locked away in the pits, closets, and institutions of enlightened societies everywhere. But there is a growing consciousness among us. . . . Because there is always an underground. Notes get passed among survivors. And the notes we are passing these days say, "There's power in difference. Power. Pass the word." Culture. It's about passing the word. And disability culture is passing the word that there's a new definition of disability and it includes power. (Wade, 1994)

LEGISLATIVE AND SOCIAL POLICY INITIATIVES EXPERIENCED BY DISABLED PEOPLE

The history of the disability rights movement has culminated in several key pieces of legislation that reify the values and rights of the movement. It is critical that occu-

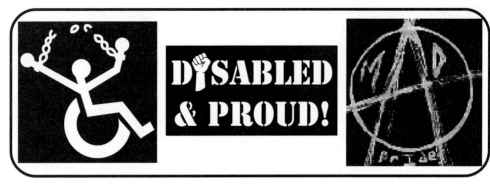

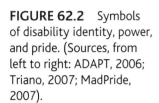

FIGURE 62.2 Symbols of disability identity, power, and pride. (Sources, from left to right: ADAPT, 2006; Triano, 2007; MadPride, 2007).

pational therapists be informed about this legislation and stay abreast of changes to it in reauthorizations, as this information is essential to advocacy. Table 62.2 summarizes many of the primary social policies and legislation within the United States that influence the rights, choices, and control of disabled people. They correspond to major areas of societal participation (e.g., transportation, work) that also represent ongoing areas of disability activism to further increase societal opportunities. Following is a brief overview of these policies, legislation, and systems:

♦ **Rehabilitation Act of 1973, Section 504:** A federal act that prohibits discrimination on the basis of disability in programs conducted by federal agencies, in programs that receive federal financial assistance, in federal employment, and in the employment practices of federal contractors. Section 504 states that "no qualified individual with a disability in the United States shall be excluded from, denied the benefits of, or be subjected to discrimination under" any program or activity that either receives federal financial assistance or is conducted by any executive agency or the U.S. Postal Service. Each federal agency has its own set of Section 504 regulations that apply to its own programs. Agencies that provide federal financial assistance also have Section 504 regulations covering entities that receive federal aid. Requirements common to these regulations include reasonable accommodation for employees with disabilities, program accessibility, effective communication with people who have hearing or vision disabilities, and accessible new construction and alterations.

♦ **Individuals with Disabilities Education Act (IDEA):** A federal program that provides funds to states and local education agencies (school districts) to support education for children with disabilities ages 3 to 21 years and supports early intervention services for children from birth to age 3 years. IDEA provides guidelines and protections for children to ensure their right to a free and appropriate public education. The principle of the law is that children with disabilities should not be denied the opportunities that are offered to everyone else; everyone gets access to public education, and therefore children with disabilities should have the same access. School

districts are obligated to prepare and implement an Individualized Education Program (IEP) for each disabled child that is designed to meet the child's unique needs.

♦ **Americans with Disabilities Act of 1990 (ADA):** A comprehensive federal civil rights law that provides protections to individuals with disabilities similar to those provided to individuals on the basis of race, color, sex, national origin, age, and religion. It guarantees equal opportunity for individuals with disabilities in public accommodations, employment, transportation, state and local government services, and telecommunications. There are five titles under the ADA:

Title I: Employment. Prohibits discrimination in all aspects of the employment process including recruitment, hiring, retention, and benefits of employment. Private employers with 15 or more employees and public employers with one or more employees are covered.

Title II: State and Local Government. Prohibits discrimination in all programs and services offered to the public and requires that all facilities where programs and services are delivered be readily accessible to and usable by people with disabilities, including transportation.

Title III: Places of Public Accommodation. Prohibits discrimination in the delivery of goods and services by places of public accommodation, including architectural accessibility and effective communication.

Title IV: Telecommunications. Requires access to the telecommunication services provided by private telecommunication companies (e.g., relay services).

Title V: Miscellaneous. Provisions for nondiscrimination in areas including insurance, retaliation based on exercising rights under the statute, availability of attorney fees, and more.

♦ **Help America Vote Act (HAVA):** A federal law that was enacted in 2002 to reform elections management and voter registration nationwide. The following issues are covered by HAVA:

1. The proper operation and maintenance of voting systems and technology

TABLE 62.2   IMPORTANT POLICIES AND LEGISLATION CORRESPONDING TO MAJOR AREAS OF SOCIETAL PARTICIPATION AND OCCUPATIONAL THERAPY PRACTICE

	Section 504	I.D.E.A.	ADA	HAVA	Medicaid/ Medicare
Transportation	Requires transportation systems owned/operated by entities that receive federal financial assistance to be accessible	Requires appropriate transportation services to be provided to students with disabilities	Requires all public and the majority of private transportation systems to be accessible to individuals with disabilities		Provision of transportation for medically related services
Employment	Prohibits discrimination against qualified individuals with disabilities in all aspects of employment		Prohibits discrimination against qualified individuals with disabilities by private employers of 15 or more employees and public employers with 1 or more employees		
Education	Requires entities that receive federal financial assistance to ensure equal access through architectural accessibility and provision of reasonable accommodations in K–12 and post-secondary education	Requires provision of a free appropriate public education for children with disabilities in the least restrictive environment	Prohibits discrimination by public and private educational entities including architectural accessibility, provision of reasonable accommodations. And effective communication		
Voting	Requires entities that receive federal financial assistance to ensure equal access, including architectural accessibility, provision of reasonable accommodations, and effective communication		Requires nondiscrimination in voting as a program of state and local government	Requires equal access to voting facilities and the voting process	

TABLE 62.2   IMPORTANT POLICIES AND LEGISLATION CORRESPONDING TO MAJOR AREAS OF SOCIETAL PARTICIPATION AND OCCUPATIONAL THERAPY PRACTICE   *Continued*

	Section 504	I.D.E.A.	ADA	HAVA	Medicaid/ Medicare
Housing	Requires entities that receive federal financial assistance to ensure nondiscrimination in housing, including construction of accessible housing units and reasonable modification of policy and procedure		Requires transient housing (i.e., hotels/motels, dormitories, social service housing) to be constructed in accordance with the ADA accessibility guidelines, reasonable modification of policy and procedure, and effective communication		Provision of institutional care and/or use of available (state by state) Medicaid Waiver Program to finance community based placement. May be used by states to meet their nonsegregation obligations under the Americans with Disabilities Act
Health care	Nondiscrimination in the provision of medical services offered by entities receiving federal financial assistance, including architectural accessibility, reasonable accommodations, and effective communication		Nondiscrimination in the provision of medical services, including architectural accessibility, reasonable accommodations, and effective communication		Financial support of basic medical services (dental, skilled nursing services, etc.).
Community Participation	Nondiscrimination in programs and services offered by entities receiving federal financial assistance including architectural accessibility, modification of policy and procedure, and effective communication		Nondiscrimination in access to goods and services offered by public and private entities, including architectural accessibility, modification of policy and procedure, and effective communication		Community Based Waiver Program can be used to support non-medical services that enhance quality of life (e.g., environmental modifications)

2. The rights of voters to cast provisional ballots, the proper processing and counting of those ballots, and how provisional voters can determine whether their votes were counted and, if not, why not

3. The nondiscriminatory application of HAVA's identification requirement for certain voters who register by mail

4. Identifying and assisting voters with disabilities, including psychiatric disabilities, in order that such voters can participate fully in the voting process independently and privately

5. The rights of minority language voters to receive language assistance at the polling place

◆ **Medicare:** A federal health insurance program for people age 65 years or older. Certain people younger than age 65 can qualify for Medicare too, including those who have disabilities and those who have permanent kidney failure or amyotrophic lateral sclerosis (Lou Gehrig's disease). The program helps with the cost of health care, but it does not cover all medical expenses or the cost of most long-term care. Medicare is financed by a portion of the payroll taxes paid by workers and their employers. It also is financed in part by monthly premiums deducted from Social Security checks. The Centers for Medicare & Medicaid Services (CMS) is the agency in charge of the Medicare program. Medicare has four parts:

1. Hospital insurance (Part A), which helps to pay for inpatient care in a hospital or skilled nursing facility (following a hospital stay), some home health care, and hospice care

2. Medical insurance (Part B), which helps to pay for doctors' services and many other medical services and supplies that are not covered by hospital insurance

3. Medicare Advantage (Part C), formerly known as Medicare + Choice plans, which is available in many areas. People with Medicare Parts A and B can choose to receive all of their health care services through one of these provider organizations under Part C.

4. Prescription drug coverage (Part D), which helps to pay for medications doctors prescribe for treatment

◆ **Medicaid:** A federal/state entitlement program established under Title XIX of the Social Security Act to pay for medical assistance for certain individuals and families with low incomes and resources. It is a cooperative venture funded jointly by the federal and state governments to assist states in furnishing medical assistance to eligible needy individuals. Medicaid is the largest source of funding for medical and health-related services for America's poorest people, including people with disabilities. Within broad national guidelines established by federal statutes, regulations, and policies, each state establishes its own eligibility standards; determines the type, amount, duration, and scope of services; sets the rate of payment for services; and administers its own program. Medicaid policies for eligibility, services, and payment are complex and vary considerably, even among states of similar size or geographic proximity. Thus, a person who is eligible for Medicaid in one state might not be eligible in another state, and the services that one state provides can differ considerably in amount, duration, or scope from services that are provided in a similar or neighboring state. In addition, state legislatures may change Medicaid eligibility, services, and/or reimbursement during the year. The Social Security Act authorizes multiple waiver and demonstration authorities to allow states flexibility in operating Medicaid programs. Each authority has a distinct purpose and distinct requirements. The waiver that is most commonly used by people with disabilities is the Home and Community-Based Services Waiver. This program allows for the waiver of Medicaid provisions to allow long-term care services to be delivered in community settings. This program is the Medicaid alternative to providing comprehensive long-term services in institutional settings.

Despite the existence of this disability and civil rights legislation, the DRM continues to face many important social policy issues and challenges to advancing the equality of disabled people. The level of sheer desperation in parts of the disability community continues to be astounding. More than 1.8 million people with disabilities remain isolated in nursing homes and institutions. The minimal income supports available for people living on Social Security condemn people with disabilities to abject poverty. Sheltered workshops remain an established system to address unemployment among disabled people at wages much lower than the already low minimum wage. Transportation is difficult for many disabled people, given that there are few lift-equipped over-the-road buses in the nation's bus fleet. In many cities, para-transit systems are consistently late, require advance notice to book, have increasingly limited budgets, and suffer frequent service cutbacks; in rural areas, such systems often are not available at all. According to the National Council on Disability (NCD), other social policy areas that have high priority among disabled people include access to high-quality health care, education, work, telecommunications and assistive technologies, voting rights, parenting rights, euthanasia/assisted suicide, and sexual identity and freedom (NCD, 2006a & b). Every single day people with disabilities face social policy issues. To illustrate what the DRM is doing to address ongoing isolation, discrimination, and impoverishment, this section will focus on one key social policy example: that of community living rights that cut across policies of long-term care, housing, access to services, and provision of community-based supports.

Long-term care (LTC) is an area of rapidly evolving change in concept, policy, and practice. As recently as 50 years ago, home care was mostly seen as a family responsibility with state-run institutions filling in where families were unable or unwilling to respond. Although "Homes for the Feeble Minded" "County Farms," and

"Institutions for Mental Disease" were at first seen as reform, it was not very long before journalists and whistle-blowers were exposing the abuse and neglect that were common in these places. Despite this exposure, they continue to exist in various forms or are being replaced by other institutions such as nursing homes and inter-mediate-care facilities.

In 1965, Medicare and Medicaid were created, and the social policy for providing LTC changed. While the state-operated institutions continued to be funded, the private nursing home industry began to also widely expand as large sums of Medicaid dollars became available to place lower-income people into a system that had been previously used by private pay middle- and upper-class citizens. The medical system also played a role in convincing families that all parties were better off when disabled family members were placed in institutions, such as nursing homes, citing benefits of health care access, safety, and socialization. Existing research on nursing homes has documented abuse, neglect, crime, and rapid declines of quality of life and health that would challenge these assertions (DePoy & Werrbach, 1996; Henderson, 1995; NCD, 2003, 2005a, 2006b; Wright, Grofein, & Owens, 2000). At the same time, emerging research on community-based alternatives has pointed to the high meaning of aging in place in the community and the positive outcomes of home and community-based waiver programs that provide supports to live in community settings on emotional and physical health and well being (CMS, 2007a; NCD, 2003, 2005a, 2005b, 2006a, 2006b). Despite this research, the struggle to rebalance LTC toward community-based alternatives continues, in large part because of the strength of the multi-billion-dollar nursing home and institutional industry and its political lobbies.

Some of the first steps for effecting a paradigm shift in LTC involved advocating for the creation of new consumer-directed models and use of nonprofessionalized personal assistant services. The many forms of alternatives to institutional care are known as home and community-based services. Critical steps in making this change in LTC social policy included the following:

1. The establishment of the Berkeley CIL with its experimentation with personal assistant services that resulted in the funding in 1980 of a national network of independent living centers as a base to build a broad advocacy campaign and recreate community-based alternatives.
2. The formation of People First, a national organization for and controlled by people with intellectual disabilities that was instrumental in filing court challenges to the forced institutionalization of their people.
3. The book and film (based on the book) *One Flew Over the Cuckoos Nest* and other literature, art, and films that promoted the liberation of people in LTC institutions in the public media, which also resulted in changes in public attitudes about disabled people.

4. The passage of the Americans with Disabilities Act, which defined unwanted institutionalization as a violation of the civil rights of people with disabilities.
5. The national campaign by ADAPT, a national disability rights organization, to pass legislation called MiCASSA (Medicaid Community Attendant Services And Supports Act), which called for mandated funding of home and community-based services at least as strong as the mandate to fund nursing homes and institutions. If passed, MiCASSA would allocate significant amounts of money to help people move from institutions to home and community settings and allow people real choice in where they would receive their long-term care.
6. The *Olmstead* decision, a Supreme Court case interpreting the Americans with Disabilities Act, which asserted that people with disabilities have a right to live in the most integrated setting that is appropriate to their needs. This decision has ignited activists and led to widespread systems change.

The rally across the street from the Supreme Court at the time the *Olmstead* case was being argued was one of the largest DRM rallies ever held in Washington, D.C. Strikingly, this activism resulted in many states changing their opinions to side with the DRM on *Olmstead* least restrictive placement rights. However, the political systems in many states are still skewed toward an institutional bias; approximately 70% of LTC spending nationally still goes to segregated institutional settings such as nursing homes, state mental hospitals, nursing homes specific to people with psychiatric disabilities, and intermediate-care facilities specific to people with intellectual disabilities (CMS, 2007a; NCD, 2003, 2005a, 2005b, 2006a, 2006b). Despite this institutional bias, many important steps were taken at the federal level to support *Olmstead* implementation under the umbrella policy and executive directive of the New Freedom Initiative. These actions included the following:

1. The CMS sent policy letters to all state Medicaid directors elaborating on what the states should be doing to be in compliance with *Olmstead* and to rebalance LTC financing toward community-based options.
2. CMS System Change Grants allowed states to apply for grant money that could be used to create home and community alternatives to segregated settings, to strengthen existing home and community infrastructure, and to experiment with consumer-directed programs to support community living. Some states have used the grants well and developed models that other states could learn from (see CMS, 2007b).
3. In 2006, CMS appropriated $1.75 billion to establish Money Follows the Person (MFP) Demonstration Projects. The MFP concept is one of the operative principles of the federally proposed MiCASSA legislation, which calls for consumer-directed management and

choice in supports with the money that would otherwise have been spent on institutional placement to "follow the person" to the community. Since MFP was implemented in Texas, more than 10,000 people have left nursing homes to live in the community with supports; this represents strong evidence for systems change (CMS, 2007a).

Now the battle for home and community-based LTC is specifically focused at the state level, in which policies and outcomes vary widely across the country. There are a few states such as Tennessee that still have almost no home and community-based service programs. They can be contrasted with other states such as Oregon, Washington, and New Mexico that spend more than 50% of their LTC dollars on home and community-based services, including access to occupational therapy, assistive technology, and environmental modifications.

LTC is an issue that the DRM is winning, albeit slowly. The DRM is also closely collaborating to apply the same philosophy of least restrictive, community-based living and consumer direction with senior citizens. Activists face a government that is trying to drop its responsibility to fund LTC for people who do not have resources to purchase it in the private marketplace. Cuts to Medicaid—and therefore to states—are likely to further hinder progress. Nursing homes, other private providers, and unions will intensify their efforts to hold onto the lion's share of the funding. Change will require greater political empowerment by disabled people and senior citizens as a coalition to counter this political power.

Ongoing policy issues still include the need to build stronger home and community-based infrastructure as baby boomers age. There is an increasing need to provide enough affordable, accessible housing that supports aging in place and can meet the demand that comes with increasing numbers of people moving out of institutions. New models of services that support consumer control and meet the needs of people with cognitive and psychiatric disabilities also require creative exploration, demonstration, and study. Occupational therapists can play key roles in these policy initiatives, as allies in the activism movement, and as contributors in the design, implementation, and evaluation of new community living environments and programs in collaboration with the disability and aging communities.

HOW MODELS OF DISABILITY, HISTORY, AND POLICY INFLUENCE INTERVENTION

Now that you have learned about disability models, disability rights history, key legislation, and some of the major social policy issues that affect disabled people as a minor-

ity group, the next step is one of praxis, that is, reflecting back on what you have learned and applying it to your everyday practice. Following are some key concerns and strategies to consider in trying to integrate social and minority group model approaches throughout the process of occupational therapy assessment and intervention.

- **The environment and contextual reasoning:** Throughout the assessment and intervention process, critically reflect on how the social, political, economic, and cultural environments are influencing an individual's choice, control, motivation, and self-efficacy. Embed environmental questions and discussions into your assessment, including asking whether a person has access to economic resources to engage in certain activities, whether the person is given opportunities and supports to engage in these activities, or whether the person is aware of supports such as waivers, vouchers, home services, adapted transportation, and assistive technology. Can you equally emphasize contextual reasoning, rather than focusing solely on your "clinical reasoning" during intervention; that is, can you collaboratively plan, strategize, and negotiate how the environment and the systems within it influence a person's occupational choice and control?

- **Consumer direction:** To what extent are you supporting consumer direction throughout the rehabilitation process and in key decision making beyond it? As a profession, we consistently voice our commitment to client-centered practice. However, research has shown that in reality, this often does not happen, and the therapist instead leads the therapy process (Bowen, 1996; C. Brown & Bowen, 1998). In contrast, the policy trend within the disability and senior activism communities is to move away from professional-directed services and to promote consumer-directed choice and control with supports to do so. What are you doing as an occupational therapist to promote not only client-centeredness, but also consumer direction? For example, can you incorporate time into your intervention so that the consumer can practice directing his or her own care, such as directing a personal attendant in how to support and communicate with him or her, practicing how to communicate with a rehabilitation counselor to justify the need for supports to live in the community, and applying for and managing a menu of community-based supports across different systems (e.g., medical, medication, housing, attendant care, home modifications). These are all occupational performance activities that disabled people have identified as critical to community living.

- **Risk with dignity:** A large part of occupational therapy involves determination of safety, as in safe performance of everyday activities. For example, a person might be deemed too unsafe to go back home and instead recommended for nursing home placement. In contrast, disabled people are bringing to the fore the concept of risk with dignity, that is, being able to take risks as the rest of society does and focusing on providing environmental supports to minimize the risk. What can you do as an occupational therapist to strategize environmental supports that would enable a person to live in the community or the least restrictive setting of his or her choice? Can you anticipate potential safety risks and work to problem-solve these in the natural home and community contexts? For example, in a home-based environmental intervention program for older adults with Alzheimer's disease and their spouses, the occupational therapist did a full home audit; collaborated with the consumer/caregiver to identify any potential safety issues; and used a problem worksheet to list the issues, assign next steps to work on between occupational therapy visits, and revisit the situation to see what worked or did not work (see examples from Corcoran & Gitlin, 1992; Gitlin, Corcoran, Winter, Boyce, & Hauck, 2001). Such a program could support people to stay in their homes and communities of highest meaning for as long as possible. Another way to do this is to work with the consumer to advocate for needed supports for personal safety and security, such as personal attendants, community safety check-ins, environment modifications, and assistive technology such as intercoms and emergency call systems.

♦ **Disability identity:** How are you framing disability in every interaction with disabled people? Do you talk about people as diagnostic labels (e.g., refer to people as *paras, quads, stroke, LD, TBI,* and the like) or as deficits (e.g., *your bad arm* or *affected arm*) versus respecting the individual's personhood and dignity? Do you treat disability as a negative deficit within the person that needs to be remediated, compensated for, or normalized? Can you instead frame disability as difference, as a different way of being and of doing that is significantly influenced by the environment? Can you link consumers with other disabled people who have been through a similar disability experience who can serve as positive role models and mentors on how to own difference and maintain a high quality of life? For example, can you link someone who is new to disability with disability advocates and peer-mentoring activities at a local CIL or start a peer-mentoring program at your own facility by inviting prior clients back to serve as mentors to new clients? Some community programs have also started intergenerational groups in which adults with disabilities mentor youths with disabilities or disabled youths mentor older adults who become disabled later in life.

♦ **Social interdependence:** How are you framing "success" in the rehabilitation process? Are you focusing on functional independence, that is, cognitive and physical ability to perform activities by oneself? Many

disabled people, and feminist scholars as well, would challenge this emphasis on individual independence. Instead, they point to the importance of social interdependence, that is, relying on each other and on other people and, in turn, giving back and supporting others within reciprocal relationships (Magasi & Hammel, 2004; Morris, 1992). This concept of interdependence and how to support it is critical for many disabled people. For example, during therapy, are you talking with consumers about prioritizing energies and options to use other supports and people, such as family, personal attendants, and homemakers? Are you strategizing with consumers about how to assertively ask for support without feeling helpless or dependent? Are you offering consumers information about options for support in the community, such as where to look for qualified personal attendants; how to hire, fire, and train them; and systems to fund them in the home, such as home and community-based waiver programs and CIL attendant pools?

♦ **Social participation, support, networking, and capital:** The concept of social interdependence extends to many other areas of social participation. Active engagement and participation in social relationships and membership in any social community are increasingly being identified as positively contributing to emotional and physical health outcomes and well-being (Barlow & Harrison, 1996; Barlow & Williams, 1999; Fawcett et al., 1994; Hernandez, 2005; Magasi & Hammel, 2004). Yet we often spend little if any time on these social issues within therapy, assuming that people will work on them after therapy or that it is not our role to do so. However, we also know that many disabled people are socially isolated and report that they are not participating in social opportunities as much as the rest of society is (National Organization on Disability/Harris, 2004). Strategizing ways to "be a part of," to express and strategize social and intimate relationships, and to develop a social network to meet different needs, such as emotional, instrumental, and thriving needs (Magasi & Hammel, 2004), is a valid focus for occupational therapy, given our emphasis on meaningful engagement as well as research pointing to the benefits of this social engagement. As an occupational therapist, you can help to facilitate this social network development by using assessments such as a role inventory or a social network map so that people can identify what their network looks like now versus what they want it to be and then working with consumers to link to community groups and organizations in which they can begin to create, or recreate, their networks of choice. For example, a consumer might identify the importance of participation in a religious community, and you as an occupational therapist could support the consumer in exploring how to do this and how to work with that community to make it a supportive environment for people with disabilities. As another example, you might invite in peer mentors during therapy sessions so that clients can meet other people with disabilities and determine whether they might want to establish a social network with the disability community.

◆ **Your role and power as a professional:** Are you aware of your own power as a professional therapist? Many therapists would reply that they work within a system that dictates what they can do and that they really do not have much power themselves. However, when you reflect on it, you have a great deal of power as a rehabilitation professional. You have power in determining whether a person is qualified to receive therapy services and the type and extent of therapy the person will receive, what goals are focused on in therapy and how therapy time is spent, discharge and transition planning and whether people are aware of and referred to follow-up services, information access and awareness of options and choices people have and how to advocate for needed supports, whether assistive technology is recommended and funding of it, and so on. You can passively abdicate your power, or you can use it creatively to be an advocacy ally with disabled people throughout and beyond the rehabilitation context.

◆ **Advocacy as a life role and the development of an advocacy network:** It is critical that occupational therapists recognize the importance of advocacy as a life role and work collaboratively with consumers to develop advocacy skills (including how to access information and systems to advocate for supports). An equally important occupational skill is the development of an advocacy network of support that people can count on when they need it or when self-advocacy is too tiring or not enough to address the bigger societal barriers they are facing. For example, you might work with a consumer to identify a primary personal attendant who will support the consumer in his or her everyday activities as well as several emergency backup strategies (e.g., signing up for an attendant pool at a local CIL or having the phone number of an attendant service if the person's attendant does not show that day). Just connecting a person with community advocacy groups, such as CILs, the Americans with Disabilities Act centers, and Protection and Advocacy or Ombudsman programs (available across the country), can offer the person an important source of support on which he or she can call when it is needed rather than having to try to find them during a crises or emergency. These groups can also link consumers to civil rights and legal assistance if needed, which can be particularly critical for someone who is living alone or in an institution.

◆ **Peer mentoring, support, and advocacy:** Recognizing your limitations and role as an occupational therapist is also important. Are you serving as a liaison or ally in linking consumers with other disabled people who can share their experiences and strategies or with disability-led community groups such as CILs that offer peer counseling and mentoring? Increasingly, research is showing the positive benefits of peer mentoring and social learning in supporting emotional and physical health, well-being, community living management, and advocacy skills (Balcazar et al., 1991; Barlow & Harrison, 1996; Barlow & Williams, 1999; Garcia, Kramer, Kramer, & Hammel, 2007; Hernandez, 2005; Lorig, Ritter, & Plant, 2005).

◆ **Collective and empowered consciousness:** One of the most powerful ways to develop self-advocacy is to become involved in collective activism; this is relevant for disabled people and for occupational therapy as a profession. The disability rights community offers many opportunities for social action on behalf of disabled people as a minority group. Do not assume that you need to already have self-advocacy skills to participate in these actions; instead, participation in such collective activism can lead to the development of self-advocacy. Above and beyond fighting for rights, however, comes the added benefit of empowered consciousness when one becomes a part of a shared community that is creating disability identity, culture, community, and pride. Exposing people, including yourself, to this social movement and to the culture and art that are produced within it can be a transformative experience and, in turn, can build community and power from within.

INCORPORATING DISABILITY EXPERIENCE INTO PRACTICE, RESEARCH, AND ADVOCACY: EXAMPLES FROM PARTICIPATORY ACTION RESEARCH

In this final section, we focus on opportunities to promote empowered consciousness via participatory action research. The disability community's history of interaction with researchers has led the community to distrust or be wary of the research process because of mistreatment, continued perpetuation of concepts of incompetence, or irrelevance of research findings and outcomes to their everyday lives (Kitchen, 2000; Zarb, 1992). As a result, the disability community has called for participatory and emancipatory research that is conducted by people with disabilities and that empowers people with disabilities (Zarb, 1992).

One way in which researchers and practitioners can engage in research that is more empowering is to collaborate with disabled people and disability-led community groups in participatory action research (PAR). PAR is an approach rather than a specific design or set of methods (Tewey, 1997). It involves a dynamic collaboration

This is a story about a PAR project that was a collaboration between the Chicago chapter of People First, the staff of El Valor of Chicago (a local community agency offering services to people with intellectual disabilities), the Rehabilitation Research and Training Center on Aging with Developmental Disability (with Joy Hammel as principal investigator), and Edurne Garcia, John Kramer, and Jessica Kramer, doctoral students in the Disability Studies Program at the University of Illinois at Chicago. People First, run by people with disabilities, is an international movement that promotes the self-advocacy of people with disabilities. The mission of People First of Illinois is as follows:

> To work together for justice by helping each other take charge of their lives and fight discrimination. It teaches us how to make decisions about choices that affect our lives so we can achieve our independence. The way we learn to become self-advocates is by supporting one another, and helping each other gain confidence in ourselves to speak out for what we believe. (http://www.peoplefirstofillinois.org/)

The Issue

Community agency staff members, who were people without disabilities who provided support to the Chicago chapter of People First as supporters, expressed concerns that people with intellectual disabilities in the group were not leading it or realizing self-advocacy and community advocacy empowerment goals within the group and the larger community. Group members also wanted to become more involved in advocacy and community participation activities.

The Community-Building Process

Disability studies and occupational therapy practitioners and researchers approached People First as a group to do a PAR project together to work on these goals of raising the critical awareness of the group in the broader community and developing the empowered consciousness of the group itself. The focus was placed on transferring power from agency staff to group members with intellectual disabilities. This focus is aligned with the concept of empowerment as defined by Fawcett and colleagues (1994) as a process by which people gain some control over valued events, outcomes, and resources of importance.

Participatory Strategies

A number of participatory strategies were used to recognize and tap into the wisdom and experience of the members with intellectual disabilities and to locate members in positions of power within the group. Rather than imposing preset therapeutic goals, the researchers observed and participated in several People First meetings to evaluate the group dynamics and identify existing strengths and concerns within the group. The People First members then engaged in a participatory focus group discussion that sought to better articulate why they liked being People First members, how they made decisions in the group, and what activities they would like to do as a group. To facili-

tate the participation of members, various strategies were used, including the use of a circular room arrangement in which participants face each other (with staff positioned outside the circle), round-robin questioning in which each person in the circle takes a turn in offering his or her perspectives, passing a microphone to designate who has the floor, the use of a timer, and the inclusion of many pictures to support the generation of ideas and concrete action plans.

Actions and Lessons Learned

This group discussion resulted in two main actions. First, the members identified that many decisions and actions were carried out by staff supporters rather than members. Second, the members identified that they would like their community to know about People First and that they wanted to publish a newspaper as a first step toward this goal. Many participatory strategies were introduced to support these actions. For example, the group used pictures and questions (such as "what do we want" and "what do we need to do") to create a picture-based logic model, or visual process guide, to guide the newsletter creation (see Figure 62.3). (Additional examples of logic models and how to use them in occupational therapy can be found in the work of Letts and colleagues 1999.) Group members took turns generating names and ideas for the newsletter, and voted by placing a sticker next to their favorite name. They used the same strategies to break down tasks and to select positions (see Figure 62.4).

Members then started to apply these strategies at every group meeting, slowly assuming control on a wider basis. To facilitate the group's reflection and growing empowerment, a group evaluation checklist was developed. Members determined who had carried out each task during each meeting. The members decided that each of them would pick one task they could assume control over and then used the group checklist after every meeting to check their progress. These strategies supported not only self-advocacy, but also group determination and power. Self-advocacy did not need to be taught on an individual basis or required as a prerequisite to group participation but could be learned and built on via a social group approach, with the added benefits of increased community activism and group-empowered consciousness. The other lesson that the group members learned was that there are many ways to participate and that functional independence was not the goal so much as "being a part of" and being a valued member of the group. To support this active participation, information needed to be offered in multiple accessible formats that could be used and owned by people with intellectual disabilities, and the professionals needed to step back, reflect on their power, and scaffold the empowerment of group members. (For more information on the project and resources developed, see Garcia et al., 2007.) Many of the participatory strategies that are featured in this example could also be applied in community-based OT practice and collaborations.

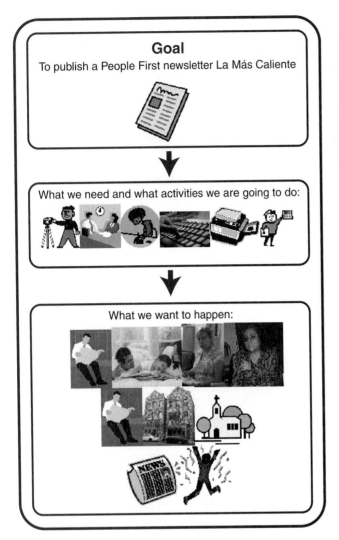

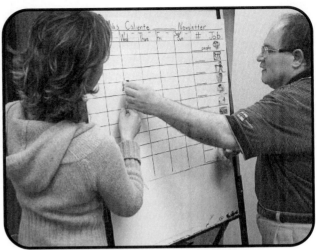

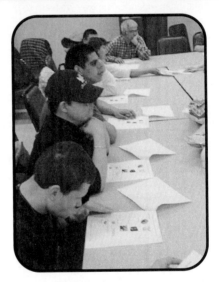

FIGURE 62.3   Picture-based logic model developed by People First group members to define their social group, membership in it, and actions they most want to do and direct.

FIGURE 62.4   Examples of action research strategies to promote access to information, decision making, and control within the People First group and empowerment activities. Top: Flipchart of tasks for newsletter with picture voting on who will take lead on each task. Bottom: Use of picture-based meeting agendas developed by participants so that they can run their own meetings.

between researchers, community partners, disabled constituents, and key stakeholders using an agenda that is driven by social issues that have been identified from within the community. PAR can result in shared knowledge that the community can use as evidence to effect social action change and to build community and empowered consciousness from within (Reason & Bradbury, 2001). It is research that is done by and with disabled people rather than for them or on their behalf. Given this applied, community-driven focus, PAR can be a useful framework for occupational therapy collaborative programming (Taylor, Braveman, & Hammel, 2004) as well as a basis for collaborating on systems change to improve participation opportunities in society. The case study provides one example of a collaborative PAR project that focused on disability rights, social justice, and empowered consciousness building with a disability community.

SUMMARY

This chapter has focused on exposing you to different ways in which you can rethink disability, specifically focusing on the perspectives, insights, and experiences of disabled people and disability advocacy organizations. Many of these perspectives may challenge you as an occupational therapist to critically examine your own power and influence as a health care professional. By understanding the history and philosophy of the disability rights movement and the sociopolitical and social justice issues that disabled people experience as a collective social group, you can begin to reframe your own practice as an occupational therapist to focus on these environmental barriers and incorporate these visions of independence, participation, citizenship, and disability identity, culture, and community building. Occupational therapists can play a critical role in shaping a person's disability experience. By serving as a facilitator and a liaison to disability groups and organizations, you can link disabled people to critical social networking and community-building opportunities. By allying with disability groups and organizations and using participatory action strategies to do so, you can also work to effect change in policies and systems to improve societal opportunities and rights.

RESOURCES

Disability Activism and Social Justice

- Locate your local centers for independent living in your area online at http://www.ilru.org/html/publications/directory/index.html
- ADAPT: http://www.adapt.org
- Disabled People's International: http://www.dpi.org/
- Disability Rights Education Defense Fund (DREDF): http://www.dredf.org
- Freedom Clearinghouse: http://www.freedomclearinghouse.org/
- Mouth: Voice of the Disability Nation: http://www.mouthmag.com/
- MadNation: People working together for social justice and human rights in mental health: http://www.madnation.cc/one.htm
- National Council on Disability (NCD): 1331 F St., NW, Suite 850, Washington, DC 20004 202-272-2004; http://www.ncd.gov/index.html
- National Council on Independent Living (NCIL): 2111 Wilson Blvd, Arlington, VA, 703-525-3406; http://www.ncil.org/
- National Empowerment Center: http://www.power2u.org/index.html
- National Organization on Disability (NOD): http://www.nod.org
- The Ragged Edge Magazine: http://www.ragged-edge-mag.com/
- Self Advocates Becoming Empowered (SABE): activists in the intellectual and developmental disability communities: http://www.sabeusa.org/ (with links to People First)

- World Institute on Disability (WID): 510 16th Street, Suite 100. Oakland, California 94612, 510-763-4100; http://www.wid.org/

Disability Policy

- Centers for Medicare & Medicaid New Freedom/Systems Change Best Practices: http://www.cms.hhs.gov/newfreedom/
- Disability and Business Technical Assistance Centers (DBTAC): regional technical assistance centers on the Americans with Disabilities Act of 1990. National toll-free number: 800-949-4232 (V/TTY). Locate the DBTAC in your region online at http://www.adata.org
- National Disability Rights Network (NDRN), Protection and Advocacy (P&A) Systems and Client Assistance Programs (CAP): http://www.napas.org/
- US Access Board:
    - ADAAG (including children's environments and additional state and local government guidelines): http://www.access-board.gov/adaag/html/adaag.htm
    - Play Areas Guidelines: http://www.access-board.gov/play/status.htm
    - Recreation Facilities Guidelines: http://www.access-board.gov/recreation/final.htm
    - UFAS (Standards for Federal Government and 504 Covered entities): http://www.access-board.gov/ufas/ufas-html/ufas.htm
    - DAAG/ABA (U.S. Access Board, Not enforceable standard under ADA): http://www.access-board.gov/ada-aba/index.htm
- ADA Accessibility Guidelines Checklist for Existing Facilities: http://www.usdoj.gov/crt/ada/checktxt.htm
- US Department of Justice:
    - ADAAG (Enforceable standards): http://www.usdoj.gov/crt/ada/reg3a.html#Anchor-42424
    - Regulations Implementing Title III of the ADA: http://www.usdoj.gov/crt/ada/reg3a.html
    - Readily Achievable Barrier Removal and Van Accessible Parking Spaces: http://www.usdoj.gov/crt/ada/adata1.htm
- Housing Policy:
    - Fair Housing Amendments of 1988 and Accessibility Guidelines: http://www.hud.gov/offices/fheo/disabilities/fhguidelines/
    - National Fair Housing Advocate: http://fairhousing.com
- Transportation Policy
    - Project Action: federally funded technical assistance project on transportation for people with disabilities: http://projectaction.easterseals.com
    - U.S. Department of Transportation: accessibility and equal access to transportation online resource: http://www.dot.gov/citizen_services/disability/disability.html

Disability History and Disability Studies

- Longmore, P., & Umansky, L. (2001). *The new disability history.* New York: New York University Press.
- Longmore, P. K. (1995). The second phase: From disability rights to disability culture. First published in *Disability*

Rag and ReSource, 16, 4–11. (Available online at: http://www.independentliving.org/docs3/longm95.html)

◆ Society for Disability Studies (international interdisciplinary organization of disability studies scholars): http://www.uic.edu/orgs/sds/

◆ The Disability Social History Project: http://www.disabilityhistory.org/

◆ The Disability Archive (excellent online library of readings from the Disability Studies community in the UK): http://www.leeds.ac.uk/disability-studies/archiveuk/index.html

Social Justice and Participatory Action References

◆ Alinsky, S. (1972). *Rules for radicals: A practical primer for realistic radicals.* New York: Vintage Books.

◆ Charlton, J. (1998). *Nothing about us without us: Disability oppression and empowerment.* Berkeley: University of California Press.

◆ Freire, P. (1970, 2000). *Pedagogy of the oppressed.* New York: Continuum International Publishing.

◆ Reason, P., & Bradbury, H. (Eds.). (2001). *Handbook of action research: Participative inquiry and practice.* Thousand Oaks, CA: Sage.

◆ Young, I. M. (1990). *Justice and the politics of difference.* Princeton, NJ: Princeton University Press.

REFERENCES

ADAPT (2006). ADAPT Home Page. Retrieved 10/31, 2006, from http://www.adapt.org/index1.html

Balcazar, F., Majors, R., Blanchard, K., Paine, A., Suarez-Balcazar, Fawcett, S., et al. (1991). Teaching minority high school students to recruit helpers to attain personal and educational goals. *Journal of Behavioral Education, 1,* 445–454.

Barlow, J., & Harrison, K. (1996). Focusing on empowerment: Facilitating self-help in young people with arthritis through a disability organization. *Disability and Society, 11*(4), 539–552.

Barlow, J., & Williams, B. (1999). 'I Now Feel That I'm Not Just a Bit of Left Luggage': The experiences of older women with arthritis attending a Personal Independence Course. *Disability and Society, 11,* 53–64.

Blumer, H. (1969). *Symbolic interaction: Perspective and method.* Englewood Cliffs, NJ: Prentice-Hall.

Bowen, R. (1996). Should occupational therapy adopt a consumer-based model of service delivery? *American Journal of Occupational Therapy, 50*(10), 899–902.

Bronfenbrenner, U. (1979). *The ecology of human development.* Cambridge, MA: Harvard University Press.

Brown, C., & Bowen, R. (1998). Including the consumer and environment in occupational therapy treatment planning. *Occupational Therapy Journal of Research, 18,* 44–62.

Brown, S. E. (1992). Creating a disability mythology. *International Journal of Rehabilitation Research, 15,* 227–233.

Centers for Medicare & Medicaid Services. (2007a). *Home & community-based waiver systems promising practices reports.* Baltimore, MD: Centers for Medicare & Medicaid Services.

(Available online at: http://www.cms.hhs.gov/Promising Practices/HCBSPPR/list.asp#TopOfPage)

Centers for Medicare & Medicaid Services. (2007b). *New Freedom Initiative overview:* Retrieved April 7, 2007, from: http://www.cms.hhs.gov/NewFreedomInitiative/01_Overview.asp#TopOfPage

Charlton, J. (1998). *Nothing about us without us.* Berkeley: University of California Press.

Corcoran, M. A., & Gitlin, L. N. (1992). Dementia management: An occupational therapy home-based intervention for caregivers. *American Journal of Occupational Therapy, 46*(9), 801–808.

DePoy, E., & Werrbach, G. (1996). Successful living placement for adults with disabilities: Considerations for social work practice. *Social Work in Health Care, 23*(4), 21–34.

Driedger, D (1989). *The last civil rights movement: Disabled Peoples' International.* New York: St. Martin's Press.

Fawcett, S. B., White, G. W., Balcazar, F. E., Suarez-Balcazar, Y., Mathews, R. M., Paine-Andrews, A, et al. (1994). A contextual-behavioral model of empowerment: Case studies with people with physical disabilities. *American Journal of Community Psychology, 22,* 475–496.

Foucault, M. (1973). *The birth of the clinic: An archaeology of medical perception.* New York: Vintage Books.

Garcia, E., Kramer, J. M., Kramer, J. C., & Hammel, J. (2007). Putting the horse before the cart: Organizational skills as a first step towards advocacy for people with intellectual disabilities. [Under Review].

Gill, C. (1999). *Models of disability.* Chicago: Chicago Center for Disability Research.

Gitlin, L. N. Corcoran, M., Winter, L., Boyce, A., & Hauck, W. W. (2001). A randomized, controlled trial of a home environmental intervention: Effect on efficacy and upset in caregivers and on daily function of persons with dementia. *Gerontologist, 41*(1):4–14.

Goffman, E. (1963). *Stigma: Notes on the management of spoiled identity.* New York: Simon & Schuster.

Goldberg, D. (Ed). (1994). *Multiculturalism: A critical reader.* Cambridge, MA: Blackwell.

Hahn, H. (1985). Disability policy and the problem of discrimination. *American Behavioral Scientist, 28*(3), 293–318.

Henderson, J. N. (1995). The culture of care in a nursing home: Effects of a medicalized model of long-term care. In J. N. Henderson & M. D. Vesperi (Eds.), *The culture of long term care: Nursing home ethnography.* Westport, CT: Bergin & Garvey.

Hernandez, B. (2005). A voice in the chorus: Perspectives of young men of color on their disabilities, identities, and peer-mentors. *Disability & Society, 20*(2), 117–133

Kitchen, R. (1997). The researched opinions on research: Disabled people and disability research. *Disability and Society, 15*(1), 25–47.

Letts, L., Law, M., Pollock, N., Stewart, D., Westmorland, M., Philpot, A., et al. (1999). Developing a programme logical model as a basis for programme evaluation. In *A programme evaluation workbook for occupational therapists: An evidence-based practice tool.* Ottawa, ON: CAOT Publications ACE.

Linton, S. (1998). *Claiming disability: Knowledge and identity.* New York: New York University Press.

Longmore, P. K. (1995). The second phase: From disability rights to disability culture. *The Disability Rag and ReSource, 16,* 4–11.

Longmore, P., & Umansky, L (2001). *The new disability history: American perspectives.* New York: New York University Press.

Lorig, K., Ritter, P. L., & Plant, K. (2005). A disease-specific self-help program compared with a generalized chronic disease self-help program for arthritis patients. *Arthritis & Rheumatism, 53,* 950–957.

MadPride (2007). MadPride Home Page. Retrieved 10/09, 2007, from http://www.ctono.freeserve.co.uk/

Magasi, S., & Hammel, J. (2004). Social support and social network mobilization in older African American women who have experienced strokes. *Disability Studies Quarterly, 24,* 4–19.

Mechanic, D. (1974). *Politics, medicine and social science.* New York: John Wiley & Sons.

Morris, J. (1992). Personal and political: A feminist perspective on researching physical disability. *Disability, Handicap, and Society, 7,* 157–166.

National Council on Disability. (2003). *Olmstead: Reclaiming institutionalized lives.* Washington DC: Author.

National Council on Disability. (2005a). *The Civil Rights of Institutionalized Persons Act: Has It fulfilled its promise?* Washington DC: Author.

National Council on Disability. (2005b). *Living independently and in the community: Implementation lessons from the United States: Quick reference guide.* Washington DC: Author.

National Council on Disability. (2006a). *National disability policy: A progress report. December 2004–December 2005.* Washington DC: Author.

National Council on Disability. (2006b). *The state of 21st century long-term services and supports: Financing and systems reform for Americans with disabilities.* Washington DC: Author.

National Organization on Disability/Harris.(2004). *2004 NOD/Harris survey of Americans with disabilities.* Washington DC: NOD.

Oliver, M. (1990). *The politics of disablement.* London: Macmillan.

Oliver, M. (1996). *Understanding disability from theory to practice.* New York: St. Martin's Press.

Reason, P., & Bradbury, H. (2001). Introduction: Inquiry and participation in search of a world worthy of human aspiration. In P. Reason & H. Bradbury (Eds.), *Handbook of Action Research.* Thousand Oaks, CA: Sage, pp. 1–14.

Rioux, M. (1997) Disability: The place of judgment in a world of fact. *Journal of Intellectual Disability Research 41*(2), 102–112.

Taylor, R., Braveman, B., & Hammel, J. (2004). Developing and evaluating community-based services through participatory action research: Three case examples. *American Journal of Occupational Therapy, 58,* 73–82

Tewey, B. P. (1997) *Building participatory action research partnerships in disability and rehabilitation research.* Washington DC: National Institute on Disability and Rehabilitation Research.

Thomas, C. (1999). *Female forms: Experiencing and understanding disability.* Philadelphia: Open University Press.

Triano, S. (2007). *Disabled and proud.* Retrieved April 5, 2007, from: http://www.disabledandproud.com/

Wade, C. M (1994). *Disability culture rap. tools for change: Disability identity and culture.* Santa Cruz, CA: Diversity World.

Wright, E. R., Gronfein, W. P., & Owens, T. J. (2000). Deinstitutionalization, social rejection, and the self-esteem of former mental patients. *Journal of Health & Social Behavior, 41,* 68–90.

Zarb, G. (1992). On the road to Damascus: First steps towards changing the relations of disability research production. *Disability, Handicap, and Society, 7,* 125–138.

XIII

THERAPISTS IN ACTION: EXAMPLES OF EXPERT PRACTICE

"The true expert, then, is someone who knows something of what lies beneath the surface of his or her practice, and spends time and effort not just understanding it but developing it further, and who can then talk about it more publicly too."

Della Fish & Colin Coles

School-Based Practice: Enabling Participation

MARY MUHLENHAUPT

Learning Objectives

After reading this chapter, you will be able to:

1. Discuss issues that occupational therapists consider to define a student's education needs and develop program plans.
2. Formulate reflective questions that are designed to contribute information to support a student's participation in the curriculum.

INTRODUCTION

Because occupational therapy services in schools are designed to enable students to participate in, and benefit from, a curriculum that prepares them for further education, employment, and independent living (Individuals With Disabilities Education Improvement Act, 2004), my practice in the schools focuses on the following:

1. The *student*—his or her motivations, interests, and functional performance in learner, friend, and player roles
2. The *curriculum*—its activities, materials, and instructional approaches
3. The *settings and situations* in which the student's school performance is expected or desired—both the human (adults and peers) and non-human environment (including physical, sensory, temporal, cultural, and legal aspects)

My work activity varies during any day. One morning begins with an impromptu meeting to discuss a teacher's concerns about one of her students. Then I go outside to the playground to complete part of an evaluation of a student who has just moved into the district. I then drive to the high school building to meet a student during her lunch period in the cafeteria. Together, we are working on ways in which she can gain independence to purchase her meal, eat at the table with her friends, and clean up after herself, all within the allotted lunch schedule. She travels around the school using an electric wheelchair and communicates with a Dynamo®, an augmentative system. Later, I implement an afternoon language arts activity with a kindergarten teacher. I focus on specific writing and drawing tasks that reinforce the phonics elements the teacher introduces. By coleading this activity, I am implementing a whole-school approach that is designed to enrich available opportunities, reduce learning challenges, and prevent failure (Gartner & Lipsky, 2002).

Throughout my school-based practice, I use occupational therapy theory and knowledge about how children develop and learn, professional reasoning and evidence, and ethical and practice standards. In addition, education philosophies, federal and state education law and regulation, state and district learning standards and curriculum, and the culture and resources of the local district influence what I do each day. I will describe my work with Davey, an 8-year-old boy, to illustrate how an occupational therapist works in a school-based setting.

REFERRAL

Davey was referred for an evaluation by the district's Child Study Team (CST). As a result of previous recommendations I had made to the district administration to streamline the evaluation process and verify educationally relevant concerns, Davey's teacher, Ms. Ray, completed a questionnaire when she initiated the evaluation request to the CST (Box 63.1).

The referral information gave me an idea of Davey's teacher's expectations as well as the challenges he was having in school, so my evaluation already had a necessary direction. A telephone interview with Davey's mother gave me an opportunity to learn her perspectives and priorities (Box 63.2). Knowing about Davey's performance over time, how he functioned in less structured and small-group or solitary situations, how he managed certain tasks at home, and what his parents, who know him best, saw as his strengths and needs would help me to individualize my evaluation.

OCCUPATIONAL PROFILE

Davey is an 8-year-old student in a third grade general education program at his neighborhood public school. He likes school, especially gym and recess. His academic strengths are in math and science. His reading skills are below grade-level expectations. His written work is often incomplete and difficult to read, and homework assignments are completed inconsistently. During classroom free choice time, he chooses games on the computer. He stumbles into things in the classroom, hurries, and trips and falls in the cafeteria and on the playground. He is distracted during many classroom routines, and Ms. Ray frequently gives him verbal reminders to refocus him back to his assignments.

Davey lives with his parents, who see him as a bright boy who needs to develop his self-control and motor coordination in order to complete his schoolwork with higher levels of independence. He needs continued prompting from his mother to stay at the kitchen table and complete his homework. He fidgets and drums with his pencil or goes off to play in the family room. Davey does not seem

---

 BOX 63.1

TEACHER QUESTIONNAIRE FOR SCHOOL-BASED OCCUPATIONAL THERAPY REFERRAL

1. What is the focus of your classroom curriculum?
General education, 3rd grade. Instructional approaches, methods, and materials have moved from the tactile-kinesthetic approaches that were emphasized in the primary grades. More emphasis on listening and following series of directions. Independent work and cooperative group work periods, initiating requests for assistance when needed.

2. How is this student managing within that curriculum?
Davey is a bright student who is very active. His written work is sloppy. Behavior difficulties interfere during parts of the day, especially when he needs to work quietly or in a small group. He pokes peers, talks about unrelated topics, asks for permission to sharpen his pencil, go to the boys'

room, etc. He is distractible and needs reminders to focus and complete assignments. Sometimes he needs extra time to settle down after "free choice" time or recess.

3. What has been tried to increase this student's participation in the curriculum? What have been the results?
Extra attention from the teacher, verbal reminders and cues, his desk is moved near to mine so I can keep an eye on him. More time in a quiet area of classroom (such as the book corner) after recess. Tried a sticker chart to motivate him to pay attention. None of these things are obviously successful. He goes to the resource room to support language arts and reading curriculum.

BOX 63.2 EXAMPLES OF PARENT INTERVIEW QUESTIONS FOR THE OCCUPATIONAL THERAPY EVALUATION

- What would you like to see Davey accomplish this year at school?
- What about Davey's performance in school and during schoolwork is of most concern to you?
- What does Davey enjoy doing at home or during free time?

to need much sleep; he has a difficult time falling asleep and wakes early each morning. He recently joined the soccer team in his community, something that his parents hope will encourage his motor skills while giving him a chance to run around and "blow off some steam."

EVALUATION PROCESS

Federal regulations determine that a school-based therapy evaluation needs to generate information that the team can use to understand the student's educational needs and plan an individualized program (IDEIA, 2004). The occupational therapist is focused on increasing competence in the student role and enabling the child to benefit from instructional activities (Muhlenhaupt, 2003). Davey was enrolled in the third grade general curriculum, a program that was already familiar to me. My next step was to learn more about the specific environments and situations in which Davey needed to participate and how he used the supports that were available to him. Several strategies accomplished this purpose:

- My direct observation of Davey's participation (both quiet, independent work and movement opportunities; solitary and group activity)
  - In the classroom during seatwork assignments (15 minutes in the classroom, beginning when the teacher gave the group instructions)
  - On the playground (15 minutes that included speaking with the recess aide about Davey's general activity during recess)
- Interview with the reading teacher to understand more about what her instruction included and how Davey functioned in the smaller group and quieter environment of the resource room
- Review of the amount and quality of Davey's finished written work completed in different settings
  - Ms. Ray provided sample homework assignments and spelling tests that Davey had completed prior to the

evaluation dates, along with samples that were representative of average work by other students in class.
- Review of Davey's educational file (social, developmental history)

While I was in the classroom for my initial observation, I asked Ms. Ray to rate Davey's performance during that time and to continue to do so during several classroom seatwork periods over the next few days, using a form I developed (see a completed form in Box 63.3). The data that Mrs. Ray recorded over nine different class periods confirmed variation in Davey's performance, his best performance being during math lessons, with lower ratings in language arts activity. When I looked further and examined these ratings against the daily class schedule, I noted that lower performance was common during classes that were held in the afternoon hours. I kept this reporting in my file and recorded the average rating over all periods (2 points) for use as a baseline against which to measure change once specific intervention strategies to enable Davey's participation were put into place.

BOX 63.3 DAVEY'S PERFORMANCE DURING ROUTINE SEATWORK ACTIVITIES

4: Completed entire task in time period, no help/reminders needed

3: Worked entire period, in seat, verbal reminders/redirection only

2: Worked entire period, but out of seat, verbal reminders and redirected to seat and task—completed assignment

1: Worked part of period, out of seat, continued redirected to task—assignment incomplete

0: Refused to work, no product turned in

Date	Class period/task	Rating
9/12	Morning board copying	2
9/12	Reading book, answering questions on paper	1
9/13	Social studies: coloring maps	3
9/14	Science: lab activity with partner	3
9/14	Language arts workbook pages	1
9/14	Spelling test	2
9/15	Math worksheets	4
9/18	Math: puzzles and sets	4
9/18	Language arts: "write a story"	1

Referral concerns did not identify any performance limitations related to fine motor difficulties in school or at home, and my observations of his work in the classroom did not lead me to suspect fine motor difficulties were a factor in his performance. Therefore, standardized measures to rate Davey's fine motor functions according to those of his peers were not indicated in this evaluation.

ANALYSIS OF OCCUPATIONAL PERFORMANCE

On the basis of the procedures I had completed to this point, I concluded that Davey understood his teacher's directions and knew what he was supposed to do in the classroom. He had the essential perceptual and motor skills needed for performance. He did not have cognitive challenges or any apparent psychosocial factors that interfered with completing the assigned work or assuming expected levels of responsibility throughout the day. Aspects of the physical environment—his desk and chair size, the writing tools and paper he used—were appropriate. I suspected that more information about his sensory processing would help me to identify whether the behavior that affected his school performance could be attributed to his unique responses to sensory information. I selected both the Sensory Profile (Dunn, 1999) and the Sensory Profile School Companion (Dunn, 2006) to provide more information.

I also scheduled an assessment period outside of the classroom so that I could observe Davey's engagement in play and learning activities. I had him participate in table-top activities and noted how he used materials, organized his work space, approached tasks, and reacted when help was needed, along with his general attention and activity level over a period of sedentary work. Then outside, I encouraged him to explore on the playground and watched his pace and choice of activity. These procedures also gave me an opportunity to implement some trial interventions. I was able to see how he responded and therefore consider some specific modifications or accommodations that might support him throughout the routines of the school day.

PROGRAM PLANNING

When compared to those of other children without disabilities, Davey's Sensory Profile results indicated definite differences in vestibular and touch systems and multisensory processing of touch, body position, and movement. Davey looked for opportunities to experience movement and touch stimuli in many situations in the classroom and across the school day. He fidgeted in his seat, and he tapped on his desk with his pencils, rulers, hands, and fingers. He left his desk and chair frequently and without permission during classroom seatwork periods and chose multiple different movement activities on the playground. When interpreted from a sensory-processing perspective

(see Chapters 59 and 60), Davey's behavior suggested that he had a high response threshold for sensory information, particularly in movement and touch systems, with difficulty modulating his responses to this type of sensory information. His preference for touch- and movement-related sensory information and the apparent challenge he faced in matching his responses to environmental demands in different situations had particular significance for Davey. Now in third grade, he faced classroom routines that incorporated less active movement and an expectation for increased focus and independent work, compared to the primary grades. Because of the difficulty of balancing this sensory information, his system became overwhelmed. I saw Davey's behavior patterns as a means to help him cope when he faced situations that challenged his sensory preferences (Dunn, 1999). This perspective helped me to explain Davey's "distractible" behavior, fidgeting, and increased activity that interfered with his listening to directions and completing a variety of assignments and tasks during the day (see Box 63.4).

THE INDIVIDUALIZED EDUCATION PROGRAM TEAM PROCESS

Collecting all of this information about Davey's strengths and needs and using occupational therapy theory and principles to develop a program plan to increase his participation made up only part of my process. As a school-based

BOX 63.4

INITIAL HYPOTHESIS TO GUIDE DAVEY'S INTERVENTION

If:

Davey's fidgeting, out-of-seat behavior, illegible penmanship, and difficulty completing assignments

Is due to:

His nervous system's unique pattern of response to sensation and difficulty modulating between too much, sufficient, or insufficient responsiveness to touch and movement sensory experiences

Then:

Considering the touch- and movement-related sensory information/events/opportunities throughout the school day and implementing specific environmental accommodations will provide sensory experiences that match his nervous system's needs and will promote optimal levels of arousal, attention, and self-regulation for effective participation in school tasks.

therapist, I then needed to convey my findings to the Individualized Education Program (IEP) team for their consideration and decision making. Recognizing that team-generated goals are the foundation for a student's school-based support services (Giangreco, 2000), the IEP team reviewed my evaluation results in relation to Davey's educational goals. The group agreed that an occupational therapy service offered new and specific strategies to support Davey's participation in the curriculum. (Box 63.5 highlights some of the information from Davey's IEP.)

In accordance with accountability requirements that are part of the IEP process (Turnbull, 2005), we targeted educational outcomes and agreed on the need to collect data in the classroom to determine whether or not Davey's behavior changed once this intervention was implemented. In keeping with IDEA provisions to support a student through a program plan that is "only as special as necessary" (Giangreco, 2000), the team acknowledged that the occupational therapist's presence in the context of Davey's school routine would not be required for an extended period over the school year. That was reflected in the way in which occupational therapy was listed in Davey's IEP: "OT services, 2 hours/month during the first marking period and 1 hour/month during the 2nd marking period" was recorded in the "Related Services" section.

IMPLEMENTING INTERVENTION

Sensory integration theory (Lane, 2002) influenced my recommendation for the availability of specific types of sensory experiences within Davey's school and homework routines. I drew on evidence suggesting that information about a child's sensory profile can be most appropriately used to design activities and environments that match the child's sensory needs rather than to guide interventions to change the child to meet the demands of specific environments (Dunn, 1999; Williams & Shellenberger, 1994).

Helping Davey to stay in his seat, sit still, and get his work done was a priority. I believed that his need for movement contributed to his distractibility and out-of-seat behavior during the language arts curriculum, which was a challenge for him, and during the long afternoon block of in-classroom activity. As a part of my school-based service, one of my visits (sessions) was a scheduled meeting with Ms. Ray to help her understand how the sequence of different activities in the school day and the demands within those activities influenced Davey's attention and activity level. Together, we identified specific tasks that incorporated movement yet fit logically within the classroom routine, such as the job of "paper passer" or "office messenger" for her to use when Davey needed a movement break. We developed a simple three-point rating scale that she used over the next week to test out whether she was more satisfied with his in-seat behavior once he took advantage of these naturally occurring movement breaks (see Box 63.6).

Until now, throughout the day, Ms. Ray had been giving Davey repeated cues and using discipline in response to his inappropriate behavior. My goal was to help him to monitor and adjust his own behavior in a variety of situations. I had some previous positive experiences with several students who had similar needs when I used the Alert Program™ (Williams & Shellenberger, 1994) (see Box 63.7). I spoke to Ms. Ray and to Davey's mother about the program, explaining the absence of published

---

BOX 63.5 **SELECTED INFORMATION FROM DAVEY'S IEP**

- Present level of academic achievement and functional performance: Mathematics at grade level. Reading at 2.0 grade level. Cognitive and motor skills at age level. He finds reasons to get out of his seat and move around the room, needs reminders to attend to, and extra time to complete, written work; written seatwork rated at 50% legible, 60% completion rate.

- IEP annual goal that occupational therapy service supported: Language arts curriculum: Davey will write paragraphs (90% legible) that include a variety of sentence types; appropriate use of the eight parts of speech; and accurate spelling, capitalization, and punctuation to complete required third grade class assignments and homework.

- Specially designed instruction: Small-group instruction in structured reading program, inclusion of second grade level reading materials for classroom use, incentives to encourage work completion and legible written production.

BOX 63.6 **TEACHER'S RATING SCALE FOLLOWING INTERVENTION IMPLEMENTATION**

+1: Student performance/participation meets classroom expectations.

0: Student performance/participation has improved but does not yet meet classroom expectations.

−1: Student performance/participation is unchanged and does not yet meet classroom expectations.

BOX 63.7 ALERT PROGRAM™

The Alert Program™ uses an engine analogy to teach children, their teachers, and their parents ways to change how alert one feels. Individuals learn to choose strategies that help to adjust behavior when they feel their "engine" is in either low or high gear, obtaining a "just-right" engine level (alert, attentive, and ready to learn).

evidence regarding the effectiveness of this approach and offering my opinion that was based on experiences with several other students. We agreed to give it a try.

During my occupational therapy sessions, I met with Davey and explained that I would show him some things he could do that would help him to follow the school rules and do his best work. I taught him some basic strategies of the Alert Program™, and we considered when he would use them. For several different days over the next three weeks, Ms. Ray again rated Davey's classroom behavior and his work completion according to the same data sheet she had used previously (see Box 63.3). The data yielded positive ratings when compared to baseline (the data that Ms. Ray had recorded during my evaluation), and that led me to recommend that Davey continue to use the Alert strategies on a regular basis. At that point, I asked Ms. Ray to record the data only once each week so that we could monitor Davey's performance. I told her to increase her data collection only if Davey's behavior and performance deteriorated. I also arranged with her for me to lead a lesson in the classroom so that she and all of the students could learn about these strategies. Davey took an active role in teaching his friends the different types of things that helped him do his best work in school. He told his friends some of the things he learned to do when "a class is going too slow and you just can't wait for recess" or when "so much is going on that it's hard to pay attention to Ms. Ray." This was an opportunity for peers to recognize Davey and learn from him. It also gave him the experience of advocating for his own needs. For Davey, this afforded a needed "self-esteem boost."

As another example of occupational therapy directed to school performance, once intervention started, Ms. Ray raised concern about Davey's protests to her when it was time to go to art. Mr. Tomkins, the art teacher, reported that Davey often refused to try projects once he arrived in the classroom. I scheduled a visit in the art room while Davey's class was in session. While there, I considered modifications or support that Davey could use

during activities that overwhelmed him, such as those with multisensory touch and smell sensations. I considered whether changes in aspects of the environment, or the demands of art room tasks and activities would enable Davey's success. On the basis of the environment and activity analysis, I recommended that rubber gloves be available for Davey to use in the art studio. With the gloves on, Davey was able to sit at the table with his peers and mold cold, wet clay.

SUMMARY

My occupational therapy intervention to support Davey's school performance was grounded in sensory integration theory. My service was directed toward adapting his environment through scheduling, task or activity supports, and modifications so that activities and environments matched Davey's sensory needs and interests and the challenging sensory aspects of his daily experiences had a less prominent influence on his performance. I used my understanding about the interaction between the student, what he or she wants and needs to do, and the influence of the situations and settings in which school performance is expected. The evaluation and intervention approaches that I used were specifically targeted to enable Davey to engage in activities and routines across the campus. As a result, he participated in, and benefited from, the third grade curriculum.

REFERENCES

Dunn, W. (1999). *Sensory Profile.* San Antonio, TX: The Psychological Corporation.

Dunn, W. (2006). *Sensory Profile school companion.* San Antonio, TX: Harcourt Assessment.

Gartner, A., & Lipsky, D. (2002). *Inclusion: A service, not a place.* Port Chester, NY: National Professional Resources.

Giangreco, M. (2000). Related services research for students with low incidence disabilities: Implications for speech-language pathologists in inclusive classrooms. *Language, Speech, and Hearing Services in Schools, 31,* 230–239.

Individuals With Disabilities Education Improvement Act. (2004). PL. 108-446, 20 U.S.C. §1400 et seq.

Lane, S. (2002). Sensory modulation. In A. Bundy, S. Lane, & E. Murray (Eds.), *Sensory integration: Theory and practice* (2nd ed., pp. 101–122). Philadelphia: F. A. Davis.

Muhlenhaupt, M. (2003). Enabling student participation through occupational therapy services in the schools. In L. Letts & D. Stewart (Eds.), *Using environments to enable occupational performance* (pp. 177–196). Thorofare, NJ: Slack.

Turnbull, R. (2005). Individuals with Disabilities Education Act Reauthorization: Accountability and personal responsibility. *Remedial and Special Education, 26,* 320–326.

Williams, M. & Shellenberger, S. (1994). *"How does your engine run?": A leader's guide to the Alert Program for Self-Regulation.* Albuquerque, NM: TherapyWorks.

There's No Place Like Home: Occupational Therapy Services for People Who Are Homeless

WINIFRED SCHULTZ-KROHN

Learning Objectives

After reading this chapter, you will be able to:

1. Describe the change in the homeless population over the past 30 years.
2. Discuss the factors contributing to homelessness.
3. Identify the role of occupational therapy for those who are homeless.
4. Identify the evidence to support occupational therapy services for those who are homeless.

Occupational therapy practitioners can serve as change agents and provide valuable services to people who are homeless (Finlayson, Baker, Rodman, & Herzberg, 2002). My introduction to working with people who are homeless came when three occupational therapy students approached me, a faculty member, to mentor their senior honors project. They were interested in providing family-centered occupational therapy intervention at a homeless shelter for families. My experiences in working with those students and the families at the shelter served as the foundation for developing an occupational therapy internship program at the shelter

MEETING THE NEEDS OF A FAMILY WHO IS HOMELESS

Dan, age 32, was employed as a janitor in a business complex for seven years. Five months ago, Dan was laid off from his janitorial position. Dan has a GED but no additional training or education and has been unable to find work. His wife Rita, age 30, works part time at a convenience store and makes minimum wage. Their daughter Emma, age 9, has asthma and regularly uses an inhaler. Their son Jacob, age 12, has a learning disability. Medical insurance was covered through Dan's job, and the extended medical coverage will end next month.

The family used to live in a studio apartment, but the rent increased, and they were no longer able to afford the apartment. They moved in with relatives a year ago. While Dan was still employed, the two families shared the costs of housing and lived in this doubled-up situation. After Dan lost his job, the relatives could not support both families. Dan's family sought housing in a homeless shelter. A shelter for women and children accepted Rita and Emma but not Dan or Jacob. Dan and Jacob searched for another shelter while Rita and Emma remained at the women's shelter.

Unfortunately, this situation is not fictitious.

and several collaborative research projects. This chapter describes occupational therapy intervention for this underserved population.

WHO ARE THE HOMELESS?

The demographics of the homeless population in the United States have changed dramatically over the past 30 years (Turner, 2004). In the past, those without a home were often single, middle-aged men with substance abuse problems (Rossi, 1990). Single men now make up only 41% of the homeless population, and homeless families, the fastest-growing segment of the homeless population, constitute 41% of the group (Turner, 2004). Single women are 13% of the homeless population, and unaccompanied youths are 5%. For adults, homelessness often presents as a series of exits and returns to being homeless (Dworsky & Piliavin, 2000). The majority of those without a home have a history of employment instability and previous episodes

of homelessness or living "doubled up," a situation in which several individuals or families are living together in housing that was designed for a smaller number of occupants. Female-headed families experienced less time being homeless and had fewer episodes of homelessness compared to both single men and single women.

WHY DOES HOMELESSNESS OCCUR?

The causes of homelessness are complex and can be conceptualized in three categories (Glasser & Bridgeman, 1999):

- **Personal deficits:** Substance abuse, mental health problems, and family violence are associated with an increased susceptibility to becoming homeless but are not definite predictors of who will become homeless.
- **External factors:** Low-paying jobs, insufficient affordable housing, and patterns of discrimination can contribute to homelessness but do not fully explain the extent or diversity in the homeless population.
- **Ecological perspective:** Personal deficits and the external factors of societal and cultural conditions may interact, leading to homelessness (Toro, Trickett, Wall, & Salem, 1991).

HOMELESSNESS IS MORE THAN LOSS OF A HOME

People who are homeless experience more than a loss of physical shelter; they experience disenfranchisement from the community (DeOllos, 1997; Toro et al., 1991). Occupational therapy intervention supports community connections by fostering social participation and is guided by two principles (Schultz-Krohn, 2004):

1. Creating an affirming environment that validates skill development can support participation in occupations (Rebeiro, 2001).
2. Participation in occupation can buffer the negative effects of stress and loss (McColl, 2002).

A shelter is not considered an affirming environment; therefore, occupational therapy practitioners focus on facilitating positive experiences for and with clients. For example, we designed an occupational therapy group for parents to help their children cope with the stress of living in a shelter. We discussed the importance of providing time for relaxing and taught stress management methods such as infant massage and relaxation techniques. Parents suggested that playing games could be used to reduce their children's level of stress. The opportunity for parents to share ideas and have those ideas endorsed within the group created a supportive environment. Parents then selected an activity that they deemed most appropriate for their children. At the next parent group, many parents shared additional relaxation ideas with each other and supported one another. The affirming and supportive environment diminished the stressful experience of living at the shelter, and parents reported having fun with their respective families.

Adults Who Are Homeless

Occupational therapy can help adults who are homeless to enhance personal attributes such as job-seeking skills and foster the living skills they need to remain housed (Davis & Kutter, 1998). A focus on instrumental activities of daily living, particularly budgeting and careful monitoring of funds, should be fostered with adults who are homeless. Although adults who are homeless might attend classes on budgeting, occupational therapy intervention helps clients to translate budgeting skills into habits (Rogers, 2000). The formation of habits enables people to focus their energy and effort on other pressing issues, such as job or housing searches. Sally, a mother who was homeless and living in a family shelter, had a habit of buying candy for her children at the store even though the shelter provided free afternoon snacks. The shelter expected Sally to save money for rent, but she had very limited funds. The occupational therapist accompanied Sally and her children to the store and provided cueing to help Sally apply budgeting skills in context. Conflicting habits, such as trying to budget funds yet buying candy, were identified and addressed through instruction and discussion and by practicing positive habits in context. When the occupational therapist accompanied Sally to the store, Sally practiced reminding her children that she could give them a snack when they returned to the shelter. The therapist supported and encouraged Sally to practice the skill of budgeting in the context where this new skill was challenged.

Adults with Mental Health Problems Who Are Homeless

People without a home often experience severe disruptions of self-esteem, self-worth, and self-efficacy (Buckner, Bassuk, & Zima 1993). Homelessness can produce depression, stress, and anxiety in parents, children, and single adults (Buckner et al., 1993; Davis & Kutter, 1998; Zima et al., 1999). Homelessness has been identified as a factor in producing mental health problems, but those who have severe and persistent mental illness, such as schizophrenia, are also at greater risk for becoming homeless. Men and women with chronic mental illnesses have a 25–50% chance of becoming homeless, particularly when there is a discontinuity of mental health support (Susser et al., 1997).

Susser and associates (1997) documented that homeless men with mental health problems who received intervention to establish networks of community support had fewer nights of homelessness than did those receiving standard mental health services. Over the course of the 18 months, the men who developed social supports maintained stability in housing and demonstrated a progressive decrease in episodes of homelessness. These findings highlight the value of community-based social ties in mitigating the risk of recurrent episodes of homelessness for men with mental illness. Promoting community connections and engagement in community activities by fostering habits related to community interaction is congruent with the occupational therapy goal of promoting healthy habits.

Kavanagh and Fares (1995) describe occupational therapy services for a woman who had depression, several episodes of homelessness, and a history of sexual abuse. Occupational therapy intervention focused on developing roles and habits that supported participation in the community. On the basis of the woman's interests and an activity analysis, the occupational therapist identified crafts that the woman could successfully complete. Previously fearful of participating in community activities, the woman was now able to attend a community fair and sell her crafts, reflecting her sense of self-efficacy—a belief that she could be successful.

Parents Who Are Homeless

Parents who are unable to provide a home for their children often experience stress, a sense of failure, loss of parental roles, and a decrease in overall family function (Thrasher & Mowbray, 1995). Living in an emergency shelter provides a family with needed housing but might not provide an environment in which a parent can exercise parental roles (Schultz-Krohn, 2004). When a family is faced with being homeless, the "structure and cohesion are severely tested by unremitting stressors and by pressing needs for basic survival" (Buckner et al., 1993, p. 385). A person's sense of self-efficacy and identity is threatened by being homeless. These combined stressors can significantly affect family functioning.

Shelter rules supersede parental authority and have been criticized as undermining the parental role of director and authority figure within the family structure. The need to perform basic child-care roles is often eliminated within the shelter (Schultz-Krohn, 2004). Meals are provided without parental input, chores are assigned by shelter staff without consulting parents, and daily routines are determined by the shelter schedule. During my study of the meaning of family routines in a homeless shelter, parents reported diminished parental authority and explained how the rules compromised their role as a parent. One parent explained, "It's not so much the rules, it's just the way it makes you feel, that you're under somebody, and you're not really the parent" (Schultz-Krohn, 2004, p. 537).

Stress, disintegration of parental roles, and conflict are related to a diminished sense of well-being in children (Vandewater & Lansford, 1998). Children who are homeless are more likely to display signs of depression,

ETHICAL DILEMMA

Maintaining Confidentiality: What Are the Risks?

You are providing occupational therapy services at a homeless shelter designed for families. A 27-year-old mother has just been reunited with her two children after completing a substance abuse program. Her children, ages 5 and 7, were both in foster care for the past year due to parental neglect. This woman, diagnosed with depression and substance abuse, has a history of being physically and sexually abused by multiple partners and receives no child support for either child. She completed her substance abuse program two months ago and became employed one month ago as a clerk at a department store. She is re-ceiving occupational therapy services to improve parenting skills, financial management, and decision-making skills. During an occupational therapy session, she reports that she went out for drinks with the other employees at work. The shelter requires that no alcohol or drugs be used while living at the shelter. Child Protective Services also stipulates that use of alcohol or drugs will result in the children being removed from the mother. She asks you not to tell anyone, and she promises that she will not go out drinking again. What do you do?

developmental delays, and physical health concerns when compared to children who live in low-income housing (Bassuk & Rosenberg, 1990). Killeen's (1993) research documents that children who felt that they performed well in the area deemed important by the parent rated their self-esteem at a higher level. Thus, helping parents to develop habits to provide specific praise for their children can support both parents and children.

To diminish the negative effects of homelessness, we developed interventions to support the interaction between parents and children. Parents were concerned about the lack of leisure and recreational activities they could engage in with their children. We acknowledged the parents' expertise and authority and explicitly identified parents as the directors of family activities. Those skills were built upon to support family interaction by providing an assortment of board games, toys, and activities that parents could use with their children. We discussed developmental play skills, and then the parents selected the toys, games, or activities that they deemed most appropriate for their children. The parents then identified the specific skill that would be praised when playing with their children. The parental skill of praising and supporting their children was fostered in the context of playtime. Follow-up sessions found parents engaging in more activities with their children and requesting additional toys, games, and activities to enhance parent-child interaction. By providing parents with guidance on how to identify behaviors they deemed important, how to provide systematic praise to their children, and how to choose activities that offer their children success, parents were better prepared to foster self-esteem and a positive self-concept in their children. The occupational therapy intervention helped parents to refine their skills of respond-ing to and controlling their children. Intervention supported the parental role, fostered positive parent-child interactions, and provided appropriate play and leisure activities for children of various ages.

Children Who Are Homeless

Occupational therapy intervention for children and adolescents may focus on fostering socioemotional developmental skills and other school-related skills (Drake, 1992; Zima, Bussing, Forness, & Benjamin, 1997). Children and adolescents who are homeless often experience disruptions in school attendance, frequent changes in schools, and a loss of school friendships, resulting in depression and anxiety manifested by poor frustration tolerance, limited decision-making skills, and poor task persistency (Zima et al., 1997, 1999). To address these needs, we provided intervention at the shelter to foster the children's engagement in activities and occupations with peers to enhance the skills needed to form and maintain friendships. For example, the environment was structured to support decision-making skills and cooperation with peers by offering a choice of cooperative activities, such as playing a board game or working on a collaborative craft project. The therapist and children discussed how a decision could be made fairly and with respect for everyone's feelings. Some children took on the role of explaining the group structure and rules to new members of the group, thereby demonstrating their sense of confidence. The structured and supported teaching, role modeling, and group facilitation provided by the occupational therapist promoted the children's acquisition and application of cooperative decision-making skills and peer relationships.

SUMMARY

Although the shelter where intervention was provided allows families to stay no longer than three months, during that brief period of time, families benefited from occupational therapy interventions designed to foster healthy habits and routines. Interventions were designed to meet the specific needs of individual clients, the parent-child dyad, and the family system. The use of affirming environments, support, and systematic encouragement facilitated self-efficacy and helped clients to develop important skills to fulfill their roles. Their skills were then practiced in various contexts to help clients develop better habits.

Many of the parents who participated in occupational therapy interventions at the shelter appreciated of the use of an affirming environment. Parents commented, "You make us feel good instead of like we don't know anything" and "You seem to really want us to succeed." Creating an environment that acknowledges a client's current skills and systematically supports the development of new skills is a foundation of occupational therapy practice. People who are homeless often face negative and demeaning situations, and occupational therapy can offer an alternative to these negative situations.

REFERENCES

Bassuk, E., & Rosenberg, L. (1990). Psychosocial characteristics of homeless children and children with homes. *Pediatrics, 85,* 257–261.

Buckner, J., Bassuk, E., & Zima, B. (1993). Mental health issues affecting homeless women: Implications for intervention. *American Journal of Orthopsychiatry, 63,* 385–399.

Davis, J., & Kutter, C. (1998). Independent living skills and posttraumatic stress disorder in women who are homeless: Implications for future practice. *American Journal of Occupational Therapy, 52,* 39–44.

DeOllos, I. (1997). *On becoming homeless: The shelterization process for homeless families.* Lanham, MD: University Press of America.

Drake, M. (1992). Level I fieldwork in a daycare for homeless children. *Occupational Therapy in Health Care, 8,* 215–223.

Dworsky, A., & Piliavin, I. (2000). Homeless spell exits and returns: Substantive and methodological elaborations on recent studies. *Social Science Review, 74,* 193–213.

Finlayson, M., Baker, M., Rodman, L., & Herzberg, G. (2002). The process and outcomes of a multimethod needs assessment at a homeless shelter. *American Journal of Occupational Therapy, 56,* 313–321.

Glasser, I., & Bridgman, R. (1999). *Braving the streets.* New York: Berghahn Books.

Kavaugh, J., & Fares, J. (1995). Using the Model of Human Occupation with homeless mentally ill clients. *British Journal of Occupational Therapy, 58,* 419–422.

Killeen, M. J. (1993). Parent influences on children's self-esteem in economically disadvantaged families. *Issues in Mental Health Nursing, 14,* 323–336.

McColl, M. A. (2002). Occupation in stressful times. *American Journal of Occupational Therapy, 56,* 350–353.

Rebeiro, K. L. (2001). Enabling occupation: The importance of an affirming environment. *Canadian Journal of Occupational Therapy, 68,* 80–89.

Rogers, J. (2000). Habits: Do we practice what we preach? *Occupational Therapy Journal of Research, Supplemental 2000, 20,* 119S–137S.

Rossi, P. (1990). The old homeless and new homelessness in historical perspective. *American Psychologist, 45,* 954–959.

Schultz-Krohn, W. (2004). The meaning of family routines in a homeless shelter. *American Journal of Occupational Therapy, 58,* 531–542.

Susser, E., Valencia, E., Conover, S., Felix, A., Tsai, W., & Wyatt, R. (1997). Preventing recurrent homelessness among mentally ill men: A "critical time" intervention after discharge from a shelter. *American Journal of Public Health, 87,* 256–262.

Thrasher, S., & Mowbray, C. (1995). A strengths perspective: An ethnographic study of homeless women with children. *Health & Social Work, 20,* 93–101.

Toro, P., Trickett, E., Wall, D., & Salem, D. (1991). Homelessness in the United States: An ecological perspective. *American Psychologist, 46,* 1208–1218.

Turner, S. M. (2004). *Homeless in America.* Farmington Hills, MI: Thomsen Learning.

Vandewater, E., & Lansford, J. (1998). Influences of family structure and parental conflict on children's well-being. *Family Relations, 47,* 323–330.

Zima, B., Bussing, R., Bystritsky, M., Widawski, M., Belin, T., & Benjamin, B. (1999). Psychosocial stressors among sheltered homeless children: Relationship to behavior problems and depressive symptoms. *American Journal of Orthopsychiatry, 69,* 127–133.

Zima, B., Bussing, R., Forness, S., & Benjamin, B. (1997). Sheltered homeless children: Their eligibility and unmet need for special education evaluations. *American Journal of Public Health, 87,* 236–240.

A Woodworker's Hand Injury: Restoring a Life

65

KAREN GARREN

It was a shock to hear that the father-in-law of a woman who worked in our building had cut his hand badly in a table saw. When he actually walked into the clinic, it was one of those moments when I could feel my heart sink. Don is a fine woodworker who built spectacular and complex crown moldings and built-ins in very upscale homes. He had indeed put his left hand through a table saw at work ten days earlier. I had just gotten a call from the hand surgeon upstairs telling me that he was sending Don down to be seen immediately for splinting and to start therapy. This doctor had not done the surgery; Don had been rushed to a hospital near where he worked some distance away and was operated on there by a plastic surgeon. The operative report was not available, but from what the doctor was able to ascertain, Don had lacerated his hand through his proximal palm and severed both flexor tendons to his long and ring fingers, amputated his small finger at the metacarpal phalangeal joint (MP), and lacerated the nerves to all his fingers. The doctor was not sure about the involvement to Don's thumb and index fingers. Don had arrived in his office bandaged and protected only by a wrist support with the fingers free to move at the proximal interphalangeal joints (PIPs). This was not good. I brought Don in immediately and told him not to move anything. He said that the doctor had just told him that but that the only thing he had been told at discharge from the hospital was to follow up in a week. He thought wiggling his fingers was good, since they were not immobilized.

There are critical elements to consider in dealing with a patient who has recently undergone reconstructive surgery of tendons and nerves. The first and foremost concern is to protect the repair and then ask questions. I knew enough history from the brief discussion with the referring surgeon to know that I needed to get Don into a protective splint as quickly as possible to reduce the tension on the tendon and nerve repairs and to stop any active motion of the repaired tendons (Culp & Taras, 2002; Duran & Houser, 1975). I also needed to assess the wound to determine the integument condition and, since no operative report was available, to visually assess the exact anatomical level of injury. At the same time, I needed to reassure Don that his zeal to get his fingers moving had probably not ruptured the repairs, since he assured me that he could wiggle them. I do not deceive patients, but informing Don of all of the possible ramifications at that point would only have distressed him, and I needed him to be focused on where we were going and what he was going to need to do. Once Don's hand was bandaged in a dry dressing and he was safely tucked into a dorsal blocking splint that positioned his wrist in 30 degrees of flexion, his MPs in 70 degrees of flexion, and his PIPs and distal phalangeal joints (DIPs) in as much extension as he could actively produce (the ideal is full extension, but he was already contracted, and applying any force could compromise the repairs), I could safely continue his evaluation. During this process, I was monitoring his reactions to the situation. It can be an extremely emotional time, and patients often have not even looked at their wounds. I keep ammonia capsules and facial tissues readily available. Don seemed to be coping by focusing on the process and asking questions.

The evaluation consisted of the following:

Subjective Examination

- Age, hand dominance
- Date and mechanism of injury
- Functional capability/work status
- Activities of daily living (ADL) status/help status
- Chief complaints: pain, loss of function, sensory changes, sleep problems
- Rehabilitation expectations/goals
- Medical management
- Awareness of pathology/precautions/contraindications/physician orders

Don was 58 years old at the time of the accident, right–handed, and married. He worked full time as a woodworker and loved his job. He wanted to return to his occupation as soon as it was possible to do so; he needed to be able to lift and carry wood supplies, hold tools and hardware, and stabilize wood with his left hand. He was unable to use his left hand for any self-care; however, over the previous week, he had become sufficiently proficient with his right hand alone to manage to dress, feed, bathe, and even drive himself. His wife managed the meals and household tasks. Initially, his chief complaints were loss of function, inability to move his hand, and numbness in all of his fingers. Don could not describe exactly how the accident had happened except that he was cutting wood on the table saw and it caught, pulling his hand down on the blade. This is a familiar story. The blade spins at an incredible speed, and when things go wrong, it is too fast to actually see or react. A table saw blade does not cut like a knife but consists of teeth that are a series of angled chisels that are an eight of an inch wide or more. It leaves a fairly wide slot when it cuts wood. The same happened to Don's hand. The blade had amputated his small finger and continued across his proximal palm in zone 3. When the tendons and nerves were cut, the result was that several millimeters of tissue were missing, as well as skin and thenar and hypothenar muscle. It follows that when the ends of the tendons and nerves were sutured together, the result was shortening of the structure, creating additional tension on the repair.

Objective Examination

- Integument
- Range of motion (ROM)
- Sensation
- Edema

To evaluate Don's hand, I needed to keep in mind the protocol that I would use to guide his physical recovery. There are multiple protocols to choose from, with extensive research supporting advantages and disadvantages. Pettengill (2005) has written a historical perspective on the research of tendon rehabilitation, with a comparison of the most recent early active motion protocols. My input is usually taken into consideration; however, it is the doctor who decides which protocol he or she wants to follow. The doctor who made this referral does not like to use any of the early active motion protocols because he thinks that research has shown that there a greater risk of rupture. In Don's case, it was not an option because his was not a clean and simple wound, we were not starting therapy three days after surgery, and we had no knowledge of what suturing technique had been used to repair the tendons. In fact, we were beginning at the tenth day, which is when research has demonstrated that the tendon tissue actually softens and is at the highest risk of rupture. The doctor was concerned about the amount of trauma and the significant amount of scarring and wanted to minimize adhesions, so I used the modified Duran protocol (Duran & Houser, 1975) to begin early passive flexion with restricted active extension of the fingers but held any active motion until the sixth week. With his wrist and MPs splinted in flexion and his interphalangeal joints (IPs) in extension, I taught Don to passively flex his fingers into his palm and actively extend his fingers as far as the splint would allow. This allowed a few millimeters of tendon excursion with minimal resistance on the repair and has been shown by research to reduce tendon adhesions. His hand was moderately swollen, and he was not able to fully flex his fingers to his palm. Don had multiple system trauma involving not only the tendons but also nerves, muscle, palmar fascia, and skin. I tested his sensation with the Semmes-Weinstein monofilaments (Bell-Krotoski, 2002) because I was not sure whether all the digital nerve branches were severed. The test revealed loss of protective sensation or complete numbness in the median and ulnar nerves to his index, long, and ring fingers.

Setting goals for Don's therapy ultimately centered on what Don wanted to accomplish. The doctor always pushes for a perfect physical outcome, and usually the patient is in agreement; however, returning the patient to his or her previous job is not automatically a goal. I often do not set a return-to-work goal in the initial evaluation when there is a traumatic injury, because it can be too early to determine what the patient wants and what the potential might be in terms of ability, time, and opportunity. Woodworking was Don's passion, not just his job. He had built something for each of his grandchildren, and he was anxious to build a rocking horse for his new grandchild.

For the next five weeks, the goals for Don were to understand the pathology, precautions, and home exercise program to increase his passive finger flexion; facilitate wound healing; and remodel scar to ensure necessary restoration of strength to the tendon tissues while safely allowing mobility through the adjacent tissues (Pettengill, 2002). The splint would not come off until the sixth week after surgery, so there could be no functional use of his hand. Don was diligent in his exercises and quickly recovered full passive finger flexion. The sutures were removed at 21 days with full skin closure. It was not until four weeks after his surgery that we finally got a copy of his original operative report revealing that there had been repair to his palmar arch, flexor pollicis longus to his thumb, and flexor digitorum superficialis (FDS) and flexor digitorum profundus (FDP) to his index finger, which had been only partially lacerated. The additional information helped me to anticipate what limitations there might be when the splint came off.

Don's treatment initially consisted of manual ROM, dressing changes, and, when the sutures were removed, moist heat, low-intensity ultrasound, and manual scar massage to increase the soft tissue extensibility and remodel the scar. His treatment was a team effort with Erin Leary (the other hand therapist in the clinic), Don, and me. This partnership required mutual attentiveness in order for Don's feelings, needs, and desires to become part of the common understanding between Don, Erin, and myself (Crepeau, 1991; Rosendahl & Ross, 1982; Tickle-Degnen, 2001).

Six weeks after surgery was the next major hurdle for Don. The splint came off, and he was allowed to move his fingers. It was hard to prepare Don for the disappointment that he felt when his fingers did not actively flex into a fist. His hope was beyond realistic expectation, but Don just wanted to move forward and do whatever it took to be able to use his hand again. He still had no sensation in his fingers.

ton his pants, hold a washcloth to bathe, and eventually hold tools to return to work. This required heat modalities; low-intensity 3-megahertz (3-MHz) ultrasound (Michlovitz, 2005); and manual therapy to facilitate healing, increase soft tissue mobility, and remodel scar. We used occupational coaching (Clark, Ennevor, & Richardson, 1996) to teach Don the skills and strategies he needed for attaining the mutually agreed-upon goals, and we created a therapeutic alliance in which we worked in the presence of one another. Erin and I served a supportive function while guiding Don in an occupation-based intervention (Tickle-Degnen, 2001). We taught Don sensory loss precautions so that he would not accidentally burn or cut himself. His home program was expanded to include paraffin and a mini-vibrator for scar remodeling and desensitization; however, he discovered that his hot tub water jets worked perfectly. Exercise and functional activities were initiated to increase his active motion and encourage grasp and pinch for pulling on clothes, holding utensils, and washing himself. He began desensitization for the scar and nerve hypersensitivity in his palm with particle immersion and vibration (Barber, 1990).

For the next six weeks, Don used the dexerciser, Chinese balls, pegboards, paper wadding, page turning, manipulating buttons, and pinching out beads in putty to regain active motion of his fingers. Experience guided the choice of these activities to promote tendon excursion through the very dense scar tissue in his palm and to train Don to begin to use his hand for light resistive functional activities. With this guided experience of how much pinch and grip force was safe, Don confidently began to try to use his hand safely at home for daily tasks. At ten weeks, the tendons had healed sufficiently to add resistance using the hand gripper to pick up checkers and the BTE (work simulator/exercise machine) to increase the force against the scar adhesions that limited tendon excursion. Sensation had begun to return in his distal palm, but his fingers remained numb.

AROM			
6 Weeks	**MP**	**PIP**	**DIP**
Index	0/60	−30/60	−10/30
Long	0/55	−30/45	−10/10
Ring	0/30	−35/45	−5/5
Thumb	−10/35		0/25
Wrist	25/60		

AROM			
10 Weeks	**MP**	**PIP**	**DIP**
Index	0/80	−20/100	−10/65
Long	0/80	−35/92	−15/45
Ring	0/30	−35/70	0/25
Thumb	−10/50		−20/75
Wrist	55/70		

His goals were to increase the active range of motion (AROM) of his fingers and wrist to pull up his pants, but-

His thumb index and long fingers progressed to full active flexion, but his ring finger had only 90 degrees of total motion. The loss of his small finger and severe limitation in active flexion of his ring finger due to adhesion of the FDP in his palm resulted in the syndrome of quadriga described by Verdan (1960), causing incomplete terminal flexion of his long and index fingers during grip. Don could not functionally grip a steering wheel or hold tools for work simulation. He was able to pinch and grip sufficiently to pull on clothes and bathe; however, buttoning and holding screws, boards, or nails were impaired by the sensory deficit.

At 12 weeks, the hand surgeon who had referred Don decided to take him back to surgery for a tenolysis or possible tendon repair, depending on what he found when he opened Don's hand, so we discharged him to a home exercise program until he returned from surgery.

Surgery revealed that the ulnar digital nerve to Don's ring finger was ruptured with a 2-cm defect between the proximal and distal ends. The proximal end of the digital nerve that had previously gone to his amputated small finger was in the immediate vicinity, so the surgeon connected that to the distal end of the ring finger ulnar digital nerve. On evaluation of the flexor tendons to the ring finger, it was discovered that both not only were extremely scarred down, but also were attached only by pseudotendons. After tenolysis of both tendons, it was decided to leave the FDS alone and excise the pseudotendon to the FDP. A primary repair to the FDP was successfully performed with minimal loss of tendon excursion.

Don was referred to therapy one week after surgery for evaluation and initiation of treatment. His original splint was modified to free his index finger and thumb, and his dressings were changed. Don was familiar with the Duran protocol and started passively ranging his long and ring fingers immediately. He required only one follow-up visit after the evaluation to achieve full passive range of motion (PROM) and was discharged to a home program until he came out of the splint to begin AROM. The biggest difference in the course of rehabilitation this time was that Don returned to work in a supervisory capacity as soon as the sutures were removed.

The doctor again decided to hold all active motion until the sixth week after surgery. Even though Don was ready this time for his finger not to move immediately, by the end of the first week of therapy, he was extremely frustrated and disappointed by the lack of progress. By the third week of therapy (nine weeks postoperative), Don was finally beginning to find it easier to do his self-care. Lack of sensation in the fingertips continued to be a problem, but Don was beginning to compensate. As patients progress through the healing process and therapy, they become more cognizant of their own physical and emotional capacity to return to previous occupations or accomplish their goals. Erin's and my goal at this juncture was to help Don begin to identify the problems that interfered with reentering or performing his occupation and to begin to plan possible solutions with him. Clark and colleagues (1996) identified this process as evoking insights in occupational storymaking. We chose many of the same activities to gain grip and pinch; however, we geared them as much as possible toward work using the nut and bolt board, pegs to simulate nails, and grasping of various-sized objects. Don had already learned how to use his hand safely for self-care tasks after the first surgery and expressed his desire to concentrate specifically on tasks that would restore function related to work,

At the tenth week, a dynamic PIP extension splint was added to reduce the flexion contracture in his ring finger and to mobilize the tendon distally through the scar adhesions (Pettengill, 2005). Don work relentlessly at home, gripping putty in an attempt to force the tendon through the thick scar, but there was still no appreciable difference in flexion, and Don was devastated. At 12 weeks, the repair site had developed enough tendon tissue growth through the anastomosis to almost eliminate the possibility of rupture. On the basis of our experience, we decided to use iontophoresis with dexamethasone to reduce the inflammation and adhesions around the healing tendon. Within one week, Don had increased his ring finger flexion and was able to flex to his central palm.

AROM			
12 Weeks (second surgery)	MP	PIP	DIP
Ring	WNL	−25/90	0/50

Don's therapeutic activities expanded to gripping tools and swinging a hammer into a pillow for controlled grip even though he was not left-handed. He began to notice a significant decrease in hypersensitivity in his palm and reported that he was picking up small pieces of wood at work with some success. At 15 weeks, he returned to full duty but was in a position to modify his activities when needed, lifting Sheetrock with his wrist instead of his fingers. At 18 weeks, he was discharged with 42 pounds of grip, 19 pounds of lateral pinch, and 12 pounds of three-point pinch; he was able to do his job and was working at home on his grandchild's rocking horse.

Over years of practice, I have learned to incorporate methods such as physical agent modalities, manual therapy techniques, and wound care into hand therapy. However, occupational therapy methods and philosophy have always been the foundation of my therapeutic approach. Helping clients to achieve occupational goals requires more than tissue healing and joint mobility. I have learned that recovery is a fabric woven from psychological, spiritual, and physical pain. Hand therapy is about restoring meaning in client's lives as well as restoring tissue function.

It has been a couple of years since Don left therapy, but he recently stopped by to drop off a *Fine Homebuild-*

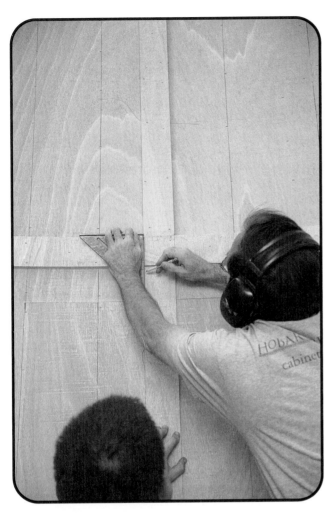

FIGURE 65.1   Don using a measuring triangle.

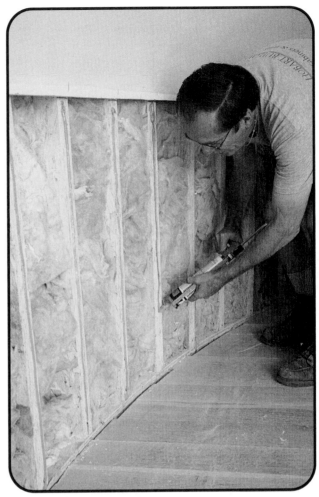

FIGURE 65.2   Don using a caulking gun.

ing magazine in which there were pictures of him building complicated wainscot on a curved stairwell. And there was his left hand holding a measuring triangle, holding a caulking gun, and supporting molding securely against the wall (Figures 65.1, 65.2, and 65.3).

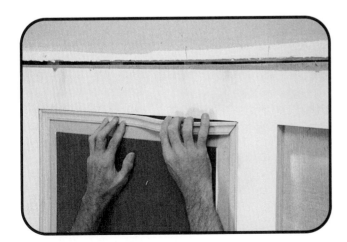

FIGURE 65.3   Don supporting molding against a wall.

REFERENCES

Barber, L. M. (1990). Desensitization of the traumatized hand. In J. Hunter, L. Schneider, E. Mackin, & A. Callahan (Eds.), *Rehabilitation of the hand* (3rd ed., pp 721–730). St. Louis: Mosby.

Bell-Krotoski, J. A. (2002). Sensibility testing with the Semmes-Weinstein monofilaments. In E. Mackin, A. Callahan, T. Skirven, L. Schneider, & A. Osterman (Eds.), *Rehabilitation of the hand and upper extremity* (5th ed., pp. 194–213). St. Louis: Mosby.

Clark, F., Ennevor, B. L., & Richardson, P. L. (1996). A grounded theory of techniques for occupational storytelling and occupational story making. In R. Zemke & F. Clark (Eds.), *Occupational science: The evolving discipline* (pp. 373–392). Philadelphia: F. A. Davis.

Crepeau, E. B. (1991). Achieving intersubjective understanding: Examples from an occupational therapy treatment session. *American Journal of Occupational Therapy, 45,* 1016–1025.

Culp, R. W., & Taras, J. S. (2002). Primary care of flexor tendon injuries. In E. Mackin, A. Callahan, T. Skirven, L. Schneider, & A. Osterman (Eds.), *Rehabilitation of the hand and upper extremity* (5th ed., pp. 415–430). St. Louis: Mosby.

Duran R, & Houser R. (1975). Controlled passive motion following flexor tendon repair in zones 2 and 3. In *AAOS Symposium on Tendon Surgery in the Hand* (pp. 105–114). St. Louis: Mosby.

Michlovitz, S. L. (2005). Is there a role for ultrasound and electrical stimulation following injury to tendon and nerve? *Journal of Hand Therapy, 18,* 292–296.

Pettengill, K. (2002). Therapist's management of the complex injury. In E. Mackin, A. Callahan, T. Skirven, L. Schneider, & A. Osterman (Eds.), *Rehabilitation of the hand and upper extremity* (5th ed., pp. 1411–1427). St. Louis: Mosby.

Pettengill, K. (2005). The evolution of early mobilization of the repaired flexor tendon. *Journal of Hand Therapy, 18,* 157–168.

Rosendahl, P. P., & Ross, V. (1982). Does your behavior affect your patient's response? *Journal of Gerontological Nursing, 8,* 572–575.

Tickle-Degnen, L. (2001). Therapeutic rapport. In C. A. Trombly & M. V. Radomski (Eds.), *Occupational therapy for physical dysfunction* (5th ed., pp. 299–311). Philadelphia: Lippincott Williams & Wilkins.

Verdan C. (1960). Syndrome of the quadriga. *Surgical Clinics of North America, 40,* 25–26.

"Mrs. W.": A Woman with Dementia

CORALIE "CORKY" GLANTZ

66

Throughout my career, I have worked with patients who have a wide variety of diagnoses. However, it is the people with dementia who have influenced me the most, personally and professionally. The work I have done with this patient population has enabled me to enhance my service delivery not only clinically but also as an educator and, more important, as an advocate. In every clinician's life, there are cases that are hard to forget. One case in particular that stands out in my mind is the work I did with a woman diagnosed with Alzheimer's disease. For this case study, she will be referred to as Mrs. W.

As you read my thoughts and memories about Mrs. W., you will recognize that a number of occupational therapy theorists and frames of reference have shaped my responses. First, I use the work of Mary Law (1998) and her colleagues in Canada for their well-developed materials on client-centered practice. Second, both the Person-Environment-Occupation Model (Law et al., 1996) and the Ecology of Human Performance (Dunn, Brown, & McGuigan, 1994) shape my emphasis on considering the person's engagement in occupations in specific contexts that either enable or handicap the person with dementia. In addition, I use research that supports the use of these frames of reference and practice models as well as the person-environment fit and quality of life for people with dementia, especially the works of Corcoran and Gitlin (1997); Davis, Hoppes, and Chesbro (2005); Dooley and Hinojosa (2004); Edelman, Fulton, and Kuhn (2004); Josephsson, Backman, Borell, Nygard, and Bernspang (1995); Nygard and Ohman (2002); Orange and Colton-Hudson (1998); and Painter (1997).

Mrs. W. was an attractive, beautifully dressed and groomed woman in her seventies who had lived her entire life in the Chicago area, although she had traveled extensively throughout the world. She had been married to the man who was described as her true love for 21 years when he suffered a heart attack and died suddenly at age 49. She remained single for the next 18 years before she married again to a doctor; her daughter described it as "a marriage of convenience." Her second husband died after 10 years of their marriage.

Mrs. W. had two children with her first husband, a boy and a girl who were 2.5 years apart in age. Her son died at age 54 of acute leukemia. The daughter married and had two children. She lived close to her mother and was quite attentive and devoted. The majority of information for the history portion of the initial evaluation was provided by Mrs. W.'s daughter. Mrs. W. was a very social person with an extensive list of close friends. She was a very giving person. Before her second marriage, she moved in with the son of her future husband in order to take care of three children after the son's wife was killed in an auto accident. Mrs. W.'s daughter indicated that Mrs. W. always made herself available to help whenever ever anyone was in need, especially her family and friends.

Mrs. W. was a wife and mother first and a homemaker second. She had not worked outside of the home since she was married. However, her time was filled with volunteer work and good deeds. Her hobbies and leisure activities included swimming and other sports; her daughter reported that Mrs. W. was an excellent athlete. It was also reported that she enjoyed reading, dancing, shopping, and some arts and crafts, including drawing and knitting. Her daughter also indicated that Mrs. W. had always loved children and spent a considerable amount of time with her grandchildren and taking care of other people's children.

I came to know Mrs. W. when she was residing in a small group home for people with dementia. Before that, she had lived in her own home, then an apartment, then a retirement home. Her daughter had instigated the moves. She felt that her mother's home was too large for her to handle and encouraged the move to the apartment. The apartment was closer to the daughter and also had a swimming pool in which her mother could swim every day. After a few years in the apartment, her daughter was concerned about her mother's memory difficulties and her safety. At this time, Mrs. W. could no longer manage her bills and her checkbook. Her daughter took her to a clinic, and her mother was diagnosed with Alzheimer's disease. Mrs. W. was aware of the diagnosis. Her daughter visited a retirement home with her mother and encouraged her to consider moving. Her mother agreed. The daughter indicated that the years when her mother lived in the retirement home went well until the other residents started to ostracize her. A number of uncomfortable situations occurred, for example, when she was playing bingo and she could not remember the numbers that were called. As a result, the other residents verbally expressed their annoyance with her. She gradually stopped participating in the activities at the retirement home and was concerned only with getting to her meals on time. She would get ready and wait hours before the dinner hour. Her daughter also reported that she would cut their excursions short because she wanted to go back to the retirement home so that she would not miss her meal. While they were on a trip together, the daughter realized that her mother was not always safe in her behavior. On one trip, her mother attempted to take a shower with scalding hot water. This and other incidents helped the daughter to make the decision to move her mother to a dementia-specific facility.

Mrs. W. was referred to occupational therapy by her physician, who had received a request by Mrs. W.'s daughter, who was concerned about her mother's decline. It was at this time that I met Mrs. W. in the small group home for people with dementia. She was socially appropriate for the initial evaluation and was able to do most of her own activities of daily living (ADLs) and some instrumental activities of daily living (IADLs) with cueing. She demonstrated difficulty with word finding, had delayed processing abilities, and had moderate immediate and short-term memory loss. She was aware of her surroundings and showed signs of sadness and depression related to her progressing disease. Her roles had changed considerably. She no longer was the helper of her friends and family, socialite, or active athlete. Her performance skills had changed; she could no longer take care of her own financial matters, take care of her home, or write letters and cards to her friends. Her motor skills were good; however, she did not have the opportunities to use them. She was able to verbalize her basic needs; however, her word-finding skills had notably declined in the past two months as reported by her daughter. Her processing skills were decreased, including her temporal organization, attention to tasks, ability to make adaptations, and ability to accommodate the method of task completion in response to a problem. Communication and interaction skills were significantly reduced, causing Mrs. W. a great deal of distress, since this was of major importance in her life.

On further evaluation, I recognized that the environment and the manner in which activities were presented caused Mrs. W. a great deal of stress. Because of her social appearance, staff often thought that she was capable of many activities that were too demanding for her. Her environment was not familiar and was quite cluttered. This caused her to have difficulty finding her way around the facility and finding things in her room. These problems appeared to complicate her daily functioning and to add to her depression, which was manifested by her starting to withdraw from the daily activities at the home. She appeared aware of the changes occurring in her life and showed signs of frustration, and as her frustrations mounted, she started to exhibit challenging behaviors. The staff reported that there were times when she would scratch them and try to bite. On further exploration, I found that the reported challenging behavior of scratching and attempted biting occurred when a male orderly was attempting to help her bathe.

I spoke with Mrs. W. and her daughter about their goals. We discussed the many strengths that Mrs. W. had and how we could use those strengths to help her to improve her situation and her quality of life in the facility. Strengths that were identified included her social awareness and enjoyment of being with other people, her love of music and dancing, her desire to be helpful and useful, her motivation to be independent, her desire to look good, caring about her clothes and jewelry, her good physical abilities, and her strong family relationships. Mrs. W. and her daughter identified their goals as (1) improving her ability to communicate with family, friends, and staff; (2) increasing her independence in ADLs and IADLs with minimum and appropriate assistance; (3) establishing a role of usefulness within the facility; (4) finding meaningful occupations that were within her abilities and did not cause frustration; and (5) participating in regular physical activity. Following are the goals as restated to make them client centered and measurable:

1. Mrs. W. will communicate her needs and thoughts to family, friends, and staff through a combination of words, gestures, and movements at least one time daily for five days.

2. Mrs. W. will increase her independence in ADLs and IADLs with minimum and appropriate assistance.
   a. She will choose her clothing and put on her own underwear and blouse and skirt or dress in the proper order with one verbal cue three mornings in succession.
   b. She will put on appropriate makeup and jewelry independently three days in one week.
   c. She will make her own bed and put clothes in the hamper or away in the closet three days in one week with minimum verbal cueing.
   d. She will safely shower independently after being escorted to the shower by a female aide two times in one week.

3. Mrs. W. will participate in helpful facility household chores of her choice two times a week for two weeks in succession.

4. Mrs. W. will participate in meaningful occupations that are within her abilities and do not cause frustration.
   a. She will have the opportunity to go shopping one time a week.
   b. She will have success in completing a craft or activity of her choice that has been broken down into appropriate steps.

5. Mrs. W. will participate in a teacher/leader role in a physical activity three times a week for three weeks.

To develop my intervention plan, I synthesized the information I had obtained from Mrs. W.'s occupational profile and the analysis of her occupational performance to focus on the specific areas of occupation and on their internal (personal and spiritual), external (physical setting, social, and virtual), and cultural contexts (American Occupational Therapy Association, 2002) that needed to be addressed. My intervention focused on the goals identified by Mrs. W. and her daughter. After analyzing Mrs. W.'s problems, strengths, and goals, I decided to focus my interventions on her ADLs and IADLs and the context in which they were being done, on her performance skills and performance patterns in relation to her roles within the facility and with her family, and on her nonverbal communication skills with family and staff of the facility.

Because Mrs. W.'s engagement in the occupation of self-care was being limited by the clutter in her room, I worked with Mrs. W., her daughter, and the facility staff in removing the clutter and organizing the room so that the necessary objects were placed within eye line of the task to be done and in the correct order. Dresser drawers were marked with line drawings and one-word descriptions of what was in them. and the clothes that she was to put on each day were hung on one hanger in the order in which she should put them on. The closet was cleared of all but a couple of favorite outfits. Jewelry was minimized to the pieces she could independently take on and off.

We also worked on grooming and bathing skills. Although Mrs. W. had to be escorted to the shower room, we worked on her being able to safely take a shower in privacy with the shower curtain closed. She was to be escorted to the shower only by a female caregiver. Because grooming, including putting on makeup, was important to her, we set up a dressing table with a seat and mirror and her necessary makeup and hair products. This setup was familiar to her, and it pleased her. Her caregiver was instructed on how to cue Mrs. W. only when necessary. In doing this, we were able to reestablish the performance skills and performance patterns in a morning routine that had been familiar to her in the past. We did have to modify the daily routine of the facility to support her cognitive abilities. We did this by allowing increased morning grooming time to compensate for her slowed processing abilities and permitting her to have a late light breakfast.

IADLs and home care had been a prevalent occupation in Mrs. W.'s life. I worked on these skills with Mrs. W. while I instructed staff in how to break the tasks down to manageable steps. Mrs. W. was then able to make her bed and clean her own room. She was also able to participate in useful tasks in the facility, such as cooking activities, setting the tables, dusting, and folding towels and linen. She was encouraged to help the staff and other residents.

Engagement in the occupation of dancing and other physical activities was another goal that we addressed. I worked with the activity director to establish a dancing class in which Mrs. W. could be not only a participant but also a leader/teacher. Mrs. W. had a wonderful sense of rhythm and retained the ability to do many dance steps. This became one of Mrs. W.'s primary roles in the facility community, and she was recognized for her abilities and for helping others to participate in an enjoyable occupation.

The final and most difficult goal that we needed to tackle dealt with communication. Because Mrs. W.'s verbal communication skills continued to decline, I referred her to speech therapy and began working with the staff and Mrs. W. on her nonverbal communication. I was surprised to find that many of the staff members did not recognize nonverbal signs of communication. Mrs. W. had exhibited very distinct and consistent signs for her most common needs, such as rubbing her stomach or a specific body part if she had pain, grimacing when she had to go to the washroom, closing her eyes or looking at the floor when she was bored or was displeased with what was happening, turning her head away when she did not want to do something, and smiling when she was pleased or wanted to do something.

A great deal of my intervention utilized therapeutic use of self (Punwar & Peloquin, 2000) and therapeutic use of occupations and activities through occupation-based activity, purposeful activity, and preparatory activity, consistent with the Occupational Therapy Practice Framework (AOTA, 2002). We collaboratively addressed all the goals set by Mrs. W., her daughter, and myself. Her participation and independence in her ADL and IADL function improved, her active engagement in occupation increased, she established roles of usefulness within the facility, and she participated in physical activities on a regular basis.

In the process of developing Mrs. W.'s occupational profile, synthesizing the information, and developing a treatment plan, I used my knowledge, critical reasoning, interpersonal abilities, performance skills, and ethical reasoning (AOTA, 2005):

- Knowledge included the integration of relevant evidence and literature on treatment of people with dementia. This included knowledge of the impact of occupational roles, habits, and routines on the day-to-day performance and well-being of older adults; the importance of involving family and caregivers; the aging process and its impact on visual, perceptual, sensory, and physical systems; normative life events, including life transitions and their impact on the older adult's occupational performance, health, and well-being; and team-building theory and teamwork models.

- The judgments and decisions I made in developing a treatment plan and in treating Mrs. W. required me to use deductive and inductive reasoning. I had to analyze Mrs. W.'s current occupational performance and how it was influenced by the context of living in the facility. Problem solving was then used to develop appropriate roles for Mrs. W. that would use her strengths (social awareness, enjoyment of being with other people, and love of music and dancing) to satisfy her need to be useful and helpful and her need for more physical exercise. Mrs. W. successfully became a leader/teacher in the facility's weekly dance program and appeared to thoroughly enjoy this new role.

- Interpersonal abilities were used in development of my professional relationships with the facility staff, Mrs. W.'s daughter, and Mrs. W. We were able to develop and sustain a team relationship to meet Mrs. W.'s goals. I received feedback from them and communicated instruction and suggestions to them regarding task segmentation, room organization, altering facility schedule to allow time for grooming activities, and nonverbal communication techniques.

- The therapeutic performance skills that I used were grounded in the core of occupational therapy; the therapeutic use of self, the therapeutic use of occupations and activities, the consultation process with family and staff, and the education process used in training staff to bring about the desired changes in Mrs. W.'s quality of life in the facility.

- Ethical reasoning was used in dealing with Mrs. W.'s grooming and bathing issues. I had to consider staff's concerns about Mrs. W.'s safety versus her rights, dignity, and desire to have privacy while taking her shower. There was also a safety issue with her mirror and makeup items and her right and desire to use these items. Mrs. W. has not presented with a challenging behavior since the changes in her bathing and grooming have occurred.

I discharged Mrs. W. from therapy after seeing her three times a week for three weeks. I had evaluated how multiple events, life transitions, and contexts had affected Mrs. W.'s occupational roles and determined optimal occupational therapy interventions, which facilitated positive outcomes in occupational performance and participation in her community within the facility.

I was called back into the facility to see Mrs. W. two years later. She had adjusted well to the facility life and was an active participant in the facility community. However, her daughter once again recognized a marked decline in her ADL abilities, her memory, and her ability to follow verbal instructions and an increase in challenging behaviors. Mrs. W.'s daughter realized that this was part of the disease progression; however, she requested occupational therapy to evaluate and determine whether anything would help to maintain her mother's abilities for a while. The physician agreed and ordered occupational therapy evaluation and two weeks of treatment. Once again, I was able to work with Mrs. W., her daughter, and the facility staff. We were able to make some adjustments in her room environment to give more cues. For example, the door of her bathroom was changed to a curtain, and receptacles that she had used as a toilet, such as the wastepaper basket, were removed. The staff were also instructed on backward chaining so that Mrs. W. still could participate in self-care activities that we altered to decrease memory demands so that she could still achieve success. We increased the use of demonstration and hand-over-hand instructions and the use of line drawings for identification of items and places, and we explored antecedents to her challenging behaviors and instructed staff to avoid the antecedents.

Mrs. W. remained an active participant in her ADLs and in some of the facility activities until about two weeks before her death. Her daughter informed me that the staff had continued to follow my suggestions and thereby had avoided precipitating Mrs. W.'s challenging behaviors. Mrs. W.'s daughter expressed her thanks and felt that occupational therapy had made a tremendous difference in her mother's transition into the facility, had helped her to make the adjustment to the facility, and thereby had improved the quality of the last years of her life.

I have learned so much from working with older adults and especially with people with dementia. Too often, I observe staff that see diseases or disabilities and do not see the person. Older adults, including people with dementia, have many strengths and abilities. They are people with wonderful knowledge and experiences, and they are people who have lived many years and have so much to give to those around them. Because I believe that they are often misunderstood, I have become active in educating staff, families, and community groups in understanding dementia. There are many ways in which therapists can help to advocate for the people and populations with whom they work. Over the years that I have been working with older adults and people with dementia, I have been involved with legislation, participating in local, state, and federal panels and consultant groups; holding workshops for facility staff and for therapists; doing presentations for local, state, and national conferences and organizations; presenting to families and seniors; and writing articles and manuals. I volunteered to do in-services and presentations. I suggested to the facilities where I was working that I would do a presentations for families and their community. I volunteered to be part of panels, and I contacted the people involved with doing the draft legislation or the studies. Being an advocate does take time, and your time is not necessarily reimbursed. However, it can bring you countless rewards. It can help you to market yourself and your profession as having knowledge in the practice area. Advocacy can also make a tremendous difference for people or populations. I pursued and participated, and I still pursue and participate. We are all busy, but we make time for what we consider important. I consider advocacy important. It has been important to me personally and professionally, and I have learned so much from doing it. It has also helped to build my practice by establishing my credibility as knowledgeable in the area of practice.

From the feedback I received from Mrs. W.'s daughter, occupational therapy enhanced the quality of Mrs. W.'s life. My experiences with Mrs. W. and other people with dementia have enhanced both my personal life and my professional outlook. These people have given me a greater understanding of how the quality of a person's life can be improved throughout the life course with appropriate intervention. I have also learned that my knowledge base can improve the quality of life for many elderly patients, not only through direct intervention but also through education of fellow clinicians and caregivers and through advocacy work. I encourage clinicians to develop a professional niche, continually increase your knowledge base, and put that knowledge base to work.

REFERENCES

American Occupational Therapy Association. (2002). Occupational Therapy Practice Framework: Domain and process. *American Journal of Occupational Therapy, 56*(6), 609–639.

Hinojosa, J., Bowen, R., Case-Smith, J., Epstein, C., Schwope, C., Moyers, P., Manoly, B., Rowley, G., (1999) *American Journal of Occupational Therapy, 53,* 599–600. Standards for continuing competence.

Corcoran, M. A., & Gitlin, L. N. (1997). *Home environmental modifications for individuals with Alzheimer's disease* (p. 149). Bethesda, MD: American Occupational Therapy Association.

Davis, L. A., Hoppes, S., & Chesbro, S. B. (2005). Cognitive-communicative and independent living skills assessment in individuals with dementia: A pilot study of environmental impact. *Topics in Geriatric Rehabilitation, 21*(2), 136–143.

Dooley, N. R., & Hinojosa, J. (2004). Improving quality of life for persons with Alzheimer's disease and their family caregivers: Brief occupational therapy intervention. *The American Journal of Occupational Therapy, 58*(5), 561–569.

Dunn, W., Brown, C., & McGuigan, A. (1994). The Ecology of Human Performance: A framework for considering the effect of context. *The American Journal of Occupational Therapy, 48*(7), 595–607.

Edelman, P., Fulton, B. R., & Kuhn, D. (2004). Comparison of dementia-specific quality of life measures in adult day centers. *Home Health Care Services Quarterly, 23*(1), 25–42.

Josephsson, S., Backman, L., Borell, L., Nygard, L., & Bernspang, B. (1995). Effectiveness of an intervention to improve occupational performance in dementia. *The Occupational Therapy Journal of Research, 15*(1), 36–49.

Law, M. (1998) *Client-centered occupational therapy.* Thorofare, NJ: Slack.

Law, M., Cooper, B., Strong, S., Stewart, D., Rigby, P., & Letts, L. (1996). The Person-Environment-Occupation Model: A transactive approach to occupational performance. *The Canadian Journal of Occupational Therapy, 63*(1), 9–23.

Nygard, L., & Ohman, A. (2002). Managing changes in everyday occupations: The experience of persons with Alzheimer's disease. *OTJR: Occupation, Participation, and Health, 22*(2), 70–81.

Orange, J. B., & Colton-Hudson, A. (1998). Enhancing communication in dementia of the Alzheimer's type. *Topics in Geriatric Rehabilitation, 14*(2), 56–75.

Painter, J. (1997). *Environmental considerations for persons with dementia of Alzheimer's type* (p. 167). Bethesda, MD: American Occupational Therapy Association.

Punwar, A. J., & Peloquin, S. M. (2000). *Occupational Therapy: Principles and practice* (3rd ed.). Baltimore: Lippincott, Williams, & Wilkins.

XIV

MANAGING PRACTICE

" In turbulent times, an enterprise has to be managed *both* to withstand sudden blows and to avail itself of sudden unexpected opportunities. This means that, in turbulent times, the fundamentals have to be managed and managed well. "

Peter F. Drucker

Management of Occupational Therapy Services

67

BRENT BRAVEMAN

Learning Objectives

After reading this chapter, you will be able to:

1. Explain the relationship and differences between administrators, managers, and supervisors in oversight of work activities in organizations.
2. Identify and give examples of the common roles, functions, and responsibilities of managers.
3. Identify and explain the areas of knowledge and skills necessary for a manager to demonstrate competency.

MANAGERS, ADMINISTRATORS, AND SUPERVISORS

One may assume a variety of professional roles over the course of a career as a practitioner. One such role is that of an *occupational therapy manager*. Management as a function of organizations and the process of managing has been the focus of considerable theory, research, publication, and other scholarly forms addressed by investigators and practitioners in a variety of fields. Consequently, many resources to guide managers in their jobs are readily available on the Internet, in bookstores, and through educational courses offered at colleges and universities or at continuing education events, such as professional conferences.

Learning to be an effective occupational therapy manager is a complicated and time-intensive process that is far beyond the scope of any single chapter or text. Therefore, this chapter will focus on helping the reader to become familiar with what an occupational therapy manager *is* and what an occupational therapy manager *does*. Chapter 69 provides a complementary discussion that focuses on supervision and the roles and functions that occupational therapy supervisors perform.

CHRISTOPHER MANAGES PRODUCTIVITY

Christopher is a new manager of an occupational therapy department in a moderate-sized community hospital who supervises eight occupational therapists and two occupational therapy assistants. His staff provides services to clients and patients across the life course who have a wide range of diagnoses, conditions, and challenges to occupational participation. Like many hospitals, the one in which Christopher is employed is facing financial challenges due to lower rates of reimbursement from the state Medicaid system, increased discounts on care provided to patients participating in managed care, and ongoing losses due to noncompensated care.

As a midlevel manager, Christopher has come under increasing pressure to raise the rates of productivity in his department and to provide less intensive service to patients such as those with Medicare for whom the hospital receives a set rate of reimbursement while achieving the same outcomes. He recognizes the challenges faced by the organization and is honestly committed to doing what he can to ensure the provision of quality care while maximizing reimbursement and minimizing costs. However, Christopher has become quite frustrated by limitations that he perceives as obstacles to making changes to have positive outcomes. There is a wide variation in the performance level of his staff, and he feels that one staff member in particular is unable to meet basic requirements for productivity despite numerous supervisory interventions. Further, Christopher questions this staff member's level of clinical competence and is concerned about patient safety. Yet Christopher has received little support from his boss or from human resources to move toward terminating this employee's

employment and has even, because of hospital policy, felt pressured to give the employee a recent raise that Christopher did not feel accurately reflected the employee's performance.

Christopher is also experiencing other frustrations, including the lack of a comprehensive set of policies and procedures to guide the work of the staff he supervises and the lack of any formal mechanism by which he can assess and document the level of competence of his staff. He is concerned that he does not have all the knowledge and skills he needs to manage the department's budget successfully. Finally, he recognizes that some of the processes and systems that are used in his department seem inefficient, frequently result in errors and rework, and lead to confusion among his staff, but he is unsure how to address these problems in an organized and strategic manner.

Questions

As you read this chapter, consider Christopher's situation and ask yourself the following questions:

1. Does Christopher appear to have the necessary authority required to manage his department and to be held responsible for the outcomes?
2. What types of managerial knowledge and skills does Christopher need to develop to help him confront the challenges he is facing?
3. How might Christopher consider the traditionally identified management functions of planning, organizing, directing, and controlling to begin to logically confront the challenges described?

Understanding the roles and functions of an occupational therapy manager requires that one consider the role of the manager in relation to administrators and supervisors. Table 67.1 provides definitions of **administration**, **management**, and **supervision**. An administrator may be defined as a member of a *governing body,* such as a Board of Directors of an organization; the top officials, such as the President or Chief Executive Officer of an organization; or that official's leadership team. Together, administrators are responsible for the overall welfare of the organization. Administrators may supervise others but often are only indirectly responsible for the oversight of the work of the organization. They frequently delegate authority for

much of the day-to-day coordination of organizational functioning to managers.

Managers are responsible for oversight of work units, such as occupational therapy departments, and of their contributions to the organization's mission. In addition to other roles and functions, managers often supervise others, but not all supervisors are managers. Supervisors contribute to meeting the mission of the organization by overseeing the daily work of front line employees.

Understanding the important concepts of **requisite managerial authority** and **power** can help us to further clarify how an occupational therapy manager is different from an organizational administrator or from an

TABLE 67.1	ADMINISTRATION, MANAGEMENT, AND SUPERVISION DEFINED
Administration	The process of guiding an organization through the authoritative control of others completed by the governing body of the organization
Management	The process of guiding a work unit by planning for future work obligations, organizing employees into functional units, directing employees in the process of completing daily work tasks, and controlling work processes and systems to assure adequate quality of work output
Supervision	The process of guiding an organization through the authoritative control of others completed by the governing body of the organization

occupational therapy supervisor. Elliot Jaques (1998) defined requisite managerial authority as "the level of control and discretion that a manager must have to be fairly held responsible for the outcomes of work groups." For example, requisite managerial authority includes the authority to hire and fire employees and to determine within reason how rewards are distributed. However, in occupational therapy, it is not uncommon for a therapist to accept a formally named position within an organization in which he or she has supervisory responsibilities but does not have requisite managerial authority. An example of such a position would be that of a *senior therapist,* an individual who might have specialized or advanced skills and who might provide clinical supervision to other therapists but who does not have the full range of managerial responsibilities.

THE FOUR TRADITIONAL MANAGERIAL FUNCTIONS

One common approach to categorizing the responsibilities of managers within an organization is to group them according to four major functions: **planning**, **organizing** (and staffing), **directing**, and **controlling**. Staffing is sometimes identified as a separate function but is often included as part of the organizing function. These functions are briefly defined and further discussed in the next sections of this chapter.

Some commonly identified functions of management are as follows:

◆ **Planning:** the process of deciding what to do by setting performance objectives and identifying the activities that need to be carried out to accomplish these objectives
◆ **Organizing and staffing:** designing workable units, determining lines of authority and communication, and developing and managing patterns of coordination
◆ **Directing:** providing guidance and leadership so that the work that is performed is congruent with goals
◆ **Controlling:** establishing performance standards, measuring, evaluating, and correcting performance

Administrators, managers, and supervisors all perform various tasks related to these four functions, but the scope of these tasks varies for the different levels of leadership. Table 67.2 provides a comparison of sample functions of administrators, managers, and supervisors organized according to the traditional four functions of management.

Planning

Planning is the process of establishing short- and long-term goals, measurable objectives, and action plans that are both congruent with the mission of the organization and consistent with the vision that current organizational leaders have established. An organization's mission is typically established by its founders and remains relatively stable. It is often expressed in the form of a mission statement that sets forth the organization's purpose, products, and services. A vision statement, by contrast, expresses an inspirational message about what a department or organization would like to become as it seeks to fulfill its mission (Hoyle, 1995).

It is common to distinguish between strategic, or long-range, planning and planning as a day-to-day management function. Strategic planning is the process of determining the long-term goals of an organization and formulating strategies to accomplish these goals (Liebler & McConnell, 2004). Goals are a reflection of the scope of the desired outcomes. Objectives are measurable steps that are taken to reach these goals. While a strategic plan may identify goals that are intended to be achieved over a three- to five-year (or longer) period of time, objectives that managers identify often are based on a one-year period that corresponds with an organization's financial cycle, or fiscal year.

Over the last several decades, strategic planning has moved in and out of favor as organizations have struggled to keep up with the frenetic pace of changes in technology, public policy, and the global economy. Operating in an environment in which change is the norm may force long-term planning, especially the related processes of mission review and visioning, to become more important (Braveman, 2006a). Because the environments in which most organizations function are constantly changing,

TABLE 67.2 COMPARISONS OF SAMPLE FUNCTIONS OF ADMINISTRATORS, MANAGERS, AND SUPERVISORS

Management Function	Organizational Administration	Occupational Therapy Managers	Occupational Therapy Supervisors
Planning	◆ Establishment of organizational mission and vision ◆ Creation of an organizational culture ◆ Strategic planning ◆ Financial forecasting ◆ Establishing organization policies and procedures	◆ Interpreting the organizational mission and vision for the staff ◆ Aligning the departmental mission and vision with the organizational mission and vision ◆ Establishing departmental objectives ◆ Creating and implementing the departmental budget ◆ Establishing departmental policies and procedures	◆ Integration of the mission and vision of the organization and department in the daily work of the department and staff ◆ Oversight of work tasks related to achievement of departmental objectives ◆ Ensuring that work is completed effectively and efficiently
Organizing and staffing	◆ Oversight of the organizational chart and determination of primary organizational structure ◆ Establishing systems for staff functions such as human resources and marketing*	◆ Recruiting, hiring, orienting, and training staff ◆ Appraising performance, determining rewards, and overseeing disciplinary actions	◆ Providing management with feedback related to the appropriateness of staffing levels ◆ Provide daily supervision, coaching, and feedback to line staff
Directing	◆ Development of parameters for staff training, education, and development ◆ Mentoring and coaching middle managers	◆ Mentoring and coaching supervisors ◆ Implementing staff training, education, and development programs	
Controlling	◆ Establishing systems to measure organizational performance and achievement of key organizational goals ◆ Setting expectations for performance for management	◆ Oversight and implementation of departmental continuous quality improvement and quality control systems ◆ Establishing performance expectations and measures for department functions and outputs	◆ Ensuring compliance with policies and procedures ◆ Measuring and recording quality indicators ◆ Alerting management to systems problems

Source: Adapted from Lyles, R. I., & Joiner, C. (1986). *Supervision in health care organizations.* New York: John Wiley & Sons.

*Staff functions relate to the overall maintenance and management of an organization (e.g., human resources, housekeeping, or marketing). Line functions relate to carrying out the primary work of the organization (e.g., occupational therapy, physical therapy, or social work in medically oriented organizations).

managers can spend a great deal of their time planning for change, employing change management strategies, and helping others to adjust to new conditions.

The scholarship on change management has focused on four principal aspects: (1) theoretical models and frameworks that reveal and guide organization members' and researchers' thinking about organization change, (2) approaches and tools for creating and managing change, (3) factors that are important to successful change management, and (4) outcomes and consequences of the process of change management (Branch, 2002). It is strongly recommended that new managers become familiar with theories of change and strategies for promoting successful change. For example, Kurt Lewin proposed a prominent and relatively simple approach to understanding change that includes three stages (Figure 67.1) (Lewin, 1997). These three stages are (1) unfreezing or recognizing the need to change, (2) changing, and (3) refreezing

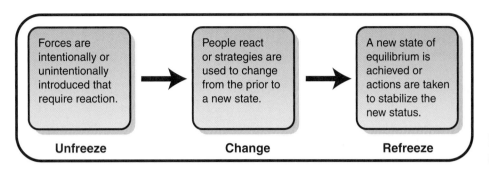

FIGURE 67.1   Lewin's three-stage model of change

or standardizing new procedures or ways of behaving. Managers can apply this theory by identifying different strategies to use with employees during each of the three stages to facilitate the change process.

In addition to establishing goals and objectives, planning includes determining the needs for the human resources, materials, supplies, facilities, and equipment required to meet goals and objectives. Both the financial planning that is involved in developing and managing a department budget and the writing of policies and procedures that guide the use of materials, supplies, facilities, and equipment and that guide staff in daily activities are also commonly considered components of planning. Another example of planning in which an occupational therapy manager might become involved is facilities planning. Planning new therapeutic spaces can be extraordinarily complex and should not be undertaken without consultation with others who have previously been through the process and should definitely not be attempted without a qualified construction team that is experienced in the design of clinical or therapeutic spaces.

Organizing and Staffing

Ideally, administrators and managers determine the structure of an organization and its departments. The structure of an organization or a department can vary in complexity. Many organizations that have existed for some time have undergone numerous restructurings that were intended to improve efficiency and effectiveness and, often, to reduce costs. These restructurings might have been planned and executed in a logical manner, or they might have happened without an overall plan as the organization grew, added new services, or had to respond to environmental influences. An organizational chart helps to facilitate understanding of an organization's structure. Liebler, Levine & Rothman (1992) described an organizational chart as a management tool that visually depicts the following aspects of an organization:

◆ Major functions, usually by department
◆ Relationships of functions or departments
◆ Channels of supervision
◆ Lines of authority and of communication
◆ Positions by job title within departments or units

When one examines an organizational chart, one must keep in mind that it is a static picture of the organization or department. It might not reflect recent changes, vacancies, or informal relationships, since written charts typically indicate only formal lines of command. The organizational chart of many large organizations support the notion that systems are often quite organic in how they grow and are restructured over time.

Although few large organizations fit the perfect theoretical profile of any formal organizational form or structure, there are a few basic structures commonly found in health care and service organizations and systems that are useful for a new manager or practitioner to understand. These structures include the dual-pyramid form of organizing: product line or service line organizations, and hybrid or matrix organizations.

The term *dual-pyramid* has been used to describe the common structure found in many medical model settings, such as acute and general hospitals. The pyramid structure is also commonly found in community-based organizations, although the second pyramid representing medical staff might be absent in these cases. A pyramid is typically used to represent an organization of personnel with upper management at the top and line staff at the bottom (Figure 67.2).

In the dual-pyramid form of organizing, the traditional relationship between medical staff and administration results in the structure shown in Figure 67.2, in which two supervisory pyramids are arranged side by side. One pyramid represents the structure of the professional staff that is organized in departments, including administration (with the chief executive officer at the top of the pyramid); allied health professionals such as occupational therapy, physical therapy and social work; and all support services such as engineering, housekeeping, and human resource personnel. A second pyramid mimics that structure but represents the organization of the medical staff with the chief medical officer at the top of the pyramid, department heads as middle management, and staff physicians as line employees (Braveman, 2006a). Although the medical staff, professional staff, and support staff all ultimately report to a board of trustees or board of directors, there are two distinct chains of command that result in the authority and accountability systems being separated on the basis of function within the organization.

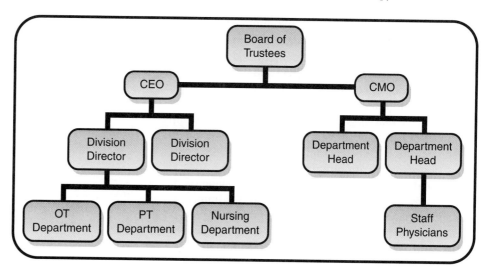

FIGURE 67.2 A sample dual-pyramid form of organizing. Source: Reprinted with permission from Braveman (2005). *Leading and managing occupational therapy services: An evidence-based approach.* Philadelphia: F. A. Davis.

A second common form of organizational structure is the *product line,* or *service line,* structure. In a product line structure, personnel are organized according to the service or product that they provide rather than according to the specific function that they complete or their departments based on education or training. A board of directors maintains ultimate authority, and the chief executive officer and chief medical officer often still maintain parallel but distinct responsibilities and authority. An example of the organizational chart for a product line form is provided in Figure 67.3.

Additional ways of structuring organizations may combine elements of the two structures described above; however, the dual-pyramid and product line structures are the most common.

Each of the methods of organization has advantages and disadvantages, and understanding how structure influences the function of an organization can help one to capitalize on the system's benefits and compensate for its limitations. For example, health care organizations that have a dual-pyramid structure rely on departments structured by discipline or professional education and training to provide for strong supervision of staff and their clinical performance. Thus, communication within a professional discipline is facilitated, and the daily work of a unit may be completed more efficiently. Because a department manager or supervisor representing each discipline has direct access to staff and to the data related to routine processes and interventions, continuous quality improvement and outcome measurement of using these data are

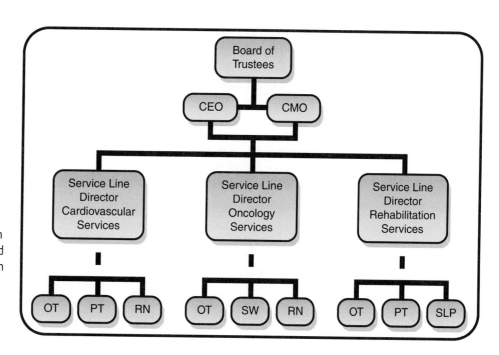

FIGURE 67.3 A sample product line management form of organizing. Source: Reprinted with permission from Braveman (2005). *Leading and managing occupational therapy services: An evidence-based approach.* Philadelphia: F. A. Davis.

also easier to measure in a dual-pyramid organization. Nonetheless, in this form of organizing, communication across disciplines might be more complicated, which can pose potential hazards for developing and managing new programs. Problem solving and process improvement in existing programming can be cumbersome when staff members feel that it is necessary to communicate up through the chains of command. The advantages and disadvantages of the dual-pyramid and the product line forms of organizing are summarized in Table 67.3.

Once decisions have been made about how an organization or a department is to be structured, administrators and managers ideally work together to develop plans for staffing and human resources management. Functions related to staffing, such as advertising or the development of policies and procedures related to employment, may be performed by a human resources department. Occupational therapy managers are frequently involved in a number of other staffing-related activities. A sample list of these activities is as follows:

- Human resources planning: collaborating with administrators and supervisors at all levels of the organization to forecast the short- and long-term personnel needs of the organization, based on the organizational mission, leadership vision, and strategic plans
- Recruitment: seeking out and attracting adequate numbers of qualified personnel to meet ongoing organizational needs, including contingencies, such as resignations and leaves of absence
- Hiring: selecting the appropriate personnel for vacant positions and associated activities, such as benefits counseling, background, and reference checks
- Orientation: introducing the new employee to organizational policies, procedures, values, personnel, and environments

TABLE 67.3 ADVANTAGES AND DISADVANTAGES OF COMMON FORMS OF ORGANIZING

	Dual Pyramid	Product Line
Communication	- Communication within a discipline is facilitated.	- Communication between disciplines becomes harder.
Planning	- Planning for activities such as professional development and clinical supervision is facilitated, but program planning becomes harder.	- Program planning and planning for interdisciplinary activities such as program evaluation is facilitated, but planning functions within disciplines becomes harder.
Budgeting	- Tracking and planning for finances related to single discipline costs are facilitated, but tracking and planning for interdisciplinary activities (e.g., cost per unit of care) are harder.	- Tracking and planning for finances related to programmatic costs are facilitated, (e.g., cost per unit of care) but tracking and planning for discipline-specific activities are harder.
Staffing	- Some needs such as providing coverage for leaves or vacancies may be easier, but the need to communicate with other managers increases. Recruitment activities are facilitated.	- Staffing activities influenced by other disciplines such as scheduling programmatic elements may be facilitated, but coverage for leaves or vacancies becomes more difficult. Recruitment of staff may be more difficult, or you might need to rely upon managers from other disciplines for assistance.
CQI, program evaluation, and outcomes	- Improving discipline-specific processes is easier, as is measuring single-discipline outcomes and indicators of program evaluation, but interdisciplinary programs require extra effort.	- Improving interdisciplinary or program processes is easier, as is measuring program outcomes and indicators of program evaluation, but discipline-specific elements require extra effort.
Professional development	- Development of discipline-specific skills related to assessment and intervention may be facilitated by the ease of access to disciplinary specialists.	- Development of interdisciplinary skills related to the needs of a population or program development or implementation may be facilitated.

Source: Reprinted with permission from Braveman, B. (2006). *Leading and managing occupational therapy services: An evidence-based approach.* Philadelphia: F. A. Davis

- Training and development: meeting the short- and long-term educational and professional development needs of employees at all levels of the organization
- Separation: terminating the employment of personnel due to resignation or inadequate job performance or that which may come about as the result of a decrease in organizational resources

Directing

Directing is the management function that involves giving guidance and leadership to subordinates so that the work that is performed is goal-oriented and contributes to meeting organizational or departmental requirements. More specifically, a director could assign and manage the workload, develop and implement policies and procedures to guide others in uniform completion of their work, provide mentoring and coaching for improved future performance, and appraise performance by providing feedback to employees about current performance.

Managing the workload is a complicated process that involves projecting the amount of work to be done, determining which resources are necessary to complete the work, and managing these resources to make certain that the appropriate person with the right skills and right equipment and space is available when needed. The workload is typically projected on a yearly basis as part of planning a departmental budget, but it may also be done on a week-to-week, day-to-day, or even hourly basis.

Writing policies and procedures to guide staff in both their daily tasks and their use of materials, supplies, facilities and equipment is a specific aspect of directing that is typically the responsibility of a department manager. Policies are statements of values that are congruent with the mission and that justify the boundaries that govern the services provided. They set parameters for making decisions about day-to-day operations. Procedures outline the specific tasks that should be completed or that provide specific direction about how a policy should be implemented. A manager should not only be able to cite a policy or procedure, but also be able to give the underlying logic for the policy's existence.

Most organizations follow a prescribed standard format that guides managers in deciding what to include in a department's Policy and Procedure Manual. If a policy and procedures format is not provided, the organization may purchase existing customizable resources on the Internet. The basic components of a policy and procedure protocol are presented in Box 67.1.

Managers also serve as mentors, coaches, and appraisers of overall work performance; and resources to develop the skills and knowledge necessary for these functions should be sought out both from within the profession of occupational therapy and from outside of it. The American Occupational Therapy Association has a number of resources related to supervisory tasks specific to occupa-

BOX 67.1 BASIC COMPONENTS OF A POLICY AND PROCEDURE

(This is not for an entire manual but the components of a single policy and procedure statement that is typically one document within a manual.)

- Policy statement(s): Brief statements of the guiding principles to be communicated
- Purpose statement(s): Brief statements that outline the reasons for inclusion of the policies or procedures
- Applicability: Lists the employee groups to which the policy and procedure applies (e.g., all occupational therapy department staff members)
- Procedures: Statements outlining the specific actions to be taken by the identified employee groups and criteria for determining adherence to the policy
- Responsibility: Identifying the individuals who are responsible for oversight of the policy and procedure (e.g., all occupational therapy team leaders)
- Review period: Lists the date of the last review and update of the policy and procedures (typically policies and procedures are reviewed on an annual basis)

tional therapy assistants or to occupational therapy aides (www.aota.org). For more generic information on models of supervision, theories of motivating others, developing effective performance appraisal systems, or providing effective mentoring or coaching; managers should look outside the occupational therapy literature. For example, associations such as the American Management Association (www.amanet.org) or the National Association for Employee Recognition (http://www.recognition.org/) provide resources about how one may become an effective supervisor.

Controlling

Controlling is a management function that relates to the processes of establishing specific work performance standards and the measurement, evaluation, and correction of performance. A key responsibility of managers is to promote the delivery of appropriate intervention through the use of quality control (QC) mechanisms and continuous quality improvement (CQI). QC and CQI are related functions, but each serves a different purpose and relies on different philosophies, strategies, tools, and techniques. The focus of QC is to intervene when the quality or quantity or work output falls below predetermined measures (indicators). The focus of CQI is to improve customer sat-

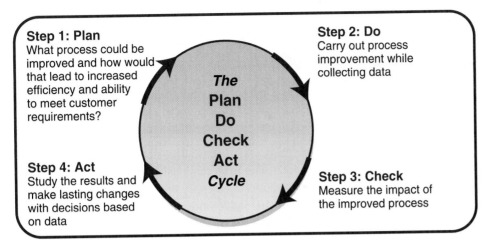

Step 1: Plan
What process could be improved and how would that lead to increased efficiency and ability to meet customer requirements?

Step 2: Do
Carry out process improvement while collecting data

Step 4: Act
Study the results and make lasting changes with decisions based on data

Step 3: Check
Measure the impact of the improved process

The Plan Do Check Act Cycle

FIGURE 67.4 The Plan, Do, Check, Act (PDCA) Cycle

isfaction by constantly striving to meet customer expectations through enhancing critical processes. A critical process is defined as any process that is performed to produce the work of an organization. Examples of occupational therapy critical processes include responding to referrals for service, administering assessments, fabricating adaptive equipment, and making postdischarge referrals.

CQI is viewed both as a philosophy of management and as an approach to managing. A CQI approach requires that managers develop a wide range of skills related to assessing tasks and people. CQI projects may be complex and time-intensive because they rely on decision making based on data and therefore require an organized and structured approach to gathering and analyzing data. Explaining CQI in depth is beyond the scope of this chapter, but Figure 67.4 provides a brief overview of commonly identified steps to choose a critical process and implementing steps that improve its performance. The Plan, Do, Check, Act (PDCA) Cycle may be invoked under other names or acronyms, but the steps of the CQI process remain constant. The most common tools and techniques and their uses are presented in Table 67.4.

FINANCIAL MANAGEMENT

An important function of most managers is the planning and controlling of a department budget. Budgets are typically planned for a calendar year or a fiscal year (e.g., many organizations operate on a fiscal year that runs from July 1 to June 30). The process of planning and managing a budget requires that a manager have a comprehensive understanding of the goals and objectives of the larger organization so that he or she can establish priorities for funding that support this mission over time.

Occupational therapy practitioners who want to become managers or directors of an occupational therapy department or to own and operate their own businesses are encouraged to learn financial planning and management and to become well versed in the use of information management technologies, such as spreadsheets or other financial management tools. Braveman (2006b) notes that effective financial planning and management requires a working knowledge of the following:

♦ Health care systems, including city, county, state, and national systems
♦ Payment and reimbursement structures, such as Medicare, Medicaid, Worker's Compensation, private insurance, and grants or foundation support
♦ Human resources systems and costs, including salary and benefit administration, training and educational costs and systems, and recruitment and retention structures
♦ Equipment and materials purchasing and management, including medical supplies, such as splinting or assistive and adaptive equipment, office supplies, and other supportive supplies
♦ Facilities management, maintenance and improvement protocols, including cleaning and maintenance of physical plant structures

Budgets may also include revenue and expense streams, although it is not uncommon for a community-based organization manager to have oversight of only expenses with no control over direct sources of revenue. Typically, the revenues and expenses associated with each department in an organization are given some sort of marker or code in the organization's accounting system that indicates how the subset of revenues and expenses relate to that department. These subsets of revenues and expenses are commonly referred to as *cost centers*. They may represent the budget of a single department or of several related services. Common examples of revenues and expenses are shown in Table 67.5 and are further explained in the following section.

Revenues may include third-party payments for services from private and public insurers, grants from government agencies or private foundations, or gifts from

TABLE 67.4   COMMON CQI CONCEPTS, TOOLS, AND TECHNIQUES

Core Concepts	Use/Importance/Summary
◆ The Plan, Do, Check, Act (PDCA) Cycle	◆ The overarching framework for guiding and ordering CQI activities
◆ Critical processes	◆ The important processes that are repeated again and again to complete the organization's or department's work
◆ Operational definitions	◆ A quantifiable description of what to measure and the steps to follow to measure it consistently
◆ Customers and customer requirements	◆ Identifying internal and external customers or individuals who receive the output of your work and their valid requirements
◆ Quality indicators	◆ Quantitative measures of compliance to valid customer requirements
◆ Variation	◆ The spread of process output over time. Discriminating between natural "common cause" variation that is inherent in a process and the uncommon "special cause" variation that you want to eliminate from a process or emulate if positive
STRATEGIES	
◆ Ground rules for meetings	◆ Explicit agreements about how a team will work together and behave as team members
◆ Roles for effective meetings	◆ Assigning roles such as the leader, scribe, facilitator, and timekeeper can lead to more effective meetings
◆ Consensus	◆ A method for reaching agreement whereby all members agree to fully support a decision even if it is not how they would act if they were acting alone
TOOLS	
◆ Process flow charts	◆ A visual representation of the steps in a process used to highlight redundancies, rework, or bottlenecks
◆ Control charts	◆ A chart with statistically determined upper and lower control limits used to determine whether a process has changed and to highlight variation
◆ Cause and effect diagrams	◆ A tool to assist in determining possible root causes to a problem.
◆ Proposed Options Matrix	◆ A tool for comparing possible options for action against a set of predetermined criteria.
TECHNIQUES	
◆ Data stratification	◆ Methods for categorizing collection of data; it is important to decide how to stratify data before you collect it
◆ Designing an effective data collection tool	◆ Tools to gather facts on how a process works or its effectiveness that allows for accurate collection of data in the simplest manner
◆ Balancing tasks and people	◆ Attending to both the needs of team members and the work to be completed to maintain team motivation
◆ Icebreakers	◆ Short activities to help team members learn about each other or to become more comfortable interacting with each other
◆ Brainstorming	◆ A method for creatively generating lists of possible causes of problems, solutions, or processes to improve
◆ Multivoting	◆ A decision-making method to narrow a larger number of options to a number that can be reasonably discussed individually

Source: Reprinted with permission from Braveman, B. (2006). *Leading and managing occupational therapy services: An evidence-based approach.* Philadelphia: F. A. Davis.

TABLE 67.5   EXAMPLES OF REVENUES AND EXPENSES

Revenue	Expenses
Individual 15 Minutes: ADL Treatment	Variable Expense—Salary
Individual 15 Minutes: Cognitive Remediation	Variable Expense—Wages
Individual 15 Minutes: Community Reintegration	Variable Expense—Office Supplies
Individual 15 Minutes: Neuromuscular Facilitation	Variable Expense—Splinting Supplies
Group 15 Minutes: Home Management	Fixed Expense—Phone
Group 15 Minutes: Communication Skills	Fixed Expense—Rent
Group 15 Minutes: Community Reintegration	Fixed Expense—Utilities

individuals or foundations. Forecasting revenues for a department requires that the manager be able to accurately predict the volume of work that a department will deliver and how that work will happen. In some settings, almost all occupational therapy intervention is provided to consumers on a one-to-one basis, while in some settings, intervention is provided to groups. By accurately predicting the total volume of work for a year, managers are able to predict the total gross revenue by multiplying the number of work units (e.g., a 15 minute unit of therapy) by the charge for each unit of service. It is important to note that in the current managed care environment, few payers reimburse at the full rate that is billed and the net revenue, or the amount of revenue after all discounts to insurers and nonreimbursed charges are accounted for, is typically much less than gross revenue.

Expenses typically include costs associated with personnel, supplies, facilities management, and equipment. As part of the process of forecasting the expense budget, managers determine the number of full-time equivalent employees that will be required to handle the projected work volume. Setting productivity standards, or the amount of work a practitioner is expected to perform in a given period, and helping staff to meet such standards is a common challenge faced by occupational therapy managers. Personnel expenses can include both salary expenses for professional staff that are exempt from the labor laws that require an organization to pay extra for overtime effort and wages for support staff that are nonexempt. Occupational therapists are often categorized as exempt, and occupational therapy assistants and occupational therapy aides are often categorized as nonexempt.

Nonpersonnel expenses; such as supplies, equipment, food, phone, continuing education, or travel allowances must also be projected. In private businesses, expenses for utilities and rent must also be considered. These expenses are categorized as either fixed or variable expenses. Fixed expenses are costs that are not directly influenced by changes in volume, such as expenses budgeted for em-

ployee continuing education. Variable expenses are those that are directly influenced by changes in volume, for example, some types of office supplies or food used for meal preparation activities. Although there might not always be a direct correlation, over time, one will be able to estimate how an increase or decrease in volume might affect expenses.

To effectively plan and control a budget, managers must learn many useful concepts and strategies Some organizations may provide training or orientation for new managers, but most often it is assumed that a new manager understands the basic information needed to develop and oversee a budget. People who are assuming their first management position would benefit from additional education or training in financial management and from networking with experienced managers. The American Occupational Therapy Association provides electronic mailing lists and other resources for managers through its Administration and Management Special Interest Section (AMSIS). More information on AMSIS and other special interest sections (SIS's) can be found at www.aota.org.

TECHNOLOGY AND MANAGEMENT

The technological advances in medicine, information management, communication, and related areas that have occurred over the last few decades are astounding. Managers must evaluate and integrate a wide range of technology into their departments, ranging from computer software programs to clinical equipment, such as driving simulators or environmental controls. Choosing and successfully integrating a new technology requires that managers synthesize information, including costs of initial purchase, maintenance, space, and training requirements and the rate at which the specific technology is advancing so that an estimate can be made of when the current technology may become outdated.

TABLE 67.6 COMMON TYPES OF DATA, SOURCES, AND POSSIBLE USES

Type of Data	Source	Use
Demographics (age, sex, educational level, etc.)	◆ Admissions records ◆ Public data sets	◆ Program planning ◆ Program evaluation
Revenue (payer source, rates, discounts)	◆ Accounting ◆ Budget reports	◆ Budgeting ◆ Program planning
Expense (accounts payable)	◆ Financial reports ◆ Purchasing records	◆ Budgeting ◆ Program planning and evaluation
Payroll (salary, benefits, leave usage)	◆ Accounting ◆ Budget reports	◆ Staffing plans ◆ Recruitment and retention
Productivity (visits, staff activity)	◆ Automated charge systems ◆ Department billing records or productivity tracking sheets	◆ Staffing plans ◆ Performance appraisal ◆ Recruitment
Personnel (licensure, competencies, professional development, performance)	◆ Human resources ◆ Departmental personnel files ◆ Professional association data sets	◆ Accreditation visits ◆ Staffing plan development ◆ Professional development plans
Clinical (diagnosis, intervention, outcomes)	◆ Medical records ◆ Outcome databases	◆ CQI ◆ Program evaluation
Legal (contracts, leases)	◆ Legal or grants and contracts department	◆ Facility planning

One major area of technology used by managers is that employed in information management, which includes the use of computers for documentation, billing, and financial management, as well as data collection and analysis for outcomes management. Table 67.6 lists common types of data and information that must be collected and managed and their possible uses. Becoming skilled at the use of software programs to organize and analyze the large amount of data available to most managers requires extra work but is well worth the effort.

MARKETING

Occupational therapy managers are often responsible for assessing the needs of the target populations served by their department or organization; determining programmatic strategies for meeting these needs; designing, implementing, and evaluating the interventions to meet identified needs; and promoting the intervention to consumers, payers, physicians, and others. These processes, collectively, are called *marketing*. Traditionally, the following four steps are identified in the marketing process:

◆ **Organizational assessment:** examination of the factors within an organization that will influence the development and promotion of a new product or service

◆ **Environmental assessment:** examination of the data and other forms of evidence, including the needs of target populations, that will guide the development and promotion of a new product or service
◆ **Market analysis:** use of the information gained during organizational and environmental assessments to validate perceptions of the wants and needs of the target populations that will receive a new product or service
◆ **Marketing communications:** packaging and promoting a product so the target populations and other key stakeholders in the new product or service have a clear understanding of what the product or service is and how it may be accessed

In larger organizations, other professionals, such as members of a marketing department, often perform portions of the marketing process, such as collecting demographic and other data about potential consumers, or may be called on to collaborate with a manager to perform these functions. However, occupational therapy managers who are also business owners or who work in community-based, nonprofit organizations might need to learn the marketing process in greater depth. These managers benefit from establishing effective networks with other managers and becoming active in professional organizations, such as their state and national occupational therapy associations and business-oriented groups such as the local Chamber of Commerce.

WHO SHOULD BE A MANAGER?

During the 1990s, numerous professions began to address managerial competencies with increasing urgency and concern, emphasizing the need to determine the initial competence of health professionals, to assess specific job competencies as professionals are hired and begin to work, and to promote the professionals' continuing development of competence (Braveman, 2006c). The assessment of initial competency and facilitation of continuing development of staff competency is a function of the occupational therapy manager.

Before assuming a role as an occupational therapy manager, one should assess one's own level of preparedness to perform the tasks associated with the role. Although the assessment of competencies for managers has not received the same attention by certifying or regulatory bodies, such as accrediting agencies, competency development and assessment have been addressed, and some empirical investigations of managerial competencies have been conducted by a number of professions (Braveman, 2006c).

Some competencies might be considered "universal" for managers. One method of identifying managerial competence is to compare their performance against the "yardstick" of previously described traditional managerial functions (e.g., planning, organizing and staffing, directing, and controlling). As a guide for this process, each of the management functions is listed below with sample areas for assessment of competency provided for each. (See Table 67.2 for additional areas for development of competencies.)

Sample Areas for Assessment of Competency for Managers

- Planning
  - Use of goal setting
  - Financial management skills
  - Understanding the changing health care environment
  - Effectiveness in decision making
- Organizing and staffing
  - Understanding team structure and flexible work design
  - Designing and leading effective teams
  - Using cooperation techniques
  - Applying coordination techniques
- Directing
  - Interpersonal competencies
    - Communication skills
    - Communicating with the boss
    - Communicating with peers and others
    - Communicating with employees
    - Being politically astute
    - Managing conflict
    - Managing diversity
  - Role model competencies
    - Demonstrating professionalism in conduct and demeanor
    - Enhancing technical competence
- Controlling
  - Empowering employees
  - Applying continuous quality improvement efforts

Other managerial competencies will depend on the nature of the manager's job. Not all managers perform the same tasks and functions, so it is important that, before accepting a management position, one understands what will be expected of one and have done a thorough assessment of readiness by identifying strengths and areas in which help might be needed. Needing supervision or help does not necessarily mean that a new manager cannot take on his or her first managerial position. But knowing when to ask for assistance is essential if one wishes to ensure success as a manager.

COMMENTARY ON THE EVIDENCE

The State of Evidence Related to Management

The existing evidence on effective managerial strategies and practices has been produced by multiple disciplines and fields such as business, organizational development, organizational psychology, social work, and nursing. The topics that have been investigated are also diverse; examples include effective leadership strategies, performance appraisal processes, factors affecting recruitment and retention, effective recognition and reward structures, change management, and continuous quality improvement.

A variety of forms of evidence, including the results of empirical studies, program descriptions, and descriptions of managerial interventions, are published widely in a range

COMMENTARY ON THE EVIDENCE *Continued*

of professional journals, Websites, and books. Although the body of evidence specifically related to management in health care organizations might be more limited, it is growing, and occupational therapy managers who wish to use an *evidence-based* approach to management will benefit from research and science conducted by other disciplines such as those mentioned.

For example, while evidence related to effective leadership is still evolving and much of the existing evidence is descriptive, there have been well designed empirical investigations of topics such as the direct impact of leader behavior on subordinate performance (Dvir, Eden, Avolio, & Shamir, 2002; Levy, Cober & Miller, 2002). Some of these studies have included randomized control-study designs.

While they are mostly descriptive, there is a plethora of reports on factors affecting the recruitment and retention of health professionals. Much of this evidence is found outside of the occupational therapy literature, but a few studies including occupational therapy practitioners or specifically on occupational therapy have been published. For example MacRae, van Diepen, and Patterson (2007) and Daniels, Vanliet, Skipper, Sanders, and Rhyne (2007) provide reports of factors that influenced students willingness to consider placement in rural underserved areas and the

implications this had for staffing in these areas. Mills and Millsteed (2002) investigated factors affecting the retention of occupational therapists in rural Australia. Painter, Akroyd, Elliot, and Adams (2003) examined burnout in a sample of 521 occupational therapists in comparison to other health care professions and Okerlund, Jackson, Parsons, and Comsa (1995) explored factors affecting recruitment and retention of occupational therapists in Utah.

While occupational therapy managers can certainly make valuable judgments by generalizing from evidence produced in other disciplines, the profession would benefit from research specifically related to occupational therapy. Questions for investigation might include the following:

◆ What factors affect long-term retention within the profession, and how might we reduce attrition from the discipline?
◆ How might occupational therapy managers influence the delivery of culturally relevant services?
◆ What factors influence the effectiveness of interdisciplinary teams?

As in most areas of occupational therapy practice, the profession will greatly benefit from the development of further evidence on management.

CONCLUSION

This chapter has provided an overview of the numerous tasks, functions, and responsibilities that an occupational therapy manager may perform. I hope that the reader has gained a perspective on the variety and complexities of a manager's responsibilities and a greater appreciation of the need for a beginning manager to get appropriate training and education. Managers work closely with the administrators and supervisors in large organizations, but small business owners and entrepreneurs also function independently as managers. Fortunately, many resources are available that are specific to occupational therapy managers, and more resources may be found in other fields, including business, psychology, and organizational development, that are useful guides for a manger performing his or her job.

REFERENCES

Branch, K. M. (2002). *Change management.* Washington, DC: U.S. Department of Energy. Retrieved November 27, 2006 from http://library.monts.cc/cm.htm

Braveman, B. (2006a). Understanding and working within organizations. In *Leading and managing occupational therapy services: An evidence-based approach* (pp. 53–80). Philadelphia: F. A. Davis.

Braveman, B. (2006b). Roles and functions of managers. In *Leading and managing occupational therapy services: An evidence-based approach* (pp. 109–139). Philadelphia: F. A. Davis.

Braveman, B. (2006c). Competency and the occupational therapy manager. In *Leading and managing occupational therapy services: An evidence-based approach* (pp. 169–195). Philadelphia: F. A. Davis.

Daniels, Z., Vanleit, B., Skipper, B., Sanders, M., & Rhyne, R. (2007). Factors in recruiting and retaining health professionals for rural practice. *Journal of Rural Health, 23*(1), 62–71.

Dvir, T., Eden, D., Avolio, B. J., & Shamir, B. (2002). Impact of transformational leadership on follower development and performance: A field experiment. *Academy of Management Journal, 45,* 735–744.

Hoyle, J. R. (1995). *Leadership and futuring: Making visions happen.* Thousand Oaks, CA: Corwin Press.

Jaques, E. (1998). *Requisite organization.* Arlington, VA: Cason Hall & Co.

Liebler, J. G., Levine, R. E., & Rothman, J. (1992). *Management principles for health professionals.* Gaithersburg, MD: Aspen Publishers.

Lewin, K. (1997). *Resolving social conflict and field theory in social sciences.* Washington, DC: American Psychological Association.

Levy, P. E., Cober, R. T., & Miller, T. (2002). The effect of transformational and transactional leadership perceptions on feedback-seeking intentions. *Journal of Applied Social Psychology, 32,* 1703–1720.

Liebler, J. G., & McConnell, C. R. (2004). *Management principles for health professionals.* Boston, MA: Jones and Bartlett.

MacRae, M., van Diepen, K., & Paterson, M. (2007). Use of clinical placements as a means of recruiting health care students to underserviced areas in Southeastern Ontario: I. Student perspectives. *Australian Journal of Rural Health, 15*(1), 21–28.

Mills, A., & Millsteed, J. (2002). Retention: An unresolved workforce issue affecting rural occupational therapy services. *Australian Occupational Therapy Journal, 49*(4), 170–181.

Okerlund, V., Jackson, P., Parsons, R., & Comsa, M. (1995). Job recruitment and retention factors for occupational therapists in Utah. *American Journal of Occupational Therapy, 49*(3), 263–265.

Painter, J., Akroyd, D., Elliot, S., & Adams, R. (2003). Burnout among occupational therapists. *Occupational Therapy in Health Care, 17*(1), 63–78.

Supervision

MARY JANE YOUNGSTROM

68

Learning Objectives

After reading this chapter, you will be able to:

1. Understand the roles and functions of supervision.
2. Differentiate types of supervision.
3. Describe supervisory processes and implementation.
4. Describe approaches to managing performance.
5. Apply AOTA guidelines for appropriate supervision of OT personnel.

Supervision is an integral part of occupational therapy service provision. The supervisory process is consciously used in our profession to ensure that our clients receive safe and effective occupational therapy services. Although the ability to supervise skillfully is developed throughout one's practice career, the entry-level practitioner must be knowledgeable about the supervisory process and have a beginning understanding of how to give and receive supervision in a manner that is consistent with the profession's values and expectations. This chapter will provide you with an overview of what supervision is and introduce you to basic information you will need to develop positive and effective supervisory relationships. Supervisory expectations and standards specific to the occupational therapy profession will be presented.

SUPERVISION EMBEDDED IN PRACTICE

The supervision process is an everyday feature of each practitioner's work experience. It is a process that supports effective job performance as well as personal growth. Read the case study about Marta, an occupational therapist (OT), and Kim an occupational therapy assistant (OTA), which describes their career experiences with supervision.

In the case scenario, supervision was a regular feature of Marta's and Kim's daily work experience. Supervision provided feedback, direction and support for Marta and Kim as they learned to carry out their responsibilities effectively and supported them in their personal professional development to gain additional competencies. Each practitioner had a designated formal supervisor, but both Marta and Kim received informal peer supervision from other therapists. The close-knit nature of the work group and everyone's interest in providing the best possible care allowed this type of supervision to occur naturally. Adding supervisory responsibilities to their jobs expanded both Marta's and Kim's job roles and offered opportunities for personal growth.

As the case study illustrates, practitioners are involved in giving as well as receiving supervision. Supervisory skills are an expected entry-level

Outline *Continued*

competency for OTs who are responsible for supervising OTAs (American Occupational Therapy Association, 2004). Entry-level OTAs may be responsible for supervising OT aides and later may move into supervisory roles with other OTAs. Both OTs and OTAs should know how to effectively provide supervision and benefit from it. Before exploring how to best provide supervision, let's first look at what supervision is and how it fits into the overall management structure of a work setting.

FORMAL SUPERVISION

Definition and Focus

Dictionaries trace the roots of the term *supervise* to the Latin roots *super-*, "over," + *videre-*, "to see" (Guralnik, 1987). Supervision is a process that involves "overseeing" or "watching" the work of another. The employer gives a supervisor formal authority to watch the work of others and ensure that the work meets the organization's goals and objectives. To effectively oversee the work of others, supervisors need to be familiar with the work of the positions they supervise. If individuals who move into supervisory positions do not have advanced knowledge or experience in the job positions they supervise, they are expected to familiarize themselves with the job tasks and responsibilities. This background allows them to provide the support and direction that supervisees need to solve work problems, to learn and grow in their jobs, and to better meet the organization's objectives (Figure 68.1).

How does the supervisor fit in the management structure of an organization? Braveman offers insight into the relationship of the two by defining *supervision* as "The control and direction of the work of one or more employees in a manner that promotes improved performance and a higher quality outcome" (Braveman, 2006, p. 142). Although supervisors may participate in all functions of management (planning, organizing, directing, and controlling), the majority of the supervisor's time is

---

CASE STUDY: *Marta and Kim: Supervision Embedded in Practice*

Marta began her career as an occupational therapist in a pediatric hospital. She worked with two other OTs and was supervised by Sarah, the senior OT in the setting. Although she met regularly with Sarah, Marta also sought and received feedback and guidance from the other OT, who was particularly experienced in working with children with head injuries. Marta used input from both OTs to expand her knowledge and develop her clinical reasoning skills. Six months after taking the job, she was given the responsibility of supervising volunteers who provided service in a playtime program for hospitalized children. She was responsible for orienting and training the volunteers. Periodically, she would observe their interactions with the children and was always available for questions. During her first year of practice, Marta was regularly involved in supervising both Level I OT and OTA students. She found these experiences to be rewarding. At the end of her second year

of work, she was assigned her first Level II clinical fieldwork student, whom she supervised on a daily basis. As the department's caseload expanded, an OTA, Kim, was hired, and Marta supervised Kim as they collaboratively worked to provide OT services to referred patients. Marta oriented Kim to the hospital and the department's policies and procedures. Initially, Marta closely observed Kim's treatments and/or cotreated with her. Kim came to the hospital with three years of experience with children, but her prior work had been in a school setting, so she was not as familiar with occupational therapy interventions involving acute medical conditions. Several months after Kim joined the department, she was given the responsibility for supervising the volunteers in the playtime program. She consulted with the recreational therapist, Terry, who worked on a different unit in the hospital, about strategies for expanding the play activities and improving volunteer participation.

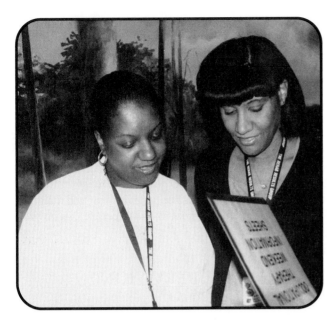

FIGURE 68.1   Discussing weekend coverage plans and how they will be implemented is a common supervisory task in hospital-based occupational therapy.

others who are in management positions. Supervisors are generally considered to be the first line of management. Although they have some management responsibilities, they are not considered to be managers.

The emphasis primarily on the directing and controlling functions of management does not diminish the importance of the supervisor's role. Formal supervisors, because of their placement within the organization, serve as a bridge between the staff and higher levels of management. In this position, the supervisor must support and interpret management decisions as well as relay staff concerns to higher management. This position can be one of the most critical in the organization (Allen, 1998, "Management Levels"). How well the supervisor can convey management concerns to staff and staff concerns to management can make or break the organization's effectiveness and ability to adapt to change.

Up to this point, we have been emphasizing the supervisor's responsibility to the organization—to oversee work to ensure the organization's success. Supervision takes on an added dimension and responsibility when people who are members of a profession (e.g., occupational therapy, nursing, psychology) take on responsibilities to supervise other members of their profession in a work setting. The provision of professional supervision that is consistent with the profession's values and standards and supports the professional growth and development of the professionals who are being supervised is integrated with the supervisor's responsibility to meet the organization's needs. For example, the supervisor must not assign tasks and responsibilities that are outside of the

typically focused on the directing and controlling functions (Allen, 1998, "Management Levels"). (See Chapter 67 for a discussion of management functions.) When we consider the supervisor's placement within the management hierarchy this becomes easier to understand (see Figure 68.2). Supervisors are placed closest to the staff level of the organization and typically do not supervise

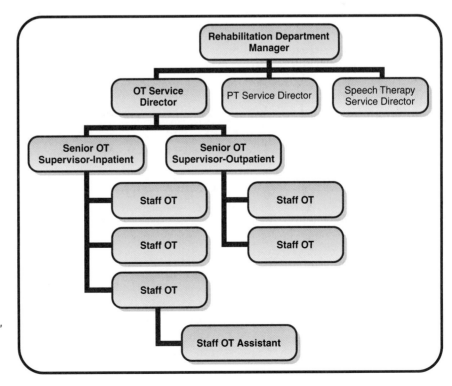

FIGURE 68.2   In this organization, the senior occupational therapists are supervisors, and the OT service director is a manager.

supervisee's professional scope of practice. The supervisor must be cognizant of the profession's standards and guidelines regarding frequency of supervision and requirements for training and competency. Overall, the supervisor must manage and supervise work in a manner that respects the profession's scope and that supports the supervisee's development of continuing competence.

The supervisor who is providing professional supervision must continually ask two related but different questions, which will guide the supervisor's observations, analysis, decisions, and actions:

1. Is the supervisee successfully accomplishing the work?
2. Is the supervisee demonstrating continued professional growth and development?

Supporting the supervisees' efforts to maintain and develop continuing competence does not conflict with supporting the supervisee to successfully accomplish the work. As individuals develop new skills and abilities, clients receive better care and organizations benefit from workers' improved expertise. The supervisor should be concurrently providing feedback on performance and assessing the supervisee's learning and professional development needs.

Functions of Supervision in a Professional Practice Setting

The supervisor's role in a professional practice setting encompasses three broad functions that are carried out under the broader management functions of directing and controlling. These functions are administrative, educational, and supportive functions (Kadushin, 1992). Table 68.1 lists examples of supervisory tasks for each function.

Administrative functions are directed toward managing the day-to-day work performance and process. Checking that all clients were seen and assigning clients to specific supervisees are examples of administrative tasks. Carrying out administrative functions ensures that the organization's day-to-day work is accomplished. The educational function is focused on the worker and is concerned with teaching and training, providing feedback about performance, and disciplining if necessary. Educational functions assist the supervisee to be effective in meeting job demands and also can help to promote the supervisee's own professional growth and development. The supportive function is directed toward relationships—both individual and group relationships within the workplace. This function focuses on developing harmonious relationships that will maintain a positive work environment in which people can be productive and successful.

INFORMAL SUPERVISION: PEER SUPERVISION

Supervision is typically understood as a formalized process that occurs in a work setting in which a person's work is supervised by a formally designated supervisor. In a health care professional practice environment where all staff members are committed to providing the best quality of service, informal peer supervision may also occur. Peer supervision is oversight that is provided by another professional who has no formal authority to provide supervision. The peer supervisor provides feedback and shares knowledge with the intent of influencing the peer professional's practices to improve client outcomes.

Peer supervision is a natural extension of each professional's responsibility to ensure that clients receive the highest quality of care. It may or may not be solicited by the "supervisee" practitioner. In the case study, Marta did seek input from her peers as a way of continuing to learn and grow as a professional, but not all practitioners seek input from others. When a peer therapist provides peer

---

TABLE 68.1 EXAMPLES OF SUPERVISORY TASKS WITHIN DIFFERENT SUPERVISORY FUNCTIONS

Administrative Function	Educational Function	Supportive Function
◆ Plan and assign workload ◆ Make schedules ◆ Set priorities for department's work activities ◆ Check performance against work standards ◆ Interpret policies and procedures ◆ Delegate work ◆ Provide written and verbal reports to managers	◆ Orient new staff ◆ Identify training needs ◆ Develop and provide training programs ◆ Identify and provide educational resources ◆ Assess performance and provide feedback ◆ Discipline	◆ Hold group meetings to allow for expression of concerns ◆ Meet individually with supervisee on a quarterly basis to check on progress toward work goals ◆ Provide informal and formal support for performance

supervision and feedback that is not requested, the intent is to improve client outcomes by offering information that could help other practitioners to improve their services.

In a professional and collegial work environment, peer supervision often occurs spontaneously and is seen as a benefit of working with others. Exchange and feedback among practitioners frequently occur as colleagues explore how to solve clinical problems and seek the best solutions for their clients. Such exchanges can be energizing for both parties. Engaging in peer supervision can be perceived as a method of mutual accountability and commitment to the profession's obligation to provide the best quality of services to clients

MENTORING

Being mentored by another professional is often confused with supervision. Mentorship and supervision are different types of relationships. In a mentor relationship, the mentor's primary concern is the personal and professional growth of the mentee (Robertson, 1992). The mentor does not necessarily have any formal authority to oversee the mentee's work. Although the mentor is interested in the work the mentee is doing, direct observation of work does not regularly occur as part of the mentoring function, and discussion does not focus on work performance per se. Instead, discussions between the mentor and mentee center on career options and decisions, identification of personal and professional growth needs and resources, and feedback about the mentee's behaviors and choices. The mentor supports the mentee in overall professional development and offers support, praise, and encouragement. The mentor is focused solely on the mentee's personal growth.

A mentor relationship may be sought by the mentee who is feeling the need of guidance and direction in professional growth and development. Sometimes mentor/mentee relationships occur spontaneously in a work environment or between two professionals who are attracted to each other. The mentee usually is attracted to the mentor's knowledge, skills, and accomplishments, and the mentor is attracted to the mentee's talent and potential as well as the opportunity to contribute to another professional's development. Generally, the mentor is an older and more experienced professional.

True mentoring relationships are acknowledged by both parties and require formal commitment of time and effort. Both parties discuss and agree on learning needs and goals for the relationship. A structure for the mentoring process is identified, whether it is periodic face-to-face meetings, written communication, or a combination of the two. Some work environments, recognizing the value of mentors, may formally assign a more experienced therapist who is not the employee's supervisor to function in a mentor role. The assigned mentor would provide support and guide the new employee in learning about and adjusting to new work situations (Allen, 1998, "Training"). Less structured or more informal mentoring relationships can also develop during the course of a practitioner's professional life. These relationships are less intense and usually of shorter duration.

It is easy to see how a mentee/mentor relationship might develop within a supervisory relationship. When this happens, both parties need to be clear about the different purposes and responsibilities of the two types of relationships. It is possible that what the mentor might counsel would not be what the supervisor would counsel. For example, a person who is functioning in the role of mentor might recognize that a mentee would benefit from staying in one clinical setting for several months to allow for solidification of learning. However, this same person, functioning as a supervisor, recognizes that staffing limitations require that the supervisee must be rotated to a new clinical setting each month. Holding both roles simultaneously can lead to role conflicts, highlighting the need to be very clear about the different responsibilities of each role. Table 68.2 offers a comparison of supervision, mentorship, and peer supervision.

Mentoring should not be confused with role modeling. A role model is usually watched and admired by a practitioner, but the role model does not have a reciprocating active interest in the person's development and might not even be aware that he or she is serving as a role model (Urish, 2004).

THE SUPERVISORY PROCESS

The overseeing of work is an *ongoing* process: It occurs repeatedly across time and is embedded in the everyday work experience. A supervisor, both formally and informally, observes and checks on the work of supervisees by talking to them about their work as well as observing them on a regular basis. A supervisor who observes the work of supervisees only occasionally and meets with them only annually to discuss performance during an annual performance review is not providing appropriate supervision. Supervisors should be regularly present in the workplace and have regular contact with their supervisees.

Supervision is an *orderly* process. A good supervisor establishes a process in which the supervisee understands when regular contacts and meetings will occur. The supervisor is clear about performance expectations and consistent in providing feedback. The supervisee learns to trust and value the supervisory process as a tool that promotes personal growth and success in the job.

The supervisory process, although orderly and expected, is also *dynamic*. It changes as people grow and work demands shift. Upon initial hiring, the supervisor might observe an employee daily and meet weekly. However, after several weeks, the employee might practice more independently without daily observation.

TABLE 68.2 COMPARISON OF SUPERVISION, MENTORSHIP, AND PEER SUPERVISION

	Supervision	Mentorship	Peer Supervision
Authority	Provided by the work organization	No formal authority	No formal authority. Supported by professional responsibility
Nature of relationship and how it is established	Formal—established by the workplace	Personal, voluntary	Informal, spontaneous
Purpose	To support growth and development that will benefit the organization	To foster personal and professional growth and development that will benefit the mentee	To support growth and development that will ensure best outcomes for clients
How established	Assigned	Sought by the mentee and mutually agreed upon	Offered by a peer or may be solicited by a practitioner
Accountability for performance	Organizational	Personal	Professional
Whose needs are met— Outcomes expected	Needs of organization: Work meets organizational objectives and needs	Needs of mentee: Mentee achieves personal and professional growth	Needs of mentee and clients: Clients receive best services

Finally, the supervision is an *interactive* process. It is based on an exchange or communication between the supervisor and the supervisee. The exchange that occurs between the occupational therapy supervisor and supervisee is central to the development and maintenance of professional competence. The AOTA document "Guidelines for Supervision, Roles, and Responsibilities During the Delivery of Occupational Therapy Services" describes supervision as "a cooperative process in which two or more people participate in a joint effort to establish, maintain, and/or elevate a level of competence and performance" (2004, p. 663).

Observe, in this description, that the profession sees supervision as a two-way street. The supervisee as well as the supervisor actively participates in the process. This is in sharp contrast to the common understanding of supervision as something that is done "to" a person and that the supervisee receives or accepts. In our profession, supervision is viewed as a cooperative process in which both parties have professional responsibility. This cooperative approach to supervision stems from the profession's ethical responsibility to demonstrate concern for the safety and well-being of their clients (Principle 1: Beneficence) and to maintain high standards of competence (Principle 4: Duty) (AOTA, 2005a).

The AOTA "Guidelines for Supervision, Roles, and Responsibilities During the Delivery of Occupational Therapy Services" describes the supervisory process as having two purposes that relate to these ethical principles: (1) to

ensure safe and effective delivery of occupational therapy services and (2) to foster professional competence and development (2004, p. 663). These objectives reflect the organizational duties of the supervisor as well as professional practice obligations. All OTs and OTAs have a common interest in providing the best possible care to their clients, and all practitioners are obligated to demonstrate continuing competence. The supervisory process is the tool that OTs and OTAs use to reach these goals.

DEVELOPING A SUPERVISORY RELATIONSHIP

The supervisory relationship is central to the supervisory process. An effective supervisory relationship is built on trust and integrity. To develop trust and integrity, the supervisor must be approachable and open to the supervisee's questions and concerns; the supervisee must feel that that his or her input is valued. The supervisor must be responsive and follow through with actions that indicate that the supervisee's concerns were considered; the supervisee will feel valued and confident in his or her personal abilities, and commitment to the organization will increase. The supervisor must be clear about expectations and provide regular objective feedback about performance; the supervisee will understand what is expected and feel more comfortable in the job. The supervisor must be consistent in the application of rewards and punishments and not play favorites; the supervisee will develop a level of trust in how he or she will be treated. When communications and actions are clear, consistent, and fair, an environment of trust develops and anxiety about performance decreases. When the supervisor is approachable and responsive, the supervisory relationship can thrive. Box 68.1 provides some additional examples of supervisory behaviors that build trust and integrity.

Both supervisee and supervisor bring their own values, beliefs, and attitudes about supervision to the relationship. Each brings past experiences with other supervisors and authority figures, which may have been positive or negative. It is the supervisor's responsibility to set the tone for the relationship in a job setting and to take actions that will support an ongoing positive relationship. The following four steps will help to ensure that a positive supervisory relationship is initiated and developed:

1. **Learn about the supervisee.** Remember that you are responsible for guiding the learning of this new employee. To do this effectively, you need to understand what your new supervisee knows and how he or she learns best. You will be particularly interested in how his or her knowledge and skills match with those that are needed for this job. Interviewing the new employee about past experiences and asking for his or her current strengths and learning needs send the message that you are interested in building on what the person knows and you value the person's experiences. You might wish to develop a skills checklist that the employee can fill out to supplement the interview process. Although the supervisor never stops learning about the supervisee's abilities, gathering this information formally during orientation to use as you begin to design training and learning experiences is very helpful. Understanding not only *what* the supervisee knows but also *how* he or she learns is also important. Does the supervisee learn best by reading, demonstration, or both? Does the supervisee prefer to work more independently with periodic review or would he or she like daily contact with you? What kind of feedback would the supervisee like, and how frequently would he or she like to receive it? Identifying the employee's learning styles and preferences can facilitate the learning process on the new job and avoid wasted time and effort for both parties.

2. **Be clear about job expectations.** During the initial orientation and training, the supervisor needs to clearly outline the performance expectations for the job. The job requirements and expectations should have been broadly discussed during the job interview and hiring process. Now is a good time to revisit this discussion and provide more specifics. Reviewing the job description is an objective method for beginning this discussion. Although job descriptions delineate major functions and lines of authority, they often do not specify in detail the quality and quantity of performance that are expected. Expectations about productivity and quality of work should be made clear to the employee. Be honest and open about consequences for various behaviors—rewards as well as punishments. In addition, organizational cultural expectations such as attitudes and behaviors employees are expected to exhibit in interdisciplinary, peer, and client/family interactions should be addressed. These expectations are often not included in a job description but are central to acceptable performance. Discuss your expectations regarding the supervisee's responsibility to learn and grow. Remember that one of your responsibilities as a professional supervising other members of your profession is to facilitate the supervisee's professional growth and competence. Share your commitment to this goal, and enlist the supervisee's commitment to it. Find out what the supervisee's personal professional goals and objectives are.

3. **Develop and implement a supervisory plan.** Our profession views the supervisory process as a collaborative one. Early in your new supervisee's employment, discuss how you view the supervisory process, and work with the employee to develop a supervisory plan that will work for both of you. Discuss topics such as frequency of supervisory contact (e.g., daily, three times per week, weekly), types of contact (e.g., informal, spontaneous, formal scheduled meeting), methods of contact (e.g., face to face, e-mail, phone, written), and preferred supervisory methods (e.g., observation, cotreatment, dialogue, documentation review). Discuss the obligations of the supervisee as well as the supervisor in supervision; for example, explain that you expect the supervisee to initiate contact with you if more frequent feedback or supervision is needed and to share his or her concerns and ideas with you openly.

BOX 68.1 KEY POSITIVE SUPERVISORY BEHAVIORS

- Praises others
- Accepts criticism and suggestion without judging
- Tells the truth
- Is supportive of supervisee—goes to bat for supervisees
- Gives credit for accomplishments
- Abides by the same rules as expects others to abide by
- Gives clear and frequent feedback
- Is dependable
- Is loyal to organization—makes decisions that are in best interest of organization
- Is respectful of differences

4. **Document supervision that is provided.** Document when you meet with your supervisee and what was discussed. A supervisory log or folder is a helpful tool that allows you to keep a record of incidents, observations, and meetings. If used routinely, the log allows you to track performance and see how it has changed. The log record provides concrete examples that can be used in your feedback and also in regular performance review meetings. Regulatory laws in some states require that supervisory logs be kept to document the supervisory process that occurs between an occupational therapist and an occupational therapy assistant to maintain current licensure.

PERFORMANCE EVALUATION: A SUPERVISORY RESPONSIBILITY

All supervisory actions are directed toward managing the supervisee's work performance. The purpose of performance management is to encourage the supervisee to meet or exceed the established job performance standards and behave safely and appropriately at work (Newstrom and Bittel, 2002, p. 335). Supervisors use a variety of methods in managing performance (e.g., incentives, job structure), but providing ongoing evaluation of performance by providing both formal and informal feedback is a central supervisory responsibility and skill.

Providing Feedback

Effective feedback is the supervisor's primary tool in influencing the employee's job performance. Employees need to know when they are meeting job performance standards and when they are not. When positive supervisory relationships have been established, feedback occurs naturally and informally throughout the work week. The supervisor comments on what he or she observes and uses the feedback to point out when performance needs to be changed as well as to verify and praise effective performance. Effective feedback needs to be descriptive rather than evaluative

> **Evaluative:** Your initial interview was poorly done.
> **Descriptive:** Your initial interview used more "closed" yes/no answer questions than open-ended questions, limiting the amount of information you were able to gather.

Effective feedback also needs to be specific rather than general.

> **General:** Your productivity performance is below our standard.
> **Specific:** We expect our therapists to see nine clients each day, and you are seeing only six.

Providing feedback that is descriptive and specific will help you to focus on the effectiveness of the supervisee's work

BOX 68.2 GUIDELINES FOR GIVING FEEDBACK

- ◆ Provide timely feedback—give feedback as close to when the behavior was observed as is possible.
- ◆ Provide balanced feedback—point out what is working as well as what needs to be changed.
- ◆ Provide feedback on behaviors that can be changed.
- ◆ Use "I" statements.
- ◆ Avoid the use of generalizations such as "always," "never," and "all."
- ◆ Ask the supervisee if he or she understood what you said; ask the supervisee to restate it in his or her own words.
- ◆ Ask for feedback about your feedback—how did you do?

behaviors and not on his or her personal characteristics or personality. This distinction is critical to the supervisee's being able to "hear" and respond to the feedback. Other suggestions for giving feedback are listed in Box 68.2.

Remember that the purpose of supervision is to support effective work performance. When supervisors evaluate employees, they are evaluating what employees do—how they behave, how they act, how effectively they are accomplishing the work. The focus of feedback in supervision—both informal and formal—is on the task, not the person. The purpose is to relay information about performance to the performer so that actions can be taken to maintain or improve performance.

Performance Evaluation and Appraisal

Newstrom and Bittel (2002, p. 293) point out four basic reasons for appraising an employee's performance:

1. To encourage good behavior or to correct and discourage below-standard performance
2. To satisfy employee's curiosity for how they are doing
3. To provide an opportunity for coaching to develop employee skills
4. To provide a firm foundation for later judgments that concern an employee's career such as promotions, pay raises, and transfers.

A supervisor should be regularly evaluating the supervisee's performance and providing feedback. However, at least once or twice a year, the supervisor should meet with the employer and provide a formal and systematic evaluation of how the person is performing, using a structured performance appraisal format. Most organizations have formal performance appraisal systems and appraisal forms.

Appraisal methods and formats may vary and could include written narratives, behaviorally anchored rating scales, management by objectives, or 360-degree feedback (Allen, 1998; Newstrom & Bittel, 2002). In a formal performance appraisal, the employee's performance is compared to established standards.

As a supervisor, you might be asked to develop job standards for occupational therapy personnel. Professional and workplace resources that can help you to identify standards include the profession's Standards of Practice (AOTA, 2005b), the "Guidelines for Supervision, Roles, and Responsibilities During the Delivery of OT Services" (AOTA, 2004), and worksite job descriptions. Standards will vary by workplace, but all standards should include *what* performance or behaviors are expected, *how* performance will be *measured,* and *when* performance is to occur. An example of a standard that includes all of these criteria is "Evaluations are completed and distributed within 24 hours of initial contact with the client."

In preparing a formal performance appraisal, the supervisor needs to complete three steps:

1. **Gather information about the employee's performance.** Review your supervisory logs, noting key incidents which you recorded. Record additional information that might have been overlooked. Review other employee records, such as attendance, training and educational records, competency check off completions. Review the previous year's performance appraisal. Talk to other members of the team both within and outside of your department to understand how the employee's performance is viewed by others. Ask the employee to perform a self-appraisal of his or her work, identifying accomplishments, strengths, and weaknesses. You can ask the employee to give this to you before the performance appraisal or have the employee bring it to the performance appraisal meeting.
2. **Compare current performance to standards.** Note areas of strength and areas in which improvement may be needed.
3. **Reflect on and synthesize information.** Consider the needs of the department as well as the professional growth needs of the supervisee. Provide feedback about the effectiveness, efficiency, and safety of performance. Note how the employee has contributed to the department's achievements. Document your comments, including both positive feedback and constructive criticism. Be careful to avoid allowing an employee's positive or negative qualities in one area to influence your assessment in other areas. Be watchful of being overly lenient or strict. Be objective and balanced, and focus feedback on task performance. Numerous websites offer information on how to perform effective performance evaluations and can alert you to additional factors to be aware of.

When the performance appraisal is completed, it is time to meet with the employee. The purpose of this meeting is to provide an opportunity for the supervisor and supervisee to discuss the employee's job performance and to collaborate on ways to improve it. Unfortunately, performance appraisal meetings are often viewed as anxiety-provoking events that focus on what the employee has done wrong. The common emphasis on the supervisor's rating of the employee tends to detract from a collaborative educational process during which supervisee and supervisor share perspectives and work together to identify barriers to improved performance. The supervisor can use several approaches to correct this problem:

1. **Demystify the process.** Make sure the employee is familiar with the evaluation process ahead of time. If a standard form is used, make sure the employee has seen it and understands any terminology or rating scales that are used. Make sure the employee is aware of the job expectations and standards. Involvement of staff members in establishing performance standards promotes adherence to and acceptance of standards. Involve the employee in the appraisal process by using a self-assessment.
2. **Plan ahead.** Notify the employee ahead of time as to when the meeting will be and allow the employee time to prepare.
3. **Establish a comfortable climate for the exchange.** Meet in private. Avoid interruptions. Allow adequate time for discussion. Put the employee at ease in the beginning, and explain that you view this time as an opportunity for mutual sharing on how to improve job performance for the benefit of the employee and the organization.

During the performance appraisal interview, be prepared to collaborate with the employee and exchange ideas. Share accomplishments, and review what has not been accomplished. If performance ratings are provided, be sure to provide reasons for your ratings that are based on actual job performance. If the employee is surprised by any of your ratings or comments, you probably have not provided enough regular feedback during the year. Take note, and work to correct that. The appraisal interview offers another opportunity to realign expectations about job performance and to target goals for the future.

Handling Work Performance Problems

Although there are numerous types of performance problems in professional practice settings, the most common ones are behavior or conduct problems in which a rule is broken, performance that falls below the standard expected, and interpersonal issues that interfere with department morale and effectiveness. Each type of problem is handled differently, but in all situations, the actions that are taken are directed toward helping the employee to improve performance and meet job expectations.

Behavior or Conduct Problems

Behavior or conduct problems are handled by disciplining. Behavior or conduct problems may include absenteeism, chronic late arrival, intoxication, insubordination, negligence in following procedures, and falsification of records. These are all serious infractions and should not be allowed to persist. Although individual facilities may adopt their own specific procedures for disciplining a variety of infractions, disciplining is generally handled in a progressive manner. In a progressive discipline approach, the employee is counseled repeatedly if performance does not improve, and the penalties for noncompliance with the rules become increasingly harsh (see Fig. 68.3).

In the first stage of progressive disciplining, the performance problem is discussed with the employee, clear expectations for acceptable performance are outlined, and consequences of not improving are described. In the second stage, the process is repeated, and this time, a written record of the exchange is documented. The employee signs it, and it is placed in his or her personnel file. If the behavior persists, in the third stage, the employee is laid off for a period of time and is told that when he or she returns to work, the behavior must be corrected or the employee will be discharged. The last stage occurs if the employee returns to work and another infraction occurs, at which time the employee is discharged.

A useful analogy for administering any discipline is the "red-hot stove" rule. The analogy likens the process of administering discipline to that of touching a red-hot stove and points out the four essential characteristics of a good disciplinary policy and practice. Discipline should be administered in the following manner:

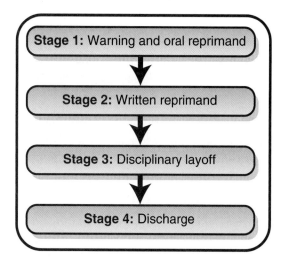

FIGURE 68.3 Using a standard sequence for dealing with performance problems is required in many formal organizations and is considered good practice in most settings.

♦ **With advance warning.** When you see a red-hot stove, you know that if you touch it, you will be burned. An employee should know what will happen if he or she breaks a rule or policy.

♦ **Immediately.** When you touch a red-hot stove, you will be burned right away. Administration of discipline should be done as soon after the occurrence of the behavior as possible.

♦ **Impartially.** No matter who touches a red-hot stove, the person will be burned. Supervisors should not play favorites in administering discipline. Everyone should receive the same penalty for the same infraction.

♦ **Consistently.** Every time you touch a red-hot stove, you get burned. Discipline should be administered the same way with each occurrence.

Performance Problems

Problems of substandard performance are more common in professional practice. When dealing with these types of problems, the supervisor needs to adopt an approach of collaborating with the supervisee and enlisting his or her help in resolving the problem. Typical steps in dealing with this type of problem after the performance problem is identified include the following:

1. Meet with supervisee and point out the performance problem. Review the standard, and describe the expected performance.
2. Collaborate with the supervisee to determine reasons for the problem. Work together to develop an action plan to improve performance.
3. Monitor performance.
4. Repeat the process if needed.
5. Inform employee of consequences if the standard is achieved and if the standard is not achieved.

Interpersonal Work Issues

Interpersonal work issues vary in scope and complexity and are common in all work groups. In a professional practice environment in which teamwork is central to the department's effectiveness and to the achievement of positive client outcomes, problems between workers should not be ignored. Interpersonal issues can arise between practitioners in the OT department or between team members from different disciplines. These types of work problems often stem from miscommunication and/or differences in communication styles or personalities. Lack of clarity about job roles or about expectations can also lead to interpersonal problems.

Just because two people are different or disagree does not mean that they cannot work effectively together. The supervisor's role in resolving these types of performance issues should focus not on personalities, individuals, or differences, but on the job tasks and mutual goals that need to be accomplished. The first approach to take when an employee complains to you about another employee is to listen carefully and encourage the person with the complaint to talk directly to the other individual. You should help the person to clarify his or her concerns and frame them in terms of how the other person's actions are affecting the person's ability to get his or her own job done. This approach often works and begins the process of opening communication.

When this approach does not work, you might need to take further action by talking to each of the parties involved. You might want to do this individually at first and then together, or you might want to approach the problem by talking to the parties at the same time. In either case, you will want to interview both to understand all of the facts and frame the issues or problems in terms of specific behavior and job performance expectations that are being affected. As the supervisor, you also must be clear about your expectations for job performance actions and attitudes and remind both of them about the department's expectations. During this discussion, each party should become more aware of his or her own behaviors as well as the behaviors of the other and how the interaction of their choices is affecting their work. Your goal in this exchange is for both parties to work out a solution that does not compromise the work of either and allows the work of the department to continue more effectively.

SUPERVISION OF OCCUPATIONAL THERAPY PERSONNEL

The profession believes that effective supervision of OT personnel is necessary to ensure safe and effective delivery of services. As was mentioned at the beginning of the chapter, supervision is embedded within the OT process. However, OT practitioners work in a broad range of work environments (medical, educational, and community-based settings). To guide practitioners in developing effective supervisory practices in these different situations, the profession has adopted supervisory guidelines that can be applied in all settings. These guidelines describe how the profession views the supervisory process, who needs to be supervised, the methods and frequency of supervision, and supervisory responsibilities of different occupational therapy personnel.

Occupational Therapists

The American Occupational Therapy Association (AOTA) describes occupational therapists as "autonomous practitioners who are able to deliver services independently" (AOTA, 2004, p. 663). Entry-level OTs are qualified to practice without supervision. The therapist's preparation to deliver services independently is based on education and training, which includes a minimum of six months of supervised fieldwork experience and successful completion of the initial certification exam. Entry-level OTs are trained as generalists and are qualified to enter general practice settings as autonomous therapists. Although entry-level therapists do not require supervision, in the past, close supervision by an intermediate or advanced level OT was recommended (AOTA, 1999). As the profession moved to entry-level master's degree preparation, thinking shifted, and responsibility is now placed on every therapist, at all levels of experience, to assess his or her personal need for supervision and seek it if needed. The current guidelines state that "Occupational therapists are encouraged to seek supervision and mentoring to develop best practice approaches and to promote professional growth" (AOTA, 2004, p. 663). This statement underscores each therapist's professional responsibility to maintain the competencies that are needed to provide safe and effective services. The therapist who enters a work setting that does not provide professional supervision should carefully compare his or her current competencies with the demands of the work setting. When this comparison reveals that current knowledge and skills may need further support or development, the therapist should seek supervision or mentoring to ensure competent practice and professional growth. Although this is not required, many entry-level therapists seek first-time jobs in which supervision will be available. These positions allow them more time to solidify clinical skills and develop confidence. Therapists beyond entry level should continue to assess their need for professional supervision if it is not provided in their work setting. Career changes, such as switching practice settings (from school to nursing home) or types of clients treated (children with autism to adults with spinal cord injuries), may challenge the therapist's current competency and alert the therapist to the need to seek supervision or mentoring (Youngstrom, 1998).

In many occupational therapy practice settings, there may be no formal supervision by another OT. This is particularly common in public school settings. In situations such as these, OTs often seek informal peer supervision from OTs in similar settings. They ask for feedback from each other and share case information, often problem solving together to plan effective interventions. This is a positive and proactive approach that helps to ensure effective professional practice and personal competence.

Occupational Therapy Assistants

Occupational therapy assistants who deliver occupational therapy services must be supervised by an occupational therapist (AOTA, 2004, 2005b). Occupational therapy assistants are trained and educated in basic occupational therapy approaches and techniques, and their role is one of assisting the occupational therapist with the delivery of services. The OT is responsible for all aspects of service delivery and works in partnership and collaboration with the OTA to provide appropriate services to clients. Entry-level OTs are expected to be able to supervise OTAs and to be knowledgeable about the collaborative supervisory relationship that the profession values (Accreditation Council for Occupational Therapy Education, 1999a). Entry-level OTAs are expected to be knowledgeable of the supervisory partnership and to seek supervision appropriately. OTAs, by virtue of their training and education, are often well qualified to take on related work roles (e.g., assistive technologists, activity program directors). When they do take jobs in these related work positions, they are not providing occupational therapy services and consequently do not need to be supervised by an occupational therapist.

Fieldwork Students

Level II fieldwork students at the therapist and assistant level both must be supervised by occupational therapy practitioners. OT students must be supervised by an OT who has at least one year of experience after being initially certified by the National Board for Certification of Occupational Therapy (ACOTE, 1999a). Occupational therapy assistant students may be supervised by either an OT or an OTA, who also must have at least one year of experience after initial certification. (ACOTE, 1999b). If an OTA is providing the Level II supervision for the OT assistant student, it is understood that the supervising assistant is supervised by an OT. According to ACOTE, personnel who are qualified to supervise Level I OT or OTA students include OTs and OTAs as well as individuals from other disciplines such as psychology, social work, and teaching (ACOTE, 1999a, 1999b).

Other Personnel

Other types of personnel who may assist with the provision of OT services or the management of services delivery, such as office personnel, OT aides, or volunteers, may be supervised by either OTs or OTAs. Table 68.3 provides an overview of whom various personnel may supervise.

TYPES OF SUPERVISION: OVERSEEING VARIOUS ASPECTS OF WORK

Work is a complex activity. The responsibility for supervising various aspects of work is sometimes assigned to different people. It is not uncommon for an occupational therapy practitioner to receive supervision from more than one person for different aspects of their work performance. Discussion of three distinct aspects of work performance and the type of supervision used to oversee that performance will help you to see how supervision in some settings may require a multifaceted approach.

Administrative Supervision

Administrative supervision is focused on monitoring performance and making sure that the supervisee's work per-

formance and professional development meet the objectives and standards of the employing organization. Administrative supervisors focus on the administrative aspects of job performance, such as attendance, schedules, benefit usage, and checking for appropriate completion of assigned job tasks. This type of supervision correlates closely with the administrative function of supervision discussed above.

Administrative supervision can be provided by an OT or an OTA to other OTs and OTAs or to members of other disciplines. Likewise, members of other disciplines can administratively supervise OTs and OTAs. This type of supervision commonly occurs in public school settings, in which school principals or special education administrators are the designated supervisors for occupational therapists. As the occupational therapist's supervisor, the principal or special education administrator would be supervising the administrative aspects of the occupational therapist's work.

Clinical or Professional Practice Supervision

Supervision that is aimed at providing support, training, and evaluation of a supervisee's professional performance and development is called **professional practice supervision** or **clinical supervision**. The term *clinical supervision* was the most commonly used term in the past to describe this type of supervision. However, as more OTs and OTAs have moved into work settings outside the clinical medical model (e.g., school settings), the term *clinical supervision* seems less appropriate than the broader term *professional practice supervision*. In professional practice supervision, the supervisor's responsibilities extend beyond the purely administrative aspects of job performance and are additionally aimed at assisting and supporting the supervisee's development of professional discipline specific-skills, such as interviewing skills, appropriate use of selected therapeutic techniques, and clinical reasoning.

Professional practice supervision can appropriately be provided only by a member of the supervisee's discipline. Consequently, it would not be appropriate for a physical therapist to provide professional practice supervision or clinical supervision to an occupational therapist. Likewise, an occupational therapist cannot be expected to provide professional practice or clinical supervision for a physical therapist. Professional practice supervision is the type of supervision that is provided by fieldwork educators during OT and OTA Level II fieldwork experiences. (Fieldwork educators also provide administrative supervision to students.) An OT may provide professional practice supervision to other OTs and OTAs, and an OTA may provide professional practice supervision to other OTAs. This type of supervision correlates closely with the educational and supportive supervisory functions.

Functional Supervision

A third type of supervision that is seen in some occupational therapy practice environments is **functional super-**

TABLE 68.3 PATTERNS OF SUPERVISION: WHO CAN SUPERVISE WHOM?

				Personnel to Supervise				
				OT Fieldwork Student		OTA Fieldwork Student		
Type of Supervisor	OTA	OT Aide	Volunteer	Level I	Level II	Level I	Level II	OT
Entry-level OT	X	X	X	X		X		
OT with more than 1 year of experience	X	X	X	X	X	X	X	X
Entry-level OTA		X	X					
OTA with more than 1 year of experience	X	X	X	X		X	X	

vision (AOTA, 1993, p. 1088). In this type of supervision, a specific aspect of work or a "function" of clinical practice is delegated to a specified individual to provide training and oversight in that aspect of work. The supervisor who is providing only functional supervision generally has advanced knowledge, skill, and competence in the area being supervised. For example, an OT supervisor of a new employee might request that another OT who is experienced in wheelchair assessment and positioning provide functional supervision to the new employee in this area. When providing functional supervision, the supervisor is not responsible for the entire supervisory process but supervises the person in relation to his or her developing specific skills or competency and the performance in only in a selected aspect of work or job function.

METHODS OF SUPERVISION

A professional practice supervisor needs to consider what supervisory methods will be most effective in developing and monitoring performance. Supervisees have different learning styles. Worksites have varying caseload demands, administrative requirements for supervision, and time available to provide supervision. Supervisory methods need to be selected to meet the supervisee's needs and the demands of the worksite.

The supervisor is responsible for initially orienting and training the supervisee and then supporting the supervisee's professional growth and development. Careful thought should be given to the type of teaching methods that will be most effective in learning new information and developing work skills. Should information be presented verbally? In writing? Via video? How interactive should the learning be? Should the learner simply observe without demonstrating his or her own skills? Should questions be encouraged? It is a good idea to vary methods and to select the ones that mesh with the learner's skill and comfort level. Involve the supervisee in the process by asking what learning approaches he or she prefers. Box 68.3 lists examples of various learning methods.

To monitor and evaluate performance, the supervisor can utilize direct and indirect approaches.

BOX 68.3 EXAMPLES OF LEARNING METHODS

- Provide written protocols or instructions.
- Have the learner report back on what he or she learned from reading.
- Provide articles or books to read or use as reference.
- Demonstrate and have the learner return the demonstration.
- Provide a verbal explanation or lecture that covers the content.
- Provide videotapes with questions about content to answer at end.
- Have the learner participate in small group discussion to problem-solve clinical situations.
- Discuss cases or problems presented, either one on one or in small groups.
- Role-play situations.
- Provide repeated practice opportunities to apply new knowledge and skills.
- Observe others carrying out tasks; ask for the learner to describe what he or she observed.
- Model desired performance and behaviors.

Direct Supervision

In direct methods of supervision, the supervisor is present when the employee is performing the job and actually observes performance. When we think of supervision methods, this approach is generally the first one that comes to mind. Direct observation gives firsthand information to the supervisor, but this approach is time consuming, and it is not always practical to use as the only method of supervision.

Indirect Supervision

Indirect methods allow the supervisor to ascertain how the job was performed by gathering this information after performance occurs. Indirect methods include communicating with the supervisee (via phone, e-mail, or written correspondence) after performance, looking at written records (attendance records, documentation), or receiving reports from others (clients, parents, other staff or team members) about the supervisee's performance. Listening to what others say provides information about the employee's performance and provides feedback about how others perceive the performance. Supervising performance in a clinical setting by reading the supervisee's documentation is a frequently used indirect method in occupational therapy practice. Reading documentation tells the supervisor what happened when clients were seen and provides insight into the supervisee's clinical reasoning and documentation skills. However, using only the indirect method of supervision without also periodically observing performance would not give the supervisor a well-rounded picture of the employee's performance in areas such as interpersonal skill, technique application, adaptability in spontaneous clinical situations, and problem solving. Both indirect and direct methods need to be used to develop an accurate and complete picture of employee performance.

FREQUENCY OF SUPERVISION

One of the first decisions a supervisor must make when developing a supervision plan is to determine how frequently to have contact with the supervisee to teach, train, monitor and evaluate performance. The members of the profession have considered this question in relation to how frequency of supervision should be determined in supervising occupational therapy assistants (see AOTA, 2004, pp. 663–664). The factors that are outlined below can be considered in all supervisory situations. In determining frequency of supervisory contact, the supervisor should consider the following:

1. **His/her own supervisory skills.** Supervisors who are new and just developing their skills might require more frequent contact with the supervisee because they are less efficient in observing and analyzing performance. They might need more time to recognize possible performance issues and to provide supervisory interventions. The supervisor who has had more experience and/or who has previously supervised in a setting might be clearer about performance expectations and able to anticipate problems and provide guidance and direction sooner.

2. **The skills of the supervisee.** New employees who come to a job with background and experience in a similar job probably bring the needed skills to the new job. Generally, these employees will require less initial training and often move very quickly to a point at which they need less frequent supervision. The supervisor, however, must individually evaluate each employee because experience does not always guarantee performance. The employee's speed and style of learning will also affect the frequency of supervision needed.

3. **The nature of the work.** Work that is more varied and complex might require more frequent supervisory contact to allow the supervisor to observe performance at different times under various conditions and levels of complexity. The new occupational therapist working in a rehab hospital whose caseload consists only of stroke patients might require less frequent supervision than the new occupational therapist who is working in an acute care setting seeing clients with orthopedic, neurological and acute medical conditions.

4. **The expectations and requirements of the work setting.** In various work settings, standards and expectations may have developed, based on experience in that setting, that require certain levels of supervision. Although an experienced supervisor might think that weekly contact is sufficient, a worksite might require daily contact.

5. **The expectations and requirements of external regulatory or legislative agencies.** Federal or state laws and regulations and accrediting agencies may specify certain methods of oversight and contact that must occur between the OT and OTA.

Frequency of supervision is generally viewed as occurring on a continuum. At the high end of the continuum, the supervisor is continually in sight of the supervisee who is working. At the low end of the continuum, the supervisor contacts the supervisee only as needed. Table 68.4 provides a description of the various levels along the continuum. In the past, the profession recommended certain frequency levels of supervision for therapists and assistants who were at various experience levels. This approach has been replaced by a more flexible approach that recognizes the variety of factors that need to contribute to the supervisory frequency decision and allows for increased flexibility in dealing with the wide variety of practice setting and supervisory demands that exist within the profession.

TABLE 68.4   CONTINUUM OF SUPERVISION

Frequency of Supervision	Definition
◆ Continuous	Supervisor is in sight of the supervisee who is working (AOTA, 1999, p. 592)
◆ Close supervision	Requires daily, direct contact at the site of work (AOTA, 1999, p. 592)
◆ Routine supervision	Requires direct contact at least every 2 weeks at the site of work, with interim supervision occurring by other methods, such as telephone or written communication (AOTA, 1999, p. 592)
◆ General supervision	At least monthly direct contact, with supervision available as needed by other methods (AOTA, 1999, p. 592)
◆ Minimal supervision	Provided only as needed and may be less than monthly (AOTA, 1999, p. 592)

There are, however, two firm directives regarding need for supervision adopted by the profession:

1. Entry-level occupational therapists do not *require* supervision. They are, however, "encouraged to seek supervision and mentoring to develop best practice approaches and promote professional growth" (AOTA, 2004, p. 663).
2. Occupational therapy assistants must *always* receive some level of regular supervision from an occupational therapist when they are providing occupational therapy services.

THE OT/OTA SUPERVISORY RELATIONSHIP

The profession perceives the supervisory relationship between the OT and OTA as a partnership. Both levels of practitioners are trained and educated within the profession but at different levels. The OT is educated at the professional knowledge and skill level and receives an entry-level graduate degree. The OTA is educated at the technical level and receives an associate of arts degree. Each level of practitioner has complementary but distinct roles. The OT is responsible for overall service provision and can carry out all facets of service provision (i.e., evaluation, intervention planning, intervention implementation and review, and outcomes assessment). The OTA's primary role is in the implementation phase of service provision. OTAs may contribute to other aspects of service provision, such as evaluation and intervention planning under the supervision of the occupational therapist.

The "Guidelines to Supervision of Occupational Therapy Personnel" (AOTA, 2004) outlines the roles and responsibilities of each level of practitioner during the delivery of services. For the partnership to be successful, the OT and OTA each must have a clear understanding of each other's role and respect and value the contribution that each practitioner makes. When the OT and OTA

work as a team, they are able to utilize and build on each other's skills and expand the number and kinds of services that can be provided to clients. When an OT partners with an OTA, the OT is often able to see more clients and to utilize the OTA's personal expertise in specific practice areas or techniques to improve client care.

Service Competency

The purpose of the supervisory process is to ensure that safe and effective services are delivered and that professional competence is fostered. The OT who carries the responsibility for overall service delivery must ensure that the OTA is performing effectively. To ensure that services provided by both levels of practitioners are safe and effective, the OT establishes service competency with the occupational therapy assistant.

> Service competency is the process of teaching, training, and evaluating in which the occupational therapist determines that the occupational therapy assistant performs tasks in the same way that the occupational therapist would and achieves the same outcomes. (AOTA, 1999)

When the OT and OTA initially start working together, the OT will establish service competency for overall job performance. In the early stages of the work relationship, the OT will need to determine what knowledge and skills the OTA has. The establishment of service competency is integrated into the normal supervisory process as the supervisor orients and trains the new employee and begins comparing the employee's performance to the established professional and worksite standards and expectations. The OT should identify the primary job tasks and skills that are needed for the OTA's job. These tasks will vary by site and service setting. The OT will observe and train the OTA and note whether the OTA can perform the identified skills and tasks and whether intervention outcomes are similar to those nor-

COMMENTARY ON THE EVIDENCE

Supervision in Occupational Therapy

The majority of research in supervision has been conducted by business and management researchers. Within the health care professions, nurses, social workers, and counseling psychologists have been the primary contributors to the research on clinical supervision. In occupational therapy, direct empirical evidence to support effective supervisory practice is lacking. The research that is available in occupational therapy is often related to management issues and/or is descriptive in focus. For example, occupational therapy managers, concerned with employee satisfaction and retention, have shown that factors such as feedback and recognition of accomplishments, realistic workloads, and autonomy and opportunities for professional growth and skill development all influence job satisfaction (Barnes, 1998; Smith, 2000). Although these studies did not directly look at supervision, the factors that were identified are all factors that a supervisor can affect, so effective supervision should attend to these factors.

Two recent studies have provided some insight into current supervisory practices. Johnson, Koenig, Piersol, Santalucia, and Wachter-Schutz (2006) reported that more fieldwork educators who supervise Level I fieldwork students are not occupational therapists than in the past. In April 2006, the National Board for Certification in Occupational Therapy reported the results of a 2005 online survey of certification OT and OTA exam candidates that included data on who the practitioner's primary supervisor was and the number of hours of direct supervision received per week (Bent & Conway, 2006). Thirty-eight percent of OTs and 23% of OTAs were supervised by members of other disciplines. Thirty-one percent of OTs and 18% of OTA received zero hours of direct supervision per week. Descriptive statistics such as these prompt us to ask other questions: How does being supervised by someone who is not an occupational therapist affect practitioners' professional growth and commitment to occupation-based practice? Does frequency of direct supervision affect the quality of services delivered and the rate of professional growth?

Both descriptive and empirical studies of supervision in occupational therapy are needed. How do supervisory practices vary by setting? What is the most efficient and effective way to establish service competency with an OTA? What supervisory approaches are most effective in supporting professional growth and development with supervisees? These are only a few of the many questions that need to be answered to provide supervisors with the evidence they need to supervise effectively.

---

mally achieved by the occupational therapist. Examples of job tasks or skills for which service competency may be established include reading the medical record, being able to record appropriate and pertinent information, and being able to appropriately grade an activity to increase its cognitive difficulty.

The concept of service competency is based on the assumption that the supervising OT is competent in the skills for which competency is being established.

Both levels of practitioners are responsible for being aware of each other's competent behaviors and providing feedback to inform each other of possible problem areas.

It is important that the supervisor establish an acceptable standard of performance or level of agreement for skills and tasks on which service competency is being established. For example, when observing client dressing performance, the OTA will rate the client's level of independence at the same level as the OT 95% of the time.

The comparison of outcomes between practitioners is an approach that helps to ensure that services clients receive are of comparable quality. It supports the validity of delegating to the OTA and ensures consistency of services. The methods the OT can use while establishing service competency could include observation, cotreatment, return demonstration of techniques or skills, review of documentation, testing for knowledge and its application, and discussion of cases to ascertain clinical reasoning and judgment.

After initial service competency is established, the OT supervisor will need to periodically recheck service competency to ensure that it is maintained. The OT may also select new tasks and skills in which to establish service competency with the OTA. For example, the OT might decide to train the OTA in how to carry out and score a particular structured assessment tool. After service competency has been established, the OT can delegate the admin-

CHANGING PRACTICE PATTERNS: TAYLOR SUPERVISES AN OTA

Taylor recently started a new job as an occupational therapist at a large long-term care facility in her community. She works with a team of two other occupational therapists and two OTAs. She is responsible for supervising Diane, one of the OTAs. Diane has been working at this facility for five years and considers herself very experienced in dealing with this population. When Taylor started the job, she met with Diane to discuss their supervisory relationship and to determine how they would conduct their OT/OTA partnership. Taylor spent time observing and working with Diane and found Diane to be very helpful in orienting her to the facility and familiarizing her with the patients and the typical occupational therapy interventions that were being used.

Taylor has now worked at the facility for over six months and is more familiar with the clients and their individual needs. She is interested in developing intervention plans that are more individualized and that use intervention activities that relate to each patient's own needs and personal lifestyle choices, whether they will return home or remain in the nursing home's long-term care wing. Interventions in the past have been focused primarily on self-care issues, and Taylor, while not wanting to ignore these occupations, would like to emphasize more instrumental activities of daily living

and leisure occupations in which patients will want to engage if they return home or that might allow them to increase their sense of self-efficacy and control if they remain in long-term care. She has communicated this goal to Diane, and when they develop intervention plans, individualized goals are developed in these areas. However, as she follows up with Diane and observes interventions and monitors patient progress, Taylor has noted that Diane is not choosing to address these goals and continues to use the routine types of tasks and activities that she was previously using.

Questions

1. How would you define the supervisory issues and problems in this situation?
2. As a supervisor in this scenario, what are Taylor's responsibilities?
3. As a supervisee in this scenario, what are Diane's responsibilities?
4. What do you think might be some of the reasons for Diane's behavior?
5. How would you suggest that Taylor approach Diane and address this problem?
6. What do you think might be some supervisory interventions that Taylor could take that would help to improve this situation?

---

istration of this assessment to the OTA and be assured that the results of the OTA's giving the test will be comparable to the results that would be obtained if the OT administered the test. Service competency does not mean that the OTA will perform the task in exactly the same manner as the OTA would—only that the outcomes will be similar.

Frequency and Type of OTA Supervision

The decisions about frequency of supervision for the OTA will vary with practice setting and should be decided on the basis of the five factors previously discussed: skills of the supervisor, skills of the supervisee, nature of the work, expectations and requirements of the work setting, and expectations and requirements of external regulatory or legislative agencies. The OTA's level of service competency and skill will influence the frequency of supervision needed. If service competency has already been established, the need for supervision might be less frequent.

When service competency is being established in a new area or skill, the supervisor will need to change the frequency of supervision until competency is established.

Work factors that can affect frequency of supervision needed by an OTA include increased complexity of client's needs and diagnoses, rapidity of client change, more involved or complex types of interventions, and increased number and diversity of clients in the assistant's caseload. When the client population is complex and/or rapidly changing, frequent reevaluation and adjustment in types of interventions and implementation plans are needed, which require the clinical reasoning and evaluation skills of the occupational therapist. Frequency of supervision needs should be regularly reassessed as workplace demands, client needs, and supervisee skills change.

Since the supervisory process with the OTA is collaborative and both practitioners are responsible for providing safe and effective services, the OT and OTA should discuss the decision about the frequency of supervision.

Supervision frequency and methods should be mutually decided upon.

Although frequency of supervision can vary, OTAs who are providing occupational therapy services will always need some level of regular supervision. Supervision of the OTA on an irregular, spontaneous, or as-needed basis is not appropriate. It does not demonstrate that the OT is providing the ongoing oversight required to ensure safe and effective services, nor does it validate that high-quality occupational therapy is being provided. Many external regulatory and legislative agencies now specify the frequency and type of supervisory contact that must take place between OT and OTA. The Centers for Medicare & Medicaid Services (CMS) states that the OTA providing services to Medicare patients under an OT working in a physician's office must have direct or on-site (in the building but not in the line of sight) supervision on the day of treatment (U.S. Department of Health and Human Services, CMS, 2006). In February 2006, CMS also clarified that the OT is required to write a progress report every 10 treatment days or once every 30-day interval and requires that the OT perform or actively participate in treatments at this frequency level if the treatments have been delegated to an OTA (Thomas, 2006). This requirement necessitates that the OT have regular contact with the client and with the OTA who is providing services. Many state regulatory agencies outline specific supervision requirements in their laws for OTA supervision. Texas requires a minimum of two hours of supervision per month consisting of real-time interaction between the OT and the OTA or direct observation of the OTA by the OT (Executive Council of Physical Therapy & Occupational Therapy Examiners, 2006). Pennsylvania states that the OT supervisor shall have supervisory contact with the OTA equal to at least 10% of the time that the OTA works in direct patient care. Face-to-face contact must occur on site at least once a month and must include direct observation of the OTA performing occupational therapy (Pennsylvania Code, 2006).

Effective OTA Supervisory Relationship

The OT supervisor has the obligation and responsibility to supervise the OTA, and the OTA has the obligation and responsibility to seek supervision. Each is open to the other. In writing about their own collaborative relationship, Barbara Hanft and Barbara Banks (1999) identified six qualities that support the development of collaborative supervisory relationships:

- "*Sensitivity,* for perceiving and responding to one another's professional and personal needs;
- *Dependability,* for keeping commitments and responding to unexpected situations;
- *Attentiveness,* for actively listening to one another;
- *Respectfulness,* for appreciating one another's distinct knowledge, experiences and judgment

BOX 68.4 SUMMARY OF STEPS TO TAKE IN SUPERVISING AN OT ASSISTANT

1. Orient OTA to worksite.
2. Share job and professional expectations.
3. Identify OTA's skill level.
4. Identify OTA's learning needs and methods of learning—ASK!
5. Establish service competency.
6. Collaborate with OTA to establish ongoing supervisory plan:
   a. Select methods.
   b. Select frequency.
7. Document ongoing supervision.

- *Collaborativeness,* for working toward a common goal and representing occupational therapy services together as a unit; and
- *Reflection,* for an ability to use self-observation to review situations objectively from different perspectives" (p. 31).

In a collaborative relationship, both parties understand their unique roles and responsibilities and respect their differences and similarities (Sands, 1998). The process of supervising the OTA will include the OTA in the decision-making process and will be individually tailored to meet the needs of the OTA and the worksite. Box 68.4 presents a summary of the primary steps that should be taken in supervising an OTA.

SUPERVISING OCCUPATIONAL THERAPY AIDES

Occupational therapy aides are individuals with no formalized education in the provision of occupational therapy services who are hired to provide supportive services to OT practitioners. Aides are trained on the job to meet the specific needs of the individual department. Aides do not provide skilled occupational therapy services, and the types of activities they can perform with clients are clearly prescribed in the "Guidelines for Supervision, Roles, and Responsibilities During the Delivery of Occupational Therapy Services" (AOTA, 2004). Aides can perform two types of tasks within the department: They can carry out (1) non–client-related tasks such as clerical work, clinic maintenance tasks, and preparation of work areas and equipment and (2) selected client-related tasks that are routine and supervised by an OT or OTA (AOTA, 2004). For a task to be considered routine, it must meet four criteria:

ETHICAL DILEMMA

Joel Supervises an Employee with Depression

Joel is a supervising occupational therapist in a large metropolitans acute care hospital. He oversees a group of three OTs and one OTA. Recently, one of his supervisees, Naomi, met with him and told him that she has been diagnosed with clinical depression. Joel is not surprised. He had noted that Naomi's work performance had changed, and he was even beginning to become concerned about the quality of Naomi's patient care decisions and her ability to handle the normally fast-paced caseload. Naomi has asked for Joel's help and support by decreasing her caseload so that she may continue to work in an effective manner.

Questions

1. Who are the different players in this scenario to whom Joel has an obligation or duty?
2. As a supervisor, what are Joel's obligations to each player?
3. How are the different needs of the players conflicting?

---

1. The outcome anticipated for the delegated task is predictable.
2. The situation of the client and the environment is stable and will not require that judgments, interpretations, or adaptations be made by the aide.
3. The client has demonstrated some previous performance ability in executing the task.
4. The task routine and process have been clearly established. (AOTA, 2004)

These criteria are based on the understanding that aides do not have the knowledge and skill to evaluate or make changes in an intervention activity but can be helpful in providing oversight or practice of selected activities when change and judgment are not anticipated.

Before a selected task can be delegated to an aide, the OT and/or OTA must be assured that the aide can carry out the task safely and effectively. They must instruct the aide and assess his or her competency in performing the delegated task. The aide also must be aware of all precautions and signs or symptoms that a particular client might demonstrate that would indicate that the aide needs to seek assistance (AOTA, 2004). Each of these requirements is intended to ensure that the aide's interaction with the client will be safe and effective. Practitioners can appropriately use aides to oversee clients who are practicing certain skills after the process has been set up (e.g., one-handed shoe tying and exercise routines). Aides can also provide another pair of hands during physical activities when additional help is needed to engage the client in an activity as when providing assistance to transfer a patient.

Aides can be supervised by either an OT or an OTA. However, when the OTA supervises the aide, the OT maintains overall responsibility for the process because of the OT's supervision of the OTA.

Frequency of supervision will vary with tasks assigned and the aide's skill. Client-related tasks may require closer supervision because of the importance of patient safety and intervention effectiveness. The supervisory plan and process need to be documented to demonstrate accountability.

SUPERVISING NON-OT PERSONNEL

The same basic guidelines and process for effective supervision should be followed in supervising non-OT personnel. The OT who assumes a supervisory or management role may supervise personnel from other disciplines who provide direct services to clients (e.g., physical therapists, psychologists, recreational therapists) as well as personnel who provide support services for the department (e.g., secretaries, reimbursement specialists, information technology specialists). The type of supervision the OT will provide to personnel from other disciplines will be administrative. OTs cannot provide professional practice supervision or clinical supervision because OTs are not trained in the other individuals' professions. Astute supervisors will ensure that their supervisees from other disciplines seek and have access to professional practice supervision and will consult with members of the supervisee's discipline to assist them in evaluating the supervisee's professional practice performance.

CONCLUSION

Supervision is a person-oriented process—much like occupational therapy. The OT supervisor must continually balance the needs of the organization with the needs of supervisees to provide safe and effective services to clients. Awareness of the basic functions of supervision and an understanding of the supervisory process make up the first step in preparing practitioners for the supervisory role.

PROVOCATIVE QUESTIONS

1. Is it possible to be both friend and supervisor?
2. How can you effectively supervise people who are older than you and have more experience?
3. Should an occupational therapist who works alone, without any other OTs, seek supervision from another OT? Why or why not?

REFERENCES

Accreditation Council for Occupational Therapy Education. (1999a). Standards for an accredited education program for the occupational therapist. *American Journal of Occupational Therapy, 53,* 575–582.

Accreditation Council for Occupational Therapy Education. (1999b). Standards for an accredited education program for the occupational therapy assistant. *American Journal of Occupational Therapy, 53,* 583–591.

Allen, G. (1998). *Supervision.* Retrieved May 15, 2006, from http://ollie.dcccd.edu/mgmt1374/book_intro.html

American Occupational Therapy Association. (1993). Occupational therapy roles. *American Journal of Occupational Therapy, 47,* 1087–1099.

American Occupational Therapy Association. (1999). Guide for the supervision of occupational therapy personnel in the delivery of occupational therapy services. *American Journal of Occupational Therapy, 53,* 592–594.

American Occupational Therapy Association. (2004). Guidelines for supervision, roles, and responsibilities during the delivery of occupational therapy services. *American Journal of Occupational Therapy, 58,* 663–667.

American Occupational Therapy Association. (2005a). Ethics: Occupational therapy code of ethics. *American Journal of Occupational Therapy 59,* 639–642.

American Occupational Therapy Association. (2005b). Standards of practice for occupational therapy. *American Journal of Occupational Therapy 59,* 663–665.

Barnes, D. S. (1998). Job satisfaction and the rehabilitation professional. *Administration and Management Special Interest Section Quarterly 14*(4), 1–2.

Bent, M. A., & Conway, S. (2006). *Results of a national study profiling the 2005 certification candidate population.* Retrieved June 19, 2006, from www.nbcot.org

Braveman, B. (2006). *Leading and managing occupational therapy services: An evidence based approach.* Philadelphia: F. A. Davis.

Executive Council of Physical Therapy & Occupational Therapy Examiners. (2006, February). *OT Newsletter.* Retrieved from http://ecptote.state.tx.us/_private/OT_February_%20newsletter%20_0206.pdf

Guralnik, D. (Ed.) (1987). *Webster's new world dictionary.* New York: Warner Books.

Hanft, B., & Banks, B. (1999). Competent supervision: a collaborative process. *OT Practice, 4*(5), 32–34.

Johnson, C. R., Koenig, K. P., Piersol, C. V., Santalucia, S. E., & Wachter-Schutz, W. (2006). Level I fieldwork today: A study of contexts and perceptions. *American Journal of Occupational Therapy, 60*(3), 275–287.

Kadushin, A. (1992). Supervision *in social work* (3rd ed.). New York: Columbia University Press.

Newstrom, J. W., & Bittel, L. R. (2002). *Supervision: Managing for results* (8th ed.). New York: Glencoe McGraw-Hill.

Pennsylvania Code. (1992). *Supervision of occupation therapy assistants.* Retrieved June 30, 2006, from www.pacode.com/secure/data/049/chapter42/s42.22.html

Robertson, S. (1992). *Find a mentor or be one.* Rockville, MD: AOTA.

Sands, M. (1998). Practitioner's perspective of the occupational therapist and occupational therapy assistant partnership. In M. E. Neistadt & E. B. Crepeau (Eds.), *Willard and Spackman's occupational therapy* (9th ed., pp. 83–89). Philadelphia: Lippincott.

Smith, V. (2000). Survey of occupational therapy job satisfaction in today's health care environment. *Administration and Management Special Interest Section Quarterly, 16*(4), 1–2.

Thomas, J. (2006, April 17). Interpreting Medicare's documentation requirements. *OT Practice, 11*(7), 8.

Urish, C. (2004, February 9). Ongoing competence through mentoring. *OT Practice, 9*(3), 10.

U.S. Department of Health and Human Services, Centers for Medicare & Medicaid Services. (2006). *11 part B billing scenarios for PTs and OTs.* Retrieved April 30, 2006, from http://www.cms.hhs.gov/TherapyServices/02_billing_scenarios.asp#TopOf Page

Youngstrom, M. J. (1998). Evolving competence in the practitioner role. *American Journal of Occupational Therapy, 52*(9), 716–720.

Payment for Services in the United States

HELENE LOHMAN AND AMY LAMB

Learning Objectives

1. Describe the historical impact of health insurance on occupational therapy practice in the United States.
2. Explain the key types of governmental and private pay insurance, as well as other methods of payment that are accessed by patients in occupational therapy practice.
3. Describe who are the uninsured in the United States and articulate issues related to lack of insurance.
4. Discuss how occupational therapists can become advocates for third-party coverage.

Susan, an occupational therapist who is a new graduate, works at an acute care hospital outpatient clinic. During her first month on the job, she had two circumstances involving reimbursement for patients that awakened her to the realities of payment. One was the case of a patient on Medicaid whom she followed for several visits. Very few patients in the clinic were on Medicaid. Susan was surprised to learn, after seeing the patient for a few sessions, that his Medicaid benefits did not reimburse for occupational therapy services in their state. He ended up paying out of pocket for some but not all of his expenses, and the hospital wrote off most of his expenses. The other patient was covered by a health maintenance organization, which required preauthorizations for therapy treatment. Not knowing the system, Susan had failed to obtain necessary preauthorization, and the patient's therapy was denied. Susan had just assumed that her manager would educate her about the specifics of payment. Susan learned from these experiences the importance of understanding the nuances of different insurance plans and methods of payment.

INTRODUCTION: OVERVIEW OF PAYMENT

Payment issues are a major force affecting occupational therapy practice (Burke & Cassidy, 1991). When major changes occur with payment sources, practice is transformed. Federal and state legislation regulating payment strongly influences the direction of these practice shifts. For example,

Medicare, Title 18 of the Social Security Act, enabled expansion of occupational therapy practice for older adults, and subsequent amendments that changed how the law was regulated resulted in shrinking practice in some areas.

In daily practice, the knowledge practitioners have about payment is often based on the typical sources that cover their patients and clients. Some therapists who handle their own billing for services are very aware of the regulations affecting the payment that they receive. Others, like Susan, depend on their billing department or their manager to keep them abreast of payment policies and procedures. We suggest that it is important for all therapists, no matter where they work, to understand payment systems that affect practice and to be proactive by being aware of changes that may affect practice. Why? Because obtaining payment is the "bread and butter" of most practices, and therapists should be involved in obtaining optimal payment. This knowledge helps to support patients in their ability to access occupational therapy services.

This chapter provides a foundation about payment systems in the United States by first providing a brief history of insurance and then reviewing the key payment sources that occupational therapists may encounter in practices. In addition, this chapter addresses the needs and issues of the growing number of uninsured people in the United States and the effect of these numbers on heath care delivery. To fully understand payment systems, knowledge is required about the legislation that affects reimbursement and associated regulations. Public policy related to payment is discussed in this chapter, supplemented by some of the information mentioned earlier in Chapter 17. Documentation, which is directly related to receiving third-party reimbursement, is discussed in Chapter 39. Therefore, it is important to consider those additional chapters to get a thorough overall picture of payment for occupational therapy services.

HISTORY OF HEALTH INSURANCE

Health insurance was introduced in the United States in the 1700s with the federal Marine Hospital Service (McCarthy & Schafermery, 2001). This insurance was an anomaly, as most people directly paid for any health care they needed until the twentieth century, when the insurance industry grew (Patel & Rushefsky, 1995). During the twentieth century, several types of insurance were introduced, which laid the foundation for insurance in the twenty-first century. Factors such as advances in medical treatment with expensive technological interventions, Americans wanting increased value for their medical care, and expanding medical costs led to the development of the insurance industry (Shi & Singh, 2004). At the beginning of the twentieth century, the first workers compensation laws were enacted. These laws were based on concerns for

the well-being of injured workers. They brought about a system that remains today of state legislation regulating the care of injured workers.

Third-Party Payment

In 1929, a model for hospital-based insurance, Blue Cross, and eventually a physician/medical services plan, Blue Shield, developed that laid the foundation for modern-day health insurance. Blue Cross/Blue Shield established a third-party payment system in which health care consumers paid a set monthly premium to receive medical services (Patel & Rushefsky, 1995). Providers were reimbursed a **fee for service** based on "reasonable and necessary" criteria with minimal restrictions on the numbers and types of interventions that consumers accessed (Sandstrom, Lohman, & Bramble, 2003). Fee-for-service type of payments occurred in **indemnity plans**, in which payments were made retrospectively to the provider.

The twentieth century also saw the growth of employer-based self-insurance plans. With self-insurance, businesses established their own internally funded plans and determined what services to include. For example, businesses could choose to include or exclude occupational therapy as a service if the insurance company from which they contracted services offered therapy in its menu of options. In 1965, federalization of health care insurance was introduced with Medicare and Medicaid. Provision of these plans paralleled the fee-for-service approach toward payment of the time. During most of the remainder of the twentieth century, health care insurance was based on a fee-for-service system with indemnity plans.

Shifting from Fee for Service to Managed Care

Legislation helped the health insurance industry to grow. Because of public policies that included tax incentives for employers and provided protection of self-insurance plans from state laws (Employment Retirement Income Security Act of 1974), the insurance industry expanded, especially in the area of self-insurance. The passage of the Health Maintenance Organization Act in 1973 laid the foundation for the development and growth of **managed care** in the insurance industry. However, it was not until the 1980s and beyond that managed care came to dominate the insurance market (Raffel & Barsukiewicz, 2002).

With the advent of managed care, a paradigm shift occurred that influenced health care payment. The insurance industry no longer focused on providing unrestricted and unlimited coverage for health care services; rather, it focused on controlling costs and coverage. An analogy of this paradigm change is like a change from having unrestricted food at a cruise ship buffet without considering the costs or amount of food being eaten (fee-for-service/indemnity plans) to knowing the food allowance before the meal and being restricted to what you can order within that predetermined amount (managed care environment). Similarly, managed care restricted payment for health care services. One result was a movement away from retrospective payment for treatments, in which payment was made on the basis of what was billed, to prospective payments, in which the amount to be paid for services was established before the treatment. In the mid-1980s, the advent of **Diagnostic Related Groups (DRGs)** for Medicare Part A patients in acute care hospitals reflected this prospective approach and the overall paradigm shift. On the whole, these measures were intended to contain the spiraling costs that resulted from Americans using their health care insurance with no limitations and thus consuming services much like those eating at a cruise ship buffet.

CONSUMER-DRIVEN HEALTH CARE

Now we are entering the age of consumer-driven health care. Some people believe that consumer-driven health care will eventually replace managed care as demand for services and costs continue to rise, especially for businesses that provide health insurance as an employee benefit. A factor that encourages this model is a large, aging baby boomer generation with high expectations for health care services (Bachman, 2004). This economically driven approach, supported by public policy, involves lowering health care expenditures while at the same time providing consumer control over health plans. Thus, decision making about health care moves to the consumer instead of to the insurer. An example of consumer-driven health care is high-deductible health plans, which are often accompanied by a **health savings account (HAS)**. These plans are also known as **health reimbursement accounts (HRA)**. HRAs or HASs allow people to save and apply pretax dollars to health related payments. Pretax dollars can be used to pay for deductibles, coinsurance, copayments, and health insurance premiums, which are traditionally paid for with after-tax dollars. The consumer can choose areas that are not always covered by some traditional insurance, such as payment for mental health services, to be reimbursed. Currently, only a small minority of Americans are enrolled in these plans (Kaiser Family Foundation, 2006). However, consumer-driven plans could grow because of regulations from the Internal Revenue Service (IRS) that allow people to roll over unused money from year to year. Regulations also include a clause to cover expenses that are not in a plan but are identified by the IRS as "qualified medical expenses under IRC Section 213 (2)" (Bachman, 2004, p. 17). Legislation will continue to push this approach forward, and the hope is that if these plans become more common, businesses will help to educate their employees about making wise choices for health care options (Anonymous, 2005).

TYPES OF PAYMENT

This section briefly describes many different methods of payment for occupational therapy services. It helps to have an overall perspective of the current status of how Americans are insured, which is presented in Figures 69.1 and 69.2. This section includes several case studies, which illustrate payment systems.

Self-Pay

In the ideal world, all people would have access to health care at a reasonable cost. Yet the reality that exists presents a very different picture. People who do not have health care insurance get sick and need therapy services. Some who do have insurance find that their plans might not cover therapy, and most plans limit the number of visits or maximum allocable charges in a given time period. For those people, self-pay is an option, and if they recognize the benefits from therapy, they might be willing to pay the bill. For example, some people choose to self-pay for occupational therapy services beyond what is offered in the school system. Some older adults or their families self-pay for therapy services if the person who needs the service does not qualify for Medicare reimbursement. Practitioners can learn from those in other fields who provide services that are not traditionally covered by medical insurance, such as

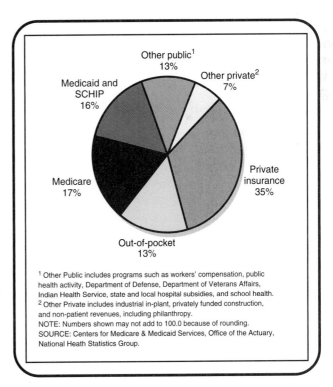

FIGURE 69.1 The nation's health dollar: where it came from, 2004. (From http://www.cms.hhs.gov/NationalHealth ExpendData/downloads/PieChartSourcesExpenditures 2004.pdf)

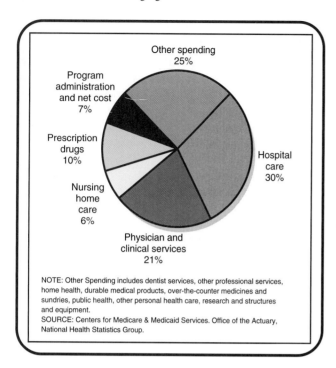

Other spending
25%

Program
administration
and net cost
7%

Prescription
drugs
10%

Nursing
home
care
6%

Physician and
clinical services
21%

Hospital
care
30%

NOTE: Other Spending includes dentist services, other professional services, home health, durable medical products, over-the-counter medicines and sundries, public health, other personal health care, research and structures and equipment.
SOURCE: Centers for Medicare & Medicaid Services. Office of the Actuary, National Health Statistics Group.

FIGURE 69.2   The nation's health dollar, where it goes, 2004. (From http://www.cms.hhs.gov/NationalHealthExpend Data/downloads/PieChartSourcesExpenditures2004.pdf)

acupuncturists or neuropaths. Many health care plans do not cover such services, but some people are willing to pay out of pocket for a perceived valuable service. Another reason for self-pay might be that a clinic does not bill insurers but requires payment up front. Thus, patients must submit their own bills to the insurer for payment.

Grants (Community Agencies)

One aspect of the American Occupational Therapy Association's Centennial Vision involves "Demonstrating and articulating our value to individuals, organizations, and communities" (AOTA, 2006, p. 3). As Case Study 69-1 illustrates, assisting communities in nontraditional settings often entails obtaining grant funding. Grant writing

is an art that involves clear documentation along with understanding the focus of the granting agency. In most cases, grant proposals must follow strict guidelines, and in all cases, they require careful documentation of the proposed program, service recipients, and expected outcomes (Braveman, 2006). Grant funding can be obtained from federal, state, or local government agencies and from private organizations. This type of "soft" payment provides funding for a prescribed time period, but when the grant is completed, practitioners need to find other sources for program support.

Costs Embedded in Larger Structures

In some instances, therapists work in settings in which the cost for their services is embedded in a larger payment structure, such as a case rate. An example of this type of coverage is by DRGs in acute care settings. With DRGs, hospitals receive from Medicare a set payment that is determined by diagnosis. All hospital services that are provided to a patient, including occupational therapy, must then be embedded in the payment structure.

Government Payment in the United States

Although we do not have universal health care in the United States, as in other major industrial countries (e.g., Canada, the United Kingdom), government funding does account for a large percentage of our health care dollar, as Figure 69.1 illustrates. The following sections outline key government programs. Note that one is a federal program (Medicare), others are federal/state programs (Medicaid, State Children's Health Insurance Program, IDEA), and one is a state program (Workers Compensation).

MEDICARE

The history of Medicare is important to consider because Medicare remains the principle financier of health care in the United States (Sandstrom et al., 2003), and changes

---

CASE STUDY: *Jeff: Paying for Services in a Homeless Shelter*

Jeff had a creative idea. He wanted to develop and administer a program to help displaced families in homeless shelters. He knew from his professional education that occupational therapy services can be provided in many nontraditional settings in the community. Jeff began a process of networking with people in his state and with professors at the local university. Through this networking, he located a state grant for which he wanted to apply to finance his idea for the program. Jeff partnered with a ther-

apist at the university, and together they wrote a proposal for a grant, which was funded for three years to develop Jeff's dream program. Jeff later reflected that he would never have been able to create this program without his university partner's mentorship. Jeff also acknowledged that it was his dream paired with his knowledge that ultimately provided access to occupational therapy for people without homes, who would not have been able to afford the services.

with the Medicare law have influenced overall health care provision and occupational therapy practice. This section includes an overview of the history of Medicare followed by a discussion of what is included in the law and how it affects current occupational therapy practice.

History

Part of the impetus for the Medicare law was to provide a solution to a growing concern about providing health care coverage for all Americans. An earlier attempt during Harry Truman's presidency to amend the Social Security act to include health insurance for all workers and their dependents as well as retired people had failed. Often with public policy, when a major bill has failed, there is an attempt to provide some type of fix to appease the American people. In this case, the fix was Medicare, as it was argued that only 15% of older adults had health insurance (Bodenheimer & Grumbach, 2005) and the older adult population had significant medical and financial needs. It was also acceptable to target older adults, because everyone inevitably would age and need health care benefits (Fein, 1986; Patel & Rushefsky, 1999). In addition, because the original Social Security law also targeted the aged, it was considered appropriate for public policy to again address the needs of that population (Fein, 1986). Another factor was that President John Kennedy was not politically strong enough to push forward a national health insurance plan, having won the election by a narrow margin (Patel & Rushefsky, 1999). One more factor that helped to push forward Medicare and other health policies was the changing composition of Congress, which had become more liberal (Lammers, 1997).

Given these factors, Medicare was passed into law during Lyndon Johnson's presidency. As with any public policy, the final bill was a compromise among different competing factions. In the U.S. system, all public policies involve compromises, which are worked out in conference committees. Thus, the final Medicare bill met the agendas of Johnson's Democratic administration by including a national health insurance for older adults funded through payroll taxes and of the Republicans by including a voluntary insurance program called Medicare Part B for physician and other services, such as occupational therapy, which was funded through general revenues (Bodenheimer & Grumbach, 1999).

Where and how many therapists practice are directly linked to the Medicare law and changes made to the law over time. Therefore, it is useful to understand an overview of key changes in the Medicare law since it was enacted in 1965. Table 69.1 highlights historical changes in the Medicare law over the years that have influenced occupational therapy practice. From the inception of Medicare in 1965 until 1983, changes in the law influenced occupational therapy practice in home health and hospice. In 1983, the introduction of a prospective payment system

(PPS) in acute care hospitals titled DRGs forever changed the landscape of Medicare reimbursement and, along with that, of occupational therapy practice. As a result of the DRGs, occupational therapists began working in larger numbers in other settings besides acute care hospitals (Swartz, 1998). DRGs resulted in shortened inpatient hospital stays and patients being discharged to other systems for additional care, such as outpatient therapy, inpatient rehabilitation units, home health care (HHC), or skilled nursing facilities (SNFs). The introduction of PPS in acute care hospitals also led to the development of new delivery systems. During the 1980s, subacute care units evolved to provide cost-efficient service to more acutely ill patients who had been discharged from hospitals with complex medical and rehabilitation needs (Griffin, 1998).

The establishment of a PPS as a cost-cutting measure spread over the next 20 years (between 1983 and 2003) into many other treatment settings covered by Medicare reimbursement. Even as early as 1984, there was discussion about launching PPS in SNFs (Scott, 1984). However, most of the system changes occurred in the late 1990s (in 1997, PPS in SNFs) or early into the next century (in 2000, HHC; in 2002, PPS in inpatient rehabilitation hospitals). In each of these settings, PPS is administered differently, but in all the systems, reimbursement for Medicare beneficiaries is allocated prospectively rather than retrospectively. Other cost-cutting measures have been introduced, such as a managed care option for Medicare beneficiaries and a cap on outpatient Part B therapy. As the large numbers of baby boomers age and qualify for Medicare coverage, one can anticipate continual cost-cutting measures. Issues of solvency are and will continue to be discussed.

How the Medicare System Works

All Medicare beneficiaries are covered under Part A, and some elect to be covered under the voluntary program of Part B. Part A covers inpatient hospitalization and critical access hospitals, SNFs, HHC, and hospice care. With Part B, the beneficiary pays a set fee per month to cover physician and outpatient services such as diagnostic tests; outpatient surgery; physical, speech, and occupational therapy; HHC; blood tests; and some preventive tests. Part B also covers some durable medical equipment. In 2006, the Medicare Prescription Drug Plans were initiated. It involves beneficiaries paying a monthly premium, a yearly deductible, and partial copayments depending on the amount that is spent out of pocket (Centers for Medicare & Medicaid Services, 2005).

As with any public policy, the original Medicare law was written very generally, with the interpretation of the law written into specific regulations, which health practitioners follow to receive payment. These regulations are governed by fiscal intermediaries located throughout the United States. Fiscal intermediaries monitor and pay

TABLE 69.1 HISTORICAL HIGHLIGHTS OF CHANGES IN THE MEDICARE LAW INFLUENCING OCCUPATIONAL THERAPY PRACTICE

Year	Amendment/Change	Impact on Occupational Therapy
July 30, 1965	Medicare or Title 18 of the Social Security Act was signed into law.	Encouraged the growth of occupational therapy practice.
1972	Medicare was extended to cover populations under age 65 with disabilities and end-stage renal disease.	Extended occupational therapy services to those who were qualified to be disabled.
1980	The Omnibus Budget Reconciliation Act included occupational therapy as a qualifying service under Part B with home health and a provision established comprehensive outpatient rehabilitation facilities to be Part B providers.	Had the potential of expanding occupational therapy services in home health as occupational therapy solely could qualify a person for skilled home health services if the person was considered to be home-bound according to the law. The second provision allowed occupational therapists to receive Part B reimbursement in freestanding rehabilitation outpatient settings, which expanded treatment coverage.
1981	The Budget Reconciliation Act eliminated occupational therapy as a qualifying service with home health.	This change required nursing, speech therapy, and physical therapy to qualify the patient for skilled care before occupational therapy. (To date, this provision remains unchanged.)
1982	In the Tax Equality and Fiscal Responsibility Act, hospice benefits were enacted on a temporary basis.	Occupational therapists began to work in hospice.
1983	Change from "reasonable cost" payment to a prospective payment system in hospitals (DRGs).	Resulted in shorter acute care hospital inpatient stays, with patients often transitioned to other settings, such as SNFs, for additional treatment. Occupational therapists began working in the systems to which patients were being discharged, such as SNFs and subacute care units.
1986	In the Consolidated Omnibus Budget Reconciliation Act of 1985, hospice benefit became permanent.	Occupational therapists work in this area.
1992	Physician services paid for on a fee schedule.	Occupational therapists also bill Medicare from the fee schedule, using Physician's Current Procedural Terminology Codes for Part B services.
1997	The Balanced Budget Act (BBA) of 1997 included a Prospective Payment System for home health beginning in 2000. The act also included a prospective payment plan for Medicare Part A in SNFs beginning in 1998. The BBA also established "caps" on Part B outpatient rehabilitation services of $1500 for occupational therapy and $1500 for speech therapy and physical therapy combined. The Balanced Budget Refinement Act called for the establishment of a PPS in inpatient rehabilitation units.	Changed the approach of practice in SNFs. Several legislative attempts were made to suspend and repeal the outpatient cap.

TABLE 69.1   HISTORICAL HIGHLIGHTS OF CHANGES IN THE MEDICARE LAW INFLUENCING OCCUPATIONAL THERAPY PRACTICE *Continued*

Year	Amendment/Change	Impact on Occupational Therapy
1999	The $1500 cap became effective in January 1999 for non-hospital-based clinics. The Medicare, Medicaid, and SCHIP Balance Budget Refinement Act of 1999 was passed, adding a two-year moratorium on therapy caps in November 1999 (became effective in 2000). Increased payment for RUGs. Added regulations for medically complex patients.	While the caps were on moratorium, OT practice with Part B remained the same.
2002	PPS was instituted in inpatient rehabilitation hospitals. (Inpatient Facility Rehabilitation Patient Assessment Instrument, IRF-PAI)	Occupational therapists participate, completing the IRF-PAI for the patient classification payment system.
2000–2005	Several acts placed moratoriums on the therapy cap (2000, 2002). Several acts were introduced to repeal the cap (2001, 2002, 2003, and 2005). The cap became effective (September 2003). Another two-year moratorium was placed on the cap December 2003.	While the caps were on moratorium, OT practice with Part B remained the same.
2006–2007	The therapy cap for hospital-based clinics was instituted. The passage of the Deficit Reduction Act of 2006 allowed for a temporary exemption process for the therapy cap for certain conditions. Legislation continues to be introduced to repeal the therapy cap.	With the exemption, occupational therapists could apply for continued treatment for some patients.

Source: Compiled from American Physical Therapy Association (2007); *Caring* (1999); Chartlinks (2005); Mallon (1981); National Association for the Support of Long Term Care (2005).

claims and perform medical reviews, audits, and investigations. Although many regulatory changes have occurred with Medicare, such as the PPS, the same guidelines remain for determining occupational therapy coverage. Reimbursement for occupational therapy treatments requires a physician's order, and treatment must be completed by a qualified occupational therapist or occupational therapy assistant under the supervision of a qualified occupational therapist. Treatment must be of reasonable duration and amount and must be appropriate for the patient's condition. Treatment must also result in practical improvements in the patient's functional performance (Centers for Medicare & Medicaid Services, 1987).

PPS in Skilled Nursing Facilities

The introduction of PPS for Part A patients in skilled nursing facilities had a significant impact on how therapists practiced in those settings. The PPS system in SNFs involves a mandated assessment structure with periodic patient reviews. The Minimal Data Set, a patient-screening form that considers the patient's status, was instituted to determine clinical care of patients and payment. Sections of this instrument help to determine the classification categories for patients and ultimately the allocation of time that patients can be followed. Patients who qualify to receive rehabilitation are divided into five resource utilization groups (RUGs) ranging from ultra-high to low. Each group has a set amount of therapy minutes that a patient receives in a week and the disciplines (ranging from one to three) that can follow the patient. For example, a patient who qualifies to be in the "very high" RUG category is followed for 500 minutes by at least one discipline (Health Care Financing Administration, 1998).

PPS in SNFs is not without controversy. When PPS was instituted, consolidations and closures of rehabilitation companies occurred, along with losses of therapy positions, salary cuts, and, in some situations, salary changes from a set amount to hourly payments (Steib, 1999). Concerns about the quality of patient care in SNFs have been voiced in pilot studies examining the impact of the PPS (Brayford et al., 2002; Kennedy, Maddock, Sporrer, &

Green, 2002). Other expressed concerns are about treatment being less client-centered, ethics of treatment, and productivity demands, as well as less evaluation, treatment, and documentation time. In addition, some therapists reported less continuing education money, reduced fieldwork placements at their worksites, downsizing of departments, and lack of job security (Brayford et al., 2002; Kennedy et al., 2002). However, practitioners can learn and have learned to work effectively with the PPS by understanding the regulations related to practice, being very time efficient, having good communication skills with other disciplines (Brayford et al., 2002), and finding a mentor (Zellis, 2001).

PPS in Home Health Settings

Often, new changes in Medicare duplicate what has been effective with earlier initiatives. Thus, similar to the PPS system, which requires use of the Minimal Data Set in skilled nursing facilities, home health practice includes an evaluation tool for Part A patients that is called the Outcome and Assessment Information Set (OASIS). The OASIS is used to evaluate patient status and monitor outcomes for quality of patient care. Occupational therapists can consult with the nurse who completes the OASIS about the primary diagnosis for which HHC is needed and about the patient's functional status. Home health agencies are paid prospectively every 60 days an established amount based on calculations. This calculation is derived from a case mix index and a clinical model from which patients are classified into groups called Home Health Resource Groups (Johnson, 2000). Other regulations that were made prior to the PPS remain intact, such as requiring home-bound status for patients under Medicare Part A and the requirement that the other health care professions of nursing, physical therapy, or speech-language pathology must skill qualify a patient to receive

the Medicare benefit before occupational therapy can be provided.

PPS in Inpatient Rehabilitation Facilities

For inpatient rehabilitation facilities, the PPS includes an evaluation tool that is called the Inpatient Rehabilitation Facility-Patient Assessment Instrument (IRF-PAI). The IRF-PAI is based on the Functional Independence Measure™. Like the requirements in skilled nursing facilities, patients are classified. However, in this system, patients are categorized in several ways: by impairment group code, by rehabilitation impairment category, by case mix group, and by the presence of comorbidities. Within this system, occupational therapy practitioners can play an important role in facilitating improved patient function from their interventions, as reflected by the scores on the IRF-PAI (Roberts, 2002).

MEDICAID

Because of an unmet societal need to help low income people, Medicaid, or Title XIX of the Social Security Act, was enacted in 1965. Medicaid insures older adults, children and parents of dependent children, pregnant women, and people with disabilities who meet the eligibility requirements. The majority of Medicaid recipients are children. Yet expenses for a small proportion of the Medicaid recipients, the older adults, account for 70% of Medicaid spending because of extensive use of acute and long-term care services (Kaiser Family Foundation, n.d.). Medicaid pays for 45% of nursing home care in the United States nationwide (Kaiser Commission on Medicaid and the Uninsured, 2007a). It is not surprising that older adults need Medicaid services, especially for nursing home care, with the average cost of nursing home care

---

CASE STUDY: *Gina: Accessing Different Payment Sources to Work in One System*

Gina's favorite population to work with was older adults. She had worked for years in skilled nursing facilities, but when assisted living facilities grew as another living alternative for older adults, Gina decided to work in an assisted living setting. She at first saw residents that qualified for therapy coverage under Medicare Part B. Gina kept current on changes in regulations about the cap on therapy charges for patients receiving Medicare Part B coverage. There were many times when the therapy cap was placed on a moratorium for therapy coverage and a point when it was enacted. When the therapy cap was enacted, Gina carefully monitored the therapy dollars that were spent

so that she did not go over the established amount. In some cases, when the client's condition warranted, Gina requested an extension from Medicare for continued therapy services. Gina's work with patients was well respected at the assisted living facility. As a result, the administrator asked her to provide some consultation, which was paid for directly out of the facility budget. As Gina's practice grew, she also began following some residents who paid out of pocket for her services (private pay). So at the same assisted living facility, Gina was able to provide a variety of types of services and receive a variety of types of payments.

in the United States being $74,095 per year (MetLife Mature Market Institute, 2005).

Medicaid also provides support to 4 in 10 children who have special needs. The Early and Periodic Screening, Diagnostic, and Treatment benefit covers a large amount of services for children (Kaiser Commission on Medicaid and the Uninsured, 2007a). Without Medicaid, many more people would join the growing ranks of Americans who are uninsured (Kaiser Commission on Medicaid and the Uninsured, 2007a).

Medicaid is a program jointly financed by federal and state governments that is regulated by each state. It is considered to be a *means tested* program as people qualify if their assets and incomes levels are below standards set by the program (Shi & Singh, 2004). States can chose to expand their baseline Medicaid coverage and income eligibility requirements beyond the federal minimal requirements. Medicaid programs vary; each state provides different services and different systems for delivery. Quite often, programs are administered by using managed care (Centers for Medicare & Medicaid Services, 2006). Each state has a plan that documents how the program is administered, eligibility requirements, and required and optional health services covered. Occupational therapy is one of the optional services; therefore, in some states, occupational therapy might not be a covered benefit. In 2004, 29 states included occupational therapy as a covered benefit, and occupational therapy was not a covered benefit in 22 states (Kaiser Family Foundation, 2004). However, states are required to reimburse occupational therapy services for children covered under the Early and Periodic Screening, Diagnostic, and Treatment benefit if ordered by a physician and deemed to be medically necessary (Mary Steiner, personal communication, June 8, 2007). It behooves occupational therapists to be aware of changes on a state level and advocate for therapy coverage in their state. Table 69.2 provides examples of required and optional Medicaid benefits.

STATE CHILDREN'S HEALTH INSURANCE PROGRAM

A more recent federal health insurance program, the State Children's Health Insurance Program (SCHIP), or Title XXI, was created in 1997 as part of the Balanced Budget Act. This program provides health insurance to children and some parents in families that are ineligible for

---

TABLE 69.2 MEDICAID SERVICES*

Examples of Required Medicaid Services	Examples of Optional Medicaid Services
• Physician, midwife, and certified nurse practitioner services • Laboratory and X-ray services • Inpatient hospital services • Outpatient hospital services • Early and Periodic Screening, Diagnostic, and Treatment services for individuals under age 21 years • Nursing home care for people over age 21 years • Home health services • Family planning and supplies • Rural health clinic/federally qualified health center services • Generally qualified health center services and any other ambulatory services offered by a federally qualified health center that are otherwise covered under the state plan	• Clinic services • Nursing facility services for those under age 21 years • Intermediate care facility/services for the developmentally disabled • Prescription drugs • Prosthetic devices and eyeglasses • Dental services • Physical therapy and related services • Personal care services • Rehabilitation services • Occupational therapy • Speech, hearing, and language services • Private duty nursing • Podiatrists' services • Chiropractic services • Transportation services • Emergency hospital services • Case management services • Respiratory care services • Home and community-based services for individuals with disabilities and chronic medical conditions

*The lists are not all-inclusive.

Source: Compiled from Kaiser Commission on Medicaid and the Uninsured. (2007b); ElderCare Online (2000); O'Connell, Watson, Butler, & Straube (2004).

ANGIE: A THERAPIST WORKING WITH A PEDIATRIC CLIENT OVER THE YEARS IN DIFFERENT SETTINGS WITH DIFFERENT PAYMENT STRUCTURES

Angie has seen Jamal, a 10-year-old child with cerebral palsy, in therapy for most of his young life. Angie has found that during the time that she had seen him, not only had her skills developed as a therapist, but she had also learned about different payment systems. Angie first saw Jamal when she was a therapist working in a neonatal intensive care unit in an inpatient acute care hospital. Jamal's hospital therapy services were reimbursed by his parent's insurance plan, a managed care organization (MCO). Angie worked with the MCO to obtain proper authorizations. Her focus for therapy with Jamal was on his medical and developmental needs. Five years later, Angie again saw Jamal, this time through the school district, where she had decided to contract part-time. There, she had to learn to change her focus from working in a traditional medical model to working in an educationally based model. Angie's treatment approach with Jamal was to help him improve his learning skills and to help him better participate in school activities. She worked with Jamal directly and consulted with his teacher on

ways to improve his writing skills and self-help skills needed to participate in the classroom and to help Jamal modify some of his behaviors that were creating problems in the classroom. Angie participated in setting goals for Jamal's Individualized Education Program (IEP). When Jamal was 7½, he fell and broke his wrist. Because Angie still provided some contractual services at the hospital, she was able to follow Jamal in outpatient therapy. Again because of the setting and the medical nature of his needs, his therapy was covered by his parent's MCO. In the hospital system, Jamal's goals were based on regaining the functional use of his upper extremity.

Questions

1. Why were the therapy goals different in the school setting than in the hospital setting?
2. What public policies regulate payment for each of the settings?
3. How could Angie learn more about the payment systems in each setting?

Medicaid and for whom health insurance is either unobtainable or cost prohibitive. Like Medicaid, SCHIP is a federal- and state-financed program in which states administer their programs (Kaiser Family Foundation, n.d.). SCHIP is quite an expansive health insurance program, covering one quarter of all children in the United States. Since its inception, SCHIP has been successful in expanding health coverage and access to care as well as in decreasing the number of uninsured children in the United States (Kaiser Commission on Medicaid and the Uninsured, 2007a).

INDIVIDUALS WITH DISABILITIES EDUCATION ACT

As of 2003, the highest percentage of occupational therapists (34.4%) were employed in school-based and early intervention practice (AOTA, 2003). In school-based practice, the Individuals with Disabilities Education Act (IDEA), a federal/state program, regulates and finances services, including occupational therapy, for children with

special needs. The specifics of school-based practice are beyond the scope of this chapter. Nevertheless, therapists working in that system will need to have a strong knowledge of the regulations related to the IDEA and the focus of occupational therapy in the school system. It is beneficial for therapists to understand how IDEA finances services for children with special needs. Because it is a federal/state program, IDEA provided some federal funding, but most of the financing for IDEA comes from taxpayers in local school districts (Baumgartner, Berry, Hojnacki, Kimball, & Leech, 2002). Thus, IDEA is really a federal, state, and school district partnership. As a result, there will be differences in services among school districts and across states. Occupational therapists' salaries, like all special education staff salaries, are figured into a special education budget. A percentage of staff salaries are paid for by state dollars, and the remainder is paid for by the school district. School districts determine whether therapists are contracted or hired as staff. Finally, states determine and regulate the payment rates for therapy and that amount can vary (Steve Milliken, personal communication, June 6, 2007).

WORKERS COMPENSATION

Workers compensation programs are state programs that pay for care of workers who have injuries or illnesses due to work-related causes. Each state has a governing body that determines the administration of the state program. Like other programs that have been discussed in this chapter (Medicaid, IDEA), workers compensation programs vary from state to state, and where they are located in the state government varies. Programs generally pay for medical services to get the person back to work, for benefits for lost wages when appropriate, and for disability. Programs may include services such as vocational rehabilitation, medical rehabilitation, job placement for someone with a permanent disability, and social services (Workers Compensation Board, n.d.). Many of these programs use a managed care approach to run their programs. How workers compensation programs are funded varies from state to state. Generally, they are financed through employer insurance, state funds, or self-insured businesses.

MANAGED CARE

Currently, managed care dominates the private health care insurance market (Dudley & Luft, 2007). Therefore, therapists in many settings will likely see patients who are covered by some type of managed care plan. There are many definitions for managed care. For example, one definition states that managed care is a "comprehensive health care which is provided to participating members of an organized health care organization through the use of a network of health care providers and facilities; it uses a delivery system that secures cost effective health care"

(Medhealthinsurance, n.d.). Another definition states that "managed care is a healthcare system in which there is administrative control over primary health care services in the medical group practice. The intention is to limit redundant facilities and services and to reduce costs" (Mosby, 2002). Thus, common to most definitions is the emphasis on controlling and reducing health care costs.

Managed care "integrates the functions of financing, insurance, delivery, and payment within one organization" (Shi & Singh, 2004, p. 326), and most managed care organizations (MCO) include primary and preventive care (Shi & Singh, 2004). **Health maintenance organizations (HMO)**, **preferred provider organizations (PPO)**, and **point of service (POS)** plans are examples of managed care options. Refer to Table 69.3 for a brief description of these services. In recent years, options such as PPO plans have proven to be the most popular because of increased consumer choice (Kaiser Family Foundation, 2006; Shi & Singh, 2004). Regardless of the type of plan, managed care includes five basic characteristics (Raffel & Barsukiewicz, 2002, p.37):

- ◆ A select panel of providers
- ◆ Comprehensive health services
- ◆ Quality tracking
- ◆ Utilization review
- ◆ Cost containment

Occupational therapy practitioners need to understand how each patient's plan works in order to receive payment. Information about a patient's plan should be obtained or provided by the patient before the initiation of treatment. Some plans require preauthorization for beginning treatment or authorization for continued treatment.

PRACTICE DILEMMA

MARK: A THERAPIST WHO LEARNED A LESSON ABOUT THE DIFFERENCES BETWEEN STATE WORKERS COMPENSATION PROGRAMS

Mark had just moved to another state and obtained a new position as an occupational therapist in a therapy clinic that specializes in orthopedics. The first patient whom he saw, Richard, had injured his right hand in a work injury. Richard's insurance coverage was workers compensation. Mark wrongly assumed that the workers compensation program would be administered in the same way as the one he had been used to working with in another state. Therefore, Mark had not been in contact with Richard's case manager.

Two weeks into therapy, the case manager called, and Mark learned from that conversation some of the differences in the state's workers compensation plan.

Questions

1. How can Mark find out what the workers compensation program in his state covers?
2. What does workers compensation cover in your state, and how is the plan administered?

TABLE 69.3 TYPES OF MANAGED CARE

Health Maintenance Organizations (HMOs)	Preferred Provider Organizations (PPOs)	Point of Service Plans (POS)
These are the most restrictive of the managed care plans. They are based on the concept of having a gatekeeper, usually a primary care provider, monitor and control all care and referrals. As much as possible, health care is provided by the primary care provider. Payment is based on a capitated predetermined fixed rate per patient.	With these plans, participants can select from a pool of a limited number of health care providers. If the enrolled person goes outside of the PPO for care, out-of-pocket costs are higher.	These plans are a hybrid of an HMO and a PPO plan. The enrolled person has a primary care health practitioner who acts as a gatekeeper to manage care and make referrals. The enrolled person also has the choice of using a group of providers like a PPO.

Source: Raffel and Barsukiewicz (2002); Sandstrom et al. (2003).

Occupational therapists work with case managers who monitor care, and good communication is essential for coordination of care (Sandstrom et al., 2003). Finally, managed care has not been without controversy with issues from consumers and health care providers alike. The Patient Bill of Rights, an attempt at federal legislation to regulate managed care organizations better, evolved because of controversies about managed care provision (Lohman, 2003).

THE UNINSURED

In the early 1990s, President Bill Clinton advocated for health care reform, proposing a universal health care plan. One of the president's arguments was the travesty of the 37 million Americans who had no health care insurance. The uninsured were not the poor or older Americans but rather the working poor, those employed in low-wage jobs. Health insurance in the United States was primarily employment based (Raffel & Barsukiewicz, 2002), and individuals in many jobs did not receive health insurance benefits. Downsizing and corporate layoffs also contributed to the uninsured pool (Johnson & Broder, 1997; Vigilante, D'Arcy, & Reina, 1999). In addition, many of the uninsured did not meet the qualifications for public insurance, such as Medicaid.

Today, over 15 years later, the problem has worsened. There are now more than 47 million uninsured Americans (DeNavas-Walt, Proctor, & Lee, 2006). As in the early 1990s, most individuals who do not have health care insurance are employed (or are dependents of people who are employed), but the employer does not provide health insurance and individual health insurance premiums are prohibitive for the individual. Young adults age 18 to 24 years are more likely than any other age group to be uninsured (DeNavas-Walt et al., 2006). The composite of uninsured people also includes immigrants, poor people without other public coverage, and even people with higher incomes (Herrick, 2006). Employees of small businesses also contribute to the pool of uninsured numbers, as approximately two out of five small businesses do not provide health care insurance (Kaiser, Family Foundation, 2006).

Lack of insurance coverage has many negative consequences. The uninsured are less likely to seek out health care or will postpone getting needed health care because of costs. The uninsured obtain less preventive care. In addition, their medical conditions are often diagnosed in later stages, and even after diagnosis, they receive less care and have higher rates of mortality than the insured population (Kaiser Commission on Medicaid and the Uninsured, 2003).

Uninsured people often end up obtaining health care in emergency rooms, which ultimately increases costs for the health care system and may be the inappropriate place to receive care (Herrick, 2006).

Occupational therapists have a moral responsibility to be aware of and consider ways to serve patients who do not have insurance. The profession's code of ethics encourages therapists to "Make every effort to advocate for recipients to obtain needed services through available means" (Commission on Standards and Ethics & Peloquin, 2005, p. 639). On a clinical level, charging reasonable fees for services and providing some pro bono service are ways to help uninsured clients. However, ultimately, the problem is a larger societal issue that will need to be solved with legislation. To date, the United States has been unsuccessful in designing a universal health care system, in spite of many efforts (Raffel & Barsukiewicz, 2002).

COBRA AND HIPAA

As was just discussed, one group that is at risk for being uninsured is people who have changed employment or have been laid off from their jobs. As a result of this major issue, the Consolidated Omnibus Budget Reconciliation Act of 1985 (COBRA) was passed. COBRA allows employees 18 months of continued insurance coverage after leaving a place of employment. However, COBRA is very costly, as individuals pay more than their group rate to obtain this insurance. High costs limit some people who cannot afford COBRA and may ultimately contribute to the number of uninsured Americans. As a result, only 7% of unemployed people get this insurance (Dalrymple, 2003, October 9).

Therapists should be familiar with the Health Insurance Portability and Accountability Act of 1996 (HIPAA) because of the privacy regulations. HIPAA also helps people who have preexisting conditions by preventing denials of insurance coverage with a new plan. HIPAA can provide continued insurance beyond the coverage of COBRA (Shi & Singh, 2004).

ADVOCACY FOR PAYMENT

Now let's return to the scenario about Susan that was presented at the beginning of the chapter. You will recall that Susan faced a number of challenges resulting from lack of coverage for the patients she was treating. As a result of experiencing these problems, Susan might become aware of her many chances to advocate for payment for her patients directly, as well as through efforts coordinated on the state level with her state occupational therapy association and even on a national level (Sandstrom et al., 2003). At the clinical level, Susan could communicate with a case manager of the patient's managed care organization to consider reversing the decision to deny coverage because of the mistake Susan had made when she failed to obtain preauthorization. If necessary, Susan could find out the process for appealing a denied claim and then help her patient to work within the managed care organization's system or possibly contact the state insurance board.

As this discussion illustrates, every time practitioners experience problems getting payment in their daily practice, they should critically consider how best to get reimbursed. Sometimes, effective communication with case managers or other key people in an insurance system make it possible to obtain payment (Sandstrom et al., 2003). Other times, simply following through with the processes in place, such as an appeals system, can work. Sometimes, going beyond the traditional system to get funds through charitable organizations might be an option. For example, therapists might consider contacting an association that specializes in a patient condition, such as the Multiple Sclerosis Association, or might find that a client's friends, family, or faith group may donate needed funds.

The second issue that Susan encountered, that of occupational therapy not being a required Medicaid benefit in her state, demonstrates an opportunity for advocacy through the state occupational therapy association's legislative committee. Susan could choose to become involved with the legislative committee. Members of the legislative committee could methodically work through an advocacy plan to obtain occupational therapy as a required Medicaid benefit in their state. There are many resources for support with such advocacy efforts through the Public Affairs Division of the American Occupational Therapy Association. This division includes a State Affairs Group, a Federal Affairs Group, and a Reimbursement and Regulatory Affairs Group. Depending on the need for advocacy support, an occupational therapist might access one or all of the groups (AOTA, n.d.). Finally, Susan could advocate on a federal level for legislation that affects payment for her practice. For example, she could advocate for possible changes in Medicaid reimbursement. Simple efforts, such as writing letters, can make a difference.

PRACTICE DILEMMA

ADVOCATING FOR SERVICE PAYMENT

Local practitioners as well as state occupational therapy associations are likely to be aware of problems related to payment for occupational therapy services. Additional issues may be posted on the AOTA Website or on the Websites of other professional and consumer groups. Take some time to find out what these concerns are, and then select one to work on to change. Then, keeping in mind the information discussed in this chapter, consider the following questions:

Questions

1. What kind of reimbursement system is related to the issue, and who controls the rules for payment?
2. What efforts have occurred over the past several years to improve the payment situation?
3. What advocacy approaches are likely to be most successful in this situation?
4. What will you do?

CONCLUSION

As the case examples and practice dilemmas in this chapter have illustrated, dealing with payment issues is a regular part of therapy practice. Practitioners may work with a variety of payment systems. On the surface, knowledge about payment systems might seem overwhelming, as the financial system in the United States is very complex. Yet it is every practitioner's professional duty to learn about these systems in order to be able to provide the right intervention and to advocate for payment when needed (Commission on Standards and Ethics & Peloquin, 2005). Payment systems change, and these changes often occur because of new or amended legislation. Keeping current with legislation that affects payment for one's area of practice is essential for successful practice.

REFERENCES

American Occupational Therapy Association. (2003, October). *Member data survey: Final report.* Bethesda, MD: Author.

American Occupational Therapy Association. (2006, January). *AOTA's centennial vision.* Retrieved on June 8, 2007, from: http://www.aota.org/nonmembers/area16/docs/vision.pdf

American Occupational Therapy Association. (n.d.). *Public affairs division.* Bethesda, MD: Author.

American Physical Therapy Association. (2007). *History of the therapy caps.* Retrieved on June 18, 2007, from: http://www.apta.org/AM/Template.cfm?Section=Home&Template=/CM/HTMLDisplay.cfm&ContentID=20959

Anderson, D. M. (2002). *Mosby's medical, nursing, & allied health dictionary* (6th ed.). St. Louis: Mosby.

Anonymous. (2005). Consumer-driven healthcare: The worthy alternative to managed care. *Health Data Management, 13*(2), 96.

Bachman, R. E. (2004). Consumer driven health care: The future is now. *Benefits Quarterly, 20*(2), 15–22.

Baumgartner, F., Berry, J., Hojnacki, M., Kimball, D., & Leech, B. (2002). *Case overview: Individuals With Disabilities Education Act.* Retrieved June 6, 2007, from: http://lobby.la.psu.edu/063_IDEA/summary_idea.htm

Bodenheimer, T. S., & Grumbach, K. (2005). *Understanding health policy: A clinical approach.* New York: McGraw-Hill.

Braveman, B. (2006). Communicating effectively in person and in writing. In B. Braveman (Ed.), *Leading and managing occupational therapy services: An evidence-based approach* (pp. 305–331). Philadelphia: F. A. Davis.

Brayford, S., Muscatine, J., Dunbar, C., Frank, A., Nguyen, P., & Fisher, G. S. (2002). A pilot study of delivery of occupational therapy in long term care settings under the Medicare Prospective Payment System. *Occupational Therapy in Health Care, 15*(2/3), 67–76.

Burke J. P., & Cassidy, J. C. (1991). Disparity between reimbursement-driven practice and humanistic values of occupational therapy. *American Journal of Occupational Therapy, 45*(2), 173–176.

Caring. (1999, September). Medicare: Past, present, and future. 16–19.

Centers for Medicare & Medicaid Services. (1987). *Coverage of services, skilled nursing facility manual.* Retrieved on July 7, 2005, from http://cms.hhs.gov.manuals/12/SNFs/SN00.asp

Centers for Medicare & Medicaid Services. (2005). *Medicare & you 2005.* Retrieved on July 7, 2005, from http://www.cms.hhs.gov/manuals/12_SNFs/sn201.asp#_1_34. http://www.medicare.gov/Publications/Search/Results.asp?dest=NAV|Home|Search|Results|SearchCriteria&version=default&browser=IE|6|WinXP&pagelist=Home&Type=PubID&PubID=10050&Language=English#TabTop

Centers for Medicare & Medicaid Services. (2006). *Medicaid managed care overview.* Retrieved on July 7, 2005, from: http://www.cms.hhs.gov/MedicaidManagCare/

Chartlinks. (2005). *Evolution of the inpatient rehabilitation facility prospective payment system.* Retrieved on June 18, 2005, from: http://www.chartlinks.com

Commission on Standards and Ethics & Peloquin, S. (2005). Occupational therapy code of ethics (2005). *American Journal of Occupational Therapy, 59*(6), 639–642.

Dalrymple, M. (2003, October 9). Senators seek tax credit for unemployed. *Associated Press Online.*

DeNavas-Walt, C. B., Proctor, B. D., & Lee, C. H. (2006, August). *Income, poverty, and health insurance coverage in the United States: 2005.* Washington, DC: U.S. Census Bureau. Retrieved on June 6, 2007, from: http://www.census.gov/prod/2006pubs/p60-231.pdf

Dudley, R. A., & Luft, H. S. (2001, April, 5). Managed care in transition. The New England Journal of Medicine, 344, 14, 1087–1092.

ElderCare Online. (2000). *Medicaid benefits.* retrieved on June 4, 2007, from: http://www.ec-online.net/Knowledge/Articles/medicaidbenefits.html

Fein, R. (1986). Medical care, medical costs: The search for a health insurance policy. Cambridge, Mass.: Harvard University Press.

Griffin, K. M. (1998). Evolution of transitional care settings: Past, present, future. *AACN Clinical Issues, 9*(3), 398–408.

Heath Care Financing Administration. (1998, May 12). *Federal register: Medicare program: Prospective payment system and consolidated billing for, final rule.* Retrieved on June 20, 2005, from: http://www.cms.hhs.gov/providers/SNFspps/fr12ma98.pdf

Herrick, D. M. (2006, September 6). *Crisis of the uninsured.* Dallas TX: Center for Policy Analysis. Retrieved on June 7, 2007, from: http://www.ncpa.org/pub/ba/ba568/ba568.pdf

Johnson, H., & Broder, D. S. (1997). *The system: The American way of politics and the breaking point.* Boston: Little, Brown.

Johnson, K. V. (2000, September, 11). Home health PPS: The new payment methodology. OT Practice, 5, 18: CE1-8.

Kaiser Commission on Medicaid and the Uninsured. (2003, September). *Access to care for the uninsured: An update.* Retrieved on June 5, 2007, from: http://www.kff.org/uninsured/upload/Access-to-Care-for-the-Uninsured-An-Update.pdf

Kaiser Family Foundation (2006, October 24) Kaiser Daily Health Policy Report: Health Care Marketplace: Consumer-Driven Health Plans Appear to Reduce Costs, But Some Plan Beneficiaries Forgo Needed Medical Care, RAND Study

Finds. Retrieved on October 2, 2007 from: http://www.kaisernetwork.org/daily_reports/rep_index.cfm?hint=3&DR_ID=40629

Kaiser Commission on Medicaid and the Uninsured. (2007a, May). *Impacts of Medicaid and SCHIP on low-income children's health.* Retrieved on June 5, 2007, from: http://www.kff.org/medicaid/upload/7645.pdf

Kaiser Commission on Medicaid and the Uninsured. (2007b, March). *Medicaid facts: The Medicaid program at glance.* Retrieved on June 4, 2007, from: http://www.kff.org/medicaid/upload/7235-02.pdf

Kaiser Family Foundation. (2004). *Benefits by service: Occupational therapy services.* Retrieved on June 4, 2007, from: http://www.kff.org/medicaid/benefits/service.jsp?gr=off&nt=on&so=0&tg=0&yr=2&cat=4&sv=25

Kaiser Family Foundation. (n.d.). *Medicaid/SCHIP.* Retrieved on May 31, 2007, from: http://www.kff.org/medicaid/index.cfm

Kennedy, J., Maddock, B., Sporrer, B., & Greene, D. (2002). Impact of Medicare changes on occupational therapy in skilled nursing facilities: Pilot study. *Physical & Occupational Therapy in Geriatrics, 21*(2), 1–13.

Lammers, W. W. (1997). Presidential leadership and health policy. In T. J. Litman & L. S. Robins (Eds.), *Health politics and policy* (3rd ed., pp. 11–35). Albany, NY: Delmar.

Lohman, H. (2003). Critical analysis of a public policy: An occupational therapist's experience with the patient bill of rights. *American Journal of Occupational Therapy, 57*(4), 468–472.

Mallon, F. J. (1981). Nationally speaking: History of occupational therapy Medicare amendments. *American Journal of Occupational Therapy, 35*(4), 231–235.

McCarthy, R. L., & Schafermery, K. W. (2001). *Introduction to health care delivery* (2nd ed.). Gaithersburg, MD: Aspen.

Medhealthinsurance. (n.d.). *Glossary of health insurance terms.* Retrieved on October 6, 2005, from: http://www.medhealthinsurance.com/glossary.htm

Metlife Mature Market Institute. (2005, September). *The Metlife market survey of nursing home & home care costs.* Retrieved on June 7, 2007, from: http://www.metlife.com/WPSAssets/41453139101127828650V1F2005%20NH%20and%20HC%20Market%20Survey.pdf

National Association for the Support of Long Term Care. (2005). *History of the Medicare Part B "therapy caps."* Retrieved on June 16, 2005, from: http://www.nasl.org/Advocacy_pages/Cap_History.htm

O'Connell, M., Watson, S., Butler, B., & Straube, D. (2004, March 24). *Introduction to Medicaid: Eligibility, federal mandates, hearings and litigation.* Retrieved on June 4, 2007, from: http://www.nls.org/conf2004/medicaid-intro.htm

Patel, K., & Rushefsky, M. E. (1999). *Health care politics and policy in America* (2nd ed). Armonk, NY: M. E. Sharpe.

Raffel, M. W. & Barsukiewicz, C. K. (2002). *The U.S. health system: Origins and functions* (5th ed). Albany, NY: Delmar.

Roberts, P. (2002, July, 8). Navigating the inpatient rehabilitation facility prospective payment system (PPS). *OT Practice,* CE1–CE8.

Sandstrom, R. W., Lohman, H., & Bramble, J. D. (2003). *Health services: Policies and systems for therapists.* Upper Saddle River, NJ, Prentice Hall.

Scott, S. J. (1984). The Medicare prospective payment system. *American Journal of Occupational Therapy, 38*(5), 330–334.

Shi; L, & Singh, D. A. (2004). Delivering health care in America: A systems approach (3rd ed). Boston: Jones and Bartlett,

Steib, P. A. (1999, March 11). Survey most practitioners holding their own. *OT Week,* 8–10.

Swartz, K. B. (1998). The history of occupational therapy. In M. E. Neistadt & E. B. Crepeau (Eds.), *Willard & Spackman's occupational therapy* (9th ed., pp. 884–865). Philadelphia: Lippincott.

Vigilante, K., D'Arcy, C., & Reina, T. (1999). Restructuring the current health insurance tax subsidy to cover the uninsured. In G. M. Arnett (Ed.), *Empowering health care consumers through tax reform* (pp. 131–145). Ann Arbor: University of Michigan Press. Retrieved June 6, 2007, from: http://www.galen.org/bookcontent.asp?p=13

Workers Compensation Board. (n.d.). *Rehabilitation and social work.* Retrieved on June 12, 2007 from: http://www.wcb.state.ny.us/content/main/workers/rehab.jsp

Zellis, S. (2001). Occupational therapy and PPS: Let's take another look. *Gerontology Special Interest Section Quarterly, 24*(4), 1–3.

RESOURCES

The Center for Medicare & Medicaid Services:
http://www.cms.hhs.gov/
The Center for Medicare & Medicaid Services provides a plethora of information and resources on these government regulations.

Families USA:
http://www.familiesusa.org/
This organization addresses issues such as Medicaid and children's health, the uninsured, Medicare, and minority health. It is very involved in the political arena.

The Kaiser Family Foundation:
http://www.kff.org/
The Kaiser Family Foundation provides a large amount of information related to health care public policy, health insurance, and the uninsured.

Kaiser Family Foundation Educational Site:
http://www.KaiserEDU.org
This is a helpful site, especially for educators. Tutorials can be obtained from
http://www.kaiseredu.org/tutorials_index.asp

Consultation

JANIE B. SCOTT

Learning Objectives

After reading this chapter, you will be able to:

1. Define terms and concepts related to consultation.
2. Identify the focus, skills, and scope of consultation services.
3. Articulate business issues that are important to consultation.
4. Identify emerging areas for consultation opportunities.

The purpose of this chapter is to discuss the individual role of the occupational therapy **consultant**. **Consultation** is a process of establishing an agreement with an individual, family, facility, community, government, or other entity to provide a discrete service that is agreed upon by all parties. Occupational therapy practitioners provide consultation services across every area of occupational therapy practice and consider every human condition. Consultants are often sought because an organization or agency is involved in a continuous quality improvement process and has determined that external consultants are needed to help improve the range of services available to meet **clients'** needs; determine ways to increase cost effectiveness; identify the type and scope of staff training needed; and create a comprehensive plan to integrate best practices throughout the department, division, or agency (Braveman, 2006).

I interviewed occupational therapy consultants (past and present), and their experiences and perspectives are interwoven throughout the chapter. The material for this chapter was based on these personal interviews, my personal experiences, and the literature on consultation in the field. Occupational therapy students and practitioners have the opportunity to learn from the experiences of others in the classroom and in practice. To communicate some real-life issues related to the consultant in the delivery of consultation services, information from the interviews will be used to underscore the elements and importance of this practice area.

BEGINNING A CONSULTATION PRACTICE

A premise of this chapter is that consultation is an advanced level of practice. Before becoming consultants, the majority of occupational therapy practitioners have years of specialized experience. Chapter 68 described the distinctions between the practices of the occupational therapy assistant and the occupational therapist. These naturally extend into occupational therapy consultation. Before starting a consultative practice, practitioners should research key aspects and then consider their own characteristics, skills, and competencies. Additionally, practitioners should reflect on the domain of the profession as it relates to opportunities to provide consultation. Each of these is discussed in the following subsections.

Research

The occupational therapy practitioner who is interested in consultation should research through his or her state board of occupational therapy practice to verify that the focus of the work the practitioner intends to do is within the occupational therapy scope of practice. Wood (2004) discussed the responsibility of striving for evidence-based practice that fulfills our passions while contributing to the profession and society. An occupation-based, evidence-based foundation in occupational therapy helps to preserve the essence of the professions' work in the community and elsewhere. Wood cautioned against practicing occupational therapy in a "decapitated" manner. As the profession assumes more of a consultative role in the community, we have the responsibility to be thoughtful in our practices, using the available evidence to support our work. This responsibility is also articulated in Principle 4 of the American Occupational Therapy Association's *Occupational Therapy Code of Ethics* (AOTA, 2005): "Occupational therapy personnel shall achieve and continually maintain high standards of **competence** (DUTY)." All principles articulated in the Code have specific relevance to the roles and responsibilities that the occupational therapy consultant assumes and performs.

Research must inform practice, particularly when the focus of the occupational therapy practice is consultation. The consultant has a responsibility to ensure that the translation of evidence to practice is delivered in a way that meets the recipient's needs, literacy level, and language competency (Hammon Kellegrew, 2005).

Skills and Competencies

Once an opportunity presents itself or you identify a potential opportunity, the next step is to assess your skills and competence. Many occupational therapy practitioners decide to venture into the consultation arena because they have amassed years of experience in a particular practice area and they want to expand the scope of their work. For example, Cindy Barrows had worked for many years with people who had mental illness. She stated:

> When I saw the opportunities to inform organizations about how occupational therapy can help address some of the behavioral and daily living issues clients and program staff faced, I offered to do presentations to community based programs. (C. Barrows, personal communication, August 17, 2006)

Later, Cindy developed a proposal that identified what occupational therapy could provide to the individual client in community-based mental health programs. A review of the information that Cindy provided led the agency to realize that they needed an occupational therapist to develop a transition program to help deinstitutionalize clients. An occupational therapist mentor suggested that Cindy provide consultation services in the area of functional and work behaviors for individuals with persistent mental illness. Cindy stepped forward and offered her services as a consultant to the agency.

Assessing your skills and competencies can be a challenging and important task in defining your potential scope of consultation. Not only do you have to consider what clinical and academic preparation you have that equips you to be an expert or consultant in a particular area, you also need to have demonstrated the competencies to perform the specific roles and duties required of a consultant in a particular situation. (See Chapter 25 for more information about assessing your own competence.) Competence may be demonstrated by advanced certifications, scholarly publications, and extensive experiences in specialty areas. The consultant has an ethical and legal obligation to the client as well as to the individuals who are served by or through the agency to offer the best, most informed services possible. Just because an opportunity sounds good, this does not necessarily mean that you should provide the consultation. An objective evaluation of your skills and careful matching of these skills to the consultation opportunities are important for success. Your **ethics** and integrity as a professional must be paramount.

Characteristics of Occupational Therapy Consultants

An analysis of information from consultants interviewed for this chapter, along with literature within the field (Braveman (2006), Dunn (1990), Epstein & Jaffee (2003), Loukas (2000), Merryman (2002), O'Connor (2000), Palisano (1989), and Scott (2006).), suggests certain characteristics that promote success in delivering occupational therapy consultation services. These include the following:

- **Expertise:** The consultant needs to have experience well beyond entry level in the area of the consultation. Consultants are experts who have the knowledge and experience to deliver their services.
- **Listening skills:** Consultants need to listen to clients and understand the corporate culture.
- **Flexibility:** Flexibility of thought is required to respond to current issues that are presented in the environment in which the consultation is occurring. That flexibility allows the consultant to customize his or her services on the basis of what the clients want to receive.
- **Awareness of opportunities relevant to occupational therapy:** Consultants maintain ongoing awareness of typical problems for clients, current occupational therapy practice relevant to these problem, the "market" or opportunities to provide services, and future trends that might affect clients.

Becky Austill-Clausen began her consultation and private practice with a sound background in occupational therapy in **contexts** that included home health, skilled nursing facilities, and school system practice. She emphasized that a consultant has to be willing to build trust with those who are involved in the **contract**:

> The occupational therapy practitioner must demonstrate a high level of ethical conduct, integrity, be a good listener and get people to talk about their problems and concerns. The consultant cannot be satisfied with the status quo. A successful consultant will collaborate with the client to determine the appropriate intervention for the environment, and be able to deliver the contract's outcomes in the good hands of the contract owner and walk away. (B. Austill-Clausen, personal communication, August 15, 2006)

Ethics and the Consultant

Awareness of the ethical obligations of occupational therapy practice is also an important characteristic of the consultant. There are many influences and temptations in fulfilling the role of a consultant. Every one of the seven principles articulated in AOTA's *Occupational Therapy Code of Ethics* (AOTA, 2005) has relevance to the occupational therapy practitioner who practices as a consultant. (Readers are encouraged to review the Code and familiarize themselves with its application to this specialized practice area.) There are temptations that need to be recognized and avoided, such as placing personal prosperity before the client's needs. Examples of this are the use of deceptive language and offering of services that the consultant does not have the competency to deliver and that could potentially harm the client physically, psychologically, or financially.

Truby LaGarde explains how she became a consultant:

> Initially, it didn't feel like I was starting a business. I was trying to find work for myself. As the shift from institutional care to home care occurred, I knew that I needed to learn more about consultation and private practice. AOTA was a great resource for me. I connected with a presenter that I heard at an AOTA conference (who became my mentor). Understanding, assertiveness, and experience equaled strength of commitment to sell ideas and inform Medicare surveyors about outcomes anticipated through occupational therapy interventions. The hospital wanted me to provide occupational therapy services for them; however, I felt that I would be more effective serving as an independent contractor/consultant. (T. LaGarde, personal communication, September 6, 2006)

In this situation, Truby recognized the good occupational therapy foundation that she had gained through her 12 years of experience. She used her grounding in ethics and her professional reasoning skills to decide on the focus of her consultation efforts.

DEFINING YOUR FOCUS

Personal interests and market demands often define the focus of consultation services. Part of the role of an entrepreneur is to "seize the day" and take advantage of available opportunities. For example, my academic background has been rich with diversity. When working at the state department for health and serving as a volunteer in my state association, I became more aware of unmet needs in my community. There was a demand for occupational therapy services for individuals with autism. The role of consultant began with clinical consultation in the direct service model for one client. Ultimately, that role expanded as the agency's needs became clear: adding in-service education to staff; identification of community resources and potential employers for the clients; and occupational staff recruitment, hiring assistance, and supervision.

DETERMINING THE SCOPE OF CONSULTATION TO INDIVIDUALS, ORGANIZATIONS, AND AGENCIES

Consultants need to differentiate the consultation services they will offer. Some consultation is provided to an individual, whereas other consultants may focus on a group or organization.

Individual Consultation

Individual consultation is a collaborative relationship that is established between a consultant and a client. Clients

---

CASE STUDY: *Determining Focus: Cindy and Truby*

Cindy Barrow's work as a consultant and her community involvement with mental health programs led to requests for her to consult on task forces and help the groups to address specific problems. Cindy developed program recommendations that included needs assessments for clients. She offered suggestions on how to organize households, create more effective milieus, and revise programming to more effectively address client needs.

Truby LaGarde's awareness of changes in **regulations** and market trends helped her to expand her consultation services through diversification. She provided consultation to home health agencies, agencies that were committed to improving the deinstitutionalization process, and individual clients.

may pay directly, or the service may be covered by a third party, such as insurance. For example, consultation services can be extended to older individuals and their families, focusing on the environment, fall prevention, or lifestyle redesign. In these situations, consultation reflects a stance of providing information or options, and the client takes the primary responsibility for adopting and implementing the suggestions.

In a somewhat different situation, the consultation arrangement may be initiated by an agency, which in turn connects the client and the consultant. In these circumstances, the agency may be the payer, receiving funding through a third party such as government funding. The client's competence may be one of the determining factors in whether the consultant has a direct relationship with the client or whether the agency manages the consultative relationship. This also touches on the importance of recognizing who the stakeholders are in the consultation. In some situations, the consultant can have responsibility to primary, secondary, and tertiary stakeholders and owe a different level of responsibility to each.

An example of consultative services mediated through an agency is those funded by the Individuals with Disabilities Education Improvement Act of 2004 (P.L. 108-446) [IDEA]. The occupational therapy consultant has opportunities to provide consultation services to the classroom teacher, the student, parents, and the school. IDEA gives the occupational therapy consultant an increased number of opportunities to address the broad range of educational possibilities for students, and the school or an educational agency serves as the arbiter.

Consultation to Organizations

Many occupational therapists have been successful in providing consultation to industries. O'Connor's work (O'Connor, 2000) focused on prevention of musculoskeletal disorders in the work environment. Fontana (1999) provides industrial consultation to analyze and advise about injury prevention, ergonomics, work hardening, and implementation of federal regulations (e.g., the Americans with Disabilities Act) in business and industry. And as was noted in the previous section, occupational therapists may provide consultation to school systems regarding maximizing educational options for students with special needs. Cindy Barrows, one of the consultants I interviewed, found consultation opportunities in mental health programs to develop new programs and revise existing ones (C. Barrows, personal communication, August 17, 2006). Home health agencies were initially Becky Austill-Clausen's consultation focus (B. Austill-Clausen, personal communication, August 15, 2006). She taught agencies how to utilize occupational therapy, physical therapy, and speech language pathology services; establish service delivery systems; develop referrals; and establish quality assurance programs. Eventually, her consultation included schools

and rehabilitation programs, often using a continuous quality improvement model.

THE EVOLUTION OF THE PRACTICE

A consultant's range and scope of services can stay focused over time or can expand. The growth of the practice can depend on the practitioner's interests and skills and the opportunities that exist or can be created. As in other areas of occupational therapy practice, the occupational therapy practitioner can specialize (e.g., providing consultation services to industry focusing on injury prevention) or may choose to provide a broader range of consultation services (e.g., to builders, contractors, and architects about incorporating accessibility and universal design concepts in to new construction and renovations, as well as working with local area agencies on aging to create fall prevention programs in senior centers, assisted living facilities, and individual homes).

MANAGING AND MARKETING THE BUSINESS OF CONSULTATION

Being a consultant often means being a business owner as well, although some individuals do provide consultation as a service offered by their employer. For those who are functioning as independent consultants, there are a number of business factors that must be addressed. For instance, the consultant needs to develop a system to document all project-related activities. Policies need to be established, such as routinely negotiating in advance if you are going to charge for missed appointments. Consultation plans must be developed that detail the services under contract, the timelines for the consultation, and anticipated income and expenditures. Adequate provisions for reserving finances for paying taxes will be required, as they often are unlikely to be deducted by the client. If you establish a home office, consult tax law and an accountant to determine the deductions that are allowable for equipment, transportation, supplies, utilities, furniture, rental expenses, and other items.

The Small Business Administration (SBA) is an excellent resource for small businesses and can answer many of the questions from consultants who are beginning new businesses or services. (See the On the Web section for the SBA website.) Mentors are sometimes available through the SBA; if one is not, new consultants should try to locate a local expert who is willing to provide guidance and assistance. These resources can assist you to lay a foundation within your community and think about how to develop the networks where you wish to provide consultation services. The more you are known and respected by those in the arena in which you wish to provide services, the more you will be able to create opportunities for yourself. If the target for consultation services will be individuals or businesses that currently are unfamiliar with occupational

---

CASE STUDY: *Growing a Consultation Business:*
Cindy, Truby, and Roxanne's Experiences

Cindy Barrows's consultation services grew as a result of her marketing efforts. Her service on committees increased her visibility in the community. She was asked to provide direct clinical consultation that focused on functional evaluations to determine the level of care a client would need in the community. Her services evolved to providing consultation to staff, making recommendations on how housing staff can optimize client's occupational performance. A further evolution occurred when the state department of mental health read Cindy's reports, recognized the quality of her recommendations, and wanted to access her expertise.

Truby LaGarde's consultation practice expanded from home health care to group homes for individuals with developmental disabilities. This **consultation process** included creating strategies for addressing some of the behavioral issues that the clients were exhibiting and recom-

mending the removal of environmental barriers that were hampering the clients' independence.

Roxanne Castaneda had formal training in consultation through graduate school in applied behavioral science with a major in organizational development. She took classes in process consultation, which provided her with techniques and models used for organizational consultation. As she states, "This was a nice complement to my OT degree" (R. Castaneda, personal communication, September 29, 2006). Roxanne recognized that her background in occupational therapy and her academic knowledge had prepared her to expand her scope of services from direct service to include consultation. She also gained consultation experience as a volunteer with the Maryland Occupational Therapy Association, contributing to her profession while gaining further knowledge that could be reflected on her resume and in practice.

---

therapy, the networking and marketing will need to be outside of traditional occupational therapy circles. Marketing plans can include presentations to community groups, publication of articles in community papers and newsletters, and teaching continuing education activities.

All consultation should begin with a structured, easy to follow plan. Boxes 70.1 and 70.2 provide some experts' advice on creating a focused and needs based consultation plan, including strategies for communicating with the agency and engaging them in the development of the plan to achieve greatest "buy in."

Sources for Reimbursement Basics

If the consultation is a client-focused role, the reimbursement for consultation services may be the traditional ones (e.g., Medicare, Medicaid, schools). Consultation to programs for individuals with developmental disabilities may be funded through state developmental disabilities programs. Organizations, agencies, and industry may have separate line funding for consultation services. Occupational therapy practitioners may also collaborate with agencies to write grants that would support the consultant and the scope of the work. Part of the preparation for providing consultation is doing one's homework to investigate where the funding streams are. AOTA can be a good source of reimbursement information that can help to connect the consultant to resources and links to others.

Some Important Elements to Include in a Contract

When the consultant has an agency as a client, the consultant has to understand the priorities of the agency, the

outcomes the agency desires, the focus of the business or service delivery, and whether or not the consultant has direct access to staff and management. It is important to clarify the length of the consultation and whether ongoing communication with staff is possible or expected. In some consultation situations, the consultant is hired to develop a product and has minimal, as opposed to regular, contact with the administrator who initiates the contract. The consultant in collaboration with the client should determine the contract focus, the communication process, the need for ongoing interactions, and whether the purpose of the consultation is to assess the environment, analyze and develop recommendations independently, and submit reports to the client at the conclusion of the consultation.

For example, in a consultation that was established with the Veterans Administration to supervise and guide the competency development of a new graduate and advise about program development, it was important to understand the lines of communication and ultimate authority. Each party to the agreement needed to know how the recommendations would be considered and adopted. Some of the questions were as follows:

1. If the consultant made recommendations to the new occupational therapy graduate, would the new graduate be expected to carry out the consultant's suggestions?
2. Who should receive recommendations about (a) performance expectations, (b) standards of occupational therapy practice, (c) treatment program suggestions—the occupational therapist, the administrator or both?
3. What obligations, if any, did the occupational therapist have to adopt and implement the program development recommendations?

BOX 70.1 THE CONSULTATION PLAN: TIPS FROM THE EXPERTS

Preplanning

- Set up a time to learn about the agency or situation from a key player in the agency.
- Obtain information about the agency and its purpose, key audiences, and goals.
- Listen for problems that might be effectively addressed by an occupational therapist.
- Explore the agency's understanding of occupational therapy.
- Ask whether you can meet again and perhaps discuss ways in which you might help.
- Send a thank you note, and call for another appointment.

Preparing the Preliminary Plan

- Develop a structured plan.
- Include concrete steps or phases.
- Develop clear goals.
- Identify ways to measure goal accomplishment.

Presenting the Plan

- Set up an appointment with key players who can make decisions about the plan.

- Present and discuss the plan.
  - Provide a written summary.
  - You might need a formal oral presentation if appropriate to the setting.
- Solicit desired adjustments to the plan and be open to changing it.
- Discuss policies that might guide implementation.

Finalizing the Plan

- Background or summary of current issues
- Focus of consultation
- Process
  - Concrete phases or steps and related time frames
  - Policies related to implementation of consultation
- Expected outcomes, including how they will be measured
- Summary of fees, related costs, and payment timelines
- Send with a letter of agreement and/or contract and cover letter.

Source: Based on information from B. Austill Clausen (personal communication, August 17, 2006), C. Barrows (personal communication August 17, 2006), R. Underwood (personal communication April 12, 2007).

BOX 70.2 RECOMMENDATIONS FOR NEW CONSULTANTS

The experienced consultants have these recommendations for those who are new to consulting.

Becky Austill-Clausen: Get the Facts

Make sure that you get the services of a lawyer and an accountant, learn the tax requirements, and understand funding streams. When questions arise, go to the top of the administration or organization so that you are sure that the information you are getting is knowledge based and reliable (B. Austill-Clausen, personal communication, August 15, 2006).

Roxanne Castaneda: Spell Out Your Needs

If verbal contracts are proposed, the consultant should summarize the understanding in writing to share with all involved parties. Administrative overhead, travel expenses, and time associated with data gathering must be taken into consideration during the contract negotiation process. Access to office space and facilities "on the road" is crucial (R. Castaneda, personal communication, September 29, 2006).

Corkey Glantz and Nancy Richman: Honor Your Promises

Always carry out promises, and do not promise what you cannot deliver (Glantz & Richmond, 2003).

The consultation can be established to deliver the services face-to-face, over the telephone, by e-mail, via video conference, or by other methods. If the consultation is delivered in a team environment, all participants should be aware of the consultation and its focus and should agree to collaborate in the process.

The language in contracts varies according to the scope of the work. Some of the elements that should be included in a contract are responsibilities of the individual or agency issuing the contract; responsibilities of the consultant, typically including the duties or expectations established between the two parties; fees and payment (e.g., what the agency agrees to pay the contractor). Include the rate or fees that will be charged and reimbursed by the hour, completion of a specific project, content of invoices, and frequency of their submissions. The section on termination will specify the starting and ending date of the agreement and the opportunity to end the contract if the conditions change, if the work is unsatisfactory, or both parties agree to end the agreement prematurely. It is useful to include in the contract language on what will occur if the agency requests extension to the scope of the work or work needs to be redone because of changes in the agency ideas and a requirement that the consultant be paid for the additional work at the same rate.

Box 70.3 lists the important elements of the contract.

IMPORTANT ISSUES IN MAINTAINING RELATIONSHIPS AND BUILDING NEW ONES

The operation of a successful consultation practice depends on establishing and maintaining good relationships with individuals and organizations. Glantz and Richman (2003) suggested that from the first phone contact to the follow-up, the consultant must have an enthusiastic, energetic attitude and philosophy. Demonstrate flexibility to promote feelings of confidence in you and the consultation services that you offer. The end of the consultation period does not mean that the relationship needs to end. Stay in contact with the individual or agency, providing information about new services offered, sending greeting cards, and supplying additional information that may meet the interests of the agents.

EMERGING AND EVOLVING PRACTICE AREAS

All of the experts agreed that the consultant needs to be aware of emerging practice areas, such as the following:

- Driving consultation services, which are expanding. The occupational therapy practitioner will have opportunities for consultation to the individual, family, the

---

BOX 70.3   ELEMENTS OF A CONTRACT

- Purpose/focus of the contract
- Timelines
- Hours per week
- Hourly rate versus flat fee
- Documentation expected
- When you will get paid
- Billing procedures
- Type of equipment: telephone access, bring own laptop versus use the equipment available on site
- Environment: Will the agency designate work space for you or will you take whatever is available?
- Contact person for agency for contractor
- Restrictions, such as consultation exclusivity
- Confidentiality clause
- The agency's right to inspect the work in progress
- Ownership: Is this a joint effort or exclusive. If joint, do both parties own and have rights to any work that is created?
- Parties in the contract: Can you hire others to assist in carrying out the deliverables
- Qualifications: Drug testing, background checks, licensure status, liability coverage
- Independent contractor versus employee
- Cancellation notice and conditions

Source: B. Austill-Clausen (personal communication, 2006).

---

primary physician, motor vehicle administrations, medical advisory boards, and others
- Consultation to local area agencies on aging to coordinate CarFit and other senior driving programs in collaboration with AAA and AARP
- Work on behalf of local businesses to modify their places of business to provide more employment opportunities for the disabled veteran
- Provision of environmental evaluations on behalf of Centers for Independent Living
- Consultation services to toy manufacturers to advise in product design to minimize repetitive motion injuries and develop appropriate packaging identifying developmental factors and age appropriateness
- Consultation to preschools in designing universal design environments and activities that promote development and social opportunities for all children
- Caregiver organizations, assisting in analyzing needs of caregivers (e.g., stress management, fall prevention, ergonomics)

CASE STUDY: *Lessons from the Experts: Becky's Advice*

What one lesson would you like to pass on to someone who is thinking about beginning to work as a consultant?

Becky Austill-Clausen has this advice (personal communication, August 15, 2006): "You need to be an expert to engage in consultation as a form of practice. This means that you must have clinical experience with clients, not just have an academic preparation. Immerse yourself in the subject area so that people will want to learn from you. Become an excellent forecaster, including awareness of current, new and innovative ideas that are state of the art."

Becky also suggested the following:

◆ Read everything, including AOTA information, business magazines, major newspapers, and best-selling books on business topics.
◆ Attend meetings and workshops to enhance the ability to forecast future trends.
◆ Be aware of what is going on legislatively.
◆ Maintain good relationships with local universities, and use faculty and sometimes students as "think tanks."
◆ Network, network, network with the community in which you are practicing and with the occupational therapy community. Be visible. Attend health fairs to promote occupational therapy and ultimately your services.

SUMMARY

Consultation is an advanced practice in the majority of circumstances. There are certain characteristics that appear to be common across individuals who are successful in their consultative roles. These include expert practice skills, knowledge of regulations governing occupational therapy practice and service payment, a strong ethical foundation, and a vision of how occupational therapy can help society. Establishing, valuing, and maintaining relationships with others is key to having the referral network that is necessary for ongoing success. Communication skills are important, and one must master the ability to communicate thoughts enthusiastically both in writing and orally. The effective consultant makes learning, knowledge acquisition, and application of that knowledge to practice a lifelong journey. Consultants must be open to possibilities, since consulting opportunities might not be labeled "occupational therapy." The innovative consultant can identify how occupational therapy can be the solution to address many organizational and business needs. At the same time, successful consultants understand the ethical and conceptual bounds of the profession.

ACKNOWLEDGMENTS

Sincere thanks are extended to my friends and colleagues who contributed their lived experiences as consultants to this chapter: Becky Austill-Clausen, Cindy Barrows, Roxanne Castaneda, Truby LaGarde, and Nancy Richman.

PRACTICE DILEMMA

RACHAEL AND HER CONSULTATION OPPORTUNITY

Rachael graduated with an entry-level degree in occupational therapy two years ago. Her first and only job has been as a staff occupational therapist in a community hospital's pediatric rehabilitation unit. A gerontology provider wants to establish community-based, aging services in Rachael's area and is recruiting occupational therapists who are qualified to serve as consultants to advise on the needs of the aging community, the services they will need, and design programs that will meet their needs. Rachael has always been interested in gerontology.

1. Should Rachael apply for this consultant position/opportunity? Why or why not?
2. What sections of the Occupational Therapy Code of Ethics are relevant to Rachael's dilemma?
3. Rachael might need to identify funding sources for these new programs. Where should she look for information?
4. What personal factors should Rachael evaluate before making a decision?

ON THE WEB

- Small Business Administration: http://www.sba.gov
- Center for Medicare and Medicaid Services: www.cms.gov
- American Occupational Therapy Association: www.aota.org
- Seabury & Smith: http://www.seaburychicago.com/
- Office of Women's Business Ownership, Online Women's Business Center: http://www.onlinewbc.gov

PROVOCATIVE QUESTIONS

1. Courtney, an occupational therapy assistant, has worked at a skilled nursing facility for the past four years. She sees opportunities in her community to support aging-in-place initiatives by becoming a home modifications consultant.

2. Craig was asked by a community developmental disability program to come and assist in a continuous quality improvement program, evaluating client programming and staff training needs and developing recommendations for improvement. Craig's seven years of experience have been in hospital-based mental health programming for adults.

REFERENCES

American Occupational Therapy Association. (2000). Fact sheet: Occupational therapy and community mental health. Retrieved September 20, 2006, from http://www.aota.org/featured/area6/links/link02ak.asp

American Occupational Therapy Association. (2005). Occupational therapy code of ethics (2005). *American Journal of Occupational Therapy, 59,* 639–642.

Braveman, B. (2006). Understanding and working within organizations. In *Leading and managing occupational therapy services: An evidence-based approach* (pp. 53–80). Philadelphia: F. A. Davis.

Dunn, W. (1990). A comparison of service provision models in school-based occupational therapy services: A pilot study. *Occupational Therapy Journal of Research, 10,* 300–320.

Epstein, C. F., & Jaffee, E. G. (2003). Consultation: Collaborative interventions for change. In G. L. McCormack, E. G. Jaffe, M Goodman-Lavey (Eds.), *The occupational therapy manager* (4th ed., pp. 259–286). Bethesda, MD: AOTA Press.

Fontana, P. A. (1999). Pushing the envelope: Entering the industrial arena. *OT Practice* December 20, 1999. Retrieved September 17, 2006, from http://www.aota.org/featured/area3/links/f-122099.asp

Glantz, C., & Richman, N. (2003). *Creativity and adaptability needed to have a successful business: OTs can do it!* Lecture presented to American Occupational Therapy Association Staff, March 25, 2003. Bethesda, MD.

Hammon Kellegrew, D. (2005). The evolution of evidence-based practice: Strategies and resources for busy practitioners. *Occupational Therapy Practice, 10*(12), 11–15.

Loukas, K. M. (2000). Emerging models of innovative community-based occupational practice. *OT Practice, 5*(14), 9–11.

Merryman, M. B. (2002). Networking as an entrée to paid community practice. *OT Practice, 7*(9), 10–13.

O'Connor, S. M. (2000). Occupational therapists and office ergonomics consulting. *OT Practice, 5*(1), 12–17.

Palisano, R. J. (1989). Comparison of two methods of service delivery fore students with learning disabilities. *Physical and Occupational Therapy in Pediatrics, 9,* 79–100.

Scott, J. B. (2006). Opportunities in home care. *OT Practice, 11*(10), 17–20.

Wood, W. (2004). The heart, mind, and soul of professionalism in occupational therapy. *American Journal of Occupational Therapy, 58,* 249–257.

XV

COMMON
CONDITIONS:
RELATED RESOURCES
AND EVIDENCE

ALCOHOLISM

Sara N. Baker

Alcoholism, or alcohol dependence, is a chronic disease characterized by the following (National Institute on Alcohol Abuse and Alcoholism, 2001):

- *Craving:* the need or compulsion to drink
- *Loss of control:* the inability to limit the amount of alcohol consumed
- *Tolerance:* an increase in amount of alcohol required to achieve the same effects
- *Physical dependence:* the presence of withdrawal symptoms if intake ceases abruptly

Alcohol abuse is the continuation of drinking when, within a 12-month period, the person's ability to fulfill the obligations of a major life role has been impaired and/or when drinking is continued despite negative life consequences such as relationship issues, legal issues, or dangerous behaviors (National Institute on Alcohol Abuse and Alcoholism, 2001).

PREVALENCE

Approximately 21.6 million American adults met the criteria for alcoholism or alcohol abuse in 2003 (National Clearinghouse for Alcohol & Drug Information, 2005). Heavy drinking is more prevalent among people who are unemployed, male, ages 18–29 years, and of American or Alaskan native, Pacific Islander, or white racial or ethnic background (Substance Abuse and Mental Health Services Administration, 2003).

COURSE AND PROGNOSIS

Alcoholism is a chronic addictive disorder that may develop over a period of years and can begin at any age. There is no cure, and the person with alcoholism may go through alternating periods of sobriety and relapse. Most people relapse at least once during recovery (National Institute on Alcohol Abuse and Alcoholism, 2001).

Symptoms of Withdrawal

Withdrawal symptoms reflect overreactivity of the autonomic nervous system; they range in severity and may include headache, nausea, anxiety, agitation, insomnia, rapid heart rate, fever, convulsions, and visual hallucinations. Withdrawal symptoms usually begin within 6–48 hours after alcohol consumption has stopped and abate within the following 24–48 hours (Myrick & Anton, 1998).

RISKS OF ALCOHOLISM

Following are some of the risks involved in alcoholism (National Institute on Alcohol Abuse and Alcoholism, 2002):

- Birth defects resulting in fetal alcohol syndrome; malformations and dysplasias of the heart, bone, kidney, visual and hearing systems; CNS neurodevelopmental abnormalities; and/or cognitive deficits
- Impaired judgment
- Job loss
- Life stress increases risk for relapse
- Medication interactions

EFFECTS OF ALCOHOL ON THE BODY

Heavy use of alcohol has been shown to negatively affect a number of body structures and systems, including the following:

- Internal organs (especially the liver and pancreas; also associated with cancers of the mouth, stomach, breast, liver, and pancreas) (National Institute on Alcohol Abuse and Alcoholism, 2000, 2002)
- The immune system (National Institute on Alcohol Abuse and Alcoholism, 2000)
- The cardiovascular system (cardiomyopathy, hypertension, stroke) (National Institute on Alcohol Abuse and Alcoholism, 2000)
- The skeletal system (decreased bone mass) (National Institute on Alcohol Abuse and Alcoholism, 2000)
- Psychosocial functioning (depression, anxiety) (Johnson-Greene, Adams, Gilman, & Junck, 2002)
- Cognitive functioning (Wernicke-Korsakoff's syndrome, alcohol-related dementia) (Hazelton, Sterns, & Chisholm, 2003)

Alcoholism co-occurs with high incidence with a number of conditions, including mental illness and traumatic injury (Johnson-Greene et al., 2002).

CONCERNS OF FAMILY AND FRIENDS

Family members and friends of people with alcohol dependence have the following concerns (National Association for Children of Alcoholics, 1998):

- Aggression and/or violence
- A variety of cognitive, physical, and psychosocial difficulties that may occur in children of people with alcoholism

◆ Concern regarding genetics of disease
◆ Marital and/or relationship conflict

OT EVALUATIONS

Occupational therapists working with adult and adolescent populations should screen for alcohol disorders. There are numerous quick, self-report screens for identifying the presence of alcohol use disorders (AUDs).

Alcohol Use Disorders Identification Test (AUDIT)

The AUDIT is a 10-question, multiple-choice screening instrument for adults that identifies people who are alcohol dependent and at risk. The score determines whether brief intervention, advice, or referral is indicated (Babor, Higgins-Biddle, Saunders, & Monteiro, 2001).

If an AUD is identified, the *Canadian Occupational Performance Measure* (COPM) may assist in identifying ADLs and/or IADLs that are being affected. Occupational performance and alcohol-specific measures available include the following:

◆ Alcohol and Drug Consequences Questionnaire (ADCQ)
◆ Alcohol Dependence Scale
◆ Barth Time Construction (BTC)
◆ Beck Depression Inventory (BDI-II)
◆ Brief Situational Confidence Questionnaire (BSCQ)
◆ Clinical Institute Withdrawal Assessment for Alcohol–Revised (CIWAA-R)
◆ Coping Behaviors Inventory (CBI)
◆ Drinker Inventory of Consequences (DrInC)
◆ Drinking Expectancy Questionnaire (DEQ)
◆ Form 90
◆ Interest Checklist
◆ Inventory of Drinking Situations (IDS)
◆ Routine Task Inventory (RTI-2)
◆ Short Alcohol Dependence Data questionnaire (SADD)

The type and method of evaluation that are used in practice will be determined by a number of factors, including the client's treatment priorities, the presence of alcohol-related cognitive impairment, comorbid disorders, and time constraints.

OT INTERVENTIONS

OT interventions that focus on reducing or stopping the intake of alcohol include the following (Stoffel & Moyers, 2004):

◆ *Brief interventions:* One or multiple short sessions providing the results of the screening, education about the risks of alcohol misuse and the benefits of moderation, provision of advice and encouragement for change, goal setting, and referral to available resources.
◆ *Cognitive-behavioral therapy (CBT):* Emphasizes the development of coping behaviors and self-efficacy to change what a person thinks and does regarding alcohol use. Relapse Prevention (RP) is a specific CBT program that targets clients who have begun abstinence.
◆ *Motivational techniques:* Identify and facilitate the client's motivation to change. Specific motivational techniques include motivational interviewing, decisional balance exercises, FRAMES, and motivational enhancement therapy.
◆ *Twelve-step program facilitation:* Social and spiritual support groups that facilitate maintenance of abstinence. Occupational therapists may work with the person to incorporate these supports into a daily routine.

Occupational therapy focuses on building and refining the skills that are needed to maximize the client's occupational and role performance and reduce the risk of relapse. Some skills that may be important to address include the following:

◆ Job skills
◆ Leisure skills and planning
◆ Life management skills, such as money management and time use
◆ Self-care skills, including eating and nutrition
◆ Social skill development, including assertiveness, communication skills, and interpersonal and social responsiveness
◆ Stress management and coping skills

Skill training and practice may be done in individual settings. However, group sessions are beneficial, as they promote drug-free socialization and are cost-effective (Cecilia, Marques, Lucia, & Formigoni, 2001). Occupational therapists' role in working with people with AUDs and their families includes education, making appropriate referrals for treatment of the disorder, and facilitating the awareness and use of community resources.

OT AND THE EVIDENCE

◆ Research indicates that brief interventions that are longer than 20 minutes reduce alcohol consumption, frequency, episodes of binge drinking, and number and length of hospitalizations for at least six months after intervention for adults who are screened for hazardous alcohol use in emergency rooms, general hospitals, and outpatient clinics (Stoffel & Moyers, 2004).
◆ CBT, including RP, appears to be most effective when used in conjunction with motivational and twelve-step strategies or pharmacological treatment. It is effective in individual and group settings and may be more effective at improving psychosocial functioning than at reducing alcohol consumption (Irvin, Bowers, Dunn, & Wang, 1999; Stoffel & Moyers, 2004).

◆ Motivational strategies are effective for people with AUD but may take longer to reduce drinking amount and frequency than other approaches (Stoffel & Moyers, 2004).

◆ Twelve-step facilitation might be most effective for people who have previously relied on external supports or who are open to spirituality; however, people who attend twelve-step programs are more likely to continue to attend meetings after cessation of formal treatment (Stoffel & Moyers, 2004).

RESOURCES

Associations

AA and Al-Anon are spiritual support group organizations with a 12-step focus for people with and family and friends of people with alcoholism in the United States, Canada, and Puerto Rico.

◆ Al-Anon/Alateen
Al-Anon World Service Office
1600 Corporate Landing Parkway
Virginia Beach, VA 23454-5617
Telephone: 1-800-4AL-ANON
Website: http://www.al-anon.alateen.org/

◆ Alcoholics Anonymous
General Service Office
Grand Central Station
P.O. Box 459
New York, NY 10163
Telephone: 1-212-870-3400
Website: http://www.aa.org/

Books for Children of Parents with AUD

◆ Black, C. (1997). *My dad loves me, my dad has a disease: A child's view: Living with addiction.* Ontario, Canada: MAC.
This book discusses addiction, feelings, and recovery.

◆ Mercury, C. (1996). *Think of wind.* Rochester, NY: One Big Press.
This story explores the feelings a child might be having while growing up in a family affected by alcoholism.

First-Person Accounts of Living with AUD

◆ Knapp, C. (1997). *Drinking: A love story.* New York: Dell.
A memoir of a woman's polished professional life and a hidden 20-year struggle with alcoholism.

◆ Burroughs, A. (2003). *Dry: A memoir.* Sydney: Picador.
One man's story of alcoholism and the impact of social and environmental context on drinking, sobriety, and relapse.

Journals

◆ *Addiction*
◆ *Alcoholism: Clinical & Experimental Research*
◆ *Drug & Alcohol Dependence*
◆ *Journal of Studies on Alcohol*

Websites

◆ American Counsel on Alcoholism
http://www.aca-usa.org/
ACA offers information and referral services for people with AUDs, their families, and health professionals.

◆ National Clearinghouse on Alcohol and Drug Information
http://www.health.org/
NCADI provides drug-specific statistical, general disorder, and research information.

◆ Substance Abuse Librarians and Information Specialists
http://salis.org/
SALIS resource page provides a listing of research-based journals and publications related to alcohol and drug addiction.

REFERENCES

Babor, T. F., Higgins-Biddle, J. C., Saunders, J. B., & Monteiro, M. G. (2001). *AUDIT: The Alcohol Use Disorders Identification Test guidelines for use in primary care* (2nd ed.). Geneva, Switzerland: World Health Organization, Department of Mental Health and Substance Dependence.

Cecilia, A., Marques, P. R., Lucia, M., & Formigoni, O. S. (2001). Comparison of individual and group cognitive-behavioral therapy for alcohol and/or drug dependent patients. *Addiction, 96,* 835–846.

Hazelton, L. D., Sterns, G. L., & Chisholm, T. (2003). Decision-making capacity and alcohol abuse: Clinical and ethical considerations in personal care choices. *General Hospital Psychiatry, 25*(2), 130–135.

Irvin, J. E., Bowers, C. A., Dunn, M. E., & Wang, M. C. (1999). Efficacy of relapse prevention: A meta-analytic review. *Journal of Consulting and Clinical Psychology, 67*(4), 563–570.

Johnson-Greene, D., Adams, K. M., Gilman, S., & Junck, L. (2002). Relationship between neuropsychosocial and emotional functioning in severe chronic alcoholism. *Clinical Neurologist, 16*(3), 300–309.

Myrick, H., & Anton, R. F. (1998). Treatment of alcohol withdrawal. *Alcohol Health & Research World, 22,* 38–43.

National Association for Children of Alcoholics. (1998). *Children of alcoholics: Important facts.* Retrieved March 1, 2005, from http://www.nacoa.net/impfacts.htm

National Clearinghouse for Alcohol & Drug Information. (2005). *Publications: April is alcohol awareness month.* Retrieved March 15, 2005, from http://www.health.org/seasonal/aprilalcohol/

National Institute on Alcohol Abuse and Alcoholism. (2000). Medical consequences of alcohol abuse. *Alcohol Research & Health, 24*(1), 27–31.

National Institute on Alcohol Abuse and Alcoholism. (2001). *Alcoholism: Getting the facts.* (NIH Publication No. 96-4153). Retrieved March 1, 2005, from http://www.niaaa.nih.gov/publications/booklet.htm

National Institute on Alcohol Abuse and Alcoholism. (2002). *Alcohol: What you don't know can harm you.* (NIH Publication No. 99-4323). Retrieved March 1, 2005, from http://www.niaaa.nih.gov/publications/harm-al.htm

Stoffel, V. C., & Moyers, P. A. (2004). An evidence-based and occupational perspective of interventions for persons with substance-use disorders. *American Journal of Occupational Therapy, 58,* 570–586.

Substance Abuse and Mental Health Services Administration. (2003). *The national survey on drug use and health.* Retrieved March 15, 2005, from http://www.oas.samhsa.gov/nhsda/2k3nsduh/2k3Results.htm#toc

ALZHEIMER'S DISEASE

Hsin-yu Kuo

Alzheimer's disease (AD), the most common form of dementia, is a progressively degenerative disorder that occurs most frequently in the elderly population. AD not only impairs an individual's broad aspects of life, but also affects the whole family and increases social burdens. With the current trend of longer life, the rates of AD have increased. It is critical to address concerns relative to maintaining the overall quality of life of individuals with AD and their families (Dooley & Hinojosa, 2004).

INCIDENCE

AD usually occurs in individuals older than 65 years of age, although in a few cases, this disorder may develop before the age of 50 years (American Psychiatric Association, 2000) or even as early as 30 years (Small et al., 1997). The incidence rate increases from approximately 1% annually among people aged 65 to 70 years to approximately 6% to 8% for people over age 85 (Mayeus, 2003).

PREVALENCE

On average, individuals with AD usually live from 3 years to 20 years after symptom onset (Mayeus, 2003). Approximately 6% to 8% of all individuals older than 65 years old have AD, and the prevalence of AD may double every 5 years after the age of 60 (Small et al., 1997). In 2000, there were 4.5 million individuals with AD in the U.S. population. Researchers estimate that the number may increase to 13.2 million by 2050 (Hebert, Scherr, Bienias, Bennett, & Evans, 2003).

SYMPTOMS

AD is characterized by gradual onset and progressive degeneration in cognition; it is accompanied by behavioral and psychological symptoms (APA, 2000; Chen, Borson, & Scanlan, 2000; Förstl & Kurz, 1999; Hart et al., 2003).

Motor declines are also usually present in later stages (APA, 2000; Förstl & Kurz, 1999).

Although the experience of symptoms and the time when symptoms may occur can vary greatly from one individual to another (Volicer, 2001), the progression of Alzheimer's symptoms can be described in terms of three stages: early/forgetfulness, middle/confusional, and late/dementia stages (Schneck, Reisberg, & Ferris, 1982).

Early/Forgetfulness Stage

- *Cognition:* Mild impairment in memory, especially short-term memory, which is often the sign that is most apparent in the early stage; lack of concentration and ability to learn new materials; mild impairment in language, including shrinking vocabulary, decreasing word fluency, or less precise expressive language
- *Behavioral and psychological:* Personality alterations; increased depression, anxiety, or irritability
- *ADL:* No significant deterioration in ADL; still able to live independently for most of the time but might need support with a variety of organizational matters

Middle/Confusional Stage

- *Cognition:* Severe impairment in recent memory; more obvious language difficulties, such as aphasia or word-finding difficulties; apraxia, agnosia, disorientation, visuospatial dysfunction, impaired judgment, and impaired executive functioning
- *Behavioral and psychological:* Increased aimless activities (e.g., wandering); disrupted sleep; delusions, hallucinations, or aggression
- *ADL:* Require extensive assistance with daily activities, including dressing, eating, and toileting

Late/Dementia Stage

- *Cognition:* Profound disturbances in orientation and memory; more distant memories are lost; unable to recognize close family members; severe intellectual

declines; language reduced to simple phrases or even single words
- *Behavioral and psychological:* Apathetic and unresponsive except for facial grimacing
- *Motor:* Severely impaired motor function; abnormal reflexes; soon progresses to a bedridden stage, with limb rigidity and incontinence of urine and feces
- *ADL:* Loss of basic daily living abilities; completely dependent in all aspects of daily living

PRECAUTIONS

As the course of AD progresses, the global functions of individuals with AD decline. These individuals become increasingly unable to take care of themselves. The following principles should be noted in order to adapt to each change in the individual's behavior and functioning as well as prevent unexpected events (Reed, 2000):

1. Avoid leaving individuals with AD alone, because they can become lost easily even in familiar environments.
2. Avoid overstimulating individuals with AD; this may exacerbate their behavioral or psychological problems.
3. Avoid arguing with individuals with AD when they do not tell the truth.
4. Minimize dangers. A safe home environment enables individuals with AD to experience increased security and more mobility.

MEDICAL MANAGEMENT

There is currently no cure or prevention for AD. However, for some individuals with early- and middle-stage AD, cholinesterase inhibitors (ChEIs), the first pharmacological treatments to be approved by the U.S. Food and Drug Administration, can assist in temporarily delaying some symptoms from worsening and in maintaining a higher level of cognitive function (Standridge, 2004). The therapeutic effect of ChEIs is associated with enhanced performance of activities of daily living, reduced behavioral disturbances, stabilized cognitive impairment, decreased caregiver stress, and delay in the first dementia-related nursing home placement (Cummings et al., 2002; Standridge, 2004). Nausea, vomiting, diarrhea, dizziness, and anorexia are the most common side effects of ChEIs and occur more frequently during dose escalation than during maintenance therapy (Standridge, 2004).

OT EVALUATIONS

The fundamental evaluation method that is used in occupational therapy for AD is observation and interview. Observe clients' involvement in activities of daily living and corroborate other information obtained from interviewing family members or caregivers (American Occupational Therapy Association, 1994). Several performance-based measures and self- or proxy-report questionnaires have been documented to assess individuals with AD as follows:

- Assessment of Motor and Process Skills (AMPS)
- Cognitive Performance Test (CPT)
- Daily Activities Questionnaire
- Disability Assessment for Dementia (DAD)
- Functional Performance Test (FPT)
- Kitchen Task Assessment (KTA)

OT INTERVENTIONS

The main purposes of OT intervention for individuals with AD are (1) to maintain functional capacity, (2) to promote participation in activities that optimize physical and mental health, and (3) to ease caregiving activities (AOTA, 1994). The OT interventions are mainly divided into two categories: the environment and the caregiver.

Environment

Environmental Modification or Adaptation

Amount of distractions, degree of safety, and level of physical and emotional comfort are crucial points that need to be incorporated into the environmental modification (Day, Carreon, & Atump, 2000). Keep environments consistent to decrease confusion, increase lighting or install ramps to promote safety, or provide a low-stimulus environment, such as painting a room in soft colors, to decrease aggression or disturbances (Dooley & Hinojosa, 2004; Gitlin & Corcoran, 1996). Putting familiar pictures or names on the door and clearly labeling physical structures with unique symbols, such as arrows for direction are also beneficial for people with AD (Nolan, Lawrence, Mathews, & Harrison, 2001).

Task Simplification

Engaging patients with dementia in familiar daily living tasks can enhance their well-being as well as lower stress on their caregivers (Hasselkus, 1998; Teri, Logdon, Uomoto, & McCurry, 1997). Task simplification is an economic way of helping people with AD to continue to engage in their ADL by diminishing the complexity of the environment and its demands on task performance. It usually involves establishing daily routines or increasing verbal, visual, or tactile cueing (Gitlin & Corcoran, 1996).

Assistive Technology and Equipment

Because users must learn how to use devices, such as medication dispensers or pill reminder boxes, to compensate for their deficits, these devices are more useful for people with mild-stage AD whose cognition and learning abilities are mildly impaired (Förstl & Kurz, 1999). Otherwise, such devices can cause further confusion and frustration (Day et al., 2000). For caregivers, monitoring systems, door alarms, grab bars, safety locks, and tub benches may be beneficial in decreasing caregiving burden (Gitlin & Corcoran, 1996).

Caregivers

Caregiver Training or Education

Through teaching or counseling of caregivers to increase their knowledge of AD, to enable them to take advantage of environmental modifications or assistive technology, to help them to deal with specific issues, such as wandering, and to enable them to cope with the stress, occupational therapists can help caregivers to alleviate their loads and increase their self-efficacy (Corcoran & Gitlin, 2001; Dooley & Hinojosa, 2004; Toth-Cohen, 2000).

Provision of Resources and Referrals

Occupational therapists have a primary role to provide information on community resources and encourage caregivers to use these resources. Resources may include respite care, in-home support services, or support groups so that the caregiver can take a break from the 24-hour-per-day care requirements (Schultz-Krohn, Foti, & Glogoski, 2001).

OT AND THE EVIDENCE

OT interventions can result in fewer declines in daily living skills and enhance the quality of life of people with AD as well as increasing caregivers' self-efficacy and decreasing their feelings of being burdened (Dooley & Hinojosa, 2004; Corcoran & Gitlin, 2001).

CAREGIVER CONCERNS

When considering the burdens of AD on society, except for financial costs, we cannot understate the emotional toll of AD on caregivers. The emotional stress on patients and their caregivers is profound and a significant source of caregiver morbidity (Small et al., 1997). Caregivers of individuals with AD may develop psychological morbidity, such as depression or anxiety (Nobili et al., 2004). Behavioral disturbances of individuals with AD seems to cause more caregiver distress than psychological symptoms do, aggression, irritability and sleep disturbance being the least well tolerated (Chen et al., 2000; Hart et al., 2003). Low income, longer hours spent caregiving, and poor functional independence of caregivers as well as younger age, lower level of education, and higher independence of individuals with AD could be predictors of caregiver depression (Covinsky et al., 2003). Unless the quality of life of both patients and their caregivers is included, any economic assessment is likely to underestimate the true cost of AD to society (Russell, Gold, Siegel, Daniels, & Weinstein, 1996).

RESOURCES

Associations

◆ Alzheimer's Association
 225 N. Michigan Avenue
 Fl.17
 Chicago, IL 60601
 Telephone: 1-800-272-3900
 Website: http://www.alz.org
◆ National Family Caregivers Association
 10400 Connecticut Avenue
 Suite 500
 Kensington, MD 20895-3944
 Telephone: 1-800-272-3900
 Website: http://www.nfcacares.org/

First-Person Accounts

◆ Cohen, E. (2003). *The house on Beartown road: A memoir of learning and forgetting.* New York: Random House.
 Cohen chronicled her caregiving experience with her aging father, who suffered from moderate-to-late-stage AD.
◆ Cooney, E. (2003). *Death in slow motion: My mother's descent into Alzheimer's.* Pittsburgh, PA: HarperCollins.
 Cooney, a freelance writer, vividly described the everyday physical and emotional stresses on her, once her mother with AD moved in with her.
◆ DeBaggio, T. (2003). *Losing my mind: An intimate look at life with Alzheimer's.* New York: Free Press.
 DeBaggio, a former journalist, professional gardener, and author of two gardening books, was diagnosed with early-onset Alzheimer's disease when he was 57 years old.
◆ McGowin, D. (1994). *Living in the labyrinth: A personal journey through the maze of Alzheimer's.* New York: Delacorte.
 McGowin, a middle-aged legal assistant, was diagnosed with early-onset AD.

Journals

◆ *Alzheimer's Disease & Associated Disorders*
◆ *American Journal of Geriatric Psychiatry*
◆ *Dementia and Geriatric Cognitive Disorders*
◆ *International Journal of Geriatric Psychiatry*
◆ *Journal of Alzheimer's Disease*
◆ *Topics in Geriatric Rehabilitation*

Websites

◆ Alzheimer's Association
http://www.alz.org
The AA offers fact sheets, news, programs, conference calendars, publications, and information on advocacy activities. Chapters nationwide provide referrals to local resources and services and sponsor support groups and educational programs.

◆ Alzheimer's Disease Education and Referral Center
http://www.alzheimers.org
The ADER Center, which is funded by the National Institute on Aging, provides fact sheets, research and technical reports, information on training programs, conference calendars, public service announcements, and online lectures. A bibliographic database of health education materials on AD and a clinical trial database are available at the site.

◆ Administration on Aging
http://www.aoa.gov
The AOA is an official federal agency that plans and delivers supportive home- and community-based services to elders and their caregivers. The AOA also provides the "Alzheimer's Resource Room" for elders, caregivers, and researchers.

◆ Family Caregiver Alliance
http://www.caregiver.org
The FCA offers fact sheets about caregiving issues, caregiver workshops, caregiving tips, and public policy conferences to keep caregivers informed. Also, the FCA provides an online discussion group for caregivers to share experiences and express emotions and frustrations.

REFERENCES

American Occupational Therapy Association. (1994). Statement: Occupational therapy services for Alzheimer's disease and other dementias. *American Journal of Occupational Therapy, 48,* 1029–1031.

American Psychiatric Association. (2000). *Diagnostic and statistical manual of mental disorders* (4th ed., text rev.). Washington, DC: Author.

Chen, J. C., Borson, S., & Scanlan, J. M. (2000). Stage-specific prevalence of behavioral symptoms in Alzheimer's disease in a multi-ethnic community sample. *American Journal of Geriatric Psychiatry, 8,* 123–133.

Corcoran, M. A., & Gitlin, L. N. (2001). Family caregiver acceptance and use of environmental strategies provided in an occupational therapy intervention. *Physical and Occupational Therapy in Geriatrics, 19,* 1–20.

Covinsky, K. E., Newcomer, R., Fox, P., Wood, J., Sands, L., Dane, K., et al. (2003). Patient and caregiver characteristics associated with depression in caregivers of patients with dementia. *Journal of General Internal Medicine, 18,* 1006–1014.

Cummings, J. L., Frank, J. C., Cherry, D., Kohatsu, N. D., Kemp, B., Hewett, L., et al. (2002). Guidelines for managing Alzheimer's disease: II. Treatment. *American Family Physician, 65,* 2525–2534.

Day, K., Carreon, D., & Atump, C. (2000). The therapeutic design of environment for people with dementia: A review of the empirical research. *Gerontologist, 40,* 397–416.

Dooley, N. R., & Hinojosa, J. (2004). Improving quality of life for persons with Alzheimer's disease and their family caregivers: A brief occupational therapy intervention. *American Journal of Occupational Therapy, 58,* 561–569.

Förstl, H., & Kurz, A. (1999). Clinical features of Alzheimer's disease. *European Archives of Psychiatry and Clinical Neuroscience, 249,* 288–290.

Gitlin, L. N., & Corcoran, M. A. (1996). Managing dementia at home: The role of home environment modification. *Topics in Geriatric Rehabilitation, 12,* 28–39.

Hart, D. J., Craig, D., Compton, S. A., Critchlow, S., Kerrigan, B. M., McIlroy, S. P., & Passmore, A. P. (2003). A retrospective study of the behavioural and psychological symptoms of mild and late phase Alzheimer's disease. *International Journal of Geriatric Psychiatry, 18,* 1037–1042.

Hasselkus, B. R. (1998). Occupation and well-being in dementia: The experience of day-care staff. *American Journal of Occupational Therapy, 52,* 423–434.

Hebert, L. E., Scherr, P. A., Bienias, J. L., Bennett, D. A., & Evans, D. A. (2003). Alzheimer disease in the US population: Prevalence estimates using the 2000 census. *Archives of Neurology, 60,* 1119–1122.

Mayeus, R. (2003). Epidemiology of neurodegeneration. *Annual Review of Neuroscience, 26,* 81–104.

Nobili, A., Riva, E., Tettamanti, M., Lucca, U., Liscio, M., Petrucci, B., et al. (2004). The effect of a structured intervention on caregivers of patients with dementia and problem behaviors: A randomized controlled pilot study. *Alzheimer's Disease & Associated Disorders, 18,* 75–82.

Nolan, B. A. D., Lawrence, K. S., Mathews, R. M., & Harrison, M. (2001). Using external memory aids to increase room finding by older adults with dementia. *American Journal of Alzheimer's disease, 16,* 251–254.

Reed, K. L. (2000). Dementia: Alzheimer's type. In K. L. Reed (Ed.), *Quick reference to occupational therapy* (2nd ed., pp. 735–745). Gaithersburg, MD: Aspen.

Russell, L. B., Gold, M. R., Siegel, J. E., Daniels, N., & Weinstein, M. S. (1996). The role of cost-effectiveness analysis in health and medicine: Panel on cost-effectiveness in health and medicine. *Journal of the American Medical Association, 276,* 1172–1177.

Schneck, M. K., Reisberg, B., & Ferris, S. H. (1982). An overview of current concepts of Alzheimer's disease. *American Journal of Psychiatry, 139,* 165–173.

Schultz-Krohn, W., Foti, D., & Glogoski, C. (2001). Degenerative disease of the central nervous system. In L. W. Pedretti & M. B. Early (Eds.), *Occupational therapy: Practice skills for physical dysfunction* (5th ed., pp. 702–729). St. Louis: Mosby.

Small, G. W., Rabins, P. V., Barry, P. P., Buckholtz, N. S., Buckholtz, N. S., & DeKosky, S. T., et al. (1997). Diagnosis and treatment of Alzheimer disease and related disorders: Consensus statement of the American Association for Geriatric Psychiatry, the Alzheimer's Association, and the American Geriatrics Society. *Journal of the American Medical Association, 278,* 1363–1371.

Standridge, J. B. (2004). Pharmacotherapeutic approach to the treatment of Alzheimer's disease. *Clinical Therapeutics, 26,* 615–630.

Teri, L., Logdon, R. G., Uomoto, J., & McCurry, S. M. (1997). Behavioral treatment of depression in dementia patients: A controlled clinical trial. *Journal of Gerontology: Psychological Sciences, 52B,* P159–P166.

Toth-Cohen, S. (2000). Role perceptions of occupational therapists providing support and education for caregivers of persons with dementia. *American Journal of Occupational Therapy, 54,* 509–515.

Volicer, L. (2001). Management of severe Alzheimer's disease and end-of-life issues. *Alzheimer's Disease & Dementia, 17,* 377–391.

AMYOTROPHIC LATERAL SCLEROSIS

Rachel Fleming, Kate-Lyn Stone, and Meredith Grimell

Amyotrophic lateral sclerosis (ALS), also referred to as Lou Gehrig's disease, is a rare, progressive, degenerative disease that affects the motor neurons in the corticospinal pathways, the motor nuclei of the brain stem, and the anterior horn cells of the spinal cord. ALS, like Parkinson's disease and multiple sclerosis, is a motor neuron disease. Decreased function of the nerve cells in the brain, brain stem, and spinal cord caused by ALS results in weakening of the muscles, which eventually leads to paralysis but does not affect personality or cognition. No known cure for ALS exists.

INCIDENCE AND PREVALENCE

- In the United States, 20,000 people currently have ALS, and 5,000 additional people are diagnosed with ALS each year.
- Individuals of all races are affected by ALS.
- The age of onset is typically between 40 and 60 years.
- More men are affected than women.
- 90–95% of all cases are of no known cause.
- 5–10% of all cases are of genetic origin.

TYPICAL COURSE

The onset of the disease varies from one individual to another. Some people experience a weakness in the arms with difficulty lifting or doing fine motor tasks or in the legs with difficulty walking or in the muscles that control speech and swallowing. Some experience generalized muscle fatigue. If the weakening begins in the hand, it will progress through the affected limb before becoming more generalized. Problems with speech or swallowing occur when motor neurons die in the brain stem. The disease progresses and eventually affects the person's ability to walk and continue performing ADL. The disease affects only the motor pathways; therefore, eye movement, bowel and bladder functions, cognition, personality, and skin sensation remain intact. Respiratory weakness ultimately is affected as the muscles deteriorate, and death usually follows unless the individual is put on a ventilator.

POTENTIAL SYMPTOMS

- Damage to lower motor neurons (in the spinal cord) leading to flaccid paralysis, decreased muscle tone, and decreased reflexes
- Damage to upper motor neurons (in the brain) and to the corticospinal tract leading to spasticity and hyperreflexia (exaggerated reflexes)
- Muscle weakness
- Muscle atrophy (distal to proximal)—a symptom that is unique to ALS
- Fatigue
- Stumbling and falling due to lower extremity weakness
- Fasciculation (muscle twitching)
- Decreased ability to regulate body temperature
- Loss of emotional control/depression
- Dysphagia (difficulty swallowing)
- Dysarthria (difficulty speaking) due to impaired cranial nerves controlling speech
- Impaired respiration due to muscle weakness
- Sialorrhea (excess drooling)
- Night cramps
- Weight loss
- Loss of endurance
- Loss of dexterity

MEDICAL MANAGEMENT

No specific assessment is used to diagnose ALS. Magnetic resonance imaging (MRI), electromyography, blood tests, and/or nerve conduction velocity are done to eliminate other diseases as possibilities. Currently, no known cure or treatment to reverse ALS exists. In 1995, the Food and Drug Administration approved Rilozule, the first drug to result in prolonging survival by several months. The drug is believed to work by decreasing damage due to the release of glutamate. The drug may extend the length of time before a person needs ventilation support.

Respiratory therapists, speech pathologists, physical therapists, occupational therapists, psychologists, and social workers typically work together to sustain the client's quality of life and to support the family. Compensatory strategies using adaptive equipment and energy conservation are common foci of treatment for an individual with ALS.

PROGNOSIS

- Most people with ALS die secondary to respiratory failure
- People who go on a ventilator generally live longer than people who do not
- 90% of people with ALS live 3–5 years after the onset of the disease
- 10% of people with ALS survive for 10 or more years after the onset

PRECAUTIONS

- Pneumonia and pulmonary emboli
- Ventilators: intermittent positive pressure ventilation (IPPV) or bilevel positive airway pressure (BiPap)
- Inability to cough to clear normal amount of mucus from airway
- Pressure sores due to decreased mobility
- Swallowing problems could lead to choking
- Posture and balance could lead to falls
- Emotional lability (outbursts of laughing or crying)
- Difficulty maintaining weight
- Shoulder subluxation
- Joint contractures

OCCUPATIONAL THERAPY EVALUATIONS

Comprehensive Evaluations

- ALS Functional Rating Scale

IADL/Leisure Evaluations

- Activity Card Sort

Upper Extremity Function Evaluation

- Purdue Pegboard
- Manual muscle testing
- Range-of-motion testing

Balance Evaluations

- Berg Balance Scale

Quality of Life/Life Satisfaction Evaluations

- COPM (Canadian Occupational Therapy Performance Measure)

OCCUPATIONAL THERAPY INTERVENTIONS

- Energy conservation: choosing which activities are most important to the client
- Compensatory strategies, such as using gravity-eliminating devices
- Use of adaptive equipment (e.g., raised toilet seat, built-up handles)
- Prevent deconditioning of remaining muscles
- Continue meaningful life roles and occupations to provide a sense of accomplishment
- Therapeutic exercise to preserve strength
- PROM (passive range of motion) and/or AROM (active range of motion) to prevent contractures at joints
- Thermoplastic resting splints for wrists and hands to assist in maintaining muscle length
- Shoulder supports to prevent subluxation
- Augmentative communication
- Postural support
- Home modifications

OT AND THE EVIDENCE

When a person is facing a life-threatening illness, the use of occupation is more powerful than ever. Occupation during this phase of life can carry many meanings. Being engaged in occupation can help to remediate physical function, challenge the mind, provide meaning in the person's new stage of life, and offer a sense of well-being to a person with ALS. Learning new skills and being challenged can be very rewarding for someone with a terminal illness, even though the person might be constrained by the illness.

Bremer, Simone, Walsh, Simmons, and Felgoise (2007) suggest that maintaining an individual's quality of life as ALS progresses should also be focused on as an important part of occupational therapy intervention. They found that two major contributing factors to good quality of life were the individual's perception of his or her health and the person's religiosity. Bello-Haas et al. (2007) examined another aspect of quality of life in their study concerning the efficacy of resistance exercise in individuals with ALS. They found that resistance exercise contributed to better function as measured by the ALS Functional Rating Scale as well as improved overall quality of life.

CAREGIVER CONCERNS

People who develop ALS experience a sudden change in life roles that can be overwhelming. Because of the rapid progression of ALS, it can be difficult for caregivers to adapt to a loved one's inability to continue life roles. Discontinuation of work after the diagnosis of ALS is common and can lead to financial strain. The sudden decrease in ADL/IADL capabilities can be difficult for the family. Caring for a family member with ALS can be physically and psychologically demanding and draining. It is important to address the issue of coping not only with the client but also with the family members. Because so much is unknown about ALS, caregivers often have many unanswered questions. Caregiver support groups can be beneficial in providing the family with necessary support and information.

RESOURCES

Associations

- ◆ ALS Association (ALSA)
  27001 Agoura Road
  Suite 150
  Calabasas Hills, CA 91301-5104
  Telephone: 818-880-9007 or 800-782-4747
  Fax: 818-880-9006
  Website: www.alsa.org
- ◆ Muscular Dystrophy Association
  3300 East Sunrise Drive
  Tucson, AZ 85718-3208
  Telephone: 520-529-2000 or 800-572-1717
  Fax: 520-529-5300
  Website: www.mdausa.org
- ◆ Les Turner ALS Foundation
  8142 North Lawndale Avenue
  Skokie, IL 60076-3322
  Telephone: 888-ALS-1107 847-679-3311
  Fax: 847-679-9109
  Website: www.lesturnerals.org
- ◆ ALSTDF
  ALS Therapy Development Institute
  215 First Street
  Cambridge, MA 02142
  Telephone: 617-441-7200
  Fax: 617-441-7299
  Website: www.als.net

First-Person Accounts

- ◆ Hanlan, A. J. (1979). *Autobiography about dying.* Garden City, NY: Doubleday.
  Through his diary writings, Allen Hanlan takes the reader on a journey from being diagnosed with ALS to facing death. A postscript by his wife about living with a dying husband is included.
- ◆ Simmons, P. (2000) *Learning to fall: The blessings of an imperfect life.* New York: Bantam Dell.
  A meditative book that is at times poetic, ironic, and humorous tells of Philip Simons's spiritual journey as he lived with ALS.

- ◆ Wakefield, D. (2005). *I remember running: The year I got everything I ever wanted—and ALS.* New York: Marlowe & Company.
  This book takes the reader on the journey of a 33-year-old woman who was diagnosed with ALS. Darcy does not allow the fatal disease to take away her dream of owning a house and having a child, and most important, the disease does not take away her will to live.

Journals

- ◆ *Amyotrophic Lateral Sclerosis and Other Motor Neuron Disorders*
- ◆ *Journal of Neurology*

Websites

- ◆ ALS Links
  www.ALSlinks.com
  This website provides an internet portal for the ALS community. It offers information about other websites that have information about ALS. It is easy to use and allows for a quick search for associations and foundations for ALS.
- ◆ National Institute of Neurological Disorders and Stroke
  http://www.ninds.nih.gov/disorders/amyotrophic lateralsclerosis
  This website provides a comprehensive fact sheet and useful information about ALS and many other diseases.

REFERENCES

Bello-Haas, V. D., Florence, J. M., Kloos, A. D., Scheirbecker, J., Lopate, G., Hayes, S. M., et al. (2007). A randomized controlled trial of resistance exercise in individuals with ALS. *Neurology, 68,* 2003–2007.

Bremer, B., Simone, A., Walsh, S., Simmons, Z., & Felgoise, S. (2004). Factors supporting quality of life over time for individuals with amyotrophic lateral sclerosis: The role of positive self-perception and religiosity. *Annals of Behavioral Medicine, 28,* 119–125.

ADDITIONAL RESOURCES

Dirette, D. K. (2000). Progressive neurological disorders. In R. A. Hanson & B. Atchison (Eds.), *Conditions in occupational therapy: Effect on occupational performance* (2nd ed., pp. 218–229). Baltimore: Lippincott Williams & Wilkins.

Gould, B. E. (2002). Chronic neurological disorders. In S. A. Kuhn (Ed.), *Pathophysiology for the health professions* (2nd ed., pp. 490–507). Philadelphia: Saunders.

Lyons, M., Orozovic, N., Davis, J., & Newman, J. (2002). Doing-being-becoming: Occupational experiences of persons with life-threatening illnesses. *American Journal of Occupational Therapy, 56,* 285–295.

Maddox, S. (2003). Amyotrophic lateral sclerosis. In *Paralysis resource guide* (pp. 3–6). Short Hills, NJ: Paralysis Resource Center.

Mitsumoto, H., & Munsat T. L. (Eds.). (2001). *Amyotrophic lateral sclerosis: A guide for patients and families*. New York: Demos Medical Publishing.

National Institute for Neurological Disorders and Stroke. (2003). *Amyotrophic lateral sclerosis fact sheet*. Retrieved March 30, 2006, from http://www.ninds.nih.gov/disorders/amyotrohiclateralsclerosis

Oliver, D., Borasio, G. D., & Walsh, D. (Eds.). (2000). *Palliative care in amyotrophic lateral sclerosis*. New York: Oxford University Press.

Reed, K. L. (2001). Amyotrophic lateral sclerosis. In R. R. Zukas (Ed.), *Quick reference to occupational therapy* (2nd ed., pp. 264–270). Gaithersburg, MD: Aspen.

Trombly, C. A. (2002). Amyotrophic lateral sclerosis. In C. A. Trombly & M. V. Radomski (Eds.), *Occupational therapy for physical dysfunction* (5th ed., pp. 899–902). Baltimore: Lippincott Williams & Wilkins.

ATTENTION DEFICIT/HYPERACTIVITY DISORDER

Ling-Yi Lin

Attention deficit/hyperactivity disorder (ADHD) is the most common childhood behavioral disorder and is probably two or three times more frequent in boys than in girls (National Institute of Mental Health, 1999). It is characterized by a persistent and frequent pattern of developmentally inappropriate inattention and impulsivity, with or without hyperactivity (American Psychiatric Association, 2000). Individuals with ADHD have impaired functioning in multiple environments, including home and school, and in relationships with peers. Some children with ADHD have sensory-processing difficulties or delayed motor skills related to performing tasks and activities.

PREVALENCE

- The prevalence of ADHD has been variously estimated as ranging from 3% to 7% in school-age children (APA, 2000).
- Up to two-thirds of children with ADHD continue to experience significant symptoms in adolescence and adulthood (Barkley, 1998).

CAUSE AND ETIOLOGY

- The cause and etiology of ADHD are not completely understood (Resnick, 2000).
- ADHD is a complex disorder that is undoubtedly the result of multiple interacting genes (NIMH, 1999).
- Other causal factors are low birth weight, prenatal maternal smoking, and additional prenatal problems (NIMH, 1999).

TYPICAL COURSE AND SYMPTOMS

ADHD symptoms arise in early childhood unless they are associated with some type of brain injury later in life. Some symptoms persist into adulthood and can pose lifelong challenges (APA, 2000). The symptom-related criteria for the three primary subtypes, adapted from *DSM-IV*, are as follows (APA, 2000):

1. *ADHD predominantly inattentive type (ADHD-I):* Individual who daydreams or seems to be in another world, is easily distracted by what is happening around him or her, and has difficulty organizing work.
2. *ADHD predominantly hyperactive-impulsive type (ADHD-HI):* Individual who acts quickly without thinking first and has difficulty remaining seated; walks, runs, or climbs around when others are seated; and talks excessively when others are talking.
3. *ADHD combined type (ADHD-C):* Individual meets both sets of inattention and hyperactive/impulsive criteria.

PRECAUTIONS

- ADHD often co-occurs with other disorders, including learning disabilities and behavioral disorders, such as oppositional defiant disorder and conduct disorder (Pliszka, Carlson, & Swanson, 1999).
- More likely to smoke, drink alcohol, and take drugs as teenagers and a higher risk of substance abuse in adults with ADHD (Resnick, 2000).
- Higher rates of various accidental injuries (Pliszka et al., 1999).
- Ritalin may have negative side effects relating to appetite, sleep, and growth (Wender, 2000).

INTERVENTION

Medication Therapy

- Stimulants, including methylphenidate, amphetamine, and pemoline, are the most widely researched and most commonly prescribed treatments for individuals with ADHD (Wender, 2000).

- Research has demonstrated that methylphenidate treatment in individuals with ADHD causes successive improvements in behaviors and cognitive tasks (Wender, 2000).

Multimodal Treatment Study of ADHD

- The comprehensive multimodal approach to treating children with ADHD requires medical, educational, behavioral, and psychological interventions and consists of parent and child education about diagnosis and treatment, specific behavior management techniques, stimulant medication, appropriate school programming, and supports (MTA Cooperative Group, 1999a, 1999b).
- An MTA study conducted by the National Institute of Mental Health and cosponsored by the U.S. Department of Education is a 14-month randomized clinical ADHD trial. The multitreatment approaches and combinations of interventions that were researched include medication management, behavioral treatment, combined medication management and behavioral therapy, and community care. The results indicated that a combination of medication and psychotherapy is particularly effective (MTA Cooperative Group, 1999a, 1999b).

Educational Management

- Other interventions for children or adolescents with ADHD include tutoring and special education.
- The direction of educational management of ADHD aims to maximize attention and concentration, counter impulsive behavior, improve self-esteem and socialization, assist in overcoming learning difficulties, and promote consistency of management between home and school (Pliszka et al., 1999; Rief, 2003).

OT EVALUATIONS

Social Skills, Home Life Routine, and Participation in Household Tasks in Family

- Children's Assessment of Participation and Enjoyment (CAPE) and Preference for Activities of Children (PAC)
- Child Routines Inventory (CRI)
- Home Situations Questionnaire (HSQ)
- Perceived Efficacy and Goal Setting System (PEGS)
- Social Skills Rating System (SSRS)

Academic Functioning

- Academic Performance Rating Scale
- School Function Assessment (SFA)
- School Situations Questionnaire (SSQ)

Marital Relationship and Family Functioning

- Dyadic Adjustment Scale (DAS)
- Locke-Wallac.nce Inventory (PAI)

Behavior

- Behavior Assessment System for Children
- Child Behavior Checklist
- Adolescent Behavior Checklist
- ADHD Behavior Checklist for Adults

Self-Perception

- Piers-Harris Children's Self Concept Scale
- Child and Adolescent Social Perception Measure
- Self-Perception Profile for Children
- Self-Perception Profile for Adolescents

Motor Coordination

- Bruinink-Oseretsky Test of Motor Proficiency
- Movement Assessment Battery for Children

Sensory and Sensory Motor Processing

- Sensory Integration and Praxis Tests (SIPT)
- Sensory Profile

Visual Motor Integration

- Beery-Buktenica Developmental Test of Visual-Motor Integration
- Test of Visual-Perceptual Skills–Revised

OT INTERVENTIONS

Behavior Modification

- Behavior modification includes strategies such as rewarding positive behavior changes and communicating clear expectations of children and adolescents with ADHD (DuPaul & Eckert, 1997).
- Parents and teachers then use the behavioral skills in their daily interactions with their children with ADHD, resulting in improvement in the children's functioning (Abramowitz & O'Leary, 1991; DuPaul & Eckert, 1997).
- Behavior modification has proven effective in children and adolescents with ADHD for improving both social and academic behaviors (MTA Cooperative Group, 1999a, 1999b; Pelham, Wheeler, & Chronis, 1998).

Cognitive Strategy Training

- Cognitive strategy training is one of the cognitive approaches that is a top-down or occupation-based approach (McCormick, Miller, & Pressley, 1989).
- Cognitive strategy training consists of five problem-solving steps: task analysis, anticipation of the difficulties, exploration and selection of task-specific strategies,

application of a strategy to the task, and evaluation of its effectiveness (McCormick et al., 1989).

♦ Cognitive strategy training teaches the child to identify, develop, and use cognitive strategies to perform daily occupations effectively (McCormick et al., 1989).

♦ Research has demonstrated that children with ADHD who were receiving cognitive strategy training (training in strategies to control impulsive behavior) and were on medication decreased their impulsivity, as reflected by performance on the delay task, which improved significantly (Brown, Wynne, & Medenis, 1985; Hall & Kataria, 1992).

Cognitive-Behavioral Therapy

♦ Cognitive-behavioral therapy (CBT) integrates the cognitive strategy training with the behavioral modification techniques. It is an action-oriented form of psychosocial therapy that assumes that maladaptive or faulty thinking patterns cause maladaptive behavior and negative emotions (Enright, 1997).

♦ Instructional strategies that are used in this kind of therapy include modeling, role-playing, and self-instruction. CBT attempts to increase self-control and problem-solving abilities by helping children with ADHD (Enright, 1997).

♦ CBT is effective in managing behavior problems in children with ADHD and can assist adults with ADHD in problem solving (Abikoff, 1987; Fehlings, Roberts, Humphries, & Dawe, 1991).

Sensory Integration

♦ Children with ADHD may have sensory modulation challenges. Sensory modulation difficulties are often the basis for interventions for children with ADHD, especially in addressing attention within the classroom (Mangeot et al., 2001).

♦ Occupational therapy for children with sensory integration dysfunction enhances their ability to process lower-level sensory information related to alertness, body movement and position, and touch. Intervention may help children pay more attention to the higher-level senses of hearing and vision (Mangeot et al., 2001).

♦ The effectiveness of the sensory integration approach has demonstrated that it can help children with ADHD to use self-regulation strategies (sensory-based activities or sensory diet) and increase their school performance such as in seated behaviors, ability to listen and attend, finishing classwork, and improvements in regulation of aggressive behavior (Arnold, Clark, Sachs, Jakim, & Smithies, 1985; Field, Quintino, Hernandez-Reif, & Koslovsky, 1998; Schilling, Washington, Billingsley, & Deitz, 2003; VandenBerg, 2001; Werry, Scaletti, & Mills, 1990).

Social Skills Training

♦ Occupational therapy practitioners working with older children, adolescents, or adults with mental health problems often use social skills groups to promote coping effectiveness and occupational performance (Case-Smith, 2001; Eklund, 1999).

♦ Current intervention approaches may also involve education and counseling (individual, couples, and family), consultation with professionals in schools and community programs, peer support and activity groups, and development of supportive social networks (Case-Smith, 2001).

♦ Social skills training can help children or adults with ADHD to learn new behaviors, problem-solving strategies, and methods of dealing with their interpersonal relationships, such as using appropriate communication skills (Ansthel & Remer, 2003; Colton & Sheridan, 1998; Frankel, Myatt, Cantwell, & Feinberg, 1997).

OT AND THE EVIDENCE

Children with ADHD may benefit from occupational therapy with a sensory integrative approach to enhance sensory processing and promote adaptive responses to environmental demands (Arnold et al., 1985; Field et al., 1998; Schilling et al., 2003; VandenBerg, 2001; Werry et al., 1990).

CAREGIVER CONCERNS

♦ Caregivers will need to provide the necessary structure and manage the environmental factors to help their children be successful, anticipating potential problems and planning accordingly (e.g., safety issues) (Rief, 2003).

♦ As with all children, the best way to manage the difficulties of those with ADHD is through watching for positive behaviors and recognizing children when they are doing well (Rief, 2003).

♦ Many adults with ADHD and parents of children with ADHD find it useful to join a local or national support group. Members of support groups share frustrations and successes, referrals to qualified specialists, and information about successful techniques (Rief, 2003).

RESOURCES

Associations

♦ Attention Deficit Disorder Association
P.O. Box 543
Pottstown, PA 19464
Telephone: 484-945-2101

Website: www.add.org

ADDA provides information, resources, and networking opportunities to help adults with ADHD lead better lives.

◆ Children and Adults with Attention-Deficit/Hyperactivity Disorder
8181 Professional Place
Suite 150
Landover, MD 20785
Telephone: 301-306-7070
Website: www.chadd.org
CHADD provides science-based, evidence-based information about ADHD to parents, educators, professionals, the media, and the general public.

◆ ADD Centers of America
30 N. Michigan Avenue, Suite 814
Chicago, IL 60602
Telephone: 312-372-4824
Website: www.addcenters.com
This organization provides information and resources to help family members and individuals with ADD or ADHD.

Books

◆ Hartmann, T., & Ratey, J. J. (1995). *ADD success stories: A guide to fulfillment for families with attention deficit disorder.* Grass Valley, CA: Underwood Books. This book is full of tips from individuals with ADD themselves about how they manage various aspects of ADD in their lives.

◆ Hallowell, E. M., & Ratey, J. J. (1995). *Driven to distraction: Recognizing and coping with attention deficit disorder from childhood through adulthood.* New York: Simon & Schuster.
This clear and valuable book dispels a variety of myths about attention deficit disorder.

◆ Kilcarr, P. J., & Quinn, P. O. (1997). *Voices from fatherhood: Fathers, sons, and ADHD.* New York: Brunner/Mazel.
This book is unique in focusing on fathers' concerns in parenting their sons with ADHD.

Journals

◆ *Journal of Attention Disorders*
◆ *Journal of Clinical Child and Adolescent Psychology*
◆ *Journal of Child Psychology & Psychiatry & Allied Disciplines*
◆ *Journal of Developmental & Behavioral Pediatrics*
◆ *Journal of the American Academy of Child & Adolescent Psychiatry*

Websites

◆ ADHD Online Community
www.adhd.com

Provides resources for family, adults with ADD, and health care professionals.

◆ Focus on ADHD
www.focusonadhd.com
Provides information and guidelines about living with people with ADHD.

◆ San Diego ADHD Webpage
www.sandiegoadhd.com
Provides a forum for communication about ADHD for parents, primary care providers, teachers, children with ADHD, and their siblings.

REFERENCES

Abikoff, H. (1987). An evaluation of cognitive behavior therapy for hyperactive children. In B. B. Lahey & A. E. Kazdin (Eds.), *Advances in clinical child psychology* (pp. 171–216). New York: Plenum Press.

Abramowitz, A. J., & O'Leary, S. G. (1991). Behavioral interventions for the classroom: Implications for student with ADHD. *School Psychology Review, 20,* 220–234.

American Psychiatric Association. (2000). *Diagnostic and statistical manual of mental disorders* (4th ed., text rev.). Washington, DC: Author.

Ansthel, K. M., & Remer, R. (2003). Social skills training in children with attention deficit hyperactivity disorder: A randomized-controlled clinical trial. *Journal of Clinical Child and Adolescent Psychology, 23,* 153–165.

Arnold, L. E., Clark, D. L., Sachs, L. A., Jakim, S., & Smithies, C. (1985). Vestibular and visual rotational stimulation as treatment for attention deficit and hyperactivity. *American Journal of Occupational Therapy, 39,* 84–91.

Barkley, R. A. (1998). *Attention-deficit-hyperactivity disorder: A handbook for diagnosis and treatment* (2nd ed.). New York: Guilford Press.

Brown, R. T., Wynne, M. E., & Medenis, R. (1985). Methylphenidate and cognitive therapy: A comparison of treatment approaches with hyperactive boys. *Journal of Abnormal Child Psychology, 13,* 69–87.

Case-Smith, J. (2001). *Occupational therapy for children.* St. Louis: Mosby.

Colton, D. L., & Sheridan, S. M. (1998). Conjoint behavioral consultation and social skill training: Enhancing the play behaviors of boys with attention deficit hyperactivity disorder. *Journal of Educational and Psychological Consultation, 9,* 3–28.

DuPaul, G. J., & Eckert, T. L. (1997). The effects of school-based interventions for attention deficit hyperactivity disorder: A meta-analysis. *School Psychology Review, 26,* 5–27.

Eklund, M. (1999). Outcome of occupational therapy in a psychiatric day care unit for long-term mentally ill patients. *Occupational Therapy in Mental Health, 14,* 21–45.

Enright, S. (1997). Cognitive behaviour therapy. *British Medical Journal, 314,* 1811–1816.

Fehlings, D. L., Roberts, W., Humphries, T., & Dawe, G. (1991). Attention deficit hyperactivity disorder: Does cognitive behavioral therapy improve home behavior? *Journal of Developmental and Behavioral Pediatrics, 12,* 223–228.

Field, T. M., Quintino, O., Hernandez-Reif, M., & Koslovsky, G. (1998). Adolescents with attention deficit hyperactivity disorder benefit from massage therapy. *Adolescence, 33,* 103–108.

Frankel, F., Myatt, R., Cantwell, D. P., & Feinberg, D. T. (1997). Parent-assisted transfer of children's social skills training: Effects on children with and without attention-deficit hyperactivity disorder. *Journal of the American Academy of Child and Adolescent Psychiatry, 36,* 1056–1064.

Hall, C. W., & Kataria, S. (1992). Effects of two treatment techniques on delay and vigilance tasks with attention deficit hyperactive disorder (ADHD) children. *Journal of Psychology, 126,* 17–25.

Mangeot, S. D., Miller, L. J., McIntosh, D. N., McGrath-Clarke, J., Simon, J., Hagerman, R. J., et al. (2001). Sensory modulation dysfunction in children with attention deficit hyperactivity disorder. *Developmental Medicine and Child Neurology, 43,* 399–406.

McCormick, C. B., Miller, G., & Pressley, M. (1989). *Cognitive strategy research: From basic research to educational application.* New York: Springer-Verlag.

MTA Cooperative Group. (1999a). A 14-month randomized clinical trial of treatment strategies for attention-deficit/hyperactivity disorder. *Archives of General Psychiatry, 56,* 1073–1086.

MTA Cooperative Group. (1999b). Moderators and mediators of treatment response for children with attention-deficit/hyperactivity disorder: The Multimodal Treatment Study of Children with Attention-Deficit/Hyperactivity Disorder. *Archives of General Psychiatry, 56,* 1088–1096.

National Institute of Mental Health. (1999). *Attention deficit hyperactivity disorder.* Retrieved March 10, 2005, from www.nimh.nih.gov/publicat/adhd.cfm

Pelham, W. E., Wheeler, T., & Chronis, A. (1998). Empirically supported psychosocial treatments for attention deficit hyperactivity disorder. *Journal of Clinical Child Psychology, 27,* 190–205.

Pliszka, S. R., Carlson, C. L., & Swanson, J. M. (1999). *ADHD with comorbid disorders: Clinical assessment and management.* New York: Guilford Press.

Resnick, R. J. (2000). *The hidden disorder: A clinician's guide to attention deficit hyperactivity disorder in adults.* Washington, DC: American Psychiatric Association.

Rief, S. F. (2003). *The ADHD book of lists: A practical guide for helping children and teens with attention deficit disorders.* San Francisco, CA: Jossey-Bass.

Schilling, D. L., Washington, K., Billingsley, F. F., & Deitz, J. (2003). Classroom seating for children with attention deficit hyperactivity disorder: Therapy balls versus chairs. *American Journal of Occupational Therapy, 57,* 534–541.

VandenBerg, N. L. (2001). The use of a weighted vest to increase on-task behavior in children with attention difficulties. *American Journal of Occupational Therapy, 55,* 621–628.

Wender, P. H. (2000). *ADHD: Attention-deficit hyperactivity disorders in children and adults.* New York: Oxford University Press.

Werry, J. S., Scaletti, R., & Mills, F. (1990). Sensory integration and teacher-judged learning problems: A controlled intervention trial. *Journal of Paediatrics & Child Health, 26,* 31–35.

BIPOLAR DISORDER

Alyssa Wells Arnold and Kate-Lyn Stone

Bipolar disorder, also known as manic-depressive illness, is a brain disorder that causes unusual shifts in a person's mood, energy, and ability to function. Bipolar disorder causes dramatic "mood" swings, or episodes of mania, hypomania, and major depression, with periods of normal mood in between. In other words, a person who has bipolar disorder may experience a mood that alternates between the "poles" of mania "highs" and depression "lows" (National Institute of Mental Health, 1999). The diagnosis of bipolar disorder is distinguished by the presence of a major depressive episode (American Psychiatric Association, 2000). Depending on the dominant mood, bipolar disorder is usually classified as either bipolar I or bipolar II (Cara, 2005).

◆ *Bipolar I:* Symptoms of major depression, coupled with the occurrence of full-blown mania or mixed symptoms

◆ *Bipolar II:* Symptoms of major depression, coupled with the reoccurrence of depressive episodes with hypomania, which is a persistent state of inflated or irritable mood that presents like symptoms of mania but are much milder (APA, 2000)

PREVALENCE

The prevalence of bipolar disorder has been estimated to affect about two million adult Americans, or about 1% of the adult population (NIMH, 1999). An equal number of men and women develop this illness: however, men tend to begin with manic episodes, and women tend to begin with depressive episodes (APA, 2000).

TYPICAL COURSE AND SIGNS AND SYMPTOMS

Bipolar symptoms usually arise in late adolescence, although they can begin in early childhood and can even initiate later in life. Episodes of mania and depression typically recur across the life course. The diagnosis of bipolar disorder is made on the basis of symptoms, course of illness, and, when available, family history (NIMH, 1999). The most prevalent symptom-related criteria for mania and depression are adapted from the DSM-IV.

Mania

- Increased physical and mental activity and energy
- Exaggerated optimism and self-confidence
- Decreased need for sleep without experiencing fatigue
- Grandiose delusions
- Impulsiveness and poor judgment
- Delusions and hallucinations in severe cases

Depression

- Prolonged sadness and persistent lethargy
- Significant changes in appetite and sleep patterns, irritability
- Feelings of guilt and worthlessness
- Inability to concentrate
- Inability to take pleasure in former interests and social withdrawal

CAUSE AND ETIOLOGY

Research suggests that bipolar disorder is linked to genetics and is most likely caused by a single gene (NIMH, 1999). Research also suggests that other factors such as biochemical, neuroendocrine, socioenvironmental, and psychosocial in combination play an active role in possible causes of bipolar disorder (Cara, 2005).

AFFILIATED PROBLEMS

Alcohol and drug abuse are very common among individuals with bipolar disorder and should be considered in the treatment plan (Strakowski & DelBello, 2000). Anxiety disorders, including posttraumatic stress disorder and obsessive-compulsive disorder, also commonly co-occur with bipolar disorder (Mueser et al., 1998).

INTERVENTIONS

Medications

Antidepressants, mood stabilizers, and antipsychotic medications such as lithium, Depakote, Risperdal, and Seroquel are the most widely researched and most commonly prescribed treatments for individuals with bipolar disorder (NIMH, 1999). Lithium is the most common mood-stabilizing medication and is often very effective in preventing the reoccurrence of both manic and depressive episodes (NIMH, 1999).

Psychoeducation

Teaching individuals with bipolar, along with their families, about the illness and its treatment includes the recognition of signs and symptoms of relapse in order to initiate early intervention (NIMH, 1999).

Electroconvulsive Therapy

If the combination of treatments proves to be ineffective, electroconvulsive therapy (ECT) is another alternative. ECT has been found to be highly effective in treatment for severe depressive, manic, and mixed episodes (NIMH, 1999).

OT EVALUATIONS

Basic and Instrumental Activity of Daily Living Skills

- Kohlman Evaluation of Living Skills (KELS)
- Milwaukee Evaluation of Daily Living Skills (MEDLS)
- Performance Assessment of Self-care Skills (PASS)
- Routine Task Inventory-2 (RTI-2)
- Assessment of Living Skills and Resources (ALSAR)
- Assessment of Motor and Process Skills (AMPS)

Psychosocial Skills

- Allen Cognitive Level Test-90 (ACLS-90)
- Role Activity Performance Scale (RAPS)
- The Assessment of Occupational Functioning (AOF)
- The Occupational Case Analysis and Interviewing Rating Scale (OCAIRS)
- The Occupational Performance History Interview II (OPHI II)

Cognitive/Perceptual Skills

- Test of Everyday Attention (TEA)
- Lowenstein Occupational Therapy Cognitive Assessment (LOTCA)
- Mini-Mental State Exam (MMSE)

Self-Perception

- The Canadian Occupational Performance Measure (COPM)
- The Occupational Questionnaire (OQ)
- The Role Checklist

OT INTERVENTIONS

Cognitive Therapy

Cognitive therapy (CT) is a technique that is used in combination with occupational therapy in order to replace negative thoughts with more realistic appraisals to reduce the impact of distorted thinking styles. This technique allows occupational therapists the opportunity to examine the meaning associated with functional activities (Giles, 2003). A recent study indicates that the combination of medication and CT has long-term positive effects with individuals who are experiencing bipolar disorder when compared to medications alone (Hensley, Nadiga, & Uhlenhuth, 2004).

Interpersonal and Social Rhythm Therapy

Interpersonal and social rhythm therapy (IPSRT) is based on the idea that disruptions in daily routines and problems in interpersonal relationships can cause reoccurrence of the manic and depressive episodes that characterize bipolar disorder. During treatment, occupational therapy practitioners help clients to understand how changes in daily routines, the quality of their relationships, and their social roles can affect their mood. Practitioners teach clients to identify triggers of mania and depression and then teach them how to better manage stressful situations and better maintain positive relationships (Frank, Swartz, & Kupfer, 2000). This intervention stresses the importance of maintaining a regular schedule of daily activities and stability in personal relationships. A recent study suggests that disruptions in an individual's medical treatment plan or routine can contribute to relapse and a worse outcome (Frank et al., 1999). Regular routines and sleep schedules can help to protect against manic and depressive episodes (NIMH, 1999)

OCCUPATIONAL THERAPY AND THE EVIDENCE

There is strong support throughout the literature for cognitive behavioral and psychosocial approaches in treating individuals with bipolar disorder. Ball, Mitchell, and Corry (2006) found cognitive behavioral therapy (CBT) to be a valuable tool for increasing behavioral self-control and increasing the amount of time between episodes in individuals with bipolar disorder. CBT used in combination with mood stabilizers (versus medication alone) has also been reported to contribute to fewer bipolar episodes, fewer hospital admissions for bipolar episodes, higher social functioning, less variability in manic symptoms, and better coping with manic symptoms (Lam et al., 2003). On the basis of the study using cognitive therapy (CT) (Hensley et al., 2004) and the study on interpersonal and social rhythm therapy (Frank et al., 1999), individuals with bipolar disorder may also benefit from occupational therapy with a cognitive behavioral approach in order to integrate the concepts of CT and IPSRT to enhance the individual's ability to self-regulate and promote improved performance patterns in the areas of habits, routines, and roles, which will improve overall participation in activities of daily living.

Psychosocial approaches used in group settings have had a positive impact on mood stabilization and preventing relapse, as well as enabling individuals to go beyond their symptoms and achieve life goals. Group psychoeducation, in addition to pharmacotherapy, improves perceived quality of life, especially concerning physical functioning, in individuals with bipolar disorder (De Andres et al., 2006; Huxley, Parikh, & Baldessarini, 2000; Michalak, Yathman, Wan, & Lam, 2005).

CAREGIVER CONCERNS

Caregivers must understand the signs and symptoms of bipolar disorder, the course of the disease, the importance of a medication schedule and good sleep hygiene, and that suicide is always a possible threat.

RESOURCES

Organizations

◆ American Psychiatric Association
1000 Wilson Boulevard
Suite 1825
Arlington, VA 22209-3901
Telephone: 703-907-7300
Website: www.psych.org
◆ Depression and Bipolar Support Alliance
730 N. Franklin Street
Suite 501
Chicago, Illinois 60610-7224
Telephone: 312-642-0049 or 800-826-3632
Fax (312) 642-7243
Website: www.dbsalliance.org
◆ National Institute of Mental Health
National Institutes of Health
6001 Executive Blvd.
Room 8184, MSC 9663
Bethesda, MD 20892-9663
Telephone: 301-443-4513/301-443-8431 (TTY) or
866-615-6464
Fax: 301-443-4279
Website: http://www.nimh.nih.gov

Books

◆ Jamison, K. R. (1995). *An unquiet mind: A memoir of moods and madness.* New York: Vintage Books.
The psychology memoir, *An Unquiet Mind,* looks into manic depressive disorder from the perspectives of both the client living with the illness and the provider who is trying to heal the client. The author recounts her own experience living with this disorder; talking about the costs of the illness and even what she found to be the benefits.

◆ Grant, R., & Ferber, E. (1999). *Why am I up, why am I down?: Understanding bipolar disorder.* New York: Dell. This informative book discusses several aspects of bipolar disorder, including: who is at risk, what causes bipolar disorder, the symptoms of both the manic and depressive phases, how to get help, the latest facts on the disorder, as well as other topics that can help lead to successful management of bipolar disorder.

◆ Miklowitz, D. J. (2002). *The bipolar disorder survival guide: What you and your family need to know.* New York: Dell.
In this book, Miklowitz covers the origins, symptoms, and treatments for bipolar disorder. It is intended for patients and has a strong emphasis on current medications used to treat bipolar disorder.

◆ Fast, J. A., & Preston, J. D. (2004). *Loving someone with bipolar disorder.* Oakland, CA: New Harbinger Publishers.
This unique book, written by someone who has bipolar disorder, provides a guide on living with someone who has the illness. It provides advice on how couples can work together as a treatment team dealing with how to live with the illness while also maintaining a loving and joyful relationship.

REFERENCES

American Psychiatric Association. (2000). *Diagnostic and statistical manual of mental disorders* (4th ed., text rev.). Washington, DC: Author.

Ball, J. R., Mitchell, P. B., & Corry, J. C. (2006). A randomized controlled trial of cognitive therapy for bipolar disorder: Focus on long-term change. *Journal of Clinical Psychiatry, 67*, 277–286.

Cara, E. (2005). Mood disorders. In E. Cara & A. MacRae (Eds.), *Psychosocial occupational therapy: A clinical practice* (2nd ed., pp. 162–192). Albany, NY: Thompson Delmar Learning.

De Andres, R. D., Aillon, N., Baridot, M. C., Bourgeois, P., Mertel, S., Nerfin, F., et al. (2006). Impact of the life goals group therapy program for bipolar patients: An open study. *Journal of Affective Disorders, 93*, 253–257.

Frank, E., Swartz, H. A., & Kupfer, D. J. (2000). Interpersonal and social rhythm therapy: Managing the chaos of bipolar disorder. *Biological Psychiatry, 48*, 593–604.

Frank, E., Swartz, H. A., Mallinger, A. G., Thase, M. E., Weaver, E. V., & Kupfer, D. J. (1999). Adjunctive psychotherapy for bipolar disorder: Effects of changing treatment modality. *Journal of Abnormal Psychology, 108*, 579–587.

Giles, G. M. (2003). Cognitive therapy. In E. Crepeau, E. S. Cohn, & B. A. B. Schell (Eds.), *Willard and Spackman's occupational therapy* (10th ed., pp. 259–260). Philadelphia: Lippincott Williams & Wilkins.

Hensley, P. L., Nadiga, D., & Uhlenhuth, E. H. (2004). Long-term effectiveness of cognitive therapy in major depressive disorder. *Depression and Anxiety, 20*, 1–7.

Huxley, N. A., Parikh, S. V., & Baldessarini, R. J. (2000). Effectiveness of psychosocial treatments in bipolar disorder: State of the evidence. *Harvard Review of Psychiatry, 8*, 126–140.

Lam, D., Watkins, E., Hayward, P., Bright, J., Wright, K., Kerr, N., et al. (2003). A randomized controlled study of cognitive therapy for relapse prevention for bipolar affective disorder: Outcome of the first year. *Archives of General Psychiatry, 60*, 145–152.

Michalak, E., Yathman, L. N., Wan, D., & Lam, R. W. (2005). Perceived quality of life in patients with bipolar disorder: Does group psychoeducation have an impact? *Canadian Journal of Psychiatry, 2005*, 95–100.

Mueser, K. T., Goodman, L. B., Trumbetta, S. L., Rosenberg, S. D., Osher, F. C., Vidaver, R., et al. (1998). Trauma and posttraumatic stress disorder in severe mental illness. *Journal of Consulting and Clinical Psychology, 66*, 493–499.

National Institute of Mental Health. (1999). *Bipolar disorder.* Retrieved April 4, 2006, from www.nimh.nih.gov/publicat/bipolar.cfm

Strakowski, S. M., & Del Bello, M. P. (2000). The co-occurrence of bipolar and substance use disorders. *Clinical Psychology Review, 20*, 191–206

CANCER

Kate-Lyn Stone

DIAGNOSIS

Cancer is characterized by the unrestrained growth and spread of abnormal cells, which develop because of damaged DNA. These cells spread throughout the body via the blood and lymph systems (National Cancer Institute, 2007). Cancer can result in death if the spread of these cells remains uncontrolled. Cancer is the second leading cause of death in the United States. Any individual of any race or gender can be diagnosed with cancer at any age; however, the rate at which cancer occurs varies from group to group. The sooner the cancer is detected and diagnosed, the better the outcome (American Cancer Society, 2007b).

INCIDENCE AND PREVALENCE

◆ Cancer is the second leading cause of death (after heart disease) in the United States (American Cancer Society, 2007a).

◆ Cancer is responsible for one of every four deaths in the United States (American Cancer Society, 2007a).

◆ Over one million people are diagnosed with cancer each year (American Cancer Society, 2007a).

◆ About 10.5 million Americans were living with a history of cancer in January 2007 (American Cancer Society, 2007a).

◆ Age is the leading risk factor for developing cancer; 56.5% of all cancers are diagnosed in individuals 65 years of age and older (Centers for Disease Control and Prevention, 2007).

◆ Breast cancer is the most common type of cancer diagnosed in women; prostate cancer is the most common type of cancer in men (American Cancer Society, 2007a).

THE CAUSE AND ETIOLOGY

Cancer can be caused by both external and internal factors. Examples of external factors include smoking cigarettes, radiation, and chemicals. Internal factors can include hormones, immune conditions, and inherited cell mutations. These factors can act alone or in combination with one another to lead to cancer (American Cancer Society, 2007b).

Risk factors for cancer can be divided into two groups: modifiable (things that are changeable) and nonmodifiable (things that cannot be altered). Major modifiable risk factors include tobacco use, unhealthy eating habits, infectious agents (such as the hepatitis B virus), ultraviolet radiation, and physical inactivity. Other modifiable risk factors can include alcohol use, occupational exposures, socioeconomic status, obesity, food contaminants, and environmental radiation. Nonmodifiable risk factors are ageing, ethnicity, race, heredity, and gender (Mackay, Jemal, Lee, & Parkin, 2006).

TYPES

There are over 100 different types of cancer that can be broken down into five main categories (National Cancer Institute, 2007):

1. *Carcinoma:* cancer in skin or tissue over internal organs
2. *Sarcoma:* cancer in bone, fat, muscle, cartilage, or blood vessels
3. *Leukemia:* cancer that begins in tissue that creates blood (e.g., bone marrow)
4. *Lymphoma and myeloma:* cancer of the immune system
5. *Central nervous system cancers:* cancers in the brain or spinal cord

An individual's prognosis, or likelihood of survival, depends on the type and stage of cancer. Precancerous abnormal cells are generally associated with the best prognosis, followed by localized cancer, then regional cancer.

Metastatic cancer is associated with the worst prognosis for survival (Mackay et al., 2006).

TYPICAL COURSE AND SYMPTOMS

All cancers, no matter what type, begin in the cells of the body. When the DNA of the cells becomes damaged, mutations are produced that affect the normal development of the cell. Because of these mutations, the cells do not die when they are supposed to and can eventually contribute to the growth of a tumor. If the tumor is malignant (cancerous), it can spread to other parts of the body (American Cancer Society, 2007b).

A symptom is an indication of a disease or condition that is noticed by the individual who experiences it but is not noticeable to other people. A sign is an indication of a disease or a condition that is observed by a health care provider. General signs and symptoms of cancer include the following:

◆ Unexplained weight loss, usually of 10 pounds or more
◆ Fever
◆ Fatigue
◆ Pain
◆ Skin changes, such as darkening, yellowing, reddening, itching, or excessive hair growth

There are, of course, specific signs and symptoms for each type of cancer. To find more information on symptoms for a specific type of cancer, the reader is referred to the American Cancer Society's Website at www.cancer.org.

SEQUENCE OF CARE

Once an individual has been diagnosed with cancer, the sooner a course of treatment is decided on, the better the outcome in most cases. The sequence of care for the treatment of cancer depends on the type of cancer, the stage of the cancer (how widespread it is in the body), and other factors for each individual, such as overall health and lifestyle. There are four major types of treatment: surgery, radiation, chemotherapy, and biologic therapies. In addition to these four, there are also hormone therapies and complementary and alternative therapies. Surgery and radiation are generally used to treat localized cancers. Chemotherapy, which involves using powerful medications, is used to treat cancer that has spread to other parts of the body. Biologic therapies, also known as immunotherapy, biotherapy, or biological response modifier therapy, use the immune system to fight cancer (American Cancer Society, 2007b).

Throughout treatment for cancer, an individual may receive services from physicians, pharmacists, counselors, physical therapists, occupational therapists, nurses, respiratory therapists, massage therapists, case managers, surgeons, and social workers. The spectrum of health care providers who are seen will depend on the type and stage of cancer.

OT ROLE

Thanks to improving and advancing technology, more and more people are surviving cancer. Because of this, the role of occupational therapists in treating cancer has also grown. Occupational therapists can work as part of a specialized team in a cancer center, in the community, and in palliative care (Crompton, 2004). In general, the goal of the occupational therapist is to improve the client's quality of life. This can be done in several ways beyond the basic self-care that is typically thought of as occupational therapy. Occupational therapists can also help the client by educating the client and his or her family, finding resources, strengthening weaknesses secondary to tumors, dealing with cognitive changes due to chemotherapy treatment, and improving endurance. Occupational therapists can also help clients with lifestyle management, fatigue management, medication management, and symptom management (Crompton, 2004).

Dr. Mack Ivy explains that "as an occupational therapist, I'm not in charge of curing cancer" (Strzelecki, 2006). What Ivy says here is important for occupational therapists to realize and remember: we cannot cure cancer, but we have the ability to improve the quality of life of individuals who are living with cancer. That can be a very powerful tool, as Ivy goes on to explain: "occupational therapy is so powerful and important because we are a discipline that addresses sensorimotor skills and cognitive and psychosocial aspects. We look at the environment and we also try to find out functional goals, as well as coping and leisure activities" (Strzelecki, 2006).

OT EVALUATIONS

Basic and Instrumental Activity of Daily Living Skills

- Kohlman Evaluation of Living Skills (KELS)
- Assessment of Motor and Process Skills (AMPS)
- Functional Independence Measure (FIM)
- Klein-Bell Activities of Daily Living Scale (Klein-Bell)
- Satisfaction With Performance Scaled Questionnaire (SPSQ)

Psychosocial Skills

- The Assessment of Occupational Functioning (AOF)
- Beck Depression Inventory (BDI)
- The Occupational Performance History Interview II (OPHI II)
- Ways of Coping Checklist (WCC)

Self-Perception

- The Canadian Occupational Performance Measure (COPM)

- The Role Checklist
- Worker Role Inventory

Other Assessments

- Manual muscle testing
- Range-of-motion testing
- Pain scales
- Home assessment

OT INTERVENTIONS

- ADL
- Energy conservation techniques
- Strengthening exercises
- Pain management
- Assistive technology
- Adaptation of the environment
- Adaptive equipment
- Patient and family education
- Home planning
- Self-management education
- Caregiver adjustment

OT AND THE EVIDENCE

Several studies discuss the benefits of psychosocial interventions for improving quality of life in individuals with cancer (Barsevick, Sweeney, Haney, & Chung, 2002; Uitterhoeve et al., 2004). More specifically, Osborn, Demoncada, and Feuerstein (2006) found cognitive behavioral therapy (CBT) to be an effective intervention for treating depression, anxiety, and quality of life in individuals with cancer. They found CBT to have short-term effects on depression and anxiety, thus reducing emotional distress, as well as short- and long-term effects on quality of life. They also found that CBT was more effective when used individually rather than in groups. Another psychosocial intervention approach that has been found to be effective in improving overall quality of life is social cognitive theory (SCT). Graves (2003) found that using SCT-based interventions improved overall quality of life in adults with cancer.

RESOURCES

Associations

- American Cancer Society
  1599 Clifton Road NE
  Atlanta, GA 30329-4251
  Telephone: 800-ACS-2345
  Website: www.cancer.org
- Lance Armstrong Foundation
  P.O. Box 161150

Austin, TX 78716-1150
Telephone: 512-236-8820
Fax: 512-236-8482
Website: www.livestrong.org

◆ National Cancer Institute
6116 Executive Boulevard
Room 3036A
Bethesda, MD 20892-8322
Telephone: 800-4-CANCER
Website: http://www.cancer.gov

◆ National Coalition for Cancer Survivorship
1010 Wayne Avenue, 5th Floor
Suite 300
Silver Spring, MD 20910
Telephone: 1-888-650-9127

Books

◆ Murray, L., & Howard, B. (2002). *Angels and monsters*. Atlanta: American Cancer Society.
This collection provides 25 accounts of children living with cancer.

◆ Dorfman, E., & Schultz, H. (2001). *Here and now: Inspiring stories of cancer survivors*. New York: Marlow.
This book provides a collection of narratives from men, women, and children who describe their life with cancer and the ways in which they coped.

Journals

◆ *British Journal of Cancer*
◆ *Cancer*
◆ *European Journal of Cancer*
◆ *International Journal of Cancer*
◆ *Supportive Care in Cancer: Official Journal of the Multinational Association of Supportive Care in Cancer*

Websites

◆ American Cancer Society
www.cancer.org
The American Cancer Society is a valuable resource for patients, family, friends, and survivors of cancer. The website provides facts, figures, and statistics about cancer as well as the latest research and clinical trials. It provides resources for making treatment decisions and how to manage life with cancer.

◆ National Cancer Institute
www.cancer.gov
The National Cancer Institute (NCI) is a component of the National Institutes of Health. NCI is the federal government's primary agency for cancer training and research. The website provides information about topics relating to cancer, cancer statistics, and clinical trials.

REFERENCES

American Cancer Society. (2007a). *Cancer facts and figures 2007.* Atlanta: American Cancer Society.

American Cancer Society. (2007b). *Detailed guide: Cancer (general information).* Retrieved October 3, 2007, from http://www.cancer.org/docroot/CRI/CRI_2_3x.asp?rnav=cridg&dt=72

Barsevick, A. M., Sweeney, C., Haney, E., & Chung, E. (2002). A systematic qualitative analysis of psychoeducational interventions for depression in patients with cancer. *Oncology Nursing Forum, 29,* 73–84.

Centers for Disease Control and Prevention. (2007). *Cancer A to Z.* Retrieved October 8, 2007, from http://www.cdc.gov/cancer/az/

Crompton, E. (2004). *Occupational therapy intervention in cancer: Guidance for professionals, managers, and decision-makers.* London: College of Occupational Therapists.

Graves, K. (2003). Social cognitive theory and cancer patients' quality of life: A meta-analysis of psychosocial intervention components. *Health Psychology, 22,* 210–219.

Mackay, J., Jemal, A., Lee, N., & Parkin, M. (2006). *The cancer atlas.* Atlanta: The American Cancer Society.

National Cancer Institute. (2007). *Cancer topics.* Retrieved September 26, 2007, from http://www.cancer.gov/cancertopics/what-is-cancer

Osborn, R. L., Demoncada, A. C., & Feuerstein, M. (2006). Psychosocial interventions for depression, anxiety, and quality of life in cancer survivors: Meta-analyses. *International Journal of Psychiatry in Medicine, 36,* 13–34.

Strzelecki, M. V. (2006). An OT approach to clients with cancer. [Electronic version]. *OT Practice, 11*(15), 7–8.

Uitterhoeve, R. J., Vernooy, M., Litjens, M., Potting, K., Bensing, J., DeMulder, P., et al. (2004). Psychosocial interventions for patients with advanced cancer: A systematic review of the literature. *British Journal of Cancer, 91,* 1050–1062.

CARDIAC CONDITIONS

Kate-Lyn Stone

DIAGNOSIS

The term *cardiac condition* is an umbrella term for several more specific heart diseases and conditions. Coronary heart disease is the most common cardiac condition in the United States (Centers for Disease Control and Prevention, 2007). The following text provides general information about cardiac conditions. For more specific information on three individual heart conditions, please refer to the resource sheets for congenital heart disease, congestive heart failure, and myocardial infarction.

INCIDENCE AND PREVALENCE

- Heart disease is the leading cause of death in the United States (Medline Plus, 2007a).
- Approximately 700,000 people in the United States die of heart disease each year, which is about 29% of all U.S. deaths each year (Centers for Disease Control and Prevention, 2007).

ETIOLOGY

There are several risk factors, which include conditions and lifestyle factors that can increase an individual's chances for developing a cardiac condition. The conditions include high levels of low-density lipoprotein (LDL) cholesterol, high blood pressure, and diabetes mellitus. Behavioral factors that contribute to the development of cardiac conditions include smoking and other tobacco use, poor diet, physical inactivity, being overweight or obese, and excessive alcohol use. One last factor that can increase an individual's chances of having a cardiac condition is heredity, since heart disease can run in a family (Centers for Disease Control and Prevention, 2007).

TYPES

As was previously noted, the term *cardiac condition* is a broad term that covers several more specific heart conditions. The following list provides more specific terminology for other heart diseases and conditions (Centers for Disease Control and Prevention, 2007):

- Acute coronary syndrome
- Arrhythmias
- Cardiomyopathy
- Congenital heart disease
- Coronary heart disease
- Heart attack (myocardial infarction)
- Heart failure
- Peripheral arterial disease
- Rheumatic heart disease

For more information on these conditions and others, the reader is referred to the Websites for the American Heart Association and the Centers for Disease Control and Prevention.

TYPICAL COURSE AND SYMPTOMS

The typical course, signs, and symptoms will vary for each condition and disease.

MEDICAL INTERVENTION

Cardiac conditions generally go unnoticed and undiagnosed until a person has chest pain, a heart attack, or a stroke. If these telltale signs do not lead to a medical emergency and the physician suspects a cardiac disease, the physician will use a variety of tests to narrow it down to a specific diagnosis. Tests that may be used include electrocardiogram, echocardiogram, stress test, catheterization, and carotid artery scan. Once a diagnosis has been determined, the individual might need to make serious lifestyle changes, take medication, undergo surgery, or a combination of the three (Dowshen, 2007).

Cardiac surgery has been made possible by two major advances in medical technology. First, the heart-lung machine takes over the work of the heart and lungs while surgery is performed, allowing blood and oxygen to be pumped throughout the body. Second, body-cooling techniques allow the heart to be stopped for longer periods of time without doing damage to the heart. If temperatures in the body are cooler, the heart requires less oxygen (Texas Heart Institute, 2007).

There are several different types of cardiac surgery. Cardiac surgery can be used to insert devices into the heart chamber, repair or replace valves, bypass or widen blocked arteries, repair aneurysms, replace weak cardiac muscles with stronger ones taken from the abdomen or back, or transplant a heart from a donor (Medline Plus, 2007b). The following are possible types of cardiac surgery that can be performed, depending on the condition that is present:

- *Coronary artery bypass:* Coronary artery bypass grafting, also known as coronary artery bypass graft surgery, coronary bypass, or bypass surgery, is the most common cardiac surgery. This surgery involves taking a vein or artery from another part of the body and replacing a section of a diseased coronary artery. This allows more blood to flow easily to the heart (Texas Heart Institute, 2007).
- *Valve repair or replacement:* In valve repair, a damaged valve is fixed so that it will work properly. In valve replacement, a damaged valve is replaced by a biological valve taken from an animal or human or by a mechanical valve made of plastic, carbon, or metal (Texas Heart Institute, 2007).
- *Arrhythmia surgery:* Arrhythmia surgery includes Maze surgery. Maze surgery is used to treat the most common type of arrhythmia, called atrial fibrillation. In Maze surgery, surgeons create a new "maze" of electrical pathways to allow electrical impulses to get through the heart easily (Texas Heart Institute, 2007).
- *Aneurysm repair:* Aneurysm repair involves using a graft, or a patch, to replace a weakened section of a blood vessel or the heart (Texas Heart Institute, 2007).

- *Transmyocardial laser revascularization:* Transmyocardial laser revascularization uses lasers to make channels in the heart muscle to allow blood to flow directly into the heart chamber (Texas Heart Institute, 2007).
- *Carotid endarterectomy:* Carotid endarterectomy involves inserting a tube above and below a blockage in the neck to reroute blood flow and then removing the fatty plaque that is causing the blockage. Carotid endarterectomy is the most common surgery to treat carotid artery disease (Texas Heart Institute, 2007).
- *Heart transplantation:* Heart transplantation is generally the last option after medicines, mechanical devices, and other therapies have failed (Texas Heart Institute, 2007).

Patients with a cardiac condition generally participate in cardiac rehabilitation after receiving their medical treatment. These rehabilitation programs usually support an individual through education and counseling services centered on increasing physical fitness, promoting health and well-being, and decreasing the risk of future cardiac conditions (American Heart Association, 2007). The physical fitness portion of the rehabilitation will be created on the basis of the type of cardiac condition that the client has and the treatment that the client has received.

PREVENTION

An individual can help to prevent the development of heart disease by following some simple guidelines (Medline Plus, 2007a):

- Maintain a good blood pressure.
- Lower cholesterol.
- Exercise on a regular basis.
- Do not smoke.
- Maintain a healthy weight.

OT ROLE

An occupational therapist will often be a member of the cardiac rehabilitation multidisciplinary team treating clients who have cardiac conditions. Occupational therapists help clients with motor and sensory skills following surgery or other medical intervention. Occupational therapists also help clients learn to break activities down into smaller parts to help in the conservation of energy (Heart and Stroke Foundation, 2006). Occupational therapists work with clients to prevent further cardiac conditions from developing by promoting healthy lifestyle routines and habits.

OT EVALUATIONS

Basic and Instrumental Activity of Daily Living Skills

- Kohlman Evaluation of Living Skills (KELS)
- Assessment of Motor and Process Skills (AMPS)
- Functional Independence Measure (FIM)
- Klein-Bell Activities of Daily Living Scale (Klein-Bell)
- Satisfaction With Performance Scaled Questionnaire (SPSQ)

Psychosocial Skills

- The Assessment of Occupational Functioning (AOF)
- The Occupational Performance History Interview II (OPHI II)

Self-Perception

- The Canadian Occupational Performance Measure (COPM)
- The Role Checklist
- Worker Role Inventory

Other Assessments

- Manual muscle testing
- Range-of-motion testing
- Pain scales
- Home assessment

OT INTERVENTIONS

- ADL
- Energy conservation techniques
- Strengthening exercises
- Pain management
- Stress management
- Assistive technology
- Adapt environment
- Adaptive equipment
- Patient and family education
- Home planning
- Self-management education

OT AND THE EVIDENCE

Cardiac rehabilitation programs conduct most of the research on interventions for cardiac conditions. Following extensive training, an occupational therapist can often be a member of the multidisciplinary team working in cardiac rehabilitation. Cardiac rehabilitation has been proven to be effective in patients of all ages. Macchi and colleagues (2007) looked at cardiac rehabilitation for individuals aged 75 and older who had undergone some kind of cardiac surgery. The researchers found positive outcomes for these individuals. Kardis, Sherman, and Barnett (2007) found similar positive improvements across all age groups in their study regarding age and quality of life after cardiac rehabilitation. They do, however, suggest that there be a greater focus on emotional support for the younger individuals participating in cardiac rehabilitation. Other studies look at the efficacy of home-based versus center-based rehabilitation. One study suggests that for low-risk clients, home-based rehabilitation is no less effective than center-based cardiac rehabilitation, on the basis of measures concerning capacity for exercise, systolic blood pressure, and total cholesterol (Jolly, Taylor, Lip & Stevens, 2006). Dalal and colleagues (2007) found results similar to those of Jolly and colleagues (2006), in that there were no significant differences between patients who received cardiac rehabilitation in the hospital versus those who received the rehabilitation at home. Dalal and colleagues (2007) used the measures of depression, anxiety, and total cholesterol levels to compare the two groups and found no statistically significant differences between the results.

RESOURCES

Associations

◆ American Heart Association
  National Center
  7272 Greenville Avenue
  Dallas, TX 75231
  Telephone: 800-AHA-USA1
  Website: www.americanheart.org/
◆ Centers for Disease Control and Prevention
  Division for Heart Disease and Stroke Prevention
  (Mail Stop K-47)
  4770 Buford Hwy, NE
  Atlanta, GA 30341-3717
  Telephone: 770-488-2424
  Website: http://www.cdc.gov/DHDSP/index.htm

Books

◆ McKibbin, S. B. (2004). *Living with a miracle: A mother and child's journey.* Lincoln, NE: iUniverse.
  This book provides a compelling and moving story about a mother fighting for her child who was born with a rare and deadly heart defect.

Journals

◆ *American Journal of Cardiology*
◆ *Heart*
◆ *International Journal of Cardiology*
◆ *Journal of Cardiovascular Nursing*

Websites

◆ American Heart Association
  http://www.americanheart.org
  The American Heart Association is dedicated to helping people build healthier lives without cardiovascular diseases or strokes. The website provides information on a range of diseases and conditions relating to the heart. It also has an in depth section about the warning signs for heart attack and stroke. It provides educational materials about how to lead a healthier lifestyle as well as the latest news on cardiac conditions of all kinds.

REFERENCES

American Heart Association. (2007). *Cardiac rehabilitation.* Retrieved October 11, 2007, from http://www.american heart.org/presenter.jhtml?identifier=3047844

Centers for Disease Control and Prevention. (2007). *Heart disease.* Retrieved October 11, 2007, from http://www.cdc. gov/HeartDisease/

Dalal, H. M., Evans, P. H., Campbell, J. L., Taylor, R. S., Watt, A., Read, K. L. Q., et al. (2007). Home-based versus hospital-based rehabilitation after myocardial infarction: A randomized trial with preference arms—Cornwall Heart Attack Rehabilitation Management Study (CHARMS). *International Journal of Cardiology, 119,* 202–211.

Dowshen, S. (2007). *Heart disease.* Retrieved October 11, 2007, from http://kidshealth.org/kid/grownup/conditions/heart_ disease.html

Heart and Stroke Foundation. (2006). *Occupational therapy.* Retrieved October 12, 2007, from http://ww1.heartand stroke.sk.ca/Page.asp?PageID=1965&ArticleID=4958&S rc=stroke&From=SubCategory

Jolly, K., Taylor, R., Lip, G. & Stevens, A. (2006). Home-based cardiac rehabilitation compared with centre-based rehabilitation and usual care: A systematic review and meta-analysis. *International Journal of Cardiology, 111,* 343–351.

Kardis, P., Sherman, M., & Barnett, S. (2007). Association of age and quality of life following phase II cardiac rehabilitation. *Journal of Nursing Care Quality, 22,* 255–259.

Macchi, C., Fattirolli, F., Lova, R. M., Conti, A., Luisi, M. L., Intini, R., et al. (2007). Early and late rehabilitation and physical training in elderly patients after cardiac surgery. *American Journal of Physical Medicine and Rehabilitation, 86,* 826–834.

Medline Plus. (2007a). *Heart diseases.* Retrieved October 11, 2007, from http://www.nlm.nih.gov/medlineplus/heart diseases.html

Medline Plus. (2007b). *Heart surgery.* Retrieved October 9, 2007, from http://www.nlm.nih.gov/medlineplus/heart surgery.html

Texas Heart Institute. (2007). *Heart surgery overview.* Retrieved October 9, 2007, from http://www.texasheartinstitute. org/HIC/Topics/Proced/

CEREBRAL PALSY

Stacey Halpern

Cerebral palsy (CP) is a term that is used to describe motor disorders that are characterized by impaired voluntary movement resulting from either prenatal developmental abnormalities or perinatal or postnatal central nervous system damage occurring before age 5 years (Merck, 1999). Common difficulties associated with CP include cognitive delays, speech difficulty, seizure disorders, feeding problems, impaired vision and hearing, abnormal sensation and perception, difficulty with bowel control, breathing problems due to poor posture, and skin conditions as a result of pressure sores (United Cerebral Palsy Association, 2001a).

CLASSIFICATION OF CEREBRAL PALSY

- *Spastic:* Results in hypertonicity ranging from mild to severe and is the most common type
- *Athetoid:* Characterized by slow, writhing, involuntary movements or abrupt, jerky movements
- *Ataxic:* Characterized by weakness, incoordination, and intentional tremor
- *Mixed:* Commonly combines spasticity and athetosis (Merck, 1999)

INCIDENCE

Approximately 8,000 infants are diagnosed with CP each year (United Cerebral Palsy Association, 2001a).

PREVALENCE

Approximately 764,000 children and adults in the United States demonstrate signs of CP (United Cerebral Palsy Association, 2001a).

COURSE AND SYMPTOMS

There are currently no interventions that can repair the damage to the areas of the brain that control muscle coordination and movement (M. Goldstein, 2004). However, medical and therapeutic interventions help to reduce the symptoms associated with CP and/or improve functional abilities in people with cerebral palsy.

Although CP is not a progressive disorder, motor abilities may decrease as the person grows and the resistance of gravity increasingly takes effect. Secondary conditions that are seen in adults with CP include pain, musculoskele-

tal deformities, overuse syndromes, fractures, and fatigue. People with CP typically live well into adulthood (Zaffuto-Sforza, 2005).

PRECAUTIONS

- Seizure disorders
- Difficulty swallowing
- Impaired vision/hearing
- Abnormal sensation/perception (United Cerebral Palsy Association, 2001a)

ALTERNATIVE TREATMENT APPROACHES

Medical Interventions

- Antispasticity medications are used to decrease nerve cell sensitivity. These medications can be given orally or through implanted pumps.
- Botulinum toxin injections can relax muscles for a period of four to six months.
- Selective dorsal rhizotomy surgery involves cutting sensory nerve fibers posterior to the spinal cord as a method for reducing muscle tone.

Complementary Alternative Medicines

These are treatment approaches that have not been accepted by mainstream practice:

- Hyperbaric oxygen therapy is believed to stimulate brain tissue by adding oxygen in increased amounts and under greater atmospheric pressure. This intervention has not been shown to produce benefits and is controversial (Hardy et al., 2002).
- Conductive education is an educational method that promotes independent functioning through practice, repetition, and verbal self-guidance. This approach has been shown to produce gains, but current research has not shown it to be better than conventional methods (Liberty, 2004; Rosenbaum, 2003).
- The Adeli suit was designed in Poland and is based on the suits from the Soviet space program. It allows for controlled exercise against resistance to strengthen muscles and increase proprioception. Research regarding this intervention is limited (Rosenbaum, 2003).
- Therapeutic electrical stimulation is believed to benefit people with CP by stimulating the increase of active movement. This approach has not been shown in re-

search to produce significant benefits (Dali et al., 2002; Sommerfelt, Markestad, Berg, & Saetesdal, 2001).

OT EVALUATIONS

The basis of occupational therapy assessment for clients with CP is to determine the client's ability to participate in society. Evaluation of the need for assistive technology is important for clients across the life course, as needs can change with age.

Pediatric Evaluations

Pediatric evaluations may include the following:

ADL

- ◆ Pediatric Evaluation of Disability Inventory
- ◆ WeeFIM

School-Specific

- ◆ School Function Assessment
- ◆ School Setting Interview

Functional Mobility

- ◆ Gross Motor Classification System

Play/Leisure

- ◆ Knox Preschool Play Scale
- ◆ Transdisciplinary Play-Based Assessment
- ◆ Play History

Adolescent/Adult Evaluations

Adolescent and adult evaluations may include the following:

General Occupational Performance

- ◆ Canadian Occupational Performance Measure
- ◆ Occupational Performance History Interview
- ◆ Occupational Circumstances Assessment Interview and Rating Scale

ADL

- ◆ Functional Independence Measure

Work

- ◆ The Work Environment Impact Scale

Leisure

- ◆ Adolescent Role Assessment
- ◆ Leisure Assessment Inventory

Additional client factors that may be assessed include cognition, tone, spasticity, sensation, fatigue, and ROM (Andren, & Grimby, 2004; Campbell, 1996; MOHO Clearinghouse, 2005).

OT INTERVENTIONS

When working with people who have CP, occupational therapy practitioners focus on adapting tasks and the environment to help enhance participation and quality of life. Occupational therapy practitioners may play a key role in helping people with CP to choose and access assistive devices and supports that will promote function. Practitioners can play an important role throughout the life course depending on the individual's needs and may be a part of early intervention, school, and rehabilitation services (D. N. Goldstein, Cohn, & Coster, 2004; Ketelaar, Vermeer, Hart, van Petegem-van Beek, & Helders, 2001; Zaffuto-Sforza, 2005).

Interventions may include the following:

- ◆ Client and caregiver education on range of motion to prevent contractures (United Cerebral Palsy Association, 2001c)
- ◆ Fabrication of orthotics or splints to align bones and maintain range of motion (M. Goldstein, 2004; United Cerebral Palsy Association, 2001b)
- ◆ Neurodevelopmental treatment (NDT), which has been associated with increased function in mobility and self-care for children with CP in small studies (Knox & Evans, 2002) but NDT has not been found to be any more effective than other approaches (Butler & Darrah, 2001)
- ◆ Constraint-induced therapy, which has been linked to gains in quality of movement and amount of use of the effected arm for young children with hemiparesis associated with CP (DeLuca, Echols, Ramey, & Taub, 2003; Taub, Ramey, DeLuca, & Echols, 2004)

OT AND THE EVIDENCE

Studies addressing the therapeutic approaches that are used by occupational therapists and other rehabilitation professionals have found that the motivation of the client, the degree of impairment, the therapist-client interaction, the intensity and duration of treatment, and the environment where therapy takes place can have more of an effect on the success of treatment than the particular intervention approach itself (M. Goldstein, 2004).

Additionally, interventions that target only physical capabilities, such as NDT, have been shown to provide only limited carryover (Law et al., 1998).

Therefore, it is most appropriate to utilize a family-centered, functional approach that promotes functional performance, identifies and changes the primary constraints of the task, and encourages practice to improve performance in all areas of occupation (Law et al., 1998).

CAREGIVER CONCERNS

- Most people with CP will need at least some type of assistance from a caregiver throughout the life course.
- It is important for caregivers to allow their loved ones to maintain as much independence as possible.
- As parents age, they might become physically unable to care for their adult children and will need to find alternatives, such as group home placement.
- It is important to make sure caregivers take care of themselves and seek assistance from others when needed. (United Cerebral Palsy Association, 2001c; Zaffuto-Sforza, 2005)

RESOURCES

Associations

- United Cerebral Palsy Association
  1660 L Street, NW
  Suite 700
  Washington, DC 20036
  Telephone: 202-776-0406 or 800-872-5827
  Fax: 202-776-0414
  Website: www.ucp.org
- American Academy for Cerebral Palsy and Developmental Medicine
  6300 North River Road
  Suite 727
  Rosemont, IL 60018-4226
  Telephone: 847-698 1635
  Fax: 847-823 0536
  Website: www.aacpdm.org

Books

- Brady, S. (2002). *Ten things I learned from Bill Porter.* Novato, CA: New World Library.
  Written by a close friend and assistant of Bill Porter, a man who worked as a door-to-door salesman despite the challenges presented to him by cerebral palsy.
- Brown, C. (1955). *My left foot.* New York: Simon & Shuster.
  The author shares his story about growing up with cerebral palsy and how he taught himself to use his foot to paint and write as a result of being unable to use his hands.
- Sienkiewicz-Mercer, R., & Kaplan, S. (1996). *I raise my eyes to say yes.* Boston: Houghton Mifflin.

This is the story of a woman who became paralyzed and unable to speak after contracting a disease during infancy. After she spent years in an institution, people around her finally realized that she was able to communicate via eye movements and facial expressions.

Journals

- *Developmental Medicine and Child Neurology*
- *Disability and Rehabilitation*

Websites

- United Cerebral Palsy Association (www.ucp.org)— This Website provides extensive information about a variety of issues and services relevant to people with cerebral palsy that is geared toward professionals as well as clients and their families.
- American Academy for Cerebral Palsy and Developmental Medicine (www.aacpdm.org)—This Website provides information about news, events, and resources for professionals as well as parents of children with cerebral palsy.

REFERENCES

Andren, E., & Grimby, G. (2004). Dependence in daily activities and life satisfaction in adult subjects with cerebral palsy or spinal bifida: A follow-up study. *Disability and Rehabilitation, 26,* 528–536.

Butler, C., & Darrah, J. (2001). AACPDM evidence report: Effects of neurodevelopmental treatment for cerebral palsy. *Developmental Medicine and Child Neurology, 43,* 778–790.

Campbell, S. K. (1996). Quantifying the effects of interventions for movement disorders resulting from cerebral palsy. *Journal of Child Neurology, 11,* S61–S70.

Dali, C., Hansen, F. J., Pedersen, S. A., Skov, L., Hilden, J., Bjornskov, I., et al. (2002). Threshold electrical stimulation (TES) in ambulant children with CP: A randomized double-blind placebo-controlled clinical trial. *Developmental Medicine and Child Neurology, 44,* 364–369.

DeLuca, S. C., Echols, K., Ramey, S. L., & Taub, E. (2003). Pediatric constraint-induced movement therapy for a young child with cerebral palsy: Two episodes of care. *Journal of the American Physical Therapy Association, 83,* 1003–1013.

Goldstein, D. N., Cohn, E., & Coster, W. (2004). Enhancing participation for children with disabilities: Application of the ICF enablement framework to pediatric physical therapy practice. *Pediatric Physical Therapy, 16,* 1–7.

Goldstein, M. (2004). The treatment of cerebral palsy: What we know, what we don't know. *Journal of Pediatrics, 145*(2, Suppl.), S42–S46.

Hardy, P., Collet, J. P., Goldberg, J., Ducruet, T., Vanasse, M., Lambert, J., et al. (2002). Neuropsychological effects of hyperbaric oxygen therapy in cerebral palsy. *Developmental Medicine and Child Neurology, 44,* 436–446.

Ketelaar, M., Vermeer, A., Hart, H., van Petegem-van Beek, E., & Helders, P. J. (2001). Effects of a functional therapy program on motor abilities of children with cerebral palsy. *Physical Therapy, 81*(9), 1534–1545.

Knox, V., & Evans, A. L. (2002). Evaluation of the functional effects of a course of Bobath therapy in children with cerebral palsy: A preliminary study. *Developmental Medicine & Child Neurology, 44,* 447–460.

Law, M., Darrah, J., Pollack, N., King, G., Rosenbaum, P., Russell, D., et al. (1998). Family-centred functional therapy for children with cerebral palsy: An emerging practice model. *Physical and Occupational Therapy in Pediatrics, 18,* 83–102.

Liberty, K. (2004). Developmental gains in early intervention based on conductive education by young children with motor disorders. *International Journal of Rehabilitation Research, 27,* 17–25.

Merck. (1999). *Cerebral palsy syndromes.* Retrieved March 25, 2005, from http://www.merck.com/mrkshared/CVM HighLight?file=/mrkshared/mmanual/section19/chapter271/271b.jsp%3Fregion%3Dmerckcom&word=Cerebral&word=Palsy&domain=www.merck.com#hl_anchor

MOHO Clearinghouse. (2005). *Assessments.* Retrieved April 6, 2005, from http://www.moho.uic.edu/assessments.html

Rosenbaum, P. (2003). Controversial treatment of spasticity: Exploring alternative therapies for motor function in children with cerebral palsy. *Journal of Child Neurology, 18,* S89–S94.

Sommerfelt, K., Markestad, T., Berg, K., & Saetesdal, I. (2001). Therapeutic electrical stimulation in cerebral palsy: A randomized, controlled crossover trial. *Developmental Medicine and Child Neurology, 43,* 609–613.

Taub, E., Ramey, S. L., DeLuca, S., & Echols, K. (2004). Efficacy of constraint-induced movement therapy for children with cerebral palsy with asymmetric motor impairment. *Pediatrics, 113,* 305–312.

United Cerebral Palsy Association. (2001a). *Facts & figures.* Retrieved March 25, 2005, from http://www.ucp.org/ucp_generaldoc.cfm/1/9/37/37-37/447

United Cerebral Palsy Association. (2001b). *The treatment of cerebral palsy.* Retrieved March 25, 2005, from http://www.ucp.org/ucp_generaldoc.cfm/1/4/11654/11654-11654/4790

United Cerebral Palsy Association. (2001c). *Caregiving basics.* Retrieved April 7, 2005, from http://www.ucp.org/ucp_channeldoc.cfm/1/11/54/54-54/2934

Zaffuto-Sforza, C. D. (2004). Aging with cerebral palsy. *Physical Medicine and Rehabilitation Clinics of North America, 16,* 235–249.

CEREBROVASCULAR ACCIDENT

Kristin Knesek

A cerebrovascular accident (CVA), also known as a *stroke,* is caused by a disruption of the blood supply to the brain, which results in anoxia and brain tissue death (World Health Organization, 2005). A CVA is characterized by a sudden or gradual onset of neurological deficits. The location of the lesion, extent of the injury, and mechanism by which the vascular injury occurred each play a role in the typical course and prognosis for recovery. Some individuals may experience small *lacunar* strokes from which they recover fully, while others may experience complete strokes from which the symptoms never fully subside. *Ischemic strokes,* which account for approximately 88% of strokes, are caused by vessel blockage secondary to arteriosclerotic or hypertensive stenosis (American Stroke Association, 2005a). *Hemorrhagic strokes,* in which recovery is often less promising, result from rupture in an arteriosclerotic blood vessel (ASA, 2005a).

INCIDENCE AND PREVALENCE

- Stroke killed an estimated 163,538 people in 2001 (the nation's third leading cause of death).
- Each year, about 700,000 people experience a new or recurrent stroke. About 500,000 are first attacks, and 200,000 are recurrent attacks.
- About 4.8 million stroke survivors live in the United States today. (ASA, 2005a)

TYPICAL COURSE

Although recovery has traditionally been thought to peak within the first three months after stroke, with slower recovery for up to one year, new evidence indicates that recovery of function is possible for many years (Liepert, Bauder, Miltner, Taub, & Weiller, 2000; Taub & Unswatte, 1998). The course of recovery is unpredictable; some individuals regain full function, and others regain very little.

POTENTIAL SYMPTOMS

- Hemiplegia/paresis: decreased function on one side of the body
- Aphasia: problems with communication
- Apraxia: motor planning problems
- Dysarthria: neuromotor speech output problems
- Visual-perceptual deficits (e.g., homonymous hemianopsia)
- Somatosensory deficits: sensory problems

◆ Cognitive deficits (e.g., decreased insight, safety awareness, and/or judgment)

◆ Psychosocial deficits (e.g., depression, decreased motivation, decreased social participation, and/or isolation)

◆ Incontinence: inability to control excretory functions

GENERAL SAFETY PRECAUTIONS

◆ *Medical status/stability:* This should be assessed daily when the individual is in the acute stage of recovery (i.e., the therapist should be familiar with symptoms of progressing/recurring stroke).

◆ *Cardiac/respiratory precautions:* Watch for blood pressure changes, dizziness, breathing difficulties, chest pain, excessive fatigue, and/or altered heart rate or rhythm.

◆ *Fall prevention:* Provide appropriate supervision and assistance during all transfers and functional mobility.

◆ *Shoulder subluxation/pain:* To avoid shoulder injury, never pull or lift an individual's affected upper extremity.

◆ *Skin integrity:* This could become an issue because of decreased sensation, visual deficits, and/or neglect; therefore, it should be monitored frequently.

◆ *Swallowing status:* Determine swallowing ability and use safe swallow techniques as needed. Refer to a speech-language pathologist as needed.

◆ *Poor safety awareness/impulsive behavior:* Provide appropriate level of supervision.

◆ *Muscle stiffness:* Range of motion should be performed on the affected upper extremity to prevent muscle stiffness and/or contractures.

◆ *General safety concerns:* Educate the individual, the family, and other health care providers regarding all precautions in order to maximize safety at all times.

MEDICAL MANAGEMENT

Medical management for stroke is as follows (Express Scripts, 2005).

Acute Treatment

1. *Thrombolytic agents ("clot busters"):* These dissolve the clot that is blocking the flow of blood through the vessel. Thrombolytics are considered a first line of treatment.
2. *Anticoagulants:* These prevent the formation of the hematoma (blood clot) or inhibit its growth. Anticoagulants are considered a second line of treatment.
3. *Antiplatelet treatments:* These work by preventing platelets in the blood from sticking together and form-

ing a clot. Antiplatelets are considered a second line of treatment and are also used to decrease the risk of a second stroke.

New drug therapies for the prevention of stroke aim to improve or reverse the effects of an acute stroke. These drugs include prostacyclin and calcium channel–blocking agents. Use of a combination of aspirin and calcium channel blockers has been used very early after ischemic stroke (during hospitalization) with encouraging initial results.

SURGERY

Carotid endarectomy is a surgical procedure that is used to treat and prevent acute ischemic stroke. This is an effective treatment for protecting against a first stroke in individuals with severe stenosis of the major blood vessels in the brain. For individuals who have intact awareness and have persistently progressing ischemic strokes, this procedure may also be utilized (Express Scripts, 2005).

Surgical treatment for hemorrhagic stroke involves removing the hematoma from the area. Individuals who remain conscious and have a small hematoma (less than 20 cc or less than 3 cm in diameter) often improve without surgery. In contrast, individuals who are in a coma secondary to a large hematoma (greater than 80 cc or 6 cm in diameter) often do poorly regardless of treatment. Individuals who have moderate to large hematomas and remain conscious are the most likely candidates for surgery (Express Scripts, 2005).

OCCUPATIONAL THERAPY EVALUATIONS

Comprehensive Evaluations

◆ American Heart Association Stroke Outcome Classification (AHA.SOC)
◆ Functional Independence Measure (FIM)
◆ National Institutes of Health Stroke Score (NIHSS)

ADL Evaluations

◆ Assessment of Motor and Process Skills (AMPS)
◆ Barthel Index (BI)

IADL/Leisure Evaluations

◆ Activity Card Sort (ACS)
◆ Frenchay Activities Index

Upper Extremity Function Evaluations

- Fugl-Meyer Upper Extremity Motor Performance Test
- The Functional Test for the Hemiplegic/Paretic Upper Extremity
- The Modified Ashworth Scale (spasticity)

Range of motion (via goniometry), strength (via manual muscle testing, dynamometer, and/or pinch meter), and edema (via volumeter) may be measured as needed.

Balance Evaluations

- Berg Balance Scale (fall predictor)
- Postural Assessment Scale for Stroke Patients (PASS)
- The Motor Assessment Scale

Cognition and/or Perception Evaluations

- Behavioral Inattention Test (BIT)
- Lowenstein Occupational Therapy Cognitive Assessment (LOTCA)

Quality of Life/Life Satisfaction Evaluations

- Canadian Occupational Therapy Performance Measure (COPM)
- Short-Form 36 Health Survey (SF-36)
- Stroke Impact Scale (SIS)
- Stroke-Specific Quality of Life Scale (SS-QOL)

OCCUPATIONAL THERAPY INTERVENTIONS

General

- ADL/IADL retraining
- Training in the use of adaptive equipment
- Environmental adaptation

Upper Extremity Function

- Constraint-induced therapy
- Modified constraint-induced therapy
- Mental imagery
- Robot-assisted rehabilitation
- Sensory stimulation
- Task-specific training utilizing shaping techniques
- Use of compensatory strategies
- Use of meaningful, purposeful, client-chosen occupations as therapeutic change agents
- Virtual reality

Cognitive/Perceptual Rehabilitation

- Cognitive retraining
- Use of compensatory strategies (e.g., verbal cueing, use of anchoring techniques for neglect)

Endurance, Balance, Functional Mobility

- Therapeutic exercise
- Use of compensatory strategies

OCCUPATIONAL THERAPY AND THE EVIDENCE

Occupational therapy effectively improves performance of ADLs/IADLs and role participation for individuals who have experienced stroke. Goal-specific teaching and practice of meaningful, client-chosen activities in a familiar context along with provision of necessary adaptations and training in the use of these adaptations has proved to be effective for improving occupational performance after stroke (Trombly & Ma, 2002). Treatments that occupational therapists use to remediate impairments are generally beneficial, especially those that involve activity and/or occupation to bring about change (Ma & Trombly, 2002).

CAREGIVER CONCERNS

According to Visser-Meily, van Heugten, Post, Schepers, and Lindeman (2005), caregiver burden is quite common after stroke, and high levels of burden are often related to deterioration of the caregiver's own health status, social life, and well-being. Jonsson, Lindgren, Hallstrom, Norrving, and Lindgren (2005) concluded from low emotional-mental scores on the SF-36 that informal caregivers are often under considerable strain. Furthermore, caregiver depression can worsen the depression of an individual who has had a stroke and may predict poor response to rehabilitation (Visser-Meily et al., 2005). Isolation from people other than the ones they are caring for is also a major concern for caregivers (ASA, 2005b). It is imperative that caregivers be educated about taking care of themselves, including their physical, emotional, mental, spiritual, interpersonal, and financial health (ASA, 2005b).

The following recommendations for informal caregivers have been adapted from the American Stroke Association (2005b):

- *Set goals and limits:* Think realistically about what you can and cannot do.
- *Be organized:* Have a "job description" in which you define what you and the one you are caring for need (i.e. assistance with housekeeping, shopping).

◆ *Recognize your own limits:* Realize when you need a break and take time for yourself.
◆ *Involve others:* Involve other family members and friends in the caregiving experience.

As occupational therapists, we can utilize these recommendations to educate and assist caregivers with regard to their role in caring for the individual who has had a stroke.

RESOURCES

Associations

◆ American Stroke Association
(Division of the American Heart Association)
7272 Greenville Avenue
Dallas, TX 75231-4596
Telephone: 800-242-8721
Fax: 214-706-1191
Website: http://www.strokeassociation.org/presenter.jhtml?identifier=1200037
◆ American Stroke Foundation
11902 Lowell
Suite 104
Overland Park, KS 66213
Telephone: 866-549-1776
Fax: 913-649-6661
Website: http://www.americanstroke.org
◆ Stroke Family Support Network
Telephone: 888-478-7653

First-Person Accounts

◆ Klein, B. S. (1998). *Slow dance: A story of stroke, love, and disability.* Berkeley, CA: Rage Mill Press.
In her mid-forties, Bonnie Klein, a brilliant filmmaker, experienced a catastrophic stroke that changed her life. She provides a moving account of her struggle first to survive, then to "reinvent" rehabilitation, and finally to accept the challenge of living with a disability. This is also a remarkable love story.
◆ Mayer, T. K. (2000). *Teaching me to run.* Boston: Prince Gallison Press.
This is an inspirational story of one middle-aged woman's struggle back from the debilitating effects of stroke. The author battles to relearn not only to walk, but also to run, against all odds.
◆ McCrum, R. (1998). *My year off, recovering life after a stroke.* New York: Avon Books.
Robert McCrum had a right CVA in 1995 at the age of 42. He presents an account of the physical and psychological effects of stroke, including impaired speech, impaired left arm and leg function, and the inability to engage in a valued life role: work.
◆ Simon, S. (2002). *A stroke of genius: Messages of hope and healing from a thriving stroke survivor.* Delray Beach, FL: The Cedars Group.

This book was written by a man who had a cerebral hemorrhage at the age of fifty-six. He explains the causes of the two major types of stroke and reveals information about other medical issues involved with stroke. Simon gives advice to his audience, including medical doctors and therapists, on how to deal with the various physical and psychosocial implications of stroke.

Journals

◆ *Archives of Physical Medicine and Rehabilitation*
◆ *Neurology*
◆ *Stroke*

Websites

◆ MedlinePlus
http://www.hlm.nih.gov/medlineplus/stroke.html
Provides links to several other helpful Websites; as such, it is a great starting place for stroke-related research. It is part of the National Institutes of Health, a well-known and stable source of health information.
◆ American Stroke Association
http://www.strokeassociation.org/presenter.jhtml?identifier=1200037
Provides user-friendly, comprehensive stroke information for both professionals and caregivers. It is easy to navigate and visually appealing. The level of readability enables individuals of many educational levels to access and understand information with regard to stroke.
◆ National Institute of Neurological Disorders and Stroke
http://www.ninds.nih.gov/about_ninds_plans.htm
Provides up-to-date research studies in the field and is quite beneficial for clinicians. This is a stable site, sponsored not only by the National Institutes of Health (NIH) but also by the U.S. Department of Health and Human Services.

REFERENCES

American Stroke Association. (2005a). *What is stroke?* Retrieved April 6, 2005, from http://www.strokeassociation.org/presenter.jhtml?identifier=2528

American Stroke Association. (2005b). *Who is a caregiver?* Retrieved April 6, 2005, from http://www.strokeassociation.org/presenter.jhtml?identifier=1022

Express Scripts. (2005). *Drug digest.* Retrieved March 15, 2005, from http://www.drugdigest.com

Jonsson, A. C., Lindgren, I., Hallstrom, B., Norrving, B., & Lindgren, A. (2005). Determinants of quality of life in stroke survivors and their informal caregivers. *Stroke, 36,* 803–808.

Liepert, J., Bauder, H., Miltner, W., Taub, E., & Weiller, C. (2000). Treatment-induced cortical reorganization after stroke in humans. *Stroke, 31,* 1210–1216.

Ma, H., & Trombly, C. A. (2002). Synthesis of the effects of occupational therapy for persons with stroke. II: Remediation. *American Journal of Occupational Therapy, 56,* 260–273.

Taub, E., & Unswatte, G. (1998). *Use-dependent cortical re-organization after brain injury.* Presented at INABIS '98: Fifth Internet World Congress on Biomedical Sciences at McMaster University, Canada, December 7–16. Invited Symposium. Retrieved December 11, 2004, from http://www.mcmaster.ca/inabis98/schallert/taub0818/two.html

Trombly, C. A., & Ma, H. (2002). Synthesis of the effects of occupational therapy for persons with stroke. I: Restora-tion of roles, tasks, and activities. *American Journal of Occupational Therapy, 56,* 250–259.

Visser-Meily, A., van Heugten, C., Post, M., Schepers, V., & Lindeman, E. (2005). Intervention studies for caregivers of stroke survivors: A critical review. *Patient Education and Counseling, 56,* 257–267.

World Health Organization. (2005). *Types of cardiovascular disease.* Retrieved April 6, 2005, from http://www.who.int/cardiovascular_diseases/en/cvd_atlas_01_types.pdf

CHRONIC OBSTRUCTIVE PULMONARY DISEASE

Kim Bennet, Kate-Lyn Stone, and Meredith Grinnell

Chronic obstructive pulmonary disease (COPD) is characterized by an obstruction to airflow that interferes with normal breathing. COPD is a permanent and progressive condition that includes both chronic bronchitis and emphysema. Chronic bronchitis is a longstanding inflammation of the mucous membranes of the bronchial airways. Chronic bronchitis is characterized by an increase of mucus secretion and a chronic productive cough for at least three months in two consecutive years for which other causes (e.g., infection, cancer, chronic heart failure) have been ruled out. Emphysema is defined by an abnormal permanent enlargement of the airspaces in the lungs, with the progressive and irreversible destruction of the alveolar walls. These changes result in loss of lung elasticity, which impairs gas exchange (oxygen, carbon dioxide) (American Lung Association, 2007).

ETIOLOGY

There are several causative factors related to COPD, of which smoking is considered to be the most significant. Other risk factors include prolonged inhalation of lung irritants such as pollution, dusts, or chemicals; passive exposure to cigarette smoking; and genetics (alpha 1 antitrypsin deficiency) (Daniel & Strickland, 1992).

INCIDENCE AND PREVALENCE

- COPD is the fourth leading cause of death in the United States for all ages and both genders.
- Approximately 16 million people in the United States have some form of COPD.
- COPD is responsible for over 13.4 million office visits per year and is the third most frequent justification for home care services.
- People with COPD commonly become symptomatic during the middle adulthood. The incidence of COPD increases with age (American Lung Association, 2007).

TYPICAL COURSE AND SYMPTOMS

COPD develops slowly and progresses in the following four stages:

- People who are at risk of COPD. At this stage, individuals have normal lung function but suffer chronic cough and sputum production.
- Mild COPD. At this stage, there is mild airflow limitation, but patients might be unaware that their lung function is abnormal.
- Moderate COPD. By this stage, the airflow limitation is causing symptoms such as shortness of breath on exertion. Patients usually seek medical attention at this stage.
- Severe COPD. By this stage, airflow limitation is severe, symptoms are severe, and exacerbations may be life threatening (National Heart Lung and Blood Institute, 2007).

TYPICAL INTERVENTIONS AND EXPECTED OUTCOMES

Management of COPD requires a long-term therapeutic approach. Treatment focuses on symptom management through education about the disease and actively engaging the patients with COPD in care management. Pulmonary rehabilitation programs are designed to address the aspects of COPD management as follows.

Education About COPD

Patients are educated in preventive care (e.g., minimizing potential irritants in the home and work environment) and optimization of medications (e.g., purpose of medication, dosage, side effects, and schedule of administration).

Smoking Cessation

Patients are encouraged to discontinue smoking because stopping smoking is the single most effective step in slowing the progression of COPD. Benefits to smoking cessation include reduction in the number of respiratory infections, improvement in the function of the mucociliary clearance of the lungs, decreased cough and dyspnea, increased appetite, and decreased sputum production. Smoking cessation programs are helpful in assisting and supporting lifestyle change.

Medication

Medications may include a broad-spectrum of antibiotics to avoid an exacerbation, flu vaccinations, and bronchodilators. Corticosteroids may be considered to control severe acute episodes of bronchospasm.

Nutrition

Patients with COPD who experience dyspnea may also experience difficulty eating, resulting in weight loss and nutritional deficits. These two factors tend to decrease respiratory muscle strength; therefore, patients need to be instructed on the benefits of eating high-fat, low-carbohydrate food in small, frequent meals.

Exercise

Exercise is an important component in pulmonary rehabilitation. Exercise reduces cardiovascular disease risks, improves musculoskeletal functioning, and may help to prevent bone loss in older patients.

Oxygen Supplementation

Oxygen therapy decreases morbidity and mortality for patients with COPD, especially when used more than 18 hours per day. Oxygen supplementation is typically used to enable daily activities and exercising.

Breathing Retraining

The goals of breathing retraining include decreasing the work of breathing, improving oxygenation, increasing the efficiency of breathing patterns, and promoting the client's control of breathing. Diaphragmatic and pursed-lip breathing are two types of breathing techniques that are used. Diaphragmatic breathing improves the efficiency of breathing and the patient's awareness of breathing patterns. Pursed-lip breathing allows patients to slow their breathing, increases the expiration pressure, improves the oxygenation, and reduces respiratory rate.

Chest Physiotherapy

Chest physiotherapy includes chest percussion, postural drainage, and vibration and rib shaking. These techniques are used to aid patients in clearing pulmonary secretions.

Pulmonary Hygiene

Pulmonary hygiene includes hydration, deep breathing exercises, and coughing techniques (Weilitz, 2000).

PROGNOSIS

COPD is a chronic disorder that cannot be totally reversed or corrected. The prognosis is dependent on the patient's present clinical status, recent functional history, and response to current functional activity. At any level of lung impairment, prognosis improves when the patient stops smoking. The best indicator of prognosis is the forced expiratory volume (FEV) or the volume of air that is forcefully expelled in 1 second. A patient with an FEV1 greater than 1.5 L has a very good prognosis, expected survival rate being 10 to 20 years. A patient with an FEV1 of 1.0–1.25 L is considered to experience moderate lung impairments with predicted survival for 6–10 years. Patients with an FEV1 less than 0.75 L are considered to have severe lung impairments and have a mortality rate of 2 to 6 years. (Daniel & Strickland, 1992).

PRECAUTIONS

1. Patients should avoid exposures to cigarette smoke, fumes, dust, odors from solvents, powders or spray aerosols, and other respiratory irritants.
2. Interventions should be stopped if the patient becomes nauseous, dizzy, or fatigued; has shortness of breath; or has chest pains.
3. If oxygen is to be administered, the patient should be informed and aware of appropriate safeguards.
4. Be aware of cyanosis and refer to the physician immediately. (Daniel & Strickland, 1992)

OT EVALUATIONS AND INTERVENTIONS AND SEQUENCE OF CARE

Occupational therapists are responsible for providing appropriate services for the patient with COPD; assisting the patient with COPD in achieving the maximal functional level of independence; educating the patient and family regarding ongoing treatment and ensuring consistent home management of the patient on discharge; and assisting the patient and the family in adjusting to disability and life changes. The following are occupational performance areas and components that are assessed. All areas are assessed in relation to functional performance. Various performance areas and skills are identified to create realistic client-centered treatment goals (Paul & Orchanian, 2003).

Assessment of Performance Areas

- Activities of daily living: basic ADL and IADL skills
- Work and productive activities: home management, care for others, and vocational activities
- Play or leisure performance (Huntley, 2002; Paul & Orchanian, 2003)

Assessment of Performance Components

- *Neuromusculoskeletal:* range of motion, muscle tone, strength, endurance, postural alignment
- *Psychosocial skills:* psychological, social, and self-management (Paul & Orchanian, 2003)

Standardized Assessment Tools

- Borg Scale of Perceived Exertion
- Klein-Bell Activities of Daily Living Scale
- Kohlman Evaluation of Daily Living Scale
- Assessment of Motor Process Skills (AMPS)
- Functional Independence Measure (FIM)
- Tinetti Test of Balance and Gait
- Berg Balance Test
- Self-Assessment of Leisure Interests
- Interest Checklist
- Self-Esteem Scale
- Tennessee Self-Concept Scale–Revised (TSCS) (Paul & Orchanian, 2003)

Other Tests

- Chronic Obstructive Pulmonary Disease Evaluation Form and Procedures
- Range-of-motion testing(AROM/PROM)
- Manual muscle testing
- Home Assessment and Recommendations Evaluation Form (Paul & Orchanian, 2003)

OT INTERVENTIONS

- Maintain or improve upper extremity strength, ROM, and tolerance
- Maximize or improve the patient's independence in ADLs
- Assist the patient and family with psychological adjustment to disease
- Ensure safety and accessibility in home
- Increase the patient's and family or caregiver's knowledge of rehabilitation process for patient with COPD
- Increase the patient's endurance to sustain daily activities and exercise
- Explore avocational interests and assess adaptations needed to allow the patient to engage in them
- Assist the patient in learning appropriate relaxation techniques to decrease tension, stress, and fear

- Increase the patient's ability to cope with cognitive deficits
- Increase the patient's independence and accessibility within the community
- Increase the patient's independence in driving and driving safety (Daniel & Strickland, 1992; Huntley, 2002)

OT AND THE EVIDENCE

Lorenzi and colleagues (2004) evaluated the effectiveness of OT as an adjunctive measure to comprehensive pulmonary rehabilitation for disabled hospitalized COPD patients. Results showed that OT for basic domestic activities during comprehensive pulmonary rehabilitation specifically improved the outcome of patients with severe COPD.

Guided imagery has been found to be an effective intervention for developing more effective breathing patterns in individuals with COPD. Louie (2004) found that these relaxation sessions, which connect the mind, body, and spirit, lead to raised oxygen saturation in the blood. Another intervention to promote the management of acute exacerbations of COPD is the development and implementation of an action plan. Action plans incorporate guidelines for independently initiating strategies if there is a change in the state of an individual's COPD that could lead to an exacerbation (Turnock, Walters, Walters, & Wood-Baker, 2007). These plans are useful to increase an individual's sense of self-efficacy in managing his or her disease.

Community-based settings offering groups for individuals with COPD have also been evaluated and found to have positive psychosocial outcomes. Woo and colleagues (2006) found that people were empowered and enthusiastic about the social support they received from the group setting. Group activities include education about COPD, breathing exercises, use of medication, nutrition, relaxation strategies, and strengthening and aerobic exercises.

CAREGIVER CONCERNS

As COPD progresses and the patient's activity becomes more restricted, many patients become more dependent on family members and develop a sense of isolation, loss of control, and depression. It is important for the health care professional to give caregivers the tools to recognize these feelings and encourage the patient to talk about them; professional support from psychiatrists or psychologists may be helpful. Gentle encouragement to exercise regularly and recognition that activities must be carefully planned in advance will help to ensure a better quality of life.

For additional information, see http://www.copd-international.com/caregivers. This Website is the COPD Caregiver Community funded by COPD-International.

RESOURCES

Associations

♦ American Lung Association of Georgia
2452 Spring Road
Smyrna, GA 30080
Telephone: 770-434-5864 or 800-LUNG-USA
Fax: 770-319-0349
Website: www.alaga.org

♦ National Heart, Lung, and Blood Institute
Building 31, Room 5A52
31 Center Drive MSC 2486
Bethesda, MD 20892
Telephone: 301-592-8573/240-629-3255 (TTY) or
800-877-8339
Website: www.nhlbi.nih.gov

First-Person Accounts

Carter, R., Nicotra, B., & Tucker, J.-V. (1999). *Courage and information for life with chronic obstructive pulmonary disease.* Peabody, MA: New Technology Publishing.

Jo-Von Tucker has taken an active role to prevent COPD from controlling her life. She passes along valuable tips, information, and details of daily living to give hope and support to those who suffer from COPD. Jo-Von Tucker combines the experience and insights as a patient with expertise of medical and rehabilitation professionals (the two other authors). The purpose of this easy-to-understand book is to help people with COPD actively manage their own health care.

Vogel, L. G. (2004). *Huffin' n' puffin': Living with COPD.* West Conshohocken, PA: Infinity Publishing.

Written by a COPD patient, this book provides realistic information about living with COPD. Using stories and poetry in a lighthearted manner, the author explains what COPD is; explores diagnosis, treatment, medications, doctors and caregivers; and describes living and coping with the disease on a daily basis. Including a glossary and COPD resource guide, the book is essential reading for every COPD patient and family member.

Journals

♦ *Journal of Respiratory Care Practitioners*
♦ *Journal of Chronic Pulmonary Rehabilitation*

Websites

♦ American Lung Association
http://www.lungusa.org
The American Lung Association is dedicated to providing current information about COPD and offering various resources for patients, caregivers, health professionals, and researchers. The American Lung Association Action Network allows volunteer activists from coast to coast to advocate to the world on preventing lung disease and promoting lung health.

♦ Global Initiative for Chronic Obstructive Lung Disease
http://goldcopd.com
GOLD works with health care professionals and public health officials around the world to raise awareness of COPD and to improve prevention and treatment of this lung disease. Through the development of evidence-based guidelines for COPD management and events such as the annual celebration of World COPD Day, GOLD is working to improve the lives of people with COPD in every corner of the globe.

♦ COPD-International
http://www.copd-international.com
COPD-International is a nonprofit organization whose purpose is to provide information and interactive support for COPD patients, caregivers, families, and concerned individuals.

REFERENCES

American Lung Association. (2007). *Chronic obstructive pulmonary disease* (COPD) fact sheet. Retrieved October 30, 2007, from http://www.lungusa.org/site/apps/nl/content3.asp?c=dvLUK9O0E&b=2058829&content_id={EE451F66-996B-4C23-874D-BF66586196FF}&notoc=1.

Daniel, M., & Strickland, L. R. (1992). Chronic obstructive pulmonary disease. In M. S. Daniel (Ed.) *Occupational therapy protocol management in adult physical dysfunction* (pp. 224–229). Gaithersburg, MD: Aspen.

Huntley, N. (2002). Cardiac and pulmonary diseases. In C. A. Trombly & M. V. Radomski (Eds.), *Occupational therapy for physical dysfunction* (5th ed., pp. 1082–1087). Philadelphia: Lippincott Williams & Wilkins.

Lorenzi, C. M., Cilione, C., Rizzardi, R., Furino, V., Bellantone, T., Lugli, D., et al. (2004). Occupational therapy and pulmonary rehabilitation of disabled COPD patients. *Respiration, 71,* 246–251. Retrieved October 30, 2007 from http://content.karger.com/produktedb/produkte.asp?typ=fulltext&file=RES2004071003246.

Louie, S. (2004). The effects of guided imagery relaxation in people with COPD. *Occupational Therapy International, 11,* 145–159.

National Heart Lung and Blood Institute. (2007). *COPD.* Retrieved October 30, 2007, from http://www.nhlbi.nih.gov/health/dci/Diseases/Copd/Copd_WhatIs.html.

Paul, S., & Orchanian, D. P. (2003). Chronic obstructive pulmonary disease. In *Pocket guide to assessment in occupational therapy* (pp. 50–52). Albany, NY: Thomson Delmar Learning.

Turnock, A. C., Walters, E. H., Walters, J. A. E., & Wood-Baker, R. (2007). Action plans for chronic obstructive pulmonary disease (Cochrane Review). In *The Cochrane Library,* Issue 2.

Weilitz, P. B. (2000). Respiratory function. In A. G. Lueckenotte (Ed.), *Gerontologic nursing* (2nd ed, pp. 495–503). St. Louis: Mosby.

Woo, J., Chan, W., Fai, Y., Chan, W., Hui, E., Lum, C., et al. (2006). A community model of group therapy for the older patients with chronic obstructive pulmonary disease: A pilot study. *Journal of Evaluation in Clinical Practice, 12,* 523–531.

CONGENITAL HEART DISEASE

Kate-Lyn Stone

DIAGNOSIS

The term *congenital heart disease,* also known as congenital heart defects, cyanotic heart disease, heart defects, or congenital cardiovascular malformation, implies that there is a defect in the heart that has been present since birth (National Heart Lung and Blood Institute, 2007). This is the most common type of birth defect (Medline Plus, 2007). The normal flow of blood through the heart is altered because of congenital heart defects (National Heart Lung and Blood Institute, 2007).

INCIDENCE AND PREVALENCE

- Approximately 8 of every 1,000 newborn babies have a congenital heart defect (Baffa, 2007).
- In the United States, more than 35,000 children are born each year with a congenital heart defect (National Heart Lung and Blood Institute, 2007).

ETIOLOGY

The cause of most congenital heart defects is unknown. It is known that these defects develop because of abnormal development in the heart of the fetus early in the pregnancy (Baffa, 2007). It is thought that heredity might play a role in some congenital heart defects; for example, a parent with a heart defect might be more likely than another parent to have a child with a heart defect at birth (National Heart Lung and Blood Institute, 2007).

TYPES

Congenital heart defects can vary from simple ones, such as a hole in an interior wall of the heart, to complex ones, which are generally a combination of simple defects (National Heart Lung and Blood Institute, 2007). There are several different names for congenital heart defects, including the following (Baffa, 2007):

- Aortic stenosis
- Atrial septal defect
- Atrioventricular canal defect
- Coarctation of the aorta
- Hypoplastic left heart syndrome
- Patent ductus arteriosus
- Pulmonary atresia
- Pulmonary stenosis
- Tetralogy of Fallot
- Total anomalous pulmonary venous connection
- Transposition of the great arteries
- Tricuspid atresia
- Truncus arteriosus
- Ventricular septal defect

For more information about these types of heart defects, the reader is referred to the Nemours Foundation Website: http://kidshealth.org/parent/medical/heart/congenital_heart_defects.html.

SIGNS AND SYMPTOMS

Telltale signs of congenital heart disease include cyanosis (a bluish color) to the skin around the mouth, on the lips, or on the tongue; increased breathing rate; heart murmur; inability to gain weight; sweating; and weak strength of pulse. Symptoms include poor appetite and difficulty breathing (Baffa, 2007).

SEQUENCE OF CARE

If it is suspected that a child has a congenital heart defect, the primary care physician will probably refer the child to a pediatric cardiologist. The cardiologist will complete a full physical examination and order a chest X-ray to look at the heart and lungs. An electrocardiogram will also be done to look at electrical signals from the heart. Cardiac catheterization, using colored dyes, allows a better look at the heart's inner structures. The catheter can also measure pressures and oxygen levels within the heart (Baffa, 2007). Once a child has been diagnosed as having a congenital heart defect, the surgeon may repair the defect with either surgery or perform another surgical procedure using a catheter. In the more severe and complex cases, a heart transplant might be the best option for the child (National Heart Lung and Blood Institute, 2007).

IMPLICATIONS FOR OT

See the resource sheet on cardiac conditions.

SEE CARDIAC CONDITIONS FOR ADDITIONAL RESOURCES

REFERENCES

Baffa, G. (2007). *Congenital heart defects.* Retrieved October 9, 2007, from http://kidshealth.org/parent/medical/heart/congenital_heart_defects.html

Medline Plus. (2007). *Congenital heart defects.* Retrieved October 9, 2007, from http://www.nlm.nih.gov/medlineplus/congenitalheartdefects.html

National Heart Lung and Blood Institute. (2007). *Congenital heart defects.* Retrieved October 9, 2007, from http://www.nhlbi.nih.gov/health/dci/Diseases/chd/chd_what.html

CONGESTIVE HEART FAILURE

Kate-Lyn Stone

DIAGNOSIS

The term *congestive heart failure,* or simply *heart failure,* is the name for the condition in which any of the four chambers of the heart—the atria, the upper chambers, the ventricles, or the lower chambers—loses its ability to keep up with the amount of blood that is flowing through the heart (American Heart Association, 2007). Heart failure is a chronic disease with no cure.

INCIDENCE AND PREVALENCE

- ◆ Approximately 5 million people are living with heart failure in the United States (American Heart Association, 2007).
- ◆ 550,000 new cases of heart failure are diagnosed in the United States each year (American Heart Association, 2007).

ETIOLOGY

Everybody's heart loses some ability to pump blood as the person ages. Heart failure occurs because of the added stress of other health conditions in addition to aging. These conditions include: coronary artery disease, past heart attacks, high blood pressure, abnormal heart valves, heart muscle disease, heart defects from birth, severe lung damage, diabetes, severe anemia, overactive thyroid, and abnormal heart rhythm (American Heart Association, 2007).

TYPES

Left-Sided Heart Failure (Left Ventricular Heart Failure)

Left-sided heart failure involves the left ventricle of the heart. Systolic failure occurs when the left ventricle loses its ability to contract normally, which means that the heart cannot pump enough blood into circulation. Diastolic failure occurs when the left ventricle cannot relax normally, which means that the heart does not adequately fill with blood between each pump. In either case, the heart's ability to circulate blood properly decreases, and fluid builds up throughout the body. This explains the term *congestive heart failure* (American Heart Association, 2007).

Right-Sided Heart Failure (Right Ventricular Heart Failure)

Right-sided heart failure usually occurs secondary to left ventricular heart failure. When the left ventricle is not working properly, blood backs up to the lungs, essentially damaging the heart's right side in the process (American Heart Association, 2007).

TYPICAL COURSE AND SYMPTOMS

Heart failure can affect the right side, the left side, or both sides of the heart; however, it generally begins in the left side. This condition generally occurs little by little over time. To compensate for the loss of ability, the heart first tries to enlarge, develop more mass, and pump faster. These are temporary changes that the body makes to address heart failure that mask the condition but do not cure it. This helps to explain why some people are not diagnosed with heart failure until several years after it first develops. Eventually, the heart can no longer mask the problem, and the symptoms of heart failure begin to emerge (American Heart Association, 2007).

Symptoms of heart failure include the following (American Heart Association, 2007):

- ◆ Shortness of breath or breathlessness
- ◆ Pain in the abdomen
- ◆ Difficulty sleeping
- ◆ Loss of appetite
- ◆ Increased fatigue

Signs of heart failure include the following (American Heart Association, 2007):

- ◆ Sudden weight gain
- ◆ Increased swelling in the lower extremities
- ◆ Swelling in the abdomen
- ◆ Frequent cough

MEDICAL INTERVENTIONS AND TREATMENTS

Medications

The following are medications that are commonly used to treat heart failure (American Heart Association, 2007):

- ◆ *ACE inhibitors (angiotensin-converting-enzyme inhibitors):* Considered the primary drug used to treat heart failure. ACE inhibitors act as vasodilators (expand blood vessels) and have been proven to slow the progression of heart failure. They lower the levels of angiotensin in the body, which is a substance that can lead to an increase in blood pressure.

- *Diuretics (water pills):* Cause the body to eliminate more fluid than usual. Diuretics help the heart to work less by decreasing the amount of fluid the heart has to pump throughout the body.
- *Vasodilators:* Expand the blood vessels, which allows blood to flow more easily through them, thus decreasing the amount of work the heart has to do.
- *Digitalis preparations (also known as digoxin):* Increases the heart's contractions as well as slowing some irregular heartbeats.
- *Beta blockers:* Decrease the heart's inclination to beat faster.
- *Blood thinners:* Thin the blood, which allows the blood to flow more easily through the vessels.
- *Angiotensin II receptor blockers:* Completely block effect of angiotensin on the heart and blood vessels.
- *Calcium channel blockers:* Used to treat high blood pressure by decreasing calcium's role in the contraction of the muscles of the heart. The muscles relax, thus allowing the heart to work less.
- *Potassium:* Helps to control the rhythm of the heart.

Valve Replacement Surgery

In valve replacement surgery, the inefficient valve is removed and replaced with a mechanical valve made from metal, plastic, or human or animal tissue or a valve taken from a donor.

Angioplasty

Angioplasty is used to open blocked blood vessels.

Coronary Artery Bypass

Coronary artery bypass is used to reroute the blood supply around a section of artery that is blocked.

Defibrillator Implantation

A defibrillator provides pacing to the heart when an abnormal rhythm is detected.

Heart Transplant

A transplant involves removing the damaged heart and replacing it with a heart from a donor.

Left Ventricular Assist Device

The left ventricular assist device is a mechanical pump that helps to maintain the pumping of the heart.

ROLE OF OT

See the resource sheet on cardiac conditions.

OTHER RESOURCES

See the resource sheet on cardiac conditions

REFERENCES

American Heart Association. (2007). *Heart failure.* Retrieved October 8, 2007, from http://www.americanheart.org/presenter.jhtml?identifier=1486

DEPRESSION

Laurie Dossett and Kate-Lyn Stone

Depression is a serious mental illness. It is a disorder that affects one's thoughts, moods, feelings, behavior, and physical health. There are two main types of depression: major depression (interferes with daily occupations) and dysthymia (less severe with chronic symptoms that do not disable but can lead to major depression) (National Institute of Mental Health, 2000).

INCIDENCE AND PREVALENCE

Depressive disorders affect approximately 9.5% of adult Americans, or about 19 million people in a given year (NIMH, 2005). Depression often begins between the ages of 15 and 30 but can occur at any age, including childhood.

Women are two times as likely as men to experience depression. Depression (not including bipolar disorder) is the leading cause of disability among men and women of all ages in the United States and worldwide, according to the World Health Organization (2001).

DIAGNOSIS

At least five of the following symptoms must be present for a diagnosis of depression (American Psychiatric Association, 2000):

- Depressed mood, nearly every day during most of the day

◆ Marked diminished interest or pleasure in almost all activities
◆ Significant weight loss (when not dieting), weight gain, or a change in appetite
◆ Insomnia or hypersomnia (excess sleep)
◆ Feelings of worthlessness or inappropriate guilt
◆ Impaired psychomotor agitation or psychomotor retardation
◆ Fatigue or loss of energy
◆ Feelings of inability to concentrate or indecisiveness
◆ Recurrent thoughts of death, recurrent suicidal ideation

These symptoms must be present during the same two-week period and must represent a change from a previous level of functioning (American Psychiatric Association, 2000, p. 356).

The diagnostic criteria for a single episode or recurrent major depression differ from the above symptoms, and a complete description of these criteria is beyond the scope of this document.

ETIOLOGY

There is no single cause of depression. Stressful life events can trigger depression, or depression can occur spontaneously with no identifiable cause. Depression can be familial, suggesting that there may be a genetic component (NIMH, 2000). Biological factors and changes in body chemistry can also be causes of depression (American Psychological Association, 2005).

AFFILIATED PROBLEMS

Depression often co-occurs with other serious illnesses, such as heart disease, stroke, diabetes, cancer, and Parkinson's disease. Depression can and should be treated when it co-occurs with other illnesses, as untreated depression can delay recovery from these other illnesses or worsen them (Agency for Healthcare Research and Quality, 2000; NIMH, 2000).

PRECAUTIONS

Individuals with severe depression are at risk for harming themselves and possibly for suicidal ideation. The primary risk factor for suicide in both the general population and the clinical population is a mood disorder such as depression (often with comorbid substance abuse) (AHRQ, 2004). Heavy drinking and other forms of substance abuse increase one's risk of a mood disorder such as depression (Ramsey, Engler, & Stein, 2005).

TREATMENT

In a time of crisis, if a person has thoughts of harming himself or herself or of committing suicide, a hospital emergency room may be able to provide temporary help (NIMH, 2000). The person with depression can then be referred to other services for long-term care, such as family doctors; mental health specialists such as psychiatrists, psychologists, social workers, or mental health counselor; community mental health centers; hospital psychiatry departments and outpatient clinics; or private clinics and facilities (NIMH, 2000).

Psychotherapy

◆ Talk therapies help clients to gain insight into and resolve their problems through verbal exchange with the therapist.
◆ Behavioral therapists help clients learn how to obtain more satisfaction and rewards through their own actions and how to unlearn the behavioral patterns that contribute to or result from their depression.
◆ Cognitive/behavioral therapists help clients to change the negative styles of thinking and behaving that are often associated with depression.

Medication

◆ Selective serotonin reuptake inhibitors (SSRIs)
◆ Tricyclic and tetracyclic antidepressants
◆ Monoamine oxidase inhibitors (MAOIs)
◆ Serotonin and norepinephrine reuptake inhibitors (SNRIs)

Electroconvulsive Therapy

Electroconvulsive therapy is used as a last resort when no other treatments have proven effective. It involves electrically inducing a seizure that causes physiological and biomechanical changes in the brain (NIMH, 2000).

OT EVALUATIONS

Observations, interviews, and history taking play a major role in evaluating depression (Cara, 2005). An occupational therapist will analyze a person's ability to perform relevant occupations (American Occupational Therapy Association, 2002). The following assessment instruments are also used when appropriate:

◆ Canadian Occupational Performance Measure (COPM)
◆ Kohlman Evaluation of Living Skills (KEHLS) (Kohlman Thompson, 1992)

- Scorable Self-Care Evaluation
- Beck Depression Inventory (Beck, 1978)

OT INTERVENTIONS

Occupational therapy often becomes involved with the depressed client in an attempt to assist in the remediation and treatment of symptoms. Group therapy is commonly used in mental health settings, and the focus of interventions may be on any number of following areas:

ADL/IADL

- Medication/time management
- Activities of daily living
- Community mobility/reentry
- Reestablishing normal routines

Social

- Expressive activities
- Social integration
- Functional behavior training
- Focuses on restoring motor and cognitive functioning

PERFORMANCE SKILLS/WORK

- Stress management (relaxation training, attention to stressors, biofeedback)
- Lifestyle alterations
- Judgment skills
- Work to increase self-esteem with attainable goals
- Instructing the individual on setting realistic goals
- Psychoeducation concerning symptoms and precursors to symptom exacerbation

OCCUPATIONAL THERAPY AND THE EVIDENCE

For children and adolescents with depression, cognitive-behavioral therapy (CBT), interpersonal psychotherapy, psychosocial intervention, antidepressants, or a combination of pharmacological options is an effective first-line treatment (Dopheide, 2006). Occupational therapists are among the many professionals who can be qualified to use CBT and interpersonal psychotherapy during interventions (Dopheide, 2006). CBT, used in conjunction with pharmacotherapy, has been observed to reduce negative thinking associated with depression, lessen residual symptoms of depression, and decrease the possibility for relapse (Beevers & Miller, 2005; Fava et al., 2004; Hensley,

Nadiga, & Uhlenhuth, 2004). Current evidence also suggests leisure activity, including exercise, cards, bingo, and church attendance, as a valuable tool for decreasing depression. Occupational therapists have experience using activity as a part of intervention to treat a variety of conditions. Therefore, using leisure activity as a modality to decrease depression would be an appropriate occupational therapy approach. Keeping a holistic approach in mind, occupational therapists not only treat the condition itself, but also seek to improve the individual's functioning and overall well-being (Babyak et al., 2000; Fine, 2000).

CAREGIVER/FAMILY CONCERNS

Having a loved one with depression can be very stressful. Individuals with mood disorders, such as depression, have a very high rate of divorce (Long, 1998). Family therapy may be beneficial when (1) the depression appears to be seriously jeopardizing the client's marriage and family functioning or (2) a client's depression appears to be promoted and maintained by marital and family interaction patterns (Long, 1998).

RESOURCES

Organizations

National Institute of Mental Health
Public Information and Communications Branch
6001 Executive Boulevard
Room 8184, MSC 9663
Bethesda, MD 20892-9663
Telephone: 301-443-5413 or 866-615-6464 (toll-free)
TTY: 301-443-8431 or 866-415-8051 (toll-free)
Fax: 301-443-4279
Website: http://www.nimh.nih.gov

American Psychiatric Association
1400 K Street, NW
Washington, DC 20005
Telephone: (202) 682-6220
Website: http://www.psych.org/

American Psychological Association
750 First Street, NE
Washington, DC 20002-4242
Telephone: (202) 336-5500
Website: http://www.apa.org/

Depression and Bipolar Support Alliance
730 North Franklin Street
Suite 501
Chicago, IL 60610-3526
Telephone: 312-642-0049 or 800-826-3632
Website: http://www.dbsalliance.org

National Foundation for Depressive Illness
P.O. Box 2257
New York, NY 10116
Telephone: (800) 248-4344 or (800) 239-1265
Website: http://www.depression.org

Journals

- *American Journal of Psychology*
- *American Journal of Psychiatry*
- *Psychiatric Rehabilitation Journal*
- *Journal of Clinical Psychiatry*
- *Behavior Modification*
- *Rehabilitation Psychology*

Websites

- National Institute of Mental Health
  http://www.nimh.nih.gov/
  A government Website that provides information on mental health–related topics and offers many free resources that are easily accessed by the public and professionals.
- Depression Alliance On-line
  http://www.depressionalliance.org
  Website of a U.K. nonprofit organization run by and for people with depression. Provides message boards, information, and other online resources for people with depression.

Books and Booklets

- National Institute of Mental Health. (2002). *Stories of depression: Does this sound like you?* Bethesda, MD: Author.
  An easy-to-read booklet with personal stories of depression that includes a checklist of symptoms and tips on getting help.
- National Institute of Mental Health. (2000). *Depression.* Bethesda, MD: Author.
  A detailed booklet that describes symptoms, causes, and treatments, with information on getting help and coping.
- Styron, W. (1992). *Darkness visible.* London: Picador.
  A personal account of the author's struggle with deep depression and his eventual recovery.
- Irwin, C. (1999). *Conquering the beast within: How I fought depression and won . . . and how you can, too.* New York: Times Books.
  The author shares her own compelling story of how she struggled with clinical depression at age 14; was hospitalized, sought therapy, found the right medication, and successfully made the long, arduous climb back to good health.

- Woolis, R. (1992). *When someone you love has a mental illness: A handbook for family, friends and caregivers.* New York: Penguin Putnam.
  This book addresses short-term, daily problems of living with someone who has a mental illness, as well as long-term planning and care.

REFERENCES

Agency for Healthcare Research and Quality. (2000). *Improving quality of care for people with depression. Translating research into practice.* Retrieved January 29, 2006, from http://www.ahrq.gov/research/deprqoc.htm

Agency for Healthcare Research and Quality. (2004). *Screening for suicide risk: A systematic evidence review for the U.S. Preventative Services Task Force.* Retrieved January 30, 2006, from http://www.ahrq.gov/downloads/pub/prevent/pdfser/suicidser.pdf

American Occupational Therapy Association. (2002). *Understanding mood disorders.* Retrieved February 4, 2006, from http://www.aota.org/featured/area6/docs/mood.pdf

American Psychiatric Association. (2000). *Diagnostic and statistical manual of mental disorders* (4th ed., text rev.). Washington, DC: Author.

American Psychological Association. (2005). *Depression and how psychotherapy and other treatments can help people recover.* Retrieved February 5, 2006, from http://www.apa.org/pubinfo/depression.html

Babyak, M., Blumenthal, J., Herman, S., Khatri, P., Doraiswamy, M., Moore, K., et al. (2000). Exercise treatment for major depression: Maintenance of therapeutic benefit at 10 months. *Psychosomatic Medicine, 62,* 633–638.

Beck, A. (1978). *Beck Depression Inventory.* San Antonio, TX: Psychological Corporation.

Beevers, C., & Miller, I. (2005). Unlinking negative cognition and symptoms of depression: Evidence of a specific treatment effect for cognitive therapy. *Journal of Consulting and Clinical Psychology, 73,* 68–77.

Cara, E. (2005). Mood disorders. In E. Cara & A. MacRae (Eds.), *Psychosocial occupational therapy: A clinical practice* (2nd ed., pp. 162–192). Albany, NY: Thomson Delmar Learning.

Dopheide, J. (2006). Recognizing and treating depression in children and adolescents. *American Journal of Health-Systems Pharmacology, 63,* 233–243.

Fava, G., Ruini, C., Rafanelli, C., Finos, L., Conti, S., & Grandi, S. (2004). Six-year outcome of cognitive behavior therapy for prevention of recurrent depression. *American Journal of Psychiatry, 161,* 1872–1876.

Fine, J. (2000). The effect of leisure activity on depression in the elderly: Implications for the field of occupational therapy. *Occupational Therapy in Health Care, 13,* 45–59.

Hensley, P. L., Nadiga, D., & Uhlenhuth, E. H. (2004). Long-term effectiveness of cognitive therapy in major depressive disorder. *Depression and Anxiety, 20,* 1–7.

Kohlman Thompson, L. (1992). *The Kohlman Evaluation of Living Skills* (3rd ed.). Bethesda, MD: American Occupational Therapy Association.

Long, P. W. (1998). *Major depression disorder.* Retrieved January 20, 2006, from http://www.mentalhealth.com/rx/p23-md01.html#Head_3d

National Institute of Mental Health. (2000). *Depression.* Retrieved January 19, 2006, from, http://www.nimh.nih.gov/publicat/depression.cfm

National Institute of Mental Health. (2005). *Stories of depression: Does this sound like you?* Retrieved January 19, 2006, from http://www.nimh.nih.gov/publicat/nimhstories depression.cfm

Ramsey, S. E., Engler, P. A., & Stein, M. D. (2005). Alcohol use among depressed patients: The need for assessment and intervention. *Professional Psychology: Research and Practice, 36*(2), 203–207.

World Health Organization. (2001). *World health report 2001: Mental health: New understanding, new hope.* Geneva: Author.

DEVELOPMENTAL COORDINATION DISORDER

Kimberly Fletcher

The *Diagnostic and Statistical Manual-IV* describes developmental coordination disorder (DCD) as "a marked impairment in the development of motor coordination that must significantly interfere with academic achievement or activities of daily living, not be due to a general medical condition or pervasive developmental disorder and if mental retardation is present the motor difficulties must be in excess of those usually associated with it" (American Psychiatric Association, 2000, p. 56). DCD has been discussed in the literature under a number of different names, including *minimal brain dysfunction, perceptual motor dysfunction, physical awkwardness, clumsy child syndrome,* and *developmental dyspraxia* (Miller, Polatajko, Missiuna, Mandich, & Macnab, 2001).

INCIDENCE

◆ Six percent of school-age children are estimated to have some degree of DCD (Dilley, 2004).

CHARACTERISTICS

Many, but not all, children with DCD have the following characteristics:

◆ Born prematurely or having low birth weight
◆ Delayed motor milestones
◆ Comorbid attentional problems or learning disabilities

COURSE

◆ Potential etiologies include brain damage, genetic predisposition, or impairment in information processing.
◆ DCD is typically diagnosed at school age when children begin to have difficulties keeping up with classroom tasks (Cermak & Larkin, 2002).
◆ There is strong empirical evidence that the motor problems associated with DCD persist into adulthood (Miller, Missiuna, et al., 2001).

SYMPTOMS

At Home

◆ Late reaching motor milestones
◆ Difficulty walking up and down stairs
◆ Difficulty with dressing
◆ Falls often
◆ Difficulty with puzzles and sorting (http://dyspraxia foundation.org.uk/an_overview.htm)

At School

◆ Avoids physical education and games
◆ Might not run, hop, catch, or kick like peers
◆ Poor pencil grip
◆ Immature artwork
◆ Might have trouble with math
◆ Difficulty copying from board (http://dyspraxiafounda tion.org.uk/an_overview.htm)
◆ Handwriting is extremely effortful
◆ Difficulty on the playground
◆ Reduced participation in unstructured physical activities
◆ Academic problems
◆ Organization problems
◆ Task completion problems (Miller, Missiuna, et al., 2001)
◆ Difficulty keeping friends

POTENTIAL RISKS

◆ DCD can lead to the development of secondary mental health and educational issues, including poor social competence, academic problems, behavioral problems, and low self-esteem (Miller, Missiuna, et al., 2001)
◆ Children with DCD tend to be less successful than other children in sports and other physical activities and games, resulting in a tendency to avoid physical activities. This withdrawal has negative effects on the

musculoskeletal and cardiopulmonary systems (Cermak & Larkin, 2002).

OT EVALUATIONS

Occupational Performance Based

◆ Perceived Efficacy and Goal Setting System (PEGS)
◆ The School Function Assessment (SFA)
◆ The Movement Assessment Battery for Children Checklist (M-ABC Checklist)
◆ Developmental Coordination Disorder Questionnaire
◆ The Pediatric Interest Profiles (PIP)
◆ The Child Routine Inventory
◆ The Children's Assessment of Participation and Enjoyment (CAPE)

Motor Skills Assessments

1. Movement Assessment Battery for Children (M-MABC)
2. Bruininks Oseretsky Test of Motor Proficiency

OT INTERVENTIONS

◆ *Cognitive strategies:* A well supported example of this approach is the CO-OP approach. The CO-OP approach is an individualized, child-centered treatment that focuses on identifying cognitive strategies for successful task performance (Miller, Polatajko, Missiuna, Mandich, & Macnab, 2001).
◆ *Neuromotor Task Training (NTT):* NTT is an approach based in motor learning theory. NTT involves direct teaching of the task to be learned, through analysis and training of motor control processes. NTT has demonstrated positive effects on handwriting and fine and gross motor skills (Niemeijer, Smits-Engelsman, Reynders, & Shoemaker, 2003).
◆ *Parent and teacher training:* Training parents and teachers to work with children around developing specific skills using a cognitive motor approach has been found to be effective for some children (Sugden & Chambers, 2003).
◆ *Activity analysis/consultation:* It is important to consider the features of an activity; for example, in intervening to increase a child's participation in the community, one would consider the amount of hand-eye coordination involved in baseball versus swimming (Chen & Cohn, 2003).

OT AND THE EVIDENCE

A small randomized clinical trial comparing the CO-OP approach to a contemporary treatment approach (including neuromuscular, multisensory and biomechanical treatments), found the CO-OP approach to be most effective (Miller, Polatajko et al., 2001).

Additionally, Polatajko, Mandich, Miller, and Macnab (2001) analyzed five studies of the effectiveness of the CO-OP approach in children with DCD. They found that all five studies supported the use of the CO-OP approach with children with DCD. Three of the five studies indicated that the effect of the CO-OP treatment was reproducible across therapists, children, and a variety of activities.

CAREGIVER CONCERNS

Caregivers of children with DCD often have the following concerns:

◆ Their child's social development and whether their child can participate in activities that are typical for the child's peer group (Chen & Cohn, 2003).
◆ The possibility that the family unit could be limited in its participation within their community and involvement in leisure activities as a result of difficulties experienced by the child with DCD (Chen & Cohn, 2003).

RESOURCES

Associations

◆ The Dyspraxia Foundation
8 West Alley
Hitchin
Hertfordshire SG5 1EG
United Kingdom
Telephone: (01462) 455016 or (01462) 45986 (Dyspraxia Helpline)
Website: http://www.dyspraxiafoundation.org.uk/
The Dyspraxia Foundation is a British institution that was founded to support individuals and families that are affected by developmental dyspraxia. The Website provides a variety of easily navigated links to information, resources, shopping, and local groups within the United Kingdom.

Books

◆ Ball, M. (2002) *Developmental coordination disorder: Hints and tips for the activities of daily living.* London: Jessica Kingsley.
This book is intended as a resource for parents and caregivers of children with DCD.
◆ Colley, M., & Dyspraxia Foundation Adult Support Group. (2000). *Living with dyspraxia: A guide for adults.* Hitchin, UK: Dyspraxia Foundation.
Includes tips and strategies from adults living with dyspraxia.

Journals

- *Human Movement Science*

Websites

- The Dyspraxia Foundation
  http://www.dyspraxiafoundation.org.uk/
  A site in the United Kingdom that is full of resources and information.
- CanChild Centre for Childhood Disability Research
  http://www.fhs.mcmaster.ca/canchild
  Canchild provides information on DCD as well as other diagnosis.

REFERENCES

American Psychiatric Association. (2000). *Diagnostic and statistical manual of mental disorders* (4th ed., text rev.). Washington, DC: Author.

Cermak, S., & Larkin, D. (2002). *Developmental coordination disorder.* Albany, NY: Thomson Delmar Learning.

Chen, H.-F., & Cohn, E. (2003). Social participation for children with developmental coordination disorder: Conceptual, evaluation and intervention considerations. *Physical and Occupational Therapy in Pediatrics, 23*(4), 61–78.

Dilley, J. (2004). *Developmental coordination disorder.* Retrieved April 20, 2005, from http://www.nlm.nih.gov/medline/ency/article/001533.htm

Miller, L., Missiuna, C., Macnab, C., Malloy-Miller, T., & Polatajko, H. (2001). Clinical description of children with developmental coordination disorder. *Canadian Journal of Occupational Therapy, 68*(1), 5–15.

Miller, L., Polatajko, H., Missiuna, C., Mandich, A., & Macnab, J. (2001). A pilot trial of a cognitive treatment for children with developmental coordination disorder. *Human Movement Science, 20,* 183–210.

Niemeijer, A., Smits-Engelsman, B., Reynders, K., & Shoemaker, M. (2003). Verbal actions of physiotherapists to enhance motor learning in children with DCD. *Human Movement Science, 22,* 567–581.

Polatajko, H., Mandich, A., Miller, L., & Macnab, J. (2001). Cognitive orientation to daily occupational performance (CO-OP): II. The evidence. *Physical & Occupational Therapy in Pediatrics, 20*(2–3), 83–106.

Sugden, D., & Chambers, M. (2003). Intervention in children with developmental coordination disorder: The role of parents and teachers. *British Journal of Educational Psychology, 73*(4), 545–561.

DOWN SYNDROME

Alisa Jordan

Down syndrome is a genetic condition that is caused by a chromosomal mutation resulting in a third chromosome 21 (trisomy 21) in 95% of cases. It can also be caused by an unbalanced translocation of genetic material or mosaicism, in which one cell line is typical and one displays trisomy 21. Down syndrome can be diagnosed through prenatal testing or shortly after birth (American Academy of Pediatrics, 2001).

INCIDENCE

Down syndrome occurs in 1 in 800 births in the United States and 1 in 400 births for women over 35 years of age. (National Institute of Child Health & Human Development, 2006).

CHARACTERISTICS

People with Down syndrome have a wide variety of physical and functional abilities. The phenotype (physical appearance) of Down syndrome typically includes the following:

- Sloping forehead
- Flat nasal bridge
- Upslanting openings between the upper and lower eyelids
- Tongue protrusion
- Broad hands with short fifth fingers
- Small head, ears, and mouth (AAP, 2001; Roizen & Patterson, 2003)

The behavioral/cognitive phenotype of people with Down syndrome has been described as follows:

- Mental retardation (of varying degrees)
- Deficits in grammar skills, expressive language, auditory memory, intelligible speech
- Strengths in receptive language, visual-spatial memory, and interest in social interactions (Chapman & Hesketh, 2001)

PRECAUTIONS AND RELATED CONDITIONS

- Congenital heart disease
- Hypotonia
- Neck joint instability or subluxation
- Hearing loss
- Vision problems
- Hypothyroidism and obesity

◆ Celiac disease (gluten allergy)
◆ Respiratory tract infections
◆ Seizures
◆ Alzheimer's disease after the age of 40 years (AAP, 2001; Roizen & Patterson, 2003)

COURSE AND LIFE EXPECTANCY

◆ Life expectancy for people with Down syndrome is currently over 50 years (Roizen & Patterson, 2003).
◆ Over 80% of children born with Down syndrome survive to the age of 5 years (Dastgiri, Gilmour, & Stone, 2003).
◆ With services and support, many children and young adults with Down syndrome are able to participate in inclusive classrooms and progress with academic and self-care skills (Turner & Alborz, 2003).
◆ After transition from school services, many individuals with Down syndrome are able to live and work in the community, either independently or, commonly, with support from family or a group home environment (Roizen & Patterson, 2003).
◆ Later in life, approximately 75% of adults over 60 years with Down syndrome show signs and symptoms of Alzheimer's disease (Roizen & Patterson, 2003).

INTERDISCIPLINARY INTERVENTIONS

Traditional medical specialties consulted may include the following:

◆ Developmental pediatrics
◆ Neurology
◆ Gastroenterology
◆ Cardiology
◆ Orthopedics
◆ Endocrinology
◆ Ophthalmology
◆ Audiology (Leshin, 2002)

Therapies and support services are often an integral part in the lives and development of individuals with Down syndrome. In addition to occupational therapy, individuals may receive the following:

◆ Physical therapy
◆ Speech therapy
◆ Nutritional counseling
◆ Special education
◆ Vocational support
◆ Residential/community living support
◆ Dementia/Alzheimer's-related services (Leshin, 2002)

Alternative therapies may also be used in treatment for individuals with Down syndrome. Research supporting these interventions in reducing the related conditions of

Down syndrome is limited or nonexistent. These therapies include the following:

◆ Cell therapy
◆ Nootropics ("smart drugs")
◆ Nutritional supplements
◆ Plastic surgery (Leshin, 2002)

OT EVALUATION

Pediatric

ADL and Adaptive Behavior

◆ Pediatric Evaluation of Disability Inventory (PEDI)
◆ Vineland Adaptive Behavior Scales (VABS)
◆ Functional Independence Measure for Children (WeeFIM)

School Participation and Functioning

◆ School Function Assessment (SFA)
◆ Occupational Therapy Psychosocial Assessment of Learning (OTPAL)

Play/Leisure

◆ Test of Playfulness

Adolescent/Adult

ADL

◆ Functional Independence Measure (FIM)

Transition Services

◆ Transition Planning Inventory (TPI)

Occupational Needs, Interests, and Environmental Fit

◆ The Volitional Questionnaire Assessment (VQ)
◆ Canadian Occupational Performance Measure (COPM)

Other Client Performance Areas

◆ Fine and gross motor skills
◆ Praxis
◆ Visual-motor and perceptual skills
◆ Sensory processing
◆ Muscle tone
◆ Cognition and safety awareness
◆ Assistive technology needs

Caregivers of Adults with Down Syndrome and Alzheimer's Issues and Needs

◆ Caregiver Activity Survey-Intellectual Disability (CAS-ID)

OT INTERVENTION

Occupational therapy can be beneficial to individuals with Down syndrome throughout the life course. Because of the variability in functional strengths and limitations in this population, client-centered services are especially essential to effectiveness.

Early Intervention for Ages 0–3 Years

Possible Client Challenges

◆ Developmental delays in many areas, especially praxis and prehension
◆ Poor motivation and poor ability to explore and learn from the environment (Duff & Charles, 2004; Fidler, Hepburn, Mankin, & Rogers, 2005; Niccols, Atkinson, & Pepler, 2003)

Possible Interventions

◆ Efficient physical, cognitive, communication, social-emotional, and adaptive skill development
◆ Facilitation of participation in environment and family routines
◆ Maintenance of development rate
◆ Environmental adaptation (American Occupational Therapy Association, 2004; Lebeer & Rijke, 2003; Mahoney, Robinson, & Fewell, 2001)

Important Considerations

◆ Most children with Down syndrome take about twice as long as typical children to reach developmental milestones (Palisano et al., 2001).
◆ No one particular frame of reference commonly used by occupational therapists in early intervention (neurodevelopmental treatment, sensory integration, etc.) has been found to be more effective than others and should be used in conjunction to address all client needs (Mahoney et al., 2001; Uyanik, Bumin, & Kayihan, 2003).

Characteristics of Effective Intervention

◆ Natural environment
◆ Involvement and education of parents and caregivers
◆ Promotion of positive caregiver-child interactions (Lebeer & Rijke, 2003; Mahoney et al., 2001; Uyanik et al., 2003)

School Services for Ages 3–22 Years

Possible Client Challenges

◆ Toilet training
◆ Complex fine motor tasks
◆ Peer play and interactions

◆ Few severe functional limitations (Dolva, Coster, & Lilja, 2004; Leonard, Msall, Bower, Tremont, & Leonard, 2002)

Possible Interventions

◆ IEP consultation
◆ Elimination of barriers to learning and inclusion through environmental modification
◆ Supports for behavioral, social skills and ADL development
◆ Educating teachers, professionals, and parents about school-age issues related to Down syndrome
◆ Integration of outpatient and school services (AOTA, 2004; Cross, Traub, Hutter-Pishgahi, & Shelton, 2004; Wolpert, 2001)

Transitioning Out of School Services

At this stage, important tasks are development of supports and planning for optimal performance after exit from school in areas including the following:

◆ ADL, IADL, related assistive technology
◆ Prevocational and vocational skills
◆ Social skills and leisure participation
◆ Environmental modification (Kardos & White, 2005; Spencer, Emery, & Schneck, 2003)

Supported Employment and Community Living for Ages 18 Years and Older

Possible Client Challenges

◆ Limited independent living skills
◆ Aggressive or agitation behaviors, potentially due to exposure to negative life events, such as the constant shift in staff or location of group homes, relationship difficulties, or illness (Owen et al., 2004)

Possible Interventions

◆ Environmental adaptation for just-right fit
◆ Cognitive, problem solving, and social skill training
◆ ADL training and adaptation
◆ Adaptive equipment
◆ Sensory and occupation-based aggressive behavior management
◆ Self-advocacy and effective communication training (Chan, Fung, Tong, & Thompson, 2005; LaVigna, Christian, Liberman, Camacho, & Willis, 2002; Siporin & Lysack, 2004)

Characteristics of Effective Intervention

◆ Foster the client's feelings of being respected
◆ Promote the client's autonomy and choice
◆ Maximize the client's competence and productivity
◆ Use concrete, simple, repetitive, and multisensory teaching approaches (LaVigna et al., 2002; Siporin & Lysack, 2004)

OT AND THE EVIDENCE

The collaboration between therapist and parent(s) has been seen as a positive, effective, and valued part of intervention by all parties involved (Hanson, 2003; Hinojosa, Sproat, Mankhetwit & Anderson, 2002; Mayer, White, Ward, & Barnaby, 2002). While the strongest therapist-parent collaboration is typically during early intervention services, continued relationships have the potential to continue to provide benefit throughout the life course.

Research suggests that benefits for parents who are involved in their child's therapy include the following:

- Feeling more engaged in the system
- Receiving more education and information about their child
- Improved ability to see the strengths and progress made by their child
- Increased parental compliance and carryover of intervention strategies
- Increased developmental gains in relation to positive parent-child interaction (Mahoney et al., 2001; Mahoney, Wheeden, & Perales, 2004)

CAREGIVER CONCERNS

Being a caregiver for an individual with Down syndrome is often a lifelong role. Parents may benefit from the following:

- Education for parents to understand and take care of their children and themselves
- Early fostering of positive parent-child relationships and interactions in service provision
- Increased support for parents as services for the child decrease after they leave school
- Interventions to address negative or aggressive behaviors
- Respite services, especially if adult children still reside at home
- Encouragement to advocate for children and family's needs throughout the life course (Abbeduto et al., 2004; Ben-Zur, Duvdevany, & Lury, 2005; Hanson, 2004)

RESOURCES

Associations

1. National Down Syndrome Society
   666 Broadway
   New York, NY 10012
   Telephone: 1-800-221-4602
   Website: http://www.ndss.org/
2. National Down Syndrome Congress
   1370 Center Drive
   Atlanta, GA 30338
   Telephone: 1-800-232-6372
   Website: http://www.ndsccenter.org

Books

- Zuckoff, M. (2002). *Choosing Naia: A family's journey.* Boston: Beacon Press.
  Follows the Fairchild family through the prenatal diagnosis of their daughter with Down syndrome to her toddler years.
- Kingley, J., & Levitz, M. (1994). *Count us in: Growing up with Down syndrome.* New York: Harcourt Brace.
  A firsthand account of life with Down syndrome written by two young men; addresses issues relating to school, friendship, intimacy, advocacy, and independence.
- Cohen, W. I., Nadel, L., & Madnick, M. E. (Eds.). (2002). *Down syndrome: Visions for the 21st century.* New York: Wiley-Liss.
  A comprehensive resource for professionals and families covering a wide range of topics with contributions by people with Down syndrome and multidisciplinary experts.

Journals

- *Journal of Intellectual Disability Research*
- *Research in Developmental Disabilities*

Websites

- Down Syndrome Educational Trust
  http://www.downsed.org/
  Access to Down syndrome–related research, information, and resources for professionals and parents
- Down syndrome.com
  http://www.downsyndrome.com/
  Provides a comprehensive list of links to other internet resources on Down syndrome

REFERENCES

Abbeduto, L., Seltzer, M. M., Shattuck, P., Krauss, M. W., Orsmond, G., & Murphy, M. M. (2004). Psychological well-being and coping in mothers of youths with autism, Down syndrome, or fragile X syndrome. *American Journal of Mental Retardation, 109,* 237–254.

American Academy of Pediatrics. (2001). Health supervision for children with Down syndrome. *Pediatrics, 107,* 442–449.

American Occupational Therapy Association. (2004). Occupational therapy services in early intervention and school-based programs. *American Journal of Occupational Therapy, 58,* 681–685.

Ben-Zur, H., Duvdevany, I., & Lury, L. (2005). Associations of social support and hardiness with mental health among mothers of adult children with intellectual disability. *Journal of Intellectual Disability Research, 49,* 54–62.

Chan, S., Fung, M. Y., Tong, C. W., & Thompson, D. (2005). The clinical effectiveness of a multisensory therapy on clients with developmental disability. *Research in Developmental Disabilities, 26,* 131–142.

Chapman, R. S., & Hesketh, L. J. (2001). Language, cognition, and short-term memory in individuals with Down syndrome. *Down Syndrome Research and Practice, 7,* 1–7.

Cross, A. F. Traub, E., Hutter-Pishgahi, L., & Shelton, G. (2004). Elements of successful inclusion for children with significant disabilities. *Topics in Early Childhood Special Education, 24,* 169–183.

Dastgiri, S., Gilmour, W. H., & Stone, D. H. (2003). Survival of children born with congenital anomalies. *Archives of Disease in Childhood, 88,* 391–394.

Dolva, A.-S., Coster, W., & Lilja, M. (2004). Functional performance in children with Down syndrome. *American Journal of Occupational Therapy, 58,* 621–628.

Duff, S. V., & Charles, J. (2004). Enhancing prehension in infants and children: Fostering neuromotor strategies. *Physical and Occupational Therapy in Pediatrics, 24,* 129–172.

Fidler, D. J., Hepburn, S. L., Mankin, G., & Rogers, S. J. (2005). Praxis skills in young children with Down syndrome, other developmental disabilities, and typically developing children. *American Journal of Occupational Therapy, 59,* 129–138.

Hanson, M. J. (2003). Twenty-five years after early intervention: A follow-up of children with Down syndrome and their families. *Infants and Young Children, 16,* 354–365.

Hinojosa, J., Sproat, C. T., Mankhetwit, S., & Anderson, J. (2002). Shifts in parent-therapist partnerships: Twelve years of change. *American Journal of Occupational Therapy, 56,* 556–563.

Kardos, M. & White, B. P. (2005). The role of the school-based occupational therapist in secondary education transition planning: A pilot-survey study. *American Journal of Occupational Therapy, 59,* 173–180.

LaVigna, G. W., Christian, L., Liberman, R. P., Camacho, E., & Willis, T. J. (2002). Training professionals in use of positive methods for community integration of persons with developmental disabilities. *Psychiatric Services, 53,* 16–18.

Lebeer, J., & Rijke, R. (2003). Ecology of development in children with brain impairment. *Child: Care, Health, & Development, 29,* 131–140.

Leonard, S., Msall, M., Bower, C., Tremont, M., & Leonard, H. (2002). Functional status of school-aged children with Down syndrome. *Journal of Paediatrics and Child Health, 38,* 160–165.

Leshin, L. (2002). Pediatric health update on Down syndrome. In W. I. Cohen, L. Nadel, & M. E. Madnick (Eds.), *Down syndrome: Visions of change for the 21st century,* New York: Wiley-Liss.

Mahoney, G., Robinson, C., & Fewell, R. R. (2001). The effects of early motor intervention on children with Down syndrome and cerebral palsy: A field-based study. *Developmental and Behavioral Pediatrics, 22,* 153–162.

Mahoney, G., Wheeden, C. A., & Perales, F. (2004). Relationship of preschool special education outcomes to instructional practices and parent-child interaction. *Research in Developmental Disabilities, 25,* 539–558.

Mayer, M. L., White, B. P., Ward, J. D., & Barnaby, E. M. (2002). Therapists' perceptions about making a difference in parent-child relationships in early intervention occupational therapy services. *American Journal of Occupational Therapy, 56,* 411–421.

National Institute of Child Health and Human Development, NIH, DHHS. (1997). Facts about Down's syndrome (97-3402). Washington, DC: U.S. Government Printing Office.

Niccols, A., Atkinson, L, & Pepler, D. (2003). Mastery motivation in young children with Down's syndrome: Relations with cognitive and adaptive competence. *Journal of Intellectual Disability Research, 47,* 121–133.

Owen, D. M., Hastings, R. P., Noone, S. J., Chin, J., Harman, K., Roberts, J., et al. (2004). Life events as correlates of problem behavior and mental health in a residential population of adults with developmental disabilities. *Research in Developmental Disabilities, 25,* 309–320.

Palisano, R. J., Walter, S., Russell, D., Rosenbaum, P., Gemus, M., Galuppi, L., et al. (2001). Gross motor function of children with Down syndrome: Creation of motor growth curves. *Archives of Physical Medicine and Rehabilitation, 82,* 494–500.

Roizen, N. J., & Patterson, D. (2003). Down's syndrome. *Lancet, 361,* 1281–1289.

Siporin, S., & Lysack, C. (2004). Quality of life and supported employment: A case study of three women with developmental disabilities. *American Journal of Occupational Therapy, 58,* 455–465.

Spencer, J. E., Emery, L. J., & Schneck, C. M. (2003). Occupational therapy in transitioning adolescents to post-secondary activities. *American Journal of Occupational Therapy, 57,* 435–441.

Turner, S., & Alborz, A. (2003). Academic attainments of children with Down's syndrome: A longitudinal study. *British Journal of Educational Psychology, 73,* 563–583.

Uyanik, M., Bumin, G., & Kayihan, H. (2003). Comparison of different therapy approaches in children with Down syndrome. *Pediatrics International, 45,* 68–73.

Wolpert, G. (2001). What general educators have to say about successfully including students with Down syndrome in their classes. *Journal of Research in Childhood Education, 16,* 28–38.

FRAGILE X SYNDROME

Laurie Dossett and Kate-Lyn Stone

Fragile X syndrome, also known simply as *fragile X,* is the most common inherited form of mental retardation. It results from a change, or mutation, in a single gene (the Fragile X Mental Retardation 1, or FMR1, gene) on the X chromosome (March of Dimes, 2003; National Institute of Child Health & Human Development, 2005). This mutation can be passed from one generation to the next. The name comes from the place on the X chromosome where the mutation appears and the fact that the affected portion looks fragile (March of Dimes, 2003).

INCIDENCE AND PREVALENCE

Fragile X affects approximately 1 in 4,000 males and about 1 in 8,000 females and occurs across all ethnic and racial groups (March of Dimes, 2003).

CAUSE

Fragile X syndrome occurs when the mutated gene cannot produce enough of a protein (fragile X mental retardation protein, or FMRP) that is needed by the body's cells, especially cells in the brain, to develop and function normally (NICHD, 2005; National Fragile X Foundation, 2006). Usually, females with fragile X either do not have the common characteristics that are seen in males or have the characteristics in a milder form (NFXF, 2006). This difference may be due to the fact that females have two X chromosomes and therefore have two sets of instructions for making FMRP, so affected females can often make enough to fill most of the body's needs (NFXF, 2006). Because males only have one X chromosome, they do not produce enough FMRP for their bodies. Mothers of affected boys are carriers of the gene.

SYMPTOMS AND CHARACTERISTICS

Young children with fragile X often have delays in developmental milestones. Many clinicians refer to some signs of fragile X as "autistic-like" (March of Dimes, 2003).

Intelligence and Learning

The most common effect of fragile X is on intelligence, more than 80% of affected males having an IQ of 75 or less, with more variable effects in females (NICHD, 2005). Some females have mental impairment, some have learning disabilities, and some have a normal IQ. Adults and children with fragile X may have varying degrees of mental retardation or learning disabilities (March of Dimes, 2003; NICHD, 2005).

Physical

Many infants and young children show no typical characteristics of fragile X, but as they enter puberty, some characteristics become more evident (NICHD, 2005). Some of these include a long, narrow face or jaw; large ears; flat feet; a high, arched palate; and hyperflexible joints (especially metatarsophalangeal joints), and children with fragile X might not be as tall as their peers (March of Dimes, 2003; NICHD, 2005). Males with fragile X may also develop enlarged testicles, a condition called macro-orchidism (NICHD, 2005). Girls with fragile X have fewer or less severe characteristics, but many do have large ears.

Social/Behavioral/Emotional

Many children who have been diagnosed with fragile X experience behavior problems, anxiety, possible depression, difficulties paying attention, and poor eye contact. They do not react well to new situations, and during adolescence, boys may exhibit aggressive behavior (March of Dimes, 2003; NFXF, 2006; NICHD, 2005). Behaviors such as hand flapping and chewing on skin, clothes, or objects are often seen in boys (March of Dimes, 2003; NFXF, 2006).

Sensory

Many children and adults with fragile X are very sensitive to certain sensations in their environments (NICHD, 2005). Sensory disorders in people with fragile X often include hyperarousal or hypoarousal, sensory overreactivity and sensory underreactivity, including motor planning issues and fine motor weaknesses, and tactile defensiveness (NFXF, 2006). Children with fragile X may also have problems with balance, coordination, and connective tissue, which cause difficulties for them as they learn to sit, stand, and walk or, later, to ride a bicycle (NICHD, 2005).

Speech and Language

Many children with fragile X begin talking later than expected; most begin to use words around age 4, but some might not talk until age 6 or 7 (NICHD, 2006). Language difficulties in children who have fragile X range from mild stuttering to more severe problems with basic language skills, boys typically have more problems and girls rarely experience severe problems (NFXF, 2006; NICHD, 2005).

DIAGNOSIS

A blood test can identify people who either have fragile X syndrome or are carriers of the disorder (March of Dimes, 2003). Prenatal tests using amniocentesis or chorionic villus sampling can determine whether a baby of a carrier mother has inherited the full mutation, but this test cannot always determine whether the baby will have mental retardation (March of Dimes, 2003).

AFFILIATED CONDITIONS

Most people with fragile X do not have serious medical problems and have a normal life expectancy, though about 20% of people with fragile X will develop seizures, which are usually controlled with medication (March of Dimes, 2003). Children with fragile X may also be at an increased risk for autism, inner ear problems, sleep disturbances, ADD/ADHD, vision problems, digestive disorders, connective tissue problems, and premature ovarian failure in females (March of Dimes, 2003; NICHD, 2005).

TREATMENT

At this time, there is no cure for fragile X syndrome. It is possible, however, that through appropriate medications and education, the potential for each person can be maximized and signs can be minimized (Fragile X Research Foundation, 2005; NICHD, 2005).

Education

Most children with fragile X will qualify for special education services (because of mental retardation) in their school, where an individualized education plan (IEP) will be designed for the child (NICHD, 2005). These services will be provided from ages 3 to 21 years (or until they graduate from high school) through the Individuals with Disabilities Education Act (IDEA), which provides for a free, appropriate, individualized education in the least restrictive environment (Fragile X Research Foundation, 2005). As students get older, vocational assessment is a related service that should be part of the IEP from the middle school or early high school level (Fragile X Research Foundation, 2005). These assessments are provided to students in middle or high school who are beginning to plan their lives after graduation and are designed to assess the adolescent's aptitudes and interests as they relate to careers. When students leave high school, IDEA requires a plan that includes a coordinated set of activities based on the individual student's needs and interests (Fragile X Research Foundation, 2005). This helps during the transition period and helps these individuals and their families to decide what vocational education or postsecondary education options are appropriate, what supported employment might be needed, and the level of independence that is needed for living arrangements and community participation (Fragile X Research Foundation, 2005).

Medication

Medications are sometimes used to treat symptoms of fragile X or affiliated problems. They are usually most effective when used in conjunction with therapeutic interventions (NICHD, 2005).

Therapeutic Options

Many children (and some adults) with fragile X will find participation in services such as speech-language therapy, occupational therapy, behavioral therapy, and physical therapy beneficial to improve functioning in many areas (NICHD, 2005).

OCCUPATIONAL THERAPY EVALUATIONS

Occupational therapists may observe chewing and swallowing; grasp; states of alertness and overload; reactions to sound, light, and touch; and other sensorimotor and fine motor areas (NFXF, 2006). Occupational therapists will often use standard assessments to test for development and functional abilities. Some of these assessments may include the following:

- Infant-Toddler Developmental Assessment (birth to 36 months)
- Hawaii Early Learning Profile (0–36 months) (HELP)
- Miller Assessment for Preschoolers (2 years, 9 months to 5 years, 8 months) (MAP)
- Bayley Scale of Infant Development (1–42 months)
- Sensory Integration and Praxis Tests (4 years to 8 years, 11 months) (SIPT)
- Peabody Developmental Motor Scales-2 (1 month to 6 years) (PDMS)
- Bruininks-Oseretsky Test of Motor Proficiency (4.5–14.5 years) (BOT-2)

OCCUPATIONAL THERAPY INTERVENTION

Occupational therapists can work with people of all ages with fragile X to make necessary modifications in tasks or environments to ensure maximum functional performance (NICHD, 2005). This may include making changes in someone's home or school environment or finding appropriate assistive devices and equipment. As children grow older, an OT in a high school may work with students to match interests and abilities to find employment or volunteer work or to develop new skills (NICHD, 2005). Occupational therapy may be provided in early intervention, early childhood, and school programs; in work settings; and through private agencies (Fragile X Research Foundation, 2005).

Early Intervention Services

The Early Intervention for Infants and Toddlers with Disabilities and Their Families program is an amendment to IDEA to encourage states to set up programs for very young children and their families. Services are jointly selected by parents and service providers and may be offered in the home, school, hospital, or center.

Occupational therapists may work with families to adjust when they bring their newborn home and teach caregivers calming strategies, massage, deep pressure, and other supportive techniques for soothing an overstimulated baby (Fragile X Research Foundation, 2005).

School System

Younger school-aged children may receive occupational therapy services involving sensory integration and assistance with fine motor skills for activities such as writing or using a computer keyboard (Fragile X Research Foundation, 2005). As students get older, occupational therapists may evaluate workplaces and provide services to help both work skills and the work environment; and when vocational planning takes place, the OT plays a role in considering what type of work would be a good match for an individual (Fragile X Research Foundation, 2005).

OT AND THE EVIDENCE

Much of the research on fragile X syndrome (FXS), which is closely linked to other types of developmental disorders, discusses the importance of early identification of FXS. Early identification allows for early intervention, which provides important services for newborns and their families. High-quality early intervention has been shown to have beneficial effects on the progress of children with developmental disabilities secondary to FXS (Bailey, 2004; Bailey, Skinner, & Sparkman, 2003). Current research also directs attention to the importance of taking the environment into consideration when planning intervention for children with FXS (Baker & Donnelly, 2001; Mirrett, Roberts & Price, 2003). Mirrett, Roberts, and Price (2003) suggest that intervention accommodations should include providing visually based learning (photographs, picture symbols, or communication books); providing stable routines for transitions; making modifications for limited attention span; and adjusting, as necessary, during treatment for sensory processing difficulties. Shaaf and Miller (2005) found occupational therapy incorporating sensory integration to be particularly helpful in guiding intervention for children with FXS who have sensory processing difficulties.

CAREGIVER/FAMILY CONCERNS

Caregivers of children with special needs have common concerns for their children and their entire families. The process of getting a diagnosis can be long and trying for many families, leading to incredible stress.

RESOURCES

Organizations

- FRAXA (The Fragile X Research Foundation)
  45 Pleasant Street
  Newburyport, MA 01950

  Telephone: 978-462-1866
  Fax: 978-463-9985
  Website: www.fraxa.org
  Run by parents, relatives, and friends of those with fragile X, as well as by medical professionals. Promotes and funds scientific research aimed at the treatment and cure of fragile X.
- National Fragile X Foundation
  P.O. Box 190488
  San Francisco, CA 94119-0488
  Telephone: 800-688-8765
  Fax: 925-938-9315
  Website: www.fragilex.org
  Provides information and support to individuals with fragile X, their families, educators, and health professionals.

Books

- Schopmeyer, B. B. & Lowe, F. (1992). *The fragile X child*. San Diego: Singular Publishing Group.
  A book covering what fragile X syndrome is, intervention options (including occupational therapy), and case studies.
- Webber, J. D. (2000). *Children with fragile X syndrome: A parent's guide*. Bethesda, MD: Woodbine House.
  Written by leading professionals in the field and experienced parents, the guide is both helpful and supportive. Information helps families to adjust, understand their child's strengths and weaknesses, and know where to seek further help and expertise.
- Griffin, E. (2004). *Fragile X, fragile hope: Finding joy in parenting a special needs child*. Bethesda, MD: Woodbine House.
  Provides a complete, sensitive introduction to fragile X syndrome, written by renowned professionals and experienced parents, who offer an in-depth look at the issues and concerns affecting children and their families. It covers diagnosis, parental emotions, therapies and medications, development, early intervention, education, daily care, legal rights, and advocacy.
- Icon Health Publications. (2005). *The official parent's sourcebook on fragile X syndrome: A directory for the internet age*. San Diego: Icon Group International.
  This book was created for parents who have decided to make education and research an integral part of the treatment process; it tells parents where and how to look for information covering virtually all topics related to fragile X syndrome.
- Busby, M., & Massey, M. (2006). *Dear Megan: Letters on life, love and fragile X*. Sterling, VA: Capital Books.
  In the form of intimate letters over the years between two mothers of different generations, this book is about dealing with the tragedy of having two mentally retarded

children as well as the privilege of joining the crusade to cure fragile X.

Websites

◆ March of Dimes
http://www.marchofdimes.com
A Website for professionals and nonprofessionals to obtain information on many different pregnancy- and birth-related topics, specifically premature births, birth defects, and prevention.

REFERENCES

Bailey, D. B. (2004). Newborn screening for fragile X syndrome. *Mental Retardation and Developmental Disabilities Research Reviews, 10,* 3–10.

Bailey, D. B., Skinner, D., & Sparkman, K. L. (2003). Discovering fragile X syndrome: Family experiences and perceptions. *Pediatrics, 111,* 407–416.

Baker, K., & Donnelly, M. (2001). The social experiences of children with disability and the influence of environment: A framework for intervention. *Disability and Society, 16,* 71–85.

Fragile X Research Foundation. (2005). *About fragile X.* Retrieved March 25, 2006, from http://www.fraxa.org/aboutFX.aspx

March of Dimes. (2003). *Fragile X syndrome.* Retrieved March 22, 2006, from http://www.marchofdimes.com/professionals/681_9266.asp

Mirrett, P., Roberts, J., & Price, J. (2003). Early intervention practices and communication intervention strategies for young males with fragile X syndrome. *Language, Speech, and Hearing Services in Schools, 34,* 320–331.

National Fragile X Foundation. (2006). *Characteristics of fragile X syndrome.* Retrieved March 24, 2006, from http://www.nfxf.org/html/characteristics.htm

National Institute of Child Health & Human Development. (2005). *Families and fragile X syndrome.* Retrieved March 22, 2006, from http://www.nichd.nih.gov/publications/pubs/fragileX/

Schaaf, R., & Miller, L. J. (2005). Occupational therapy using a sensory integrative approach for children with developmental disabilities. *Mental Retardation and Developmental Disabilities: Research Reviews, 11,* 143–148.

HIP AND KNEE REPLACEMENTS

Jennifer Keller and Kate-Lyn Stone

DESCRIPTION OF CONDITION

Knee Replacements (Total Knee Arthroplasty)

The largest joint in the body is the knee. Nearly normal knee joint function is vital to the performance of several routine daily activities. Disease or injury can compromise the function of the knee. Knee replacements are generally performed to decrease pain and muscle weakness and to improve limited function secondary to arthritis (the leading cause of knee pain and loss of function) or injury (American Academy of Orthopedic Surgeons, 2006b). Mezey (2001) states that knee replacements involve replacing the joint with an implant attaching to the tibia and femur. The surfaces are prepared by cutting the bones and flattening the surfaces prior to attaching the implant.

Hip Replacements (Total Hip Arthroplasty)

One of the largest weight-bearing joints in the body is the hip (AAOS, 2006a). When medications, changes in activities, and walking aids are no longer decreasing hip pain and stiffness secondary to arthritis, injury, or fracture, total hip replacements may be the next reasonable solution (AAOS, 2006). Total hip replacements are the most common hip procedure (Gann, 2001). Fagerson (1998) notes that total hip replacements are frequently performed on individuals who have rheumatoid arthritis and osteoarthri-

tis. In this procedure, the joint is removed and replaced with an implant. Recovery after surgery can last anywhere from 6 to 12 weeks (Fagerson, 1998).

INCIDENCE AND PREVALENCE

◆ More than 300,000 knee replacements are performed each year in the United States (Mayo Clinic, 2006).
◆ More than 193,000 total hip replacements are performed each year in the United States (AAOS, 2006a).
◆ Approximately 85–97% of patients experience no pain after having a total hip replacement (Daniel & Strickland, 1992).

SEQUENCE OF CARE

Hip Replacement/Knee Replacement

Physicians conduct an initial assessment of the injury, including pain level and ability to function, and collect information regarding medical history and current health status (AAOS, 2006a). A physical examination is used to evaluate joint strength, stability, and range of motion. X-rays, CT scans, or MRIs are used to determine the specific diagnosis. Surgery is conducted to stabilize the joint and structures (Merck, 2005).

SYMPTOMS

The following symptoms may indicate a need for knee replacement:

- Severe pain that limits participation in everyday activities
- Moderate pain while at rest
- Inflammation and swelling that does not improve with medication
- Knee deformity
- Limited range of motion, knee stiffness
- Limited function
- Limited ability to perform ADL

The following symptoms may indicate a need for hip replacement:

- Hip pain that limits activities such as walking and bending
- Pain that continues even when not in use
- Stiffness
- Limited function
- Limited range of motion
- Limited mobility and strength
- Limited weight bearing
- Limited ability to perform ADL

GENERAL PRECAUTIONS AND CONSIDERATIONS

These general precautions and considerations are taken immediately following joint replacement surgery:

- *Medical status:* Each day, the client must be assessed by the physician, whose orders determine the course of therapy (Daniel & Strickland, 1992).
- *Cardiac/respiratory:* Watch for risks related to anesthesia, including heart attack, stroke, pneumonia, and blood clots. Blood clots can occur in the legs, but usually appear a few days after surgery. These can be dangerous because they may move from the leg to the lungs causing shortness of breath, chest pain, and even death. It is recommended that a patient get out of bed shortly after surgery to decrease the risk of forming blood clots (The Patient Education Institute, 2004).
- *Fall prevention:* Provide supervision when the client is performing tasks. The client needs to follow all precautions to prevent further injury or damage to the repaired or replaced joint (Bear-Lehman, 2002).
- *Skin integrity:* Watch for signs of skin breakdown, especially if the client is bed-bound for long periods. Frequent weight shifts will prevent bedsores. Follow wound care protocol for incisions (Daniel & Strickland, 1992).
- *Muscle stiffness:* Range of motion frequently is limited because of periods of immobility. PROM/AROM will minimize the stiffness and increase range in the muscles (Bear-Lehman, 2002).
- *Safety concerns:* The client needs to be safe within his or her environment. Frequently, these clients need assistance when maneuvering in the environment (Bear-Lehman, 2002).

PRECAUTIONS

Always consider incision management and weight-bearing status for all orthopedic conditions of the lower extremity as prescribed by the physician's order.

Knee precautions for the first six to eight weeks after surgery include the following (AAOS, 2006b):

- Follow the physician's orders.
- Follow range of motion guidelines.
- Avoid high-impact activities, such as running.
- Avoid excessive activity or weight gain, as this may hasten normal wear.

Hip precautions for the first six to eight weeks after surgery include the following (Dolhi, Leibold, & Schreiber, 2003):

- Follow the physician's orders.
- Avoid extreme hip internal or external rotation.
- Avoid hip adduction.
- No hip flexion beyond 90 degrees.
- No crossing legs, knees, or ankles
- No lying or rolling on the affected side.

Long-term precautions for joint replacement surgeries include the following (Huddleston, 2005):

- Prophylactic antibiotic use prior to dental work or other medical procedures or surgeries.
- Being cautious of infection. After a joint replacement, if an individual gets an infection in the body, it can travel through the bloodstream to the replaced joint. This can eventually lead to a systemic infection.

POSTSURGICAL MEDICAL INTERVENTIONS

Following are typical postsurgical medical interventions for knee and hip replacements (Fagerson, 1998; Paul & Orchanian, 2003; WebMD, 2006):

- Surgery to repair, replace, or remove the joint. The surgeon removes the diseased tissue and cartilage from the joint and replaces the removed parts with new, artificial parts
- Pain medications for pain management
- Antibiotics to prevent infection
- Anticoagulants to prevent blood clots

- Catheter for urination
- Compression stockings or a compression pump to maintain circulation
- Impatient and outpatient rehabilitation

TYPICAL OT EVALUATIONS

Following are typical occupational therapy evaluations for knee and hip replacements (Paul & Orchanian, 2003):

Comprehensive Assessments

- Functional Independence Measure (FIM)
- Assessment of Motor and Process Skills (AMPS)
- Barthel Index
- Katz ADL
- Berg Balance Test

Quality of Life or Life Satisfaction Assessments

- Canadian Occupational Performance Measure (COPM)
- Role/interest Checklist
- Short Form-36 Health Survey (SF-36)
- Worker Role Inventory

Psychosocial Assessments

- Peiers-Harris Coping Inventory
- Geriatric Depression Scale

Other Assessments

- Manual muscle testing
- Range-of-motion testing using a goniometer
- Pain scales
- Home assessment

TYPICAL OT INTERVENTION

- The primary goal is to restore functional status to the client (Bear-Lehman, 2002).
- When the client is cleared medically, the therapist needs to conduct a careful analysis of functional activities (Bear-Lehman, 2002).
- Follow protocols for wound care (Dolhi et al., 2003). Avoid soaking the wound in water until the incision has thoroughly sealed and dried (AAOS, 2006a, 2006b).
- In treatment, consider weight-bearing status and precautions (Bear-Lehman, 2002).

OT INTERVENTIONS

- ADLs
- Energy conservation techniques
- Strengthening exercises
- Pain management
- Assistive technology
- Adapt environment
- Adaptive equipment
- IADL
- Safety, hip and other precautions, and fall prevention
- Patient and family education
- Home planning, including installing grab bars in showers, handrails in stairways, a toilet seat riser, and a shower bench; removing loose carpets; and preparing a temporary living space on the ground floor if possible

OT AND EVIDENCE

Novalis, Messenger, and Morris (2000) examined critical pathways regarding hip injuries. The researchers obtained eight critical pathways from various rehabilitation facilities. The pathways included functional transfers, adaptive equipment, and length of patient stay. Benchmarks differed depending on the facility. It was found that the array of occupational therapy benchmarks suggests a broad scope for the role of occupational therapists in enhancing clients' functional outcomes (Novalis et al., 2000).

Coudeyre and colleagues (2007) found that a preoperative rehabilitation program consisting of education and preparation was effective in contributing to a decrease in length of hospital stay following total hip and knee replacements. It is suggested that the program consist of a multidisciplinary approach of at least physical therapy, education, and occupational therapy home visits. Crowe and Henderson (2003) discovered similar results with their preoperative, individually tailored rehabilitation program with an interdisciplinary approach that helped to reduce average length of stay following surgery.

CAREGIVER ISSUES

Hip and knee replacements engender the following issues among family members and caregivers (Merck, 2005):

- The patient is vulnerable to secondary complications due to surgery.
- Swelling, pressure sores, stiffness, and functional changes affect the patient.
- Patients often are reliant on caregivers for assistance with ADL and IADL.

RESOURCES

Associations

- American Orthopaedic Association
  6300 N. River Road
  Suite 505
  Rosemont, IL 60018
  Telephone: 847-318-7330
  Fax: 847-318-7339
  Website: http://aoassn.org
  This organization provides information on orthopedic conditions and surgeons.

- American Academy of Orthopedic Surgeons
  6300 North River Road
  Rosemont, Illinois 60018-4262
  Telephone: 847-823-7186
  Fax: 847-823-8125
  Website: http://www.aaos.org/
  This organization provides information for patients regarding procedures and rehabilitation and has a listing of orthopedic surgeons.

Books

- Nohava, A. G. (2001). *My bilateral knee replacement: A personal story.* Lincoln, NE: iUniverse.
  This book gives a woman's account of her bilateral knee replacements.

OT Journals

- *Rheumatology*
- *Journal of Bone & Joint Surgery*
- *Disability & Rehabilitation*
- *Clinical Rehabilitation*

Websites

- The National Center for Injury Prevention and Control (NCIPC)
  http://www.cdc.gov/ncipc/default.htm
  This site works to reduce morbidity, disability, mortality, and costs associated with injuries. It has information regarding falls and fall prevention.
- The American Orthopaedic Association
  http://aoassn.org
  This site provides information on orthopedic conditions and surgeons.
- Journal of Bone & Joint Surgery
  http://www.ejbjs.org/
  This site has information articles on various orthopedic surgeries.

REFERENCES

American Academy of Orthopedic Surgeons. (2006a). *Total hip replacement.* Retrieved August 26, 2007, from http://orthoinfo.aaos.org/fact/thr_report.cfm?Thread_ID=50&topcategory=Hip

American Academy of Orthopedic Surgeons. (2006b). *Total knee replacement.* Retrieved August 26, 2007, from http://orthoinfo.aaos.org/fact/thr_report.cfm?Thread_ID=513&topcategory=Knee

Bear-Lehman, J. (2002). Orthopaedic conditions. In C. A. Trombly & M. V. Radomski (Eds.), *Occupational therapy for physical dysfunction* (5th ed., pp. 909–924). Philadelphia: Lippincott Williams & Wilkins.

Coudeyre, E., Jardin, C., Givron, P., Ribinik, P., Revel, M., & Rannou, F. (2007). Could preoperative rehabilitation modify postoperative outcomes after total hip and knee arthroplasty?: Elaboration of French clinical practice guidelines. *Annales de Readaptation et de Medecine Physique, 50,* 189–197.

Crowe, J., & Henderson, J. (2003). Pre-arthroplasty rehabilitation is effective in reducing hospital stay. *Canadian Journal of Occupational Therapy, 70,* 88–96.

Daniel, M. S. & Strickland, L. R. (1992). *Occupational therapy protocol management in adult dysfunction.* Gaithersburg, MD: Aspen.

Dolhi, C., Leibold, M. L., & Schreiber, J. (2003). Adult orthopedic dysfunction. In E. B. Crepeau, E. S. Cohn & B. A. B. Schell (Eds.), *Willard and Spackman's occupational therapy* (10th ed., pp. 789–796). Philadelphia: Lippincott Williams & Wilkins.

Fagerson, T. (1998). *The hip handbook.* Boston: Butterworth-Heinemann.

Gann, N. (2001). *Orthopedics at a glance.* Thorofare, NJ: Slack.

Huddleston, H. D. (2005). *Arthritis of the knee joint.* Retrieved September 12, 2007, from http://www.hipsandknees.com/knee/kneecare.htm

Mayo Clinic. (2006). *Knee replacement: Surgery can relieve pain.* Retrieved August 24, 2007, from http://www.mayoclinic.com/health/knee-replacement/HQ00977

Merck. (2005). *The Merck manual of geriatrics.* Retrieved March 28, 2006, from http://www.merck.com/mrkshared/mmg/sec2/ch22/ch22a.jsp

Mezey, M. D. (2001) *Encyclopedia of elder care.* New York: Springer.

Novalis, S. N., Messenger, M. F., & Morris, L. (2000). Occupational therapy benchmarks within orthopedic (hip) critical pathways. *American Journal of Occupational Therapy, 54,* 155–158.

The Patient Education Institute. NLM. NIH. (2004). X-plain hip replacement surgery: Reference summary. Retrieved October 30, 2007, from http://www.nlm.nih.gov/medlineplus/tutorials/hipreplacement/htm/index.htm.

Paul, S., & Orchanian, D. P. (2003). *Pocket guide to assessment in occupational therapy.* Clifton Park, NY: Thomson Learning.

WebMD. (2006). *Hip fracture.* Retrieved March 23, 2006, from http://webmd.com/hw/trauma_first_aid/aa6976.asp?printing=ture

HIV/AIDS

Alyssa Wells Arnold and Kate-Lyn Stone

DIAGNOSIS

Acquired immunodeficiency syndrome (AIDS) is caused by the human immunodeficiency virus (HIV) (National Institutes of Health, 2005). The diagnosis of HIV is determined by testing blood for the presence of antibodies (disease-fighting proteins) to HIV by using two different types of antibody tests: ELISA and Western blot. HIV antibodies generally do not reach noticeable levels in the blood for one to three months following infection (NIH, 2005). HIV progressively destroys the body's ability to fight infections and certain cancers by damaging and killing the T helper cells (T4 cells) that are responsible for fighting diseases in the body's immune system. Individuals with a T4 level count below 200 are diagnosed with an AIDS-defining opportunistic infection (Copperman, Forwell, & Hugos, 2002).

PREVALENCE

The Centers for Disease Control and Prevention (2005) estimates the prevalence of HIV/AIDS in the United States at the end of 2003 to be 1,039,000–1,185,000. Of these, approximately 25% of HIV-positive individuals remain unaware of their HIV infection (Glynn & Rhodes, 2005). The CDC has estimated that approximately 40,000 people in the United States become infected with HIV each year. HIV can affect both males and females; however, in 2004, almost three quarters of HIV/AIDS diagnoses were for male adolescents and adults. Females make up 27% of new HIV diagnoses (CDC, 2005). HIV can affect all ethnicities; however, in 2004, half the people in the United States who were diagnosed with HIV/AIDS were African Americans. Caucasians make up 30%, Hispanics 18%, and Asian/Pacific Islander and Native American/Alaskan Native 2% of the HIV/AIDS population (CDC, 2005).

TYPICAL COURSE AND SYMPTOMS

According to NIH (2005), individuals begin to present with flulike symptoms within one to two months after exposure to HIV/AIDS. During this period, people are very infectious, and HIV is present in large quantities in genital fluids. More persistent or severe symptoms might not appear for 10 years or more after HIV first enters the body in adults or within two years in children who are born HIV-positive (NIH, 2005). As the immune system deteri-

orates, the first signs of infection occur in the large lymph nodes. According to the NIH, the most prevalent symptoms prior to the onset of AIDS include the following:

◆ Lack of energy
◆ Weight loss
◆ Frequent fevers and sweats
◆ Persistent or frequent yeast infections (oral or vaginal)
◆ Persistent skin rashes or flaky skin
◆ Pelvic inflammatory disease in women that does not respond to treatment
◆ Short-term memory loss

According to the NIH (2005), symptoms related to the onset of opportunistic illness include the following:

◆ Coughing and shortness of breath
◆ Seizures and lack of coordination
◆ Difficult or painful swallowing
◆ Mental symptoms such as confusion and forgetfulness
◆ Severe and persistent diarrhea, nausea, abdominal cramps, and vomiting
◆ Vision loss
◆ Weight loss and extreme fatigue
◆ Severe headaches
◆ Coma

CAUSE AND ETIOLOGY

HIV is most commonly transmitted through sexual contact. HIV can also be transmitted through the use of contaminated needles or blood transfusions and prenatally from mother to fetus (NIH, 2005).

AFFILIATED PROBLEMS

Depression is very common among individuals with HIV/AIDS and should be considered in the treatment plan (Copperman et al., 2002). HIV is also associated with many neurological complications, such as cognitive and motor changes (Copperman, 2003), which can affect an individual's ability to complete activities of daily living. Alcohol use increases the risk of developing some infections that can occur as complications of AIDS. Tuberculosis, pneumonia caused by *Streptococcus pneumoniae,* and hepatitis C are three infections that are associated with both alcohol and AIDS. Alcohol may also exacerbate damage to the brain caused by AIDS (National Institute on Alcohol Abuse and Alcoholism, 2002).

INTERVENTIONS

Medications

Health care providers must use a combination of medications to effectively suppress HIV. When the multiple drugs (three or more) are used in combination, this type of treatment is referred to as highly active antiretroviral therapy (HAART). HAART is the most common form of treatment for individuals with HIV or AIDS. HAART is not a cure for AIDS; however, it has greatly improved the health of many people with AIDS, and it reduces the amount of virus circulating in the blood to nearly undetectable levels (NIH, 2005).

Psychoeducation

Teaching individuals with HIV/AIDS and their families about the disease and how to prevent transmission is extremely important. This includes avoiding behaviors that put a person at risk of infection, such as sharing needles and having unprotected sex (NIH, 2005).

OT EVALUATIONS

Basic and Instrumental Activity of Daily Living Skills

- Kohlman Evaluation of Living Skills (KELS)
- Assessment of Motor and Process Skills (AMPS)
- Functional Independence Measure (FIM)
- Klein-Bell Activities of Daily Living Scale (Klein-Bell)
- Satisfaction With Performance Scaled Questionnaire (SPSQ)

Psychosocial Skills

- Allen Cognitive Level Test-90 (ACLS-90)
- The Assessment of Occupational Functioning (AOF)
- The Occupational Performance History Interview II (OPHI II)

Cognitive/Perceptual Skills

- Test of Everyday Attention (TEA)
- Lowenstein Occupational Therapy Cognitive Assessment (LOCTA)
- Mini-Mental State (MMSE)

Self-Perception

- The Canadian Occupational Performance Measure (COPM)
- The Role Checklist

Somatic Sensory Evaluations

- Primary somatic system
  1. Light touch
  2. Pain
  3. Temperature
- Discriminative somatic system
  1. Tactile localization
  2. Two-point discrimination
  3. Stereognosis
  4. Proprioception
  5. Kinesthesia

OT INTERVENTIONS

- ADL
- Energy conservation techniques
- Strengthening exercises
- Assistive technology
- IADL
- Patient and family education
- Dietary concerns regarding weight management
- Medication management, including scheduling
- Prevention education
- Group therapy
- Coping

OT AND THE EVIDENCE

Group therapy can be beneficial for individuals with HIV/AIDS. Group therapy has been applied to concepts such as symptom management, self-management and coping skills, psychoeducational support, and cognitive behavioral psychotherapy (Chiou et al., 2004; Inouye, Flannelly, & Flannelly, 2001; Nokes, Chew, & Altman 2003; Rousaud et al., 2007). Nokes, Chew, and Altman (2003) found that group therapy enables individuals with HIV/AIDS to develop connections with other individuals who are coping with the same illness.

Exercise is also a key management strategy to address impairments, limitations, and restrictions in individuals with HIV/AIDS. O'Brien, Nixon, Glazier, and Tynan (2004) found progressive resistive exercise to have several benefits, including increases in body weight and composition, improvements in cardiopulmonary fitness, and improvements in psychological status. Constant or interval aerobic exercise or a combination of aerobic exercise and progressive resistive exercise has been found to lead to significant reductions in depression and improvements in cardiopulmonary fitness (Nixon, O'Brien, Glazier, & Tynan, 2007). Overall, exercise as an intervention strategy appears to be safe and beneficial for individuals with HIV/AIDS.

REFERENCES

Centers for Disease Control and Prevention. (2005). *A glance at the AIDS epidemic.* Retrieved May 6, 2006, from http://www.cdc.gov/hiv/resources/factsheets/At-A-Glance.htm

Chiou, P. Y., Kuo, B. I. T., Lee, M. B., Chen, Y. M., Wu, S. I., & Lin, L. C. (2004). Program of symptom management for improving self-care for patients with HIV/AIDS. *AIDS Patient Care and STDs, 18,* 539–547.

Copperman, L. F., Forwell, S. J., & Hugos, L. (2002). Neuro-degenerative diseases. In C. A. Trombly & M. A. Radomski (Eds.), *Occupational therapy for physical dysfunction* (5th ed., pp. 903–905). Philadelphia: Lippincott Williams & Wilkins.

Glynn, M., & Rhodes, P. (2005). *Estimated HIV prevalence in the United States at the end of 2003.* National HIV Prevention Conference, Atlanta, June 2005.

Inouye, J., Flannelly, L., & Flannelly, K. J. (2001). The effectiveness of self-management training for individuals with HIV/AIDS. *Journal of the Association of Nurses in AIDS Care, 12,* 71–82.

National Institutes of Health. (2005). *HIV infection and AIDS: An overview.* Retrieved May 6, 2006, from http://www.niaid.nih.gov/factsheets/hivinf.htm

National Institutes on Alcohol Abuse and Alcoholism. (2002). Alcohol Alert, 57. Retrieved October 30, 2007, from http://www.nlm.nih.gov/medlineplus/aids.html

Nixon, S., O'Brien, K., Glazier, R. H., & Tynan, A. M. Aerobic exercise interventions for adults living with HIV/AIDS (Cochrane Review). In *The Cochrane Library,* Issue 2, 2007.

Nokes, K. M., Chew, L., & Altman, C. (2003). Using a telephone support group for HIV-positive persons aged 50+ to increase social support and health-related knowledge. *AIDS Patient Care and STDs, 17,* 345–351.

O'Brien K., Nixon S., Glazier R. H., & Tynan A. M. Progressive resistive exercise interventions for adults living with HIV/AIDS. *Cochrane Database of Systematic Reviews* 2004, Issue 4. Art. No. CD004248. DOI: 10.1002/14651858. CD004248.pub2

Rousaud, A., Blanch, J., Hautzinger, M., Lazzari, E., Peri, J. M., Puig, O., et al. (2007). Improvement of psychosocial adjustment to HIV-1 infection through a cognitive-behavioral oriented group psychotherapy program: A pilot study. *AIDS Patient Care and STDs, 21,* 212–222.

JUVENILE RHEUMATOID ARTHRITIS

Kate-Lyn Stone

The information that is presented in this resource sheet is specific to juvenile rheumatoid arthritis (JRA). For general information on rheumatoid arthritis and additional information regarding JRA, please refer to the resource sheet for rheumatoid arthritis.

DESCRIPTION

Juvenile rheumatoid arthritis (JRA) is the most common type of arthritis in children. JRA causes joint stiffness or inflammation in children aged 16 years old or younger. According to the definition of JRA provided by the National Institute of Arthritis and Musculoskeletal and Skin Diseases (2001), the joint inflammation and stiffness that lead to a diagnosis of JRA last for at least six weeks. There are three types of JRA: pauciartricular (four or fewer joints involved), polyartricular (five or more joints involved), and systemic onset (at least one joint involved as well as inflammation in internal organs). JRA has no known cause or cure (Arthritis Foundation, 2007). In terms of etiology, some researchers are considering a two-step process as a cause. The researchers speculate that something in the child's genetics leads to the tendency to develop JRA, and an environmental factor triggers the JRA to emerge (National Institute of Arthritis and Musculoskeletal and Skin Diseases, 2001).

INCIDENCE AND PREVALENCE

◆ Approximately 300,000 children in the United States have some form of arthritis (Nemours Foundation, 2005).

◆ The most prevalent form of arthritis in children is JRA, which affects approximately 50,000 children in the United States (Nemours Foundation, 2005).

SIGNS

The four most common symptoms of JRA are as follows (Arthritis Foundation, 2007):

◆ Joint inflammation
◆ Joint contracture
◆ Joint damage
◆ Alteration/change in growth most evident by impaired mandibular growth resulting in altered morphology and position of the facial skeleton

Other signs of JRA can include the following:

◆ Stiffness, especially after rest or decreased activity level (also called gelling)
◆ Weakness in muscles surrounding the involved joints
◆ Skin erythema and rash

Symptoms include the following:

- Pain
- Fatigue

An important fact to remember about signs and symptoms is that they are different for each child and can vary from day to day in the same child.

TYPES OF JRA

Pauciartricular JRA

About half of all children with JRA have the pauciartricular type. The literal meaning of pauciartricular is "few joints." Knees, ankles, and elbows are the most commonly involved joints in this type of JRA. Rather than being a symmetrical arthritis like adult RA, pauciartricular JRA generally affects a joint on only one side of the body (Arthritis Foundation, 2007).

Polyartricular JRA

About 30% of children with JRA have this type (National Institute of Arthritis and Musculoskeletal and Skin Diseases, 2001). Girls are more commonly affected than boys by polyartricular (meaning "many joints") JRA. Generally, the small joints of the fingers and hands are affected, but JRA can also affect weight-bearing joints such as the ankles, knees, and hips. The neck and jaw can also be affected. Polyartricular JRA is a symmetrical arthritis, meaning that joints on both sides of the body are involved. Signs of JRA can include fever; a positive blood test for rheumatoid factor; nodules on points of the body that receive pressure from chairs, shoes, or other objects; and anemia. Children with polyartricular JRA are at risk for developing damage to joints, which can influence how they grow (Arthritis Foundation, 2007).

Systemic Onset JRA

Systemic onset JRA is the least common form of JRA, only 20% of all children with JRA being affected (National Institute of Arthritis and Musculoskeletal and Skin Diseases, 2001). Boys and girls have equal chances of developing this form of JRA, which is a systemic illness that can affect the child's entire body. Signs of systemic onset JRA include high fevers; rash; arthritis (joint pain and inflammation); inflammation of internal organs; anemia; high white blood cell and platelet counts; and enlarged lymph nodes, liver, or spleen. The disease seems to disappear about one year after onset for about 50% of children with systemic onset JRA (Arthritis Foundation, 2007).

RESOURCES

Associations

- American Juvenile Arthritis Organization
  1330 West Peachtree Street
  Suite 100
  Atlanta, GA 30309
  Telephone: 404-872-7100 or 800-568-4045
  Website: www.arthritis.org
- Kids on the Block, Inc.
  9385-C Gerwig Lane
  Columbia, MD 21046
  Telephone: 410-290-9095 or 800-368-5437
  Website: www.kotb.com

Books

- Parker, J. M. & Parker, P. M. (Eds.) (2002). *The official patient's sourcebook on juvenile rheumatoid arthritis: A revised and updated directory for the internet age.* San Diego: Icon Health Publications.
  This book provides information on virtually all topics related to JRA. It directs individuals living with JRA on where and how to find resources and answers to the many questions that they may have. This book provides research from the most basic to the most advanced levels and draws from sources such as public, academic, and peer-reviewed research.
- Gray, S. H. & Bloch, S. (2002). *Living with juvenile rheumatoid arthritis.* Mankota: World.
  This book is written for younger children and meant to be read aloud. This is a helpful book for children who are trying to deal with living with JRA. It begins with an anecdote from a child and then explains what JRA is and what the disease does to the body.

Journals

- *Journal of Clinical Rheumatology*
- *Annals of the Rheumatic Diseases*
- *Arthritis and Rheumatism*
- *Arthritis Care and Research*

Websites

Please refer to the Arthritis Resource Sheet for helpful websites regarding JRA.

REFERENCES

Arthritis Foundation. (2007). *Juvenile rheumatoid arthritis.* Retrieved September 23, 2007, from, http://ww2.arthritis.org/conditions/DiseaseCenter/jra.asp

National Institute of Arthritis and Musculoskeletal and Skin Diseases. (2001). *Questions and answers about juvenile rheumatoid arthritis.* Bethesda, MD: National Institutes of Health.

Nemours Foundation. (2005). *Juvenile rheumatoid arthritis.* Retrieved September 23, 2007, from, http://www.kidshealth.org/parent/medical/arthritis/jra.html

MULTIPLE SCLEROSIS

Jennifer Keller and Kate-Lyn Stone

Multiple sclerosis (MS) is a progressive neurological condition that is characterized by patches of demyelination of nerves in areas of the brain and the spinal cord, which result in distorted or interrupted transmission of nerve impulses to and from the brain (Beers & Berkow, 1999). MS is considered to be an autoimmune disease. The body's own defense system attacks the myelin sheath that surrounds and protects the nerve fibers of the CNS. The sites where myelin is lost appear as hardened sclerotic (scarred) areas in the CNS and cause a variety of physical and neurological symptoms (Reed, 2001).

PREVALENCE/INCIDENCE

Approximately 400,000 Americans have MS, and every week, about 200 people are diagnosed. Worldwide, MS may affect 2.5 million individuals. Most people with MS are diagnosed between the ages of 20 and 50 years. It affects twice as many women as men.

COURSE

People with MS can expect one of four clinical courses of disease, each of which might be mild, moderate, or severe (National Multiple Sclerosis Society, 2004).

Relapsing-Remitting

In the relapsing-remitting course, the person experiences clearly defined exacerbations (relapses) and episodes of acute worsening of neurological function that are followed by partial or complete recovery periods (remissions) free of disease progression. This is the most common form of MS at time of initial diagnosis (~85%).

Primary-Progressive

In the primary-progressive course, the person experiences a slow but nearly continuous worsening of the disease from the onset, with no distinct relapses or remissions. However, there are variations in rates of progression over time, occasional plateaus, and temporary minor improvements. This course is relatively rare (~10%).

Secondary-Progressive

In the secondary-progressive course, the person experiences an initial period of relapsing-remitting disease followed by a steadily worsening, unpredictable disease course. About 50% of people with relapsing-remitting MS developed this form of the disease within 10 years of their initial diagnosis. However, there is preliminary research to suggest that disease-modifying treatments may significantly delay this progression.

Progressive-Relapsing

In the progressive-relapsing course, the person experiences a steadily worsening disease from the onset but also has clear acute relapses, with or without recovery. In contrast to relapsing-remitting MS, the periods between relapses are characterized by continuing disease progression. This course is relatively rare (~5%).

PROGNOSIS

According to Dirette (2007), approximately 60% of individuals with MS can continue to be fully functional for up to 10 years following their first exacerbation. In addition to this, approximately 30% of individuals with MS continue to be able to function 30 years after their first exacerbation. The fact that an individual is diagnosed with MS does not mean that his or her life expectancy is significantly decreased. There are some individuals, however, who do become quite disabled secondary to MS, and some even die prematurely from infections or complications (Dirette, 2007).

SYMPTOMS

Primary Signs as a Result of Demyelination of the CNS

◆ Muscle stiffness (spasticity) or weakness
◆ Tremulousness in extremities
◆ Paresthesias, numbness, and blunting of sensation (e.g., reduced pain or temperature sense, disturbances of vibratory or position sense)

- Partial or complete paralysis of extremities
- Visual deficits (vision loss, blurred or double vision)
- Extended periods of fatigue
- Interruptions in sexual functioning
- Problems with memory, concentration, information processing, or rapid problem-solving skills
- Visual-spatial deficits
- Difficulty articulating speech
- Fluctuation in mood/depression
- Emotional lability

Secondary Signs

- Pain
- Staggering gait and/or loss of balance
- Poor coordination
- Loss of bladder or bowel control; frequent urinary tract infections
- Anxiety and sleep disturbances
- Contractures and pressure sores
- Decreased ADL skills

Tertiary Signs

- Shift in roles, changing responsibilities
- Social isolation
- Divorce
- Loss of independence
- Stigma of disability (Shapiro, 2003)

INTERDISCIPLINARY TREATMENT

Medications

- Corticosteroids are used to shorten acute attacks, reduce inflammation, and ease symptoms.
- Disease-modifying treatment with injections of the protein interferon-beta reduces the frequency of relapses in MS and might help to delay eventual disability. These medications have shown effectiveness in modifying the natural course of relapsing MS by altering the rate and/or extent of disease progression. Medication management with these "disease modifiers" is recommended as early as possible for individuals with a relapsing course.
- More potent medications are being developed that are effective in slowing down MS that is rapidly worsening or becoming progressive (Beers & Berkow, 1999).

Rehabilitation

- *Physical therapy:* Physical therapy focuses primarily on mobility and the use of mobility aids, spasticity of the muscles, and physical fitness. Personalized exercise programs may help people recover muscle control and

strength after an exacerbation. There is significant evidence associating aerobic exercise with improved quality of life, mobility, endurance, and reduction in fatigue (Mostert & Kesselring, 2002). Hydrotherapy is a popular form of aerobic exercise that addresses the fatigue and weakness experienced by individuals with MS.
- *Occupational therapy:* Occupational therapy focuses on strength, coordination, and fine motor control of the upper extremities. Fatigue and pain management techniques have been well supported as a means to improve occupational performance and satisfaction. Psychosocial intervention is embedded in the treatment plan to address cognitive, emotional, and self-concept issues.
- *Speech therapy:* In progressive forms of MS, problems with speech or swallowing due to muscle weakness or a lack of coordination may need to be addressed.
- *Psychosocial support/counseling:* Individual or group therapy can help individuals with MS and their families to deal with depression, anxiety, and the unpredictability of the disease process. Evidence suggests that a personalized psychosocial rehabilitation program encourages active participation, increased autonomy, and improved quality of life (Ferriani et al., 2002).

OCCUPATIONAL THERAPY EVALUATIONS

Comprehensive Evaluations

- The Functional Assessment of Multiple Sclerosis (FAMS)
- Functional Independence Measure (FIM)
- Multiple Sclerosis Impact Scale (MSIS-29)

ADL Evaluations

- Assessment of Motor and Process Skills (AMPS)
- Barthel Index (BI)

Fatigue Evaluations

- Fatigue Severity Scale (FSS)
- Modified Fatigue Impact Scale (MFIS)

Psychosocial Evaluations

- Beck Depression Inventory (BDI)
- Self-Perceived Burden Scale (SPBS)
- Ways of Coping Checklist (WCC)

Quality of Life/Life Satisfaction Evaluations

- Canadian Occupational Therapy Performance Measure (COPM)
- Health Status Questionnaire (SF-36)

- Multiple Sclerosis QOL Inventory (MSQLI)
- Multiple Sclerosis Quality of Life-54 (MSQOL-54)
- Occupational Performance History Interview (OPHI)

Other Areas to Address

- Balance and coordination
- Caregiver adjustment
- Cognition and memory
- Coping skills
- Daily living skills
- Driving skills
- Environmental barriers
- Fine motor skills
- Leisure interests
- Locus of control
- Muscle strength and spasticity
- Pain and sensation
- Self-concept
- Sexuality
- Vision and perception

OT INTERVENTIONS

- ADL training
- Assistive technology
- Cognitive retraining
- Employment modifications
- Energy conservation
- Environmental modifications
- Home management
- Pain treatment
- ROM/endurance/strengthening for functional activity
- Safety awareness
- Splinting
- Stress management

OT AND THE EVIDENCE

Meta-analysis suggests that occupational therapy–related treatments are effective in treating the deficits associated with MS, particularly for outcomes in the capacity and ability (e.g., muscle strength, ROM, mood) and task and activity (e.g., dressing, bathing, ambulation) levels of performance. The effect sizes for the capacities and abilities outcomes were generally large for studies that examined a specific intervention method, such as exercise, fatigue management, cooling, and transcutaneous electrical nerve stimulator application for pain. A smaller effect size has been shown for emotional and cognitive outcomes, such as stress management, skills training in socialization, and attention training (Baker & Tickle-Degnen, 2001). Alternative therapies including acupuncture, massage,

yoga, meditation, and dietary modifications have shown encouraging results as part of the treatment program for individuals with MS (MS Australia, 2001).

Fatigue is one of the most common targets of OT intervention. It impedes an affected person's ability to fully engage in desired occupational performance and roles. There is significant evidence to support the use of energy conservation education within both community-based and inpatient rehabilitation settings to reduce the impact of fatigue among people with MS and possible positive change associated with peer support (Vanage, Gilbertson, & Mathiowetz, 2003). Energy conservation courses, including education about rest and delegation of tasks to others, have been found to be effective interventions (Holberg & Finlayson, 2007; Matuska, Mathiowetz, & Finlayson, 2007; Vanage et al., 2006).

Coping involves cognitive and behavioral efforts to master, reduce or tolerate an external or internal demand created by a stressful situation. Certain types of coping strategies have been shown to be associated with better or worse adjustment in MS. Many studies in the chronic illness literature have demonstrated that high levels of increasing feelings of self-efficacy, improving quality of life, and lower levels of depression are associated with emotion-focused coping. In contrast, problem-focused coping has been shown to be associated with lower levels of depression and higher levels of adjustment. OT intervention should involve teaching successful coping and integrating it into daily life (Artnett, Higginson, Voss, Randolph, & Grandey, 2002).

CAREGIVER CONCERNS

MS affects people in their most productive years: young adults readying themselves to leave home in pursuit of academic, vocational, or social goals; men and women starting their careers and families of their own; and those in middle age who are enjoying their productive years and planning for retirement. In each of these age groups, the diagnosis of MS has a significant impact on the individual and the family members and/or loved ones in his or her life. Challenges to family coping include the following:

- Individual needs and coping styles
- Disruption in family rhythm
- Disruption in family communication
- Uncertainty and anxiety
- Adaptation and adjustment
- Impact of cognitive changes

Approximately 100,000 people who have MS require help with daily activities or personal care. They receive most of their help from spouses, who typically have major additional responsibilities, including employment and child care. Caregiver burnout has many different causes, including physical strain and emotional stress. Some ways to address these issues include the following:

♦ Effective communication
♦ Relieving pressures of caregiving
♦ Planning and decision making for the future (Kalb, 1998)

RESOURCES

Associations

♦ MS ActiveSource
14 Cambridge Center
Cambridge, MA 02142
Telephone: 800-456-2255
Website: www.msactivesource.com
♦ The National Multiple Sclerosis Society
733 Third Avenue
New York, NY 10017
Telephone: 800-344-4867
Website: www.nmss.org
♦ Through the Looking Glass (for parents)
2198 Sixth St.
Suite 100
Berkeley, CA 94710
Telephone: 800-644-2666
TTY: 800-804-1616
Website: http://lookingglass.org

Journals

♦ *Multiple Sclerosis*
♦ *Disability and Rehabilitation*

First-Person Accounts

♦ Davis, A. (2004). *My story: A photographic essay on life with multiple sclerosis.* New York: Demos Medical Publishing.
Photographs and personal stories of people living with MS, their families, and friends.
♦ Williams, M. (2004). *Climbing higher.* New York: NAL Trade.
In 1999, after almost 20 years of mysterious symptoms that he tried to ignore, Montel Williams, a decorated former naval intelligence officer and Emmy award–winning talk show host, was finally diagnosed with MS. In his personal account, he describes his resourceful approach to the challenges he faced and divergent roads a life can take when diagnosed with MS.
♦ Mackie, C. (1999). *Me and my shadow.* London: Aurum Press.

Mackie was in her early twenties and a flight attendant with British Airways when she was stricken with MS. This book tells about MS and its effects on living, loving, and working. Although it is a moving, personal story of love and loss, it is also profoundly educative.
♦ Mairs, N. (1996). *Waist-high world: A life among the non-disabled.* Boston: Beacon Press.
Nancy Mairs is a gifted essayist who landed in a wheelchair years ago because of degenerative MS that had significantly affected her strength and mobility. In her exploratory essays, there is genuine humor as Mairs addresses issues that range from physical intimacy and a spouse's health problems to concerns with public facilities and her advocacy achievements.

Websites

♦ National Multiple Sclerosis Society
www.nationalmssociety.org
This website provides accurate and current information on diagnosis, treatment, and resources and supports for individuals with MS, their families, and health care providers.
♦ Multiple Sclerosis International Federation
www.msif.org
Comprehensive, international, and ongoing resource developed by experts worldwide. An easily navigated Website that is useful for a variety of audiences and available in many languages.
♦ MS Neighborhood
www.msneighborhood.com
Support and practical advice for individuals with MS. Additional information on clinical trials, treatment, current news, and message board for questions.
♦ Understanding MS
www.understandingms.com
Educational resource for patients and families living with MS, including video transcripts for each topic to reach individuals who are unable to access written material.

REFERENCES

Baker, N., & Tickle-Degnen, L. (2001). The effectiveness of physical, psychological, and functional interventions in treating clients with multiple sclerosis: A meta-analysis. *The American Journal of Occupational Therapy, 55,* 324–331.

Beers, M., & Berkow, R. (1999). The *Merck manual of diagnosis and therapy* (17th ed). Whitehouse Station, NJ: Merck Research Laboratories.

Dirette, D. (2007). Progressive neurological disorders. In B. A. Atchison & D. K. Dirette (Eds.), *Conditions in Occupational*

Therapy (3rd ed., pp. 261–274). Philadelphia: Lippincott Williams and Wilkins.

Ferriani, E., Ravaioli, C., Trombetti, M., Balugani, R., Battaglia, S., & Stecchi, S. (2002). Psychological rehabilitation: An integrated approach to provide the best quality of life in multiple sclerosis patients. *Multiple Sclerosis, 8,* S129–S129.

Holberg, C., & Finlayson, M. (2007). Factors influencing the use of energy conservation strategies by persons with multiple sclerosis. *American Journal of Occupational Therapy, 61,* 96–107.

Kalb, R. (1998). *Multiple sclerosis: A guide for families.* New York: Demos Vermande.

National Multiple Sclerosis Society. (2004). *What is multiple sclerosis?* Retrieved April 4, 2005, from http://www.nationalmssociety.org/What%20is%20MS.asp

Matuska, K., Mathiowetz, V., & Finlayson, M. (2007). Use and perceived effectiveness of energy conservation strategies for managing multiple sclerosis fatigue. *American Journal of Occupational Therapy, 61,* 62–69.

Mostert, S., & Kesselring, J. (2002). Effects of a short-term exercise training program on aerobic fitness, fatigue, health perception and activity level of subjects with multiple sclerosis. *Multiple Sclerosis, 8,* 161–168.

MS Australia. (2001). *Multiple sclerosis: Alternative therapies.* Retrieved April 8, 2005, from http://www.betterhealth.vic.gov.au/bhcv2/bhcarticles.nsf/pages/Multiple_sclerosis_and_alternative_therapies?open

Reed, K. (2001). *Quick reference to occupational therapy* (2nd ed). Gaithersburg, MD: Aspen

Shapiro, R. (2003). *Managing the symptoms of multiple sclerosis.* New York: Demos.

Vanage, S., Gilbertson, K., & Mathiowetz, V. (2003). Effects of an energy conservation course on fatigue impact for persons with progressive multiple sclerosis. *American Journal of Occupational Therapy, 57,* 315–323.

MYOCARDIAL INFARCTION

Kate-Lyn Stone

DIAGNOSIS

Myocardial infarction (MI) is also referred to as *heart attack, acute MI, acute coronary syndrome, coronary thrombosis,* or *coronary occlusion* (National Heart Lung and Blood Institute, 2007). It occurs when the heart is starved of oxygen because of a lack of blood supply. This causes the heart muscle to die or to become permanently damaged (Weinrauch, 2007). The most common site of a myocardial infarction is the left ventricle (American Heart Association, 2007).

INCIDENCE AND PREVALENCE

◆ Approximately one of every five deaths in the United States is caused by a heart attack (Weinrauch, 2007).
◆ In the United States, about 1.1 million people have a heart attack each year, and about 50% of these people die (National Heart Lung and Blood Institute, 2007).

ETIOLOGY

The coronary arteries are the arteries that are responsible for bringing blood, and thus oxygen, to the heart. When a coronary artery becomes blocked by a blood clot, blood cannot get to the heart. This starves the heart of oxygen, and a myocardial infarction is generally the result (Weinrauch, 2007). The most common underlying cause of myocardial infarction is atherosclerotic heart disease (American Heart Association, 2007).

Risk factors for myocardial infarction include the following (Weinrauch, 2007):

◆ Hereditary factors
◆ Gender, males being more likely to suffer a heart attack
◆ Diabetes
◆ Aging
◆ High blood pressure
◆ Smoking
◆ Poor eating habits
◆ High LDL cholesterol levels
◆ Abnormally high levels of homocysteine (an amino acid), C-reactive protein (related to inflammation), and fibrinogen (involved in blood clotting)
◆ In some cases, extremely high levels of stress can lead to a heart attack

SIGNS AND SYMPTOMS

Symptoms of a myocardial infarction include the following (Weinrauch, 2007):

◆ Chest pain, usually lasting longer than 20 minutes; can be mild or severe and can feel like heavy pressure, squeezing, or bad indigestion
◆ Shortness of breath
◆ Nausea
◆ Anxiety

◆ Dizziness
◆ Palpations in the heart

Signs of a myocardial infarction include the following:

◆ Sweating
◆ Fainting
◆ Cough

SEQUENCE OF CARE

A myocardial infarction is a medical emergency that can result in death if health care is not sought immediately once symptoms begin to appear. Individuals have the best prognosis if they begin to receive treatment within the first hour after symptoms occur (National Heart Lung and Blood Institute, 2007). On admission, the physician will conduct a physical examination, including examination of the client's heart and lungs. Pulse and blood pressure may also be monitored. Tests that look specifically at the heart are then administered. Such tests include coronary angiography, CT scan, echocardiography, electrocardiogram, MRI, and nuclear ventriculography. Blood tests may also be used to look for substances that are indicative of heart tissue damage (Weinrauch, 2007).

If diagnosed with a heart attack, the individual will need to stay in the hospital. Oxygen will be administered, regardless of whether levels are normal or abnormal, to decrease cardiac load. Some clients will receive thrombolytic therapy, which involves giving the clients blood thinners within the first 12 hours of the onset of chest pain. Thrombolytic therapy is not appropriate for all clients, especially women who are pregnant, people who have had a stroke or head injury in the past three months, people with high blood pressure, or people with a history of using blood thinners. Angioplasty, a surgery to open blocked arteries, may be used instead of thrombolytic therapy. Other medicines that are used for myocardial infarction include nitroglycerin (to decrease chest pain), antiplatelet medicines (to prevent clot formations), beta-blockers (to reduce strain on the heart), and ACE inhibitors (to prevent heat failure). In some cases, the patient might need emergency coronary artery bypass surgery (Weinrauch, 2007).

PREVENTION

There are several ways in which people can decrease their chances of having a myocardial infarction, or heart attack. These include the following (Weinrauch, 2007):

◆ Maintain good blood pressure and cholesterol levels.
◆ Do not smoke.
◆ Eat a well-balanced, low-fat diet.
◆ Exercise consistently.
◆ If overweight, lose weight safely, but consult your health care provider before doing so.
◆ Use aspirin therapy, but consult your physician before beginning this on your own.

ROLE OF OT

See the resource list sheet in cardiac conditions.

RESOURCES

Please refer to the resource sheet on cardiac conditions for further information on resources for myocardial infarction.

REFERENCES

American Heart Association. (2007). *Myocardial ischemia, injury, and infarction.* Retrieved October 9, 2007, from http://www.americanheart.org/presenter.jhtml?identifier=251

National Heart Lung and Blood Institute. (2007). *What is heart attack?* Retrieved October 9, 2007, from http://www.nhlbi.nih.gov/health/dci/Diseases/HeartAttack/HeartAttack_WhatIs.html

Weinrauch, L. (2007). *Heart attack. Medline Plus.* Retrieved October 8, 2007, from http://www.nlm.nih.gov/medlineplus/ency/article/000195.htm

OPPOSITIONAL DEFIANT DISORDER

Karen Marticello

Oppositional defiant disorder (ODD) is a recurrent pattern of negativistic, defiant, disobedient, and hostile behavior toward authority figures that persists for at least six months (American Psychiatric Association, 2000).

PREVALENCE

The prevalence rate of ODD is 2–16%. After puberty, this condition is as prevalent in girls as in boys (Prairienet Community Resources, 2005).

ETIOLOGY AND RISK FACTORS

Biological factors have been supported by the demonstration of genetic correlations, atypical frontal lobe activation patterns, and underarousal of the physiological factors, such as lower heart rate. Child functional factors including temperament and intensity of reactions to negative stimuli may contribute to ODD. Psychosocial factors include family instability, economic stress, parental mental illness, harsh punitive behaviors, inconsistent parenting practices, multiple moves, and divorce (Burke, Loeber, & Birmaher, 2002).

COURSE AND SYMPTOMS

The course of ODD is different in different people. It is a disorder of childhood and adolescence that usually begins by age 8, if not earlier. Symptoms include the following:

- Losing one's temper
- Arguing with adults
- Actively defying requests
- Refusing to follow rules
- Deliberately annoying other people
- Blaming others for one's mistakes
- Being touchy, easily angered or annoyed, resentful, spiteful, or vindictive (American Psychiatric Association, 2000).

Symptoms may change. Younger children are likely to engage in defiant behaviors, and older children are likely to engage in covert behavior such as stealing. In some children, ODD evolves into a conduct disorder or mood disorder. Later in life, this condition may evolve into antisocial personality disorder.

COMORBID CONDITIONS

Diagnosis is complicated by relatively high rates of comorbid disruptive behavior disorders. Some symptoms of attention-deficit/hyperactivity (ADHD) disorder and conduct disorder overlap. In some children, ODD may be the developmental precursor for conduct disorder. Comorbidity of ODD with ADHD has been reported to occur in 50–65% of children with ODD. ODD commonly occurs with anxiety and depressive disorders, as well as with learning disabilities and academic difficulties (Greene et al., 2002). ODD is often misdiagnosed in children with a history of trauma whose behaviors are related to neural disorders, that is, sensory-processing disorders (B. Atchison, personal communication, July 28, 2007).

PRECAUTIONS

In problem situations, children with ODD are more likely to react with aggressive physical actions than verbal ones. Professionals should be aware of their own safety and the safety of those around them (eMedicine, 2005).

INTERDISCIPLINARY TREATMENT

Multidimensional Intervention Foster Care

A broad based-intervention that targets many family and extrafamilial factors while the child is on out-of-home placement. This intervention involves placing a child or adolescent in the home of a foster parent who has been trained in behavior management skills. The foster parent establishes an individualized plan to reinforce desired self-management, academic, and social behaviors (Woolfenden, Williams, & Peat, 2005).

Pharmacotherapy

Medication treatment alone appears to be an ineffective method of treating ODD. However, it can be effective for treating some symptoms of comorbid disorders.

OT EVALUATIONS

Home

- Children Helping Out: Responsibilities, Expectations, and Supports (CHORES)
- Behavior Assessment Rating Scale (BASC)
- Test of Environmental Supportiveness (TOES)

Community

- Social Skills Rating System (SSRS)
- The Work Environmental Impact Scale (WEIS)

School

- School Function Assessment (SFA)
- Occupational Therapy Psychosocial Assessment of Learning (OTPAC)

Individual

- Toddler Behavior Assessment Questionnaire
- Coping Inventory
- Children's Assessment of Participation and Enjoyment (CAPE)
- Pediatric Interest Profile (PIP)
- Play History

♦ Preferences for Activities of Children (PAC)
♦ Sensory Profile

Family

♦ Stress Management Questionnaire
♦ Parenting Stress Index (PSI)

OT INTERVENTION

Intervention for ODD is complex and challenging. Children with ODD are frequently uncooperative and experience feelings of fear and mistrust toward authority. Intervention involves a multimodal, psychosocial approach that includes parent training, social skills training, and group therapy.

Interventions with the Child

Social Skills Training, Problem Solving, and Anger Management

Children with ODD and conduct problems show cognitive and behavioral deficits with peers. These children often have limited social and conflict resolution skills, loneliness and negative attributions, inability to empathize or understand others' perspectives, and limited use of feeling language.

Cognitive behavioral intervention activities may include the following:

♦ Videotape modeling and role-plays to provide opportunities to reenact conflict situations using coping skills and acceptable solutions.
♦ Read and discuss stories depicting children solving social problems and then sharing feelings about the stories.
♦ Strategies to strengthen motivation, hold attention, and reinforce key concepts and newly acquired skills (Webster-Stratton, Reid, & Hammond, 2001).

Child-Centered Intervention

The child initiates activities while the therapist creates a positive environment. This intervention is useful for building rapport.

Interest Groups

Interest groups assist the child in developing interests that can be used during frustrating times or for practicing social skills.

Socratic Questioning

This intervention involves asking questions to guide a child through a problem situation, such as "Why did you choose to do that?" (Garlikov, 2003).

Behavior Management

Use of behavior-recording charts, a time-out process, and alternating liked and disliked activities.

Interventions with Parents

Behavioral Parent Training

This intervention is based on the assumption that the child's behavior is related to past and current interactions with significant others and that the behavior of these significant people must be changed to change the child's behavior (Nixon, 2002).

Intervention strategies include the following:

♦ Teaching parents to attend to and praise their child's appropriate behaviors through the use of techniques such as providing simple and clear commands and using time-outs.
♦ Labeled praise involves describing enthusiastically what the child is doing whenever possible to inform the child of what is clearly appropriate behavior.
♦ Role-playing of techniques to generalize strategies to different environments (e.g., going to the grocery store or visiting friends).

Stress Management

♦ Coping skills training provides resources for parent support groups and instruction in time management instruction, cognitive restructuring, and social skills and assertive training.
♦ Other stress management techniques include exercise, deep breathing, meditation, verbalization, and exploration of leisure interests and participation (Mindtools, 2005).

Interventions in the Environment

A sensory integration approach adapts aspects of the environment to promote self-regulation and attention (i.e., limit distractions) and to decrease hyperactivity. This approach also includes developing structure and routines as well as successful transitions within home and school activities.

OT AND THE EVIDENCE

The occupational therapy literature does not contain recent and relevant evidence regarding this topic; therefore, evidence from other peer-reviewed journals is presented here.

Results from a social skills and problem-solving training group indicate that this intervention was successful in producing clinically and statistically significant improvements in child conduct problems (i.e., aggression) and in children's cognitive social problem-solving strategies after treatment. Parent and teacher reports and independent observations indicated that these changes were produced both at home and in the classroom, suggesting generalized improvements across settings (Webster-Stratton, Reid, & Hammond, 2001).

CAREGIVER CONCERNS

ODD can have a negative effect on the family environment, leading to less cohesion, more conflict, and increased parental stress. However, this relationship is reciprocal, since many parental factors have been identified as risk factors for ODD. Parental mental illness (including substance abuse, depression, and antisocial personality disorder), physical punishment, marital discord and divorce, and socioeconomic status have all been correlated with ODD. Therefore, effective treatment of ODD may include services for the parents such as mental health services, vocational and money management skills training, and education regarding community resources to address these concerns (Burke et al., 2002; eMedicine, 2005).

RESOURCES

Associations

- The American Academy of Child and Adolescent Psychiatry
  3615 Wisconsin Avenue
  Washington, D.C. 20016
  Telephone: 202-966-7300
  Website: www.aacap.org
- The National Mental Health Association
  2001 N. Beauregard Street
  12th Floor
  Alexandria, VA 22311
  Telephone 703-684-7722
  Website: www.nmha.org

Books

- Greene, R. (2001). *The explosive child: A new approach for understanding and parenting easily frustrated, chronically inflexible children.* New York: HarperCollins.
  This book provides parents with many examples of children with behavior problems and an approach for managing these behavioral problems.
- Keith, D. V., Connell, G. M., & Connell, L. C. (2000). *Defiance in the family: Finding hope in therapy.* Philadelphia: Taylor & Francis.
  Written primarily for therapists, this book describes how family therapy can rebuild family relationships.

Journals

- *American Journal of Psychiatry*
- *Journal of the American Academy of Child and Adolescent Psychiatry*
- *Journal of Child Psychology and Psychiatry*

Websites

- Dore Frances: Oppositional Defiant Disorder
  http://www.dorefrances.com/articles.php?id=14
  Contains up-to-date information for parents about ODD and schooling options for their child. Also provides help hotlines for both parents and adolescents.
- Dr. Grohol's Psych Central: Oppositional Defiant Disorder
  http://psychcentral.com/disorders/sx73.htm
  Provides information about diagnosis, symptoms, and treatment. Also contains links to chat rooms and support forums.

REFERENCES

American Psychiatric Association. (2000). *Diagnostic and statistical manual of mental disorders* (4th ed., text rev.). Washington, DC: Author.

Burke, J. D., Loeber, R., & Birmaher, B. (2002). Oppositional defiant disorder and conduct disorder: A review of the past 10 years, part II. *Journal of the American Academy of Child and Adolescent Psychiatry, 41*(11), 1275–1293.

eMedicine. (2005). *Oppositional defiant disorder.* Retrieved February 24, 2005, from http://emedicine.com/ped/topic2791.htm

Garlikov, R. (2003). *The Socratic method: Teaching by asking instead of by telling.* Retrieved April 11, 2005, from http://www.garlikov.com/Soc_Meth.html

Greene, R. W., Biederman, J., Zerwas, S., Monuteaux, M. C., Goring, J. C., & Faraone, S. V. (2002). Psychiatric comorbidity, family dysfunction, and social impairment in referred youth with oppositional defiant disorder. *American Journal of Psychiatry, 159,* 1214–1224.

Mindtools. (2005). *Stress management techniques.* Retrieved April 1, 2005, from http://www.mindtools.com/smpage.html

Nixon, R. D. (2002). Treatment of behavior problems in preschoolers: A review of parent training programs. *Clinical Psychology Review, 22*(4), 525–546.

Prairienet Community Resources. (2005). *Conduct disorder and oppositional defiant disorder.* Retrieved April 1, 2005, from http://dcfwebresource.prairienet.org/resources/conduct disorder_guide.php

Webster-Stratton, C., Reid, J., & Hammond, M. (2001). Social skills and problem solving training for children with early onset conduct problems: Who benefits? *Journal of Child Psychology & Psychiatry & Allied Disciplines, 42*(7), 943–952.

Webster-Stratton, C., Reid, J., & Hammond, M. (2004). Treating children with early-onset conduct problems: Intervention outcomes for parent, child, and teacher training. *Journal of Clinical Child and Adolescent Psychology, 33*(1), 105–124.

Woolfenden, S. R., Williams, K., & Peat, J. (2005). Family and parenting interventions in children and adolescents with conduct disorder and delinquency aged 10–17. *The Cochrane Database of Systematic Reviews,* Issue 1.

ASSESSMENT REFERENCES

Coster, W. J., Deeney, T., Haltiwanger, J., & Haley, S. M. (1998). *School Function Assessment.* San Antonio, TX: Psychological Corporation/Therapy Skill Builders.

Dunn, L. (2004). Validation of the CHORES: A measure of school-aged children's participation in household tasks. *Scandinavian Journal of Occupational Therapy, 11,* 179–190.

Dunn, W. (1999). *Sensory profile: User's manual.* San Antonio, TX: Psychological Corporation.

Gresham, F. M., & Elliot, S. N. (1990). *Social Skills Rating System: Manual.* Circle Pines, MN: American Guidance Service.

Goldsmith, H. H. (1996). Studying temperament via construction of the Toddler Behavior Assessment Questionnaire. *Child Development, 67,* 218–235.

Henry, A. D. (2000). *Pediatric Interest Profiles: Surveys of play for children and adolescents.* Therapy Skill Builders.

Kielhofner, G. (2002). *A model of human occupation: Theory and application* (3rd ed., pp. 257–258) Baltimore: Lippincott, Williams & Wilkins.

Reynolds, C. R., & Kamphaus, R. W. (1992). *Behavior assessment system for children: Manual.* Circle Pines, MN: American Guidance.

OSTEOARTHRITIS

Kate-Lyn Stone

Osteoarthritis (OA) is the most common form of arthritis. It is also the oldest form; evidence of the disease has been found in Ice Age skeletons (Arthritis Foundation, 2007). OA can also be referred to as *degenerative joint disease, hypertrophic arthritis,* and *degenerative arthritis.* OA is a chronic condition that is commonly known as "wear-and-tear" arthritis because of the breakdown of the cartilage in the joints. When the cartilage wears away in this fashion, the bones of the joint rub together, causing stiffness and pain. The cause of OA is still unknown, and there is no cure (Arthritis Foundation, 2007).

There are two types of OA: primary and secondary. Primary OA is the "wear-and-tear" arthritis that is generally associated with aging. Secondary OA classifies all osteoarthritis that is not associated with aging. With secondary OA, there is an evident cause such as injury, heredity, or obesity.

INCIDENCE AND PREVALENCE

- Twenty-one million Americans live with OA (Arthritis Foundation, 2007).
- The incidence of OA increases with age; in other words, the older a person is, the more likely he or she is to develop OA.
- Under age 55, men are more likely to get OA than women are. Over age 55, women are more likely to have the condition (Arthritis Foundation, 2007).
- OA is the number one cause of disability in industrialized nations (Medline Plus, 2005).

TYPICAL COURSE OF DISEASE

There are several stages of OA including the following (Arthritis Foundation, 2007):

- The cartilage begins to break down and lose elasticity. It becomes more easily damaged by injury or overuse.
- The bone lying beneath the cartilage begins to change because of the breakdown of the cartilage. The bone may thicken, cysts may form, or bony growths known as spurs may appear at the end of the bone.
- Small pieces of bone or cartilage may detach from the joint and float loosely in the joint space.
- The synovium (the joint lining) becomes inflamed, causing inflammation proteins, known as cytokines, to further damage the already worn cartilage.

The knees, lower back, hips, fingers, and neck are the most common areas of the body to develop OA. The base of the thumb and the big toe can also be affected by OA.

SEQUENCE OF CARE

The primary care physician will begin by taking the individual's medical history and completing a thorough physical examination. During the physical exam, the physician looks for common signs of OA, such as joint swelling or tenderness, decreased range of motion, and joint damage. The physician may choose to have X-rays taken to confirm a diagnosis of OA. Joint aspiration, or draining fluid from the joint to look for crystals, is another tool that is used to rule out other conditions or diseases. Once the diagnosis has been confirmed, the patient may be referred to a rheumatologist, a doctor who specializes in arthritis, depending on the severity of the case.

Goals of a plan to treat OA include decreasing pain, increasing the ability to function on a day-to-day basis, and decreasing the speed at which the disease is progressing. A drug regime may be prescribed to begin combating OA, but ultimately, it is the lifestyle changes that the individual makes that determine how well he or she lives with the condition. Treatment plans may also include exercise, diet modification for weight control, joint protection, physical therapy, and occupational therapy. Surgery may be considered for severe cases that do not seem to be improving with other interventions (Arthritis Foundation, 2007).

SYMPTOMS

Several or all of the following symptoms may occur for an individual with OA. It is important to remember that each individual is affected by the disease differently, so symptoms will vary. The most common symptoms of OA are as follows:

- Soreness, especially after inactivity or overuse
- Stiffness
- Morning stiffness, which generally goes away within half an hour
- Pain, which is usually caused by the weakening of the muscles surrounding the joint secondary to inactivity
- Pain in the joint that generally increases over the course of the day because of the day's activities
- Irritation
- Grating of the joint
- Decreased ability of the joints to absorb shock
- Limited use of joint
- Limited range of motion
- Decreased coordination, poor posture, and difficulty walking because of pain and stiffness

For more detailed information about symptoms in each area of the body, refer to the Arthritis Foundation's Website (http://www.arthritis.org/).

ETIOLOGY

The cause of OA is unknown. There are, however, several risk factors that are thought to play a role in whether or not an individual develops OA, including age, obesity, genetics, muscle weakness, overuse of the joint, injury, other disease, or forms of arthritis. For more information on how each factor relates to the risk of developing OA, refer to http://www.arthritis.org/. An individual could acquire OA as a result of two or several of these factors combined (Arthritis Foundation, 2007). Knowing and understanding what the risk factors are can help to decrease the chances of developing this chronic condition.

INTERVENTIONS

There are several treatment options that may be beneficial in slowing the progress of OA, decreasing pain, and increasing function. These interventions include the following (Arthritis Foundation. 2007):

- Medications, generally nonsteroidal, anti-inflammatory drugs (NSAIDs)
- Physical therapy
- Occupational therapy
- Chiropractic services
- Surgery
- Glucosamine, an amino sugar, and chondroitin sulfate, part of a protein (both dietary supplements), for pain relief
- Vitamins to help ease some symptoms
- Exercise to reduce pain, increase muscle strength, and improve movement
- Weight control to reduce stress on joints
- Education about self-management for OA, including information about taking breaks, pacing oneself, keeping active, using proper body mechanics, and setting realistic goals

PREVENTION

Primary Prevention: Stop OA Before It Develops

Maintaining a healthy weight reduces the risk of an individual's developing osteoarthritis, especially in the knees. Keeping active in general reduces the risk for obesity, which in turn lessens the stress on joints and keeps them healthy (Sacks & Sniezek, 2003).

Secondary Prevention: Early Diagnosis and Good Management

By diagnosing OA early, an individual can begin to take appropriate medication to positively affect the course of the disease. Medications can also decrease pain (Sacks & Sniezek, 2003).

Tertiary Prevention: Increase Self-Management

Self-management education, weight control, and physical activity all help an individual who has been diagnosed with OA have a better sense of control over his or her life. This improves overall quality of life while one is living with OA (Sacks & Sniezek, 2003).

TYPICAL OT EVALUATION

Comprehensive Assessments

- Functional Independence Measure (FIM)
- Assessment of Motor and Process Skills (AMPS)

Quality of Life/Life Satisfaction Assessments

- Canadian Occupational Performance Measure (COPM)
- Role Interest Checklist

- Short Form-36 Health Survey (SF-36)
- Worker Role Inventory

Psychosocial Assessments

- Geriatric Depression Scale

Other Assessments

- Manual muscle testing
- Range-of-motion testing
- Pain scales
- Home assessment

TYPICAL OT INTERVENTION

Because each individual is affected by OA differently, the occupational therapist should take a top-down approach to ensure focus on each client's unique needs (Mallinson et al., 2005). This means that there is a focus on a broad range of barriers to functioning versus a focus on specific symptoms that are blocking function.

Occupational therapy programs for treating OA generally focus on the following:

- ADL
- Energy conservation techniques
- Strengthening exercises
- Pain management
- Assistive technology
- Adapt environment
- Adaptive equipment
- Patient and family education
- Home planning
- Splinting to support limbs
- Education about self-management, including learning techniques to reduce pain, proper exercise, weight management, and joint protection (National Center for Chronic Disease Prevention and Health Promotion, 2007)

OT AND EVIDENCE

Egan and Brousseau (2007) found splinting to be an effective intervention for decreasing pain and increasing function in individuals with carpometacarpal OA. They did not find one splint to be superior to the other for providing pain relief other than in terms of patient preference. Because of this, the researchers suggest taking a client-centered approach when choosing a splint for a client with OA.

Lorig, Ritter, and Plant (2005) compared the disease-specific Arthritis Self-Management Program (ASMP) with the generalized Chronic Disease Self-Management Program (CDSMP) for individuals with arthritis. They found that the ASMP should be considered as a first choice of self-management programs, since individ-

uals with arthritis at four months showed improvements in conditions. At one year, there was no difference between the ASMP and the CDSMP, suggesting that both programs are effective in improving the quality of life for individuals with arthritis.

RESOURCES

Associations

- American College of Rheumatology
  1800 Century Place, Suite 250
  Atlanta, GA 30345-4300
  Telephone: 404-633-3777
  Fax: 404-633-1870
  Website: http://www.rheumatology.org/
- Arthritis Foundation
  P.O. Box 7669
  Atlanta, GA 30357-0669
  Telephone: 1-800-283-7800
  Website: http://www.arthritis.org/
- Centers for Disease Control and Prevention
  National Center for Chronic Disease Prevention and Health Promotion
  Arthritis Section
  Mailstop K-51
  4770 Buford Highway NE
  Atlanta, GA 30341-3724
  Telephone: 770-488-5464
  Fax: 770-488-5964
  Website: http://www.cdc.gov/arthritis/
- National Institute of Arthritis and Musculoskeletal and Skin Diseases
  Information Clearinghouse
  National Institutes of Health
  1 AMS Circle
  Bethesda, MD 20892-3675
  Telephone: 1-877-226-4267
  Fax: 301-718-6366
  Website: http://www.niams.nih.gov/

Programs

- Arthritis Foundation Self-Help Program (AFSHP)
  This six-week program helps individuals with arthritis learn how to manage their condition on a day-to-day basis. It was developed by Dr. Kate Lorig of Stanford University. Studies done on this intervention report that participants experience a 20% decrease in pain and a 40% decrease in doctors' visits. As of 2007, there were 36 CDC-funded state arthritis programs.
- Chronic Disease Self-Management Program (CDSMP). This six-week program teaches self-management education for individuals with chronic diseases or conditions, including arthritis, diabetes, heart disease, and lung disease. This program was created and developed at Stan-

ford University. As of 2007, there were 36 CDC-funded state chronic disease programs.

- Arthritis Foundation Exercise Program (AFEP)
This program, developed by the Arthritis Foundation, is a community-based, recreational program that focuses on range of motion exercises, endurance building, stress management, relaxation techniques, and other topics related to health. This program is unique in that it can be tailored to meet each participant's individual needs.
- Arthritis Foundation Aquatic Program (AFAP)
This exercise program, developed by the Arthritis Foundation, is an aquatic program that works to increase flexibility, endurance, and range of motion while decreasing pain because there is less impact on the joints in the water environment.
- EnhanceFitness
Formerly known as Lifetime Fitness, this program is an evidence-based, community exercise program. It has been proven to increase strength and activity levels in individuals with arthritis.

Books

- Sharma, L. (2007). *Osteoarthritis*. Philadelphia: Elsevier Health Sciences.
- Klippel, J. H., Stone, J. H., Crofford, L. J., & White, P. (Eds.), (2001). *Primer on the rheumatic diseases*. New York: Arthritis Foundation.

Journals

- *Annals of the Rheumatic Diseases*
- *Arthritis and Rheumatism*
- *Arthritis Care and Research*
- *Journal of Rheumatology*

Websites

- Arthritis Foundation
http://www.arthritis.org/
The Arthritis Foundation is dedicated to improving the lives of individuals with arthritis through providing leadership in the prevention, control, and cure of this disease and its related conditions. The Foundation's website provides information about arthritis, medication used to treat the illness, as well as the latest research regarding arthritis.
- Centers for Disease Control and Prevention
http://www.cdc.gov/arthritis/
This website is the CDC's Arthritis Program. This program is working to measure the incidence and prevalence of arthritis, strengthen the science and research behind arthritis, increase awareness of the disease, and build state arthritis programs. The website contains a wealth of information in all of these topics as well as information about the state programs and links to these sites and other resources regarding arthritis.

REFERENCES

Arthritis Foundation. (2007). *Osteoarthritis*. Retrieved September 4, 2007, from http://www.arthritis.org/disease-center.php?disease_id=32

Egan, M., & Brousseau, L. (2007). Splinting for osteoarthritis of the carpometacarpal joint: A review of the evidence. *American Journal of Occupational Therapy, 61,* 70–78.

Lorig, K., Ritter, P. L., & Plant, K. (2005). A disease-specific self-help program compared with a generalized chronic disease self-help program for arthritis patients. *Arthritis and Rheumatism, 53,* 950–957.

Mallinson, T., Waldinger, H., Semanik, P., Lyons, J., Feinglass, J., & Chang, R. (2005). Promoting physical activity in persons with arthritis. *OT Practice, 10,* 10.

Medline Plus. (2005). *Osteoarthritis*. Retrieved September 4, 2007, from http://www.nlm.nih.gov/medlineplus/ency/article/000423.htm

National Center for Chronic Disease Prevention and Health Promotion. (2007). *Arthritis*. Retrieved September 3, 2007, from http://www.cdc.gov/arthritis/

Sacks, J. J, & Sniezek, J. E. (2003). Targeting arthritis: The nation's leading cause of disability. In *Promising Practices in Chronic Disease Prevention and Control: A Public Health Framework for Action* (pp. 5–19). Atlanta: Centers for Disease Control and Prevention.

OSTEOPOROSIS

Stephanie Grant

Osteoporosis is a disease that involves low bone mass and microarchitectural deterioration of bone tissue that leads to bone fragility and increased fracture risk particularly at the hip, spine, and wrist (Osteoporosis, 2005).

INCIDENCE AND PREVALENCE

Osteoporosis is a major public health threat for 44 million Americans, with more than 200 million people affected worldwide (International Osteoporosis Foundation, 2007; National Osteoporosis Foundation, 2007). It is estimated that 50% of women and 20% of men over 50 in the United States will have an osteoporosis related fracture during their lifetime (NOF, 2007). Risk for osteoporosis increases with age but can affect any age group. Osteoporotic fractures are associated with significant morbidity and disability leading to substantial burden on the individual, the person's family, and society (Hallberg, 2004).

DIAGNOSTIC CRITERIA, SIGNS AND SYMPTOMS

Osteoporosis is classified as either primary or secondary. Primary osteoporosis, the most common form of the disease, is the loss of bone mineral density because of altered bone remodeling that occurs within the bone itself and appears to be influenced by total bone accrual at the time of peak bone density and, in women, estrogen decline (IOF, 2007; NOF, 2007). Secondary osteoporosis is bone loss due to another cause outside of the skeletal system, such as medication-induced bone loss (including corticosteroids, anticonvulsants, or cancer therapies), rheumatoid arthritis or malabsorption syndromes (IOF, 2007; NOF, 2007).

In 1994, the World Health Organization published the WHO Diagnostic Criteria for Osteoporosis (World Health Organization Study Group, 1994):

- *Normal:* Bone mineral density (BMD) value within 1 standard deviation (S.D.) of the young-adult mean (T-score at or above −1)
- *Osteopenia:* BMD value between 1 and 2.5 S.D. below the young-adult mean (T-score between −1 and −2.5)
- *Osteoporosis:* BMD value at least 2.5 S.D. below the young adult mean (T-score at or below −2.5)
- *Severe osteoporosis:* BMD value at least 2.5 S.D. below the young adult mean and presence of fracture

While these criteria remain an important diagnostic element, research in the field has indicated that the T-score is one of many factors contributing to fracture risk, so a thorough assessment of fracture risk is important in making a diagnosis.

Fracture risk assessment is critical for individuals over the age of 65 and should include a thorough history to determine whether the individual has the following risks: is on medications that cause bone loss, smokes, sustained a fracture after age 50, has a family history of osteoporosis or parental hip fracture. Next, fracture risk assessment should examine risk to fall, low body weight or low body mass index, and inability to stand from a seated position without help or the use of the hands (Black et al., 2001; Kanis et al., 2005).

COURSE AND PROGNOSIS

Osteoporosis is not a disease of aging. In fact, it is a geriatric disease with an adolescent onset. Peak bone mass occurs in early adulthood. Therefore, accrual of bone and prevention of bone loss are essential in childhood and adolescence. This process can be negatively affected by many childhood nutrition and activity habits as well as by diseases such as anorexia nervosa, cancer, and cystic fibrosis (Bachrach, 2001).

The early stage of this disease is typically silent in nature, with few, if any, symptoms. Often, the first symptom of osteoporosis is a fracture. Early diagnosis can lead to a significantly reduced risk for fracture and loss of independence. In later stages, osteoporosis can be associated with or cause loss of height; postural changes, including kyphosis; muscle weakness, pain, particularly at the back; balance impairment; decreased health-related quality of life; and eventual loss of independence (NOF, 2007).

MEDICAL TREATMENT

Medical intervention for osteoporosis is targeted at reducing fracture risk. Increasing bone density and improving bone microarchitecture can be addressed with pharmacotherapy such as antiresorptives or anabolic agents. Antiresorptives assist in preventing additional bone loss and come in the form of bisphosphonates, selective estrogen receptor modulators, calcitonin, and estrogens. The anabolic agent teriparitide assists the body to rebuild bone. All individuals with low bone density should be counseled to take calcium (1,500 mg/day) and vitamin D (800 IU/day). In some cases, individuals may have such low vitamin D levels that they need to have vitamin D injections before beginning a pharmacotherapy regimen (NOF, 2007).

OT EVALUATION

Because osteoporosis affects so many areas of physical functioning, occupational therapists have used many assessment tools with this population.

- Canadian Occupational Performance Measure (COPM) (Law et al., 1990)
  Semistructured interview. A client-centered outcome measure that examines a client's perceptions with regard to an occupation's importance as well as performance and satisfaction with occupations. This is an effective assessment tool to use with individuals who have severe osteoporosis and related physical symptoms but has been found to have a ceiling effect in individuals with the disease who have few or no symptoms (Edwards, Baptiste, Stratford, & Law, 2007; Randles, Randolph, Schell, & Grant, 2004).
- The FRACTURE Index (Black et al., 2001)
  Evaluates and predicts an individual's fracture risk at the spine, hip, and other nonvertebral areas over the next five years.
- The Mini-Osteoporosis Quality of Life Questionnaire (Mini-OQLQ) (Ioannidis, Adachi, & Guyatt, 1999)

Self-administered and quickly completed. Examines five domains: symptoms, physical function, activities of daily living, emotional function, and leisure.

♦ The Bone Safety Evaluation (Recknor et al., 2005)
A comprehensive assessment and an osteoporosis database registry. Qualitatively and quantitatively evaluates a client's risk for fracture. A physical functional performance measure that analyzes spinal compression forces, balance, strength, flexibility, and physical symptoms with valued activities and quality of life. Calculates musculoskeletal functioning with health-related quality of life.

Occupational therapists who work with children can help to identify children who are at risk for bone loss and design intervention strategies to optimize nutrition and weight-bearing activity.

OT INTERVENTION

Occupational therapy intervention in this population focuses on rehabilitating individuals who have sustained a fracture and on fracture risk reduction for these clients as well as for individuals who are not currently coping with a new fracture. Because rehabilitation of specific fractures is beyond the scope of this resource sheet, the reader is referred to the Resources section below for where to locate this information. Occupational therapy should aim to maximize an individual's occupational performance as it relates to the person's current elevated fracture risk state. The occupational therapist should determine the activities that both are highly valued by the client and pose a risk for fracture.

♦ *Education:* Education on the osteoporosis condition to build awareness is important because this disease begins silently (Munch & Shapiro, 2006).
♦ *Safe movement:* The occupational therapist should focus on occupation-specific instruction in safe movement patterns to reduce spinal compression forces during daily activities (Meeks, 1999; NOF, 2007). Clients can learn about the safety precautions associated with osteoporosis by reading a fact sheet but are often unsure how to apply these precautions to daily activity without the help of an occupational therapist (Randles et al., 2004).
♦ *Quality of life:* When the osteoporosis condition is more severe, a client is likely to present with back pain, weakness, unsteadiness, dizziness, and fatigue (Ioannidis, Gordon, & Adachi, 2001).

The occupational therapist should address these conditions in light of their influence on the client's quality of life. Offering compensatory strategies, adaptive equipment, and alternative methods for accomplishing daily activity can significantly improve quality of life and motivate a client to engage in treatment.

♦ *Fall risk and balance:* Fall risk should be addressed and should include interventions for both intrinsic and extrinsic factors. Because fall is a leading cause of fracture, clients who present with balance impairment should be treated for the underlying cause, such as vestibular dysfunction, decreased proximal muscle strength, or postural changes (Meeks, 1999; NOF, 2007).
♦ *Posture:* Clients can benefit from postural correction techniques to minimize kyphosis and improve lordotic curve. Techniques include interventions such as weighted kyphosis bracing, visual feedback with mirrors, and use of exercise balls or air cushions (Meeks, 1999; NOF, 2007; Pfeifer et al., 2004).
♦ *Strength and flexibility:* Paraspinal, scapular, and lower body strengthening exercises as well as flexibility programs can help to reduce back pain and the risk of vertebral fracture (Meeks, 1999; NOF, 2007; Sinaki et al., 2002).
♦ *Function and occupational performance:* Adults with osteoporosis may benefit from occupational therapy for remediation or modification of basic or IADL because of disease-related physical impairments. (Hagsten, Svensson, & Gardulf, 2006). Alternatively, in the early stages of the disease, a customized blend of exercise and occupation paired with disease awareness education is an effective method (Randles et al., 2004). The unique approach that occupational therapists have with this population is to both improve physical functional performance and modify performance for fracture risk reduction as it relates to a client's occupations.

OT AND THE EVIDENCE

Although occupational therapists have treated clients with this disease concurrently with other impairments for decades, specific focus on osteoporosis as a primary disease is new in recent years.

♦ Two randomized, controlled trials found that balance training improves functional and static balance and mobility and reduces fall frequency in elderly women and in elderly women with osteoporosis (Madureira et al., 2007; Steadman, Donaldson, & Kalra, 2003).
♦ A randomized, controlled trial found that low-intensity back-strengthening exercise improves quality of life and back extensor strength in patients with osteoporosis (Hongo et al., 2007).
♦ A randomized controlled trial found that strengthened back muscles significantly reduce incidence of vertebral fractures in estrogen-deficient women (Sinaki et al., 2002).
♦ A randomized, controlled trial found that individualized occupational therapy improved the ability to perform

instrumental activities of daily living and health-related quality of life in patients with hip fracture (Hagsten et al., 2006).

RESOURCES

Associations

♦ National Osteoporosis Foundation (NOF)
1232 22nd Street N.W.
Washington, DC 20037-1202
Phone: 800-231-4222
Website: www.nof.org
This organization offers information that is geared to both consumers and professionals.

♦ International Osteoporosis Foundation (IOF)
9. re Juste-Oliver
CH-1260
Nyon, Switzerland
Phone: +41 22 994 0100
Website: www.iofbonehealth.org
This is the largest global nongovernmental organization to address this worldwide disease. Its Website addresses the needs of patients and health professionals.

Books

♦ Daniel, M. S., & Strickland, R. L. (1992). *Occupational therapy protocol management in adult physical dysfunction.* New York: Aspen.
Protocols for treatment of osteoporosis-related fractures such as hip, wrist or spine fractures.

♦ Meeks, S. (1999). *Walk Tall!* Gainesville, FL: Triad.
An exercise, postural correction, and safe movement program for individuals with bone loss.

♦ U.S. Department of Health and Human Services. (2004). *Bone health and osteoporosis: A report of the surgeon general.* Rockville, MD: Office of the Surgeon General.
Available in consumer and full-length professional versions

Journals

♦ *Journal of Bone and Mineral Research*
♦ *Osteoporosis International*

Websites

♦ For consumer-level articles on osteoporosis and bone health:
www.about.com
www.webmd.com

♦ For the consumer who wants to learn more about this disease in detail and an excellent student reference:
courses.washington.edu/bonephys/

REFERENCES

Bachrach, L. K. (2001). Acquisition of optimal bone mass in childhood and adolescence. *Trends in Endocrinology and Metabolism, 12*(1), 22–28.

Black, D. M., Steinbuch, M., Palermo, L., Dargent-Molina, P., Lindsay, R., Hoseyni, M. S., et al. (2001). An assessment tool for predicting fracture risk in postmenopausal women. *Osteoporosis International, 12,* 519–528.

Edwards, M., Baptiste, S., Stratford, P. W., & Law, M. (2007). Recovery after hip fracture: What can we learn from the Canadian Occupational Performance Measure? *American Journal of Occupational Therapy, 61,* 335–344.

Hagsten, B., Svensson, O., & Gardulf, A. (2006). Health-related quality of life and self-reported ability concerning ADL and IADL after hip fracture: A randomized trial. *Acta Orthopaedica, 77,* 114–119.

Hallberg, I., Rosenqvist, A. M., Kartous, L., Lofman, O., Wahlstrom, O., & Toss, G. (2004). Health-related quality of life after osteoporotic fractures *Osteoporosis International, 15,* 834–841.

Hongo, M., Itoi, E., Sinaki, M., Miyakoshi, N., Shimada, Y., Maekawa, S., et al. (2007). Effect of low-intensity back exercise on quality of life and back extensor strength in patients with osteoporosis: A randomized controlled trial. *Osteoporosis International, 18,* 1389–1395.

International Osteoporosis Foundation. (2007). What is osteoporosis? Retrieved October 30, 2007, from http://www.iofbonehealth.org/patients-public/about-osteoporosis/what-is-osteoporosis.html.

Ioannidis, G., Adachi, J. D., & Guyatt, G. H. (1999). Development and validation of the Mini-Osteoporosis Quality of Life Questionnaire (OQLQ) in osteoporotic women with back pain due to vertebral fractures: Osteoporosis Quality of Life Study Group. *Osteoporosis International, 10,* 207–213.

Ioannidis, G., Gordon, M., & Adachi, J. D. (2001). Quality of life in osteoporosis. *Nursing Clinics of North America, 36,* 481–489.

Kanis, J. A., Borgstrom, F., De Laet, C., Johansson, H., Johnell, O., Jonsson, B., et al. (2005). Assessment of fracture risk. *Osteoporosis International, 16,* 581–589.

Law, M., Baptiste, S., McColl, M. A., Opzoomer, A., Polatajko, H., & Pollock, N. (1990). The Canadian Occupational Performance Measure: An outcome measure for occupational therapy. *Canadian Journal of Occupational Therapy, 57,* 82–87.

Madureira, M. M., Takayama, L., Gallinaro, A. L., Caparbo, V. F., Costa, R. A., & Pereira, R. M. (2007). Balance training program is highly effective in improving functional status and reducing the risk of falls in elderly women with osteoporosis: A randomized controlled trial. *Osteoporosis International, 18,* 419–425.

Meeks, S. (1999). *Walk Tall!* Gainesville, FL: Triad.

Munch, S., & Shapiro, S. (2006). The silent thief: Osteoporosis and women's health care across the life span. *Health and Social Work, 31*(1), 44–53.

National Osteoporosis Foundation. (2007). *Fast facts on osteoporosis.* Retrieved July 21, 2007, from, http://www.nof.org/osteoporosis/diseasefacts.htm

Osteoporosis. (2005). Retrieved October 31, 2007 from http://www.merck.com/mmpe/print/sec04/ch036/ch036a.html

Pfeifer, M., Sinaki, M., Geusens, P., Boonen, S., Preisinger, E., & Minne, H. W. (2004). Musculoskeletal rehabilitation in osteoporosis: A review. *Journal of Bone and Mineral Research; 19,* 1208–1214.

Randles, N., Randolph, E., Schell, B., & Grant, S. (2004). The impact of occupational therapy intervention on adults with osteoporosis: A pilot study. *Physical & Occupational Therapy in Geriatrics, 22*(2), 43–56.

Recknor, C., Grant, S., Catanzarite, J., Mohr, K., Benson, L., & Bateman, T. (2005). *Bone safety evaluation and functional risk for fracture index.* Retrieved July 21, 2007, from http://nof.confex.com/nof/2005/techprogram/P314.htm

Sinaki, M., Itoi, E., Wahner., H. W., Wollan, P., Gelzcer, R., Mullan, B. P., et al. (2002). Stronger back muscles reduce the incidence of vertebral fractures: A prospective 10 year follow-up of postmenopausal women. *Bone, 30,* 836–841.

Steadman, J., Donaldson, N., & Kalra, L. (2003). A randomized controlled trial of an enhanced balance training program to improve mobility and reduce falls in elderly patients. *Journal of the American Geriatric Society, 51,* 847–852.

World Health Organization Study Group. (1994). *Assessment of fracture risk and its application to screening for postmenopausal osteoporosis* (Technical Report Series, Vol. 843, pp. 1–129). Geneva, Switzerland: Author.

PARKINSON'S DISEASE

Kayoko Takahashi and Pai-Chuan Huang

Parkinson's disease (PD) is an idiopathic, slowly progressive, degenerative disorder of the basal ganglia in the central nervous system. It is the second most common neurodegenerative disease. Symptoms usually appear after the age of 50 years.

INCIDENCE

Incidence increases with age from 0.3–8.3 per 1,000 of the population in age 55–79 years in Western countries. Although perhaps less frequent in China and Africa, the disease is seen worldwide. Men seem to have a higher risk than women for PD (de Lau et al., 2004).

DIAGNOSIS, SYMPTOMS, AND AFFILIATED PROBLEMS

The cause of PD remains unknown. Diagnosis is based on clinical signs, including tremor, cogwheel rigidity, bradykinesia (slowness of movement), hypokinesia (reduction of movement), akinesia (loss of movement), and postural abnormalities. The criteria are: bradykinesia plus one of the following: a classic resting tremor, unilateral onset, progressive persistent asymmetry, and excellent response to levodopa (>70%), levodopa-induced dyskinesia, and continued response to levodopa for at least five years (Marsden, 1994). Problems affiliated with PD include insomnia, depression, and medication fluctuations ("on-off" state).

HOEHN AND YAHR STAGING OF PARKINSON'S DISEASE

- *Stage I:* Unilateral; no or minimal functional impairment; resting tremor
- *Stage II:* Midline or bilateral; mild functional impairment related to trunk mobility and postural reflexes
- *Stage III:* Impairment of balance; mild to moderate functional impairment
- *Stage IV:* Increased impairment of balance but still able to walk; functional impairment increased, especially difficulties with manipulation and dexterity, which interfere with eating, dressing, and washing
- *Stage V:* Confined to a wheelchair or bed (Hoehn & Yahr, 1967)

OT EVALUATIONS

PD reduces control of muscular movements, strength, endurance, cognitive, speech, and psychosocial functions and affects all ADL. PD-specific and some general OT assessments could be appropriate.

Participation Level

- Parkinson's Disease Quality of Life Questionnaire-39 Item Version (PDQ-39)
  Self-report that includes the following:
  - Five-point Likert scale, from "always" to "never" have a problem with ADL during the past 30 days because of PD.

- Eight subscales
  1. Mobility
  2. ADL
  3. Emotional well-being
  4. Stigma
  5. Social support
  6. Cognition
  7. Communication
  8. Bodily discomfort
- Higher scores characterize lower quality of life.
- Adequate reliability has been demonstrated cross-culturally (Jenkinson, Fitzpatrick, Norquist, Findley, & Hughes, 2003).
- Canadian Occupational Performance Measure (COPM)

Activity Level

- Unified Parkinson's Disease Rating Scale (UPDRS), a rating tool that follows the longitudinal course of PD. It includes these categories:
  - Mentation, behavior, and mood
  - ADL
  - Motor sections
- Functional Independence Measure (FIM)

Client Factor Level

- Hoehn and Yahr staging of PD
- Unified Parkinson's Disease Rating Scale Balance Test
- Range-of-motion test
- Manual muscle testing
- Rigidity testing
- Cognitive tests
- Geriatric Depression Scale (GDS)

INTERVENTIONS FOR PARKINSON'S DISEASE

Medications

The following current therapies aim to replace dopamine and decrease the symptoms of PD:

- L-dopa (levodopa)
- Dopamine agonists

Surgery

Surgical interventions include the following (Clinical Neuroscience, 2005):

- Pallidotomy
- Thalamotomy
- Deep brain stimulation
- Tissue transplants

Therapies

- *Physical therapy:* Improve ADL, stride length, and walking speed (de Goede, Samyra, Kwakkel, & Wagennar, 2001; Ellis et al., 2005).
- *Speech therapy:* Improve voice and speech function (de Swart, Willemse, Maassen, & Horstink, 2003; Schulz & Grant, 2002).

OT INTERVENTION

Intervention focuses on accommodative, remedial, compensatory, preventive, and environmental adaptation approaches, involving learning to identify the fluctuation in the symptoms and adjusting or grading activities accordingly.

Self-Care

- Teach adaptive techniques and tools to reduce the effect of tremors (Lyons, 2003; Montgomery, Lieberman, Singh, & Fries, 1994).
- Provide strategies to assist with medication routines.
- Encourage maximum functional level in all activities of daily living as long as possible.

Sensorimotor

- Maintain range of motion, prevent contractures by stretching.
- Improve motor planning and increase speed by adding cues, such as music with beats (Majsak, Kaminski, Gentile, & Flanagan, 1998; Marchese, Diverio, Zucchi, Lentino, & Abbruzzese, 2000; McIntosh, Brown, Rice, & Thaut, 1997).
- Encourage the client to increase voice volume through speaking and singing activities (Pacchetti et al., 2000).

Psychosocial

- Group approach to achieve therapy objectives, especially exercise and teaching groups to improve mood and socialization (Gauthier, Dalziel, & Gauthier, 1987).
- Educate in self-management skills, such as how to respond to changing symptom displays and when to seek medical help and how to improve self-efficacy in believing that the person can control their symptoms (Lyons, 2003).
- Encourage continuation of productive activities and leisure with suitable challenges (Sunvisson & Ekman, 2001).
- Encourage the person to discuss roles within the family and living unit.

◆ Educate the family to understand how the social interaction is affected by PD, such as facial masking and oral rigidity (Lyons & Tickle-Degnen, 2003).

Environment

◆ Change the home or work environment to reduce the impact of immobility, such as a barstool for sitting and a striped pattern floor for the visual cue.
◆ Encourage the person and family to participate in a self-help or support group.
◆ Help the person and family to explore the community for resources.

OT AND THE EVIDENCE

◆ Meta-analysis found that 37% of clients had positive results without therapy but that 67% had positive results with OT-related intervention, particularly with respect to improving basic abilities and ADL (Murphy & Tickle-Degnen, 2001).
◆ Health education and exercise promotion for PD (six months) improved significantly on ADL and self-efficacy in believing that they could control their symptoms (Montgomery et al., 1994).
◆ Group occupational therapy is effective as an adjunct to drug treatment with people who have PD. At one-year follow-up, the participants who had not received the therapy had experienced a significant decline. By contrast, those who had received the therapy had maintained their functional status (Gauthier et al., 1987).

RESOURCES

Associations

For patients and caregiver, focusing on education, support, research, and raising public awareness of the disease.

◆ American Parkinson Disease Association, Inc.
1250 Hylan Boulevard
Suite 4B
Staten Island, NY 10305
Telephone: 800-223-2732
Fax: 718-981-4399
◆ Michael J. Fox Foundation for Parkinson's Research
Grand Central Station
P.O. Box 4777
New York, NY 10163
Telephone: 800-708-7644
Website: http://www.michaeljfox.org/
◆ National Parkinson Foundation:
1501 N.W. 9th Avenue
Bob Hope Road

Miami, Florida 33136-1494
Telephone: 800-327-4545
Fax: 305-243-5595
◆ Parkinson's Action Network:
1025 Vermont Ave, NW
Suite 1120
Washington, DC 20005
Telephone: 800-850-4726
Fax: 202-638-7257
Website: http://www.parkinsonsaction.org/

Books

◆ Fox, Michael J. (2002). *Lucky man.* New York: Hyperion.
Autobiography by a 43-year-old actor who has PD.
◆ Havemann, J. (2002). *A life shaken: My encounter with Parkinson's disease.* Baltimore: Johns Hopkins University Press.
True story with scientific and medical information by a man with PD.
◆ Kondracke, M. (2001). *Saving Milly: Love, politics, and Parkinson's disease.* New York: Ballantine Books.
Autobiography by a man whose wife had PD.
◆ Newsom, H (2002). *Hope: Four keys to a better quality of life for Parkinson's people.* Mercer Island, WA: The Northwest Parkinson's Foundation.
Personal guidelines and tips how to live with PD by a man who has PD.

Journals

◆ *Archives of Neurology*
◆ *Journals of Gerontology*
◆ *Journal of Neurology, Neurosurgery, and Psychiatry*
◆ *Movement Disorders*
◆ *Neurology*
◆ *Parkinsonism and Rehabilitation*

Websites

◆ American Parkinson Disease Association Inc.
http://www.apdaparkinson.org/
◆ Parkinson's Action Network
http://www.parkinsonsaction.org/

REFERENCES

Clinical Neuroscience. (n.d.) *Parkinson's disease.* Retrieved March 27, 2005, from www.pallidotomy.com

de Goede, C. J. T., Samyra, H. J. K., Kwakkel, G., & Wagennar, R. W. (2001). The effects of physical therapy in Parkinson's disease: A research synthesis. *Archives of Physical Medicine & Rehabilitation, 82,* 509–515.

de Lau, L. M. L., Giesbergen, P. C. L. M., de Rijk, M. C., Hofman, A., Koudstaal, P. J., & Breteler, M. M. B. (2004). Incidence of Parkinsonism and Parkinson disease in a general population: The Rotterdam study. *Neurology, 63,* 1240–1244.

de Swart, B. J. M., Willemse, S. C., Maassen, B. A. M., & Horstink, M. W. I. M. (2003). Improvement of voicing in patients with Parkinson's disease by speech therapy. *Neurology, 60,* 498–500.

Ellis, T., de Goede, C. J., Feldman, R. G., Wolters, E. C., Kwakkel, G., & Wagenaar, R. C. (2005). Efficacy of a physical therapy program in patients with Parkinson's disease: A randomized controlled trial. *Archives of Physical Medicine and Rehabilitation, 86,* 626–632.

Gauthier, L., Dalziel, S., & Gauthier, S. (1987). The benefits of group occupational therapy for patients with Parkinson's disease. *American Journal of Occupational Therapy, 41,* 360–365.

Hoehn, M. M., & Yahr, M. D. (1967). Parkinsonism: Onset, progression, and mortality. *Neurology, 17,* 427–442.

Jenkinson, C., Fitzpatrick, R., Norquist, J., Findley, L., & Hughes, K. (2003). Cross-cultural evaluation of the Parkinson's Disease Questionnaire: Tests of data quality, score reliability, response rate, and scaling assumptions in the United States, Canada, Japan, Italy, and Spain. *Journal of Clinical Epidemiology, 56,* 843–847.

Lyons, K. D. (2003). Self-management of Parkinson's disease: Guidelines for program development and evaluation. *Physical & Occupational Therapy in Geriatrics, 21,* 17–31.

Lyons, K. D., & Tickle-Degnen, L. (2003). Dramaturgical challenge of Parkinson's disease. *Occupational Therapy Journal of Research, 23,* 27–34.

Majsak, M. J., Kaminski, T., Gentile, A. M., & Flanagan, J. R. (1998). The reaching movements of patients with Parkin-son's disease under self-determined maximal speed and visually cued conditions. *Brain, 121,* 755–766.

Marchese, R., Diverio, M., Zucchi, F., Lentino, C., & Abbruzzese, G. (2000). The role of sensory cues in the rehabilitation of Parkinsonian patients: A comparison of two physical therapy protocols. *Movement Disorders, 15,* 879–883.

Marsden, C. D. (1994). Parkinson's disease. *Journal of Neurology, Neurosurgery, and Psychiatry, 57,* 672–681.

McIntosh, G. C., Brown, S. H., Rice, R. R., & Thaut, M. H. (1997). Rhythmic auditory-motor facilitation of gait patterns in patients with Parkinson's disease. *Journal of Neurology, Neurosurgery, and Psychiatry, 62,* 22–26.

Montgomery, E. B., Lieberman, A., Singh, G., & Fries, J. F. (1994). Patient education and health promotion can be effective in Parkinson's disease: A randomized controlled trial. *American Journal of Medicine, 97,* 429–435.

Murphy, S., & Tickle-Degnen, L. (2001). The effectiveness of occupational therapy-related treatment for persons with Parkinson's disease: A meta-analytic review. *American Journal of Occupational Therapy, 55,* 385–392.

Pacchetti, G., Mangini, F., Aglieri, R., Fundaro, C., Martignoni, E., & Nappi, G. (2000). Active music therapy in Parkinson's disease: An integrative method for motor and emotional rehabilitation. *Psychosomatic Medicine, 62,* 386–393.

Schulz, G. M., & Grant, M. K. (2002). The effects of speech therapy and pharmacological treatments on voice and speech in Parkinson's disease: a review of the literature. *Current Medicinal Chemistry, 9,* 1359–1366.

Sunvisson, H., & Ekman, S. (2001). Environmental influences on the experiences of people with Parkinson's disease. *Nursing Inquiry, 8,* 41–50.

PRENATAL DRUG EXPOSURE

Laurie Dossett and Kate-Lyn Stone

Prenatal drug exposure results from a woman using illicit drugs such as cocaine, heroin, marijuana, methamphetamines, and ecstasy (MDMA) during pregnancy. This exposure can affect a developing fetus as well as the health and development of children after birth (U.S. Department of Health and Human Services, 1994). Some effects of prenatal drug exposure are severe, while others are more subtle (National Institute on Drug Abuse, 1998).

INCIDENCE AND PREVALENCE

Although the actual number of children born each year with prenatal drug exposure can be difficult to determine, it is known that exposure occurs in all racial, ethnic, and socioeconomic groups. It is estimated that approximately 3% of pregnant women use illicit drugs (March of Dimes, 2004).

DIAGNOSIS

It can be difficult to determine whether problems experienced by some children are caused by prenatal drug exposure or result from other factors such as poor prenatal and/or postnatal care, poor nutrition or poverty (NIDA, 1998). Also, because many women who use illicit drugs during pregnancy also use tobacco products and consume alcohol, it can be difficult to determine whether problems were specifically caused by the illicit drugs (March of Dimes, 2004). Newborns who were prenatally exposed to different illicit drugs are more likely to be born prematurely, with microcephaly and low height and weight measures, than other infants who were not exposed (NIDA, 1998).

SIGNS

Note that symptoms are not applicable to infants.

Infancy (0–15 months)

◆ Unpredictable sleeping patterns
◆ Feeding difficulties
◆ Irritability
◆ Atypical social interactions
◆ Delayed language development
◆ Increased muscle tone and poor fine motor development

Toddlerhood (15–36 months)

◆ Atypical social interactions
◆ Delayed language development
◆ Minimal play strategies (USDHHS, 1994)

SIGNS AND SYMPTOMS BASED ON SPECIFIC TYPE OF DRUG EXPOSURE

There are also signs and symptoms that are specific to the illicit drug to which a child was exposed in the womb (March of Dimes, 2004):

Cocaine

◆ Increased risk of urinary tract and heart defects
◆ May be jittery or irritable (as infants)
◆ Not easily consolable (as infants)
◆ Behavior problems: inability to control emotions
◆ Learning problems: difficulty paying attention

Marijuana

◆ Postnatal withdrawal symptoms such as excessive crying and trembling (with regular exposure during the pregnancy)
◆ Subtle effects on attention abilities and solving visual problems

Ecstasy (and Other Amphetamines)

◆ Possible increase in congenital heart defects and club-foot (in females only)
◆ Postnatal: possible jitteriness, drowsiness and breathing problems

Methamphetamines

◆ Increased risk of birth defects such as cleft palate and heart and limb defects
◆ Postnatal: possible jitteriness, drowsiness, and breathing problems

Heroin

◆ Most babies who were exposed to heroin experience postnatal withdrawal signs, including fever, sneezing, trembling, irritability, diarrhea, vomiting, continual crying, and occasionally seizures
◆ May be at risk for low IQ and serious behavior problems

CAUSE

Prenatal drug exposure is caused by the use of illicit drugs by a woman during pregnancy.

AFFILIATED PROBLEMS

Other than medical problems, many children with prenatal exposure to drugs can have learning difficulties, along with trouble paying attention and staying focused (NIDA, 1998). There are also indications that these children can have difficulties in social interactions and emotional regulation (NIDA, 1998).

PRECAUTIONS

Infants who were exposed to opiates in utero may exhibit postnatal withdrawal signs, and those who were exposed to cocaine may experience increased tone, hyperexcitability, and tremors (Agency for Healthcare Research and Quality, n.d.). Children who were exposed to drugs in the womb are more likely to be vulnerable to substance abuse themselves, especially in the adolescent years (NIDA, 2004).

TREATMENT

Treatment for these children will begin at birth, especially since many drug-exposed babies will be born prematurely and might need treatment for some of the common issues associated with prematurity (March of Dimes, 2004). Sleep disturbances, difficulties in self-consoling, and feeding disorders can be treated in different ways, including teaching the caregiver to read behavioral cues, modifying the environment, and providing support for the infant's attempts at self-regulation (Cole, 1996).

OT EVALUATION

Many different assessments can be used to evaluate the development of infants and children with prenatal exposure to illicit drugs. These may include some of the common pediatric developmental screening and assessments such as the following:

◆ Infant-Toddler Developmental Assessment (birth to 36 months)
◆ Hawaii Early Learning Profile (0–36 months) (HELP)

- Miller Assessment for Preschoolers (2 years, 9 months to 5 years, 8 months) (MAP)
- Bayley Scale of Infant Development (1–42 months)
- Sensory Integration and Praxis Tests (4 years to 8 years, 11 months) (SIPT)
- Peabody Developmental Motor Scales–2 (1 month to 6 years)
- Neonatal Behavioral Assessment Scale (infants)

OT INTERVENTION

Neonatal Intensive Care Unit

- Family education and support
- Work with infants on nipple feeding to promote active suck reflex
- Infant sensory stimulation protocols (National Institutes of Health, 2004)

Early Intervention

- Feeding skills
- Sensory processing
- Motor development
- Play skills
- Adaptive behavior
- Environmental exploration
- Child-caregiver interactions (American Occupational Therapy Association, 2005)

School Systems

- Sensory integration
- Fine and gross motor development
- Classroom participation

OT AND THE EVIDENCE

Infants who have been exposed to substances while in utero have been found to have difficulty attending to books and toys, abnormalities in sleep cycles, trouble with pinpointing sound, problems with visually tracking an object, disruption in mother-infant interactions, and difficulty participating in social games (Osborn, Jeffery, & Cole, 2007; Singer et al., 2000). Early identification of such deficits is crucial in facilitating early intervention services as soon as possible to promote more normal development (Singer et al., 2000). Belcher, Butz, Hoon, Reeves, and Pulsifer (2005) found that early intervention can reduce the effects of maternal substance abuse on the exposed child. Early intervention can also have several positive benefits on the development of the child and family. Early intervention should be family-oriented, meaning that it should be directed at both the child and caregivers, as well as culturally relevant

in order to be most constructive (Dudek-Shriber, 2004). Brown, Bakeman, Coles, Platzman, and Lynch (2004) suggest that early intervention should carefully analyze and consider the effects of the caregiving environment on the development of the exposed infant.

CAREGIVER CONCERNS

Prenatal drug exposure often results in premature birth. This means that the baby will most likely spend a lot of time in the hospital, which can be very physically and emotionally stressful for caregivers. Many children will also have special needs, which will create whole new experiences for parents and other caregivers. Caregivers must also learn to be aware of subtle signs and symptoms to prevent hyperarousal and understand that often these infants are not easily consolable (Cole, 1996).

RESOURCES

Books

- Chandler, L. S., & Lane, S. J. (1996) *Children with prenatal drug exposure.* New York: Haworth Press.
  Written by clinicians who are intimately involved in the care of children exposed to drugs prenatally and their families.
- Thomas, J. Y. (2004) *Educating drug-exposed children: The aftermath of the crack-baby crisis.* New York: RoutledgeFalmer.
  This book uses teachers' experiences to understand how prenatal drug exposure affects children's development and how social construction of the problem influences perceptions within schools.
- Bullock, A., Grimes, E., & McNamara, J. (1994) *Bruised before birth: Parenting children exposed to parental substance abuse.* Greensboro, NC: Family Resources.
  Experts in special needs adoptions, these authors relate fetal alcohol syndrome and drug exposure effects to stages of development and long-range prognoses to help each child reach his or her own best capability potential.

Journals

- *Infants and Young Children*
- *Clinical Pediatrics*
- *Pediatrics International*
- *Physical & Occupational Therapy in Pediatrics*

Websites

- March of Dimes
  http://www.marchofdimes.com

A Website for professionals and nonprofessionals to obtain information on many different pregnancy- and birth-related topics, specifically premature births, birth defects, and prevention.

REFERENCES

Agency for Healthcare Research and Quality. (n.d.) *Screening for drug abuse.* Retrieved February 20, 2006, from http://www.ahrq.gov/clinic/2ndcps/drugab.pdf

American Occupational Therapy Association. (2005). *Occupational therapy for children: Birth to 3 years of age.* Fact sheet. Retrieved February 20, 2006, from http://www.aota.org/featured/area6/docs/Child0-3.pdf

Belcher, H. M. E., Butz, A. M., Hoon, A. H., Reeves, S. A., & Pulsifer, M. B. (2005). Spectrum of early intervention services for children with intrauterine drug exposure. *Infants and Young Children, 18,* 2–15.

Brown, J., Bakeman, R., Coles, C., Platzman, K., & Lynch, M. E. (2004). Prenatal cocaine exposure: A comparison of 2-year-old children in parental and nonparental care. *Child Development, 75,* 1282–1295.

Cole, J. G. (1996). Intervention strategies for infants with prenatal drug exposure. *Infants and Young Children, 8*(3), 35–39.

Dudek-Shriber, L. (2004). Parent stress in the neonatal intensive care unit and the influence of parent and infant char-

acteristics. *American Journal of Occupational Therapy, 58,* 509–520.

March of Dimes. (2004). *Illicit drug use during pregnancy.* Retrieved March 1, 2006, from http://www.marchofdimes.com/professionals/14332_1169.asp

National Institute on Drug Abuse. (2004). *Drug-related damage that occurs before birth.* Retrieved February 18, 2006, from http://www.drugabuse.gov/NIDA_notes/NNvol19N4/DirRepVol19N4.html

National Institute on Drug Abuse. (1998). *Prenatal exposure to drugs of abuse may affect later behavior and learning.* Retrieved February 17, 2006, from http://www.drugabuse.gov/NIDA_Notes/NNVol13N4/Prenatal.html.

National Institutes of Health. (2004). *NICU consultants and support staff.* Retrieved March 6, 2006, from http://www.nlm.nih.gov/medlineplus/ency/article/007249.htm

Osborn, D. A., Jeffery, H. E., & Cole, M. (2007). Opiate treatment for opiate withdrawal in newborn infants (Cochrane Review). *The Cochrane Library,* Issue 2.

Singer, L., Arendt, R., Minnes, S., Salvator, A., Siegel, C., & Lewis, B. (2000). Developing language skills of cocaine-exposed infants. *Pediatrics, 107,* 1057–1064.

U.S. Department of Health and Human Services. (1994). *Protecting children in substance-abusing families.* Retrieved March 3, 2006, from http://nccanch.acf.hhs.gov/pubs/usermanuals/subabuse/subabused.cfm

RHEUMATOID ARTHRITIS

Kate-Lyn Stone

DIAGNOSIS

Rheumatoid arthritis (RA) is a systemic, inflammatory, chronic condition. It is also considered an autoimmune disease because of the fact that people who have RA have an irregular immune response. Basically, this means that the immune system in people with RA attacks the body's healthy tissue as if the tissue were a foreign invader. RA is generally characterized by the inflammation of the synovium, or lining, of the joints (Arthritis Foundation, 2007). It generally occurs in a symmetrical way, meaning that if an individual has RA in his or her left hand, he or she is likely also to have RA in the right hand. The disease causes pain, swelling, discomfort, and loss of function in the joints (National Institute of Arthritis and Musculoskeletal and Skin Diseases, 2004). The cause of RA is unknown, and there is no cure.

INCIDENCE AND PREVALENCE

- 2.1 million Americans, approximately 1% of the population, are affected by RA (Arthritis Foundation, 2007).
- Women are two to three times more likely to develop RA than their male counterparts (Arthritis Foundation, 2007).

- Rheumatoid nodules appear in about 20% of the population with RA (Arthritis Foundation, 2007).
- People with RA generally begins to show symptoms during middle age; however, children and adolescents can also develop the disease (for more information on this condition, see the resource sheet for juvenile rheumatoid arthritis).

THE CAUSE AND ETIOLOGY

The cause of RA is unknown. There are several theories as to what could cause this disease, including theories involving the immune system, gender, genetics, or infection (Arthritis Foundation, 2007; NIAMS, 2004).

TYPICAL COURSE AND SYMPTOMS

Rheumatoid arthritis can affect any joint in the body, but it most commonly starts in the joints of the fingers, hands, and wrists. The disease process of RA generally has three stages:

1. The synovial lining begins to swell, which results in pain, stiffness, and swelling around the joint.
2. The synovium thickens because of the rapid division and growth of cells.

3. The inflamed cells in the joint begin to release enzymes that digest bone and cartilage. This often results in the joint's losing its shape and an increase in pain and loss of movement (Arthritis Foundation, 2007).

Signs include the following:

- Stiffness
- Weakness
- Flulike symptoms
- Rheumatoid nodules (bumps under the skin)
- Depression
- Weight loss
- Cold and/or sweaty hands and feet
- Decreased production of tears and saliva because of involvement of the glands that produce these secretions
- Deformity of joints
- Instability of joints
- Limited range of motion
- Decreased strength
- Decreased ability to function
- Anemia

Symptoms include the following:

- Pain
- Fatigue
- Loss of appetite

SEQUENCE OF CARE

Early diagnosis is critical in RA because it can lead to early intervention, which allows an individual with RA to continue living a productive and meaningful life. The physician makes a diagnosis based on medical history, physical examination, and X-rays and confirmed by lab tests (Arthritis Foundation, 2007). During the medical history, the physician will look for information, including, but not limited to, pain level, amount of stiffness and when the stiffness is most prevalent, and presence of fatigue. During the physical examination, the physician will look for the common signs of RA, such as swelling, tenderness, and misalignment. In addition to the medical history and the physical exam, the physician may choose to use lab tests to confirm the diagnosis. Possible lab tests include complete blood count (checking red blood cells, white blood cells, or platelets for abnormalities), erythrocyte sedimentation rate (to detect the amount of inflammation in the body), C-reactive protein (also to detect inflammation), and rheumatoid factor (the higher the amount of rheumatoid factor, the more severe the RA is). Imaging tests may also be used, such as X-rays, MRI, bone densitometry (measuring bone density), and joint ultrasound (Arthritis Foundation, 2007). Once RA has been diagnosed, appropriate treatment can begin. Refer to the following section for information on different types of treatment and the medical professionals who may be involved.

MEDICAL INTERVENTIONS

Aggressive treatment of RA can decrease the amount of damage that is done to the joint, which in turn leads to a decrease in pain and an increase in range of motion. Because each person is affected differently by RA, treatment methods differ from person to person. The overarching goals for treatment include decreasing pain, inflammation, and damage and increasing function (NIAMS, 2004). In general, treatment will include the following:

- Medications, including nonsteroidal anti-inflammatory drugs (NSAIDs), analgesic drugs, glucocorticoids or prednisone, disease-modifying antirheumatic drugs (DMARDs), biologic response modifiers, and protein-A immunoadsorption therapy (Arthritis Foundation, 2007). For more information on these drugs, visit the Arthritis Foundation's website at http://www.arthritis.org/
- Physical therapy
- Occupational therapy
- Surgery
- Proper rest
- Joint care
- Stress management
- Exercise to reduce pain and improve movement
- Weight control to reduce stress on joints

Health professionals that may be involved in treating an individual with RA include a general practitioner, a rheumatologist, a physical therapist, an occupational therapist, a nurse, a psychologist/psychiatrist, an orthopedic surgeon, and a social worker (Arthritis Foundation, 2007).

OT EVALUATIONS

Basic and Instrumental Activity of Daily Living Skills

- Kohlman Evaluation of Living Skills (KELS)
- Assessment of Motor and Process Skills (AMPS)
- Functional Independence Measure (FIM)
- Klein-Bell Activities of Daily Living Scale (Klein-Bell)
- Satisfaction With Performance Scaled Questionnaire (SPSQ)

Psychosocial Skills

- The Assessment of Occupational Functioning (AOF)
- The Occupational Performance History Interview II (OPHI II)
- Geriatric Depression Scale

Self-Perception

- The Canadian Occupational Performance Measure (COPM)

- ◆ The Role Checklist
- ◆ Worker Role Inventory

Somatic Sensory Evaluations

- ◆ Primary somatic system
  - ◆ Light touch
  - ◆ Pain
  - ◆ Temperature
- ◆ Discriminative somatic system
  - ◆ Tactile localization
  - ◆ Two-point discrimination

Other Assessments

- ◆ Manual muscle testing
- ◆ Range-of-motion testing
- ◆ Pain scales
- ◆ Home assessment

OT INTERVENTIONS

- ◆ ADL
- ◆ Energy conservation techniques
- ◆ Strengthening exercises
- ◆ Pain management
- ◆ Assistive technology
- ◆ Adapt environment
- ◆ Adaptive equipment
- ◆ Patient and family education
- ◆ Home planning
- ◆ Splinting to support limbs
- ◆ Self-management education

OT AND THE EVIDENCE

Steultjens and colleagues (2004) found that instruction and education on joint protection as an occupational therapy intervention for individuals with RA improved their functional ability. These researchers also found that splinting the involved joints led to a decrease in pain both immediately and over time as well as an immediate improvement in grip strength following splinting. Hammond and Freeman (2004) found results similar to those of Steultjens and colleagues in that an OT-administered educational joint protection program improved functional ability and improved adherence to joint protection strategies for individuals with RA. Hammond and Freeman (2004) credit the success of their program to the applied educational, behavioral, and motor learning aspects of the training instilling the clients with a greater sense of self-efficacy. Kennedy (2006) looked into the effectiveness of aerobic exercise programs for individuals with RA. She found that the exercise programs did not increase the disease progression and aided in decreasing the loss of bone mineral in the hip joint. Overall, aerobic exercise programs seem to be safe and effective for individuals with RA.

RESOURCES

Programs

- ◆ Arthritis Foundation Self-Help Program (AFSHP) (Centers for Disease Control and Prevention, 2004) This six-week program helps individuals with arthritis learn how to manage their condition on a day-to-day basis. It was developed by Dr. Kate Lorig of Stanford University. Studies done on this intervention report that participants experience a 20% decrease in pain and a 40% decrease in doctors' visits. As of 2007, there were 36 CDC-funded state arthritis programs.
- ◆ Chronic Disease Self-Management Program (CDSMP) (Centers for Disease Control and Prevention, 2004) This six-week program teaches self-management education for individuals with chronic diseases or conditions, including arthritis, diabetes, heart disease, and lung disease. This program was created and developed at Stanford University. As of 2007, there were 36 CDC-funded state chronic disease programs.
- ◆ Arthritis Foundation Exercise Program (AFEP) This program, developed by the Arthritis Foundation, is a community-based, recreational program that focuses on range-of-motion exercises, endurance building, stress management, relaxation techniques, and other topics related to health. This program is unique in that it can be tailored to meet each participant's individual needs.
- ◆ Arthritis Foundation Aquatic Program (AFAP) This exercise program, developed by the Arthritis Foundation, is an aquatic program that works to increase flexibility, endurance, and range of motion while decreasing pain because there is less impact on the joints in the water environment.
- ◆ EnhanceFitness Formerly known as Lifetime Fitness, this program is an evidence-based, community exercise program. It has been proven to increase strength and activity levels in individuals with arthritis.

Associations

- ◆ American College of Rheumatology 1800 Century Place, Suite 250 Atlanta, GA 30345-4300 Telephone: 404-633-3777 Fax: 404-633-1870 Website: http://www.rheumatology.org/
- ◆ Arthritis Foundation P.O. Box 7669 Atlanta, GA 30357-0669 Telephone: 1-800-283-7800 Website: http://www.arthritis.org/
- ◆ Centers for Disease Control and Prevention National Center for Chronic Disease Prevention and Health Promotion

Arthritis Section
Mailstop K-51
4770 Buford Highway NE
Atlanta, GA 30341-3724
Telephone: 770-488-5464
Fax: 770-488-5964
Website: http://www.cdc.gov/arthritis/
◆ National Institute of Arthritis and Musculoskeletal and
Skin Diseases
Information Clearinghouse
National Institutes of Health
1 AMS Circle
Bethesda, MD 20892-3675
Telephone: 1-877-226-4267
Fax: 301-718-6366
Website: http://www.niams.nih.gov/

Books

◆ Klippel, J. H., Stone, J. H., Crofford, L. J., & White, P.
(Eds.). (2001). *Primer on the rheumatic diseases.* New
York: Arthritis Foundation.

Journals

◆ *Annals of the Rheumatic Diseases*
◆ *Arthritis and Rheumatism*
◆ *Arthritis Care and Research*
◆ *Journal of Rheumatology*

Websites

◆ American College of Rheumatology
http://www.rheumatology.org
The American College of Rheumatology is an organization for physicians, health professionals, and scientists.
It provides programs of education, research, advocacy, and practice support. The website offers information about professional education, research and
publications regarding rheumatology.
◆ Arthritis Foundation
http://www.arthritis.org/
The Arthritis Foundation is dedicated to improving the
lives of individuals with arthritis through providing
leadership in the prevention, control, and cure of this
disease and its related conditions. The Foundation's

website provides information about arthritis, medication used to treat the illness, as well as the latest research
regarding arthritis.
◆ Centers for Disease Control and Prevention
http://www.cdc.gov/arthritis/
This website is the CDC's Arthritis Program. This program is working to measure the incidence and prevalence of arthritis, strengthen the science and research
behind arthritis, increase awareness of the disease, and
build state arthritis programs. The website contains a
wealth of information in all of these topics as well as
information about the state programs and links to
these sites and other resources regarding arthritis.
◆ National Institute of Arthritis and Musculoskeletal and
Skin Diseases
http://www.niams.nih.gov
The National Institute of Arthritis and Musculoskeletal and Skin Diseases is dedicated to supporting
research in the areas of cause, treatment, and prevention of arthritis and musculoskeletal and skin diseases.
The website contains the latest news about arthritis as
well as other health related information and research.

REFERENCES

Arthritis Foundation. (2007). *Rheumatoid arthritis.* Retrieved
September 11, 2007, from http://www.arthritis.org/disease-
center.php?disease_id=31
Centers for Disease Control and Prevention. (2004). National
Arthritis Month: May 2004. *Morbidity and Mortality Weekly
Report 53*(18), 383.
Hammond, A., & Freeman, K. (2004). The long-term outcomes
from a randomized controlled trial of an educational-
behavioural joint protection programme for people with
rheumatoid arthritis. *Clinical Rehabilitation, 18,* 520–528.
Kennedy, N. (2006). Exercise therapy for patients with rheuma-
toid arthritis: Safety of intensive programmes and effects
upon bone mineral density and disease activity: A literature
review. *Physical Therapy Reviews, 11,* 263–268.
National Institute of Arthritis and Musculoskeletal and Skin Dis-
eases. (2004). *Rheumatoid arthritis.* Bethesda, MD: National
Institutes of Health.
Steultjens, E. M. J., Bouter, L. M., Dekker, J., Kuyk, M. A. H.,
Schaardenburg, D., & Van den Ende, C. H. M. (2004).
Occupational therapy for rheumatoid arthritis. *The
Cochrane Database of Systematic Reviews,* Issue 1. Art.
No. CD003114. DOI:10.1002/14651858.CD003114.pub2.

SCHIZOPHRENIA

Grace M. Trudeau

Schizophrenia is a psychotic disorder that typically
occurs in late adolescence or adulthood and affects an
individual's perceptions and behaviors in all facets of
life. Disturbed thought patterns or psychotic symptoms
leading to severe difficulties in social or occupational
functioning must be present for a minimum of six months
for diagnosis (American Psychiatric Association, 2000).

PREVALENCE

◆ Schizophrenia affects 1% of the world's population
(National Institute of Mental Health, 2005a).
◆ Between one third and one half of Americans who are
homeless have schizophrenia (PyschologyNet.org,
2003).

ETIOLOGY AND RISK FACTORS

The etiology of schizophrenia is unknown, but theories include organic or neurological causes, events during development, environmental factors, or genetics. It is possible that "schizophrenia" is actually a collection of different underlying causes that present similarly (NIMH, 2005b).

POTENTIAL SYMPTOMS

Symptoms can be divided into two categories: negative symptoms, resulting in trait "loss," and positive symptoms, which "add" traits.

Negative Symptoms

- Flat affect
- Inattention
- Lack of interest or energy
- Impoverished thought process
- Inability to experience pleasure

Positive Symptoms

- Hallucinations
- Delusions
- Disordered or disorganized thinking
- Language disturbances
- Self-neglect
- Paranoia
- Inappropriate emotion (NIMH, 2005a; Psychology Net.org, 2003)

Typical Course

Schizophrenia may progress in three typical courses:

- Single episode of symptoms with almost complete recovery
- Repeated episodes of symptoms with moderate recovery between
- Progressive slide into long-term disability (Stevens, 1997)

OT EVALUATION

Client, Caregiver, and Staff Perceptions of Impact

- Canadian Occupational Performance Measure (COPM)
- Client Assessment of Strengths, Interests, and Goals/ Staff Observations and Client Information (CASIG/ SOCI)

- Illness Perception Questionnaire for Schizophrenia/ Illness Perception Questionnaire for Schizophrenia– Relatives Version (IPQS/IPQS-Relatives)

Activities of Daily Living/Instrumental Activities of Daily Living (ADL/IADL)

- Global Assessment of Functioning (GAF) Scale
- Kohlman Evaluation of Living Skills (KELS)
- Milwaukee Evaluation of Daily Living Skills (MEDLS)
- The Test of Grocery Shopping Skills (TOG-SS)

Cognitive Assessment

- Allen's Cognitive Levels (ACL)
- Assessment of Motor and Process Skills (AMPS)

NON-OT TREATMENTS

Antipsychotic Medications

Antipsychotic medications are generally used as the first treatment of schizophrenia to help clients establish a stable base from which other treatments may be beneficial. However, while medications have been shown to be effective in preventing psychotic relapse, with the exception of clozapine, there is no evidence that they effect change in other domains (e.g., social functioning) (Bustillo, Lauriello, Horan, & Keith, 2001; Hargreaves, Gibson & Gibson, 2005; PsychologyNet.org, 2003).

Major Side Effects of Typical Antipsychotic Medication

- Chlorpromazine (anticholinergic, sedation, hypotension)
- Thioridazine (anticholinergic, sedation, hypotension)
- Trifluoperazine (extrapyramidal)
- Thiothixene (extrapyramidal)
- Fluphenazine (extrapyramidal)
- Haloperidol (extrapyramidal)

Major Side Effects of Atypical Antipsychotic Medication

- Risperidone (limited side effects)
- Olanzapine (limited side effects)
- Clozapine (anticholinergic, sedation, hypotension, risk of agranulocytosis)

Other Side Effects

- *Anticholinergic:* Dry mouth, constipation, blurred vision, urinary retention
- *Extrapyramidal:* Dystonia, parkinsonism, akathisisa, tardive dyskinesia
- With both typical and atypical antipsychotic medications, adverse reactions may include neuroleptic malignant syndrome, malignant hyperthermia, and tardive dyskinesia.

INTERVENTION

Assertive Community Treatment (ACT)

Rehabilitation teams provide comprehensive, 24-hour, 7-day-a-week case management and active treatment. Teams support individuals in ADL, work, and leisure activities. ACT has clear effects on the prevention of psychotic relapse and rehospitalization (Bustillo et al., 2001; Russell Teske, 2000).

Clubhouses and Supported Living

Clubhouses provide support as clients move through a continuum of dependency to independence. Although clubhouses vary from one program to the next, most offer a variety of self-help and skills programs. Likewise, supported living programs enable individuals to move from supervised to independent community living (Russell Teske, 2000).

Cognitive Behavioral Treatment

Cognitive behavioral therapy (CBT) treatments target changing thought patterns in order to change behavior and increase attention, memory, planning, and decision-making skills. Following CBT, some studies have shown decreases in delusional thinking and hallucinations (Bustillo et al., 2001; Russell Teske, 2000).

Family Therapy

When individuals are returned to their families following discharge, behavioral and psychoeducational interventions are employed with the whole family. Such interventions have been shown to be effective in preventing psychotic relapse and hospitalization (Bustillo et al., 2001).

Psychoeducation

In psychoeducation, which is sometimes termed *personal therapy,* therapists teach functional living skills, symptom management, health and safety awareness, and assertiveness training in individual treatment sessions. Preliminary research shows that psychoeducation may improve social functioning (Bustillo et al., 2001; MacRae, 2005).

Social Skills Training

In social skills training, training is provided in social adaptation, self-care, and interpersonal relationships using modeling, feedback, reinforcement, and role-play. Although it is not clear that effects generalize, improvements in social skills have been shown to last after one year. There is no effect on relapse prevention, psychopathology, or employment status (Bustillo et al., 2001; Russell Teske, 2000).

Supported Employment

Supported employment programs help individuals to obtain and maintain employment. Training is completed in searching for jobs and job skills, and support is provided throughout the job acquisition and employment processes. Employment may occur in a continuum from sheltered workshops to community settings. Best evidence shows that the place-and-train vocational model is most effective in obtaining competitive employment (Bustillo et al., 2000).

OT AND THE EVIDENCE

Family therapy and assertive community treatment have clear effects on the prevention of psychotic relapse and hospitalization but no consistent effects on other outcome measures. Social skills training has been shown to improve social skills but has not been shown to have a direct impact on other areas of outcome, including relapse or employment. Supportive employment programs that use place-and-train models demonstrate a positive effect on the obtainment of competitive employment. In some studies, cognitive behavior therapy has been shown to improve delusions and hallucinations (Bustillo et al., 2001).

RESOURCES

Associations

♦ National Alliance on Mental Illness (NAMI)
   Colonial Place Three
   2107 Wilson Boulevard
   Suite 300
   Arlington, VA 22201-3042
   Telephone: 800-950-NAMI
   Website: http://www.nami.org/
   Local addresses and telephone numbers may be obtained from the Website.
♦ National Alliance for Research on Schizophrenia and Depression (NARSAD)
   60 Cutter Mill Road
   Suite 404
   Great Neck, NY 11021
   Telephone: 800-829-8289
   Website: http://www.narsad.org/
♦ National Institute of Mental Health (NIMH): Public Communications and Information
   6001 Executive Boulevard
   Room 8184, MSC 9663
   Bethesda, MD 20892-9663
   Telephone: 866-651-6464
   Website: http://www.nimh.nih.gov/
♦ World Fellowship for Schizophrenia & Allied Disorders (WFSAD):
   124 Merton Street
   Suite 507
   Toronto, Ontario, M4S 2Z2, Canada
   Telephone: 416-961-2855
   Website: http://www.world-schizophrenia.org

Websites

- British Columbia Schizophrenia Society
  http://www.bcss.org/
  Well-organized Website with information on facts, interventions, research, and resources.
- Mental Wellness.com
  http://www.mentalwellness.com
  Information on schizophrenia, bipolar disorder, and mental health. Includes everyday tips, programs, and inspirational stories.
- Schizophrenia Society of Canada
  http://www.schizophrenia.ca/
  English and French advocacy and support website.

First-Person Accounts

- Earley, P. (2006). *Crazy: A father's search through America's mental health madness.* New York: Penguin. A journalist of more than 30 years, Pete Earley writes of his experience with his son, who was diagnosed with schizophrenia, and of the mental health care system and its ties to the criminal justice system.
- Simon, C. (1998). *Mad house: Growing up in the shadow of mentally ill siblings.* New York: Penguin Books. Simon recounts the experience of growing up with two siblings with schizophrenia and the effect on her family.
- Spiro Wagner, P., & Spiro, C. (2005). *Divided minds: Twin sisters and their journey through schizophrenia.* Lancaster, UK, St. Martin's Press. A vivid description of the experiences of a woman with schizophrenia and her psychiatrist twin sister.
- Steele, K., & Berman, C. (2002). *The day the voices stopped: A memoir of madness and hope.* New York: Basic Books. An inspiring story of how advocacy and activism helped the author to retain control while living with schizophrenia for over 30 years.

Journals

- *Journal of Clinical Psychiatry*
- *Journal of Mental Health*
- *Mental Health Today*
- *Schizophrenia Bulletin*
- *Schizophrenia Research*

REFERENCES

American Psychiatric Association. (2000). *Diagnostic and statistical manual of mental disorders* (4th ed., text rev.). Washington, DC: Author.

Bustillo, J. R., Lauriello, J., Horan, W. P., & Keith, S. J. (2001). The psychosocial treatment of schizophrenia: An update. *American Journal of Psychiatry, 158,* 163–175.

Hargreaves, W. A., Gibson, P. J., & Gibson, J. P. (2005). The effectiveness and cost of risperidone and olanzapine for schizophrenia: A systematic review. *CNS Drugs, 19,* 393–410.

MacRae, A. (2005). Demonstrating effectiveness in occupational therapy. In E. Cara & A. MacRae (Eds.), *Psychosocial occupational therapy: A clinical practice* (2nd ed., 687–709). Clifton Park, NY: Thomson Delmar Learning.

National Institute of Mental Health. (2005a). *Schizophrenia.* Retrieved April 4, 2006, from http://www.nimh.nih.gov/publicat/schizoph.cfm

National Institute of Mental Health. (2005b). *Schizophrenia research at the National Institute of Mental Health.* Retrieved April 4, 2006, from http://www.nimh.nih.gov/publicat/schizresfact.cfm

PsychologyNet.org. (2003). *Schizophrenia.* Retrieved March 11, 2004, from http://psychologynet.org/schiz.html

Russell Teske, Y. (2000). Schizophrenia. In R. A. Hansen & B. Atchinson (Eds.), *Conditions in occupational therapy: Effect on occupational performance* (2nd ed., pp. 54–74). Philadelphia: Lippincott Williams & Wilkins.

Stevens, J. R. (1997). Anatomy of schizophrenia revisited. *Schizophrenia Bulletin, 23,* 373–383.

SPINA BIFIDA AND NEURAL TUBE DEFECTS

Bridget A. Kane

Neural tube defects are malformations of the central nervous system that occur in utero within the first four weeks of gestation. There are three major forms of neural tube defects:

- Anencephaly is the absence of growth of the cerebral hemispheres. Newborns with this condition either are stillborn or die shortly after birth (Beers & Berkow, 1999).
- Encephalocele includes brain protrusion in the occipital region, often resulting in motor impairments, seizures, hydrocephalus, and mental retardation (Liptak, 1997).
- Spina bifida is a defect in the vertebral arches and the spinal column that occurs most commonly in the lower thoracic, lumbar, or sacral regions (Beers & Berkow, 1999).

The exact cause of spina bifida remains unknown. Genetics, environmental factors, certain medications, and maternal nutritional deficiency are suspected to influence neural tube development (National Institute of Neurological Disorders and Stroke, 2004; Spina Bifida Association of America, 2001).

INCIDENCE AND PREVALENCE

Spina bifida is reportedly "the most frequently occurring permanently disabling birth defect," affecting 1 in every 1,000 births in the United States. It is estimated that up to 70,000 people are living with spina bifida in the United States (SBAA, 2001, p. 1).

Prognosis

Approximately 90% of infants who are born with spina bifida will live into adulthood (SBAA, 2001). The cause of death for older individuals with spina bifida is usually loss of renal function and/or shunt complications (Beers & Berkow, 1999).

Common Characteristics

Signs vary based on the extent of the condition and may include the following:

- Paralysis, including sensory and motor impairments below the level of the lesion
- Hydrocephalus
- Cognitive impairments ranging from learning disabilities to mental retardation
- Sensory-processing and perceptual deficits
- Bladder and bowel dysfunction
- Psychosocial and sexual concerns
- Orthopedic conditions, including club foot, dislocated hip, scoliosis, kyphosis, and joint abnormalities due to overuse or muscle imbalance (Beers & Berkow, 1999; Brown, 2001; National Dissemination Center for Children with Disabilities, 2004; Simeonsson, McMillen, & Huntington, 2002; Snow, 1999; Wills, 1993)

HEALTH MANAGEMENT

Integrated, multidisciplinary services that are comprehensive, coordinated, and longitudinal are most effective in promoting health and participation in the community for individuals with spina bifida (Bent et al., 2002; Kinsman, Levey, Ruffing, Stone, & Warren, 2000). Interventions may include the following:

- Neurologic and orthopedic surgery
  - Surgical repair of open lesions is completed within 24 hours of birth to decrease the risk of infection and preserve existing spinal cord function.
  - Shunt implantation to manage hydrocephalus
  - Antibiotics and/or neurosurgical intervention to treat cerebrospinal fluid (CSF) abnormalities and meningeal or ventricular infection
- Urologic care with possible catheterization, along with bowel and bladder programs
- Radiographic imaging to monitor the integrity of spine, skull, hips, and lower extremities

- Orthotic and mobility interventions
- Screening for scoliosis, pathological fractures, and pressure sores
- Nutritional counseling (Beers & Berkow, 1999; Brown, 2001; NINDS, 2004)

PRECAUTIONS

Precautions involved in spina bifida include the following (Brown, 2001; Dias, 2003; McLone & Dias, 2001; Rekate, 2001; Scoggin & Parks, 1997):

- Contractures
- Joint protection
- Pressure sores and skin breakdown
- Seizures
- Latex sensitivity/allergy, with adverse reactions to latex that may include the following:
  - Itchy, watery eyes
  - Sneezing and coughing
  - Rash or hives
  - Swelling of trachea
  - Wheezing or shortness of breath
  - Anaphylactic shock
- Shunt malfunction: Signs of shunt malfunction include the following:
  - Headaches
  - Vomiting
  - Seizures
  - Behavioral and cognitive changes
  - Progressive decline in motor performance
  - Gagging or difficulty swallowing
  - Change in urinary or bowel function
  - "Setting sun" eyes
  - Increased head size
- Shunt infection, with signs that include those of shunt malfunction and the following:
  - Fever
  - Neck stiffness
  - Pain and tenderness
  - Skin redness
  - Abdominal pain
  - Drainage from shunt tract

OCCUPATIONAL THERAPY EVALUATION

Pediatric Evaluations

Daily Living Skills

- Functional Independence Measure for Children (WeeFIM)
- Hawaii Early Learning Profile (HELP)
- Pediatric Evaluation of Disability Inventory (PEDI)
- Vineland Adaptive Behavior Scales

School-Specific

◆ School Function Assessment (SFA)

Play/Leisure and Social Skills

◆ Children's Assessment of Participation and Enjoyment (CAPE)
◆ Play History
◆ Social Skills Rating System
◆ Test of Playfulness

Transition Planning and Goal Setting

◆ Canadian Occupational Performance Measure (COPM)
◆ Choosing Outcomes and Accommodations for Children (COACH)
◆ Making Action Plans (MAPS)
◆ Perceived Efficacy and Goal Setting (PEGS)
◆ Transition Planning Inventory

Additional assessments that target specific areas, including feeding, handwriting and academic performance, driving, and employment, may also be appropriate.

Adult Evaluations

Occupational Performance

◆ Canadian Occupational Performance Measure (COPM)
◆ Occupational Performance History Interview

Daily Living Skills

◆ Functional Independence Measure (FIM)

Additional assessments for adults may address employment, driving, accessing the community, IADL, and home safety.

Throughout the life course, body structure and function factors that can influence occupational performance should also be assessed. These factors can include range of motion, muscle strength and tone, postural deviations, sensation, visual perception, and sensory processing (Razma, 2001).

OT INTERVENTION

OT may address the physical, cognitive, neurological, social, and environmental factors that affect participation in daily activities for individuals with spina bifida. Changes in levels of dependence over time and the additional effects of aging support the need for continued assessment and intervention throughout the life course (Andren & Grimby, 2004; Brown, 2001; Klingbeil, Baer, & Wilson, 2004). Intervention may address accessibility, assistive technology and adaptive equipment, family and caregiver education and training, energy conservation and proper body mechanics, fitness and recreation, disability awareness, social skills, community integration, splinting and

orthotics, skin care, positioning, and, most important, transition planning.

OT AND THE EVIDENCE

◆ Children with developmental disabilities whose mothers participated in a one-hour intervention addressing caregiver-child interaction demonstrated significant improvement in playfulness, as measured by the Test of Playfulness, compared to children with developmental disabilities who participated in a one-hour neurodevelopmental treatment session (Okimoto, Bundy, & Hanzlik, 2000). These results reinforce the importance of occupation-based and family-focused OT services to support improved participation in meaningful activities for children with disabilities.
◆ A 12-week psychoeducational group for children with spina bifida that focused on didactic teaching, personal goal setting, social interaction, and homework was found to be effective in improving self-care skills (Engelman, Loomis, & Kleiback, 1994).
◆ Participation in a short-term, inpatient rehabilitative program that provides interdisciplinary services can be effective in increasing independence in ADL for children and adolescents with spina bifida (Bolding & Llorens, 1991).
◆ The incorporation of leisure in the lives of individuals with congenital disabilities has been found to provide enjoyment; physical and mental health benefits; and opportunities to develop self-concept, self-worth, and friendships (Specht, King, Brown, & Foris, 2002).
◆ The use of word prediction programs have the potential to improve written production and task performance for school-aged children with spina bifida based on a consideration of individual skills and task requirements (Tam, Reid, Naumann, & O'Keefe, 2002).

There is a significant need to expand on the research that is currently available regarding occupational therapists' role in working with individuals with spina bifida and their families. The Spina Bifida Association of America identified a number of clinical questions that require further research (Liptak, 2003). Research priorities that relate to occupational therapy practice include independence, self-care, sexuality, education, employment, socialization, family functioning, mobility, behavioral and mental health, learning, orthopedics, and skin care.

FAMILY AND CAREGIVER CONCERNS

Family-centered and culturally competent care is essential in providing services for individuals with spina bifida. Because spina bifida is a chronic condition, lifelong planning is necessary for the individual and his or her family. The Needs Assessment Questionnaire developed by Kennedy and colleagues (1998) may assist in identifying the needs for the individual with spina bifida and the individual's family. Needs are considered in the following areas:

- Transportation
- Accessibility
- Independence
- Finances
- Medical resources
- Communication
- Family and socialization
- Education of others
- School services
- Vocational training

Preliminary use of the Needs Assessment Questionnaire indicated that children with spina bifida and their families identified priorities and needs differently. Parents perceived greater needs than their children did (Buran, McDaniel, & Brei, 2002; Kennedy et al., 1998).

RESOURCES

Associations

- Easter Seals
  230 West Monroe Street
  Suite 1800
  Chicago, IL 60606
  Telephone: 800-221-6827
  Website: http://www.easterseals.com
  Local addresses and telephone numbers may be obtained from the Website.
- March of Dimes
  1275 Mamaroneck Avenue
  White Plains, NY 10605
  Website: http://www.marchofdimes.com
  Local addresses and telephone numbers can be obtained from the Website.

Articles and Books

- Lutkenhoff, M., & Oppenheimer, S. (1997). *SPINAbilities: A young person's guide to spina bifida.* Bethesda, MD: Woodbine.
  A practical guide for youth with spina bifida that addresses increasing independence and managing health
- Lutkenhoff, M. (1999). *Children with spina bifida: A parent's guide.* Bethesda, MD: Woodbine.
  Designed to address common questions and concerns parents have about their child's condition and development
- Neville-Jan, A. (2003). Encounters in a world of pain: An autoethnography. *American Journal of Occupational Therapy, 57,* 88–98.
  Presents the author's personal narrative of her experience living with chronic pain and spina bifida, along with

a reflection on the concept of pain and the role of OT in working with individuals with chronic pain.

- Sandler, A. (2004). *Living with spina bifida: A guide for families and professionals.* Chapel Hill, NC: University of North Carolina Press.
  Addresses clients' biopsychosocial and developmental needs from birth through adolescence and into adulthood. Parent insights, a glossary, a list of spina bifida associations, and suggested readings are included.

Journals

- *The Journal of Special Education*
- *The Journal of Developmental and Physical Disabilities*

Websites

- Spina Bifida Association of America
  http://www.sbaa.org.
  This Website provides an overview of symptoms, treatment options and programs, current research, support services, publication lists, and many more resources. This site is also presented in Spanish.
- National Institute of Neurological Disorders and Stroke
  http://www.ninds.nih.gov
  The National Institute of Neurological Disorders and Stroke (NINDS) conducts and supports research on brain and nervous system disorders. This Website provides information on condition descriptions, treatment, prognosis, and research.

REFERENCES

Andren, E., & Grimby, G. (2004). Dependence in daily activities and life satisfaction in adult subjects with cerebral palsy or spina bifida: A follow-up study. *Disability and Rehabilitation, 26,* 528–536.

Beers, M. H., & Berkow, R. (Eds.). (1999). *The Merck manual of diagnosis and therapy* (17th ed.). Whitehouse Station, NJ: Merck Research Laboratories.

Bent, N., Tennant, A. Swift, T., Posnett, J., Scuffham, P., & Chamberlain, M. A. (2002). Team approach versus ad hoc health services for young people with physical disabilities: A retrospective cohort study. *Lancet, 360,* 1280–1286.

Bolding, D. J., & Llorens, L. A. (1991). The effects of habilitative hospital admission on self-care, self-esteem, and frequency of physical care. *American Journal of Occupational Therapy, 45,* 796–800.

Brown, J. P. (2001). Orthopaedic care of children with spina bifida: You've come a long way, baby. *Orthopaedic Nursing, 20,* 51–58.

Buran, C. F., McDaniel, A. M., & Brei, T. J. (2002). Needs assessment in a spina bifida program: A comparison of the perceptions by adolescents with spina bifida and their parents. *Clinical Nurse Specialist, 16,* 256–262.

Dias, M. S. (2003). *Hydrocephalus and shunts in the person with spina bifida.* Retrieved February 2, 2005, from http://www.sbaa.org/site/PageServer?pagename=asb_hydrocephalus

Engelman, B. E., Loomis, J. W., & Kleiback, L. (1994). A psychoeducational group addressing self-care, self-esteem, and social skills in children with spina bifida. *European Journal of Pediatric Surgery, 4,* 38–39.

Kennedy, S. E., Garcia Martin, S. D., Kelley, J. M., Walton, B., Vleck, C. K., Hassanein, R. S., et al. (1998). Identification of medical and nonmedical needs of adolescents and young adults with spina bifida and their families: A preliminary study. *Children's Health Care, 27,* 47–61.

Kinsman, S. L., Levey, E., Ruffing, V., Stone, J., & Warren, L. (2000). Beyond multidisciplinary care: A new conceptual model for spina bifida services. *European Journal of Pediatric Surgery, 10,* 35–38.

Klingbeil, H., Baer, H. R., & Wilson, P. E. (2004). Aging with disability. *Archives of Physical Medicine and Rehabilitation, 85,* S68–S73.

Liptak, G. S. (1997). Neural tube defects. In M. L. Batshaw (Ed.), *Children with disabilities,* (4th ed., pp. 529–552). Baltimore: Brooks.

Liptak, G. S. (Ed.). (2003). *Spina bifida: Developing a research agenda.* Retrieved March 10, 2005, from http://www.sbaa.org/site/DocServer/Evidence-based_practice_in_SB1.pdf?docID=121

McLone, D. G., & Dias, M. S. (2001). Hydrocephalus and the Chiari II malformation in myelomeningocele. In J. F. Sarwark & J. P. Lubicky (Eds.), *Caring for the child with spina bifida* (pp. 29–42). Rosemont, IL: American Academy of Orthopaedic Surgeons.

National Dissemination Center for Children with Disabilities. (2004). *Spina bifida.* Retrieved February 9, 2005, from http://www.nichcy.org/pubs/factshe/fs12txt.htm

National Institute of Neurological Disorders and Stroke. (2004). *NINDS spina bifida information page.* Retrieved February 5, 2005, from http://www.ninds.nih.gov/disorders/spina_bifida/spina_bifida.htm

Okimoto, A. M., Bundy, A., & Hanzlik, J. (2000). Playfulness in children with and without disability: Measurement and intervention. *American Journal of Occupational Therapy, 54,* 73–82.

Razma, K. G. (2001). Occupational therapy evaluation and treatment: Considerations in patients with myelomeningocele. In J. F. Sarwark & J. P. Lubicky (Eds.), *Caring for the child with spina bifida* (pp. 533–549). Rosemont, IL: American Academy of Orthopaedic Surgeons.

Rekate, H. L. (2001). Pathophysiology and management of hydrocephalus in spina bifida. In J. F. Sarwark & J. P. Lubicky (Eds.), *Caring for the child with spina bifida* (pp. 395–407). Rosemont, IL: American Academy of Orthopaedic Surgeons.

Scoggin, A. E., & Parks, K. M. (1997). Latex sensitivity in children with spina bifida: Implications for occupational therapy practitioners. *American Journal of Occupational Therapy, 51,* 608–611.

Simeonsson, R. J., McMillen, J. S., & Huntington, G. S. (2002). Secondary conditions in children with disabilities: Spina bifida as a case example. *Mental Retardation and Developmental Disabilities, 8,* 198–205.

Snow, J. H. (1999). Executive processes for children with spina bifida. *Children's Health Care, 28,* 241–253.

Specht, J., King, G., Brown, E., & Foris, C. (2002). The importance of leisure in the lives of persons with congenital physical disabilities. *American Journal of Occupational Therapy, 56,* 436–445.

Spina Bifida Association of America. (2001). *Spotlight on spina bifida.* Retrieved February 9, 2005, from http://www.sbaa.org/site/DocServer/Spotlight_on_Spina_Bifida.doc?docID=1181

Tam, C., Reid, D., Naumann, S., & O'Keefe, B, 2002. Perceived benefits of word prediction intervention on written productivity in children with spinal bifida and hydrocephalus. *Occupational Therapy International, 9,* 237–255.

Wills, K. E. (1993). Neuropsychological functioning in children with spina bifida and/or hydrocephalus. *Journal of Clinical Child Psychology, 22,* 247–265.

SPINAL CORD INJURY

Kirsten Protos, Kate-Lyn Stone, and Meredith Grinnell

DEFINITION

Spinal cord injury (SCI) involves damage to the spinal nerves through compression, bruising, or severing of the spinal cord, which results in paralysis and loss of sensory and motor function based on the level at which the injury occurs.

ETIOLOGY

SCI is most often caused by trauma, such as car accidents or gunshot wounds, but can also be the result of tumors or acquired diseases.

CLASSIFICATION

A *complete injury* indicates that there is no sensory or motor function below the level of injury. When there is some remaining sensory or motor function below the level of injury, it is considered an *incomplete injury*. SCI is categorized as tetraplegia or paraplegia. *Tetraplegia* involves a loss of function in both the upper and lower extremities; *paraplegia* involves a loss of function in the lower extremities only.

INCIDENCE AND PREVALENCE

There are approximately 250,000 people living with a SCI in the United States today, with 11,000 new cases occurring each year. There is a higher incidence of SCI among people ages 18–25, males being at a significantly higher risk than females (National SCI Statistical Center, 2005; Reed, 2001; Spinal Cord Injury Resource Center, 2006b).

TYPICAL COURSE

Half of all people with SCI have associated injuries, especially if the injury was due to trauma. The length of stay in an acute care hospital depends on the severity of the SCI and the related injuries. When patients are medically stable, they are transferred to an inpatient rehabilitation hospital, where the average length of stay is about 44 days. Individuals with higher-level injuries often require longer and more intensive treatment than do individuals with lower-level injuries. After leaving inpatient rehab, most patients continue their therapy at an outpatient facility. Patients who survive the initial 24 hours after their injury have an 85% chance of surviving 10 years or more, younger survivors and those with lower and incomplete injuries having a better chance for survival (Shepherd Center, 2000; Spinal Cord Injury Recovery Center, 2006b).

SYMPTOMS AND COMPLICATIONS

Major Signs

- Paralysis: no motor function at and below the level of injury for individuals with complete SCIs; weakness and decreased range of motion in the partially affected muscles
- Paresis: impaired motor function at or below the level of injury for individuals with incomplete SCIs
- Sensory deficits: no sensory function at and below the level of injury for individuals with complete SCIs; impaired sensory function at or below level of injury for individuals with incomplete SCIs
- Spasticity: strong involuntary muscle spasms in the impaired limbs
- Respiratory dysfunction: loss of function or weakness in the respiratory muscles for individuals with high injury levels (C1–C3)
- Bladder and bowel dysfunction
- Orthostatic hypotension: drops in blood pressure on movement during the acute phase of the injury
- Pain
- Reproductive and sexual dysfunction

Complications

- Autonomic dysreflexia: a potentially fatal condition that causes blood pressure to rise dangerously high because of a noxious stimulus to the body below the level of injury
- Skin breakdown and pressure sores
- Pain
- Urinary tract infections
- Pneumonia
- Heterotopic ossification: abnormal bone growth at large joints
- Deep vein thrombosis
- Cardiovascular disease

(National Institute of Neurological Disorders and Stroke, 2003; Reed, 2001; Spinal Cord Injury Resource Center, 2006b)

TYPICAL INTERVENTIONS

- *Immobilization:* The spine and/or neck are immobilized to prevent further injury immediately following injury and surgery.
- *Medication:* In the first 24 hours following injury corticosteroid medications, such as methylprednisolone, are given to reduce swelling in the spinal cord. Medications are also used for pain management, because many patients with SCIs are in a great deal of pain during the acute period.
- *Surgery:* It is often necessary to perform surgery to remove or repair broken bones and ligaments of the spine caused by a traumatic injury. Fractured vertebrae are often fused or grafted to normal vertebrae by using metal rods or screws to prevent movement of the fractured vertebrae.
- *Rehabilitation:* In rehabilitation, a patient with a SCI will receive continuing medical care; physical, occupational, and recreational therapies; speech therapy if necessary; counseling services; and patient and caregiver education. The focus is on restoring strength and function and developing compensatory strategies to help the patient gain as much independence as possible. (Spinal Cord Injury Recovery Center, 2006a).

PROGNOSIS

Survivors of SCI will continue to live with functional limitations based on their level and type of injury. They may also continue to deal with pain and other secondary complications, depending on how they handle their daily care (NINDS, 2003). People with paraplegia and/or incomplete injuries tend to do better than those with tetraplegia and/or complete injuries. Advances in treatment, rehabilitation, and assistive technology have made it possible to improve some of the functional capabilities of people with SCIs.

PRECAUTIONS

- Monitor the patient's skin for redness or ulcers; individuals with SCI must perform pressure relief every 30 minutes to reduce the risk of skin breakdown.
- Monitor blood pressure and check for dizziness to prevent orthostatic hypotension.
- Observe body temperature; people with SCI, especially high level and in the acute phase, can have problems with temperature regulation.
- Watch for signs indicating autonomic dysreflexia (headache, sweating, congestion, hypertension, bradycardia); if these signs are observed, immediately place the patient in an upright position and remove any restricting materials or obvious noxious stimuli.
- Monitor the respiration of patients with a C1–C4 injury, especially if the patient is on a ventilator.
- Assess the patient for pain, spasticity, muscle stiffness/hypertonia, decreased range of motion, and subluxation to prevent further injury during treatment. (NINDS, 2003; Reed, 2001).

OCCUPATIONAL THERAPY EVALUATIONS

Motor and Sensory Function Evaluations

- American Spinal Injury Association (ASIA) Impairment Scale
- Manual muscle testing
- Range-of-motion testing using a goniometer

ADL and IADL Evaluations

- Functional Independence Measure (FIM)
- Barthel Index
- Klein-Bell ADL Scale
- Quadriplegic Index of Function (Reed, 2001)

OCCUPATIONAL THERAPY INTERVENTIONS

In rehabilitation of individuals with SCI, occupational therapists use a combination of biomechanical and rehabilitative (compensatory) treatment models.

- *Biomechanical model:* Used to help the patient improve strength, range of motion, endurance, balance, mobility, and energy conservation.
- *Rehabilitative model:* Used to improve the patient's functional performance to be as independent as possible; compensatory strategies and assistive technology are used to improve function in occupational performance areas such as ADL/IADL, leisure, and work and productivity.

- Occupational therapists also often address patients' cognitive and psychosocial needs in their intervention as well as providing patient and caregiver education and home modification suggestions (Dolhi, 2001; Reed, 2001).

FAMILY AND CAREGIVER CONCERNS

Caregivers have a responsibility to care for and perform the activities that their loved one with a SCI cannot do independently. Individuals with higher-level injuries require more work and diligence to prevent complications. Some concerns of caregivers can include the following:

- Financial coverage for medical bills, services, and equipment
- Physical and emotional support for caregivers—support groups are important
- Being able to perform the daily medical tasks to keep the loved one healthy
- Having a good quality of life

OCCUPATIONAL THERAPY AND THE EVIDENCE

Occupational therapists are the most appropriate service providers to address function in the performance areas of patients with SCI. According to the AOTA's practice guidelines for adults with spinal cord injury (Dolhi, 2001), occupational therapy intervention focuses on ADL, work, and leisure activities. Occupational therapists are also involved in education of family members and caregivers, environmental adaptation, assistive technology and equipment, and driving evaluation and training. Occupational therapists enable their clients to perform activities that are meaningful by building a trusting relationship with the client, being flexible and creative with resources and approaches to treatment, and adapting the environment (Guidetti & Tham, 2002).

Spinal cord injury has several different aspects that have been reviewed in current research. Functional electrical therapy, which is used to restore useful movements, has been found to be effective for both grasping exercises and gait training for individuals with spinal cord injury (Popovic et al., 2006; Thrasher, Flett, & Popovic, 2006). Kennedy, Duff, Evans, and Beedie (2003) found programs that use cognitive behavioral techniques in a group setting to be successful in reducing depression and anxiety associated with spinal cord injury. Participants found the shared problem solving among the group members to be particularly helpful. Guidetti and Tham (2002) addressed strategies that occupational therapists use in self-care training and suggested that occupational therapists, through understanding each individual person, vary their strategies to meet the needs of each person's unique experience with spinal cord injury. Last, a weight management program involving education about nutrition, exercise, and behavior modification was effective for obese and overweight individuals with spinal cord injury to safely lose weight without compromising lean body mass and overall well-being (Chen, Henson, Jackson, & Richards, 2006).

RESOURCES

Associations

- The National Spinal Cord Injury Association
  6701 Democracy Boulevard
  Suite 300-9
  Bethesda, MD 20817
  Helpline: 800-962-9629
  Fax: (301) 990-0445
  Website: http://www.spinalcord.org/
- United Spinal Association
  75-20 Astoria Boulevard
  Jackson Heights, New York 11370
  Telephone: 718-803-3782
  Fax: (718) 803-0414
  Website: http://www.unitedspinal.org
- Christopher Reeve Paralysis Foundation
  636 Morris Turnpike
  Suite 3A
  Short Hills, NJ 07078
  Telephone: 800-225-0292
  Website: http://www.christopherreeve.org

First-Person Accounts

- Reeve, C. (1999). *Still me.* New York: Ballantine Books. This is Christopher Reeve's first book after the riding accident that left him a high tetraplegic. The moving autobiography chronicles his recovery and journey to reclaim his life.
- Reeve, C. (2005). *Nothing is impossible: Reflections on a new life.* New York: Ballantine Books.
  Christopher Reeve's follow-up book to *Still Me* reveals a more inspirational side of him as it addresses aspects of successful living with a SCI and dealing with major life issues.
- Ellison, J., & Ellison, B. (2004). *The Brooke Ellison story: One mother, one daughter, one journey.* New York: Hyperion Books.
  This book is a heartfelt and courageous story of how Brooke Ellison overcame impossible odds as young girl living with a SCI who went on to graduate from Harvard University. The book is written by both Brooke and her mother about their journey together.

Journals

- *Spinal Cord*
- *Journal of Rehabilitation Research & Development*
- *Journal of Neurotrauma*

Websites

- Spinal Cord Injury Information Network
  http://www.spinalcord.uab.edu
  This Website is run by the University of Alabama at Birmingham and the UAB Model SCI Care System. It provides a wealth of information related to SCI, facts and statistics, research, and other links.
- The Foundation for Spinal Cord Injury Prevention, Care, and Cure
  http://www.fscip.org/index.html
  This Website is a great place for individuals living with SCI and their family members to get vital information and links for support groups and discussion sites.
- National Institute of Neurological Disorders and Stroke
  http://www.ninds.nih.gov/disorders/sci/sci.htm
  This Website, which is run by the U.S. Department of Health and Human Services and the National Institutes of Health, is a good resource for up-to-date research information and links to publications and patient recruitment for SCI studies.
- MedlinePlus
  http://www.nlm.nih.gov/medlineplus/spinalcordin
  juries.html
  This is another Website run by the U.S. Department of Health and Human Services and the National Institutes of Health. It has a lot of links to important medical information related to SCI and secondary complications and prevention.

REFERENCES

Chen, Y., Henson, S., Jackson, A. B., & Richards, J. S. (2006). Obesity intervention in persons with spinal cord injury. *Spinal Cord, 44,* 82–91.

Dolhi, C. D. (2001). *Occupational therapy practice guidelines for adults with spinal cord injury* (3rd ed.). Bethesda, MD: The American Occupational Therapy Association.

Guidetti, S., & Tham, K. (2002). Therapeutic strategies used by occupational therapists in self-care training: A qualitative study. *Occupational Therapy International, 9,* 257–276.

Kennedy, P., Duff, J., Evans, M., & Beedie, A. (2003). Coping effectiveness training reduces depression and anxiety following traumatic spinal cord injuries. *The British Psychology Society, 42,* 41–52.

National Institute of Neurological Disorders and Stroke. NIH. DHHS (2003). Spinal cord injury: Hope through research (03-160). Bethesda: National Institutes of Health.

National SCI Statistical Center. (2005). *Spinal cord injury: Facts and figures at a glance.* Retrieved April 3, 2006, from http://www.spinalcord.uab.edu/show.asp?durki=21446

Popovic, M. R., Thrasher, T. A., Adams, M. E., Takes, V., Zivanovic, V., & Tonack, M. I. (2006). Functional electrical therapy: Retraining grasping in spinal cord injury. *Spinal Cord, 44,* 143–151.

Reed, K. L. (2001). Spinal cord injuries: Adult. In *Quick reference to occupational therapy* (2nd ed., pp. 538–553). Austin, Texas: Pro-Ed.

Shepherd Center. (2000). *Spinal cord injury: Facts & figures.* Retrieved April 2, 2006, from http://www.shepherd.org

Spinal Cord Injury Recovery Center. (2006a). *SCI treatment.* Retrieved March 20, 2006, from http://www.sci-recovery.org/sci-help.htm

Spinal Cord Injury Resource Center. (2006b). *Spinal cord 101.* Retrieved March 31, 2006, from http://www.spinalinjury.net

Thrasher, T. A., Flett, H. M., & Popovic, H. R. (2006). Gait training regimen for incomplete spinal cord injury using functional electrical stimulation. *Spinal Cord, 44,* 357–361.

TRAUMATIC BRAIN INJURY

Justina Hsu

A traumatic brain injury (TBI) is an insult to the brain that is not of a degenerative or congenital nature, but caused by an external physical force. A TBI may produce a diminished or altered state of consciousness that results in impairment of cognitive abilities or physical functioning as well as disturbances of behavioral or emotional function. These impairments may be either temporary or permanent and may cause partial or total functional disability or psychosocial maladjustment (Brain Injury Association of America).

TWO TYPES OF TRAUMATIC BRAIN INJURY:

- Penetrating or missile (open) injuries, which result from penetration of the skull
- Nonpenetrating, closed head injuries, which result from rapid acceleration or deceleration of the brain within the skull, causing damage at the point of impact (coup injuries) or at the opposite pole (contrecoup injuries)

INCIDENCE AND PREVALENCE

- Each year, an estimated 1.5 million Americans sustain a TBI.
- An estimated 5.3 million Americans currently live with disabilities resulting from a TBI.
- TBIs cause more death and disability than any other neurological condition before the age of 50 years.
- The majority of TBI is seen primarily in males between the ages of 18 and 25 years (Brain Injury Association of America).

PRIMARY CAUSES

The primary causes leading to TBI are motor vehicle, motorcycle, or off-road vehicle accidents; falls; sports-related accidents; objects falling on the head; and interpersonal violence.

TYPICAL COURSE/PROGNOSIS

No two brain injuries are exactly the same; the course of a TBI is complex and can vary greatly between individuals. Early prediction of outcome and prognosis is difficult because of the complex interaction of various factors, including the cause, location, and severity of injury; age; length of posttraumatic amnesia; increased intracranial pressure; and/or alteration of consciousness. Accurate prognosis requires repeated observations over weeks or months to predict the level of recovery.

POSSIBLE SYMPTOMS/DEFICITS

Depending on the location and severity of the injury, deficits may be present in the areas of cognitive, behavioral/emotional, physical, and/or sensory impairments.

RANCHO LOS AMIGOS LEVELS OF COGNITIVE FUNCTIONING SCALE

The Rancho Los Amigos Scale, a nonstandardized method of organizing and describing clinical observations of cognitive performance in individuals with TBI, allows for better assessment of recovery and improved communication with families. The Rancho Los Amigos Scale is a widely used tool that divides stages of recovery into 10 levels of cognitive functioning that are useful for documenting and assessing progress.

- Level I: No response
- Level II: Generalized response
- Level III: Localized response
- Level IV: Confused, agitated
- Level V: Confused, inappropriate
- Level VI: Confused, appropriate
- Level VII: Automatic, appropriate
- Level VIII: Purposeful, appropriate, with stand-by assistance

- Level IX: Purposeful, appropriate, with stand-by assistance on request
- Level X: Purposeful, appropriate, modified independence

OT EVALUATIONS

- Rancho Los Amigos Levels of Cognitive Functioning Scale

Acute Stages of Recovery

- Glasgow Coma Scale (GCS): Not administered by occupational therapists but important for quantifying level of consciousness and predicting recovery with early treatment and prognostic indicators.
- Western Neuro Sensory Stimulation Profile (WNSSP)
- Coma Recovery Scale

Inpatient Rehabilitation

- Functional Independence Measure (FIM)
- Functional Assessment Measure (FAM)
- Assessment of Motor and Process Skills (AMPS)
- Loewenstein Occupational Therapy Cognitive Assessment (LOTCA)
- Kitchen Task Assessment (KTA)

Postacute Rehabilitation

- Canadian Occupational Performance Measure (COPM)
- Safety Assessment of Function and the Environment for Rehabilitation (SAFER)
- Interest Checklist

OT INTERVENTION

Acute Stages of Recovery

- Positioning
- AROM, AAROM, PROM exercises
- Sensory stimulation
- Splinting and casting
- Patient and family education and support

Inpatient Rehabilitation

- Optimize gross and fine motor functioning and abilities through meaningful tasks and activities
- Optimize visual-perceptual functioning and abilities through environmental adaptations, compensatory techniques, and assistive devices such as low-vision aids
- Maximize cognitive functioning and abilities with compensatory or remedial strategies that optimize the areas of orientation, attention, and memory

- Increase independence in ADL and IADL
- Patient and family education and support

Postacute Rehabilitation

- Community reintegration
- Maximize cognitive abilities in natural environments by teaching compensatory and adaptive cognitive strategies
- Environmental modifications and adaptive equipment
- Restore competence in ADL and IADL
- Participation in previous or new leisure activities
- Patient and family education and support

OT AND THE EVIDENCE

Occupational therapy plays an integral role as a part of an interdisciplinary rehabilitation team for individuals with TBI in multiple settings, including inpatient, outpatient, and community settings. Evidence has shown occupational therapy to be effective in improving occupational performance through participation in functional tasks and activities for individuals with TBI. Trombly, Radomski, Trexel, and Burnett-Smith (2002) concluded that participation in goal-specific outpatient occupational therapy that focuses on teaching compensatory strategies is strongly associated with the achievement of self-identified goals and the reduction of disability in adults with mild to moderate brain injury. Trombly, Radomski and Davis (1998) found that people with TBI who participated in outpatient occupational therapy showed a significant achievement of self-identified goals, independence, and satisfaction with their tasks performance after treatment. A study by Neistadt (1994) concluded that functional activities may be more effective than tabletop activities in promoting fine motor coordination in persons with TBI. Dirette (2002) found that clients with brain injury slowly developed awareness of their deficits when they were in situations that enabled then to compare current performance to performance prior to brain injury.

CAREGIVER CONCERNS

Families and caregivers require education and support for the many behavioral, emotional, and personality changes that can occur in an individual following a TBI. A study by Groom, Shaw, O'Connor, Howard, and Pickens (1998) concluded that caregiver stress level is significantly related to the presence of the neurobehavioral symptoms of inappropriateness, depression, and indifference that are often seen in individuals with TBI. The possible issues caregivers may encounter during recovery with an individual following TBI include the following:

- Management of agitation
- Personality and behavioral changes following injury
- Difficulty with community reintegration and adaptation
- Lack of awareness of deficits/denial
- Deficits in higher-level cognitive functions, including orientation, attention, and memory
- Disinhibition of inappropriate behavior
- Depression
- Long-term need for assistance/care
- Change in family and societal roles
- Safety concerns/awareness

RESOURCES

Associations

- Brain Trauma Foundation
  523 East 72nd Street
  8th Floor
  New York, NY 10021
  Telephone: 212-772-0608
  Fax: 212-772-0357
  Website: http://www.braintrauma.org
- Brain Injury Association of America
  105 North Alfred Street
  Alexandria, VA 22314
  Telephone: 800-444-6443
  Family Helpline: 703-236-6000
  Fax: 703-236-6001
  Website: http://www.biausa.org
- Family Caregiver Alliance
  690 Market Street
  Suite 600
  San Francisco, CA 94104
  Telephone: 415-434-3388 or 800-445-8106
  Fax: 415-434-3508
  Website: http://www.caregiver.org

First-Person Accounts

- Crimmins, C. (2001). *Where Is the Mango Princess?* New York: Random House.
  Crimmins tells her personal story of the victories and losses she endured as the caregiver of an individual recovering from a severe brain injury. She describes issues ranging from the frustrations of dealing with doctors and insurance plans to the pain of caregiver issues.
- Meili, T. (2003). *I am the Central Park jogger: A story of hope and possibility.* Waterville, ME: Thorndike Press.
  Meili tells her personal experience of recovery from a violence-related TBI following an attack in Central Park. She focuses her book on the rehabilitation process, how brain injury affected her personal and professional life, and her outlook on living with a brain injury.

- Osborn, C. (2000). *Over my head: A doctor's own story of head injury from the inside looking out.* Riverside, NJ: Andrews McMeel.
  Dr. Osborn chronicles her rehabilitation process following a brain injury from the struggle to remaster basic skills to the pain of parting with her old identity as a young doctor and the challenge of building a new life.

Journals

- *Brain*
- *TBI Challenge!*
- *Journal of Head Trauma Rehabilitation.*

Websites

- Brain Injury Association of America
  www.biusa.org
  This is a thorough and accessible Website that provides information and resources relating to TBI for families, professionals, and individuals with brain injuries.
- Traumatic Brain Injury Resource Guide
  www.neuroskills.com
  This Website is a source of information, services, and products relating to TBI, brain injury recovery, and postacute rehabilitation.
- National Institute of Neurological Disorders and Stroke: Traumatic Brain Injury Information
  http://www.ninds.nih.gov/disorders/tbi/tbi.htm
  This Webpage from the NINDS is easily accessible and provides basic and fundamental information on the treatment, prognosis, research and resources related to TBI.

REFERENCES

Brain Injury Association of American. (2005). *Facts about traumatic brain injury.* Retrieved October 30, 2007, from http://www.biausa.org/elements/aboutbi.htm/factsheets/factsaboutBI.8.29.05.pdf

Dirette, D. (2002). The development of awareness and the use of compensatory strategies for cognitive deficits. *Brain Injury, 16,* 861–871.

Groom, K. N., Shaw, T. G., O'Connor, M. E., Howard, N. I., & Pickens, A. (1998). Neurobehavioral symptoms and family dysfunctioning in traumatically brain-injured adults. *Archives of Clinical Neuropsychology, 13,* 695–711.

Neistadt, M. E. (1994). The effects of different treatment activities on functional fine motor coordination in adults with brain injury. *American Journal of Occupational Therapy, 48,* 877–882.

Trombly, C. A., Radomski, M. V., & Davis, E. S. (1998). Achievement of self-identified goals by adults with traumatic brain injury: Phase I. *American Journal of Occupational Therapy, 52,* 810–818.

Trombly, C. A., Radomski, M. V., Trexel, C., & Burnett-Smith, S. E. (2002). Occupational therapy and achievement of self-identified goals by adults with acquired brain injury: Phase II. *American Journal of Occupational Therapy, 56*, 489–498.

REFERENCES FOR ASSESSMENTS

Ansell, B. J., & Keenan, J. E. (1989). The Western Neuro Sensory Stimulation Profile: A tool for assessing slow-to-recover head-injured patients. *Archives of Physical Medicine and Rehabilitation, 70*, 104–108.

Carswell, A., McColl, M. A., Baptiste, S., Law, M., Polatajko, H., & Pollock, N. (2004). The Canadian Occupational Performance Measure: A research and clinical literature review. *Canadian Journal of Occupational Therapy, 71*, 210–222.

Cup, E. H., Scholte op Reimer, W. J., Thijssen, M. C., & van Kuyks-Minis, M. A. (2003). Reliability and validity of the Canadian Occupational Performance Measure in stroke patients. *Clinical Rehabilitation, 17*, 402–409.

Dedding, C., Cardol, M., Eyssen, I. C., Dekker, J., & Beelen, A. (2004). Validity of the Canadian Occupational Performance Measure: A client-centered outcome measurement. *Clinical Rehabilitation, 18*, 660–667.

Dodds, T. A., Matrin, D. P., Stolov, W. C., & Deyo, R. A. (1993). A validation of the Functional Independence Measurement and its performance among rehabilitation inpatients. *Archives of Physical Medicine and Rehabilitation, 74*, 531–536.

Giacino, J. T., Kezmarsky, M. A., DeLuca, J., & Cicerone, K. D. (1991). Monitoring rate of recovery to predict outcome in minimally responsive patients. *Archives of Physical Medicine and Rehabilitation, 72*, 897–901.

Katz, N., Itzovish, M., Averbuch, S., & Elazar, B. (1989). Loewenstein Occupational Therapy Cognitive Assessment battery for brain injured patients: Reliability and validity. *American Journal of Occupational Therapy, 43*, 184–192.

Klyczek, J. P., Bauer-Yox, N., & Fiedler, R. C. (1997). The Interest Checklist: A factor analysis. *American Journal of Occupational Therapy, 51*, 815–823.

Linden, A., Boschian, K., Eker, C., Schalen, W., & Nordstrom, C. H. (2005). Assessment of Motor and Process Skills reflects brain injured patients' ability to resume independent living better than neuropsychological tests. *Acta Neurologica Scandinavica, 111*, 364–369.

Oliver, R., Blathwayt, J., Brackley, C., & Tamaki, T. (1993). Development of the Safety Assessment of Function and the Environment for Rehabilitation (SAFER) tool. *Canadian Journal of Occupational Therapy, 60*, 78–82.

Ottenbacher, K. J., Hsu, Y., Granger, C. V., & Fiedler, R. C. (1996). The reliability of the Functional Independence Measure: A quantitative review. *Archives of Physical Medicine and Rehabilitation, 77*, 1226–1232.

Pentland, B., Hellawell, D. J., & Benjamin, J. (1999). The Functional Assessment Measure (FIM+ FAM) as part of the hospital discharge summary after brain injury rehabilitation. *Clinical Rehabilitation, 13*, 498–502.

Zafonte, R. D., Hammond, F. M., Mann, N. R., Wood, D. L., Black, K. L., & Millis, S. R. (1996). Relationship between Glasgow Coma Scale and functional outcome. *American Journal Physical and Medical Rehabilitation, 75*, 364–369.

XVI

Occupational Therapy Resource Summaries: Practice Settings

Settings Providing Medical and Psychiatric Services

PAMELA ROBERTS AND MARY EVENSON

ACUTE MEDICAL/SURGICAL CARE

Persons Most Likely to Benefit from Type of Care

- Need for medical or surgical stabilization, 24-hour physician and nursing care
- Typical diagnoses include: cerebral palsy, stroke, brain injury, spinal cord injury, neurological disease, cardiac disease, pulmonary disease, orthopedics, and cancer

Requirements for Admission to Setting

- Need for medical or surgical diagnosis or intervention
- Admitted from emergency room, direct admission, or transfer from another facility

Typical Setting

- Private hospital
- Community hospital
- Veteran's Administration hospital
- Specialty hospital

Typical Length of Stay

- Varies based on diagnosis
- Diagnostic related groups (DRGs)
- Short term, usually 1–2 weeks or less

Typical Services

- Trauma services
- Intensive care unit

1074

- Medical services
- Surgical services
- Consultations by allied health care providers

Type of Occupational Therapy Service

- Direct or consultation

Role of Occupational Therapy

- OT role for trauma services and ICU may be direct or consultation including positioning, range of motion, splinting/casting, and sensory stimulation
- OT role for medical and surgical services may be direct or consultation. Safety assessment; assessment of client's abilities, roles, habits and routines. Functional survival skills such as eating/dysphagia, grooming, dressing, bathing, and toileting, functional transfers and mobility
- Recommendations for continued services at next level of care
- Discharge planning

Typical Precautions

- Evaluation and monitoring of vital signs (respiratory, cardiac, neurological, gastrointestinal, and immune systems)
- Monitor and evaluate vital signs as indicated (heart rate, blood pressure, and respirations)
- Postsurgical protocols as applicable
- Dietary restrictions per individual needs
- Fall prevention protocols

Discharge Disposition

- Home
- Board and care
- Retirement home
- Assisted living
- Skilled nursing facility
- Hospice
- Inpatient rehabilitation unit or hospital
- Community discharge with home health
- Community discharge with outpatient rehabilitation

Legislation and Funding/Payment

- Prospective payment system
- Private insurance or self-pay
- Managed care (PPO or HMO)
- Indemnity
- Workers' compensation
- Medicare
- Medicaid

INPATIENT REHABILITATION

Persons Most Likely to Benefit from Type of Care

- People who require a comprehensive rehabilitation program
- 75% of clients must have a diagnosis within the Centers for Medicare and Medicaid Services (CMS) thirteen diagnostic groups. CMS-13 Diagnostic Groups include: (1) Stroke, (2) Spinal Cord Injury, (3) Congenital Deformity, (4) Amputation, (5) Major Multiple Trauma, (6) Fracture of Femur, (7) Brain Injury, (8) Neurological Disorders, (9) Burns, (10) Active Polyarticular Rheumatoid Arthritis, Psoriatic Arthritis, and Seronegative Arthropathies, (11) Systemic Vasculidities with Joint Inflammation, (12) Severe or Advanced Osteoarthritis, (13) Knee or Hip Replacement if one of the following conditions are met: (a) Patient underwent bilateral knee or bilateral hip joint replacement surgery immediately preceding the IRF admission, (b) patient is extremely obese with a body mass index of at least 50 at the time of admission to the IRF, and (c) patient is age 85 or older at the time of the admission to the IRF

Requirements for Admission to Setting

- Transfer from a hospital, nursing home, or home
- Must be able to tolerate intensive therapy for a minimum of 3 hours of therapy for 5 out of 7 days
- Must require care from a multidisciplinary team with at least two disciplines
- Must meet medical necessity
- Must require 24–7 rehabilitation nursing
- Must require close monitoring by a physician with training in rehabilitation

Typical Setting

- Free-standing rehabilitation center
- Unit within hospital
- Veteran's Administration rehabilitation unit

Typical Length of Stay

- 2–4 weeks
- Target length of stay by case mix groups (CMGs)

Typical Services

- Rehabilitation physician, rehabilitation nursing, physical therapy, occupational therapy, speech-language pathology, therapeutic recreation, neuropsychology or psychology, social services, respiratory therapy, dietary, pharmacy, and other services by consultation

Type of Occupational Therapy Service

- Direct

Role of Occupational Therapy

- Comprehensive evaluation
- Participation in functional outcomes such as the Inpatient Rehabilitation Facility Patient Assessment Instrument (IRF-PAI)
- Self-care skills
- Functional mobility
- Functional mobility during ADL
- Communication during ADL
- Cognition during ADL
- Home management skills
- Community reintegration
- Discharge planning
- Recommendations for continued services at next level of care

Typical Precautions

- Monitor and evaluate vital signs as indicated (heart rate, blood pressure, and respirations)
- Postsurgical protocols as applicable
- Dietary restrictions per individual needs
- Fall prevention protocols

Discharge Disposition

- Home
- Board and care
- Retirement home
- Assisted living
- Skilled nursing facility
- Hospice
- Community discharge with home health
- Community discharge with outpatient rehabilitation

Legislation and Funding/Payment

- Prospective payment system
- Private insurance or self-pay
- Managed care (PPO or HMO)
- Indemnity
- Workers' compensation
- Medicare
- Medicaid

SKILLED NURSING/ TRANSITIONAL CARE

Persons Most Likely to Benefit from Type of Care

- People who require special, 24-hour care for either a short or extended period of time
- Same diagnoses as acute medical/surgical care

Requirements for Admission to Setting

- Bridge the gap with another level of care
- Admitted from acute care hospital
- Skilled intervention such as intravenous medication, wound care, etc.
- Disability with a new functional deficit

Typical Setting

- Unit in a hospital
- Free-standing nursing home

Typical Length of Stay

- Short term: variable not to exceed 100 days
- Long term: indefinite or as needed

Typical Services

- Physician, nursing, social services, activity therapy and/ or therapeutic recreation
- Physical therapy, occupational therapy, speech-language pathology
- Other services by consultation

Type of Occupational Therapy Service

- Direct
- Consultation
- Participation in the Minimal Data Set (MDS)

Role of Occupational Therapy

- Short-term care is more intensive with specified frequency
- Long-term care is by consultation
- Self-care skills such as eating/dysphagia, grooming, upper and lower body dressing, bathing, and toileting
- Mobility skills during ADL such as bed, chair, wheelchair transfers, toilet and tub/shower transfers, and functional mobility
- Home management and community skills such as car transfers, kitchen activities, public dining, care of pets, etc.

Typical Precautions

- Monitor and evaluate vital signs as indicated (heart rate, blood pressure, and respirations)
- Post surgical protocols as applicable
- Dietary restrictions per individual needs
- Fall prevention protocols

Discharge Disposition

- Home
- Board and care

- Retirement home
- Assisted living
- Inpatient rehabilitation
- Hospice
- Community discharge with home health
- Community discharge with outpatient rehabilitation

Legislation and Funding/Payment

- Prospective payment system
- Private insurance or self-pay
- Managed care (PPO or HMO)
- Indemnity
- Workers' compensation
- Medicare
- Medicaid

OUTPATIENT REHABILITATION

Persons Most Likely to Benefit from Type of Care

- Children or adults who can benefit from rehabilitation services due to functional limitations that interfere with abilities to participate in social roles and activities

Requirements for Admission to Setting

- Need for medical or surgical diagnosis or need for skilled intervention
- Admitted from a variety of places including institutional care or home

Typical Setting

- May be part of free-standing rehabilitation center, unit within the hospital, or Veteran's Administration hospital
- May be a satellite clinic (affiliated with a health care institution) or an independent, privately owned clinic

Typical Length of Stay

- Need for skilled intervention
- Number of visits varies depending on skilled need

Typical Services

- Physician referral may be required
- Self-referral for self-pay services

Type of Occupational Therapy Service

- Direct

Role of Occupational Therapy

- Self-care skills such as eating/dysphagia, grooming, upper and lower body dressing, bathing, and toileting

- Home management, community skills, work skills, driving
- Social participation such as student, worker, caregiver roles
- Therapeutic activities/exercise to remediate body structure/body function impairments

Typical Precautions

- Varies based on diagnosis

Discharge Disposition

- Incorporation into home and community activities

Legislation and Funding/Payment

- Prospective payment system
- Private insurance or self-pay
- Managed care (PPO or HMO)
- Indemnity
- Workers' compensation
- Medicare
- Medicaid

INPATIENT PSYCHIATRY

Persons Most Likely to Benefit from Type of Care

- People who require special, 24-hour care for either a short or extended period of time
- Some typical diagnoses based on the *DSM IV-TR* include depression, schizoaffective disorders, mood disorders, obsessive-compulsive disorders, anxiety, eating, and phobic disorders, etc.

Requirements for Admission to Setting

- Need for psychiatric diagnosis or intervention
- Admitted from the emergency room
- Direct admit
- Transfer from another facility
- Person who requires 24-hour monitoring for safety
- May be court ordered as in the case of forensic cases in which client's require secured (locked) units due to safety risk to self or others

Typical Setting

- Free-standing hospital
- Private hospital
- Unit within hospital
- State hospital
- Veteran's Administration hospital

Typical Length of Stay

- 1–3 weeks

Typical Services

- Psychiatry
- Psychology
- Nursing
- Mental health workers
- Social services
- Occupational therapy
- Therapeutic recreation
- Art therapy
- Expressive or music therapy
- Behavior management
- Other services by consultation

Type of Occupational Therapy Service

- Direct
- Consultation

Role of Occupational Therapy

- Assessment of client's abilities, roles, habits, and routines
- Safety assessment
- May administer the Allen Assessment of Cognitive Levels
- Recommendations for continued services at next level of care; discharge planning
- Individual and/or group intervention
- Functional skills such as self-care, home and community function
- Reinforce behavioral or therapeutic plan as indicated

Typical Precautions

- Unit may be locked
- 'Sharps' precautions to prevent self-injury
- Individualized medication/prescription plans and dietary or nutritional care plans
- Suicide precautions as relevant
- Behavioral guidelines for program participation per institution procedures

Discharge Disposition

- Home
- Skilled nursing facility
- Community discharge with partial hospitalization
- Community discharge with home health
- Community discharge with outpatient
- Outpatient

Legislation and Funding/Payment

- Private insurance or self-pay
- Medicare
- Medicaid
- SSI

PARTIAL HOSPITALIZATION

Persons Most Likely to Benefit from Type of Care

- People who require episodic focused psychiatric intervention
- Same diagnoses as inpatient psychiatry

Requirements for Admission to Setting

- Transition from inpatient or as an alternative to acute psychiatric hospitalization
- Structured program

Typical Setting

- Free-standing hospital
- Private hospital
- Unit within hospital
- Veteran's Administration hospital

Typical Length of Stay

- Usually 1–3 months

Typical Services

- Psychiatry
- Psychology
- Mental health workers
- Social services
- Occupational therapy
- Therapeutic recreation

Type of Occupational Therapy Service

- Direct
- Consultation

Role of Occupational Therapy

- Assessment of client's abilities, roles, habits, and routines
- Continuity of care for self-management goals with emphasis on productive living for home, community, and work
- Individual and/or group treatment
- Recommendations for continued services at next level of care

Typical Precautions

- Behavioral guidelines for program participation per institution procedures
- Requirements might include mandatory attendance or remaining drug-free

Discharge Disposition

◆ Outpatient

Legislation and Funding/Payment

◆ Private insurance or self-pay
◆ Medicare
◆ Medicaid
◆ SSI

LONG-TERM CARE (PHYSICAL AND MENTAL HEALTH)

Persons Most Likely to Benefit from Type of Care

◆ For people who require special, 24-hour care for an indefinite period of time and for whom a functional recovery may not be possible or lack of resources to be safe at home
◆ Same diagnoses as acute medical/surgical and inpatient psychiatry plus mental retardation

Requirements for Admission to Setting

◆ Transfer from a hospital, nursing home, or home
◆ Bridge gap between inpatient setting and home versus determine need for permanent placement
◆ Person needs assistance with activities of daily living

Typical Setting

◆ Free-standing hospital
◆ Private hospital
◆ State hospital
◆ Veteran's Administration hospital
◆ Free-standing nursing home
◆ Private nursing home
◆ Custodial care such as eating/dysphagia, grooming and bathing

Typical Length of Stay

◆ Variable
◆ Indefinite

Typical Services

◆ Physician/psychiatrists
◆ Nursing
◆ Mental health workers
◆ Therapy consultation as indicated for safety assessment, self-care skills and routines, positioning, functional mobility during ADL, adaptations, and caregiver training.

Type of Occupational Therapy Service

◆ Direct
◆ Consultation

Role of Occupational Therapy

◆ Individual assessment and interventions as indicated
◆ Consultant to program for activities of daily living, environmental adaptations, and behavior management

Typical Precautions

◆ Unit may be locked
◆ 'Sharps' precautions to prevent self-injury
◆ Fall prevention protocols as indicated

Discharge Disposition

◆ Home
◆ Community-based placement such as group home

Legislation and Funding/Payment

◆ Medicare Part B
◆ Medicaid
◆ Private insurance or self-pay supplement

Community-Based Settings for Children

LOU ANN GRISWOLD, MARY EVENSON, AND PAMELA ROBERTS

EARLY INTERVENTION

Type of Setting

Services are provided in the child's natural environment, where the child spends most of his/her time, e.g., home or child-care. The therapist may be employed by a profit or not-for-profit agency or hospital.

Recipients of Service

Infants and toddlers, up to 3 years of age and their families

Eligibility

Children who

- Have developmental delay in one or more areas of development or have a diagnosis that is likely to result in developmental delay
- Have an identified disability or condition or are at risk for developing a disability
- Demonstrate atypical behaviors noted by family members and a qualified professional
- Have circumstances that place the child and/or parent that places the child at risk for developmental delay

Each state also has its own specific eligibility criteria.

Length of Services

Depending on when the child enters early intervention, services may last for up to 3 years, at which time the child transitions to another setting of services. Progress is monitored and goals are rewritten annually.

Focus of Services

A team approach to enable family members to promote early child development including sensory-motor development, gross and fine motor skills, communication, cognitive, and social-emotional development for their child. Services not only address the child's needs, as identified in collaboration with the child's family, but also include support for family members, using a family-centered model for service delivery.

Model of Service Delivery

The OT may see the child directly or provide indirect services through consultation to another team member who provides direct services to a child and family, using a transdisciplinary model of service delivery.

Role of Occupational Therapy

Collaborate with family and other professional team members to provide services that address the family's needs in promoting the young child's development. OT focuses on promoting parent-child interaction, activities of daily living—particularly feeding and play skills—while enhancing all aspects of development. OT expertise includes sensory-motor development leading to gross and fine motor skills, self-help skills, and social-emotional development.

Intervention Approach

- ◆ Establish performance skills, performance patterns, and client factors using occupation-based activities
- ◆ Prevent disability

Discharge

Transition to a preschool program or from all supports and services occurs by the child's 3rd birthday. Transition planning is essential to ensure continuity of services.

Legislation and Funding

Individuals with Disabilities Education Act (IDEA) ensures that infants and young children who meet eligibility requirements receive services. IDEA specifies that services address families' needs through development of a Family Service Plan, and that services are provided in natural settings (e.g., home or child care). Early intervention services are primarily funded by federal (IDEA) and state money. Private insurance and Medicaid also fund services.

PRESCHOOL

Type of Setting

Preschool provided through the public school system or private child-care/preschool setting. The preschool may be for all children, including those with identified special needs, or a preschool that provides education and related services to children with special needs.

Recipients of Service

Children who are 3 years and older, until they enter elementary school. The child's preschool teacher, who is a colleague, may also be a secondary recipient of service as she or he learns new strategies to support a child in the classroom.

Eligibility

Children who have an identified disability that fits one of the categories specified under IDEA are eligible for special education. Eligibility is determined using multiple sources of evaluation information gathered by qualified examiners. Children are eligible for occupational therapy if services will assist the child to participate in preschool activities.

Length of Services

Depending on when the child enters preschool, services may last for up to 3 years, at which time the child transitions to another setting of services. Progress is monitored and goals are rewritten annually.

Focus of Services

In the natural environment of preschool, the focus of preschool education typically is on pre-academic skills and social-emotional development. Some preschool teachers also include gross motor development in their early childhood education curriculum.

Model of Service Delivery

- ◆ Direct individual or group services to support a child's education and development
- ◆ Direct services to the whole class so that all children benefit from developmentally appropriate activities
- ◆ Consultation to the teacher to provide strategies that support the child's performance in the preschool program

Role of Occupational Therapy

The OT supports the child's preschool education program by carrying out or suggesting activities that promote the child's overall development and ability to fully participate in preschool activities. Often the OT will work closely with the other members of the preschool team to determine activities that address multiple areas of development simultaneously, based on a theme of learning determined by the teacher (e.g., dinosaurs, oceans, seasons of the year). OT expertise includes sensory-motor development leading to gross and fine motor skills and social-emotional development.

Intervention Approach

♦ Establish performance skills, performance patterns, and client factors using occupation-based activities
♦ Promote development
♦ Modify the environment or activity demands for better occupational performance

Discharge

Preschool services end when a child transitions into kindergarten or elementary school.

Legislation and Funding

Individuals with Disabilities Education Act (IDEA) specifies that occupational therapy services remain educationally relevant and support the child's ability to participate in preschool activities. IDEA also mandates that all eligible children receive a free and appropriate education to meet their needs and that special education and services should be provided in the least restrictive environment. Medicaid funds may also help support services, particularly assistive technology, for qualified children.

SCHOOLS

Type of Setting

Public or private schools: kindergarten through elementary school; middle school or junior high; high school

Recipients of Service

The student is the primary recipient of OT services. The student's teacher, who is a colleague, may also be a secondary recipient of service as she or he learns new strategies to support a student in the classroom.

Eligibility

Students who have an identified disability that fits one of the categories specified under IDEA are eligible for special education. Eligibility is determined using multiple sources of evaluation information gathered by qualified examiners. Students are eligible for occupational therapy if services will assist the student benefit from the special education program. All eligibility and service decisions are made by a student's individual education program (IEP) team, of which the student's parents are part. Students in private schools are not entitled to services under IDEA. Special education is provided in accordance with the school's mission.

Length of Services

Students may receive OT services, as determined eligible, for any number of years, until they graduate from high school or turn 21 years of age. Need for service is monitored and goals are rewritten annually. Every 3 years, a student must be re-evaluated for eligibility for special education and all related services, including occupational therapy.

Focus of Services

Occupational therapy is a related service, that is, OT supports a student's special education program. Services may focus on performing schoolwork tasks, organizing the student's daily schedule and materials, negotiating the cafeteria, or participating in recess and physical education. As students reach the point of planning for transition out of the school system, the focus of their special education program and occupational therapy broadens to include independent living and community participation needs after high school such as education, vocational training, employment, and activities of daily living. Some school districts are using OT services to support population needs within the school to address broad existing student needs or to prevent future problems.

Model of Service Delivery

♦ Direct individual or group services to support a student's special education program
♦ Direct services to the whole class so that all students benefit from activities
♦ Consultation to teachers or staff to provide strategies that supports the student's performance in schoolwork tasks and in participating in school activities (lunch, recess, physical education)

Role of Occupational Therapy

The OT supports the student's education program by carrying out or suggesting activities that promote the student's performance throughout the school day and ability to fully participate in school activities. In addition to knowledge of development, OT expertise includes performance analysis and task analysis and modification of activity demands and the environment.

Intervention Approach

♦ Establish performance skills, performance patterns, and client factors using occupation-based activities
♦ Modify the environment or activity demands for better occupational performance

Discharge

School-based OT services end when a student is no longer eligible for services or special education or when he or she transitions to community living by graduating or turning 21 years old.

Legislation and Funding

Individuals with Disabilities Education Act (IDEA) specifies that occupational therapy services remain educationally relevant and support the student's ability to participate in educational activities. IDEA mandates that all eligible students receive a free and appropriate education to meet their needs and that special education and services should be provided in the least restrictive environment. No Child Left Behind (NCLB) legislation also requires schools to be accountable for students' outcomes, including those with disabilities, and requires evidence-based practices be used. Medicaid funds may also help support services, particularly assistive technology, for qualified students.

PRIVATE PRACTICE

Type of Setting

Private clinic

Recipients of Service

Children of all ages may receive private services. Typically private occupational therapists provide services to augment those provided by the school-based therapist to address needs that extend beyond those related to education. Children may have needs that do not impede education and consequently do not qualify for OT services in school, so parents may seek private services.

Eligibility

Decreased performance in daily tasks or desired activities; decreased body function, such as poor processing of sensory input, delayed gross or fine motor development, or low self-esteem. The payer of services may have specific eligibility requirements to include standard scores on assessments. Out-of-pocket payment for services does not have eligibility stipulations.

Length of Services

Determined by the payer of services and may be limited to the number of visits based on the diagnosis. Unlimited length of services for out-of-pocket payment. Services may last from six months to several years.

Focus of Services

In the clinic setting, the focus is typically on enhancing occupational performance related to play, engaging in household chores, and performing personal activities of daily living. Enhanced performance is most often addressed through improving body function such as improving sensory processing or motor development.

Model of Service Delivery

- Direct individual or small group services
- Consultation to the parents to provide strategies that support the child's performance at home

Role of Occupational Therapy

Occupational therapy addresses the child's needs that may not be met at school. OT expertise includes sensory-motor development leading to gross and fine motor skills and social-emotional development. In private practice, the OT may focus more on body functions such as sensory processing, motor planning, and visual perception that provide a foundation for skills needed in school, activities of daily living, and play.

Intervention Approach

- Establish performance skills, performance patterns, and client factors using occupation-based activities, purposeful activities, and preparatory methods
- Promote development
- Modify the environment or activity demands for better occupational performance

Discharge

Children may be discharged to school-based occupational therapy services or to extracurricular activities that will continue to address their needs such as tai-kwon-do, horseback riding, soccer, and gymnastics.

Legislation and Funding

Funding sources include Medicaid, health insurance, federal grants and private pay. Each funding source has its own regulations and policies for reimbursement, including the diagnostic code to be used, number of visits allowed, or a dollar cap for services.

Community-Based Settings for Adults

LOU ANN GRISWOLD, MARY EVENSON, AND PAMELA ROBERTS

ADULT DAY SERVICES (SOCIAL, MEDICAL, DEMENTIA)

Community-based settings are for adults living at home with the need for socialization and supervision, medical services, and/or dementia supports.

Setting

Usually free-standing, but may be associated with other community programs or health agencies such as senior centers, mental health centers, rehabilitation centers, nursing homes, or hospitals

Goals of Setting

- Provide social/medical programming to increase the quality of life and health status of day care participants via three different types of programs:
  - **Social:** Day programs with social goals provide social/recreational activities, meals, and some health supports.
  - **Medical:** Medical day programs provide rehabilitation and medical services to enhance health status and independence for people with more severe health problems. The goal is to provide sufficient supports to forestall nursing home placement.
  - **Dementia:** Day programs designed to meet the needs for people with Alzheimer's disease and related disorders focus on providing programming with cognitive supports that improve the quality of life for program participants

Occupational Therapy Role

- Consultative services including assistance with modifying and adapting activity programming for all three types of day programs
- Direct service including assessment of individuals related to ADL, IADL, safety, cognitive function, etc. OT intervention may be provided in medical and dementia oriented day programs to maintain a person's skills and performance patterns.

- Educational services to staff and family members regarding ADL, IADL, safety, fall prevention, etc.

Legislation and Funding

Day programs are regulated by state governments and may be funded through federal, state, county, city, or town budgets. Some may be funded through churches or other charitable organizations. Medicaid may fund participants who meet financial guidelines and require medical or dementia services. Some long-term care policies provide reimbursement for day programs. Scholarships and sliding fees may also be available.

ASSISTED LIVING FACILITIES

Population

Assisted living facilities provide residential care for elders who can no longer live independently but do not require the medical services of a skilled nursing facility. They may experience difficulty with ADL, IADL, safety, etc. caused by dementia, neurological impairment, or other medical problem.

Setting

Assisted living facilities are residential in nature with single or double rooms, small suites, or apartments. Common areas for meals and social activities are provided. Typically these facilities are small with fewer than 50 residents.

Goals of Setting

- Improve quality of life by providing a safe, supportive environment that enhances autonomy and choice
- Provide supervision and support for self-care and instrumental ADL, as needed
- Provide activity programming to foster social engagement and participation

Occupational Therapy Role

- Consultation to activity program to assure that the program engages residents in occupations of their choice, assist facility personnel to modify the physical and social environment to promote safety and independence
- Direct services including evaluation and intervention to increase independence in ADL and IADL, prevent falls, and enhance participation in social activities by restoring performance skills and patterns or modifying the environment or task demands
- Education of direct service staff regarding issues related to aging, occupation, and health promotion

Legislation and Funding

Medicare and Medicaid may be available for people with dementia or certain medical conditions. Long-term care insurance may cover assisted living. Private pay.

COMMUNITY MENTAL HEALTH PROGRAMS

Population

Community mental health programs serve clients who have chronic mental illness such as schizophrenia, bipolar disorder, borderline personality, etc.

Setting

Day programs are usually free-standing but are sometimes part of a larger community health facility.

Goals of Setting

- Provide ongoing support and structure to people who have mental health diagnoses to live in the community by promoting daily routine, a sense of belonging to the program community as well as the community at large
- Participants may come and go based on program interests or may be expected to participate all day, for a certain number of days per week, as determined by the participant, a case manager, desired long-term goals, and the protocol of the setting
- A variety of professionals provide daily programming to address participants' needs such as social workers, recreational therapists, art therapists, and dance movement therapists. Many programs focus on participants supporting one another.

Occupational Therapy Role

- Direct services to establish or restore performance skills for work, self-care, and leisure including coping strategies, interpersonal skills, time management, and decision-making. Services are often offered within a natural context of task expectations (e.g., using a budget to grocery shop), preparing a balanced meal, and cleaning up.
- Consultative role with other staff regarding strategies to support participants' behavior and ability to cope with challenges in social environments and adapt tasks for participant success

Legislation and Funding

Community mental health is primarily funded through state money and Medicaid.

GROUP HOMES

Population

Group homes serve adults with chronic mental illness, cognitive dysfunction, or developmental disabilities who need 24-hour residential care.

Setting

Small residential facilities (typically 3 to 10 residents) designed to create support, structure, and stability in a home-like setting. A full-time staff supervises and supports residents.

Goals of Setting

◆ Provide quality of life with maximum independence and autonomy

◆ Residents are involved in choices regarding their care, rehabilitation programs, work settings, leisure opportunities, etc. Residents are encouraged to take responsibility for their home, health, and hygiene.

◆ Group homes are designed to foster the development of social networks within the facility itself and in the community. Many residents work in sheltered workshops or supported employment during the day.

Occupational Therapy Role

◆ Consultative role with staff regarding behavioral management techniques, development of social and recreational programs in the home and facilitating independence in ADLs and IADLs by establishing performance patterns or modifying environment or activity demands.

◆ Direct services, primarily evaluation, to identify skills and develop behavioral plans and involvement in social, recreational, and work-related activities.

Legislation and Funding

Group homes are largely funded through Medicaid, state and local support.

SHELTERED WORKSHOPS AND VOCATIONAL TRAINING PROGRAMS

Population

Sheltered workshops and vocational training programs are for adults, usually who have developmental disability or cognitive limitation, who work together in a facility to complete work tasks obtained by facility staff.

Setting

Usually free-standing facility

Goals of Setting

◆ Provide support to workers as they perform work tasks such as parts assembly, packing, sorting, etc. Workers paid at percent of work output based on their performance in relation to typical work performance.

◆ Provide social opportunities for workers during the day and after work hours

◆ Goal setting and supports for transition to supported or independent employment in the community

Occupational Therapy Role

Evaluate workers' performance skills to match the activity demands of various possible jobs. For intervention, occupational therapists serve as consultants to other staff at the sheltered workshop or vocational training program to:

◆ Modify the work environment or activity demands for more efficient performance

◆ Establish performance patterns and new performance skills

◆ Maintain performance skills that workers have acquired

Legislation and Funding

Revenue primarily comes from the contracting company for which the work is being done. State funding and grants from nonprofit agencies may help support the programs.

SUPPORTED EMPLOYMENT

Population

Supported employment is for people with severe chronic mental illness, mental retardation, learning disabilities, traumatic brain injury, and other severe disabilities who desire to work but have disabilities sufficient to preclude their employment in traditional settings without ongoing support to perform their job.

Setting

Work environments in the community

Goals of Setting

Supported employment is designed to enable people with severe disabilities to work in work settings in their community by providing job coaches, assistive technology, job training, transportation, and supervision. By working in the community, people with disabilities are more effectively integrated in work, social networks, and community life.

Job coaches assist the employee to work effectively to meet the demands of the job and work environment. Natural supports from co-workers and supervisors further enable social integration. The employee is paid and receives the same benefits as other workers and receives ongoing support to maintain employment as long as this is necessary.

Occupational Therapy Role

◆ Consultation with work sites to assure integration of the employee and to provide education regarding adaptation of the work site environment and activity demands.

◆ Direct services in the role of job coach to assist the employee to adapt to the work site and to function effectively by learning job skills and interacting appropriately with other employees at the work site. May be involved in matching prospective worker to potential work sites.

Legislation and Funding

Funding varies from state to state via Vocational Rehabilitation, Division of Mental Health, and Medicaid

WORK-RELATED PROGRAMS

Population

Work-related programs serve people with acquired disability who require rehabilitation to return to the workforce, either to their previous job or a new one that better fits their current functional capacity. Common problems of clients relate to work-related injuries such as repetitive trauma disorders, shoulder, back, hand injuries, acquired brain injury, or stroke.

Setting

Work or vocational programs may be in free-standing or a part of other facilities such as a hospital, rehabilitation center, or community program.

Goals of Setting

Provide rehabilitation services to enable the client to return to work. Physical therapists, occupational therapists and employment specialists work together to achieve client-related goals. Referral for certified vocational evaluation may be appropriate.

Occupational Therapy Role

◆ Evaluation of work tolerance including medical history, worker interview, job description, pain assessment, physical assessment, lifting/carrying ability, pushing/pulling, stopping, bending, kneeling, crawling, sitting, and standing

◆ Intervention focuses on the development of work related skills primarily using purposeful activities such as work simulation, and preparatory methods, e.g., work conditioning, work hardening, and exercise programs

◆ Modification of job demands when necessary and possible to better match the current skills of the client

Legislation and Funding

Division of Vocational Rehabilitation at the state level, workers' compensation, income from litigation, and private insurance.

XVII

Table of Assessments: Listed Alphabetically by Title

CHERYL BOOP

Assessment Title	Author(s)	Publisher and/or Contact Information	Ages	Stated Purpose	Areas Assessed
Academic Performance Rating Scale	DuPaul, G. J., Rapport, M. D., and Perriello, L. M.	DuPaul, G. J., Rapport, M. D., & Perriello, L. M. (1991). Teacher Ratings of Academic Skills: The Development of the Academic Performance Rating Scale. *School Psychology Review, 20*(2), 284–300.	School age	Measure academic performance on three factors	Academic success; impulse control; academic productivity
Accessibility Checklist	Goltsman, S., Gilbert, T., and Wohlford, S.	Goltsman, S., Gilbert, T., & Wohlford, S. (1993). *The accessibility checklist: An evaluation system for buildings and outdoor settings* (2nd ed.). Berkeley, CA: M.I.G. Communications.	Adults	Identify problems in community accessibility; a comprehensive system for achieving compliance with current access laws.	Community environment
Activity Index & Meaningfulness of Activity Scale	Nystrom, E. P., and Gregory, M. D.	Gregory, M. D. (1983). Occupational behavior and life satisfaction among retirees. *American Journal of Occupational Therapy, 37,* 548–553. Nystrom, E. P. (1974). Activity patterns and leisure concepts among the elderly. *American Journal of Occupational Therapy, 28,* 337–345.	Older adults	Examine the meaning and significance of activity and activity patterns among the elderly	Activity/leisure
Action Research Arm Test (ARAT)	Carroll, D.	Carroll, D. (1965). A quantitative test of upper extremity function. *Journal of Chronic Diseases, 18,* 479–491. http://www.strokecenter.org/trials/scales/action_research_arm_test.pdf	Adults	Measures the ability to grasp, move, and release objects of different size, weight and shape	Grasp strength; pinch strength; grip strength
Actual Amount of Use Test (AAUT)	Taub, E., DeLuca, S., and Cargo, J. E.	Uswatte, G., Taub, E., Pearson, S., Light, K., & Thompson, P. (2004). Validity of the Actual Amount of Use Test: evidence from a multisite, national clinical trial of CI therapy for persons with subacute stroke. Manuscript in preparation. Taub E, DeLuca S, Cargo JE, inventors. Actual amount of use test (AAUT); 1996	Adults	Measures spontaneous use of a limb	Motor function

Title	Author	Source	Population	Purpose	Domain
ADHD Behavior Checklist for Adults	Barkley, R. A., and Murphy, K. R.	Barkley, R. A., & Murphy, K. R. (1998) *Attention deficit hyperactivity disorder: A clinical workbook* (2nd ed.). New York: Guilford Publications.	Adults	A self-report symptom checklist to help diagnose ADHD in adults	Attention
Adolescent Behavior Checklist	Demb, H. B., Brier, N., Huron, R., and Tomor, E.	Demb, H. B., Brier, N., Huron, R., & Tomor, E. (1994). The Adolescent Behavior Checklist: Normative Data and Sensitivity and Specificity of a Screening Tool for Diagnosable Psychiatric Disorders in Adolescents with Mental Retardation and Other Developmental Disabilities. *Research in Developmental Disabilities, 15*(2), 151–65	12–21 years "with mild mental retardation or borderline intelligence"	To identify adolescents at risk for having a diagnosable psychiatric disturbance	Behavior
Adolescent Role Assessment (ARA)	Black, M. M.	Black, M. M. (1976). Adolescent role assessment. *American Journal of Occupational Therapy, 30*(2), 73–79.	Adolescents	Gathers information on the adolescent's occupational role involvement over time and across domains	Childhood play; socialization with family; socialization with peers; school functioning; occupational choice; anticipated adult work
Adolescent/Adult Sensory Profile	Brown, C., and Dunn, W.	Harcourt Assessment, Inc. Attn: Customer Service P.O. Box 599700 San Antonio, TX 78259 (800)211-8378 Fax: (800) 232-1223	11 years and up	To determine how well a subject processes sensory information in everyday situations and to profile the sensory system's effect on functional performance	Sensory processing; modulation; and behavioral and emotional responses
Adult Nowicki Strickland Internal External Control Scale (ANSIE)	Nowicki, S., and Duke, M. P.	Educational Testing Service (ETS) Test Collection Library Rosedale and Carter Roads Princeton, NJ 08541 609-734-5689 http://www.ets.org/testcoll/	Adults	Identifies a client's locus of control	Locus of control

Continued

Continued

Assessment Title	Author(s)	Publisher and/or Contact Information	Ages	Stated Purpose	Areas Assessed
Adult Playfulness Scale	Glynn, M. A., and Webster, J.	Glynn, M. A., & Webster, J. (1992). The adult playfulness scale: An initial assessment. *Psychological Reports, 71*, 83–103	Adults	Measures adult play behavior in the workplace.	Play/leisure
Alberta Infant Motor Scale (AIMS)	Piper, M. C., and Darrah, J.	Elsevier Customer Service Department 11830 Westline Industrial Drive St. Louis, MO 63146 800-545-2522	Birth to 18 months	To provide a performance-based, norm-referenced measure of infant motor maturation	Progressive development and integration of antigravity muscular control in the prone, supine, sitting and standing positions
Allen Battery	Allen, C. K.	385 Coquina Ave Ormond Beach, FL 32174 800-853-2472 jim@allen-cognitive-levels.com	All ages	To assess cognitive disability and suggest treatment approach	Problem-solving; following directions
Allen Cognitive Level Screen-5 (ACLS-5)	Allen, C. K., Austin, S. L., David, S. K., Earhart, C. A., McCraith, D. B., & Riska-Williams, L.	Allen, C. K., Austin, S. L., David, S. K., Earhart, C. A., McCraith, D. B, & Riska-Williams, L. (2007). *Manual for the Allen cognitive level screen-5 (ACLS-5) and Large Allen cognitive level screen-5 (LACLS-5).* Camarillo, CA: ACLS and LACLS Committee. ACLS and LACLS Committee P.O. Box 3144 Camarillo, CA 93011	All ages	To provide a quick measure of learning potential, global cognitive processing capacities and performance abilities	Problem-solving; following directions
Allen Diagnostic Module Instruction Manual (ADMIM)	Earhart, C, Allen, C., and Blue, T.	385 Coquina Ave Ormond Beach, FL 32174 800-853-2472 jim@allen-cognitive-levels.com	All ages	To assess cognitive disability and suggest treatment approach	Problem-solving; following directions
Allen Semantic Differential Scale	Allen, L.	Allen, L. (1986). Measuring attitudes toward computer assisted instruction: The development of a semantic differential tool. *Computers in Nursing, 4*(4), 144–151.	Adults	Evaluates individual's responses to webpage interventions	Comfort; creativity; function of webpage healthcare intervention

ALS Functional Rating Scale (ALSFRS)	Cedarbaum, J.	http://www.outcomes-umassmed.org/als/alsscale.cfm ALS CNTF Treatment Study (ACTS) Phase I-II Study Group. (1996). The Amyotrophic Lateral Sclerosis Functional Rating Scale. Assessment of activities of daily living in patients with Amyotrophic Lateral Sclerosis. *Archives of Neurology, 53,* 141–147.	Adults	Evaluates the functional status of individuals diagnosed with ALS	ADLs; IADLs
Americans with Disabilities Act (ADA) Accessibility Guidelines Checklist for Buildings and Facilities	U.S. Architectural and Transportation Barriers Compliance Board	U.S. Architectural & Transportation Barriers Compliance Board. (1992). *Americans with Disabilities Act accessibility guidelines checklist for buildings and facilities.* Washington, D.C.: Author	Adults	Identifies accessibility in the community	Community environment; workplace environment
Americans with Disabilities (ADA) Worksite Assessment	Jacobs, K.	Jacobs, K. (1999). (Ed.) *Ergonomics for Therapists.* (2nd ed.). Newton, MA: Butterworth Heinemann.	Adults	To assess worksite compliance with ADA regulations and ergonomics	Workplace environment
Arm Motor Ability Test (AMAT)	Kopp, B., Kunkel, A., Flor, H., Platz, T., Rose, U., Mauritz, K. H., Gresser, K., McCulloch, K. L., and Taub, E.	Kopp, B., Kunkel, A., Flor, H., Platz, T., Rose, U., Mauritz, K. H., Gresser, K., McCulloch, K. L., and Taub, E. (1997). The Arm Motor Ability Test: Reliability, validity, and sensitivity to change of an instrument for assessing disabilities in activities of daily living. *Archives of Physical Medicine and Rehabilitation, 78*(6), 615–620.	Adults	Measures upper extremity movement using daily activity tasks	ADLs; IADLs
The Arthritis Hand Function Test	Backman, C., Mackie, H., and Harris, J.	Backman C., Mackie H., Harris J. (1991). Arthritis hand function test: development of a standardized assessment tool. *The Occupational Therapy Journal of Research* July/Aug. 11, 4, 245–256. The School of Rehabilitation Sciences University of British Columbia T325-2211 Wesbrook Mall Vancouver, BC Canada V6T 2B5	Adults	Assesses pure and applied strength and dexterity of both hands in adults with rheumatoid arthritis and osteoarthritis	Hand strength and dexterity; ADLs

Continued

Continued

Assessment Title	Author(s)	Publisher and/or Contact Information	Ages	Stated Purpose	Areas Assessed
Assessment of Awareness of Disability (AAD)	Tham, K., Bernspang, B., and Fisher, A. G.	Kottorp, A. (2006). The Assessment of Awareness of Disability (AAD). Manual for Administration and Scoring. Karolinska Institutet, Stockholm, Sweden. Tham, K., Bernspang, B., & Fisher, A. G. (1999). Development of the assessment of awareness of disability. *Scandinavian Journal of Occupational Therapy, 6,* 184–190.	Adults	To assess an individual's awareness of their disability and its affects on performance of activities of daily living	ADLs
Assessment of Communication and Interaction Skills (ACIS)	Salamy, M., Simon, S., and Kielhofner, G..	www.moho.uic.edu	Adults	Assess the communication/interaction skills of adults who have physical or mental illness	Communication; social interaction skills
Assessment of Living Skills and Resources (ALSAR)	Williams, J. H., Drinka, T. J. K., Greenberg, J. R., Farrell-Holtan, J., Euhardy, R., and Schram, M	Drinka, T. J. K., Williams, J., Schram, M., Farrell-Holtan, J., & Euhardy, M. Assessment of Living Skills and Resources (ALSAR) an instrumental activities of daily living assessment instrument. In: Osterweil, D., Brummel-Smith, K., Beck, & J., Eds. (2000). *Comprehensive geriatric Assessment.* New York: McGraw-Hill, pp. 726–729. Williams, J. H., Drinka, T. J. K., Greenberg, J. R., Farrell-Holtan, J., Euhardy, R., and Schram, M. (1991). Development and Testing of the Assessment of Living Skills and Resources (ALSAR) in Elderly Community-Dwelling Veterans. *Gerontologist, 31*(1) 84–91.	Adults	An interview that assesses a person's level of independence	IADL

				Play/leisure
Assessment of Ludic Behavior (ALB)	Ferland, F.	Ferland, F. (1997). *Play, children with physical disabilities and occupational therapy: The Ludic model.* Ottawa, ON: University of Ottawa Press	Children	Assess play behaviors of children with disabilities
Assessment of Motor and Process Skills (AMPS)	Fisher, A. G.	Fisher, A. G. (2006). *Assessment of motor and process skills. vol. 1: Development, standardization, and administration manual* (6th ed.). Fort Collins, CO: Three Star Press. http://www.ampsintl.com/	3 years and up	Provides an objective assessment of motor and process skills in the context of performing several familiar functional tasks of the subject's choice	Process skills, such as the ability to initiate, inquire, notice and respond, pace, sequence, organize, and terminate
Assessment of Occupational Functioning (AOF)—second revision	Watts, J. H., Brollier, C., Bauer, D., and Schmidt, W.	Watts, J. H., Brollier, C., Bauer, D., & Schmidt, W. (1989). The Assessment of Occupation Functioning: The Second Revision. In J. H. Watts & C. Brollier (Eds.). *Instrument development in occupational therapy* (pp. 61–88). New York: Haworth.	Adults	Screens overall occupational function of residents in long-term care settings	Volition; habituation; performance; values; personal causation; interests; roles; habits; skills; school and job history
Assessment of Occupational Functioning—Collaborative Version (AOF-CV)	Watts, J. H.	www.moho.uic.edu Janet H. Watts, PhD, OTR/L Virginia Commonwealth University / Department of OT VCU Box 980008 Richmond, VA 23298-0008 jhwatts@hsc.vcu.edu	Adults	Used to inform intervention by indicating the factors likely to influence a person's ability to function	Personal causation; values; roles; habits; skills
Assimilation, Integration, Marginalization, Segregation (AIMS) Interview	Minnes, P., Buell, K., Feldman, M. A., McColl, M. A., and McCreary, B.	Minnes, P., Buell, K., Feldman, M. A., McColl, M. A., & McCreary, B. (2002). Community Integration as Acculturation: Preliminary Validation of the AIMS Interview. *Journal of Applied Research in Intellectual Disabilities, 15*(4), 377–387	Adults	Measures community integration for adults with disabilities	Community integration

Continued

Continued

Assessment Title	Author(s)	Publisher and/or Contact Information	Ages	Stated Purpose	Areas Assessed
Assistive Technology Evaluation	Cook, A. M., and Hussey, S. M.	Cook, A. M., & Hussey, S. M. (1996). *Assistive technology: Principles and Practice.* St. Louis: Mosby.	Adults	To determine which, if any, assistive technology devices can allow an individual to maximize efficient performance of activities	Demographic and referral information; medical and health information; sensory and perceptual abilities; ADL; social interaction; learning and behavior; functional abilities; motor skills; mobility and positioning; and communication skills
Awareness Questionnaire (AQ)	Sherer, M., Boake, C., Levin, E., Silver, B. V., Ringholz, G., and High, W. M.	Sherer, M. (2004). The Awareness Questionnaire. *The Center for Outcome Measurement in Brain Injury.* http://www.tbims.org/combi/aq	Adults	Measures impaired self-awareness after traumatic brain injury (TBI); it may also be appropriate for use with persons with other types of acquired brain injury.	Self-awareness; ADLs
Balcones Sensory Integration Screening Kit		Texas Occupational Therapy Association, Inc. P.O. Box 15576 Austin, TX 78761-5576 512-454-8682 mary@tota.org	Children in K–12	To assist in identifying special neuro-behavioral, behavioral, and/or classroom performance	Ocular-motor control; proprioception; primitive reflex-brain stem midline interaction; vestibular; tactile perception; stereognosis; visual-motor perception; lateralization

The Baking Tray Task	Tham, K. and Tegner, R.	Tham, K. & Tegner, R. (1996). The Baking Tray Task: A Test of Spatial Neglect. *Neuropsychological Rehabilitation, 6*(1), 19–26(8)	Adults	Assesses unilateral neglect	Unilateral neglect
The Balloons Test	Edgeworth, J., Robertson, I., McMillan, T.	Harcourt Assessment, Inc. Attn: Customer Service P.O. Box 599700 San Antonio, TX 78259 (800)211-8378 Fax: (800) 232-1223	Adults	To detect visual inattention following brain injury	Visual attention
BTE Work Simulator	BTE Technologies, Inc.	BTE Technologies, Inc. 7455-L New Ridge Road Hanover, MD 21076-3105 800-331-8845	Adults	Used in work capacity evaluations to determine whether clients have the capabilities to return to work	Physical strength and endurance using a variety of attachments simulating tools
Barthel Index	Mahoney, F. I., and Barthel, D. W.	Mahoney, F. I., & Barthel, D. W. (1965). Functional Evaluation: The Barthel Index. *Maryland State Medical Journal, 14*, 61–65.	Adults	Reflects the functional status of hospital patients in activities of daily living and to assess change	Activities of daily living
Bay Area Functional Performance Evaluation (BaFPE)	Williams, S. L., and Bloomer, J.	Sammons Preston P.O. Box 5071 Bolingbrook, IL 60440-5071 (800) 323-5547 www.sammonspreston.com	Late adolescence to adult	To assess cognitive, affective, and performance skills in daily living tasks and social interaction skills; evaluate the effectiveness of OT	Social interaction/behavior; ADL skills, cognitive, affective and performance skills
Bayley Scales of Infant Development®, 2nd Edition (BSID-II)	Bayley, N.	Harcourt Assessment, Inc. Attn: Customer Service P.O. Box 599700 San Antonio, TX 78259 (800)211-8378 Fax: (800) 232-1223	Birth to 42 months	To assess the current developmental functioning of infants and children	Mental, cognitive, motor and adaptive behaviors
Beck Depression Inventory®—II (BDI®-II)	Beck, A. T., Steer, R. A., and Brown, G. K.	Harcourt Assessment, Inc. Attn: Customer Service P.O. Box 599700 San Antonio, TX 78259 (800)211-8378 Fax: (800) 232-1223	13 to 80 years	To assess the intensity of depression	Depression

Continued

Continued

Assessment Title	Author(s)	Publisher and/or Contact Information	Ages	Stated Purpose	Areas Assessed
Beery–Buktenica Developmental Test of Visual-Motor Integration, 5th Edition (BEERY VMI™)	Beery, K. E., Buktenica, N. A., and Beery, N. A.	Pearson Assessments P.O. Box 1416 Minneapolis, MN 55440 (800) 627-7271	2 to 18 years	Helps to assess the extent to which individuals can integrate their visual and motor abilities	Visual-motor integration skills; visual perceptual skills; motor coordination skills
Behavior Assessment Rating Scale, 2nd Edition (BASC-2)	Reynolds, C. R., and Kamphaus, R. W.	Pearson Assessments P.O. Box 1416 Minneapolis, MN 55440 (800) 627-7271	2.0 to 21.11 years	Teacher rating; parent rating; self-rating; student observation; structured developmental history	Behaviors, thoughts, and emotions of children and adolescents
Behavioral Assessment of the Dysexecutive Syndrome (BADS)	Wilson, B. A., Alderman, N., Burgess, P., Emslie, H., and Evans, J. J.	Psychological Assessment Resources, Inc. 16204 N. Florida Avenue Lutz, FL 33549 813-968-3003/ 800-383-6595	16 years and up	To assess problem-solving, planning, and organizational skills over time	Temporal judgment; ability to change response patterns; problem-solving; strategizing
Behavioral Assessment of the Dysexecutive Syndrome for Children (BADS-C)	Emslie, H., Wilson, F. C., Burden, V., Nimmo-Smith, I., and Wilson, B. A.	Psychological Assessment Resources, Inc. 16204 N. Florida Avenue Lutz, FL 33549 813-968-3003/ 800-383-6595	8 to 16 years	Assists in early identification of deficits in executive functioning in children	Inflexibility and perseveration; novel problem solving; impulsivity; planning; the ability to utilize feedback and moderate one's behaviour accordingly
Behavioral Inattention Test (BIT)	Wilson, B., Cockburn, J., and Halligan, P.	Harcourt Assessment, Inc. Attn: Customer Service P.O. Box 599700 San Antonio, TX 78259 (800)211-8378 Fax: (800) 232-1223	Adults	To identify unilateral visual neglect and how it affects daily life	9 subtests reflecting daily life activities; 6 conventional pencil-and-paper tasks

Title	Author	Source	Population	Purpose	Area
Behavior Rating Inventory of Executive Function—Adult Version (Brief-A)	Roth, R., Isquith, P., and Gioia, G.	Psychological Assessment Resources, Inc. 16204 N. Florida Avenue Lutz, FL 33549 813-968-3003/ 800-383-6595	Adults and elder adults	To assess adult executive functioning/self-regulation in individuals ages 18 to 90 years	Executive functioning
The Bells Test	Gauthier, L., Dehaut, F., and Joanette, Y.	Gauthier, L., Dehaut, F., & Joanette, Y. (1989). The bells test: a quantitative and qualitative test for visual neglect. *The International Journal of Clinical Neuropsychology* 11(2), 49–54.	Adults	To assess visual neglect	Visual attention
Bennett Hand Tool Dexterity Test (H-TDT)	Bennett, G. K.	Harcourt Assessment, Inc. Attn: Customer Service P.O. Box 599700 San Antonio, TX 78259 (800)211-8378 Fax: (800) 232-1223	Adults	To assess dexterity and basic hand-tool skills for manual jobs	Tool skills; safety skills
Benton Constructional Praxis Test	Benton, A. L., Hamsher, K., Varney, N. R., and Spreen, O.	Benton, A. L., Hamsher, K., Varney, N. R., & Spreen, O. *Contributions to neuropsychological assessment: Clinical manual.* New York: Oxford University Press. 1983.	All ages	To assess three-dimensional visual motor and constructional skills	Visual motor and construction skills
Berg Balance Scale	Berg, K., Wood-Dauphinee, S., Williams, J. I., and Gayton, D.	The Center for Gerontology and Health Care Research Brown University Box G-B213 171 Meeting Street Providence, Rhode Island 02912 401-863-1560 http://www.chcr.brown.edu/GERIATRIC_ASSESSMENT_TOOL_KIT.PDF	Adults	To measure balance in 14 activities performed in standing	Balance
Blessed Dementia Rating Scale (DRS)	Blessed, G., Tomlinson, B., Roth, M., and Wade, D. T.	Blessed dementia rating scale (1968). Blessed G; Tomlinson B; Roth M. Wade DT (1992). *Measurement in neurological rehabilitation.* New York: Oxford University Press, pp. 126–129	Adults	To assess the functional capacity of individuals with dementia during daily activity skills	ADLs

Continued

Continued

Assessment Title	Author(s)	Publisher and/or Contact Information	Ages	Stated Purpose	Areas Assessed
Bone Safety Evaluation (BSE)	Grant, S. L., and Recknor, C. P.	United Osteoporosis Centers IONmed Systems 2350 Limestone Parkway Gainesville, GA 30501 www.ionmed.us	Adults	Comprehensive performance-based bone health and fracture risk assessment	Spine compression; balance; strength; flexibility; medication/therapy adherence; valued activities; quality of life
Borg Numerical Pain Scale	Borg, G.	Borg, G. *Borg's Perceived Exertion and Pain Scale.*, Champaign, IL: Human Kinetics. 1998.	Adults	Self-assessment of pain	Pain
Borg Scale of Rating Perceived Exertion (RPE)	Borg, G.	Borg, G. *Borg's Perceived Exertion and Pain Scale.*, Champaign, IL: Human Kinetics. 1998.	Adults	Self-assessment of exertion during activities	Perceived exertion
Boston Diagnostic Aphasia Examination, 3rd Edition (BDAE-3)	Goodglass, H., Kaplan, E., and Barresi, B.	Harcourt Assessment, Inc. Attn: Customer Service P.O. Box 599700 San Antonio, TX 78259 (800)211-8378 Fax: (800) 232-1223	Adults	To evaluate a broad range of language impairments that often arise as a consequence of organic brain dysfunction	Perceptual modalities; processing functions; and response modalities
Box and Block Test	Mathiowetz, V., Vollard, G., Kashman, N., and Weber, K.	Sammons Preston P.O. Box 5071 Bolingbrook, IL 60440-5071 (800) 323-5547 www.sammonspreston.com	7 years and up	To provide a baseline for upper extremity manual dexterity and gross motor coordination	Manual dexterity
Brain Injury Visual Assessment Battery for Adults (BiVABA)	Warren, M.	visABILITIES Rehab Services Inc 1634-A Montgomery Hwy / #195 Hoover, AL 35216 Toll Free: (888) 752-4364	Adults with acquired brain injury	Focuses on identification of the functional limitations experienced by an individual as the result of visual impairment	Visual acuity (distant and reading); contrast sensitivity function; visual field; oculomotor function; visual attention and scanning

Title	Author	Reference/Source	Age	Description	Domain
Brief Pain Inventory	Cleeland, C. S.	Cleeland, C. S. (1991). Research in cancer pain: What we know and what we need to know. *Cancer, 67,* 823–827.	Adults	How much pain interferes with occupational performance and mood	Pain and relationship to occupational performance
Brief Test of Head Injury (BTHI)	Helm-Estabrooks, N. and Hotz, G.	PRO-ED, Inc. 8700 Shoal Creek Blvd. Austin, TX 78757 (800) 897-3202	Adults	Designed to provide information about cognitive, linguistic, and communicative abilities of patients with severe head trauma	Cognition; linguistics, communication
Bruininks-Oseretsky Test of Motor Proficiency, 2nd Edition (BOT-2)	Bruininks, R. H., and Bruininks, B. D.	Pearson Assessments P.O. Box 1416 Minneapolis, MN 55440 (800) 627-7271	4 to 21 years	To assess the gross and fine motor functioning of school-age clients	Fine motor control; manual dexterity; body coordination; strength and agility
Canadian Occupational Performance Measure (COPM)©, 4th Edition	Law, M., Baptiste, S., Carswell, A., McColl, M. A., Polatajko, H., and Pollock, N.	Canadian Association of Occupational Therapists 110 Eglinton Avenue West 3rd Floor Toronto, Ontario M4R 1A3 Canada 416-487-5404 http://www.caot.ca/copm/index.htm	7 years and up	Measures client's perception of his/her occupational performance over time	Self-care; productivity; leisure
Caregiver Activity Survey—Intellectual Disability (CAS-ID)	McCarron, M., Gill, M., Lawlor, B., and Beagly, C.	McCarron, M., Gill, M., Lawlor, B., & Beagly, C. (2002). A Pilot Study of the Reliability and Validity of the Caregiver Activity Survey—Intellectual Disability (CAS-ID) *Journal of Intellectual Disability Research, 46,* 605–612	Adults	Identifies and measures care and resource requirements for people experiencing decline associated with dementia	ADLs
Child and Adolescent Social Perception Measure (CASP)	Magill-Evans, J., Koning, C., Cameron-Sadava, A., and Manyk, K.	Magill-Evans, J., Koning, C., Cameron-Sadava, A., & Manyk, K. (1995). The Child and Adolescent Social Perception Measure. *Journal of Nonverbal Behavior, 19,* 151–169.	6 to 15 years	To measure a child's sensitivity to non-verbal aspects of communication	Ability to interpret nonverbal aspects of communication

Continued

Continued

Assessment Title	Author(s)	Publisher and/or Contact Information	Ages	Stated Purpose	Areas Assessed
Child Behavior Checklist for Ages 6–18 (CBCL/6–18)	Achenbach, T. M.	ASEBA Research Center for Children, Youth, and Families 1 South Prospect Street Burlington, VT 05401-3456 802-264-6433 www.ASEBA.org	4 to 18 years	To record a child's competencies and problems as reported by parent or caregiver	Internalizing and externalizing psychological symptoms for children and adolescents
Child Behaviors Inventory of Playfulness (CBI)	Rogers, C. S., Impara, J. C., Frary, R. B, Harris, T., Meeks, A., Semanic-Lauth, S., and Reynolds, M. R.	Rogers, C. S., Impara, J. C., Frary, R. B., Harris, T., Meeks, A., Semanic-Lauth, S., & Reynolds, M. R. (1998). Measuring playfulness: Development of the child behaviors inventory of playfulness. In M. C. Duncan, G. Chick, & A. Aycock (Eds.), *Play & culture studies. Volume 1: Diversions and divergences in fields of play*. Greenwich, CT: Ablex Publishing.	Children	Examines playful behaviors of children	Play/leisure
Child Occupational Self Assessment (COSA)	Keller, J., Kafkes, A., Basu, S., Federico, J., and Kielhofner, G.	www.moho.uic.edu	Children and youth	To understand how a child/youth perceives their own sense of occupational competence in everyday activities as well as the importance of those activities in their life	Activities of daily living
Child Routines Inventory (CRI)	Sytsma, S. E., Kelley, M. L., and Wymer, J. H.	Sytsma, S. E., Kelley, M. L., & Wymer, J. H. (2001). Development and initial validation of the Child Routines Inventory. *Journal of Psychopathology and Behavioral Assessment, 23*(4), 241–251.	5 to 12 years	To assess commonly occurring routines in school-age children	ADLs; IADLs

Title	Authors	Publisher/Contact	Age	Purpose	Focus
Children's Assessment of Participation and Enjoyment (CAPE)	King, G., Law, M., King, S., Harms, S., Kertoy, M., Rosenbaum, P., and Young, N.	Harcourt Assessment, Inc. Attn: Customer Service P.O. Box 599700 San Antonio, TX 78259 (800)211-8378 Fax: (800) 232-1223	6 years and up	Gathers information on child's participation in everyday activities outside of mandated school activities	Social participation in non-school activities
Children's Handwriting Evaluation Scale (CHES)	Texas Scottish Rite Hospital	CHES 5530 Farquhar Dallas, TX 75209 214-366-3667	Grades 3–8	Provides a reliable measure of handwriting rate and quality	Letter size consistency; letter formation; letters on the line; spacing between letters and words
Children's Handwriting Evaluation Scale for Manuscript Writing (CHES-M)	Texas Scottish Rite Hospital	CHES 5530 Farquhar Dallas, TX 75209 214-366-3667	Grades 1–2	Provides a reliable measure of handwriting rate and quality	Copying; taking notes; presenting ideas in writing
Children Helping Out: Responsibilities, Expectations, and Supports (CHORES)	Dunn, L.	Dunn. L. (2004). Validation of the CHORES: A measure of school-aged children's participation in household tasks. *Scandinavian Journal of Occupational Therapy, 11*(4), 179–190	School age children and adolescents	To assess a child's participation in household tasks and changes in the amount of assistance needed to participate	ADLs; IADLs
Children's Paced Auditory Serial Addition Test (CHIPASAT)	Dyche, G., and Johnson, D.	Dyche, G., & Johnson, D. (1991). Development and evaluation of CHIPASAT, an attentional test for children: II test-retest reliability and practice effect for a normal sample. *Perceptual Motor Skills, 72*, 563–572.	Children	To detect subtle impairments in attention and speed of processing, functional observation of everyday activities	Attention and speed of processing
Choosing Outcomes and Accommodations for Children (COACH), 2nd Edition	Giangreco, M. F., Cloninger, C. J., and Iverson, V. S.	Customer Service Department Brookes Publishing Co. P.O. Box 10624 Baltimore, MD 21285-0624 1-800-638-3775 custserv@brookespublishing.com	3 to 21 years	Used to develop an appropriate, individualized education program	Family interview; learning outcomes; general supports; annual goals

Continued

Continued

Assessment Title	Author(s)	Publisher and/or Contact Information	Ages	Stated Purpose	Areas Assessed
Classroom Observation Guide	Griswold, L.	Griswold, L. (1994). Ethnographic analysis: A study of classroom environments. *American Journal of Occupational Therapy, 48,* 397–402.	Children	Helps therapists understand classroom context	Activities of classroom settings; people in classroom settings; communication in classroom settings
Clinical Test of Sensory Integration and Balance (CTSIB)	Shumway-Cook, A., and Horak, F. B.	Shumway-Cook, A., & Horak, F. B. (1986). Assessing the influence of sensory interaction on balance: Suggestions from the field. *Physical Therapy, 66,* 1548–1550.	All	To assess a patient's ability to tolerate varied surfaces and sensory conditions	Balance; interaction of ocular, vestibular, and musculoskeletal systems
Cognitive Assessment of Minnesota (CAM)	Rustad, R. A., DeGroot, T. L., Jungkunz, M. L., Freeberg, K. S., Borowick, L. G., and Wanttie, A. M.	Harcourt Assessment, Inc. Attn: Customer Service P.O. Box 599700 San Antonio, TX 78259 (800)211-8378 Fax: (800) 232-1223	Adults	Screens a wide range of cognitive skills in order to identify general problem areas	Attention; memory; visual neglect; math; ability to follow directions; judgment
Cognitive Performance Test (CPT)	Burns, T.	Theressa Burns, OTR GRECC 11G Veterans Affairs Medical Center One Veterans Drive Minneapolis, MN 55417	Adults	Assesses how cognitive processing deficits affect performance of common activities	Cognitive processing
Community Adaptive Planning Assessment	Spencer, J., and Davidson, H.	Spencer, J. & Davidson, J. (1998). The Community Adaptive Planning Assessment: A clinical tool for documenting future planning with clients. *American Journal of Occupational Therapy, 52*(1), 19–30.	Adults	Examines major occupations of an individual at times of expected change	Activities involved in occupation; persons involved and their roles; physical setting; value of the occupation to self and others

Title	Author(s)	Reference	Age	Purpose	Content
Community Integration Measure	McColl, M. A., Davies, D., Carlson, P., Johnston, J., and Minnes, P.	McColl, M. A., Davies, D., Carlson, P., Johnston, J., & Minnes, P. (2001). The community integration measure: development and preliminary validation. *Archives of Physical Medicine and Rehabilitation, 82,* 429–34.	Adults	Appraise an individual's views about connecting to community	Integration into community
Community Integration Questionnaire	Willer, B., Rosenthal, M., Kreutzer, J., Gordon, W., and Rempel, R.	Centre for Research on Community Integration at the Ontario Brain Injury Association 3550 Schmon Parkway Thorold, Ontario L2V 4Y6, Canada	Adults	Helps clients examine the extent of their community participation	Household activities; shopping; errands; leisure activities; visiting friends; social events; productive activities
Competency Rating Scale	Prigatano, G.	Prigatano, G. P. *Neuropsychological rehabilitation after brain injury.* Baltimore, MD: Johns Hopkins University Press. 1986. For more information, contact: Tessa Hart, PhD. MossRehab TBI Model System Philadelphia, PA 215-456-5925.	Adult	Self-report instrument asks the client to rate his/her degree of difficulty in a variety of tasks and functions	Self-awareness following traumatic brain injury
Comprehensive Trail-Making Test (CTMT)	Reynolds, C. R.	PRO-ED, Inc. 8700 Shoal Creek Blvd. Austin, TX 78757 (800) 897-3202	11 to 74 years	To evaluate and diagnose of brain injury and other forms of central nervous system compromise	Visual search and sequencing; attention; concentration; resistance to distraction; and cognitive flexibility (or set-shifting)
Computer Attitude Scale	Loyd, B. H., and Gressard, C.	Loyd, B. H., & Gressard, C. (1984). The effects of sex, age, and computer experience on computer attitudes, *AEDS Journal, 18,* 67–77.	Adults	Assesses general attitudes toward computers	Computer anxiety; computer confidence; computer liking
Computer System Usability Questionnaire	Lewis, J.	Lewis, J. R. (1995) *IBM Computer Usability Satisfaction Questionnaires: Psychometric Evaluation and Instructions for Use. International Journal of Human-Computer Interaction, 7*(1), 57–78	All ages	Can be used to evaluate specific software programs for individuals	Usefulness; information quality; interface quality

Continued

Continued

Assessment Title	Author(s)	Publisher and/or Contact Information	Ages	Stated Purpose	Areas Assessed
Contextual Memory Test (CMT)	Toglia, J. P.	Harcourt Assessment, Inc. Attn: Customer Service P.O. Box 599700 San Antonio, TX 78259 (800)211-8378 Fax: (800) 232-1223	18 years and up	To assess awareness of memory capacity, use of strategy, and recall	Memory strategies for task completion
Coping Inventory	Zeitlin, S.	Scholastic Testing Service 480 Meyer Road Bensonville, IL 60106-1617 (800) 642-6787	Observation form for 3 to 16 years; self-rated form for 15 years to adult	To assess adaptive and maladaptive coping habits, skills, and behaviors	Coping with self; coping with environment; use of personal resources; initiation of activity
Cost of Care Index	Kosberg, J., and Cairl, R.	Kosberg, J. & Cairl, R. (1986). The cost of care index: A case management tool for screening informal care providers. *The Gerontological Society of America, 26*, 273–278.	Adults	Identifies concerns of families providing care to elders	Personal and social restrictions; physical and emotional health; value placed on caregiving; characteristics of care recipient; and economic costs
Craig Handicap Assessment and Report Technique (CHART)	Whiteneck, G., Charlifue, S., Gerhart, K., Overholser, J., and Richardson, G.	Craig Hospital Research Department 3425 S. Clarkson Street Englewood, Colorado 80113 (303) 789-8202 Dave Mellick, MA	Adult	Assess behaviors related to participation	Orientation; physical independence; mobility; occupation; social integration; economic self-sufficiency

Title	Author(s)	Reference/Source	Age	Description	Domains
Craig Hospital Inventory of Environmental Factors (CHIEF and CHIEF short form)	Craig Hospital	Harrison-Felix, C. (2001). The Craig Hospital Inventory of Environmental Factors. *The Center for Outcome Measurement in Brain Injury.* http://www.tbims.org/combi/chief http://www.craighospital.org/Research/Disability/CHIEF%20Manual.pdf	16 to 95 years	Designed to assess the frequency and magnitude of perceived physical, attitudinal, and policy barriers that keep people with disabilities from doing what they want or need to do	ADLs; IADLs
Crawford Small Parts Dexterity Test (CSPDT)	Crawford, J.	Harcourt Assessment, Inc. Attn: Customer Service P.O. Box 599700 San Antonio, TX 78259 (800)211-8378 Fax: (800) 232-1223	Adult	Assess dexterity and fine motor skills in handling small tools and parts; determine whether your applicant has the skills vital in positions requiring agility and strong dexterity	Eye-hand coordination; fine motor skills
Daily Activities Checklist	Brown, C., Hamera, E., and Long, C.	Brown, C., Hamera, E., & Long, C. (1996). The Daily Activities Checklist: A functional assessment for consumers with mental illness living in the community. *Occupational Therapy in Health Care, 10*(3), 33–44.	Adults	Examines engagement of persons with mental illness in social settings	ADLS; community living skills; socialization; quality of daily life
Daily Activities Questionnaire (DAQ)	Oakley, F., Sunderland, T., Hill, J. L., Phillips, S. L., Makahon, R., and Ebner, J. D.	Oakley, F., Sunderland, T., Hill, J. L., Phillips, S. L., Makahon, R., & Ebner, J. D. (1991). The Daily Activities Questionnaire: a functional assessment for people with Alzheimer's disease. *Physical and Occupational Therapy in Geriatrics, 10,* 67–81.	Adults	Assesses instrumental and self-care activities of daily living of people diagnosed with Alzheimer disease	ADLs; IADLs
Daily Activity Diary	Follick, M. J., Ahern, D. K., and Laser-Wolston, N.	Follick, M. J., Ahern, D. K., & Laser-Wolston, N. (1984). Evaluation of a daily activity diary for chronic pain patients. *Pain, 19,* 373–382.	Adults	To examine time use in relation to pain	Time spent sitting, standing, reclining and in productive activities
DeGangi-Berk Test of Sensory Integration	Berk, R. A., and DeGangi, G. A.	Western Psychological Services 12031 Wilshire Boulevard Los Angeles, CA 90025 800-648-8857	3 to 5 years	To measure sensory integration in preschoolers and to detect sensory integrative dysfunction	Postural control; bilateral motor integration; reflex integration

Continued

Continued

Assessment Title	Author(s)	Publisher and/or Contact Information	Ages	Stated Purpose	Areas Assessed
The Denver II	Frankenberg, W. K., Dodds, J., Archer, P., Shapiro, H., and Bresnick, B.	Denver Developmental Materials, Inc. P.O. Box 371075 Denver, CO 80237-5075 (800) 419-4729	Birth to 6 years	To screen for developmental delays	Personal-social; fine motor adaptive; language; gross motor; behavior during testing
Developmental Coordination Disorder Questionnaire (DCDQ)	Wilson, Dewey, and Campbell	Wilson, B., Dewey, D., & Campbell, A. (1998). *The Developmental Coordination Disorder Questionnaire*. Calgary: Author.	5 to 7 years	Uses parental reports to identify developmental coordination disorder	Motor coordination skills
Developmental Test of Visual Perception, 2nd Edition (DTVP-2)	Hammill, D. D., Pearson, N. A., and Voress, J. K.	PRO-ED, Inc. 8700 Shoal Creek Blvd. Austin, TX 78757 (800) 897-3202	4 to 10 years	Identifies disturbances of visual perception and visual-motor integration	Eye-hand coordination; copying; spatial relationships; position in space; figure-ground; visual closure; visual-motor speed; form constancy
Digit Span (portion of WAIS-R)	Kaplan, E., Fein, D., Morris, R., and Delis, D. C.	Harcourt Assessment, Inc. Attn: Customer Service P.O. Box 599700 San Antonio, TX 78259 (800)211-8378 Fax: (800) 232-1223	All ages	To assess short-term auditory memory	Involves auditory attention, concentration, and memory tracking
Disability Assessment for Dementia (DAD)	Gelinas, I., Gauthier, L. and McIntyre, M.	Gelinas, I., Gauthier, L. & McIntyre, M. (1999) Development of a functional measure for persons with Alzheimer's disease: the Disability Assessment for Dementia. *American Journal of Occupational Therapy, 53*, 471–481.	Adults	Assesses basic and instrumental activities of daily living of people diagnosed with Alzheimer's disease	ADLs; IADLs
Disability Rights Guide	National Council on Disability	National Council on Disability 1331 F Street, NW, Suite 850 Washington, DC 20004 (202) 272-2004	Adults	Identifies problems in accessing community resources	Community integration

				Social interaction
Disability Social Distance Scale	Tringo, J.	Tringo, J. L. Disability social distance scale [DSDS] (1970). In R. F. Antonak & H. Livne (Eds.) (1998). *Measurement of attitudes toward people with disabilities: Methods, psychometrics and scale* (pp. 153–156). Springfield, IL: Charles Thomas	Adults	To identify whether attitudes toward persons with disabilities are affected by the type of disability	
Dyadic Adjustment Scale (DAS)	Spanier, G.	MHS Inc P.O. Box 950 North Tonawanda, NY 14120-0950 800-456-3003	Adults	Assesses both partners perceptions of relationship adjustment	Relationship satisfaction
Early Coping Inventory	Zeitlin, S., Williamson, G. G., and Szczepanski, M.	Scholastic Testing Service 480 Meyer Road Bensonville, IL 60106-1617 (800) 642-6787	Birth to 3 years	To measure adaptive behavior	Sensorimotor organization; reactive behavior; self-initiated behavior
EASE 3.2 Basic and EASE 3.2 Deluxe	Christenson, M.	http://www.lifease.com/lifease-ease.html#Basic	Adult	To identify potential home environment problems and to list the best possible solutions and items based on an individual's home setting and functional capability	ADLs; IADLs
Erhardt Developmental Prehension Assessment (EDPA©)	Erhardt, R. P.	Erhardt Developmental Products® 2379 Snowshoe Court Maplewood, MN 55119	Birth to 6 years	To measure components and skills of hand function development in children with disabilities	Arm and hand development
Erhardt Developmental Vision Assessment, Revised (EDVA©)	Erhardt, R. P.	Erhardt Developmental Products® 2379 Snowshoe Court Maplewood, MN 55119	Birth to 6 years	To measure visual-motor development	Involuntary visual patterns; voluntary eye movements
Evaluation Tool of Children's Handwriting (ETCH)	Amundson, S. J.	O.T. KIDS P.O. Box 1118 Homer, AK 99603 907-235-0688	Grades 1–3	Evaluates a child's speed and legibility of writing in various manuscript and cursive writing tasks	Writing speed; writing legibility; sensorimotor skills

Continued

Continued

Assessment Title	Author(s)	Publisher and/or Contact Information	Ages	Stated Purpose	Areas Assessed
Everyday Memory Questionnaire	Sunderland, A., Harris, J. E., and Gleave, J.	Sunderland, A., Harris, J. E., Gleave, J. (1983). Everyday memory questionnaire. In D. T. Wade (Ed.). (1992). *Measurement in neurological rehabilitation* (pp. 140–141). New York: Oxford University Press.	Adults	To assess a client's general awareness of memory capabilities and knowledge about the functioning of memory and memory strategies	Memory during ADL tasks
Executive Function Performance Test (EFPT)	Baum, C., Edwards, D., Morrison, T., and Hahn, M., 2003	Baum, C., Edwards, D., Morrison, T., & Hahn, M. (2003). *Executive Function Performance Test.* St. Louis, MO: Washington University School of Medicine.	Adults	Assesses everyday functional status	ADLs; IADLs
Executive Function Route Finding Task (EFRT)	Boyd, T. M., and Sautter, S. W.	Boyd, T. M., & Sautter, S. W. (1993). Route-Finding: A measure of everyday executive functioning in the head-injured adult. *Applied Cognitive Psychology, 7,* 171–181.	Adults	To assess a person's ability to get from point A to point B in a familiar environment	Understanding the task; seeking information; remembering instructions; detecting errors; correcting errors; ability to stick with the task
Fatigue Severity Scale (FSS)	Krupp, L. B., LaRocca, N. G., Muir-Nash, J., and Steinberg, A. D.	Krupp, L. B., LaRocca, N. G., Muir-Nash, J., & Steinberg, A. D. (1989). The Fatigue Severity Scale: Application to patients with multiple sclerosis and systemic lupus erythematosus. *Archives of Neurology, 46,* 1121–1123.	Adults	Evaluates the impact of fatigue on activities of daily living	ADLs
Feasibility Evaluation Checklist (FEC)	Matheson, L.	EPIC 188 Woodlands Place Court St. Charles, MO 63303 Telephone: 636-724-4556 Fax: 636-898-0954 http://www.epicrehab.com/FreeResources/FEC.pdf	Adults	To assess a person's ability to perform job functions	Productivity; safety; interpersonal behavior

Fine Dexterity Test	The Morrisby Organisation	The Morrisby Organisation, Focus 31 North, Cleveland Road, Hemel Hempstead, Hertfordshire, HP2 7EY Tel: 01442 215521—Fax: 01442 240531. info@morrisby.com	Ages 16 to adult	To assess candidates for small parts assembly	To measure fine motor and small tool dexterity
Fine Motor Task Assessment	McHale, K., and Cermak, S. A.	McHale, K. & Cermak, S. A. (1992). Fine motor activities in elementary school: Preliminary findings and provisional implications for children with fine motor problems. *American Journal of Occupational Therapy, 46*(10), 898–903.	School age	Provides a detailed picture of fine motor skills of children	Fine motor tasks; integrated fine motor tasks; other academic tasks; and nonacademic activities
FirstSTEP Developmental Screening Test	Miller, L. J.	Harcourt Assessment, Inc. Attn: Customer Service P.O. Box 599700 San Antonio, TX 78259 (800)211-8378 Fax: (800) 232-1223	2.9 to 6.2 years	Identifies preschoolers at risk for developmental delays	Cognition; communication; motor skills
The FRACTURE Index (FI)	Black, D. M., Steinbuch, M., Palermo, L., Dargent-Molina, P., Lindsay, R., and Hoseyni, M. S.	Black, D. M., Steinbuch, M., Palermo, L., Dargent-Molina, P., Lindsay, R., & Hoseyni, M. S. (2001). An assessment tool for predicting fracture risk in postmenopausal women. *Osteoporosis International, (12),* 519–528.	Adults	Evaluates and predicts an individual's fracture risk at the spine, hip, and other non-vertebral areas over the next 5 years	Bone strength
Frenchay Activities Index	Holbrook, M. and Skilbeck, C. E.	Holbrook, M., & Skilbeck, C. E. (1983). An activities index for use with stroke patients. *Age and Ageing, 12*(2), 166–170	Adults	To assess functional status post-stroke	ADLs; IADLs
Fugl-Meyer Evaluation of Physical Performance	Fugl-Meyer, A. R., Jaasko, L., Leyman, ll, Olsson, S., and Steglind, S.	Fugl-Meyer, A. R., Jaasko, L., Leyman, ll, Olsson, S., & Steglind, S. (1975). The post-stroke hemiplegic patient. I. A method for evaluation of physical performance. *Scandinavian Journal of Rehabilitation Medicine, 7,* 13–31. Fugl-Meyer, A. R., Jaasko, L., Leyman, ll, Olsson, S., & Steglind, S. (1975). Post-stroke hemiplegic patient: Assessment of physical properties. *Scandinavian Journal of Rehabilitation Medicine, 7,* 83–93.	Adults	To quantify motor recovery stages based on the Brunnstrom and Twitchell scales	Motor recovery; balance; sensation; range of motion; pain

Continued

Continued

Assessment Title	Author(s)	Publisher and/or Contact Information	Ages	Stated Purpose	Areas Assessed
Functional Assessment Measure (FAM)	Rehabilitation Research Center for TBI & SCI at Santa Clara Valley Medical Center	Wright, J. (2000). The Functional Assessment Measure. *The Center for Outcome Measurement in Brain Injury.* http://www.tbims.org/combi/FAM http://www.birf.info/home/bi-tools/tests/fam.html	Adults	An adjunct to the FIM™—the areas addressed in the FAM are to be added to the scores from the FIM™. The FAM does not stand alone.	Cognition; behavior; communication; community functioning
Functional Assessment of Multiple Sclerosis (FAMS)	Cella, D. F., Dineen, K., Arnason, B., Reder, A., Webster, K. A., Karabatsos, G., Chang, C., Lloyd, S., Mo, F., Stewart, J., and Stefoski, D.	Cella, D. F., Dineen, K., Arnason, B., Reder, A., Webster, K. A., Karabatsos, G., Chang, C., Lloyd, S., Mo, F., Stewart, J., & Stefoski, D. (1996). Validation of the Functional Assessment of Multiple Sclerosis quality of life instrument. *Neurology, 47,* 129–139	Adults	Measures quality of life in people diagnosed with multiple sclerosis	Mobility; symptoms; emotional well-being (depression); general contentment; thinking/fatigue; family/social well-being
Functional Independence Measure (FIM)™	The Center for Functional Assessment Research at SUNY Buffalo	Uniform Data System for Medical Rehabilitation 270 Northpointe Parkway Suite 300 Amherst, NY 14228 (716) 817-7800	Adults with various physical impairments	Measures functional status; reflects the impact of disability on the individual and on human and economic resources in the community	18 activities, 13 with a motor emphasis related to self-care; 5 with a cognitive emphasis involving communication
Functional Reach Test	Duncan, P. W., Weiner, D. K., Chandler, J., and Studenski, S.	Pamela W. Duncan Graduate Program in Physical Therapy P.O. Box 3965, Duke University Medical Center Durham, NC 27710 http://www.ohcponline.com/tools/functionalreach.html	Adults	To assess balance impairment, detect chance in balance performance over time, and to aid in designing modified environments for impaired persons	Balance and maximum forward reach
Galveston Orientation and Amnesia Test (GOAT)	Levin, H. S., O'Donnell, V. M., and Grossman, R. G.	The University of Texas Medical Branch at Galveston 301 University Boulevard Galveston, Texas 77555-1028 409-772-9576 http://www.utmb.edu/psychology/Adultrehab/GOAT.htm	Adolescents and adults	To assess orientation and memory over time to measure progress	Orientation; memory

Assessment	Author(s)	Source	Age	Purpose	Areas Assessed
Glasgow Coma Scale	Teasdale, G., and Jennett, B.	Teasdale, G., & Jennett, B. (1994). Assessment of coma and impaired consciousness: practical scale. *Lancet, 2,* 81–84.	Adult	To monitor levels of consciousness in people with traumatic brain injury	Motor, verbal and eye-opening responses
Global Assessment of Functioning (GAF) Scale		DSM—IV-TR, page 32 American Psychiatric Association, Division of Research, 1000 Wilson Boulevard, Arlington, Va. 22209-3901.	Adults	To rate the social, occupational, and psychological functioning of adults	ADLs; social skills
Grooved Peg Board Test	Trites, R.	Lafayette Instrument Co. 3700 Sagamore Parkway North— PO Box 5729 Lafayette, IN 47903-5729 Phone 765-423-1505 Fax 765-423-4111 Toll Free 800-428-7545	Ages 5 to adult	To test manipulative dexterity; this test requires more complex visual-motor coordination than other pegboard tests	Eye-hand coordination; fine motor dexterity
Gross Motor Function Measure	Russell, D., Rosenbaum, P., Gowland, C., Hardy, S., Lane, M., Plews, N., McGavin, H., Cadman, D., and Jarvis, S.	Blackwell Publishing AIDC PO Box 20 Williston, VT 05495-9957 800-216-2522 www.blackwellpublishing.com	5 months to 16 years	Evaluates change in motor function for children with cerebral palsy (has also been used for children with Down syndrome)	Lying and rolling; sitting; crawling and kneeling; standing; walking; and running, jumping
Gross Motor Function Classification System (GMFCS)	Palisano, R., Rosenbaum, P., Walter, S., Russell, D., Wood, E., and Galuppi, B.	Palisano, R., Rosenbaum, P., Walter, S., Russell, D., Wood, E., & Galuppi, B. (1997). Development and reliability of a system to classify gross motor function in children with cerebral palsy. *Developmental Medicine and Child Neurology, 39,* 214–223	2 to 12 years	To provide a standardized system to classify the gross motor function of children with cerebral palsy	Gross motor function
Hawaii Early Learning Profile (HELP)	Furuno, S., O'Reilly, K. A., Hosaka, C. M., Inatsuka, T. T., Zeistloft-Falbey, B., and Allman, T.	VORT Corporation P.O. Box 60132-W Palo Alto, CA 94306 650-322-8282	Birth to 3 years	To assess developmental skills and behaviors	Cognitive; language; gross motor; fine motor; social; and self-help skills
Holmes-Rahe Life Change Index	Holmes, T. H., and Rahe, R. H.	Holmes, T. H., & Rahe, R. H. (1967). The social readjustment rating scale. *Journal of Psychosomatic Research, 11,* 213–218	Adults	Self-assessment to identify stressors in the client's life	Social adjustment

Continued

Continued

Assessment Title	Author(s)	Publisher and/or Contact Information	Ages	Stated Purpose	Areas Assessed
Home and Community Environment Instrument (HACE)	Keysor, J. J., Jette, A. M., and Haley, S. M.	Keysor, J. J., Jette, A. M., & Haley, S. M. (2005). Development of the home and community environment (HACE) instrument. *Journal of Rehabilitation Medicine, 37*(1), 37–44	Adults	Assesses factors in the home and community that affect mobility, communication, and interaction	Mobility; communication; social interaction; ADLs
Home-Based Intervention for Caregivers of Elders with Dementia	Corcoran, M. A., and Gitlin, L. N.	Corcoran, M. A., & Gitlin, L. N. (1992). Dementia management: An occupational therapy home-based intervention for caregivers. *American Journal of Occupational Therapy, 46*(9), 801–808.	Adults	Strategy to modify household culture to support optimal occupational performance of elderly persons and caregivers	Home environment of older adults
Home Falls and Accidents Screening Tool (HOME-FAST)	Mackenzie, L.	Can be obtained from Dr MacKenzie at Lynette.Mackenzie@newcastle.edu.au	Older adults at risk of falling	To identify environmental and functional safety in the home	Fall and accident risk; safety
Home Modification Workbook	Adaptive Environments Center	Adaptive Environment Center. (1988). *Home modification workbook.* Boston: Author.	Adults	Identify architectural barriers in the home	Home environment
Home Observation and Measurement of the Environment (HOME), 3rd Edition	Caldwell, B.	Lorraine Coulson CRTL Room 205 University of Arkansas at Little Rock 2801 S. University Little Rock, AR 72204 501-565-7627 http://www.ualr.edu/COEDEPT/case/ent/home.html lrcoulson@ualr.edu	Birth to 3 years; other inventories available for 3 to 15 years	To assess the stimulation potential of the child's developmental environment; used primarily as a screening instrument	Human environmental properties; nonhuman environmental properties
Home Situations Questionnaire (HSQ)	Barkley, R.	Barkley, R. A., & Murphy, K. R. (1998) *Attention deficit hyperactivity disorder: A clinical workbook* (2nd ed.). New York: Guilford Publications.	School age	Identifies how symptoms of ADD/ADHD disrupt the home environment and the child's ability to participate in ADLs	ADLs

Hopkins Verbal Learning Test—Revised (HVLT-R)	Brandt, J. and Benedict, R.	Psychological Assessment Resources, Inc. 16204 N. Florida Avenue Lutz, FL 33549 813-968-3003	16 years to adult	Assesses verbal learning and memory	Immediate recall; delayed recall; delayed recognition
Housing Enabler	Steinfeld, E., Iwarsson, S., and Isacsson, A.	Susanne Iwarsson Veten & Skapen HB Pl 2532 SE-288 93 Nävlinge Sweden http://www.enabler.nu	Adults	Identifies potential problems, severe problems, or impossibility of use of assistive devices for an individual	Limitations and use of assistive devices; potential environmental barriers inside or outside the home
Illness Perception Questionnaire for Schizophrenia (IPQS)	Lobban, F., Barrowclough, C. and Jones, S.	Lobban, F., Barrowclough, C. & Jones, S. (2005). Assessing cognitive representations of mental health problems. I. The illness perception questionnaire for schizophrenia. *British Journal of Clinical Psychology, 44*(2), 147–162.	Adults	To assess how an individual diagnosed with schizophrenia perceives themselves and the impact of their perceptions on their health and performance	Self-perception
Illness Perception Questionnaire for Schizophrenia—Relatives' Version (IPQS-Relatives)	Lobban, F., Barrowclough, C. and Jones, S.	Lobban, F., Barrowclough, C. & Jones, S. (2005). Assessing cognitive representations of mental health problems. II. The illness perception questionnaire for schizophrenia: Relatives' version. *British Journal of Clinical Psychology, 44*(2), 163–179.	Adults	To assess the perceptions of relatives of individuals diagnosed with schizophrenia to understand how they impact the individual's health and performance	
Indented Paragraph Test	Caplan, B.	Caplan, B. (1987). Assessment of unilateral neglect: A new reading test. *Journal of Clinical and Experimental Neuropsychology, 9,* 359–364.	Adults	Uses variable left margin to assess subtle unilateral neglect	Scanning; reading, unilateral neglect
Independent Living Scales (ILS)	Loeb, P. A.	Harcourt Assessment, Inc. Attn: Customer Service P.O. Box 599700 San Antonio, TX 78259 (800) 211-8378 Fax: (800) 232-1223	Adults	Determine to what degree adults are capable of caring for themselves and their property	Memory and orientation; managing money; managing home and transportation; health and safety; and social adjustment

Continued

Continued

Assessment Title	Author(s)	Publisher and/or Contact Information	Ages	Stated Purpose	Areas Assessed
Individual Differences Questionnaire	Paivio, A.	Paivio, A. (1971). *Imagery and Verbal Processes.* New York: Holt Rinehart & Winston.	Adults	Identifies and helps therapist create virtual contexts that are able to be used by individuals with different thinking and learning styles	Imagery and verbal thinking habits and skills
Infant/Toddler Sensory Profile	Dunn, W.	Harcourt Assessment, Inc. Attn: Customer Service P.O. Box 599700 San Antonio, TX 78259 (800)211-8378 Fax: (800) 232-1223	Birth to 3 years	To determine how well a subject processes sensory information in everyday situations and to profile the sensory system's effect on functional performance	Sensory processing, modulation, and behavioral and emotional responses
Inpatient Rehabilitation Facility—Patient Assessment Instrument (IRF-PAI)	Uniform Data System for Medical Rehabilitation	Uniform Data System for Medical Rehabilitation 270 Northpointe Parkway Suite 300 Amherst, NY 14228 (716) 568-0037 www.cms.hhs.gov/InpatientRehabFacPPS/downloads/irfpai-manual040104.pdf	Adults with various physical impairments	Essentially the FIM™ with quality indicators; used with PPS	18 activities, 13 with a motor emphasis related to self-care; 5 with a cognitive emphasis involving communication; quality indicators include respiratory status, pain, PUSH scale, and safety
Interest Checklist/NPI Interest Checklist	Matsutsuyu, J. revised by Rogers, J., Weinstein J., and Figone, J.	Matsutsuyu J. S. (1969). The interest check list, *American Journal of Occupational Therapy*, 23(4):323–328. Rogers, J. C., Weinstein, J. M., & Figone, J. J. (1978). The Interest Checklist: An empirical assessment. *American Journal of Occupational Therapy*, 32, 628–630.	Adolescents to adult	Gathers data about a person's interest patterns and characteristics	ADL; manual skills; cultural and educational activities; physical sports; social and recreational activities

			Adults	Allows a person to articulate personal environmental meanings and priorities	Meaning of personal environment
Interview-In-Place	Lifchez, R.	Lifchez, R. (1987). *Rethinking architecture: Design students and physically disabled people.* Berkeley, CA: University of California Press.			
Jebsen Hand Function Test	Jebsen, R. H., Taylor, N., Trieschmann, R. B., Trotter, M. J., and Howard, L. A.	Sammons Preston, Inc. PO Box 50710 Bolingbrook, IL 60440-5071 800-323-5547 www.sammonspreston.com	5 years and up	To assess effective use of the hands in everyday activity by performing tasks representative of functional manual activities	Writing; card turning; picking up small objects; simulated feeding; stacking checkers; picking up light and heavy objects
Kitchen Task Assessment (KTA)	Baum, C., and Edwards, D. F.	Baum, C., & Edwards, D. F. (1993). Cognitive performance in senile dementia of the Alzheimer's type: The Kitchen Task Assessment, *American Journal of Occupational Therapy, 47,* 431–436.	Adults	Measures the level of cognitive support required by a person diagnosed with dementia	ADLs
Klein-Bell Activities of Daily Living Scale	Klein, R. M., and Bell, B.	Marie Gary HSCER Distribution HSBT 281 SB 56 University of Washington Seattle, Washington 98195	Children and adults	Measure ADL independence to determine current status, change in status, and subactivities to focus on in rehabilitation	Dressing, mobility, elimination, bathing and hygiene, eating, and emergency communication
Knox Cube Test	Stone, M. H., and B. D. Wright	Stoelting Co. 620 Wheat Lane Wood Dale, IL 60191 630-860-9700 www.stoeltingco.com/tests	2 to 8 years; 8 years and up	Nonverbal mental test to measure attention span and memory	Attention span; short-term memory
Knox Preschool Play Scale (PPS-R)	Knox, S.	Knox, S. (1997). Development and current use of the Knox Preschool Play Scale. In L. Parham & L. Fazio (Eds.) *Play in occupational therapy for children.* (pp. 35–51). St. Louis: Mosby.	Birth to 6 years	Observational assessment of play skills	Space management; material management; pretense or symbolic play; participation in play

Continued

Continued

Assessment Title	Author(s)	Publisher and/or Contact Information	Ages	Stated Purpose	Areas Assessed
Kohlman Evaluation of Living Skills (KELS)	McGourty, L. K., (1979, 1999)	AOTA Products PO Box 0151 Annapolis Junction, MD 20701-0151 877-404-AOTA www.aota.org	Adults with cognitive impairments	Evaluate the ability to live independently and safely in the community	Self-care, safety and health, money management, transportation and telephone, work and leisure; tends to emphasize the knowledge component of activities
Large Allen Cognitive Level (ACLS-5) Screen	[See p. 1092, Allen Cognitive Level Screen-5 (ACLS-5)]	[See p. 1092, Allen Cognitive Level Screen-5 (ACLS-5)]	[See p. 1092, Allen Cognitive Level Screen-5 (ACLS-5)]	[See p. 1092, Allen Cognitive Level Screen-5 (ACLS-5)]	[See p. 1092, Allen Cognitive Level Screen-5 (ACLS-5)]
Leisure Activities Finder (LAF)	Holmberg, K., Rosen, D., and Holland, J. L.	Psychological Assessment Resources, Inc. 16204 N. Florida Avenue Lutz, FL 33549 813-968-3003	Adults	Assists clients with finding leisure activities	Play/leisure
Leisure Assessment Inventory (LAI)	Hawkins, B. A., Ardovino, P., Brattain Rogers, N., Foose, A., and Ohlsen, N.	Idyll Arbor 39129 264th Ave SE Enumclaw, WA 98022 voice: 360-825-7797 fax: 360-825-5670 sales@idyllarbor.com	Adults	Measures the leisure behavior of adults through its four components: 1. The Leisure Activity Participation Index (LAP), 2. the Leisure Preference Index (L-PREF), 3. the Leisure Interest Index (L-INT), and 4. the Leisure Constraints Index (L-CON)	Leisure skill; social skills

Title	Author	Reference/Contact	Age	Purpose	Play/leisure
Leisure Boredom Scale (LBS)	Iso-Ahola, S. E., and Weissinger, E.	Iso-Ahola, S. E., & Weissinger, E. (1990). Perceptions of boredom in leisure: conceptualization, reliability and validity of the leisure boredom scale. *Journal of Leisure Research, 22,* 17–25.	All ages	Measures constraints on achieving enjoyment from leisure activities	
Leisure Competence Measure	Kloseck, M., and Crilly, R.	Dr. Marita Kloseck, CTRS Division of Geriatric Medicine, Parkwood Hospital 801 Commissioners Road East London, Ontario, Canada N6C SJl 519-859-1232 mkloseck@execulink.com.	All ages	Measures outcomes in leisure/play activities	Leisure awareness; leisure attitude; leisure skills; cultural/social behaviors; interpersonal skills; community integration skills; social contact; and community participation
Leisure Diagnostic Battery	Witt, P., and Ellis, G.	Venture Publishing, Inc. 1999 Cato Avenue State College, PA 16801 814-234-4561	Adolescents and adults	Assesses an individual's "leisure functioning"	Perceived Leisure Competency Scale; Perceived Leisure Control Scale; Leisure Needs Scale; Depth of Involvement in Leisure Scale; Playfulness Scale; Perceived Freedom in Leisure—Total Score; Barriers to Leisure Involvement Scale; Knowledge of Leisure Opportunities Test; and Leisure Preference Inventory

Continued

Continued

Assessment Title	Author(s)	Publisher and/or Contact Information	Ages	Stated Purpose	Areas Assessed
Leisure Satisfaction Scale	Beard, J. G., and Ragheb, M. G.	Beard, J. G., & Ragheb, M. G. (1980). The leisure satisfaction measure. _Journal of Leisure Research, 12_(1), 20–33	All ages	Measures a client's level of satisfaction in leisure activities	Play/leisure
Limits of Stability (LOS)	Nashner, L. M.	NeuroCom 9570 SE Lawnfield Road Clackamas, OR 97015 800-767-6744	Adult	To assess dynamic balance	Reaction time; directional control; movement velocity; movement distance; ankle range of motion
Lincoln-Oseretsky Motor Development Scale	Sloan, W.	Stoelting Company 620 Wheat Lane Wood Dale, Illinois 60191 630-860-9700	6 to 14 years	To measure unilateral and bilateral motor development	Static coordination; dynamic coordination; speed of movement; finger dexterity; eye-hand coordination; gross motor skills
Line Cancellation Test	Albert, M. L.	Albert, M. L. (1973). A simple test of visual neglect. _Neurology, 23,_ 658–665.	Adults	To measure hemispatial neglect	Visual attention
Locke-Wallace Marital Adjustment Scale (MAT)	Locke, H. J. and Wallace, K. M. (1959)	Corcoran, K., & Fischer, J. (2000). _Measures for clinical practice: A sourcebook._ 3rd Ed. Volume 1 (pp. 133–135). New York: Free Press.	Adults	To measure marital adjustment	Relationship
Lowenstein Occupational Therapy Cognitive Assessment (LOTCA™), 2nd Edition	Itzkovich, M., Elazar, B., Averbuch, S., and Katz, N.	Therapro, Inc. 225 Arlington Street Framingham, MA 01702-8723 508-872-9494	6 years and up	To identify abilities and limitations in areas of cognitive processing	Orientation; perception; visuomotor organization; thinking operations
Lowenstein Occupational Therapy Cognitive Assessment—Geriatric (LOTCA™-G)	Elazar, B., Itzkovich, M., and Katz, N.	Therapro, Inc. 225 Arlington Street Framingham, MA 01702-8723 508-872-9494	Older adults	To identify abilities and limitations in areas of cognitive processing	Orientation; perception; visuomotor organization; thinking operations

Maintaining Seniors' Independence through Home Adaptation: A self-assessment guide	Canadian Mortgage and Housing Corporation	http://www.cmhc.ca/en/co/maho/adse/masein/index.cfm	Older adults	Identifies the types of difficulties that seniors can experience and describes types of adaptations that can help overcome these difficulties	ADLs; home safety
Making Action Plans (MAPs)	Forest, M., and Lusthaus, E.	Inclusion Press/Centre for Integrated Education and Community 24 Thome Crescent Toronto, ON., Canada, M6H 2S5 416-658-5363 http://www.inclusion.com	3 to 21 years	Provides a framework to more fully integrate students; to be used in conjunction with the IEP	Personal history; fears; wishes; strengths; needs; "ideal day"
Marital Satisfaction Inventory	Snyder, D. K.	Psychological Assessment Resources, Inc. 16204 N. Florida Avenue Lutz, FL 33549 813-968-3003/ 800-383-6595	18 years and up	To assess conflict within a relationship between individuals ages 18 and older	Relationships; communication
Matson Evaluation of Social Skills in Individuals with Severe Retardation (MESSIER)	Matson, J. L., and LeBlanc, L. A.	Matson, J. L. (1995). *Matson Evaluation of Social Skills for Individuals with Severe Retardation.* Baton Rouge: Scientific Publisher.	All ages	To measure social skills of people with severe developmental delays	Social skills
Maximum Voluntary Efforts Tests (MVE)	Hildreth, D., Breidenbach, W., Lister, G., and Hodges, A.	Hildreth, D., Breidenbach, W., Lister, G., & Hodges, A. (1989). Detection of submaximal effort by use of rapid exchange grip. *Journal of Hand Surgery, 14A(4),* 742–745.	Adults	Uses client's intra-task consistency as an indication of whether the person has exerted maximal effort	Effort in physical strength tasks
Mayo-Portland Adaptability Inventory (MPAI-4)	Malec, J. F., and Lezak, M. D.	http://www.tbims.org/combi/mpai/ Malec, J. F. (2004). Comparability of Mayo-Portland Adaptability Inventory ratings by staff, significant others, and people with acquired brain injury. *Brain Injury, 18,* 563–575.	Adolescents to adults	To measure long-term outcomes of brain injury	Emotions; behavior; functional abilities; physical disabilities; and societal participation

Continued

Continued

Assessment Title	Author(s)	Publisher and/or Contact Information	Ages	Stated Purpose	Areas Assessed
McCarthy Scale of Children's Abilities	McCarthy, D.	Harcourt Assessment, Inc. Attn: Customer Service P.O. Box 599700 San Antonio, TX 78259 800-211-8378 fax: 800-232-1223	2.6 to 8.6 years	To determine a child's intellectual level, strengths, and weaknesses	Verbal; perceptual-performance; quantitative; general cognitive; memory; and motor skills
McGill Pain Questionnaire	Melzack, R.	Melzack, R. (1983). The McGill pain questionnaire. In Melzack, R. (Ed.) *Pain measurement and assessment* (pp. 41–48). New York: Raven Press.	Adults	Self-assessment of pain	Pain
McMaster Family Assessment Device	Epstein, N. B., Baldwin, L. M., and Bishop, D. S.	Brown University Butler Hospital Family Research Program Butler Hospital 345 Blackstone Road Providence, RI 02906	Adults	Evaluates adaptation to having a child with a head injury	General family functioning; problem-solving; communication; roles; affective responsiveness; affective involvement; behavior control
Measure of the Quality of Environment (MQE), Version 2	Fougeyrollas, P., Noreau, L., Michel, G., and Boschen, K.	Fougeyrollas, P., Noreau, L., Michel, G., & Boschen, K. (1999). Measure of the quality of environment (MQE) Version 2. Charles, (Quebec), Canada: INDCP-C.P. 225	Adults	To evaluate the influence of environmental factors on the quality of participation in activities of daily living in relation to an individual's functional capabilities	ADLs; IADLs
Melbourne Assessment of Unilateral Upper Limb Function	Randall, M. J., Johnson, L. M., and Reddihough, D. S.	Randall, M. J., Johnson, L. M., & Reddihough, D. S. (1999) *The Melbourne Assessment of Unilateral Upper Limb Function: Test administration manual.* Melbourne: Royal Children's Hospital.	5 to 15 years	Measures quality of upper extremity movement	Upper extremity movement

Melville-Nelson Self-Care Assessment (SCA)	Nelson, D. L. and Melville, L. L	Nelson, D. L., Melville, L. L., Wilkerson, J. D., Magness, R. A., Grech, J. L., & Rosenberg, J. A. (2002). Interrater reliability, concurrent validity, responsiveness, and predictive validity of the Melville-Nelson Self-Care Assessment. *American Journal of Occupational Therapy, 56,* 51–59. http://hsc.utoledo.edu/allh/ot/melville.html lmelville@meduohio.edu	Adults in sub-acute rehab and nursing homes	To objectively assess self-care skills	Bed mobility; transfers; dressing; eating; toileting; personal hygiene; and bathing
Middlesex Elderly Assessment of Mental State (MEAMS)	Golding, E.	National Rehabilitation Services 117 North Elm Street PO Box 1247 Gaylord, MI 49735 517-732-3866	Older adults	To assess gross impairment of specific cognitive skills; designed to differentiate between organically-based cognitive impairments and functional illnesses	12 simple cognitive tasks
Miller Assessment for Preschoolers (MAP)	Miller, L. J.	Harcourt Assessment, Inc. Attn: Customer Service P.O. Box 599700 San Antonio, TX 78259 800-211-8378 fax: 800-232-1223	2 to 6 years	To identify children who exhibit moderate "preacademic problems"	Sensory, motor, and cognitive skills through verbal and nonverbal tasks
Milwaukee Evaluation of Daily Living Skills (MEDLS)	Leonardelli, C.	SLACK, Inc. 6900 Grove Road Thorofare, NJ 08086 800-257-8290	Adults with chronic mental health problems	Establish baseline behaviors to develop treatment objectives related to daily living skills	Communication, personal care, clothing care, home and community safety, money management, personal health care, medication management, telephone use,

Continued

Continued

Assessment Title	Author(s)	Publisher and/or Contact Information	Ages	Stated Purpose	Areas Assessed
					transportation usage, time awareness; subtests can be used individually or in combination
Mini Mental State Exam (MMSE)	Folstein, M. F., Folstein, S. E., and McHugh, P. R.	Folstein, M. F., Folstein, S. E., & McHugh, P. R. (1975). Minimental state: A practical method for grading the cognitive-state of patients for the clinician. *Journal of Psychiatric Research, 12,* 89–198.	Adolescents and adults	To quantitatively measure cognitive performance	Orientation; memory; attention; calculation; recall; language
Mini-Osteoporosis Quality of Life Questionnaire (OQLQ)	Ioannidid, G., Adachi, J. D., and Guyatt, G. H.	Ioannidid, G., Adachi, J. D., & Guyatt, G. H. (1999). Development and validation of the Mini-Osteoporosis Quality of Life Questionnaire (OQLQ) in osteoporotic women with back pain due to vertebral fractures. *Osteoporosis International, 10*(3), 207–213.	Adults	Measures quality of life in individuals with osteoporosis	Symptoms; physical function; ADLs; emotional function; leisure
Minimum Data Set—Section G. Physical Functioning and Structural Problems Scale, Version 2.0	Health Care Financing Administration	US Government Printing Office Washington, D.C. http://www.cms.hhs.gov/Nursing HomeQualityInits/downloads/MDS20MDSAllForms.pdf	Residents in long-term care; clients in home care	To describe baseline ADL and track changes in ADL	Bed mobility, transfer, walk in room, walk in corridor, locomotion on unit, locomotion off unit, dressing, eating, toilet use, personal hygiene and bathing
Minnesota Handwriting Assessment	Reisman, J.	Harcourt Assessment, Inc. Attn: Customer Service P.O. Box 599700 San Antonio, TX 78259 800-211-8378 fax: 800-232-1223	5 to 7 years	To analyze handwriting skills and demonstrate progress resulting from intervention	Legibility; form; alignment; size; spacing

Title	Author(s)	Source/Citation	Age	Purpose	Areas Assessed
Minnesota Rate of Manipulation Tests (MRMT)		Matheson P.O. Box 492 Keene, NH 03431 800-443-7690	13 years and up	To measure manual dexterity (speed of gross arm and hand movements during rapid eye-hand coordination tasks)	Placing test; turning test; displacing test; one-hand turning and placing; two handed turning and placing
Model of Human Occupation Screening Tool (MOHOST), Version 2.0	Parkinson, S., Forsyth, K., and Kielhofner, G.	www.moho.uic.edu	Adults	To assess an individual's capacity for occupational functioning	Volition; habituation; motor skills; and environment
Models of Media Representation of Disability	Haller, B.	Haller, B. (1995). Rethinking models of media representation of disability. *Disability Studies Quarterly, 15*(2), 26–30.	Adults	Identify ways in which societal beliefs and values shape an individual's views	Attitudes toward disability
Modified Dynamic Visual Processing Assessment (M-DVPA)	Toglia, J. P., and Finkelstein, N.	Toglia, J. P. & Finkelstein, N. (1991). *Manual for the Dynamic Visual Processing Assessment,* unpublished manuscript.	Adults	To assess visual processing in a dynamic interaction	Visual processing
Modified Mini-Mental Examination [3MS] (Teng & Chui, 1987)	Teng, E. L. and Chui, H. C.	Teng, E. L. & Chui, H. C. (1987). The Modified Mini-Mental State (3MS) Examination. *Journal of Clinical Psychiatry. 48*(8): 314–318.	Adolescents and adults	To quantitatively measure cognitive performance	Orientation; memory; attention; calculation; recall; language
Mother-Child Interaction Checklist	Barrera, M., and Vella, D.	Barrera, M. & Vella, D. (1987). Disabled and nondisabled infants' interactions with their mothers. *American Journal of Occupational Therapy, 41,* 168–172.	Infants and adults	Structured format to allow observation of interactions between mothers and children	Maternal behaviors; infant behaviors; reciprocal behaviors
Motor Activity Log: Amount of Use Scale (AOU)	Uswatte, G., Taub, E., Morris, D., Light, K., and Thompson, P. A.	Uswatte, G., Taub, E., Morris, D., Light, K., & Thompson, P. A. (2006). The Motor Activity Log-28: Assessing daily use of the hemiparetic arm after stroke. *Neurology, 67,* 1189–1194	Adults	Provides information about actual use of the limb in everyday life situations	ADLs; IADLs

Continued

Continued

Assessment Title	Author(s)	Publisher and/or Contact Information	Ages	Stated Purpose	Areas Assessed
Motor-Free Visual Perception Test, 3rd Edition (MVPT-3)	Colarusso, R. P., and Hammill, D. D.	Academic Therapy Publications 20 Commercial Blvd. Novato, CA 94949 800-422-7249	4 to 11 years	To test visual perception without motor involvement	Spatial relationships; visual discrimination; visual figure ground; visual closure; and visual memory
Movement Assessment Battery for Children (Movement ABC)	Henderson, S. E., and Sugden, D. A.	Harcourt Assessment, Inc. Attn: Customer Service P.O. Box 599700 San Antonio, TX 78259 800-211-8378 fax: 800-232-1223	4 to 12 years	To assess children's motor skills in children with motor impairments	Static balance; dynamic balance; manual dexterity; speed of movement; eye-hand coordination; problem-solving skills
Movement Assessment for Infants (MAI)	Chandler, L., Andrews, M., Swanson, M., and Larson, A.	Chandler, L., Andrews, M., Swanson, M., & Larson, A. (1980). *Movement assessment of infants: A manual.* Rolling Bay, WA: Authors.	Birth to 12 months	To differentiate between normal variance among developing infants versus developmental delay	Motor function; neurological function
Multidimensional Functional Assessment Questionnaire	Duke University Center for the Study of Aging and Human Development	Duke University Center for the Study of Aging and Human Development. (1978). *Multidimensional functional assessment: The OARS methodology.* Durham, NC: Author.	Adults	Plan optimal community living arrangements	Functional level of individual; community service use and perceived need for services
Multiphasic Environmental Assessment Procedure—Architectural Features Checklist (MEAP)	Moos, R., and Lemke, S.	Moos, R. & Lemke, S. (1979). Multi-Phasic Environmental Assessment Procedures (MEAP): Preliminary Manual, Palo Alto, CA, *Social Ecology Laboratory,* Stanford University School of Medicine.	Older adults	To evaluate care settings for older adults	Accessibility; safety

Multiple Errands Test	Shallice, T., and Burgess, P. W.	To assess the executive function that allows an individual to act on their own initiative and to solve problems in a relatively open ended situation	Adolescents to adults	Executive function, initiation and problem solving involved in activities of daily living
Multiple Sclerosis Impact Scale (MSIS-29)	Fitzpatrick, R., Hobart, J., Lamping, D. L., Riazi, A. and Thompson, A.	To measure the physical and the psychological impact of multiple sclerosis from the patient's perspective	Adults	Disability/physical functioning; quality of life
Multiple Sclerosis Quality of Life—54 Instrument (MSQOL-54)	Vickrey, B. G., Hays, R. D., Harooni, R., Myers, L. W., and Ellison, G. W.	Measures quality of life in people diagnosed with multiple sclerosis	Adults	Physical function; role limitations-physical; role limitations-emotional; pain; emotional well-being; energy; health perceptions; social function; cognitive function; health distress; overall quality of life; sexual function
Multiple Sclerosis Quality of Life Inventory (MSQLI)	National Multiple Sclerosis Society Consortium of Multiple Sclerosis Centers	Measures quality of life in adults with multiple sclerosis	Adults	Quality of life

Sources:
Shallice, T., & Burgess, P. W. (1991). Deficits in strategy application following frontal lobe damage in man. *Brain, 114*, 727–741.

Hobart, J., Lamping, D., Fitzpatrick, R., Riazi, A., & Thompson, A. (2001). The Multiple Sclerosis Impact Scale (MSIS-29): A new patient-based outcome measure. *Brain, 124*, 962–973.

Dr. Barbara Vickrey, Health Services Research Center, UCLA Wilshire Center, 10920 Wilshire Blvd., Suite 300, Los Angeles, CA 90024-6505, bvickrey@ucla.edu.

Director of Health Care Delivery and Policy Research, National Multiple Sclerosis Society, Nicholas LaRocca, PhD, 733 Third Avenue, 3rd floor, New York, NY 10017, 212.476.0414, nicholas.larocca@nmss.org, http://www.nationalmssociety.org/docs/HOM/MSQLI_Manual_and_Forms.pdf

Continued

Continued

Assessment Title	Author(s)	Publisher and/or Contact Information	Ages	Stated Purpose	Areas Assessed
Neighborhood Mobility Survey	Cantor, M.	Cantor, M. (1979). Life space and social support. In Byerts, T., Jowell, S., & Pastalan, L. (Eds.), *Environmental context of aging: Lifestyles, environmental quality, and living arrangements* (pp. 33–61). New York: Garland STPM Press.	Adults	Provides a framework for evaluating how far and by what methods people travel on a regular basis to important resources in their environment	Mobility within community
Neurobehavioral Cognitive Status Screening Examination (COGNISTAT)	Northern California Neurobehavioral Group, Inc	NCNG, Inc. P.O. Box 460 Fairfax, CA 94978 (800) 922-5840 www.cognistat.com	12 years and up	To screen individuals who cannot tolerate more complicated or lengthier neuropsychological tests; assesses intellectual functioning in five areas	Language; memory; arithmetic; attention; judgment; and reasoning
NIH Activity Record	Gloria Furst, OTR, MPH	National Institutes of Health Building 10, Room 6s235 10 Center Drive MSC 1604 Bethesda, MD 20892-1604 Gfurst@cc.nih.gov	Adolescents to adults	To identify changes in role activities	Activities of daily living
Orientation Log (O-log)	Novack, T.	Novack, T. (2000). The Orientation Log. *The Center for Outcome Measurement in Brain Injury.* http://www.tbims.org/combi/olog	Adolescents to adults	To measure orientation to time, place, and circumstance in a rehabilitation population; can measure change over time	Orientation
Rolyan ® 9-Hole Peg Test	Mathiowetz, V., Weber, K., Kashman, N., and Volland, G.	Sammons Preston P.O. Box 5071 Bolingbrook, IL 60440-5071 800-323-5547 www.sammonspreston.com	Adults	To measure finger dexterity; can be more applicable to neurologically involved patients	Fine motor dexterity

Title	Authors	Source	Age	Purpose	Focus
Nowicki-Strickland Locus of Control Scale for Children (TIM(C))	Nowicki, S., and Strickland, B.	Educational Testing Service (ETS) Test Collection Library Rosedale and Carter Roads Princeton, NJ 08541 609-734-5689	Grades 3–12	Identifies a child's locus of control	Locus of control
Nursing Child Assessment Satellite Training (NCAST) feeding and teaching scales	Barnard, K. E., and Sumner, G.	University of Washington Center on Human Development and Disability Box 357920 Seattle, WA 98195-7920 206-543-8528 www.ncast.org	All ages	Measures caregiver-child interaction	Six constructs of caregiver-child interaction
Occupational Circumstances Assessment—Interview Rating Scale (OCAIRS), version 4.0	Forsyth, K., Deshpande, S., Kielhofner, G., Henriksson, C., Haglund, L., Olson, L., Skinner, S., and Kulkarni, S.	www.moho.uic.edu	Adolescents to adults	Gathers data on a client's occupational adaptation	Personal causation; values and goals; interests; roles; habits; skills; previous experiences; physical and social environments; overall occupation participation and adaptation
Occupational Performance History Intervie, Second Version (OPHI-II)	Kielhofner, G., Mallinson, T., Crawford, C., Nowak, M., Rigby, M., Henry, A., Walens, D.	www.moho.uic.edu	Adolescents and adults	Gathers data on a client's occupational adaptation over time	Activity/occupational choices; critical life events; daily routines; occupational roles; occupational behavior settings
Occupational Questionnaire (OQ)	Smith, N. R., Kielhofner, G., and Watts, J. H.	www.moho.uic.edu Use link for "Other instruments based on MOHO"	Adults	Gathers data on time use patterns and feelings about time use	Time use

Continued

Continued

Assessment Title	Author(s)	Publisher and/or Contact Information	Ages	Stated Purpose	Areas Assessed
Occupational Self-Assessment (OSA), version 2.2	Baron, K., Kielhofner, G., Iyenger, A., Gold-hammer, V., and Wolenski, J.	www.moho.uic.edu	14 years and up	Self-report of client's perception of his/her occupational competence on their occupational adaptation.	Volition; habituation; performance; values; personal causation; interests; roles; habits; skills
Occupational Therapy Psychosocial Assessment of Learning (OT PAL)	Townsend, S. C., Carey, P. D., Hollins, N. L., Helfrich, C., Blondis, M., Hoffman, A., Collins, L., Knudson, J., and Blackwell, A.	Townsend, S. C., Carey, P. D., Hollins, N. L., Helfrich, C., Blondis, M., Hoffman, A., Collins, L., Knudson, J., & Blackwell, A. (2001). *The Occupational Therapy Psychosocial Assessment of Learning (OT PAL).* Chicago: University of Illinois, Department of Occupational Therapy, Model of Human Occupation Clearinghouse. http://www.moho.uic.edu/assess/otpal.html	Children	Assists clinicians in identifying a child's strengths and limitations within the school environment	Student's volition (the ability to make choices); habituation (roles and routines); and environmental fit within the classroom setting
Oswestry Low Back Pain Disability Questionnaire	Fairbank, J. C. T., Couper Mbaot, J., Davies, J. B., and O'Brien, J. P.	Fairbank, J. C. T., Couper Mbaot, J., Davies, J. B., & O'Brien, J. P. (1980). The Oswestry Low Back Pain Disability Questionnaire. *Physiotherapy, 66,* 271–272.	Adults	Self-assessment of pain	Pain
OT ADL Neurobehavioral Evaluation (A-ONE)	Arnadottir, G.	Arnadottir, G. (1990). *The brain and behavior: Assessing cortical dysfunction through activities of daily living.* Philadelphia: Mosby. http://www.glengillen.com/A-One.htm Guðrún Árnadóttir: a-one@islandia.is	16 years and up	Identifies neurobehavioral deficits, the impact they have on functional performance of ADL, and how they relate to the location of cortical lesions	ADL performance in dressing, grooming and hygiene, transfers and mobility, feeding, and communication

Outcome and Assessment Information Set, B-1, M0640-M0800 (OASIS)	Center for Health Services and Policy Research	http://homehealth101.com/OASIS Draftb1.pdf	Adults	Measures the ability to perform ADL and IADL in people in home care	Dressing; toileting; transferring; ambulation/locomotion; feeding/eating; grooming Meal preparation; transportation; laundry; housekeeping; using telephone; medication management
Paced Auditory Serial Addition Test (PASAT)	Gronwall, D. M. A.	Gronwall, D. M. A. (1977). Paced Auditory Serial Addition Task: A measure of recovery from concussion. *Perceptual and Motor Skills, 44,* 367–373. http://www.pasat.us/	Adults	To detect subtle impairments in attention and speed of processing	Auditory attention and processing during everyday activities
Pain Behavior Checklist	Turk, D. C., Wack, J. T., and Kerns, R. D.	Turk, D. C., Wack, J. T., & Kerns, R. D. (1985). An empirical examination of the "pain behavior" construct. *Journal of Behavioral Medicine, 8,* 119–130.	Adults	Documenting overt pain behaviors	Behavior related to pain
Parenting Alliance Measure (PAM)	Abidin, R. R., and Konold, T. R.	Psychological Assessment Resources, Inc. 16204 N. Florida Avenue Lutz, FL 33549 813-968-3003 800-383-6595	Adults	Measures the strength of the child-rearing alliance between parents of children ages 1 to 19 years	Relationship
Parenting Stress Index (PSI), 3rd Edition	Abidin, R. R.	Psychological Assessment Resources, Inc. 16204 N. Florida Avenue Lutz, FL 33549 813-968-3003 800-383-6595	Adults	To identify stressors experienced by parents that are related to dysfunctional parenting	Coping skills; parenting skills

Continued

Continued

Assessment Title	Author(s)	Publisher and/or Contact Information	Ages	Stated Purpose	Areas Assessed
Parkinson's Disease Quality of Life Questionnaire (PDQ-39)	University of Oxford Health Services Research Unit	Jenkinson, C., Fitzpatrick, R., & Peto, V. (1998). *The Parkinson's Disease Questionnaire: User Manual for the PDQ-39, PDQ-8 and the PDQ Summary Index.* Oxford: Health Services Research Unit. http://www.publichealth.ox.ac.uk/units/hsru/PDQ/Intro%20pdq	Adults with Parkinson's disease	To measure health related quality of life in patients diagnosed with Parkinson's disease	Activities of daily living; emotions; stigma; social support; cognition; communication; bodily discomfort
Participation Objective, Participation Subjective (POPS)	Brown, M., Dijkers, M. P. J. M., Gordon, W. A., Ashman, T., Charatz, H., and Cheng, Z.	Brown, M., Dijkers, M. P. J. M., Gordon, W. A., Ashman, T., Charatz, H., & Cheng, Z. (2004). Participation Objective, Participation Subjective: A measure of participation combining insider and outsider perspectives. *Journal of Head Trauma Rehabilitation, 19,* 459–481.		Uses two perspectives (the person with a disability and a normative "outsider") to measure participation in ADLs and IADLs	ADLs; IADLs; community integration
Patient Competency Rating Scale (PCRS)	Hart, T.	Hart, T. (2000). The Patient Competency Rating Scale. *The Center for Outcome Measurement in Brain Injury.* http://www.tbims.org/combi/pcrs (accessed August 18, 2007).	Adults	To evaluate self-awareness (the ability to appraise one's current strengths and weaknesses) following traumatic brain injury	ADLs; behavioral and emotional function; cognitive abilities; and physical function
Peabody Developmental Motor Scales, 2nd Edition (PDMS-2)	Folio, M. R., and Fewell, R. R.	PRO-ED, Inc. 8700 Shoal Creek Blvd. Austin, TX 78757 (800) 897-3202	Birth to 7 years	To quantitatively assess motor development of children	Gross and fine motor skills
Pediatric Evaluation of Disability Inventory (PEDI)	Haley, S. M., Coster, W. J., Ludlow, L. H., Haltiwanger, J. T., and Andrellos, P. J.	Harcourt Assessment, Inc. Attn: Customer Service P.O. Box 599700 San Antonio, TX 78259 800-211-8378 Fax: (800) 232-1223	6 months to 7.5 years	To assess functional skills of young children, monitor progress, or evaluate the outcome of a therapeutic program	Self-care; mobility; social function

Pediatric Interest Profiles (PIPs): Kid's Play Profile Preteen Play Profile Adolescent Leisure Interest Profile	Henry, A. D.	www.moho.uic.edu Harcourt Assessment, Inc. Attn: Customer Service P.O. Box 599700 San Antonio, TX 78259 800-211-8378 fax: 800-232-1223 www.moho.uic.edu	Kid's Play: 6 to 9 years; Preteen Play: 9 to 12 years; Adolescent Leisure Interest: 12 to 21 years	To select specific play/ leisure activities with which to engage a child by assessing the child's interest and participation in play and leisure activities	Interest and partici-pation in play and leisure activities
Pediatric Volitional Questionnaire, version 2.0 2002	Basu, S., Kafkes, A., Geist, R., and Kielhofner, G.	www.moho.uic.edu	2 to 7 years	Play-based observational assessment designed to evaluate a young child's volition	Motivation; personal causation; values; and interests
Perceived Efficacy and Goal Setting System (PEGS)	Missiuna, C., Pollock, N., and Law, M.	Harcourt Assessment, Inc. Attn: Customer Service P.O. Box 599700 San Antonio, TX 78259 800-211-8378 fax: 800-232-1223	5 to 10 years	To assess a child's daily activities in the home, school, and commu-nity environments	ADLs; IADLs
Performance Assess-ment of Self-Care Skills—Version 3.1 (PASS)	Holm, M. B., and Rogers, J. C.	University of Pittsburgh School of Health and Rehabilitation Sciences Pittsburgh, PA 15260	Adults with various impairments	Evaluate independent living skills in client's home and in the clinic, and to assess change	Functional mobil-ity; personal care; home management
Piers-Harris Children's Self Concept Scale, 2nd Edition	Piers, E. V., Harris, D. B., and Herzberg, D. S.	Western Psychological Services 12031 Wilshire Blvd. Los Angeles, CA 90025-1251 310-478-2061 www.wpspublish.com	7 to 18 years	Measures psychological health in children and adolescents	Coping; emotional health
Planning Alternative Tomorrows with Hope (PATH)	Pearpoint, J., O'Brien, J., and Forest, M.	Inclusion Press/Centre for Integrated Education and Community 24 Thome Crescent Toronto, ON, Canada M6H 2S5 416-658-5363 http://www.inclusion.com	All ages	Helps clients reach their life goals, identify their strengths	Client goals

Continued

Continued

Assessment Title	Author(s)	Publisher and/or Contact Information	Ages	Stated Purpose	Areas Assessed
Play History	Takata, N.	Behnke, C. & Fetkovich, M. (1984). Examining the reliability and validity of the Play History. *American Journal of Occupational Therapy, 38,* 94–100.	Children and adolescents	To identify a child's play experiences and play opportunities	Previous play experiences; actual play and opportunity for play
Preferences for Activities of Children (PAC)	CanChild Centre for Childhood Disability Research	Harcourt Assessment, Inc. Attn: Customer Service P.O. Box 599700 San Antonio, TX 78259 800-211-8378 fax: 800-232-1223	6 years and up	Examines a child's preferences for activities	Child's preference for activities
Preschool and Kindergarten Behavior Scales, 2nd Edition (PKBS-2)	Merrell, K. W.	PRO-ED, Inc. 8700 Shoal Creek Blvd. Austin, TX 78757 800-897-3202	3 to 6 years	To identify social skills and behaviors of children	Social skills
Preschool Play Scale	Please see "Knox Preschool Play Scale"				
Profile of Executive Control System (PRO-EX)	Branswell, D., Hartry, A., Hoornbeek, S., Johansen, A., Johnson, L., Schultz, J., and Sohlberg, M. M.	NO LONGER AVAILABLE as of 8/2007 Lash and Associates Publishing/ Training, Inc. 708 Young Forest Drive Wake Forest, NC 27587 919-562-0015	Adults	To assess the executive control system in order to identify deficits in the subject's ability to plan, organize, and self-evaluate	Planning; organizing; self-evaluation
Prospective Memory Screening (PROMS)	Sohlberg, M. M. and Mateer, C.	Sohlberg, M. M., & Mateer, C. (1989). *Introduction to cognitive rehabilitation: Theory and practice.* New York: Guilford Press.	Adults	To assess the ability to design and carry out planned actions appropriately	Motor and process skills in relation to activity demands
Purdue Peg Board	Tiffin, J.	Lafayette Instrument Company 3700 Sagamore Parkway North PO Box 5729 Lafayette, IN 47903 800-428-7545	5 years and up	To measure dexterity of fingertip activity and finger/hand/arm activity	Finger dexterity, fine motor coordination and speed

Quick Neurological Screening Test-II (QNST-II)	Mutti, M., Sterling, H. M., Martin, N. A. and Spalding, N. V.	Academic Therapy Publications 20 Commercial Blvd. Novato, CA 94949-6191 800-422-7249 fax: 415-883-3720 www.academictherapy.com	5 to 18 years	To assess a child's maturity and developmental skills	Large and small muscle control; motor planning; sequencing; sense of rate and rhythm; spatial organization; visual and auditory perceptual skills; balance; cerebellar-vestibular function; disorders of attention
Rabideau Kitchen Evaluation-Revised (RKE-R)	Neistadt, M. E.	Neistadt, M. E. (1994). A meal preparation treatment protocol for adults with brain injury. *American Journal of Occupational Therapy, 48*(5). 431–438.	Adults	To evaluate the use of a meal preparation treatment protocol based on cognitive-perceptual information processing theory for adults with traumatic or anoxic acquired brain injury	Meal preparation skills
Ransford Pain Drawing	Ransford, A., Cairns, D., and Mooney, V.	Ransford, A., Cairns, D., & Mooney, V. (1979). The pain drawing as an aid to the psychological evaluation of patients with low back pain. *Spine, 1*, 127–134.	Adults	Self-assessment of pain	Pain
Readily Achievable Checklist	Cronburg, J., Barnett, J., and Goldman, N.	Cronburg, J., Barnett, J., & Goldman, N. (1993). *Readily achievable checklist: A survey for accessibility.* Boston: Adaptive Environments. http://www.adaptiveenvironments.org	Adults	To assess accessibility in the community	Community environment
Rehabilitation Institute of Chicago Functional Assessment Scale: Version V	Cichowski, K. C.	Rehabilitation Institute of Chicago 345 East Superior St Chicago, Il 60611-4496 312-238-5433 http://lifecenter.ric.org/	Adults	To evaluate client's ability to complete instrumental activities of daily living	Instrumental activities of daily living

Continued

Continued

Assessment Title	Author(s)	Publisher and/or Contact Information	Ages	Stated Purpose	Areas Assessed
Reintegration to Normal Living (RNL)	Wood-Dauphinee, S., Opzoomer, M. A., Williams, J. I., Marchand, J., and Spitzer, W. O.	Wood-Dauphinee, S., Opzoomer, A., Williams, J. I., Marchand, B., & Spitzer, W. O. (1988). Assessment of global function: The Reintegration to Normal Living Index. *Archives of Physical Medicine and Rehabilitation, 69,* 583–590.	Adults	To assess how well individuals return to normal living patterns following incapacitating diseases or injury	ADLs
Repeatable Battery for the Assessment of Neuropsychological Status (RBANS™)	Randolph, C.	Harcourt Assessment, Inc. Attn: Customer Service P.O. Box 599700 San Antonio, TX 78259 800-211-8378 fax: 800-232-1223	20 to 89 years	To measure cognitive decline in individuals who have neurologic injury or disease such as dementia, head injury, and stroke; can measure change over time.	Cognition
Revised Observed Tasks of Daily Living (OTDL-R)	Diehl, M. K., Marsiske, M, Horgas, A. L., Rosenberg, A., Saczynski, J. S., and Willis, S. L.	Diehl, M. K., Marsiske, M., Horgas, A. L., Rosenberg, A., Saczynski, J. S., & Willis, S. L. (2005). The Revised Observed Tasks of Daily Living: A performance-based assessment of everyday problem solving in older adults. *The Journal of Applied Gerontology, 24*(3), 211–230. http://marsiskelab.phhp.ufl.edu/otdl/otdl.html	Older adults	Measures everyday problem solving skills	ADLs
Risk Factor Checklist	UC Davis	Biological and Agricultural Engineering Department University of California One Shields Avenue Davis, CA 95616-5294 530-752-0102 http://ag-ergo.ucdavis.edu/help/	Adults	Identifies specific workplace risks	Risks in workplace

Rivermead Behavioral Memory Test—extended version (RBMT-E)	Wilson, B., Cockburn, J., and Baddeley, A.	Harcourt Assessment, Inc. Attn: Customer Service P.O. Box 599700 San Antonio, TX 78259 800-211-8378 fax: 800-232-1223	All	To detect and identify memory impairments that occur in every activity, with a broader cultural sensitivity	Memory
Rivermead Behavioral Memory Test, 2nd Edition (RBMT-2)	Wilson, B., Cockburn, J., and Baddeley, A.	Harcourt Assessment, Inc. Attn: Customer Service P.O. Box 599700 San Antonio, TX 78259 800-211-8378 fax: 800-232-1223	Adults, 16 to 96 years	Detects and identifies memory impairments	Memory
Rivermead Behavioral Memory Test for Children (RBMT-C)	Alrich, F. K., and Wilson, B.	Harcourt Assessment, Inc. Attn: Customer Service P.O. Box 599700 San Antonio, TX 78259 800-211-8378 fax: 800-232-1223	Children, 5 to 10 years; 5 years and up	To detect and identify memory impairments that occur in every activity	Verbal recall; remember to do a task later in the test; remember and identify pictures; remember and retell a story; retrace a route around the room; memory
Role Activity Performance Scale (RAPS)	Good-Ellis, M. A.	Good-Ellis, M. A. (1999). Chapter 14: The Role Activity Performance Scale. In Hemphill-Pearson, B. J. (Ed.). *Assessments in occupational therapy mental health: An integrative approach.* Thorofare, NJ: Slack.	Adults	Assesses role activity performance history over time (up to 18 months)	ADLs; IADLs

Continued

Continued

Assessment Title	Author(s)	Publisher and/or Contact Information	Ages	Stated Purpose	Areas Assessed
Role Checklist (RC)	Oakley, F.	Frances Oakley, MS, OTR/L, FAOTA Occupational Therapy Service National Institutes of Health Building 10, Room 6S-235 10 Center Drive MSC 1604 Bethesda, MD 20892-1604 Email Fran Oakley to request the Role Checklist at foakley@nih.gov. Please include the following information in your email request: First and Last Name, Type of facility in which you work, Type of clients served, City, State, and Country of Residence.	Adults	To assess productive roles in adult life	Roles significant to the client; motivation to engage in tasks necessary to those roles; perceptions of role shifting
Routine Task Inventory	Heimann, N. E., and Allen, C. K., and Yerxa, E. J.	Heimann, N. E. & Allen, C. K. (1989). The routine task inventory: A tool for describing the functional behavior of the cognitively disabled. *Occupational Therapy Practice 1*(1), 67–74. In Chapter 7 of Allen, C. K., Earhart, C. A., and Blue, T. (1992). *Occupational Therapy Treatment Goals for the Physically and Cognitively Disabled.* American Occupational Therapy Association, Bethesda, MD. Available from: 385 Coquina Ave Ormond Beach, FL 32174 800-853-2472 jim@allen-cognitive-levels.com	Adults	To assess functional behavior during typical tasks using self-report or observation	Self-awareness (e.g., grooming, dressing, bathing), situational awareness (e.g., housekeeping, spending money, shopping), occupational role (e.g., planning/ doing major role activities, pacing and timing actions), social role (e.g., communicating meaning, following directions)

Safety Assessment of Function and the Environment for Rehabilitation (SAFER)	Oliver R., Blathwayt J., Brackley C., and Tamaki T.	Oliver, R., Blathwayt, J., Brackley, C., & Tamaki, T. (1993). Development of the Safety Assessment of Function and the Environment for Rehabilitation (SAFER) tool. *Canadian Journal of Occupational Therapy* 60(2), 78–82.	Older adults	To evaluate home safety for elders	Evaluates risks in various rooms of the home as well as general risks such as fire hazards; examines safety issues in how the individual performs various self-care and household tasks; examines the potential for wandering and the use of memory aids; and identifies how help could be summoned
Scales of Cognitive Ability for Traumatic Brain Injury (SCATBI)	Adamovich, B., and Henderson, J.	PRO-ED, Inc. 8700 Shoal Creek Blvd. Austin, TX 78757 800-897-3202	Adolescent and adult	To assess cognitive and linguistic abilities in people with head injury; to gauge severity and chart progress during recovery	Perception/discrimination; orientation; organization; recall; reasoning
School Function Assessment	Coster, W., Deeney, T., Haltiwanger, J., and Haley, S.	Harcourt Assessment, Inc. Attn: Customer Service P.O. Box 599700 San Antonio, TX 78259 800-211-8378 fax: 800-232-1223	Kindergarten to 6th grade	To evaluate and monitor a student's performance of functional tasks and activities that support his/her participation in elementary school	Participation in elementary school setting; task supports; activity performance

Continued

Continued

Assessment Title	Author(s)	Publisher and/or Contact Information	Ages	Stated Purpose	Areas Assessed
School Setting Interview (SSI), Version 3.0	Hemmingsson, H., Egilson, S., Hoffman, O. R., and Kielhofner, G.	www.moho.uic.edu	9 years to high school	Allows children and adolescents with disabilities to describe the impact of the environment on their functioning in multiple school settings	Impact of school environment on functional performance of children and adolescents with disability
School Situations Questionnaire (HSQ)	Barkley, R.	Barkley, R. A., & Murphy, K. R. (1998) *Attention deficit hyperactivity disorder: A clinical workbook.* 2nd ed. New York: Guilford.	School age	Identifies how symptoms of ADD/ADHD disrupt the school environment and the child's ability to participate in ADLs	ADLs
Self-Assessment of Leisure Interests	Kautzmann, L. N.	Kautzmann L. N. (1984): Identifying leisure interests: a self-assessment approach for adults with arthritis. *Occupational Therapy Assessment, 45.*	Adults	Assesses the leisure interests of adults with rheumatoid arthritis or degenerative joint disease	Leisure interests
Self-Awareness of Deficits Interview (SADI)	Fleming, J. M., Strong, J., and Ashton, R. Also cited: Levine, M. J., Van Horn, K. R., and Curtis, A. B.	Fleming, J. M., Strong, J., & Ashton, R. (1996). Self-awareness of deficits in adults with traumatic brain injury: How best to measure? *Brain Injury, 10,* 1–15. Levine, M. J., Van Horn, K. R., & Curtis, A. B. (1993). Developmental models of social cognition in assessing psychosocial adjustments in head injury. *Brain Injury, 7*(2), 153–167.	Adults	To assess self-awareness after brain injury	Self-awareness
Self-Directed Search	Holland, J. L.	Psychological Assessment Resources, Inc. 16204 N. Florida Avenue Lutz, FL 33549 813-968-3003 http://www.self-directed-search.com/	14 years and up	Assesses career interests	Aspirations; activities; competencies; occupations

Self-Perception Profile for Children	Harter, S.	Harter, S. (1985). *The Self-Perception Profile for Children: Revision of the Perceived Competence Scale for Children*. Denver, CO: University of Denver.	Children 8 years and older	To measure self-esteem and perceived competence in children	Scholastic competence; social acceptance; athletic competence; physical appearance; behavioral conduct; self-worth.
Self-Perception Profile for Adolescents	Harter, S.	Harter, S. (1988). *Manual for the Adolescent Self-Perception Profile*. Denver, CO: Author.	Adolescents	To measure self-esteem and perceived competence in adolescents	Scholastic competence; social acceptance; athletic competence; physical appearance; behavioral conduct; self-worth.
Semmes–Weinstein Monofilament Test	Weinstein, S.	Weinstein, S. (1993). Fifty years of somatosensory research: From the Semmes-Weinstein monofilaments to the Weinstein Enhanced Sensory Test. *Journal of Hand Therapy, 6,* 11–22.	All	Identifies skin pressure thresholds useful in determining degree of normal and protective sensation	Skin sensation
Sensory Integration and Praxis Tests (SIPT)	Ayres, A. J.	Western Psychological Services 12031 Wilshire Boulevard Los Angeles, CA 90025 800-648-8857	4 to 8.11 years	To assess praxis and sensory processing and integration of vestibular, proprioceptive, tactile, kinesthetic, and visual systems	Sensory processing; visual-spatial perception; coordination; motor planning
Sensory Organization Test (SOT)	Nashner, L. M.	NeuroCom 9570 SE Lawnfield Road Clackamas, OR 97015 800-767-6744	Adult	To objectively identify abnormalities in a patient's use of somatosensory, visual and vestibular systems that contribute to postural control	Postural stability in various sensory conditions/ environments

Continued

Continued

Assessment Title	Author(s)	Publisher and/or Contact Information	Ages	Stated Purpose	Areas Assessed
Sensory Processing Measure (SPM) Home Form	Parham, L. D. and Ecker, C.	Western Psychological Services 12031 Wilshire Boulevard Los Angeles, CA 90025 800-648-8857	5 to 12 years	To provide a complete picture of a child's sensory processing difficulties in the home	Visual; auditory; tactile; proprioceptive; vestibular
Sensory Processing Measure (SPM) School Form	Miller-Kuhaneck, H., Henry, D., and Glennon, T.	Western Psychological Services 12031 Wilshire Boulevard Los Angeles, CA 90025 800-648-8857	5 to 12 years	To provide a complete picture of a child's sensory processing difficulties at school	Visual; auditory; tactile; proprioceptive; vestibular
Sensory Profile; Adolescent/Adult Sensory Profile; Infant/Toddler Sensory Profile	Dunn, W.	Harcourt Assessment, Inc. Attn: Customer Service P.O. Box 599700 San Antonio, TX 78259 800-211-8378 fax: 800-232-1223	Sensory Profile: 3 to 10 years; Adolescent/Adult: 10 years and up; Infant/Toddler: 0 to 36 months	To determine how well a subject processes sensory information in everyday situations and to profile the sensory system's effect on functional performance	Sensory processing, modulation, and behavioral and emotional responses
Short Child Occupational Profile (SCOPE)	Bowyer, P., Ross, M., Schwartz, O., Kielhofner, G., & Kramer, J	www.moho.uic.edu	2 to 21 years	To assess a child's capacity for occupational functioning	Volition; habituation; motor skills; and environment
Skills Assessment Module (SAM)	Rosinek, M.	Rosinek, M. (1985). *Skills Assessment Module.* Athens, GA: Piney Mountain Press.	Adults	To attain a baseline of a client's ability to perform job-simulated tasks	Motor and process skills in relation to job tasks
Social Interaction Scale (SIS)	Trower, P., Bryant, B., and Argyle, M.	Trower, P., Bryant, B., & Argyle, M. (1978). *Social skills and mental health.* London: Methuen.	Adults	To rate social behavior that is exhibited during a semi-structured interview	Social competence; voice quality; nonverbal communication; conversation

Title	Author	Source	Age	Description	Domain
Social Skills Rating System	Gresham, F. M., and Elliot, S. N.	Pearson Assessments P.O. Box 1416 Minneapolis, MN 55440 800-627-7271	3 to 18 years	Rates social behaviors believed to affect areas such as teacher-student relationships, peer acceptance, and academic performance	Social skills (cooperation, assertion, responsibility, empathy, and self-control); problem behaviors; and academic competence (teacher ratings of reading, math performance, general cognitive functioning, motivation, and parental support)
Sociospatial Support Inventory	Rowles, G.	Rowles, G. (1983). Geographical dimensions of social support in rural Appalachia (pp. 111–130). In G. Rowles & R. Ohta (Eds.), *Aging and milieu: Environmental perspectives on growing old*. New York: Academic Press.	Adults	Catalyst for examining how an individual can evaluate alternative ways to manage community living support arrangements	Perception of support in environment
Source Book	Kelly, C., and Snell, K.	Kelly, C. & Snell, K. (1989). *The source book: Architectural guidelines for barrier free design*. Toronto, ON: Barrier-Free Design Centre.	Adults	To identify architectural barriers in the home, work, and community	Home, work, community environments
Spinal Functions Sort	Matheson, L. N., and Matheson, M. L.	EPIC 188 Woodlands Place Court St. Charles, MO 63303 636-724-4556 fax: 636-898-0954	Adult	To quantify the subject's perception of ability to perform work tasks that involve the spine	Perception of work tasks
Spiritual Well-Being Scale	Bufford, R., Paloutzian, R., and Ellison, C.	Ellison, C. (1983). Spiritual well-being: Conceptualization and measurement. *Journal of Psychology and Technology, 11*(4), 330–340. http://www.lifeadvance.com/	All ages	Catalyst to explore various forms of spirituality	Spirituality

Continued

Continued

Assessment Title	Author(s)	Publisher and/or Contact Information	Ages	Stated Purpose	Areas Assessed
Stress Management Questionnaire	Stein, F., and Nikolic, S.	Stein, F., & Nikolic, S. (1989). Teaching stress management techniques to a schizophrenic person. *American Journal of Occupational Therapy, 43,* 162–169. http://www.delmarlearning.com	Adults	Self-assessment to identify stressors in the subject's daily life	Perceptions of stress in daily life
Stroke Impact Scale (SIS)	Landon Center on Aging, University of Kansas Medical Center	Landon Center on Aging University of Kansas Medical Center Mail Stop 1005 3901 Rainbow Boulevard Kansas City, KS 66160 913-588-1203 http://www2.kumc.edu/coa/SIS/Stroke-Impact-Scale.htm	Adults	Measures stroke recovery in eight domains: strength, hand function, mobility, activities of daily living, emotion, memory, communication, social participation	Strength; hand function; mobility; activities of daily living; emotion; memory; communication; social participation
Stroke Specific Quality of Life Scale (SS-QOL)	Williams, L. S., Weinberger, M., Harris, L. E., Clark, D. O., and Biller, J.	Williams, L. S., Weinberger, M., Harris, L. E., Clark, D. O., & Biller, J. (1999). Development of a stroke-specific quality of life scale. *Stroke, 30*(7), 1362–1369. http://www.strokecenter.org/trials/scales/ssqol.html	Adults	To measure quality of life of individuals post-stroke	Mobility; energy; upper extremity function; work/productivity; mood; self-care; social roles; family roles; vision; language; thinking; personality
Subjective Index of Physical and Social Outcomes (SIPSO)	Trigg, R. and Wood, V. A.	Trigg, R. & Wood, V. A. (2000). The Subjective Index of Physical and Social Outcome (SIPSO): A new measure for use with stroke patients. *Clinical Rehabilitation, 14*(3), 288–299.	Adults	Measures social integration after stroke	ADLS; IADLS; community integration; social skills
Tennessee Self-Concept Scale, 2nd Edition (TSCS:2)	Fitts, W. H. and Warren, W. L.	Western Psychological Services 12031 Wilshire Boulevard Los Angeles, CA 90025 800-648-8857	7 to 90 years	Measures self-concept across the lifespan	Motor skills; values; social skills; academics

Title	Author	Source	Population	Purpose	Construct
Test d'Évaluation des Membres supérieurs des Personnes Agées (TEMPA)	Desrosiers Hébert Dutil and Bravo	Desrosiers, J., Hébert, J., Dutil, É., Bravo, G., & Mercier, L. (1994). Validity of a measurement instrument for upper extremity performance: the TEMPA. *Occupational Therapy Journal of Research 14*, 267–281.	Adults	Measures upper extremity performance using ADLs	Upper extremity performance
Test of Environmental Supportiveness	Bundy, A.	School of Occupation and Leisure Sciences Faculty of Health Sciences The University of Sydney PO Box 170 Lidcombe, NSW 1825 Australia	Children	Assesses the extent to which the environment supports an individual's play	Caregiver's actions, rules, and boundaries; peer, younger, and older playmates' use of cues and domination of interaction; natural and fabricated objects; amount and configuration of space; sensory environment; safety and accessibility of space
Test of Everyday Attention (TEA)	Robertson, I., Ward, T., Ridgeway, V., and Nimmo-Smith, I.	Harcourt Assessment, Inc. Attn: Customer Service P.O. Box 599700 San Antonio, TX 78259 800-211-8378 fax: 800-232-1223	18 years and up	To test attention systems serving different functions in everyday behavior	Selective attention; sustained attention; attentional switching; divided attention
Test of Everyday Attention for Children (TEA–Ch)	Manly, T., Robertson, I., Anderson, V., and Nimmo-Smith, I.	Harcourt Assessment, Inc. Attn: Customer Service P.O. Box 599700 San Antonio, TX 78259 800-211-8378 fax: 800-232-1223	6 to 16 years	To test attention systems serving different functions in everyday behavior	Selective attention; sustained attention; attentional switching; divided attention
Test of Grocery Shopping Skills (TOGSS©)	Brown, T., Rempfer, M., and Hamera, E.	Attention: Tana Brown University of Kansas Medical Center 3033 Robinson 3901 Rainbow Blvd. Kansas City, KS 66160	Adults	Measures a consumer's ability to complete a grocery shopping task	IADLs

Continued

Continued

Assessment Title	Author(s)	Publisher and/or Contact Information	Ages	Stated Purpose	Areas Assessed
Test of Gross Motor Development, 2nd Edition (TGMD-2)	Ulrich, D. A.	PRO-ED, Inc. 8700 Shoal Creek Blvd. Austin, TX 78757 800-897-3202	3 to 11 years	Measures common gross motor skills	Locomotor; object control
Test of Handwriting Skills–Revised (THS-R)	Gardner, M. A.	Therapro, Inc. 225 Arlington Street Framingham, MA 01702-8723 508-872-9494 or 800-257-5376	5 to 18.11 years	Standardized assessment of manuscript and cursive handwriting skills	Manuscript and cursive; writing from memory; writing from dictation; copying upper case and lower case selected letters and numbers; copying words and sentences; speed of writing; reversals; spacing, etc.
Test of Oral and Limb Apraxia (TOLA)	Helm-Estabrooks, N.	NOTE: Test is no longer in print as of December 2001. PRO-ED, Inc. 8700 Shoal Creek Blvd. Austin, TX 78757 800-897-3202	Adults	Designed to identify, measure, and evaluate the presence of oral and limb apraxia in individuals with developmental or acquired neurologic disorders	Motor planning
Test of Orientation for Rehabilitation Patients (TORP)	Dietz, J., Beeman, C., and Thorn, D.	Harcourt Assessment, Inc. Attn: Customer Service P.O. Box 599700 San Antonio, TX 78259 800-211-8378 fax: 800-232-1223	Adolescents and adults	To determine the existence and extent of disorientation, establish a baseline level of performance, plan intervention, monitor progress, assess effectiveness of treatment	Orientation to person and personal situation, place, time, schedule, and temporal continuity

Title	Author	Source	Age	Purpose	Area
Test of Playfulness (ToP)	Bundy, A.	School of Occupation and Leisure Sciences Faculty of Health Sciences The University of Sydney PO Box 170 Lidcombe, NSW 1825 Australia	15 months to 10 years	Assesses a child's play behavior based on playfulness rather than on motor, cognitive, or language skills	Playfulness
Test of Visual-Perceptual Skills-3 (TVPS-3)	Martin, N.	Psychological and Educational Publications, Inc. 1477 Rollins Road Burlingame, CA 94010 800-523-5775	4 to 18.11 years	To determine visual-perceptual strengths and weaknesses without the use of motor responses	Visual discrimination; visual memory; visual-spatial relations; visual form constancy; visual sequential memory; visual figure-ground; visual closure
Test of Visual-Motor Skills-Revised (TVMS-R)	Gardner, M.	Psychological and Educational Publications, Inc. 1477 Rollins Road Burlingame, CA 94010 800-523-5775	3 to 14 years	To assess how a child visually perceives nonlanguage forms and translates what is perceived through hand function	Copy 23 geometric forms
Test of Visual-Motor Skills: Upper Level Adolescents and Adults (TVMS:UL)	Gardner, M.	Psychological and Educational Publications, Inc. 1477 Rollins Road Burlingame, CA 94010 800-523-5775	12 to 40 years	To assess how an adolescent or adult visually perceives nonlanguage forms and translates what is perceived through hand function	Copy 26 geometric forms
The Experience of Leisure Scale (TELS)	Meakins, C., and Bundy, A.	Meakins, C., & Bundy, A. The Experience of Leisure Scale (TELS). In press.	Adolescents and adults	Examines play and leisure experiences of adults and adolescents	Play/leisure
Tinetti Assessment Tool	Tinetti, M.	Dr. Mary Tinetti Yale Medical Group 300 George Street, 6th Floor New Haven, CT 06511 203-688-5238 http://www.sgim.org/TinettiTool.PDF	Adult	To measure fall-risk in adult and geriatric populations	Gait; balance

Continued

Continued

Assessment Title	Author(s)	Publisher and/or Contact Information	Ages	Stated Purpose	Areas Assessed
Toddler and Infant Motor Evaluation (TIME)	Miller, L. J., and Roid, G. H.	Harcourt Assessment, Inc. Attn: Customer Service P.O. Box 599700 San Antonio, TX 78259 800-211-8378 fax: 800-232-1223	Birth to 4 years	To be used as a comprehensive assessment of children who are suspected to have motor delays or deviations	Mobility; stability; motor organization; social-emotional; functional performance
Toddler Behavior Assessment Questionnaire (TBAQ)	Goldsmith, H. H.	Goldsmith, H. H. (1996). Studying temperament via construction of the Toddler Behavior Assessment Questionnaire. *Child Development, 67*, 218–235. University of Wisconsin—UW Twin Center http://psych.wisc.edu/goldsmith/Researchers/GEO/TBAQ.htm	16 to 36 months	To examine temperament-related behavior	Activity level (motor skills); anger; fear; pleasure; interest
Toglia Category Assessment (TCA)	Toglia, J. P.	Maddak Inc. 6 Industrial Road Pequannock, NJ 07440-199	All ages	To assess category flexibility	Categorization; strategies; problem-solving
Transdisciplinary Play-Based Assessment (TPBA-2) and Transdisciplinary Play-Based Intervention (TPBI-2)	Linder, T. W.	Customer Service Department Brookes Publishing Co. P.O. Box 10624 Baltimore, MD 21285-0624 800-638-3775	0 to 6 years	Uses play to assess a child's development	Cognition; communication; language; movement skills; social and emotional development
Transition Planning Inventory (TPI)—Updated Version	Clark, G. M. and Patton, J. R.	PRO-ED, Inc. 8700 Shoal Creek Blvd. Austin, TX 78757 800-897-3202	14 to 22 years	To identify and plan for the comprehensive transitional needs of students. Designed to provide school personnel with a systematic way to address mandates of the *Individuals with Disabilities Education Act (IDEA)*	School skills; interests; environmental requirements

Unified Parkinson's Disease Rating Scale	Fahn S, Elton R, Members of the UPDRS Development Committee	http://www.mdvu.org/pdf/updrs.pdf http://www.mdvu.org/pdf/upddf.pdf Fahn, S., Marsden, C. D., Calne, D. B., & Goldstein, M. (Eds.). (1987). *Recent developments in Parkinson's disease, Vol 2.* (pp. 153–163, 293–304). Florham Park, NJ: Macmillan Health Care Information.	Adults	Follows the longitudinal course of Parkinson's disease	Mentation, behavior and mood; ADLs; motor skills
Valpar Component Work Samples	Valpar Corporation	Valpar Corporation 3801 East 34th Street Suite 105 Tucson, AZ 85713 800-528-7070	Adults	To generate clinical and actuarial data on universal worker characteristics	Mechanical and clerical work skills
Verbal and Nonverbal Cancellation Tasks	Mesulam, M.	Mesulam, M. (1985). Attention, confusional states and neglect. In M. Mesulam (Ed.), *Principles of behavioral neurology* (pp. 125–68). Philadelphia: F. A. Davis.	All ages	To detect the presence of neglect	Attention, visual neglect
Vermont Interdependent Services Team Approach (VISTA)	Giangreco, M. F.	Giangreco, M. F. (1996). *VISTA: Vermont Interdependent Services Team Approach. A guide to coordinating support services.* Baltimore: Paul H. Brookes.	3 to 21 years	To facilitate cross-disciplinary, inter dependent, support service/related service decision-making and implementation for students with disabilities in schools	Support services in the school system
Vineland Adaptive Behavior Scales, Revised (VABS)	Sparrow, S. S., Balla, D. A., and Cicchetti, D. V.	American Guidance Service, Inc. Publisher's Building Circle Pines, MN 55014 800-328-2560	Birth to 19 years	To assess personal and social sufficiency of individuals from birth to adulthood	Communication; activities of daily living; socialization; motor skills; adaptive behavior; maladaptive behavior

Continued

Continued

Assessment Title	Author(s)	Publisher and/or Contact Information	Ages	Stated Purpose	Areas Assessed
Volitional Questionnaire, Version 4.0	de las Heras, C. G., Geist, R., Kielhofner, G., and Li, Y.	www.moho.uic.edu	Adults	Assesses volition by observation	Motivation; values; interests
Waddell Signs	Waddell, G., McCulloch, J., Kummel, E., and Venner, R.	Waddell, G., McCulloch, J., Kummel, E., & Venner, R. (1980). Nonorganic physical signs in low-back pain. *Spine, 5,* 117–125.	Adult	To help the therapist detect abnormal illness behavior or symptoms not consistent with typical anatomy and physiology	Back pain symptom magnification
Ways of Coping Checklist (WCC)	Folkman, S., and Lazarus, R. S.	Lazarus, R. S., & Folkman, S. (1984). *Stress, appraisal, and coping.* New York: Springer.	Adults	Assesses coping strategies	Problem-solving skills; emotion-regulation
WeeFIM™ (Guide for the Uniform Data Set for Medical Rehabilitation for Children), Version 6.0	The Center for Functional Assessment Research	Uniform Data System for Medical Rehabilitation, 2005. The WeeFIM II System Clinical Guide, Version 6.0. Buffalo: UDSMR. Information Resource Center Uniform Data System for Medical Rehabilitation 270 Northpointe Parkway, Suite 300 Amherst, NY 14228 716-817-7800 info@udsmr.org	Children from 6 months to 7 years	Measure disability severity related to physical impairment, across health, development, educational, and community settings	18 activities, 13 with a motor emphasis related to self-care; 5 with a cognitive emphasis involving communication
Westmead Home Safety Assessment (WeHSA)	Clemson, L.	Clemson L. (1997). *Home fall hazards: A guide to identifying fall hazards in the homes of elderly people and an accompaniment to the assessment tool, the Westmead home safety assessment (WeHSA).* West Brunswick, Victoria: Coordinates Publications.	Older adults	To evaluate potential fall hazards in the home	Fall risk; safety

Title	Author	Source	Population	Purpose	Domain
WEST Tool Sort	Matheson, L.	Matheson L. Work Evaluation Systems Technology, 1981 WEST Tool Sort Signal Hill, CA	Adults	Self-assessment of a subject's ability to use specific tools to perform ADL and work tasks	Motor and process skills in relation to ADL and work tasks
Western Neuro Sensory Stimulation Profile (WNSSP)	Ansell, B. J., and Keenan, J. E.	Ansell, B. J. & Keenan, J. E. (1989). The Western Neuro Sensory Stimulation Profile: a tool for assessing slow-to-recover head-injured patients. *Archives of Physical Medical Rehabilitation, 70*(2), 104–108.	Adults	To assess cognitive function in severely impaired head-injured adults (Rancho levels II–V) and to monitor and predict change in slow-to-recover patients	Arousal/attention; expressive communication; response to auditory, visual, tactile, and olfactory stimulation
Work Environment Impact Scale (WEIS), Version 2.0	Moore-Corner, R., Kielhofner, G., and Olson, L.	www.moho.uic.edu	Adults	Examines how individuals with disabilities experience the work environment	Work environment factors and their impact on performance; satisfaction; physical, social, and emotional well-being of the worker
Work Environments Scale	Moos, R.	CPP, Inc., and Davies-Black Publishing 1055 Joaquin Road, 2nd Floor Mountain View, CA 94043 650-969-8901 or 800-624-1765	Adults	Examines the interpersonal environment of a workplace	Workplace environment
Work Experience Survey (WES)	Roesller, R. T., Reed, C. A., and Rumrill, P. D.	Roesller, R. T., Reed, C. A., & Rumrill, P. D. (1995). *The Work Experience Survey (WES) Manual: A structured interview for identifying barriers to career maintenance. A service provider's guide.* Arkansas Research and Training Center in Vocational Rehabilitation Arkansas University P.O. Box 1358 Hot Springs, AR 71902 501-624-4411	Adults	To help individuals with disabilities direct their own accommodation planning in the workplace	Workplace environment

Continued

Continued

Assessment Title	Author(s)	Publisher and/or Contact Information	Ages	Stated Purpose	Areas Assessed
Worker Role Interview (WRI), Version 10.0	Braveman, B., Robson, M., Velozo, C., Kielhofner, G., Fisher, G., Forsyth, K., and Kerschbaum, J.	www.moho.uic.edu	Adults	Gathers data on psychosocial and environmental factors related to work	Personal causation; values; interests; roles and habits related to work; influence of the environment
Workplace Workbook 2.0	Mueller, J.	Mueller, J. L. (1992). *The workplace workbook 2.0: An illustrated guide to workplace accommodation and technology.* Amherst, MA: Human Resource Development Press.	Adults	To identify barriers in the workplace	Workplace environment

ADL, activity of daily living; *AOTA*, American Occupational Association; *IADL*, instrumental activity of daily living; *IEP*, individualized education program; *NIH*, National Institute of Health.

Glossary

The following definitions are drawn from the chapters in this book and are intended as a resource for understanding. Chapter numbers appear in parentheses at the end of each definition so that readers can refer to the cited chapters for concepts and definitions listed here. The Glossary also includes definitions from the draft Occupational Therapy Practice Framework. These definitions are indicated by the abbreviation OTPF-II. Readers should cite the appropriate chapter authors or original citations when referring to these constructs.

Accreditation Council of Occupational Therapy Education of the American Occupational Therapy Association (ACOTE)   Maintains standards and accredits occupational therapy education programs primarily in the United States.

Active Range of Motion (AROM)   Arc of motion through which the joint passes when moved by muscles acting on the joint (54).

Activities of Daily Living (ADL)   Activities oriented toward taking care of one's own body, also is referred to as basic activities of daily living (BADLs)/ and /personal activities of daily living (PADLs); activities are essential for survival and well-being (OTPF-II).

Activity   Abstract idea about the kinds of things individuals do and the way they typically do them in a given culture (35).

Activity Analysis   Analysis of how an activity is perceived to be typically done in the relevant culture, identifying typical demands and performance skills for an activity (35).

Activity Choices   Activities that are engaged in during play and leisure. Activities that individuals or groups select to enact (52).

Activity Interests   Affective responses to play and leisure activities and perceptions and awareness of self and environments in relation to play and leisure activities. Affective and intellectual responses to options for engagement (52).

Adaptation   Changing task demands so they are consistent with the individual's ability level; may involve modification by reducing demands, use of assistive devices, or changes in the physical or social environment (35). Internal change in the functional state of the person as a result of increased relative mastery over occupational challenges (45). A change in response approach that the client makes when encountering an occupational challenge (OTPF-II).

Adaptation Gestalt   Relative balance of sensorimotor, cognitive, and psychosocial functioning that the individual creates internally in order to carry out an adaptive response (45).

Adaptive Capacity   Apparent capability of the individual to perceive the need for change and draw from a repertoire of adaptive responses that will enable him or her to experience mastery over the environment (45).

Adaptive Response or Adaptive Interaction   An appropriate action in which the individual responds successfully to some environmental demand; interactions between an individual and the environment in which the individual meets the demands of the task (59).

Adaptive Response Subprocess   Internal process through which an individual generates, evaluates, and integrates new adaptations into his or her person (45).

Adaptiveness   Ability the individual demonstrates in response to challenging, novel situations that call for an adaptive response (45).

Adequacy   Measure of performance indicating the efficiency of the action or process used to execute tasks and the acceptability of the outcome or product of that action (46).

Administration   Process of guiding an organization through the authoritative control of others completed by the governing body of the organization (67).

Administrative Controls   Changes in the nature of work such as scheduling, worker rotation, or assignment of work tasks (51).

Administrative Supervision Aspect of supervision directed toward managing the day-to-day work performance and process; includes tasks such as scheduling, monitoring performance, and delegating (68).

Adrenal glands Organs resting on top of the kidneys that produce the majority of hormones in the body linked to stress responses and arousal, including epinephrine, norepinephrine, and cortisol (56).

Advocacy Active support or pursuit of public policy and resource allocation decisions within political, economic, and social systems and institutions to directly affect people's lives (OTPF-II).

Ageism Stereotypic and often negative bias against older adults; a form of discrimination based on age (7).

Agnosia Inability to recognize familiar objects in spite of intact sensory capacities (57).

Allostasis (allostatic) A state of change and refers to active body responses and adaptations to environmental demands; the human stress response is an example of allostasis (56).

Allostatic Load (See also *Stress.*) A state of chronic stress (chronic allostasis) (56).

Alpha-Amylase Digestive enzyme, linked with sympathetic nervous system/sympathetic adrenomedullary system (SNS/SAM) activation (56).

American Occupational Therapy Association (AOTA) National professional association for occupational therapy with voluntary membership that represents and promotes members' interests.

American Occupational Therapy Foundation (AOTF) Nonprofit organization dedicated to expanding and refining the knowledge base of occupational therapy; provides support to research and education through grants and scholarships.

Antigroup Destructive forces in groups with potential for creative resolution (37).

Apraxia Inability to perform motor activities although sensory motor function is intact and the individual understands the requirements of the task (57).

Arena Place in which activities occur (35).

Arousal Level of alertness and responsiveness to stimuli (59).

Assessment Specific method, tool, or strategy that is utilized as part of the evaluation process (48, 50).

Assessment Evidence Research findings that test the quality of clinical assessment procedures (30).

Attention The cognitive ability to focus on a task, issue, or object (57).

Auditory Scanning Method of scanning used for a person who cannot see in which each option is announced aloud prior to selection (61).

Autonomic Nervous System (ANS) Portion of the nervous system that regulates smooth muscle activity, including heart and other organ functions, as well as both allostatic and homeostatic activities, including breathing, cardiac activity, cell repair, digestion, sleep, metabolic activity, and stress responding. The ANS has two branches, sympathetic and parasympathetic, that generally exert opposite effects on body organs and systems (56).

Aversion to Movement A type of sensory modulation dysfunction characterized by autonomic nervous system reactions to movements that most individuals would consider nonnoxious; thought to be the result of poor processing of vestibular information (59).

Balance Ability to maintain the body in equilibrium (synonym: *Stability*) (55).

Balance of Excitation and Inhibition Mediates input and output in the brain. Too much excitation leads to overreaction; too much inhibition leads to failure to notice and respond to the world. At each synapse and within neuron systems, there is a continuous negotiation between the excitation and inhibition messages that are available. There has to be enough excitation to override the inhibition in order to get an action (58).

Being in Place Sense of comfort and belonging stemming from the totality of physical, cognitive, emotional, imaginative, and historical habitation of an environment (8).

Beliefs Any cognitive content that an individual holds as true (OTPF-II).

Bilateral Motor Coordination Using both sides of the body in a smooth, coordinated way (59).

Biofeedback Use of instruments that help individuals to recognize how their bodies are working and teach them how to control patterns of physiological functioning (56).

Biological Needs Things that are essential to individual and species survival, including sustenance, self-care, shelter, and safety (5).

Biomarker Biologic or physiologic characteristic that can be objectively measured by using specialized machines (e.g., PET scanners) or assay procedures (e.g., salivary cortisol); assumed to be a window into the structural and physiological processes of a functioning body (56).

Blocked Practice Rote schedule of practice that involves repetition of one task before the next task is introduced (54).

Body Functions Physiological processes of the body (53).

Body Scheme Unconscious mechanism underlying spatial motor coordination that provides the central nervous system with information abut the relationship of the body and its parts to environmental space (59).

Body Structures Anatomical parts of the body such as bones and organs (53).

Boundary Crossing Ways in which people who come from different lived worlds and have different life experiences find commonalities and areas of mutual interest, bridge differences, negotiate multiple and diverse perspectives, develop understandings, and respect multiple and, at times, divergent perspectives (4).

Capacities Grounded in the biological features of *Homo sapiens* shaped by genetic heritage and occupational history; include strength, speed, dexterity, agility, gracefulness, cardiovascular fitness, insight, cunning, know-how, wisdom, thoughtfulness, tenderness, and so on (5). Generic abilities (e.g., attention, proprioception, joint mobility) inherent to people and task-specific skills such as dressing, meal preparation, Website designing, and playing wheelchair basketball (46).

Case Management Collaborative process of assessing, planning, implementing, coordinating, monitoring, and evaluating options and services to meet an individual's health needs through communication and available resources to promote high-quality cost effective outcomes (51).

Catecholamines Epinephrine (also known as adrenaline), norepinephrine (also known as noradrenaline), and dopamine; also known as biogenic amines, a type of amino acid, catecholamines are hormones produced by the adrenal glands, sympathetic nervous system, and brain; exert effects on organs and structures throughout the body and brain (56).

Centers for Disease Control (CDC) Principal agency in the U.S. government for protecting the health and safety of all Americans and for providing essential human services, especially for those people who are least able to help themselves (17).

Centers for Medicaid and Medicare Services (CMS) U.S. government agency whose mission is to ensure effective, up-to-date health care and coverage and to promote quality care for beneficiaries (17).

Central Tendency Average or majority attribute (e.g., mean, median, mode) among individuals in a population (30).

Centrifugal Control Most basic central nervous system operation; the brain's ability to regulate its own input; accomplished suppression, divergence, and convergence (58).

Class Ranking of people into a hierarchy within a culture, arising from interdependent economic relationships such as "middle class," "upper class," or "lower class" (7).

Client Individual, agency, organization, or government entity that contract with the consultant for a specific scope of work (70). Recipients of service may include individuals and other people relevant to the individual's life, including family, caregivers, teachers, employers, and others who may also help or be served indirectly; organizations such as business, industries, or agencies; and populations within a community (OTPF-II).

Client-Centered Philosophy of service committed to respect for and partnership with people receiving services (18). Emphasizes the individual recipient of service and a focus on developing, restoring, or adapting the individual's skills and organizing and using assistance available in natural supports from family and friends (19).

Clinical Reasoning Process used by practitioners to plan, direct, perform, and reflect on client care. See *Professional Reasoning* for a term that is considered to be broader (32).

Clinical Supervision (synonym: *Supervision*) (68).

Clinical Utility Ease and efficiency in the use of a test and the clinical relevance and meaning of the information that it provides (47).

Clonus Movement disorder characterized by rapid successive contractions and relaxations (55).

Closed Skills Stereotypical tasks with little trial variability and low information processing demands (55).

Coaching Providing verbal expectations and support to help an individual engage in therapy and sustain growth or changes (35).

Cognition Mental processes including attention, memory, motivation, emotional control, motor control, sensory processing, and thinking (55). Ability to think and reason to solve problems (57).

Collaboration Process through which practitioners and clients discuss client priorities, set goals, make decisions about intervention options, and work together in mutual effort and partnership toward goals (33).

Collaborative Supervision Involves one or more supervisors working with multiple students with all participants viewed as more equal partners in the learning process (26).

Collusion Working with others in a closed or secretive fashion, often to avoid a perceived negative consequence (37).

Community Sharing of an area, interests, and interactions, as well as a sense of shared identity (19).

Community Based Emphasizes delivery of services in locations within a client's local places or environments of community living (19).

Community Centered Emphasizes the community as a recipient of intervention and a focus on accessibility and acceptance within physical, social, and cultural environments (19).

Community Development Community consultation, deliberation, and action to promote individual, family, and communitywide responsibility for self-sustaining development, health, and well-being (18).

Community Supervision (synonym: *supervision*) (68).

Competence Developed and maintained practitioner knowledge, critical reasoning, interpersonal abilities, performance skills, and ethical reasoning (70).

Competencies Explicit statements that define specific areas of practitioner expertise and are related to effective or superior performance in a job (25).

Competency Characteristics Intrinsic to the practitioner; include such aspects as expert knowledge and skills, motivation to change performance, positive self-concept to become proficient, attitudes conducive to learning, and valuing of learning (25).

Competent Successfully performing a behavior or task as measured according to a specific criterion (25).

Conditioning Designing situations that increase or decrease the likelihood of a behavior being performed (36).

Construction Ability Ability to perform the sequences of movement involved in producing two- or three-dimensional representations as in drawing or assembling tasks (59).

Consultant Individual retained by an individual, group, agency, organization, or government entity to provide expert advice and recommendations according to an established agreement between two parties (70).

Consultation Process Type of intervention in which practitioners use their knowledge and expertise to collaborate with the client; involves identifying the problem, creating possible solutions, trying solutions, and altering them as necessary for greater effectiveness; consultant is not directly responsible for the outcome of the intervention (70).

Context Variety of interrelated conditions (cultural, physical, social, spiritual, temporal, and virtual) within and surrounding the client that influence performance (57, 70).

Contextual Features Cultural, physical, social, personal, spiritual, temporal, and virtual aspects of home, school, work, and community settings that facilitate or hinder participation (52).

Continuing Competence A practitioner's evolving or lifelong capacity to perform changing responsibilities as a part of professional role performance (25).

Continuing Competency Focuses on the regularity of meeting standards for current role performance regardless of the dynamic nature of professional practice (25).

Contract Agreement or promise to perform certain work (70).

Contraindications A therapeutic procedure that could potentially harm a client because of the client's condition or medications (39).

Control Enhancers Means of extending the capabilities of a client with an assistive device so as to preserve the ability to use a direct selection method (61).

Controlling Establishing performance standards, measuring, evaluating, and correcting performance (67).

Convergence Bringing input together from many sources; in the sensory systems, input from multiple sensory inputs converge so that the brain can create a more organized response (59).

Co-occupation Shared occupations in which participants are active agents (35).

Coordination An automatic response that is monitored primarily through proprioceptive sensory feedback (55).

Coordinative Structure Aggregate of subsystems organized around a specific goal directed movement (55).

Cortisol Corticosteroid hormone released from the adrenal glands via a complex system, the hypothalamic-pituitary-adrenal axis (HPA); sustains metabolic activity, increased vigilance, and increased blood pressure, among other processes, such that the individual can adapt to environmental challenges that last longer than a few minutes (56).

Countertransference Therapist's subjective and objective responses to group members (37).

Credentialing Process of authentication of qualifications in order to have the authority to perform a skilled service within specified limits (25).

Credentials Abbreviations after a person's name that designate that person's educational level and/or professional designation (39).

Cultural Myth Unfounded or poorly founded belief about a human group that is given uncritical acceptance by members of another group and that operates in support of existing or traditional practices and institutions (6).

Cultural Practices Familiar or repeated activities shared with others in a community; carry normative expectations and are given significance beyond the immediate goal of the activity (2). Familiar occupations carried out in similar ways by members of a community; occupations are given significance beyond their immediate outcome (3).

Cultural Relativism Perspective that holds that there is no single truth, yielding multiple truths and a situation-based ethic (27).

Cultural Stereotype Mental picture based on myth that leads people to associate a characteristic or set of characteristics with a particular group of others (6).

Degrees of Freedom The individual components (cells, tissues, organs, subsystems) of a system (e.g., human being) that can define that system and can be controlled and organized in any number of ways (55).

Descriptive Evidence Research findings that describe the experiences and needs of individuals in a clinical population (30).

Determinants of Health Range of personal, social, economic, and environmental factors that determine the health status of individuals or populations (18).

Developmental Model of Supervision Framework that outlines four different phases of the learner and supervisor relationship: directive, coaching, supportive, and delegation (26).

Dexterity Type of fine coordination that is mostly demonstrated in the use of the upper extremity (55).

Diagnostic Related Groups (DRGs) Classification system for Medicare Part A payments based on groups of diagnoses and procedures (69).

Direct Selection Selection from a set that contains all options as in a computer keyboard or a number pad (61).

Directing Providing guidance and leadership so that the work that is performed is congruent with goals (67).

Disability Impairments, limitations of activity and function, and activity restrictions (19, 55).

Discontinuation Summary Discharge summary; written at the termination of services to summarize the course of a client's intervention (39).

Discrete Tasks Actions that have a recognizable beginning and end (55).

Divergence Ability of the brain to transmit sensory input to many parts of the brain so that the input can affect multiple places at once; allows an entire muscle to work rather than one muscle fiber (59).

Dynamometer Instrument used to measure grip strength (54).

Dyspnea Shortness of breath (48).

Dyspraxia A developmental condition in which the ability to plan unfamiliar motor tasks is impaired (59).

Early Intervening Services Academic and behavior support to succeed in general education, not part of special education (50).

Effectiveness Evidence Research findings that evaluate the effectiveness of interventions (30).

Efficacy Expectations A person's belief about how successful or unsuccessful he or she will be at performing a skill or occupation (36).

Electrocardiogram (ECG/EKG) Test using attached wires (or wireless) to leads placed on the chest that document the pattern of electrical activity of the heart (56).

Electrodermal Response (EDR)/Galvanic Skin Response (GSR) Measurement of the electrical conductance of skin via skin-placed sensors designed to detect sweat gland activity (56).

Electroencephalograph (EEG) Noninvasive method of looking at electrical brain activity through wires and sensors that are placed on a person's head (56).

Electronic Aids to Daily Living (EADLs) Provide the user with control over appliances and other electronic devices (e.g., a door opener) within the environment; a wide variety of switches interface with EADLs to allow individuals with a variety of skills and impairments to use them (48).

Emergent Performance Combination of abilities put together in unpredictable ways to generate organized patterns of occupational behavior that is consistent with a particular situation (2). Investment of personal capacities put together in unpredictable ways to generate organized patterns of occupational behavior that fit the perceived affordances as well as children's reasons for doing the activity (3).

Empathic Competence Practitioner's emotional discernment to accurately perceive and respond to clients and their experiences in order to finely tune the therapy process (18).

Empathy Awareness of and insight into the feelings, emotions, and behavior of another person and their meaning and significance; not the same as sympathy, which is usually nonobjective and noncritical (33).

Endurance Ability to sustain a given activity over time (54).

Energy Conservation Modifying or adapting the environment or method of doing a task to increase efficiency and reduce stress on the respiratory system (54).

Engineering Controls Equipment and workplace designs or changes that reduce the human efforts needed (51).

Environment Physical, social, and cultural milieu that provides the stage on which lives are lived (8). Particular physical, social, cultural, economic, and political features within a person's context that affects the motivation, organization, and performance of occupation (44). The context for everyday living, including physical, social, cultural, economic, and institutional dimensions (60).

Environmental Affordance All action possibilities latent in the environment that within context invites or elicits interaction (59).

Environmental Demands Requirements that environments place on people during task performance (46).

Environmental Modifications Making minor or major alterations or changes to the environment to support the occupational performance of individuals or groups (60).

Environmental Press Demand characteristics of an environment that influence an individual's ability to perform an activity (60).

Epinephrine (adrenaline) Catecholamine produced by the adrenal glands that exerts effects on organs and structures throughout the body including the brain; primary purposes are to increase heart rate and blood pressure, facilitate efficient breathing, divert blood to large muscles, and mobilize blood sugars and fats so that an individual is prepared to respond to environmental challenges; acts as a neurotransmitter in the brain and as a hormone in blood circulation (56).

Ergonomics Scientific discipline concerned with the understanding of interactions among humans and other elements of a system; profession that applies theory, principles, data, and methods to design in order to optimize human well-being and overall system performance (51).

Essential Tasks Basic job duties that all employees must be able to perform with or without reasonable accommodation (51).

Ethnicity Socially constructed and potentially dynamic group membership based on subjective belief in common descent because of similarities of physical type and/or customs that may be self-selected or imposed from outside the group (6). Identification of a group (by group itself or others) on the basis of a boundary that distinguishes them from other groups—racial, cultural, linguistic, economic, religious, political—may be more or less porous; members of an ethnic group are often presumed to be culturally or biologically similar, although this is not necessarily the case (7).

Evaluation Process of gathering and interpreting qualitative and/or quantitative data to understand client needs and desires, describe function, predict future function, plan intervention, or measure outcome of OT intervention (39, 46, 47, 48, 50).

Evidence-Based Practice Use of research study findings, client values and practitioner expertise during clinical reasoning to support the process of making wise practice decisions (30).

Excitation Arousal of the nervous system (55).

Executive Function Ability to organize, problem-solve, and engage in independent behavior (57).

Exteroception Sensations from outside the body; information from touch, taste, sight, sound, and smell (59).

Facilitation Stimuli generated or information relayed following an action or interaction; often used to modify and refine future behavior (59).

Fading Systematic reduction of support (scaffold) to clients so that task demands increase; used when clients improve their skills (35).

Fair Testing Practice of determining potential sources of bias, irrelevant to the content of a test, that might negatively influence the performance of a person because of culture, age, disability, or some other trait and making modifications or accommodations to the test or test situation to minimize this bias without undue influence on reliability or validity (47).

Family-Centered Care Effective and compassionate attention to the concerns of family members; addressing the needs hopes of people and their families (4).

Fee for Service Retrospective reimbursement for medical services based on "reasonable and necessary" criteria (69).

Feedback Information that the learner receives about performance; critical for learning (54). Information arising from the response itself (productions feedback) or from changes that occur in the environment as a result of the response (outcome feedback) (59).

Fidelity Faithfulness of intervention to underlying therapeutic principles (59).

Fieldwork Work done or firsthand observations made in the field as opposed to those done or observed in a controlled environment (26).

Fine Coordination Smooth and harmonious action of groups of muscles working together to produce a desired finely controlled motion (55).

Formal Authority Right to issue orders or direct action by virtue of one's formal position (67).

Formal Theory Explanation of observable events or relationships by stating a series of abstract propositions or principles (42).

Fraud The act of intentionally being deceptive in relation to the provision of services; can include fabricating documentation for services that were not really rendered, billing for more services than were provided in a visit, or accepting bribes or kickbacks for referrals (39).

Free Appropriate Public Education (FAPE) Special education and related services provided at public expense that meets the standards of the state education agency (SEA) (50).

Function Processes, actions, and behavior of the various organs and systems of the body (55).

Functional Capacity Evaluation Measurement of an individual's abilities and/or limitations in the context of safe, productive work tasks (51).

Functional Group Group process procedure in which time and energy are used in purposeful action to promote adaptation through occupation (37).

Functional Supervision Supervision over a specific aspect of work or job function (69).

Functioning Extent to which people are able to engage in occupations, influenced by health conditions and the physical, social, and attitudinal context (5).

Gemeinschaft Characterizes the relationships between individuals in community that are private and based on shared interests with kin or family, neighborhoods, and groups of friends (19).

General Education Environment, curriculum, and activities available to all students (50).

General Schema Implicit cognitive map of the world as known, which can be evoked and mentally constituted at diverse scales and in diverse manifestations that vary according to the circumstances in which it is invoked (8).

Generalization Spontaneous ability to transfer what is learned in one situation to a different situation (57).

Genotype Actual genetic inheritance of an individual; a collection of specific alleles (6).

Gesellschaft Characterizes social actions in community that are a public expression or response to a duty or to an organization within society (19).

Goniometer Instrument that is used to measure joint range of motion (54).

Grading Sequentially increasing demands of an occupation to stimulate improved function or reducing the demands to respond to client difficulties in performance (35).

Gravitational Insecurity Type of sensory modulation dysfunction that is thought to result from poor processing of vestibular and proprioceptive sensation; manifested as fear of moving, being out of the upright, or having one's feet off the ground that is out of proportion to any danger; also refers to any postural deficits the individual has (59).

Gross Coordination The combined activity of many muscles into smooth patterns and sequences of motion; smooth, directed, and fluid actions supporting everyday activities (55).

Group Cohesiveness Attraction of members for their group and for the other members; members of a cohesive group accept one another, provide support, and form meaningful relationships in the group; may be a significant factor in successful group therapy outcome (37).

Group Process A complex set of interdependent variables acting on and within a group and its members (37).

Habits Acquired tendencies to automatically respond and perform in certain, consistent ways in familiar environments or situations (44). Automatic behavior that is integrated into more complex patterns that enable people to function on a day-to-day basis; may be useful, dominat-

ing, or impoverished and either support or interfere with performance in areas of occupation (OTPF-II).

Habituation Internalized readiness to exhibit consistent patterns of behavior guided by habits and roles and fitted to the characteristics of routine temporal, physical, and social environments (44).

Health A state of being that is usually associated with the absence of illness or injury but increasingly is taken to mean the extent to which a person participates in age-appropriate mobility, self-care, domestic, educational, vocational, and community occupations (5). State of complete physical, mental, and social well-being and not merely the absence of disease or infirmity (18).

Health Disparities Gaps in the quality of health and health care across racial and ethnic groups, population-specific differences in the presence of disease, health outcomes, or access to health care (7).

Health Maintenance Organization (HMO) Managed care system in which health care providers are gatekeepers who oversee patient treatment within the system (69).

Health Promotion Process of enabling people to increase control over and improve their health (18). Movement toward optimal health and high-level wellness (51).

Health Reimbursement Accounts (HRA) Savings account used for medical bills that is not subject to income tax (synonym: *Health Savings Accounts*) (69).

Health Resources and Services Administration (HRSA) Primary federal agency for improving access to health care services for people who are uninsured, isolated, or medically vulnerable (17).

Health Savings Account (HSA) Savings account used for medical bills that is not subject to income tax (synonym: *Health Reimbursement Accounts*) (69).

Here-and-Now Spontaneous action that focuses on the present (37).

Heterarchical Approach Suggests that therapists consider a network of factors for clinical decision making instead of a hierarchy of levels (27).

Home Abiding place of affection, provides a sense of centering, permanence, ownership, responsibility, control, self-expression, privacy, refuge, comfort (familiarity), emotional affiliation, and belonging (8).

Homeostasis Maintenance of internal environment, describes periods in which the body grows and regenerates in order to maintain balance and health among body systems, involves conservation and restoration of energy, the digestion and absorption of nutrients, body repair and healing, sexual reproduction, and excretion of waste (56).

Homophobia Unreasonable fear or hatred of gay or lesbian people (6).

Hypertonia Excessive muscle tension in a muscle (55).

Hypothalamic-Pituitary-Adrenal Axis (HPA) Also referred to as the limbic-hypothalamic-pituitary-adrenal axis (LHPA), a pathway that describes connections between brain structures and the organ responsible for the production of cortisol (56).

Hypothalamus Brain structure in the diencephalon section of the brain, oversees the autonomic nervous system, receives input from multiple regions of the brain, including the cerebral cortex and limbic system, to provide both internal and external sources of information that are necessary to regulate the internal environment of the human body (56).

Hypotonia Decrease in a muscle's resistance to stretch as the joint is moved through the range of motion, client's inability to recruit adequate force to move against gravity (55).

Ideation Conceptualizing an action; knowing what to do (59).

Impairment Any problem with a normal psychological or physiological function, such as concentration or respiration, or with a body structure such as a limb, joint, or organ (5).

Incompetence Acting without appropriate knowledge, skill, or ability (39).

Incoordination Extraneous, uneven, or inaccurate movements (55).

Indemnity Plans Insurance plans that pay for costs associated with a medical condition or injury; associated with fee-for-service method of payment (69).

Independence Measure of performance indicating the ability to perform a task independently with or without adaptive equipment (46). Ability to participate in self-directed, necessary, and preferred occupations in a satisfying manner irrespective of the amount or kind of external assistance desired or required (OTPF-II).

Independent Living Movement Organized approach by those with disability that incorporates ideas about managing their personal life, participating in community life, fulfilling social roles, sustaining self-determination; and minimizing physical or psychological dependence on others; emphasizes a person being physically located in a community setting and participating in community activities with consumer direction and control (19).

Indirect Selection Also called scanning; the user uses a switch to choose from subsets of all options, which are offered sequentially in a scanning array (61).

Individual Controls Physical, cognitive, and social skills and performance of the workers; safe, efficient job design depends on coordination of all aspects of the system (51).

Individual Education Program (IEP) Written plan for the delivery of educationally related services to children ages 3–21 years with disabilities, as mandated by IDEA (39, 50).

Individual Family Service Plan (IFSP) Written plan for the delivery of services to children with disabilities ages birth through 2 years; prepares children with disabilities to enter the educational system at age 3 years (39).

Individual Variation Differences among individuals in their attributes (e.g., range, standard deviation) (30).

Individuals with Disabilities Education Act (IDEA) Federal law that mandates that educational services must be provided to a child with a disability from birth to age 21 years (39).

Information Processing The processing of information that includes registration of sensory information, perception or interpretation of the data, identification or memory, and cognition (59).

Inhibition Release of a neurotransmitter at the synapse makes it less likely that the postsynaptic neuron will reach threshold (signal level) required for an action potential to occur and therefore for the sensory or motor information to be transmitted (59).

Inner Drive Motivation and self-direction that come from within a child to develop sensory integration (59).

Institutional Bias Financial support for institutional care, nursing home care, or other segregated settings rather than community-based settings (17).

Instrumental ADLs (IADLs) Activities to support daily life within the home and community that often require more complex interactions than self-care used in ADLs (OTPF-II).

Integrated Practitioner Considers the best scientific evidence while simultaneously attending to the humanistic aspects of the client's narrative and lived experience (27).

Interagency Model of Fieldwork Development of a new role for occupational therapy by collaborating with a community agency or industry to create a fieldwork experience for students (26).

Interdependence Mutual dependence, people's reliance on each other as a natural consequence of living (OTPF-II).

Interests What one finds enjoyable or satisfying to do (44).

Internalized Role Incorporation of a socially and/or personally defined status and a related cluster of attitudes and actions (44).

International Classification of Function [ICF] Model proposed by the World Health Organization that describes a person's level of ability along a continuum of impairment to participation (55).

Interoception Sensation originating from inside the body; perception of visceral sensations arising from internal organs (59).

Intervention Process and skilled actions taken by occupational therapy practitioners in collaboration with the client to facilitate engagement in occupations related to health and participation. The intervention process includes the plan, implementation, and review (OTPF-II).

Isokinetic Exercise Exercise in which speed of the muscle contraction is controlled and maximum exertion occurs at the end of the range; contraction can be eccentric or concentric (54).

Isometric Exercise Exercise involving a muscle contraction in which there is no lengthening or shortening of a muscle (54).

Isotonic Exercise Exercise in which the muscles actively lengthen and shorten during the contraction (54).

Job Analysis Formal methodology that details the interaction between the worker and the equipment of a system (51).

Job Description Defines the essential functions of the job and how the job relates to other jobs and to the workplace (51).

Joint Protection Techniques to reduce stress on joints, pain and inflammation, and deformity during performance of daily tasks (54).

Just-Right Challenge A task that is manageably demanding; promotes central nervous system integration (59).

Least Restrictive Environment (LRE) Environment that provides maximum interaction with nondisabled peers and is consistent with the needs of the child/student (50).

Leisure Nonobligatory activity that is intrinsically motivated and engaged in during discretionary time (OTPF-II).

Level I Fieldwork Experiences designed to enrich didactic course work through directed observation and participation in selected aspects of the occupational therapy process (26).

Level II Fieldwork In-depth experience in delivering occupational therapy services to clients, focusing on the application of purposeful and meaningful occupation, as integral to the academic program's curriculum design (26).

Life World Phenomenological spatiotemporal context of human experience (8).

Limbic System Cluster of brain structures that are responsible for emotion formation and emotional behavior as well as complex cognitive thought processing (e.g., memory) (56).

Low Registration High thresholds and a passive self-regulation strategy. People with a low registration pattern of sensory processing do not detect sensory input that others notice readily (59).

Malpractice Misconduct on the part of a professional that results in harm to a client (39).

Managed Care Comprehensive health care system that provides a variety of health services and facilities with a focus on controlling costs (69).

Management Process of guiding a work unit by planning for future work obligations, organizing employees into functional units, directing employees in the process of completing daily work tasks, and controlling work processes and systems to ensure adequate quality of work output (67).

Marginal Functions Tasks that are not essential to the specific job or tasks that could, if necessary, be completed by another worker (51).

Measurement Process of assigning numbers to represent quantities of a trait, attribute, or characteristic or to classify objects (47).

Memory Ability to register, retain, and recall past experience, knowledge, and sensation (57).

Mental Status Examination Formal procedure to examine and diagnose mental functioning, including a general description of a person, notation of emotional expression, identification of perceptual disturbances, and exploration of thought processes and thought content (57).

Metacognitive Cognitive processes in which one thinks about one's own thinking (32).

Modification Changes in the form or character of a task (35)

Motor Control Ability to direct the movement (static or dynamic) of the body through conscious or unconscious motor and sensory processes (55).

Motor Learning Set of processes associated with practice or experience leading to permanent changes in the capability for skilled acts (54, 55).

Motor Planning Ability to carry out a skilled, nonhabitual motor activity (57). Process that bridges ideation and motor execution to enable an adaptive response (59).

Motor Program Abstract representation that prescribes the movements required to perform a given motor task (55).

Motor Skill Learned and goal directed movement requiring some degree of precision and accuracy (55).

Movement Motor action that is reflexive and/or controlled (55).

Multimedia Mode of communication using a computer and requiring human interaction (41).

Muscle Strength Ability to produce movement or resist an external force (54).

Myth An unfounded or poorly founded belief that is given uncritical acceptance by members of a group (6).

Negligence Failing to do something that ought to be done to prevent harm to a client (39).

Nervous System Thresholds Amount of excitatory input necessary to activate neurons; thresholds for responding occur along a continuum rather than at extremes; may be lower thresholds for some inputs and higher thresholds for other inputs (59).

Neural Map Sensory information "stored" as a consequence of active movement, with more variations of movement enabling the development of more accurate "maps" (59).

Neurohormone Hormone that influences brain (neural) structures (56).

Neuroplasticity Brain's ability to reorganize itself by forming new neural connections throughout life; in development, it entails the activity-dependent shaping of connections at synapses where information is transferred from one nerve cell to another; is influenced profoundly by sensory experience during childhood (59).

New Poor Unexpected poverty with inability to meet most basic needs; major factors contributing to growing numbers of new poor are job layoffs, family breakdown, and sudden illness (7).

Norepinephrine (noradrenaline) Another catecholamine (see *Epinephrine*) produced by both the adrenal glands and neurons in the sympathetic nervous system neurons; Although similar in structure and influence to epinephrine, norepinephrine has its own receptor sites on the same and sometimes different organs (56).

Normative Expectations Activities or occupations that are viewed as standard behavior expected of other people in the same circumstances; may be encouraged by members of the community (3).

Objective Observation Measurement or compilation of data in ways that others can easily replicate (53).

Occupation Ordinary and extraordinary things people do in their day-to-day lives that occupy time, modify the environment, ensure survival, maintain well-being, nurture others, contribute to society, and pass on cultural meanings and through which people develop skills, knowledge, and capacity for doing and fulfilling their potential (5). Personal activities that individuals choose to engage in and the ways in which each individual experiences them (35). An activity that has three inextricably linked properties: (a) active involvement of the person, (b) meaning to the person, and (c) a process with a product that may be either tangible or intangible (45). Meaningful, purposeful activity (51).

Occupation-Based Intervention A client-centered intervention in which the occupational therapy practitioner and client collaboratively select and design activities that have specific relevance or meaning to the client and support the client's interests, needs, health, and participation in daily life (OTPF-II).

Occupational Activities Tasks that are directly related to the individual's preferred occupational role. Such tasks must have personal meaning and occupational relevance; the individual must be the primary actor in the activity (45).

Occupational Adaptation Constructing a positive occupational identity and achieving occupational competence over time in the context of one's environment (44). Normative process, internal to the person, by which competence in occupational functioning develops (45).

Occupational Adaptation Model of Professional Development Conceptualizes three classes of adaptive response behaviors—primitive, transitional, and mature—that are typically demonstrated among all students; students tend to revert to lower-level behaviors when faced with situations that they perceive as too difficult or too unfamiliar (26).

Occupational Adaptation Process Normative internal process that is activated by the individual when approaching and adapting to challenges in life (45).

Occupational Analysis Analysis of an occupation that is relevant to an individual within the actual context of performance (35).

Occupational Apartheid Separation between those who have meaningful, useful occupations and those who are deprived of, isolated from, or otherwise constrained in their daily life occupations (7, 27).

Occupational Challenge What the individual experiences when circumstances create significant difficulty in carrying out his or her occupational roles (45).

Occupational Competence Degree to which one is able to sustain a pattern of occupational participation that reflects one's occupational identity (44).

Occupational Deprivation Situations in which people's needs for meaningful and health-promoting occupations go unmet or are systematically denied (27).

Occupational Engagement Clients' doing, thinking, and feeling under certain environmental conditions in the midst of or as a planned consequence of therapy (44).

Occupational Environment One of the three primary elements in the theory of occupational adaptation. In contrast with other environments, the occupational environment calls for an occupational response from the individual in the context of either work, play/leisure, or self-maintenance. The contexts are shaped by unique physical, social, and cultural influences (45).

Occupational Identity Composite sense of who one is and who one wishes to become as an occupational being generated from one's history of occupational participation (44).

Occupational Justice Concept to guide humans as occupational beings who need and want to participate in occupations in order to develop and thrive and the political, social, economic, and cultural factors that may influence such participation (7). Right of every individual to be able to meet basic needs and to have equal opportunities and life chances to reach toward her or his potential but specific to the individual's engagement in diverse and meaningful occupations (20).

Occupational Orchestration The capacity of individuals to enact their occupations on a daily basis to meet their needs and those in their social world; rhythmic, harmonious composition of daily life (35).

Occupational Participation Engagement in work, play, or activities of daily living that are part of one's sociocultural context and that are desired and/or necessary to one's well-being (44).

Occupational Performance Doing a task related to participation in a major life area (44).

Occupational Profile A summary of the client's occupational history and experiences as described by the client; includes the client's patterns of living, interests, values, and needs relative to the current situation (39).

Occupational Readiness A term that characterizes interventions that are designed to affect the individual's sensorimotor, cognitive, and/or psychosocial deficits (e.g., strengthening, endurance, and ROM activities; memory training; stress management) (45).

Occupational Response Outcome; the observable by-product of the adaptive response; the individual's action or behavior in response to an occupational challenge (45).

Occupational Role The occupations that an individual assigns to particular roles (35).

Occupational Role Expectations Product of both the individual's personal desires for performance and demands that stem from the occupational environment and its respective physical, social, and cultural influences; the internal and external expectations shape the uniqueness of the challenge the person experiences (45).

Occupational Science A basic science concerned with the study of occupation and human life, particularly related to health, well-being, and social participation (1).

Occupational Therapist (OTR) Graduate of an accredited occupational therapy program who has completed fieldwork and passed the certification examination administered by the National Board for Certification of Occupational Therapy (NBCOT); also referred to as a certified occupational therapist or registered occupational therapist (25).

Occupational Therapy Aide An individual who is assigned by a certified occupational therapist to perform delegated, selected, skilled tasks in specific situations under intense close supervision by an occupational therapy practitioner (25).

Occupational Therapy Assistant (OTA) Graduate of an accredited occupational therapy assistant program who has completed fieldwork and passed the certification examination by the National Board for Certification of Occupational Therapy; also referred to as a certified occupational therapy assistant (COTA) (25).

Occupational Therapy Practitioner Occupational therapist or occupational therapy assistant (25).

Occupational Therapy Process Problem-solving method used by occupational therapy practitioners to help clients improve their occupational performance; consists of theory selection, evaluation, problem definition, intervention planning, intervention implementation, and reevaluation (46).

Office of the Surgeon General The Surgeon General is the chief health educator in the United States, giving Americans the best scientific information available on how to improve their health and reduce the risk of illness and injury (17).

Open Skills Motor skills that are performed in a constantly changing environment, have high information-processing demands, and are attention demanding (55).

Operational Definition Clear description of a concept or term that contains sufficient detail to enable uniform interpretation of the concept or term by many individuals (48).

Organizing Designing workable units, determining lines of authority and communication, and developing and managing patterns of coordination (67).

Orientation Awareness of self in relation to time, place, and identification of others (57).

Orthotic Relatively permanent device worn to substitute for impaired or lost muscle function (54).

Outcome Result(s) or consequence(s) of occupational therapy intervention (46).

Oxytocin Primarily a neurohormone produced in the hypothalamus and released into the bloodstream by the pituitary gland; primary role is regulation of social emotions and reproductive behavior; supports caregiving behavior, including stimulating milk production for breast-feeding; released during orgasm; measured through blood and cerebral spinal fluid samples (56).

Parasympathetic Branch of the Autonomic Nervous System (PNS) System that is mostly concerned with generalized homeostasis (56).

Participation Taking part in any occupation, whether by oneself or as part of a group, regardless of the reason for taking part, involvement in life situations, which encompasses all aspects of human functioning that involve learning and applying knowledge, completing tasks, communication, mobility, self-care, domestic life, interpersonal relationships, major life areas such as education and employment, and community, social, and civic life (5).

Passive Range of Motion (PROM) Arc of motion through which the joint passes when moved by an outside force (54).

Peer Supervision Oversight provided by another professional who does not have any formal authority to provide supervision but participates in providing feedback or sharing knowledge with another professional with the intent of influencing the other person's practices to improve client outcomes (68).

Perception Integration of impressions from the different sensory sources into psychological, meaningful information (55). Meaning that the brain gives to sensory input; consists of "maps" of every part of our body that are stored in the nervous system as the sensations from the skin, muscles, joints, and gravity and movement receptors are organized and sorted during the person's daily activities (59).

Performance Capacity Underlying mental and physical abilities and how they are used and experienced in performance (44). Ability for doing things provided by the status of underlying objective physical and mental components and corresponding subjective experience (46).

Performance Discrepancy Performance problems that occur when performance demands exceed a person's capacities (46).

Performance Parameters Variables or characteristics of task performance that can be observed and/or measured, such as independence, pain, and satisfaction (46, 48).

Perseveration Unnecessary and prolonged repetition of a word, phase, or movement (57).

Person-Environment-Occupation Fit The goodness of fit or congruence in the relationship that exists between the person, his or her occupation, and the environment in which the occupation is being performed (60).

Personal Causation Individual's sense of competence and effectiveness (44).

Personal Factors Aspects of the human condition such as body structures and body functions (53).

Personal Meaning Satisfaction of conscious or unconscious needs and/or attribution of benefits derived from activities (52).

Personal Theory Private understanding based on experience (42).

Phases of Group Development Theoretical, predictable periods in the life cycle of a group (37).

Phenotype Appearance of an individual that has a relationship to genotype but not a direct correspondence because it reflects variation in expression of alleles (6).

Physical Agent Modality (PAM) Treatment that uses energy in the form of heat, light, sound, cold, electricity, or mechanical devices (54).

Physical Environment Includes human-made environments, natural environments, equipment, and technology (60).

Place Space or location that is given meaning through habitation and the accumulation of location-based life experiences (8).

Plan of Care A written document that that describes the client's occupational therapy goals and how those goals will be achieved; also be called a care plan, intervention plan, or treatment plan (39).

Planning Process of deciding what to do by setting performance objectives and identifying the activities needed to accomplish these objectives (67).

Play Any spontaneous or organized activity that provides enjoyment, entertainment, amusement, or diversion (OTPF-II).

Point of Service Plans Managed care option consisting of a hybrid of an HMO and a PPO plan (69).

Policies Written statements of direction and responsibility (39).

Political Activities of Daily Living Adoption by mainstream therapists of concepts and practices related to occupational justice, such as political action to resolve occupational injustice, including understanding the political nature of human relations and societies (27).

Population Group of people who collectively possess the specific traits or characteristics of interest for a particular study or intervention (47).

Population Health Health outcomes of a group of individuals, including the distribution of such outcomes within the group (18).

Portfolio Archive of self-assessment processes, learning plans, evidence of engagement in selected learning methods, reflection on the learning process, and outcomes of the application of learning to practice (25).

Postural Adaptation Ability of the body to maintain balance automatically and remain upright during alterations in positions and challenges to stability (55).

Postural Alignment A bodily position in which the center of gravity of each body segment is over the supporting base of the body (55).

Postural Control Controlling or regulating the body's position in space to maintain stability and orientation (55, 59).

Posture Composite of the positions of all the joints of the body at any given time (55).

Power Ability to force compliance with one's wishes through coercion despite resistance (67).

Praxis Engaging in a new or nonhabitual motor act; in addition to executing the motor act, praxis requires the cognitive ability to come up with the idea for action (ideation) and the ability to plan the action to be performed (59).

Precautions Actions to prevent harm to an individual (39).

Preferred Provider Organization (PPO) Flexible form of managed care consisting of a group of health care providers and hospitals that the consumer can choose to access health services at a reduced cost (69).

Present Levels of Educational Performance Information from the special education evaluation that describe a student's current school performance; includes how the student's disability affects involvement and progress in the general education curriculum (50).

Prevention Measures not only to prevent the occurrence of disease such as risk factor reduction, but also to arrest its progress and reduce its consequences once established. Prevention can also apply to injury prevention (18).

Primary Health Care Essential health care made accessible at a cost a country and community can afford, with methods that are practical, scientifically sound, and socially acceptable (18).

Primary Prevention Aimed at preventing the disease or injury from ever occurring (18).

Primary Reflexes Innate motor reactions that do not require cognitive processing and are elicited automatically in response to a stimulus (55).

Problem Definition Component of the occupational therapy process describing the performance problem to be addressed by occupational therapy interventions (46).

Procedures Written statements that describe how policies should be implemented (39).

Professional Development Process involving planning and achievement of excellence or establishing expertise in seeking a change in responsibilities or when assuming more complex professional roles (25).

Professional Practice Supervision Supervision of others in the same profession, undertaken with an understanding of the profession's values, standards, and ethics aimed at providing support, training, and evaluation of the supervisie's professional performance (68).

Professional Reasoning Process used by practitioners to plan, direct, perform, and reflect on client care. Includes processes by supervisors, fieldwork educators, and occupational therapy managers as they conceptualize occupational therapy practice (32).

Progress Notes Any note written about a client that explains what the client did in occupational therapy. It may be written in a narrative (paragraph form), SOAP, or other format (39).

Project-Focused Fieldwork Managing a project, such as developing new programs or resources or evaluating an existing program, including conducting a needs assessment/analysis, proposal preparation, and development of reporting structures and timelines (26).

Projective Identification Experiencing a feeling or experience in common and disavowing it while at the same time displacing the feeling onto another individual (37).

Proportional Controls Linking direction and speed within the same controller such as a joystick or in an option for setting up a mouse (61).

Proprioception Sensations derived from movement (i.e., speed, rate, sequencing, timing, and force) and joint position; Derived from stimulation to muscle and, to a lesser extent, joint receptors, especially from resistance to movement (59).

Prosthesis Device that substitutes for a lost body part (54).

Psychometrics Properties Estimates of aspects of a test or the outcomes of a test score, such as reliability or validity, that provide evidence that it measures what it is intended to measure in a consistent and stable manner for a specific purpose (47).

Public Health Science and art of promoting health, preventing disease, and prolonging life through the organized efforts of society (18). Dealing with the protection and improvement of community health through organized efforts of preventive medicine, as well as environmental and social sciences (19).

Punishment A response to an undesired behavior (36).

Purposeful Activities Goal-directed behaviors leading to an occupation that are designed or graded to help a client develop, recover from an impairment, or learn an adaptive approach (35).

Random Practice Schedule of practice that involves nonsystematic but repetitive practice of the same set of tasks (54).

Range of Motion (ROM) Arc of motion through which a joint moves (54).

Reaction Time Time from when a stimulus is given to the time when a movement begins in reaction to the stimulus (55).

Reading Level Grade level at which an individual reads; academic level and reading level are often not equivalent (41).

Reductionism Whole is understood in terms of its parts. In occupational therapy, reductionism means focusing intervention on the parts of the person (physical, emotional, or cognitive) or parts of the occupation (2).

Regulations Rules or laws issued by a government that guide conduct (70).

Reinforcement Something that causes a behavior to be strengthened and performed again (36).

Related Services In a school setting, services that help a child with a disability to benefit from special education, such as those provided by occupational or physical therapy practitioners, school nurse, psychologist, or social worker or special transportation services (39).

Reliability Consistency and repeatability of the outcome of administration of a test across time, parallel forms of the test, and raters. It also refers to the consistency of the internal structure of the test (47).

Religion Corporate beliefs with its attendant practices (9).

Requisite Managerial Authority The level of control and discretion that a manager must have to be fairly held responsible for the outcomes of work groups (67).

Response The reaction to the stimulus (36).

Response to Intervention (RtI) An integrated approach to service delivery that includes both general and special education and includes high-quality instruction, interventions matched to student need, frequent progress monitoring, and data-based decision making (50).

Responsiveness Evidence Research findings that test the quality of progress-monitoring procedures (30).

Rigidity Simultaneous increases of muscle tone in the agonist and antagonist muscle that result in increased resistance to passive motion in any direction (55).

Risk Factors Characteristics associated with individuals who have a health condition that may include demographic variables, behavioral risk factors, and environmental factors (19).

Rituals Highly symbolic actions with a strong affective component and representative of a collection of events that are performed at regular intervals or on specific occasions (OTPF-II).

Role Normative models shaped by the culture (35). Set of behaviors expected by society, shaped by culture and

further conceptualized and defined by the individual (OTPF-II).

Role-Emerging Supervision Occurs in a placement where there is no occupational therapist on-site with opportunities for students to be more autonomous and independent, promoting increased professional growth (26).

Role Lock Fixed perceptions of others' view of someone's position and function in a group (37).

Routines Patterns of behavior that are observable, regular, and repetitive and that provide structure for daily life; may be satisfying, promoting, or damaging; require momentary time commitment; and are embedded in cultural and ecological contexts (OTPF-II).

Safety Measure of task performance indicating that a person can perform a task without risk to himself or herself or to the task environment (46).

Same Site Model of Fieldwork Entails students completing a Level I and Level II fieldwork experience at the same training site (26).

Sample A group of individuals selected to represent the theoretical population (47).

Satisfaction with Experience Overall feelings and perceptions related to experience (52).

Scaffolding Providing help or support to an individual to enable task completion (35, 59).

Scapegoating Individuals displacing common feelings and attitudes, usually negative, onto someone else in a group (37).

Screening Obtaining and reviewing data that are relevant to a potential client to determine the need for further evaluation and intervention (39).

Secondary Prevention aimed at changing unhealthy lifestyles or behaviors to reduce risk (18).

Self-Appraisal Examination of competencies and client outcomes in order to make decisions about how best to learn; once learning is implemented, selecting the evidence of learning that best indicates achievement of the competency statement (25).

Self-Assessment Provides the means to assess performance, abilities, and skills; to analyze demands and resources of the work environment; to interpret information about clients' outcomes; to reassess current learning goals; and to develop goals and plans for professional growth and continuing competence and competency (25).

Self-Determination Combination of skills, knowledge, and beliefs that enable a person to engage in goal-directed, self-regulated, autonomous behavior and to make choices and control one's life (OTPF-II).

Self-Efficacy Beliefs of individuals in their capabilities to organize and execute the courses of action required to deal with prospective situations (OTPF-II).

Self-Regulation Ability to adapt emotional expression, behavioral activity level, and attention/arousal level effectively in response to the contextual demands of the environment (56, 59).

Self-Regulation Strategies Strategies that individuals use to control the amount of sensory input they receive, whereas other people are passive, letting things happen and then responding. Self-regulation also occurs along a continuum rather than as only active or passive responding (58, 59).

Sensation Avoiding Low thresholds and an active self-regulation strategy. People with a sensation avoiding pattern of sensory processing actively work to limit the sensory input that they have to encounter throughout the day (59).

Sensation Seeking High thresholds and an active self-regulation strategy. People with a sensation seeking pattern of sensory processing create more sensory input for themselves, and derive pleasure from sensation (59).

Sensory Defensiveness Fight-or-flight reaction to sensation that most others would consider nonnoxious (59).

Sensory Detection Sensory registration; first step of sensory processing within the central nervous system (59).

Sensory Discrimination Discerning the qualities, similarities and differences of stimuli (59).

Sensory Integration and Praxis Tests A battery of 17 tests designed to evaluate several aspects of praxis as well as some aspects of somatosensory and visual discrimination and postural control in children 4 through 8 years of age with mild to moderate learning or motor difficulties; contributes to understanding a child's difficulties and planning intervention (59).

Sensory Modulation The ability to regulate and organize reactions to sensory input in a graded and adaptive manner; the balancing of excitatory and inhibitory inputs and adapting to environmental changes (59).

Sensory Processing Functions related to sensation occurring in the central nervous system; includes reception, modulation, integration, and organization of sensory stimuli; also includes the behavioral responses to sensory input (59).

Sensory Registration Noticing sensory stimuli in the environment (59).

Sensory Sensitivity Represents low thresholds and a passive self regulation strategy. People with a sensory sensitivity pattern of sensory processing notice many sensory experiences around them, and detect details of sensory input that others might not notice (58).

Serial Tasks Several discrete movements performed in a structured sequence (55).

Service Coordinator The person responsible for managing a student's IFSP or IEP (39).

Services on Behalf of the Child Includes supports for parents and school personnel that can include specialized training that helps them to work more effectively with the child (50).

Shaping A strategy to develop closer and closer approximations of behavior (36).

Shear Parallel but opposing forces that injure soft tissue (61).

Sheltered Workshop Noncompetitive employment setting that is intended to provide many of the positive benefits of a work atmosphere for individuals with disabilities (51).

Skill Observable, goal-directed action that a person uses while performing (44).

Skill Acquisition Process of learning a skill (55).

SOAP (Subjective, Objective, Assessment, Plan) A type of progress note written in a standard format so that specific information is easy to find (39).

Social Determinants of Health Factors that go beyond inherited biology and access to health care services but still exert a major influence on human health and well-being, including income and social status, social support networks, education and literacy, social and physical environment, personal health practices and coping skills, discrimination, and social exclusion; also used to describe a branch of public health and epidemiology (7).

Social Gradient Concept that higher standing in the social hierarchy leads to improved health status (7).

Social Inequality Unequal rewards and opportunities that accrue to different individuals and groups, particularly rewards and opportunities that are judged to be unfair, unjust, avoidable, and unnecessary; often linked to unequal distribution of economic assets and power within a society (7).

Social Justice Ethical distribution and sharing of resources, rights, and responsibilities between people recognizing their equal worth as citizens (OTPF-II).

Social Mobility The degree to which, in a given society, an individual's social status can change throughout the life course or the degree to which that individual's offspring and subsequent generations move up and down the class system (7).

Socioeconomic Position Includes both resource-based and prestige-based measures as linked to both childhood and adult social class position; gives greater weight to the role of material resources in shaping life chances, including health, as compared to socioeconomic status (7).

Socioeconomic Status (SES) Status- or prestige-based measure of place in the social hierarchy; measurement of SES includes occupational attainment, education, and income (7).

Somatodyspraxia A relatively severe form of sensory-integrative-based dyspraxia characterized by difficulty with both easy (feedback-dependent) and more difficult (feedforward-dependent) motor tasks; thought to be based in poor processing (59).

Spasticity Velocity-dependent resistance to muscle stretch as the joint is moved through the range of motion (55).

Special Education Educational services that are designed to help a child with a disability learn in a way that is consistent with that child's unique needs; provided with no cost to parents (39, 50).

Specially Designed Instruction Instruction that has been individualized to meet the unique needs of a student in order to receive free and appropriate education in the least restrictive environment (50).

Spirituality A deep experience of meaning by engaging in occupations that involve the enacting of personal ideologies, reflection, and intention within a supportive contextual environment (9). Personal quest for understanding answers to ultimate questions about life, about meaning, and about relationship with the sacred or transcendent, which may (or may not) lead to or arise from the development of religious rituals and the formation of community (OTPF-II).

Splint Temporary device that is used to facilitate recover from an injury or to enhance function (54).

Stability Ability to maintain the body in equilibrium (synonym: *Balance*) (55).

Standardized Test Measurement instrument that has been developed in a rigorous, scientific manner for a defined construct and population with a prescribed process of administration and scoring and with demonstrated psychometric properties (47).

Stimulus Something that prompts a behavior (36).

Stress Heightened state of action or arousal in the mind and body; can be positive (e.g., falling in love) or negative (e.g., a state of wear and tear on the body), as well as physical (e.g., exercise) and psychological (e.g., a state of worry) (56).

Subgrouping Dyads or clusters of members who consciously or unconsciously band together in a group for the purpose of avoiding something displeasing (37).

Subjective Experience State of mind with which activities are approached and affective experience of engaging in them (53).

Sundowning Increased confusion or disorientation that occurs at the end of the day; typically seen in people with Alzheimer's disease or other dementias (57).

Supervision Process of guiding an organization through the authoritative control of others completed by the governing body of the organization (67). Providing support, training, and evaluation of a supervisee's professional performance and development (68).

Supplemental Aids and Services Aids and services, in addition to specially designed instruction or related services, that are provided for a student in order to receive free and appropriate education in the least restrictive environment (50).

Supported Employment Competitive work in an integrated work environment consistent with the individual's strengths, resources, priorities, concerns, abilities, capabilities, interests, and informed choice (51).

Suppression Ability to dampen some stimuli so that other stimuli are easier to detect; ability to filter through all the input to the brain to determine which stimuli warrant attention and which stimuli can be ignored safely (59).

Surveillance Zone Space within the visual field of a person's residence (8).

Sympathetic Branch of the Autonomic Nervous System (SNS) Drives the fear, flight, or fight responses with increased respiration, cardiac activity, and metabolic activity, among others (56).

Synaptic Activity Transfer of information from one cell to another at a synapse, which can be facilitated if the firing of the presynaptic cell increases the likelihood that the postsynaptic cell will reach threshold and fire an action potential (excitatory synapse) or inhibited if the firing of the presynaptic cell reduces the likelihood of the postsynaptic cell firing (inhibitory synapse) (59).

Synaptic Function Entails the transfer of information from one cell (presynaptic neuron) to another (postsynaptic neuron) at the synaptic cleft; commonly referred to as synaptic transmission (59).

Synergy Functional coupling of groups of muscles constrained to act as a unit (55).

Systems Approach Views the properties of the whole, or system, as arising from interactions and relationships among the parts (51).

Tactile Defensiveness A sensory integrative dysfunction in which tactile sensations cause excessive emotional reactions, hyperactivity, or other behavior problems (59).

Target Condition The public health or disease outcome that the preventive care intervention avoids (primary prevention) or identifies early (secondary prevention) or treats effectively (tertiary prevention) (19).

Task Analysis Systematic process of determining task demands (51).

Task Demands Action requirements that a task puts on people (46).

Terminal Device Prosthetic hand or hook that is attached to the wrist unit of a prosthesis (54).

Tertiary Prevention Aimed at reducing the effect of a disease or injury or preventing the person from becoming more ill or dying (18).

Third-Party Payer Private company or government agency (such as Medicare) that provides payment for medical expenses (48).

Tone Amount of tension within a muscle (55).

Transaction As used in reference to the person-task-environment transaction, the balance or equilibrium achieved between person (client) and task and environment factors that optimally supports occupational performance (46). Process that involves two or more individuals or elements that reciprocally and continually influence and affect one another through an ongoing relationship (OTPF-II).

Transference Negative and positive feelings, attitudes, and responses to others based on an individual's psychological and social history (37).

Transition Planning Preparation of the student to leave the school setting and enter employment; education and rehabilitation team involved in this preparation (51).

Underresponsiveness A type of sensory modulation response pattern characterized by fewer or flattened overt responses to sensation compared to the responses of people with normal sensory modulation (59).

Unilateral Neglect Lack of awareness of stimuli presented to the side opposite the cerebral lesion in individuals who do not have primary sensory or motor impairments (57).

Universal Design Design of environments and products to be usable by all people to the greatest extent possible without the need for special arrangements or adaptations (19). The intent of universal design is to simplify life for everyone by making products, communications, and the built environment more usable by as many people as possible at little or no extra cost (60, 61).

Validity Evidence from theory and scientific study that supports the meaning, utility, and appropriateness of inferences and actions resulting from test scores, congruent with the defined purposes of the test (47).

Values What one finds important and meaningful to do (44).

Vasopressin Hormone produced in the hypothalamus and released by the pituitary gland; regulates water and salt concentrations in the blood, as well as blood pressure; also believed to play a key role in the regulation of social behavior; measured in blood and cerebral spinal fluid (56).

Vestibular Sensation derived from stimulation to the vestibular mechanism in the inner ear that occurs through movement and position of the head; contributes to posture and the maintenance of a stable visual field (59).

Visitability Home construction practices offering specific features that make the home easier for people with a mobility impairment to visit (e.g., zero-step entrance, 32-inch doorways, main floor bathroom) (19). Movement to change home construction practices so that new homes, whether or not designated for residents who currently have disabilities, offer a few specific features that make the home easier for people who develop a mobility impairment to live in and visit (60).

Visual Perceptual Cognitive process of obtaining and interpreting visual information from the environment; includes discrimination, memory, spatial relationships, form constancy, sequential memory, figure-ground, and closure (59).

Volition Pattern of thoughts and feelings about oneself as an actor in one's world that occur as one anticipates, chooses, experiences, and interprets what one does (44).

Well-Being Extent to which individuals experience a sense of vitality and satisfaction with their life and circumstances; subjective perceptions of occupational performance, rather than objective measurements of the frequency or extent of participation in valued occupations (5).

Wellness Process of taking responsibility for realizing one's maximum health potential (51).

Work Exertion or effort directed to produce or accomplish something (51).

Work Conditioning Emphasizes physical conditioning; addresses issues of strength, endurance, flexibility, motor control, and cardiopulmonary function (51).

Work Hardening Highly structured, goal-oriented, individualized treatment program designed to maximize the individual's ability to return to work (51).

Work Integration Programs Coordination of the clinical features of the injured worker into the organizational and ergonomic aspects of the system (56).

Working Poor People who maintain full-time jobs but remain in relative poverty according to government-established poverty standards; may have negative net worth and lack the ability to escape their situations (7).

World Federation of Occupational Therapists (WFOT) Key international representative for occupational therapy and the official international organization for the promotion of occupational therapy (23, 24).

Xenophobia An unreasonable fear or hatred of those who are different from oneself (6).

Index

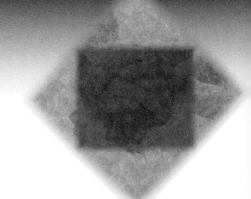

Page numbers in *italics* denote figures; those followed by a t denote tables; those with an n denote footnotes.